OPTUM360°®

CODING COMPANION

AF753654

Cardiology/Cardiothoracic/ Vascular Surgery

A comprehensive illustrated guide to coding and reimbursement

2020

Publisher's Notice

Coding Companion for Cardiology/Cardiothoracic/Vascular Surgery is designed to be an authoritative source of information about coding and reimbursement issues affecting cardiology, cardiovascular surgery, and vascular surgery procedures. Every effort has been made to verify accuracy and all information is believed reliable at the time of publication. Absolute accuracy cannot be guaranteed, however. This publication is made available with the understanding that the publisher is not engaged in rendering legal or other services that require a professional license.

American Medical Association Notice

Fee schedules, relative value units, conversion factors and/or related components are not assigned by the AMA, are not part of CPT, and the AMA is not recommending their use. The AMA does not directly or indirectly practice medicine or dispense medical services. The AMA assumes no liability for data contained or not contained herein.

CPT is a registered trademark of the American Medical Association.

The responsibility for the content of any "National Correct Coding Policy" included in this product is with the Centers for Medicare and Medicaid Services and no endorsement by the AMA is intended or should be implied. The AMA disclaims responsibility for any consequences or liability attributable to or related to any use, nonuse or interpretation of information contained in this product.

Our Commitment to Accuracy

Optum360 is committed to producing accurate and reliable materials.

To report corrections, please email accuracy@optum.com. You can also reach customer service by calling 1.800.464.3649, option 1.

Copyright

Made in the USA

ISBN 978-1-62254-570-4

Acknowledgments

Marianne Randall, CPC, *Product Manager*
Karen Schmidt, BSN, *Technical Director*
Stacy Perry, *Manager, Desktop Publishing*
Lisa Singley, *Project Manager*
Loraine Hewitt, *Clinical/Technical Editor*
Leanne Patterson, CPC, *Clinical/Technical Editor*
Tracy Betzler, *Senior Desktop Publishing Specialist*
Hope M. Dunn, *Senior Desktop Publishing Specialist*
Katie Russell, *Desktop Publishing Specialist*
Kimberli Turner, *Editor*

Technical Editors

Leanne Patterson, CPC

Ms. Patterson has more than 10 years of experience in the health care profession. She has an extensive background in professional component coding, with expertise in E/M coding and auditing, and HIPAA compliance. Her experience includes general surgery coding, serving as Director of Compliance, conducting chart-to-claim audits and physician education. She has been responsible for coding and denial management in large multi-specialty physician practices, and most recently served as a practice manager where she supervised implementation of a new EHR system. Ms. Patterson is credentialed by the American Academy of Professional Coders (AAPC) as a Certified Professional Coder (CPC).

Contents

Getting Started with Coding Companion

Coding Companion for Cardiology/Cardiothoracic/Vascular Surgery is designed to be a guide to the specialty procedures classified in the CPT® book. It is structured to help coders understand procedures and translate physician narrative into correct CPT codes by combining many clinical resources into one, easy-to-use source book.

The book also allows coders to validate the intended code selection by providing an easy-to-understand explanation of the procedure and associated conditions or indications for performing the various procedures. As a result, data quality and reimbursement will be improved by providing code-specific clinical information and helpful tips regarding the coding of procedures.

CPT Codes

For ease of use, evaluation and management codes related to Cardiology/Cardiothoracic/Vascular Surgery are listed first in the *Coding Companion*. All other CPT codes in *Coding Companion* are listed in ascending numeric order. Included in the code set are all surgery, radiology, laboratory, and medicine codes pertinent to the specialty. Each CPT code is followed by its official CPT code description.

Resequencing of CPT Codes

The American Medical Association (AMA) employs a resequenced numbering methodology. According to the AMA, there are instances where a new code is needed within an existing grouping of codes, but an unused code number is not available to keep the range sequential. In the instance where the existing codes were not changed or had only minimal changes, the AMA assigned a code out of numeric sequence with the other related codes being grouped together. The resequenced codes and their descriptions have been placed with their related codes, out of numeric sequence.

CPT codes within the Optum360 *Coding Companion* series display in their resequenced order. Resequenced codes are enclosed in brackets for easy identification.

ICD-10-CM

Overall, the 10th revision goes into greater clinical detail than did ICD-9-CM and addresses information about previously classified diseases, as well as those diseases discovered since the last revision. Conditions are grouped with general epidemiological purposes and the evaluation of health care in mind. New features have been added, and conditions have been reorganized, although the format and conventions of the classification remain unchanged for the most part.

Detailed Code Information

One or more columns are dedicated to each procedure or service or to a series of similar procedures/services. Following the specific CPT code and its narrative, is a combination of features. A sample is shown on page ii. The black boxes with numbers in them correspond to the information on the pages following the sample.

Appendix Codes and Descriptions

Some CPT codes are presented in a less comprehensive format in the appendix. The CPT codes appropriate to the specialty are included in the appendix with the official CPT code description. The codes are presented in numeric order, and each code is followed by an easy-to-understand lay description of the procedure.

The codes in the appendix are presented in the following order:

- HCPCS
- Surgery
- Radiology
- Pathology and Laboratory
- Medicine Services
- Category III

Category II codes are not published in this book. Refer to the CPT book for code descriptions.

CCI Edit Updates

The *Coding Companion* series includes the list of codes from the official Centers for Medicare and Medicaid Services' National Correct Coding Policy Manual for Part B Medicare Contractors that are considered to be an integral part of the comprehensive code or mutually exclusive of it and should not be reported separately. The codes in the Correct Coding Initiative (CCI) section are from version 25.3, the most current version available at press time. The CCI edits are located in a section at the back of the book. Optum360 maintains a website to accompany the Coding Companions series and posts updated CCI edits on this website so that current information is available before the next edition. The website address is http://www.optum360coding.com/ProductUpdates/. The 2020 edition password is: **CODING20**. Log in each quarter to ensure you receive the most current updates. An email reminder will also be sent to you to let you know when the updates are available.

Index

A comprehensive index is provided for easy access to the codes. The index entries have several axes. A code can be looked up by its procedural name or by the diagnoses commonly associated with it. Codes are also indexed anatomically. For example:

32800 Repair lung hernia through chest wall

could be found in the index under the following main terms:

Hernia
 Repair
  Lung, 32800

Repair
 Lung
  Hernia, 32800

General Guidelines

Providers

The AMA advises coders that while a particular service or procedure may be assigned to a specific section, it is not limited to use only by that specialty group (see paragraphs two and three under "Instructions for Use of the CPT Codebook" on page xiii of the CPT Book). Additionally, the procedures and services listed throughout the book are for use by any qualified physician or other qualified health care professional or entity (e.g., hospitals, laboratories, or home health agencies). Keep in mind that there may be other policies or guidance that can affect who may report a specific service.

Supplies

Some payers may allow physicians to separately report drugs and other supplies when reporting the place of service as office or other nonfacility setting. Drugs and supplies are to be reported by the facility only when performed in a facility setting.

Professional and Technical Component

Radiology and some pathology codes often have a technical and a professional component. When physicians do not own their own equipment and send their patients to outside testing facilities, they should append modifier 26 to the procedural code to indicate they performed only the professional component.

31515 1

31515 Laryngoscopy direct, with or without tracheoscopy; for aspiration

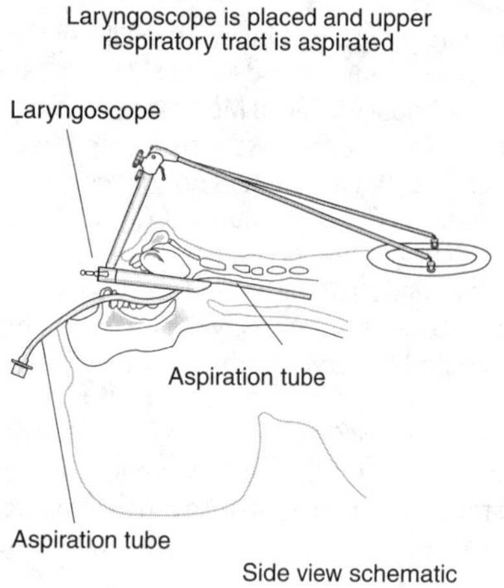

2

Explanation 3

The physician uses an aspirator to remove excess saliva or semi-solid foreign material from the larynx. After applying topical anesthesia to the oral cavity and pharynx, the physician inserts the laryngoscope through the patient's mouth. An aspirator is fed through the laryngoscope and the larynx is cleared of saliva and semi-solid foreign material. If a tracheoscopy is performed, a bronchoscope is inserted through the laryngoscope for microscopic visualization of the trachea and bronchi. No other procedure is performed.

Coding Tips 4

Laryngoscopy code selection is dependent on two variables. Laryngoscopy procedures may be either direct or indirect, and they may be performed with either a rigid or flexible scope. A direct laryngoscopy allows the physician to see the larynx through a scope in the throat. In contrast, when an indirect laryngoscopy is performed, the physician uses mirrors to visualize the larynx. Code 31515 refers to direct visualization with a rigid laryngoscope. Report the appropriate endoscopy for each anatomic site examined. Surgical endoscopy includes a diagnostic endoscopy; however, diagnostic endoscopy can be identified separately when performed at the same surgical session as an open procedure.

ICD-10-CM Diagnostic Codes 5

J04.0	Acute laryngitis
J05.0	Acute obstructive laryngitis [croup]
J38.3	Other diseases of vocal cords
J38.7	Other diseases of larynx
J39.0	Retropharyngeal and parapharyngeal abscess
J39.8	Other specified diseases of upper respiratory tract
J69.0	Pneumonitis due to inhalation of food and vomit
J69.1	Pneumonitis due to inhalation of oils and essences
J69.8	Pneumonitis due to inhalation of other solids and liquids
J95.01	Hemorrhage from tracheostomy stoma
J95.02	Infection of tracheostomy stoma
J95.09	Other tracheostomy complication
J95.859	Other complication of respirator [ventilator]
J95.88	Other intraoperative complications of respiratory system, not elsewhere classified
J95.89	Other postprocedural complications and disorders of respiratory system, not elsewhere classified
O89.01	Aspiration pneumonitis due to anesthesia during the puerperium
P24.01	Meconium aspiration with respiratory symptoms
P24.11	Neonatal aspiration of (clear) amniotic fluid and mucus with respiratory symptoms
P24.21	Neonatal aspiration of blood with respiratory symptoms
P24.31	Neonatal aspiration of milk and regurgitated food with respiratory symptoms
P24.81	Other neonatal aspiration with respiratory symptoms
R04.1	Hemorrhage from throat
R04.2	Hemoptysis
R04.81	Acute idiopathic pulmonary hemorrhage in infants
R04.89	Hemorrhage from other sites in respiratory passages
R09.3	Abnormal sputum
T81.41XA	Infection following a procedure, superficial incisional surgical site, initial encounter
T81.42XA	Infection following a procedure, deep incisional surgical site, initial encounter
T81.43XA	Infection following a procedure, organ and space surgical site, initial encounter
T81.44XA	Sepsis following a procedure, initial encounter
T81.49XA	Infection following a procedure, other surgical site, initial encounter

Associated HCPCS Codes 6

A4305 Disposable drug delivery system, flow rate of 50 ml or greater per hour

AMA: 31515 1998,Nov,1 7

Relative Value Units/Medicare Edits 8

Non-Facility RVU	Work	PE	MP	Total
31515	1.8	3.76	0.23	5.79
Facility RVU	**Work**	**PE**	**MP**	**Total**
31515	1.8	1.09	0.23	3.12

	FUD	Status	MUE	Modifiers				IOM Reference
31515	0	A	1(3)	51	N/A	N/A	N/A	None

* with documentation

Terms To Know 9

direct laryngoscopy. Endoscopic instrument, such as a flexible or rigid fiberoptic scope, inserted into the larynx for direct viewing capabilities of the voice box and vocal cords.

larynx. Musculocartilaginous structure between the trachea and the pharynx that functions as the valve preventing food and other particles from entering the respiratory tract, as well as the voice mechanism. Also called the voicebox, the larynx is composed of three single cartilages: cricoid, epiglottis, and thyroid; and three paired cartilages: arytenoid, corniculate, and cuneiform.

trachea. Tube descending from the larynx and branching into the right and left main bronchi.

1. CPT Codes and Descriptions

This edition of *Coding Companion* is updated with CPT codes for year 2020.

The following icons are used in *Coding Companion:*

- ● This CPT code is new for 2020.
- ▲ This CPT code description is revised for 2020.
- + This CPT code is an add-on code.

Add-on codes are not subject to bilateral or multiple procedure rules, reimbursement reduction, or appending modifier 50 or 51. Add-on codes describe additional intraservice work associated with the primary procedure performed by the same physician on the same date of service and are not reported as stand-alone procedures. Add-on codes for procedures performed on bilateral structures are reported by listing the add-on code twice.

[ ] CPT codes enclosed in brackets are resequenced and may not appear in numerical order.

2. Illustrations

The illustrations that accompany the *Coding Companion* series provide coders a better understanding of the medical procedures referenced by the codes and data. The graphics offer coders a visual link between the technical language of the operative report and the cryptic descriptions accompanying the codes. Although most pages will have an illustration, there will be some pages that do not.

3. Explanation

Every CPT code or series of similar codes is presented with its official CPT code description. However, sometimes these descriptions do not provide the coder with sufficient information to make a proper code selection. In *Coding Companion*, an easy-to-understand step-by-step clinical description of the procedure is provided. Technical language that might be used by the physician is included and defined. *Coding Companion* describes the most common method of performing each procedure.

4. Coding Tips

Coding tips provide information on how the code should be used, provides related CPT codes, and offers help concerning common billing errors, modifier usage, and anesthesia. This information comes from consultants and technical editors at Optum360 and from the coding guidelines provided in the CPT book and by the Centers for Medicare and Medicaid Services (CMS).

5. ICD-10-CM Diagnostic Codes

ICD-10-CM diagnostic codes listed are common diagnoses or reasons the procedure may be necessary. This list in most cases is inclusive to the specialty. Please note that in some instances the ICD-10-CM codes for only one side of the body (right) have been listed with the CPT code. The associated ICD-10-CM codes for the other side and/or bilateral may also be appropriate. Codes that refer to the right or left are identified with the ☑ icon to alert the user to check for laterality. In some cases, not every possible code is listed and the ICD-10-CM book should be referenced for other valid codes.

6. Associated HCPCS Codes

Medicare and some other payers require the use of HCPCS Level II codes and not CPT codes when reporting certain services. The HCPCS codes and their description are displayed in this field. If there is not a HCPCS code for this service, this field will not be displayed.

7. AMA References

The AMA references for *CPT Assistant* are listed by CPT code, with the most recent reference listed first. Generally only the last six years of references are listed.

8. Relative Value Units/Medicare Edits

Medicare edits are provided for most codes. These 2020 Medicare edits were current as of November 2019.

Relative Value Units

In a resource based relative value scale (RBRVS), services are ranked based on the relative costs of the resources required to provide those services as opposed to the average fee for the service, or average prevailing Medicare charge. The Medicare RBRVS defines three distinct components affecting the value of each service or procedure:

- Physician work component, reflecting the physician's time and skill
- Practice expense (PE) component, reflecting the physician's rent, staff, supplies, equipment, and other overhead
- Malpractice (MP) component, reflecting the relative risk or liability associated with the service
- Total RVUs are a sum of the work, PE, and MP RVUs

There are two groups of RVUs listed for each CPT code. The first RVU group is for facilities (Facility RVU), which includes services provided in hospitals, ambulatory surgical centers, or skilled nursing facilities. The second RVU group is for nonfacilities (Non-Facility RVU), which represents services provided in physician offices, patient's homes, or other nonhospital settings. The appendix includes RVU components for facility and non-facility. Because no values have been established by CMS for the Category III codes, no relative value unit/grids are identified. Refer to the RBRVS tool or guide for the RVUs when the technical (modifier TC) or professional (modifier26) component of a procedure is provided.

Medicare Follow-Up Days (FUD)

Information on the Medicare global period is provided here. The global period is the time following a surgery during which routine care by the physician is considered postoperative and included in the surgical fee. Office visits or other routine care related to the original surgery cannot be separately reported if they occur during the global period.

Status

The Medicare status indicates if the service is separately payable by Medicare. The Medicare RBRVS includes:

- A Active code—separate payment may be made
- B Bundled code—payment is bundled into other service
- C Carrier priced—individual carrier will price the code
- I Not valid—Medicare uses another code for this service
- N Non-covered—service is not covered by Medicare
- R Restricted—special coverage instructions apply
- T Injections—separately payable if no other services on same date
- X Statutory exclusion—no RVUs or payment

Medically Unlikely Edits

This column provides the maximum number of units allowed by Medicare. However, it is also important to note that not every code has a Medically Unlikely Edit (MUE) available. Medicare has assigned some MUE values that are not publically available. If there is no information in the MUE column for a particular code, this doesn't mean that there is no MUE. It may simply mean that CMS has not released information on that MUE. Watch the remittance advice for possible details on MUE denials related to those codes. If there is not a published MUE, a dash will display in the field.

An additional component of the MUE edit is the MUE Adjudication Indicator (MAI). This edit is the result of an audit by the Office of the Inspector General (OIG) that identified inappropriate billing practices that bypassed the MUE edits. These included inappropriate reporting of bilateral services and split billing.

There are three MUE Adjudication Indicators.

- 1 Line Edit
- 2 Date of Service Edit: Policy
- 3 Date of Service Edit: Clinical

The MUE will be listed following the MAI value. For example code 11446 has a MUE value of 3 and a MAI value of 1. This will display in the MUE field as "3(1)."

Modifiers

Medicare identifies some modifiers that are required or appropriate to report with the CPT code. When the modifiers are not appropriate, it will be indicated with N/A. Four modifiers are included.

51 Multiple Procedure
Medicare and other payers reduce the reimbursement of second and subsequent procedures performed at the same session to 50 percent of the allowable. For endoscopic procedures, the reimbursement is reduced by the value of the endoscopic base code.

50 Bilateral Procedures
This modifier is used to identify when the same procedure is performed bilaterally. Medicare requires one line with modifier 50 and the reimbursement is 50 percent of the allowable. Other payers may require two lines and will reduce the second procedure.

62* Two Surgeons
Medicare identifies procedures that may be performed by co-surgeons. The reimbursement is split between both providers. Both surgeons must report the same code when using this modifier.

80* Assistant Surgeon
An assistant surgeon is allowed if modifier 80 is listed. Reimbursement is usually 20 percent of the allowable. For Medicare it is 16 percent to account for the patient's co-pay amount.

* with documentation

Modifiers 62 and 80 may require supporting documentation to justify the co- or assistant surgeon.

Medicare Official Regulatory Information

Medicare official regulatory information provides official regulatory guidelines. Also known as the CMS Online Manual System, the Internet-only Manuals (IOM) contain official CMS information pertaining to program issuances, instructions, policies, and procedures based on statutes, regulations, guidelines, models, and directives. Optum360 has provided the reference for the surgery codes. The full text of guidelines can be found online at http://www.cms.gov/Regulations-and-Guidance/Guidance/Manuals/.

9. Terms to Know

Some codes are accompanied by general information pertinent to the procedure, labeled "Terms to Know." This information is not critical to code selection, but is a useful supplement to coders hoping to expand their knowledge of the specialty.

99201-99205

99201 Office or other outpatient visit for the evaluation and management of a new patient, which requires these 3 key components: A problem focused history; A problem focused examination; Straightforward medical decision making. Counseling and/or coordination of care with other physicians, other qualified health care professionals, or agencies are provided consistent with the nature of the problem(s) and the patient's and/or family's needs. Usually, the presenting problem(s) are self limited or minor. Typically, 10 minutes are spent face-to-face with the patient and/or family.

99202 Office or other outpatient visit for the evaluation and management of a new patient, which requires these 3 key components: An expanded problem focused history; An expanded problem focused examination; Straightforward medical decision making. Counseling and/or coordination of care with other physicians, other qualified health care professionals, or agencies are provided consistent with the nature of the problem(s) and the patient's and/or family's needs. Usually, the presenting problem(s) are of low to moderate severity. Typically, 20 minutes are spent face-to-face with the patient and/or family.

99203 Office or other outpatient visit for the evaluation and management of a new patient, which requires these 3 key components: A detailed history; A detailed examination; Medical decision making of low complexity. Counseling and/or coordination of care with other physicians, other qualified health care professionals, or agencies are provided consistent with the nature of the problem(s) and the patient's and/or family's needs. Usually, the presenting problem(s) are of moderate severity. Typically, 30 minutes are spent face-to-face with the patient and/or family.

99204 Office or other outpatient visit for the evaluation and management of a new patient, which requires these 3 key components: A comprehensive history; A comprehensive examination; Medical decision making of moderate complexity. Counseling and/or coordination of care with other physicians, other qualified health care professionals, or agencies are provided consistent with the nature of the problem(s) and the patient's and/or family's needs. Usually, the presenting problem(s) are of moderate to high severity. Typically, 45 minutes are spent face-to-face with the patient and/or family.

99205 Office or other outpatient visit for the evaluation and management of a new patient, which requires these 3 key components: A comprehensive history; A comprehensive examination; Medical decision making of high complexity. Counseling and/or coordination of care with other physicians, other qualified health care professionals, or agencies are provided consistent with the nature of the problem(s) and the patient's and/or family's needs. Usually, the presenting problem(s) are of moderate to high severity. Typically, 60 minutes are spent face-to-face with the patient and/or family.

Explanation

Providers report these codes for new patients being seen in the doctor's office, a multispecialty group clinic, or other outpatient environment. Services are reported based on meeting all three key components—history, exam, and medical decision making (MDM)—within each level of service. The most basic service is represented by 99201, which describes a problem focused history and exam with straightforward medical decision making encompassing approximately 10 minutes of face-to-face time with the patient and/or family. Mid-level services describe problems involving an expanded problem focused history and exam or a detailed history and exam as represented by 99202 and 99203, respectively. Medical decision making for 99202 is the same as for a level one visit (straightforward) and is designated as low complexity for the level three services. At these levels of service, the encounter can involve face-to-face time of 20 (99202) to 30 minutes (99203). The last two levels of service in this category represent moderate to severe problems; both services involve comprehensive history and examination components. The differentiating factor between the two levels is the medical decision making; 99204 involves moderate complexity MDM and approximately 45 minutes of face-to-face time with the patient and/or family while the highest level of service in this category (99205) involves MDM of high complexity and one hour of face-to-face time.

Coding Tips

These codes are used to report office or other outpatient services for a new patient. All three key components (history, exam, and medical decision making) must be met or exceeded for the level of service selected. Time may be used to select the level of service when counseling and coordination of care are documented as at least half of the time spent face-to-face with the patient. Codes may be selected based upon the 1995 or the 1997 Evaluation and Management Guidelines. For office or other outpatient services for an established patient, see 99211-99215. For observation care services, see 99217-99226. For patients admitted and discharged from observation or inpatient status on the same date, see 99234-99236.

ICD-10-CM Diagnostic Codes

The application of this code is too broad to adequately present ICD-10-CM diagnostic code links here. Refer to your ICD-10-CM book.

AMA: **99201** 2019,Jan,3; 2019,Feb,3; 2018,Sep,14; 2018,Mar,7; 2018,Jan,8; 2018,Apr,10; 2018,Apr,9; 2017,Jun,6; 2017,Jan,8; 2017,Aug,3; 2016,Sep,6; 2016,Mar,10; 2016,Jan,13; 2016,Jan,7; 2016,Dec,11; 2015,Oct,3; 2015,Jan,12; 2015,Jan,16; 2015,Dec,3; 2014,Oct,3; 2014,Oct,8; 2014,Nov,14; 2014,Jan,11; 2014,Aug,3; 2013,Jun,3-5; 2013,Jan,9-10; 2013,Aug,13 **99202** 2019,Jan,3; 2019,Feb,3; 2018,Sep,14; 2018,Mar,7; 2018,Jan,8; 2018,Apr,9; 2018,Apr,10; 2017,Jun,6; 2017,Jan,8; 2017,Aug,3; 2016,Sep,6; 2016,Mar,10; 2016,Jan,13; 2016,Jan,7; 2016,Dec,11; 2015,Oct,3; 2015,Jan,12; 2015,Jan,16; 2015,Dec,3; 2014,Oct,3; 2014,Oct,8; 2014,Nov,14; 2014,Jan,11; 2014,Aug,3; 2013,Jun,3-5; 2013,Jan,9-10; 2013,Aug,13 **99203** 2019,Jan,3; 2019,Feb,3; 2018,Sep,14; 2018,Mar,7; 2018,Jan,8; 2018,Apr,10; 2018,Apr,9; 2017,Jun,6; 2017,Jan,8; 2017,Aug,3; 2016,Sep,6; 2016,Mar,10; 2016,Jan,13; 2016,Jan,7; 2016,Dec,11; 2015,Oct,3; 2015,Jan,16; 2015,Jan,12; 2015,Dec,3; 2014,Oct,8; 2014,Oct,3; 2014,Nov,14; 2014,Jan,11; 2014,Aug,3; 2013,Jun,3-5; 2013,Jan,9-10; 2013,Aug,13 **99204** 2019,Jan,3; 2019,Feb,3; 2018,Sep,14; 2018,Mar,7; 2018,Jan,8; 2018,Apr,9; 2018,Apr,10; 2017,Jun,6; 2017,Jan,8; 2017,Aug,3; 2016,Sep,6; 2016,Mar,10; 2016,Jan,13; 2016,Jan,7; 2016,Dec,11; 2015,Oct,3; 2015,Jan,16; 2015,Jan,12; 2015,Dec,3; 2014,Oct,8; 2014,Oct,3; 2014,Nov,14; 2014,Jan,11; 2014,Aug,3; 2013,Jun,3-5; 2013,Jan,9-10; 2013,Aug,13 **99205** 2019,Jan,3; 2019,Feb,3; 2018,Sep,14; 2018,Mar,7; 2018,Jan,8; 2018,Apr,9; 2018,Apr,10; 2017,Jun,6; 2017,Jan,8; 2017,Aug,3; 2016,Sep,6; 2016,Mar,10; 2016,Jan,13; 2016,Jan,7; 2016,Dec,11; 2015,Oct,3; 2015,Jan,16; 2015,Jan,12; 2015,Dec,3; 2014,Oct,8; 2014,Oct,3; 2014,Nov,14; 2014,Jan,11; 2014,Aug,3; 2013,Jun,3-5; 2013,Jan,9-10; 2013,Aug,13

Relative Value Units/Medicare Edits

Non-Facility RVU	Work	PE	MP	Total
99201	0.48	0.76	0.05	1.29
99202	0.93	1.14	0.08	2.15
99203	1.42	1.49	0.14	3.05
99204	2.43	1.99	0.21	4.63
99205	3.17	2.38	0.27	5.82
Facility RVU	**Work**	**PE**	**MP**	**Total**
99201	0.48	0.23	0.05	0.76
99202	0.93	0.42	0.08	1.43
99203	1.42	0.59	0.14	2.15
99204	2.43	1.0	0.21	3.64
99205	3.17	1.31	0.27	4.75

	FUD	Status	MUE	Modifiers				IOM Reference
99201	N/A	A	1(2)	N/A	N/A	N/A	80*	100-04,11,40.1.3; 100-04,12,30.6.4; 100-04,12,30.6.7; 100-04,12,30.6.10; 100-04,12,30.6.15.1; 100-04,12,100.1.1; 100-04,12,190.7; 100-04,12,230; 100-04,12,230.1; 100-04,18,80.2; 100-04,32,12.1; 100-04,32,130.1
99202	N/A	A	1(2)	N/A	N/A	N/A	80*	
99203	N/A	A	1(2)	N/A	N/A	N/A	80*	
99204	N/A	A	1(2)	N/A	N/A	N/A	80*	
99205	N/A	A	1(2)	N/A	N/A	N/A	80*	

* with documentation

Terms To Know

new patient. Patient who is receiving face-to-face care from a provider/qualified health care professional or another physician/qualified health care professional of the exact same specialty and subspecialty who belongs to the same group practice for the first time in three years. For OPPS hospitals, a patient who has not been registered as an inpatient or outpatient, including off-campus provider based clinic or emergency department, within the past three years.

outpatient visit. Encounter in a recognized outpatient facility.

99211-99215

99211 Office or other outpatient visit for the evaluation and management of an established patient, that may not require the presence of a physician or other qualified health care professional. Usually, the presenting problem(s) are minimal. Typically, 5 minutes are spent performing or supervising these services.

99212 Office or other outpatient visit for the evaluation and management of an established patient, which requires at least 2 of these 3 key components: A problem focused history; A problem focused examination; Straightforward medical decision making. Counseling and/or coordination of care with other physicians, other qualified health care professionals, or agencies are provided consistent with the nature of the problem(s) and the patient's and/or family's needs. Usually, the presenting problem(s) are self limited or minor. Typically, 10 minutes are spent face-to-face with the patient and/or family.

99213 Office or other outpatient visit for the evaluation and management of an established patient, which requires at least 2 of these 3 key components: An expanded problem focused history; An expanded problem focused examination; Medical decision making of low complexity. Counseling and coordination of care with other physicians, other qualified health care professionals, or agencies are provided consistent with the nature of the problem(s) and the patient's and/or family's needs. Usually, the presenting problem(s) are of low to moderate severity. Typically, 15 minutes are spent face-to-face with the patient and/or family.

99214 Office or other outpatient visit for the evaluation and management of an established patient, which requires at least 2 of these 3 key components: A detailed history; A detailed examination; Medical decision making of moderate complexity. Counseling and/or coordination of care with other physicians, other qualified health care professionals, or agencies are provided consistent with the nature of the problem(s) and the patient's and/or family's needs. Usually, the presenting problem(s) are of moderate to high severity. Typically, 25 minutes are spent face-to-face with the patient and/or family.

99215 Office or other outpatient visit for the evaluation and management of an established patient, which requires at least 2 of these 3 key components: A comprehensive history; A comprehensive examination; Medical decision making of high complexity. Counseling and/or coordination of care with other physicians, other qualified health care professionals, or agencies are provided consistent with the nature of the problem(s) and the patient's and/or family's needs. Usually, the presenting problem(s) are of moderate to high severity. Typically, 40 minutes are spent face-to-face with the patient and/or family.

Explanation

Providers report these codes for established patients being seen in the doctor's office, a multispecialty group clinic, or other outpatient environment. Services are reported based on meeting two of the three key components—history, exam, and medical decision making (MDM)—within each level of service excluding the most basic service represented by 99211 that describes an encounter not requiring the presence of a clinician. Presenting problems are typically very minimal and the encounter usually only takes five minutes. Code 99212 describes a problem focused history and exam with straightforward medical decision making encompassing approximately 10 minutes of face-to-face time with the patient and/or family. The mid-level services describe problems involving an expanded problem focused history and exam or a detailed history and exam as represented by 99213 and 99214, respectively. Medical decision making for 99213 is designated as low complexity and for a

 ● New ▲ Revised + Add On AMA: CPT Assist [Resequenced] ☑ Laterality

level four service (99214), MDM would involve moderate complexity. At these levels of service, the encounter can involve face-to-face time of 15 (99213) to 25 minutes (99214). The last level of service in this category, 99215, represents moderate to high severity problems that consist of a comprehensive history and examination, as well as high complexity medical decision making. This encounter involves approximately 40 minutes of face-to-face time with the patient and/or family.

Coding Tips

These codes are used to report office or other outpatient services for an established patient. Two of the three key components (history, exam, and medical decision making) must be met or exceeded for the level of service selected. Time may be used to select the level of service when counseling and coordination of care are documented as at least half of the time spent face-to-face with the patient. Codes may be selected based upon the 1995 or the 1997 Evaluation and Management Guidelines. Code 99211 does not require the presence of a physician or other qualified health care professional. For office or other outpatient services for a new patient, see 99201-99205. For observation care services, see 99217-99226. For patients admitted and discharged from observation or inpatient status on the same date, see 99234-99236.

ICD-10-CM Diagnostic Codes

The application of this code is too broad to adequately present ICD-10-CM diagnostic code links here. Refer to your ICD-10-CM book.

AMA: 99211 2019,Jan,3; 2019,Feb,3; 2018,Sep,14; 2018,Mar,7; 2018,Jan,8; 2018,Apr,10; 2018,Apr,9; 2017,Mar,10; 2017,Jun,6; 2017,Jan,8; 2017,Aug,3; 2016,Sep,6; 2016,Mar,10; 2016,Jan,7; 2016,Jan,13; 2016,Dec,11; 2015,Oct,3; 2015,Jan,12; 2015,Jan,16; 2015,Dec,3; 2014,Oct,8; 2014,Oct,3; 2014,Nov,14; 2014,Mar,13; 2014,Jan,11; 2014,Aug,3; 2013,Nov,3; 2013,Mar,13; 2013,Jun,3-5; 2013,Jan,9-10; 2013,Aug,13 **99212** 2019,Jan,3; 2019,Feb,3; 2018,Sep,14; 2018,Mar,7; 2018,Jan,8; 2018,Apr,10; 2018,Apr,9; 2017,Oct,5; 2017,Jun,6; 2017,Jan,8; 2017,Aug,3; 2016,Sep,6; 2016,Mar,10; 2016,Jan,13; 2016,Jan,7; 2016,Dec,11; 2015,Oct,3; 2015,Jan,12; 2015,Jan,16; 2015,Dec,3; 2014,Oct,3; 2014,Oct,8; 2014,Nov,14; 2014,Jan,11; 2014,Aug,3; 2013,Nov,3; 2013,Mar,13; 2013,Jun,3-5; 2013,Jan,9-10; 2013,Aug,13 **99213** 2019,Jan,3; 2019,Feb,3; 2018,Sep,14; 2018,Mar,7; 2018,Jan,8; 2018,Apr,10; 2018,Apr,9; 2017,Jun,6; 2017,Jan,8; 2017,Aug,3; 2016,Sep,6; 2016,Mar,10; 2016,Jan,13; 2016,Jan,7; 2016,Dec,11; 2015,Oct,3; 2015,Jan,12; 2015,Jan,16; 2015,Dec,3; 2014,Oct,8; 2014,Oct,3; 2014,Nov,14; 2014,Jan,11; 2014,Aug,3; 2013,Nov,3; 2013,Mar,13; 2013,Jun,3-5; 2013,Jan,9-10; 2013,Aug,13 **99214** 2019,Jan,3; 2019,Feb,3; 2018,Sep,14; 2018,Mar,7; 2018,Jan,8; 2018,Apr,9; 2018,Apr,10; 2017,Jun,6; 2017,Jan,8; 2017,Aug,3; 2016,Sep,6; 2016,Mar,10; 2016,Jan,13; 2016,Jan,7; 2016,Dec,11; 2015,Oct,3; 2015,Jan,12; 2015,Jan,16; 2015,Dec,3; 2014,Oct,3; 2014,Oct,8; 2014,Nov,14; 2014,Jan,11; 2014,Aug,3; 2013,Nov,3; 2013,Mar,13; 2013,Jun,3-5; 2013,Jan,9-10; 2013,Aug,13 **99215** 2019,Jan,3; 2019,Feb,3; 2018,Sep,14; 2018,Mar,7; 2018,Jan,8; 2018,Apr,9; 2018,Apr,10; 2017,Jun,6; 2017,Jan,8; 2017,Aug,3; 2016,Sep,6; 2016,Mar,10; 2016,Jan,13; 2016,Jan,7; 2016,Dec,11; 2015,Oct,3; 2015,Jan,12; 2015,Jan,16; 2015,Dec,3; 2014,Oct,8; 2014,Oct,3; 2014,Nov,14; 2014,Jan,11; 2014,Aug,3; 2013,Nov,3; 2013,Mar,13; 2013,Jun,3-5; 2013,Jan,9-10; 2013,Aug,13

Relative Value Units/Medicare Edits

Non-Facility RVU	Work	PE	MP	Total
99211	0.18	0.45	0.01	0.64
99212	0.48	0.75	0.04	1.27
99213	0.97	1.05	0.07	2.09
99214	1.5	1.46	0.1	3.06
99215	2.11	1.84	0.15	4.1
Facility RVU	**Work**	**PE**	**MP**	**Total**
99211	0.18	0.07	0.01	0.26
99212	0.48	0.2	0.04	0.72
99213	0.97	0.4	0.07	1.44
99214	1.5	0.62	0.1	2.22
99215	2.11	0.87	0.15	3.13

	FUD	Status	MUE	Modifiers				IOM Reference
99211	N/A	A	1(3)	N/A	N/A	N/A	80*	None
99212	N/A	A	2(3)	N/A	N/A	N/A	80*	
99213	N/A	A	2(3)	N/A	N/A	N/A	80*	
99214	N/A	A	2(3)	N/A	N/A	N/A	80*	
99215	N/A	A	1(3)	N/A	N/A	N/A	80*	

* with documentation

Terms To Know

established patient. Patient who has received professional services in a face-to-face setting within the last three years from the same physician/qualified health care professional or another physician/qualified health care professional of the exact same specialty and subspecialty who belongs to the same group practice. If the patient is seen by a physician/qualified health care professional who is covering for another physician/qualified health care professional, the patient will be considered the same as if seen by the physician/qualified health care professional who is unavailable.

other qualified health care professional. Individual who is qualified by education, training, licensure/regulation, and facility privileging to perform a professional service within his or her scope of practice and independently (or as incident-to) report the professional service without requiring physician supervision. Payers may state exemptions in writing or state and local regulations may not follow this definition for performance of some services. Always refer to any relevant plan policies and federal and/or state laws to determine who may perform and report services.

qualified health care professional. Educated, licensed or certified, and regulated professional operating under a specified scope of practice to provide patient services that are separate and distinct from other clinical staff.

99217

99217 Observation care discharge day management (This code is to be utilized to report all services provided to a patient on discharge from outpatient hospital "observation status" if the discharge is on other than the initial date of "observation status." To report services to a patient designated as "observation status" or "inpatient status" and discharged on the same date, use the codes for Observation or Inpatient Care Services [including Admission and Discharge Services, 99234-99236 as appropriate.])

Explanation

This code describes the final processes associated with discharging a patient from outpatient hospital observation status and includes a patient exam, a discussion about the hospital stay, instructions for ongoing care, as well as preparing the medical discharge records. Report this code only when the patient has been discharged from observation services on a date other than the initial date of observation care. There are no key components or time estimates associated with this service.

Coding Tips

This code is used to report hospital outpatient observation discharge services. This code includes patient examination, discharge and follow-up care instructions, and preparation of all medical records. Time is not a factor when selecting this E/M service. For patients admitted and discharged from observation or inpatient status on the same date, see 99234-99236; for hospital inpatient discharge services, see 99238-99239.

ICD-10-CM Diagnostic Codes

The application of this code is too broad to adequately present ICD-10-CM diagnostic code links here. Refer to your ICD-10-CM book.

AMA: **99217** 2019,Jul,10; 2018,Jan,8; 2017,Jun,6; 2017,Jan,8; 2017,Aug,3; 2016,Jan,13; 2016,Jan,7; 2016,Dec,11; 2015,Jan,16; 2015,Dec,3; 2014,Oct,8; 2014,Nov,14; 2014,Jan,11; 2013,Jun,3-5; 2013,Jan,9-10

Relative Value Units/Medicare Edits

Non-Facility RVU	Work	PE	MP	Total
99217	1.28	0.69	0.09	2.06
Facility RVU	**Work**	**PE**	**MP**	**Total**
99217	1.28	0.69	0.09	2.06

	FUD	Status	MUE	Modifiers				IOM Reference
99217	N/A	A	1(2)	N/A	N/A	N/A	80*	100-04,11,40.1.3; 100-04,12,30.6.4; 100-04,12,30.6.8; 100-04,12,100; 100-04,32,130.1

* with documentation

99218-99220

99218 Initial observation care, per day, for the evaluation and management of a patient which requires these 3 key components: A detailed or comprehensive history; A detailed or comprehensive examination; and Medical decision making that is straightforward or of low complexity. Counseling and/or coordination of care with other physicians, other qualified health care professionals, or agencies are provided consistent with the nature of the problem(s) and the patient's and/or family's needs. Usually, the problem(s) requiring admission to outpatient hospital "observation status" are of low severity. Typically, 30 minutes are spent at the bedside and on the patient's hospital floor or unit.

99219 Initial observation care, per day, for the evaluation and management of a patient, which requires these 3 key components: A comprehensive history; A comprehensive examination; and Medical decision making of moderate complexity. Counseling and/or coordination of care with other physicians, other qualified health care professionals, or agencies are provided consistent with the nature of the problem(s) and the patient's and/or family's needs. Usually, the problem(s) requiring admission to outpatient hospital "observation status" are of moderate severity. Typically, 50 minutes are spent at the bedside and on the patient's hospital floor or unit.

99220 Initial observation care, per day, for the evaluation and management of a patient, which requires these 3 key components: A comprehensive history; A comprehensive examination; and Medical decision making of high complexity. Counseling and/or coordination of care with other physicians, other qualified health care professionals, or agencies are provided consistent with the nature of the problem(s) and the patient's and/or family's needs. Usually, the problem(s) requiring admission to outpatient hospital "observation status" are of high severity. Typically, 70 minutes are spent at the bedside and on the patient's hospital floor or unit.

Explanation

Initial hospital observation service codes describe the first visit of the patient's admission for hospital outpatient observation care by the supervising qualified clinician. Hospital outpatient observation status includes the supervision of the care plan for observation as well as periodic reassessments. The patient is not required to be physically located in a designated observation area within a hospital; however, if such an area is utilized, these codes should be reported. When a patient is admitted to observation status during the course of another encounter from a different site of service, such as the physician's office, a nursing home, or the emergency department, all of the E/M services rendered by the supervising clinician as part of the observation status are considered part of the initial observation care services when they are performed on the same day; the level of initial observation code reported by the clinician should incorporate the other services related to the hospital outpatient observation admission that were provided in any other sites of services as well as those provided in the actual observation setting. Codes are reported per day and do not differentiate between new or established patients. Under the initial observation care category, there are three levels represented by 99218, 99219, and 99220. These levels require all three key components to be documented. The lowest level of care within this category, 99218, requires a detailed or comprehensive history and exam as well as straightforward or low complexity medical decision making (MDM) with approximately 30 minutes time being spent at the patient's bedside and on the patient's floor or unit. For the mid-level and highest level observation care codes, a comprehensive history and examination are required. Medical decision making is the differentiating factor for these two levels. For moderate complexity, report 99219. For observation care requiring MDM of high complexity, report 99220. The clinician typically spends 50 (99219) to 70 (99220) minutes at the patient's bedside or on the unit accordingly.

Coding Tips

These codes are used to report initial hospital outpatient observation services. All three key components (history, exam, and medical decision making) must be met or exceeded for the level of service selected. Time may be used to select the level of service when counseling and coordination of care are documented as at least half of the time spent face-to-face with the patient. All evaluation and management services provided by the clinician leading up to the initiation of the observation status are considered to be part of the patient's initial observation care when performed on the same date of service. The designation of "observation status" refers to the initiation of observation care and not to a specific area of the facility. CPT guidelines indicate these services are reported only by the admitting/supervising provider; all other providers should report 99224-99226 or 99241-99245. Medicare and some payers may allow providers of different specialties to report initial hospital services and require the admitting/supervising provider to append modifier AI. For observation discharge on a different date of service than the admission, see 99217. For patients admitted and discharged from observation or inpatient status on the same date, see 99234-99236.

ICD-10-CM Diagnostic Codes

The application of this code is too broad to adequately present ICD-10-CM diagnostic code links here. Refer to your ICD-10-CM book.

AMA: **99218** 2019,Jul,10; 2018,Jan,8; 2018,Dec,8; 2018,Dec,8; 2017,Jun,6; 2017,Jan,8; 2017,Aug,3; 2016,Jan,13; 2016,Jan,7; 2016,Dec,11; 2015,Mar,3; 2015,Jul,3; 2015,Jan,16; 2015,Dec,3; 2014,Oct,8; 2014,Nov,14; 2014,Jan,11; 2013,Jun,3-5; 2013,Jan,9-10; 2013,Aug,13 **99219** 2019,Jul,10; 2018,Jan,8; 2018,Dec,8; 2018,Dec,8; 2017,Jun,6; 2017,Jan,8; 2017,Aug,3; 2016,Jan,13; 2016,Jan,7; 2016,Dec,11; 2015,Jul,3; 2015,Jan,16; 2015,Dec,3; 2014,Oct,8; 2014,Nov,14; 2014,Jan,11; 2013,Jun,3-5; 2013,Jan,9-10; 2013,Aug,13 **99220** 2019,Jul,10; 2018,Jan,8; 2018,Dec,8; 2018,Dec,8; 2017,Jun,6; 2017,Jan,8; 2017,Aug,3; 2016,Jan,13; 2016,Jan,7; 2016,Dec,11; 2015,Jul,3; 2015,Jan,16; 2015,Dec,3; 2014,Oct,8; 2014,Nov,14; 2014,Jan,11; 2013,Jun,3-5; 2013,Jan,9-10; 2013,Aug,13

Relative Value Units/Medicare Edits

Non-Facility RVU	Work	PE	MP	Total
99218	1.92	0.73	0.16	2.81
99219	2.6	1.04	0.19	3.83
99220	3.56	1.42	0.25	5.23
Facility RVU	**Work**	**PE**	**MP**	**Total**
99218	1.92	0.73	0.16	2.81
99219	2.6	1.04	0.19	3.83
99220	3.56	1.42	0.25	5.23

	FUD	Status	MUE	Modifiers				IOM Reference
99218	N/A	A	1(2)	N/A	N/A	N/A	80*	100-04,12,100
99219	N/A	A	1(2)	N/A	N/A	N/A	80*	
99220	N/A	A	1(2)	N/A	N/A	N/A	80*	

* with documentation

[99224, 99225, 99226]

99224 Subsequent observation care, per day, for the evaluation and management of a patient, which requires at least 2 of these 3 key components: Problem focused interval history; Problem focused examination; Medical decision making that is straightforward or of low complexity. Counseling and/or coordination of care with other physicians, other qualified health care professionals, or agencies are provided consistent with the nature of the problem(s) and the patient's and/or family's needs. Usually, the patient is stable, recovering, or improving. Typically, 15 minutes are spent at the bedside and on the patient's hospital floor or unit.

99225 Subsequent observation care, per day, for the evaluation and management of a patient, which requires at least 2 of these 3 key components: An expanded problem focused interval history; An expanded problem focused examination; Medical decision making of moderate complexity. Counseling and/or coordination of care with other physicians, other qualified health care professionals, or agencies are provided consistent with the nature of the problem(s) and the patient's and/or family's needs. Usually, the patient is responding inadequately to therapy or has developed a minor complication. Typically, 25 minutes are spent at the bedside and on the patient's hospital floor or unit.

99226 Subsequent observation care, per day, for the evaluation and management of a patient, which requires at least 2 of these 3 key components: A detailed interval history; A detailed examination; Medical decision making of high complexity. Counseling and/or coordination of care with other physicians, other qualified health care professionals, or agencies are provided consistent with the nature of the problem(s) and the patient's and/or family's needs. Usually, the patient is unstable or has developed a significant complication or a significant new problem. Typically, 35 minutes are spent at the bedside and on the patient's hospital floor or unit.

Explanation

Subsequent hospital observation service codes describe visits that occur after the first encounter of the patient's admission for observation care by the supervising qualified clinician. Observation status includes supervision of the care plan for observation as well as periodic reassessments. The patient is not required to be physically located in a designated observation area within a hospital; however, if such an area is utilized, these codes are reported. Codes are reported per day and, as with the initial observation care codes, do not differentiate between new or established patients. Under the subsequent observation care category, there are three levels represented by resequenced codes 99224, 99225, and 99226. All three of these levels require at least two out of the three key components to be documented. The lowest level of care, 99224, describes a problem-focused interval history as well as a problem-focused examination with straightforward or low complexity medical decision making and involves approximately 15 minutes of time by the provider at the patient's bedside or on the unit. For mid-level observation care code 99225, an expanded problem-focused history and examination are required with moderate medical decision making. Time associated with this level usually involves 25 minutes at the bedside or on the patient's floor. The third and highest level of follow-up observation care, 99226, requires a detailed history and exam as well as medical decision making of high complexity; the provider typically spends around 35 minutes with the patient or on the unit. All three levels of subsequent observation care involve the clinician reviewing the patient's medical record, results from diagnostic studies, as well as any changes to the patient's status such as the condition, response to treatments, or changes in health history since the last assessment.

Coding Tips

These codes are used to report subsequent hospital outpatient observation services. Two of the three key components (history, exam, and medical decision making) must be met or exceeded for the level of service selected. Time may be used to select the level of service when counseling and coordination of care are documented as at least half of the time spent face-to-face with the patient. Subsequent hospital outpatient observation care services include review of the medical record, including all diagnostic studies, as well as changes noted in the patient's condition and response to treatment since the last evaluation. The designation of "observation status" refers to the initiation of observation care and not to a specific area of the facility. For initial observation care, see 99218-99220; for observation discharge on a different date of service than the admission, see 99217. For patients admitted and discharged from observation or inpatient status on the same date, see 99234-99236.

ICD-10-CM Diagnostic Codes

The application of this code is too broad to adequately present ICD-10-CM diagnostic code links here. Refer to your ICD-10-CM book.

AMA: **99224** 2019,Jul,10; 2018,Jan,8; 2017,Jun,6; 2017,Jan,8; 2017,Aug,3; 2016,Jan,13; 2016,Jan,7; 2016,Dec,11; 2015,Jan,16; 2015,Dec,3; 2014,Oct,8; 2014,Nov,14; 2014,Jan,11; 2013,Jun,3-5; 2013,Jan,9-10; 2013,Aug,13 **99225** 2019,Jul,10; 2018,Jan,8; 2017,Jun,6; 2017,Jan,8; 2017,Aug,3; 2016,Jan,13; 2016,Jan,7; 2016,Dec,11; 2015,Jan,16; 2015,Dec,3; 2014,Oct,8; 2014,Nov,14; 2014,Jan,11; 2013,Jun,3-5; 2013,Jan,9-10; 2013,Aug,13 **99226** 2019,Jul,10; 2018,Jan,8; 2017,Jun,6; 2017,Jan,8; 2017,Aug,3; 2016,Jan,13; 2016,Jan,7; 2016,Dec,11; 2015,Jan,16; 2015,Dec,3; 2014,Oct,8; 2014,Nov,14; 2014,Jan,11; 2013,Jun,3-5; 2013,Jan,9-10; 2013,Aug,13

Relative Value Units/Medicare Edits

Non-Facility RVU	Work	PE	MP	Total
99224	0.76	0.3	0.06	1.12
99225	1.39	0.57	0.1	2.06
99226	2.0	0.82	0.13	2.95
Facility RVU	**Work**	**PE**	**MP**	**Total**
99224	0.76	0.3	0.06	1.12
99225	1.39	0.57	0.1	2.06
99226	2.0	0.82	0.13	2.95

	FUD	Status	MUE	Modifiers				IOM Reference
99224	N/A	A	1(2)	N/A	N/A	N/A	80*	None
99225	N/A	A	1(2)	N/A	N/A	N/A	80*	
99226	N/A	A	1(2)	N/A	N/A	N/A	80*	

* with documentation

99221-99223

99221 Initial hospital care, per day, for the evaluation and management of a patient, which requires these 3 key components: A detailed or comprehensive history; A detailed or comprehensive examination; and Medical decision making that is straightforward or of low complexity. Counseling and/or coordination of care with other physicians, other qualified health care professionals, or agencies are provided consistent with the nature of the problem(s) and the patient's and/or family's needs. Usually, the problem(s) requiring admission are of low severity. Typically, 30 minutes are spent at the bedside and on the patient's hospital floor or unit.

99222 Initial hospital care, per day, for the evaluation and management of a patient, which requires these 3 key components: A comprehensive history; A comprehensive examination; and Medical decision making of moderate complexity. Counseling and/or coordination of care with other physicians, other qualified health care professionals, or agencies are provided consistent with the nature of the problem(s) and the patient's and/or family's needs. Usually, the problem(s) requiring admission are of moderate severity. Typically, 50 minutes are spent at the bedside and on the patient's hospital floor or unit.

99223 Initial hospital care, per day, for the evaluation and management of a patient, which requires these 3 key components: A comprehensive history; A comprehensive examination; and Medical decision making of high complexity. Counseling and/or coordination of care with other physicians, other qualified health care professionals, or agencies are provided consistent with the nature of the problem(s) and the patient's and/or family's needs. Usually, the problem(s) requiring admission are of high severity. Typically, 70 minutes are spent at the bedside and on the patient's hospital floor or unit.

Explanation

Initial hospital inpatient service codes describe the first encounter with the patient by the admitting physician or qualified clinician. For initial encounters by a physician other than the admitting physician, see the initial inpatient consultation codes or subsequent inpatient care codes. When the patient is admitted to the hospital under inpatient status during the course of another encounter from a different site of service, such as the physician's office, a nursing home, or the emergency department, all of the E/M services rendered by the supervising clinician as part of the inpatient admission status are considered part of the initial inpatient care services when they are performed on the same day. The level of initial inpatient care reported by the clinician should incorporate the other services related to the hospital admission that were provided in any other sites of services as well as those provided in the actual inpatient setting. Codes are reported per day and do not differentiate between new or established patients. Under the initial inpatient care category, there are three levels represented by 99221, 99222, and 99223. All of these levels require all three key components—history, exam, and medical decision making—to be documented. The lowest level of care within this category, 99221, requires a detailed or comprehensive history and exam as well as straightforward or low complexity medical decision making with approximately 30 minutes time being spent at the patient's bedside and on the patient's floor or unit. For the mid-level and highest level initial inpatient care codes, a comprehensive history and examination are required. Medical decision making is the differentiating factor for these two levels; for moderate complexity, report 99222 and for initial inpatient care requiring MDM of high complexity, report 99223. The clinician typically spends 50 (99222) to 70 (99223) minutes at the patient's bedside or on the unit accordingly. Note that these codes include services provided to patients in a "partial hospital" setting.

Coding Tips

These codes are used to report initial hospital inpatient services. All three key components (history, exam, and medical decision making) must be met or exceeded for the level of service selected. Time may be used to select the level of service when counseling and coordination of care are documented as at least half of the floor/unit time spent with the patient. Evaluation and management services provided by the clinician leading up to the initiation of observation status or inpatient admission are considered to be part of the patient's initial hospital care when performed on the same date of service. Codes may be selected based upon the 1995 or the 1997 Evaluation and Management Guidelines. CPT guidelines indicate these services are reported only by the admitting/supervising provider; all other providers should report 99231-99233 or 99251-99255. Medicare and some payers may allow providers of different specialties to report initial hospital services and require the admitting/supervising provider to append modifier AI. For subsequent inpatient care, see 99231-99233. For discharge from an inpatient stay on a different date of service than the admission, see 99238-99239. For patients admitted and discharged from observation or inpatient status on the same date, see 99234-99236.

ICD-10-CM Diagnostic Codes

The application of this code is too broad to adequately present ICD-10-CM diagnostic code links here. Refer to your ICD-10-CM book.

AMA: **99221** 2018,Jan,8; 2018,Dec,8; 2018,Dec,8; 2017,Jun,6; 2017,Jan,8; 2017,Aug,3; 2016,Mar,10; 2016,Jan,13; 2016,Jan,7; 2016,Dec,11; 2015,Jul,3; 2015,Jan,16; 2015,Dec,3; 2015,Dec,18; 2014,Oct,8; 2014,Nov,14; 2014,Jan,11; 2013,Jun,3-5; 2013,Jan,9-10; 2013,Aug,13 **99222** 2018,Jan,8; 2018,Dec,8; 2018,Dec,8; 2017,Jun,6; 2017,Jan,8; 2017,Aug,3; 2016,Mar,10; 2016,Jan,13; 2016,Jan,7; 2016,Dec,11; 2015,Mar,3; 2015,Jul,3; 2015,Jan,16; 2015,Dec,3; 2015,Dec,18; 2014,Oct,8; 2014,Nov,14; 2014,Jan,11; 2013,Jun,3-5; 2013,Jan,9-10; 2013,Aug,13 **99223** 2018,Jan,8; 2018,Dec,8; 2018,Dec,8; 2017,Jun,6; 2017,Jan,8; 2017,Aug,3; 2016,Mar,10; 2016,Jan,13; 2016,Jan,7; 2016,Dec,11; 2015,Jul,3; 2015,Jan,16; 2015,Dec,3; 2015,Dec,18; 2014,Oct,8; 2014,Nov,14; 2014,Jan,11; 2013,Jun,3-5; 2013,Jan,9-10; 2013,Aug,13

Relative Value Units/Medicare Edits

Non-Facility RVU	Work	PE	MP	Total
99221	1.92	0.75	0.19	2.86
99222	2.61	1.04	0.21	3.86
99223	3.86	1.56	0.28	5.7
Facility RVU	**Work**	**PE**	**MP**	**Total**
99221	1.92	0.75	0.19	2.86
99222	2.61	1.04	0.21	3.86
99223	3.86	1.56	0.28	5.7

	FUD	Status	MUE	Modifiers				IOM Reference
99221	N/A	A	1(3)	N/A	N/A	N/A	80*	100-04,12,30.6.4; 100-04,12,30.6.9; 100-04,12,30.6.9.1; 100-04,12,30.6.15.1; 100-04,12,100
99222	N/A	A	1(3)	N/A	N/A	N/A	80*	
99223	N/A	A	1(3)	N/A	N/A	N/A	80*	

* with documentation

99231-99233

99231 Subsequent hospital care, per day, for the evaluation and management of a patient, which requires at least 2 of these 3 key components: A problem focused interval history; A problem focused examination; Medical decision making that is straightforward or of low complexity. Counseling and/or coordination of care with other physicians, other qualified health care professionals, or agencies are provided consistent with the nature of the problem(s) and the patient's and/or family's needs. Usually, the patient is stable, recovering or improving. Typically, 15 minutes are spent at the bedside and on the patient's hospital floor or unit.

99232 Subsequent hospital care, per day, for the evaluation and management of a patient, which requires at least 2 of these 3 key components: An expanded problem focused interval history; An expanded problem focused examination; Medical decision making of moderate complexity. Counseling and/or coordination of care with other physicians, other qualified health care professionals, or agencies are provided consistent with the nature of the problem(s) and the patient's and/or family's needs. Usually, the patient is responding inadequately to therapy or has developed a minor complication. Typically, 25 minutes are spent at the bedside and on the patient's hospital floor or unit.

99233 Subsequent hospital care, per day, for the evaluation and management of a patient, which requires at least 2 of these 3 key components: A detailed interval history; A detailed examination; Medical decision making of high complexity. Counseling and/or coordination of care with other physicians, other qualified health care professionals, or agencies are provided consistent with the nature of the problem(s) and the patient's and/or family's needs. Usually, the patient is unstable or has developed a significant complication or a significant new problem. Typically, 35 minutes are spent at the bedside and on the patient's hospital floor or unit.

Explanation

Subsequent hospital inpatient service codes describe visits that occur after the first encounter of the patient's inpatient hospital admission by the supervising physician or qualified clinician. Codes are reported per day and do not differentiate between new or established patients. Under the subsequent inpatient care category, there are three levels represented by 99231, 99232, and 99233. All of these levels require at least two out of the three key components—history, exam, and medical decision making—to be documented. The lowest level of care within this category, 99231, describes a problem-focused interval history as well as a problem-focused examination with straightforward or low complexity medical decision making and involves approximately 15 minutes of time by the provider at the patient's bedside or on the unit. For the mid-level subsequent inpatient care code, 99232, an expanded problem-focused history and examination are required with moderate medical decision making. Time associated with this level usually involves 25 minutes at the bedside or on the patient's floor. The third and highest level of subsequent inpatient care, 99233, requires a detailed history and exam as well as medical decision making of high complexity. For this level of care, the provider typically spends around 35 minutes with the patient or on the unit. All three levels of subsequent inpatient care involve the clinician reviewing the patient's medical record, results from diagnostic studies, as well as any changes to the patient's status such as physical condition, response to treatments, or changes in health history since the last assessment.

Coding Tips

These codes are used to report subsequent hospital inpatient services. Two of the three key components (history, exam, and medical decision making) must be met or exceeded for the level of service selected. Time may be used to select the level of service when counseling and coordination of care are documented as at least half of the floor/unit time spent with the patient. Codes may be selected based upon the 1995 or the 1997 Evaluation and Management Guidelines. Subsequent inpatient care services include review of the medical record, including all diagnostic studies, as well as changes noted in the patient's condition and response to treatment since the last evaluation. For initial inpatient care, see 99221-99223. For discharge from an inpatient stay on a different date of service than the admission, see 99238-99239. For patients admitted and discharged from observation or inpatient status on the same date, see 99234-99236.

ICD-10-CM Diagnostic Codes

The application of this code is too broad to adequately present ICD-10-CM diagnostic code links here. Refer to your ICD-10-CM book.

AMA: **99231** 2018,Jan,8; 2018,Dec,8; 2018,Dec,8; 2017,Jun,6; 2017,Jan,8; 2017,Aug,3; 2016,Jan,13; 2016,Jan,7; 2016,Dec,11; 2015,Jul,3; 2015,Jan,16; 2015,Dec,3; 2014,Oct,8; 2014,Nov,14; 2014,May,4; 2014,Jan,11; 2013,Sep,17; 2013,Jun,3-5; 2013,Jan,9-10; 2013,Aug,13 **99232** 2018,Jan,8; 2018,Dec,8; 2018,Dec,8; 2017,Jun,6; 2017,Jan,8; 2017,Aug,3; 2016,Oct,8; 2016,Jan,13; 2016,Jan,7; 2016,Dec,11; 2015,Jul,3; 2015,Jan,16; 2015,Dec,3; 2014,Oct,8; 2014,Nov,14; 2014,Jan,11; 2013,Jun,3-5; 2013,Jan,9-10; 2013,Aug,13 **99233** 2018,Jan,8; 2018,Dec,8; 2018,Dec,8; 2017,Jun,6; 2017,Jan,8; 2017,Aug,3; 2016,Oct,8; 2016,Jan,7; 2016,Jan,13; 2016,Dec,11; 2015,Jul,3; 2015,Jan,16; 2015,Dec,3; 2014,Oct,8; 2014,Nov,14; 2014,May,4; 2014,Jan,11; 2013,Jun,3-5; 2013,Jan,9-10; 2013,Aug,13

Relative Value Units/Medicare Edits

Non-Facility RVU	Work	PE	MP	Total
99231	0.76	0.29	0.06	1.11
99232	1.39	0.56	0.1	2.05
99233	2.0	0.79	0.14	2.93
Facility RVU	**Work**	**PE**	**MP**	**Total**
99231	0.76	0.29	0.06	1.11
99232	1.39	0.56	0.1	2.05
99233	2.0	0.79	0.14	2.93

	FUD	Status	MUE	Modifiers				IOM Reference
99231	N/A	A	1(3)	N/A	N/A	N/A	80*	100-04,12,30.6.9.2; 100-04,12,100
99232	N/A	A	1(3)	N/A	N/A	N/A	80*	
99233	N/A	A	1(3)	N/A	N/A	N/A	80*	

* with documentation

99234-99236

99234 Observation or inpatient hospital care, for the evaluation and management of a patient including admission and discharge on the same date, which requires these 3 key components: A detailed or comprehensive history; A detailed or comprehensive examination; and Medical decision making that is straightforward or of low complexity. Counseling and/or coordination of care with other physicians, other qualified health care professionals, or agencies are provided consistent with the nature of the problem(s) and the patient's and/or family's needs. Usually the presenting problem(s) requiring admission are of low severity. Typically, 40 minutes are spent at the bedside and on the patient's hospital floor or unit.

99235 Observation or inpatient hospital care, for the evaluation and management of a patient including admission and discharge on the same date, which requires these 3 key components: A comprehensive history; A comprehensive examination; and Medical decision making of moderate complexity. Counseling and/or coordination of care with other physicians, other qualified health care professionals, or agencies are provided consistent with the nature of the problem(s) and the patient's and/or family's needs. Usually the presenting problem(s) requiring admission are of moderate severity. Typically, 50 minutes are spent at the bedside and on the patient's hospital floor or unit.

99236 Observation or inpatient hospital care, for the evaluation and management of a patient including admission and discharge on the same date, which requires these 3 key components: A comprehensive history; A comprehensive examination; and Medical decision making of high complexity. Counseling and/or coordination of care with other physicians, other qualified health care professionals, or agencies are provided consistent with the nature of the problem(s) and the patient's and/or family's needs. Usually the presenting problem(s) requiring admission are of high severity. Typically, 55 minutes are spent at the bedside and on the patient's hospital floor or unit.

Explanation

Hospital observation or inpatient care service in cases where the patient is admitted and discharged on the same date of service by the supervising or qualified clinician is reported with 99234-99236. Observation status includes the supervision of the care plan for observation as well as the periodic reassessments. The patient is not required to be physically located in a designated observation area within a hospital; however, if such an area is utilized, these codes should be reported. When a patient is admitted to the hospital from observation status on the same date of service, the clinician should only report the appropriate level of initial hospital care code. The level of care reported should reflect all of the other services from the observation status services the clinician rendered to the patient on the same date of service as well as those provided in the actual inpatient setting. Codes do not differentiate between new or established patients. Under this care category, there are three levels represented by 99234, 99235, and 99236. All of these levels require all three key components—history, exam, and medical decision making—to be documented. The lowest level of care within this category, 99234, requires a detailed or comprehensive history and exam as well as straightforward medical decision making or that of low complexity with approximately 40 minutes time being spent at the patient's bedside and on the patient's floor or unit. For the mid-level and highest level observation or inpatient care codes, a comprehensive history and examination are required. Medical decision making is the differentiating factor for these two levels; for moderate complexity, report 99235 and for observation or inpatient care requiring MDM of high complexity, report 99236. The clinician typically spends 50 (99235) to 55 (99236) minutes at the patient's bedside or on the unit accordingly. Note that these codes should be reported only when the patient has been admitted and discharged on the same date of service.

Coding Tips

These codes are used to report observation or initial hospital services for the patient admitted and discharged on the same date of service. All three key components (history, exam, and medical decision making) must be met or exceeded for the level of service selected. Evaluation and management services provided by the clinician leading up to the initiation of observation status or inpatient admission are considered to be part of the patient's initial hospital care when performed on the same date of service. The designation of "observation status" refers to the initiation of observation care and not to a specific area of the facility. For patients admitted to observation status, initial care, see 99218-99220; subsequent observation care, see 99224-99226; for observation discharge on a different date of service than the admission, see 99217. For initial inpatient care, see 99221-99223; subsequent inpatient care, see 99231-99233. For discharge from an inpatient stay on a different date of service than the admission, see 99238-99239.

ICD-10-CM Diagnostic Codes

The application of this code is too broad to adequately present ICD-10-CM diagnostic code links here. Refer to your ICD-10-CM book.

AMA: 99234 2018,Jan,8; 2018,Dec,8; 2018,Dec,8; 2018,Apr,10; 2017,Jun,6; 2017,Jan,8; 2017,Aug,3; 2016,Jan,13; 2016,Dec,11; 2015,Jul,3; 2015,Jan,16; 2014,Oct,8; 2014,Jan,11; 2013,Jun,3-5 **99235** 2018,Jan,8; 2018,Dec,8; 2018,Dec,8; 2018,Apr,10; 2017,Jun,6; 2017,Jan,8; 2017,Aug,3; 2016,Jan,13; 2016,Dec,11; 2015,Jul,3; 2015,Jan,16; 2014,Oct,8; 2014,Jan,11; 2013,Jun,3-5 **99236** 2018,Jan,8; 2018,Dec,8; 2018,Dec,8; 2018,Apr,10; 2017,Jun,6; 2017,Jan,8; 2017,Aug,3; 2016,Jan,13; 2016,Dec,11; 2015,Jul,3; 2015,Jan,16; 2014,Oct,8; 2014,Jan,11; 2013,Jun,3-5

Relative Value Units/Medicare Edits

Non-Facility RVU	Work	PE	MP	Total
99234	2.56	0.99	0.2	3.75
99235	3.24	1.3	0.23	4.77
99236	4.2	1.65	0.28	6.13
Facility RVU	**Work**	**PE**	**MP**	**Total**
99234	2.56	0.99	0.2	3.75
99235	3.24	1.3	0.23	4.77
99236	4.2	1.65	0.28	6.13

	FUD	Status	MUE	Modifiers				IOM Reference
99234	N/A	A	1(3)	N/A	N/A	N/A	80*	100-04,12,30.6.4; 100-04,12,30.6.9; 100-04,12,30.6.9.1; 100-04,12,30.6.9.2; 100-04,12,100
99235	N/A	A	1(3)	N/A	N/A	N/A	80*	
99236	N/A	A	1(3)	N/A	N/A	N/A	80*	

* with documentation

99238-99239

99238 Hospital discharge day management; 30 minutes or less
99239 more than 30 minutes

Explanation

Hospital discharge services are time-based codes that, when reported, describe the amount of time spent by the qualified clinician during all final steps involved in the discharge of a patient from the hospital on a date that differs from the date of admission, including the last patient exam, discussing the hospital stay, instructions for ongoing care as it relates to all pertinent caregivers, as well as preparing the medical discharge records, prescriptions, and/or referrals as applicable. Time reported should be for the total duration of time spent by the provider even when the time spent on that date is not continuous. For a hospital discharge duration of 30 minutes or less, report 99238; for a duration of greater than 30 minutes, report 99239. There are no key components associated with these services.

Coding Tips

These codes are used to report all discharge day services for the hospital inpatient, including patient examination, discharge and follow-up care instructions, and preparation of all medical records. These are time-based codes and time spent with the patient must be documented in the medical record. For observation discharge on a different date of service than the admission, see 99217. For patients admitted and discharged from observation or inpatient status on the same date, see 99234-99236.

ICD-10-CM Diagnostic Codes

The application of this code is too broad to adequately present ICD-10-CM diagnostic code links here. Refer to your ICD-10-CM book.

AMA: 99238 2018,Jan,8; 2018,Dec,8; 2018,Dec,8; 2017,Jun,6; 2017,Jan,8; 2017,Aug,3; 2016,Jan,13; 2016,Dec,11; 2015,Jan,16; 2014,Oct,8; 2014,Jan,11; 2013,Jun,3-5; 2013,Aug,13 **99239** 2018,Jan,8; 2018,Dec,8; 2018,Dec,8; 2017,Jun,6; 2017,Jan,8; 2017,Aug,3; 2016,Jan,13; 2016,Dec,11; 2015,Jan,16; 2014,Oct,8; 2014,Jan,11; 2013,Jun,3-5; 2013,Aug,13

Relative Value Units/Medicare Edits

Non-Facility RVU	Work	PE	MP	Total
99238	1.28	0.69	0.09	2.06
99239	1.9	1.0	0.12	3.02
Facility RVU	**Work**	**PE**	**MP**	**Total**
99238	1.28	0.69	0.09	2.06
99239	1.9	1.0	0.12	3.02

	FUD	Status	MUE	Modifiers				IOM Reference
99238	N/A	A	1(2)	N/A	N/A	N/A	80*	100-04,12,30.6.4; 100-04,12,30.6.9; 100-04,12,30.6.9.1; 100-04,12,30.6.9.2; 100-04,12,100
99239	N/A	A	1(2)	N/A	N/A	N/A	80*	

* with documentation

 ● New ▲ Revised + Add On AMA: CPT Assist [Resequenced] ☑ Laterality

99241-99245

99241 Office consultation for a new or established patient, which requires these 3 key components: A problem focused history; A problem focused examination; and Straightforward medical decision making. Counseling and/or coordination of care with other physicians, other qualified health care professionals, or agencies are provided consistent with the nature of the problem(s) and the patient's and/or family's needs. Usually, the presenting problem(s) are self limited or minor. Typically, 15 minutes are spent face-to-face with the patient and/or family.

99242 Office consultation for a new or established patient, which requires these 3 key components: An expanded problem focused history; An expanded problem focused examination; and Straightforward medical decision making. Counseling and/or coordination of care with other physicians, other qualified health care professionals, or agencies are provided consistent with the nature of the problem(s) and the patient's and/or family's needs. Usually, the presenting problem(s) are of low severity. Typically, 30 minutes are spent face-to-face with the patient and/or family.

99243 Office consultation for a new or established patient, which requires these 3 key components: A detailed history; A detailed examination; and Medical decision making of low complexity. Counseling and/or coordination of care with other physicians, other qualified health care professionals, or agencies are provided consistent with the nature of the problem(s) and the patient's and/or family's needs. Usually, the presenting problem(s) are of moderate severity. Typically, 40 minutes are spent face-to-face with the patient and/or family.

99244 Office consultation for a new or established patient, which requires these 3 key components: A comprehensive history; A comprehensive examination; and Medical decision making of moderate complexity. Counseling and/or coordination of care with other physicians, other qualified health care professionals, or agencies are provided consistent with the nature of the problem(s) and the patient's and/or family's needs. Usually, the presenting problem(s) are of moderate to high severity. Typically, 60 minutes are spent face-to-face with the patient and/or family.

99245 Office consultation for a new or established patient, which requires these 3 key components: A comprehensive history; A comprehensive examination; and Medical decision making of high complexity. Counseling and/or coordination of care with other physicians, other qualified health care professionals, or agencies are provided consistent with the nature of the problem(s) and the patient's and/or family's needs. Usually, the presenting problem(s) are of moderate to high severity. Typically, 80 minutes are spent face-to-face with the patient and/or family.

Explanation

Office and other outpatient consultation service codes describe encounters where another qualified clinician's advice or opinion regarding diagnosis and treatment or determination to accept transfer of care of a patient is rendered at the request of the primary treating provider. Consultations may also be requested by another appropriate source; for example, a third-party payer may request a second opinion. The request for a consultation must be documented in the medical record, as well as a written report of the consultation findings. During the course of a consultation, the physician consultant can initiate diagnostic or therapeutic services at the same encounter or at a follow-up visit. Other separately reportable procedures or services performed in conjunction with the consultation may be reported separately. Codes do not differentiate between new or established patients. Services are reported based on meeting all three key components—history, exam, and medical decision making (MDM)—within each level of service. The most basic service, 99241, describes a problem focused history and exam with straightforward medical decision making encompassing approximately 15 minutes of face-to-face time with the patient and/or family discussing a minor or self-limiting complaint. The mid-level services describe problems involving an expanded problem focused history and exam or a detailed history and exam as represented by 99242 and 99243, respectively. Medical decision making for 99242 is the same as for a level one visit (straightforward) and is designated as low complexity for the level three service (99243). At these levels of service, the encounter can involve face-to-face time of 30 (99242) to 40 (99243) minutes involving minimal to low severity concerns. The last two levels of service in this category represent moderate to high severity problems and both services involve comprehensive history and examination components. The differentiating factor between the two levels is the medical decision making; code 99244 involves moderate complexity MDM and approximately 60 minutes of face-to-face time with the patient and/or family while the highest level of service in this category, 99245, involves MDM of high complexity and approximately 80 minutes of face-to-face time.

Coding Tips

These codes are used to report consultations in the office or outpatient setting. All three key components (history, exam, and medical decision making) must be met or exceeded for the level of service selected. Time may be used to select the level of service when counseling and coordination of care are documented as at least half of the time spent face-to-face with the patient. Codes may be selected based upon the 1995 or the 1997 Evaluation and Management Guidelines. Consultation codes are not covered by Medicare and some payers. Report new or established outpatient E/M codes for consultation services. Consultation services should not be reported when the care and management of a problem or condition is assumed prior to the initial examination of the patient. In these situations the appropriate initial or subsequent evaluation and management service should be reported. For office or other outpatient services for a new patient, see 99201-99205; for an established patient, see 99211-99215. For inpatient consultation services, see 99251-99255.

ICD-10-CM Diagnostic Codes

The application of this code is too broad to adequately present ICD-10-CM diagnostic code links here. Refer to your ICD-10-CM book.

AMA: 99241 2018,Mar,7; 2018,Jan,8; 2018,Apr,10; 2018,Apr,9; 2017,Jun,6; 2017,Jan,8; 2017,Aug,3; 2016,Sep,6; 2016,Jan,13; 2016,Jan,7; 2016,Dec,11; 2015,Jan,16; 2015,Jan,12; 2014,Sep,13; 2014,Oct,8; 2014,Nov,14; 2014,Jan,11; 2014,Aug,3; 2013,Jun,3-5; 2013,Jan,9-10 **99242** 2018,Mar,7; 2018,Jan,8; 2018,Apr,10; 2018,Apr,9; 2017,Jun,6; 2017,Jun,8; 2017,Jan,8; 2017,Aug,3; 2016,Sep,6; 2016,Jan,7; 2016,Jan,13; 2016,Dec,11; 2015,Jan,16; 2015,Jan,12; 2014,Sep,13; 2014,Oct,8; 2014,Nov,14; 2014,Jan,11; 2014,Aug,3; 2013,Jun,3-5; 2013,Jan,9-10 **99243** 2018,Mar,7; 2018,Jan,8; 2018,Apr,10; 2018,Apr,9; 2017,Jun,6; 2017,Jan,8; 2017,Aug,3; 2016,Sep,6; 2016,Jan,13; 2016,Jan,7; 2016,Dec,11; 2015,Jan,12; 2015,Jan,16; 2014,Sep,13; 2014,Oct,8; 2014,Nov,14; 2014,Jan,11; 2014,Aug,3; 2013,Jun,3-5; 2013,Jan,9-10 **99244** 2018,Mar,7; 2018,Jan,8; 2018,Apr,10; 2018,Apr,9; 2017,Jun,6; 2017,Jan,8; 2017,Aug,3; 2016,Sep,6; 2016,Jan,13; 2016,Jan,7; 2016,Dec,11; 2015,Jan,12; 2015,Jan,16; 2014,Sep,13; 2014,Oct,8; 2014,Nov,14; 2014,Jan,11; 2014,Aug,3; 2013,Jun,3-5; 2013,Jan,9-10; 2013,Aug,12 **99245** 2018,Mar,7; 2018,Jan,8; 2018,Apr,10; 2018,Apr,9; 2017,Jun,6; 2017,Jan,8; 2017,Aug,3; 2016,Sep,6; 2016,Jan,13; 2016,Jan,7; 2016,Dec,11; 2015,Jan,16; 2015,Jan,12; 2014,Sep,13; 2014,Oct,8; 2014,Nov,14; 2014,Jan,11; 2014,Aug,3; 2013,Jun,3-5; 2013,Jan,9-10

Relative Value Units/Medicare Edits

Non-Facility RVU	Work	PE	MP	Total
99241	0.64	0.66	0.04	1.34
99242	1.34	1.1	0.08	2.52
99243	1.88	1.46	0.11	3.45
99244	3.02	1.96	0.18	5.16
99245	3.77	2.3	0.22	6.29
Facility RVU	**Work**	**PE**	**MP**	**Total**
99241	0.64	0.24	0.04	0.92
99242	1.34	0.51	0.08	1.93
99243	1.88	0.71	0.11	2.7
99244	3.02	1.14	0.18	4.34
99245	3.77	1.38	0.22	5.37

	FUD	Status	MUE	Modifiers				IOM Reference
99241	N/A	I	0(3)	N/A	N/A	N/A	N/A	100-04,4,160; 100-04,12,30.6.4; 100-04,12,30.6.10; 100-04,12,30.6.15.1; 100-04,12,100
99242	N/A	I	0(3)	N/A	N/A	N/A	N/A	
99243	N/A	I	0(3)	N/A	N/A	N/A	N/A	
99244	N/A	I	0(3)	N/A	N/A	N/A	N/A	
99245	N/A	I	0(3)	N/A	N/A	N/A	N/A	

* with documentation

Terms To Know

consultation. Advice or opinion regarding diagnosis and treatment or determination to accept transfer of care of a patient rendered by a medical professional at the request of the primary care provider.

key components. Three components of history, examination, and medical decision making are considered the keys to selecting the correct level of E/M codes. In most cases, all three components must be addressed in the documentation. However, in established, subsequent, and follow-up categories, only two of the three must be met or exceeded for a given code.

99251-99255

99251 Inpatient consultation for a new or established patient, which requires these 3 key components: A problem focused history; A problem focused examination; and Straightforward medical decision making. Counseling and/or coordination of care with other physicians, other qualified health care professionals, or agencies are provided consistent with the nature of the problem(s) and the patient's and/or family's needs. Usually, the presenting problem(s) are self limited or minor. Typically, 20 minutes are spent at the bedside and on the patient's hospital floor or unit.

99252 Inpatient consultation for a new or established patient, which requires these 3 key components: An expanded problem focused history; An expanded problem focused examination; and Straightforward medical decision making. Counseling and/or coordination of care with other physicians, other qualified health care professionals, or agencies are provided consistent with the nature of the problem(s) and the patient's and/or family's needs. Usually, the presenting problem(s) are of low severity. Typically, 40 minutes are spent at the bedside and on the patient's hospital floor or unit.

99253 Inpatient consultation for a new or established patient, which requires these 3 key components: A detailed history; A detailed examination; and Medical decision making of low complexity. Counseling and/or coordination of care with other physicians, other qualified health care professionals, or agencies are provided consistent with the nature of the problem(s) and the patient's and/or family's needs. Usually, the presenting problem(s) are of moderate severity. Typically, 55 minutes are spent at the bedside and on the patient's hospital floor or unit.

99254 Inpatient consultation for a new or established patient, which requires these 3 key components: A comprehensive history; A comprehensive examination; and Medical decision making of moderate complexity. Counseling and/or coordination of care with other physicians, other qualified health care professionals, or agencies are provided consistent with the nature of the problem(s) and the patient's and/or family's needs. Usually, the presenting problem(s) are of moderate to high severity. Typically, 80 minutes are spent at the bedside and on the patient's hospital floor or unit.

99255 Inpatient consultation for a new or established patient, which requires these 3 key components: A comprehensive history; A comprehensive examination; and Medical decision making of high complexity. Counseling and/or coordination of care with other physicians, other qualified health care professionals, or agencies are provided consistent with the nature of the problem(s) and the patient's and/or family's needs. Usually, the presenting problem(s) are of moderate to high severity. Typically, 110 minutes are spent at the bedside and on the patient's hospital floor or unit.

Explanation

Inpatient consultation service codes describe encounters with patients admitted to the hospital, residing in nursing facilities, or to patients in a partial hospital setting where another qualified clinician's advice or opinion regarding diagnosis and treatment or determination to accept transfer of care of a patient is rendered at the request of the primary treating provider. The request for a consultation must be documented in the patient's medical record, as well as a written report of the findings of the consultation to the primary treating physician. During the course of a consultation, the physician consultant can initiate diagnostic or therapeutic services at the same encounter or at a follow-up visit. Other procedures or services performed in conjunction with the consultation may be reported separately. Codes do not differentiate between new or established patients and only one inpatient consultation services code should be reported per admission. Services are reported based on meeting all three key components—history, exam, and medical decision making (MDM)—within each level of service. The most basic service, as represented by 99251, describes a problem focused history and exam with straightforward medical decision making for a minor or self-limiting complaint encompassing approximately 20 minutes of time at the patient's bedside or on the unit. The mid-level services describe problems involving an expanded problem focused history and exam or a detailed history and exam as represented by 99252 and 99253, respectively. Medical decision making for 99252 is the same (straightforward) as for a level one visit (99251) and is designated as low complexity for the level three service (99253). At these levels of service, the encounter can involve time at the patient's bedside or on the unit of 40 (99252) to 55 (99253) minutes involving minimal to low severity concerns. The last two levels of service in this category represent moderate to high severity problems and both services involve comprehensive history and examination components. The differentiating factor between the two levels is the medical decision making. Code 99254 involves moderate complexity MDM and approximately 80 minutes of time at the patient's bedside or on the unit while the highest level of service in this category, 99255, involves MDM of high complexity and approximately 110 minutes at the patient's bedside or on the unit.

Coding Tips

These codes are used to report consultations in the inpatient setting. All three key components (history, exam, and medical decision making) must be met or exceeded for the level of service selected. Time may be used to select the level of service when counseling and coordination of care are documented as at least half of the time spent face-to-face with the patient. Consultation codes are not covered by Medicare and some payers. Report new or established inpatient E/M codes for consultation services. Consultation services should not be reported when the care and management of a problem or condition is assumed prior to the initial examination of the patient. In these situations the appropriate initial or subsequent evaluation and management service should be reported. Do not report an inpatient and outpatient consultation when both are related to the same inpatient admission. For initial hospital care services, see 99221-99223; for subsequent hospital care services, see 99231-99233. For office or other outpatient consultation services, see 99241-99245.

ICD-10-CM Diagnostic Codes

The application of this code is too broad to adequately present ICD-10-CM diagnostic code links here. Refer to your ICD-10-CM book.

AMA: 99251 2018,Jan,8; 2017,Jun,6; 2017,Jan,8; 2017,Aug,3; 2016,Jan,7; 2016,Jan,13; 2016,Dec,11; 2015,Jan,16; 2014,Oct,8; 2014,Nov,14; 2014,Jan,11; 2013,Jun,3-5; 2013,Jan,9-10 **99252** 2018,Jan,8; 2017,Jun,6; 2017,Jan,8; 2017,Aug,3; 2016,Jan,7; 2016,Jan,13; 2016,Dec,11; 2015,Jan,16; 2014,Oct,8; 2014,Nov,14; 2014,Jan,11; 2013,Jun,3-5; 2013,Jan,9-10 **99253** 2018,Jan,8; 2017,Jun,6; 2017,Jan,8; 2017,Aug,3; 2016,Jan,13; 2016,Jan,7; 2016,Dec,11; 2015,Jan,16; 2014,Oct,8; 2014,Nov,14; 2014,Jan,11; 2013,Jun,3-5; 2013,Jan,9-10 **99254** 2018,Jan,8; 2017,Jun,6; 2017,Jan,8; 2017,Aug,3; 2016,Jan,7; 2016,Jan,13; 2016,Dec,11; 2015,Jan,16; 2014,Oct,8; 2014,Nov,14; 2014,Jan,11; 2013,Jun,3-5; 2013,Jan,9-10 **99255** 2018,Jan,8; 2017,Jun,6; 2017,Jan,8; 2017,Aug,3; 2016,Jan,7; 2016,Jan,13; 2016,Dec,11; 2015,Jan,16; 2014,Oct,8; 2014,Nov,14; 2014,Jan,11; 2013,Jun,3-5; 2013,Jan,9-10

Relative Value Units/Medicare Edits

Non-Facility RVU	Work	PE	MP	Total
99251	1.0	0.32	0.06	1.38
99252	1.5	0.52	0.09	2.11
99253	2.27	0.84	0.14	3.25
99254	3.29	1.23	0.2	4.72
99255	4.0	1.44	0.24	5.68
Facility RVU	**Work**	**PE**	**MP**	**Total**
99251	1.0	0.32	0.06	1.38
99252	1.5	0.52	0.09	2.11
99253	2.27	0.84	0.14	3.25
99254	3.29	1.23	0.2	4.72
99255	4.0	1.44	0.24	5.68

	FUD	Status	MUE	Modifiers				IOM Reference
99251	N/A	I	0(3)	N/A	N/A	N/A	N/A	100-04,12,30.6.4; 100-04,12,30.6.10; 100-04,12,100
99252	N/A	I	0(3)	N/A	N/A	N/A	N/A	
99253	N/A	I	0(3)	N/A	N/A	N/A	N/A	
99254	N/A	I	0(3)	N/A	N/A	N/A	N/A	
99255	N/A	I	0(3)	N/A	N/A	N/A	N/A	

* with documentation

Terms To Know

consultation. Advice or opinion regarding diagnosis and treatment or determination to accept transfer of care of a patient that is rendered by a medical professional at the request of the primary care provider. Consultations may also be requested by another appropriate source. A request for consultation must be documented in the medical record, as well as a written report of the findings of the consultation. Since January 1, 2010, Medicare no longer recognizes CPT consultation codes; however, telehealth consultation services reported with HCPCS Level II codes are a paid service under the Medicare Physician Fee Schedule (MPFS).

key components. Three components of history, examination, and medical decision making are considered the keys to selecting the correct level of E/M codes. In most cases, all three components must be addressed in the documentation. However, in established, subsequent, and follow-up categories, only two of the three must be met or exceeded for a given code.

99281-99285

99281 Emergency department visit for the evaluation and management of a patient, which requires these 3 key components: A problem focused history; A problem focused examination; and Straightforward medical decision making. Counseling and/or coordination of care with other physicians, other qualified health care professionals, or agencies are provided consistent with the nature of the problem(s) and the patient's and/or family's needs. Usually, the presenting problem(s) are self limited or minor.

99282 Emergency department visit for the evaluation and management of a patient, which requires these 3 key components: An expanded problem focused history; An expanded problem focused examination; and Medical decision making of low complexity. Counseling and/or coordination of care with other physicians, other qualified health care professionals, or agencies are provided consistent with the nature of the problem(s) and the patient's and/or family's needs. Usually, the presenting problem(s) are of low to moderate severity.

99283 Emergency department visit for the evaluation and management of a patient, which requires these 3 key components: An expanded problem focused history; An expanded problem focused examination; and Medical decision making of moderate complexity. Counseling and/or coordination of care with other physicians, other qualified health care professionals, or agencies are provided consistent with the nature of the problem(s) and the patient's and/or family's needs. Usually, the presenting problem(s) are of moderate severity.

99284 Emergency department visit for the evaluation and management of a patient, which requires these 3 key components: A detailed history; A detailed examination; and Medical decision making of moderate complexity. Counseling and/or coordination of care with other physicians, other qualified health care professionals, or agencies are provided consistent with the nature of the problem(s) and the patient's and/or family's needs. Usually, the presenting problem(s) are of high severity, and require urgent evaluation by the physician, or other qualified health care professionals but do not pose an immediate significant threat to life or physiologic function.

99285 Emergency department visit for the evaluation and management of a patient, which requires these 3 key components within the constraints imposed by the urgency of the patient's clinical condition and/or mental status: A comprehensive history; A comprehensive examination; and Medical decision making of high complexity. Counseling and/or coordination of care with other physicians, other qualified health care professionals, or agencies are provided consistent with the nature of the problem(s) and the patient's and/or family's needs. Usually, the presenting problem(s) are of high severity and pose an immediate significant threat to life or physiologic function.

Explanation

Emergency department services codes describe E/M services provided to patients in the emergency department (ED). ED codes are typically reported per day and do not differentiate between new or established patients. Under the emergency department services category, there are five levels represented by 99281-99285. All levels require the three key components—history, exam, and medical decision making—to be documented. The lowest level of care, 99281, requires a problem focused history and exam with straightforward medical decision making involving a minor or self-limiting complaint. Mid-level services describe an expanded problem focused history and exam with medical decision making of low or moderate complexity as represented by 99282 and 99283, respectively. At these levels of service, the encounter typically addresses low to moderate severity health concerns. The last two levels of service in this category represent high severity problems. Code 99284 describes a high severity health concern that does not pose an immediate threat to life or physiologic function; a detailed history and exam in conjunction with moderate complexity medical decision making are required for reporting this level of service. The highest level of service, 99285, requires a comprehensive history and examination with high complexity medical decision making for high severity health issues that pose an immediate threat to the life or physiologic function of the patient. Time is not listed as a component in the code descriptors for emergency department services as these types of services are provided based on the varying intensity of the patient's condition and may involve emergency providers caring for several patients over an extended period of time involving multiple encounters making it difficult for the clinician to accurately detail the amount of time spent face-to-face with the patient.

Coding Tips

These codes are used to report emergency department services for the new or established patient. All three key components (history, exam, and medical decision making) must be met or exceeded for the level of service selected. Time is not a factor when selecting this E/M service. An emergency department is typically described as an organized hospital-based facility available 24 hours a day, providing unscheduled episodic services to patients in need of urgent medical attention. For critical care services provided in the emergency department, see 99291-99292. For observation care services provided to a patient located in the emergency department, see 99217-99220. For patients admitted and discharged from observation or inpatient status on the same date, see 99234-99236. Report place of service code 23 for services provided in the hospital emergency room.

ICD-10-CM Diagnostic Codes

The application of this code is too broad to adequately present ICD-10-CM diagnostic code links here. Refer to your ICD-10-CM book.

AMA: **99281** 2019,Jul,10; 2018,Jan,8; 2017,Jun,6; 2017,Jan,8; 2017,Aug,3; 2016,Jan,13; 2016,Jan,7; 2015,Jan,16; 2015,Jan,12; 2014,Oct,8; 2014,Nov,14; 2014,Jan,11; 2013,Jun,3-5; 2013,Jan,9-10 **99282** 2019,Jul,10; 2018,Jan,8; 2017,Jun,6; 2017,Jan,8; 2017,Aug,3; 2016,Jan,13; 2016,Jan,7; 2015,Jan,12; 2015,Jan,16; 2014,Oct,8; 2014,Nov,14; 2014,Jan,11; 2013,Jun,3-5; 2013,Jan,9-10 **99283** 2019,Jul,10; 2018,Jan,8; 2017,Jun,6; 2017,Jan,8; 2017,Aug,3; 2016,Jan,13; 2016,Jan,7; 2015,Jan,16; 2015,Jan,12; 2014,Oct,8; 2014,Nov,14; 2014,Jan,11; 2013,Jun,3-5; 2013,Jan,9-10 **99284** 2019,Jul,10; 2018,Jan,8; 2017,Jun,6; 2017,Jan,8; 2017,Aug,3; 2016,Jan,13; 2016,Jan,7; 2015,Jan,12; 2015,Jan,16; 2014,Oct,8; 2014,Nov,14; 2014,Jan,11; 2013,Jun,3-5; 2013,Jan,9-10 **99285** 2019,Jul,10; 2018,Jan,8; 2017,Jun,6; 2017,Jan,8; 2017,Aug,3; 2016,Jan,13; 2016,Jan,7; 2015,Jan,12; 2015,Jan,16; 2014,Oct,8; 2014,Nov,14; 2014,Jan,11; 2013,Jun,3-5; 2013,Jan,9-10

Relative Value Units/Medicare Edits

Non-Facility RVU	Work	PE	MP	Total
99281	0.45	0.11	0.04	0.6
99282	0.88	0.21	0.08	1.17
99283	1.34	0.29	0.12	1.75
99284	2.56	0.53	0.23	3.32
99285	3.8	0.74	0.35	4.89
Facility RVU	**Work**	**PE**	**MP**	**Total**
99281	0.45	0.11	0.04	0.6
99282	0.88	0.21	0.08	1.17
99283	1.34	0.29	0.12	1.75
99284	2.56	0.53	0.23	3.32
99285	3.8	0.74	0.35	4.89

	FUD	Status	MUE	Modifiers				IOM Reference
99281	N/A	A	1(3)	N/A	N/A	N/A	80*	100-04,4,160; 100-04,12,30.6.4; 100-04,12,30.6.11; 100-04,12,100
99282	N/A	A	1(3)	N/A	N/A	N/A	80*	
99283	N/A	A	1(3)	N/A	N/A	N/A	80*	
99284	N/A	A	1(3)	N/A	N/A	N/A	80*	
99285	N/A	A	1(3)	N/A	N/A	N/A	80*	

* with documentation

Terms To Know

detailed physical examination. Under the 1995 guidelines, examination of two to seven organ systems, with at least one system documented in detail. Under the 1997 guidelines, an examination of at least six organ systems or body areas, including at least two bullet point elements for each system/area or at least 12 bullet point elements from at least two organ systems or body areas.

expanded problem focused physical examination. Under the 1995 guidelines, examination of two to seven organ systems. Under the 1997 guidelines, examination of at least six bullet point elements in one or more organ systems from the general multisystem examination OR examination of at least six of the bullet point elements from one of the 10 single organ system exams.

problem focused physical examination. Under the 1995 guidelines, an examination of one organ system or body area. Under the 1997 guidelines, examination of one to five bullet point elements in one or more organ system or body areas.

99288

99288 Physician or other qualified health care professional direction of emergency medical systems (EMS) emergency care, advanced life support

Explanation

This code is used to report qualified clinician direction of emergency medical systems (EMS) emergency care or advanced life support in the emergency department (ED). This can involve the clinician communicating via a two-way voice system with emergency medical technicians in an ambulance or with other rescue personnel who are outside of the hospital emergency department. Clinician direction of the performance of medically necessary procedures includes, but is not limited to, telemetry of cardiac rhythm; cardiac and/or pulmonary resuscitation; endotracheal or esophageal obturator airway intubation; administration of intravenous (IV) fluids and/or intramuscular (IM), intra-tracheal, or subcutaneous drugs; and/or electrical conversion of cardiac arrhythmia.

Coding Tips

This code is used by a facility-based practitioner (emergency department, critical care unit) who is directing remote emergency care or advanced life support in the urgent care of the patient. Time is not a factor when selecting this E/M service. This service may be reported in addition to other E/M services on the same date when documented in the patient record.

ICD-10-CM Diagnostic Codes

The application of this code is too broad to adequately present ICD-10-CM diagnostic code links here. Refer to your ICD-10-CM book.

AMA: **99288** 2018,Jan,8; 2017,Jun,6; 2017,Jan,8; 2017,Aug,3; 2016,Jan,13; 2015,Jan,16; 2014,Oct,8; 2014,Jan,11; 2013,May,6-7

Relative Value Units/Medicare Edits

Non-Facility RVU	Work	PE	MP	Total
99288	0.0	0.0	0.0	0.0
Facility RVU	**Work**	**PE**	**MP**	**Total**
99288	0.0	0.0	0.0	0.0

	FUD	Status	MUE	Modifiers				IOM Reference
99288	N/A	B	0(3)	N/A	N/A	N/A	N/A	100-04,12,100

* with documentation

Terms To Know

emergency department. Organized hospital-based facility for the provision of unscheduled episodic services to patients who present for immediate medical attention. The facility must be available 24 hours a day.

qualified health care professional. Educated, licensed or certified, and regulated professional operating under a specified scope of practice to provide patient services that are separate and distinct from other clinical staff.

99291-99292

99291 Critical care, evaluation and management of the critically ill or critically injured patient; first 30-74 minutes

\+ **99292** each additional 30 minutes (List separately in addition to code for primary service)

Explanation

Critical care services are reported by a physician or other qualified health care provider for critically ill or injured patients. Critical illnesses or injuries are defined as those with impairment to one or more vital organ systems with an increased risk of rapid or imminent health deterioration. Critical care services require direct patient/provider involvement with highly complex decision making in order to evaluate, control, and support vital systems functions to treat one or more vital organ system failures and/or to avoid further decline of the patient's condition. Vital organ system failure includes, but is not limited to, failure of the central nervous, circulatory, or respiratory systems; kidneys; liver; shock; and other metabolic processes. Generally, critical care services necessitate the interpretation of many physiologic parameters and/or other applications of advanced technology as available in a critical care unit, pediatric intensive care unit, respiratory care unit, in an emergency facility, patient room or other hospital department; however, in emergent situations, critical care may be provided where these elements are not available. Critical care may be provided so long as the patient's condition continues to warrant the level of care according to the criteria described. Care provided to patients residing in a critical care unit but not fitting the criteria for critical care is reported using other E/M codes, as appropriate. These codes are time based codes, meaning the total time spent must be documented and includes direct patient care bedside or time spent on the patient's floor or unit (reviewing laboratory results or imaging studies and discussing the patient's care with medical staff, time spent with family members, caregivers, or other surrogate decision makers to gather information on the patient's medical history, reviewing the patient's condition or prognosis, and discussing various treatment options or limitations of treatment), as long as the clinician is immediately available and not providing services to any other patient during the same time period. Time spent outside of the patient's unit or floor, including telephone calls, caregiver discussions, or time spent in actions that do not directly contribute to the patient's care rendered in the critical unit are not reported as critical care. Report these codes for attendance of the patient during transport for patients 24 months of age or older to or from a facility. Code 99291 represents the first 30 to 74 minutes of critical care and is reported once per day. Additional time beyond the first 74 minutes is reported in 30 minute increments with 99292.

Coding Tips

These codes are used to report critical care services. These are time-based services and the total time spent providing critical care must be documented in the medical record. All time spent providing critical care on the same date of service is added together and does not need to be contiguous. Time is reported for practitioner time spent in care of the critically ill or injured patient at the patient's bedside and on the floor/unit. Time spent off the patient unit, even if related to patient care, is not counted. Do not report critical care for patients who may be in the critical care unit but are not currently critically ill. The following services are considered inclusive to the critical care codes when reported by the clinician: interpretation of cardiac output measurements, chest x-rays, pulse oximetry, blood gases, collection and interpretation of physiologic data, computer data such as ECGs, gastric intubation, vascular access, and ventilation management. Code 99291 is reported once per day. Code 99292 is reported in addition to code 99291. Medicare and some other payers may allow 99292 to be reported alone when critical care is reported by another physician of the same group and specialty the same date as another provider reporting 99291. For care of the critically ill neonate, see 99468-99469; for patients 29 days through 24 months, see 99471-99472; and for patients 2 through 5 years, see 99475-99476.

ICD-10-CM Diagnostic Codes

The application of this code is too broad to adequately present ICD-10-CM diagnostic code links here. Refer to your ICD-10-CM book.

AMA: **99291** 2019,Jul,10; 2019,Aug,8; 2018,Jun,9; 2018,Jan,8; 2018,Dec,8; 2018,Dec,8; 2017,Jun,6; 2017,Jan,8; 2017,Aug,3; 2016,Oct,8; 2016,May,3; 2016,Jan,13; 2016,Aug,9; 2015,Jul,3; 2015,Jan,16; 2015,Feb,10; 2014,Oct,8; 2014,Oct,14; 2014,May,4; 2014,Jan,11; 2014,Aug,5; 2013,May,6-7; 2013,Feb,16-17 **99292** 2019,Jul,10; 2019,Aug,8; 2018,Jun,9; 2018,Jan,8; 2018,Dec,8; 2018,Dec,8; 2017,Jun,6; 2017,Jan,8; 2017,Aug,3; 2016,May,3; 2016,Jan,13; 2016,Aug,9; 2015,Jul,3; 2015,Jan,16; 2015,Feb,10; 2014,Oct,14; 2014,Oct,8; 2014,May,4; 2014,Jan,11; 2014,Aug,5; 2013,May,6-7; 2013,Feb,16-17

Relative Value Units/Medicare Edits

Non-Facility RVU	Work	PE	MP	Total
99291	4.5	2.93	0.39	7.82
99292	2.25	1.01	0.2	3.46
Facility RVU	**Work**	**PE**	**MP**	**Total**
99291	4.5	1.39	0.39	6.28
99292	2.25	0.7	0.2	3.15

	FUD	Status	MUE	Modifiers				IOM Reference
99291	N/A	A	1(2)	N/A	N/A	N/A	80*	100-04,4,160; 100-04,12,30.6.9; 100-04,12,100
99292	N/A	A	8(3)	N/A	N/A	N/A	80*	

* with documentation

E/M Services

99304-99306

99304 Initial nursing facility care, per day, for the evaluation and management of a patient, which requires these 3 key components: A detailed or comprehensive history; A detailed or comprehensive examination; and Medical decision making that is straightforward or of low complexity. Counseling and/or coordination of care with other physicians, other qualified health care professionals, or agencies are provided consistent with the nature of the problem(s) and the patient's and/or family's needs. Usually, the problem(s) requiring admission are of low severity. Typically, 25 minutes are spent at the bedside and on the patient's facility floor or unit.

99305 Initial nursing facility care, per day, for the evaluation and management of a patient, which requires these 3 key components: A comprehensive history; A comprehensive examination; and Medical decision making of moderate complexity. Counseling and/or coordination of care with other physicians, other qualified health care professionals, or agencies are provided consistent with the nature of the problem(s) and the patient's and/or family's needs. Usually, the problem(s) requiring admission are of moderate severity. Typically, 35 minutes are spent at the bedside and on the patient's facility floor or unit.

99306 Initial nursing facility care, per day, for the evaluation and management of a patient, which requires these 3 key components: A comprehensive history; A comprehensive examination; and Medical decision making of high complexity. Counseling and/or coordination of care with other physicians, other qualified health care professionals, or agencies are provided consistent with the nature of the problem(s) and the patient's and/or family's needs. Usually, the problem(s) requiring admission are of high severity. Typically, 45 minutes are spent at the bedside and on the patient's facility floor or unit.

Explanation

Initial nursing facility service codes describe the first encounter with the patient by the admitting physician to nursing facilities, formerly referred to as skilled nursing facilities (SNF), intermediate care facilities (ICF), or long term care facilities (LTCF). These facilities provide specialized care to its residents, such as convalescent, rehabilitative, or long-term care. These codes are also reported for services rendered to patients in a psychiatric residential treatment center—a 24-hour live-in facility, a standalone facility, or separate part of a psychiatric facility, staffed with medical professionals in a structured therapeutic environment. When the patient is admitted to the nursing facility during the course of another encounter from a different site of service, such as the physician's office or the emergency department, all of the E/M services rendered by the supervising clinician are considered part of the initial nursing facility care services when performed on the same day and the level of care reported for that date is inclusive of these services. Physician services may also include information necessary to complete the Resident Assessment Instrument (RAI). Every RAI is comprised of the Minimum Data Set (MDS), Resident Assessment Protocols (RAP), and the utilization guidelines. Initial nursing facility codes do not differentiate between new or established patients. Under the initial nursing facility care category, there are three levels represented by 99304, 99305, and 99306. All of these levels require all three key components—history, exam, and medical decision making—to be documented. The lowest level of care within this category, 99304, requires a detailed or comprehensive history and exam as well as straightforward medical decision making or that of low severity with approximately 25 minutes being spent at the patient's bedside and on the patient's floor or unit. The midlevel and highest level initial nursing facility care codes require a comprehensive history and examination. Medical decision making is the differentiating factor for these two levels; for moderate complexity, report 99305 and for initial nursing facility care requiring MDM of high complexity, report 99306. The clinician typically spends 35 (99305) to 45 (99306) minutes at the patient's bedside or on the unit accordingly.

Coding Tips

These codes are used to report the initial encounter in the nursing facility setting or psychiatric residential treatment center. All three key components (history, exam, and medical decision making) must be met or exceeded for the level of service selected. Time may be used to select the level of service when counseling and coordination of care are documented as at least half of the floor/unit time spent with the patient. CPT guidelines indicate these services are reported only by the admitting/supervising provider; all other providers should report 99307-99310 or 99251-99255. Medicare and some payers may allow providers of different specialties to report initial nursing facility services and require the admitting/supervising provider to append modifier AI. All evaluation and management services provided in other settings (e.g., office, emergency department) leading up to the nursing facility admission are considered to be part of the patient's initial nursing facility admission when performed on the same date of service and should be reflected in the code selection. These codes are used to report the initial evaluation of a patient including the Resident Assessment Instrument (RAI). The major components of the RAI include the Minimum Data Set (MDS), a screening and assessment tool, the Resident Assessment Protocols (RAPs) that identify potential problems, and follow-up assessment guidelines. Hospital inpatient or observation discharge services may be reported separately when performed on the same date of service. For care plan oversight services provided to nursing facility residents, see 99379-99380. For subsequent nursing facility care services, see 99307-99310. For nursing facility discharge services, see 99315-99316.

ICD-10-CM Diagnostic Codes

The application of this code is too broad to adequately present ICD-10-CM diagnostic code links here. Refer to your ICD-10-CM book.

AMA: **99304** 2018,Jan,8; 2017,Jun,6; 2017,Jan,8; 2017,Aug,3; 2016,Jan,13; 2016,Jan,7; 2016,Dec,11; 2015,Jan,16; 2014,Oct,8; 2014,Nov,14; 2014,Jan,11; 2013,Jun,3-5; 2013,Jan,9-10 **99305** 2018,Jan,8; 2017,Jun,6; 2017,Jan,8; 2017,Aug,3; 2016,Jan,7; 2016,Jan,13; 2016,Dec,11; 2015,Jan,16; 2014,Oct,8; 2014,Nov,14; 2014,Jan,11; 2013,Jun,3-5; 2013,Jan,9-10 **99306** 2018,Jan,8; 2017,Jun,6; 2017,Jan,8; 2017,Aug,3; 2016,Jan,13; 2016,Jan,7; 2016,Dec,11; 2015,Jan,16; 2014,Oct,8; 2014,Nov,14; 2014,Jan,11; 2013,Jun,3-5; 2013,Jan,9-10

Relative Value Units/Medicare Edits

Non-Facility RVU	Work	PE	MP	Total
99304	1.64	0.78	0.12	2.54
99305	2.35	1.16	0.16	3.67
99306	3.06	1.45	0.19	4.7
Facility RVU	**Work**	**PE**	**MP**	**Total**
99304	1.64	0.78	0.12	2.54
99305	2.35	1.16	0.16	3.67
99306	3.06	1.45	0.19	4.7

	FUD	Status	MUE	Modifiers				IOM Reference
99304	N/A	A	1(2)	N/A	N/A	N/A	80*	100-04,12,30.6.4; 100-04,12,30.6.13
99305	N/A	A	1(2)	N/A	N/A	N/A	80*	
99306	N/A	A	1(2)	N/A	N/A	N/A	80*	

* with documentation

99307-99310

99307 Subsequent nursing facility care, per day, for the evaluation and management of a patient, which requires at least 2 of these 3 key components: A problem focused interval history; A problem focused examination; Straightforward medical decision making. Counseling and/or coordination of care with other physicians, other qualified health care professionals, or agencies are provided consistent with the nature of the problem(s) and the patient's and/or family's needs. Usually, the patient is stable, recovering, or improving. Typically, 10 minutes are spent at the bedside and on the patient's facility floor or unit.

99308 Subsequent nursing facility care, per day, for the evaluation and management of a patient, which requires at least 2 of these 3 key components: An expanded problem focused interval history; An expanded problem focused examination; Medical decision making of low complexity. Counseling and/or coordination of care with other physicians, other qualified health care professionals, or agencies are provided consistent with the nature of the problem(s) and the patient's and/or family's needs. Usually, the patient is responding inadequately to therapy or has developed a minor complication. Typically, 15 minutes are spent at the bedside and on the patient's facility floor or unit.

99309 Subsequent nursing facility care, per day, for the evaluation and management of a patient, which requires at least 2 of these 3 key components: A detailed interval history; A detailed examination; Medical decision making of moderate complexity. Counseling and/or coordination of care with other physicians, other qualified health care professionals, or agencies are provided consistent with the nature of the problem(s) and the patient's and/or family's needs. Usually, the patient has developed a significant complication or a significant new problem. Typically, 25 minutes are spent at the bedside and on the patient's facility floor or unit.

99310 Subsequent nursing facility care, per day, for the evaluation and management of a patient, which requires at least 2 of these 3 key components: A comprehensive interval history; A comprehensive examination; Medical decision making of high complexity. Counseling and/or coordination of care with other physicians, other qualified health care professionals, or agencies are provided consistent with the nature of the problem(s) and the patient's and/or family's needs. The patient may be unstable or may have developed a significant new problem requiring immediate physician attention. Typically, 35 minutes are spent at the bedside and on the patient's facility floor or unit.

Explanation

Subsequent nursing facility care services codes describe visits that occur after the first encounter of the patient's nursing facility admission by the supervising qualified clinician. Codes are reported per day and do not differentiate between new or established patients. Under the subsequent nursing facility care category, there are four levels of service represented by 99307, 99308, 99309, and 99310. Each level requires at least two out of the three key components—history, exam, and medical decision making—to be documented. The lowest level of care within this category, 99307, describes a problem-focused interval history as well as a problem-focused examination with straightforward medical decision making involving approximately 10 minutes of time by the provider at the patient's bedside or on the unit. For the mid-level subsequent nursing facility care code, 99308, an expanded problem-focused history and examination are required with low complexity medical decision making. Time associated with this level usually involves 15 minutes at the bedside or on the patient's floor. The third level of follow-up nursing facility care, 99309, requires a detailed history and exam as well as medical decision making of moderate complexity; for this level of care, the provider typically spends approximately 25 minutes at the bedside or on the patient's floor or unit. The fourth and highest level of nursing facility care is reported with 99310 and requires a comprehensive history and examination with high complexity medical decision making. The provider generally spends 35 minutes at the patient's bedside or on the unit or floor. All four levels of subsequent nursing facility care involve the clinician reviewing the patient's medical record, results from diagnostic studies, as well as any changes to the patient's status such as physical condition, response to treatments, or changes in health history since the last assessment.

Coding Tips

These codes are used to report the subsequent encounters in the nursing facility setting or psychiatric residential treatment center. Two of the three key components (history, exam, and medical decision making) must be met or exceeded for the level of service selected. Time may be used to select the level of service when counseling and coordination of care are documented as at least half of the floor/unit time spent with the patient. Codes may be selected based upon the 1995 or the 1997 Evaluation and Management Guidelines. Subsequent nursing facility services include review of the medical record, including all diagnostic studies, as well as changes noted in the patient's condition and response to treatment since the last evaluation. For care plan oversight services provided to nursing facility residents, see 99379-99380. For initial nursing facility care services, see 99304-99306; for nursing facility discharge services, see 99315-99316. Report place of service (POS) code 31 for the skilled nursing facility; report POS code 32 for the nursing facility; and report POS code 56 for the psychiatric residential treatment center.

ICD-10-CM Diagnostic Codes

The application of this code is too broad to adequately present ICD-10-CM diagnostic code links here. Refer to your ICD-10-CM book.

AMA: **99307** 2018,Jan,8; 2017,Jun,6; 2017,Jan,8; 2017,Aug,3; 2016,Jan,13; 2016,Jan,7; 2016,Dec,11; 2015,Jan,16; 2014,Oct,8; 2014,Nov,14; 2014,Jan,11; 2013,Jun,3-5; 2013,Jan,9-10 **99308** 2018,Jan,8; 2017,Jun,6; 2017,Jan,8; 2017,Aug,3; 2016,Jan,13; 2016,Jan,7; 2016,Dec,11; 2015,Jan,16; 2014,Oct,8; 2014,Nov,14; 2014,Jan,11; 2013,Jun,3-5; 2013,Jan,9-10 **99309** 2018,Jan,8; 2017,Jun,6; 2017,Jan,8; 2017,Aug,3; 2016,Jan,13; 2016,Jan,7; 2016,Dec,11; 2015,Jan,16; 2014,Oct,8; 2014,Nov,14; 2014,Jan,11; 2013,Jun,3-5; 2013,Jan,9-10 **99310** 2018,Jan,8; 2017,Jun,6; 2017,Jan,8; 2017,Aug,3; 2016,Jan,13; 2016,Jan,7; 2016,Dec,11; 2015,Jan,16; 2014,Oct,8; 2014,Nov,14; 2014,Jan,11; 2013,Jun,3-5; 2013,Jan,9-10

Relative Value Units/Medicare Edits

Non-Facility RVU	Work	PE	MP	Total
99307	0.76	0.43	0.05	1.24
99308	1.16	0.7	0.08	1.94
99309	1.55	0.92	0.11	2.58
99310	2.35	1.31	0.16	3.82
Facility RVU	**Work**	**PE**	**MP**	**Total**
99307	0.76	0.43	0.05	1.24
99308	1.16	0.7	0.08	1.94
99309	1.55	0.92	0.11	2.58
99310	2.35	1.31	0.16	3.82

	FUD	Status	MUE	Modifiers				IOM Reference
99307	N/A	A	1(2)	N/A	N/A	N/A	80*	None
99308	N/A	A	1(2)	N/A	N/A	N/A	80*	
99309	N/A	A	1(2)	N/A	N/A	N/A	80*	
99310	N/A	A	1(2)	N/A	N/A	N/A	80*	

* with documentation

Terms To Know

counseling. Discussion with a patient and/or family concerning one or more of the following areas: diagnostic results, impressions, and/or recommended diagnostic studies; prognosis; risks and benefits of management (treatment) options; instructions for management (treatment) and/or follow-up; importance of compliance with chosen management (treatment) options; risk factor reduction; and patient and family education.

medical decision making. Consideration of the differential diagnoses, the amount and/or complexity of data reviewed and considered (medical records, test results, correspondence from previous treating physicians, etc.), current diagnostic studies ordered, and treatment or management options and risk (complications of the patient's condition, the potential for complications, continued morbidity, risk of mortality, any comorbidities associated with the patient's disease process).

subsequent encounter. Denotes encounters by any provider after the initial encounter by the admitting or supervising provider, even if it is the first time the provider is seeing the patient.

99315-99316

99315 Nursing facility discharge day management; 30 minutes or less
99316 more than 30 minutes

Explanation

Nursing facility discharge services are time-based codes that describe the amount of time spent by the clinician during all final steps involved in the discharge of a patient from the nursing facility, including the last patient exam, discussing the nursing facility stay, instructions for ongoing care as it relates to all pertinent caregivers, and preparing the medical discharge records, prescriptions, and/or referrals as applicable. Time reported should be for the total duration of time spent by the provider even when the time spent on that date is not continuous. For a nursing facility discharge duration of 30 minutes or less, report 99315; for a duration of greater than 30 minutes, report 99316. These codes are reported following initial and subsequent nursing facility care codes 99304-99306 and 99307-99310.

Coding Tips

These codes are used to report all discharge day services for the nursing facility resident. These codes include patient examination, follow-up care instructions to appropriate caregivers, prescriptions, referrals, and preparation of all medical records. These are time-based codes and floor unit time spent caring for the patient must be documented in the medical record. All time spent providing discharge services on the same date of service is added together and does not need to be contiguous. For initial nursing facility care services, see 99304-99306; for subsequent nursing facility care services, see 99307-99310. Report place of service (POS) code 31 for the skilled nursing facility; report POS code 32 for the nursing facility; and report POS code 56 for the psychiatric residential treatment center.

ICD-10-CM Diagnostic Codes

The application of this code is too broad to adequately present ICD-10-CM diagnostic code links here. Refer to your ICD-10-CM book.

AMA: **99315** 2018,Jan,8; 2017,Jun,6; 2017,Jan,8; 2017,Aug,3; 2016,Jan,13; 2016,Jan,7; 2016,Dec,11; 2015,Jan,16; 2014,Oct,8; 2014,Nov,14; 2014,Jan,11; 2013,Jun,3-5; 2013,Jan,9-10 **99316** 2018,Jan,8; 2017,Jun,6; 2017,Jan,8; 2017,Aug,3; 2016,Jan,13; 2016,Jan,7; 2016,Dec,11; 2015,Jan,16; 2014,Oct,8; 2014,Nov,14; 2014,Jan,11; 2013,Jun,3-5; 2013,Jan,9-10

Relative Value Units/Medicare Edits

Non-Facility RVU	Work	PE	MP	Total
99315	1.28	0.7	0.09	2.07
99316	1.9	0.95	0.13	2.98
Facility RVU	**Work**	**PE**	**MP**	**Total**
99315	1.28	0.7	0.09	2.07
99316	1.9	0.95	0.13	2.98

	FUD	Status	MUE	Modifiers				IOM Reference
99315	N/A	A	1(2)	N/A	N/A	N/A	80*	100-04,12,30.6.4; 100-04,12,30.6.13; 100-04,12,100
99316	N/A	A	1(2)	N/A	N/A	N/A	80*	

* with documentation

99324-99328

99324 Domiciliary or rest home visit for the evaluation and management of a new patient, which requires these 3 key components: A problem focused history; A problem focused examination; and Straightforward medical decision making. Counseling and/or coordination of care with other physicians, other qualified health care professionals, or agencies are provided consistent with the nature of the problem(s) and the patient's and/or family's needs. Usually, the presenting problem(s) are of low severity. Typically, 20 minutes are spent with the patient and/or family or caregiver.

99325 Domiciliary or rest home visit for the evaluation and management of a new patient, which requires these 3 key components: An expanded problem focused history; An expanded problem focused examination; and Medical decision making of low complexity. Counseling and/or coordination of care with other physicians, other qualified health care professionals, or agencies are provided consistent with the nature of the problem(s) and the patient's and/or family's needs. Usually, the presenting problem(s) are of moderate severity. Typically, 30 minutes are spent with the patient and/or family or caregiver.

99326 Domiciliary or rest home visit for the evaluation and management of a new patient, which requires these 3 key components: A detailed history; A detailed examination; and Medical decision making of moderate complexity. Counseling and/or coordination of care with other physicians, other qualified health care professionals, or agencies are provided consistent with the nature of the problem(s) and the patient's and/or family's needs. Usually, the presenting problem(s) are of moderate to high severity. Typically, 45 minutes are spent with the patient and/or family or caregiver.

99327 Domiciliary or rest home visit for the evaluation and management of a new patient, which requires these 3 key components: A comprehensive history; A comprehensive examination; and Medical decision making of moderate complexity. Counseling and/or coordination of care with other physicians, other qualified health care professionals, or agencies are provided consistent with the nature of the problem(s) and the patient's and/or family's needs. Usually, the presenting problem(s) are of high severity. Typically, 60 minutes are spent with the patient and/or family or caregiver.

99328 Domiciliary or rest home visit for the evaluation and management of a new patient, which requires these 3 key components: A comprehensive history; A comprehensive examination; and Medical decision making of high complexity. Counseling and/or coordination of care with other physicians, other qualified health care professionals, or agencies are provided consistent with the nature of the problem(s) and the patient's and/or family's needs. Usually, the patient is unstable or has developed a significant new problem requiring immediate physician attention. Typically, 75 minutes are spent with the patient and/or family or caregiver.

Explanation

Providers report domiciliary, rest home, or custodial care services codes for E/M services rendered to new patients residing in a facility, usually long-term, that offers room and board as well as other personal assistance services. These codes may also be reported for patients residing in an assisted living facility. Services are reported based on meeting all three key components—history, exam, and medical decision making (MDM)—within each level of service. The most basic service, 99324, describes a problem focused history and exam with straightforward medical decision making for low severity problems encompassing approximately 20 minutes of time with the patient and/or family or caregiver. Mid-level services require an expanded problem focused history and exam or a detailed history and exam, represented by 99325 and 99326, respectively. Medical decision making for 99325 is designated as low complexity; moderate complexity for 99326. At these levels of service, the encounter can involve physician time spent with the patient and/or family or caregiver of 30 (99325) to 45 minutes (99326). The last two levels of service in this category require documenting comprehensive history and examination components. The differentiating factor between the two levels is the medical decision making; 99327 involves moderate complexity MDM and approximately 60 minutes of time with the patient and/or family or caregiver for high severity problems, while the highest level of service in this category, 99328, involves MDM of high complexity and 75 minutes of time with the patient and/or family or caregiver as a result of the patient being unstable or having developed a significant, new problem necessitating the immediate attention of the clinician.

Coding Tips

These codes are used to report services provided in a domiciliary setting for a new patient, including services provided in a group home, assisted living facility, intermediate care, or custodial care facilities. All three key components (history, exam, and medical decision making) must be met or exceeded for the level of service selected. Time may be used to select the level of service when counseling and coordination of care are documented as at least half of the time spent face-to-face with the patient. Codes may be selected based upon the 1995 or the 1997 Evaluation and Management Guidelines. These services are reported by the admitting/supervising provider; all other providers should report other E/M services. For care plan oversight services provided to a patient residing in a domiciliary facility under the care of a hospice agency, see 99377-99378; for a home health agency, see 99374-99375. For care plan oversight services provided to a patient under home, domiciliary, or rest home (assisted living) care, see 99339-99340.

ICD-10-CM Diagnostic Codes

The application of this code is too broad to adequately present ICD-10-CM diagnostic code links here. Refer to your ICD-10-CM book.

AMA: 99324 2018,Jan,8; 2018,Apr,9; 2017,Jun,6; 2017,Jan,8; 2017,Aug,3; 2016,Jan,13; 2016,Jan,7; 2016,Dec,11; 2015,Jan,16; 2014,Oct,8; 2014,Oct,3; 2014,Nov,14; 2014,Jan,11; 2013,Jun,3-5; 2013,Jan,9-10 **99325** 2018,Jan,8; 2018,Apr,9; 2017,Jun,6; 2017,Jan,8; 2017,Aug,3; 2016,Jan,13; 2016,Jan,7; 2016,Dec,11; 2015,Jan,16; 2014,Oct,8; 2014,Oct,3; 2014,Nov,14; 2014,Jan,11; 2013,Jun,3-5; 2013,Jan,9-10 **99326** 2018,Jan,8; 2018,Apr,9; 2017,Jun,6; 2017,Jan,8; 2017,Aug,3; 2016,Jan,7; 2016,Jan,13; 2016,Dec,11; 2015,Jan,16; 2014,Oct,8; 2014,Oct,3; 2014,Nov,14; 2014,Jan,11; 2013,Jun,3-5; 2013,Jan,9-10 **99327** 2018,Jan,8; 2018,Apr,9; 2017,Jun,6; 2017,Jan,8; 2017,Aug,3; 2016,Jan,13; 2016,Jan,7; 2016,Dec,11; 2015,Jan,16; 2014,Oct,8; 2014,Oct,3; 2014,Nov,14; 2014,Jan,11; 2013,Jun,3-5; 2013,Jan,9-10 **99328** 2018,Jan,8; 2018,Apr,9; 2017,Jun,6; 2017,Jan,8; 2017,Aug,3; 2016,Jan,13; 2016,Jan,7; 2016,Dec,11; 2015,Jan,16; 2014,Oct,8; 2014,Oct,3; 2014,Nov,14; 2014,Jan,11; 2013,Jun,3-5; 2013,Jan,9-10

Relative Value Units/Medicare Edits

Non-Facility RVU	Work	PE	MP	Total
99324	1.01	0.48	0.07	1.56
99325	1.52	0.64	0.1	2.26
99326	2.63	1.12	0.17	3.92
99327	3.46	1.57	0.23	5.26
99328	4.09	1.83	0.27	6.19
Facility RVU	**Work**	**PE**	**MP**	**Total**
99324	1.01	0.48	0.07	1.56
99325	1.52	0.64	0.1	2.26
99326	2.63	1.12	0.17	3.92
99327	3.46	1.57	0.23	5.26
99328	4.09	1.83	0.27	6.19

	FUD	Status	MUE	Modifiers				IOM Reference
99324	N/A	A	1(2)	N/A	N/A	N/A	80*	100-04,12,30.6.4; 100-04,12,30.6.14
99325	N/A	A	1(2)	N/A	N/A	N/A	80*	
99326	N/A	A	1(2)	N/A	N/A	N/A	80*	
99327	N/A	A	1(2)	N/A	N/A	N/A	80*	
99328	N/A	A	1(2)	N/A	N/A	N/A	80*	

* with documentation

Terms To Know

domiciliary. Facility, such as an assisted living, group home, custodial care, or an intermediate care facility, that provides room and board on a long-term basis and may include personal assistance services.

new patient. Patient who is receiving face-to-face care from a provider/qualified health care professional or another physician/qualified health care professional of the exact same specialty and subspecialty who belongs to the same group practice for the first time in three years. For OPPS hospitals, a patient who has not been registered as an inpatient or outpatient, including off-campus provider based clinic or emergency department, within the past three years.

99334-99337

99334 Domiciliary or rest home visit for the evaluation and management of an established patient, which requires at least 2 of these 3 key components: A problem focused interval history; A problem focused examination; Straightforward medical decision making. Counseling and/or coordination of care with other physicians, other qualified health care professionals, or agencies are provided consistent with the nature of the problem(s) and the patient's and/or family's needs. Usually, the presenting problem(s) are self-limited or minor. Typically, 15 minutes are spent with the patient and/or family or caregiver.

99335 Domiciliary or rest home visit for the evaluation and management of an established patient, which requires at least 2 of these 3 key components: An expanded problem focused interval history; An expanded problem focused examination; Medical decision making of low complexity. Counseling and/or coordination of care with other physicians, other qualified health care professionals, or agencies are provided consistent with the nature of the problem(s) and the patient's and/or family's needs. Usually, the presenting problem(s) are of low to moderate severity. Typically, 25 minutes are spent with the patient and/or family or caregiver.

99336 Domiciliary or rest home visit for the evaluation and management of an established patient, which requires at least 2 of these 3 key components: A detailed interval history; A detailed examination; Medical decision making of moderate complexity. Counseling and/or coordination of care with other physicians, other qualified health care professionals, or agencies are provided consistent with the nature of the problem(s) and the patient's and/or family's needs. Usually, the presenting problem(s) are of moderate to high severity. Typically, 40 minutes are spent with the patient and/or family or caregiver.

99337 Domiciliary or rest home visit for the evaluation and management of an established patient, which requires at least 2 of these 3 key components: A comprehensive interval history; A comprehensive examination; Medical decision making of moderate to high complexity. Counseling and/or coordination of care with other physicians, other qualified health care professionals, or agencies are provided consistent with the nature of the problem(s) and the patient's and/or family's needs. Usually, the presenting problem(s) are of moderate to high severity. The patient may be unstable or may have developed a significant new problem requiring immediate physician attention. Typically, 60 minutes are spent with the patient and/or family or caregiver.

Explanation

Providers report domiciliary, rest home, or custodial care services codes for E/M services rendered to established patients residing in a facility, usually long-term, that offers room and board as well as other personal assistance services. These codes may also be reported for patients residing in an assisted living facility. Services in this category are reported based on meeting at least two of the three key components—history, exam, and medical decision making (MDM)—within each level of service. The most basic service, 99334, describes a problem-focused interval history and problem-focused exam with straightforward medical decision making for problems considered minimal and generally involves approximately 15 minutes of time with the patient and/or family or caregiver. Mid-level services require an expanded problem focused history and exam or a detailed history and exam as represented by 99335 and 99336, respectively. Medical decision making for 99335 is designated as low complexity; moderate complexity for 99336. At these levels of service, the encounter can involve clinician time spent with the patient and/or family or caregiver of 25 (99335) to 40 minutes (99336) for problems considered to be of a low to moderate or moderate to high severity. The last level of service in this category, 99337, consists of a comprehensive history and examination, as well as medical decision making of moderate to high complexity. The clinician can expect to spend approximately 60 minutes duration with the patient and/or family or caregiver for moderate to high severity problems as a result of the patient being unstable or having developed a significant, new problem necessitating the immediate attention of the provider.

Coding Tips

These codes are used to report services provided in a domiciliary setting for an established patient, including services provided in a group home, assisted living facility, intermediate care, or custodial care facilities. Two of the three key components (history, exam, and medical decision making) must be met or exceeded for the level of service selected. Time may be used to select the level of service when counseling and coordination of care are documented as at least half of the time spent face-to-face with the patient. Codes may be selected based upon the 1995 or the 1997 Evaluation and Management Guidelines. For care plan oversight services provided to a patient residing in a domiciliary facility under the care of a hospice agency, see 99377-99378; provided under the care of a home health agency, see 99374-99375. For care plan oversight services provided to a patient under home, domiciliary, or rest home (assisted living) care, see 99339-99340.

ICD-10-CM Diagnostic Codes

The application of this code is too broad to adequately present ICD-10-CM diagnostic code links here. Refer to your ICD-10-CM book.

AMA: **99334** 2018,Jan,8; 2018,Apr,9; 2017,Jun,6; 2017,Jan,8; 2017,Aug,3; 2016,Jan,13; 2016,Jan,7; 2016,Dec,11; 2015,Jan,16; 2014,Oct,8; 2014,Oct,3; 2014,Nov,14; 2014,Jan,11; 2013,Nov,3; 2013,Jun,3-5; 2013,Jan,9-10 **99335** 2018,Jan,8; 2018,Apr,9; 2017,Jun,6; 2017,Jan,8; 2017,Aug,3; 2016,Jan,13; 2016,Jan,7; 2016,Dec,11; 2015,Jan,16; 2014,Oct,8; 2014,Oct,3; 2014,Nov,14; 2014,Jan,11; 2013,Nov,3; 2013,Jun,3-5; 2013,Jan,9-10 **99336** 2018,Jan,8; 2018,Apr,9; 2017,Jun,6; 2017,Jan,8; 2017,Aug,3; 2016,Jan,13; 2016,Jan,7; 2016,Dec,11; 2015,Jan,16; 2014,Oct,8; 2014,Oct,3; 2014,Nov,14; 2014,Jan,11; 2013,Nov,3; 2013,Jun,3-5; 2013,Jan,9-10 **99337** 2018,Jan,8; 2018,Apr,9; 2017,Jun,6; 2017,Jan,8; 2017,Aug,3; 2016,Jan,13; 2016,Jan,7; 2016,Dec,11; 2015,Jan,16; 2014,Oct,8; 2014,Oct,3; 2014,Nov,14; 2014,Jan,11; 2013,Nov,3; 2013,Jun,3-5; 2013,Jan,9-10

Relative Value Units/Medicare Edits

Non-Facility RVU	Work	PE	MP	Total
99334	1.07	0.56	0.07	1.7
99335	1.72	0.85	0.11	2.68
99336	2.46	1.19	0.17	3.82
99337	3.58	1.65	0.24	5.47
Facility RVU	**Work**	**PE**	**MP**	**Total**
99334	1.07	0.56	0.07	1.7
99335	1.72	0.85	0.11	2.68
99336	2.46	1.19	0.17	3.82
99337	3.58	1.65	0.24	5.47

	FUD	Status	MUE	Modifiers				IOM Reference
99334	N/A	A	1(3)	N/A	N/A	N/A	80*	None
99335	N/A	A	1(3)	N/A	N/A	N/A	80*	
99336	N/A	A	1(3)	N/A	N/A	N/A	80*	
99337	N/A	A	1(3)	N/A	N/A	N/A	80*	

* with documentation

99339-99340

99339 Individual physician supervision of a patient (patient not present) in home, domiciliary or rest home (eg, assisted living facility) requiring complex and multidisciplinary care modalities involving regular physician development and/or revision of care plans, review of subsequent reports of patient status, review of related laboratory and other studies, communication (including telephone calls) for purposes of assessment or care decisions with health care professional(s), family member(s), surrogate decision maker(s) (eg, legal guardian) and/or key caregiver(s) involved in patient's care, integration of new information into the medical treatment plan and/or adjustment of medical therapy, within a calendar month; 15-29 minutes

99340 30 minutes or more

Explanation

Care plan oversight (CPO) services are reported for the primary supervising health care provider's time in reviewing and adjusting treatment plans. These services may include review of multiple modalities; patient status' relevant laboratory tests; communication with other health care team members, family members, and/or patient advocates; and developing a new course of action or any adjustments to the current plan. Codes are reported within one calendar month and are classified according to the place of service. The initial service for each location is approximately 15 to 29 minutes in duration; each additional 30 minutes is reported separately. Report 99339-99340 when the patient is in a domiciliary or rest home; 99374-99375 for patients in a home health setting; 99377-99378 for hospice patients; and 99379-99380 for patients residing in a nursing facility. Note that only one clinician is eligible to report CPO services for a specific time period in order to demonstrate the singular or lead role the clinician has with a particular patient.

Coding Tips

These codes are used to report care plan oversight services provided in the home, domiciliary, or rest home (assisted living) setting. These codes are reported separately from other E/M services provided in these settings. The sum of total time for services provided over the 30-day period determines the code selection. Only one physician may report these services for a given period of time. These are time-based codes and time spent involved in care plan activities must be documented in the medical record. For care plan oversight services provided to hospice, home health, and nursing facility patients, see 99374-99380. Do not report these codes with 99487-99489 or 99495-99496 for the same month.

ICD-10-CM Diagnostic Codes

The application of this code is too broad to adequately present ICD-10-CM diagnostic code links here. Refer to your ICD-10-CM book.

AMA: **99339** 2019,Jan,6; 2018,Oct,9; 2018,Jan,8; 2017,Jun,6; 2017,Jan,8; 2017,Aug,3; 2016,Jan,13; 2015,Jan,16; 2014,Oct,8; 2014,Oct,3; 2014,Jan,11; 2013,Sep,15-16; 2013,Nov,3; 2013,Jun,3-5; 2013,Apr,3-4 **99340** 2019,Jan,6; 2018,Oct,9; 2018,Jan,8; 2017,Jun,6; 2017,Jan,8; 2017,Aug,3; 2016,Jan,13; 2015,Jan,16; 2014,Oct,3; 2014,Oct,8; 2014,Jan,11; 2013,Sep,15-16; 2013,Nov,3; 2013,Jun,3-5; 2013,Apr,3-4

Relative Value Units/Medicare Edits

Non-Facility RVU	Work	PE	MP	Total
99339	1.25	0.85	0.07	2.17
99340	1.8	1.14	0.11	3.05
Facility RVU	**Work**	**PE**	**MP**	**Total**
99339	1.25	0.85	0.07	2.17
99340	1.8	1.14	0.11	3.05

	FUD	Status	MUE	Modifiers				IOM Reference
99339	N/A	B	0(3)	N/A	N/A	N/A	N/A	100-04,12,30.6.4;
99340	N/A	B	0(3)	N/A	N/A	N/A	N/A	100-04,12,30.6.14; 100-04,12,180; 100-04,12,180.1

* with documentation

Terms To Know

care plan oversight services. Physician's ongoing review and revision of a patient's care plan involving complex or multidisciplinary care modalities.

domiciliary. Facility, such as an assisted living, group home, custodial care, or an intermediate care facility, that provides room and board on a long-term basis and may include personal assistance services.

99341-99345

99341 Home visit for the evaluation and management of a new patient, which requires these 3 key components: A problem focused history; A problem focused examination; and Straightforward medical decision making. Counseling and/or coordination of care with other physicians, other qualified health care professionals, or agencies are provided consistent with the nature of the problem(s) and the patient's and/or family's needs. Usually, the presenting problem(s) are of low severity. Typically, 20 minutes are spent face-to-face with the patient and/or family.

99342 Home visit for the evaluation and management of a new patient, which requires these 3 key components: An expanded problem focused history; An expanded problem focused examination; and Medical decision making of low complexity. Counseling and/or coordination of care with other physicians, other qualified health care professionals, or agencies are provided consistent with the nature of the problem(s) and the patient's and/or family's needs. Usually, the presenting problem(s) are of moderate severity. Typically, 30 minutes are spent face-to-face with the patient and/or family.

99343 Home visit for the evaluation and management of a new patient, which requires these 3 key components: A detailed history; A detailed examination; and Medical decision making of moderate complexity. Counseling and/or coordination of care with other physicians, other qualified health care professionals, or agencies are provided consistent with the nature of the problem(s) and the patient's and/or family's needs. Usually, the presenting problem(s) are of moderate to high severity. Typically, 45 minutes are spent face-to-face with the patient and/or family.

99344 Home visit for the evaluation and management of a new patient, which requires these 3 key components: A comprehensive history; A comprehensive examination; and Medical decision making of moderate complexity. Counseling and/or coordination of care with other physicians, other qualified health care professionals, or agencies are provided consistent with the nature of the problem(s) and the patient's and/or family's needs. Usually, the presenting problem(s) are of high severity. Typically, 60 minutes are spent face-to-face with the patient and/or family.

99345 Home visit for the evaluation and management of a new patient, which requires these 3 key components: A comprehensive history; A comprehensive examination; and Medical decision making of high complexity. Counseling and/or coordination of care with other physicians, other qualified health care professionals, or agencies are provided consistent with the nature of the problem(s) and the patient's and/or family's needs. Usually, the patient is unstable or has developed a significant new problem requiring immediate physician attention. Typically, 75 minutes are spent face-to-face with the patient and/or family.

Explanation

Home services codes are reported by providers for E/M services rendered to new patients residing in a personal residence. Services are reported based on meeting all three key components—history, exam, and medical decision making (MDM)—within each level of service. The most basic service, 99341, describes a problem focused history and exam with straightforward medical decision making for low severity problems encompassing approximately 20 minutes of time with the patient and/or family or caregiver. Mid-level services require an expanded problem focused history and exam or a detailed history and exam as represented by 99342 and 99343, respectively. Medical decision making for 99342 is designated as low complexity; moderate complexity for 99343. At these levels of service, the encounter can involve face-to-face time spent with the patient and/or family or caregiver of 30 (99342) to 45 minutes (99343). The last two levels of service in this category require documenting comprehensive history and examination components. The differentiating factor between the two levels is the medical decision making; 99344 involves moderate complexity MDM and approximately 60 minutes of face-to-face time with the patient and/or family or caregiver for high severity problems, while the highest level of service in this category, 99345, involves MDM of high complexity and 75 minutes of face-to-face time with the patient and/or family or caregiver as a result of the patient being unstable or having developed a significant, new problem necessitating the immediate attention of the clinician.

Coding Tips

These codes are used to report evaluation and management services provided in a private residence, temporary lodging, or short-term accommodation such as a hotel, campground, hostel, or cruise ship for a new patient. All three key components (history, exam, and medical decision making) must be met or exceeded for the level of service selected. Time may be used to select the level of service when counseling and coordination of care are documented as at least half of the time spent face-to-face with the patient. For commercial payers, consider assigning the appropriate consultation code instead of these codes when an opinion or advice about a specific problem has been requested by another qualified provider. Consultation codes are not covered by Medicare and some payers. Report the appropriate new or established outpatient E/M code for consultation services. For care plan oversight provided in the home under the care of a hospice agency, see 99377-99378; provided under the care of a home health agency, see 99374-99375. For care plan oversight services provided to a patient under home, domiciliary, or rest home (assisted living) care, see 99339-99340. Report place of service (POS) code 12 for services rendered in a private residence.

ICD-10-CM Diagnostic Codes

The application of this code is too broad to adequately present ICD-10-CM diagnostic code links here. Refer to your ICD-10-CM book.

AMA: 99341 2018,Jan,8; 2018,Apr,9; 2017,Jun,6; 2017,Jan,8; 2017,Aug,3; 2016,Jan,13; 2016,Jan,7; 2016,Dec,11; 2015,Jan,16; 2014,Oct,3; 2014,Oct,8; 2014,Nov,14; 2014,Jan,11; 2013,Jun,3-5; 2013,Jan,9-10 **99342** 2018,Jan,8; 2018,Apr,9; 2017,Jun,6; 2017,Jan,8; 2017,Aug,3; 2016,Jan,7; 2016,Jan,13; 2016,Dec,11; 2015,Jan,16; 2014,Oct,8; 2014,Oct,3; 2014,Nov,14; 2014,Jan,11; 2013,Jun,3-5; 2013,Jan,9-10 **99343** 2018,Jan,8; 2018,Apr,9; 2017,Jun,6; 2017,Jan,8; 2017,Aug,3; 2016,Jan,13; 2016,Jan,7; 2016,Dec,11; 2015,Jan,16; 2014,Oct,8; 2014,Oct,3; 2014,Nov,14; 2014,Jan,11; 2013,Jun,3-5; 2013,Jan,9-10 **99344** 2018,Jan,8; 2018,Apr,9; 2017,Jun,6; 2017,Jan,8; 2017,Aug,3; 2016,Jan,13; 2016,Jan,7; 2016,Dec,11; 2015,Jan,16; 2014,Oct,8; 2014,Oct,3; 2014,Nov,14; 2014,Jan,11; 2013,Jun,3-5; 2013,Jan,9-10 **99345** 2018,Jan,8; 2018,Apr,9; 2017,Jun,6; 2017,Jan,8; 2017,Aug,3; 2016,Jan,13; 2016,Jan,7; 2016,Dec,11; 2015,Jan,16; 2014,Oct,8; 2014,Oct,3; 2014,Nov,14; 2014,Jan,11; 2013,Jun,3-5; 2013,Jan,9-10

Relative Value Units/Medicare Edits

Non-Facility RVU	Work	PE	MP	Total
99341	1.01	0.48	0.07	1.56
99342	1.52	0.62	0.11	2.25
99343	2.53	0.96	0.18	3.67
99344	3.38	1.53	0.23	5.14
99345	4.09	1.88	0.28	6.25
Facility RVU	**Work**	**PE**	**MP**	**Total**
99341	1.01	0.48	0.07	1.56
99342	1.52	0.62	0.11	2.25
99343	2.53	0.96	0.18	3.67
99344	3.38	1.53	0.23	5.14
99345	4.09	1.88	0.28	6.25

	FUD	Status	MUE	Modifiers				IOM Reference
99341	N/A	A	1(2)	N/A	N/A	N/A	80*	100-04,12,30.6.4;
99342	N/A	A	1(2)	N/A	N/A	N/A	80*	100-04,12,30.6.14;
99343	N/A	A	1(2)	N/A	N/A	N/A	80*	100-04,12,30.6.14.1;
99344	N/A	A	1(2)	N/A	N/A	N/A	80*	100-04,12,30.6.15.1
99345	N/A	A	1(2)	N/A	N/A	N/A	80*	

* with documentation

Terms To Know

comprehensive physical examination. Under the 1995 guidelines, examination of at least eight organ systems or one comprehensive single-system examination. Under the 1997 guidelines, an examination of at least nine organ systems or body areas, which must include all bullet point elements within each of the nine systems/areas for the multisystem exam or examination of all bullet point elements from one of the 10 single organ system exams.

new patient. Patient who is receiving face-to-face care from a provider/qualified health care professional or another physician/qualified health care professional of the exact same specialty and subspecialty who belongs to the same group practice for the first time in three years. For OPPS hospitals, a patient who has not been registered as an inpatient or outpatient, including off-campus provider based clinic or emergency department, within the past three years.

99347-99350

99347 Home visit for the evaluation and management of an established patient, which requires at least 2 of these 3 key components: A problem focused interval history; A problem focused examination; Straightforward medical decision making. Counseling and/or coordination of care with other physicians, other qualified health care professionals, or agencies are provided consistent with the nature of the problem(s) and the patient's and/or family's needs. Usually, the presenting problem(s) are self limited or minor. Typically, 15 minutes are spent face-to-face with the patient and/or family.

99348 Home visit for the evaluation and management of an established patient, which requires at least 2 of these 3 key components: An expanded problem focused interval history; An expanded problem focused examination; Medical decision making of low complexity. Counseling and/or coordination of care with other physicians, other qualified health care professionals, or agencies are provided consistent with the nature of the problem(s) and the patient's and/or family's needs. Usually, the presenting problem(s) are of low to moderate severity. Typically, 25 minutes are spent face-to-face with the patient and/or family.

99349 Home visit for the evaluation and management of an established patient, which requires at least 2 of these 3 key components: A detailed interval history; A detailed examination; Medical decision making of moderate complexity. Counseling and/or coordination of care with other physicians, other qualified health care professionals, or agencies are provided consistent with the nature of the problem(s) and the patient's and/or family's needs. Usually, the presenting problem(s) are moderate to high severity. Typically, 40 minutes are spent face-to-face with the patient and/or family.

99350 Home visit for the evaluation and management of an established patient, which requires at least 2 of these 3 key components: A comprehensive interval history; A comprehensive examination; Medical decision making of moderate to high complexity. Counseling and/or coordination of care with other physicians, other qualified health care professionals, or agencies are provided consistent with the nature of the problem(s) and the patient's and/or family's needs. Usually, the presenting problem(s) are of moderate to high severity. The patient may be unstable or may have developed a significant new problem requiring immediate physician attention. Typically, 60 minutes are spent face-to-face with the patient and/or family.

Explanation

Home services codes are reported by providers for E/M services rendered to established patients residing in a personal residence. Services are reported based on meeting two out of the three key components—history, exam, and medical decision making (MDM)—within each level of service. The most basic service, 99347, describes a problem focused history and exam with straightforward medical decision making for problems that are self-limiting or minor encompassing approximately 15 minutes of face-to-face time with the patient and/or family or caregiver. Mid-level services require an expanded problem focused history and exam or a detailed history and exam as represented by 99348 and 99349, respectively. Medical decision making for 99348 is designated as low complexity; moderate complexity for 99349. At these levels of service, the encounter can involve face-to-face time spent with the patient and/or family or caregiver of 25 (99348) to 40 minutes (99349) for low to moderate or moderate to high severity problems. The last level of service in this category, 99350, consists of a comprehensive history and examination as well as medical decision making of moderate to high complexity. The clinician can expect to spend approximately 60 minutes face-to-face duration with the patient and/or family or caregiver for moderate to high severity problems as a result of the patient being unstable or having developed a significant, new problem necessitating the immediate attention of the clinician.

Coding Tips

These codes are used to report evaluation and management services provided in a private residence for an established patient. Two of the three key components (history, exam, and medical decision making) must be met or exceeded for the level of service selected. Time may be used to select the level of service when counseling and coordination of care are documented as at least half of the time spent face-to-face with the patient. For commercial payers, consider assigning the appropriate consultation code instead of these codes when an opinion or advice about a specific problem has been requested by another qualified provider. Consultation codes are not covered by Medicare and some payers. Report new or established outpatient E/M codes for consultation services. For care plan oversight provided in the home under the care of a hospice agency, see 99377-99378; provided under the care of a home health agency, see 99374-99375. For care plan oversight services provided to a patient under home, domiciliary, or rest home (assisted living) care, see 99339-99340. Report place of service (POS) code 12 for services rendered in a private residence.

ICD-10-CM Diagnostic Codes

The application of this code is too broad to adequately present ICD-10-CM diagnostic code links here. Refer to your ICD-10-CM book.

AMA: **99347** 2018,Jan,8; 2018,Apr,9; 2017,Jun,6; 2017,Jan,8; 2017,Aug,3; 2016,Jan,13; 2016,Jan,7; 2016,Dec,11; 2015,Jan,16; 2014,Oct,8; 2014,Oct,3; 2014,Nov,14; 2014,Jan,11; 2013,Nov,3; 2013,Jun,3-5; 2013,Jan,9-10 **99348** 2018,Jan,8; 2018,Apr,9; 2017,Jun,6; 2017,Jan,8; 2017,Aug,3; 2016,Jan,13; 2016,Jan,7; 2016,Dec,11; 2015,Jan,16; 2014,Oct,8; 2014,Oct,3; 2014,Nov,14; 2014,Jan,11; 2013,Nov,3; 2013,Jun,3-5; 2013,Jan,9-10 **99349** 2018,Jan,8; 2018,Apr,9; 2017,Jun,6; 2017,Jan,8; 2017,Aug,3; 2016,Jan,13; 2016,Jan,7; 2016,Dec,11; 2015,Jan,16; 2014,Oct,8; 2014,Oct,3; 2014,Nov,14; 2014,Jan,11; 2013,Nov,3; 2013,Jun,3-5; 2013,Jan,9-10 **99350** 2018,Jan,8; 2018,Apr,9; 2017,Jun,6; 2017,Jan,8; 2017,Aug,3; 2016,Jan,13; 2016,Jan,7; 2016,Dec,11; 2015,Jan,16; 2014,Oct,8; 2014,Oct,3; 2014,Nov,14; 2014,Jan,11; 2013,Nov,3; 2013,Jun,3-5; 2013,Jan,9-10

Relative Value Units/Medicare Edits

Non-Facility RVU	Work	PE	MP	Total
99347	1.0	0.49	0.07	1.56
99348	1.56	0.7	0.11	2.37
99349	2.33	1.15	0.16	3.64
99350	3.28	1.54	0.23	5.05
Facility RVU	**Work**	**PE**	**MP**	**Total**
99347	1.0	0.49	0.07	1.56
99348	1.56	0.7	0.11	2.37
99349	2.33	1.15	0.16	3.64
99350	3.28	1.54	0.23	5.05

	FUD	Status	MUE	Modifiers				IOM Reference
99347	N/A	A	1(3)	N/A	N/A	N/A	80*	None
99348	N/A	A	1(3)	N/A	N/A	N/A	80*	
99349	N/A	A	1(3)	N/A	N/A	N/A	80*	
99350	N/A	A	1(3)	N/A	N/A	N/A	80*	

* with documentation

99354-99359

+ **99354** Prolonged evaluation and management or psychotherapy service(s) (beyond the typical service time of the primary procedure) in the office or other outpatient setting requiring direct patient contact beyond the usual service; first hour (List separately in addition to code for office or other outpatient Evaluation and Management or psychotherapy service)
+ **99355** each additional 30 minutes (List separately in addition to code for prolonged service)
+ **99356** Prolonged service in the inpatient or observation setting, requiring unit/floor time beyond the usual service; first hour (List separately in addition to code for inpatient Evaluation and Management service)
+ **99357** each additional 30 minutes (List separately in addition to code for prolonged service)

99358 Prolonged evaluation and management service before and/or after direct patient care; first hour

+ **99359** each additional 30 minutes (List separately in addition to code for prolonged service)

Explanation

Prolonged services involve face-to-face patient contact or psychotherapy services beyond the typical service time and should only be reported once per day. Direct patient contact also includes additional non-face-to-face time, such as time spent on the patient's floor or unit in the hospital or nursing facility setting. For prolonged services rendered in the office or outpatient setting for the first 30 to 74 minutes, report 99354; for each additional 30 minutes, report 99355. For prolonged services rendered in the inpatient or observation setting for the first 30 to 74 minutes, report 99356; for each additional 30 minutes, report 99357. Codes should be reported using the total duration of face-to-face time spent by the clinician on the date of service even when the time spent is not continuous. Report prolonged service without direct patient contact with 99358-99359.

Coding Tips

These codes are used to report prolonged services, with direct patient contact (99354-99357) or without direct patient contact (99358-99359) beyond the usual service. These are time-based codes and time spent with the patient must be documented in the medical record. Codes 99354-99357 are only reported in addition to other time-based E/M services. Time spent on other separately reported services excluding the E/M service should not be counted toward the prolonged service time. Code selection is based on whether the service is provided in the office or other outpatient setting or the inpatient setting. For prolonged services provided by a physician or other qualified health care professional involving direct face-to-face time with the patient in the office or other outpatient setting, see 99354-99355. For prolonged services provided by a physician or other qualified health care professional involving total time spent at the patient's bedside and on the floor/unit in the hospital or nursing facility, see 99356-99357. For prolonged services provided by a physician or other qualified health care professional without face-to-face contact or unit/floor time, see 99358-99359. Codes 99358-99359 may be reported on a different date of service than the primary service and do not require the primary service to have an established time. Prolonged service of less than 30 minutes should not be reported separately. Report 99354, 99356, and 99358 only once per day for the initial hour of prolonged service care; for each additional 30 minute block of time beyond the initial hour, see 99355, 99357, and 99359. For prolonged services provided by clinical staff, see 99415-99416. Do not report 99354-99355 with 99415 or 99416. Report 99354 in addition to 90837, 90847, 99201-99215, 99241-99245, 99324-99337, 99341-99350, and 99483. Report 99355 in addition to 99354. Report 99356 in addition to 90837, 90847, 99218-99220, 99221-99223, 99224-99226, 99231-99233, 99234-99236, 99251-99255, and 99304-99310. Report 99357 in addition to 99356. Do not report 99358-99359 in the same month when reporting 99484, 99487-99489, or 99490-99494. Do not report 99358 or 99359 for time spent performing the following E/M or monitoring services: 93792-93793, 99339, 99340, 99374-99380, 99366-99368, or 99421-99423. Report 99359 in addition to 99358.

ICD-10-CM Diagnostic Codes

The application of this code is too broad to adequately present ICD-10-CM diagnostic code links here. Refer to your ICD-10-CM book.

AMA: **99354** 2019,Jun,7; 2018,Jan,8; 2017,Jan,8; 2016,Jan,13; 2016,Dec,11; 2015,Oct,9; 2015,Oct,3; 2015,Jan,16; 2014,Oct,8; 2014,Jun,14; 2014,Jan,11; 2014,Apr,6; 2013,Oct,11; 2013,May,12; 2013,Jun,3-5 **99355** 2019,Jun,7; 2018,Jan,8; 2017,Jan,8; 2016,Jan,13; 2016,Dec,11; 2015,Oct,3; 2015,Oct,9; 2015,Jan,16; 2014,Oct,8; 2014,Jun,14; 2014,Jan,11; 2014,Apr,6; 2013,Oct,11; 2013,May,12; 2013,Jun,3-5 **99356** 2019,Jun,7; 2018,Jan,8; 2017,Jan,8; 2016,Jan,13; 2016,Dec,11; 2015,Oct,3; 2015,Oct,9; 2015,Jan,16; 2014,Oct,8; 2014,Jun,14; 2014,Jan,11; 2014,Apr,6; 2013,Oct,11; 2013,May,12; 2013,Jun,3-5 **99357** 2019,Jun,7; 2018,Jan,8; 2017,Jan,8; 2016,Jan,13; 2016,Dec,11; 2015,Oct,3; 2015,Oct,9; 2015,Jan,16; 2014,Oct,8; 2014,Jun,14; 2014,Jan,11; 2014,Apr,6; 2013,Oct,11; 2013,May,12; 2013,Jun,3-5 **99358** 2019,Jun,7; 2019,Jan,13; 2018,Oct,9; 2018,Jan,8; 2017,Jan,8; 2016,Jan,13; 2015,Jan,16; 2014,Oct,8; 2014,Oct,3; 2014,Jan,11; 2013,Oct,11; 2013,Nov,3; 2013,Apr,3-4 **99359** 2019,Jun,7; 2019,Jan,13; 2018,Oct,9; 2018,Jan,8; 2017,Jan,8; 2016,Jan,13; 2015,Jan,16; 2014,Oct,8; 2014,Oct,3; 2014,Jan,11; 2013,Oct,11; 2013,Nov,3; 2013,Apr,3-4

Relative Value Units/Medicare Edits

Non-Facility RVU	Work	PE	MP	Total
99354	2.33	1.18	0.16	3.67
99355	1.77	0.91	0.12	2.8
99356	1.71	0.78	0.11	2.6
99357	1.71	0.79	0.11	2.61
99358	2.1	0.9	0.15	3.15
99359	1.0	0.45	0.07	1.52
Facility RVU	**Work**	**PE**	**MP**	**Total**
99354	2.33	0.95	0.16	3.44
99355	1.77	0.71	0.12	2.6
99356	1.71	0.78	0.11	2.6
99357	1.71	0.79	0.11	2.61
99358	2.1	0.9	0.15	3.15
99359	1.0	0.45	0.07	1.52

	FUD	Status	MUE	Modifiers				IOM Reference
99354	N/A	A	1(2)	N/A	N/A	N/A	80*	100-04,11,40.1.3; 100-04,12,30.6.4; 100-04,12,30.6.13; 100-04,12,30.6.14; 100-04,12,30.6.15.1; 100-04,12,30.6.15.2; 100-04,12,100
99355	N/A	A	4(3)	N/A	N/A	N/A	80*	
99356	N/A	A	1(2)	N/A	N/A	N/A	80*	
99357	N/A	A	4(3)	N/A	N/A	N/A	80*	
99358	N/A	A	1(2)	N/A	N/A	N/A	80*	
99359	N/A	A	2(3)	N/A	N/A	N/A	80*	

* with documentation

 ● New ▲ Revised + Add On AMA: CPT Assist [Resequenced] ☑ Laterality

[99415, 99416]

\+ **99415** Prolonged clinical staff service (the service beyond the typical service time) during an evaluation and management service in the office or outpatient setting, direct patient contact with physician supervision; first hour (List separately in addition to code for outpatient Evaluation and Management service)

\+ **99416** Prolonged clinical staff service (the service beyond the typical service time) during an evaluation and management service in the office or outpatient setting, direct patient contact with physician supervision; each additional 30 minutes (List separately in addition to code for prolonged service)

Explanation

Prolonged clinical staff services are reported with resequenced codes that were added to describe special situations in which the physician's staff provided assistance to a patient beyond the usual time associated with circumstances requiring observation of the patient, such as in cases where the patient was administered a new medication or inhaled drug requiring monitoring to ensure patient safety in the office or outpatient setting. Such cases do not necessitate the clinician being face-to-face with the patient throughout the entire time period; observation and monitoring of the patient can be performed by a member of the clinician's staff under the provider's supervision. Report these codes in conjunction with the designated E/M service code along with any other service provided at the same encounter. Codes in this category should report the total amount of face-to-face time spent with the patient by the clinical staff on the same date of service even if the time is not continuous; time spent rendering other separately reportable services other than the E/M service do not count toward the prolonged services time. The average face-to-face time described in the primary E/M service code descriptor is used to define when these prolonged service codes should begin. For example 99214 Office or other outpatient visit, established patient, level 4, has an average time period of 25 minutes; therefore, prolonged services would commence after another 45 minutes had passed. Report the first 45 to 74 minutes of prolonged services using 99415. For each additional 30 minutes of prolonged services, report 99416.

Coding Tips

These codes are used to report prolonged face-to-face services provided by the clinical staff in the office or outpatient setting. These are time-based codes and time spent with the patient must be documented in the medical record. Time spent on other separately reported services excluding the E/M service should not be counted toward the prolonged service time. These codes are reported in addition to the other E/M service provided on the same date of service. A provider must be available to provide direct supervision of the clinical staff. Report 99415 only once per day for the initial hour of prolonged service care; for each additional 30 minute block of time beyond the initial hour, see 99416. Prolonged service of less than 45 minutes should not be reported separately. For prolonged services involving direct face-to-face time with the physician or other qualified healthcare provider in the office or other outpatient setting, see 99354-99355. Do not report 99415-99416 with 99354 or 99355. Report 99415 in addition to 99201-99205 and 99211-99215. Report 99416 in addition to 99415.

ICD-10-CM Diagnostic Codes

The application of this code is too broad to adequately present ICD-10-CM diagnostic code links here. Refer to your ICD-10-CM book.

AMA: 99415 2018,Jan,8; 2017,Jan,8; 2016,Mar,8; 2016,Jan,13; 2016,Feb,13; 2015,Oct,3 **99416** 2018,Jan,8; 2017,Jan,8; 2016,Mar,8; 2016,Jan,13; 2016,Feb,13; 2015,Oct,3

Relative Value Units/Medicare Edits

Non-Facility RVU	Work	PE	MP	Total
99415	0.0	0.27	0.01	0.28
99416	0.0	0.12	0.0	0.12
Facility RVU	**Work**	**PE**	**MP**	**Total**
99415	0.0	0.27	0.01	0.28
99416	0.0	0.12	0.0	0.12

	FUD	Status	MUE	Modifiers				IOM Reference
99415	N/A	A	1(2)	N/A	N/A	N/A	80*	None
99416	N/A	A	3(3)	N/A	N/A	N/A	80*	

* with documentation

Terms To Know

add-on code. Code representing a procedure performed in addition to the primary procedure and is represented with a + in the CPT book. Add-on codes are never reported for stand-alone services but are reported secondarily in addition to the primary procedure.

clinical staff. Someone who works for, or under, the direction of a physician or qualified health care professional and does not bill services separately. The person may be licensed or regulated to help the physician perform specific duties.

99360

99360 Standby service, requiring prolonged attendance, each 30 minutes (eg, operative standby, standby for frozen section, for cesarean/high risk delivery, for monitoring EEG)

Explanation

Standby services are those requested of a qualified clinician that involves prolonged attendance without face-to-face contact with the patient (e.g., operative or cesarean/high-risk delivery standby, EEG monitoring, or standby to obtain a frozen section specimen). The clinician on standby is not permitted to provide care or services to other patients during the standby period. This code should not be used to report time spent proctoring another individual nor should it be used if the standby period ends with the standby clinician performing a procedure that is subject to the surgical package. This code encompasses the total duration of time spent on standby on a given date; standby services of less than 30 minutes total duration are not reported separately. A second and subsequent period of standby, after the initial 30 minutes, may be reported contingent that each unit of standby service equates to a full 30 minutes.

Coding Tips

This code is used to report standby services requested by another clinician for prolonged attendance without face-to-face patient contact. This is a time-based code representing the total duration of time spent providing standby services and must be documented in the medical record. Standby services of less than 30 minutes should not be reported separately. Report each additional 30 minutes of time beyond the initial time only when a full 30-minute period is provided. Report this code with 99460 or 99465, if applicable. Do not report 99360 in addition to 99464.

ICD-10-CM Diagnostic Codes

The application of this code is too broad to adequately present ICD-10-CM diagnostic code links here. Refer to your ICD-10-CM book.

AMA: **99360** 2018,Jan,8; 2017,Jan,8; 2016,Jan,13; 2015,Jan,16; 2014,Oct,8; 2014,Jan,11; 2014,Apr,5; 2013,May,8-10

Relative Value Units/Medicare Edits

Non-Facility RVU	Work	PE	MP	Total
99360	1.2	0.46	0.07	1.73
Facility RVU	**Work**	**PE**	**MP**	**Total**
99360	1.2	0.46	0.07	1.73

	FUD	Status	MUE	Modifiers				IOM Reference
99360	N/A	X	1(3)	N/A	N/A	N/A	N/A	100-04,12,30.6.4; 100-04,12,30.6.15.3

* with documentation

99366-99368

99366 Medical team conference with interdisciplinary team of health care professionals, face-to-face with patient and/or family, 30 minutes or more, participation by nonphysician qualified health care professional

99367 Medical team conference with interdisciplinary team of health care professionals, patient and/or family not present, 30 minutes or more; participation by physician

99368 participation by nonphysician qualified health care professional

Explanation

A medical team conference is defined as a service where at least three qualified health care professionals from different specialties or disciplines, each of whom provides direct care to the patient, actively engage in the evolution, revision, coordination, and implementation of health care services needed by the patient. The conferences may or may not involve the presence of the patient, family members, community agencies, surrogate decision makers/legal guardians, and/or caregivers. Medical team clinicians should report the time spent in a team conference with the patient and/or family present with the appropriate E/M code, using time as a key controlling factor for selecting a code when counseling and/or coordination of care dominates the service. The individual clinician must be directly involved with rendering face-to-face services outside of the conference visit with other clinicians or agencies. All medical professionals participating on the medical team must document their own individual participation in the team conference, in addition to their contributed information and follow-up treatment recommendations. However, only one individual from the same specialty may report a code from this category at the same encounter. No individuals may report a code from range 99366-99368 if participation in the medical team conference is a part of a facility or organizational service contractually provided by the facility or organization. Team conferences commence upon review of the individual patient case and conclude once the review has come to a conclusion. Record keeping and report generation time is not reportable. The clinician must report all time for which he or she was present. Reportable time is not limited to the time that the clinician is communicating with other team members, the patient, and/or the patient's family. Note that time spent in medical team conferences should not be used toward determining other E/M services such as care plan oversight services, home, domiciliary, or rest home care plan oversight, prolonged services, psychotherapy, or any other E/M service. Nonphysician qualified health care professionals may report 99366, medical team conference, direct (face-to-face) contact with patient and/or family, when the patient is present for any or all of the medical conference with a duration of at least 30 minutes. This includes such providers as speech-language pathologists, physical therapists, occupational therapists, social workers, and dieticians. Medical conferences of less than 30 minutes duration are not reported. Codes 99367-99368 describe team conferences without direct, face-to-face patient and/or family contact.

Coding Tips

These codes are used to report medical team conferences, with direct patient and/or family contact (99366) or without direct patient and/or family contact (99367-99368). For medical team participation by a nonphysician healthcare professional with direct patient and/or family contact, see 99366; without direct patient or family contact, see 99368. For medical team participation by the physician without direct patient and/or family contact, see 99367. Medical team meetings of less than 30 minutes should not be reported separately. For physician participation with face-to-face patient contact, report the appropriate E/M code. Do not report medical team conference codes in the same month as complex chronic care coordination services 99487-99489 or transitional care management services 99495-99496.

ICD-10-CM Diagnostic Codes

The application of this code is too broad to adequately present ICD-10-CM diagnostic code links here. Refer to your ICD-10-CM book.

AMA: **99366** 2018,Jan,8; 2018,Apr,9; 2017,Jan,8; 2016,Jan,13; 2015,Jan,16; 2014,Oct,3; 2014,Oct,8; 2014,Jun,3; 2014,Jan,11; 2013,Nov,3; 2013,Apr,3-4 **99367** 2018,Jan,8; 2018,Apr,9; 2017,Jan,8; 2016,Jan,13; 2015,Jan,16; 2014,Oct,8; 2014,Jun,3; 2014,Jan,11; 2013,Nov,3; 2013,Apr,3-4 **99368** 2018,Jan,8; 2018,Apr,9; 2017,Jan,8; 2016,Jan,13; 2015,Jan,16; 2014,Oct,8; 2014,Oct,3; 2014,Jun,3; 2014,Jan,11; 2013,Nov,3; 2013,Apr,3-4

Relative Value Units/Medicare Edits

Non-Facility RVU	Work	PE	MP	Total
99366	0.82	0.34	0.05	1.21
99367	1.1	0.43	0.07	1.6
99368	0.72	0.28	0.04	1.04
Facility RVU	**Work**	**PE**	**MP**	**Total**
99366	0.82	0.32	0.05	1.19
99367	1.1	0.43	0.07	1.6
99368	0.72	0.28	0.04	1.04

	FUD	Status	MUE	Modifiers				IOM Reference
99366	N/A	B	0(3)	N/A	N/A	N/A	N/A	100-02,15,230.4; 100-04,11,40.1.3
99367	N/A	B	0(3)	N/A	N/A	N/A	N/A	
99368	N/A	B	0(3)	N/A	N/A	N/A	N/A	

* with documentation

99374-99380

99374 Supervision of a patient under care of home health agency (patient not present) in home, domiciliary or equivalent environment (eg, Alzheimer's facility) requiring complex and multidisciplinary care modalities involving regular development and/or revision of care plans by that individual, review of subsequent reports of patient status, review of related laboratory and other studies, communication (including telephone calls) for purposes of assessment or care decisions with health care professional(s), family member(s), surrogate decision maker(s) (eg, legal guardian) and/or key caregiver(s) involved in patient's care, integration of new information into the medical treatment plan and/or adjustment of medical therapy, within a calendar month; 15-29 minutes

99375 30 minutes or more

99377 Supervision of a hospice patient (patient not present) requiring complex and multidisciplinary care modalities involving regular development and/or revision of care plans by that individual, review of subsequent reports of patient status, review of related laboratory and other studies, communication (including telephone calls) for purposes of assessment or care decisions with health care professional(s), family member(s), surrogate decision maker(s) (eg, legal guardian) and/or key caregiver(s) involved in patient's care, integration of new information into the medical treatment plan and/or adjustment of medical therapy, within a calendar month; 15-29 minutes

99378 30 minutes or more

99379 Supervision of a nursing facility patient (patient not present) requiring complex and multidisciplinary care modalities involving regular development and/or revision of care plans by that individual, review of subsequent reports of patient status, review of related laboratory and other studies, communication (including telephone calls) for purposes of assessment or care decisions with health care professional(s), family member(s), surrogate decision maker(s) (eg, legal guardian) and/or key caregiver(s) involved in patient's care, integration of new information into the medical treatment plan and/or adjustment of medical therapy, within a calendar month; 15-29 minutes

99380 30 minutes or more

Explanation

Care plan oversight (CPO) services are reported for the primary supervising health care provider's time in reviewing and adjusting treatment plans. These services may include review of multiple modalities; patient status' relevant laboratory tests; communication with other health care team members, family members, and/or patient advocates; and developing a new course of action or any adjustments to the current plan. Codes are reported within one calendar month and are classified according to the place of service. The initial service for each location is approximately 15 to 29 minutes in duration; each additional 30 minutes is reported separately. Report 99374-99375 for patients in a home health setting; 99377-99378 for hospice patients; and 99379-99380 for patients residing in a nursing facility. Note that only one clinician is eligible to report CPO services for a specific time period in order to demonstrate the singular or lead role the clinician has with a particular patient.

Coding Tips

These codes are used to report care plan oversight (CPO) services of the physicians' supervision of patients in nursing facilities, under the care of home health agencies, or hospice benefits that require complex or multidisciplinary care modalities requiring ongoing provider involvement in the plan of care. These are time-based codes and time spent with the patient must be documented in the medical record. Total time for care plan oversight provided within a 30-day period determines code selection. Only one clinician is eligible to report CPO services for a specific time period in order to demonstrate the singular or lead role the clinician has with a particular patient. CPO services should not be reported until after the end of the month in which the services are performed. Coverage of these services varies by payer. Check with the payer for their specific coverage guidelines. For care plan oversight services provided to patients in the home, domiciliary, or rest home (assisted living), see 99339-99340. Do not report 99374-99378 with complex chronic care coordination services 99487-99489 for the same month. Do not report 99374-99380 when transitional care services 99495-99496 are reported during the same service time or for time reported with 98966-98968, 99421-99423, or 99441-99443.

ICD-10-CM Diagnostic Codes

The application of this code is too broad to adequately present ICD-10-CM diagnostic code links here. Refer to your ICD-10-CM book.

AMA: **99374** 2019,Jan,6; 2018,Jan,8; 2017,Jan,8; 2016,Jan,13; 2015,Jan,16; 2014,Oct,3; 2014,Oct,8; 2014,Jan,11; 2013,Sep,15-16; 2013,Nov,3; 2013,Jul,11-12; 2013,Apr,3-4 **99375** 2019,Jan,6; 2018,Jan,8; 2017,Jan,8; 2016,Jan,13; 2015,Jan,16; 2014,Oct,3; 2014,Oct,8; 2014,Jan,11; 2013,Sep,15-16; 2013,Nov,3; 2013,Jul,11-12; 2013,Apr,3-4 **99377** 2019,Jan,6; 2018,Jan,8; 2017,Jan,8; 2016,Jan,13; 2015,Jan,16; 2014,Oct,8; 2014,Oct,3; 2014,Jan,11; 2013,Sep,15-16; 2013,Nov,3; 2013,Jul,11-12; 2013,Apr,3-4 **99378** 2019,Jan,6; 2018,Jan,8; 2017,Jan,8; 2016,Jan,13; 2015,Jan,16; 2014,Oct,8; 2014,Oct,3; 2014,Jan,11; 2013,Sep,15-16; 2013,Nov,3; 2013,Jul,11-12; 2013,Apr,3-4 **99379** 2019,Jan,6; 2018,Jan,8; 2017,Jan,8; 2016,Jan,13; 2015,Jan,16; 2014,Oct,8; 2014,Oct,3; 2014,Jan,11; 2013,Sep,15-16; 2013,Nov,3; 2013,Jul,11-12; 2013,Apr,3-4 **99380** 2019,Jan,6; 2018,Jan,8; 2017,Jan,8; 2016,Jan,13; 2015,Jan,16; 2014,Oct,8; 2014,Oct,3; 2014,Jan,11; 2013,Sep,15-16; 2013,Nov,3; 2013,Jul,11-12; 2013,Apr,3-4

Relative Value Units/Medicare Edits

Non-Facility RVU	Work	PE	MP	Total
99374	1.1	0.79	0.07	1.96
99375	1.73	1.11	0.1	2.94
99377	1.1	0.79	0.07	1.96
99378	1.73	1.11	0.1	2.94
99379	1.1	0.79	0.07	1.96
99380	1.73	1.11	0.1	2.94
Facility RVU	**Work**	**PE**	**MP**	**Total**
99374	1.1	0.43	0.07	1.6
99375	1.73	0.67	0.1	2.5
99377	1.1	0.43	0.07	1.6
99378	1.73	0.67	0.1	2.5
99379	1.1	0.43	0.07	1.6
99380	1.73	0.67	0.1	2.5

	FUD	Status	MUE	Modifiers				IOM Reference
99374	N/A	B	0(3)	N/A	N/A	N/A	N/A	100-04,11,10; 100-04,11,40.1.3.1; 100-04,12,30.6.4; 100-04,12,180; 100-04,12,180.1
99375	N/A	I	0(3)	N/A	N/A	N/A	N/A	
99377	N/A	B	0(3)	N/A	N/A	N/A	N/A	
99378	N/A	I	0(3)	N/A	N/A	N/A	N/A	
99379	N/A	B	0(3)	N/A	N/A	N/A	N/A	
99380	N/A	B	0(3)	N/A	N/A	N/A	N/A	

* with documentation

99381-99387

99381 Initial comprehensive preventive medicine evaluation and management of an individual including an age and gender appropriate history, examination, counseling/anticipatory guidance/risk factor reduction interventions, and the ordering of laboratory/diagnostic procedures, new patient; infant (age younger than 1 year)

99382 early childhood (age 1 through 4 years)

99383 late childhood (age 5 through 11 years)

99384 adolescent (age 12 through 17 years)

99385 18-39 years

99386 40-64 years

99387 65 years and older

Explanation

Initial preventive medicine services are typically well-patient examinations for new patients with code selection dependent upon the patient's age. These services include applicable patient history and examination, guidance/recommendation regarding personal risk factors, and any laboratory and/or diagnostic procedures ordered. Clinicians are not required to report minor or self-limiting problems or complaints noted during the course of the preventive examination when those problems do not require any additional work or necessitate performing the key components of a problem oriented E/M service. Report 99381 for infants younger than 1 year of age; 99382 for children 1 to 4 years of age; 99383 for children 5 to 11 years of age; 99384 for adolescents12 to 17 years of age; 99385 for adult patients 18 to 39 years of age; 99386 for patients 40 to 64 years of age; and 99387 for patients 65 years of age and older.

Coding Tips

These codes are used to report preventive medicine services for a new patient. Time is not a factor when selecting this E/M service. Code selection is determined based on whether the patient is new or established and the age of the patient. When documentation supports that a significant, separately identifiable problem-oriented evaluation and management (E/M) service is rendered, the appropriate code for the E/M service may be reported separately. Append modifier 25 to the service code selected to indicate that a separately identifiable E/M service was provided on the same date of service as the preventive medicine service. Immunizations and ancillary services, including laboratory, radiology, or screening tests, performed at the time of the preventive service may be reported separately. Preventive medicine services are not covered by Medicare. For preventive services provided to an established patient, see 99391-99397.

ICD-10-CM Diagnostic Codes

The application of this code is too broad to adequately present ICD-10-CM diagnostic code links here. Refer to your ICD-10-CM book.

AMA: **99381** 2018,Jan,8; 2017,Jan,8; 2016,Mar,8; 2016,Jan,13; 2015,Jan,16; 2014,Oct,8; 2014,Jan,11; 2013,Jan,9-10 **99382** 2018,Jan,8; 2017,Jan,8; 2016,Mar,8; 2016,Jan,13; 2015,Jan,16; 2014,Oct,8; 2014,Jan,11; 2013,Jan,9-10 **99383** 2018,Jan,8; 2017,Jan,8; 2016,Mar,8; 2016,Jan,13; 2015,Jan,16; 2014,Oct,8; 2014,Jan,11; 2013,Jan,9-10 **99384** 2018,Jan,8; 2017,Jan,8; 2016,Mar,8; 2016,Jan,13; 2015,Jan,12; 2015,Jan,16; 2014,Oct,8; 2014,Jan,11; 2013,Jan,9-10 **99385** 2018,Jan,8; 2017,Jan,8; 2016,Mar,8; 2016,Jan,13; 2015,Jan,12; 2015,Jan,16; 2014,Oct,8; 2014,Jan,11; 2013,Jan,9-10 **99386** 2018,Jan,8; 2017,Jan,8; 2016,Mar,8; 2016,Jan,13; 2015,Jan,12; 2015,Jan,16; 2014,Oct,8; 2014,Jan,11; 2013,Jan,9-10 **99387** 2018,Jan,8; 2017,Jan,8; 2016,Mar,8; 2016,Jan,13; 2015,Jan,16; 2014,Oct,8; 2014,Jan,11; 2013,Jan,9-10

● New ▲ Revised + Add On AMA: CPT Assist [Resequenced] ☑ Laterality

Relative Value Units/Medicare Edits

Non-Facility RVU	Work	PE	MP	Total
99381	1.5	1.54	0.09	3.13
99382	1.6	1.58	0.1	3.28
99383	1.7	1.61	0.1	3.41
99384	2.0	1.73	0.12	3.85
99385	1.92	1.69	0.11	3.72
99386	2.33	1.85	0.14	4.32
99387	2.5	2.03	0.15	4.68
Facility RVU	**Work**	**PE**	**MP**	**Total**
99381	1.5	0.58	0.09	2.17
99382	1.6	0.62	0.1	2.32
99383	1.7	0.66	0.1	2.46
99384	2.0	0.76	0.12	2.88
99385	1.92	0.73	0.11	2.76
99386	2.33	0.89	0.14	3.36
99387	2.5	0.96	0.15	3.61

	FUD	Status	MUE	Modifiers				IOM Reference
99381	N/A	N	0(3)	N/A	N/A	N/A	N/A	100-04,12,30.6.2;
99382	N/A	N	0(3)	N/A	N/A	N/A	N/A	100-04,12,30.6.4
99383	N/A	N	0(3)	N/A	N/A	N/A	N/A	
99384	N/A	N	0(3)	N/A	N/A	N/A	N/A	
99385	N/A	N	0(3)	N/A	N/A	N/A	N/A	
99386	N/A	N	0(3)	N/A	N/A	N/A	N/A	
99387	N/A	N	0(3)	N/A	N/A	N/A	N/A	

* with documentation

Terms To Know

preventive medicine service. Evaluation and management service provided as a periodic health screening and/or prophylactic service that does not typically include management of new or existing diagnoses or problems.

99391-99397

99391 Periodic comprehensive preventive medicine reevaluation and management of an individual including an age and gender appropriate history, examination, counseling/anticipatory guidance/risk factor reduction interventions, and the ordering of laboratory/diagnostic procedures, established patient; infant (age younger than 1 year)

99392 early childhood (age 1 through 4 years)

99393 late childhood (age 5 through 11 years)

99394 adolescent (age 12 through 17 years)

99395 18-39 years

99396 40-64 years

99397 65 years and older

Explanation

Periodic comprehensive preventive medicine services are typically well-patient examinations for established patients presenting for reevaluations and/or management of overall health condition with code selection dependent upon the patient's age. These services include applicable patient history and examination, guidance/recommendation regarding personal risk factors, and any laboratory and/or diagnostic procedures ordered. Clinicians are not required to report minor or self-limiting problems or complaints noted during the course of the preventive examination when those problems do not require any additional work or necessitate performing the key components of a problem oriented E/M service. Report 99391 for infants younger than 1 year of age; 99392 for children 1 to 4 years of age; 99393 for children 5 to 11 years of age; 99394 for adolescents12 to 17 years of age; 99395 for adult patients 18 to 39 years of age; 99396 for patients 40 to 64 years of age; and 99397 for patients 65 years of age and older.

Coding Tips

These codes are used to report preventive medicine services for an established patient. Time is not a factor when selecting this E/M service. Code selection is determined based on whether the patient is new or established and the age of the patient. When documentation supports that a significant, separately identifiable problem-oriented evaluation and management (E/M) service is rendered, the appropriate code for the E/M service may be reported separately. Append modifier 25 to the service code selected to indicate that a separately identifiable E/M service was provided on the same date of service as the preventive medicine service. Immunizations and ancillary services, including laboratory, radiology, or screening tests, performed at the time of the preventive service may be reported separately. Preventive medicine services are not covered by Medicare. For preventive services provided to a new patient, see 99381-99387.

ICD-10-CM Diagnostic Codes

The application of this code is too broad to adequately present ICD-10-CM diagnostic code links here. Refer to your ICD-10-CM book.

AMA: **99391** 2018,Jan,8; 2017,Jan,8; 2016,Mar,8; 2016,Jan,13; 2015,Jan,16; 2014,Oct,8; 2014,Jan,11; 2013,Jan,9-10 **99392** 2018,Jan,8; 2017,Jan,8; 2016,Mar,8; 2016,Jan,13; 2015,Jan,16; 2014,Oct,8; 2014,Jan,11; 2013,Jan,9-10 **99393** 2018,Jan,8; 2017,Jan,8; 2016,Mar,8; 2016,Jan,13; 2015,Jan,16; 2014,Oct,8; 2014,Jan,11; 2013,Jan,9-10 **99394** 2018,Jan,8; 2017,Jan,8; 2016,Mar,8; 2016,Jan,13; 2015,Jan,12; 2015,Jan,16; 2014,Oct,8; 2014,Jan,11; 2013,Jan,9-10 **99395** 2018,Jan,8; 2017,Jan,8; 2016,Mar,8; 2016,Jan,13; 2015,Jan,16; 2015,Jan,12; 2014,Oct,8; 2014,Jan,11; 2013,Jan,9-10 **99396** 2018,Jan,8; 2017,Sep,11; 2017,Jan,8; 2016,Mar,8; 2016,Jan,13; 2015,Jan,12; 2015,Jan,16; 2014,Oct,8; 2014,Jan,11; 2013,Jan,9-10 **99397** 2018,Jan,8; 2017,Jan,8; 2016,Mar,8; 2016,Jan,13; 2015,Jan,16; 2014,Oct,8; 2014,Jan,11; 2013,Jan,9-10

Relative Value Units/Medicare Edits

Non-Facility RVU	Work	PE	MP	Total
99391	1.37	1.37	0.08	2.82
99392	1.5	1.42	0.09	3.01
99393	1.5	1.41	0.09	3.0
99394	1.7	1.49	0.1	3.29
99395	1.75	1.51	0.1	3.36
99396	1.9	1.57	0.11	3.58
99397	2.0	1.73	0.12	3.85
Facility RVU	**Work**	**PE**	**MP**	**Total**
99391	1.37	0.53	0.08	1.98
99392	1.5	0.58	0.09	2.17
99393	1.5	0.58	0.09	2.17
99394	1.7	0.66	0.1	2.46
99395	1.75	0.68	0.1	2.53
99396	1.9	0.73	0.11	2.74
99397	2.0	0.76	0.12	2.88

	FUD	Status	MUE	Modifiers				IOM Reference
99391	N/A	N	0(3)	N/A	N/A	N/A	N/A	None
99392	N/A	N	0(3)	N/A	N/A	N/A	N/A	
99393	N/A	N	0(3)	N/A	N/A	N/A	N/A	
99394	N/A	N	0(3)	N/A	N/A	N/A	N/A	
99395	N/A	N	0(3)	N/A	N/A	N/A	N/A	
99396	N/A	N	0(3)	N/A	N/A	N/A	N/A	
99397	N/A	N	0(3)	N/A	N/A	N/A	N/A	

* with documentation

Terms To Know

preventive medicine service. Evaluation and management service provided as a periodic health screening and/or prophylactic service that does not typically include management of new or existing diagnoses or problems.

99401-99404

99401 Preventive medicine counseling and/or risk factor reduction intervention(s) provided to an individual (separate procedure); approximately 15 minutes

99402 approximately 30 minutes

99403 approximately 45 minutes

99404 approximately 60 minutes

Explanation

Preventive medicine individual counseling services are face-to-face services performed by a qualified clinician in order to foster healthy living and/or avert illness/injury. Risk factor counseling may be utilized in the absence of illness. These services may include counseling/evaluation of family issues, appropriate diet and exercise, high-risk behavior, avoidance of injury, dental issues, and discussion of available laboratory and/or diagnostic results. Report 99401 for encounters lasting 15 minutes; 99402 for 30 minutes; 99403 for 45 minutes; and 99404 for a duration of 60 minutes.

Coding Tips

These codes are used to report counseling services provided to patients to support healthy living and reduce risk of illness or injury. These services are provided face-to-face by the physician or other qualified healthcare provider. These are time-based codes and time spent with the patient must be documented in the medical record. These separate procedures by definition are usually a component of a more complex service and are not identified separately. When performed alone or with other unrelated procedures/services they may be reported. When documentation supports that a significant, separately identifiable problem-oriented evaluation and management (E/M) service is rendered, the appropriate code for the E/M service may be reported separately. Append modifier 25 to the service code selected to indicate that a separately identifiable E/M service was provided on the same date of service as the counseling service. Do not report 96156-96159 or 96164-96171 in addition to 99401-99404 on the same date of service. For preventive medicine counseling provided in a group setting, see 99411-99412. For behavior change intervention services, see 99406-99409.

ICD-10-CM Diagnostic Codes

The application of this code is too broad to adequately present ICD-10-CM diagnostic code links here. Refer to your ICD-10-CM book.

AMA: **99401** 2018,Jan,8; 2017,Jan,8; 2016,Mar,8; 2016,Jan,13; 2015,Jan,16; 2014,Oct,8; 2014,Jan,11; 2014,Aug,5; 2013,Jan,9-10 **99402** 2018,Jan,8; 2017,Jan,8; 2016,Mar,8; 2016,Jan,13; 2015,Jan,16; 2014,Oct,8; 2014,Jan,11; 2014,Aug,5; 2013,Jan,9-10 **99403** 2018,Jan,8; 2017,Jan,8; 2016,Mar,8; 2016,Jan,13; 2015,Jan,16; 2014,Oct,8; 2014,Jan,11; 2014,Aug,5; 2013,Jan,9-10 **99404** 2018,Jan,8; 2017,Jan,8; 2016,Mar,8; 2016,Jan,13; 2015,Jan,16; 2014,Oct,8; 2014,Jan,11; 2014,Aug,5; 2013,Jan,9-10

Relative Value Units/Medicare Edits

Non-Facility RVU	Work	PE	MP	Total
99401	0.48	0.59	0.03	1.1
99402	0.98	0.77	0.06	1.81
99403	1.46	0.96	0.09	2.51
99404	1.95	1.14	0.12	3.21
Facility RVU	**Work**	**PE**	**MP**	**Total**
99401	0.48	0.19	0.03	0.7
99402	0.98	0.38	0.06	1.42
99403	1.46	0.57	0.09	2.12
99404	1.95	0.74	0.12	2.81

	FUD	Status	MUE	Modifiers				IOM Reference
99401	N/A	N	0(3)	N/A	N/A	N/A	N/A	100-04,12,30.6.4
99402	N/A	N	0(3)	N/A	N/A	N/A	N/A	
99403	N/A	N	0(3)	N/A	N/A	N/A	N/A	
99404	N/A	N	0(3)	N/A	N/A	N/A	N/A	

* with documentation

Terms To Know

counseling. Discussion with a patient and/or family concerning one or more of the following areas: diagnostic results, impressions, and/or recommended diagnostic studies; prognosis; risks and benefits of management (treatment) options; instructions for management (treatment) and/or follow-up; importance of compliance with chosen management (treatment) options; risk factor reduction; and patient and family education.

preventive medicine service. Evaluation and management service provided as a periodic health screening and/or prophylactic service that does not typically include management of new or existing diagnoses or problems.

99406-99409

99406 Smoking and tobacco use cessation counseling visit; intermediate, greater than 3 minutes up to 10 minutes

99407 intensive, greater than 10 minutes

99408 Alcohol and/or substance (other than tobacco) abuse structured screening (eg, AUDIT, DAST), and brief intervention (SBI) services; 15 to 30 minutes

99409 greater than 30 minutes

Explanation

Individual behavior change intervention services are counseling and/or intervention services directed at high-risk behaviors such as tobacco, alcohol, and substance abuse. These services can be reported as treatment of the condition or in relation to the condition that has the potential of causing illness or injury. Additionally, the encounter uses validated instruments to determine the patient's opinion related to behavior change and providing input on a plan to change behavior with appropriate actions and motivation. Report 99406 for smoking and tobacco cessation counseling requiring three to 10 minutes of time and 99407 for counseling requiring more than ten minutes. Report 99408 for alcohol and/or substance abuse screening utilizing such instruments as AUDIT, DAST, and intervention services requiring 15 to 30 minutes; for more than 30 minutes, report 99409.

Coding Tips

These codes are used to report interventional counseling services provided to patients to promote behavioral change when the behavior is considered an illness itself or to change the behavior before it results in an illness. These are time-based codes and time spent with the patient must be documented in the medical record. When documentation supports that a significant, separately identifiable problem-oriented evaluation and management (E/M) service is rendered, the appropriate code for the E/M service may be reported separately. Append modifier 25 to the service code selected to indicate that a separately identifiable E/M service was provided on the same date of service as the counseling service. Codes 99408 and 99409 should only be reported for the initial screening and brief intervention. Do not report 99407 in addition to 99406. Do not report 99409 in addition to 99408. Do not report 96156-96159 or 96164-96171 in addition to 99406-99409 on the same date of service. For preventive medicine counseling provided to an individual, see 99401-99404. For preventive medicine counseling provided in a group setting, see 99411-99412.

ICD-10-CM Diagnostic Codes

The application of this code is too broad to adequately present ICD-10-CM diagnostic code links here. Refer to your ICD-10-CM book.

AMA: 99406 2018,Jan,8; 2017,Nov,3; 2017,Jan,8; 2016,Mar,8; 2016,Jan,13; 2015,Jan,16; 2014,Oct,8; 2014,Jan,11; 2013,Jan,9-10 **99407** 2018,Jan,8; 2017,Nov,3; 2017,Jan,8; 2016,Mar,8; 2016,Jan,13; 2015,Jan,16; 2014,Oct,8; 2014,Jan,11; 2013,Jan,9-10 **99408** 2018,Jan,8; 2017,Nov,3; 2017,Jan,8; 2016,Nov,5; 2016,Mar,8; 2016,Jan,13; 2015,Jan,16; 2014,Oct,8; 2014,Jan,11; 2013,Jan,9-10 **99409** 2018,Jan,8; 2017,Nov,3; 2017,Jan,8; 2016,Nov,5; 2016,Mar,8; 2016,Jan,13; 2015,Jan,16; 2014,Oct,8; 2014,Jan,11; 2013,Jan,9-10

Relative Value Units/Medicare Edits

Non-Facility RVU	Work	PE	MP	Total
99406	0.24	0.16	0.02	0.42
99407	0.5	0.26	0.04	0.8
99408	0.65	0.32	0.04	1.01
99409	1.3	0.57	0.08	1.95
Facility RVU	**Work**	**PE**	**MP**	**Total**
99406	0.24	0.09	0.02	0.35
99407	0.5	0.19	0.04	0.73
99408	0.65	0.25	0.04	0.94
99409	1.3	0.5	0.08	1.88

	FUD	Status	MUE	Modifiers				IOM Reference
99406	N/A	A	1(2)	N/A	N/A	N/A	80*	None
99407	N/A	A	1(2)	N/A	N/A	N/A	80*	
99408	N/A	N	0(3)	N/A	N/A	N/A	N/A	
99409	N/A	N	0(3)	N/A	N/A	N/A	N/A	

* with documentation

Terms To Know

AUDIT. Alcohol use disorder identification test.

DAST. Drug abuse screening test.

99411-99412

99411 Preventive medicine counseling and/or risk factor reduction intervention(s) provided to individuals in a group setting (separate procedure); approximately 30 minutes

99412 approximately 60 minutes

Explanation

Preventive medicine group counseling services are face-to-face services performed by a qualified clinician in order to foster healthy living and/or avert illness/injury. Risk factor counseling may be utilized in the absence of illness in a group setting. These services may include counseling/evaluation of family issues, appropriate diet and exercise, high-risk behavior, avoidance of injury, dental issues, and discussion of available laboratory and/or diagnostic results. Report 99411 for encounters of 30 minutes duration and 99412 for encounters lasting 60 minutes.

Coding Tips

These codes are used to report counseling services provided to patients to support healthy living and reduce risk of illness or injury. These services are provided face-to-face by the physician or other qualified healthcare provider. These are time-based codes and time spent with the patient must be documented in the medical record. These separate procedures by definition are usually a component of a more complex service and are not identified separately. When performed alone or with other unrelated procedures/services they may be reported. When documentation supports that a significant, separately identifiable problem-oriented evaluation and management (E/M) service is rendered, the appropriate code for the E/M service may be reported separately. Append modifier 25 to the service code selected to indicate that a separately identifiable E/M service was provided on the same date of service as the counseling service. Do not report 96156-96159 or 96164-96171 in addition to 99411-99412 on the same date of service. For group counseling of patients with symptoms or established illness, see 99078. For preventive medicine counseling provided to an individual, see 99401-99404. For behavior change intervention services, see 99406-99409.

ICD-10-CM Diagnostic Codes

The application of this code is too broad to adequately present ICD-10-CM diagnostic code links here. Refer to your ICD-10-CM book.

AMA: **99411** 2018,Jan,8; 2017,Jan,8; 2016,Mar,8; 2016,Jan,13; 2015,Jan,16; 2014,Oct,8; 2014,Jan,11; 2013,Jan,9-10 **99412** 2018,Jan,8; 2017,Jan,8; 2016,Mar,8; 2016,Jan,13; 2015,Jan,16; 2014,Oct,8; 2014,Jan,11; 2013,Jan,9-10

Relative Value Units/Medicare Edits

Non-Facility RVU	Work	PE	MP	Total
99411	0.15	0.39	0.01	0.55
99412	0.25	0.43	0.01	0.69
Facility RVU	**Work**	**PE**	**MP**	**Total**
99411	0.15	0.06	0.01	0.22
99412	0.25	0.1	0.01	0.36

	FUD	Status	MUE	Modifiers				IOM Reference
99411	N/A	N	0(3)	N/A	N/A	N/A	N/A	None
99412	N/A	N	0(3)	N/A	N/A	N/A	N/A	

* with documentation

99441-99443

99441 Telephone evaluation and management service by a physician or other qualified health care professional who may report evaluation and management services provided to an established patient, parent, or guardian not originating from a related E/M service provided within the previous 7 days nor leading to an E/M service or procedure within the next 24 hours or soonest available appointment; 5-10 minutes of medical discussion

99442 11-20 minutes of medical discussion

99443 21-30 minutes of medical discussion

Explanation

Telephone services are non-face-to-face encounters originating from the established patient for evaluation or management of a problem provided by a qualified clinician. The problem may not be related to an E/M encounter that occurred within the previous seven days nor can the problem lead to an E/M encounter or other service within the following 24 hours or next available in-office appointment opening. Report 99441 for services lasting five to 10 minutes; 99442 for services lasting 11 to 20 minutes; and 99443 for calls lasting 21 to 30 minutes.

Coding Tips

These codes are used to report non-face-to-face patient services initiated by an established patient via the telephone. These are time-based codes and time spent with the patient must be documented in the medical record. These codes should not be reported if the provider decides to see the patient within 24 hours or by the next available urgent visit appointment, or if the provider performed a related E/M service within the previous seven days or the call is initiated within a postoperative period. Medicare and other payers may not reimburse separately for these services. Check with the specific payer to determine coverage. Do not report 99441-99443 when the same provider has reported 99421-99423 for the same problem in the previous seven days. For nonphysician telephone medical services, see 98966-98968. Do not report these services when performed concurrently with other billable services, such as 99339-99340, 99374-99380, 99487-99489, or 99495-99496. Do not report these services for INR monitoring when reporting 93792 or 93793.

ICD-10-CM Diagnostic Codes

The application of this code is too broad to adequately present ICD-10-CM diagnostic code links here. Refer to your ICD-10-CM book.

AMA: **99441** 2019,Mar,8; 2018,Mar,7; 2018,Jan,8; 2017,Jan,8; 2016,Jan,13; 2015,Jan,16; 2014,Oct,8; 2014,Oct,3; 2014,Jan,11; 2013,Oct,11; 2013,Nov,3; 2013,Apr,3-4 **99442** 2019,Mar,8; 2018,Mar,7; 2018,Jan,8; 2017,Jan,8; 2016,Jan,13; 2015,Jan,16; 2014,Oct,3; 2014,Oct,8; 2014,Jan,11; 2013,Oct,11; 2013,Nov,3; 2013,Apr,3-4 **99443** 2019,Mar,8; 2018,Mar,7; 2018,Jan,8; 2017,Jan,8; 2016,Jan,13; 2015,Jan,16; 2014,Oct,8; 2014,Oct,3; 2014,Jan,11; 2013,Oct,11; 2013,Nov,3; 2013,Apr,3-4

Relative Value Units/Medicare Edits

Non-Facility RVU	Work	PE	MP	Total
99441	0.25	0.13	0.01	0.39
99442	0.5	0.23	0.03	0.76
99443	0.75	0.33	0.04	1.12
Facility RVU	**Work**	**PE**	**MP**	**Total**
99441	0.25	0.1	0.01	0.36
99442	0.5	0.19	0.03	0.72
99443	0.75	0.29	0.04	1.08

	FUD	Status	MUE	Modifiers				IOM Reference
99441	N/A	N	0(3)	N/A	N/A	N/A	N/A	None
99442	N/A	N	0(3)	N/A	N/A	N/A	N/A	
99443	N/A	N	0(3)	N/A	N/A	N/A	N/A	

* with documentation

Terms To Know

established patient. Patient who has received professional services in a face-to-face setting within the last three years from the same physician/qualified health care professional or another physician/qualified health care professional of the exact same specialty and subspecialty who belongs to the same group practice. If the patient is seen by a physician/qualified health care professional who is covering for another physician/qualified health care professional, the patient will be considered the same as if seen by the physician/qualified health care professional who is unavailable.

other qualified health care professional. Individual who is qualified by education, training, licensure/regulation, and facility privileging to perform a professional service within his or her scope of practice and independently (or as incident-to) report the professional service without requiring physician supervision. Payers may state exemptions in writing or state and local regulations may not follow this definition for performance of some services. Always refer to any relevant plan policies and federal and/or state laws to determine who may perform and report services. ***Synonym(s):*** *OQHCP.*

[99421, 99422, 99423]

- ● **99421** Online digital evaluation and management service, for an established patient, for up to 7 days, cumulative time during the 7 days; 5-10 minutes
- ● **99422** Online digital evaluation and management service, for an established patient, for up to 7 days, cumulative time during the 7 days; 11-20 minutes
- ● **99423** Online digital evaluation and management service, for an established patient, for up to 7 days, cumulative time during the 7 days; 21 or more minutes

Explanation

On-line medical evaluation services are non-face-to-face encounters originating from the established patient to the physician or other qualified health care professional for evaluation or management of a problem utilizing internet resources. The service includes all communication, prescription, and laboratory orders with permanent storage in the patient's medical record. The service may include more than one provider responding to the same patient and is only reportable once during seven days for the same encounter. Do not report these codes if the online patient request is related to an E/M service that occurred within the previous seven days or within the global period following a procedure. Report 99421 if the cumulative time during the seven-day period is five to 10 minutes; 99422 for 11 to 20 minutes; and 99423 for 21 or more minutes.

Coding Tips

These codes are used to report non-face-to-face patient services initiated by an established patient via an on-line inquiry. Providers must provide a timely response to the inquiry and the encounter must be stored permanently to report this service. These services are reported once in a seven-day period and are reported for the cumulative time devoted to the service over the seven days. Cumulative time of less than five minutes should not be reported. A new/unrelated problem initiated within seven days of a previous E/M visit that address a different problem may be reported separately. Medicare and other payers may not reimburse separately for these services. Check with the specific payer to determine coverage. For nonphysician on-line medical services, see 98970, 98971, and 98972. Do not report these services when performed concurrently with other billable services, such as 99091, 99339-99340, 99374-99380, 99487-99489, or 99495-99496. Do not report these services for INR monitoring when reporting 93792 or 93793.

ICD-10-CM Diagnostic Codes

The application of this code is too broad to adequately present ICD-10-CM diagnostic code links here. Refer to your ICD-10-CM book.

Relative Value Units/Medicare Edits

Non-Facility RVU	Work	PE	MP	Total
99421				
99422				
99423				

Facility RVU	Work	PE	MP	Total
99421				
99422				
99423				

	FUD	Status	MUE	Modifiers				IOM Reference
99421	N/A		-	N/A	N/A	N/A	N/A	None
99422	N/A		-	N/A	N/A	N/A	N/A	
99423	N/A		-	N/A	N/A	N/A	N/A	

* with documentation

Terms To Know

established patient. 1) Patient who has received professional services in a face-to-face setting within the last three years from the same physician/qualified health care professional or another physician/qualified health care professional of the exact same specialty and subspecialty who belongs to the same group practice. 2) For OPPS hospitals, patient who has been registered as an inpatient or outpatient in a hospital's provider-based clinic or emergency department within the past three years.

other qualified health care professional. Individual who is qualified by education, training, licensure/regulation, and facility privileging to perform a professional service within his or her scope of practice and independently (or as incident-to) report the professional service without requiring physician supervision. Payers may state exemptions in writing or state and local regulations may not follow this definition for performance of some services. Always refer to any relevant plan policies and federal and/or state laws to determine who may perform and report services.

 ● New ▲ Revised + Add On AMA: CPT Assist [Resequenced] ☑ Laterality

99446-99449 [99451, 99452]

99446 Interprofessional telephone/Internet/electronic health record assessment and management service provided by a consultative physician, including a verbal and written report to the patient's treating/requesting physician or other qualified health care professional; 5-10 minutes of medical consultative discussion and review

99447 11-20 minutes of medical consultative discussion and review

99448 21-30 minutes of medical consultative discussion and review

99449 31 minutes or more of medical consultative discussion and review

99451 Interprofessional telephone/Internet/electronic health record assessment and management service provided by a consultative physician, including a written report to the patient's treating/requesting physician or other qualified health care professional, 5 minutes or more of medical consultative time

99452 Interprofessional telephone/Internet/electronic health record referral service(s) provided by a treating/requesting physician or other qualified health care professional, 30 minutes

Explanation

Interprofessional telephone/internet/electronic health record consultation services are utilized when the attending qualified clinician requests the input of another provider with specific knowledge of the condition. This specialist may assist in diagnosis or treatment of the patient without seeing the patient and often occurs when the situation is urgent and/or complex in nature. The patient may be a new or established patient with a new problem or exacerbation of a current problem in the eyes of the consulting physician; however, the consultant may not have seen the patient within the previous 14 days. This code may not be reported for transfer of care or to schedule a face-to-face with the consultant within the next 14 days or next available appointment opening. This discussion includes appropriate review of medical records, laboratory and radiology results, medication review/tolerance, and pathology results. The consult should account for more than 50 percent of the time in discussion; if more than one discussion is necessary, the time is cumulative with the code reported one time. The patient's medical record should contain a request for consult with an explanation as to the medical necessity of the request and the consulting physician should provide a verbal and written report to the requesting/treating clinician. These codes are not reportable if the discussion requires less than five minutes of time. Report 99446 for encounters of five- to 10 minutes duration; 99447 for 11 to 20 minutes; 99448 for 21 to 30 minutes; and 99449 for encounters of more than 30 minutes duration. Report 99451 for encounters of five or more minutes that include a written report only from the consulting physician. The attending qualified clinician can report 99452 when 16 to 30 minutes of the clinician's time is spent preparing for or communicating with the consultant; 99452 can only be reported once during a 14-day period.

Coding Tips

These codes are used to report an assessment and management service requested by the patient's treating clinician for guidance from a specialist in treating the patient. These are time-based codes and time spent in medical consultation must be documented in the medical record. These codes do not differentiate between a new or established patient. Do not report these codes for the sole purpose of arranging a transfer of care or other face-to-face services. Report 99446-99449 for time spent in telephone/internet/electronic health record assessment and review with verbal and written report of findings. Report 99451-99452 for written report of findings without a verbal report. Prolonged service codes 99354-99357 may be reported by the treating/requesting provider in addition to these services when the patient is present (on-site) and the telephone/internet/electronic health record discussion with the consultant exceeds 30 minutes. Prolonged service codes 99358-99359 may be reported by the treating/requesting provider in addition to these services when the patient is on site and the telephone/internet discussion with the consultant exceeds 30 minutes. For telephone services conducted by the physician directly with the patient, see 99441-99443. For on-line digital medical evaluation and management services provided by the physician directly with the patient, see 99421-99423. For nonphysician telephone or online medical services, see 98966-98968.

ICD-10-CM Diagnostic Codes

The application of this code is too broad to adequately present ICD-10-CM diagnostic code links here. Refer to your ICD-10-CM book.

AMA: **99446** 2019,Jun,7; 2019,Jan,3; 2018,Jan,8; 2017,Jan,8; 2016,Jan,13; 2015,Jan,16; 2014,Oct,8; 2014,Jun,14; 2013,Oct,11 **99447** 2019,Jun,7; 2019,Jan,3; 2018,Jan,8; 2017,Jan,8; 2016,Jan,13; 2015,Jan,16; 2014,Oct,8; 2014,Jun,14; 2013,Oct,11 **99448** 2019,Jun,7; 2019,Jan,3; 2018,Jan,8; 2017,Jan,8; 2016,Jan,13; 2015,Jan,16; 2014,Oct,8; 2014,Jun,14; 2013,Oct,11 **99449** 2019,Jun,7; 2019,Jan,3; 2018,Jan,8; 2017,Jan,8; 2016,Jan,13; 2015,Jan,16; 2014,Oct,8; 2014,Jun,14; 2013,Oct,11 **99451** 2019,Jun,7; 2019,Jan,3 **99452** 2019,Jun,7; 2019,Jan,3

Relative Value Units/Medicare Edits

Non-Facility RVU	Work	PE	MP	Total
99446	0.35	0.14	0.02	0.51
99447	0.7	0.27	0.04	1.01
99448	1.05	0.41	0.06	1.52
99449	1.4	0.54	0.08	2.02
99451	0.7	0.29	0.05	1.04
99452	0.7	0.29	0.05	1.04
Facility RVU	**Work**	**PE**	**MP**	**Total**
99446	0.35	0.14	0.02	0.51
99447	0.7	0.27	0.04	1.01
99448	1.05	0.41	0.06	1.52
99449	1.4	0.54	0.08	2.02
99451	0.7	0.29	0.05	1.04
99452	0.7	0.29	0.05	1.04

	FUD	Status	MUE	Modifiers				IOM Reference
99446	N/A	A	1(2)	N/A	N/A	N/A	80*	None
99447	N/A	A	1(2)	N/A	N/A	N/A	80*	
99448	N/A	A	1(2)	N/A	N/A	N/A	80*	
99449	N/A	A	1(2)	N/A	N/A	N/A	80*	
99451	N/A	A	1(2)	N/A	N/A	N/A	80*	
99452	N/A	A	1(2)	N/A	N/A	N/A	80*	

* with documentation

[99453, 99454]

99453 Remote monitoring of physiologic parameter(s) (eg, weight, blood pressure, pulse oximetry, respiratory flow rate), initial; set-up and patient education on use of equipment

99454 Remote monitoring of physiologic parameter(s) (eg, weight, blood pressure, pulse oximetry, respiratory flow rate), initial; device(s) supply with daily recording(s) or programmed alert(s) transmission, each 30 days

Explanation

A physician or other qualified health care professional orders an FDA-defined remote patient monitoring (RPM) device that is used by a patient for the purposes of collecting, monitoring, and reporting health-related data to the provider, including, but not limited to, weight, blood pressure, or pulse oximetry. This technology allows for the gathering of health data from the patient in one location and the electronic transmission of that data to a provider in a different location for review and subsequent recommendations, particularly in patients with ongoing and/or chronic disease processes. Code 99453 reports the work involved with orienting the patient to the RPM process, the initial device set-up, and patient instruction and training for each episode of care. An episode of care is described as starting at the time the RPM device service begins and is complete when the established treatment goal has been reached. Code 99454 reports the supply of the actual device including the daily recordings and program alert transmissions for a 30-day period. These codes should not be reported for monitoring if the duration is less than 16 days.

Coding Tips

These codes are used to report the remote physiological monitoring services of a medically approved device ordered by the physician or other qualified health care professional. Code 99453 is used to report initial patient education with set up and instruction. Code 99454 is used to report each 30 days of device recording and transmission. For self-measured blood pressure monitoring, see 99473-99474.

ICD-10-CM Diagnostic Codes

The application of this code is too broad to adequately present ICD-10-CM diagnostic code links here. Refer to your ICD-10-CM book.

AMA: 99453 2019,Mar,10; 2019,Jan,6; 2019,Jan,3 **99454** 2019,Mar,10; 2019,Jan,3; 2019,Jan,6

Relative Value Units/Medicare Edits

Non-Facility RVU	Work	PE	MP	Total
99453	0.0	0.53	0.01	0.54
99454	0.0	1.77	0.01	1.78
Facility RVU	**Work**	**PE**	**MP**	**Total**
99453	0.0	0.53	0.01	0.54
99454	0.0	1.77	0.01	1.78

	FUD	Status	MUE	Modifiers				IOM Reference
99453	N/A	A	1(2)	N/A	N/A	N/A	80*	None
99454	N/A	A	1(2)	N/A	N/A	N/A	80*	

* with documentation

[99091]

99091 Collection and interpretation of physiologic data (eg, ECG, blood pressure, glucose monitoring) digitally stored and/or transmitted by the patient and/or caregiver to the physician or other qualified health care professional, qualified by education, training, licensure/regulation (when applicable) requiring a minimum of 30 minutes of time, each 30 days

Explanation

A physician or other qualified health care professional collects and interprets physiologic data. The data (e.g., blood pressure) is stored digitally and may be transmitted by the patient and/or the caregiver to the provider. The report should contain the time it took the provider to acquire the physiologic data, review and interpret the data, and modify any care plan due to the additional data acquisition. A minimum of 30 minutes every 30 days must be spent in the collection and interpretation of data to report this service.

Coding Tips

This code is used to report the collection and interpretation of physiological data. The data is stored or transmitted from a patient based device and reviewed by a qualified provider. Report 99091 once per 30 days when at least 30 minutes of provider time is spent. When performed on the same day the patient presents for another E/M service, do not report 99091 separately.

ICD-10-CM Diagnostic Codes

The application of this code is too broad to adequately present ICD-10-CM diagnostic code links here. Refer to your ICD-10-CM book.

AMA: 99091 2019,Jun,3; 2019,Jan,6; 2018,Mar,5; 2018,Jun,6; 2018,Jan,8; 2018,Feb,7; 2018,Dec,10; 2018,Dec,10; 2017,Jan,8; 2016,Jan,13; 2015,Jan,16; 2014,Oct,3; 2014,Jan,11; 2013,Nov,3; 2013,Apr,3-4

Relative Value Units/Medicare Edits

Non-Facility RVU	Work	PE	MP	Total
99091	1.1	0.45	0.07	1.62
Facility RVU	**Work**	**PE**	**MP**	**Total**
99091	1.1	0.45	0.07	1.62

	FUD	Status	MUE	Modifiers				IOM Reference
99091	N/A	A	1(2)	N/A	N/A	N/A	80*	None

* with documentation

[99473, 99474]

- ● **99473** Self-measured blood pressure using a device validated for clinical accuracy; patient education/training and device calibration
- ● **99474** Self-measured blood pressure using a device validated for clinical accuracy; separate self-measurements of two readings one minute apart, twice daily over a 30-day period (minimum of 12 readings), collection of data reported by the patient and/or caregiver to the physician or other qualified health care professional, with report of average systolic and diastolic pressures and subsequent communication of a treatment plan to the patient

Explanation

Self-measured blood pressure monitoring (SMBP) has been shown to be an effective approach to lowering blood pressure (BP), improving control in patients with hypertension, and increasing patient compliance with antihypertensive therapy. Also known as out-of-office BP measurement or home BP monitoring, the practice involves the use of devices that have been validated for clinical accuracy. Devices that measure blood pressure over the upper arm remain the most accurate choice compared to other available options, and remain the standard for proper BP measurement over finger, wrist, mobile health, and wearable devices. Report 99473 for patient education/training and device calibration. Report 99474 for separate self-measurements of two readings, one minute apart, twice daily over a 30-day period with a minimum of 12 readings. This includes collection of data reported by the patient and/or caregiver to the physician or other qualified health care professional, with a report of average systolic and diastolic pressures and subsequent communication of a treatment plan to the patient.

Coding Tips

These codes are used to report patient measured blood pressure using a medically validated device. Code 99473 is used to report initial patient education and device calibration. Code 99474 is used to report each 30 days of collected data reported by the patient and an appropriate treatment plan provided to the patient. Code 99473 may only be reported once per device and code 99474 may only be reported once per calendar month. These codes should not be reported in the same calendar month as 93784, 93786, 93788, 93790, 99091, 99453, 99454, 99457, 99487, or 99489-99491.

ICD-10-CM Diagnostic Codes

The application of this code is too broad to adequately present ICD-10-CM diagnostic code links here. Refer to your ICD-10-CM book.

Relative Value Units/Medicare Edits

Non-Facility RVU	Work	PE	MP	Total
99473				
99474				
Facility RVU	**Work**	**PE**	**MP**	**Total**
99473				
99474				

	FUD	Status	MUE	Modifiers				IOM Reference
99473	N/A		-	N/A	N/A	N/A	N/A	None
99474	N/A		-	N/A	N/A	N/A	N/A	

* with documentation

[99457, 99458]

- ▲ **99457** Remote physiologic monitoring treatment management services, clinical staff/physician/other qualified health care professional time in a calendar month requiring interactive communication with the patient/caregiver during the month; first 20 minutes
- + ● **99458** Remote physiologic monitoring treatment management services, clinical staff/physician/other qualified health care professional time in a calendar month requiring interactive communication with the patient/caregiver during the month; each additional 20 minutes (List separately in addition to code for primary procedure)

Explanation

The provider or clinical staff utilizes the results obtained from an FDA-defined remote patient physiologic monitoring (RPM) device to oversee the patient's treatment plan. The device is ordered by a physician or other qualified health care provider and used by the patient for the purposes of collecting, monitoring, and reporting health-related data, including, but not limited to, weight, blood pressure, or pulse oximetry. This technology allows for the gathering of health data from the patient in one location and the electronic transmission of that data to a provider in a different location for review and subsequent recommendations, particularly in patients with ongoing and/or chronic disease processes. Report these codes to identify time spent managing care when the patient or the practice does not meet requirements for reporting a more specific service. These codes may be reported simultaneously with chronic care management, transitional care management, and behavioral health integration services. Time involved in performing this service should remain separate and distinct from other services and does not count toward the required time for both services in a single month. Live and interactive communication with the patient and/or caregiver is required. Report 99457 for the first 20 minutes of clinician time per calendar month and 99458 for each additional 20 minutes.

Coding Tips

These codes are used to report treatment management of a patient currently monitored remotely for physiological parameters. Report 99457 once per calendar month when at least 20 minutes of live interactive communication is provided, regardless of the number of modalities performed. Report 99458 for each additional 20 minutes minimum of monitoring during the same month. Use 99457-99458 only when another more specific code is not available. Codes 99457 and 99458 may be reported with 99487, 99489, 99490, 99495, 99496, 99484, and 99492-99494, but may not be performed concurrently. Do not report 99457 or 99458 with 99201-99205, 99211-99215, 99221-99223, 99231-99233, 99251-99255, 99324-99328, 99334-99337, or 99341-99350. Do not report 99457 with 93264, 99091, or in the same month as 99473-99474.

ICD-10-CM Diagnostic Codes

The application of this code is too broad to adequately present ICD-10-CM diagnostic code links here. Refer to your ICD-10-CM book.

AMA: **99457** 2019,Jun,3; 2019,Jan,3; 2019,Jan,6

Relative Value Units/Medicare Edits

Non-Facility RVU	Work	PE	MP	Total
99457	0.61	0.78	0.04	1.43
99458				
Facility RVU	**Work**	**PE**	**MP**	**Total**
99457	0.61	0.25	0.04	0.9
99458				

	FUD	Status	MUE	Modifiers				IOM Reference
99457	N/A	A	1(2)	N/A	N/A	N/A	80*	None
99458	N/A		-	N/A	N/A	N/A	N/A	

* with documentation

Terms To Know

monitoring. Recording of events; keep track, regulate, or control patient activities and record findings.

other qualified health care professional. Individual who is qualified by education, training, licensure/regulation, and facility privileging to perform a professional service within his or her scope of practice and independently (or as incident-to) report the professional service without requiring physician supervision. Payers may state exemptions in writing or state and local regulations may not follow this definition for performance of some services. Always refer to any relevant plan policies and federal and/or state laws to determine who may perform and report services.

treatment plan. Plan of care established by the provider outlining specific deficits and planned treatment that may be submitted to the case manager when seeking certification for a plan member.

99464-99465

99464 Attendance at delivery (when requested by the delivering physician or other qualified health care professional) and initial stabilization of newborn

99465 Delivery/birthing room resuscitation, provision of positive pressure ventilation and/or chest compressions in the presence of acute inadequate ventilation and/or cardiac output

Explanation

Delivery/birthing room attendance and resuscitation services are reported when special newborn circumstances require additional attendance and/or care. Report 99464 when attendance during delivery is requested by the delivering health care professional with newborn stabilization. Report 99465 for delivery/birthing room resuscitation, including any positive pressure ventilation and/or chest compression when required due to unsatisfactory ventilation or cardiac output.

Coding Tips

These codes are used to report stabilization or resuscitation services provided to a newborn in the delivery or birthing center. Additional services performed as a necessary part of the resuscitation service, including intubation and vascular lines, may be reported in addition to 99465. These additional services should only be reported when necessary for resuscitation not as a convenience prior to admission to a neonatal intensive care unit. These codes may be reported in addition to 99460, 99468, and 99477. Do not report 99465 with 99464.

ICD-10-CM Diagnostic Codes

The application of this code is too broad to adequately present ICD-10-CM diagnostic code links here. Refer to your ICD-10-CM book.

AMA: **99464** 2018,Jan,8; 2017,Jan,8; 2016,Jan,13; 2015,Jan,16; 2014,Oct,8; 2014,Jan,11 **99465** 2018,Jan,8; 2017,Jan,8; 2016,Jan,13; 2015,Jan,16; 2014,Oct,8; 2014,Jan,11

Relative Value Units/Medicare Edits

Non-Facility RVU	Work	PE	MP	Total
99464	1.5	0.52	0.1	2.12
99465	2.93	1.01	0.19	4.13
Facility RVU	**Work**	**PE**	**MP**	**Total**
99464	1.5	0.52	0.1	2.12
99465	2.93	1.01	0.19	4.13

	FUD	Status	MUE	Modifiers				IOM Reference
99464	N/A	A	1(2)	N/A	N/A	N/A	80*	None
99465	N/A	A	1(2)	N/A	N/A	N/A	80*	

* with documentation

99468-99476

99468 Initial inpatient neonatal critical care, per day, for the evaluation and management of a critically ill neonate, 28 days of age or younger

99469 Subsequent inpatient neonatal critical care, per day, for the evaluation and management of a critically ill neonate, 28 days of age or younger

99471 Initial inpatient pediatric critical care, per day, for the evaluation and management of a critically ill infant or young child, 29 days through 24 months of age

99472 Subsequent inpatient pediatric critical care, per day, for the evaluation and management of a critically ill infant or young child, 29 days through 24 months of age

99475 Initial inpatient pediatric critical care, per day, for the evaluation and management of a critically ill infant or young child, 2 through 5 years of age

99476 Subsequent inpatient pediatric critical care, per day, for the evaluation and management of a critically ill infant or young child, 2 through 5 years of age

Explanation

Inpatient neonatal and pediatric critical care services are reported for neonates (28 days of age or younger) and pediatric patients (29 days through less than 6 years of age) beginning with the date of admission to the critical care unit and for all following days that the patient remains in the unit. Codes are only reportable once daily, per patient, by a single provider within the admission range of the specific facility. Several services are included in the care of these patients and are not separately reportable by the provider, such as monitoring vital signs, any required vascular access, ventilation oversight, blood gas, pulse oximetry measurement, evaluation of car seat, blood transfusion, oral/nasogastric tube insertion, suprapubic bladder aspiration and/or bladder catheter placement, and lumbar puncture. Facilities, however, may report these services separately. Report 99468 for initial inpatient neonates; 99469 for subsequent inpatient neonates; 99471 for initial inpatient pediatric patients aged 29 days to 24 months; 99472 for subsequent inpatient pediatric patients aged 29 days to 24 months; 99475 for initial inpatient pediatric patients 2 to 5 years of age; and 99476 for subsequent inpatient pediatric patients 2 to 5 years of age.

Coding Tips

These codes are used to report inpatient neonatal and pediatric critical care services. Code selection is determined based on whether the service is an initial or subsequent encounter and the age of the patient. These codes are reported on a per day basis. Report an initial critical care code for the first day of service and a subsequent critical care code for the following day(s) of service for the same patient admission. These codes may only be reported by one physician and only once per day, per patient. The following services are considered inclusive to the critical care codes when reported by the physician: airway management, ventilation management, blood gases, blood transfusion, nasogastric tube placement, bladder aspiration, catheterization, lumbar puncture, vascular access, and car seat evaluation. Codes 99468, 99471, and 99475 for initial critical care services should only be reported once per hospital stay. For initiation of selective head or total body hypothermia, see 99184. For neonatal and pediatric patients that receive critical care services in the outpatient setting, see 99291-99292. For critical care provided to patients 6 years of age or older, see 99291-99292. For neonatal patients that are not critically ill but require intensive monitoring or other intensive care, see 99477-99480.

ICD-10-CM Diagnostic Codes

The application of this code is too broad to adequately present ICD-10-CM diagnostic code links here. Refer to your ICD-10-CM book.

AMA: **99468** 2018,Jun,9; 2018,Jan,8; 2018,Dec,8; 2018,Dec,8; 2017,Jan,8; 2016,May,3; 2016,Jan,13; 2015,Oct,8; 2015,Jul,3; 2015,Jan,16; 2015,Feb,10; 2014,Oct,8; 2014,May,4; 2014,Jan,11 **99469** 2018,Jun,9; 2018,Jan,8; 2018,Dec,8; 2018,Dec,8; 2017,Jan,8; 2016,May,3; 2016,Jan,13; 2015,Oct,8; 2015,Jul,3; 2015,Jan,16; 2015,Feb,10; 2014,Oct,8; 2014,May,4; 2014,Jan,11 **99471** 2018,Jun,9; 2018,Jan,8; 2018,Dec,8; 2018,Dec,8; 2017,Jan,8; 2016,May,3; 2016,Jan,13; 2015,Jul,3; 2015,Jan,16; 2015,Feb,10; 2014,Oct,8; 2014,Jan,11 **99472** 2018,Jun,9; 2018,Jan,8; 2018,Dec,8; 2018,Dec,8; 2017,Jan,8; 2016,May,3; 2016,Jan,13; 2015,Jul,3; 2015,Jan,16; 2015,Feb,10; 2014,Oct,8; 2014,Jan,11 **99475** 2018,Jun,9; 2018,Jan,8; 2018,Dec,8; 2018,Dec,8; 2017,Jan,8; 2016,May,3; 2016,Jan,13; 2015,Jul,3; 2015,Jan,16; 2015,Feb,10; 2014,Oct,8; 2014,Jan,11 **99476** 2018,Jun,9; 2018,Jan,8; 2018,Dec,8; 2018,Dec,8; 2017,Jan,8; 2016,May,3; 2016,Jan,13; 2015,Jul,3; 2015,Jan,16; 2015,Feb,10; 2014,Oct,8; 2014,Jan,11

Relative Value Units/Medicare Edits

Non-Facility RVU	Work	PE	MP	Total
99468	18.46	6.36	1.18	26.0
99469	7.99	2.75	0.5	11.24
99471	15.98	5.51	1.02	22.51
99472	7.99	2.93	0.61	11.53
99475	11.25	3.88	0.71	15.84
99476	6.75	2.55	0.56	9.86
Facility RVU	**Work**	**PE**	**MP**	**Total**
99468	18.46	6.36	1.18	26.0
99469	7.99	2.75	0.5	11.24
99471	15.98	5.51	1.02	22.51
99472	7.99	2.93	0.61	11.53
99475	11.25	3.88	0.71	15.84
99476	6.75	2.55	0.56	9.86

	FUD	Status	MUE	Modifiers				IOM Reference
99468	N/A	A	1(2)	N/A	N/A	N/A	80*	100-04,12,30.6.4
99469	N/A	A	1(2)	N/A	N/A	N/A	80*	
99471	N/A	A	1(2)	N/A	N/A	N/A	80*	
99472	N/A	A	1(2)	N/A	N/A	N/A	80*	
99475	N/A	A	1(2)	N/A	N/A	N/A	80*	
99476	N/A	A	1(2)	N/A	N/A	N/A	80*	

* with documentation

99487-99489 [99490, 99491]

99490 Chronic care management services, at least 20 minutes of clinical staff time directed by a physician or other qualified health care professional, per calendar month, with the following required elements: multiple (two or more) chronic conditions expected to last at least 12 months, or until the death of the patient; chronic conditions place the patient at significant risk of death, acute exacerbation/decompensation, or functional decline; comprehensive care plan established, implemented, revised, or monitored.

99491 Chronic care management services, provided personally by a physician or other qualified health care professional, at least 30 minutes of physician or other qualified health care professional time, per calendar month, with the following required elements: multiple (two or more) chronic conditions expected to last at least 12 months, or until the death of the patient; chronic conditions place the patient at significant risk of death, acute exacerbation/decompensation, or functional decline; comprehensive care plan established, implemented, revised, or monitored

99487 Complex chronic care management services, with the following required elements: multiple (two or more) chronic conditions expected to last at least 12 months, or until the death of the patient, chronic conditions place the patient at significant risk of death, acute exacerbation/decompensation, or functional decline, establishment or substantial revision of a comprehensive care plan, moderate or high complexity medical decision making; 60 minutes of clinical staff time directed by a physician or other qualified health care professional, per calendar month

\+ **99489** each additional 30 minutes of clinical staff time directed by a physician or other qualified health care professional, per calendar month (List separately in addition to code for primary procedure)

Explanation

Care management services are defined as the management and support services rendered by clinical staff under the supervision of a qualified clinician for patients living in a personal residence, domiciliary, rest home, or assisted living facility. Some components of case management services include, but are not limited to, creating, implementing, altering, or monitoring a care plan; coordinating with other professionals and/or agencies; and providing education to the patient or caregiver on the patient's medical condition, care plan, and prognosis. The clinician is also responsible for the oversight of those services, as well as for the patient's other medical conditions, psychosocial needs, and normal activities of daily living (ADL). Care plans address all of the patient's health issues and are based on a thorough evaluation involving assessment of the patient's physical, mental, cognitive, social, and functional health, as well as an environmental review, and are revised as necessary. Codes may only be reported by the clinician who has the role of care manager with a particular patient for that one-month period. Time spent face-to-face or non-face-to-face with clinical staff communicating with the patient, family, caregivers, other health care professionals, and agencies revising, documenting, and putting into action the care plan or teaching the patient self-management skills or techniques may be used to determine the care management staff time for that one-month time period. Time with clinical staff is reported only when there are two or more staff members meeting regarding the specific patient. Additionally, time with clinical staff should not be counted if the clinician has reported an E/M service for that same date. Generally, services provided by clinical staff involve such activities as ongoing review of the patient's status, including reviewing laboratory or other test results that are not reported as part of an E/M service, evaluating whether the patient is following the treatment regime, and medication management. Chronic care management services are represented by resequenced codes 99490 and 99491 and describe services provided to patients with medical and/or psychosocial needs that necessitate creating, implementing, changing, or monitoring the care plan. Typically patients receiving this care have a minimum of two and possibly more chronic ongoing or episodic health conditions that are anticipated to last at least one year or until the patient expires and put the patient at increased risk of death, exacerbation, or functional decline. Code 99490 should be reported once per calendar month and involve a minimum of 20 minutes of clinical staff time. Code 99491 is also reported monthly and represents at least 30 minutes of the physician or other qualified health care professional involved with care management activities. Complex chronic care management services represented by 99487 and add-on code 99489 differ from chronic care management in that the adult patient generally has at least two or more complex chronic conditions being treated by three or more prescription medications and generally receives other types of interventions including physical or occupational therapy; pediatric patients usually receive three or more interventions that may include medications, nutritional support, or respiratory therapy. Report 99487 when approximately one hour of clinical staff time overseen by a clinician is rendered during a single calendar month. Report 99489 for each additional 30 minutes.

Coding Tips

These codes are used to report care management services provided by the clinical staff under the direction of a qualified healthcare professional to a patient residing at home or in an assisted living facility, domiciliary, or rest home. These are time-based codes and total time spent performing care management services during the calendar month should be documented in the patient record. Do not report these codes if all elements listed in the code description are not performed. If the physician provides face-to-face E/M visits in the same calendar month, these visits may be reported separately. Do not count clinical staff time for a particular day if the physician reports an E/M service on that day. These codes may only be reported once per calendar month by the provider that assumes the care management role for the patient. Code 99489 should only be reported in addition to 99487. Do not report 99490 if less than 20 minutes of chronic care management is provided in the calendar month. Report 99491 when more than 30 minutes of chronic care management is provided in the same calendar month. Do not report both 99490 and 99491 during the same calendar month, or with 99487 or 99489. Do not report 99487 if less than 60 minutes of complex chronic care management is provided in a calendar month. Do not report 99489 if less than 30 minutes of additional time beyond the first 60 minutes of complex chronic care is provided. Do not report these codes in addition to 90951-90970 for ESRD services or in the postoperative period of a reported surgery. Do not report these codes in addition to 90951-90970 in the same calendar month. Do not report 99487, 99489, or 99490 with 93792-93793, 98960-98962, 98966-98968, 99071, 99078, 99080, 99091, 99339-99340, 99358-99359, 99366-99368, 99374-99380, 99441-99443, 99495-99496, or 99605-99607 in the same calendar month. Do not report 99487-99489 or 99490 with 99421-99423 for the same time period. For psychiatric care management services, see 99492-99494.

ICD-10-CM Diagnostic Codes

The application of this code is too broad to adequately present ICD-10-CM diagnostic code links here. Refer to your ICD-10-CM book.

AMA: 99487 2019,Jan,6; 2018,Oct,9; 2018,Mar,5; 2018,Mar,7; 2018,Jul,12; 2018,Jan,8; 2018,Feb,7; 2018,Apr,9; 2017,Jan,8; 2017,Apr,9; 2016,Jan,13; 2015,Jan,16; 2014,Oct,3; 2014,Oct,8; 2014,Jun,3; 2014,Jan,11; 2014,Feb,3;

2013,Sep,15-16; 2013,Nov,3; 2013,Jan,3-5; 2013,Apr,3-4 **99489** 2019,Jan,6; 2018,Oct,9; 2018,Mar,7; 2018,Mar,5; 2018,Jul,12; 2018,Jan,8; 2018,Feb,7; 2018,Apr,9; 2017,Jan,8; 2017,Apr,9; 2016,Jan,13; 2015,Jan,16; 2014,Oct,8; 2014,Oct,3; 2014,Jun,3; 2014,Jan,11; 2013,Sep,15-16; 2013,Nov,3; 2013,Jan,3-5; 2013,Apr,3-4 **99490** 2019,Jan,6; 2018,Oct,9; 2018,Mar,7; 2018,Mar,5; 2018,Jul,12; 2018,Jan,8; 2018,Feb,7; 2018,Apr,9; 2017,Jan,8; 2016,Jan,13; 2015,Jan,16; 2015,Feb,3; 2014,Oct,3

Relative Value Units/Medicare Edits

Non-Facility RVU	Work	PE	MP	Total
99490	0.61	0.52	0.04	1.17
99491	1.45	0.79	0.09	2.33
99487	1.0	1.52	0.06	2.58
99489	0.5	0.76	0.03	1.29
Facility RVU	**Work**	**PE**	**MP**	**Total**
99490	0.61	0.25	0.04	0.9
99491	1.45	0.79	0.09	2.33
99487	1.0	0.41	0.06	1.47
99489	0.5	0.21	0.03	0.74

	FUD	Status	MUE	Modifiers				IOM Reference
99490	N/A	A	1(2)	N/A	N/A	N/A	80*	None
99491	N/A	A	1(2)	N/A	N/A	N/A	80*	
99487	N/A	A	1(2)	N/A	N/A	N/A	80*	
99489	N/A	A	10(3)	N/A	N/A	N/A	80*	

* with documentation

99495-99496

99495 Transitional Care Management Services with the following required elements: Communication (direct contact, telephone, electronic) with the patient and/or caregiver within 2 business days of discharge Medical decision making of at least moderate complexity during the service period Face-to-face visit, within 14 calendar days of discharge

99496 Transitional Care Management Services with the following required elements: Communication (direct contact, telephone, electronic) with the patient and/or caregiver within 2 business days of discharge Medical decision making of high complexity during the service period Face-to-face visit, within 7 calendar days of discharge

Explanation

Transitional care management services are reported for patients requiring moderate to high complex medical decision making who are transitioning from an inpatient facility to a home or community type setting, such as a domiciliary or assisted living facility. The start date is the day of discharge from the inpatient setting and lasts through the following 29 days. These services include one face-to-face encounter in addition to other services performed within the specific timeframe by licensed clinical staff. These services are provided under direct qualified clinician supervision and may include communication with family and care givers, evaluation of treatment and medication, education on resources with assistance to available care, and review of discharge information, follow-up appointments, and interaction with other qualified health care professionals. To report these services, the initial direct contact (includes telephone/electronic) must occur within two days of discharge with review of medication regimen by the date of the initial face-to-face encounter. The date of the direct contact and medical decision making drives the code selection. Report 99495 when MDM is at least moderate complexity in addition to the face-to-face encounter within 14 days of hospital discharge. Report 99496 when MDM is high complexity in addition to the face-to-face encounter within seven days of hospital discharge.

Coding Tips

These codes are used to report services provided to a new or established patient whose medical or psychological issues necessitate a moderate or high level of medical decision making while transitioning from an inpatient facility, partial hospital, observation status, or skilled nursing facility to an assisted living facility, home, domiciliary, or rest home. Transitional care management (TCM) services require a face-to-face visit, initial patient contact, and medication reconciliation all within a specific timeframe. Do not report these codes if all elements listed in the code description are not performed. These codes may only be reported one time within 30 days of discharge and by only one provider. Code 99495 requires the face-to-face visit within 14 calendar days of discharge. Code 99496 requires one face-to-face visit within seven calendar days of discharge. If the physician or other qualified health care professional provides more than one face-to-face E/M visit within the 30 days, these visits may be reported separately. Do not repot 99495 or 99496 in addition to 93792 or 93793. Do not report these codes when reporting 90951-90970, 98960-98962, 98966-98968, 99071, 99078, 99080, 99091, 99339, 99340, 99358, 99359, 99366-99368, 99374-99380, 99441-99443, 99487-99489, or 99605-99607 when performed within the same 30-day period of 99495 or 99496.

ICD-10-CM Diagnostic Codes

The application of this code is too broad to adequately present ICD-10-CM diagnostic code links here. Refer to your ICD-10-CM book.

AMA: 99495 2019,Jan,6; 2018,Mar,5; 2018,Mar,7; 2018,Jul,12; 2018,Jan,8; 2018,Feb,7; 2018,Apr,9; 2017,Jan,8; 2016,Jan,13; 2015,Jan,16; 2014,Oct,3;

2014,Oct,8; 2014,Mar,13; 2014,Jan,11; 2013,Sep,15-16; 2013,Nov,3; 2013,Jul,11-12; 2013,Jan,3-5; 2013,Dec,11; 2013,Aug,13; 2013,Apr,3-4 **99496** 2019,Jan,6; 2018,Mar,5; 2018,Mar,7; 2018,Jul,12; 2018,Jan,8; 2018,Feb,7; 2018,Apr,9; 2017,Jan,8; 2016,Jan,13; 2015,Jan,16; 2014,Oct,3; 2014,Oct,8; 2014,Mar,13; 2014,Jan,11; 2013,Sep,15-16; 2013,Nov,3; 2013,Jul,11-12; 2013,Jan,3-5; 2013,Aug,13; 2013,Apr,3-4

Relative Value Units/Medicare Edits

Non-Facility RVU	Work	PE	MP	Total
99495	2.11	2.38	0.13	4.62
99496	3.05	3.27	0.2	6.52
Facility RVU	**Work**	**PE**	**MP**	**Total**
99495	2.11	0.87	0.13	3.11
99496	3.05	1.26	0.2	4.51

	FUD	Status	MUE	Modifiers				IOM Reference
99495	N/A	A	1(2)	N/A	N/A	N/A	80*	None
99496	N/A	A	1(2)	N/A	N/A	N/A	80*	

* with documentation

Terms To Know

medical decision making. Consideration of the differential diagnoses, the amount and/or complexity of data reviewed and considered (medical records, test results, correspondence from previous treating physicians, etc.), current diagnostic studies ordered, and treatment or management options and risk (complications of the patient's condition, the potential for complications, continued morbidity, risk of mortality, any comorbidities associated with the patient's disease process).

other qualified health care professional. Individual who is qualified by education, training, licensure/regulation, and facility privileging to perform a professional service within his or her scope of practice and independently (or as incident-to) report the professional service without requiring physician supervision. Payers may state exemptions in writing or state and local regulations may not follow this definition for performance of some services. Always refer to any relevant plan policies and federal and/or state laws to determine who may perform and report services.

99497-99498

99497 Advance care planning including the explanation and discussion of advance directives such as standard forms (with completion of such forms, when performed), by the physician or other qualified health care professional; first 30 minutes, face-to-face with the patient, family member(s), and/or surrogate

\+ **99498** each additional 30 minutes (List separately in addition to code for primary procedure)

Explanation

Advance care planning services are reported for the discussion and explanation of advanced directives by a qualified clinician. These services are time-based services that do not involve any active management of problems during the course of the face-to-face service between the provider and a patient, family member, or surrogate and may be reported on the same day as another E/M service. Report 99497 for the first 30 minutes of advance care planning and 99498 for each additional 30 minutes.

Coding Tips

These codes are used to report counseling and discussion of advance care directives face-to-face with the patient, family member, or surrogate. An advance directive document appointing an agent and/or recording of the wishes of the patient's medical treatment should be recorded in the medical record. These codes may be reported separately when performed on the same day as another E/M service. Use 99498 in addition to 99497. These codes may be reported in addition to the following E/M codes when performed on the same date of service: 99201-99215, 99217-99226, 99231-99236, 99238-99239, 99241-99245, 99251-99255, 99281-99285, 99304-99310, 99315-99316, 99318, 99324-99328, 99334-99337, 99341-99345, 99347-99350, 99381-99397, and 99495-99496. Do not report these codes when reporting 99291-99292, 99468-99469, 99471-99472, 99475-99480, or 99483 on the same date of service.

ICD-10-CM Diagnostic Codes

The application of this code is too broad to adequately present ICD-10-CM diagnostic code links here. Refer to your ICD-10-CM book.

AMA: **99497** 2018,Jan,8; 2018,Apr,9; 2017,Jan,8; 2016,Jan,13; 2016,Feb,7; 2015,Jan,16; 2014,Dec,11 **99498** 2018,Jan,8; 2018,Apr,9; 2017,Jan,8; 2016,Jan,13; 2016,Feb,7; 2015,Jan,16; 2014,Dec,11

Relative Value Units/Medicare Edits

Non-Facility RVU	Work	PE	MP	Total
99497	1.5	0.8	0.1	2.4
99498	1.4	0.62	0.09	2.11
Facility RVU	**Work**	**PE**	**MP**	**Total**
99497	1.5	0.63	0.1	2.23
99498	1.4	0.61	0.09	2.1

	FUD	Status	MUE	Modifiers				IOM Reference
99497	N/A	A	1(2)	N/A	N/A	N/A	80*	None
99498	N/A	A	3(3)	N/A	N/A	N/A	80*	

* with documentation

 ● New ▲ Revised + Add On AMA: CPT Assist [Resequenced] ☑ Laterality

20101

20101 Exploration of penetrating wound (separate procedure); chest

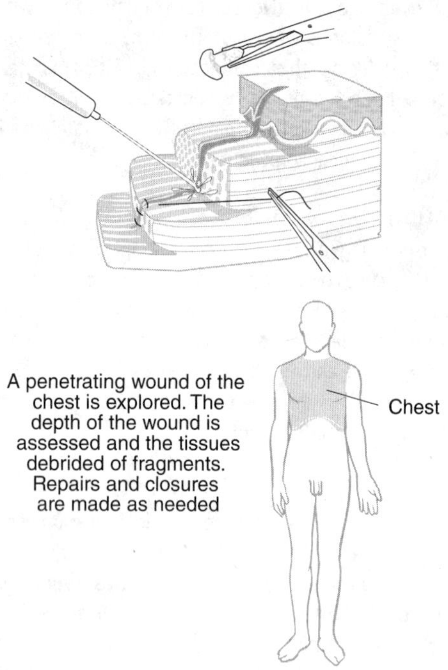

Explanation

The physician explores a penetrating wound of the chest in the operating room, such as a gunshot or stab wound, to help identify damaged structures. Nerve, organ, and blood vessel integrity is assessed. The wound may be enlarged to help assess the damage. Debridement, removal of foreign bodies, and ligation or coagulation of minor blood vessels in the subcutaneous tissues, fascia, and muscle are also included in this code. Damaged tissues are debrided and repaired when possible. The wound is closed (if clean) or packed open if contaminated by the penetrating body.

Coding Tips

This separate procedure by definition is usually a component of a more complex service and is not identified separately. When performed alone or with other unrelated procedures/services, it may be reported. If performed alone, list the code; if performed with other procedures/services, list the code and append modifier 59 or an X{EPSU} modifier. This code includes debridement, enlargement of the wound (to determine penetration), removal of foreign body, and minor blood vessel ligation or coagulation. If major repair is performed on a major structure or major blood vessel, requiring thoracotomy, then 20101 is not reported separately. For simple, intermediate, or complex repair that does not require enlargement of the wound, report the specific codes for repair instead of 20101. Surgical trays, A4550, are not separately reimbursed by Medicare; however, other third-party payers may cover them. Check with the specific payer to determine coverage.

ICD-10-CM Diagnostic Codes

S21.111A Laceration without foreign body of right front wall of thorax without penetration into thoracic cavity, initial encounter ☑
S21.112A Laceration without foreign body of left front wall of thorax without penetration into thoracic cavity, initial encounter ☑
S21.121A Laceration with foreign body of right front wall of thorax without penetration into thoracic cavity, initial encounter ☑
S21.122A Laceration with foreign body of left front wall of thorax without penetration into thoracic cavity, initial encounter ☑
S21.131A Puncture wound without foreign body of right front wall of thorax without penetration into thoracic cavity, initial encounter ☑
S21.132A Puncture wound without foreign body of left front wall of thorax without penetration into thoracic cavity, initial encounter ☑
S21.141A Puncture wound with foreign body of right front wall of thorax without penetration into thoracic cavity, initial encounter ☑
S21.142A Puncture wound with foreign body of left front wall of thorax without penetration into thoracic cavity, initial encounter ☑
S21.151A Open bite of right front wall of thorax without penetration into thoracic cavity, initial encounter ☑
S21.152A Open bite of left front wall of thorax without penetration into thoracic cavity, initial encounter ☑
S21.211A Laceration without foreign body of right back wall of thorax without penetration into thoracic cavity, initial encounter ☑
S21.212A Laceration without foreign body of left back wall of thorax without penetration into thoracic cavity, initial encounter ☑
S21.221A Laceration with foreign body of right back wall of thorax without penetration into thoracic cavity, initial encounter ☑
S21.222A Laceration with foreign body of left back wall of thorax without penetration into thoracic cavity, initial encounter ☑
S21.231A Puncture wound without foreign body of right back wall of thorax without penetration into thoracic cavity, initial encounter ☑
S21.232A Puncture wound without foreign body of left back wall of thorax without penetration into thoracic cavity, initial encounter ☑
S21.241A Puncture wound with foreign body of right back wall of thorax without penetration into thoracic cavity, initial encounter ☑
S21.242A Puncture wound with foreign body of left back wall of thorax without penetration into thoracic cavity, initial encounter ☑
S21.251A Open bite of right back wall of thorax without penetration into thoracic cavity, initial encounter ☑
S21.252A Open bite of left back wall of thorax without penetration into thoracic cavity, initial encounter ☑
S29.021A Laceration of muscle and tendon of front wall of thorax, initial encounter
S29.022A Laceration of muscle and tendon of back wall of thorax, initial encounter
S29.091A Other injury of muscle and tendon of front wall of thorax, initial encounter
S29.092A Other injury of muscle and tendon of back wall of thorax, initial encounter
S29.8XXA Other specified injuries of thorax, initial encounter

AMA: 20101 2018,Jan,8; 2017,Jan,8; 2016,Jan,13; 2015,Jan,16; 2014,Jan,11

Relative Value Units/Medicare Edits

Non-Facility RVU	Work	PE	MP	Total
20101	3.23	8.96	0.78	12.97
Facility RVU	**Work**	**PE**	**MP**	**Total**
20101	3.23	2.04	0.78	6.05

	FUD	Status	MUE	Modifiers				IOM Reference
20101	10	A	2(3)	51	N/A	N/A	N/A	None

* with documentation

+ **20985** Computer-assisted surgical navigational procedure for musculoskeletal procedures, image-less (List separately in addition to code for primary procedure)

Explanation

Imageless computer-assisted surgery (CAS) is an adjunct process used in conjunction with certain orthopaedic procedures. Using such tools as markers, reference frames, intraoperative sensing, and computer workstations, imageless computer-assisted navigational procedures increase visualization of the surgical field and aid in precise navigation with minimally invasive approaches. Imageless navigation uses angles and measurements (kinematics) for anatomy determination. Through direct imageless applications, landmarks are established on a universal limb model. This application requires touch-pointing the anatomic landmarks, which are then registered in the computer for use in accurate navigation and measurement in relation to any bone or instrument movement as the surgery is performed. This application provides a way to establish coordinates as an aid for precisely locating anatomical structures in open or percutaneous procedures without the use of preoperative or intraoperative images. Code 20985 is reported in addition to the procedure code when the physician uses an imageless system to help determine coordinates.

Coding Tips

Do not report 20985 with 61781–61783. For computer-assisted navigational procedures with image guidance based on images that are acquired preoperatively and intraoperatively, see 0054T and 0055T.

ICD-10-CM Diagnostic Codes

This/these CPT code(s) are add on code(s). See the primary procedure code that this code is performed with for your ICD-10-CM code selections.

AMA: **20985** 2018,Jan,8; 2017,Jan,8; 2016,Jan,13; 2015,Jan,16; 2014,Jan,11

Relative Value Units/Medicare Edits

Non-Facility RVU	Work	PE	MP	Total
20985	2.5	1.25	0.49	4.24
Facility RVU	**Work**	**PE**	**MP**	**Total**
20985	2.5	1.25	0.49	4.24

	FUD	Status	MUE	Modifiers				IOM Reference
20985	N/A	A	2(3)	N/A	N/A	N/A	80*	None

* with documentation

Terms To Know

CT. Computed tomography.

fluoroscopy. Radiology technique that allows visual examination of part of the body or a function of an organ using a device that projects an x-ray image on a fluorescent screen.

ultrasound. Imaging using ultra-high sound frequency bounced off body structures.

21501-21502

21501 Incision and drainage, deep abscess or hematoma, soft tissues of neck or thorax;
21502 with partial rib ostectomy

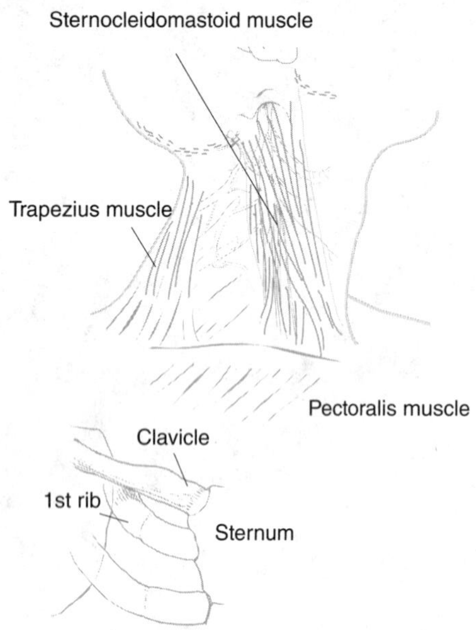

A deep abscess or hematoma of the soft tissues of the neck or thorax is incised and drained

Explanation

The physician performs surgery to remove or drain an abscess or hematoma from the deep soft tissues of the neck or thorax. With proper anesthesia administered, the physician makes an incision overlying the site of the abscess or hematoma of the neck or thorax. Dissection is carried down through the deep subcutaneous tissues and may be continued into the fascia or muscle to expose the abscess or hematoma. The incision may be extended if the mass is larger than expected. The abscess or hematoma is incised and the contents are drained. The area is irrigated and the incision is repaired in layers with sutures, staples, and/or Steri-strips; closed with drains in place; or simply left open to further facilitate drainage of infection. Report 21502 if a partial rib ostectomy is performed during this procedure.

Coding Tips

If significant additional time and effort are documented, append modifier 22 and submit a cover letter and operative report. For a biopsy of the soft tissue of the neck or thorax, see 21550.

ICD-10-CM Diagnostic Codes

L03.221	Cellulitis of neck
L03.312	Cellulitis of back [any part except buttock]
L03.313	Cellulitis of chest wall
S10.83XA	Contusion of other specified part of neck, initial encounter
S20.211A	Contusion of right front wall of thorax, initial encounter ☑
S20.212A	Contusion of left front wall of thorax, initial encounter ☑
S20.221A	Contusion of right back wall of thorax, initial encounter ☑
S20.222A	Contusion of left back wall of thorax, initial encounter ☑
T81.41XA	Infection following a procedure, superficial incisional surgical site, initial encounter
T81.42XA	Infection following a procedure, deep incisional surgical site, initial encounter
T81.43XA	Infection following a procedure, organ and space surgical site, initial encounter
T81.44XA	Sepsis following a procedure, initial encounter
T81.49XA	Infection following a procedure, other surgical site, initial encounter

AMA: 21501 2018,Sep,7; 2018,Jan,8; 2017,Jan,8; 2016,Jan,13; 2015,Jan,16; 2014,Dec,16; 2014,Dec,16 **21502** 2018,Sep,7

Relative Value Units/Medicare Edits

Non-Facility RVU	Work	PE	MP	Total
21501	3.98	8.42	0.78	13.18
21502	7.55	5.22	1.79	14.56
Facility RVU	**Work**	**PE**	**MP**	**Total**
21501	3.98	4.53	0.78	9.29
21502	7.55	5.22	1.79	14.56

	FUD	Status	MUE	Modifiers				IOM Reference
21501	90	A	3(3)	51	N/A	N/A	N/A	None
21502	90	A	1(3)	51	N/A	N/A	80	

* with documentation

Terms To Know

abscess. Circumscribed collection of pus resulting from bacteria, frequently associated with swelling and other signs of inflammation.

cellulitis. Infection of the skin and subcutaneous tissues, most often caused by Staphylococcus or Streptococcus bacteria secondary to a cutaneous lesion. Progression of the inflammation may lead to abscess and tissue death, or even systemic infection-like bacteremia.

contusion. Superficial injury (bruising) produced by impact without a break in the skin.

drain. Device that creates a channel to allow fluid from a cavity, wound, or infected area to exit the body.

hematoma. Tumor-like collection of blood in some part of the body caused by a break in a blood vessel wall, usually as a result of trauma.

incision and drainage. Cutting open body tissue for the removal of tissue fluids or infected discharge from a wound or cavity.

infected postoperative seroma. Infection within a pocket of serum following surgery.

ostectomy. Excision of bone.

secondary. Second in order of occurrence or importance, or appearing during the course of another disease or condition.

soft tissue. Nonepithelial tissues outside of the skeleton that includes subcutaneous adipose tissue, fibrous tissue, fascia, muscles, blood and lymph vessels, and peripheral nervous system tissue.

21510

21510 Incision, deep, with opening of bone cortex (eg, for osteomyelitis or bone abscess), thorax

A deep, surgical incision extends to the bone and into the bone cortex

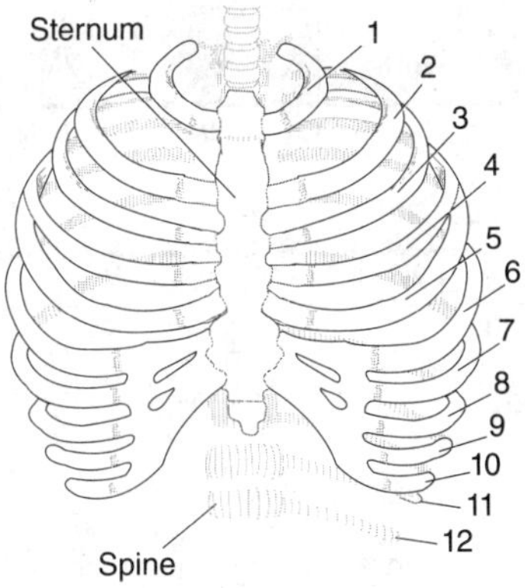

Explanation

The physician incises the bone cortex of infected bone in the thorax to treat an abscess or osteomyelitis. The physician makes an incision over the affected area. Dissection is carried down through the soft tissues to expose the bone. The periosteum is split and reflected from the bone overlying the infected area. A curette may be used to scrape away the abscess or infected portion down to healthy bony tissue or drill holes may be made through the cortex into the medullary canal in a window outline around the infected or abscessed bone. The area is drained and debrided of infected bony and soft tissue. The physician irrigates the area with antibiotic solution, the periosteum is closed over the bone, and the soft tissues are sutured closed; or the wound is packed and left open, allowing the area to drain. Secondary closure is performed approximately three weeks later. Dressings are changed daily.

Coding Tips

If significant additional time and effort are documented, append modifier 22 and submit a cover letter and operative report. When 21510 is performed with another separately identifiable procedure, the highest dollar value code is listed as the primary procedure, and subsequent procedures are appended with modifier 51.

ICD-10-CM Diagnostic Codes

L03.313	Cellulitis of chest wall
M46.23	Osteomyelitis of vertebra, cervicothoracic region
M46.24	Osteomyelitis of vertebra, thoracic region
M46.25	Osteomyelitis of vertebra, thoracolumbar region
M86.08	Acute hematogenous osteomyelitis, other sites
M86.18	Other acute osteomyelitis, other site
M86.28	Subacute osteomyelitis, other site
M86.38	Chronic multifocal osteomyelitis, other site
M86.48	Chronic osteomyelitis with draining sinus, other site
M86.58	Other chronic hematogenous osteomyelitis, other site
M86.68	Other chronic osteomyelitis, other site
M86.8X8	Other osteomyelitis, other site
T81.41XA	Infection following a procedure, superficial incisional surgical site, initial encounter
T81.42XA	Infection following a procedure, deep incisional surgical site, initial encounter
T81.43XA	Infection following a procedure, organ and space surgical site, initial encounter
T81.44XA	Sepsis following a procedure, initial encounter
T81.49XA	Infection following a procedure, other surgical site, initial encounter

AMA: 21510 2018,Sep,7

Relative Value Units/Medicare Edits

Non-Facility RVU	Work	PE	MP	Total
21510	6.2	5.13	1.46	12.79
Facility RVU	**Work**	**PE**	**MP**	**Total**
21510	6.2	5.13	1.46	12.79

	FUD	Status	MUE	Modifiers				IOM Reference
21510	90	A	1(3)	51	N/A	N/A	80*	None

* with documentation

Terms To Know

abscess. Circumscribed collection of pus resulting from bacteria, frequently associated with swelling and other signs of inflammation.

cellulitis. Infection of the skin and subcutaneous tissues, most often caused by Staphylococcus or Streptococcus bacteria secondary to a cutaneous lesion. Progression of the inflammation may lead to abscess and tissue death, or even systemic infection-like bacteremia.

debride. To remove all foreign objects and devitalized or infected tissue from a burn or wound to prevent infection and promote healing.

dissect. Cut apart or separate tissue for surgical purposes or for visual or microscopic study.

infected postoperative seroma. Infection within a pocket of serum following surgery.

osteomyelitis. Inflammation of bone that may remain localized or spread to the marrow, cortex, or periosteum, in response to an infecting organism, usually bacterial and pyogenic.

osteotomy. Surgical cutting of a bone.

periosteum. Double-layered connective membrane on the outer surface of bone.

secondary. Second in order of occurrence or importance, or appearing during the course of another disease or condition.

sequestrectomy. Surgical excision of a nonviable piece of bone that has become walled off, or sequestered, away from living bone during necrosis.

21550

21550 Biopsy, soft tissue of neck or thorax

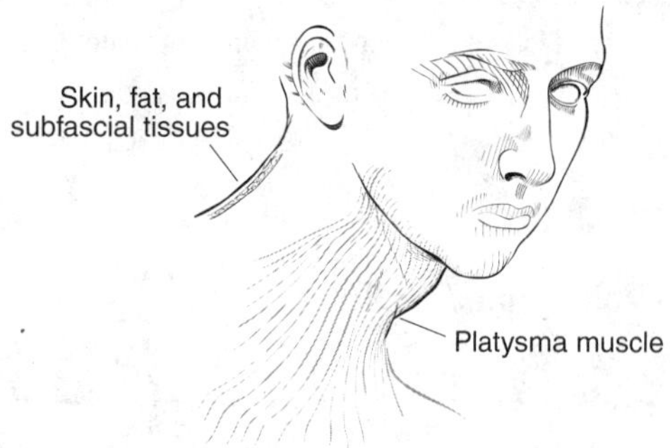

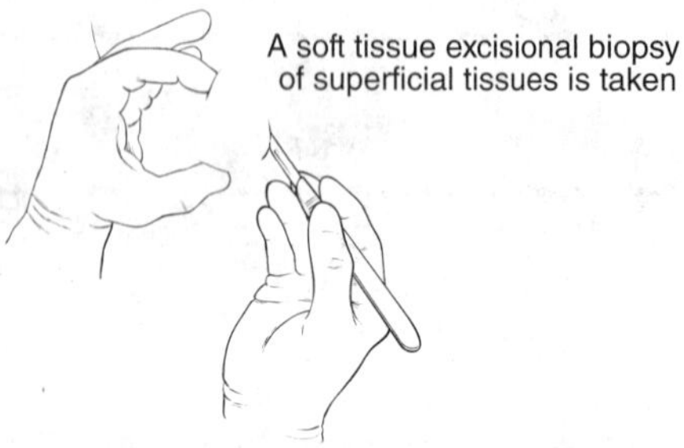

Explanation

The physician performs a biopsy of the soft tissues of the neck or thorax. With proper anesthesia administered, the physician identifies the mass through palpation and x-ray (reported separately), if needed. An incision is made over the site and dissection is taken down to the subcutaneous fat or further into the fascia or muscle to reach the lesion. A portion of the tissue mass is excised and submitted for pathology. The area is irrigated and the incision is closed with layered sutures.

Coding Tips

Note that 21550 is for incisional biopsy. A biopsy is not reported separately when followed by an excisional removal during the same operative session. When 21550 is performed with another separately identifiable procedure, the highest dollar value code is listed as the primary procedure, and subsequent procedures are appended with modifier 51. If a needle biopsy of soft tissue is needed, see 20206. Surgical trays, A4550, are not separately reimbursed by Medicare; however, other third-party payers may cover them. Check with the specific payer to determine coverage.

ICD-10-CM Diagnostic Codes

C49.0	Malignant neoplasm of connective and soft tissue of head, face and neck
C49.3	Malignant neoplasm of connective and soft tissue of thorax
C76.0	Malignant neoplasm of head, face and neck
C76.1	Malignant neoplasm of thorax
C79.89	Secondary malignant neoplasm of other specified sites
D09.8	Carcinoma in situ of other specified sites
D21.0	Benign neoplasm of connective and other soft tissue of head, face and neck
D21.3	Benign neoplasm of connective and other soft tissue of thorax
D49.89	Neoplasm of unspecified behavior of other specified sites
L03.221	Cellulitis of neck
L03.313	Cellulitis of chest wall
R22.1	Localized swelling, mass and lump, neck
R22.2	Localized swelling, mass and lump, trunk

AMA: **21550** 2018,Sep,7

Relative Value Units/Medicare Edits

Non-Facility RVU	Work	PE	MP	Total
21550	2.11	5.04	0.31	7.46
Facility RVU	**Work**	**PE**	**MP**	**Total**
21550	2.11	2.09	0.31	4.51

	FUD	Status	MUE	Modifiers				IOM Reference
21550	10	A	2(3)	51	N/A	N/A	N/A	None

* with documentation

Terms To Know

benign. Mild or nonmalignant in nature.

biopsy. Tissue or fluid removed for diagnostic purposes through analysis of the cells in the biopsy material.

carcinoma in situ. Malignancy that arises from the cells of the vessel, gland, or organ of origin that remains confined to that site or has not invaded neighboring tissue.

incision. Act of cutting into tissue or an organ.

irrigation. To wash out or cleanse a body cavity, wound, or tissue with water or other fluid.

malignant. Any condition tending to progress toward death, specifically an invasive tumor with a loss of cellular differentiation that has the ability to spread or metastasize to other body areas.

neoplasm. New abnormal growth, tumor.

palpate. Examination by feeling with the hand.

secondary. Second in order of occurrence or importance, or appearing during the course of another disease or condition.

soft tissue. Nonepithelial tissues outside of the skeleton that includes subcutaneous adipose tissue, fibrous tissue, fascia, muscles, blood and lymph vessels, and peripheral nervous system tissue.

suture. Numerous stitching techniques employed in wound closure.

21555-21556 [21552, 21554]

21555 Excision, tumor, soft tissue of neck or anterior thorax, subcutaneous; less than 3 cm

21552 Excision, tumor, soft tissue of neck or anterior thorax, subcutaneous; 3 cm or greater

21556 Excision, tumor, soft tissue of neck or anterior thorax, subfascial (eg, intramuscular); less than 5 cm

21554 Excision, tumor, soft tissue of neck or anterior thorax, subfascial (eg, intramuscular); 5 cm or greater

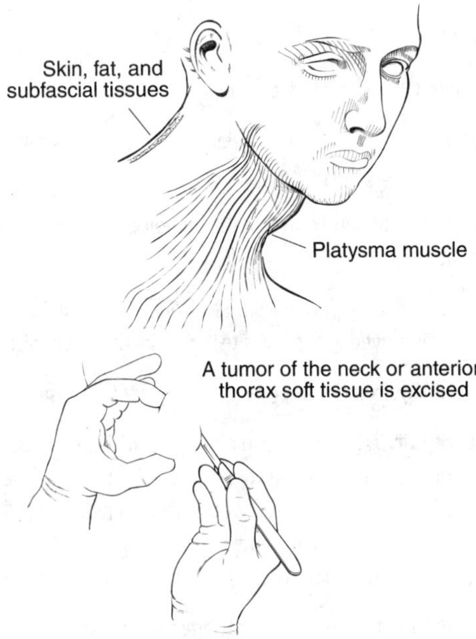

Explanation

The physician removes a tumor from the soft tissue of the neck or anterior thorax (chest) that is located in the subcutaneous tissue in 21552 or 21555 and in the deep soft tissue, below the fascial plane or within the muscle, in 21554 or 21556. With the proper anesthesia administered, the physician makes an incision in the skin overlying the mass and dissects down to the tumor. The extent of the tumor is identified and a dissection is undertaken all the way around the tumor. A portion of neighboring soft tissue may also be removed to ensure adequate removal of all tumor tissue. A drain may be inserted and the incision is repaired with layers of sutures, staples, or Steri-strips. Report 21555 for excision of subcutaneous tumors whose resected area is less than 3 cm and 21552 for excision of subcutaneous tumors 3 cm or greater. Report 21556 for excision of subfascial or intramuscular tumors whose resected area is less than 5 cm and 21554 for excision of subfascial or intramuscular tumors 5 cm or greater.

Coding Tips

If significant additional time and effort are documented, append modifier 22 and submit a cover letter and operative report. When 21555 is performed with another separately identifiable procedure, the highest dollar value code is listed as the primary procedure, and subsequent procedures are appended with modifier 51. A biopsy is not identified separately when followed by an excisional removal during the same operative session. Report any free grafts or flaps separately. For excision of a chest wall tumor involving ribs, see 21601–21603. Surgical trays, A4550, are not separately reimbursed by Medicare; however, other third-party payers may cover them. Check with the specific payer to determine coverage.

ICD-10-CM Diagnostic Codes

C49.0	Malignant neoplasm of connective and soft tissue of head, face and neck
C49.3	Malignant neoplasm of connective and soft tissue of thorax
C76.0	Malignant neoplasm of head, face and neck
C76.1	Malignant neoplasm of thorax
D17.1	Benign lipomatous neoplasm of skin and subcutaneous tissue of trunk
D17.39	Benign lipomatous neoplasm of skin and subcutaneous tissue of other sites
D21.0	Benign neoplasm of connective and other soft tissue of head, face and neck
D21.3	Benign neoplasm of connective and other soft tissue of thorax
D48.1	Neoplasm of uncertain behavior of connective and other soft tissue

AMA: 21552 2018,Sep,7 **21554** 2018,Sep,7 **21555** 2018,Sep,7; 2018,Jan,8; 2017,Jan,8; 2016,Jan,13; 2015,Jan,16; 2014,Jan,11 **21556** 2018,Sep,7

Relative Value Units/Medicare Edits

Non-Facility RVU	Work	PE	MP	Total
21555	3.96	7.31	0.8	12.07
21552	6.49	4.93	1.44	12.86
21556	7.66	6.09	1.44	15.19
21554	11.13	7.6	2.33	21.06
Facility RVU	**Work**	**PE**	**MP**	**Total**
21555	3.96	4.02	0.8	8.78
21552	6.49	4.93	1.44	12.86
21556	7.66	6.09	1.44	15.19
21554	11.13	7.6	2.33	21.06

	FUD	Status	MUE	Modifiers				IOM Reference
21555	90	A	2(3)	51	N/A	N/A	N/A	None
21552	90	A	2(3)	51	N/A	N/A	80	
21556	90	A	2(3)	51	N/A	N/A	N/A	
21554	90	A	2(3)	51	N/A	N/A	80	

* with documentation

Terms To Know

fascia. Fibrous sheet or band of tissue that envelops organs, muscles, and groupings of muscles.

flap. Mass of flesh and skin partially excised from its location but retaining its blood supply that is moved to another site to repair adjacent or distant defects.

free graft. Unattached piece of skin and tissue moved to another part of the body and sutured into place to repair a defect.

Merkel cell carcinoma. Rare form of skin cancer that typically presents on the face, head, or neck as a flesh-colored or bluish-red lesion. This neoplasm is fast growing and can metastasize quickly to other areas of the body. Risk factors include older patients with weakened immune systems and/or long-term exposure to the sun.

21557-21558

21557 Radical resection of tumor (eg, sarcoma), soft tissue of neck or anterior thorax; less than 5 cm

21558 5 cm or greater

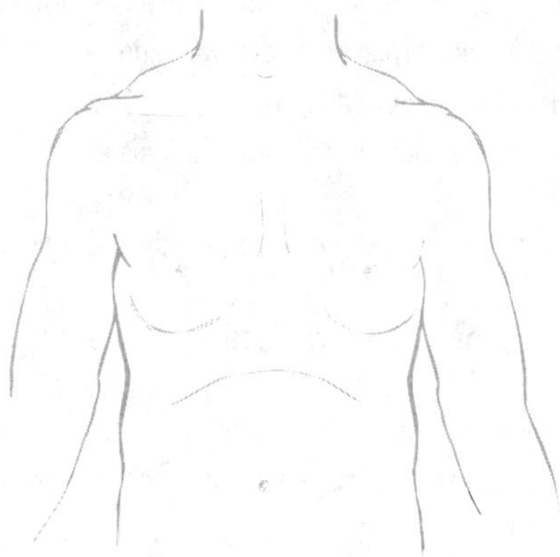

Radical resection of soft tissue tumor of the neck or anterior thorax

Explanation

The physician performs a radical resection of a malignant soft tissue tumor (i.e., sarcoma) from the neck or anterior thorax, not involving bone. An incision is made over the tumor and dissection exposes it. The tumor and any adjacent tissue that may be affected by the spread of the neoplasm are excised. Large resections may be needed. The type and stage of the lesion determines the extent of the tumor margin resection area. Muscle or fascia may need to be repaired and drains may be placed. The surgical wound may be closed using simple or intermediate repair or separately reportable complex closure, adjacent tissue transfer, or graft. Report 21557 for excision of tumors whose resected area is less than 5 cm and 21558 for excision of tumors 5 cm or greater.

Coding Tips

An excisional biopsy is not reported separately when a therapeutic excision is performed during the same surgical session. Report any free grafts or flaps separately. Surgical trays, A4550, are not separately reimbursed by Medicare; however, other third-party payers may cover them. Check with the specific payer to determine coverage. For radical resection of cutaneous tumors, see 11600–11620.

ICD-10-CM Diagnostic Codes

C49.0 Malignant neoplasm of connective and soft tissue of head, face and neck

C49.3 Malignant neoplasm of connective and soft tissue of thorax

C76.0 Malignant neoplasm of head, face and neck

C76.1 Malignant neoplasm of thorax

AMA: **21557** 2018,Sep,7; 2018,Jan,8; 2017,Jan,8; 2016,Jan,13; 2015,Jan,16; 2014,Jan,11 **21558** 2018,Sep,7

Relative Value Units/Medicare Edits

Non-Facility RVU	Work	PE	MP	Total
21557	14.75	9.82	2.91	27.48
21558	21.58	12.77	4.41	38.76
Facility RVU	**Work**	**PE**	**MP**	**Total**
21557	14.75	9.82	2.91	27.48
21558	21.58	12.77	4.41	38.76

	FUD	Status	MUE	Modifiers				IOM Reference
21557	90	A	1(3)	51	N/A	62*	80	None
21558	90	A	1(3)	51	N/A	62*	80	

* with documentation

Terms To Know

anterior. Situated in the front area or toward the belly surface of the body.

complex. Composite or collection of related things, such as symptoms, anatomical parts, or surgical procedures.

fascia. Fibrous sheet or band of tissue that envelops organs, muscles, and groupings of muscles.

flap. Mass of flesh and skin partially excised from its location but retaining its blood supply that is moved to another site to repair adjacent or distant defects.

graft. Tissue implant from another part of the body or another person.

intermediate repair. ***1)*** Surgical closure of a wound requiring closure of one or more of the deeper subcutaneous tissue and non-muscle fascia layers in addition to the skin. ***2)*** Contaminated wounds with single layer closure that need extensive cleaning or foreign body removal. ***3)*** Wounds with limited undermining less than the width of the wound.

malignant. Any condition tending to progress toward death, specifically an invasive tumor with a loss of cellular differentiation that has the ability to spread or metastasize to other body areas.

radical. Extensive surgery.

resection. Surgical removal of a part or all of an organ or body part.

soft tissue. Nonepithelial tissues outside of the skeleton.

21600

21600 Excision of rib, partial

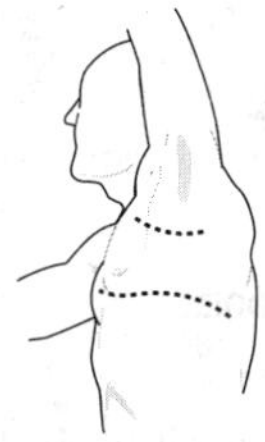

A portion of a single rib is surgically removed

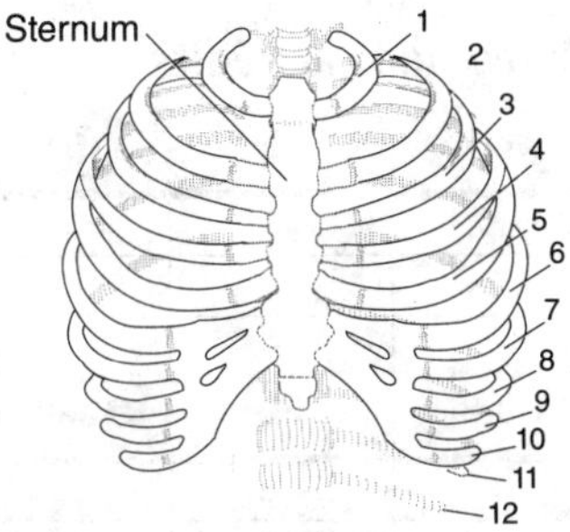

The ribs are the framework of the thoracic cage. Ten pairs connect anteriorly to the sternum and two pairs (11 and 12) float. Ribs numbered 7 to 10 fuse to form the costal margin before attaching to the sternum

Explanation

The physician removes part of one rib. With the patient under anesthesia, the physician makes an incision in the skin of the chest overlying the rib. The tissues are dissected deep to the rib itself. The rib is identified. The physician removes the desired part of the rib using a saw and other instruments. The remaining pieces of the rib and the wound itself are irrigated and debrided. The incision is sutured in layers.

Coding Tips

If this procedure is a component of a more complex service, it is not reported separately. When 21600 is performed with another separately identifiable procedure, the highest dollar value code is listed as the primary procedure, and subsequent procedures are appended with modifier 51. For an excision of the first and/or cervical rib, see 21615–21616. For resection of the cervical rib with division of scalenus anticus, see 21705. For an excision of a chest wall tumor involving the ribs, see 21601–21603. For radical chest wall or rib cage debridement due to an injury that includes bone, skin, and subcutaneous tissue, see 11044 and 11047.

ICD-10-CM Diagnostic Codes

C41.3	Malignant neoplasm of ribs, sternum and clavicle
D16.7	Benign neoplasm of ribs, sternum and clavicle
M86.38	Chronic multifocal osteomyelitis, other site
M86.48	Chronic osteomyelitis with draining sinus, other site
M86.58	Other chronic hematogenous osteomyelitis, other site
M86.68	Other chronic osteomyelitis, other site
Q76.6	Other congenital malformations of ribs
Q76.8	Other congenital malformations of bony thorax

AMA: 21600 2018,Sep,7; 2018,Jan,8; 2017,Jan,8; 2016,Jan,13; 2015,Jan,16; 2014,Jan,11; 2013,Mar,13

Relative Value Units/Medicare Edits

Non-Facility RVU	Work	PE	MP	Total
21600	7.26	7.04	1.55	15.85
Facility RVU	**Work**	**PE**	**MP**	**Total**
21600	7.26	7.04	1.55	15.85

	FUD	Status	MUE	Modifiers				IOM Reference
21600	90	A	5(3)	51	N/A	62*	80	None

* with documentation

Terms To Know

benign. Mild or nonmalignant in nature.

debride. To remove all foreign objects and devitalized or infected tissue from a burn or wound to prevent infection and promote healing.

dissect. Cut apart or separate tissue for surgical purposes or for visual or microscopic study.

excision. Surgical removal of an organ or tissue.

infection. Presence of microorganisms in body tissues that may result in cellular damage.

irrigation. To wash out or cleanse a body cavity, wound, or tissue with water or other fluid.

malignant. Any condition tending to progress toward death, specifically an invasive tumor with a loss of cellular differentiation that has the ability to spread or metastasize to other body areas.

ostectomy. Excision of bone.

osteomyelitis. Inflammation of bone that may remain localized or spread to the marrow, cortex, or periosteum, in response to an infecting organism, usually bacterial and pyogenic.

primary. Principal or first in the order of occurrence or importance.

secondary. Second in order of occurrence or importance, or appearing during the course of another disease or condition.

21601-21603

- **21601** Excision of chest wall tumor including rib(s)
- **21602** Excision of chest wall tumor involving rib(s), with plastic reconstruction; without mediastinal lymphadenectomy
- **21603** with mediastinal lymphadenectomy

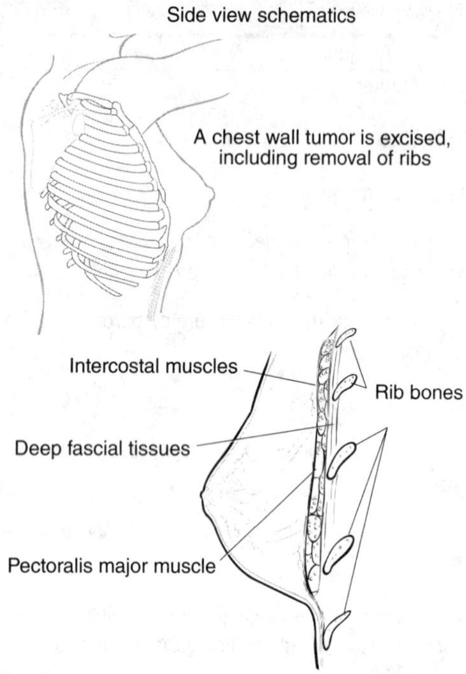

Explanation

The physician excises a chest wall tumor, including ribs. An incision in the skin of the chest overlying the site of the tumor is made. The tumor and surrounding tissue are excised. The tissue removed includes at least one adjacent rib above or below the tumor site and any associated intercostal muscles. It may also include rib cage resection and/or an en bloc resection of muscles, including the pectoralis minor or major, the serratus anterior, or the latissimus dorsi. The physician ligates or cauterizes bleeding vessels. A chest tube may be placed to re-expand the lung. The incision is repaired with layered closure and a pressure dressing is applied to the wound. In 21602, the physician excises a chest wall tumor, involving ribs, with plastic reconstruction. The tumor and surrounding tissue are excised and includes at least one adjacent rib above and below the tumor site and all intervening intercostal muscles. It may also include an en bloc resection of muscles, including the pectoralis minor or major, the serratus anterior, or the latissimus dorsi. In 21603, lymphatic tissue lying within the mediastinum is also removed. The physician ligates or cauterizes bleeding vessels. A chest tube may be placed to re-expand the lung. Plastic reconstruction is done and may involve rib grafts and/or a myocutaneous flap. A pressure dressing is applied to the wound.

Coding Tips

For a tumor of the neck or thorax not involving the ribs, see 21555–21557. An excisional biopsy is not reported separately when a therapeutic excision is performed during the same surgical session. Do not report 21601–21603 with 32100, 32503, 32504, 32551, 32554, or 32555.

ICD-10-CM Diagnostic Codes

C41.3	Malignant neoplasm of ribs, sternum and clavicle
C49.3	Malignant neoplasm of connective and soft tissue of thorax
C76.1	Malignant neoplasm of thorax
C79.51	Secondary malignant neoplasm of bone
C79.89	Secondary malignant neoplasm of other specified sites
D09.8	Carcinoma in situ of other specified sites
D16.7	Benign neoplasm of ribs, sternum and clavicle
D21.3	Benign neoplasm of connective and other soft tissue of thorax
D36.0	Benign neoplasm of lymph nodes
D36.7	Benign neoplasm of other specified sites
D48.0	Neoplasm of uncertain behavior of bone and articular cartilage
D48.1	Neoplasm of uncertain behavior of connective and other soft tissue
D48.7	Neoplasm of uncertain behavior of other specified sites
R22.2	Localized swelling, mass and lump, trunk

Relative Value Units/Medicare Edits

Non-Facility RVU	Work	PE	MP	Total
21601				
21602				
21603				
Facility RVU	**Work**	**PE**	**MP**	**Total**
21601				
21602				
21603				

	FUD	Status	MUE	Modifiers				IOM Reference
21601	N/A		-	N/A	N/A	N/A	N/A	None
21602	N/A		-	N/A	N/A	N/A	N/A	
21603	N/A		-	N/A	N/A	N/A	N/A	

* with documentation

Terms To Know

cautery. Destruction or burning of tissue by means of a hot instrument, an electric current, or a caustic chemical, such as silver nitrate.

en bloc removal. Take out as a whole or all in one mass.

lymphadenectomy. Dissection of lymph nodes free from the vessels and removal for examination by frozen section in a separate procedure to detect early-stage metastases.

mediastinum. Collection of organs and tissues that separate the pleural sacs. Located between the sternum and spine above the diaphragm, it contains the heart and great vessels, trachea and bronchi, esophagus, thymus, lymph nodes, and nerves.

21610

21610 Costotransversectomy (separate procedure)

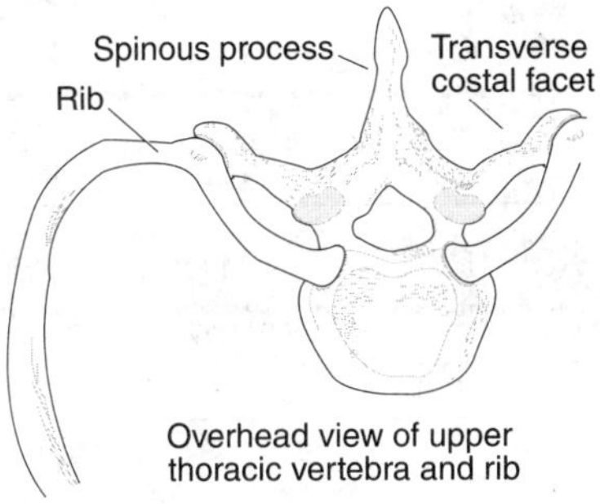

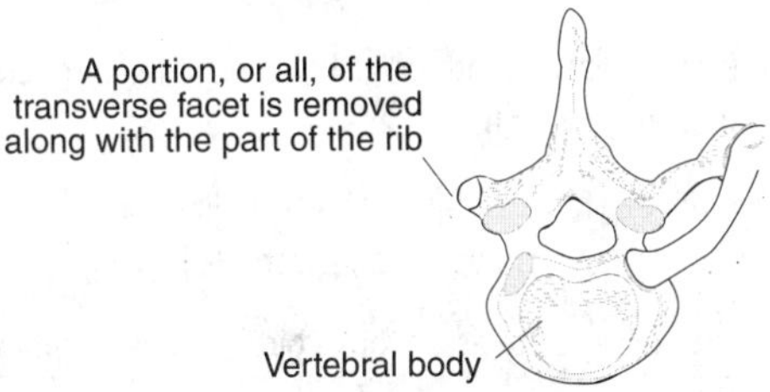

Explanation

The physician resects the costovertebral joint. The physician makes a posterior incision overlying the joint. The tissues are dissected from the joint and the transverse process is cut from the vertebral body. The physician removes all or a portion of the adjacent rib. The incision is closed in sutured layers.

Coding Tips

This separate procedure by definition is usually a component of a more complex service and is not identified separately. When performed alone or with other unrelated procedures/services, it may be reported. If performed alone, list the code; if performed with other procedures/services, list the code and append modifier 59 or an X{EPSU} modifier. This procedure involves partial or complete excision of the affected rib at the costovertebral joint.

ICD-10-CM Diagnostic Codes

A18.01	Tuberculosis of spine
C41.2	Malignant neoplasm of vertebral column
C41.3	Malignant neoplasm of ribs, sternum and clavicle
C79.51	Secondary malignant neoplasm of bone
C7B.03	Secondary carcinoid tumors of bone
D16.6	Benign neoplasm of vertebral column
D16.7	Benign neoplasm of ribs, sternum and clavicle
M86.38	Chronic multifocal osteomyelitis, other site
M86.48	Chronic osteomyelitis with draining sinus, other site
M86.58	Other chronic hematogenous osteomyelitis, other site
M86.68	Other chronic osteomyelitis, other site
M86.8X8	Other osteomyelitis, other site
Q76.6	Other congenital malformations of ribs
Q76.8	Other congenital malformations of bony thorax

AMA: 21610 2018,Sep,7

Relative Value Units/Medicare Edits

Non-Facility RVU	Work	PE	MP	Total
21610	15.91	12.6	6.59	35.1
Facility RVU	**Work**	**PE**	**MP**	**Total**
21610	15.91	12.6	6.59	35.1

	FUD	Status	MUE	Modifiers				IOM Reference
21610	90	A	1(3)	51	N/A	N/A	80	None

* with documentation

Terms To Know

anomaly. Irregularity in the structure or position of an organ or tissue.

benign. Mild or nonmalignant in nature.

congenital. Present at birth, occurring through heredity or an influence during gestation up to the moment of birth.

dissect. Cut apart or separate tissue for surgical purposes or for visual or microscopic study.

facet. Smooth surface area where the transverse and articular processes of certain vertebrae articulate with another vertebra.

incision. Act of cutting into tissue or an organ.

malignant. Any condition tending to progress toward death, specifically an invasive tumor with a loss of cellular differentiation that has the ability to spread or metastasize to other body areas.

neoplasm. New abnormal growth, tumor.

ostectomy. Excision of bone.

osteoarthrosis. Most common form of a noninflammatory degenerative joint disease with degenerating articular cartilage, bone enlargement, and synovial membrane changes.

osteomyelitis. Inflammation of bone that may remain localized or spread to the marrow, cortex, or periosteum, in response to an infecting organism, usually bacterial and pyogenic.

resect. Cutting out or removing a portion or all of a bone, organ, or other structure.

transverse. Crosswise at right angles to the long axis of a structure or part.

vertebral body. Disc-shaped portion of a vertebra that is anteriorly located and bears weight.

21615-21616

21615 Excision first and/or cervical rib;
21616 with sympathectomy

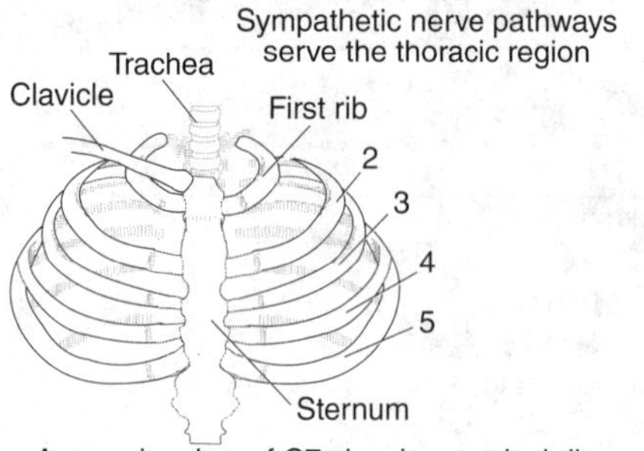

A superior view of C7 showing cervical rib; attachment anteriorly may be to the first rib, or its costal cartilage (Type II), or even the sternum (Type IV); no anterior attachment is also found (Type I)

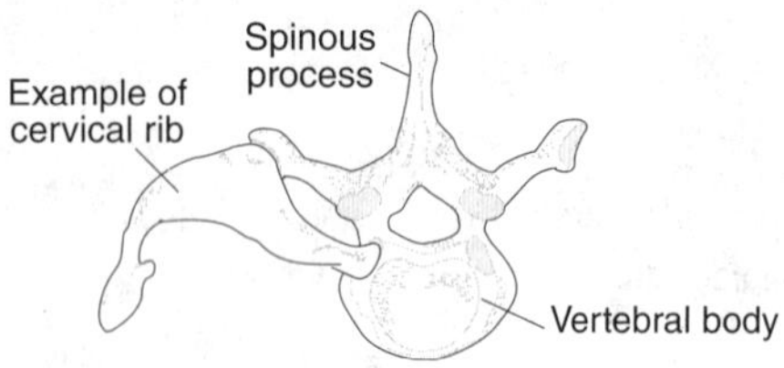

A cervical rib is present on the seventh vertebra in about 1 percent of the population

Explanation

The physician performs surgery to remove the first rib and/or an extraneous cervical rib. With the patient under anesthesia, an incision is made in the skin just above the clavicle on the affected side and carried deep to the rib. The rib is identified and the attached soft tissues are dissected from the bone. The physician excises the rib using a saw and other surgical instruments. The rib is freed from its articulation and removed. The wound is irrigated and closed in layers. A dressing is applied. Report 21616 if a sympathetic nerve pathway is cut during the procedure.

Coding Tips

These are unilateral procedures. If performed bilaterally, some payers require that the service be reported twice with modifier 50 appended to the second code, while others require identification of the service only once with modifier 50 appended. Check with individual payers. Modifier 50 identifies a procedure performed identically on the opposite side of the body (mirror image). For a partial rib excision, see 21600. For resection of a cervical rib with division scalenus anticus, see 21705.

ICD-10-CM Diagnostic Codes

G54.0	Brachial plexus disorders
I74.2	Embolism and thrombosis of arteries of the upper extremities
M54.12	Radiculopathy, cervical region
M95.4	Acquired deformity of chest and rib
Q76.5	Cervical rib

AMA: 21615 2018,Sep,7; 2018,Jan,8; 2017,Jan,8; 2016,Jan,13; 2015,Jan,16; 2014,Mar,13 **21616** 2018,Sep,7

Relative Value Units/Medicare Edits

Non-Facility RVU	Work	PE	MP	Total
21615	10.45	4.75	2.38	17.58
21616	12.69	4.93	2.94	20.56
Facility RVU	**Work**	**PE**	**MP**	**Total**
21615	10.45	4.75	2.38	17.58
21616	12.69	4.93	2.94	20.56

	FUD	Status	MUE	Modifiers				IOM Reference
21615	90	A	1(2)	51	50	62*	80	None
21616	90	A	1(2)	51	50	N/A	80	

* with documentation

Terms To Know

cervicalgia. Pain localized to the cervical region, generally referring to the posterior or lateral regions of the neck.

debride. To remove all foreign objects and devitalized or infected tissue from a burn or wound to prevent infection and promote healing.

dissect. Cut apart or separate tissue for surgical purposes or for visual or microscopic study.

embolism. Obstruction of a blood vessel resulting from a clot or foreign substance.

excision. Surgical removal of an organ or tissue.

irrigate. Washing out, lavage.

lesion. Area of damaged tissue that has lost continuity or function, due to disease or trauma. Lesions may be located on internal structures such as the brain, nerves, or kidneys, or visible on the skin.

neuritis. Inflammation of a nerve or group of nerves, often manifested by loss of function and reflexes, pain, and numbness or tingling.

ostectomy. Excision of bone.

radiculitis. Pain along an inflamed nerve, with inflammation of the root of the associated spinal nerve.

Raynaud's phenomenon. Vascular disorder resulting in bilateral decreased circulation of the fingers and toes causing a pale or bluish appearance, numbness, tingling, and pain brought on by cold or emotions and relieved with heat.

resection. Surgical removal of a part or all of an organ or body part.

sympathectomy. Surgical interruption or transection of a sympathetic nervous system pathway.

thrombosis. Condition arising from the presence or formation of blood clots within a blood vessel that may cause vascular obstruction and insufficient oxygenation.

21620

21620 Ostectomy of sternum, partial

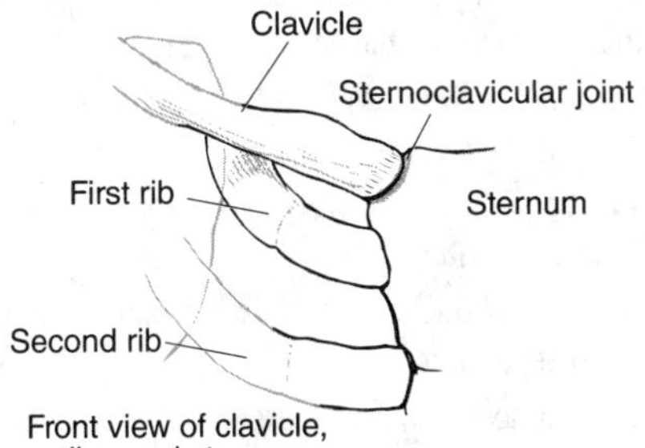

Front view of clavicle, ribs, and sternum

The sternum is the flat, elongated bone that makes up the anterior structure of the thoracic cage. It has three parts: the manubrium (uppermost), the body, and the xiphoid process (lowermost)

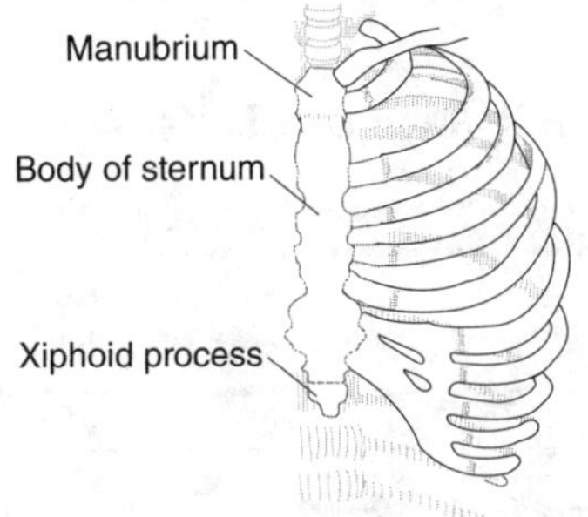

Explanation

The physician removes a portion of the sternum from the chest. With the patient under anesthesia, the physician makes an incision in the skin overlying the sternum. This is carried deep through the subcutaneous tissues to the bone. The sternum is identified and the attached soft tissues are carefully dissected from the bone. The physician marks the portion of the sternum to be removed. The bone is cut in the appropriate places using a saw and other surgical instruments. The remaining portion of the bone is irrigated and smoothed as needed. The wound is closed in layers and a dressing is applied.

Coding Tips

When this procedure is performed to access the chest cavity for open heart surgery, it is incidental to that procedure and is not reported separately. If significant additional time and effort are documented, append modifier 22 and submit a cover letter and operative report. When 21620 is performed with another separately identifiable procedure, the highest dollar value code is listed as the primary procedure, and subsequent procedures are appended with modifier 51.

ICD-10-CM Diagnostic Codes

C41.3	Malignant neoplasm of ribs, sternum and clavicle
D16.7	Benign neoplasm of ribs, sternum and clavicle
Q76.7	Congenital malformation of sternum

AMA: 21620 2018,Sep,7

Relative Value Units/Medicare Edits

Non-Facility RVU	Work	PE	MP	Total
21620	7.28	5.65	1.59	14.52
Facility RVU	**Work**	**PE**	**MP**	**Total**
21620	7.28	5.65	1.59	14.52

	FUD	Status	MUE	Modifiers				IOM Reference
21620	90	A	1(2)	51	N/A	62*	80	None

* with documentation

Terms To Know

aseptic necrosis. Death of bone tissue resulting from a disruption in the vascular supply, caused by a noninfectious disease process, such as a fracture or the administration of immunosuppressive drugs.

benign. Mild or nonmalignant in nature.

chronic. Persistent, continuing, or recurring.

debridement. Removal of dead or contaminated tissue and foreign matter from a wound.

incision. Act of cutting into tissue or an organ.

irrigate. Washing out, lavage.

malignant. Any condition tending to progress toward death, specifically an invasive tumor with a loss of cellular differentiation that has the ability to spread or metastasize to other body areas.

ostectomy. Excision of bone.

osteomyelitis. Inflammation of bone that may remain localized or spread to the marrow, cortex, or periosteum, in response to an infecting organism, usually bacterial and pyogenic.

secondary. Second in order of occurrence or importance, or appearing during the course of another disease or condition.

soft tissue. Nonepithelial tissues outside of the skeleton that includes subcutaneous adipose tissue, fibrous tissue, fascia, muscles, blood and lymph vessels, and peripheral nervous system tissue.

21627

21627 Sternal debridement

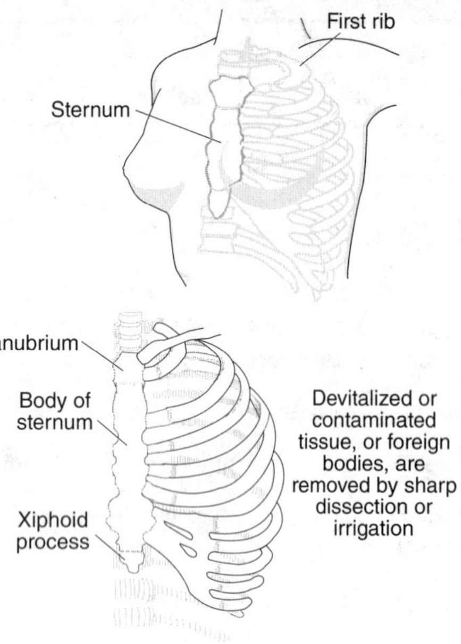

There are three parts of the sternum: the manubrium (uppermost), the body, and the xiphoid process

Explanation

The physician performs a debridement of the sternum. With the patient under anesthesia, the physician makes an incision in the skin overlying the sternum. The incision is carried deep to the bone. The sternum is debrided as warranted using any of a variety of hand or powered surgical instruments. Irrigation is used so that debridement can be completed as extensively as indicated. The wound may be loosely packed and a dressing applied or it may be closed in layers and a dressing applied.

Coding Tips

This procedure is usually performed to treat postoperative infection following open thoracic surgery. It may also be performed following open injury complicated by infection. For closure of sternotomy separation with or without debridement, see 21750.

ICD-10-CM Diagnostic Codes

C41.3 Malignant neoplasm of ribs, sternum and clavicle
D16.7 Benign neoplasm of ribs, sternum and clavicle
S21.121A Laceration with foreign body of right front wall of thorax without penetration into thoracic cavity, initial encounter ☑
S21.122A Laceration with foreign body of left front wall of thorax without penetration into thoracic cavity, initial encounter ☑
S21.141A Puncture wound with foreign body of right front wall of thorax without penetration into thoracic cavity, initial encounter ☑
S21.142A Puncture wound with foreign body of left front wall of thorax without penetration into thoracic cavity, initial encounter ☑
S21.321A Laceration with foreign body of right front wall of thorax with penetration into thoracic cavity, initial encounter ☑
S21.322A Laceration with foreign body of left front wall of thorax with penetration into thoracic cavity, initial encounter ☑
S21.341A Puncture wound with foreign body of right front wall of thorax with penetration into thoracic cavity, initial encounter ☑
S21.342A Puncture wound with foreign body of left front wall of thorax with penetration into thoracic cavity, initial encounter ☑
S21.351A Open bite of right front wall of thorax with penetration into thoracic cavity, initial encounter ☑
S21.352A Open bite of left front wall of thorax with penetration into thoracic cavity, initial encounter ☑
T81.41XA Infection following a procedure, superficial incisional surgical site, initial encounter
T81.42XA Infection following a procedure, deep incisional surgical site, initial encounter
T81.43XA Infection following a procedure, organ and space surgical site, initial encounter
T81.44XA Sepsis following a procedure, initial encounter
T81.49XA Infection following a procedure, other surgical site, initial encounter

AMA: 21627 2018,Sep,7; 2018,Jan,8; 2017,Jan,8; 2016,Jan,13; 2015,Jan,16; 2014,Jan,11

Relative Value Units/Medicare Edits

Non-Facility RVU	Work	PE	MP	Total
21627	7.3	6.6	1.59	15.49
Facility RVU	**Work**	**PE**	**MP**	**Total**
21627	7.3	6.6	1.59	15.49

	FUD	Status	MUE	Modifiers				IOM Reference
21627	90	A	1(2)	51	N/A	N/A	80	None

* with documentation

Terms To Know

aseptic necrosis. Death of bone tissue resulting from a disruption in the vascular supply, caused by a noninfectious disease process, such as a fracture or the administration of immunosuppressive drugs.

chronic. Persistent, continuing, or recurring.

debridement. Removal of dead or contaminated tissue and foreign matter from a wound.

infected postoperative seroma. Infection within a pocket of serum following surgery.

irrigation. To wash out or cleanse a body cavity, wound, or tissue with water or other fluid.

lesion. Area of damaged tissue that has lost continuity or function, due to disease or trauma.

malignant. Any condition tending to progress toward death, specifically an invasive tumor with a loss of cellular differentiation that has the ability to spread or metastasize to other body areas.

secondary. Second in order of occurrence or importance, or appearing during the course of another disease or condition.

soft tissue. Nonepithelial tissues outside of the skeleton that includes subcutaneous adipose tissue, fibrous tissue, fascia, muscles, blood and lymph vessels, and peripheral nervous system tissue.

21630-21632

21630 Radical resection of sternum;
21632 with mediastinal lymphadenectomy

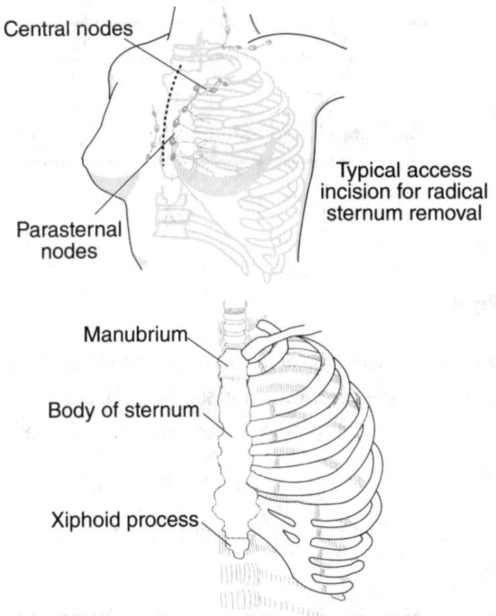

The sternum is the flat, elongated bone that makes up the anterior structure of the thoracic cage

Explanation

The physician removes most or all of the sternum from the chest. With the patient under anesthesia, the physician makes a long incision overlying the sternum and anterior chest. This is carried deep to the bone. Dissection is performed around the sternum. Ribs are disarticulated as needed and thorough debridement is accomplished. Using saws and other surgical instruments, the physician removes the bone. Internal fixation devices (reported separately) are often needed to support the ribs and chest wall. The wound is thoroughly irrigated and closed in layers. Report 21632 if a mediastinal lymphadenectomy is performed during the procedure.

Coding Tips

Debridement, irrigation, and closure are not reported separately. If significant additional time and effort are documented, append modifier 22 and submit a cover letter and operative report. When 21630 or 21632 is performed with another separately identifiable procedure, the highest dollar value code is listed as the primary procedure, and subsequent procedures are appended with modifier 51. If internal fixation devices are necessary, report separately; see 21825.

ICD-10-CM Diagnostic Codes

C41.3 Malignant neoplasm of ribs, sternum and clavicle
C77.1 Secondary and unspecified malignant neoplasm of intrathoracic lymph nodes
C78.1 Secondary malignant neoplasm of mediastinum
D16.7 Benign neoplasm of ribs, sternum and clavicle
S21.121A Laceration with foreign body of right front wall of thorax without penetration into thoracic cavity, initial encounter ☑
S21.122A Laceration with foreign body of left front wall of thorax without penetration into thoracic cavity, initial encounter ☑
S21.129A Laceration with foreign body of unspecified front wall of thorax without penetration into thoracic cavity, initial encounter
S21.141A Puncture wound with foreign body of right front wall of thorax without penetration into thoracic cavity, initial encounter ☑
S21.142A Puncture wound with foreign body of left front wall of thorax without penetration into thoracic cavity, initial encounter ☑
S21.149A Puncture wound with foreign body of unspecified front wall of thorax without penetration into thoracic cavity, initial encounter
S21.92XA Laceration with foreign body of unspecified part of thorax, initial encounter
S21.94XA Puncture wound with foreign body of unspecified part of thorax, initial encounter
T81.41XA Infection following a procedure, superficial incisional surgical site, initial encounter
T81.42XA Infection following a procedure, deep incisional surgical site, initial encounter
T81.43XA Infection following a procedure, organ and space surgical site, initial encounter
T81.44XA Sepsis following a procedure, initial encounter
T81.49XA Infection following a procedure, other surgical site, initial encounter

AMA: 21630 2018,Sep,7 **21632** 2018,Sep,7

Relative Value Units/Medicare Edits

Non-Facility RVU	Work	PE	MP	Total
21630	19.18	12.4	3.86	35.44
21632	19.68	10.55	4.66	34.89
Facility RVU	**Work**	**PE**	**MP**	**Total**
21630	19.18	12.4	3.86	35.44
21632	19.68	10.55	4.66	34.89

	FUD	Status	MUE	Modifiers				IOM Reference
21630	90	A	1(2)	51	N/A	62*	80	None
21632	90	A	1(2)	51	N/A	62*	80	

* with documentation

Terms To Know

aseptic necrosis. Death of bone tissue resulting from a disruption in the vascular supply, caused by a noninfectious disease process, such as a fracture or the administration of immunosuppressive drugs.

lymphadenectomy. Dissection of lymph nodes free from the vessels and removal for examination by frozen section in a separate procedure to detect early-stage metastases.

malignant. Any condition tending to progress toward death, specifically an invasive tumor with a loss of cellular differentiation that has the ability to spread or metastasize to other body areas.

neoplasm. New abnormal growth, tumor.

resection. Surgical removal of a part or all of an organ or body part.

21700-21705

21700 Division of scalenus anticus; without resection of cervical rib
21705 with resection of cervical rib

Numerous structures cross or attach to the first rib, including the anterior scalenus

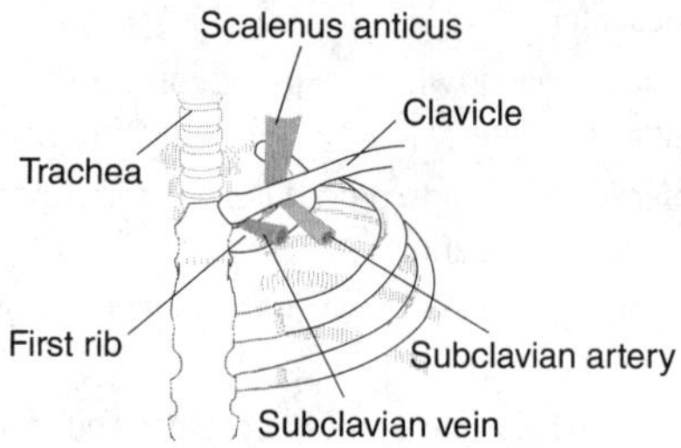

Superior view of C7 showing cervical rib, which usually occurs bilaterally

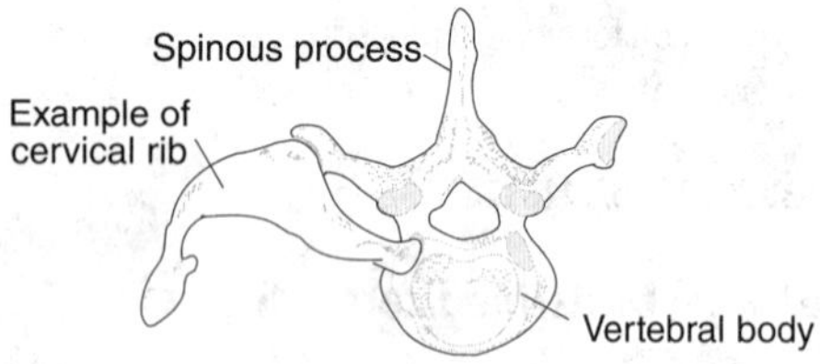

Explanation

The physician performs a surgical procedure where the scalenus anticus muscle is divided, usually for the purpose of treating thoracic outlet syndrome. With the patient under anesthesia, the physician makes an incision overlying the scalene muscle. This incision is carried deep to the muscle. The muscle is exposed and identified. A discission of the muscle is performed in line of the fibers. This relieves the pressure on the neurovascular structures. The wound is thoroughly irrigated and closed in layers. Report 21700 if the procedure does not include resection of the cervical rib. Report 21705 if resection of the cervical rib is performed during the procedure.

Coding Tips

When 21700 or 21705 is performed with another separately identifiable procedure, the highest dollar value code is listed as the primary procedure, and subsequent procedures are appended with modifier 51. For resection of the cervical rib without division of scalenus anticus, see 21615–21616.

ICD-10-CM Diagnostic Codes

G54.0	Brachial plexus disorders
Q76.5	Cervical rib

AMA: **21700** 2018,Sep,7 **21705** 2018,Sep,7; 2018,Jan,8; 2017,Jan,8; 2016,Jan,13; 2015,Jan,16; 2014,Mar,13

Relative Value Units/Medicare Edits

Non-Facility RVU	Work	PE	MP	Total
21700	6.31	2.54	1.45	10.3
21705	9.92	3.23	2.29	15.44
Facility RVU	**Work**	**PE**	**MP**	**Total**
21700	6.31	2.54	1.45	10.3
21705	9.92	3.23	2.29	15.44

	FUD	Status	MUE	Modifiers				IOM Reference
21700	90	A	1(2)	51	50	N/A	80	None
21705	90	A	1(2)	51	50	N/A	80	

* with documentation

Terms To Know

brachial plexus. Large bundle of nerves originating in the C5 to T2 spinal segments, located in the neck, axilla, and subclavicular area, and an anatomic landmark and site of administration of medication for pain management.

cervical. Relation to the cervical spine or to the cervix.

clavicle. Bone located between the sternum and scapula, connecting the arm to the body.

dissection. Separating by cutting tissue or body structures apart.

incision. Act of cutting into tissue or an organ.

irrigate. Washing out, lavage.

lesion. Area of damaged tissue that has lost continuity or function, due to disease or trauma.

ostectomy. Excision of bone.

resection. Surgical removal of a part or all of an organ or body part.

scalenus anticus syndrome. Disorder presenting symptoms similar to Raynaud's, caused by pressure of brachial plexus and subclavian artery against first thoracic rib.

scapula. Triangular bone commonly referred to as the shoulder blade.

soft tissue. Nonepithelial tissues outside of the skeleton that includes subcutaneous adipose tissue, fibrous tissue, fascia, muscles, blood and lymph vessels, and peripheral nervous system tissue.

spasm. Involuntary muscle contraction.

vertebral body. Disc-shaped portion of a vertebra that is anteriorly located and bears weight.

21740

21740 Reconstructive repair of pectus excavatum or carinatum; open

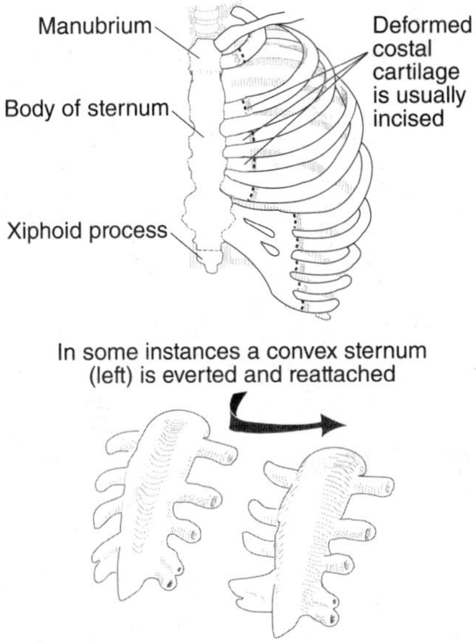

Explanation

The physician performs surgery on the anterior chest to correct pectus excavatum (a depression in the chest wall) or pectus carinatum (a forward projection of the chest wall). With the patient under anesthesia, the physician makes an incision overlying the anterior sternum. This is carried deep to the bone. The costal cartilages are exposed and deformed rib ends are freed from their sternal attachments. The sternum is mobilized and restored to its normal position. Internal fixation devices are employed to hold the sternum in corrected alignment. The physician irrigates the wound and closes it in layers with sutures.

Coding Tips

If significant additional time and effort are documented, append modifier 22 and submit a cover letter and operative report. Internal fixation devices are not reported separately. Report radiological services separately. For minimally invasive approach, see 21742 and 21743.

ICD-10-CM Diagnostic Codes

Q67.6 Pectus excavatum
Q67.7 Pectus carinatum

AMA: **21740** 2018,Sep,7

Relative Value Units/Medicare Edits

Non-Facility RVU	Work	PE	MP	Total
21740	17.57	8.1	4.17	29.84
Facility RVU	**Work**	**PE**	**MP**	**Total**
21740	17.57	8.1	4.17	29.84

	FUD	Status	MUE	Modifiers				IOM Reference
21740	90	A	1(2)	51	N/A	62*	80	None

* with documentation

21742-21743

21742 Reconstructive repair of pectus excavatum or carinatum; minimally invasive approach (Nuss procedure), without thoracoscopy

21743 minimally invasive approach (Nuss procedure), with thoracoscopy

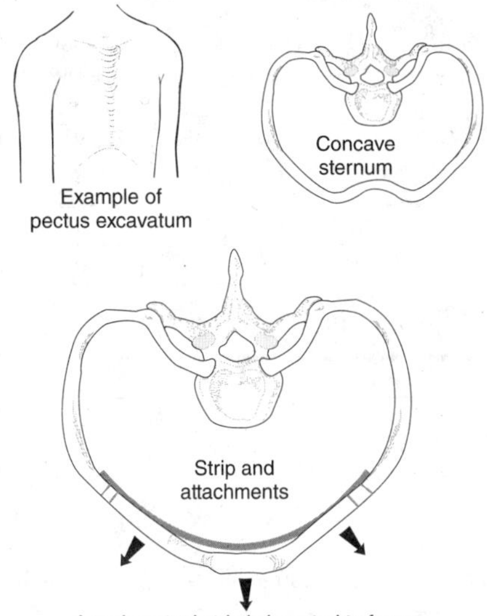

A spring steel strip is inserted to force the sternum into normal anatomic shape

Explanation

The physician performs a Nuss procedure, also known as minimally invasive repair of pectus excavatum (MIRPE), without thoracoscopy in 21742 and with thoracoscopy in 21743. Pectus excavatum is a depression of the sternum and chest, giving a sunken appearance. The chest is first marked at strategic points and the length of a curved steel bar, called the Lorenz pectus bar, to be inserted into the sternum is measured and shaped to fit the individual's chest. Midaxillary line incisions are made on the right and left side aligned with the deepest depression point. A skin tunnel is raised from the incisions and another small lateral incision is made for insertion of a thoracoscope. The skin incisions are elevated and a long introducer instrument is inserted through the right intercostal space at the top of the pectus ridge and slowly advanced across the anterior mediastinal space with videoscopic guidance. The sternum is forcefully lifted as the introducer is passed to the other side. Once behind the sternum, the tip is pushed through the intercostal space at the top of the pectus ridge on the left side and brought out through that skin incision. Umbilical tape is pulled through the tunnel and used to guide the prepared bar. The bar is inserted with the convex curve facing posteriorly and rotated with a flipping instrument until the convex curve faces anteriorly. The bar can be pulled back out and bent in a more ideal curvature for correction as many times as needed. Usually only one bar is placed. With the bar in position, a stabilizing bar is sutured around the pectus bar and to the muscle. Sutures are placed in the lateral chest wall musculature as well as one other fixation point to the side of the sternum around one rib and the pectus bar. Wounds are closed and the patient is extubated while deeply anesthetized and kept well sedated for a few days with pain management therapy.

Coding Tips

If significant additional time and effort are documented, append modifier 22 and submit a cover letter and operative report. Internal fixation devices are not reported separately. Radiological services are not reported separately. For reconstructive repair of the pectus excavatum or carinatum, invasive approach, see 21740.

ICD-10-CM Diagnostic Codes

Q67.6	Pectus excavatum
Q67.7	Pectus carinatum

AMA: **21742** 2018,Sep,7 **21743** 2018,Sep,7

Relative Value Units/Medicare Edits

Non-Facility RVU	Work	PE	MP	Total
21742	0.0	0.0	0.0	0.0
21743	0.0	0.0	0.0	0.0
Facility RVU	**Work**	**PE**	**MP**	**Total**
21742	0.0	0.0	0.0	0.0
21743	0.0	0.0	0.0	0.0

	FUD	Status	MUE	Modifiers				IOM Reference
21742	90	C	1(2)	51	N/A	62*	80	None
21743	90	C	1(2)	51	N/A	62*	80	

* with documentation

Terms To Know

alignment. Establishment of a straight line or harmonious relationship between structures.

anterior. Situated in the front area or toward the belly surface of the body; an anatomical reference point used to show the position and relationship of one body structure to another.

congenital. Present at birth, occurring through heredity or an influence during gestation up to the moment of birth.

incision. Act of cutting into tissue or an organ.

invasive. Insertion of an instrument, device, or foreign matter into the body or requiring puncture or incision of the skin.

lateral. On/to the side.

pectus carinatum. Congenital abnormality of the anterior chest wall with protrusion of the sternum, rounding the appearance of the chest.

pectus excavatum. Congenital abnormality of the anterior chest wall with depression of the sternum, sinking the appearance of the chest.

posterior. Located in the back part or caudal end of the body.

reconstruction. Recreating, restoring, or rebuilding a body part or organ.

21750

21750 Closure of median sternotomy separation with or without debridement (separate procedure)

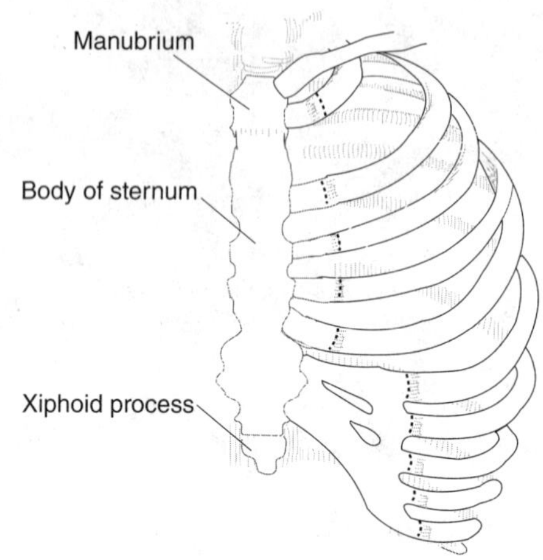

Explanation

The physician performs surgery on the sternum bone to put the bone back together following previous surgical separation. With the patient under anesthesia, the physician makes an incision overlying the sternum. The incision is carried deep to the bone and the separated pieces are identified. The physician may debride soft tissue or bone. The bony fragments are manipulated back together and held in place. The physician uses wire or other internal fixation devices to maintain the bone in appropriate position. The wound is irrigated and closed in layers.

Coding Tips

This separate procedure by definition is usually a component of a more complex service and is not identified separately. When performed alone or with other unrelated procedures/services, it may be reported. If performed alone, list the code; if performed with other procedures/services, list the code and append modifier 59 or an X{EPSU} modifier. Sternal debridement is included in this procedure and should not be reported separately. For sternal debridement only, see 21627. When 21750 is performed with another separately identifiable procedure, the highest dollar value code is listed as the primary procedure, and subsequent procedures are appended with modifier 51.

ICD-10-CM Diagnostic Codes

I97.88	Other intraoperative complications of the circulatory system, not elsewhere classified
I97.89	Other postprocedural complications and disorders of the circulatory system, not elsewhere classified
J95.89	Other postprocedural complications and disorders of respiratory system, not elsewhere classified
T81.32XA	Disruption of internal operation (surgical) wound, not elsewhere classified, initial encounter
T81.41XA	Infection following a procedure, superficial incisional surgical site, initial encounter
T81.42XA	Infection following a procedure, deep incisional surgical site, initial encounter

T81.43XA Infection following a procedure, organ and space surgical site, initial encounter

T81.44XA Sepsis following a procedure, initial encounter

T81.49XA Infection following a procedure, other surgical site, initial encounter

T81.89XA Other complications of procedures, not elsewhere classified, initial encounter

AMA: 21750 2018,Sep,7; 2018,Jan,8; 2017,Jan,8; 2016,Jan,13; 2015,Jan,16; 2014,Jan,11

Relative Value Units/Medicare Edits

Non-Facility RVU	Work	PE	MP	Total
21750	11.4	5.69	2.62	19.71
Facility RVU	**Work**	**PE**	**MP**	**Total**
21750	11.4	5.69	2.62	19.71

	FUD	Status	MUE	Modifiers				IOM Reference
21750	90	A	1(2)	51	N/A	62*	80	None

* with documentation

Terms To Know

debridement. Removal of dead or contaminated tissue and foreign matter from a wound.

infection. Presence of microorganisms in body tissues that may result in cellular damage.

irrigate. Washing out, lavage.

lesion. Area of damaged tissue that has lost continuity or function, due to disease or trauma. Lesions may be located on internal structures such as the brain, nerves, or kidneys, or visible on the skin.

malunion. Fracture that has united in a faulty position due to inadequate reduction of the original fracture, insufficient holding of a previously well-reduced fracture, contracture of the soft tissues, or comminuted or osteoporotic bone causing a slow disintegration of the fracture.

manipulation. Skillful treatment by hand to reduce fractures and dislocations or provide therapy through forceful passive movement of a joint beyond its active limit of motion.

median sternotomy. Standard incision for open chest cardiac surgeries, from above the bellybutton to just under the chin, down the center of the chest through the sternum into the thoracic cavity.

nonunion. Failure of two ends of a fracture to mend or completely heal.

soft tissue. Nonepithelial tissues outside of the skeleton that includes subcutaneous adipose tissue, fibrous tissue, fascia, muscles, blood and lymph vessels, and peripheral nervous system tissue.

21811-21813

21811 Open treatment of rib fracture(s) with internal fixation, includes thoracoscopic visualization when performed, unilateral; 1-3 ribs

21812 4-6 ribs

21813 7 or more ribs

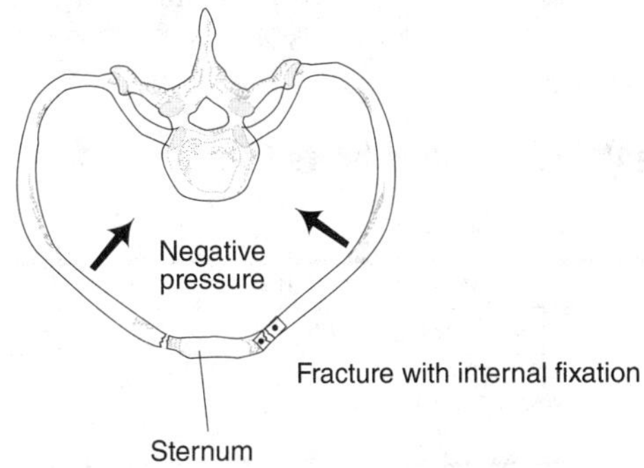

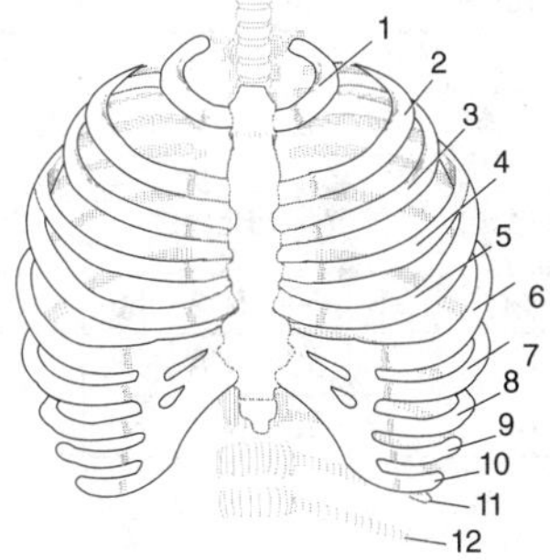

Explanation

The physician performs surgery on one or more unilateral rib fractures requiring internal fixation. With the patient under anesthesia, the physician makes an incision overlying the fractured rib. This is carried deep to the bone. The fracture is found, the pieces are identified, and dead tissue is debrided as needed. The physician manipulates and aligns the fracture fragments into an acceptable position and stabilizes the fragments using devices such as pins, rods, screws, or wires. The wound is irrigated and closed in layers. Report 21811 for treatment of one to three ribs; 21812 for four to six ribs; and 21813 for seven or more ribs. This includes thoracoscopic visualization when utilized.

Coding Tips

These codes are unilateral procedures. If performed bilaterally, some payers require that the service be reported twice with modifier 50 appended to the second code while others require identification of the service only once with modifier 50 appended. Check with individual payers. Modifier 50 identifies a procedure performed identically on the opposite side of the body (mirror image).

ICD-10-CM Diagnostic Codes

S22.31XA Fracture of one rib, right side, initial encounter for closed fracture ☑

S22.31XB Fracture of one rib, right side, initial encounter for open fracture ☑

S22.31XG Fracture of one rib, right side, subsequent encounter for fracture with delayed healing ☑

S22.31XK Fracture of one rib, right side, subsequent encounter for fracture with nonunion ☑

S22.41XA Multiple fractures of ribs, right side, initial encounter for closed fracture ☑

S22.41XB	Multiple fractures of ribs, right side, initial encounter for open fracture ☑
S22.41XG	Multiple fractures of ribs, right side, subsequent encounter for fracture with delayed healing ☑
S22.41XK	Multiple fractures of ribs, right side, subsequent encounter for fracture with nonunion ☑

AMA: 21811 2018,Sep,7; 2018,Jan,8; 2017,Jan,8; 2016,Jan,13; 2015,Aug,3 **21812** 2018,Sep,7; 2018,Jan,8; 2017,Jan,8; 2016,Jan,13; 2015,Aug,3 **21813** 2018,Sep,7; 2018,Jan,8; 2017,Jan,8; 2016,Jan,13; 2015,Aug,3

Relative Value Units/Medicare Edits

Non-Facility RVU	Work	PE	MP	Total
21811	10.79	4.0	2.39	17.18
21812	13.0	5.17	2.9	21.07
21813	17.61	6.79	4.27	28.67
Facility RVU	**Work**	**PE**	**MP**	**Total**
21811	10.79	4.0	2.39	17.18
21812	13.0	5.17	2.9	21.07
21813	17.61	6.79	4.27	28.67

	FUD	Status	MUE	Modifiers				IOM Reference
21811	0	A	1(2)	51	50	N/A	80	None
21812	0	A	1(2)	51	50	N/A	80	
21813	0	A	1(2)	51	50	N/A	80	

* with documentation

Terms To Know

debride. To remove all foreign objects and devitalized or infected tissue from a burn or wound to prevent infection and promote healing.

manipulate. Treatment by hand.

manubrium. Sternum.

21820

21820 Closed treatment of sternum fracture

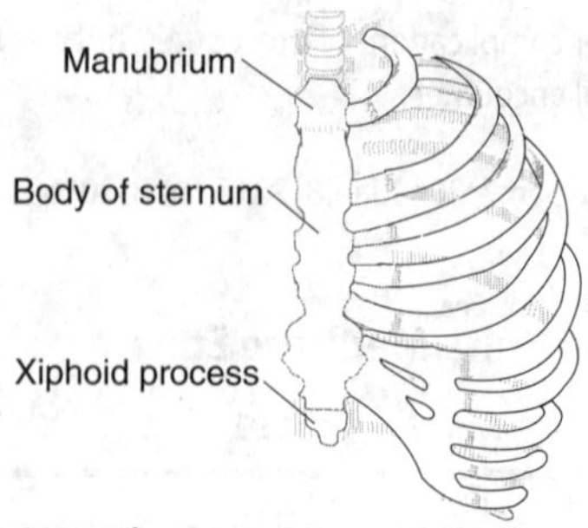

Fractures often occur at or near the juncture of the manubrium and the body of the sternum

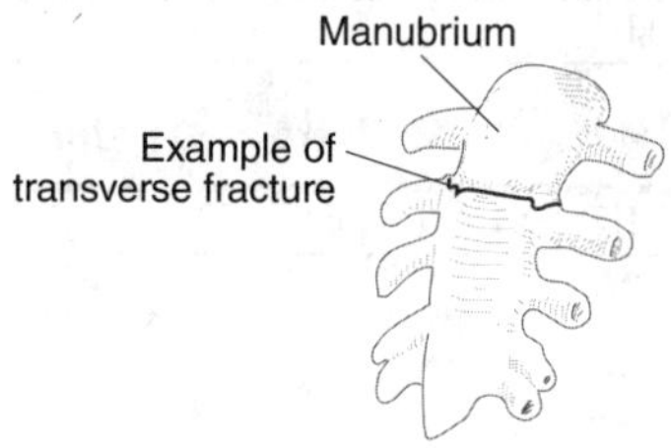

Explanation

Separately reportable x-rays are used to identify if a fracture of the sternum is present. If the fracture is non-displaced and stable, closed treatment is initiated. Braces or splints are not used. The patient's activity is modified while the fracture heals.

Coding Tips

Closed treatment may be reported even for nondisplaced sternum fractures requiring no splinting or bracing. When 21820 is performed with another separately identifiable procedure, the highest dollar value code is listed as the primary procedure, and subsequent procedures are appended with modifier 51. For open treatment, see 21825.

ICD-10-CM Diagnostic Codes

S22.20XA	Unspecified fracture of sternum, initial encounter for closed fracture
S22.21XA	Fracture of manubrium, initial encounter for closed fracture
S22.22XA	Fracture of body of sternum, initial encounter for closed fracture
S22.23XA	Sternal manubrial dissociation, initial encounter for closed fracture
S22.24XA	Fracture of xiphoid process, initial encounter for closed fracture

AMA: 21820 2018,Sep,7

Relative Value Units/Medicare Edits

Non-Facility RVU	Work	PE	MP	Total
21820	1.36	2.48	0.24	4.08
Facility RVU	**Work**	**PE**	**MP**	**Total**
21820	1.36	2.5	0.24	4.1

	FUD	Status	MUE	Modifiers				IOM Reference
21820	90	A	1(2)	51	N/A	N/A	N/A	None

* with documentation

21825

21825 Open treatment of sternum fracture with or without skeletal fixation

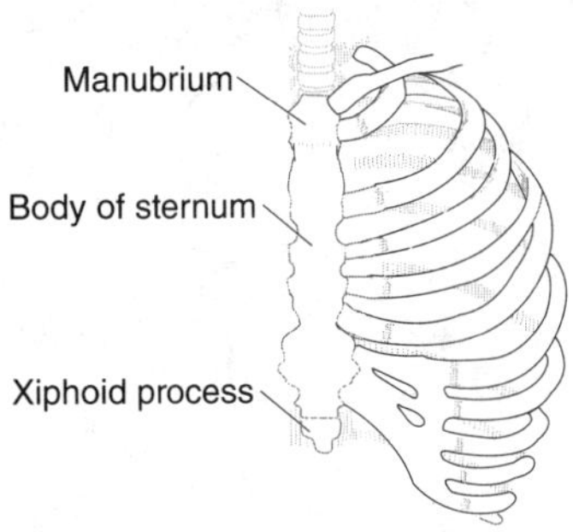

Fractures often occur at or near the juncture of the manubrium and the body of the sternum

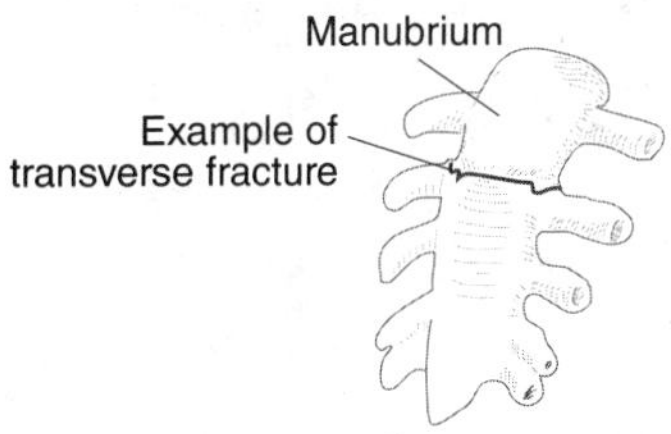

Explanation

The physician performs an open surgical reduction of a sternum fracture. The patient is positioned supine on the operating table. A longitudinal incision is made along the midportion of the sternum. Dissection exposes the fractured sternum. The surgeon reduces the fracture. If fixation is needed to keep the fracture stable, the physician drills holes on either side of the fracture. Wire is passed through the holes and around the fracture and the wire ends are twisted together to immobilize the fracture. The incision is repaired in layers with sutures, staples, or Steri-strips.

Coding Tips

Any wiring or internal fixation is not reported separately. Report open treatment of rib fractures separately, see 21811–21813. When 21825 is performed with another separately identifiable procedure, the highest dollar value code is listed as the primary procedure, and subsequent procedures are appended with modifier 51. For closed treatment of a sternum fracture, see 21820.

ICD-10-CM Diagnostic Codes

S22.21XA	Fracture of manubrium, initial encounter for closed fracture
S22.21XB	Fracture of manubrium, initial encounter for open fracture
S22.22XA	Fracture of body of sternum, initial encounter for closed fracture
S22.22XB	Fracture of body of sternum, initial encounter for open fracture
S22.23XA	Sternal manubrial dissociation, initial encounter for closed fracture
S22.23XB	Sternal manubrial dissociation, initial encounter for open fracture
S22.24XA	Fracture of xiphoid process, initial encounter for closed fracture
S22.24XB	Fracture of xiphoid process, initial encounter for open fracture

AMA: 21825 2018,Sep,7

Relative Value Units/Medicare Edits

Non-Facility RVU	Work	PE	MP	Total
21825	7.76	6.07	1.76	15.59
Facility RVU	**Work**	**PE**	**MP**	**Total**
21825	7.76	6.07	1.76	15.59

	FUD	Status	MUE	Modifiers				IOM Reference
21825	90	A	1(2)	51	N/A	62*	80	None

* with documentation

Terms To Know

closed fracture. Break in a bone without a concomitant opening in the skin.

dissection. Separating by cutting tissue or body structures apart.

fixation. Act or condition of being attached, secured, fastened, or held in position.

immobilizer. Device used to restrain a part of the body, keeping the body part from moving.

incision. Act of cutting into tissue or an organ.

internal skeletal fixation. Repair involving wires, pins, screws, and/or plates placed through or within the fractured area to stabilize and immobilize the injury.

malunion. Fracture that has united in a faulty position due to inadequate reduction of the original fracture, insufficient holding of a previously well-reduced fracture, contracture of the soft tissues, or comminuted or osteoporotic bone causing a slow disintegration of the fracture.

nonunion. Failure of two ends of a fracture to mend or completely heal.

open fracture. Exposed break in a bone, always considered compound due to its high risk of infection from the open wound leading to the fracture. Broken bone ends may protrude through the skin and contaminants or foreign bodies are often embedded in the tissues.

open reduction. Treatment of a fracture or dislocation by surgically exposing the site and manipulating the fracture fragments or bone ends into proper alignment under direct vision.

reduction. Correction of a fracture, dislocation, or hernia to the correct place and alignment, manually or by surgery.

stabilization. Fixed, firm state that is resistant to change.

31500

31500 Intubation, endotracheal, emergency procedure

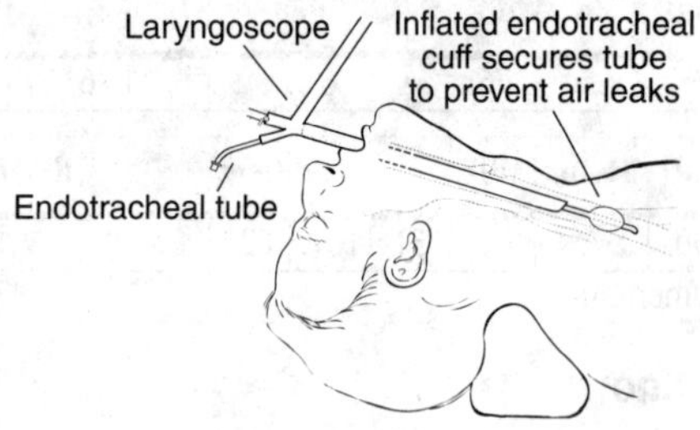

An emergency endotracheal intubation is performed

Explanation

The physician places an endotracheal tube to provide air passage in emergency situations. The patient is ventilated with a mask and bag and positioned by extending the neck anteriorly and the head posteriorly. The physician places the laryngoscope into the patient's mouth and advances the blade toward the epiglottis until the vocal cords are visible. An endotracheal tube is inserted between the vocal cords and advanced to the proper position. The cuff of the endotracheal tube is inflated.

Coding Tips

As exempt from modifier 51, 31500 has not been designated in CPT as an add-on service/procedure. However, codes identified as exempt from modifier 51 are not subject to multiple procedure rules. No reimbursement reduction or modifier 51 is applied. Emergency endotracheal intubation may be reported separately when performed in connection with critical care; see 99291 or 99292 and notes for definitions of critical care and other procedures that may be reported. Code 31500 is included in bundled pediatric and neonatal critical care service codes 99468–99472, 99475, and 99476 and intensive care service codes 99477–99480.

ICD-10-CM Diagnostic Codes

The application of this code is too broad to adequately present ICD-10-CM diagnostic code links here. Refer to your ICD-10-CM book.

AMA: **31500** 2018,Jan,8; 2017,Jan,8; 2016,Oct,8; 2016,May,3; 2016,Jan,13; 2015,Jan,16; 2014,Jan,11

Relative Value Units/Medicare Edits

Non-Facility RVU	Work	PE	MP	Total
31500	3.0	0.71	0.36	4.07
Facility RVU	**Work**	**PE**	**MP**	**Total**
31500	3.0	0.71	0.36	4.07

	FUD	Status	MUE	Modifiers				IOM Reference
31500	0	A	2(3)	N/A	N/A	N/A	N/A	None

* with documentation

31515

31515 Laryngoscopy direct, with or without tracheoscopy; for aspiration

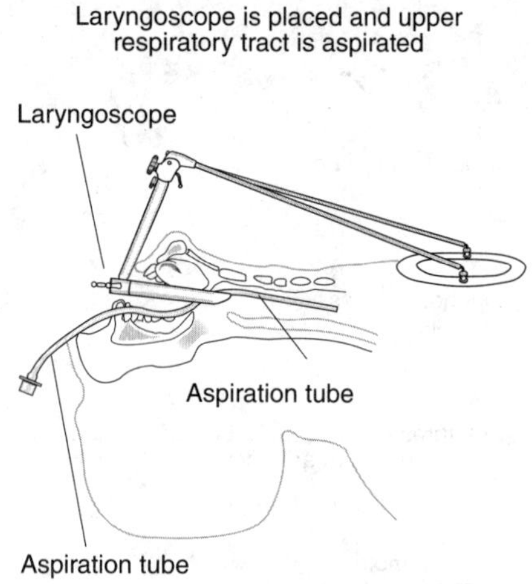

Side view schematic

Explanation

The physician uses an aspirator to remove excess saliva or semi-solid foreign material from the larynx. After applying topical anesthesia to the oral cavity and pharynx, the physician inserts the laryngoscope through the patient's mouth. An aspirator is fed through the laryngoscope and the larynx is cleared of saliva and semi-solid foreign material. If a tracheoscopy is performed, a bronchoscope is inserted through the laryngoscope for microscopic visualization of the trachea and bronchi. No other procedure is performed.

Coding Tips

Laryngoscopy code selection is dependent on two variables. Laryngoscopy procedures may be either direct or indirect, and they may be performed with either a rigid or flexible scope. A direct laryngoscopy allows the physician to see the larynx through a scope in the throat. In contrast, when an indirect laryngoscopy is performed, the physician uses mirrors to visualize the larynx. Code 31515 refers to direct visualization with a rigid laryngoscope. Report the appropriate endoscopy for each anatomic site examined. Surgical endoscopy includes a diagnostic endoscopy; however, diagnostic endoscopy can be identified separately when performed at the same surgical session as an open procedure.

ICD-10-CM Diagnostic Codes

J04.0	Acute laryngitis
J05.0	Acute obstructive laryngitis [croup]
J38.3	Other diseases of vocal cords
J38.7	Other diseases of larynx
J39.0	Retropharyngeal and parapharyngeal abscess
J39.8	Other specified diseases of upper respiratory tract
J69.0	Pneumonitis due to inhalation of food and vomit
J69.1	Pneumonitis due to inhalation of oils and essences
J69.8	Pneumonitis due to inhalation of other solids and liquids
J95.01	Hemorrhage from tracheostomy stoma
J95.02	Infection of tracheostomy stoma
J95.09	Other tracheostomy complication
J95.859	Other complication of respirator [ventilator]

J95.88	Other intraoperative complications of respiratory system, not elsewhere classified
J95.89	Other postprocedural complications and disorders of respiratory system, not elsewhere classified
O89.01	Aspiration pneumonitis due to anesthesia during the puerperium
P24.01	Meconium aspiration with respiratory symptoms
P24.11	Neonatal aspiration of (clear) amniotic fluid and mucus with respiratory symptoms
P24.21	Neonatal aspiration of blood with respiratory symptoms
P24.31	Neonatal aspiration of milk and regurgitated food with respiratory symptoms
P24.81	Other neonatal aspiration with respiratory symptoms
R04.1	Hemorrhage from throat
R04.2	Hemoptysis
R04.81	Acute idiopathic pulmonary hemorrhage in infants
R04.89	Hemorrhage from other sites in respiratory passages
R09.3	Abnormal sputum
T81.41XA	Infection following a procedure, superficial incisional surgical site, initial encounter
T81.42XA	Infection following a procedure, deep incisional surgical site, initial encounter
T81.43XA	Infection following a procedure, organ and space surgical site, initial encounter
T81.44XA	Sepsis following a procedure, initial encounter
T81.49XA	Infection following a procedure, other surgical site, initial encounter

Associated HCPCS Codes

A4305	Disposable drug delivery system, flow rate of 50 ml or greater per hour

AMA: 31515 1998,Nov,1

Relative Value Units/Medicare Edits

Non-Facility RVU	Work	PE	MP	Total
31515	1.8	3.76	0.23	5.79
Facility RVU	**Work**	**PE**	**MP**	**Total**
31515	1.8	1.09	0.23	3.12

	FUD	Status	MUE	Modifiers				IOM Reference
31515	0	A	1(3)	51	N/A	N/A	N/A	None

* with documentation

Terms To Know

direct laryngoscopy. Endoscopic instrument, such as a flexible or rigid fiberoptic scope, inserted into the larynx for direct viewing capabilities of the voice box and vocal cords.

larynx. Musculocartilaginous structure between the trachea and the pharynx that functions as the valve preventing food and other particles from entering the respiratory tract, as well as the voice mechanism. Also called the voicebox, the larynx is composed of three single cartilages: cricoid, epiglottis, and thyroid; and three paired cartilages: arytenoid, corniculate, and cuneiform.

trachea. Tube descending from the larynx and branching into the right and left main bronchi.

31520-31526

31520 Laryngoscopy direct, with or without tracheoscopy; diagnostic, newborn

31525 diagnostic, except newborn

31526 diagnostic, with operating microscope or telescope

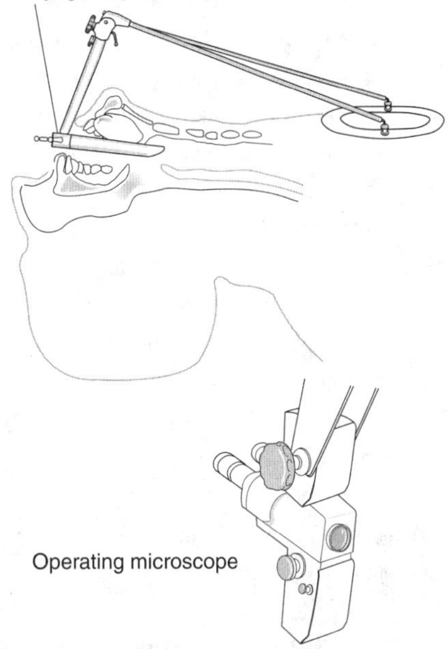

Explanation

The physician places a rigid laryngoscope to examine the patient's larynx. The physician administers a topical anesthetic to the oral cavity, pharynx, and larynx and inserts the laryngoscope through the patient's mouth. The interior of the larynx of a newborn is examined in 31520 and of a patient other than a newborn in 31525. In 31526, the physician uses an operating microscope or a telescope to examine the interior of the larynx. For all procedures, if a tracheoscopy is performed, a bronchoscope is inserted through the laryngoscope for microscopic visualization of the trachea and bronchi. No other procedure is performed at this time.

Coding Tips

Laryngoscopy code selection is dependent on two variables. Laryngoscopy procedures may be either direct or indirect, and they may be performed with either a rigid or flexible scope. A direct laryngoscopy allows the physician to see the larynx through a scope in the throat. In contrast, when an indirect laryngoscopy is performed, the physician uses mirrors to visualize the larynx. Report the appropriate endoscopy for each anatomic site examined. Surgical endoscopy includes a diagnostic endoscopy; however, diagnostic endoscopy can be identified separately when performed at the same surgical session as an open procedure. Do not append modifier 63 to 31520 as the description or nature of the procedure includes infants up to 4 kg. Use of an operating microscope is included in 31526. Do not report 69990 separately.

ICD-10-CM Diagnostic Codes

A36.0	Pharyngeal diphtheria
A36.1	Nasopharyngeal diphtheria
A36.2	Laryngeal diphtheria
C05.0	Malignant neoplasm of hard palate
C05.2	Malignant neoplasm of uvula

C06.2 Malignant neoplasm of retromolar area
C09.0 Malignant neoplasm of tonsillar fossa
C09.1 Malignant neoplasm of tonsillar pillar (anterior) (posterior)
C10.0 Malignant neoplasm of vallecula
C10.1 Malignant neoplasm of anterior surface of epiglottis
C10.2 Malignant neoplasm of lateral wall of oropharynx
C10.3 Malignant neoplasm of posterior wall of oropharynx
C10.4 Malignant neoplasm of branchial cleft
C11.0 Malignant neoplasm of superior wall of nasopharynx
C11.1 Malignant neoplasm of posterior wall of nasopharynx
C11.2 Malignant neoplasm of lateral wall of nasopharynx
C11.3 Malignant neoplasm of anterior wall of nasopharynx
C12 Malignant neoplasm of pyriform sinus
C13.0 Malignant neoplasm of postcricoid region
C13.1 Malignant neoplasm of aryepiglottic fold, hypopharyngeal aspect
C13.2 Malignant neoplasm of posterior wall of hypopharynx
C15.3 Malignant neoplasm of upper third of esophagus
C32.0 Malignant neoplasm of glottis
C32.1 Malignant neoplasm of supraglottis
C32.2 Malignant neoplasm of subglottis
C32.3 Malignant neoplasm of laryngeal cartilage
C33 Malignant neoplasm of trachea
D02.0 Carcinoma in situ of larynx
D02.1 Carcinoma in situ of trachea
I69.091 Dysphagia following nontraumatic subarachnoid hemorrhage
I69.191 Dysphagia following nontraumatic intracerebral hemorrhage
I69.391 Dysphagia following cerebral infarction
J04.11 Acute tracheitis with obstruction
J04.2 Acute laryngotracheitis
J05.0 Acute obstructive laryngitis [croup]
J05.11 Acute epiglottitis with obstruction
J06.0 Acute laryngopharyngitis
J31.2 Chronic pharyngitis
J37.1 Chronic laryngotracheitis
J38.01 Paralysis of vocal cords and larynx, unilateral
J38.1 Polyp of vocal cord and larynx
J38.2 Nodules of vocal cords
J38.4 Edema of larynx
J38.5 Laryngeal spasm
J38.6 Stenosis of larynx
J39.0 Retropharyngeal and parapharyngeal abscess
P24.01 Meconium aspiration with respiratory symptoms
P24.11 Neonatal aspiration of (clear) amniotic fluid and mucus with respiratory symptoms
P24.21 Neonatal aspiration of blood with respiratory symptoms
P26.0 Tracheobronchial hemorrhage originating in the perinatal period
P28.3 Primary sleep apnea of newborn
Q31.0 Web of larynx
Q31.1 Congenital subglottic stenosis
Q31.2 Laryngeal hypoplasia
Q31.3 Laryngocele
Q31.5 Congenital laryngomalacia
Q32.0 Congenital tracheomalacia
R04.1 Hemorrhage from throat
R04.2 Hemoptysis
R06.03 Acute respiratory distress
R47.02 Dysphasia
R47.1 Dysarthria and anarthria
R47.81 Slurred speech
R49.0 Dysphonia
R49.1 Aphonia
S11.014A Puncture wound with foreign body of larynx, initial encounter
S11.022A Laceration with foreign body of trachea, initial encounter
S11.024A Puncture wound with foreign body of trachea, initial encounter
T27.0XXA Burn of larynx and trachea, initial encounter
T27.1XXA Burn involving larynx and trachea with lung, initial encounter

AMA: **31525** 2018,Jan,8; 2017,Jan,8; 2016,Jan,13; 2015,Jan,16; 2014,Jan,11 **31526** 2018,Jan,8; 2017,Jun,10; 2016,Feb,12

Relative Value Units/Medicare Edits

Non-Facility RVU	Work	PE	MP	Total
31520	2.56	1.55	0.37	4.48
31525	2.63	4.13	0.36	7.12
31526	2.57	1.55	0.37	4.49
Facility RVU	**Work**	**PE**	**MP**	**Total**
31520	2.56	1.55	0.37	4.48
31525	2.63	1.57	0.36	4.56
31526	2.57	1.55	0.37	4.49

	FUD	Status	MUE	Modifiers				IOM Reference
31520	0	A	1(3)	51	N/A	N/A	80*	None
31525	0	A	1(3)	51	N/A	N/A	N/A	
31526	0	A	1(3)	51	N/A	N/A	N/A	

* with documentation

Terms To Know

apnea. Absence of breathing or breath.

atresia. Congenital closure or absence of a tubular organ or an opening to the body surface.

larynx. Musculocartilaginous structure between the trachea and the pharynx that functions as the valve preventing food and other particles from entering the respiratory tract, as well as the voice mechanism.

meconium aspiration syndrome. Newborn respiratory complications resulting from the passage and subsequent aspiration of meconium (fetal intestinal waste material) prior to or during delivery.

polyp. Small growth on a stalk-like attachment projecting from a mucous membrane.

respiratory distress syndrome. Premature neonates with respiratory distress and associated with reduced amounts of lung surfactant. Frequently fatal.

trachea. Tube descending from the larynx and branching into the right and left main bronchi.

31527-31529

31527 Laryngoscopy direct, with or without tracheoscopy; with insertion of obturator

31528 with dilation, initial

31529 with dilation, subsequent

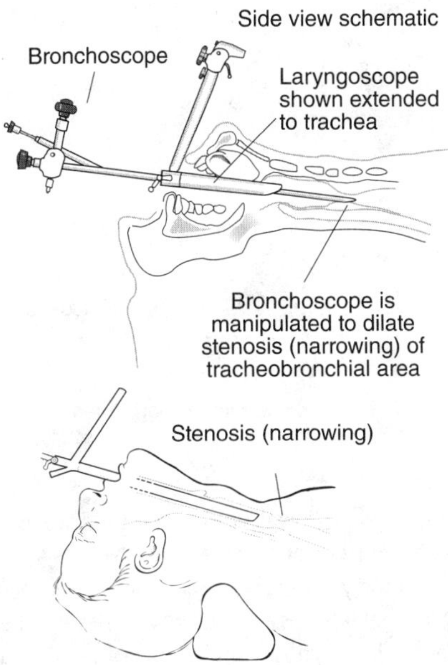

Explanation

In 31527, the physician administers a topical anesthetic to the oral cavity, pharynx, and larynx and inserts the laryngoscope through the patient's mouth. The interior of the larynx is examined. An obturator is an object that is used to close an opening. A wire is threaded through a cannulated needle that has been placed into the larynx. The end of the wire is grasped with forceps and drawn out through the laryngoscope. The wire is drawn through the obturator and threaded through another needle in the supraglottic space. The external ends of the wire are knotted over a stent. In 31528, the physician dilates the tracheobronchial stenosis. The physician administers a topical or general anesthetic and inserts the laryngoscope into the patient's mouth. The interior of the larynx is examined. The physician manipulates the laryngoscope to dilate areas of the tracheobronchial stenosis. Use 31529 to report subsequent dilations. If a tracheoscopy is performed, a bronchoscope is inserted through the laryngoscope for visualization of the trachea and bronchi.

Coding Tips

Laryngoscopy code selection is dependent on two variables. Laryngoscopy procedures may be either direct or indirect, and they may be performed with either a rigid or flexible scope. Codes 31527–31529 refer to direct visualization with a rigid laryngoscope. Report the appropriate endoscopy for each anatomic site examined. Surgical endoscopy includes a diagnostic endoscopy; however, diagnostic endoscopy can be identified separately when performed at the same surgical session as an open procedure.

ICD-10-CM Diagnostic Codes

C12	Malignant neoplasm of pyriform sinus
C13.0	Malignant neoplasm of postcricoid region
C13.1	Malignant neoplasm of aryepiglottic fold, hypopharyngeal aspect
C32.0	Malignant neoplasm of glottis
C32.1	Malignant neoplasm of supraglottis
C32.2	Malignant neoplasm of subglottis
C32.3	Malignant neoplasm of laryngeal cartilage
C32.8	Malignant neoplasm of overlapping sites of larynx
D02.0	Carcinoma in situ of larynx
D10.7	Benign neoplasm of hypopharynx
D14.1	Benign neoplasm of larynx
D38.0	Neoplasm of uncertain behavior of larynx
D38.1	Neoplasm of uncertain behavior of trachea, bronchus and lung
J05.0	Acute obstructive laryngitis [croup]
J05.11	Acute epiglottitis with obstruction
J37.0	Chronic laryngitis
J37.1	Chronic laryngotracheitis
J38.01	Paralysis of vocal cords and larynx, unilateral
J38.02	Paralysis of vocal cords and larynx, bilateral
J38.1	Polyp of vocal cord and larynx
J38.2	Nodules of vocal cords
J38.3	Other diseases of vocal cords
J38.5	Laryngeal spasm
J38.6	Stenosis of larynx
J38.7	Other diseases of larynx
J95.5	Postprocedural subglottic stenosis
Q31.0	Web of larynx
Q31.1	Congenital subglottic stenosis
Q31.2	Laryngeal hypoplasia
Q31.3	Laryngocele
Q31.5	Congenital laryngomalacia
Q31.8	Other congenital malformations of larynx
Q32.0	Congenital tracheomalacia
Q32.1	Other congenital malformations of trachea
S10.0XXA	Contusion of throat, initial encounter
S11.011A	Laceration without foreign body of larynx, initial encounter
S11.012A	Laceration with foreign body of larynx, initial encounter
S11.013A	Puncture wound without foreign body of larynx, initial encounter
S11.014A	Puncture wound with foreign body of larynx, initial encounter
S11.015A	Open bite of larynx, initial encounter
S11.032A	Laceration with foreign body of vocal cord, initial encounter
S11.034A	Puncture wound with foreign body of vocal cord, initial encounter
S12.8XXA	Fracture of other parts of neck, initial encounter
S17.0XXA	Crushing injury of larynx and trachea, initial encounter
S19.81XA	Other specified injuries of larynx, initial encounter
S19.83XA	Other specified injuries of vocal cord, initial encounter
T17.320A	Food in larynx causing asphyxiation, initial encounter
T17.328A	Food in larynx causing other injury, initial encounter
T17.390A	Other foreign object in larynx causing asphyxiation, initial encounter
T17.398A	Other foreign object in larynx causing other injury, initial encounter
T27.0XXA	Burn of larynx and trachea, initial encounter
T27.1XXA	Burn involving larynx and trachea with lung, initial encounter
T27.4XXA	Corrosion of larynx and trachea, initial encounter
T27.5XXA	Corrosion involving larynx and trachea with lung, initial encounter

AMA: 31528 2002,May,7 **31529** 2002,May,7

Relative Value Units/Medicare Edits

Non-Facility RVU	Work	PE	MP	Total
31527	3.27	1.85	0.46	5.58
31528	2.37	1.42	0.34	4.13
31529	2.68	1.55	0.39	4.62
Facility RVU	**Work**	**PE**	**MP**	**Total**
31527	3.27	1.85	0.46	5.58
31528	2.37	1.42	0.34	4.13
31529	2.68	1.55	0.39	4.62

	FUD	Status	MUE	Modifiers				IOM Reference
31527	0	A	1(2)	51	N/A	N/A	80*	None
31528	0	A	1(2)	51	N/A	N/A	80*	
31529	0	A	1(3)	51	N/A	N/A	80*	

* with documentation

Terms To Know

dilation. Artificial increase in the diameter of an opening or lumen made by medication or by instrumentation.

direct laryngoscopy. Endoscopic instrument, such as a flexible or rigid fiberoptic scope, inserted into the larynx for direct viewing capabilities of the voice box and vocal cords.

larynx. Musculocartilaginous structure between the trachea and the pharynx that functions as the valve preventing food and other particles from entering the respiratory tract, as well as the voice mechanism. Also called the voicebox, the larynx is composed of three single cartilages: cricoid, epiglottis, and thyroid; and three paired cartilages: arytenoid, corniculate, and cuneiform.

obturator. Prosthesis used to close an acquired or congenital opening in the palate that aids in speech and chewing.

stenosis. Narrowing or constriction of a passage.

trachea. Tube descending from the larynx and branching into the right and left main bronchi.

31592

31592 Cricotracheal resection

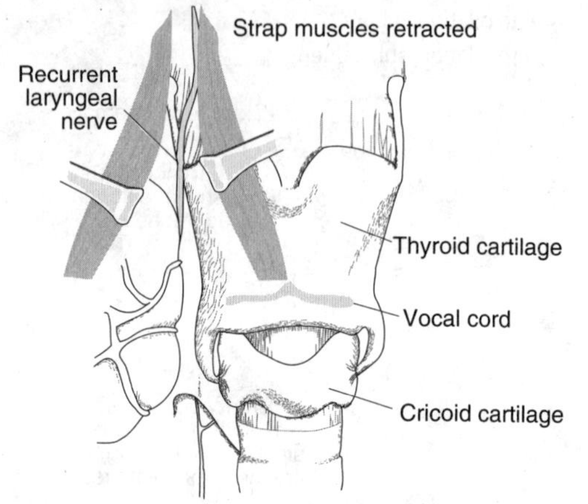

Cricotracheal resection is performed

Explanation

The physician removes a narrowed portion of the trachea usually below the larynx. A horizontal skin incision is made across the base of the neck or, in some cases, a sternotomy may be necessary. The prior tracheotomy stoma is removed when applicable. Flaps are lifted from the level of the hyoid bone to the suprasternal notch. The cricoid cartilage is split vertically and examined to be certain one intact ring between the area of resection and stoma is available in order for appropriate anastomosis between the trachea and larynx. Sutures are placed on both sides of the trachea just under the lowest level of the resection. Portions of the cricoid cartilage are removed from the anterior and lateral positions, avoiding the cricoarytenoid joint. The area of stenosis is removed with focus on avoiding the underlying esophagus. Upon removal of the narrowed portion, the ends are tied with absorbable sutures within the tracheal wall. Skin incisions are closed with sutures or staples. Sutures join the skin on the lower chin to the chest to prevent backward movement of the head or a neck brace may be utilized to keep sutures intact. This procedure may be performed as a single or double stage procedure depending on the exact location of the stenosis. In a single stage (SSCTR) procedure, a previously placed tracheotomy tube is removed and an endotracheal tube inserted. In a double stage (DSCTR) procedure, a stent may be inserted above the tracheotomy tube or a T-tube may be utilized instead of the tracheotomy tube. This allows the airway to remain open and is removed four to six weeks postop.

Coding Tips

Harvesting of the graft and rotational or advancement flaps performed through the same incision are not reported separately. For tracheostomy, see 31600–31610. For excision of a tracheal stenosis and anastomosis, see 31780 and 31781.

ICD-10-CM Diagnostic Codes

J38.01	Paralysis of vocal cords and larynx, unilateral
J38.02	Paralysis of vocal cords and larynx, bilateral
J38.3	Other diseases of vocal cords
J38.6	Stenosis of larynx

AMA: 31592 2018,Jan,8; 2017,Mar,10; 2017,Jul,7; 2017,Feb,14; 2017,Apr,5

Relative Value Units/Medicare Edits

Non-Facility RVU	Work	PE	MP	Total
31592	25.0	19.98	4.26	49.24
Facility RVU	**Work**	**PE**	**MP**	**Total**
31592	25.0	19.98	4.26	49.24

	FUD	Status	MUE	Modifiers				IOM Reference
31592	90	A	1(2)	51	N/A	62*	80*	None

* with documentation

Terms To Know

larynx. Musculocartilaginous structure between the trachea and the pharynx that functions as the valve preventing food and other particles from entering the respiratory tract, as well as the voice mechanism.

stenosis. Narrowing or constriction of a passage.

sternotomy. Incision into the sternum, the bone that forms the front of the chest cavity and connects with the ribs.

trachea. Tube descending from the larynx and branching into the right and left main bronchi.

tracheotomy. Formation of a tracheal opening on the neck surface with tube insertion to allow for respiration in cases of obstruction or decreased patency. A tracheotomy may be planned or performed on an emergency basis for temporary or long-term use.

31600-31610

31600 Tracheostomy, planned (separate procedure);
31601 younger than 2 years
31603 Tracheostomy, emergency procedure; transtracheal
31605 cricothyroid membrane
31610 Tracheostomy, fenestration procedure with skin flaps

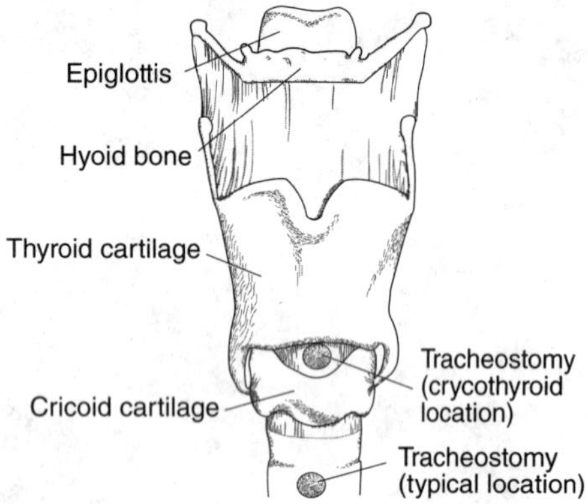

A tracheostomy is often performed just below the first tracheal ring and provides the patient with a controllable airway

Explanation

The physician creates a tracheostomy. The physician makes a horizontal neck incision and dissects the muscles to expose the trachea. The thyroid isthmus is cut if necessary. The trachea is incised and an airway is inserted. After bleeding is controlled, a stoma is created by suturing the skin to the tissue layers. In 31600, the tracheostomy is a planned procedure. In 31601, it is a planned procedure performed on patients younger than 2 years of age. In 31603, it is performed under emergency conditions by puncturing the trachea and inserting a cannula. In 31605, it is performed under emergency conditions by puncturing the cricothyroid membrane located just above the cricoid and inserting a cannula. This is not a true tracheostomy and is usually converted to a tracheostomy once the situation is no longer emergent. In 31610, skin flaps are used to create a more permanent stoma.

Coding Tips

Note that 31600 and 31601, separate procedures by definition, are usually a component of a more complex service and are not identified separately. When performed alone or with other unrelated procedures/services, they may be reported. If performed alone, list the code; if performed with other procedures/services, list the code and append modifier 59 or an X{EPSU} modifier. For endotracheal intubation, see 31500. For tracheal aspiration under direct vision, see 31515.

ICD-10-CM Diagnostic Codes

C01	Malignant neoplasm of base of tongue
C02.4	Malignant neoplasm of lingual tonsil
C09.0	Malignant neoplasm of tonsillar fossa
C09.1	Malignant neoplasm of tonsillar pillar (anterior) (posterior)
C10.0	Malignant neoplasm of vallecula
C10.1	Malignant neoplasm of anterior surface of epiglottis
C10.2	Malignant neoplasm of lateral wall of oropharynx
C10.3	Malignant neoplasm of posterior wall of oropharynx
C10.4	Malignant neoplasm of branchial cleft
C12	Malignant neoplasm of pyriform sinus
C13.0	Malignant neoplasm of postcricoid region
C13.1	Malignant neoplasm of aryepiglottic fold, hypopharyngeal aspect
C13.2	Malignant neoplasm of posterior wall of hypopharynx
C32.0	Malignant neoplasm of glottis
C32.1	Malignant neoplasm of supraglottis
C32.2	Malignant neoplasm of subglottis
C32.3	Malignant neoplasm of laryngeal cartilage
G12.0	Infantile spinal muscular atrophy, type I [Werdnig-Hoffman]
G12.21	Amyotrophic lateral sclerosis
G12.22	Progressive bulbar palsy
G12.23	Primary lateral sclerosis
G12.24	Familial motor neuron disease
G12.25	Progressive spinal muscle atrophy
G46.3	Brain stem stroke syndrome
G80.0	Spastic quadriplegic cerebral palsy
G93.1	Anoxic brain damage, not elsewhere classified
J38.02	Paralysis of vocal cords and larynx, bilateral
J38.6	Stenosis of larynx
J80	Acute respiratory distress syndrome
J95.821	Acute postprocedural respiratory failure
J95.822	Acute and chronic postprocedural respiratory failure
J96.01	Acute respiratory failure with hypoxia
J96.02	Acute respiratory failure with hypercapnia
J96.11	Chronic respiratory failure with hypoxia
J96.12	Chronic respiratory failure with hypercapnia
J96.21	Acute and chronic respiratory failure with hypoxia
J96.22	Acute and chronic respiratory failure with hypercapnia
P22.0	Respiratory distress syndrome of newborn
P27.0	Wilson-Mikity syndrome
P27.1	Bronchopulmonary dysplasia originating in the perinatal period
P28.2	Cyanotic attacks of newborn
P28.5	Respiratory failure of newborn
Q31.1	Congenital subglottic stenosis
Q31.2	Laryngeal hypoplasia
Q31.3	Laryngocele
Q31.5	Congenital laryngomalacia
Q32.0	Congenital tracheomalacia
Q32.2	Congenital bronchomalacia
Q32.3	Congenital stenosis of bronchus
R06.03	Acute respiratory distress
S11.012A	Laceration with foreign body of larynx, initial encounter
S11.014A	Puncture wound with foreign body of larynx, initial encounter
S17.0XXA	Crushing injury of larynx and trachea, initial encounter
T27.0XXA	Burn of larynx and trachea, initial encounter
T27.4XXA	Corrosion of larynx and trachea, initial encounter

AMA: 31600 2019,Sep,10; 2017,Apr,5 **31601** 2017,Apr,5 **31603** 2017,Apr,5 **31605** 2017,Apr,5 **31610** 2017,Apr,5

Relative Value Units/Medicare Edits

Non-Facility RVU	Work	PE	MP	Total
31600	5.56	2.31	1.04	8.91
31601	8.0	3.83	1.15	12.98
31603	6.0	2.27	1.04	9.31
31605	6.45	2.02	1.14	9.61
31610	12.0	13.39	1.85	27.24
Facility RVU	**Work**	**PE**	**MP**	**Total**
31600	5.56	2.31	1.04	8.91
31601	8.0	3.83	1.15	12.98
31603	6.0	2.27	1.04	9.31
31605	6.45	2.02	1.14	9.61
31610	12.0	13.39	1.85	27.24

	FUD	Status	MUE	Modifiers				IOM Reference
31600	0	A	1(2)	51	N/A	N/A	N/A	None
31601	0	A	1(2)	51	N/A	62*	80	
31603	0	A	1(2)	51	N/A	N/A	N/A	
31605	0	A	1(2)	51	N/A	N/A	N/A	
31610	90	A	1(2)	51	N/A	N/A	N/A	

* with documentation

Terms To Know

apnea. Absence of breathing or breath.

atresia. Congenital closure or absence of a tubular organ or an opening to the body surface.

cyanosis. Bluish discoloration due to an excessive amount of deoxygenated hemoglobin in the blood.

dyspnea. Difficult or labored breathing.

fenestration. Presence of small openings from piercing or perforations.

intubation. Insertion of a tube into a hollow organ, canal, or cavity within the body.

respiratory distress syndrome. Premature neonates with respiratory distress and associated with reduced amounts of lung surfactant. Frequently fatal.

stoma. Opening created in the abdominal wall from an internal organ or structure for diversion of waste elimination, drainage, and access.

stridor. Harsh, high-pitched sound produced when breathing with an obstructed airway, like the inspiratory sound heard when laryngeal obstruction is present or heard in patients with lung or esophageal cancers that have grown to sizes that compress the airway.

trachea. Tube descending from the larynx and branching into the right and left main bronchi.

tracheostomy. Formation of a tracheal opening on the neck surface with tube insertion to allow for respiration in cases of obstruction or decreased patency. A tracheostomy may be planned or performed on an emergency basis for temporary or long-term use.

31611

31611 Construction of tracheoesophageal fistula and subsequent insertion of an alaryngeal speech prosthesis (eg, voice button, Blom-Singer prosthesis)

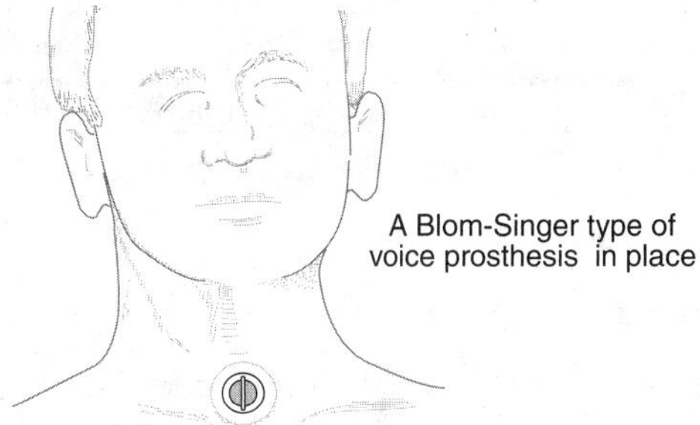

A tracheoesophageal fistula is created in order to fit a "voice button" device, usually following a laryngectomy

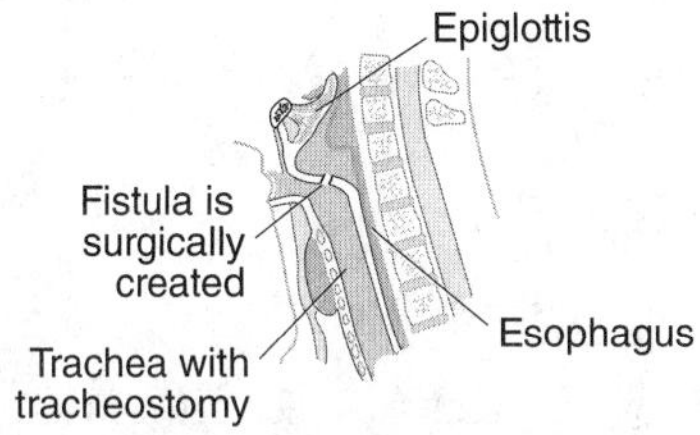

Explanation

The physician constructs a tracheal esophageal fistula for vocalization. The physician makes a horizontal neck incision and dissects the tissues between the tracheostoma and the esophagus. The esophagus is incised and a laryngeal speech prosthesis is inserted between the esophagus and the trachea, creating a fistula. The prosthesis, called a voice button or a Blom-Singer prosthesis, is a one-way valve enabling the patient to phonate. The physician closes the incision around the prosthesis.

Coding Tips

Construction of a tracheoesophageal fistula, also referred to as fistulization, should not be confused with fistula repair. Fistulization involves creation of a communication between two structures, whereas fistula repair involves closure of a communication. For repair of a tracheoesophageal fistula, thoracic approach, see 43312.

ICD-10-CM Diagnostic Codes

C12	Malignant neoplasm of pyriform sinus
C13.0	Malignant neoplasm of postcricoid region
C13.1	Malignant neoplasm of aryepiglottic fold, hypopharyngeal aspect
C32.0	Malignant neoplasm of glottis
C32.1	Malignant neoplasm of supraglottis
C32.2	Malignant neoplasm of subglottis
C32.3	Malignant neoplasm of laryngeal cartilage
C32.8	Malignant neoplasm of overlapping sites of larynx
Q31.2	Laryngeal hypoplasia
Q31.8	Other congenital malformations of larynx
Z85.21	Personal history of malignant neoplasm of larynx

Relative Value Units/Medicare Edits

Non-Facility RVU	Work	PE	MP	Total
31611	6.0	8.35	0.87	15.22
Facility RVU	**Work**	**PE**	**MP**	**Total**
31611	6.0	8.35	0.87	15.22

	FUD	Status	MUE	Modifiers				IOM Reference
31611	90	A	1(2)	51	N/A	62*	80	None

* with documentation

Terms To Know

anomaly. Irregularity in the structure or position of an organ or tissue.

congenital. Present at birth, occurring through heredity or an influence during gestation up to the moment of birth.

dissect. Cut apart or separate tissue for surgical purposes or for visual or microscopic study.

esophagus. Muscular tube that carries swallowed liquids and foods from the pharynx to the stomach.

fistula. Abnormal tube-like passage between two body cavities or organs or from an organ to the outside surface.

fistulization. Creation of a communication between two structures that were not previously connected.

incision. Act of cutting into tissue or an organ.

malignant. Any condition tending to progress toward death, specifically an invasive tumor with a loss of cellular differentiation that has the ability to spread or metastasize to other body areas.

neoplasm. New abnormal growth, tumor.

prosthesis. Man-made substitute for a missing body part.

reconstruction. Recreating, restoring, or rebuilding a body part or organ.

trachea. Tube descending from the larynx and branching into the right and left main bronchi.

tracheostomy. Formation of a tracheal opening on the neck surface with tube insertion to allow for respiration in cases of obstruction or decreased patency. A tracheostomy may be planned or performed on an emergency basis for temporary or long-term use.

31612

31612 Tracheal puncture, percutaneous with transtracheal aspiration and/or injection

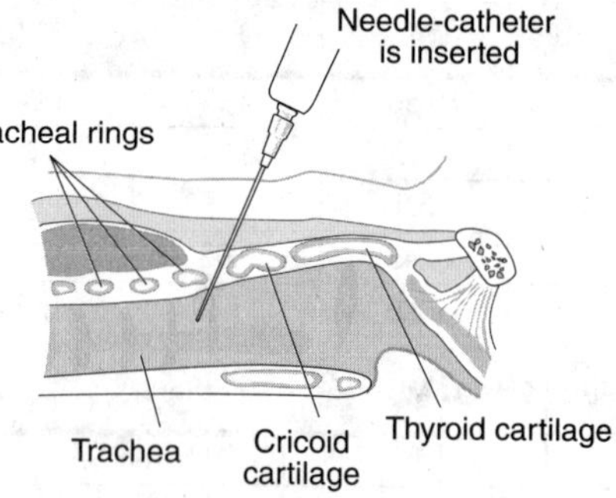

Midsagittal view showing needle placement

Explanation

The physician punctures the trachea with a needle to aspirate secretions or inject a therapeutic agent. The physician palpates the site and inserts a hollow point needle. Secretions are aspirated or a therapeutic agent is injected. The needle is removed.

Coding Tips

For tracheal aspiration under direct vision, see 31515. For catheter aspiration of tracheobronchial tree, see 31725.

ICD-10-CM Diagnostic Codes

A48.1	Legionnaires' disease
J44.0	Chronic obstructive pulmonary disease with (acute) lower respiratory infection
J44.1	Chronic obstructive pulmonary disease with (acute) exacerbation
J45.20	Mild intermittent asthma, uncomplicated
J45.21	Mild intermittent asthma with (acute) exacerbation
J45.22	Mild intermittent asthma with status asthmaticus
J45.31	Mild persistent asthma with (acute) exacerbation
J45.32	Mild persistent asthma with status asthmaticus
J45.41	Moderate persistent asthma with (acute) exacerbation
J45.42	Moderate persistent asthma with status asthmaticus
J45.51	Severe persistent asthma with (acute) exacerbation
J45.52	Severe persistent asthma with status asthmaticus
J68.0	Bronchitis and pneumonitis due to chemicals, gases, fumes and vapors
J69.0	Pneumonitis due to inhalation of food and vomit
J69.8	Pneumonitis due to inhalation of other solids and liquids
O74.0	Aspiration pneumonitis due to anesthesia during labor and delivery
O74.1	Other pulmonary complications of anesthesia during labor and delivery
O89.01	Aspiration pneumonitis due to anesthesia during the puerperium
O89.09	Other pulmonary complications of anesthesia during the puerperium
P24.01	Meconium aspiration with respiratory symptoms

P24.11 Neonatal aspiration of (clear) amniotic fluid and mucus with respiratory symptoms

P24.21 Neonatal aspiration of blood with respiratory symptoms

P24.31 Neonatal aspiration of milk and regurgitated food with respiratory symptoms

P24.81 Other neonatal aspiration with respiratory symptoms

AMA: 31612 1994,Win,1

Relative Value Units/Medicare Edits

Non-Facility RVU	Work	PE	MP	Total
31612	0.91	1.34	0.14	2.39
Facility RVU	**Work**	**PE**	**MP**	**Total**
31612	0.91	0.34	0.14	1.39

	FUD	Status	MUE	Modifiers				IOM Reference
31612	0	A	1(3)	51	N/A	N/A	80*	None

* with documentation

Terms To Know

anomaly. Irregularity in the structure or position of an organ or tissue.

aspirate. To withdraw fluid or air from a body cavity by suction.

congenital. Present at birth, occurring through heredity or an influence during gestation up to the moment of birth.

meconium aspiration syndrome. Newborn respiratory complications resulting from the passage and subsequent aspiration of meconium (fetal intestinal waste material) prior to or during delivery.

trachea. Tube descending from the larynx and branching into the right and left main bronchi.

31613-31614

31613 Tracheostoma revision; simple, without flap rotation

31614 complex, with flap rotation

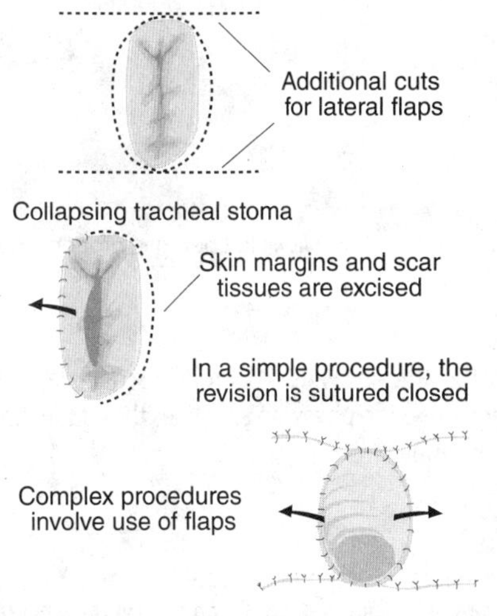

An existing tracheal stoma is surgically revised

Explanation

The physician revises a tracheal stoma. The physician incises the stoma area and resects redundant scar tissue or a poorly healing wound. The skin is re-anastomosed and sewn to the stoma in sutured layers. Report 31613 for performance of a simple revision and 31614 if a complex procedure is performed with flap rotation.

Coding Tips

These procedure codes are reported for revision only. For an initial tracheostomy, see 31600–31610.

ICD-10-CM Diagnostic Codes

J95.00 Unspecified tracheostomy complication

J95.01 Hemorrhage from tracheostomy stoma

J95.02 Infection of tracheostomy stoma

J95.03 Malfunction of tracheostomy stoma

J95.04 Tracheo-esophageal fistula following tracheostomy

J95.09 Other tracheostomy complication

Z85.21 Personal history of malignant neoplasm of larynx

Relative Value Units/Medicare Edits

Non-Facility RVU	Work	PE	MP	Total
31613	4.71	7.19	0.77	12.67
31614	8.63	11.14	1.29	21.06
Facility RVU	**Work**	**PE**	**MP**	**Total**
31613	4.71	7.19	0.77	12.67
31614	8.63	11.14	1.29	21.06

	FUD	Status	MUE	Modifiers				IOM Reference
31613	90	A	1(2)	51	N/A	N/A	N/A	None
31614	90	A	1(2)	51	N/A	N/A	N/A	

* with documentation

Trachea and Bronchi

31615

31615 Tracheobronchoscopy through established tracheostomy incision

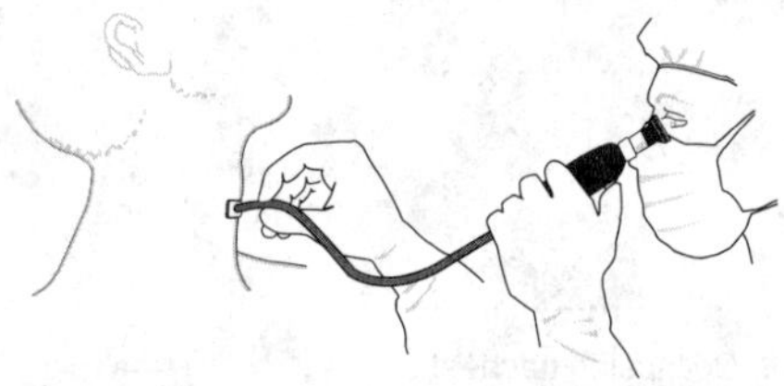

Examination using flexible fiberoptic bronchoscope

Explanation

The physician views the airway using a bronchoscope placed through an existing tracheostomy. The physician examines the conducting airways. The bronchoscope is removed.

Coding Tips

When medically necessary, report moderate (conscious) sedation provided by the performing physician with 99151-99153. When provided by another physician, report 99155-99157. This procedure is similar to a diagnostic bronchoscopy, 31622, except that in 31615 the endoscope is passed through an existing tracheostomy instead of through the oral or nasal cavity. Report the appropriate endoscopy for each anatomic site examined. Surgical endoscopy includes a diagnostic endoscopy; however, diagnostic endoscopy can be identified separately when performed at the same surgical session as an open procedure. For tracheoscopy, see 31515–31574. Report any additional therapeutic procedures separately. Surgical trays, A4550, are not separately reimbursed by Medicare; however, other third-party payers may cover them. Check with the specific payer to determine coverage.

ICD-10-CM Diagnostic Codes

B25.0	Cytomegaloviral pneumonitis
B44.0	Invasive pulmonary aspergillosis
B59	Pneumocystosis
C33	Malignant neoplasm of trachea
C34.01	Malignant neoplasm of right main bronchus ☑
C34.02	Malignant neoplasm of left main bronchus ☑
C34.11	Malignant neoplasm of upper lobe, right bronchus or lung ☑
C34.12	Malignant neoplasm of upper lobe, left bronchus or lung ☑
C34.2	Malignant neoplasm of middle lobe, bronchus or lung
C34.81	Malignant neoplasm of overlapping sites of right bronchus and lung ☑
C34.82	Malignant neoplasm of overlapping sites of left bronchus and lung ☑
C78.01	Secondary malignant neoplasm of right lung ☑
C78.02	Secondary malignant neoplasm of left lung ☑
C78.39	Secondary malignant neoplasm of other respiratory organs
C7A.090	Malignant carcinoid tumor of the bronchus and lung
D02.1	Carcinoma in situ of trachea
D02.21	Carcinoma in situ of right bronchus and lung ☑
D02.22	Carcinoma in situ of left bronchus and lung ☑
D14.2	Benign neoplasm of trachea
D14.31	Benign neoplasm of right bronchus and lung ☑
D14.32	Benign neoplasm of left bronchus and lung ☑
D38.1	Neoplasm of uncertain behavior of trachea, bronchus and lung
D3A.090	Benign carcinoid tumor of the bronchus and lung
D86.0	Sarcoidosis of lung
D86.1	Sarcoidosis of lymph nodes
E84.0	Cystic fibrosis with pulmonary manifestations
J10.08	Influenza due to other identified influenza virus with other specified pneumonia
J11.08	Influenza due to unidentified influenza virus with specified pneumonia
J12.0	Adenoviral pneumonia
J12.1	Respiratory syncytial virus pneumonia
J12.2	Parainfluenza virus pneumonia
J12.3	Human metapneumovirus pneumonia
J12.81	Pneumonia due to SARS-associated coronavirus
J12.89	Other viral pneumonia
J15.212	Pneumonia due to Methicillin resistant Staphylococcus aureus
J17	Pneumonia in diseases classified elsewhere
J44.0	Chronic obstructive pulmonary disease with (acute) lower respiratory infection
J44.1	Chronic obstructive pulmonary disease with (acute) exacerbation
J47.0	Bronchiectasis with acute lower respiratory infection
J47.1	Bronchiectasis with (acute) exacerbation
J47.9	Bronchiectasis, uncomplicated
J67.7	Air conditioner and humidifier lung
J67.8	Hypersensitivity pneumonitis due to other organic dusts
J68.0	Bronchitis and pneumonitis due to chemicals, gases, fumes and vapors
J68.4	Chronic respiratory conditions due to chemicals, gases, fumes and vapors
J69.0	Pneumonitis due to inhalation of food and vomit
J69.1	Pneumonitis due to inhalation of oils and essences
J69.8	Pneumonitis due to inhalation of other solids and liquids
J70.2	Acute drug-induced interstitial lung disorders
J70.3	Chronic drug-induced interstitial lung disorders
J70.5	Respiratory conditions due to smoke inhalation
J95.851	Ventilator associated pneumonia
J95.859	Other complication of respirator [ventilator]
J95.89	Other postprocedural complications and disorders of respiratory system, not elsewhere classified
J96.01	Acute respiratory failure with hypoxia
J96.02	Acute respiratory failure with hypercapnia
J96.11	Chronic respiratory failure with hypoxia
J96.12	Chronic respiratory failure with hypercapnia
J96.21	Acute and chronic respiratory failure with hypoxia
J96.22	Acute and chronic respiratory failure with hypercapnia
J98.09	Other diseases of bronchus, not elsewhere classified
J98.4	Other disorders of lung
J98.8	Other specified respiratory disorders
Q32.0	Congenital tracheomalacia
Q32.1	Other congenital malformations of trachea
Q32.2	Congenital bronchomalacia
T17.510A	Gastric contents in bronchus causing asphyxiation, initial encounter

T17.518A Gastric contents in bronchus causing other injury, initial encounter

T17.520A Food in bronchus causing asphyxiation, initial encounter

T17.528A Food in bronchus causing other injury, initial encounter

T17.590A Other foreign object in bronchus causing asphyxiation, initial encounter

T17.598A Other foreign object in bronchus causing other injury, initial encounter

T17.810A Gastric contents in other parts of respiratory tract causing asphyxiation, initial encounter

T17.818A Gastric contents in other parts of respiratory tract causing other injury, initial encounter

T17.820A Food in other parts of respiratory tract causing asphyxiation, initial encounter

T17.828A Food in other parts of respiratory tract causing other injury, initial encounter

T17.890A Other foreign object in other parts of respiratory tract causing asphyxiation, initial encounter

T17.898A Other foreign object in other parts of respiratory tract causing other injury, initial encounter

T17.910A Gastric contents in respiratory tract, part unspecified causing asphyxiation, initial encounter

T17.918A Gastric contents in respiratory tract, part unspecified causing other injury, initial encounter

T17.920A Food in respiratory tract, part unspecified causing asphyxiation, initial encounter

T17.928A Food in respiratory tract, part unspecified causing other injury, initial encounter

T17.990A Other foreign object in respiratory tract, part unspecified in causing asphyxiation, initial encounter

T17.998A Other foreign object in respiratory tract, part unspecified causing other injury, initial encounter

AMA: **31615** 2018,Jan,8; 2017,Jan,8; 2016,Jan,13; 2015,Jan,16; 2014,Jan,11; 2013,Mar,8-9

Relative Value Units/Medicare Edits

Non-Facility RVU	Work	PE	MP	Total
31615	1.84	2.74	0.25	4.83
Facility RVU	**Work**	**PE**	**MP**	**Total**
31615	1.84	1.2	0.25	3.29

	FUD	Status	MUE	Modifiers				IOM Reference
31615	0	A	1(3)	51	N/A	N/A	N/A	None

* with documentation

31622-31624

31622 Bronchoscopy, rigid or flexible, including fluoroscopic guidance, when performed; diagnostic, with cell washing, when performed (separate procedure)

31623 with brushing or protected brushings

31624 with bronchial alveolar lavage

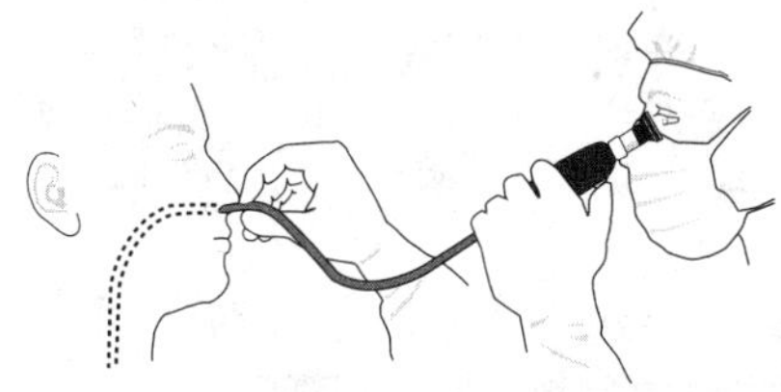

Examination using flexible fiberoptic bronchoscope

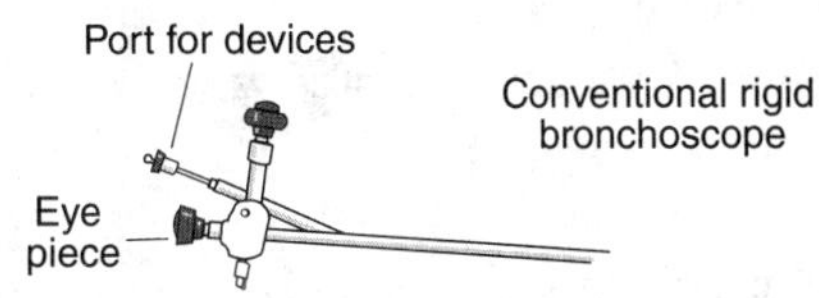

Explanation

The physician views the airway using a flexible fiberoptic or rigid bronchoscope that is introduced through the nasal or oral cavity. The airway is anesthetized. The bronchoscope is inserted and advanced through the nasal or oral cavity, past the larynx to inspect the bronchus. In 31622, after diagnostic visualization of the bronchus, cell washings may be obtained through the bronchoscope. In 31623, sample lung tissue is obtained with brushings or protected brushing through the scope. In 31624, the bronchoscopy includes bronchial alveolar lavage, which allows lung tissue to be sampled by irrigating with saline followed by suctioning the fluid. The bronchoscope is removed. These codes include fluoroscopic guidance, when performed.

Coding Tips

When medically necessary, report moderate (conscious) sedation provided by the performing physician with 99151-99153. When provided by another physician, report 99155-99157. Note that 31622, a separate procedure by definition, is usually a component of a more complex service and is not identified separately. When performed alone or with other unrelated procedures/services, it may be reported. If performed alone, list the code; if performed with other procedures/services, list the code and append modifier 59 or an X{EPSU} modifier. Report the appropriate endoscopy for each anatomic site examined. Surgical endoscopy includes a diagnostic endoscopy; however, diagnostic endoscopy can be identified separately when performed at the same surgical session as an open procedure. Fluoroscopic guidance is not reported separately.

ICD-10-CM Diagnostic Codes

B25.0 Cytomegaloviral pneumonitis

B44.0 Invasive pulmonary aspergillosis

B59 Pneumocystosis

C34.01 Malignant neoplasm of right main bronchus ☑

C34.02 Malignant neoplasm of left main bronchus ☑

C34.11 Malignant neoplasm of upper lobe, right bronchus or lung ☑

C34.12 Malignant neoplasm of upper lobe, left bronchus or lung ☑

C34.2 Malignant neoplasm of middle lobe, bronchus or lung

C34.31 Malignant neoplasm of lower lobe, right bronchus or lung ☑

C34.32 Malignant neoplasm of lower lobe, left bronchus or lung ☑

C34.81 Malignant neoplasm of overlapping sites of right bronchus and lung ☑
C34.82 Malignant neoplasm of overlapping sites of left bronchus and lung ☑
C78.01 Secondary malignant neoplasm of right lung ☑
C78.02 Secondary malignant neoplasm of left lung ☑
C78.39 Secondary malignant neoplasm of other respiratory organs
C7A.090 Malignant carcinoid tumor of the bronchus and lung
D02.1 Carcinoma in situ of trachea
D02.21 Carcinoma in situ of right bronchus and lung ☑
D02.22 Carcinoma in situ of left bronchus and lung ☑
D14.2 Benign neoplasm of trachea
D86.0 Sarcoidosis of lung
E84.0 Cystic fibrosis with pulmonary manifestations
J10.08 Influenza due to other identified influenza virus with other specified pneumonia
J11.08 Influenza due to unidentified influenza virus with specified pneumonia
J12.0 Adenoviral pneumonia
J12.1 Respiratory syncytial virus pneumonia
J12.2 Parainfluenza virus pneumonia
J12.3 Human metapneumovirus pneumonia
J12.81 Pneumonia due to SARS-associated coronavirus
J12.89 Other viral pneumonia
J15.212 Pneumonia due to Methicillin resistant Staphylococcus aureus
J17 Pneumonia in diseases classified elsewhere
J41.0 Simple chronic bronchitis
J41.1 Mucopurulent chronic bronchitis
J43.0 Unilateral pulmonary emphysema [MacLeod's syndrome]
J43.1 Panlobular emphysema
J43.2 Centrilobular emphysema
J43.8 Other emphysema
J44.0 Chronic obstructive pulmonary disease with (acute) lower respiratory infection
J44.1 Chronic obstructive pulmonary disease with (acute) exacerbation
J47.0 Bronchiectasis with acute lower respiratory infection
J47.1 Bronchiectasis with (acute) exacerbation
J60 Coalworker's pneumoconiosis
J63.0 Aluminosis (of lung)
J63.1 Bauxite fibrosis (of lung)
J63.2 Berylliosis
J63.3 Graphite fibrosis (of lung)
J63.4 Siderosis
J63.5 Stannosis
J65 Pneumoconiosis associated with tuberculosis
J66.0 Byssinosis
J66.1 Flax-dressers' disease
J66.2 Cannabinosis
J70.2 Acute drug-induced interstitial lung disorders
J70.3 Chronic drug-induced interstitial lung disorders
J70.5 Respiratory conditions due to smoke inhalation
J84.114 Acute interstitial pneumonitis
J84.115 Respiratory bronchiolitis interstitial lung disease
J84.2 Lymphoid interstitial pneumonia
J85.0 Gangrene and necrosis of lung
J85.1 Abscess of lung with pneumonia
J95.4 Chemical pneumonitis due to anesthesia
J95.821 Acute postprocedural respiratory failure
J95.822 Acute and chronic postprocedural respiratory failure
J95.851 Ventilator associated pneumonia
J95.859 Other complication of respirator [ventilator]
J95.89 Other postprocedural complications and disorders of respiratory system, not elsewhere classified
J96.01 Acute respiratory failure with hypoxia
J96.02 Acute respiratory failure with hypercapnia
J96.11 Chronic respiratory failure with hypoxia
J96.12 Chronic respiratory failure with hypercapnia
J96.21 Acute and chronic respiratory failure with hypoxia
J96.22 Acute and chronic respiratory failure with hypercapnia
J98.09 Other diseases of bronchus, not elsewhere classified
J98.11 Atelectasis
J98.19 Other pulmonary collapse
J98.4 Other disorders of lung
J98.8 Other specified respiratory disorders
J99 Respiratory disorders in diseases classified elsewhere
M32.13 Lung involvement in systemic lupus erythematosus
M33.01 Juvenile dermatomyositis with respiratory involvement
M35.02 Sicca syndrome with lung involvement
P27.0 Wilson-Mikity syndrome
P27.1 Bronchopulmonary dysplasia originating in the perinatal period
Q32.2 Congenital bronchomalacia

AMA: **31622** 2018,Jan,8; 2017,Jan,8; 2016,Jan,13; 2016,Apr,5; 2015,Jan,16; 2014,Jan,11; 2013,Mar,8-9 **31623** 2018,Jan,8; 2017,Jan,8; 2016,Jan,13; 2016,Apr,5; 2015,Jan,16; 2014,Jan,11; 2013,Mar,8-9 **31624** 2018,Jan,8; 2017,Jun,10; 2017,Jan,8; 2016,Jan,13; 2016,Apr,5; 2015,Jan,16; 2014,Jan,11; 2013,Mar,8-9

Relative Value Units/Medicare Edits

Non-Facility RVU	Work	PE	MP	Total
31622	2.53	4.04	0.27	6.84
31623	2.63	4.66	0.22	7.51
31624	2.63	4.24	0.23	7.1
Facility RVU	**Work**	**PE**	**MP**	**Total**
31622	2.53	0.98	0.27	3.78
31623	2.63	0.96	0.22	3.81
31624	2.63	1.0	0.23	3.86

	FUD	Status	MUE	Modifiers				IOM Reference
31622	0	A	1(3)	51	N/A	N/A	N/A	None
31623	0	A	1(3)	51	N/A	N/A	N/A	
31624	0	A	1(3)	51	N/A	N/A	N/A	

* with documentation

31625

31625 Bronchoscopy, rigid or flexible, including fluoroscopic guidance, when performed; with bronchial or endobronchial biopsy(s), single or multiple sites

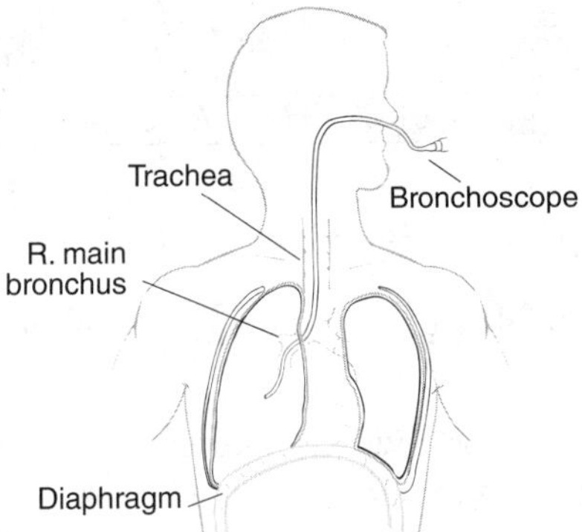

Examination using flexible fiberoptic bronchoscope

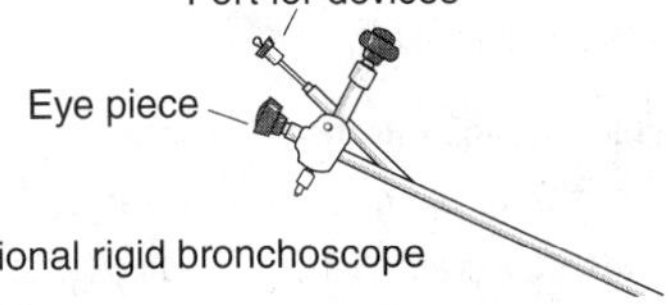

Conventional rigid bronchoscope

Explanation

The physician views the airway using a flexible fiberoptic or rigid bronchoscope that is introduced through the nasal or oral cavity. The airway is anesthetized. The bronchoscope is inserted and advanced through the nasal or oral cavity, past the larynx to inspect the bronchus, including fluoroscopic guidance, if used. After diagnostic visualization of the bronchus, a sample of bronchial or endobronchial tissue is removed for study. More than one site may be biopsied. Bleeding is assessed and controlled, and the bronchoscope is removed.

Coding Tips

When medically necessary, report moderate (conscious) sedation provided by the performing physician with 99151-99153. When provided by another physician, report 99155-99157. Surgical endoscopy includes a diagnostic endoscopy; however, diagnostic endoscopy can be identified separately when performed at the same surgical session as an open procedure. Fluoroscopic guidance is not reported separately.

ICD-10-CM Diagnostic Codes

B59	Pneumocystosis
C33	Malignant neoplasm of trachea
C34.01	Malignant neoplasm of right main bronchus ☑
C34.02	Malignant neoplasm of left main bronchus ☑
C34.11	Malignant neoplasm of upper lobe, right bronchus or lung ☑
C34.12	Malignant neoplasm of upper lobe, left bronchus or lung ☑
C34.2	Malignant neoplasm of middle lobe, bronchus or lung
C34.31	Malignant neoplasm of lower lobe, right bronchus or lung ☑
C34.32	Malignant neoplasm of lower lobe, left bronchus or lung ☑
C34.81	Malignant neoplasm of overlapping sites of right bronchus and lung ☑
C34.82	Malignant neoplasm of overlapping sites of left bronchus and lung ☑
C77.1	Secondary and unspecified malignant neoplasm of intrathoracic lymph nodes
C78.01	Secondary malignant neoplasm of right lung ☑
C78.02	Secondary malignant neoplasm of left lung ☑
C78.39	Secondary malignant neoplasm of other respiratory organs
C79.89	Secondary malignant neoplasm of other specified sites
C7A.090	Malignant carcinoid tumor of the bronchus and lung
C81.02	Nodular lymphocyte predominant Hodgkin lymphoma, intrathoracic lymph nodes
C81.12	Nodular sclerosis Hodgkin lymphoma, intrathoracic lymph nodes
C81.22	Mixed cellularity Hodgkin lymphoma, intrathoracic lymph nodes
C81.32	Lymphocyte depleted Hodgkin lymphoma, intrathoracic lymph nodes
C81.42	Lymphocyte-rich Hodgkin lymphoma, intrathoracic lymph nodes
C81.72	Other Hodgkin lymphoma, intrathoracic lymph nodes
C82.02	Follicular lymphoma grade I, intrathoracic lymph nodes
C82.12	Follicular lymphoma grade II, intrathoracic lymph nodes
C82.32	Follicular lymphoma grade IIIa, intrathoracic lymph nodes
C82.52	Diffuse follicle center lymphoma, intrathoracic lymph nodes
C83.02	Small cell B-cell lymphoma, intrathoracic lymph nodes
C83.12	Mantle cell lymphoma, intrathoracic lymph nodes
C83.32	Diffuse large B-cell lymphoma, intrathoracic lymph nodes
C83.52	Lymphoblastic (diffuse) lymphoma, intrathoracic lymph nodes
C83.72	Burkitt lymphoma, intrathoracic lymph nodes
D02.1	Carcinoma in situ of trachea
D02.21	Carcinoma in situ of right bronchus and lung ☑
D02.22	Carcinoma in situ of left bronchus and lung ☑
D14.2	Benign neoplasm of trachea
D14.31	Benign neoplasm of right bronchus and lung ☑
D14.32	Benign neoplasm of left bronchus and lung ☑
D38.1	Neoplasm of uncertain behavior of trachea, bronchus and lung
D3A.090	Benign carcinoid tumor of the bronchus and lung
D49.1	Neoplasm of unspecified behavior of respiratory system
D86.0	Sarcoidosis of lung
D86.1	Sarcoidosis of lymph nodes
D86.2	Sarcoidosis of lung with sarcoidosis of lymph nodes
J15.212	Pneumonia due to Methicillin resistant Staphylococcus aureus
J18.0	Bronchopneumonia, unspecified organism
J18.2	Hypostatic pneumonia, unspecified organism
J18.8	Other pneumonia, unspecified organism
J18.9	Pneumonia, unspecified organism
J39.8	Other specified diseases of upper respiratory tract
J60	Coalworker's pneumoconiosis
J61	Pneumoconiosis due to asbestos and other mineral fibers
J62.0	Pneumoconiosis due to talc dust
J62.8	Pneumoconiosis due to other dust containing silica
J63.0	Aluminosis (of lung)
J63.1	Bauxite fibrosis (of lung)
J63.2	Berylliosis
J63.3	Graphite fibrosis (of lung)
J63.4	Siderosis
J63.5	Stannosis
J63.6	Pneumoconiosis due to other specified inorganic dusts

J65	Pneumoconiosis associated with tuberculosis
J66.0	Byssinosis
J66.1	Flax-dressers' disease
J66.2	Cannabinosis
J66.8	Airway disease due to other specific organic dusts
J67.8	Hypersensitivity pneumonitis due to other organic dusts
J68.0	Bronchitis and pneumonitis due to chemicals, gases, fumes and vapors
J68.4	Chronic respiratory conditions due to chemicals, gases, fumes and vapors
J69.0	Pneumonitis due to inhalation of food and vomit
J69.1	Pneumonitis due to inhalation of oils and essences
J69.8	Pneumonitis due to inhalation of other solids and liquids
J70.1	Chronic and other pulmonary manifestations due to radiation
J70.2	Acute drug-induced interstitial lung disorders
J70.3	Chronic drug-induced interstitial lung disorders
J82	Pulmonary eosinophilia, not elsewhere classified
J84.01	Alveolar proteinosis
J84.02	Pulmonary alveolar microlithiasis
J84.03	Idiopathic pulmonary hemosiderosis
J84.09	Other alveolar and parieto-alveolar conditions
J84.112	Idiopathic pulmonary fibrosis
J84.113	Idiopathic non-specific interstitial pneumonitis
J84.114	Acute interstitial pneumonitis
J84.115	Respiratory bronchiolitis interstitial lung disease
J84.116	Cryptogenic organizing pneumonia
J84.117	Desquamative interstitial pneumonia
J84.17	Other interstitial pulmonary diseases with fibrosis in diseases classified elsewhere
J84.2	Lymphoid interstitial pneumonia
J84.82	Adult pulmonary Langerhans cell histiocytosis
J84.83	Surfactant mutations of the lung
J84.841	Neuroendocrine cell hyperplasia of infancy
J84.842	Pulmonary interstitial glycogenosis
J84.848	Other interstitial lung diseases of childhood
J84.89	Other specified interstitial pulmonary diseases
J85.0	Gangrene and necrosis of lung
J85.1	Abscess of lung with pneumonia
J85.2	Abscess of lung without pneumonia
J98.11	Atelectasis
M32.13	Lung involvement in systemic lupus erythematosus
M33.01	Juvenile dermatomyositis with respiratory involvement
M33.11	Other dermatomyositis with respiratory involvement
M33.21	Polymyositis with respiratory involvement
M35.02	Sicca syndrome with lung involvement

AMA: 31625 2018,Jan,8; 2017,Jan,8; 2016,Jan,13; 2016,Apr,5; 2015,Jan,16; 2014,Jan,11; 2013,Mar,8-9

Relative Value Units/Medicare Edits

Non-Facility RVU	Work	PE	MP	Total
31625	3.11	6.21	0.27	9.59
Facility RVU	**Work**	**PE**	**MP**	**Total**
31625	3.11	1.11	0.27	4.49

	FUD	Status	MUE	Modifiers				IOM Reference
31625	0	A	1(2)	51	N/A	N/A	N/A	None

* with documentation

Terms To Know

biopsy. Tissue or fluid removed for diagnostic purposes through analysis of the cells in the biopsy material.

bronchoscope. Endoscopic instrument used for the diagnosis, inspection, and treatment of the tracheobronchial tree.

fluoroscopy. Radiology technique that allows visual examination of part of the body or a function of an organ using a device that projects an x-ray image on a fluorescent screen.

larynx. Musculocartilaginous structure between the trachea and the pharynx that functions as the valve preventing food and other particles from entering the respiratory tract, as well as the voice mechanism.

31626

31626 Bronchoscopy, rigid or flexible, including fluoroscopic guidance, when performed; with placement of fiducial markers, single or multiple

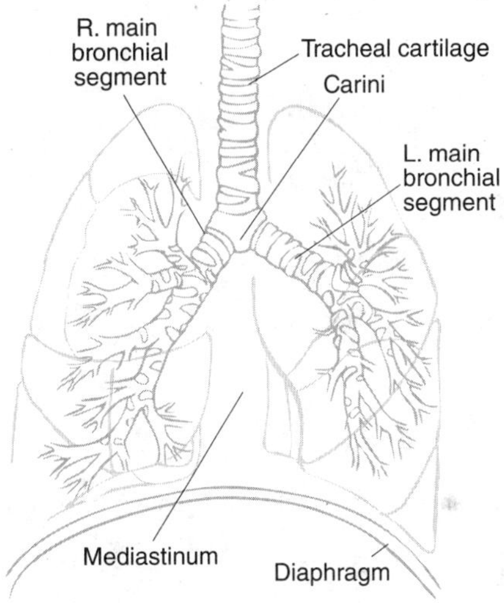

Explanation

The physician views the airway using a flexible fiberoptic or rigid bronchoscope that is introduced through the nasal or oral cavity. The airway is anesthetized. The bronchoscope is inserted and advanced through the nasal or oral cavity, past the larynx to inspect the bronchus, including fluoroscopic guidance, if used. After diagnostic visualization of the bronchus, one or more fiducial markers are placed.

Coding Tips

When medically necessary, report moderate (conscious) sedation provided by the performing physician with 99151-99153. When provided by another physician, report 99155-99157. Supplies used when providing this procedure may be reported with the appropriate HCPCS Level II code. Check with the specific payer to determine coverage.

ICD-10-CM Diagnostic Codes

C33	Malignant neoplasm of trachea
C34.01	Malignant neoplasm of right main bronchus ☑
C34.02	Malignant neoplasm of left main bronchus ☑
C34.11	Malignant neoplasm of upper lobe, right bronchus or lung ☑
C34.12	Malignant neoplasm of upper lobe, left bronchus or lung ☑
C34.2	Malignant neoplasm of middle lobe, bronchus or lung
C34.31	Malignant neoplasm of lower lobe, right bronchus or lung ☑
C34.32	Malignant neoplasm of lower lobe, left bronchus or lung ☑
C34.81	Malignant neoplasm of overlapping sites of right bronchus and lung ☑
C34.82	Malignant neoplasm of overlapping sites of left bronchus and lung ☑
C77.1	Secondary and unspecified malignant neoplasm of intrathoracic lymph nodes
C78.01	Secondary malignant neoplasm of right lung ☑
C78.02	Secondary malignant neoplasm of left lung ☑
C78.39	Secondary malignant neoplasm of other respiratory organs
C7A.090	Malignant carcinoid tumor of the bronchus and lung
D02.1	Carcinoma in situ of trachea
D02.21	Carcinoma in situ of right bronchus and lung ☑
D02.22	Carcinoma in situ of left bronchus and lung ☑

AMA: 31626 2018,Jan,8; 2017,Jun,10; 2017,Jan,8; 2016,Jan,13; 2016,Apr,5; 2015,Jun,6; 2015,Jan,16; 2014,Jan,11; 2013,Mar,8-9

Relative Value Units/Medicare Edits

Non-Facility RVU	Work	PE	MP	Total
31626	3.91	19.59	0.44	23.94
Facility RVU	**Work**	**PE**	**MP**	**Total**
31626	3.91	1.37	0.44	5.72

	FUD	Status	MUE	Modifiers				IOM Reference
31626	0	A	1(2)	51	N/A	N/A	80*	None

* with documentation

Terms To Know

fluoroscopy. Radiology technique that allows visual examination of part of the body or a function of an organ using a device that projects an x-ray image on a fluorescent screen.

larynx. Musculocartilaginous structure between the trachea and the pharynx that functions as the valve preventing food and other particles from entering the respiratory tract, as well as the voice mechanism.

malignant. Any condition tending to progress toward death, specifically an invasive tumor with a loss of cellular differentiation that has the ability to spread or metastasize to other body areas.

mediastinum. Collection of organs and tissues that separate the pleural sacs. Located between the sternum and spine above the diaphragm, it contains the heart and great vessels, trachea and bronchi, esophagus, thymus, lymph nodes, and nerves.

31627

+ 31627 Bronchoscopy, rigid or flexible, including fluoroscopic guidance, when performed; with computer-assisted, image-guided navigation (List separately in addition to code for primary procedure[s])

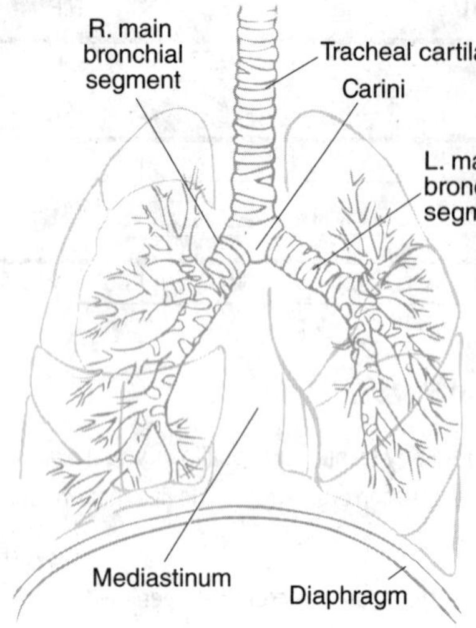

Explanation

The physician views the airway using a flexible fiberoptic or rigid bronchoscope that is introduced through the nasal or oral cavity. The airway is anesthetized. The bronchoscope is inserted and advanced through the nasal or oral cavity, past the larynx to inspect the bronchus, including fluoroscopic guidance, if used. This code reports the use of computer-assisted, image-guided navigation, and includes 3D reconstruction.

Coding Tips

Use 31627 in addition to 31615, 31622–31626, 31628–31631, 31635, 31636, and 31638–31643. Do not report 31627 with 76376 and 76377. When medically necessary, report moderate (conscious) sedation provided by the performing physician with 99151-99153. When provided by another physician, report 99155-99157.

ICD-10-CM Diagnostic Codes

This/these CPT code(s) are add on code(s). See the primary procedure code that this code is performed with for your ICD-10-CM code selections. Diagnostic code(s) would be the same as the actual procedure performed.

AMA: 31627 2018,Jan,8; 2017,Jan,8; 2016,Jan,13; 2015,Jan,16; 2014,Jan,11; 2013,Mar,8-9

Relative Value Units/Medicare Edits

Non-Facility RVU	Work	PE	MP	Total
31627	2.0	35.62	0.2	37.82
Facility RVU	**Work**	**PE**	**MP**	**Total**
31627	2.0	0.6	0.2	2.8

	FUD	Status	MUE	Modifiers				IOM Reference
31627	N/A	A	1(3)	N/A	N/A	N/A	80*	None

* with documentation

31628-31629

31628 Bronchoscopy, rigid or flexible, including fluoroscopic guidance, when performed; with transbronchial lung biopsy(s), single lobe

31629 with transbronchial needle aspiration biopsy(s), trachea, main stem and/or lobar bronchus(i)

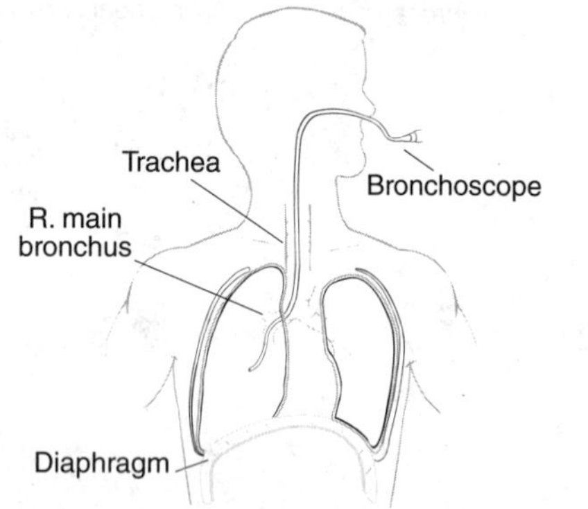

Examination using flexible fiberoptic bronchoscope

Explanation

The physician views the airway using a flexible fiberoptic or rigid bronchoscope that is introduced through the nasal or oral cavity. The airway is anesthetized. The bronchoscope is inserted and advanced through the nasal or oral cavity, past the larynx to inspect the bronchus, including fluoroscopic guidance, if used. After diagnostic visualization of the bronchus, the physician passes closed biopsy forceps (31628) through a channel in the bronchoscope and through the bronchial wall to obtain one or more lung tissue samples from a single lobe. Alternately, the physician passes a needle (31629) through a channel in the bronchoscope and through the bronchial wall to obtain one or more aspiration biopsies of the trachea, main stem, and/or lobar bronchi. Bleeding is assessed and controlled, and the bronchoscope is removed.

Coding Tips

When these procedures are performed with another separately identifiable procedure, the highest dollar value code is listed as the primary procedure, and subsequent procedures are appended with modifier 51. When medically necessary, report moderate (conscious) sedation provided by the performing physician with 99151-99153. When provided by another physician, report 99155-99157. Report the appropriate endoscopy for each anatomic site examined. Surgical endoscopy includes a diagnostic endoscopy; however, diagnostic endoscopy can be identified separately when performed at the same surgical session as an open procedure. Fluoroscopic guidance is not reported separately. Codes 31628 and 31629 are reported only once regardless of how many biopsies are performed in the lobe or upper airway. For transbronchial lung biopsies performed on an additional lobe, see 31632.

ICD-10-CM Diagnostic Codes

B59	Pneumocystosis
C33	Malignant neoplasm of trachea
C34.01	Malignant neoplasm of right main bronchus ☑
C34.02	Malignant neoplasm of left main bronchus ☑
C34.11	Malignant neoplasm of upper lobe, right bronchus or lung ☑
C34.12	Malignant neoplasm of upper lobe, left bronchus or lung ☑
C34.2	Malignant neoplasm of middle lobe, bronchus or lung
C34.31	Malignant neoplasm of lower lobe, right bronchus or lung ☑
C34.32	Malignant neoplasm of lower lobe, left bronchus or lung ☑

C34.81 Malignant neoplasm of overlapping sites of right bronchus and lung ☑
C34.82 Malignant neoplasm of overlapping sites of left bronchus and lung ☑
C77.1 Secondary and unspecified malignant neoplasm of intrathoracic lymph nodes
C78.01 Secondary malignant neoplasm of right lung ☑
C78.02 Secondary malignant neoplasm of left lung ☑
C78.39 Secondary malignant neoplasm of other respiratory organs
C79.89 Secondary malignant neoplasm of other specified sites
C7A.090 Malignant carcinoid tumor of the bronchus and lung
C81.02 Nodular lymphocyte predominant Hodgkin lymphoma, intrathoracic lymph nodes
C81.12 Nodular sclerosis Hodgkin lymphoma, intrathoracic lymph nodes
C81.22 Mixed cellularity Hodgkin lymphoma, intrathoracic lymph nodes
C81.32 Lymphocyte depleted Hodgkin lymphoma, intrathoracic lymph nodes
C81.42 Lymphocyte-rich Hodgkin lymphoma, intrathoracic lymph nodes
C81.72 Other Hodgkin lymphoma, intrathoracic lymph nodes
C82.02 Follicular lymphoma grade I, intrathoracic lymph nodes
C82.12 Follicular lymphoma grade II, intrathoracic lymph nodes
C82.32 Follicular lymphoma grade IIIa, intrathoracic lymph nodes
C82.52 Diffuse follicle center lymphoma, intrathoracic lymph nodes
C83.02 Small cell B-cell lymphoma, intrathoracic lymph nodes
C83.12 Mantle cell lymphoma, intrathoracic lymph nodes
C83.32 Diffuse large B-cell lymphoma, intrathoracic lymph nodes
C83.52 Lymphoblastic (diffuse) lymphoma, intrathoracic lymph nodes
C83.72 Burkitt lymphoma, intrathoracic lymph nodes
D02.1 Carcinoma in situ of trachea
D02.21 Carcinoma in situ of right bronchus and lung ☑
D02.22 Carcinoma in situ of left bronchus and lung ☑
D14.2 Benign neoplasm of trachea
D14.31 Benign neoplasm of right bronchus and lung ☑
D14.32 Benign neoplasm of left bronchus and lung ☑
D19.0 Benign neoplasm of mesothelial tissue of pleura
D38.1 Neoplasm of uncertain behavior of trachea, bronchus and lung
D3A.090 Benign carcinoid tumor of the bronchus and lung
D49.1 Neoplasm of unspecified behavior of respiratory system
D86.0 Sarcoidosis of lung
D86.1 Sarcoidosis of lymph nodes
D86.2 Sarcoidosis of lung with sarcoidosis of lymph nodes
J15.212 Pneumonia due to Methicillin resistant Staphylococcus aureus
J39.8 Other specified diseases of upper respiratory tract
J60 Coalworker's pneumoconiosis
J61 Pneumoconiosis due to asbestos and other mineral fibers
J62.0 Pneumoconiosis due to talc dust
J62.8 Pneumoconiosis due to other dust containing silica
J63.0 Aluminosis (of lung)
J63.1 Bauxite fibrosis (of lung)
J63.2 Berylliosis
J63.3 Graphite fibrosis (of lung)
J63.4 Siderosis
J63.5 Stannosis
J63.6 Pneumoconiosis due to other specified inorganic dusts
J65 Pneumoconiosis associated with tuberculosis
J66.0 Byssinosis
J66.1 Flax-dressers' disease
J66.2 Cannabinosis
J66.8 Airway disease due to other specific organic dusts
J67.8 Hypersensitivity pneumonitis due to other organic dusts
J68.0 Bronchitis and pneumonitis due to chemicals, gases, fumes and vapors
J68.4 Chronic respiratory conditions due to chemicals, gases, fumes and vapors
J69.0 Pneumonitis due to inhalation of food and vomit
J69.1 Pneumonitis due to inhalation of oils and essences
J69.8 Pneumonitis due to inhalation of other solids and liquids
J70.1 Chronic and other pulmonary manifestations due to radiation
J70.2 Acute drug-induced interstitial lung disorders
J70.3 Chronic drug-induced interstitial lung disorders
J82 Pulmonary eosinophilia, not elsewhere classified
J84.01 Alveolar proteinosis
J84.02 Pulmonary alveolar microlithiasis
J84.03 Idiopathic pulmonary hemosiderosis
J84.09 Other alveolar and parieto-alveolar conditions
J84.112 Idiopathic pulmonary fibrosis
J84.113 Idiopathic non-specific interstitial pneumonitis
J84.114 Acute interstitial pneumonitis
J84.115 Respiratory bronchiolitis interstitial lung disease
J84.116 Cryptogenic organizing pneumonia
J84.117 Desquamative interstitial pneumonia
J84.17 Other interstitial pulmonary diseases with fibrosis in diseases classified elsewhere
J84.2 Lymphoid interstitial pneumonia
J84.82 Adult pulmonary Langerhans cell histiocytosis
J84.83 Surfactant mutations of the lung
J84.841 Neuroendocrine cell hyperplasia of infancy
J84.842 Pulmonary interstitial glycogenosis
J84.848 Other interstitial lung diseases of childhood
J84.89 Other specified interstitial pulmonary diseases
J85.0 Gangrene and necrosis of lung
J85.1 Abscess of lung with pneumonia
J85.2 Abscess of lung without pneumonia
J98.11 Atelectasis
M32.13 Lung involvement in systemic lupus erythematosus
M33.01 Juvenile dermatomyositis with respiratory involvement
M33.11 Other dermatomyositis with respiratory involvement
M33.21 Polymyositis with respiratory involvement
M35.02 Sicca syndrome with lung involvement

AMA: **31628** 2018,Jan,8; 2017,Jun,10; 2017,Jan,8; 2016,Jan,13; 2016,Apr,5; 2015,Jan,16; 2014,Jan,11; 2013,Mar,8-9 **31629** 2018,Jan,8; 2017,Jan,8; 2016,Jan,13; 2016,Apr,5; 2015,Jan,16; 2014,Jan,11; 2013,Mar,8-9

Relative Value Units/Medicare Edits

Non-Facility RVU	Work	PE	MP	Total
31628	3.55	6.35	0.28	10.18
31629	3.75	8.51	0.33	12.59

Facility RVU	Work	PE	MP	Total
31628	3.55	1.23	0.28	5.06
31629	3.75	1.3	0.33	5.38

	FUD	Status	MUE	Modifiers				IOM Reference
31628	0	A	1(2)	51	N/A	N/A	N/A	None
31629	0	A	1(2)	51	N/A	N/A	N/A	

* with documentation

Terms To Know

atelectasis. Collapse of lung tissue affecting part or all of one lung, preventing normal oxygen absorption to healthy tissues.

bronchoscope. Endoscopic instrument used for the diagnosis, inspection, and treatment of the tracheobronchial tree.

histiocytosis. Blood disease in which there is an abnormal multiplication of white blood cells.

sarcoidosis. Clustering of immune cells resulting in granuloma formation. Often affects the lungs and lymphatic system but can occur in other body sites.

31630-31631

31630 Bronchoscopy, rigid or flexible, including fluoroscopic guidance, when performed; with tracheal/bronchial dilation or closed reduction of fracture

31631 with placement of tracheal stent(s) (includes tracheal/bronchial dilation as required)

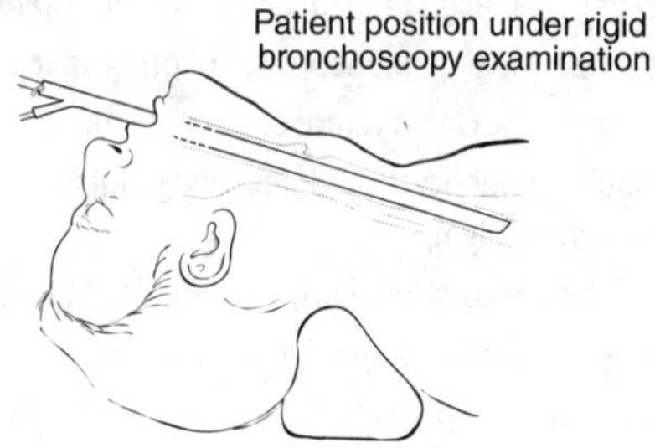

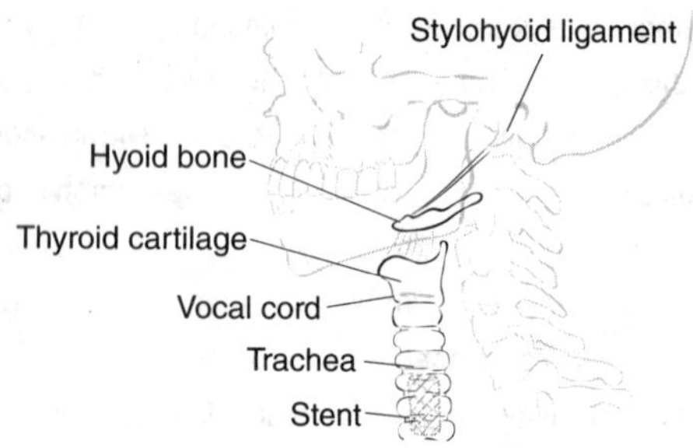

Explanation

The physician performs tracheal/bronchial dilation or closed fracture reduction using a flexible fiberoptic or rigid bronchoscope introduced through the nasal or oral cavity. The physician uses the views obtained through the bronchoscope to identify any narrowing or fracture of the trachea or bronchus. The physician introduces a wire through the narrowed or fractured part of the airway and removes the bronchoscope. A series of dilators or stents are passed over the wire to open the airway until sufficient dilation or closed reduction of the stricture or fracture is accomplished. This may be done with or without fluoroscopic guidance. In 31631, the physician places a tracheal stent or stents using a flexible fiberoptic or rigid bronchoscope introduced through the nasal or oral cavity, using local anesthesia of the patient's airway. The physician uses the views obtained through the bronchoscope to identify any narrowing or area of the trachea that requires stenting for support. The physician introduces a wire through the narrowed part of the trachea and removes the bronchoscope. If dilation is first required, a series of dilators are passed over the wire to open the airway until sufficient tracheal/bronchial dilation is accomplished. A stent is passed over the wire to the target area in the trachea and positioned in place to maintain an open airway.

Coding Tips

When 31630 or 31631 is performed with another separately identifiable procedure, the highest dollar value code is listed as the primary procedure, and subsequent procedures are appended with modifier 51. When endoscopic procedures are performed, report the appropriate endoscopy of each anatomic site examined. Surgical endoscopy includes a diagnostic endoscopy; however, diagnostic endoscopy can be reported separately when performed at the same surgical session as an open procedure. For bronchial stent placement, see 31636 and 31637. For tracheal/bronchial stent revision, see 31638.

ICD-10-CM Diagnostic Codes

C33 Malignant neoplasm of trachea

C34.01	Malignant neoplasm of right main bronchus ☑
C34.02	Malignant neoplasm of left main bronchus ☑
C34.11	Malignant neoplasm of upper lobe, right bronchus or lung ☑
C34.12	Malignant neoplasm of upper lobe, left bronchus or lung ☑
C34.2	Malignant neoplasm of middle lobe, bronchus or lung
C34.31	Malignant neoplasm of lower lobe, right bronchus or lung ☑
C34.32	Malignant neoplasm of lower lobe, left bronchus or lung ☑
C34.81	Malignant neoplasm of overlapping sites of right bronchus and lung ☑
C34.82	Malignant neoplasm of overlapping sites of left bronchus and lung ☑
C78.01	Secondary malignant neoplasm of right lung ☑
C78.02	Secondary malignant neoplasm of left lung ☑
C81.02	Nodular lymphocyte predominant Hodgkin lymphoma, intrathoracic lymph nodes
C81.12	Nodular sclerosis Hodgkin lymphoma, intrathoracic lymph nodes
C81.22	Mixed cellularity Hodgkin lymphoma, intrathoracic lymph nodes
C81.32	Lymphocyte depleted Hodgkin lymphoma, intrathoracic lymph nodes
C81.42	Lymphocyte-rich Hodgkin lymphoma, intrathoracic lymph nodes
C81.72	Other Hodgkin lymphoma, intrathoracic lymph nodes
C82.32	Follicular lymphoma grade IIIa, intrathoracic lymph nodes
C82.52	Diffuse follicle center lymphoma, intrathoracic lymph nodes
C83.12	Mantle cell lymphoma, intrathoracic lymph nodes
C83.32	Diffuse large B-cell lymphoma, intrathoracic lymph nodes
C83.52	Lymphoblastic (diffuse) lymphoma, intrathoracic lymph nodes
C83.72	Burkitt lymphoma, intrathoracic lymph nodes
D14.2	Benign neoplasm of trachea
D14.31	Benign neoplasm of right bronchus and lung ☑
D14.32	Benign neoplasm of left bronchus and lung ☑
D38.1	Neoplasm of uncertain behavior of trachea, bronchus and lung
D3A.090	Benign carcinoid tumor of the bronchus and lung
D86.0	Sarcoidosis of lung
D86.1	Sarcoidosis of lymph nodes
D86.2	Sarcoidosis of lung with sarcoidosis of lymph nodes
J39.8	Other specified diseases of upper respiratory tract
J98.09	Other diseases of bronchus, not elsewhere classified
Q32.0	Congenital tracheomalacia
Q32.1	Other congenital malformations of trachea
S12.8XXA	Fracture of other parts of neck, initial encounter

AMA: 31630 2018,Jan,8; 2017,Jan,8; 2016,Jan,13; 2015,Jan,16; 2014,Jan,11; 2013,Mar,8-9 **31631** 2018,Jan,8; 2017,Jan,8; 2016,Jan,13; 2015,Jan,16; 2014,Jan,11; 2013,Mar,8-9

Relative Value Units/Medicare Edits

Non-Facility RVU	Work	PE	MP	Total
31630	3.81	1.45	0.45	5.71
31631	4.36	1.65	0.57	6.58
Facility RVU	**Work**	**PE**	**MP**	**Total**
31630	3.81	1.45	0.45	5.71
31631	4.36	1.65	0.57	6.58

	FUD	Status	MUE	Modifiers				IOM Reference
31630	0	A	1(3)	51	N/A	N/A	N/A	None
31631	0	A	1(2)	51	N/A	N/A	N/A	

* with documentation

Terms To Know

closed reduction. Treatment of a fracture by manipulating it into proper alignment without opening the skin.

dilation. Artificial increase in the diameter of an opening or lumen made by medication or by instrumentation.

hyoid bone. Single, U-shaped bone palpable in the neck above the larynx and below the mandible (lower jaw) with various muscles attached but not articulating with any other bone.

stent. Tube to provide support in a body cavity or lumen.

31632-31633

+ 31632 Bronchoscopy, rigid or flexible, including fluoroscopic guidance, when performed; with transbronchial lung biopsy(s), each additional lobe (List separately in addition to code for primary procedure)

+ 31633 with transbronchial needle aspiration biopsy(s), each additional lobe (List separately in addition to code for primary procedure)

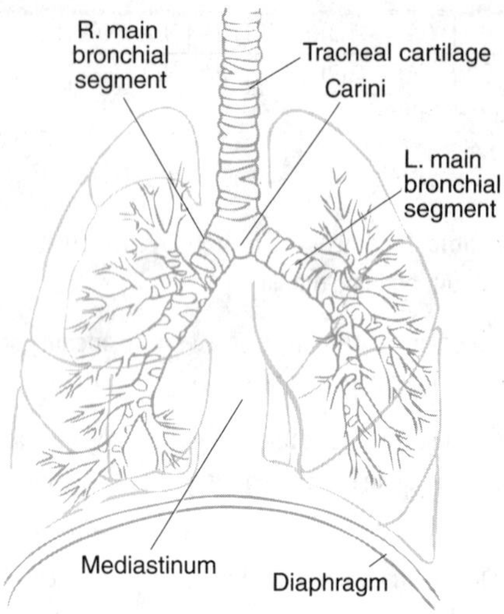

Explanation

The physician views the airway using a flexible fiberoptic or rigid bronchoscope that is introduced through the nasal or oral cavity. The airway is anesthetized. The bronchoscope is inserted. It is advanced through the larynx to the bronchus. Fluoroscopy (x-ray) may be used to assist with navigation of the bronchoscope tip to the abnormal tissue to be biopsied. In 31632, the physician passes closed biopsy forceps through a channel in the bronchoscope, through the bronchial wall, and obtains tissue samples in one lobe. Report 31632 for each additional lobe in which this is done. In 31633, a needle is passed through a channel in the bronchoscope, into the trachea, main stem, and/or a lobe of the bronchus, and an aspiration biopsy is obtained. Report 31633 for each additional lobe in which this is done.

Coding Tips

Use 31632 in addition to 31628. Use 31633 in addition to 31629. When medically necessary, report moderate (conscious) sedation provided by the performing physician with 99151-99153. When provided by another physician, report 99155-99157. These codes should only be reported once regardless of how many transbronchial needle aspiration biopsies are performed in the trachea or the additional lobe.

ICD-10-CM Diagnostic Codes

This/these CPT code(s) are add on code(s). See the primary procedure code that this code is performed with for your ICD-10-CM code selections. Diagnostic code(s) would be the same as the actual procedure performed.

AMA: 31632 2018,Jan,8; 2017,Jan,8; 2016,Jan,13; 2015,Jan,16; 2014,Jan,11; 2013,Mar,8-9 **31633** 2018,Jan,8; 2017,Jan,8; 2016,Jan,13; 2015,Jan,16; 2014,Jan,11; 2013,Mar,8-9

Relative Value Units/Medicare Edits

Non-Facility RVU	Work	PE	MP	Total
31632	1.03	0.7	0.08	1.81
31633	1.32	0.84	0.11	2.27
Facility RVU	**Work**	**PE**	**MP**	**Total**
31632	1.03	0.3	0.08	1.41
31633	1.32	0.4	0.11	1.83

	FUD	Status	MUE	Modifiers				IOM Reference
31632	N/A	A	2(3)	N/A	N/A	N/A	N/A	None
31633	N/A	A	2(3)	N/A	N/A	N/A	N/A	

* with documentation

Terms To Know

anesthesia. Loss of feeling or sensation, usually induced to permit the performance of surgery or other painful procedures.

aspiration. Drawing fluid out by suction.

biopsy. Tissue or fluid removed for diagnostic purposes through analysis of the cells in the biopsy material.

bronchoscopy. Endoscopic procedure used for the diagnosis, inspection, and treatment of the tracheobronchial tree.

flexible fiberoptic bronchoscope. Small, flexible endoscope with an external diameter between 3.0 and 6.0 mm composed of four channels: two light channels, one vision channel, and one open channel that accommodates biopsy forceps, cytology brush, suction tube, lavage tube, anesthetic, or oxygen.

fluoroscopy. Radiology technique that allows visual examination of part of the body or a function of an organ using a device that projects an x-ray image on a fluorescent screen.

forceps. Tool used for grasping or compressing tissue.

larynx. Musculocartilaginous structure between the trachea and the pharynx that functions as the valve preventing food and other particles from entering the respiratory tract, as well as the voice mechanism.

trachea. Tube descending from the larynx and branching into the right and left main bronchi.

31634

31634 Bronchoscopy, rigid or flexible, including fluoroscopic guidance, when performed; with balloon occlusion, with assessment of air leak, with administration of occlusive substance (eg, fibrin glue), if performed

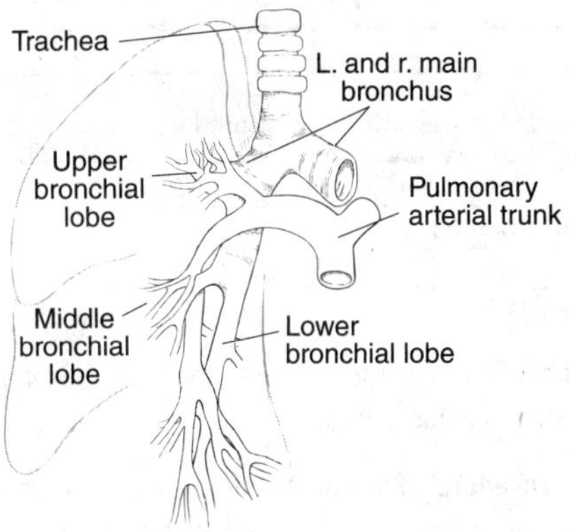

Explanation

The physician treats a bronchopleural fistula (BPF) with bronchoscopic balloon occlusion. BPF is often a serious postoperative complication of thoracic surgery, although it can also occur as a complication in a diseased lung or a previously normal lung. The physician views the airway using a flexible fiberoptic or rigid bronchoscope that is introduced through the nasal or oral cavity. The airway is anesthetized. The bronchoscope is inserted. It is advanced through the larynx to the bronchus. Fluoroscopy (x-ray) may be used to assist with navigation of the bronchoscope tip to the area of the air leak, which is then assessed. A balloon catheter is placed at the site of the leak and inflated until the leak is occluded. Keeping the inflated catheter in this position, an appropriate sealant (e.g., fibrin) may be injected. Once effective sealing is verified, the catheter and bronchoscope are removed.

Coding Tips

When medically necessary, report moderate (conscious) sedation provided by the performing physician with 99151-99153. When provided by another physician, report 99155-99157. Report the appropriate endoscopy for each anatomic site examined. Surgical endoscopy includes a diagnostic endoscopy; however, diagnostic endoscopy can be identified separately when performed at the same surgical session as an open procedure. Do not report 31634 in addition to 31647 or 31651 when performed at the same surgical session.

ICD-10-CM Diagnostic Codes

E84.0	Cystic fibrosis with pulmonary manifestations
J84.81	Lymphangioleiomyomatosis
J93.0	Spontaneous tension pneumothorax
J93.11	Primary spontaneous pneumothorax
J93.12	Secondary spontaneous pneumothorax
J93.81	Chronic pneumothorax
J93.82	Other air leak
J93.83	Other pneumothorax
J94.8	Other specified pleural conditions
J95.811	Postprocedural pneumothorax
J95.812	Postprocedural air leak
P25.1	Pneumothorax originating in the perinatal period
S27.0XXA	Traumatic pneumothorax, initial encounter
S27.1XXA	Traumatic hemothorax, initial encounter
S27.2XXA	Traumatic hemopneumothorax, initial encounter
S27.311A	Primary blast injury of lung, unilateral, initial encounter
S27.312A	Primary blast injury of lung, bilateral, initial encounter ☑
S27.321A	Contusion of lung, unilateral, initial encounter
S27.322A	Contusion of lung, bilateral, initial encounter ☑
S27.331A	Laceration of lung, unilateral, initial encounter
S27.332A	Laceration of lung, bilateral, initial encounter ☑
S27.391A	Other injuries of lung, unilateral, initial encounter
S27.392A	Other injuries of lung, bilateral, initial encounter ☑

AMA: 31634 2018,Jan,8; 2017,Jan,8; 2016,Jan,13; 2015,Jan,16; 2014,Jan,11; 2013,Mar,8-9

Relative Value Units/Medicare Edits

Non-Facility RVU	Work	PE	MP	Total
31634	3.75	45.26	0.39	49.4

Facility RVU	Work	PE	MP	Total
31634	3.75	1.39	0.39	5.53

	FUD	Status	MUE	Modifiers				IOM Reference
31634	0	A	1(3)	51	N/A	N/A	80	None

* with documentation

Terms To Know

bronchoscope. Endoscopic instrument used for the diagnosis, inspection, and treatment of the tracheobronchial tree.

fistula. Abnormal tube-like passage between two body cavities or organs or from an organ to the outside surface.

occlusion. Constriction, closure, or blockage of a passage.

31635

31635 Bronchoscopy, rigid or flexible, including fluoroscopic guidance, when performed; with removal of foreign body

The airway is viewed through a bronchoscope and a foreign body is excised

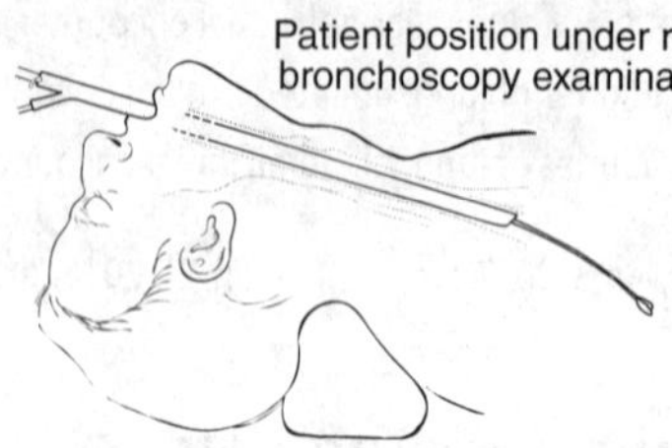

Explanation

The physician views the airway using a flexible fiberoptic or rigid bronchoscope introduced through the nasal or oral cavity, using local anesthesia of the patient's airway. The physician uses the views obtained through the bronchoscope to locate the foreign body within the airway. The physician passes a snare, basket, or biopsy forceps through a channel in the bronchoscope to grasp the foreign body. The bronchoscope and foreign body are removed. This may be done with or without fluoroscopic guidance.

Coding Tips

When medically necessary, report moderate (conscious) sedation provided by the performing physician with 99151-99153. When provided by another physician, report 99155-99157. Report the appropriate endoscopy for each anatomic site examined. Surgical endoscopy includes a diagnostic endoscopy; however, diagnostic endoscopy can be identified separately when performed at the same surgical session as an open procedure. For removal of previously implanted bronchial valves, see 31648 and 31649.

ICD-10-CM Diagnostic Codes

- T17.510A Gastric contents in bronchus causing asphyxiation, initial encounter
- T17.518A Gastric contents in bronchus causing other injury, initial encounter
- T17.520A Food in bronchus causing asphyxiation, initial encounter
- T17.528A Food in bronchus causing other injury, initial encounter
- T17.590A Other foreign object in bronchus causing asphyxiation, initial encounter
- T17.598A Other foreign object in bronchus causing other injury, initial encounter
- T17.810A Gastric contents in other parts of respiratory tract causing asphyxiation, initial encounter
- T17.818A Gastric contents in other parts of respiratory tract causing other injury, initial encounter
- T17.820A Food in other parts of respiratory tract causing asphyxiation, initial encounter
- T17.828A Food in other parts of respiratory tract causing other injury, initial encounter
- T17.890A Other foreign object in other parts of respiratory tract causing asphyxiation, initial encounter
- T17.898A Other foreign object in other parts of respiratory tract causing other injury, initial encounter

AMA: 31635 2018,Jan,8; 2017,Jan,8; 2016,Jan,13; 2015,Jan,16; 2014,Jan,11; 2013,Mar,8-9

Relative Value Units/Medicare Edits

Non-Facility RVU	Work	PE	MP	Total
31635	3.42	4.26	0.35	8.03
Facility RVU	**Work**	**PE**	**MP**	**Total**
31635	3.42	1.29	0.35	5.06

	FUD	Status	MUE	Modifiers				IOM Reference
31635	0	A	1(3)	51	N/A	N/A	N/A	None

* with documentation

Terms To Know

bronchoscope. Endoscopic instrument used for the diagnosis, inspection, and treatment of the tracheobronchial tree.

diagnostic procedures. Procedure performed on a patient to obtain information to assess the medical condition of the patient or to identify a disease and to determine the nature and severity of an illness or injury.

endoscopy. Visual inspection of the body using a fiberoptic scope.

flexible fiberoptic bronchoscope. Small, flexible endoscope with an external diameter between 3.0 and 6.0 mm composed of four channels: two light channels, one vision channel, and one open channel that accommodates biopsy forceps, cytology brush, suction tube, lavage tube, anesthetic, or oxygen.

snare. Wire used as a loop to excise a polyp or lesion.

Trachea and Bronchi

● New ▲ Revised + Add On AMA: CPT Assist [Resequenced] ☑ Laterality

31636-31638

31636 Bronchoscopy, rigid or flexible, including fluoroscopic guidance, when performed; with placement of bronchial stent(s) (includes tracheal/bronchial dilation as required), initial bronchus

\+ **31637** each additional major bronchus stented (List separately in addition to code for primary procedure)

31638 with revision of tracheal or bronchial stent inserted at previous session (includes tracheal/bronchial dilation as required)

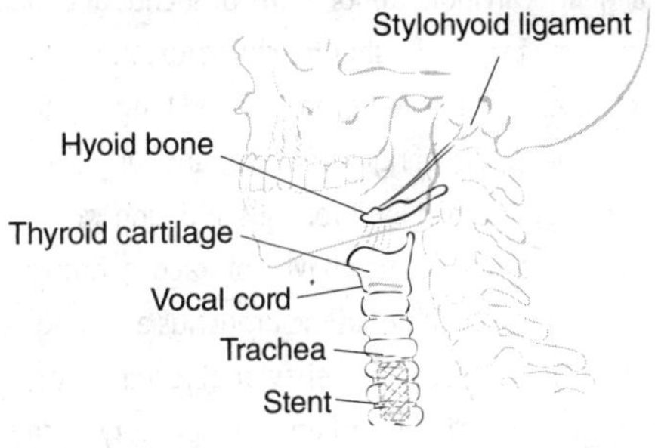

Explanation

A rigid or flexible bronchoscopy is performed, with or without fluoroscopic guidance, to place a bronchial stent. The type of stent used, as well as the level of patency vs. obstruction in the airway, will vary the placement technique. Initial assessment with the bronchoscope is done to determine the lesion's size and location. If fluoroscopy is used, the distal target position for stent placement is marked with a radiopaque object, such as a treated paperclip taped to the chest. If the airway is near completely occluded, a flexible tipped guidewire is placed through the bronchoscope, a balloon catheter is fed over the guidewire, and initial dilation is done. With the bronchoscope removed and the wire still in place, the stent, such as woven mesh or single wire stent with polyurethane covering, is passed over the guidewire by a stent catheter just past the obstruction. The stent is deployed by slowly sliding the plastic sheath covering back until it is snugly fitted. Report 31636 for the initial bronchial stent placement, 31637 for each additional major bronchus stented, and 31638 for the revision of a stent inserted in a previous session.

Coding Tips

Use 31637 in addition to 31636. Fluoroscopy is included in these procedures and should not be reported separately.

ICD-10-CM Diagnostic Codes

C33	Malignant neoplasm of trachea
C34.01	Malignant neoplasm of right main bronchus ☑
C34.02	Malignant neoplasm of left main bronchus ☑
C34.11	Malignant neoplasm of upper lobe, right bronchus or lung ☑
C34.12	Malignant neoplasm of upper lobe, left bronchus or lung ☑
C34.2	Malignant neoplasm of middle lobe, bronchus or lung
C34.31	Malignant neoplasm of lower lobe, right bronchus or lung ☑
C34.32	Malignant neoplasm of lower lobe, left bronchus or lung ☑
C34.81	Malignant neoplasm of overlapping sites of right bronchus and lung ☑
C34.82	Malignant neoplasm of overlapping sites of left bronchus and lung ☑
C77.1	Secondary and unspecified malignant neoplasm of intrathoracic lymph nodes
C78.01	Secondary malignant neoplasm of right lung ☑
C78.02	Secondary malignant neoplasm of left lung ☑
C7A.090	Malignant carcinoid tumor of the bronchus and lung
C81.02	Nodular lymphocyte predominant Hodgkin lymphoma, intrathoracic lymph nodes
C81.12	Nodular sclerosis Hodgkin lymphoma, intrathoracic lymph nodes
C81.22	Mixed cellularity Hodgkin lymphoma, intrathoracic lymph nodes
C81.32	Lymphocyte depleted Hodgkin lymphoma, intrathoracic lymph nodes
C81.42	Lymphocyte-rich Hodgkin lymphoma, intrathoracic lymph nodes
C81.72	Other Hodgkin lymphoma, intrathoracic lymph nodes
C82.32	Follicular lymphoma grade IIIa, intrathoracic lymph nodes
C82.52	Diffuse follicle center lymphoma, intrathoracic lymph nodes
C83.02	Small cell B-cell lymphoma, intrathoracic lymph nodes
C83.12	Mantle cell lymphoma, intrathoracic lymph nodes
C83.32	Diffuse large B-cell lymphoma, intrathoracic lymph nodes
C83.52	Lymphoblastic (diffuse) lymphoma, intrathoracic lymph nodes
C83.72	Burkitt lymphoma, intrathoracic lymph nodes
D14.2	Benign neoplasm of trachea
D14.31	Benign neoplasm of right bronchus and lung ☑
D14.32	Benign neoplasm of left bronchus and lung ☑
D38.1	Neoplasm of uncertain behavior of trachea, bronchus and lung
D3A.090	Benign carcinoid tumor of the bronchus and lung
D86.0	Sarcoidosis of lung
D86.1	Sarcoidosis of lymph nodes
D86.2	Sarcoidosis of lung with sarcoidosis of lymph nodes
J39.8	Other specified diseases of upper respiratory tract
J98.09	Other diseases of bronchus, not elsewhere classified
Q32.0	Congenital tracheomalacia
Q32.1	Other congenital malformations of trachea
Q32.2	Congenital bronchomalacia
Q32.3	Congenital stenosis of bronchus
Q32.4	Other congenital malformations of bronchus

AMA: **31636** 2018,Jan,8; 2017,Jan,8; 2016,Jan,13; 2015,Jan,16; 2014,Jan,11; 2013,Mar,8-9 **31637** 2018,Jan,8; 2017,Jan,8; 2016,Jan,13; 2015,Jan,16; 2014,Jan,11; 2013,Mar,8-9 **31638** 2018,Jan,8; 2017,Jan,8; 2016,Jan,13; 2015,Jan,16; 2014,Jan,11; 2013,Mar,8-9

Relative Value Units/Medicare Edits

Non-Facility RVU	Work	PE	MP	Total
31636	4.3	1.56	0.49	6.35
31637	1.58	0.49	0.15	2.22
31638	4.88	1.78	0.55	7.21
Facility RVU	**Work**	**PE**	**MP**	**Total**
31636	4.3	1.56	0.49	6.35
31637	1.58	0.49	0.15	2.22
31638	4.88	1.78	0.55	7.21

	FUD	Status	MUE	Modifiers				IOM Reference
31636	0	A	1(2)	51	N/A	N/A	N/A	None
31637	N/A	A	2(3)	N/A	N/A	N/A	N/A	
31638	0	A	1(3)	51	N/A	N/A	N/A	

* with documentation

31640-31641

31640 Bronchoscopy, rigid or flexible, including fluoroscopic guidance, when performed; with excision of tumor

31641 with destruction of tumor or relief of stenosis by any method other than excision (eg, laser therapy, cryotherapy)

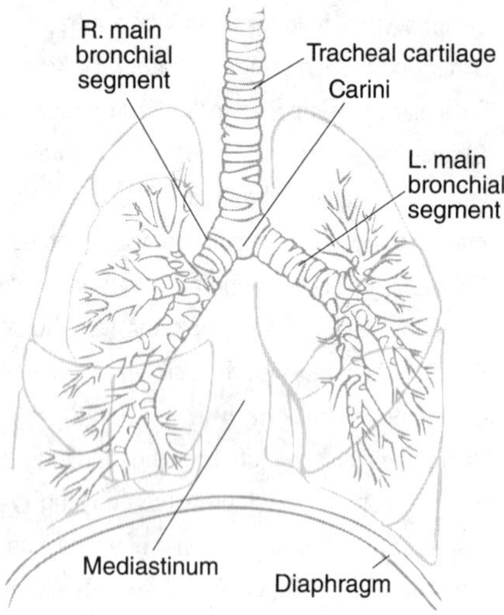

The airway is viewed through a bronchoscope

Explanation

In 31640, the physician views the airway using a flexible fiberoptic or rigid bronchoscope introduced through the nasal or oral cavity, using local anesthesia of the patient's airway. The physician uses the views obtained through the bronchoscope to identify the tumor from within the airway. The physician may use fluoroscopy (x-ray) to assist with navigation of the bronchoscope tip to the abnormal tissue. The physician passes forceps through channels in the bronchoscope to grasp and excise the tumor. The bronchoscope is removed. This may be done with or without fluoroscopic guidance. In 31641, the physician views the airway using a bronchoscope introduced through the nasal or oral cavity, using local anesthesia of the patient's airway. The physician uses the views obtained through the bronchoscope to identify the tumor and/or area of stenosis from within the airway. Fluoroscopy (x-ray) may be used to assist with navigation of the bronchoscope tip to the abnormal tissue and is included when performed. The physician passes a laser or freezing (cryo) probe through a channel in the bronchoscope to destroy the tumor or any areas of stenosis. The bronchoscope is removed.

Coding Tips

Report the appropriate endoscopy for each anatomic site examined. Surgical endoscopy includes a diagnostic endoscopy; however, diagnostic endoscopy can be identified separately when performed at the same surgical session as an open procedure. A biopsy is not reported separately when followed by an excisional removal during the same operative session. Bronchoscopic photodynamic therapy (96570–96571) is reported separately when performed with 31641.

ICD-10-CM Diagnostic Codes

C34.01 Malignant neoplasm of right main bronchus ☑
C34.02 Malignant neoplasm of left main bronchus ☑
C34.11 Malignant neoplasm of upper lobe, right bronchus or lung ☑
C34.12 Malignant neoplasm of upper lobe, left bronchus or lung ☑
C34.2 Malignant neoplasm of middle lobe, bronchus or lung
C34.31 Malignant neoplasm of lower lobe, right bronchus or lung ☑
C34.32 Malignant neoplasm of lower lobe, left bronchus or lung ☑
C34.81 Malignant neoplasm of overlapping sites of right bronchus and lung ☑
C34.82 Malignant neoplasm of overlapping sites of left bronchus and lung ☑
C78.01 Secondary malignant neoplasm of right lung ☑
C78.02 Secondary malignant neoplasm of left lung ☑
C78.39 Secondary malignant neoplasm of other respiratory organs
C7A.090 Malignant carcinoid tumor of the bronchus and lung
D02.21 Carcinoma in situ of right bronchus and lung ☑
D02.22 Carcinoma in situ of left bronchus and lung ☑
D14.31 Benign neoplasm of right bronchus and lung ☑
D14.32 Benign neoplasm of left bronchus and lung ☑
D38.1 Neoplasm of uncertain behavior of trachea, bronchus and lung
D3A.090 Benign carcinoid tumor of the bronchus and lung
D49.1 Neoplasm of unspecified behavior of respiratory system
J39.8 Other specified diseases of upper respiratory tract
J98.09 Other diseases of bronchus, not elsewhere classified

AMA: **31640** 2018,Jan,8; 2017,Jan,8; 2016,Jan,13; 2016,Apr,5; 2015,Jan,16; 2014,Jan,11; 2013,Mar,8-9 **31641** 2018,Jan,8; 2017,Jan,8; 2016,Jan,13; 2015,Jan,16; 2014,Jan,11; 2013,Mar,8-9; 2013,Apr,8-9

Relative Value Units/Medicare Edits

Non-Facility RVU	Work	PE	MP	Total
31640	4.93	1.77	0.52	7.22
31641	5.02	1.84	0.53	7.39
Facility RVU	**Work**	**PE**	**MP**	**Total**
31640	4.93	1.77	0.52	7.22
31641	5.02	1.84	0.53	7.39

	FUD	Status	MUE	Modifiers				IOM Reference
31640	0	A	1(3)	51	N/A	N/A	N/A	None
31641	0	A	1(3)	51	N/A	N/A	N/A	

* with documentation

31643

31643 Bronchoscopy, rigid or flexible, including fluoroscopic guidance, when performed; with placement of catheter(s) for intracavitary radioelement application

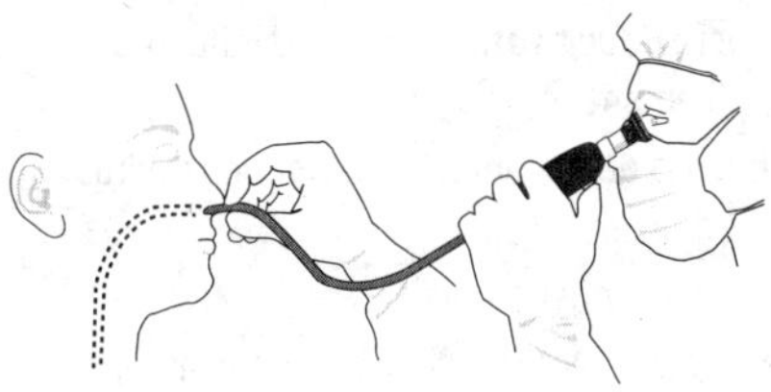

Examination using flexible bronchoscope

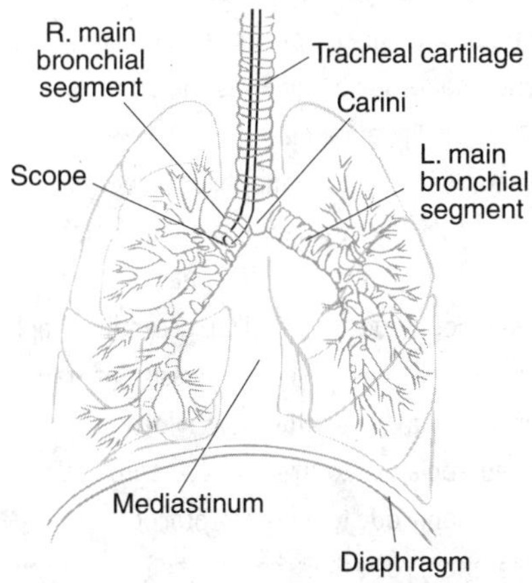

A catheter is advanced through the bronchoscope and contrast or other media is released for intracavity radiography studies

Explanation

The physician views the airway using a bronchoscope with a fiberoptic camera and operating device. The airway is anesthetized and the bronchoscope is introduced through the nasal or oral cavity and advanced through the bronchus. A catheter is inserted through the bronchoscope into a lung cavity and is placed at the site where, in a separately reportable procedure, intracavitary radioelements will be applied. This code includes the use of fluoroscopic guidance, when performed.

Coding Tips

When 31643 is performed with another separately identifiable procedure, the highest dollar value code is listed as the primary procedure, and subsequent procedures are appended with modifier 51. Report the appropriate endoscopy for each anatomic site examined. Surgical endoscopy includes a diagnostic endoscopy; however, diagnostic endoscopy can be identified separately when performed at the same surgical session as an open procedure. Report intracavitary radioelement application separately, see 77761–77763 and 77770–77772. Fluoroscopic guidance is not reported separately.

ICD-10-CM Diagnostic Codes

C34.01 Malignant neoplasm of right main bronchus ☑
C34.02 Malignant neoplasm of left main bronchus ☑
C34.11 Malignant neoplasm of upper lobe, right bronchus or lung ☑
C34.12 Malignant neoplasm of upper lobe, left bronchus or lung ☑
C34.2 Malignant neoplasm of middle lobe, bronchus or lung
C34.31 Malignant neoplasm of lower lobe, right bronchus or lung ☑
C34.32 Malignant neoplasm of lower lobe, left bronchus or lung ☑
C34.81 Malignant neoplasm of overlapping sites of right bronchus and lung ☑
C34.82 Malignant neoplasm of overlapping sites of left bronchus and lung ☑
C78.01 Secondary malignant neoplasm of right lung ☑
C78.02 Secondary malignant neoplasm of left lung ☑
C7A.090 Malignant carcinoid tumor of the bronchus and lung
D02.21 Carcinoma in situ of right bronchus and lung ☑
D02.22 Carcinoma in situ of left bronchus and lung ☑

AMA: 31643 2018,Jan,8; 2017,Jan,8; 2016,Jan,13; 2016,Apr,5; 2015,Jan,16; 2014,Jan,11; 2013,Mar,8-9

Relative Value Units/Medicare Edits

Non-Facility RVU	Work	PE	MP	Total
31643	3.49	1.3	0.3	5.09
Facility RVU	**Work**	**PE**	**MP**	**Total**
31643	3.49	1.3	0.3	5.09

	FUD	Status	MUE	Modifiers				IOM Reference
31643	0	A	1(2)	51	N/A	N/A	N/A	None

* with documentation

Terms To Know

carcinoma in situ. Malignancy that arises from the cells of the vessel, gland, or organ of origin that remains confined to that site or has not invaded neighboring tissue.

flexible fiberoptic bronchoscope. Small, flexible endoscope with an external diameter between 3.0 and 6.0 mm composed of four channels: two light channels, one vision channel, and one open channel that accommodates biopsy forceps, cytology brush, suction tube, lavage tube, anesthetic, or oxygen.

fluoroscopy. Radiology technique that allows visual examination of part of the body or a function of an organ using a device that projects an x-ray image on a fluorescent screen.

malignant. Any condition tending to progress toward death, specifically an invasive tumor with a loss of cellular differentiation that has the ability to spread or metastasize to other body areas.

radioactive substances. Materials used in the diagnosis and treatment of disease that emit high-speed particles and energy-containing rays.

31645-31646

31645 Bronchoscopy, rigid or flexible, including fluoroscopic guidance, when performed; with therapeutic aspiration of tracheobronchial tree, initial

31646 with therapeutic aspiration of tracheobronchial tree, subsequent

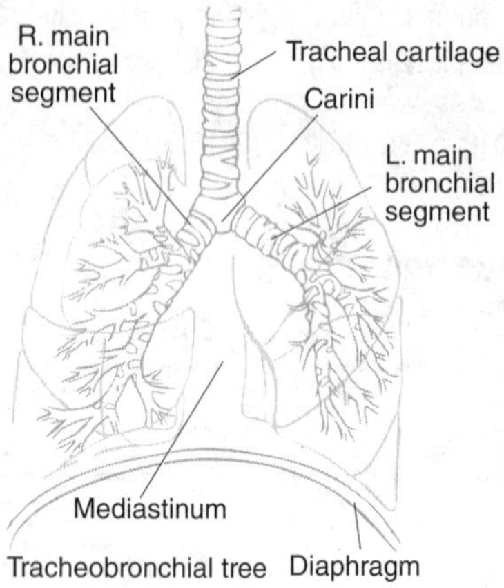

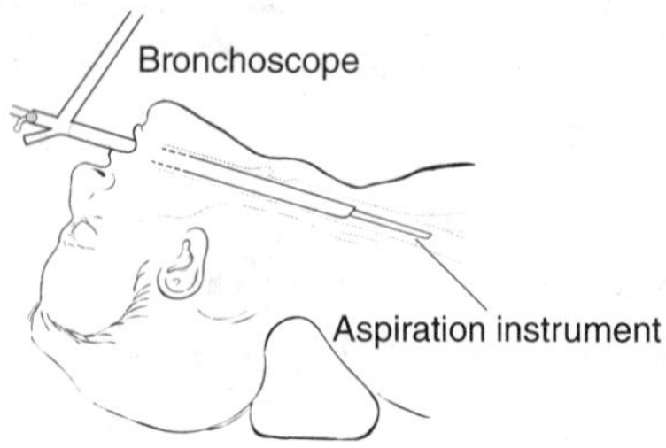

Explanation

The physician views the airway using a bronchoscope introduced through the nasal or oral cavity, using local anesthesia of the patient's airway. The physician uses the views obtained through the bronchoscope to identify the closest approach to the fluid collection from within the airway. The physician may use fluoroscopy (x-ray) to assist with navigation of the bronchoscope tip to the fluid collection. The physician passes a catheter through a channel in the bronchoscope and aspirates the tracheobronchial tree. Alternately, the physician passes a needle through a channel in the bronchoscope into the fluid collection and aspirates fluid through the needle. The bronchoscope is removed. Report 31645 for the initial treatment only. Report 31646 for any subsequent aspiration procedures performed during the same hospital stay. These codes include the use of fluoroscopic guidance, when performed.

Coding Tips

When medically necessary, report moderate (conscious) sedation provided by the performing physician with 99151-99153. When provided by another physician, report 99155-99157. Report the appropriate endoscopy for each anatomic site examined. Surgical endoscopy includes a diagnostic endoscopy; however, diagnostic endoscopy can be identified separately when performed at the same surgical session as an open procedure. For a bedside catheter aspiration of the tracheobronchial tree, see 31725.

ICD-10-CM Diagnostic Codes

A06.5	Amebic lung abscess
A22.1	Pulmonary anthrax
A37.01	Whooping cough due to Bordetella pertussis with pneumonia
A37.11	Whooping cough due to Bordetella parapertussis with pneumonia
A37.81	Whooping cough due to other Bordetella species with pneumonia
B25.0	Cytomegaloviral pneumonitis
B44.0	Invasive pulmonary aspergillosis
B77.81	Ascariasis pneumonia
E84.0	Cystic fibrosis with pulmonary manifestations
J10.08	Influenza due to other identified influenza virus with other specified pneumonia
J11.08	Influenza due to unidentified influenza virus with specified pneumonia
J12.0	Adenoviral pneumonia
J12.1	Respiratory syncytial virus pneumonia
J12.2	Parainfluenza virus pneumonia
J12.3	Human metapneumovirus pneumonia
J12.81	Pneumonia due to SARS-associated coronavirus
J12.89	Other viral pneumonia
J14	Pneumonia due to Hemophilus influenzae
J15.0	Pneumonia due to Klebsiella pneumoniae
J15.1	Pneumonia due to Pseudomonas
J15.211	Pneumonia due to Methicillin susceptible Staphylococcus aureus
J15.212	Pneumonia due to Methicillin resistant Staphylococcus aureus
J15.29	Pneumonia due to other staphylococcus
J15.3	Pneumonia due to streptococcus, group B
J15.4	Pneumonia due to other streptococci
J15.5	Pneumonia due to Escherichia coli
J15.6	Pneumonia due to other Gram-negative bacteria
J15.7	Pneumonia due to Mycoplasma pneumoniae
J15.8	Pneumonia due to other specified bacteria
J16.0	Chlamydial pneumonia
J16.8	Pneumonia due to other specified infectious organisms
J17	Pneumonia in diseases classified elsewhere
J41.0	Simple chronic bronchitis
J41.1	Mucopurulent chronic bronchitis
J41.8	Mixed simple and mucopurulent chronic bronchitis
J43.0	Unilateral pulmonary emphysema [MacLeod's syndrome]
J43.1	Panlobular emphysema
J43.2	Centrilobular emphysema
J43.8	Other emphysema
J44.0	Chronic obstructive pulmonary disease with (acute) lower respiratory infection
J44.1	Chronic obstructive pulmonary disease with (acute) exacerbation
J47.0	Bronchiectasis with acute lower respiratory infection
J47.1	Bronchiectasis with (acute) exacerbation
J85.0	Gangrene and necrosis of lung
J85.1	Abscess of lung with pneumonia
J85.2	Abscess of lung without pneumonia
J85.3	Abscess of mediastinum
J86.0	Pyothorax with fistula
J86.9	Pyothorax without fistula
J95.851	Ventilator associated pneumonia
J98.11	Atelectasis
J98.19	Other pulmonary collapse

AMA: 31645 2018,Jan,8; 2017,Jan,8; 2016,Jan,13; 2016,Apr,5; 2015,Jan,16; 2014,Jan,11; 2013,Mar,8-9 **31646** 2018,Sep,3; 2018,Jan,8; 2017,Jan,8; 2016,Jan,13; 2016,Apr,5; 2015,Jan,16; 2014,Jan,11; 2013,Mar,8-9

Relative Value Units/Medicare Edits

Non-Facility RVU	Work	PE	MP	Total
31645	2.88	4.28	0.26	7.42
31646	2.78	1.05	0.26	4.09
Facility RVU	**Work**	**PE**	**MP**	**Total**
31645	2.88	1.07	0.26	4.21
31646	2.78	1.05	0.26	4.09

	FUD	Status	MUE	Modifiers				IOM Reference
31645	0	A	1(2)	51	N/A	N/A	N/A	None
31646	0	A	2(3)	51	N/A	N/A	N/A	

* with documentation

Terms To Know

aspiration. Drawing fluid out by suction.

diaphragm. Muscular wall separating the thorax and its structures from the abdomen.

fluoroscopy. Radiology technique that allows visual examination of part of the body or a function of an organ using a device that projects an x-ray image on a fluorescent screen.

mediastinum. Collection of organs and tissues that separate the pleural sacs. Located between the sternum and spine above the diaphragm, it contains the heart and great vessels, trachea and bronchi, esophagus, thymus, lymph nodes, and nerves.

trachea. Tube descending from the larynx and branching into the right and left main bronchi.

31717

31717 Catheterization with bronchial brush biopsy

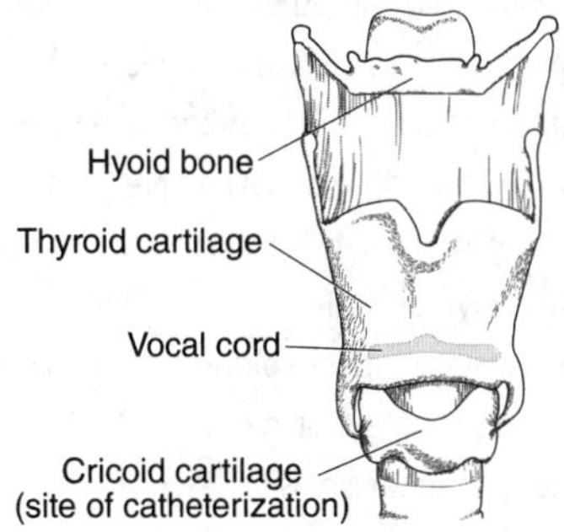

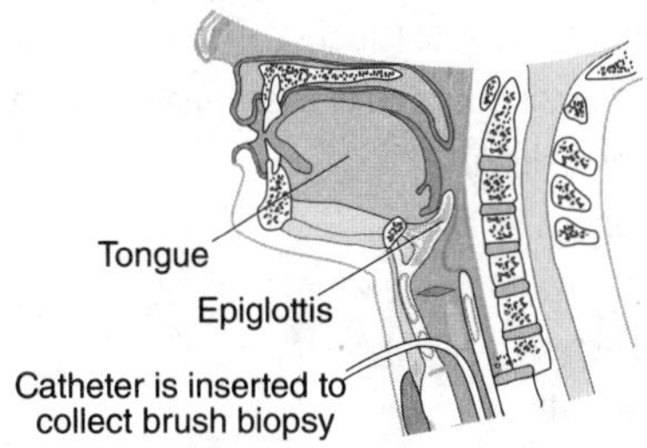

Explanation

The physician catheterizes the trachea to obtain a bronchial brush biopsy. The physician inserts a needle through the cricoid cartilage or the trachea. A catheter is passed over the needle and a brush is placed through the catheter to obtain bronchial tissue. A bronchoscope may be used to guide the brush. The brush is withdrawn through the catheter and both are removed. The incision may be closed with sutures.

Coding Tips

Brush biopsy is included in this procedure and should not be reported separately. For tracheal aspiration using direct vision, see 31515. For endotracheal intubation, see 31500.

ICD-10-CM Diagnostic Codes

B25.0	Cytomegaloviral pneumonitis
B44.0	Invasive pulmonary aspergillosis
B59	Pneumocystosis
C34.01	Malignant neoplasm of right main bronchus ☑
C34.02	Malignant neoplasm of left main bronchus ☑
C34.11	Malignant neoplasm of upper lobe, right bronchus or lung ☑
C34.12	Malignant neoplasm of upper lobe, left bronchus or lung ☑
C34.2	Malignant neoplasm of middle lobe, bronchus or lung
C34.31	Malignant neoplasm of lower lobe, right bronchus or lung ☑
C34.32	Malignant neoplasm of lower lobe, left bronchus or lung ☑
C34.81	Malignant neoplasm of overlapping sites of right bronchus and lung ☑
C34.82	Malignant neoplasm of overlapping sites of left bronchus and lung ☑
C78.01	Secondary malignant neoplasm of right lung ☑
C78.02	Secondary malignant neoplasm of left lung ☑
C78.2	Secondary malignant neoplasm of pleura
C7A.090	Malignant carcinoid tumor of the bronchus and lung

D02.21	Carcinoma in situ of right bronchus and lung ☑
D02.22	Carcinoma in situ of left bronchus and lung ☑
D14.31	Benign neoplasm of right bronchus and lung ☑
D14.32	Benign neoplasm of left bronchus and lung ☑
D19.0	Benign neoplasm of mesothelial tissue of pleura
D38.1	Neoplasm of uncertain behavior of trachea, bronchus and lung
D3A.090	Benign carcinoid tumor of the bronchus and lung
D49.1	Neoplasm of unspecified behavior of respiratory system
D86.0	Sarcoidosis of lung
D86.1	Sarcoidosis of lymph nodes
D86.2	Sarcoidosis of lung with sarcoidosis of lymph nodes
J15.212	Pneumonia due to Methicillin resistant Staphylococcus aureus
J60	Coalworker's pneumoconiosis
J61	Pneumoconiosis due to asbestos and other mineral fibers
J62.0	Pneumoconiosis due to talc dust
J62.8	Pneumoconiosis due to other dust containing silica
J63.0	Aluminosis (of lung)
J63.1	Bauxite fibrosis (of lung)
J63.2	Berylliosis
J63.3	Graphite fibrosis (of lung)
J63.4	Siderosis
J63.5	Stannosis
J63.6	Pneumoconiosis due to other specified inorganic dusts
J65	Pneumoconiosis associated with tuberculosis
J66.0	Byssinosis
J66.1	Flax-dressers' disease
J66.2	Cannabinosis
J66.8	Airway disease due to other specific organic dusts
J68.4	Chronic respiratory conditions due to chemicals, gases, fumes and vapors
J69.0	Pneumonitis due to inhalation of food and vomit
J70.1	Chronic and other pulmonary manifestations due to radiation
J82	Pulmonary eosinophilia, not elsewhere classified
J84.01	Alveolar proteinosis
J84.02	Pulmonary alveolar microlithiasis
J84.03	Idiopathic pulmonary hemosiderosis
J84.09	Other alveolar and parieto-alveolar conditions
J84.112	Idiopathic pulmonary fibrosis
J84.113	Idiopathic non-specific interstitial pneumonitis
J84.114	Acute interstitial pneumonitis
J84.115	Respiratory bronchiolitis interstitial lung disease
J84.116	Cryptogenic organizing pneumonia
J84.117	Desquamative interstitial pneumonia
J84.17	Other interstitial pulmonary diseases with fibrosis in diseases classified elsewhere
J84.2	Lymphoid interstitial pneumonia
J84.89	Other specified interstitial pulmonary diseases
J85.0	Gangrene and necrosis of lung
J85.1	Abscess of lung with pneumonia
J85.2	Abscess of lung without pneumonia
J86.0	Pyothorax with fistula
J86.9	Pyothorax without fistula
J90	Pleural effusion, not elsewhere classified
J98.11	Atelectasis
J98.19	Other pulmonary collapse
J98.4	Other disorders of lung
M32.13	Lung involvement in systemic lupus erythematosus
M33.01	Juvenile dermatomyositis with respiratory involvement
M33.11	Other dermatomyositis with respiratory involvement
M33.21	Polymyositis with respiratory involvement
M35.02	Sicca syndrome with lung involvement
P27.0	Wilson-Mikity syndrome

AMA: 31717 2018,Jan,8; 2017,Jan,8; 2016,Jan,13; 2015,Jan,16; 2014,Jan,11

Relative Value Units/Medicare Edits

Non-Facility RVU	Work	PE	MP	Total
31717	2.12	5.69	0.17	7.98
Facility RVU	**Work**	**PE**	**MP**	**Total**
31717	2.12	0.89	0.17	3.18

	FUD	Status	MUE	Modifiers				IOM Reference
31717	0	A	1(3)	51	N/A	N/A	N/A	None

* with documentation

Terms To Know

cricoid. Circular cartilage around the trachea.

epiglottis. Lid-like cartilaginous tissue that covers the entrance to the larynx and blocks food from entering the trachea.

hyoid bone. Single, U-shaped bone palpable in the neck above the larynx and below the mandible (lower jaw) with various muscles attached but not articulating with any other bone.

trachea. Tube descending from the larynx and branching into the right and left main bronchi.

31720-31725

31720 Catheter aspiration (separate procedure); nasotracheal
31725 tracheobronchial with fiberscope, bedside

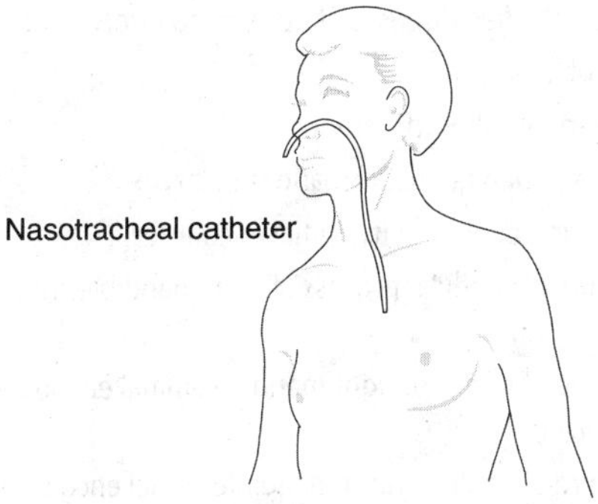

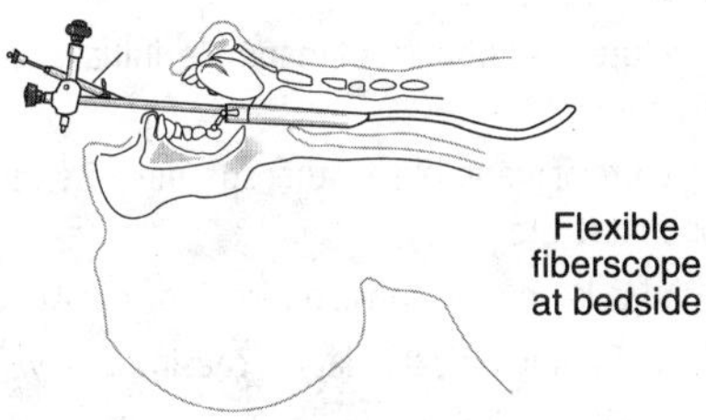

Side view schematic

Explanation

The physician aspirates sputum from the lungs using a nasal tracheal catheter. The physician passes a suction catheter through the nose into the trachea. Saline may be used to liquify secretions. The secretions are removed with suction and the catheter is removed. Report 31725 if a tracheobronchial approach with fiberscope is used at bedside.

Coding Tips

These separate procedures by definition are usually a component of a more complex service and are not identified separately. When performed alone or with other unrelated procedures/services, they may be reported. If performed alone, list the code; if performed with other procedures/services, list the code and append modifier 59 or an X{EPSU} modifier. When medically necessary, report moderate (conscious) sedation provided by the performing physician with 99151-99153. When provided by another physician, report 99155-99157.

ICD-10-CM Diagnostic Codes

B25.0	Cytomegaloviral pneumonitis
B44.0	Invasive pulmonary aspergillosis
E84.0	Cystic fibrosis with pulmonary manifestations
J10.08	Influenza due to other identified influenza virus with other specified pneumonia
J11.08	Influenza due to unidentified influenza virus with specified pneumonia
J12.0	Adenoviral pneumonia
J12.1	Respiratory syncytial virus pneumonia
J12.2	Parainfluenza virus pneumonia
J12.3	Human metapneumovirus pneumonia
J12.81	Pneumonia due to SARS-associated coronavirus
J12.89	Other viral pneumonia
J17	Pneumonia in diseases classified elsewhere
J41.0	Simple chronic bronchitis
J41.1	Mucopurulent chronic bronchitis
J41.8	Mixed simple and mucopurulent chronic bronchitis
J43.0	Unilateral pulmonary emphysema [MacLeod's syndrome]
J43.1	Panlobular emphysema
J43.2	Centrilobular emphysema
J43.8	Other emphysema
J44.1	Chronic obstructive pulmonary disease with (acute) exacerbation
J47.0	Bronchiectasis with acute lower respiratory infection
J47.1	Bronchiectasis with (acute) exacerbation
J82	Pulmonary eosinophilia, not elsewhere classified
J84.01	Alveolar proteinosis
J84.02	Pulmonary alveolar microlithiasis
J84.03	Idiopathic pulmonary hemosiderosis
J84.09	Other alveolar and parieto-alveolar conditions
J84.112	Idiopathic pulmonary fibrosis
J84.113	Idiopathic non-specific interstitial pneumonitis
J84.114	Acute interstitial pneumonitis
J84.115	Respiratory bronchiolitis interstitial lung disease
J84.117	Desquamative interstitial pneumonia
J84.17	Other interstitial pulmonary diseases with fibrosis in diseases classified elsewhere
J84.2	Lymphoid interstitial pneumonia
J84.89	Other specified interstitial pulmonary diseases
J85.0	Gangrene and necrosis of lung
J85.1	Abscess of lung with pneumonia
J85.2	Abscess of lung without pneumonia
J95.851	Ventilator associated pneumonia
J98.11	Atelectasis
J98.19	Other pulmonary collapse

AMA: **31720** 1994,Win,1

Relative Value Units/Medicare Edits

Non-Facility RVU	Work	PE	MP	Total
31720	1.06	0.29	0.08	1.43
31725	1.71	0.41	0.17	2.29
Facility RVU	**Work**	**PE**	**MP**	**Total**
31720	1.06	0.29	0.08	1.43
31725	1.71	0.41	0.17	2.29

	FUD	Status	MUE	Modifiers				IOM Reference
31720	0	A	1(3)	51	N/A	N/A	N/A	None
31725	0	A	1(3)	51	N/A	N/A	N/A	

* with documentation

31730

31730 Transtracheal (percutaneous) introduction of needle wire dilator/stent or indwelling tube for oxygen therapy

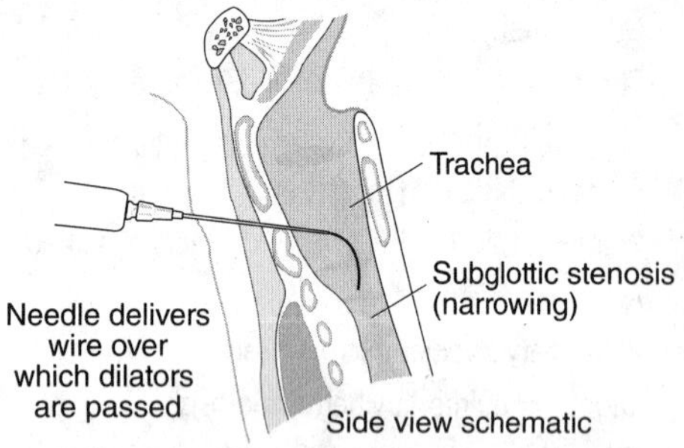

A percutaneous approach is used to introduce a wire and dilator to relieve stenosis in the tracheal tract. An indwelling stent or tube may be left in place following the procedure

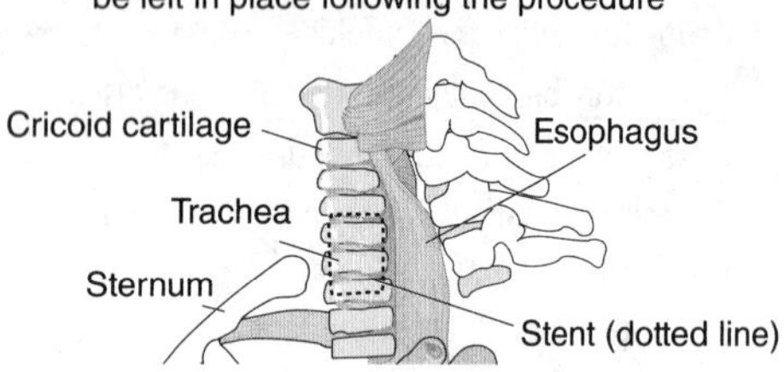

Explanation

The physician introduces a needle wire dilator/stent into the trachea to relieve a subglottic stenosis. The physician places a needle through the cricoid membrane or trachea. A wire is passed through the needle and the needle is removed. A series of dilators or stents are passed over the wire to open the trachea. When sufficient dilation is gained, a stent or indwelling tube for oxygen therapy is left in place to maintain patency.

Coding Tips

For endotracheal intubation, see 31500. For tracheal or bronchial dilation and/or stent placement performed endoscopically, see 31630–31631.

ICD-10-CM Diagnostic Codes

C10.0	Malignant neoplasm of vallecula
C10.1	Malignant neoplasm of anterior surface of epiglottis
C10.2	Malignant neoplasm of lateral wall of oropharynx
C10.3	Malignant neoplasm of posterior wall of oropharynx
C10.4	Malignant neoplasm of branchial cleft
C10.8	Malignant neoplasm of overlapping sites of oropharynx
C12	Malignant neoplasm of pyriform sinus
C13.0	Malignant neoplasm of postcricoid region
C13.1	Malignant neoplasm of aryepiglottic fold, hypopharyngeal aspect
C13.2	Malignant neoplasm of posterior wall of hypopharynx
C13.8	Malignant neoplasm of overlapping sites of hypopharynx
C14.2	Malignant neoplasm of Waldeyer's ring
C14.8	Malignant neoplasm of overlapping sites of lip, oral cavity and pharynx
C32.0	Malignant neoplasm of glottis
C32.1	Malignant neoplasm of supraglottis
C32.2	Malignant neoplasm of subglottis
J05.11	Acute epiglottitis with obstruction
J38.4	Edema of larynx
J38.6	Stenosis of larynx
J38.7	Other diseases of larynx
J39.8	Other specified diseases of upper respiratory tract
Q31.0	Web of larynx
Q31.1	Congenital subglottic stenosis
Q31.8	Other congenital malformations of larynx
S00.532A	Contusion of oral cavity, initial encounter
S02.611B	Fracture of condylar process of right mandible, initial encounter for open fracture ☑
S02.641B	Fracture of ramus of right mandible, initial encounter for open fracture ☑
S02.651B	Fracture of angle of right mandible, initial encounter for open fracture ☑
S02.66XB	Fracture of symphysis of mandible, initial encounter for open fracture
S02.69XB	Fracture of mandible of other specified site, initial encounter for open fracture
T17.320A	Food in larynx causing asphyxiation, initial encounter
T17.390A	Other foreign object in larynx causing asphyxiation, initial encounter

AMA: **31730** 1992,Win,1

Relative Value Units/Medicare Edits

Non-Facility RVU	Work	PE	MP	Total
31730	2.85	30.85	0.54	34.24
Facility RVU	**Work**	**PE**	**MP**	**Total**
31730	2.85	0.93	0.54	4.32

	FUD	Status	MUE	Modifiers				IOM Reference
31730	0	A	1(3)	51	N/A	N/A	N/A	None

* with documentation

Terms To Know

dilation. Artificial increase in the diameter of an opening or lumen made by medication or by instrumentation.

lumen. Space inside an intestine, artery, vein, duct, or tube.

percutaneous. Through the skin.

stenosis. Narrowing or constriction of a passage.

31760

31760 Tracheoplasty; intrathoracic

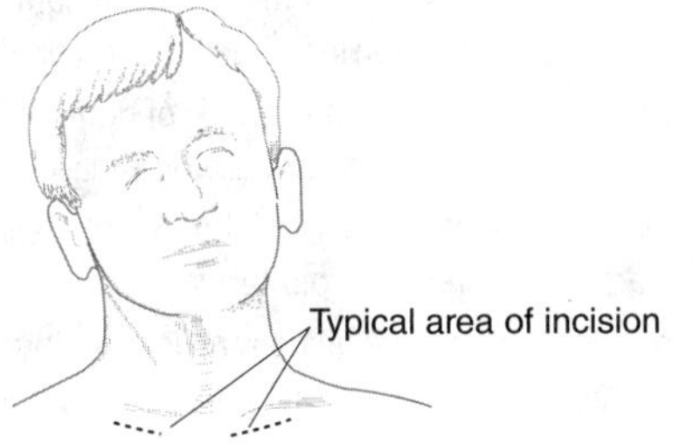

Any of a wide variety of surgical repairs may be made to the tracheopharyngeal area using an intrathoracic surgical approach

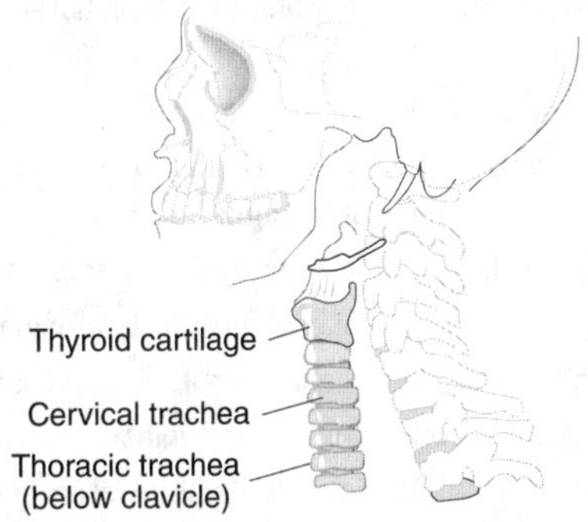

Explanation

The physician makes an incision in the thorax and approaches the trachea by opening the rib cage. An airway is inserted and the trachea is incised. Surgical repair of the trachea is undertaken. End-to-end anastomosis of the trachea may be performed. For satisfactory reconstruction, it may be necessary for the physician to surgically repair the trachea using splints constructed from rib or costal cartilage to patch the length of the trachea. Once repair is achieved, the airway is removed and the incisions are closed.

Coding Tips

When 31760 is performed with another separately identifiable procedure, the highest dollar value code is listed as the primary procedure, and subsequent procedures are appended with modifier 51. Report any free grafts or flaps separately.

ICD-10-CM Diagnostic Codes

C33	Malignant neoplasm of trachea
C78.39	Secondary malignant neoplasm of other respiratory organs
D02.1	Carcinoma in situ of trachea
D14.2	Benign neoplasm of trachea
D38.1	Neoplasm of uncertain behavior of trachea, bronchus and lung
Q32.0	Congenital tracheomalacia
Q32.1	Other congenital malformations of trachea
Q39.1	Atresia of esophagus with tracheo-esophageal fistula
Q39.2	Congenital tracheo-esophageal fistula without atresia
S11.021A	Laceration without foreign body of trachea, initial encounter
S11.022A	Laceration with foreign body of trachea, initial encounter
S11.023A	Puncture wound without foreign body of trachea, initial encounter
S11.024A	Puncture wound with foreign body of trachea, initial encounter
S11.025A	Open bite of trachea, initial encounter
S17.0XXA	Crushing injury of larynx and trachea, initial encounter
T27.0XXA	Burn of larynx and trachea, initial encounter
T27.1XXA	Burn involving larynx and trachea with lung, initial encounter
T27.4XXA	Corrosion of larynx and trachea, initial encounter
T27.5XXA	Corrosion involving larynx and trachea with lung, initial encounter
Z85.12	Personal history of malignant neoplasm of trachea

Relative Value Units/Medicare Edits

Non-Facility RVU	Work	PE	MP	Total
31760	23.48	10.63	5.57	39.68
Facility RVU	**Work**	**PE**	**MP**	**Total**
31760	23.48	10.63	5.57	39.68

	FUD	Status	MUE	Modifiers				IOM Reference
31760	90	A	1(2)	51	N/A	62*	80	None

* with documentation

Terms To Know

anastomosis. Surgically created connection between ducts, blood vessels, or bowel segments to allow flow from one to the other.

cartilage. Variety of fibrous connective tissue that is inherently nonvascular. Usually found in the joints, it aids in movement and provides a cushion to absorb jolts and shocks.

free graft. Unattached piece of skin and tissue moved to another part of the body and sutured into place to repair a defect.

malignant. Any condition tending to progress toward death, specifically an invasive tumor with a loss of cellular differentiation that has the ability to spread or metastasize to other body areas.

reconstruction. Recreating, restoring, or rebuilding a body part or organ.

tracheoesophageal fistula. Abnormal opening between the trachea and the esophagus. There are three types of tracheoesophageal fistulas; congenital, formed from a previous tracheostomy, and fistula not caused by previous surgery.

31770-31775

31770 Bronchoplasty; graft repair
31775 excision stenosis and anastomosis

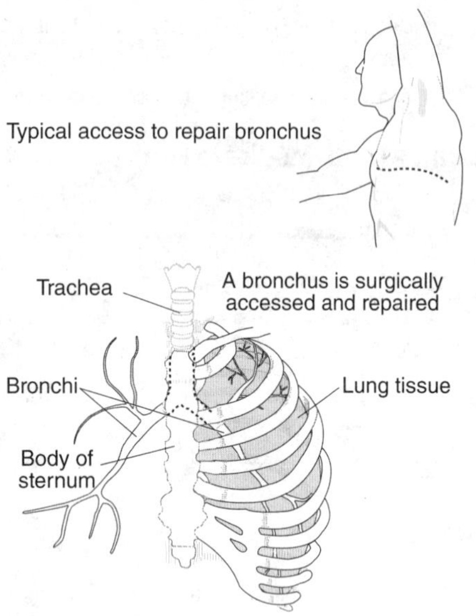

Explanation

The physician repairs a bronchus. The physician makes a lateral thoracotomy incision to access the bronchus. An autograft or Silastic stent may be used to repair the bronchus in 31770. A chest tube is inserted and the wound is closed in sutured layers. Report 31775 if an excision stenosis and anastomosis are performed with this procedure.

Coding Tips

Codes 31770 and 31775 should be reported when a bronchoplasty is performed without concurrent lobectomy or segmentectomy. When bronchoplasty is performed with lobectomy/segmentectomy, report the code for lobectomy/segmentectomy with 32480, 32482, or 32484; and the bronchoplasty with 32501.

ICD-10-CM Diagnostic Codes

C34.01 Malignant neoplasm of right main bronchus ☑
C34.11 Malignant neoplasm of upper lobe, right bronchus or lung ☑
C34.2 Malignant neoplasm of middle lobe, bronchus or lung
C34.31 Malignant neoplasm of lower lobe, right bronchus or lung ☑
C34.81 Malignant neoplasm of overlapping sites of right bronchus and lung ☑
C78.01 Secondary malignant neoplasm of right lung ☑
C78.1 Secondary malignant neoplasm of mediastinum
C7A.090 Malignant carcinoid tumor of the bronchus and lung
D02.21 Carcinoma in situ of right bronchus and lung ☑
D14.31 Benign neoplasm of right bronchus and lung ☑
D38.1 Neoplasm of uncertain behavior of trachea, bronchus and lung
D3A.090 Benign carcinoid tumor of the bronchus and lung
D86.0 Sarcoidosis of lung
D86.1 Sarcoidosis of lymph nodes
D86.2 Sarcoidosis of lung with sarcoidosis of lymph nodes
Q32.3 Congenital stenosis of bronchus
Q32.4 Other congenital malformations of bronchus
S21.311A Laceration without foreign body of right front wall of thorax with penetration into thoracic cavity, initial encounter ☑
S21.321A Laceration with foreign body of right front wall of thorax with penetration into thoracic cavity, initial encounter ☑
S21.331A Puncture wound without foreign body of right front wall of thorax with penetration into thoracic cavity, initial encounter ☑
S21.341A Puncture wound with foreign body of right front wall of thorax with penetration into thoracic cavity, initial encounter ☑
S21.351A Open bite of right front wall of thorax with penetration into thoracic cavity, initial encounter ☑
S21.411A Laceration without foreign body of right back wall of thorax with penetration into thoracic cavity, initial encounter ☑
S21.421A Laceration with foreign body of right back wall of thorax with penetration into thoracic cavity, initial encounter ☑
S21.431A Puncture wound without foreign body of right back wall of thorax with penetration into thoracic cavity, initial encounter ☑
S21.441A Puncture wound with foreign body of right back wall of thorax with penetration into thoracic cavity, initial encounter ☑
S21.451A Open bite of right back wall of thorax with penetration into thoracic cavity, initial encounter ☑
S27.411A Primary blast injury of bronchus, unilateral, initial encounter
S27.412A Primary blast injury of bronchus, bilateral, initial encounter ☑
S27.421A Contusion of bronchus, unilateral, initial encounter
S27.422A Contusion of bronchus, bilateral, initial encounter ☑
S27.431A Laceration of bronchus, unilateral, initial encounter
S27.432A Laceration of bronchus, bilateral, initial encounter ☑
S27.491A Other injury of bronchus, unilateral, initial encounter
S27.492A Other injury of bronchus, bilateral, initial encounter ☑
Z85.118 Personal history of other malignant neoplasm of bronchus and lung

Relative Value Units/Medicare Edits

Non-Facility RVU	Work	PE	MP	Total
31770	23.54	9.4	5.58	38.52
31775	24.59	10.06	5.83	40.48
Facility RVU	**Work**	**PE**	**MP**	**Total**
31770	23.54	9.4	5.58	38.52
31775	24.59	10.06	5.83	40.48

	FUD	Status	MUE	Modifiers				IOM Reference
31770	90	A	2(3)	51	N/A	62*	80	None
31775	90	A	1(3)	51	N/A	N/A	80	

* with documentation

Terms To Know

anastomosis. Surgically created connection between ducts, blood vessels, or bowel segments to allow flow from one to the other.

autograft. Tissue harvested from the same individual at one anatomical site and grafted to another separate anatomical site.

stenosis. Narrowing or constriction of a passage.

31781

31781 Excision tracheal stenosis and anastomosis; cervicothoracic

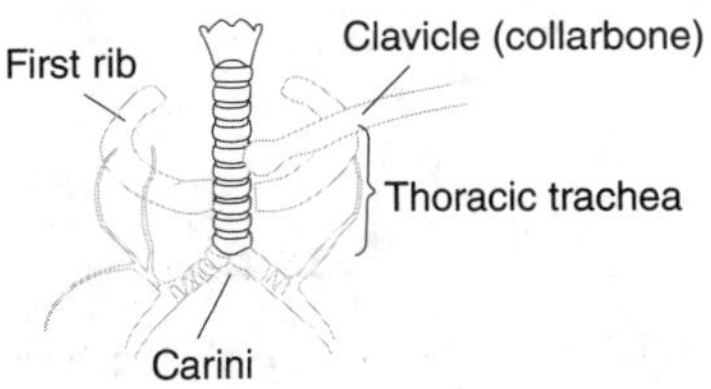

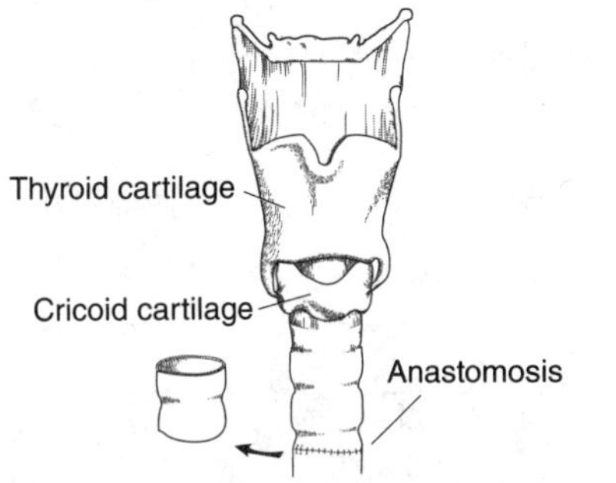

A section of stenosed trachea is removed via a cervicothoracic approach; the two ends are then anastomosed together

Explanation

The physician excises a tracheal stenosis and re-anastomoses the trachea. The physician makes a cervicothoracic incision to access the stenosis. The trachea is incised and the stenosis is resected. The proximal and distal portions of the trachea are brought together and closed with sutures. The wound is closed in sutured layers.

Coding Tips

If significant additional time and effort are documented, append modifier 22 and submit a cover letter and operative report. When 31781 is performed with another separately identifiable procedure, the highest dollar value code is listed as the primary procedure, and subsequent procedures are appended with modifier 51.

ICD-10-CM Diagnostic Codes

J39.8	Other specified diseases of upper respiratory tract
J95.03	Malfunction of tracheostomy stoma
Q32.1	Other congenital malformations of trachea
Z85.12	Personal history of malignant neoplasm of trachea

AMA: 31781 2018,Jan,8; 2017,Feb,14; 2017,Apr,5

Relative Value Units/Medicare Edits

Non-Facility RVU	Work	PE	MP	Total
31781	24.85	9.37	5.9	40.12
Facility RVU	**Work**	**PE**	**MP**	**Total**
31781	24.85	9.37	5.9	40.12

	FUD	Status	MUE	Modifiers				IOM Reference
31781	90	A	1(2)	51	N/A	62*	80	None

* with documentation

31786

31786 Excision of tracheal tumor or carcinoma; thoracic

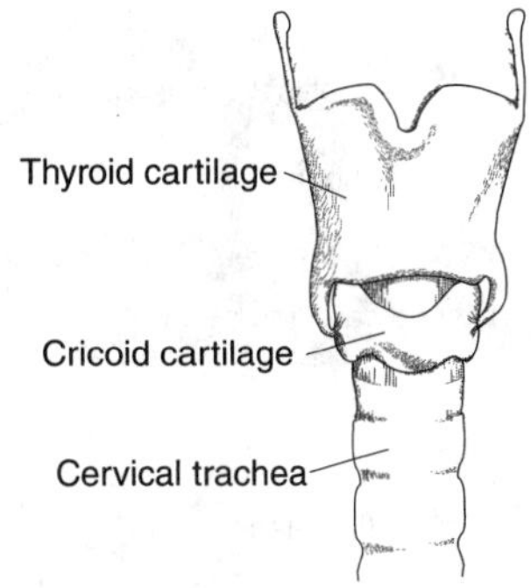

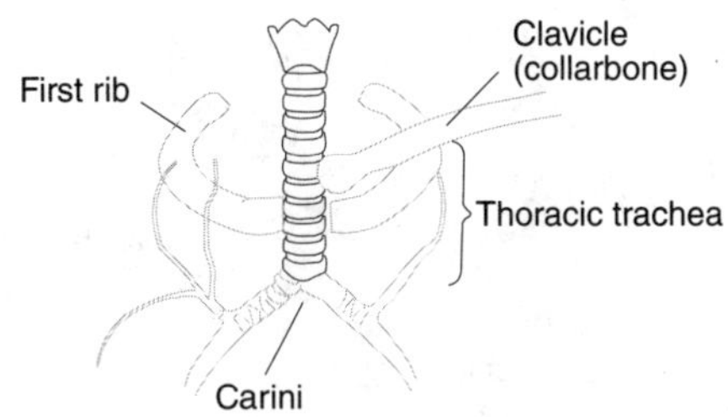

Explanation

The physician excises a tracheal tumor or carcinoma. The physician makes a thoracic approach to access the mass. The trachea is incised and the mass is resected. If necessary, the proximal and distal portions of the trachea are brought together and closed with sutures. The wound is sutured in layers.

Coding Tips

If significant additional time and effort are documented, append modifier 22 and submit a cover letter and operative report. When 31786 is performed with another separately identifiable procedure, the highest dollar value code is listed as the primary procedure, and subsequent procedures are appended with modifier 51. Report any free grafts or flaps separately.

ICD-10-CM Diagnostic Codes

C33	Malignant neoplasm of trachea
C78.39	Secondary malignant neoplasm of other respiratory organs
D02.1	Carcinoma in situ of trachea
D14.2	Benign neoplasm of trachea
D38.1	Neoplasm of uncertain behavior of trachea, bronchus and lung
D3A.090	Benign carcinoid tumor of the bronchus and lung

Relative Value Units/Medicare Edits

Non-Facility RVU	Work	PE	MP	Total
31786	25.42	10.29	6.03	41.74
Facility RVU	**Work**	**PE**	**MP**	**Total**
31786	25.42	10.29	6.03	41.74

	FUD	Status	MUE	Modifiers				IOM Reference
31786	90	A	1(3)	51	N/A	62*	80	None

* with documentation

 ● New ▲ Revised + Add On AMA: CPT Assist [Resequenced] ☑ Laterality

31805

31805 Suture of tracheal wound or injury; intrathoracic

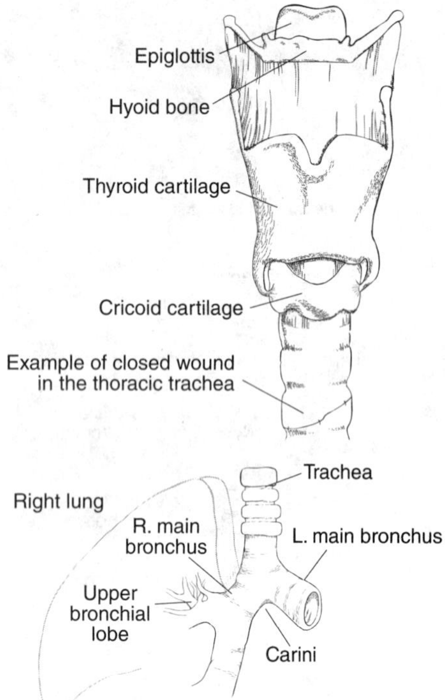

Explanation

The physician closes a wound or injury of the intrathoracic trachea. The physician debrides the wound and closes the trachea with sutures. The tissues are sutured in layers.

Coding Tips

If significant additional time and effort are documented, append modifier 22 and submit a cover letter and operative report.

ICD-10-CM Diagnostic Codes

S27.50XA	Unspecified injury of thoracic trachea, initial encounter
S27.51XA	Primary blast injury of thoracic trachea, initial encounter
S27.52XA	Contusion of thoracic trachea, initial encounter
S27.53XA	Laceration of thoracic trachea, initial encounter
S27.59XA	Other injury of thoracic trachea, initial encounter
T27.1XXA	Burn involving larynx and trachea with lung, initial encounter
T27.5XXA	Corrosion involving larynx and trachea with lung, initial encounter

Relative Value Units/Medicare Edits

Non-Facility RVU	Work	PE	MP	Total
31805	13.42	6.95	3.19	23.56
Facility RVU	**Work**	**PE**	**MP**	**Total**
31805	13.42	6.95	3.19	23.56

	FUD	Status	MUE	Modifiers				IOM Reference
31805	90	A	1(3)	51	N/A	62*	80	None

* with documentation

31820-31825

31820 Surgical closure tracheostomy or fistula; without plastic repair
31825 with plastic repair

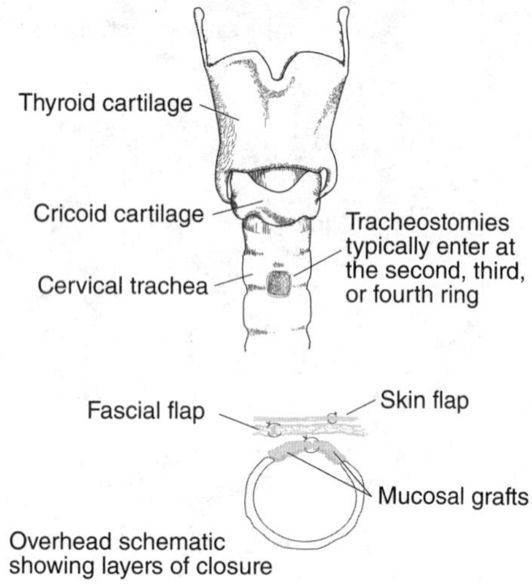

Explanation

The physician closes a tracheostomy or fistula. The physician excises the scarred tissue forming the tracheostomy or fistula. If the trachea has healed, it is closed with sutures. The remaining tissues of the tracheostomy or fistula are pulled together and the wound is sutured in layers. Report 31820 if the tracheostomy or fistula is closed without plastic repair; report 31825 if the tracheostomy or fistula is closed with plastic repair of the skin made to hide the repair.

Coding Tips

Fistula repairs may be performed for a variety of reasons and code selection is dependent on the nature of the fistula. Codes 31820 and 31825 should be reported for closure of a surgically created tracheostomy or fistula originally performed to establish an open airway. Repair of a fistula that is a complication of another surgical procedure is not reported with these codes. For repair of a tracheoesophageal fistula, see 43305 and 43312. Report any free grafts or flaps separately.

ICD-10-CM Diagnostic Codes

Z42.8	Encounter for other plastic and reconstructive surgery following medical procedure or healed injury
Z43.0	Encounter for attention to tracheostomy

Relative Value Units/Medicare Edits

Non-Facility RVU	Work	PE	MP	Total
31820	4.64	7.04	0.69	12.37
31825	7.07	9.04	1.05	17.16
Facility RVU	**Work**	**PE**	**MP**	**Total**
31820	4.64	4.02	0.69	9.35
31825	7.07	5.59	1.05	13.71

	FUD	Status	MUE	Modifiers				IOM Reference
31820	90	A	1(2)	51	N/A	N/A	80*	None
31825	90	A	1(2)	51	N/A	N/A	80*	

* with documentation

32035-32036

32035 Thoracostomy; with rib resection for empyema
32036 with open flap drainage for empyema

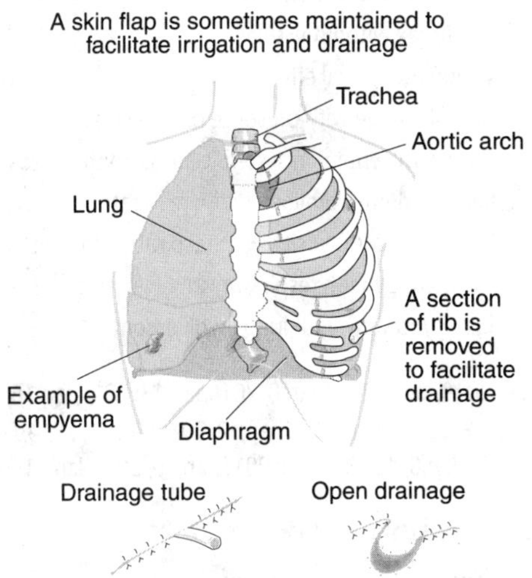

Explanation

The physician removes the purulent fluid of an empyema by creating a drainage wound in the chest. Using a scalpel, an incision is made through the skin of the chest and the incision is deepened to expose a portion of a rib. In 32035, to enter the chest cavity, a short segment of the exposed rib is removed using rib cutters. The resulting defect in the chest wall allows for the continuous release of pus from the empyema (abscess in the chest cavity). In 32036, to create a drainage site, a short segment of the rib is removed using rib cutters. The resulting defect in the chest wall allows for the continuous release of pus from the empyema. To ensure that the drainage wound stays open, a flap is created in the skin and subcutaneous tissues.

Coding Tips

Open flap drainage (32036) requires a subsequent procedure for closure once the empyema has resolved. For closure of the chest wall following open flap drainage for empyema, see 32810. For tube thoracostomy for empyema, see 32551. Wound exploration resulting from penetrating trauma without thoracotomy is reported with 20101.

ICD-10-CM Diagnostic Codes

J86.0 Pyothorax with fistula
J86.9 Pyothorax without fistula

Relative Value Units/Medicare Edits

Non-Facility RVU	Work	PE	MP	Total
32035	11.29	6.94	2.69	20.92
32036	12.3	7.29	2.8	22.39
Facility RVU	**Work**	**PE**	**MP**	**Total**
32035	11.29	6.94	2.69	20.92
32036	12.3	7.29	2.8	22.39

	FUD	Status	MUE	Modifiers				IOM Reference
32035	90	A	1(2)	51	50	62*	80	None
32036	90	A	1(3)	51	50	62*	80	

* with documentation

32096-32098

32096 Thoracotomy, with diagnostic biopsy(ies) of lung infiltrate(s) (eg, wedge, incisional), unilateral
32097 Thoracotomy, with diagnostic biopsy(ies) of lung nodule(s) or mass(es) (eg, wedge, incisional), unilateral
32098 Thoracotomy, with biopsy(ies) of pleura

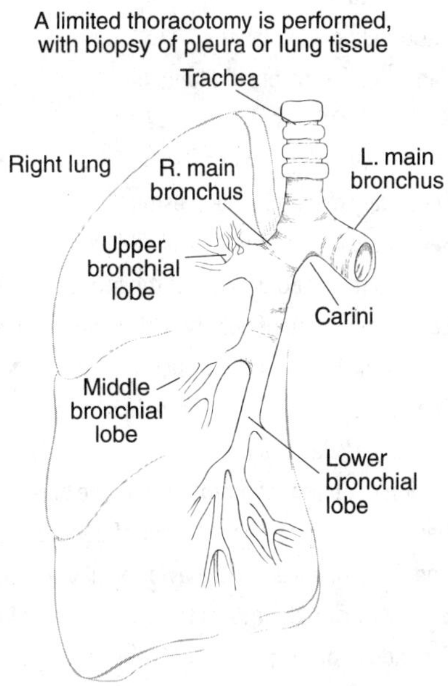

Explanation

The physician removes a sample of tissue from the lung or the pleura. Using a scalpel, the skin between two ribs is incised and the tissues separated to expose the inside of the chest cavity. A representative sample of tissue is removed from the lung or pleura using a biopsy needle or by cutting with a scalpel or scissors. The surgical wound is closed by suturing. Report 32096 when the biopsy is performed to sample unilateral lung infiltrates. Report 32097 when the biopsy is of a unilateral lung nodule or mass. Report 32098 when the tissue biopsied is the pleura.

Coding Tips

Note that 32096 and 32097 are unilateral procedures. If performed bilaterally, some payers require that the service be reported twice with modifier 50 appended to the second code while others require identification of the service only once with modifier 50 appended. Check with individual payers. Modifier 50 identifies a procedure performed identically on the opposite side of the body (mirror image). Codes 32096 and 32097 should only be reported once per lung. Do not report 32096 or 32097 with 32440, 32442, 32445, or 32488. A diagnostic wedge biopsy is characterized by removing tissue without concern for resection margins. A therapeutic wedge resection involves close attention to resection margins and complete resection. For wound exploration as a result of penetrating trauma not by thoracotomy, see 20101.

ICD-10-CM Diagnostic Codes

A15.6 Tuberculous pleurisy
B59 Pneumocystosis
C34.01 Malignant neoplasm of right main bronchus ☑
C34.02 Malignant neoplasm of left main bronchus ☑
C34.11 Malignant neoplasm of upper lobe, right bronchus or lung ☑
C34.12 Malignant neoplasm of upper lobe, left bronchus or lung ☑
C34.2 Malignant neoplasm of middle lobe, bronchus or lung
C34.31 Malignant neoplasm of lower lobe, right bronchus or lung ☑

C34.32 Malignant neoplasm of lower lobe, left bronchus or lung ☑
C34.81 Malignant neoplasm of overlapping sites of right bronchus and lung ☑
C34.82 Malignant neoplasm of overlapping sites of left bronchus and lung ☑
C38.4 Malignant neoplasm of pleura
C38.8 Malignant neoplasm of overlapping sites of heart, mediastinum and pleura
C45.0 Mesothelioma of pleura
C46.51 Kaposi's sarcoma of right lung ☑
C46.52 Kaposi's sarcoma of left lung ☑
C78.01 Secondary malignant neoplasm of right lung ☑
C78.02 Secondary malignant neoplasm of left lung ☑
C78.2 Secondary malignant neoplasm of pleura
C7A.090 Malignant carcinoid tumor of the bronchus and lung
D02.21 Carcinoma in situ of right bronchus and lung ☑
D02.22 Carcinoma in situ of left bronchus and lung ☑
D14.31 Benign neoplasm of right bronchus and lung ☑
D14.32 Benign neoplasm of left bronchus and lung ☑
D19.0 Benign neoplasm of mesothelial tissue of pleura
D38.1 Neoplasm of uncertain behavior of trachea, bronchus and lung
D38.2 Neoplasm of uncertain behavior of pleura
D3A.090 Benign carcinoid tumor of the bronchus and lung
D86.0 Sarcoidosis of lung
J60 Coalworker's pneumoconiosis
J61 Pneumoconiosis due to asbestos and other mineral fibers
J62.0 Pneumoconiosis due to talc dust
J62.8 Pneumoconiosis due to other dust containing silica
J63.0 Aluminosis (of lung)
J63.1 Bauxite fibrosis (of lung)
J63.2 Berylliosis
J63.3 Graphite fibrosis (of lung)
J63.4 Siderosis
J63.5 Stannosis
J63.6 Pneumoconiosis due to other specified inorganic dusts
J66.0 Byssinosis
J66.1 Flax-dressers' disease
J66.2 Cannabinosis
J66.8 Airway disease due to other specific organic dusts
J67.8 Hypersensitivity pneumonitis due to other organic dusts
J67.9 Hypersensitivity pneumonitis due to unspecified organic dust
J68.0 Bronchitis and pneumonitis due to chemicals, gases, fumes and vapors
J68.4 Chronic respiratory conditions due to chemicals, gases, fumes and vapors
J70.2 Acute drug-induced interstitial lung disorders
J82 Pulmonary eosinophilia, not elsewhere classified
J84.112 Idiopathic pulmonary fibrosis
J84.113 Idiopathic non-specific interstitial pneumonitis
J84.115 Respiratory bronchiolitis interstitial lung disease
J84.117 Desquamative interstitial pneumonia
J84.17 Other interstitial pulmonary diseases with fibrosis in diseases classified elsewhere
J84.2 Lymphoid interstitial pneumonia
J84.82 Adult pulmonary Langerhans cell histiocytosis
J84.848 Other interstitial lung diseases of childhood
J84.89 Other specified interstitial pulmonary diseases
J85.0 Gangrene and necrosis of lung
J86.0 Pyothorax with fistula
J86.9 Pyothorax without fistula
J91.0 Malignant pleural effusion
J92.0 Pleural plaque with presence of asbestos
M32.13 Lung involvement in systemic lupus erythematosus
M33.01 Juvenile dermatomyositis with respiratory involvement
M33.11 Other dermatomyositis with respiratory involvement
M33.21 Polymyositis with respiratory involvement
M35.02 Sicca syndrome with lung involvement

AMA: 32096 2018,Jan,8; 2017,Jan,8; 2016,Jan,13; 2015,Jan,16; 2014,Jan,11 **32097** 2018,Jan,8; 2017,Jan,8; 2016,Jan,13; 2015,Jan,16; 2014,Jan,11 **32098** 2018,Jan,8; 2017,Jan,8; 2016,Jan,13; 2015,Jan,16; 2014,Jan,11

Relative Value Units/Medicare Edits

Non-Facility RVU	Work	PE	MP	Total
32096	13.75	6.31	3.14	23.2
32097	13.75	6.29	3.15	23.19
32098	12.91	6.12	2.94	21.97
Facility RVU	**Work**	**PE**	**MP**	**Total**
32096	13.75	6.31	3.14	23.2
32097	13.75	6.29	3.15	23.19
32098	12.91	6.12	2.94	21.97

	FUD	Status	MUE	Modifiers				IOM Reference
32096	90	A	1(3)	51	N/A	62*	80	None
32097	90	A	1(3)	51	N/A	62*	80	
32098	90	A	1(2)	51	N/A	62*	80	

* with documentation

Terms To Know

effusion. Escape of fluid from within a body cavity.

hemoptysis. Coughing up or spitting out blood or blood-streaked sputum.

pleura. One of the two membranes that surround the lungs. The visceral pleura encases the lung and the parietal pleura lines the inner chest walls.

pleurisy. Inflammation of the serous membrane that lines the lungs and the thoracic cavity. Pleurisy may cause effusion within the cavity or have exudate in the pleural space or on the membrane surface.

thoracotomy. Surgical procedure for opening the chest wall in order to access the lungs, esophagus, trachea, aorta, heart, and diaphragm.

32100

32100 Thoracotomy; with exploration

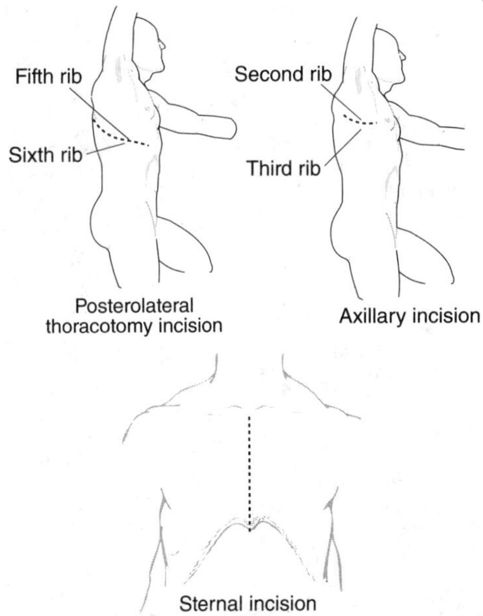

Any of a number of access incisions may be used

Explanation

The physician opens the chest cavity widely to directly visualize and assess the organs and structures in the chest. Using a scalpel, the surgeon makes a long incision around the side of the chest between two of the ribs. The incision is carried through all of the tissue layers into the chest cavity. Rib spreaders are inserted into the wound and the ribs are spread apart exposing the lung, heart, and other structures. Alternately, the chest cavity can be opened and the operation performed through a vertical incision in the center of the chest through the sternum. The skin incision is carried down to the sternum bone and a saw is used to split the sternum. With the sternum split in half, the chest is entered by spreading the sternum apart with a set of rib spreaders. The chest cavity is explored and the anatomy visualized using a gloved hand and large gauze sponges. The surgical instruments are removed. A chest tube(s) may be used to provide drainage for the chest cavity. When the procedure is complete, if applicable, the sternotomy is repaired using wires to bring the two halves of the sternum together, and the operative wound is closed by sutures or staples.

Coding Tips

Report 32100 for a major thoracotomy when the chest cavity is opened to fully explore any lesions. For a thoracotomy with a biopsy, see 32096, 32097, and 32098. For exploration of a chest wound not requiring thoracotomy, see 20101. Do not report 32100 with 21601-21603, 32503, 32504, 33955-33957, 33963, or 33964.

ICD-10-CM Diagnostic Codes

C34.01	Malignant neoplasm of right main bronchus ☑
C34.02	Malignant neoplasm of left main bronchus ☑
C34.11	Malignant neoplasm of upper lobe, right bronchus or lung ☑
C34.12	Malignant neoplasm of upper lobe, left bronchus or lung ☑
C34.2	Malignant neoplasm of middle lobe, bronchus or lung
C34.31	Malignant neoplasm of lower lobe, right bronchus or lung ☑
C34.32	Malignant neoplasm of lower lobe, left bronchus or lung ☑
C34.81	Malignant neoplasm of overlapping sites of right bronchus and lung ☑
C34.82	Malignant neoplasm of overlapping sites of left bronchus and lung ☑
C46.51	Kaposi's sarcoma of right lung ☑
C46.52	Kaposi's sarcoma of left lung ☑
D14.31	Benign neoplasm of right bronchus and lung ☑
D14.32	Benign neoplasm of left bronchus and lung ☑
D3A.090	Benign carcinoid tumor of the bronchus and lung
S26.01XA	Contusion of heart with hemopericardium, initial encounter
S26.020A	Mild laceration of heart with hemopericardium, initial encounter
S26.021A	Moderate laceration of heart with hemopericardium, initial encounter
S26.022A	Major laceration of heart with hemopericardium, initial encounter
S26.09XA	Other injury of heart with hemopericardium, initial encounter
S26.11XA	Contusion of heart without hemopericardium, initial encounter
S26.12XA	Laceration of heart without hemopericardium, initial encounter
S26.19XA	Other injury of heart without hemopericardium, initial encounter
S27.0XXA	Traumatic pneumothorax, initial encounter
S27.1XXA	Traumatic hemothorax, initial encounter
S27.2XXA	Traumatic hemopneumothorax, initial encounter
S27.311A	Primary blast injury of lung, unilateral, initial encounter
S27.312A	Primary blast injury of lung, bilateral, initial encounter ☑
S27.321A	Contusion of lung, unilateral, initial encounter
S27.322A	Contusion of lung, bilateral, initial encounter ☑
S27.331A	Laceration of lung, unilateral, initial encounter
S27.332A	Laceration of lung, bilateral, initial encounter ☑
S27.391A	Other injuries of lung, unilateral, initial encounter
S27.392A	Other injuries of lung, bilateral, initial encounter ☑
S27.411A	Primary blast injury of bronchus, unilateral, initial encounter
S27.412A	Primary blast injury of bronchus, bilateral, initial encounter ☑
S27.421A	Contusion of bronchus, unilateral, initial encounter
S27.422A	Contusion of bronchus, bilateral, initial encounter ☑
S27.431A	Laceration of bronchus, unilateral, initial encounter
S27.432A	Laceration of bronchus, bilateral, initial encounter ☑
S27.491A	Other injury of bronchus, unilateral, initial encounter
S27.492A	Other injury of bronchus, bilateral, initial encounter ☑
S27.51XA	Primary blast injury of thoracic trachea, initial encounter
S27.52XA	Contusion of thoracic trachea, initial encounter
S27.53XA	Laceration of thoracic trachea, initial encounter
S27.59XA	Other injury of thoracic trachea, initial encounter
S27.63XA	Laceration of pleura, initial encounter
S27.69XA	Other injury of pleura, initial encounter
S27.802A	Contusion of diaphragm, initial encounter
S27.803A	Laceration of diaphragm, initial encounter
S27.808A	Other injury of diaphragm, initial encounter
S27.812A	Contusion of esophagus (thoracic part), initial encounter
S27.813A	Laceration of esophagus (thoracic part), initial encounter
S27.818A	Other injury of esophagus (thoracic part), initial encounter
S27.892A	Contusion of other specified intrathoracic organs, initial encounter
S27.893A	Laceration of other specified intrathoracic organs, initial encounter

S27.898A Other injury of other specified intrathoracic organs, initial encounter

S28.0XXA Crushed chest, initial encounter

AMA: **32100** 2018,Jan,8; 2017,Jan,8; 2016,Jan,13; 2015,Jul,3; 2015,Jan,16; 2014,Jan,11; 2013,Jan,6-8

Relative Value Units/Medicare Edits

Non-Facility RVU	Work	PE	MP	Total
32100	13.75	6.46	3.18	23.39
Facility RVU	**Work**	**PE**	**MP**	**Total**
32100	13.75	6.46	3.18	23.39

	FUD	Status	MUE	Modifiers				IOM Reference
32100	90	A	1(3)	51	N/A	62*	80	None

* with documentation

Terms To Know

sternotomy. Incision into the sternum, the bone that forms the front of the chest cavity and connects with the ribs.

thoracotomy. Surgical procedure for opening the chest wall in order to access the lungs, esophagus, trachea, aorta, heart, and diaphragm.

32110

32110 Thoracotomy; with control of traumatic hemorrhage and/or repair of lung tear

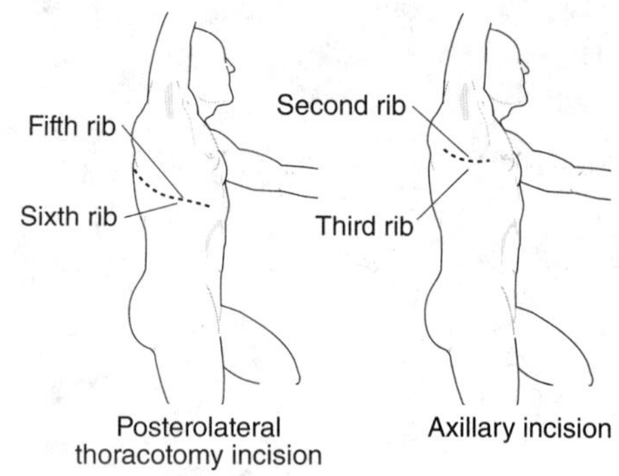

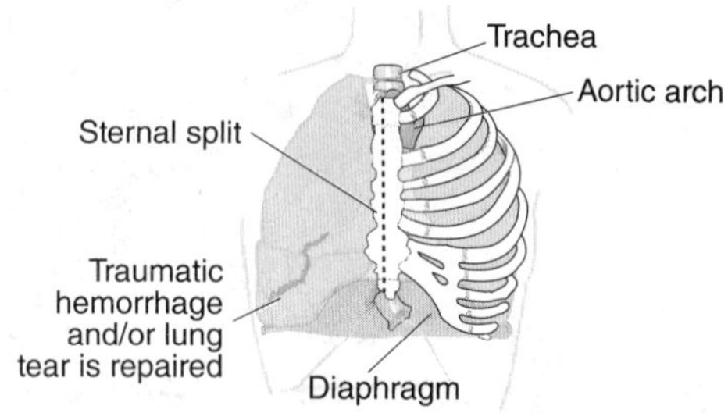

Explanation

The physician opens the chest cavity widely to directly visualize and assess the organs and structures in the chest. Using a scalpel, the surgeon makes a long incision around the side of the chest between two of the ribs. The incision is carried through all of the tissue layers into the chest cavity. Rib spreaders are inserted into the wound and the ribs are spread apart exposing the lung, heart, and other structures. Alternately, the chest cavity can be opened and the operation performed through a vertical incision in the center of the chest through the sternum. The skin incision is carried down to the sternum bone and a saw is used to split the sternum. With the sternum split in half, the chest is entered by spreading the sternum apart with a set of rib spreaders. The chest cavity is explored and the anatomy visualized using a gloved hand and large gauze sponges. The site of the hemorrhage or lung tear is identified and repaired. The surgical instruments are removed. A chest tube(s) may be used to provide drainage for the chest cavity. When the procedure is complete, if applicable, the sternotomy is repaired using wires to bring the two halves of the sternum together, and the operative wound is closed by sutures or staples.

Coding Tips

When 32110 is performed with another separately identifiable procedure, the highest dollar value code is listed as the primary procedure, and subsequent procedures are appended with modifier 51. If traumatic hemorrhage is controlled through a thoracoscope, not open thoracotomy, see 32654.

ICD-10-CM Diagnostic Codes

S21.311A Laceration without foreign body of right front wall of thorax with penetration into thoracic cavity, initial encounter ☑

S21.312A Laceration without foreign body of left front wall of thorax with penetration into thoracic cavity, initial encounter ☑

S21.321A Laceration with foreign body of right front wall of thorax with penetration into thoracic cavity, initial encounter ☑

S21.322A Laceration with foreign body of left front wall of thorax with penetration into thoracic cavity, initial encounter ☑

S21.331A Puncture wound without foreign body of right front wall of thorax with penetration into thoracic cavity, initial encounter ☑

S21.332A Puncture wound without foreign body of left front wall of thorax with penetration into thoracic cavity, initial encounter ☑

S21.341A Puncture wound with foreign body of right front wall of thorax with penetration into thoracic cavity, initial encounter ☑

S21.342A Puncture wound with foreign body of left front wall of thorax with penetration into thoracic cavity, initial encounter ☑

S21.351A Open bite of right front wall of thorax with penetration into thoracic cavity, initial encounter ☑

S21.352A Open bite of left front wall of thorax with penetration into thoracic cavity, initial encounter ☑

S21.411A Laceration without foreign body of right back wall of thorax with penetration into thoracic cavity, initial encounter ☑

S21.412A Laceration without foreign body of left back wall of thorax with penetration into thoracic cavity, initial encounter ☑

S21.421A Laceration with foreign body of right back wall of thorax with penetration into thoracic cavity, initial encounter ☑

S21.422A Laceration with foreign body of left back wall of thorax with penetration into thoracic cavity, initial encounter ☑

S21.431A Puncture wound without foreign body of right back wall of thorax with penetration into thoracic cavity, initial encounter ☑

S21.432A Puncture wound without foreign body of left back wall of thorax with penetration into thoracic cavity, initial encounter ☑

S21.441A Puncture wound with foreign body of right back wall of thorax with penetration into thoracic cavity, initial encounter ☑

S21.442A Puncture wound with foreign body of left back wall of thorax with penetration into thoracic cavity, initial encounter ☑

S21.451A Open bite of right back wall of thorax with penetration into thoracic cavity, initial encounter ☑

S21.452A Open bite of left back wall of thorax with penetration into thoracic cavity, initial encounter ☑

S25.411A Minor laceration of right pulmonary blood vessels, initial encounter ☑

S25.412A Minor laceration of left pulmonary blood vessels, initial encounter ☑

S25.421A Major laceration of right pulmonary blood vessels, initial encounter ☑

S25.422A Major laceration of left pulmonary blood vessels, initial encounter ☑

S25.491A Other specified injury of right pulmonary blood vessels, initial encounter ☑

S25.492A Other specified injury of left pulmonary blood vessels, initial encounter ☑

S25.811A Laceration of other blood vessels of thorax, right side, initial encounter ☑

S25.812A Laceration of other blood vessels of thorax, left side, initial encounter ☑

S25.891A Other specified injury of other blood vessels of thorax, right side, initial encounter ☑

S25.892A Other specified injury of other blood vessels of thorax, left side, initial encounter ☑

S27.0XXA Traumatic pneumothorax, initial encounter

S27.1XXA Traumatic hemothorax, initial encounter

S27.2XXA Traumatic hemopneumothorax, initial encounter

S27.311A Primary blast injury of lung, unilateral, initial encounter

S27.312A Primary blast injury of lung, bilateral, initial encounter ☑

S27.321A Contusion of lung, unilateral, initial encounter

S27.322A Contusion of lung, bilateral, initial encounter ☑

S27.331A Laceration of lung, unilateral, initial encounter

S27.332A Laceration of lung, bilateral, initial encounter ☑

S27.391A Other injuries of lung, unilateral, initial encounter

S27.392A Other injuries of lung, bilateral, initial encounter ☑

S28.0XXA Crushed chest, initial encounter

AMA: 32110 2018,Jan,8; 2017,Jan,8; 2016,Jan,13; 2015,Jan,16; 2014,Jan,11

Relative Value Units/Medicare Edits

Non-Facility RVU	Work	PE	MP	Total
32110	25.28	11.46	5.7	42.44
Facility RVU	**Work**	**PE**	**MP**	**Total**
32110	25.28	11.46	5.7	42.44

	FUD	Status	MUE	Modifiers				IOM Reference
32110	90	A	1(3)	51	N/A	62*	80	None

* with documentation

Terms To Know

spontaneous tension pneumothorax. Air leaking from the lung and trapped in the lung lining.

thoracotomy. Surgical procedure for opening the chest wall in order to access the lungs, esophagus, trachea, aorta, heart, and diaphragm.

32120

32120 Thoracotomy; for postoperative complications

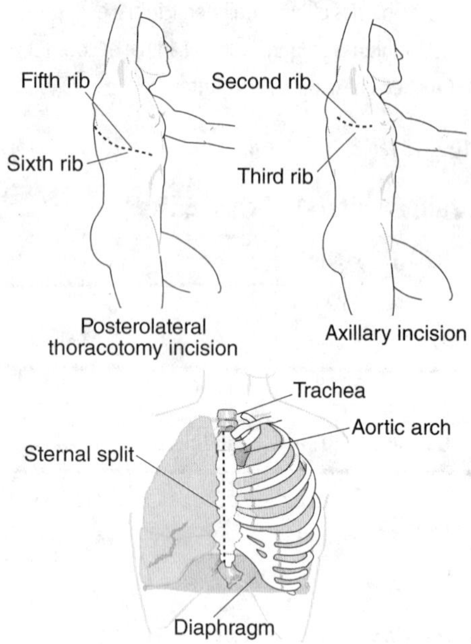

Explanation

The physician performs a thoracotomy to identify any thoracic postoperative complications. The physician opens the chest cavity widely to directly visualize and assess the organs and structures in the chest. Using a scalpel, the surgeon makes a long incision around the side of the chest between two of the ribs. The incision is carried through all of the tissue layers into the chest cavity. Rib spreaders are inserted into the wound and the ribs are spread apart exposing the lung, heart, and other structures. Alternately, the chest cavity can be opened and the operation performed through a vertical incision in the center of the chest through the sternum. The skin incision is carried down to the sternum bone and a saw is used to split the sternum. With the sternum split in half, the chest is entered by spreading the sternum apart with a set of rib spreaders. The chest cavity is explored and the anatomy visualized using a gloved hand and large gauze sponges. The surgical instruments are removed. A chest tube(s) may be used to provide drainage for the chest cavity. When the procedure is complete, if applicable, the sternotomy is repaired using wires to bring the two halves of the sternum together, and the operative wound is closed by sutures or staples.

Coding Tips

When 32120 is performed with another separately identifiable procedure, the highest dollar value code is listed as the primary procedure, and subsequent procedures are appended with modifier 51.

ICD-10-CM Diagnostic Codes

J95.811 Postprocedural pneumothorax
J95.812 Postprocedural air leak
J95.830 Postprocedural hemorrhage of a respiratory system organ or structure following a respiratory system procedure
J95.831 Postprocedural hemorrhage of a respiratory system organ or structure following other procedure
J95.860 Postprocedural hematoma of a respiratory system organ or structure following a respiratory system procedure
J95.861 Postprocedural hematoma of a respiratory system organ or structure following other procedure
J95.862 Postprocedural seroma of a respiratory system organ or structure following a respiratory system procedure
J95.863 Postprocedural seroma of a respiratory system organ or structure following other procedure
J95.89 Other postprocedural complications and disorders of respiratory system, not elsewhere classified
T81.41XA Infection following a procedure, superficial incisional surgical site, initial encounter
T81.42XA Infection following a procedure, deep incisional surgical site, initial encounter
T81.43XA Infection following a procedure, organ and space surgical site, initial encounter
T81.44XA Sepsis following a procedure, initial encounter
T81.49XA Infection following a procedure, other surgical site, initial encounter
T81.510A Adhesions due to foreign body accidentally left in body following surgical operation, initial encounter
T81.520A Obstruction due to foreign body accidentally left in body following surgical operation, initial encounter
T81.530A Perforation due to foreign body accidentally left in body following surgical operation, initial encounter
T81.538A Perforation due to foreign body accidentally left in body following other procedure, initial encounter

Relative Value Units/Medicare Edits

Non-Facility RVU	Work	PE	MP	Total
32120	14.39	7.46	3.32	25.17
Facility RVU	**Work**	**PE**	**MP**	**Total**
32120	14.39	7.46	3.32	25.17

	FUD	Status	MUE	Modifiers				IOM Reference
32120	90	A	1(3)	51	N/A	62*	80	None

* with documentation

Terms To Know

empyema. Accumulation of pus within the respiratory or pleural cavity.

fistula. Abnormal tube-like passage between two body cavities or organs or from an organ to the outside surface.

thoracotomy. Surgical procedure for opening the chest wall in order to access the lungs, esophagus, trachea, aorta, heart, and diaphragm.

32124

32124 Thoracotomy; with open intrapleural pneumonolysis

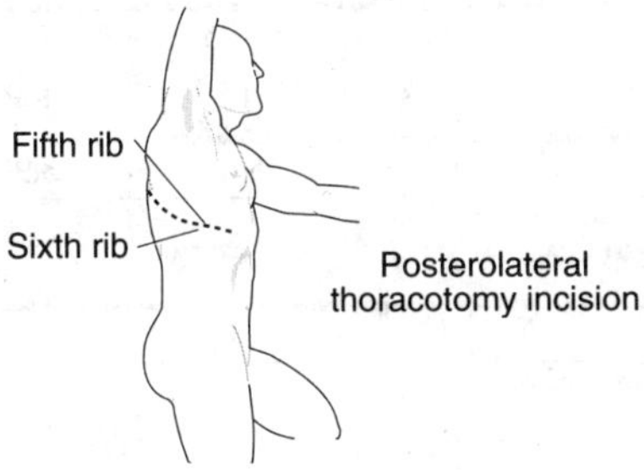

Adhesions between lung tissue and the inside surface of the chest cavity are released

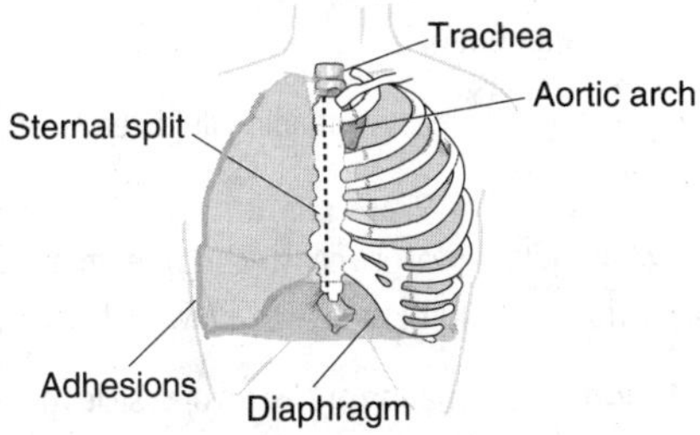

Explanation

The physician opens the chest cavity widely to directly visualize and separate the surface of the lung, which has become adherent to the inside surface of the chest cavity. Using a scalpel, the surgeon makes a long incision around the side of the chest between two of the ribs. The incision is carried through all of the tissue layers into the chest cavity. Rib spreaders are inserted into the wound and the ribs are spread apart exposing the lung. Alternately, the chest cavity can be opened and the operation performed through a vertical incision in the center of the chest through the sternum. The skin incision is carried down to the sternum bone and a saw is used to split the sternum. With the sternum split in half, the chest is entered by spreading the sternum apart with a set of rib spreaders. Using a gloved hand and a large moist gauze sponge, the surgeon manually divides the tissues attaching the lung to the wall of the chest cavity. When the procedure is complete, the instruments and gauze sponges are removed. A chest tube(s) may be used to provide drainage for the chest cavity. If applicable, the sternotomy is repaired using wires to bring the two halves of the sternum together, and the operative wound is closed by sutures or staples.

Coding Tips

If total decortication, including intrapleural pneumonolysis, is performed via thoracoscopy, see 32652.

ICD-10-CM Diagnostic Codes

A15.0	Tuberculosis of lung
A15.6	Tuberculous pleurisy
B90.9	Sequelae of respiratory and unspecified tuberculosis

AMA: 32124 2018,Jan,8; 2017,Jan,8; 2016,Jan,13; 2015,Jan,16; 2014,Jan,11

Relative Value Units/Medicare Edits

Non-Facility RVU	Work	PE	MP	Total
32124	15.45	7.7	3.56	26.71
Facility RVU	**Work**	**PE**	**MP**	**Total**
32124	15.45	7.7	3.56	26.71

	FUD	Status	MUE	Modifiers				IOM Reference
32124	90	A	1(3)	51	N/A	62*	80	None

* with documentation

Terms To Know

adhesion. Abnormal fibrous connection between two structures, soft tissue or bony structures, that may occur as the result of surgery, infection, or trauma.

complication. Condition arising after the beginning of observation and treatment that modifies the course of the patient's illness or the medical care required, or an undesired result or misadventure in medical care.

decortication of lung. Removal of a constricting membrane or layer of pleural tissue from a portion of the lung surface to allow for lung expansion.

effusion. Escape of fluid from within a body cavity.

empyema. Accumulation of pus within the respiratory or pleural cavity.

fistula. Abnormal tube-like passage between two body cavities or organs or from an organ to the outside surface.

iatrogenic. Adversely induced in the patient; caused by medical treatment.

incision. Act of cutting into tissue or an organ.

late effect. Abnormality, dysfunction, or other residual condition produced after the acute phase of an illness, injury, or disease is over. There is no time limit on when late effects can appear.

pleurisy. Inflammation of the serous membrane that lines the lungs and the thoracic cavity. Pleurisy may cause effusion within the cavity or have exudate in the pleural space or on the membrane surface.

thoracotomy. Surgical procedure for opening the chest wall in order to access the lungs, esophagus, trachea, aorta, heart, and diaphragm.

32140

32140 Thoracotomy; with cyst(s) removal, includes pleural procedure when performed

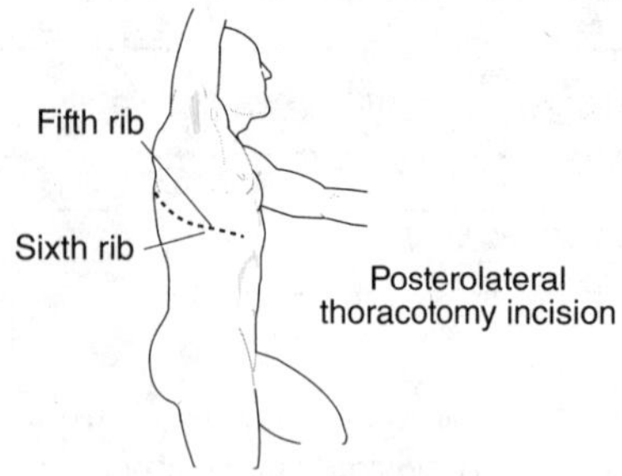

Lung cysts are removed

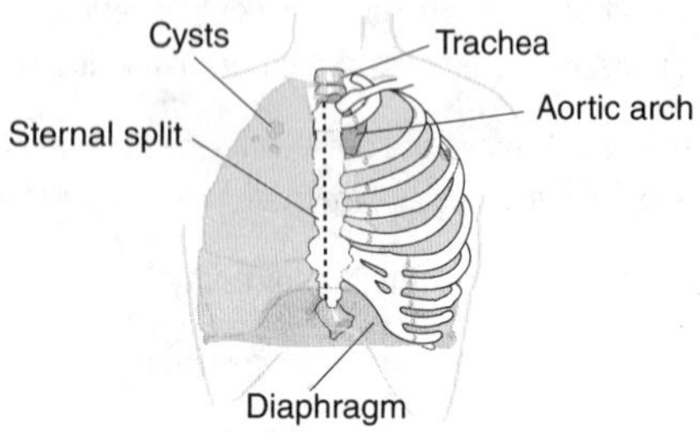

Explanation

The physician opens the chest cavity widely to remove one or more lung cysts. Using a scalpel, the surgeon makes a long incision around the side of the chest between two of the ribs. The incision is carried through all of the tissue layers into the chest cavity. Rib spreaders are inserted into the wound and the ribs are spread apart exposing the lung. Alternately, the chest cavity can be opened and the operation performed through a vertical incision in the center of the chest through the sternum. The skin incision is carried down to the sternum bone and a saw is used to split the sternum. With the sternum split in half, the chest is entered by spreading the sternum apart with a set of rib spreaders. Space is made in the chest by packing the uninvolved lung away from the operative field by using large moist gauze sponges. In order to perform the procedure, the pleural surface may require an operative procedure such as pneumonolysis (separation of the surface of the lung that has become adherent to the inside surface of the chest cavity). The lung cyst is located and removed by sharp and blunt dissection of the tissues. When the procedure is complete, the instruments and gauze sponges are removed. A chest tube(s) may be used to provide drainage for the chest cavity. If applicable, the sternotomy is repaired using wires to bring the two halves of the sternum together, and the operative wound is closed by sutures or staples.

Coding Tips

For surgical thoracoscopy with excision of a pericardial cyst, tumor, or mass, see 32661; with excision of a mediastinal cyst, tumor, or mass, see 32662. Supplies used when providing this procedure may be reported with the appropriate HCPCS Level II codes. Check with the specific payer to determine coverage.

ICD-10-CM Diagnostic Codes

B67.1	Echinococcus granulosus infection of lung
J98.4	Other disorders of lung
Q33.0	Congenital cystic lung

AMA: 32140 2018,Jan,8; 2017,Jan,8; 2016,Jan,13; 2015,Jan,16; 2014,Jan,11

Relative Value Units/Medicare Edits

Non-Facility RVU	Work	PE	MP	Total
32140	16.66	8.05	3.96	28.67
Facility RVU	**Work**	**PE**	**MP**	**Total**
32140	16.66	8.05	3.96	28.67

	FUD	Status	MUE	Modifiers				IOM Reference
32140	90	A	1(3)	51	N/A	62*	80	None

* with documentation

Terms To Know

congenital. Present at birth, occurring through heredity or an influence during gestation up to the moment of birth.

cyst. Elevated encapsulated mass containing fluid, semisolid, or solid material with a membranous lining.

decortication of lung. Removal of a constricting membrane or layer of pleural tissue from a portion of the lung surface to allow for lung expansion.

emphysematous bleb. Formation of blisters or vesicles greater than 1.0 mm within an emphysematous lung, containing serum or blood.

excision. Surgical removal of an organ or tissue.

fibrosis. Formation of fibrous tissue as part of the restorative process.

incision. Act of cutting into tissue or an organ.

lesion. Area of damaged tissue that has lost continuity or function, due to disease or trauma.

thoracotomy. Surgical procedure for opening the chest wall in order to access the lungs, esophagus, trachea, aorta, heart, and diaphragm.

32141

32141 Thoracotomy; with resection-plication of bullae, includes any pleural procedure when performed

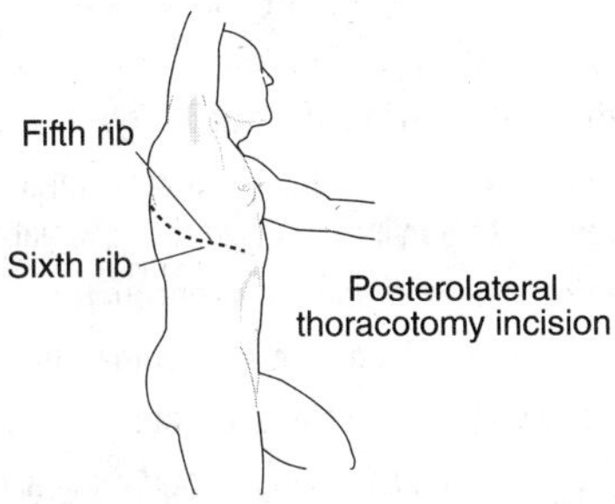

Lung cysts are removed

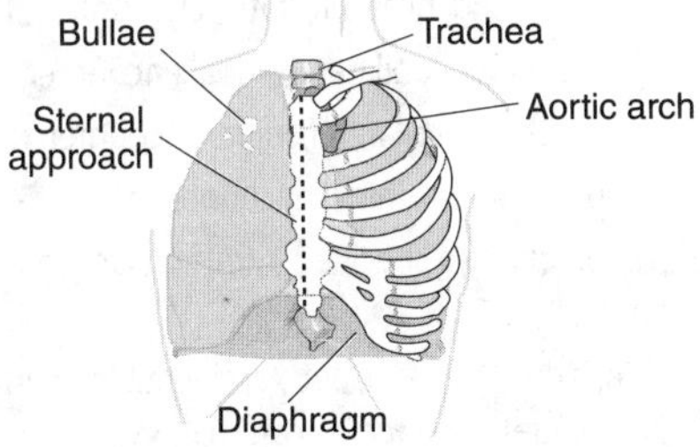

Explanation

The physician opens the chest cavity widely to remove one or more lung bullae (large non-functional air sacs). Using a scalpel, the surgeon makes a long incision around the side of the chest between two of the ribs. The incision is carried through all of the tissue layers into the chest cavity. Rib spreaders are inserted into the wound and the ribs are spread apart exposing the lung. Alternately, the chest cavity can be opened and the operation performed through a vertical incision in the center of the chest through the sternum. The skin incision is carried down to the sternum bone and a saw is used to split the sternum. With the sternum split in half, the chest is entered by spreading the sternum apart with a set of rib spreaders. Space is made in the chest by packing the uninvolved lung away from the operative field using large moist gauze sponges. In order to perform the procedure, the pleural surface may require an operative procedure such as pneumonolysis (separation of the surface of the lung that has become adherent to the inside surface of the chest cavity). The lung bullae is located and removed by sharp and blunt dissection of the tissues and often by folding and suturing of the tissues (plication). When the procedure is complete, the instruments and gauze sponges are removed. A chest tube(s) may be used to provide drainage for the chest cavity. If applicable, the sternotomy is repaired using wires to bring the two halves of the sternum together, and the operative wound is closed by sutures or staples.

Coding Tips

To report thoracoscopy with excision or plication of bullae, including any pleural procedure, see 32655. For excision/plication of emphysematous lungs for lung volume reduction, see 32491. Supplies used when providing this procedure may be reported with the appropriate HCPCS Level II codes. Check with the specific payer to determine coverage.

ICD-10-CM Diagnostic Codes

J43.0	Unilateral pulmonary emphysema [MacLeod's syndrome]
J43.1	Panlobular emphysema
J43.2	Centrilobular emphysema
J43.8	Other emphysema
J43.9	Emphysema, unspecified

AMA: 32141 2018,Jan,8; 2017,Jan,8; 2016,Jan,13; 2015,Jan,16; 2014,Jan,11

Relative Value Units/Medicare Edits

Non-Facility RVU	Work	PE	MP	Total
32141	27.18	10.67	6.2	44.05
Facility RVU	**Work**	**PE**	**MP**	**Total**
32141	27.18	10.67	6.2	44.05

	FUD	Status	MUE	Modifiers				IOM Reference
32141	90	A	1(3)	51	N/A	62*	80	None

* with documentation

Terms To Know

blunt dissection. Surgical technique used to expose an underlying area by separating along natural cleavage lines of tissue, without cutting.

emphysematous bleb. Formation of blisters or vesicles greater than 1.0 mm within an emphysematous lung, containing serum or blood.

excision. Surgical removal of an organ or tissue.

lesion. Area of damaged tissue that has lost continuity or function, due to disease or trauma.

pleura. One of the two membranes that surround the lungs. The visceral pleura encases the lung and the parietal pleura lines the inner chest walls.

plication. Surgical technique involving folding, tucking, or pleating to reduce the size of a hollow structure or organ.

sternotomy. Incision into the sternum, the bone that forms the front of the chest cavity and connects with the ribs.

thoracotomy. Surgical procedure for opening the chest wall in order to access the lungs, esophagus, trachea, aorta, heart, and diaphragm.

32150-32151

32150 Thoracotomy; with removal of intrapleural foreign body or fibrin deposit

32151 with removal of intrapulmonary foreign body

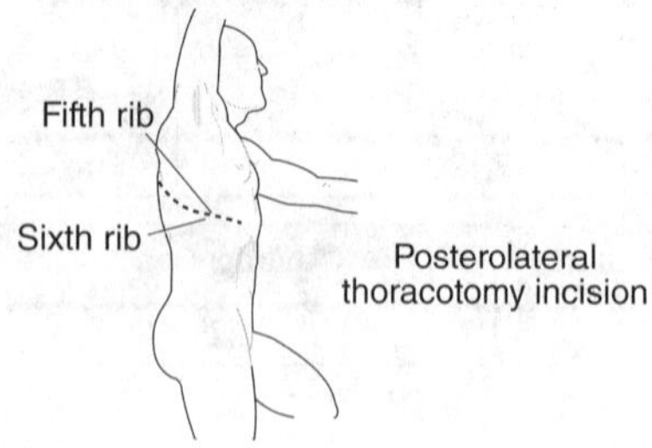

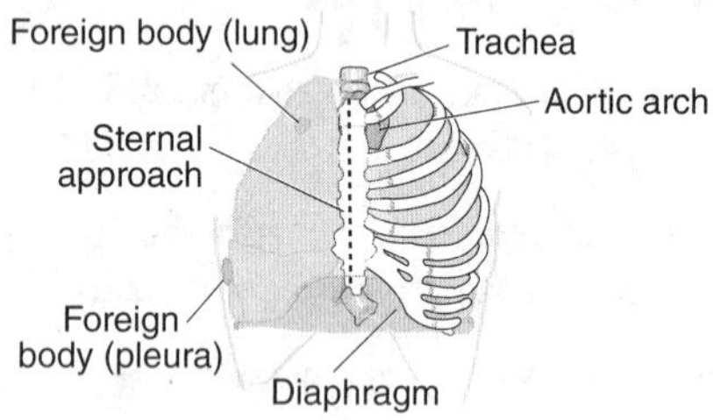

Explanation

The physician opens the chest cavity widely to remove a foreign body or fibrin deposit (thick insoluble protein deposit formed after the clotting of blood). Using a scalpel, the surgeon makes a long incision around the side of the chest between two of the ribs. The incision is carried through all of the tissue layers into the chest cavity. Rib spreaders are inserted into the wound and the ribs are spread apart exposing the lung. Alternately, the chest cavity can be opened and the operation performed through a vertical incision in the center of the chest through the sternum. The skin incision is carried down to the sternum bone and a saw is used to split the sternum. With the sternum split in half, the chest is entered by spreading the sternum apart with a set of rib spreaders. Space is made in the chest by packing the uninvolved lung away from the operative field using large moist gauze sponges. The foreign body or fibrin deposit is located and removed by sharp and blunt dissection. When the procedure is complete, the instruments and gauze sponges are removed. A chest tube(s) may be used to provide drainage for the chest cavity. If applicable, the sternotomy is repaired using wires to bring the two halves of the sternum together, and the operative wound is closed by sutures or staples. Report 32150 for removal of an intrapleural foreign body or fibrin deposits and 32151 for removal of an intrapulmonary foreign body.

Coding Tips

If removal of an intrapleural foreign body or a fibrin deposit is achieved by thoracoscopy, see 32653.

ICD-10-CM Diagnostic Codes

J92.0 Pleural plaque with presence of asbestos
J92.9 Pleural plaque without asbestos
J94.2 Hemothorax
S21.321A Laceration with foreign body of right front wall of thorax with penetration into thoracic cavity, initial encounter ☑
S21.322A Laceration with foreign body of left front wall of thorax with penetration into thoracic cavity, initial encounter ☑
S21.341A Puncture wound with foreign body of right front wall of thorax with penetration into thoracic cavity, initial encounter ☑
S21.342A Puncture wound with foreign body of left front wall of thorax with penetration into thoracic cavity, initial encounter ☑
S21.421A Laceration with foreign body of right back wall of thorax with penetration into thoracic cavity, initial encounter ☑
S21.422A Laceration with foreign body of left back wall of thorax with penetration into thoracic cavity, initial encounter ☑
S21.441A Puncture wound with foreign body of right back wall of thorax with penetration into thoracic cavity, initial encounter ☑
S21.442A Puncture wound with foreign body of left back wall of thorax with penetration into thoracic cavity, initial encounter ☑
S27.1XXA Traumatic hemothorax, initial encounter
S27.2XXA Traumatic hemopneumothorax, initial encounter
S27.311A Primary blast injury of lung, unilateral, initial encounter
S27.312A Primary blast injury of lung, bilateral, initial encounter ☑
S27.321A Contusion of lung, unilateral, initial encounter
S27.322A Contusion of lung, bilateral, initial encounter ☑
S27.331A Laceration of lung, unilateral, initial encounter
S27.332A Laceration of lung, bilateral, initial encounter ☑
S27.63XA Laceration of pleura, initial encounter
S27.893A Laceration of other specified intrathoracic organs, initial encounter
T81.510A Adhesions due to foreign body accidentally left in body following surgical operation, initial encounter
T81.520A Obstruction due to foreign body accidentally left in body following surgical operation, initial encounter
T81.530A Perforation due to foreign body accidentally left in body following surgical operation, initial encounter
T81.590A Other complications of foreign body accidentally left in body following surgical operation, initial encounter

AMA: 32150 2018,Jan,8; 2017,Jan,8; 2016,Jan,13; 2015,Jan,16; 2014,Jan,11

Relative Value Units/Medicare Edits

Non-Facility RVU	Work	PE	MP	Total
32150	16.82	8.34	3.82	28.98
32151	16.94	8.12	4.02	29.08
Facility RVU	**Work**	**PE**	**MP**	**Total**
32150	16.82	8.34	3.82	28.98
32151	16.94	8.12	4.02	29.08

	FUD	Status	MUE	Modifiers				IOM Reference
32150	90	A	1(3)	51	N/A	62*	80	None
32151	90	A	1(3)	51	N/A	62*	80	

* with documentation

Terms To Know

blunt dissection. Surgical technique used to expose an underlying area by separating along natural cleavage lines of tissue, without cutting.

effusion. Escape of fluid from within a body cavity.

fibrin. Main fibrous composition of blood clots.

pleura. One of the two membranes that surround the lungs. The visceral pleura encases the lung and the parietal pleura lines the inner chest walls.

thoracotomy. Surgical procedure for opening the chest wall in order to access the lungs, esophagus, trachea, aorta, heart, and diaphragm.

32160

32160 Thoracotomy; with cardiac massage

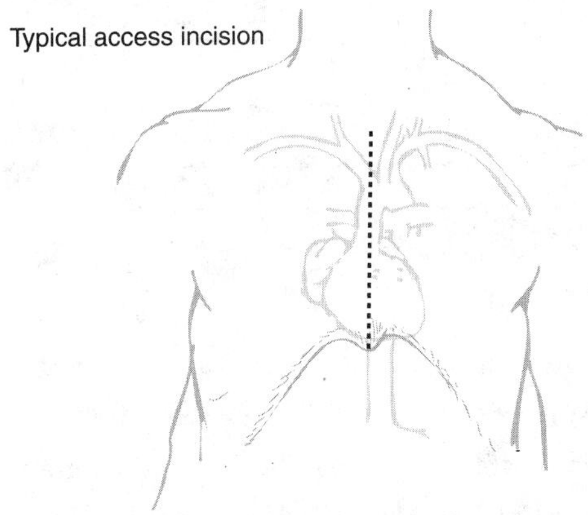

The heart is accessed through a major thoracotomy and direct cardiac massage is initiated

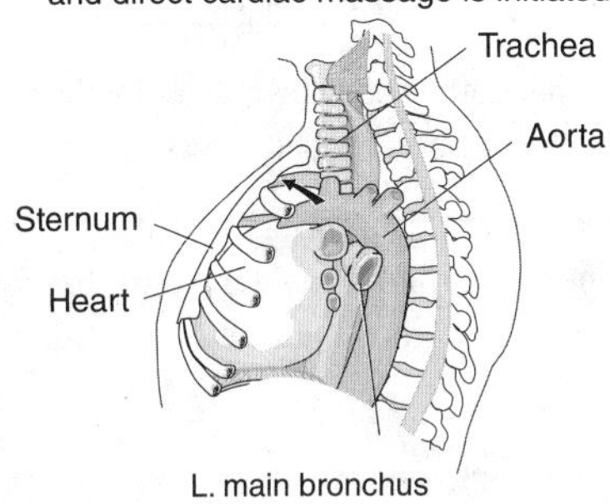

Explanation

The physician opens the chest cavity widely to perform manual cardiac massage in the case of cardiac arrest. Using a scalpel, the surgeon makes a long incision around the side of the chest between two of the ribs. The incision is carried through all of the tissue layers into the chest cavity. Rib spreaders are inserted into the wound and the ribs are spread apart exposing the lung. Alternately, the chest cavity can be opened and the operation performed through a vertical incision in the center of the chest through the sternum. The skin incision is carried down to the sternum bone and a saw is used to split the sternum. With the sternum split in half, the chest is entered by spreading the sternum apart with a set of rib spreaders. Space is made in the chest by packing the uninvolved lung away from the operative field using large moist gauze sponges. The heart is exposed and squeezed rhythmically to mimic cardiac contractions, thus pumping blood through the body. The heart may be directly contra-shocked to produce spontaneous heartbeats. When the procedure is complete, the instruments and gauze sponges are removed. A chest tube(s) may be used to provide drainage for the chest cavity. If applicable, the sternotomy is repaired using wires to bring the two halves of the sternum together, and the operative wound is closed by sutures or staples.

Coding Tips

For closed cardiopulmonary resuscitation, see 92950. For other resections of the lung, see 32480–32504.

ICD-10-CM Diagnostic Codes

I46.2	Cardiac arrest due to underlying cardiac condition
I46.8	Cardiac arrest due to other underlying condition
I46.9	Cardiac arrest, cause unspecified
I97.120	Postprocedural cardiac arrest following cardiac surgery
I97.121	Postprocedural cardiac arrest following other surgery
I97.710	Intraoperative cardiac arrest during cardiac surgery
I97.711	Intraoperative cardiac arrest during other surgery

Relative Value Units/Medicare Edits

Non-Facility RVU	Work	PE	MP	Total
32160	13.1	6.91	2.94	22.95
Facility RVU	Work	PE	MP	Total
32160	13.1	6.91	2.94	22.95

	FUD	Status	MUE	Modifiers				IOM Reference
32160	90	A	1(3)	51	N/A	62*	80	None

* with documentation

Terms To Know

cardiac arrest. Sudden, unexpected cessation of cardiac action, including absence of heart sounds and/or blood pressure.

incision. Act of cutting into tissue or an organ.

massage. Systematic and patterned stroking, kneading, and therapeutic friction applied to soft tissue by hand.

resuscitation. Restoration to life or consciousness of one apparently dead, it includes such measures as artificial respiration and cardiac massage or electrical shock.

sternotomy. Incision into the sternum, the bone that forms the front of the chest cavity and connects with the ribs.

suture. Numerous stitching techniques employed in wound closure.

thoracotomy. Surgical procedure for opening the chest wall in order to access the lungs, esophagus, trachea, aorta, heart, and diaphragm.

32200

32200 Pneumonostomy, with open drainage of abscess or cyst

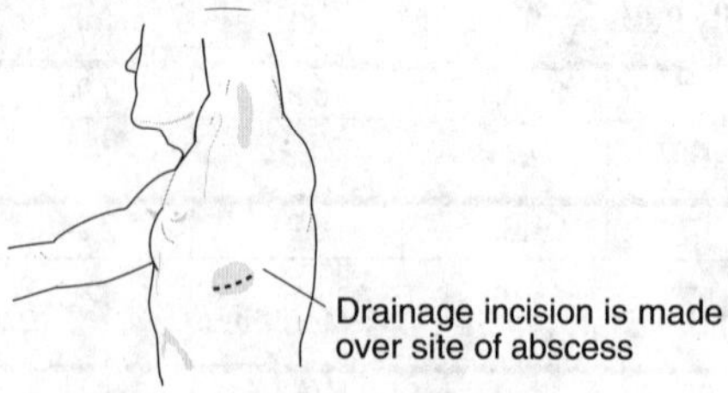

A stoma, or opening, into the abscess in the chest cavity allows it to drain to the outside

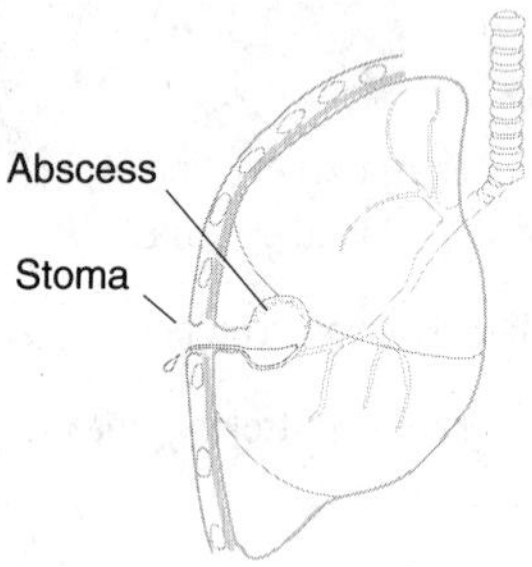

Explanation

The physician treats an abscess or cyst in the lung by draining the pus or fluid directly through the chest wall. Using a scalpel, the skin between two ribs is incised and the tissues separated to expose the inside of the chest cavity. The lung is cut with scissors or a scalpel down to the abscess or the cyst. The abscess or cyst is opened and the fluid is allowed to drain through the wound created in the lung and the chest wall. A rubber drainage tube may be left in place to maintain or facilitate drainage. The incision is not sutured closed. The outside incision is dressed with bulky gauze dressing to absorb the drainage.

Coding Tips

A pneumonostomy is performed for abscess or cyst within the lung. For empyema, an accumulation of pus in the pleural space, see 32035–32036. For drainage of an abscess in the thoracic cavity by tube thoracostomy, see 32551. For a percutaneous image-guided drainage of an abscess or cyst of the lungs by catheter placement, see 49405.

ICD-10-CM Diagnostic Codes

B67.1	Echinococcus granulosus infection of lung
J85.0	Gangrene and necrosis of lung
J85.1	Abscess of lung with pneumonia
J85.2	Abscess of lung without pneumonia
J86.0	Pyothorax with fistula
J86.9	Pyothorax without fistula
J98.4	Other disorders of lung
Q33.0	Congenital cystic lung

AMA: **32200** 2013,Nov,9

Relative Value Units/Medicare Edits

Non-Facility RVU	Work	PE	MP	Total
32200	18.68	9.75	4.44	32.87
Facility RVU	**Work**	**PE**	**MP**	**Total**
32200	18.68	9.75	4.44	32.87

	FUD	Status	MUE	Modifiers				IOM Reference
32200	90	A	2(3)	51	N/A	62*	80	None

* with documentation

Terms To Know

abscess. Circumscribed collection of pus resulting from bacteria, frequently associated with swelling and other signs of inflammation.

emphysematous bleb. Formation of blisters or vesicles greater than 1.0 mm within an emphysematous lung, containing serum or blood.

empyema. Accumulation of pus within the respiratory or pleural cavity.

incision and drainage. Cutting open body tissue for the removal of tissue fluids or infected discharge from a wound or cavity.

mediastinum. Collection of organs and tissues that separate the pleural sacs. Located between the sternum and spine above the diaphragm, it contains the heart and great vessels, trachea and bronchi, esophagus, thymus, lymph nodes, and nerves.

percutaneous. Through the skin.

pneumonotomy. Surgical incision into a lung.

thoracostomy. Creation of an opening in the chest wall for drainage.

32215

32215 Pleural scarification for repeat pneumothorax

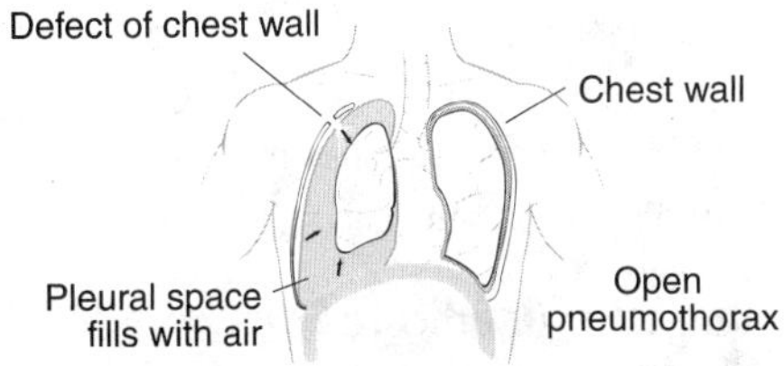

Pneumothorax is the presence of air in the pleural space. The lung may collapse, as shown, and a life-threatening situation arise

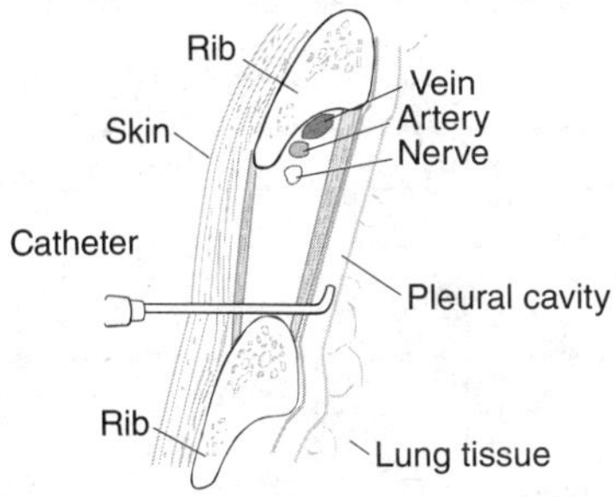

Injecting an abrasive chemical solution into the pleural space causes it to scar and adhere to the cavity walls. The pleural space is effectively eliminated, preventing pneumothorax

Explanation

The physician treats repeat pneumothorax by producing adhesions between the surface of the lung and the inside surface of the chest cavity. To create the adhesions, a chemical solution is injected into the chest cavity and allowed to circulate over the surface of the lung and the inside surface of the chest cavity. The physicians injects the solution by passing a tube into the chest cavity. The physician passes a trocar over the top of a rib and punctures through the chest tissues between the ribs and enters the pleural cavity. With the end of the trocar in the chest cavity, the physician advances the plastic tube into the chest cavity. The sharp instrument is removed leaving one end of the plastic catheter in place within the chest cavity. A syringe is attached to the outside end of the catheter and fluid is injected into the chest cavity. The fluid selected is design to cause the formation of adhesive scar tissue between the surface of the lung and the inside surface of the chest cavity. Once the lung adheres to the chest wall it can no longer collapse and allow the formation of a pneumothorax.

Coding Tips

Supplies used when providing this procedure may be reported with the appropriate HCPCS Level II codes. Check with the specific payer to determine coverage. To report chemical pleurodesis for recurrent or persistent pneumothorax, see 32560.

ICD-10-CM Diagnostic Codes

J93.0	Spontaneous tension pneumothorax
J93.11	Primary spontaneous pneumothorax
J93.12	Secondary spontaneous pneumothorax
J93.81	Chronic pneumothorax
J93.83	Other pneumothorax
J95.811	Postprocedural pneumothorax
J95.812	Postprocedural air leak
P25.1	Pneumothorax originating in the perinatal period

Relative Value Units/Medicare Edits

Non-Facility RVU	Work	PE	MP	Total
32215	13.05	6.92	2.97	22.94
Facility RVU	**Work**	**PE**	**MP**	**Total**
32215	13.05	6.92	2.97	22.94

	FUD	Status	MUE	Modifiers				IOM Reference
32215	90	A	1(2)	51	50	62*	80	None

* with documentation

Terms To Know

adhesion. Abnormal fibrous connection between two structures, soft tissue or bony structures, that may occur as the result of surgery, infection, or trauma.

catheter. Flexible tube inserted into an area of the body for introducing or withdrawing fluid.

iatrogenic pneumothorax. Air trapped in the lining of the lung following surgery.

pleura. One of the two membranes that surround the lungs. The visceral pleura encases the lung and the parietal pleura lines the inner chest walls.

scarification. Process of making scratches or small cuts in the skin or tissue.

spontaneous tension pneumothorax. Air leaking from the lung and trapped in the lung lining.

trocar. Cannula or a sharp pointed instrument used to puncture and aspirate fluid from cavities.

32220-32225

32220 Decortication, pulmonary (separate procedure); total
32225 partial

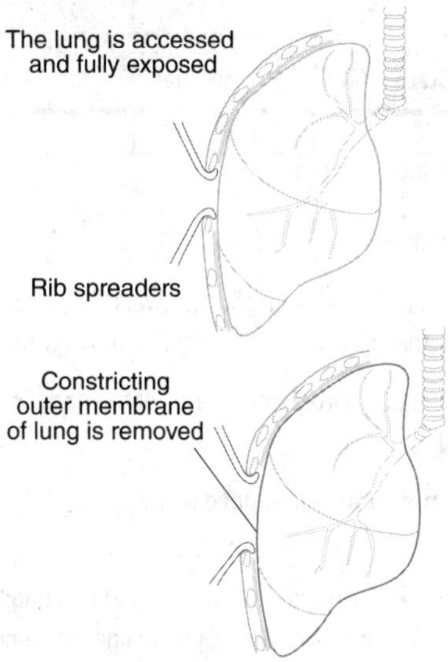

Explanation

The physician removes a constricting membrane or layer of tissue from the surface of the lung (decortication) in order to permit the lung to fully expand. The physician opens the chest cavity widely. Using a scalpel, the surgeon makes a long incision around the side of the chest between two of the ribs. The incision is carried through all the tissue layers into the chest cavity. Rib spreaders are inserted into the wound and the ribs are spread apart exposing the lung. The constricting membrane is stripped off the surface of the lung. In 32225, only a portion of the lung surface is removed. The chest wall incision is sutured closed in layers. A chest tube(s) may be used to provide drainage for the chest cavity. Alternately, the chest cavity can be opened by a vertical incision in the front of the chest through the sternum. The skin incision is carried down to the sternum bone and a saw is used to split the sternum. With the sternum split in half, the chest is entered by spreading the sternum apart with a set of rib spreaders. When the procedure is complete, the wound is closed by using wires to bring the two halves of the sternum together and the skin is closed by suturing.

Coding Tips

These separate procedures by definition are usually a component of a more complex service and are not identified separately. When performed alone or with other unrelated procedures/services, they may be reported. If performed alone, list the code; if performed with other procedures/services, list the code and append modifier 59 or an X{EPSU} modifier. If the procedure is attempted thoracoscopically, but requires major thoracotomy for completion, report 32220 or 32225 for the open portion of the procedure and report a diagnostic thoracoscopy, 32601, as a secondary procedure. For decortication and parietal pleurectomy, see 32320. For surgical thoracoscopy with partial pulmonary decortication, see 32651; with total decortication, including intrapleural pneumonolysis, see 32652.

ICD-10-CM Diagnostic Codes

A15.0	Tuberculosis of lung
A15.6	Tuberculous pleurisy
C38.4	Malignant neoplasm of pleura
C45.0	Mesothelioma of pleura
C78.2	Secondary malignant neoplasm of pleura
J86.0	Pyothorax with fistula
J86.9	Pyothorax without fistula
J91.0	Malignant pleural effusion
J94.1	Fibrothorax
J94.2	Hemothorax
S27.1XXA	Traumatic hemothorax, initial encounter
S27.2XXA	Traumatic hemopneumothorax, initial encounter

Relative Value Units/Medicare Edits

Non-Facility RVU	Work	PE	MP	Total
32220	26.65	13.02	6.12	45.79
32225	16.75	8.12	3.81	28.68
Facility RVU	**Work**	**PE**	**MP**	**Total**
32220	26.65	13.02	6.12	45.79
32225	16.75	8.12	3.81	28.68

	FUD	Status	MUE	Modifiers				IOM Reference
32220	90	A	1(2)	51	50	62*	80	None
32225	90	A	1(2)	51	50	62*	80	

* with documentation

Terms To Know

abscess. Circumscribed collection of pus resulting from bacteria, frequently associated with swelling and other signs of inflammation.

fibrosis. Formation of fibrous tissue as part of the restorative process.

incision. Act of cutting into tissue or an organ.

malignant. Any condition tending to progress toward death, specifically an invasive tumor with a loss of cellular differentiation that has the ability to spread or metastasize to other body areas.

neoplasm. New abnormal growth, tumor.

secondary. Second in order of occurrence or importance, or appearing during the course of another disease or condition.

32310

32310 Pleurectomy, parietal (separate procedure)

The parietal pleura, a membranous tissue lining the inside of the chest cavity, is removed

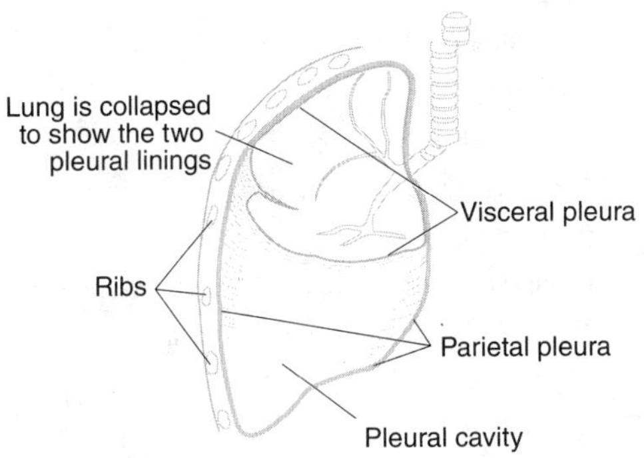

Explanation

The physician removes the membranous tissue lining the inside surface of the chest cavity (the parietal pleura). The physician opens the chest cavity widely to gain access to the inside surface of the chest. Using a scalpel, the surgeon makes a long incision around the side of the chest between two of the ribs. The incision is carried through all the tissue layers into the chest cavity. Rib spreaders are inserted into the wound and the ribs are spread apart exposing the lung. The parietal pleura is stripped from the inside surface of the chest. The chest wall incision is sutured closed in layers. A chest tube(s) may be used to provide drainage for the chest cavity. Alternately, the chest cavity can be opened and the operation performed through a vertical incision in the center of the chest through the sternum. The skin incision is carried down to the sternum bone and a saw is used to split the sternum. With the sternum split in half, the chest is entered by spreading the sternum apart with a set of rib spreaders. When the procedure is complete, the wound is closed by using wires to bring the two halves of the sternum together and the skin is closed over the sternum by suturing.

Coding Tips

This separate procedure by definition is usually a component of a more complex service and is not identified separately. When performed alone or with other unrelated procedures/services, it may be reported. If performed alone, list the code; if performed with other procedures/services, list the code and append modifier 59 or an X{EPSU} modifier. If the procedure is attempted thoracoscopically, but requires major thoracotomy for completion, report 32310 for the open portion of the procedure and report a diagnostic thoracoscopy, 32601, as a secondary procedure. For surgical thoracoscopy with parietal pleurectomy, see 32656.

ICD-10-CM Diagnostic Codes

A15.0	Tuberculosis of lung
C38.4	Malignant neoplasm of pleura
C45.0	Mesothelioma of pleura
C78.2	Secondary malignant neoplasm of pleura
J86.0	Pyothorax with fistula
J86.9	Pyothorax without fistula
J91.0	Malignant pleural effusion
J93.0	Spontaneous tension pneumothorax
J93.11	Primary spontaneous pneumothorax
J93.12	Secondary spontaneous pneumothorax
J93.81	Chronic pneumothorax
J93.82	Other air leak
J93.83	Other pneumothorax
J94.1	Fibrothorax
J94.2	Hemothorax
J94.8	Other specified pleural conditions
J95.811	Postprocedural pneumothorax
J95.812	Postprocedural air leak
P25.1	Pneumothorax originating in the perinatal period
S27.2XXA	Traumatic hemopneumothorax, initial encounter

AMA: 32310 1994,Win,1

Relative Value Units/Medicare Edits

Non-Facility RVU	Work	PE	MP	Total
32310	15.28	7.54	3.51	26.33
Facility RVU	**Work**	**PE**	**MP**	**Total**
32310	15.28	7.54	3.51	26.33

	FUD	Status	MUE	Modifiers				IOM Reference
32310	90	A	1(3)	51	N/A	62*	80	None

* with documentation

Terms To Know

diaphragm. Muscular wall separating the thorax and its structures from the abdomen.

pleura. One of the two membranes that surround the lungs. The visceral pleura encases the lung and the parietal pleura lines the inner chest walls.

pneumothorax. Collapsed lung due to air or gas trapped in the pleural space formed by the membrane that encloses the lungs and lines the thoracic cavity.

32320

32320 Decortication and parietal pleurectomy

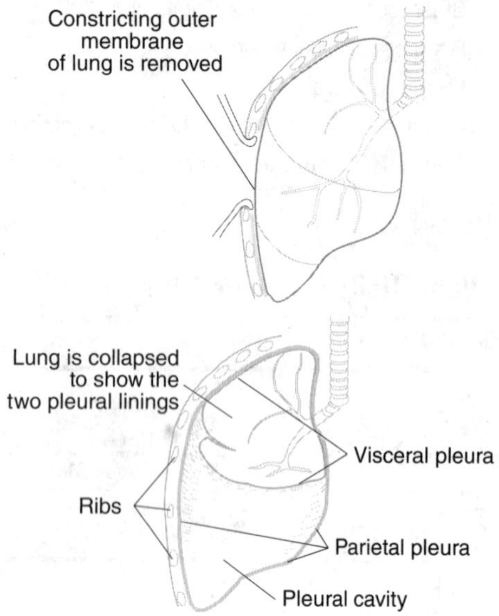

Explanation

The physician removes a constricting membrane or layer of tissue from a portion of the surface of the lung (decortication) in order to permit the lung to fully expand and also removes the membranous tissue lining the inside surface of the chest cavity (the parietal pleura). The physician opens the chest cavity widely. Using a scalpel, the surgeon makes a long incision around the side of the chest between two of the ribs. The incision is carried through all the tissue layers into the chest cavity. Rib spreaders are inserted into the wound and the ribs are spread apart exposing the lung. The constricting membrane is stripped off the surface of the lung. The parietal pleura is stripped from the inside surface of the chest. The chest wall incision is sutured closed in layers. A chest tube(s) may be used to provide drainage for the chest cavity. Alternately, the chest cavity can be opened and the operation performed through a vertical incision in the center of the chest through the sternum. The skin incision is carried down to the sternum bone and a saw is used to split the sternum. With the sternum split in half, the chest is entered by spreading the sternum apart with a set of rib spreaders. When the procedure is complete, the wound is closed by using wires to bring the two halves of the sternum together and the skin is closed over the sternum by suturing.

Coding Tips

For partial decortication only, see 32225. For total decortication only, see 32220. For parietal pleurectomy only, see 32310. For surgical thoracoscopy with partial pulmonary decortication, see 32651. For surgical thoracoscopy with parietal pleurectomy, see 32656.

ICD-10-CM Diagnostic Codes

A15.0	Tuberculosis of lung
A15.6	Tuberculous pleurisy
C38.4	Malignant neoplasm of pleura
C45.0	Mesothelioma of pleura
C78.2	Secondary malignant neoplasm of pleura
J86.0	Pyothorax with fistula
J86.9	Pyothorax without fistula
J91.0	Malignant pleural effusion
J93.0	Spontaneous tension pneumothorax
J93.11	Primary spontaneous pneumothorax
J93.12	Secondary spontaneous pneumothorax
J93.81	Chronic pneumothorax
J93.82	Other air leak
J93.83	Other pneumothorax
J94.1	Fibrothorax
J94.2	Hemothorax
J94.8	Other specified pleural conditions
J95.811	Postprocedural pneumothorax
J95.812	Postprocedural air leak
P25.1	Pneumothorax originating in the perinatal period
S27.2XXA	Traumatic hemopneumothorax, initial encounter

AMA: 32320 1994,Fal,1

Relative Value Units/Medicare Edits

Non-Facility RVU	Work	PE	MP	Total
32320	27.25	12.58	6.3	46.13
Facility RVU	**Work**	**PE**	**MP**	**Total**
32320	27.25	12.58	6.3	46.13

	FUD	Status	MUE	Modifiers				IOM Reference
32320	90	A	1(3)	51	N/A	62*	80	None

* with documentation

Terms To Know

decortication of lung. Removal of a constricting membrane or layer of pleural tissue from a portion of the lung surface to allow for lung expansion.

pleura. One of the two membranes that surround the lungs. The visceral pleura encases the lung and the parietal pleura lines the inner chest walls.

pleural effusion. Collection of lymph and other fluid within the pleural space.

pneumothorax. Collapsed lung due to air or gas trapped in the pleural space formed by the membrane that encloses the lungs and lines the thoracic cavity.

32400

32400 Biopsy, pleura, percutaneous needle

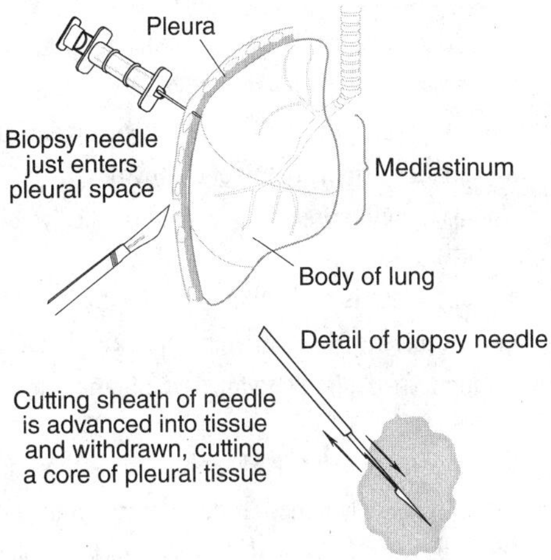

Explanation

The physician obtains a sample of the lining of the lung and/or the lining of the inside of the chest cavity by needle biopsy. Using a pleural biopsy needle, the physician passes the needle over the top of a rib, punctures through the chest tissues between two ribs, enters the pleural cavity and slightly punctures the surface of the lung. With the end of the needle in the chest cavity, the physician withdraws a piece of tissue. The needle is withdrawn and the puncture site covered with a bandage. The procedure is often done under radiological guidance to assure more precise placement of the needle.

Coding Tips

For fine needle aspiration, see 10004-10012 and 10021. For percutaneous biopsy, lung or mediastinum, see 32405. For a diagnostic thoracoscopy with biopsy of the lungs and pleural space, see 32607, 32608, and/or 32609. For open biopsy of the pleura, see 32098. If imaging guidance is performed, see 76942, 77002, 77012, or 77021.

ICD-10-CM Diagnostic Codes

A15.6	Tuberculous pleurisy
C38.4	Malignant neoplasm of pleura
C38.8	Malignant neoplasm of overlapping sites of heart, mediastinum and pleura
C45.0	Mesothelioma of pleura
C78.2	Secondary malignant neoplasm of pleura
D19.0	Benign neoplasm of mesothelial tissue of pleura
D38.2	Neoplasm of uncertain behavior of pleura
J86.0	Pyothorax with fistula
J86.9	Pyothorax without fistula
J90	Pleural effusion, not elsewhere classified
J91.0	Malignant pleural effusion
J91.8	Pleural effusion in other conditions classified elsewhere
J92.0	Pleural plaque with presence of asbestos
J92.9	Pleural plaque without asbestos
J94.0	Chylous effusion
J94.1	Fibrothorax
J94.2	Hemothorax
J94.8	Other specified pleural conditions
M32.13	Lung involvement in systemic lupus erythematosus
Q34.0	Anomaly of pleura

AMA: 32400 2019,Apr,4; 2018,Jan,8; 2017,Jan,8; 2016,Jan,13; 2015,Jan,16; 2014,Jan,11

Relative Value Units/Medicare Edits

Non-Facility RVU	Work	PE	MP	Total
32400	1.76	2.49	0.16	4.41
Facility RVU	**Work**	**PE**	**MP**	**Total**
32400	1.76	0.58	0.16	2.5

	FUD	Status	MUE	Modifiers				IOM Reference
32400	0	A	2(3)	51	N/A	N/A	N/A	None

* with documentation

Terms To Know

effusion. Escape of fluid from within a body cavity.

percutaneous approach. Method used to gain access to a body organ or specific area by puncture or minor incision through the skin or mucous membrane and/or any other body layers necessary to reach the procedure site.

pleura. One of the two membranes that surround the lungs. The visceral pleura encases the lung and the parietal pleura lines the inner chest walls.

32405

32405 Biopsy, lung or mediastinum, percutaneous needle

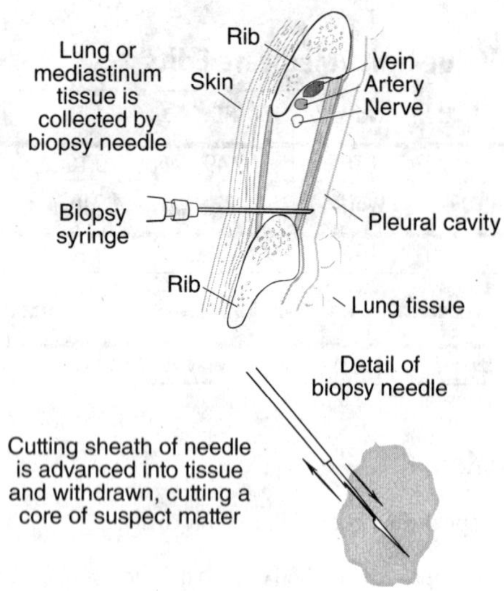

Explanation

The physician obtains a sample of the lung or the mediastinum (the tissues in the center of the chest between the two lung cavities) by puncturing through the space between two of the ribs with a needle. The procedure is often done under radiological guidance to assure more precise placement of the needle. Using a biopsy needle, the physician passes the needle over the top of a rib, punctures through the chest tissues, enters the pleural cavity, and punctures into the area of concern in the lung or the mediastinum. With the end of the needle in the chest cavity, the physician withdraws a piece of tissue. The needle is withdrawn and the puncture site covered with a bandage.

Coding Tips

When medically necessary, report moderate (conscious) sedation provided by the performing physician with 99151-99153. When provided by another physician, report 99155-99157. For fine needle aspiration, see 10004-10012 and 10021. For biopsy of the lung, open, see 32096 or 32097. For biopsy of the mediastinum, open, see 39000 or 39010. For thoracoscopic (VATS) biopsy of the lung, pleura, pericardium, or mediastinal space, see 32604, 32606, 32607, 32608, or 32609. If imaging guidance is performed, see 76942, 77002, 77012, or 77021.

ICD-10-CM Diagnostic Codes

C34.01 Malignant neoplasm of right main bronchus ☑
C34.02 Malignant neoplasm of left main bronchus ☑
C34.11 Malignant neoplasm of upper lobe, right bronchus or lung ☑
C34.12 Malignant neoplasm of upper lobe, left bronchus or lung ☑
C34.2 Malignant neoplasm of middle lobe, bronchus or lung
C34.31 Malignant neoplasm of lower lobe, right bronchus or lung ☑
C34.32 Malignant neoplasm of lower lobe, left bronchus or lung ☑
C34.81 Malignant neoplasm of overlapping sites of right bronchus and lung ☑
C34.82 Malignant neoplasm of overlapping sites of left bronchus and lung ☑
C37 Malignant neoplasm of thymus
C38.1 Malignant neoplasm of anterior mediastinum
C38.2 Malignant neoplasm of posterior mediastinum
C38.8 Malignant neoplasm of overlapping sites of heart, mediastinum and pleura
C46.51 Kaposi's sarcoma of right lung ☑
C46.52 Kaposi's sarcoma of left lung ☑
C78.01 Secondary malignant neoplasm of right lung ☑
C78.02 Secondary malignant neoplasm of left lung ☑
C78.1 Secondary malignant neoplasm of mediastinum
C7A.090 Malignant carcinoid tumor of the bronchus and lung
C7A.091 Malignant carcinoid tumor of the thymus
C81.02 Nodular lymphocyte predominant Hodgkin lymphoma, intrathoracic lymph nodes
C81.12 Nodular sclerosis Hodgkin lymphoma, intrathoracic lymph nodes
C81.22 Mixed cellularity Hodgkin lymphoma, intrathoracic lymph nodes
C81.32 Lymphocyte depleted Hodgkin lymphoma, intrathoracic lymph nodes
C81.42 Lymphocyte-rich Hodgkin lymphoma, intrathoracic lymph nodes
C81.72 Other Hodgkin lymphoma, intrathoracic lymph nodes
C82.02 Follicular lymphoma grade I, intrathoracic lymph nodes
C82.12 Follicular lymphoma grade II, intrathoracic lymph nodes
C82.32 Follicular lymphoma grade IIIa, intrathoracic lymph nodes
C82.52 Diffuse follicle center lymphoma, intrathoracic lymph nodes
C83.02 Small cell B-cell lymphoma, intrathoracic lymph nodes
C83.12 Mantle cell lymphoma, intrathoracic lymph nodes
C83.32 Diffuse large B-cell lymphoma, intrathoracic lymph nodes
C83.52 Lymphoblastic (diffuse) lymphoma, intrathoracic lymph nodes
C83.72 Burkitt lymphoma, intrathoracic lymph nodes
D02.21 Carcinoma in situ of right bronchus and lung ☑
D02.22 Carcinoma in situ of left bronchus and lung ☑
D14.31 Benign neoplasm of right bronchus and lung ☑
D14.32 Benign neoplasm of left bronchus and lung ☑
D15.2 Benign neoplasm of mediastinum
D17.4 Benign lipomatous neoplasm of intrathoracic organs
D38.1 Neoplasm of uncertain behavior of trachea, bronchus and lung
D38.3 Neoplasm of uncertain behavior of mediastinum
D38.4 Neoplasm of uncertain behavior of thymus
D3A.090 Benign carcinoid tumor of the bronchus and lung

AMA: 32405 2019,Apr,4; 2018,Jan,8; 2017,Jan,8; 2016,Jan,13; 2015,Jan,16; 2014,Jan,11

Relative Value Units/Medicare Edits

Non-Facility RVU	Work	PE	MP	Total
32405	1.68	9.32	0.15	11.15
Facility RVU	**Work**	**PE**	**MP**	**Total**
32405	1.68	0.78	0.15	2.61

	FUD	Status	MUE	Modifiers				IOM Reference
32405	0	A	2(3)	51	N/A	N/A	N/A	None

* with documentation

32440

32440 Removal of lung, pneumonectomy;

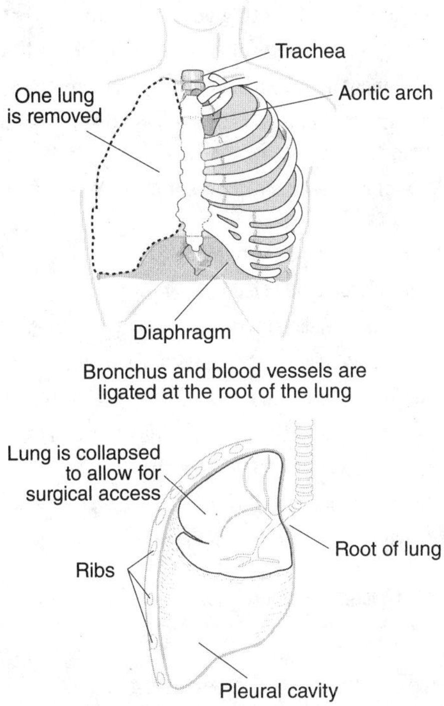

Explanation

The physician removes one lung in its entirety. The physician opens the chest cavity widely to gain access to the lung to be removed. Using a scalpel, the surgeon makes a long incision around the side of the chest between two of the ribs. The incision is carried through all of the tissue layers into the chest cavity. Rib spreaders are inserted into the wound and the ribs are spread apart exposing the lung, heart, and other structures. Alternately, the chest cavity can be opened and the operation performed through a vertical incision in the center of the chest through the sternum. The skin incision is carried down to the sternum bone and a saw is used to split the sternum. With the sternum split in half, the chest is entered by spreading the sternum apart with a set of rib spreaders. The root of the lung is found by pushing aside the deflated lung with a gloved hand and large moist gauze sponges. Within the root of the lung, the blood vessels and bronchial tubes are clamped, tied off, and cut. The lung is removed through the wide chest incision. The instruments and gauze sponges are removed. A chest tube(s) may be used to provide drainage for the chest cavity. When the procedure is complete, if applicable, the sternotomy is repaired using wires to bring the two halves of the sternum together, and the operative wound is closed by sutures or staples.

Coding Tips

For total pneumonectomy, extrapleural, see 32445. For single lobectomy, see 32480; bilobectomy, see 32482; for removal of partial lobe by segmentectomy, see 32484. For lung transplantation, see 32850–32856. For heart-lung transplant, including recipient cardiectomy-pneumonectomy, see 33935.

ICD-10-CM Diagnostic Codes

C34.01 Malignant neoplasm of right main bronchus ☑
C34.02 Malignant neoplasm of left main bronchus ☑
C34.11 Malignant neoplasm of upper lobe, right bronchus or lung ☑
C34.12 Malignant neoplasm of upper lobe, left bronchus or lung ☑
C34.2 Malignant neoplasm of middle lobe, bronchus or lung
C34.31 Malignant neoplasm of lower lobe, right bronchus or lung ☑
C34.32 Malignant neoplasm of lower lobe, left bronchus or lung ☑
C34.81 Malignant neoplasm of overlapping sites of right bronchus and lung ☑
C34.82 Malignant neoplasm of overlapping sites of left bronchus and lung ☑
C46.51 Kaposi's sarcoma of right lung ☑
C46.52 Kaposi's sarcoma of left lung ☑
C78.01 Secondary malignant neoplasm of right lung ☑
C78.02 Secondary malignant neoplasm of left lung ☑
C7A.090 Malignant carcinoid tumor of the bronchus and lung
D02.21 Carcinoma in situ of right bronchus and lung ☑
D02.22 Carcinoma in situ of left bronchus and lung ☑
D38.1 Neoplasm of uncertain behavior of trachea, bronchus and lung
J85.0 Gangrene and necrosis of lung

AMA: **32440** 2018,Jan,8; 2017,Jan,8; 2016,Jan,13; 2015,Jan,16; 2014,Jan,11

Relative Value Units/Medicare Edits

Non-Facility RVU	Work	PE	MP	Total
32440	27.28	11.64	6.25	45.17
Facility RVU	**Work**	**PE**	**MP**	**Total**
32440	27.28	11.64	6.25	45.17

	FUD	Status	MUE	Modifiers				IOM Reference
32440	90	A	1(2)	51	N/A	62*	80	None

* with documentation

Terms To Know

ligate. To tie off a blood vessel or duct with a suture or a soft, thin wire (ligature wire).

sternotomy. Incision into the sternum, the bone that forms the front of the chest cavity and connects with the ribs.

32442

32442 Removal of lung, pneumonectomy; with resection of segment of trachea followed by broncho-tracheal anastomosis (sleeve pneumonectomy)

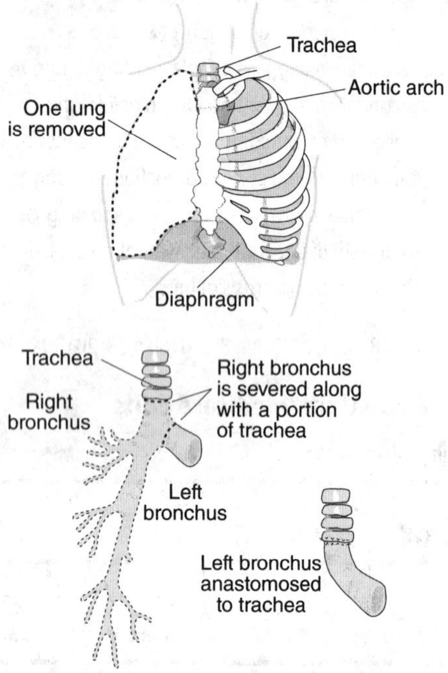

A total pneumonectomy is performed along with resection of a segment of the trachea followed by anastomosis

Explanation

The physician removes one lung in its entirety. The physician opens the chest cavity widely to gain access to the lung to be removed. Using a scalpel, the surgeon makes a long incision around the side of the chest between two of the ribs. The incision is carried through all of the tissue layers into the chest cavity. Rib spreaders are inserted into the wound and the ribs are spread apart exposing the lung, heart, and other structures. Alternately, the chest cavity can be opened and the operation performed through a vertical incision in the center of the chest through the sternum. The skin incision is carried down to the sternum bone and a saw is used to split the sternum. With the sternum split in half, the chest is entered by spreading the sternum apart with a set of rib spreaders. The root of the lung is found by pushing aside the deflated lung with a gloved hand and large moist gauze sponges. Within the root of the lung, the blood vessels and bronchial tubes are clamped, tied off, and cut. The lung and a segment of the trachea are removed through the wide chest incision. The trachea is sutured to the main bronchial tube of the remaining lung in the other half of the chest. The instruments and gauze sponges are removed. A chest tube(s) may be used to provide drainage for the chest cavity. When the procedure is complete, if applicable, the sternotomy is repaired using wires to bring the two halves of the sternum together, and the operative wound is closed by sutures or staples.

Coding Tips

For removal of lung, other than total pneumonectomy with circumferential resection of segment of bronchus followed by broncho-bronchial anastomosis (sleeve lobectomy), see 32486.

ICD-10-CM Diagnostic Codes

C33	Malignant neoplasm of trachea
C34.01	Malignant neoplasm of right main bronchus ☑
C34.02	Malignant neoplasm of left main bronchus ☑
C34.11	Malignant neoplasm of upper lobe, right bronchus or lung ☑
C34.12	Malignant neoplasm of upper lobe, left bronchus or lung ☑
C34.2	Malignant neoplasm of middle lobe, bronchus or lung
C34.31	Malignant neoplasm of lower lobe, right bronchus or lung ☑
C34.32	Malignant neoplasm of lower lobe, left bronchus or lung ☑
C34.81	Malignant neoplasm of overlapping sites of right bronchus and lung ☑
C34.82	Malignant neoplasm of overlapping sites of left bronchus and lung ☑
C46.51	Kaposi's sarcoma of right lung ☑
C46.52	Kaposi's sarcoma of left lung ☑
C78.01	Secondary malignant neoplasm of right lung ☑
C78.02	Secondary malignant neoplasm of left lung ☑
C7A.090	Malignant carcinoid tumor of the bronchus and lung
D02.21	Carcinoma in situ of right bronchus and lung ☑
D02.22	Carcinoma in situ of left bronchus and lung ☑
D38.1	Neoplasm of uncertain behavior of trachea, bronchus and lung
D3A.090	Benign carcinoid tumor of the bronchus and lung

AMA: 32442 2018,Jan,8; 2017,Jun,10; 2017,Jan,8; 2016,Jan,13; 2015,Jan,16; 2014,Jan,11

Relative Value Units/Medicare Edits

Non-Facility RVU	Work	PE	MP	Total
32442	56.47	18.92	13.51	88.9
Facility RVU	**Work**	**PE**	**MP**	**Total**
32442	56.47	18.92	13.51	88.9

	FUD	Status	MUE	Modifiers				IOM Reference
32442	90	A	1(2)	51	N/A	62*	80	None

* with documentation

Terms To Know

carcinoma in situ. Malignancy that arises from the cells of the vessel, gland, or organ of origin that remains confined to that site or has not invaded neighboring tissue.

Kaposi's sarcoma. Malignant neoplasm caused by vascular proliferation of cutaneous tumors characterized by channels lined with endothelial tissue containing vascular spaced.

resection. Surgical removal of a part or all of an organ or body part.

32445

32445 Removal of lung, pneumonectomy; extrapleural

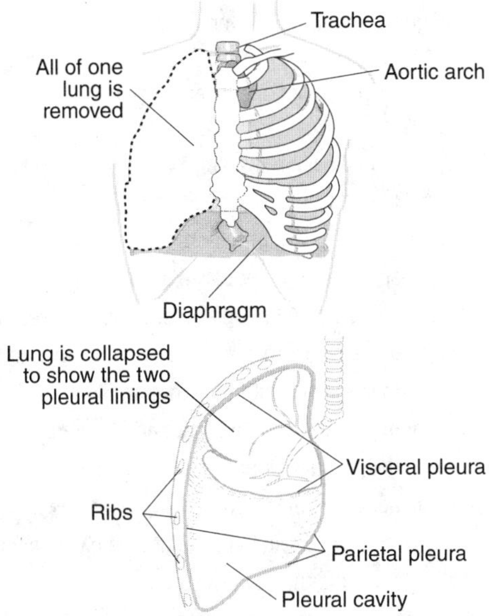

A total pneumonectomy is performed along with removal of the parietal pleura of that lobe

Explanation

The physician removes one lung in its entirety and the pleural membranes covering the lung and the inside surface of the chest cavity (the parietal pleura). The physician opens the chest cavity widely to gain access to the lung to be removed. Using a scalpel, the surgeon makes a long incision around the side of the chest between two of the ribs. The incision is carried through all of the tissue layers down to the membrane lining the chest cavity. Rib spreaders are inserted into the wound and the ribs are spread apart, taking care to preserve the integrity of the chest lining. Holding a gauze sponge, the surgeon strips away the lining inside the chest all the way around to the root of the lung. This creates a sac of the parietal pleura that contains the lung. Within the root of the lung, the blood vessels and bronchial tubes are clamped, tied off, and cut. The lung and the pleural tissues of the inside of the chest wall are removed through the wide chest incision. After the removal of the instruments and gauze sponges, the chest incision is sutured closed in layers. A chest tube(s) may be used to provide drainage for the chest cavity.

Coding Tips

If extrapleural pneumonectomy with empyectomy is performed, report 32540 in addition to 32445. For chest wall tumor resection performed with lung resection, see 21601-21603. For a single lobectomy, see 32480; bilobectomy, see 32482. For removal of a partial lobe by segmentectomy, see 32484. For lung transplantation, see 32850–32856. For a heart-lung transplant, including recipient cardiectomy-pneumonectomy, see 33935.

ICD-10-CM Diagnostic Codes

C45.0 Mesothelioma of pleura

AMA: 32445 2018,Jan,8; 2017,Jan,8; 2016,Jan,13; 2015,Jan,16; 2014,Jan,11

Relative Value Units/Medicare Edits

Non-Facility RVU	Work	PE	MP	Total
32445	63.84	23.39	15.34	102.57
Facility RVU	**Work**	**PE**	**MP**	**Total**
32445	63.84	23.39	15.34	102.57

	FUD	Status	MUE	Modifiers				IOM Reference
32445	90	A	1(2)	51	N/A	62*	80	None

* with documentation

Terms To Know

carcinoma in situ. Malignancy that arises from the cells of the vessel, gland, or organ of origin that remains confined to that site or has not invaded neighboring tissue.

empyectomy. Removal of an accumulation of pus.

Kaposi's sarcoma. Malignant neoplasm caused by vascular proliferation of cutaneous tumors characterized by channels lined with endothelial tissue containing vascular spaced.

lobectomy. Excision of a lobe of an organ such as the liver, thyroid, lung, or brain.

pulmonary congestion. Excessive retention of interstitial fluid in the lungs and pulmonary vessels.

32480-32482

32480 Removal of lung, other than pneumonectomy; single lobe (lobectomy)
32482 2 lobes (bilobectomy)

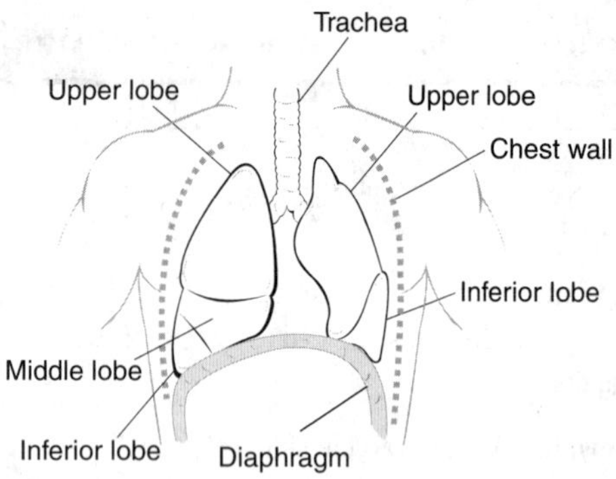

Explanation

The physician opens the chest cavity widely to gain access to the lung to be removed. Using a scalpel, the surgeon makes a long incision around the side of the chest between two of the ribs. The incision is carried through all of the tissue layers into the chest cavity. Rib spreaders are inserted into the wound and the ribs are spread apart exposing the lung. Alternately, the chest cavity can be opened and the operation performed through a vertical incision in the center of the chest through the sternum. The skin incision is carried down to the sternum bone and a saw is used to split the sternum. With the sternum split in half, the chest is entered by spreading the sternum apart with a set of rib spreaders. The lobe(s) to be removed is identified and isolated in the operative field by pushing aside the deflated lung with a gloved hand and large moist gauze sponges. Within the lobe(s) of the lung, the main blood vessels and bronchial tubes are clamped, tied off, and cut. The lobe(s) is removed through the wide chest incision. The instruments and gauze sponges are removed. A chest tube(s) may be used to provide drainage for the chest cavity. When the procedure is complete, if applicable, the sternotomy is repaired using wires to bring the two halves of the sternum together, and the operative wound is closed by sutures or staples. Report 32480 when one lobe is removed and 32482 when two lobes are removed.

Coding Tips

Diagnostic lung biopsies with intraoperative pathology that determines the need for resection or other definitive procedures should be reported using only the most complex service performed. If lung resection is performed with chest wall tumor resection, report the appropriate chest wall tumor resection code (21601–21603) in addition to 32480 or 32482. When concurrent decortication is performed with a lobectomy or segmentectomy, report 32320 in addition to 32480 or 32482. If bronchoplasty is performed at the time of a lobectomy, report 32501 in addition to 32480 or 32482. For removal of a single segment, see 32484; with circumferential resection of bronchus and reanastomosis, see 32486; for completion pneumonectomy, see 32488. For total pneumonectomy, see 32440. For surgical thoracoscopy, with total or segmental lobectomy, see 32663.

ICD-10-CM Diagnostic Codes

A15.0 Tuberculosis of lung
B44.0 Invasive pulmonary aspergillosis
B44.1 Other pulmonary aspergillosis
C34.01 Malignant neoplasm of right main bronchus ☑
C34.02 Malignant neoplasm of left main bronchus ☑
C34.11 Malignant neoplasm of upper lobe, right bronchus or lung ☑
C34.12 Malignant neoplasm of upper lobe, left bronchus or lung ☑
C34.2 Malignant neoplasm of middle lobe, bronchus or lung
C34.31 Malignant neoplasm of lower lobe, right bronchus or lung ☑
C34.32 Malignant neoplasm of lower lobe, left bronchus or lung ☑
C34.81 Malignant neoplasm of overlapping sites of right bronchus and lung ☑
C34.82 Malignant neoplasm of overlapping sites of left bronchus and lung ☑
C46.51 Kaposi's sarcoma of right lung ☑
C46.52 Kaposi's sarcoma of left lung ☑
C78.01 Secondary malignant neoplasm of right lung ☑
C78.02 Secondary malignant neoplasm of left lung ☑
C79.89 Secondary malignant neoplasm of other specified sites
C7A.090 Malignant carcinoid tumor of the bronchus and lung
D02.21 Carcinoma in situ of right bronchus and lung ☑
D02.22 Carcinoma in situ of left bronchus and lung ☑
D14.31 Benign neoplasm of right bronchus and lung ☑
D14.32 Benign neoplasm of left bronchus and lung ☑
D38.1 Neoplasm of uncertain behavior of trachea, bronchus and lung
D3A.090 Benign carcinoid tumor of the bronchus and lung
J43.0 Unilateral pulmonary emphysema [MacLeod's syndrome]
J43.1 Panlobular emphysema
J43.2 Centrilobular emphysema
J43.8 Other emphysema
J47.0 Bronchiectasis with acute lower respiratory infection
J47.1 Bronchiectasis with (acute) exacerbation
J85.0 Gangrene and necrosis of lung
J85.1 Abscess of lung with pneumonia
J85.2 Abscess of lung without pneumonia
J98.4 Other disorders of lung
Q33.2 Sequestration of lung

AMA: **32480** 2018,Jan,8; 2017,Jan,8; 2016,Jan,13; 2015,Jan,16; 2014,Jan,11
32482 2018,Jan,8; 2017,Jan,8; 2016,Jan,13; 2015,Jan,16; 2014,Jan,11

Relative Value Units/Medicare Edits

Non-Facility RVU	Work	PE	MP	Total
32480	25.82	10.93	5.92	42.67
32482	27.44	11.91	6.28	45.63
Facility RVU	**Work**	**PE**	**MP**	**Total**
32480	25.82	10.93	5.92	42.67
32482	27.44	11.91	6.28	45.63

	FUD	Status	MUE	Modifiers				IOM Reference
32480	90	A	1(2)	51	N/A	62*	80	None
32482	90	A	1(2)	51	N/A	62*	80	

* with documentation

Terms To Know

bronchiectasis. Dilation of the bronchi with mucous production and persistent cough due to infection or chronic conditions that causes diminished lung capacity and frequent infections of the lung.

32484

32484 Removal of lung, other than pneumonectomy; single segment (segmentectomy)

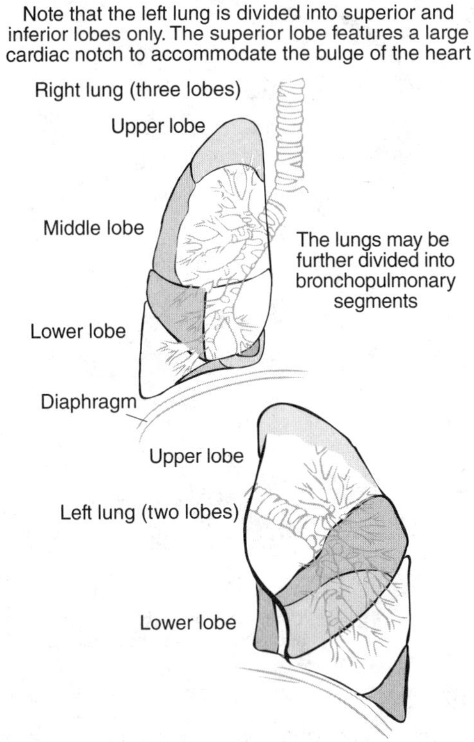

Explanation

The physician removes a segment of a lobe of one lung. The physician opens the chest cavity widely to gain access to the lung to be removed. Using a scalpel, the surgeon makes a long incision around the side of the chest between two of the ribs. The incision is carried through all of the tissue layers into the chest cavity. Rib spreaders are inserted into the wound and the ribs are spread apart exposing the lung. Alternately, the chest cavity can be opened and the operation performed through a vertical incision in the center of the chest through the sternum. The skin incision is carried down to the sternum bone and a saw is used to split the sternum. With the sternum split in half, the chest is entered by spreading the sternum apart with a set of rib spreaders. The segment to be removed is identified and isolated in the operative field by pushing aside the deflated lung with a gloved hand and large moist gauze sponges. Within the segment of the lung, the main blood vessels and bronchial tubes are clamped, tied off, and cut. The segment is removed through the wide chest incision. The instruments and gauze sponges are removed. A chest tube(s) may be used to provide drainage for the chest cavity. When the procedure is complete, if applicable, the sternotomy is repaired using wires to bring the two halves of the sternum together, and the operative wound is closed by sutures or staples.

Coding Tips

Diagnostic lung biopsies with intraoperative pathology that determines the need for resection or other definitive procedures should be reported using only the most complex service performed. If lung resection is performed with chest wall tumor resection, report the appropriate chest wall tumor resection code (21601–21603) in addition to 32484. When concurrent decortication is performed with lobectomy or segmentectomy, report 32320 in addition to 32484. If bronchoplasty is performed at the time of a segmentectomy, report 32501 in addition to 32484. For removal of a single lobe, see 32480; two lobes, see 32482; with circumferential resection of bronchus and reanastomosis, see 32486; for completion pneumonectomy, see 32488. For total pneumonectomy, see 32440. For surgical thoracoscopy, with total or segmental lobectomy, see 32663.

ICD-10-CM Diagnostic Codes

A15.0	Tuberculosis of lung
B44.0	Invasive pulmonary aspergillosis
B44.1	Other pulmonary aspergillosis
C34.01	Malignant neoplasm of right main bronchus ☑
C34.02	Malignant neoplasm of left main bronchus ☑
C34.11	Malignant neoplasm of upper lobe, right bronchus or lung ☑
C34.12	Malignant neoplasm of upper lobe, left bronchus or lung ☑
C34.2	Malignant neoplasm of middle lobe, bronchus or lung
C34.31	Malignant neoplasm of lower lobe, right bronchus or lung ☑
C34.32	Malignant neoplasm of lower lobe, left bronchus or lung ☑
C34.81	Malignant neoplasm of overlapping sites of right bronchus and lung ☑
C34.82	Malignant neoplasm of overlapping sites of left bronchus and lung ☑
C46.51	Kaposi's sarcoma of right lung ☑
C46.52	Kaposi's sarcoma of left lung ☑
C78.01	Secondary malignant neoplasm of right lung ☑
C78.02	Secondary malignant neoplasm of left lung ☑
C79.89	Secondary malignant neoplasm of other specified sites
C7A.090	Malignant carcinoid tumor of the bronchus and lung
D02.21	Carcinoma in situ of right bronchus and lung ☑
D02.22	Carcinoma in situ of left bronchus and lung ☑
D14.31	Benign neoplasm of right bronchus and lung ☑
D14.32	Benign neoplasm of left bronchus and lung ☑
D38.1	Neoplasm of uncertain behavior of trachea, bronchus and lung
D3A.090	Benign carcinoid tumor of the bronchus and lung
J43.0	Unilateral pulmonary emphysema [MacLeod's syndrome]
J43.1	Panlobular emphysema
J43.2	Centrilobular emphysema
J43.8	Other emphysema
J47.0	Bronchiectasis with acute lower respiratory infection
J47.1	Bronchiectasis with (acute) exacerbation
J85.0	Gangrene and necrosis of lung
J85.1	Abscess of lung with pneumonia
J85.2	Abscess of lung without pneumonia
J98.4	Other disorders of lung
Q33.2	Sequestration of lung

AMA: 32484 2018,Jan,8; 2017,Jan,8; 2016,Jan,13; 2015,Jan,16; 2014,Jan,11

Relative Value Units/Medicare Edits

Non-Facility RVU	Work	PE	MP	Total
32484	25.38	10.14	5.83	41.35
Facility RVU	**Work**	**PE**	**MP**	**Total**
32484	25.38	10.14	5.83	41.35

	FUD	Status	MUE	Modifiers				IOM Reference
32484	90	A	2(3)	51	N/A	62*	80	None

* with documentation

Terms To Know

aspergillosis. Infection by Aspergillus species, mainly A. Fumigatus, A. flavus group, or A. terreus group.

bronchiectasis. Dilation of the bronchi with mucous production and persistent cough due to infection or chronic conditions that causes diminished lung capacity and frequent infections of the lung.

clamp. Tool used to grip, compress, join, or fasten body parts.

emphysema. Pathological condition in which there is destructive enlargement of the air sacs in the lungs resulting in damage and lack of elasticity to the alveolar walls, commonly seen in long-term smokers.

Kaposi's sarcoma. Malignant neoplasm caused by vascular proliferation of cutaneous tumors characterized by channels lined with endothelial tissue containing vascular spaced.

pneumonectomy. Surgical removal of a lung or lung tissue.

resection. Surgical removal of a part or all of an organ or body part.

segmentectomy. Removal of a segment of a gland or an organ.

thoracostomy. Creation of an opening in the chest wall for drainage.

tuberculosis. Bacterial infection that typically spreads by inhalation of an airborne agent that usually attacks the lungs, but may also affect other organs.

32486

32486 Removal of lung, other than pneumonectomy; with circumferential resection of segment of bronchus followed by broncho-bronchial anastomosis (sleeve lobectomy)

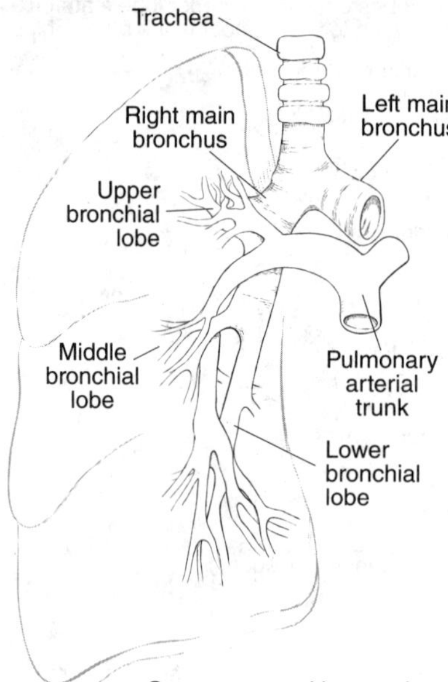

One segment with resection of bronchus and anastomosis

Explanation

The physician removes a portion (lobectomy, bilobectomy, or segmentectomy) of one lung and repairs a bronchial tube that has been partially resected. The physician opens the chest cavity widely to gain access to the lung to be removed. Using a scalpel, the surgeon makes a long incision around the side of the chest between two of the ribs. The incision is carried through all of the tissue layers into the chest cavity. Rib spreaders are inserted into the wound and the ribs are spread apart exposing the lung. Alternately, the chest cavity can be opened and the operation performed through a vertical incision in the center of the chest through the sternum. The skin incision is carried down to the sternum bone and a saw is used to split the sternum. With the sternum split in half, the chest is entered by spreading the sternum apart with a set of rib spreaders. The portion of lung to be removed is identified and isolated in the operative field by pushing aside the deflated lung with a gloved hand and large moist gauze sponges. Within the lung, main blood vessels and bronchial tubes are clamped, tied off, and cut. The resected part of the lung is removed through the wide chest incision. The segment of diseased or damaged bronchial tube is removed. The healthy end of the smaller bronchial tube in the remaining lobe is sutured to the main bronchial tube in the root of the lung. The instruments and gauze sponges are removed. A chest tube(s) may be used to provide drainage for the chest cavity. When the procedure is complete, if applicable, the sternotomy is repaired using wires to bring the two halves of the sternum together, and the operative wound is closed by sutures or staples.

Coding Tips

Diagnostic lung biopsies with intraoperative pathology that determines the need for resection or another definitive procedure should be reported using only the most complex service performed. When a diagnostic wedge resection is performed and followed by a more complex procedure on the same anatomic location, report add-on codes 32507 or 32668 with the more complex procedure. When a therapeutic wedge resection is performed on a different lobe than a more complex lung resection, append modifier 59 or an X{EPSU} modifier. If a lung resection is performed with chest wall tumor resection, report the appropriate chest wall tumor resection code (21601–21603) in addition to 32486. When concurrent decortication is performed with a lobectomy or segmentectomy, report 32320 in addition to 32486. If bronchoplasty is performed at the time of a lobectomy, bilobectomy, or segmentectomy, report 32501 in addition to the applicable procedure: 32480–32484. For removal of a single lobe, see 32480; two lobes, see 32482; single segment, see 32484; for completion pneumonectomy, see 32488. For total pneumonectomy, see 32440. For surgical thoracoscopy, with total or segmental lobectomy, see 32663.

ICD-10-CM Diagnostic Codes

A15.0	Tuberculosis of lung
B44.0	Invasive pulmonary aspergillosis
B44.1	Other pulmonary aspergillosis
C34.01	Malignant neoplasm of right main bronchus ☑
C34.02	Malignant neoplasm of left main bronchus ☑
C34.11	Malignant neoplasm of upper lobe, right bronchus or lung ☑
C34.12	Malignant neoplasm of upper lobe, left bronchus or lung ☑
C34.2	Malignant neoplasm of middle lobe, bronchus or lung
C34.31	Malignant neoplasm of lower lobe, right bronchus or lung ☑
C34.32	Malignant neoplasm of lower lobe, left bronchus or lung ☑
C34.81	Malignant neoplasm of overlapping sites of right bronchus and lung ☑
C34.82	Malignant neoplasm of overlapping sites of left bronchus and lung ☑
C46.51	Kaposi's sarcoma of right lung ☑
C46.52	Kaposi's sarcoma of left lung ☑
C78.01	Secondary malignant neoplasm of right lung ☑
C78.02	Secondary malignant neoplasm of left lung ☑
C79.89	Secondary malignant neoplasm of other specified sites
C7A.090	Malignant carcinoid tumor of the bronchus and lung
D02.21	Carcinoma in situ of right bronchus and lung ☑
D02.22	Carcinoma in situ of left bronchus and lung ☑
D14.31	Benign neoplasm of right bronchus and lung ☑
D14.32	Benign neoplasm of left bronchus and lung ☑
D38.1	Neoplasm of uncertain behavior of trachea, bronchus and lung
D3A.090	Benign carcinoid tumor of the bronchus and lung
J43.0	Unilateral pulmonary emphysema [MacLeod's syndrome]
J43.1	Panlobular emphysema
J43.2	Centrilobular emphysema
J43.8	Other emphysema
J47.0	Bronchiectasis with acute lower respiratory infection
J47.1	Bronchiectasis with (acute) exacerbation
J85.0	Gangrene and necrosis of lung
J85.1	Abscess of lung with pneumonia
J85.2	Abscess of lung without pneumonia
J98.4	Other disorders of lung
Q33.2	Sequestration of lung

AMA: 32486 2018,Jan,8; 2017,Jun,10; 2017,Jan,8; 2016,Jan,13; 2015,Jan,16; 2014,Jan,11

Relative Value Units/Medicare Edits

Non-Facility RVU	Work	PE	MP	Total
32486	42.88	15.24	10.01	68.13
Facility RVU	**Work**	**PE**	**MP**	**Total**
32486	42.88	15.24	10.01	68.13

	FUD	Status	MUE	Modifiers				IOM Reference
32486	90	A	1(3)	51	N/A	62*	80	None

* with documentation

Terms To Know

anastomosis. Surgically created connection between ducts, blood vessels, or bowel segments to allow flow from one to the other.

circumferential. Pertaining to the perimeter of an object or body.

Kaposi's sarcoma. Malignant neoplasm caused by vascular proliferation of cutaneous tumors characterized by channels lined with endothelial tissue containing vascular spaced.

lobectomy. Excision of a lobe of an organ such as the liver, thyroid, lung, or brain.

pneumonectomy. Surgical removal of a lung or lung tissue.

resect. Cutting out or removing a portion or all of a bone, organ, or other structure.

sternotomy. Incision into the sternum, the bone that forms the front of the chest cavity and connects with the ribs.

tuberculosis. Bacterial infection that typically spreads by inhalation of an airborne agent that usually attacks the lungs, but may also affect other organs.

32488

32488 Removal of lung, other than pneumonectomy; with all remaining lung following previous removal of a portion of lung (completion pneumonectomy)

Note that the left lung is divided into superior and inferior lobes only. The superior lobe features a large cardiac notch to accommodate the bulge of the heart

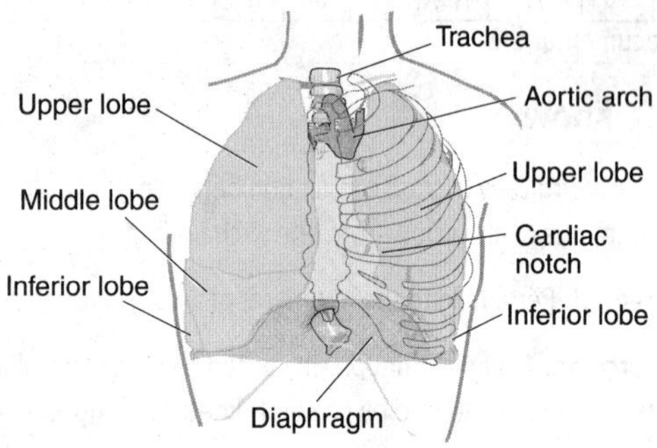

Explanation

The physician removes the remaining portion(s) of a lung from a prior partial lung removal. The physician opens the chest cavity widely to gain access to the lung to be removed. Using a scalpel, the surgeon makes a long incision around the side of the chest between two of the ribs. The incision is carried through all of the tissue layers into the chest cavity. Rib spreaders are inserted into the wound and the ribs are spread apart exposing the lung. Alternately, the chest cavity can be opened and the operation performed through a vertical incision in the center of the chest through the sternum. The skin incision is carried down to the sternum bone and a saw is used to split the sternum. With the sternum split in half, the chest is entered by spreading the sternum apart with a set of rib spreaders. The remaining portion of lung is isolated in the operative field by pushing aside the deflated lung with a gloved hand and large moist gauze sponges. Within the root of the lung, the blood vessels and bronchial tubes are clamped, tied off, and cut. The lung is removed through the wide chest incision. The instruments and gauze sponges are removed. A chest tube(s) may be used to provide drainage for the chest cavity. When the procedure is complete, if applicable, the sternotomy is repaired using wires to bring the two halves of the sternum together, and the operative wound is closed by sutures or staples.

Coding Tips

If a lung resection is performed with chest wall tumor resection, report the appropriate chest wall tumor resection code (21601–21603) in addition to 32488. When concurrent decortication is performed with a lobectomy or segmentectomy, report 32320 in addition to 32488. For removal of a single lobe, see 32480; two lobes, see 32482; single segment, see 32484; with circumferential resection of bronchus and reanastomosis, see 32486. For a total pneumonectomy, see 32440. For a surgical thoracoscopy, with a total or segmental lobectomy, see 32663. For lobectomy or segmentectomy with concomitant decortication, see 32320 in addition to the code for lung removal.

ICD-10-CM Diagnostic Codes

A15.0	Tuberculosis of lung
B44.0	Invasive pulmonary aspergillosis
B44.1	Other pulmonary aspergillosis
C34.01	Malignant neoplasm of right main bronchus ☑
C34.02	Malignant neoplasm of left main bronchus ☑
C34.11	Malignant neoplasm of upper lobe, right bronchus or lung ☑
C34.12	Malignant neoplasm of upper lobe, left bronchus or lung ☑
C34.2	Malignant neoplasm of middle lobe, bronchus or lung
C34.31	Malignant neoplasm of lower lobe, right bronchus or lung ☑
C34.32	Malignant neoplasm of lower lobe, left bronchus or lung ☑
C34.81	Malignant neoplasm of overlapping sites of right bronchus and lung ☑
C34.82	Malignant neoplasm of overlapping sites of left bronchus and lung ☑
C46.51	Kaposi's sarcoma of right lung ☑
C46.52	Kaposi's sarcoma of left lung ☑
C78.01	Secondary malignant neoplasm of right lung ☑
C78.02	Secondary malignant neoplasm of left lung ☑
C79.89	Secondary malignant neoplasm of other specified sites
C7A.090	Malignant carcinoid tumor of the bronchus and lung
D02.21	Carcinoma in situ of right bronchus and lung ☑
D02.22	Carcinoma in situ of left bronchus and lung ☑
D14.31	Benign neoplasm of right bronchus and lung ☑
D14.32	Benign neoplasm of left bronchus and lung ☑
D38.1	Neoplasm of uncertain behavior of trachea, bronchus and lung
D3A.090	Benign carcinoid tumor of the bronchus and lung
J43.0	Unilateral pulmonary emphysema [MacLeod's syndrome]
J43.1	Panlobular emphysema
J43.2	Centrilobular emphysema
J43.8	Other emphysema
J47.0	Bronchiectasis with acute lower respiratory infection
J47.1	Bronchiectasis with (acute) exacerbation
J85.0	Gangrene and necrosis of lung
J85.1	Abscess of lung with pneumonia
J85.2	Abscess of lung without pneumonia
J98.4	Other disorders of lung
Q33.2	Sequestration of lung

AMA: 32488 2018,Jan,8; 2017,Jan,8; 2016,Jan,13; 2015,Jan,16; 2014,Jan,11

Relative Value Units/Medicare Edits

Non-Facility RVU	Work	PE	MP	Total
32488	42.99	16.15	10.25	69.39
Facility RVU	**Work**	**PE**	**MP**	**Total**
32488	42.99	16.15	10.25	69.39

	FUD	Status	MUE	Modifiers				IOM Reference
32488	90	A	1(2)	51	N/A	62*	80	None

* with documentation

Terms To Know

aspergillosis. Infection by Aspergillus species, mainly A. Fumigatus, A. flavus group, or A. terreus group.

bronchiectasis. Dilation of the bronchi with mucous production and persistent cough due to infection or chronic conditions that causes diminished lung capacity and frequent infections of the lung.

32491

32491 Removal of lung, other than pneumonectomy; with resection-plication of emphysematous lung(s) (bullous or non-bullous) for lung volume reduction, sternal split or transthoracic approach, includes any pleural procedure, when performed

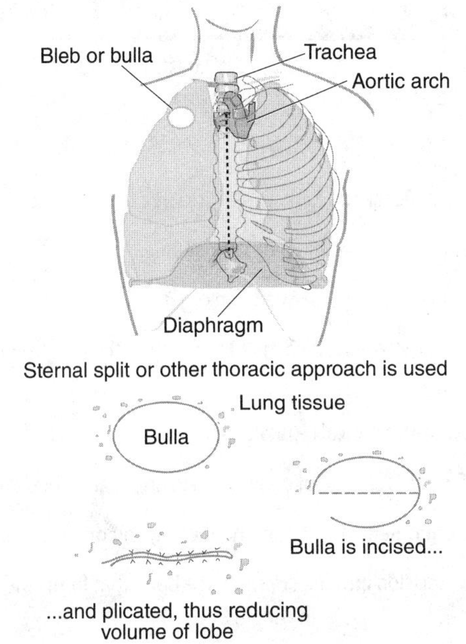

Emphysematous lungs may develop open areas of damaged tissue called blebs or bullae. Removal or plication of a bleb reduces lung volume

Explanation

The physician removes part of an emphysematous lung. Using a scalpel, the surgeon makes a long incision around the side of the chest between two of the ribs. The incision is carried through all of the tissue layers into the chest cavity. Rib spreaders are inserted into the wound and the ribs are spread apart exposing the lung. Alternately, the chest cavity can be opened and the operation performed through a vertical incision in the center of the chest through the sternum. The skin incision is carried down to the sternum bone and a saw is used to split the sternum. With the sternum split in half, the chest is entered by spreading the sternum apart with a set of rib spreaders. Space is made in the chest by packing the uninvolved lung away from the operative field using large moist gauze sponges. In order to perform the procedure, the pleural surface may require an operative procedure such as pneumonolysis (separation of the surface of the lung that has become adherent to the inside surface of the chest cavity). The lung tissue to be removed is identified and isolated in the operative field by pushing aside the deflated lung with a gloved hand and large moist gauze sponges. The lung tissue may be further isolated using a row of staples. The emphysematous lung tissue is removed by sharp and blunt dissection and often by folding and suturing of the tissues (plication). When the procedure is complete, the instruments and gauze sponges are removed. A chest tube(s) may be used to provide drainage for the chest cavity. If applicable, the sternotomy is repaired using wires to bring the two halves of the sternum together, and the operative wound is closed by sutures or staples.

Coding Tips

Diagnostic lung biopsies with intraoperative pathology that determines the need for resection or another definitive procedure should be reported using only the most complex service performed. When a diagnostic wedge resection is performed and followed by a more complex procedure on the same anatomic location, report add-on codes 32507 or 32668 with the more complex procedure. When a therapeutic wedge resection is performed on a different lobe than a more complex lung resection, append modifier 59 or an X{EPSU} modifier. For a thoracotomy with excision or plication of bullae, with or without any pleural procedure, see 32141. For a surgical thoracoscopy with excision-plication of bullae, including any pleural procedure, see 32655. For open wedge resection of the lung, see 32505, 32506, or 32507. When lung resection is performed with chest wall tumor resection, use 21601-21603 to report the appropriate chest wall tumor resection, in addition to lung resection codes 32480, 32482, 32484, 32486, 32488, 32505, 32506, and 32507. Supplies used when providing this procedure may be reported with the appropriate HCPCS Level II codes. Check with the specific payer to determine coverage.

ICD-10-CM Diagnostic Codes

J43.0	Unilateral pulmonary emphysema [MacLeod's syndrome]
J43.1	Panlobular emphysema
J43.2	Centrilobular emphysema
J43.8	Other emphysema
J43.9	Emphysema, unspecified
J98.2	Interstitial emphysema
J98.3	Compensatory emphysema
T79.7XXA	Traumatic subcutaneous emphysema, initial encounter

AMA: **32491** 2018,Jan,8; 2017,Jan,8; 2016,Jan,13; 2015,Jan,16; 2014,Jan,11

Relative Value Units/Medicare Edits

Non-Facility RVU	Work	PE	MP	Total
32491	25.24	11.59	5.81	42.64
Facility RVU	**Work**	**PE**	**MP**	**Total**
32491	25.24	11.59	5.81	42.64

	FUD	Status	MUE	Modifiers				IOM Reference
32491	90	R	1(2)	51	50	62*	80	100-04,3,100.7

* with documentation

Terms To Know

emphysema. Pathological condition in which there is destructive enlargement of the air sacs in the lungs resulting in damage and lack of elasticity to the alveolar walls, commonly seen in long-term smokers.

emphysematous bleb. Formation of blisters or vesicles greater than 1.0 mm within an emphysematous lung, containing serum or blood.

excision. Surgical removal of an organ or tissue.

plication. Surgical technique involving folding, tucking, or pleating to reduce the size of a hollow structure or organ.

thoracotomy. Surgical procedure for opening the chest wall in order to access the lungs, esophagus, trachea, aorta, heart, and diaphragm.

32501

+ 32501 Resection and repair of portion of bronchus (bronchoplasty) when performed at time of lobectomy or segmentectomy (List separately in addition to code for primary procedure)

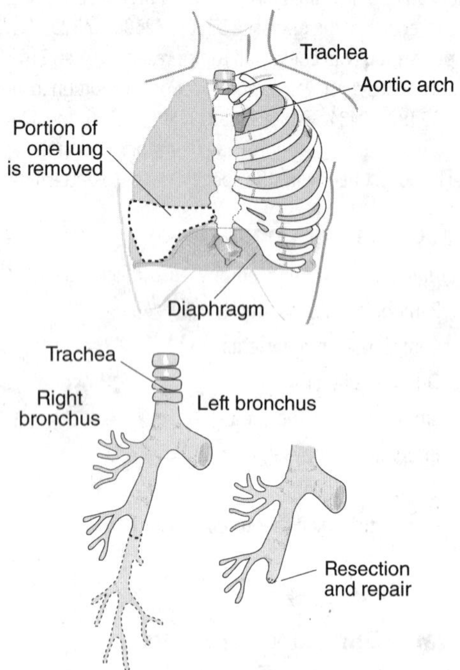

A portion of bronchus is resected and repaired

Explanation

During lobectomy or segmentectomy, the physician repairs part of a bronchus. After removing the lobes or lobe segments (see codes 32480, 32482, 32484 for procedure description), the segment of diseased or damaged bronchial tube is repaired and sutured to the main bronchial tube in the root of the lung. The remaining instruments and gauze sponges are removed from the chest cavity. The chest incision is sutured closed in layers (sternal wires are used if the chest was entered through a midline sternal incision). A chest tube(s) may be used to provide drainage for the chest cavity. List this code separately in addition to the primary procedure.

Coding Tips

Use 32501 in addition to 32480, 32482, and 32484. Also report 32501 when plastic closure is required to preserve function of a lung following the removal of a portion of that lung. It is not to be used in the instance of closure of the proximal end of a bronchus resection. For removal of lung, other than total pneumonectomy, with circumferential resection of segment of bronchus followed by broncho-bronchial anastomosis (sleeve lobectomy), see 32486.

ICD-10-CM Diagnostic Codes

This/these CPT code(s) are add on code(s). See the primary procedure code that this code is performed with for your ICD-10-CM code selections. Diagnostic code(s) would be the same as the actual procedure performed.

AMA: 32501 1995,Win,1

Relative Value Units/Medicare Edits

Non-Facility RVU	Work	PE	MP	Total
32501	4.68	1.32	1.07	7.07
Facility RVU	**Work**	**PE**	**MP**	**Total**
32501	4.68	1.32	1.07	7.07

	FUD	Status	MUE	Modifiers				IOM Reference
32501	N/A	A	1(3)	N/A	N/A	62*	80	None

* with documentation

Terms To Know

bronchoplasty. Reconstruction or plastic repair of the bronchus.

excision. Surgical removal of an organ or tissue.

incision. Act of cutting into tissue or an organ.

lobectomy. Excision of a lobe of an organ such as the liver, thyroid, lung, or brain.

pneumonectomy. Surgical removal of a lung or lung tissue.

resection. Surgical removal of a part or all of an organ or body part.

segmentectomy. Removal of a segment of a gland or an organ.

sternotomy. Incision into the sternum, the bone that forms the front of the chest cavity and connects with the ribs.

trachea. Tube descending from the larynx and branching into the right and left main bronchi.

32503-32504

32503 Resection of apical lung tumor (eg, Pancoast tumor), including chest wall resection, rib(s) resection(s), neurovascular dissection, when performed; without chest wall reconstruction(s)

32504 with chest wall reconstruction

A Pancoast tumor is a tumor at the apex of the lung

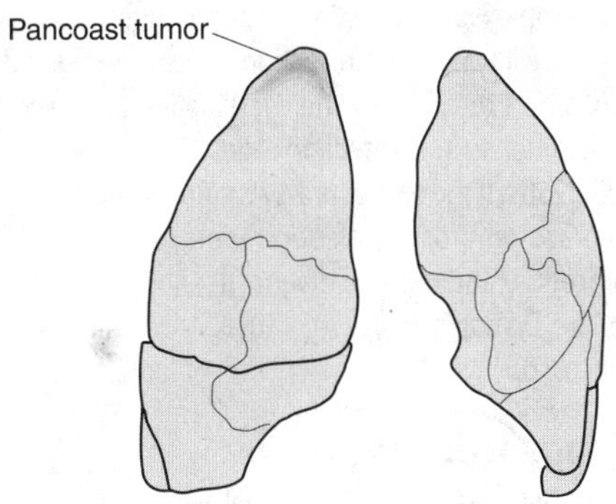

Explanation

The physician removes a tumor from the apex of the lung, such as a Pancoast tumor, as well as a portion of the chest wall. The patient may be intubated with a double lumen endotracheal tube to verify correct positioning and to evaluate endobronchial disease. The chest cavity is entered using an anterior or posterior incision. The posterior incision is made along the outline of the scapula, entering the pleural space at the third or fourth intercostal space. In some cases, an anterior transcervical approach is used. The necessary extended en bloc resection of the chest wall includes posterior portions of the first three ribs, part of the upper thoracic vertebrae (including the transverse process), the intercostal nerves, the lower trunk of the brachial plexus, the stellate ganglion, a section of the dorsal sympathetic ganglion, and the portion of the involved lung. For tumors that are situated peripherally, the apical segment of the upper lobe of the lung is separated from the remaining superior lobe. The apex of the lung is left attached to the chest wall. The first through third, fourth, or fifth ribs are sectioned anteriorly. The subclavian artery is sharply dissected from the surrounding structures. A subperiosteal dissection is performed around the first rib, which is transected, and the subclavian vessels are mobilized superiorly. If preoperative magnetic resonance imaging demonstrated vessel involvement, an initial anterior approach is performed to dissect or graft the vessels. The ribs are disarticulated and the tumor, along with the involved chest wall, is gradually mobilized. Next, the segmental vessels are identified, doubly ligated, and transected. The parietal pleura are bluntly dissected along the anterior border of the spinal column. The tumor and the involved chest wall that has remained attached to the inferior trunk of the brachial plexus is excised, using caution to spare the T1 nerve root as it crosses beneath the angle of the first rib to join the C8 nerve root. If a tumor has invaded the vertebral bodies, the subclavian artery, or the C8 to T1 nerve routes, a multidisciplinary approach may be necessary. At the completion of the procedure, two large chest tubes are placed: one at the apex of the chest to drain any residual air and the other to drain fluids. Report 32504 when chest wall reconstruction is performed.

Coding Tips

When a diagnostic wedge resection is performed and followed by a more complex procedure on the same anatomic location, report add-on codes 32507 or 32668 with the more complex procedure. When a therapeutic wedge resection is performed on a different lobe than a more complex lung resection, append modifier 59 or an X{EPSU} modifier. Do not report 32503 or 32504 with 21601-21603, 32100, 32551, 32554, or 32555.

ICD-10-CM Diagnostic Codes

C34.10 Malignant neoplasm of upper lobe, unspecified bronchus or lung

C34.11 Malignant neoplasm of upper lobe, right bronchus or lung ☑

C34.12 Malignant neoplasm of upper lobe, left bronchus or lung ☑

AMA: 32503 2012,Sep,3-8; 2012,Oct,9-11 **32504** 2012,Sep,3-8; 2012,Oct,9-11

Relative Value Units/Medicare Edits

Non-Facility RVU	Work	PE	MP	Total
32503	31.74	12.76	7.55	52.05
32504	36.54	14.1	8.7	59.34
Facility RVU	**Work**	**PE**	**MP**	**Total**
32503	31.74	12.76	7.55	52.05
32504	36.54	14.1	8.7	59.34

	FUD	Status	MUE	Modifiers				IOM Reference
32503	90	A	1(2)	51	N/A	62*	80	None
32504	90	A	1(2)	51	N/A	62*	80	

* with documentation

Terms To Know

apex. Highest point of a root end of a tooth, or the end of any organ.

en bloc removal. Take out as a whole or all in one mass.

ligate. To tie off a blood vessel or duct with a suture or a soft, thin wire (ligature wire).

Pancoast syndrome. Neoplasm of upper lobe of the lung.

pleura. One of the two membranes that surround the lungs. The visceral pleura encases the lung and the parietal pleura lines the inner chest walls.

transection. Transverse dissection; to cut across a long axis; cross section.

32505-32507

32505 Thoracotomy; with therapeutic wedge resection (eg, mass, nodule), initial

\+ **32506** with therapeutic wedge resection (eg, mass or nodule), each additional resection, ipsilateral (List separately in addition to code for primary procedure)

\+ **32507** with diagnostic wedge resection followed by anatomic lung resection (List separately in addition to code for primary procedure)

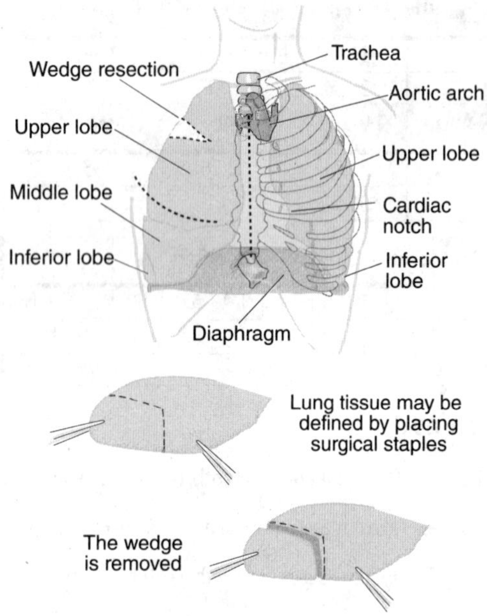

A wedge resection, single or multiple, is taken from a lung

Explanation

The physician removes a wedge-shaped portion(s) of a lobe(s) on one or both lungs. The physician opens the chest cavity widely to gain access to the lung to be removed. Using a scalpel, the surgeon makes a long incision around the side of the chest between two of the ribs. The incision is carried through all of the tissue layers into the chest cavity. Rib spreaders are inserted into the wound and the ribs are spread apart exposing the lung. Alternately, the chest cavity can be opened and the operation performed through a vertical incision in the center of the chest through the sternum. The skin incision is carried down to the sternum bone and a saw is used to split the sternum. With the sternum split in half, the chest is entered by spreading the sternum apart with a set of rib spreaders. The area to be removed is identified and isolated in the operative field by pushing aside the deflated lung with a gloved hand and large moist gauze sponges. The healthy portions of the lung surrounding the area(s) to be removed are clamped and the unhealthy portion is removed by cutting the lung tissue isolated by the clamps. Sutures or surgical clips are used to repair the cut portion of the remaining lung tissue. The instruments and gauze sponges are removed. A chest tube(s) may be used to provide drainage for the chest cavity. When the procedure is complete, if applicable, the sternotomy is repaired using wires to bring the two halves of the sternum together and the operative wound is closed by sutures or staples. Report 32505 for the initial therapeutic wedge resection and 32506 for each additional wedge resection on the same side. Report 32507 when the wedge resection is followed by a lung resection.

Coding Tips

Report 32506 in addition to 32505. Report 32507 in addition to 32440, 32442, 32445, 32480, 32482, 32484, 32486, 32488, 32503, and 32504. Therapeutic wedge resection codes (32505, 32506, 32666, or 32667) should not be reported in addition to the more complex lung procedures (lobectomy) unless wedge resection is performed on a different lobe or lung. When a diagnostic wedge resection is performed and followed by a more complex procedure on the same anatomic location, report 32507 or 32668 with the more complex procedure. When a therapeutic wedge resection is performed on a different lobe than a more complex lung resection, append modifier 59 or X{EPSU}. If lung resection and chest wall tumor resection are performed at the same operative session, report the appropriate chest wall tumor resection code (21601-21603) in addition to lung resection codes 32480, 32482, 32484, 32486, 32488, and 32505-32507. If the procedure is attempted thoracoscopically, but requires major thoracotomy for completion, report 32505-32507 for the open portion of the procedure and report a diagnostic thoracoscopy, 32601, as a secondary procedure. Do not report 32505 with 32440, 32442, 32445, or 32488. For surgical thoracoscopy with wedge resection of lung, see 32666-32668.

ICD-10-CM Diagnostic Codes

A15.0	Tuberculosis of lung
B44.0	Invasive pulmonary aspergillosis
B44.1	Other pulmonary aspergillosis
C34.11	Malignant neoplasm of upper lobe, right bronchus or lung ☑
C34.12	Malignant neoplasm of upper lobe, left bronchus or lung ☑
C34.2	Malignant neoplasm of middle lobe, bronchus or lung
C34.31	Malignant neoplasm of lower lobe, right bronchus or lung ☑
C34.32	Malignant neoplasm of lower lobe, left bronchus or lung ☑
C34.81	Malignant neoplasm of overlapping sites of right bronchus and lung ☑
C34.82	Malignant neoplasm of overlapping sites of left bronchus and lung ☑
C46.51	Kaposi's sarcoma of right lung ☑
C46.52	Kaposi's sarcoma of left lung ☑
C78.01	Secondary malignant neoplasm of right lung ☑
C78.02	Secondary malignant neoplasm of left lung ☑
C7A.090	Malignant carcinoid tumor of the bronchus and lung
D02.21	Carcinoma in situ of right bronchus and lung ☑
D02.22	Carcinoma in situ of left bronchus and lung ☑
D14.31	Benign neoplasm of right bronchus and lung ☑
D14.32	Benign neoplasm of left bronchus and lung ☑
D38.1	Neoplasm of uncertain behavior of trachea, bronchus and lung
D3A.090	Benign carcinoid tumor of the bronchus and lung
D86.0	Sarcoidosis of lung
J43.0	Unilateral pulmonary emphysema [MacLeod's syndrome]
J43.1	Panlobular emphysema
J43.2	Centrilobular emphysema
J47.0	Bronchiectasis with acute lower respiratory infection
J47.1	Bronchiectasis with (acute) exacerbation
J85.0	Gangrene and necrosis of lung
J85.1	Abscess of lung with pneumonia
J85.2	Abscess of lung without pneumonia
J98.4	Other disorders of lung
Q33.2	Sequestration of lung

AMA: 32505 2018,Jan,8; 2017,Jan,8; 2016,Jan,13; 2015,Jan,16; 2014,Jan,11 **32506** 2018,Jan,8; 2017,Jan,8; 2016,Jan,13; 2015,Jan,16; 2014,Jan,11 **32507** 2018,Jan,8; 2017,Jan,8; 2016,Jan,13; 2015,Jan,16; 2014,Jan,11

Relative Value Units/Medicare Edits

Non-Facility RVU	Work	PE	MP	Total
32505	15.75	7.5	3.63	26.88
32506	3.0	0.84	0.69	4.53
32507	3.0	0.84	0.68	4.52
Facility RVU	**Work**	**PE**	**MP**	**Total**
32505	15.75	7.5	3.63	26.88
32506	3.0	0.84	0.69	4.53
32507	3.0	0.84	0.68	4.52

	FUD	Status	MUE	Modifiers				IOM Reference
32505	90	A	1(2)	51	N/A	62*	80	None
32506	N/A	A	3(3)	N/A	N/A	62*	80	
32507	N/A	A	2(3)	N/A	N/A	62*	80	

* with documentation

Terms To Know

resection. Surgical removal of a part or all of an organ or body part.

sternotomy. Incision into the sternum, the bone that forms the front of the chest cavity and connects with the ribs.

therapeutic procedure. Manner of effecting change through the application of clinical skills and/or services that attempt to improve function.

thoracotomy. Surgical procedure for opening the chest wall in order to access the lungs, esophagus, trachea, aorta, heart, and diaphragm.

wedge excision. Surgical removal of a section of tissue that is thick at one edge and tapers to a thin edge.

32540

32540 Extrapleural enucleation of empyema (empyemectomy)

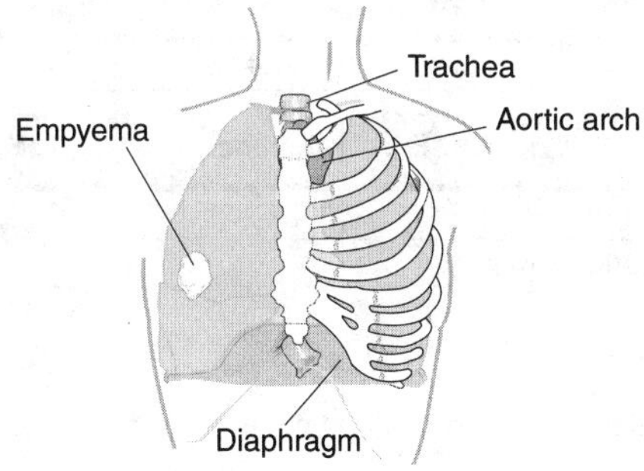

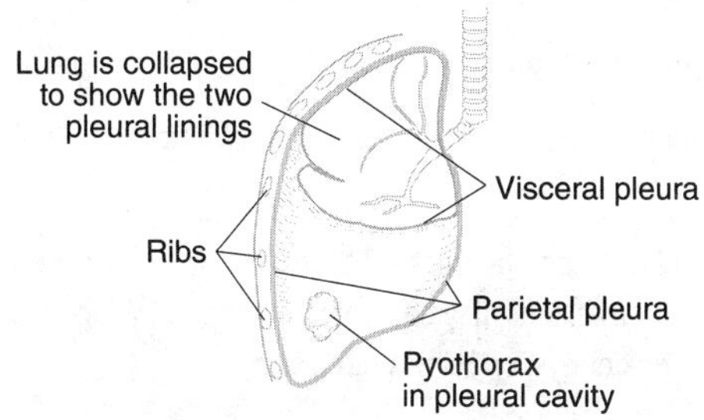

An empyema is a pocket of pus within a body cavity and may also be referred to as a pyothorax, or pus in the pleural cavity

Explanation

The physician removes an empyema (an abscess in the chest cavity between the lung and the chest wall) in its entirety, including the pleural membranes surrounding the abscess. The physician opens the chest cavity to gain access to the abscess. Using a scalpel, the surgeon makes an incision around the side of the chest between two of the ribs. The incision is carried through all the tissue layers down to the membrane lining the chest cavity. Rib spreaders are inserted into the wound and the ribs are spread apart exposing the tissues, taking care to preserve the integrity of the chest lining. Holding a gauze sponge, the surgeon strips away the lining adherent to the chest wall and the abscess and carries this all the way around the abscess. This creates a sac that contains the abscess. The intact mass is shelled out through the chest incision. After the removal of the instruments and gauze sponges, the chest incision is sutured closed in layers leaving a drainage tube or the wound is partially closed to allow drainage.

Coding Tips

When performed at the time of a lung excision, report 32540 with the appropriate lung removal code, 32440–32491. For tube thoracotomy with or without water seal for abscess, hemothorax, or empyema (separate procedure), see 32551. For thoracostomy, with rib resection for empyema, see 32035; with open flap drainage for empyema, see 32036. For pneumonostomy with open drainage of abscess or cyst, see 32200.

ICD-10-CM Diagnostic Codes

A15.6	Tuberculous pleurisy
J86.0	Pyothorax with fistula
J86.9	Pyothorax without fistula

AMA: 32540 1994,Fal,1

Relative Value Units/Medicare Edits

Non-Facility RVU	Work	PE	MP	Total
32540	30.35	12.4	6.94	49.69
Facility RVU	**Work**	**PE**	**MP**	**Total**
32540	30.35	12.4	6.94	49.69

	FUD	Status	MUE	Modifiers				IOM Reference
32540	90	A	1(3)	51	N/A	62*	80	None

* with documentation

Terms To Know

abscess. Circumscribed collection of pus resulting from bacteria, frequently associated with swelling and other signs of inflammation.

empyema. Accumulation of pus within the respiratory or pleural cavity.

fistula. Abnormal tube-like passage between two body cavities or organs or from an organ to the outside surface.

lesion. Area of damaged tissue that has lost continuity or function, due to disease or trauma. Lesions may be located on internal structures such as the brain, nerves, or kidneys, or visible on the skin.

resection. Surgical removal of a part or all of an organ or body part.

thoracostomy. Creation of an opening in the chest wall for drainage.

thoracotomy. Surgical procedure for opening the chest wall in order to access the lungs, esophagus, trachea, aorta, heart, and diaphragm.

32550

32550 Insertion of indwelling tunneled pleural catheter with cuff

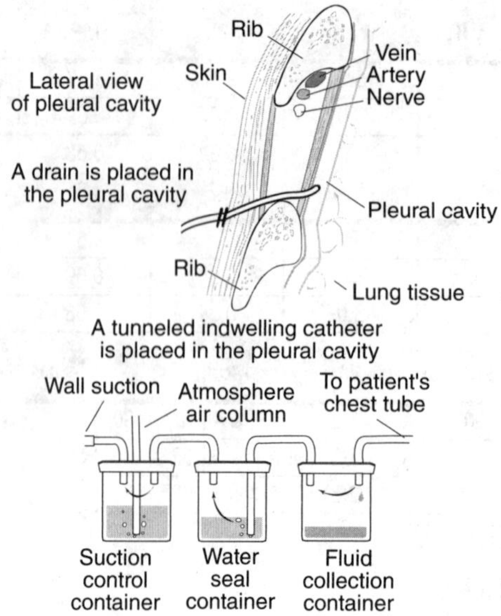

Explanation

The physician inserts a tunneled, indwelling pleural catheter to aid quality of life and long-term management of malignant effusion. The catheter allows drainage on an outpatient or home basis and consists of flexible rubber tubing with a safety drainage valve to provide access to the pleural cavity and prevent air and fluid entering. A polyester cuff secures the catheter in place and helps prevent infection. Using separately reportable imaging guidance, the physician inserts the catheter percutaneously through a small incision in the anterior axillary area. The pleural catheter is threaded over a guidewire to access the pleural cavity, tunneled under the skin along the chest wall, and brought out that side in the lower chest. After placement, the patient may drain pleural fluid at home periodically into vacuum bottles by connecting the matching drainage line access tip to the valve.

Coding Tips

When medically necessary, report moderate (conscious) sedation provided by the performing physician with 99151-99153. When provided by another physician, report 99155-99157. Supplies used when providing this procedure may be reported with the appropriate HCPCS Level II codes. Check with the specific payer to determine coverage. If performed on the same side of the chest, do not report 32550 with 32554–32557. If imaging guidance is performed, see 75989.

ICD-10-CM Diagnostic Codes

A15.6	Tuberculous pleurisy
A15.7	Primary respiratory tuberculosis
J90	Pleural effusion, not elsewhere classified
J91.0	Malignant pleural effusion
J91.8	Pleural effusion in other conditions classified elsewhere
J94.0	Chylous effusion
M32.13	Lung involvement in systemic lupus erythematosus

AMA: 32550 2018,Jan,8; 2017,Jan,8; 2016,Jan,13; 2015,Jan,16; 2014,May,3; 2014,Mar,13; 2014,Jan,11

Relative Value Units/Medicare Edits

Non-Facility RVU	Work	PE	MP	Total
32550	3.92	16.83	0.54	21.29
Facility RVU	**Work**	**PE**	**MP**	**Total**
32550	3.92	1.52	0.54	5.98

	FUD	Status	MUE	Modifiers				IOM Reference
32550	0	A	2(3)	N/A	N/A	N/A	N/A	None

* with documentation

Terms To Know

carcinoma in situ. Malignancy that arises from the cells of the vessel, gland, or organ of origin that remains confined to that site or has not invaded neighboring tissue.

malignant neoplasm. Any cancerous tumor or lesion exhibiting uncontrolled tissue growth that can progressively invade other parts of the body with its disease-generating cells.

pleura. One of the two membranes that surround the lungs. The visceral pleura encases the lung and the parietal pleura lines the inner chest walls.

secondary. Second in order of occurrence or importance, or appearing during the course of another disease or condition.

32551

32551 Tube thoracostomy, includes connection to drainage system (eg, water seal), when performed, open (separate procedure)

The conventional three-bottle water seal system evacuates the pleural space without backpressure. The negative pressure works to reinflate the lung and seal any leakage

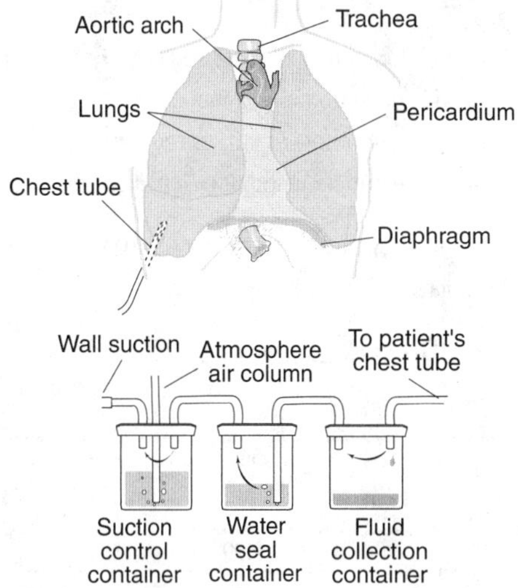

Explanation

The physician removes fluid and/or air from the chest cavity by puncturing through the space between the ribs. To enter the chest cavity, the physician passes a trocar over the top of a rib, punctures through the chest tissues between the ribs, and enters the pleural cavity. Separately reportable imaging guidance may be used. With the end of the trocar in the chest cavity, the physician advances the plastic tube into the chest cavity. The sharp trocar is removed leaving one end of the plastic catheter in place within the chest cavity. A large syringe is attached to the outside end of the catheter and the fluid (blood or pus) is removed from the chest cavity by pulling back on the plunger of the syringe. The outside end of the tube may be connected to a drainage system, such as a water seal, to prevent air from being sucked into the chest cavity and to allow continuous or intermittent removal of air or fluid.

Coding Tips

When medically necessary, report moderate (conscious) sedation provided by the performing physician with 99151-99153. When provided by another physician, report 99155-99157. Do not report 32551 with 33020 or 33025 if a pleural drain is placed on the same side. For pleural drainage, percutaneous, with insertion of an indwelling catheter, see 32556–32557. Do not report 32551 with 43287 or 43288. For radiological supervision and interpretation, see 75989.

ICD-10-CM Diagnostic Codes

J86.0	Pyothorax with fistula
J86.9	Pyothorax without fistula
J90	Pleural effusion, not elsewhere classified
J91.0	Malignant pleural effusion
J91.8	Pleural effusion in other conditions classified elsewhere
J93.0	Spontaneous tension pneumothorax
J93.11	Primary spontaneous pneumothorax
J93.12	Secondary spontaneous pneumothorax
J93.81	Chronic pneumothorax

J93.82	Other air leak
J93.83	Other pneumothorax
J94.0	Chylous effusion
J94.2	Hemothorax
J94.8	Other specified pleural conditions
J95.811	Postprocedural pneumothorax
P26.0	Tracheobronchial hemorrhage originating in the perinatal period
P26.1	Massive pulmonary hemorrhage originating in the perinatal period
P26.8	Other pulmonary hemorrhages originating in the perinatal period
S27.0XXA	Traumatic pneumothorax, initial encounter
S27.1XXA	Traumatic hemothorax, initial encounter
S27.2XXA	Traumatic hemopneumothorax, initial encounter

AMA: 32551 2018,Jul,7; 2018,Jan,8; 2017,Jun,10; 2017,Jan,8; 2016,Jan,13; 2015,Jan,16; 2014,May,3; 2014,Jan,11

Relative Value Units/Medicare Edits

Non-Facility RVU	Work	PE	MP	Total
32551	3.04	0.99	0.5	4.53
Facility RVU	**Work**	**PE**	**MP**	**Total**
32551	3.04	0.99	0.5	4.53

	FUD	Status	MUE	Modifiers				IOM Reference
32551	0	A	2(3)	51	50	N/A	N/A	None

* with documentation

Terms To Know

hemothorax. Blood collecting in the pleural cavity.

pneumothorax. Collapsed lung due to air or gas trapped in the pleural space formed by the membrane that encloses the lungs and lines the thoracic cavity.

thoracostomy. Creation of an opening in the chest wall for drainage.

trocar. Cannula or a sharp pointed instrument used to puncture and aspirate fluid from cavities.

32552

32552 Removal of indwelling tunneled pleural catheter with cuff

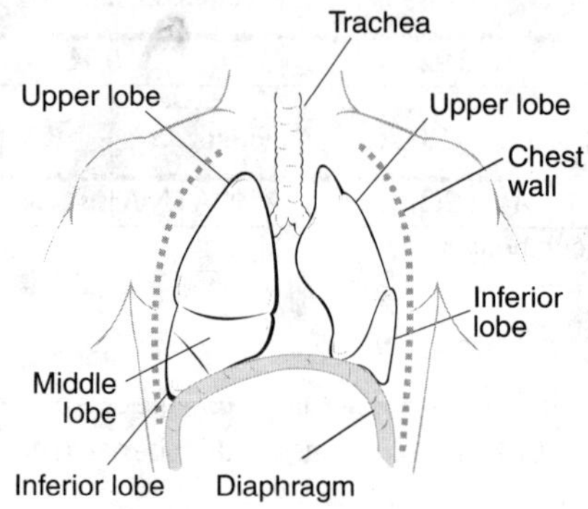

Explanation

The physician removes a previously placed, indwelling tunneled pleural catheter with cuff. Following administration of local anesthesia along the subcutaneous catheter tunnel, blunt dissection is used to release the cuff and the catheter is meticulously withdrawn. Conscious sedation may be required.

Coding Tips

For insertion of an indwelling tunneled pleural catheter with cuff, see 32550. For insertion of a chest tube, see 32551.

ICD-10-CM Diagnostic Codes

T85.79XA	Infection and inflammatory reaction due to other internal prosthetic devices, implants and grafts, initial encounter
Z48.03	Encounter for change or removal of drains

AMA: 32552 2018,Jan,8; 2017,Jan,8; 2016,Jan,13; 2015,Jan,16; 2014,Jan,11

Relative Value Units/Medicare Edits

Non-Facility RVU	Work	PE	MP	Total
32552	2.53	2.37	0.36	5.26
Facility RVU	**Work**	**PE**	**MP**	**Total**
32552	2.53	1.66	0.36	4.55

	FUD	Status	MUE	Modifiers				IOM Reference
32552	10	A	2(2)	51	N/A	N/A	80*	None

* with documentation

Lungs and Pleura

32553

32553 Placement of interstitial device(s) for radiation therapy guidance (eg, fiducial markers, dosimeter), percutaneous, intra-thoracic, single or multiple

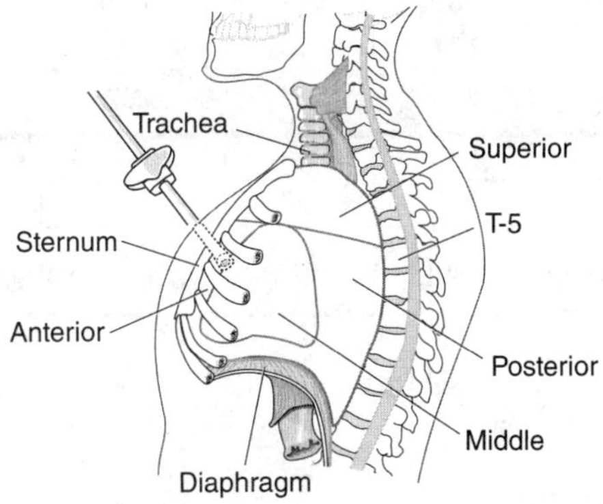

Percutaneous placement of interstitial device into the thorax

Explanation

The physician places one or more interstitial devices such as gold seeds (fiducial markers) for radiation therapy guidance or a dosimeter to gauge the amount of radiation received. Implanted percutaneously in and/or around an intrathoracic soft tissue tumor, these act as radiographic landmarks to define the position of the target lesion. Under CT or other image guidance, the physician injects a small capsule or seed into the intrathoracic tissue using a needle injection device. Allowing for precision in targeting radiation and/or for measuring the radiation doses received, an injected fiducial marker is visible by ultrasound and fluoroscopy and permits accurate triangulation of the tissue to be treated. An injected capsule dosimeter relays radiation dose information so that the clinical team can monitor for any deviation between the radiation plan and the actual radiation received.

Coding Tips

Report the device separately. When medically necessary, report moderate (conscious) sedation provided by the performing physician with 99151-99153. When provided by another physician, report 99155-99157. For radiology services, see 76942, 77002, 77012, and 77021. When percutaneous placement of interstitial devices related to intra-abdominal, intrapelvic, and/or retroperitoneal radiation therapy guidance is required, see 49411.

ICD-10-CM Diagnostic Codes

C33	Malignant neoplasm of trachea
C34.01	Malignant neoplasm of right main bronchus ☑
C34.02	Malignant neoplasm of left main bronchus ☑
C34.11	Malignant neoplasm of upper lobe, right bronchus or lung ☑
C34.12	Malignant neoplasm of upper lobe, left bronchus or lung ☑
C34.2	Malignant neoplasm of middle lobe, bronchus or lung
C34.31	Malignant neoplasm of lower lobe, right bronchus or lung ☑
C34.32	Malignant neoplasm of lower lobe, left bronchus or lung ☑
C34.81	Malignant neoplasm of overlapping sites of right bronchus and lung ☑
C34.82	Malignant neoplasm of overlapping sites of left bronchus and lung ☑
C38.4	Malignant neoplasm of pleura
C45.0	Mesothelioma of pleura
C46.51	Kaposi's sarcoma of right lung ☑
C46.52	Kaposi's sarcoma of left lung ☑
C76.1	Malignant neoplasm of thorax
C78.01	Secondary malignant neoplasm of right lung ☑
C78.02	Secondary malignant neoplasm of left lung ☑
C78.2	Secondary malignant neoplasm of pleura
C79.89	Secondary malignant neoplasm of other specified sites
C7A.090	Malignant carcinoid tumor of the bronchus and lung
D02.21	Carcinoma in situ of right bronchus and lung ☑
D02.22	Carcinoma in situ of left bronchus and lung ☑
D09.3	Carcinoma in situ of thyroid and other endocrine glands
D09.8	Carcinoma in situ of other specified sites
D14.31	Benign neoplasm of right bronchus and lung ☑
D14.32	Benign neoplasm of left bronchus and lung ☑
D19.0	Benign neoplasm of mesothelial tissue of pleura
D38.1	Neoplasm of uncertain behavior of trachea, bronchus and lung
D38.2	Neoplasm of uncertain behavior of pleura
D3A.090	Benign carcinoid tumor of the bronchus and lung

AMA: **32553** 2018,Jan,8; 2017,Jan,8; 2016,Jun,3; 2016,Jan,13; 2015,Jun,6; 2015,Jan,16; 2014,Jan,11

Relative Value Units/Medicare Edits

Non-Facility RVU	Work	PE	MP	Total
32553	3.55	11.02	0.32	14.89
Facility RVU	**Work**	**PE**	**MP**	**Total**
32553	3.55	1.31	0.32	5.18

	FUD	Status	MUE	Modifiers				IOM Reference
32553	0	A	1(2)	51	N/A	N/A	80	None

* with documentation

Terms To Know

in situ. Located in the natural position or contained within the origin site, not spread into neighboring tissue.

Kaposi's sarcoma. Malignant neoplasm caused by vascular proliferation of cutaneous tumors characterized by channels lined with endothelial tissue containing vascular spaced.

ultrasound. Imaging using ultra-high sound frequency bounced off body structures.

32554-32555

32554 Thoracentesis, needle or catheter, aspiration of the pleural space; without imaging guidance

32555 with imaging guidance

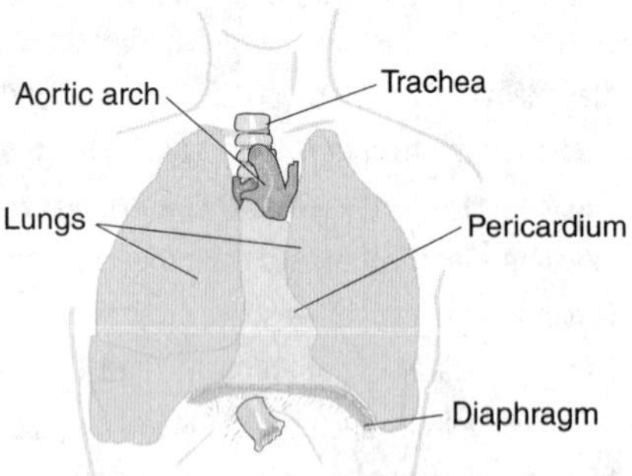

The pleural space is aspirated

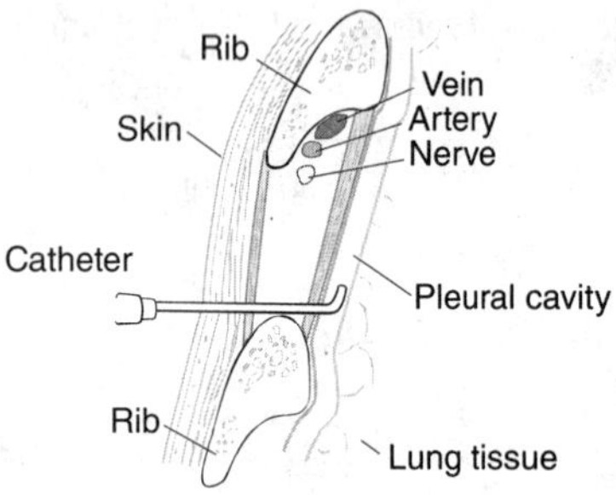

Explanation

The physician removes fluid and/or air from the chest cavity by puncturing through the space between the ribs with a hollow needle (cannula) and entering the chest cavity. The fluid (blood or pus) is removed from the chest cavity by pulling back on the plunger of the syringe attached to the cannula. Report 32554 if the procedure is performed without imaging guidance. Report 32555 when imaging guidance is used during the procedure.

Coding Tips

Do not report 32554 or 32555 with 32550, 32551, 76942, 77002, 77012, 77021, or 75989. For percutaneous insertion of a pleural catheter, see 32556 and 33557.

ICD-10-CM Diagnostic Codes

A15.6	Tuberculous pleurisy
J86.0	Pyothorax with fistula
J86.9	Pyothorax without fistula
J90	Pleural effusion, not elsewhere classified
J91.0	Malignant pleural effusion
J91.8	Pleural effusion in other conditions classified elsewhere
J93.0	Spontaneous tension pneumothorax
J93.11	Primary spontaneous pneumothorax
J94.0	Chylous effusion
J94.2	Hemothorax
J94.8	Other specified pleural conditions
J95.4	Chemical pneumonitis due to anesthesia
M32.13	Lung involvement in systemic lupus erythematosus
M35.02	Sicca syndrome with lung involvement

AMA: 32554 2018,Jan,8; 2017,Jan,8; 2016,Jan,13; 2015,Jan,16; 2014,Jan,11; 2013,Nov,9 **32555** 2018,Jan,8; 2017,Jan,8; 2016,Jan,13; 2015,Jan,16; 2014,Jan,11; 2013,Nov,9

Relative Value Units/Medicare Edits

Non-Facility RVU	Work	PE	MP	Total
32554	1.82	4.0	0.19	6.01
32555	2.27	6.05	0.19	8.51
Facility RVU	**Work**	**PE**	**MP**	**Total**
32554	1.82	0.57	0.19	2.58
32555	2.27	0.76	0.19	3.22

	FUD	Status	MUE	Modifiers				IOM Reference
32554	0	A	2(3)	51	50	N/A	N/A	None
32555	0	A	2(3)	51	50	N/A	N/A	

* with documentation

Terms To Know

aspirate. To withdraw fluid or air from a body cavity by suction.

cannula. Tube inserted into a blood vessel, duct, or body cavity to facilitate passage.

effusion. Escape of fluid from within a body cavity.

percutaneous. Through the skin.

pleura. One of the two membranes that surround the lungs. The visceral pleura encases the lung and the parietal pleura lines the inner chest walls.

32556-32557

32556 Pleural drainage, percutaneous, with insertion of indwelling catheter; without imaging guidance

32557 with imaging guidance

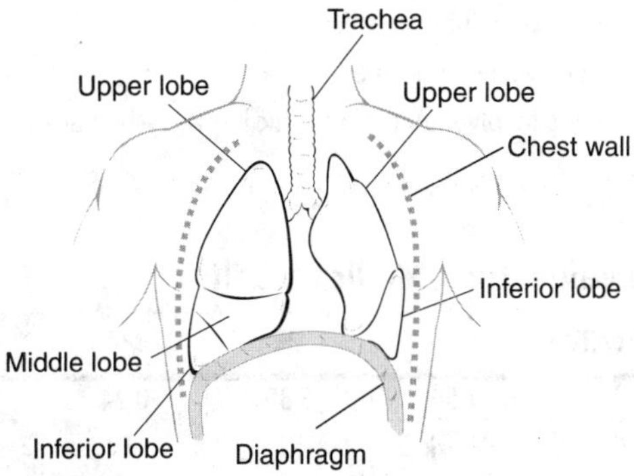

Explanation

The physician removes fluid and/or air from the chest cavity. The patient is positioned dependent upon the location of the fluid (blood or pus) on preprocedural imaging. The chest cavity is accessed by puncturing through the space between the ribs with a needle. Once the fluid is accessed via the needle(s), a guidewire is inserted to the most distal point of the fluid in the pleural cavity. A catheter (i.e., pigtail catheter) is inserted the length of the guidewire and the chest cavity is drained. In some instances, the catheter is connected to a water seal system. Report 32556 if the procedure is performed without imaging guidance. Report 32557 when imaging guidance is used during the procedure.

Coding Tips

Do not report 32556 or 32557 with 32550, 32551, 76942, 77002, 77012, 77021, or 75989. For an open procedure, see 32551. For needle or catheter aspiration of the pleural space via thoracentesis, see 32554 and 32555. For insertion of an indwelling tunneled pleural catheter with a cuff, see 32550.

ICD-10-CM Diagnostic Codes

A15.6	Tuberculous pleurisy
J86.0	Pyothorax with fistula
J86.9	Pyothorax without fistula
J90	Pleural effusion, not elsewhere classified
J91.0	Malignant pleural effusion
J91.8	Pleural effusion in other conditions classified elsewhere
J94.0	Chylous effusion
J94.2	Hemothorax
M32.13	Lung involvement in systemic lupus erythematosus
S27.0XXA	Traumatic pneumothorax, initial encounter
S27.1XXA	Traumatic hemothorax, initial encounter

AMA: **32556** 2018,Jan,8; 2017,Jan,8; 2016,Jan,13; 2015,Jan,16; 2014,Jan,11; 2013,Nov,9 **32557** 2018,Jan,8; 2017,Jan,8; 2016,Jan,13; 2015,Jan,16; 2014,May,3; 2014,Jan,11; 2013,Nov,9

Relative Value Units/Medicare Edits

Non-Facility RVU	Work	PE	MP	Total
32556	2.5	14.63	0.28	17.41
32557	3.12	12.66	0.27	16.05
Facility RVU	**Work**	**PE**	**MP**	**Total**
32556	2.5	0.77	0.28	3.55
32557	3.12	1.0	0.27	4.39

	FUD	Status	MUE	Modifiers				IOM Reference
32556	0	A	2(3)	51	50	N/A	N/A	None
32557	0	A	2(3)	51	50	N/A	N/A	

* with documentation

Terms To Know

fistula. Abnormal tube-like passage between two body cavities or organs or from an organ to the outside surface.

pleural effusion. Collection of lymph and other fluid within the pleural space.

pyothorax. Collection of pus in the pleural space that is commonly caused by an infection that spreads from the lung, such as bacterial pneumonia or a lung abscess.

Lungs and Pleura

32560

32560 Instillation, via chest tube/catheter, agent for pleurodesis (eg, talc for recurrent or persistent pneumothorax)

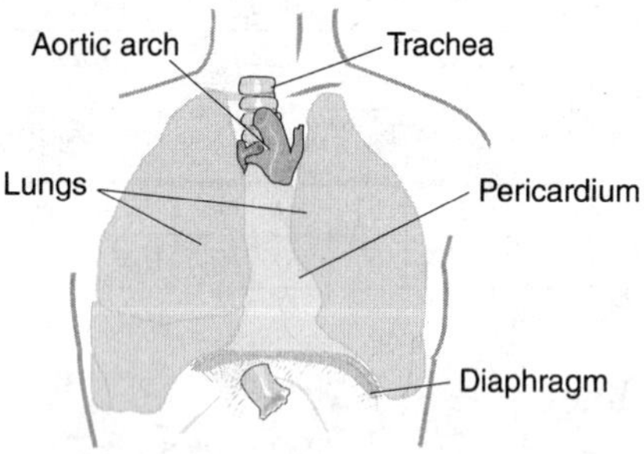

Pleurodesis is the insertion of a caustic chemical into the pleural space, inducing inflammation to eliminate repeated Reffusion and/or pneumothorax

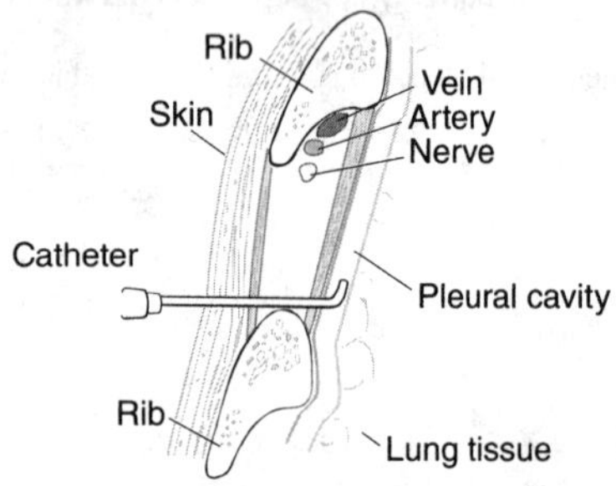

Explanation

The physician instills an agent for pleurodesis, such as talc for recurrent or persistent pneumothorax, into the chest cavity via a chest tube or catheter by puncturing through the space between the ribs. The physician passes a trocar over the top of a rib, punctures through the chest tissues, and enters the pleural cavity. With the end of the trocar, the physician advances the plastic tube into the chest cavity within the pleural space, specifically between the layers of the visceral and parietal pleura. The sharp instrument is removed leaving one end of the plastic catheter in place. A syringe is attached to the outside end of the catheter and the agent is injected into the pleural space. The agent selected is designed to eradicate the pleural space preventing reoccurrence of pleural effusion.

Coding Tips

For thoracentesis with aspiration of the pleural space, see 32554 and 32555. For treatment of pneumothorax with thoracentesis, with insertion of an indwelling catheter, see 32556 and 32557. For pleural scarification by other methods, see 32215. For insertion of a chest tube, see 32551. For thoracoscopy with pleurodesis, see 32650.

ICD-10-CM Diagnostic Codes

J86.0	Pyothorax with fistula
J86.9	Pyothorax without fistula
J90	Pleural effusion, not elsewhere classified
J91.0	Malignant pleural effusion
J91.8	Pleural effusion in other conditions classified elsewhere
J93.0	Spontaneous tension pneumothorax
J93.11	Primary spontaneous pneumothorax
J93.12	Secondary spontaneous pneumothorax
J93.81	Chronic pneumothorax
J93.82	Other air leak
J93.83	Other pneumothorax
J94.0	Chylous effusion
J94.8	Other specified pleural conditions
J95.811	Postprocedural pneumothorax
J95.812	Postprocedural air leak
L60.5	Yellow nail syndrome
M32.13	Lung involvement in systemic lupus erythematosus

AMA: 32560 2018,Jan,8; 2017,Jan,8; 2016,Jan,13; 2015,Jan,16; 2014,Jan,11

Relative Value Units/Medicare Edits

Non-Facility RVU	Work	PE	MP	Total
32560	1.54	5.39	0.24	7.17
Facility RVU	**Work**	**PE**	**MP**	**Total**
32560	1.54	0.47	0.24	2.25

	FUD	Status	MUE	Modifiers				IOM Reference
32560	0	A	1(3)	51	N/A	N/A	N/A	None

* with documentation

Terms To Know

dyspnea. Difficult or labored breathing.

effusion. Escape of fluid from within a body cavity.

emphysematous bleb. Formation of blisters or vesicles greater than 1.0 mm within an emphysematous lung, containing serum or blood.

fistula. Abnormal tube-like passage between two body cavities or organs or from an organ to the outside surface.

pleurisy. Inflammation of the serous membrane that lines the lungs and the thoracic cavity. Pleurisy may cause effusion within the cavity or have exudate in the pleural space or on the membrane surface.

pleurisy. Inflammation of the serous membrane that lines the lungs and the thoracic cavity. Pleurisy may cause effusion within the cavity or have exudate in the pleural space or on the membrane surface.

spontaneous tension pneumothorax. Air leaking from the lung and trapped in the lung lining.

thoracentesis. Surgical puncture of the chest cavity with a specialized needle or hollow tubing to aspirate fluid from within the pleural space for diagnostic or therapeutic reasons.

trocar. Cannula or a sharp pointed instrument used to puncture and aspirate fluid from cavities.

32561-32562

32561 Instillation(s), via chest tube/catheter, agent for fibrinolysis (eg, fibrinolytic agent for break up of multiloculated effusion); initial day

32562 subsequent day

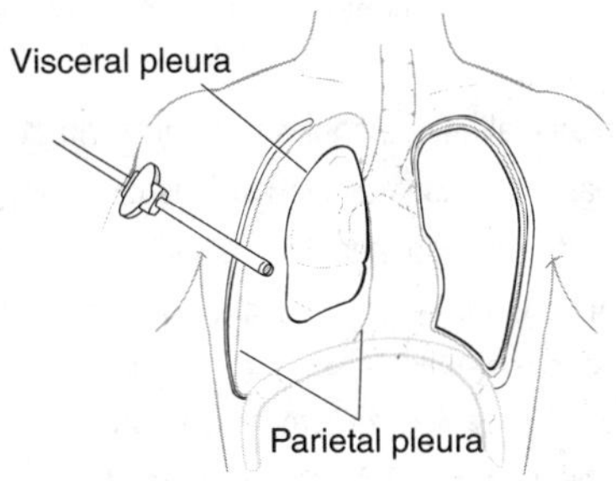

Explanation

The physician instills a fibrinolytic agent (one that breaks up fibrinous adhesions) into the chest cavity via a chest tube or catheter by puncturing through the space between the ribs. To enter the chest cavity, the physician passes a trocar over the top of a rib, punctures through the chest tissues, and enters the pleural cavity. With the end of the trocar in the chest cavity, the physician advances the plastic tube into the chest cavity. The sharp instrument is removed, leaving one end of the plastic catheter in place within the chest cavity. A syringe is attached to the outside end of the catheter and a fibrinolytic agent, such as a saline mixture with Streptokinase or urokinase, is injected into the chest cavity. The agent selected is designed to break up multiloculated pleural effusions and facilitate adequate drainage. Report 32561 for the first day of instillation and 32562 for each subsequent day.

Coding Tips

These codes should be reported only once per day even if multiple instillations are performed. For insertion of a chest tube, see 32551.

ICD-10-CM Diagnostic Codes

A15.6	Tuberculous pleurisy
J90	Pleural effusion, not elsewhere classified
J91.0	Malignant pleural effusion
J91.8	Pleural effusion in other conditions classified elsewhere
J94.0	Chylous effusion
J94.2	Hemothorax
J94.8	Other specified pleural conditions
M32.13	Lung involvement in systemic lupus erythematosus

AMA: 32561 2018,Jan,8; 2017,Jan,8; 2016,Jan,13; 2015,Jan,16; 2014,Jan,11
32562 2018,Jan,8; 2017,Jan,8; 2016,Jan,13; 2015,Jan,16; 2014,Jan,11

Relative Value Units/Medicare Edits

Non-Facility RVU	Work	PE	MP	Total
32561	1.39	1.12	0.15	2.66
32562	1.24	1.0	0.14	2.38
Facility RVU	**Work**	**PE**	**MP**	**Total**
32561	1.39	0.43	0.15	1.97
32562	1.24	0.38	0.14	1.76

	FUD	Status	MUE	Modifiers				IOM Reference
32561	0	A	1(2)	51	N/A	N/A	80	None
32562	0	A	1(2)	51	N/A	N/A	80	

* with documentation

Terms To Know

effusion. Escape of fluid from within a body cavity.

fistula. Abnormal tube-like passage between two body cavities or organs or from an organ to the outside surface.

pleural effusion. Collection of lymph and other fluid within the pleural space.

pleurisy. Inflammation of the serous membrane that lines the lungs and the thoracic cavity. Pleurisy may cause effusion within the cavity or have exudate in the pleural space or on the membrane surface.

trocar. Cannula or a sharp pointed instrument used to puncture and aspirate fluid from cavities.

32601

32601 Thoracoscopy, diagnostic (separate procedure); lungs, pericardial sac, mediastinal or pleural space, without biopsy

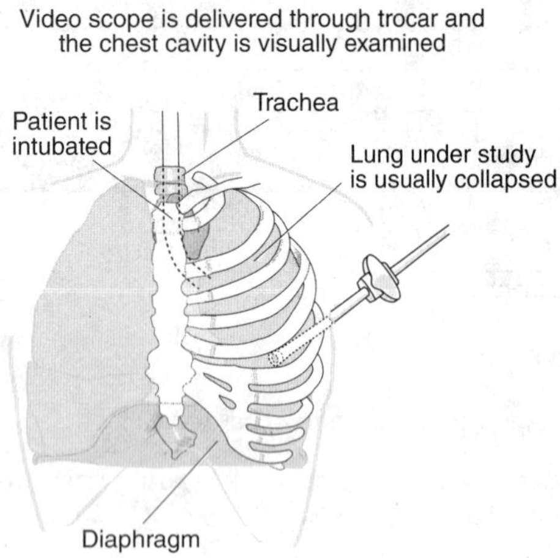

Explanation

The physician examines the inside of the chest cavity through a rigid or flexible fiberoptic endoscope. The procedure can be done under local or general anesthesia. The surgeon makes a small incision between two ribs and by blunt dissection and the use of a trocar enters the thoracic cavity. The endoscope is passed through the trocar and into the chest cavity. The lung is usually partially collapsed by instilling air into the chest through the trocar, or if general anesthesia is used, the lung may be collapsed through a double lumen endotracheal tube inserted through the mouth into the trachea. The contents of the chest cavity are examined by direct visualization and/or the use of a video camera. Still photographs may be taken as part of the procedure. At the conclusion of the procedure, the endoscope and the trocar are removed. A chest tube for drainage and re-expansion of the lung is usually inserted through the wound used for the thoracoscopy.

Coding Tips

This separate procedure by definition is usually a component of a more complex service and not identified separately. When performed alone or with other unrelated procedures/services, it may be reported. If performed alone, list the code; if performed with other procedures/services, list the code and append modifier 59 or an X{EPSU} modifier. Report the appropriate endoscopy for each anatomic site examined. Surgical thoracoscopy (video-assisted thoracic surgery or VATS) always includes diagnostic thoracoscopy. For thoracoscopic biopsies of lung infiltrates, lung nodules, or masses, or for pleural biopsies, see 32607–32609. For a thoracotomy to biopsy lung or pleura, see 32096, 32097, or 32098. Supplies used when providing this procedure may be reported with the appropriate HCPCS Level II codes. Check with the specific payer to determine coverage.

ICD-10-CM Diagnostic Codes

A18.84	Tuberculosis of heart
A39.53	Meningococcal pericarditis
A54.83	Gonococcal heart infection
B33.23	Viral pericarditis
C34.01	Malignant neoplasm of right main bronchus ☑
C34.02	Malignant neoplasm of left main bronchus ☑
C34.2	Malignant neoplasm of middle lobe, bronchus or lung
C34.31	Malignant neoplasm of lower lobe, right bronchus or lung ☑
C34.32	Malignant neoplasm of lower lobe, left bronchus or lung ☑
C38.0	Malignant neoplasm of heart
C38.1	Malignant neoplasm of anterior mediastinum
C38.2	Malignant neoplasm of posterior mediastinum
C38.4	Malignant neoplasm of pleura
C45.0	Mesothelioma of pleura
C46.51	Kaposi's sarcoma of right lung ☑
C76.1	Malignant neoplasm of thorax
C78.01	Secondary malignant neoplasm of right lung ☑
C78.1	Secondary malignant neoplasm of mediastinum
C78.2	Secondary malignant neoplasm of pleura
C81.02	Nodular lymphocyte predominant Hodgkin lymphoma, intrathoracic lymph nodes
C81.12	Nodular sclerosis Hodgkin lymphoma, intrathoracic lymph nodes
C81.22	Mixed cellularity Hodgkin lymphoma, intrathoracic lymph nodes
C81.32	Lymphocyte depleted Hodgkin lymphoma, intrathoracic lymph nodes
C81.42	Lymphocyte-rich Hodgkin lymphoma, intrathoracic lymph nodes
C82.02	Follicular lymphoma grade I, intrathoracic lymph nodes
C82.12	Follicular lymphoma grade II, intrathoracic lymph nodes
C82.32	Follicular lymphoma grade IIIa, intrathoracic lymph nodes
C82.52	Diffuse follicle center lymphoma, intrathoracic lymph nodes
C82.62	Cutaneous follicle center lymphoma, intrathoracic lymph nodes
C83.02	Small cell B-cell lymphoma, intrathoracic lymph nodes
C83.12	Mantle cell lymphoma, intrathoracic lymph nodes
C83.32	Diffuse large B-cell lymphoma, intrathoracic lymph nodes
C83.52	Lymphoblastic (diffuse) lymphoma, intrathoracic lymph nodes
C83.72	Burkitt lymphoma, intrathoracic lymph nodes
C84.02	Mycosis fungoides, intrathoracic lymph nodes
C84.12	Sezary disease, intrathoracic lymph nodes
C85.22	Mediastinal (thymic) large B-cell lymphoma, intrathoracic lymph nodes
I01.0	Acute rheumatic pericarditis
I09.2	Chronic rheumatic pericarditis
I30.0	Acute nonspecific idiopathic pericarditis
I30.1	Infective pericarditis
I31.0	Chronic adhesive pericarditis
I31.1	Chronic constrictive pericarditis
I31.3	Pericardial effusion (noninflammatory)
J85.0	Gangrene and necrosis of lung
J85.1	Abscess of lung with pneumonia
J85.3	Abscess of mediastinum
J86.0	Pyothorax with fistula
J90	Pleural effusion, not elsewhere classified
J91.0	Malignant pleural effusion
J91.8	Pleural effusion in other conditions classified elsewhere
J93.0	Spontaneous tension pneumothorax
J93.11	Primary spontaneous pneumothorax
J93.12	Secondary spontaneous pneumothorax
J93.81	Chronic pneumothorax
J94.0	Chylous effusion
J94.1	Fibrothorax
J94.2	Hemothorax

M32.12	Pericarditis in systemic lupus erythematosus
M32.13	Lung involvement in systemic lupus erythematosus

AMA: 32601 2018,Jan,8; 2017,Jan,8; 2016,Jan,13; 2015,Jan,16; 2014,Jan,11; 2013,Aug,13

Relative Value Units/Medicare Edits

Non-Facility RVU	Work	PE	MP	Total
32601	5.5	2.17	1.23	8.9
Facility RVU	**Work**	**PE**	**MP**	**Total**
32601	5.5	2.17	1.23	8.9

	FUD	Status	MUE	Modifiers				IOM Reference
32601	0	A	1(3)	51	N/A	N/A	80*	None

* with documentation

Terms To Know

blunt dissection. Surgical technique used to expose an underlying area by separating along natural cleavage lines of tissue, without cutting.

cannula. Tube inserted into a blood vessel, duct, or body cavity to facilitate passage.

pleura. One of the two membranes that surround the lungs. The visceral pleura encases the lung and the parietal pleura lines the inner chest walls.

trocar. Cannula or a sharp pointed instrument used to puncture and aspirate fluid from cavities.

VATS. Video-assisted thoracic surgery. Less invasive technique than open thoracic surgery for various procedures on the heart and lungs. The surgeon typically gains access to the chest cavity using trocars (slender tube-like instruments), through which an endoscope and the surgical instruments are passed. The patient's internal organs can then be viewed intraoperatively on a monitor.

32604

32604 Thoracoscopy, diagnostic (separate procedure); pericardial sac, with biopsy

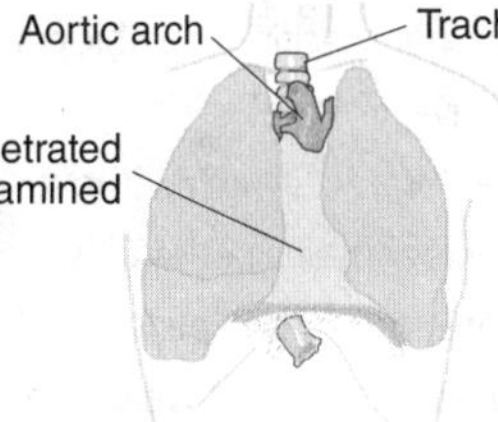

Video scope is delivered through trocar and the pericardial sac is visually examined

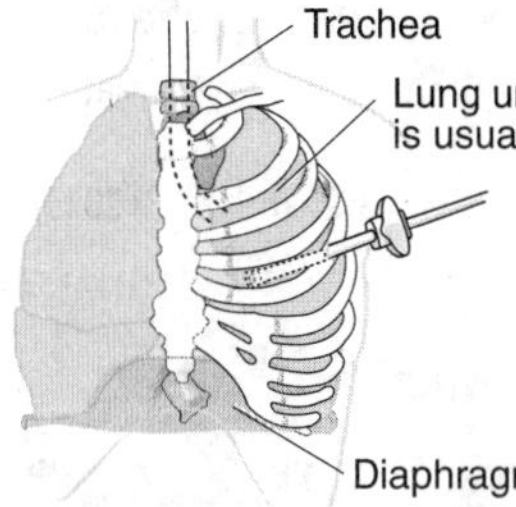

Explanation

The physician examines the pericardial sac using a rigid or flexible fiberoptic endoscope. The procedure can be done under local or general anesthesia. The physician makes a small incision between two ribs and by blunt dissection and the use of a trocar enters the thoracic cavity. The endoscope is passed through the trocar and into the chest cavity. The lung is usually partially collapsed by instilling air into the chest through the trocar or, if general anesthesia is used, the lung may be collapsed through a double lumen endotracheal tube inserted through the mouth into the trachea. The endoscope is advanced to and into the pericardial sac as the physician views the structures and the anatomy of the area through the scope. The contents of the pericardial sac are examined by direct visualization and/or the use of a video camera. Still photographs may be taken as part of the procedure. The pericardial tissue selected for biopsy is identified and the biopsy is taken using a device inserted through the endoscope. At the conclusion of the procedure, the endoscope and the trocar are withdrawn. A chest tube for drainage and re-expansion of the lung is usually inserted through the wound used for the thoracoscopy.

Coding Tips

This separate procedure by definition is usually a component of a more complex service and is not identified separately. When performed alone or with other unrelated procedures/services, it may be reported. If performed alone, list the code; if performed with other procedures/services, list the code and append modifier 59 or X{EPSU}. Report the appropriate endoscopy for each anatomic site examined. Surgical thoracoscopy (video-assisted thoracic surgery or VATS) always includes diagnostic thoracoscopy. For diagnostic thoracoscopy of the pericardial sac without biopsy, see 32601. To report pericardial biopsy, open, see 39010.

ICD-10-CM Diagnostic Codes

A18.84	Tuberculosis of heart
A39.53	Meningococcal pericarditis
A52.06	Other syphilitic heart involvement
A54.83	Gonococcal heart infection

A69.29	Other conditions associated with Lyme disease
B33.23	Viral pericarditis
C38.0	Malignant neoplasm of heart
C45.2	Mesothelioma of pericardium
I01.0	Acute rheumatic pericarditis
I09.2	Chronic rheumatic pericarditis
I30.0	Acute nonspecific idiopathic pericarditis
I30.1	Infective pericarditis
I30.8	Other forms of acute pericarditis
I31.0	Chronic adhesive pericarditis
I31.1	Chronic constrictive pericarditis
I31.2	Hemopericardium, not elsewhere classified
I31.3	Pericardial effusion (noninflammatory)
I31.8	Other specified diseases of pericardium
I32	Pericarditis in diseases classified elsewhere
M32.12	Pericarditis in systemic lupus erythematosus

AMA: 32604 2018,Jan,8; 2017,Jan,8; 2016,Jan,13; 2015,Jan,16; 2014,Jan,11; 2013,Aug,13

Relative Value Units/Medicare Edits

Non-Facility RVU	Work	PE	MP	Total
32604	8.77	3.09	2.09	13.95
Facility RVU	**Work**	**PE**	**MP**	**Total**
32604	8.77	3.09	2.09	13.95

	FUD	Status	MUE	Modifiers				IOM Reference
32604	0	A	1(3)	51	N/A	N/A	80*	None

* with documentation

Terms To Know

biopsy. Tissue or fluid removed for diagnostic purposes through analysis of the cells in the biopsy material.

diagnostic procedures. Procedure performed on a patient to obtain information to assess the medical condition of the patient or to identify a disease and to determine the nature and severity of an illness or injury.

pericarditis. Inflammation affecting the pericardium, the fibroserous membrane that surrounds the heart.

Lungs and Pleura

32606

32606 Thoracoscopy, diagnostic (separate procedure); mediastinal space, with biopsy

Video scope is delivered through trocar and the mediastinal space is visually examined

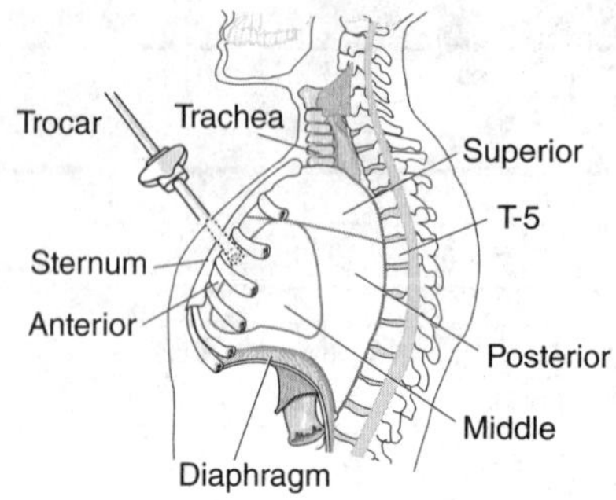

The mediastinal space is the general region between the left and right lungs

Explanation

The physician examines the inside of the mediastinal space through a rigid or flexible fiberoptic endoscope. The procedure can be done under local or general anesthesia. The physician makes a small incision between two ribs and by blunt dissection and the use of a trocar enters the thoracic cavity. The endoscope is passed through the trocar and into the chest cavity. The lung is usually partially collapsed by instilling air into the chest through the trocar or, if general anesthesia is used, the lung may be collapsed through a special double lumen endotracheal tube inserted through the mouth into the trachea. As the physician views the structures and the anatomy of the area through the endoscope, the endoscope is advanced into the mediastinum (area inside the center of the chest cavity between the lungs). The contents of the mediastinal space are examined by direct visualization and/or by the use of a video camera. Still photographs may be taken as part of the procedure. The tissue selected for biopsy is identified and a biopsy taken using a device inserted through the endoscope. At the conclusion of the procedure, the endoscope and the trocar are withdrawn. A chest tube for drainage and re-expansion of the lung is usually inserted through the wound used for the thoracoscopy.

Coding Tips

This separate procedure by definition is usually a component of a more complex service and is not identified separately. When performed alone or with other unrelated procedures/services, it may be reported. If performed alone, list the code; if performed with other procedures/services, list the code and append modifier 59 or an X{EPSU} modifier. Report the appropriate endoscopy for each anatomic site examined. Surgical thoracoscopy (video-assisted thoracic surgery or VATS) always includes diagnostic thoracoscopy. For diagnostic thoracoscopy in the mediastinal space, see 32601. For a biopsy of the lung or mediastinum by percutaneous needle, see 32405. For mediastinoscopy, with or without biopsy, see 39401.

ICD-10-CM Diagnostic Codes

C33	Malignant neoplasm of trachea
C34.01	Malignant neoplasm of right main bronchus ☑
C34.02	Malignant neoplasm of left main bronchus ☑
C38.0	Malignant neoplasm of heart
C38.1	Malignant neoplasm of anterior mediastinum
C38.2	Malignant neoplasm of posterior mediastinum

C38.8	Malignant neoplasm of overlapping sites of heart, mediastinum and pleura
C78.1	Secondary malignant neoplasm of mediastinum
C7A.090	Malignant carcinoid tumor of the bronchus and lung
C81.02	Nodular lymphocyte predominant Hodgkin lymphoma, intrathoracic lymph nodes
C81.12	Nodular sclerosis Hodgkin lymphoma, intrathoracic lymph nodes
C81.22	Mixed cellularity Hodgkin lymphoma, intrathoracic lymph nodes
C81.32	Lymphocyte depleted Hodgkin lymphoma, intrathoracic lymph nodes
C81.42	Lymphocyte-rich Hodgkin lymphoma, intrathoracic lymph nodes
C81.72	Other Hodgkin lymphoma, intrathoracic lymph nodes
C82.02	Follicular lymphoma grade I, intrathoracic lymph nodes
C82.12	Follicular lymphoma grade II, intrathoracic lymph nodes
C82.32	Follicular lymphoma grade IIIa, intrathoracic lymph nodes
C82.52	Diffuse follicle center lymphoma, intrathoracic lymph nodes
C82.62	Cutaneous follicle center lymphoma, intrathoracic lymph nodes
C82.82	Other types of follicular lymphoma, intrathoracic lymph nodes
C83.02	Small cell B-cell lymphoma, intrathoracic lymph nodes
C83.12	Mantle cell lymphoma, intrathoracic lymph nodes
C83.32	Diffuse large B-cell lymphoma, intrathoracic lymph nodes
C83.52	Lymphoblastic (diffuse) lymphoma, intrathoracic lymph nodes
C83.72	Burkitt lymphoma, intrathoracic lymph nodes
C84.02	Mycosis fungoides, intrathoracic lymph nodes
C84.12	Sezary disease, intrathoracic lymph nodes
C84.Z2	Other mature T/NK-cell lymphomas, intrathoracic lymph nodes
C85.22	Mediastinal (thymic) large B-cell lymphoma, intrathoracic lymph nodes
C85.82	Other specified types of non-Hodgkin lymphoma, intrathoracic lymph nodes
D14.31	Benign neoplasm of right bronchus and lung ☑
D14.32	Benign neoplasm of left bronchus and lung ☑
D15.0	Benign neoplasm of thymus
D15.2	Benign neoplasm of mediastinum
D38.3	Neoplasm of uncertain behavior of mediastinum
D38.4	Neoplasm of uncertain behavior of thymus
D3A.090	Benign carcinoid tumor of the bronchus and lung

AMA: 32606 2018,Jan,8; 2017,Jan,8; 2016,Jan,13; 2015,Jan,16; 2014,Jan,11; 2013,Aug,13

Relative Value Units/Medicare Edits

Non-Facility RVU	Work	PE	MP	Total
32606	8.39	3.05	1.91	13.35
Facility RVU	**Work**	**PE**	**MP**	**Total**
32606	8.39	3.05	1.91	13.35

	FUD	Status	MUE	Modifiers				IOM Reference
32606	0	A	1(3)	51	N/A	N/A	80*	None

* with documentation

32607

32607 Thoracoscopy; with diagnostic biopsy(ies) of lung infiltrate(s) (eg, wedge, incisional), unilateral

Video scope is delivered through trocar and the chest cavity is visually examined

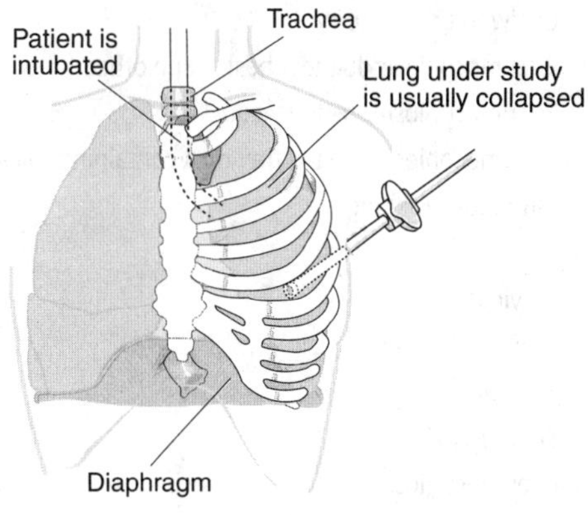

Lung infiltrates are biopsied

Explanation

The physician biopsies lung infiltrates through a rigid or flexible fiberoptic endoscope. This procedure can be done under local or general anesthesia. The surgeon makes a small incision between two ribs and by blunt dissection and the use of a trocar enters the thoracic cavity. The endoscope is passed through the trocar and into the chest cavity. One lung is usually partially collapsed by instilling air into the chest through the trocar or, if general anesthesia is used, the lung may be collapsed through a double lumen endotracheal tube inserted through the mouth into the trachea. The contents of the chest cavity are examined by direct visualization and/or the use of a video camera. Still photographs may be taken as part of the procedure. The lung infiltrates selected for biopsy are identified and the biopsy is taken using a device inserted through the endoscope. At the conclusion of the procedure, the endoscope and the trocar are removed. A chest tube for drainage and re-expansion of the lung is usually inserted through the wound used for the thoracoscopy.

Coding Tips

This is a unilateral procedure. If performed bilaterally, some payers require that the service be reported twice with modifier 50 appended to the second code while others require identification of the service only once with modifier 50 appended. Check with the individual payers. Modifier 50 identifies a procedure performed identically on the opposite side of the body (mirror image). This code should only be reported once per lung. Do not report 32607 with 32440, 32442, 32445, 32488, or 32671.

ICD-10-CM Diagnostic Codes

C34.11	Malignant neoplasm of upper lobe, right bronchus or lung ☑
C34.12	Malignant neoplasm of upper lobe, left bronchus or lung ☑
C34.2	Malignant neoplasm of middle lobe, bronchus or lung
C34.31	Malignant neoplasm of lower lobe, right bronchus or lung ☑
C34.32	Malignant neoplasm of lower lobe, left bronchus or lung ☑
C34.81	Malignant neoplasm of overlapping sites of right bronchus and lung ☑
C34.82	Malignant neoplasm of overlapping sites of left bronchus and lung ☑
C78.01	Secondary malignant neoplasm of right lung ☑

C78.02	Secondary malignant neoplasm of left lung ☑
D02.21	Carcinoma in situ of right bronchus and lung ☑
D02.22	Carcinoma in situ of left bronchus and lung ☑
D14.31	Benign neoplasm of right bronchus and lung ☑
D14.32	Benign neoplasm of left bronchus and lung ☑
D38.1	Neoplasm of uncertain behavior of trachea, bronchus and lung
D86.0	Sarcoidosis of lung
J60	Coalworker's pneumoconiosis
J61	Pneumoconiosis due to asbestos and other mineral fibers
J62.0	Pneumoconiosis due to talc dust
J62.8	Pneumoconiosis due to other dust containing silica
J63.0	Aluminosis (of lung)
J63.1	Bauxite fibrosis (of lung)
J63.2	Berylliosis
J63.3	Graphite fibrosis (of lung)
J63.4	Siderosis
J63.5	Stannosis
J63.6	Pneumoconiosis due to other specified inorganic dusts
J66.0	Byssinosis
J66.1	Flax-dressers' disease
J66.2	Cannabinosis
J66.8	Airway disease due to other specific organic dusts
J67.8	Hypersensitivity pneumonitis due to other organic dusts
J68.0	Bronchitis and pneumonitis due to chemicals, gases, fumes and vapors
J68.4	Chronic respiratory conditions due to chemicals, gases, fumes and vapors
J70.2	Acute drug-induced interstitial lung disorders
J82	Pulmonary eosinophilia, not elsewhere classified
J84.112	Idiopathic pulmonary fibrosis
J84.113	Idiopathic non-specific interstitial pneumonitis
J84.115	Respiratory bronchiolitis interstitial lung disease
J84.117	Desquamative interstitial pneumonia
J84.17	Other interstitial pulmonary diseases with fibrosis in diseases classified elsewhere
J84.2	Lymphoid interstitial pneumonia
J84.82	Adult pulmonary Langerhans cell histiocytosis
J84.848	Other interstitial lung diseases of childhood
J84.89	Other specified interstitial pulmonary diseases
M32.13	Lung involvement in systemic lupus erythematosus
M33.01	Juvenile dermatomyositis with respiratory involvement
M33.11	Other dermatomyositis with respiratory involvement
M33.21	Polymyositis with respiratory involvement
M35.02	Sicca syndrome with lung involvement

AMA: 32607 2018,Jan,8; 2017,Jan,8; 2016,Jan,13; 2015,Jan,16; 2014,Jan,11; 2013,Aug,13

Relative Value Units/Medicare Edits

Non-Facility RVU	Work	PE	MP	Total
32607	5.5	2.16	1.23	8.89
Facility RVU	**Work**	**PE**	**MP**	**Total**
32607	5.5	2.16	1.23	8.89

	FUD	Status	MUE	Modifiers				IOM Reference
32607	0	A	1(3)	51	N/A	N/A	80*	None

* with documentation

Terms To Know

hemoptysis. Coughing up or spitting out blood or blood-streaked sputum.

pleural effusion. Collection of lymph and other fluid within the pleural space.

pleurisy. Inflammation of the serous membrane that lines the lungs and the thoracic cavity. Pleurisy may cause effusion within the cavity or have exudate in the pleural space or on the membrane surface.

tuberculosis. Bacterial infection that typically spreads by inhalation of an airborne agent that usually attacks the lungs, but may also affect other organs.

32608

32608 Thoracoscopy; with diagnostic biopsy(ies) of lung nodule(s) or mass(es) (eg, wedge, incisional), unilateral

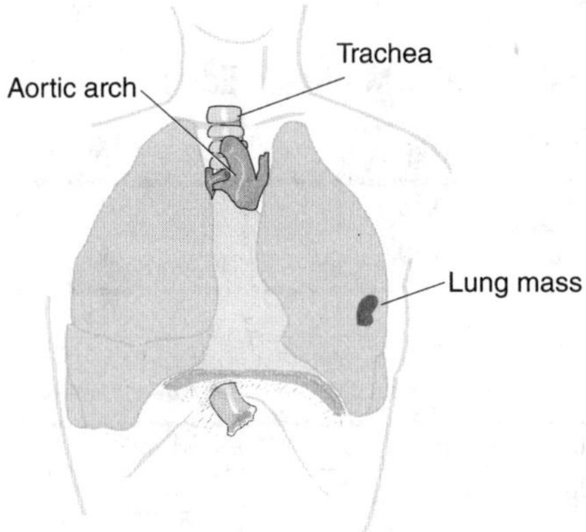

Video scope is delivered through trocar, and the pericardial sac is visually examined and nodules or masses are biopsied

Explanation

The physician biopsies a lung nodule or mass through a rigid or flexible fiberoptic endoscope. This procedure can be done under local or general anesthesia. The surgeon makes a small incision between two ribs and by blunt dissection and the use of a trocar enters the thoracic cavity. The endoscope is passed through the trocar and into the chest cavity. One lung is usually partially collapsed by instilling air into the chest through the trocar or, if general anesthesia is used, the lung may be collapsed through a double lumen endotracheal tube inserted through the mouth into the trachea. The contents of the chest cavity are examined by direct visualization and/or the use of a video camera. Still photographs may be taken as part of the procedure. The lung nodule(s) or mass(es) selected for biopsy is identified and the biopsy is taken using a device inserted through the endoscope. At the conclusion of the procedure, the endoscope and the trocar are removed. A chest tube for drainage and re-expansion of the lung is usually inserted through the wound used for the thoracoscopy.

Coding Tips

This is a unilateral procedure. If performed bilaterally, some payers require that the service be reported twice with modifier 50 appended to the second code while others require identification of the service only once with modifier 50 appended. Check with individual payers. Modifier 50 identifies a procedure performed identically on the opposite side of the body (mirror image). This code may only be reported once per lung. Do not report 32608 with 32440, 32442, 32445, 32488, or 32671.

ICD-10-CM Diagnostic Codes

B67.1	Echinococcus granulosus infection of lung
C34.11	Malignant neoplasm of upper lobe, right bronchus or lung ☑
C34.12	Malignant neoplasm of upper lobe, left bronchus or lung ☑
C34.2	Malignant neoplasm of middle lobe, bronchus or lung
C34.31	Malignant neoplasm of lower lobe, right bronchus or lung ☑
C34.32	Malignant neoplasm of lower lobe, left bronchus or lung ☑
C34.81	Malignant neoplasm of overlapping sites of right bronchus and lung ☑
C34.82	Malignant neoplasm of overlapping sites of left bronchus and lung ☑
C46.51	Kaposi's sarcoma of right lung ☑
C46.52	Kaposi's sarcoma of left lung ☑
C78.01	Secondary malignant neoplasm of right lung ☑
C78.02	Secondary malignant neoplasm of left lung ☑
D02.21	Carcinoma in situ of right bronchus and lung ☑
D02.22	Carcinoma in situ of left bronchus and lung ☑
D14.31	Benign neoplasm of right bronchus and lung ☑
D14.32	Benign neoplasm of left bronchus and lung ☑
D38.1	Neoplasm of uncertain behavior of trachea, bronchus and lung
D86.0	Sarcoidosis of lung
J85.0	Gangrene and necrosis of lung
R91.1	Solitary pulmonary nodule

AMA: 32608 2018,Jan,8; 2017,Jan,8; 2016,Jan,13; 2015,Jan,16; 2014,Jan,11; 2013,Aug,13

Relative Value Units/Medicare Edits

Non-Facility RVU	Work	PE	MP	Total
32608	6.84	2.54	1.53	10.91
Facility RVU	**Work**	**PE**	**MP**	**Total**
32608	6.84	2.54	1.53	10.91

	FUD	Status	MUE	Modifiers				IOM Reference
32608	0	A	1(3)	51	N/A	N/A	80*	None

* with documentation

Terms To Know

dissection. Separating by cutting tissue or body structures apart.

endoscopy. Visual inspection of the body using a fiberoptic scope.

general anesthesia. State of unconsciousness produced by an anesthetic agent or agents, inducing amnesia by blocking the awareness center in the brain, and rendering the patient unable to control protective reflexes, such as breathing.

32609

32609 Thoracoscopy; with biopsy(ies) of pleura

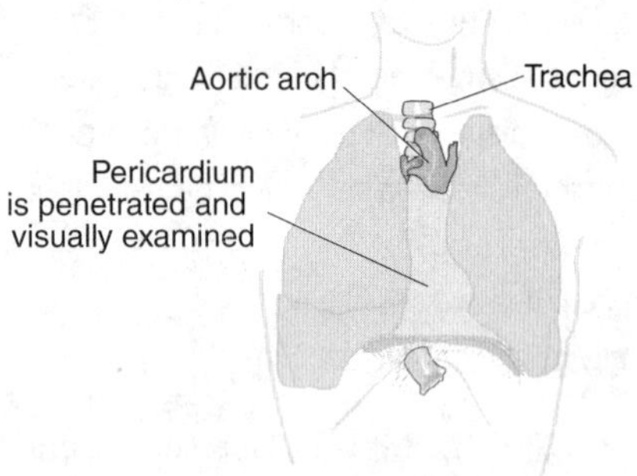

Video scope is delivered through trocar and the pericardial sac is visually examined in and biopsies obtained

Explanation

The physician biopsies the pleura through a rigid or flexible fiberoptic endoscope. This procedure can be done under local or general anesthesia. The surgeon makes a small incision between two ribs and by blunt dissection and the use of a trocar enters the thoracic cavity. The endoscope is passed through the trocar and into the chest cavity. One lung is usually partially collapsed by instilling air into the chest through the trocar or, if general anesthesia is used, the lung may be collapsed through a double lumen endotracheal tube inserted through the mouth into the trachea. The contents of the chest cavity are examined by direct visualization and/or the use of a video camera. Still photographs may be taken as part of the procedure. The area of the pleura selected for biopsy is identified and the biopsy is taken using a device inserted through the endoscope. At the conclusion of the procedure, the endoscope and the trocar are removed. A chest tube for drainage and re-expansion of the lung is usually inserted through the wound used for the thoracoscopy.

Coding Tips

Surgical thoracoscopy (video-assisted thoracic surgery or VATS) always includes diagnostic thoracoscopy.

ICD-10-CM Diagnostic Codes

A15.6	Tuberculous pleurisy
C38.4	Malignant neoplasm of pleura
C38.8	Malignant neoplasm of overlapping sites of heart, mediastinum and pleura
C45.0	Mesothelioma of pleura
C78.2	Secondary malignant neoplasm of pleura
D19.0	Benign neoplasm of mesothelial tissue of pleura
D38.2	Neoplasm of uncertain behavior of pleura
J86.0	Pyothorax with fistula
J86.9	Pyothorax without fistula
J90	Pleural effusion, not elsewhere classified
J91.0	Malignant pleural effusion
J91.8	Pleural effusion in other conditions classified elsewhere
J92.0	Pleural plaque with presence of asbestos
J92.9	Pleural plaque without asbestos
J94.0	Chylous effusion
J94.1	Fibrothorax
J94.2	Hemothorax
J94.8	Other specified pleural conditions
M32.13	Lung involvement in systemic lupus erythematosus
Q34.0	Anomaly of pleura

AMA: 32609 2018,Jan,8; 2017,Jan,8; 2016,Jan,13; 2015,Jan,16; 2014,Jan,11; 2013,Aug,13

Relative Value Units/Medicare Edits

Non-Facility RVU	Work	PE	MP	Total
32609	4.58	1.9	0.97	7.45
Facility RVU	**Work**	**PE**	**MP**	**Total**
32609	4.58	1.9	0.97	7.45

	FUD	Status	MUE	Modifiers				IOM Reference
32609	0	A	1(3)	51	N/A	N/A	80*	None

* with documentation

Terms To Know

dissection. Separating by cutting tissue or body structures apart.

hemoptysis. Coughing up or spitting out blood or blood-streaked sputum.

pleura. One of the two membranes that surround the lungs. The visceral pleura encases the lung and the parietal pleura lines the inner chest walls.

pleural effusion. Collection of lymph and other fluid within the pleural space.

pleurisy. Inflammation of the serous membrane that lines the lungs and the thoracic cavity. Pleurisy may cause effusion within the cavity or have exudate in the pleural space or on the membrane surface.

trachea. Tube descending from the larynx and branching into the right and left main bronchi.

trocar. Cannula or a sharp pointed instrument used to puncture and aspirate fluid from cavities.

32650

32650 Thoracoscopy, surgical; with pleurodesis (eg, mechanical or chemical)

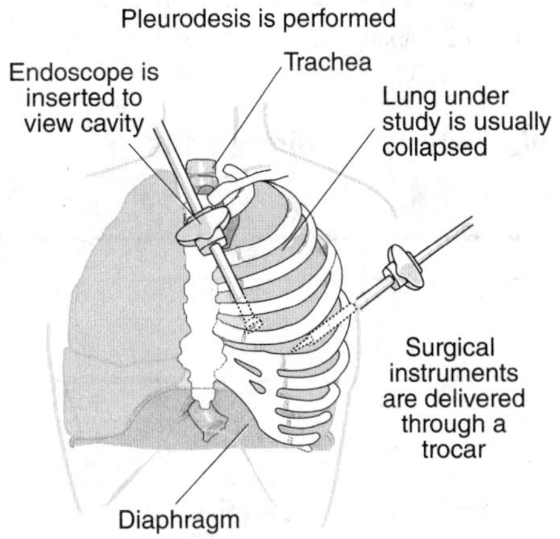

Explanation

The physician examines the inside of the chest cavity through a rigid or flexible fiberoptic endoscope and induces adhesion of the surface of the lung to the inside surface of the chest cavity. The procedure can be done under local or general anesthesia. The physician makes a small incision between two ribs and by blunt dissection and the use of a trocar enters the thoracic cavity. The endoscope is passed through the trocar and into the chest cavity. The lung is usually partially collapsed by instilling air into the chest through the trocar or, if general anesthesia is used, the lung may be collapsed through a double lumen endotracheal tube inserted through the mouth into the trachea. The contents of the chest cavity are examined by direct visualization and/or by the use of a video camera. Still photographs may be taken as part of the procedure. A second trocar and instruments may be inserted into the chest cavity through a second wound in the chest. Adhesion may be induced in one of two ways: by abrading the surfaces of the lung and the inside of the chest cavity or by the instillation of chemicals into the chest cavity that bath the surfaces of the lung and the inside of the chest cavity. Most commonly, a chemical solution is instilled into the chest through the endoscope or second puncture site. At the conclusion of the procedure, the endoscope and the trocar are removed. A chest tube for drainage and re-expansion of the lung is usually inserted through the wound used for the thoracoscopy.

Coding Tips

Surgical thoracoscopy always includes diagnostic thoracoscopy. For percutaneous chemical pleurodesis, see 32560. For pleural scarification for repeat pneumothorax, see 32215.

ICD-10-CM Diagnostic Codes

J86.0	Pyothorax with fistula
J86.9	Pyothorax without fistula
J90	Pleural effusion, not elsewhere classified
J91.0	Malignant pleural effusion
J91.8	Pleural effusion in other conditions classified elsewhere
J93.0	Spontaneous tension pneumothorax
J93.11	Primary spontaneous pneumothorax
J93.12	Secondary spontaneous pneumothorax
J93.81	Chronic pneumothorax
J93.82	Other air leak
J93.83	Other pneumothorax
J94.0	Chylous effusion
J94.8	Other specified pleural conditions
J95.811	Postprocedural pneumothorax
J95.812	Postprocedural air leak
L60.5	Yellow nail syndrome
M32.13	Lung involvement in systemic lupus erythematosus

AMA: 32650 2018,Jan,8; 2017,Jan,8; 2016,Jan,13; 2015,Jan,16; 2014,Jan,11; 2013,Aug,13

Relative Value Units/Medicare Edits

Non-Facility RVU	Work	PE	MP	Total
32650	10.83	5.92	2.44	19.19
Facility RVU	**Work**	**PE**	**MP**	**Total**
32650	10.83	5.92	2.44	19.19

	FUD	Status	MUE	Modifiers				IOM Reference
32650	90	A	1(2)	51	50	62*	80	None

* with documentation

Terms To Know

emphysematous bleb. Formation of blisters or vesicles greater than 1.0 mm within an emphysematous lung, containing serum or blood.

pleurodesis. Injection of a sclerosing agent into the pleural space for creating adhesions between the parietal and the visceral pleura to treat a collapsed lung caused by air trapped in the pleural cavity, or severe cases of pleural effusion.

32651-32652

32651 Thoracoscopy, surgical; with partial pulmonary decortication
32652 with total pulmonary decortication, including intrapleural pneumonolysis

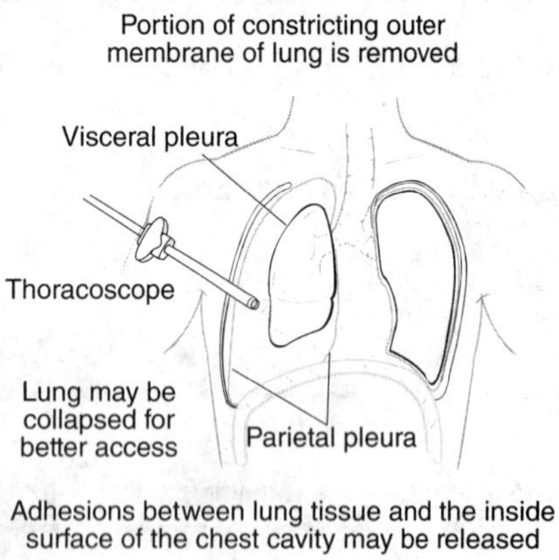

Explanation

The physician examines the inside of the chest cavity through a rigid or flexible fiberoptic endoscope and removes a portion of the tissue covering the surface of the lung. The procedure can be done under local or general anesthesia. The physician makes a small incision between two ribs and by blunt dissection and the use of a trocar enters the thoracic cavity. The endoscope is passed through the trocar and into the chest cavity. The lung is usually partially collapsed by instilling air into the chest through the trocar or, if general anesthesia is used, the lung may be collapsed through a double lumen endotracheal tube inserted through the mouth into the trachea. The contents of the chest cavity are examined by direct visualization and/or by the use of a video camera. Still photographs may be taken as part of the procedure. A second and/or third trocar and instruments may be inserted into the chest cavity through a second and/or third wound in the chest. Under direct visualization through the endoscope, the physician strips away the membranous tissues covering a portion of the lung (or all of the lung ins 32652) using instruments inserted into the chest through the secondary sites. Code 32652 includes intrapleural pneumonolysis in which the physician divides the tissues attaching the lung to the wall of the chest cavity. At the conclusion of the procedure, the endoscope and the trocar are removed. A chest tube for drainage and re-expansion of the lung is usually inserted through the wound used for the thoracoscopy.

Coding Tips

Surgical thoracoscopy always includes diagnostic thoracoscopy. For a major thoracotomy with open intrapleural pneumonolysis, see 32124. For total pulmonary decortication (separate procedure), see 32220; partial, see 32225. For decortication and parietal pleurectomy, see 32320.

ICD-10-CM Diagnostic Codes

A15.6	Tuberculous pleurisy
C38.4	Malignant neoplasm of pleura
C38.8	Malignant neoplasm of overlapping sites of heart, mediastinum and pleura
C45.0	Mesothelioma of pleura
C78.2	Secondary malignant neoplasm of pleura
D19.0	Benign neoplasm of mesothelial tissue of pleura
J86.0	Pyothorax with fistula
J86.9	Pyothorax without fistula
J92.0	Pleural plaque with presence of asbestos
J92.9	Pleural plaque without asbestos
J94.1	Fibrothorax

AMA: 32651 2018,Jan,8; 2017,Jan,8; 2016,Jan,13; 2015,Jan,16; 2014,Jan,11; 2013,Aug,13 **32652** 2018,Jan,8; 2017,Jan,8; 2016,Jan,13; 2015,Jan,16; 2014,Jan,11; 2013,Aug,13

Relative Value Units/Medicare Edits

Non-Facility RVU	Work	PE	MP	Total
32651	18.78	8.49	4.33	31.6
32652	29.13	12.12	6.72	47.97
Facility RVU	**Work**	**PE**	**MP**	**Total**
32651	18.78	8.49	4.33	31.6
32652	29.13	12.12	6.72	47.97

	FUD	Status	MUE	Modifiers				IOM Reference
32651	90	A	1(2)	51	50	62*	80	None
32652	90	A	1(2)	51	50	62*	80	

* with documentation

Terms To Know

decortication. Removal of the cortical substance, the encapsulating or encasing material, of an organ, such as the kidneys or lungs.

effusion. Escape of fluid from within a body cavity.

pneumothorax. Collapsed lung due to air or gas trapped in the pleural space formed by the membrane that encloses the lungs and lines the thoracic cavity.

32653

32653 Thoracoscopy, surgical; with removal of intrapleural foreign body or fibrin deposit

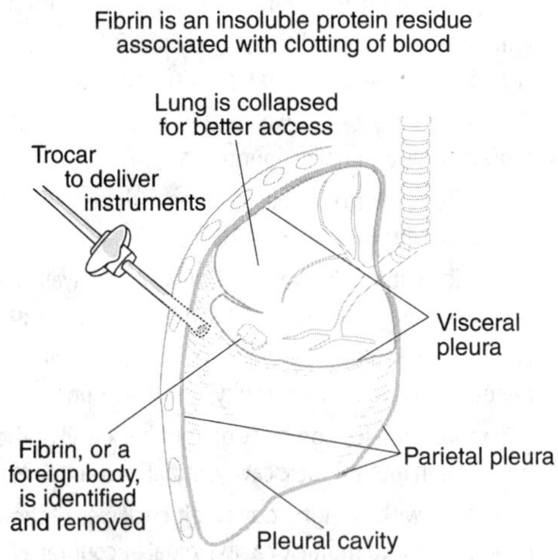

Surgical thoracoscopy is performed

Explanation

The physician examines the inside of the chest cavity through either a rigid or flexible fiberoptic endoscope and removes a foreign body or a fibrin deposit (the thick tissue much like remains of a blood clot). The procedure can be done under local or general anesthesia. The surgeon makes a small incision between two ribs and, by blunt dissection and the use of a trocar, enters the thoracic cavity. The endoscope is passed through the trocar and into the chest cavity. The lung is usually partially collapsed by instilling air into the chest through the trocar or, if general anesthesia is used, the lung may be collapsed through a special double lumen endotracheal tube inserted through the mouth into the trachea. The contents of the chest cavity are examined by direct visualization and/or by the use of a video camera. Still photographs may be taken as part of the procedure. A second and/or third trocar and instruments may be inserted into the chest cavity through a second and/or third wound in the chest. The foreign body or fibrin deposit is located and removed using instruments through the scope or the secondary sites. At the conclusion of the procedure, the endoscope and the trocar are removed. A chest tube for drainage and re-expansion of the lung is usually inserted through the wound used for the thoracoscopy.

Coding Tips

Surgical thoracoscopy always includes diagnostic thoracoscopy. For a thoracotomy with removal of an intrapleural foreign body or a fibrin deposit, see 32150.

ICD-10-CM Diagnostic Codes

J94.2 Hemothorax
S21.321A Laceration with foreign body of right front wall of thorax with penetration into thoracic cavity, initial encounter ☑
S21.322A Laceration with foreign body of left front wall of thorax with penetration into thoracic cavity, initial encounter ☑
S21.341A Puncture wound with foreign body of right front wall of thorax with penetration into thoracic cavity, initial encounter ☑
S21.342A Puncture wound with foreign body of left front wall of thorax with penetration into thoracic cavity, initial encounter ☑
S21.421A Laceration with foreign body of right back wall of thorax with penetration into thoracic cavity, initial encounter ☑
S21.422A Laceration with foreign body of left back wall of thorax with penetration into thoracic cavity, initial encounter ☑
S21.441A Puncture wound with foreign body of right back wall of thorax with penetration into thoracic cavity, initial encounter ☑
S21.442A Puncture wound with foreign body of left back wall of thorax with penetration into thoracic cavity, initial encounter ☑
S27.1XXA Traumatic hemothorax, initial encounter
S27.2XXA Traumatic hemopneumothorax, initial encounter
S27.311A Primary blast injury of lung, unilateral, initial encounter
S27.312A Primary blast injury of lung, bilateral, initial encounter ☑
S27.321A Contusion of lung, unilateral, initial encounter
S27.322A Contusion of lung, bilateral, initial encounter ☑
S27.331A Laceration of lung, unilateral, initial encounter
S27.332A Laceration of lung, bilateral, initial encounter ☑
S27.63XA Laceration of pleura, initial encounter
S27.893A Laceration of other specified intrathoracic organs, initial encounter
T81.510A Adhesions due to foreign body accidentally left in body following surgical operation, initial encounter
T81.518A Adhesions due to foreign body accidentally left in body following other procedure, initial encounter
T81.520A Obstruction due to foreign body accidentally left in body following surgical operation, initial encounter
T81.528A Obstruction due to foreign body accidentally left in body following other procedure, initial encounter
T81.530A Perforation due to foreign body accidentally left in body following surgical operation, initial encounter
T81.538A Perforation due to foreign body accidentally left in body following other procedure, initial encounter
T81.590A Other complications of foreign body accidentally left in body following surgical operation, initial encounter
T81.598A Other complications of foreign body accidentally left in body following other procedure, initial encounter

AMA: 32653 2018,Jan,8; 2017,Jan,8; 2016,Jan,13; 2015,Jan,16; 2014,Jan,11; 2013,Aug,13

Relative Value Units/Medicare Edits

Non-Facility RVU	Work	PE	MP	Total
32653	18.17	8.29	4.15	30.61
Facility RVU	**Work**	**PE**	**MP**	**Total**
32653	18.17	8.29	4.15	30.61

	FUD	Status	MUE	Modifiers				IOM Reference
32653	90	A	1(3)	51	N/A	62*	80	None

* with documentation

32654

32654 Thoracoscopy, surgical; with control of traumatic hemorrhage.

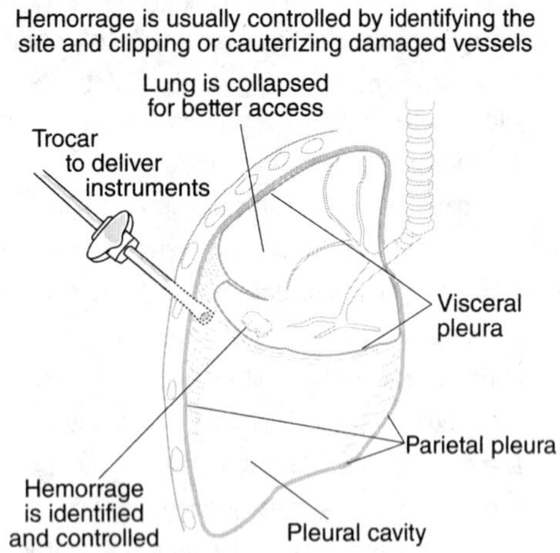

Surgical thoracoscopy is performed

Explanation

The physician examines the inside of the chest cavity through either a rigid or flexible fiberoptic endoscope and controls bleeding from a wound to the chest. The procedure can be done under local or general anesthesia. The physician makes a small incision between two ribs and, by blunt dissection and the use of a trocar, enters the thoracic cavity. The endoscope is passed through the trocar and into the chest cavity. The lung is usually partially collapsed by instilling air into the chest through the trocar or, if general anesthesia is used, the lung may be collapsed through a special double lumen endotracheal tube inserted through the mouth into the trachea. The contents of the chest cavity are examined by direct visualization and/or by the use of a video camera. Still photographs may be taken as part of the procedure. A second and/or third trocar and instruments may be inserted into the chest cavity through a second and/or third wound in the chest. Under direct visualization through the endoscope, the physician manipulates the instruments inserted through the secondary sites and localizes the site of the bleeding. The hemorrhage is controlled by clipping or cauterizing the damaged blood vessel. At the conclusion of the procedure, the endoscope and the trocar(s) are removed. A chest tube for drainage and re-expansion of the lung is usually inserted through the wound used for the thoracoscopy.

Coding Tips

Surgical thoracoscopy always includes diagnostic thoracoscopy. Code 32654 should not be billed with thoracoscopic intervention codes. It is intended to be used only when bleeding occurs spontaneously or as the result of trauma, not when it results from another surgical intervention. For a major thoracotomy with control of a traumatic hemorrhage and/or repair of a lung tear, see 32110.

ICD-10-CM Diagnostic Codes

S21.311A Laceration without foreign body of right front wall of thorax with penetration into thoracic cavity, initial encounter ☑

S21.312A Laceration without foreign body of left front wall of thorax with penetration into thoracic cavity, initial encounter ☑

S21.321A Laceration with foreign body of right front wall of thorax with penetration into thoracic cavity, initial encounter ☑

S21.322A Laceration with foreign body of left front wall of thorax with penetration into thoracic cavity, initial encounter ☑

S21.331A Puncture wound without foreign body of right front wall of thorax with penetration into thoracic cavity, initial encounter ☑

S21.332A Puncture wound without foreign body of left front wall of thorax with penetration into thoracic cavity, initial encounter ☑

S21.341A Puncture wound with foreign body of right front wall of thorax with penetration into thoracic cavity, initial encounter ☑

S21.342A Puncture wound with foreign body of left front wall of thorax with penetration into thoracic cavity, initial encounter ☑

S21.351A Open bite of right front wall of thorax with penetration into thoracic cavity, initial encounter ☑

S21.352A Open bite of left front wall of thorax with penetration into thoracic cavity, initial encounter ☑

S21.411A Laceration without foreign body of right back wall of thorax with penetration into thoracic cavity, initial encounter ☑

S21.412A Laceration without foreign body of left back wall of thorax with penetration into thoracic cavity, initial encounter ☑

S21.421A Laceration with foreign body of right back wall of thorax with penetration into thoracic cavity, initial encounter ☑

S21.422A Laceration with foreign body of left back wall of thorax with penetration into thoracic cavity, initial encounter ☑

S21.431A Puncture wound without foreign body of right back wall of thorax with penetration into thoracic cavity, initial encounter ☑

S21.432A Puncture wound without foreign body of left back wall of thorax with penetration into thoracic cavity, initial encounter ☑

S21.441A Puncture wound with foreign body of right back wall of thorax with penetration into thoracic cavity, initial encounter ☑

S21.442A Puncture wound with foreign body of left back wall of thorax with penetration into thoracic cavity, initial encounter ☑

S21.451A Open bite of right back wall of thorax with penetration into thoracic cavity, initial encounter ☑

S21.452A Open bite of left back wall of thorax with penetration into thoracic cavity, initial encounter ☑

S25.491A Other specified injury of right pulmonary blood vessels, initial encounter ☑

S25.492A Other specified injury of left pulmonary blood vessels, initial encounter ☑

S25.811A Laceration of other blood vessels of thorax, right side, initial encounter ☑

S25.812A Laceration of other blood vessels of thorax, left side, initial encounter ☑

S25.891A Other specified injury of other blood vessels of thorax, right side, initial encounter ☑

S25.892A Other specified injury of other blood vessels of thorax, left side, initial encounter ☑

S27.0XXA Traumatic pneumothorax, initial encounter

S27.1XXA Traumatic hemothorax, initial encounter

S27.2XXA Traumatic hemopneumothorax, initial encounter

S27.311A Primary blast injury of lung, unilateral, initial encounter

S27.312A Primary blast injury of lung, bilateral, initial encounter ☑

S27.321A Contusion of lung, unilateral, initial encounter

S27.322A Contusion of lung, bilateral, initial encounter ☑

S27.331A Laceration of lung, unilateral, initial encounter

S27.332A Laceration of lung, bilateral, initial encounter ☑

S27.391A Other injuries of lung, unilateral, initial encounter

S27.392A Other injuries of lung, bilateral, initial encounter ☑

S28.0XXA Crushed chest, initial encounter

AMA: 32654 2018,Jan,8; 2017,Jan,8; 2016,Jan,13; 2015,Jan,16; 2014,Jan,11; 2013,Aug,13

Relative Value Units/Medicare Edits

Non-Facility RVU	Work	PE	MP	Total
32654	20.52	8.71	4.06	33.29
Facility RVU	**Work**	**PE**	**MP**	**Total**
32654	20.52	8.71	4.06	33.29

	FUD	Status	MUE	Modifiers				IOM Reference
32654	90	A	1(3)	51	50	62*	80	None

* with documentation

Terms To Know

cauterize. Heat or chemicals used to burn or cut.

dissection. Separating by cutting tissue or body structures apart.

hemoptysis. Coughing up or spitting out blood or blood-streaked sputum.

hemorrhage. Internal or external bleeding with loss of significant amounts of blood.

trocar. Cannula or a sharp pointed instrument used to puncture and aspirate fluid from cavities.

32655-32656

32655 Thoracoscopy, surgical; with resection-plication of bullae, includes any pleural procedure when performed

32656 with parietal pleurectomy

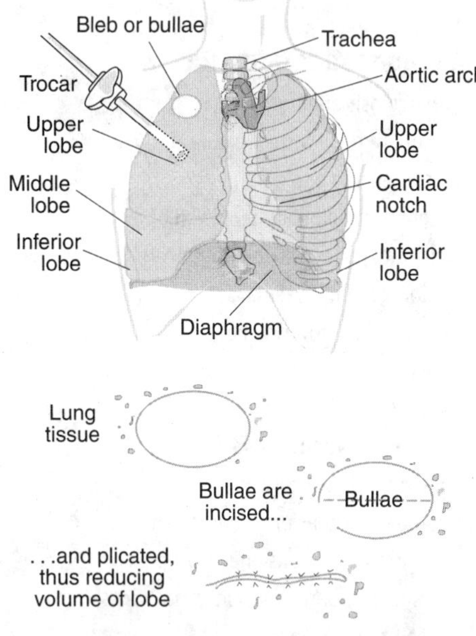

Emphysematous lungs may develop open areas of damaged tissue called blebs or bullaes

Explanation

The physician examines the inside of the chest cavity through a rigid or flexible fiberoptic endoscope and removes one or more lung bullae (large nonfunctional air sacs) in 32655 and removes the inside lining of the chest cavity (the parietal pleura) in 32656. The physician makes a small incision between two ribs and by blunt dissection and the use of a trocar enters the thoracic cavity. The endoscope is passed through the trocar and into the chest cavity. The lung is usually partially collapsed by instilling air into the chest through the trocar or the lung may be collapsed through a double lumen endotracheal tube inserted through the mouth into the trachea. The contents of the chest cavity are examined by direct visualization and/or by the use of a video camera. Still photographs may be taken as part of the procedure. A second and/or third trocar and instruments may be inserted into the chest cavity through a second and/or third wound in the chest. Under direct visualization through the endoscope, the physician manipulates the instruments inserted through the secondary sites and localizes the items to be removed. In 32655, the bulla(e) is removed by sharp and blunt dissection of the tissues, which often requires folding and suturing of the tissues (plication). In order to perform the procedure, the pleural surface may require an operative procedure such as pneumonolysis (separation of the surface of the lung that has become adherent to the inside surface of the chest cavity). In 32656, the physician manipulates the instruments inserted through the secondary sites and strips away the parietal pleura from the inside surface of the chest. At the conclusion of the procedure, the endoscope and the trocar(s) are removed. A chest tube for drainage and re-expansion of the lung is usually inserted through the wound used for the thoracoscopy.

Coding Tips

When a diagnostic wedge resection is performed and followed by a more complex procedure on the same anatomic location, report add-on codes 32507 or 32668 with the more complex procedure. When a therapeutic wedge resection is performed on a different lobe than a more complex lung resection, append modifier 59 or an X{EPSU} modifier. Surgical thoracoscopy always includes diagnostic thoracoscopy. For thoracoscopic lung volume reduction, see 32672. For thoracoscopic wedge resection, see 32666, 32667, or 32668. For a major thoracotomy with excision-plication of bullae, with or without any pleural procedure, see 32141. For open parietal pleurectomy (separate procedure), see 32310. For open decortication and parietal pleurectomy, see 32320.

ICD-10-CM Diagnostic Codes

A15.0	Tuberculosis of lung
C38.4	Malignant neoplasm of pleura
C45.0	Mesothelioma of pleura
C78.2	Secondary malignant neoplasm of pleura
J43.0	Unilateral pulmonary emphysema [MacLeod's syndrome]
J43.1	Panlobular emphysema
J43.2	Centrilobular emphysema
J43.8	Other emphysema
J86.0	Pyothorax with fistula
J86.9	Pyothorax without fistula
J91.0	Malignant pleural effusion
J93.0	Spontaneous tension pneumothorax
J93.11	Primary spontaneous pneumothorax
J93.12	Secondary spontaneous pneumothorax
J93.81	Chronic pneumothorax
J94.1	Fibrothorax
J94.2	Hemothorax
J95.811	Postprocedural pneumothorax
J95.812	Postprocedural air leak
P25.1	Pneumothorax originating in the perinatal period
S27.0XXA	Traumatic pneumothorax, initial encounter
S27.2XXA	Traumatic hemopneumothorax, initial encounter

AMA: 32655 2018,Jan,8; 2017,Jan,8; 2016,Jan,13; 2015,Jan,16; 2014,Jan,11; 2013,Aug,13 **32656** 2018,Jan,8; 2017,Jan,8; 2016,Jan,13; 2015,Jan,16; 2014,Jan,11; 2013,Aug,13

Relative Value Units/Medicare Edits

Non-Facility RVU	Work	PE	MP	Total
32655	16.17	7.67	3.73	27.57
32656	13.26	6.78	3.05	23.09
Facility RVU	**Work**	**PE**	**MP**	**Total**
32655	16.17	7.67	3.73	27.57
32656	13.26	6.78	3.05	23.09

	FUD	Status	MUE	Modifiers				IOM Reference
32655	90	A	1(3)	51	50	62*	80	None
32656	90	A	1(2)	51	50	62*	80	

* with documentation

32658

32658 Thoracoscopy, surgical; with removal of clot or foreign body from pericardial sac

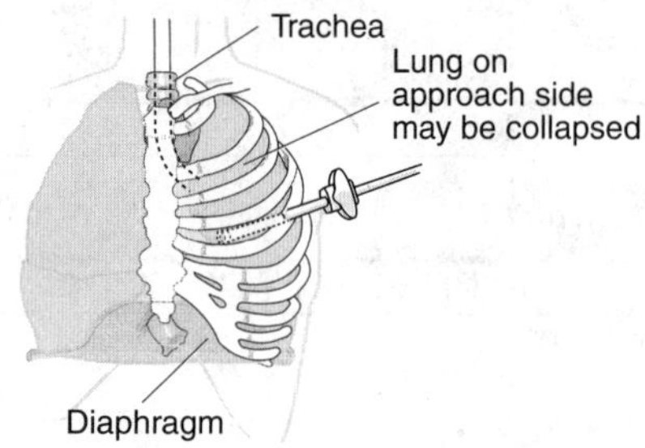

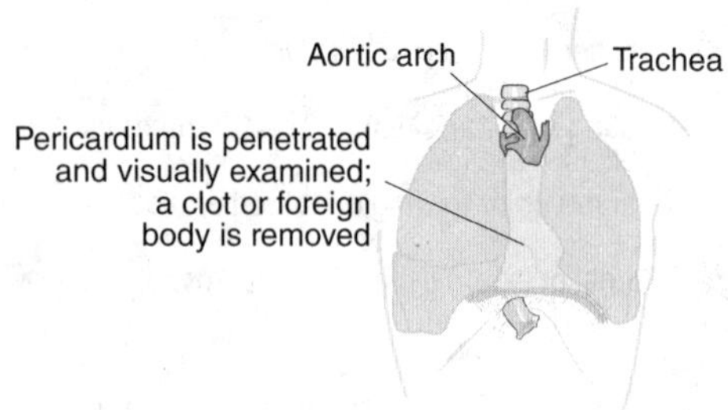

Explanation

The physician examines the inside of the pericardial sac through either a rigid or flexible fiberoptic endoscope and removes a blood clot or foreign body. The procedure can be done under local or general anesthesia. The physician makes a small incision between two ribs and, by blunt dissection and the use of a trocar, enters the thoracic cavity. The endoscope is passed through the trocar and into the chest cavity. The lung is usually partially collapsed by instilling air into the chest through the trocar or, if general anesthesia is used, the lung may be collapsed through a special double lumen endotracheal tube inserted through the mouth into the trachea. The endoscope is advanced to and into the pericardial sac as the physician views the structures and the anatomy of the area through the scope. The contents of the pericardial sac are examined by direct visualization and/or by the use of a video camera. Still photographs may be taken as part of the procedure. The clot and/or foreign body is identified and removed using a device through the endoscope or using a second instrument introduced into the area through a second insertion site in the chest. At the conclusion of the procedure, the endoscope and the trocar are withdrawn. A chest tube for drainage and re-expansion of the lung is usually inserted through the wound used for the thoracoscopy.

Coding Tips

Surgical thoracoscopy always includes diagnostic thoracoscopy. For an open pericardiotomy for the removal of a clot or foreign body (primary procedure), see 33020.

ICD-10-CM Diagnostic Codes

I23.0	Hemopericardium as current complication following acute myocardial infarction
I31.2	Hemopericardium, not elsewhere classified
I31.4	Cardiac tamponade
S26.01XA	Contusion of heart with hemopericardium, initial encounter
S26.020A	Mild laceration of heart with hemopericardium, initial encounter
S26.021A	Moderate laceration of heart with hemopericardium, initial encounter

● New ▲ Revised + Add On AMA: CPT Assist [Resequenced] ☑ Laterality

S26.022A Major laceration of heart with hemopericardium, initial encounter

S26.09XA Other injury of heart with hemopericardium, initial encounter

AMA: 32658 2018,Jan,8; 2017,Jan,8; 2016,Jan,13; 2015,Jan,16; 2014,Jan,11; 2013,Aug,13

Relative Value Units/Medicare Edits

Non-Facility RVU	Work	PE	MP	Total
32658	11.71	6.13	2.79	20.63
Facility RVU	**Work**	**PE**	**MP**	**Total**
32658	11.71	6.13	2.79	20.63

	FUD	Status	MUE	Modifiers				IOM Reference
32658	90	A	1(3)	51	N/A	62*	80	None

* with documentation

Terms To Know

contusion. Superficial injury (bruising) produced by impact without a break in the skin.

dissection. Separating by cutting tissue or body structures apart.

foreign body. Any object or substance found in an organ and tissue that does not belong under normal circumstances.

infection. Presence of microorganisms in body tissues that may result in cellular damage.

trocar. Cannula or a sharp pointed instrument used to puncture and aspirate fluid from cavities.

32659-32661

32659 Thoracoscopy, surgical; with creation of pericardial window or partial resection of pericardial sac for drainage

32661 with excision of pericardial cyst, tumor, or mass

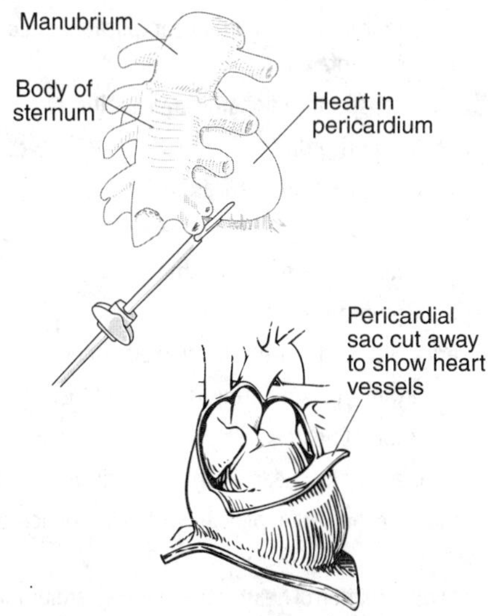

The pericardial sac is accessed through the use of a variety of endoscopic techniques

Explanation

The physician operates on the pericardial sac (the sac surrounding the heart) through a rigid or flexible fiberoptic endoscope and creates a hole in the pericardial sac for drainage. The procedure can be done under local or general anesthesia. The physician makes a small incision between two ribs and by blunt dissection and the use of a trocar enters the thoracic cavity. The endoscope is passed through the trocar and into the chest cavity. The lung is usually partially collapsed by instilling air into the chest through the trocar or, if general anesthesia is used, the lung may be collapsed through a double lumen endotracheal tube inserted through the mouth into the trachea. The endoscope is advanced to and into the pericardial sac as the physician views the structures and the anatomy of the area through the scope. The contents of the pericardial sac are examined by direct visualization and/or by the use of a video camera. Still photographs may be taken as part of the procedure. Using an instrument introduced through the endoscope or through a second wound in the chest, the physician creates an opening in the pericardial sac to allow constant drainage from the sac. The drainage opening is made by the creation of a window (a flap) in the pericardium or by resecting (cutting away) a portion of the pericardium. At the conclusion of the procedure, the endoscope and the trocar are withdrawn. A chest tube for drainage and re-expansion of the lung is usually inserted through the wound used for the thoracoscopy. In 32661, a cyst, tumor, or mass lesion inside the pericardial sac is also excised.

Coding Tips

Surgical thoracoscopy always includes diagnostic thoracoscopy. For an open creation of a pericardial window or partial resection for drainage, see 33025. For open pericardiectomy, see 33030–33031. For open excision of a pericardial cyst or tumor, see 33050.

ICD-10-CM Diagnostic Codes

A18.84 Tuberculosis of heart

A39.53 Meningococcal pericarditis

A52.06 Other syphilitic heart involvement

A54.83 Gonococcal heart infection

A69.29	Other conditions associated with Lyme disease
B33.23	Viral pericarditis
C38.0	Malignant neoplasm of heart
C45.2	Mesothelioma of pericardium
I01.0	Acute rheumatic pericarditis
I09.2	Chronic rheumatic pericarditis
I23.0	Hemopericardium as current complication following acute myocardial infarction
I30.0	Acute nonspecific idiopathic pericarditis
I30.1	Infective pericarditis
I30.8	Other forms of acute pericarditis
I31.2	Hemopericardium, not elsewhere classified
I31.3	Pericardial effusion (noninflammatory)
I31.4	Cardiac tamponade
I32	Pericarditis in diseases classified elsewhere
M32.12	Pericarditis in systemic lupus erythematosus
S26.01XA	Contusion of heart with hemopericardium, initial encounter
S26.020A	Mild laceration of heart with hemopericardium, initial encounter
S26.021A	Moderate laceration of heart with hemopericardium, initial encounter
S26.022A	Major laceration of heart with hemopericardium, initial encounter
S26.09XA	Other injury of heart with hemopericardium, initial encounter

AMA: 32659 2018,Jan,8; 2017,Jan,8; 2016,Jan,13; 2015,Jan,16; 2014,Jan,11; 2013,Aug,13 **32661** 2018,Jan,8; 2017,Jan,8; 2016,Jan,13; 2015,Jan,16; 2014,Jan,11; 2013,Aug,13

Relative Value Units/Medicare Edits

Non-Facility RVU	Work	PE	MP	Total
32659	11.94	6.4	2.76	21.1
32661	13.33	6.57	3.16	23.06
Facility RVU	**Work**	**PE**	**MP**	**Total**
32659	11.94	6.4	2.76	21.1
32661	13.33	6.57	3.16	23.06

	FUD	Status	MUE	Modifiers				IOM Reference
32659	90	A	1(2)	51	N/A	62*	80	None
32661	90	A	1(3)	51	N/A	62*	80	

* with documentation

32662

32662 Thoracoscopy, surgical; with excision of mediastinal cyst, tumor, or mass

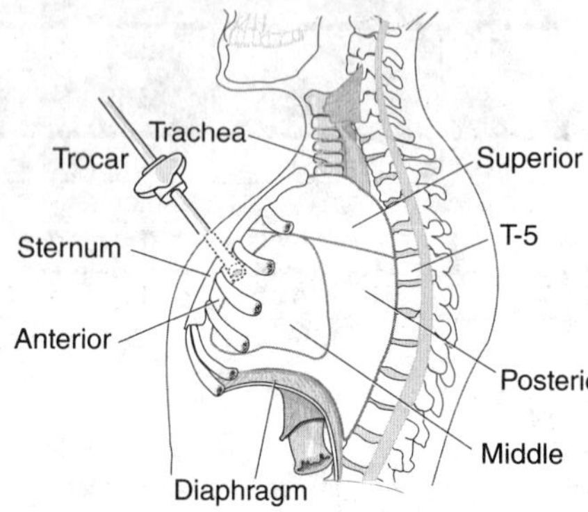

Explanation

The physician removes a cyst, tumor, or mass from the mediastinum through either a rigid or flexible fiberoptic endoscope. The procedure can be done under local or general anesthesia. The physician makes a small incision between two ribs and by blunt dissection and the use of a trocar enters the thoracic cavity. The endoscope is passed through the trocar and into the chest cavity. The lung is usually partially collapsed by instilling air into the chest through the trocar or, if general anesthesia is used, the lung may be collapsed through a special double lumen endotracheal tube inserted through the mouth into the trachea. As the physician views the structures and the anatomy of the area through the endoscope, the endoscope is advanced to and into the mediastinum (area inside the center of the chest cavity between the lungs). The contents of the mediastinal space are examined by direct visualization and/or by the use of a video camera. Still photographs may be taken as part of the procedure. The cyst, tumor, or mass is identified and removed using instruments guided through the endoscope or by using instruments introduced into the area through a second and/or third insertion site in the chest. At the conclusion of the procedure, the endoscope and the trocar are withdrawn. A chest tube for drainage and re-expansion of the lung is usually inserted through the wound used for the thoracoscopy.

Coding Tips

Surgical thoracoscopy always includes diagnostic thoracoscopy. For open excision of a mediastinal cyst, see 39200. For open excision of a mediastinal tumor, see 39220.

ICD-10-CM Diagnostic Codes

C33	Malignant neoplasm of trachea
C34.01	Malignant neoplasm of right main bronchus ☑
C34.02	Malignant neoplasm of left main bronchus ☑
C38.0	Malignant neoplasm of heart
C38.1	Malignant neoplasm of anterior mediastinum
C38.2	Malignant neoplasm of posterior mediastinum
C38.8	Malignant neoplasm of overlapping sites of heart, mediastinum and pleura
C78.1	Secondary malignant neoplasm of mediastinum
C7A.090	Malignant carcinoid tumor of the bronchus and lung

C81.02	Nodular lymphocyte predominant Hodgkin lymphoma, intrathoracic lymph nodes
C81.12	Nodular sclerosis Hodgkin lymphoma, intrathoracic lymph nodes
C81.22	Mixed cellularity Hodgkin lymphoma, intrathoracic lymph nodes
C81.32	Lymphocyte depleted Hodgkin lymphoma, intrathoracic lymph nodes
C81.42	Lymphocyte-rich Hodgkin lymphoma, intrathoracic lymph nodes
C81.72	Other Hodgkin lymphoma, intrathoracic lymph nodes
C82.02	Follicular lymphoma grade I, intrathoracic lymph nodes
C82.12	Follicular lymphoma grade II, intrathoracic lymph nodes
C82.32	Follicular lymphoma grade IIIa, intrathoracic lymph nodes
C82.52	Diffuse follicle center lymphoma, intrathoracic lymph nodes
C82.62	Cutaneous follicle center lymphoma, intrathoracic lymph nodes
C82.82	Other types of follicular lymphoma, intrathoracic lymph nodes
C83.02	Small cell B-cell lymphoma, intrathoracic lymph nodes
C83.12	Mantle cell lymphoma, intrathoracic lymph nodes
C83.32	Diffuse large B-cell lymphoma, intrathoracic lymph nodes
C83.52	Lymphoblastic (diffuse) lymphoma, intrathoracic lymph nodes
C83.72	Burkitt lymphoma, intrathoracic lymph nodes
C84.02	Mycosis fungoides, intrathoracic lymph nodes
C84.12	Sezary disease, intrathoracic lymph nodes
C84.Z2	Other mature T/NK-cell lymphomas, intrathoracic lymph nodes
C85.22	Mediastinal (thymic) large B-cell lymphoma, intrathoracic lymph nodes
C85.82	Other specified types of non-Hodgkin lymphoma, intrathoracic lymph nodes
D14.31	Benign neoplasm of right bronchus and lung ☑
D14.32	Benign neoplasm of left bronchus and lung ☑
D15.0	Benign neoplasm of thymus
D15.2	Benign neoplasm of mediastinum
D38.3	Neoplasm of uncertain behavior of mediastinum
D38.4	Neoplasm of uncertain behavior of thymus
D3A.090	Benign carcinoid tumor of the bronchus and lung

AMA: 32662 2018,Jan,8; 2017,Jan,8; 2016,Jan,13; 2015,Jan,16; 2014,Jan,11; 2013,Aug,13

Relative Value Units/Medicare Edits

Non-Facility RVU	Work	PE	MP	Total
32662	14.99	7.3	3.46	25.75
Facility RVU	**Work**	**PE**	**MP**	**Total**
32662	14.99	7.3	3.46	25.75

	FUD	Status	MUE	Modifiers				IOM Reference
32662	90	A	1(3)	51	N/A	62*	80	None

* with documentation

32663

32663 Thoracoscopy, surgical; with lobectomy (single lobe)

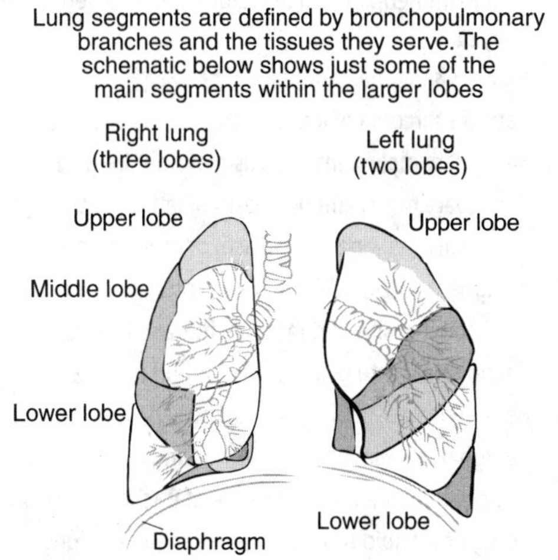

The major lobes of the lung differ from right to left. The right lung has three lobes and the left two, due to the space given over to the heart and pericardium

Explanation

The physician removes an entire lobe of one lung through a rigid or flexible fiberoptic endoscope. The physician makes a small incision between two ribs and by blunt dissection and the use of a trocar enters the thoracic cavity. The endoscope is passed through the trocar and into the chest cavity. The lung is usually partially collapsed by instilling air into the chest through the trocar or the lung may be collapsed through a double lumen endotracheal tube inserted through the mouth into the trachea. The contents of the chest cavity are examined by direct visualization and/or by the use of a video camera. Still photographs may be taken as part of the procedure. Additional instruments may be inserted into the chest cavity through a second and/or third wound in the chest. Under direct visualization through the endoscope, the physician manipulates the instruments inserted through the secondary sites and clamps the blood vessels and bronchial tubes going to the lobe of the lung to be removed. With the clamps in place, the lobe is removed by dividing the vessel and bronchial tubes isolated by the clamps. Any cut portions of the remaining lung tissue are repaired by suturing or clipping with surgical clips. At the conclusion of the procedure, the endoscope and the trocar(s) are removed. A chest tube for drainage and re-expansion of the lung is usually inserted through the wound used for the thoracoscopy.

Coding Tips

Surgical thoracoscopy always includes diagnostic thoracoscopy. For a thorascopic segmentectomy, see 32669. For open lung resections, see 32480-32488.

ICD-10-CM Diagnostic Codes

A15.0	Tuberculosis of lung
B44.0	Invasive pulmonary aspergillosis
B44.1	Other pulmonary aspergillosis
C34.01	Malignant neoplasm of right main bronchus ☑
C34.02	Malignant neoplasm of left main bronchus ☑
C34.11	Malignant neoplasm of upper lobe, right bronchus or lung ☑
C34.12	Malignant neoplasm of upper lobe, left bronchus or lung ☑
C34.2	Malignant neoplasm of middle lobe, bronchus or lung

C34.31	Malignant neoplasm of lower lobe, right bronchus or lung ☑
C34.32	Malignant neoplasm of lower lobe, left bronchus or lung ☑
C34.81	Malignant neoplasm of overlapping sites of right bronchus and lung ☑
C34.82	Malignant neoplasm of overlapping sites of left bronchus and lung ☑
C46.51	Kaposi's sarcoma of right lung ☑
C46.52	Kaposi's sarcoma of left lung ☑
C78.01	Secondary malignant neoplasm of right lung ☑
C78.02	Secondary malignant neoplasm of left lung ☑
C79.89	Secondary malignant neoplasm of other specified sites
C7A.090	Malignant carcinoid tumor of the bronchus and lung
D02.21	Carcinoma in situ of right bronchus and lung ☑
D02.22	Carcinoma in situ of left bronchus and lung ☑
D14.31	Benign neoplasm of right bronchus and lung ☑
D14.32	Benign neoplasm of left bronchus and lung ☑
D38.1	Neoplasm of uncertain behavior of trachea, bronchus and lung
D3A.090	Benign carcinoid tumor of the bronchus and lung
J43.0	Unilateral pulmonary emphysema [MacLeod's syndrome]
J43.1	Panlobular emphysema
J43.2	Centrilobular emphysema
J43.8	Other emphysema
J47.0	Bronchiectasis with acute lower respiratory infection
J47.1	Bronchiectasis with (acute) exacerbation
J85.0	Gangrene and necrosis of lung
J85.1	Abscess of lung with pneumonia
J85.2	Abscess of lung without pneumonia
J98.4	Other disorders of lung
Q33.2	Sequestration of lung

AMA: **32663** 2018,Jan,8; 2017,Jan,8; 2016,Jan,13; 2015,Jan,16; 2014,Jan,11; 2013,Aug,13

Relative Value Units/Medicare Edits

Non-Facility RVU	Work	PE	MP	Total
32663	24.64	10.12	5.66	40.42
Facility RVU	**Work**	**PE**	**MP**	**Total**
32663	24.64	10.12	5.66	40.42

	FUD	Status	MUE	Modifiers				IOM Reference
32663	90	A	1(3)	51	N/A	62*	80	None

* with documentation

Terms To Know

bronchiectasis. Dilation of the bronchi with mucous production and persistent cough due to infection or chronic conditions that causes diminished lung capacity and frequent infections of the lung.

32664

32664 Thoracoscopy, surgical; with thoracic sympathectomy

A thoracic sympathectomy is performed using thoracoscopic technique

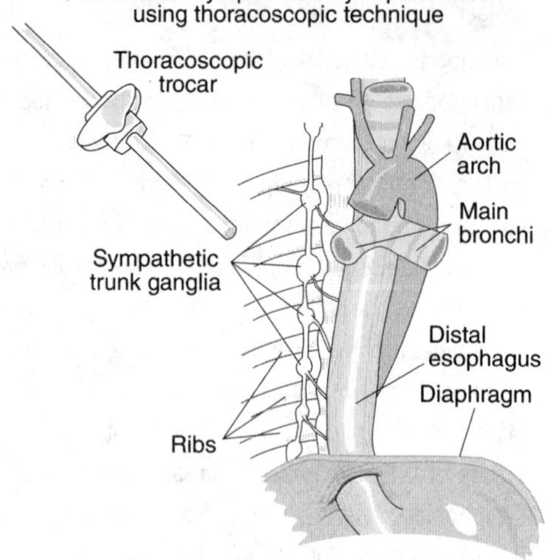

Schematic showing sympathetic nerve trunk in relation to select thoracic structures. The sympathetic trunk ganglia lie on the juncture of the rib and spine and there are usually about 10 on each side

Explanation

The physician performs a sympathectomy inside of the chest cavity through a rigid or flexible fiberoptic endoscope. The procedure can be done under local or general anesthesia. The physician makes a small incision between two ribs and by blunt dissection and the use of a trocar enters the thoracic cavity. The endoscope is passed through the trocar and into the chest cavity. The lung is usually partially collapsed by instilling air into the chest through the trocar or, if general anesthesia is used, the lung may be collapsed through a double lumen endotracheal tube inserted through the mouth into the trachea. The contents of the chest cavity are examined by direct visualization and/or by the use of a video camera. Still photographs may be taken as part of the procedure. A second and/or third trocar and instruments may be inserted into the chest cavity through a second and/or third wound in the chest. Under direct visualization through the endoscope, the physician manipulates the instruments inserted through the secondary sites and localizes and isolates a portion of the sympathetic nerves as they course deeply through the chest. The sympathectomy is accomplished by clipping and/or cutting the nerves. At the conclusion of the procedure, the endoscope and the trocar(s) are removed. A chest tube for drainage and re-expansion of the lung is usually inserted through the wound used for the thoracoscopy.

Coding Tips

Surgical thoracoscopy always includes a diagnostic thoracoscopy. For open cervicothoracic sympathectomy, see 64804. For thoracolumbar sympathectomy, see 64809.

ICD-10-CM Diagnostic Codes

G90.511	Complex regional pain syndrome I of right upper limb ☑
G90.512	Complex regional pain syndrome I of left upper limb ☑
G90.513	Complex regional pain syndrome I of upper limb, bilateral ☑
G90.521	Complex regional pain syndrome I of right lower limb ☑
G90.522	Complex regional pain syndrome I of left lower limb ☑
G90.523	Complex regional pain syndrome I of lower limb, bilateral ☑
G90.59	Complex regional pain syndrome I of other specified site

I73.00	Raynaud's syndrome without gangrene
I73.01	Raynaud's syndrome with gangrene
L74.510	Primary focal hyperhidrosis, axilla
L74.511	Primary focal hyperhidrosis, face
L74.512	Primary focal hyperhidrosis, palms
L74.513	Primary focal hyperhidrosis, soles
L74.52	Secondary focal hyperhidrosis

AMA: **32664** 2018,Jan,8; 2017,Jan,8; 2016,Jan,13; 2015,Jan,16; 2015,Dec,16; 2014,Jan,11; 2013,Aug,13

Relative Value Units/Medicare Edits

Non-Facility RVU	Work	PE	MP	Total
32664	14.28	6.84	3.4	24.52
Facility RVU	**Work**	**PE**	**MP**	**Total**
32664	14.28	6.84	3.4	24.52

	FUD	Status	MUE	Modifiers				IOM Reference
32664	90	A	1(2)	51	50	62*	80	None

* with documentation

Terms To Know

dissection. Separating by cutting tissue or body structures apart.

endoscopy. Visual inspection of the body using a fiberoptic scope.

ganglion. Fluid-filled, benign cyst appearing on a tendon sheath or aponeurosis, frequently connecting to an underlying joint.

hyperhidrosis. Condition of excessive perspiration beyond what the body requires for normal temperature control.

instillation. Administering a liquid slowly over time, drop by drop.

manipulation. Skillful treatment by hand to reduce fractures and dislocations or provide therapy through forceful passive movement of a joint beyond its active limit of motion.

sympathectomy. Surgical interruption or transection of a sympathetic nervous system pathway.

sympathetic nerves. Self-regulating nerves that are part of the autonomic nervous system and that innervate the involuntary motor systems that prepare the body for intense activity.

trocar. Cannula or a sharp pointed instrument used to puncture and aspirate fluid from cavities.

32665

32665 Thoracoscopy, surgical; with esophagomyotomy (Heller type)

An esophagomyotomy is perfomed using thoracoscopic technique

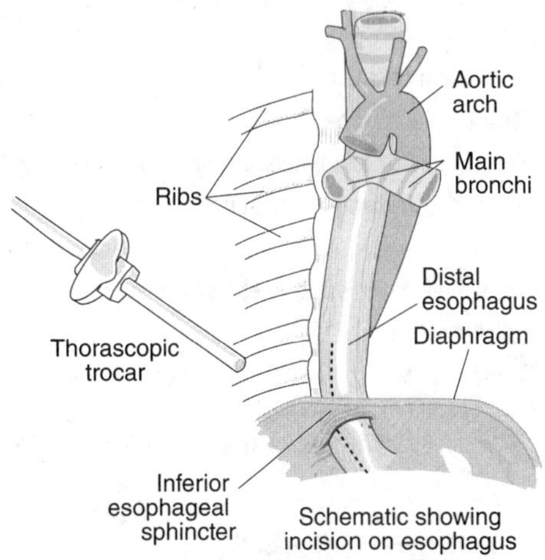

The failure of the distal esophagus to relax during swallowing is called achalasia and this procedure is a treatment for the condition. Heller procedure involves incising just the outer muscle layers of the esophagus

Explanation

The physician repairs a diseased and malfunctioning esophagus by operating through a series of several ports through the chest wall, guided under direct visualization through an endoscope introduced into the chest cavity. The physician makes a small incision between two ribs and by blunt dissection and the use of a trocar enters the thoracic cavity. The endoscope is passed through the trocar and into the chest cavity. The lung is usually partially collapsed by instilling air into the chest through the trocar or the lung may be collapsed through a special double lumen endotracheal tube inserted through the mouth into the trachea. The contents of the chest cavity are examined by direct visualization and/or by the use of a video camera. Still photographs may be taken as part of the procedure. Several other trocars and instruments are inserted into the chest cavity through a series of similar puncture wounds placed at various locations in the chest. A second fiberoptic endoscope is passed through the mouth and guided into the esophagus just above the stomach to assist in the procedure. Under direct visualization through the chest endoscope, the physician manipulates the instruments inserted through the secondary chest sites and operates on the esophagus just above its junction with the stomach. The esophagus is presented to the physician by flexing the tip of the scope inside the esophagus. The outer longitudinal muscle of the esophagus is identified, and cut in a longitudinal fashion and the incision is carried down through the circular muscle layer of the esophagus. The length of the incision is carried onto the surface of the stomach about one centimeter. The depth of the incision in the esophageal wall is down to but not through the mucosal tissues lining the inside of the esophagus. Care is taken not to enter the inside of the esophagus. The incision relaxes the esophagus just above the stomach and allows food to more easily enter the stomach in those patients who have difficulty swallowing due to disease in this area of the esophagus. At the conclusion of the procedure, the endoscope and the trocar(s) are removed. A chest tube for drainage and re-expansion of the lung is usually inserted through the wound used for the thoracoscopy.

Coding Tips

Surgical thoracoscopy always includes a diagnostic thoracoscopy. For open esophagomyotomy (Heller type), thoracic approach, see 43331. For exploratory thoracoscopy with or without biopsy, see 32601–32609.

ICD-10-CM Diagnostic Codes

K22.0	Achalasia of cardia
K22.2	Esophageal obstruction
K22.4	Dyskinesia of esophagus
K22.5	Diverticulum of esophagus, acquired
Q39.0	Atresia of esophagus without fistula
Q39.1	Atresia of esophagus with tracheo-esophageal fistula
Q39.3	Congenital stenosis and stricture of esophagus
Q39.4	Esophageal web
Q39.6	Congenital diverticulum of esophagus

AMA: 32665 2018,Jan,8; 2017,Jan,8; 2016,Jan,13; 2015,Jan,16; 2014,Jan,11; 2013,Aug,13

Relative Value Units/Medicare Edits

Non-Facility RVU	Work	PE	MP	Total
32665	21.53	9.04	5.11	35.68
Facility RVU	**Work**	**PE**	**MP**	**Total**
32665	21.53	9.04	5.11	35.68

	FUD	Status	MUE	Modifiers				IOM Reference
32665	90	A	1(2)	51	N/A	62*	80	None

* with documentation

Terms To Know

achalasia. Failure of the smooth muscles within the gastrointestinal tract to relax at points of junction; most commonly referring to the esophagogastric sphincter's failure to relax when swallowing.

blunt dissection. Surgical technique used to expose an underlying area by separating along natural cleavage lines of tissue, without cutting.

dyskinesia of esophagus. Difficult or impaired voluntary muscle movement of the esophagus.

fistula. Abnormal tube-like passage between two body cavities or organs or from an organ to the outside surface.

instillation. Administering a liquid slowly over time, drop by drop.

stenosis. Narrowing or constriction of a passage.

trocar. Cannula or a sharp pointed instrument used to puncture and aspirate fluid from cavities.

32666-32667

32666 Thoracoscopy, surgical; with therapeutic wedge resection (eg, mass, nodule), initial unilateral

\+ **32667** with therapeutic wedge resection (eg, mass or nodule), each additional resection, ipsilateral (List separately in addition to code for primary procedure)

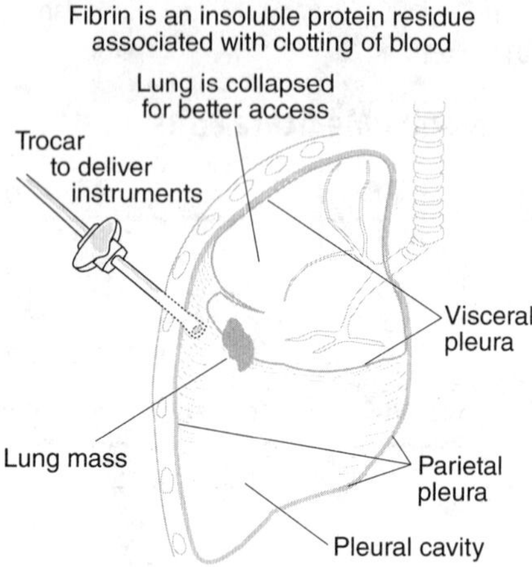

Surgical thoracoscopy is performed. The pleural cavity is visualized and a mass or nodule is removed via wedge resection

Explanation

The physician performs a wedge resection of a lung mass or nodule through a rigid or flexible fiberoptic endoscope. The physician makes a small incision between two ribs and by blunt dissection and the use of a trocar enters the thoracic cavity. The endoscope is passed through the trocar and into the chest cavity. The lung is usually partially collapsed by instilling air into the chest through the trocar or the lung may be collapsed through a double lumen endotracheal tube inserted through the mouth into the trachea. The contents of the chest cavity are examined by direct visualization and/or by the use of a video camera. Still photographs may be taken as part of the procedure. Additional instruments may be inserted into the chest cavity through a second and/or third wound in the chest. Under direct visualization through the endoscope, the physician manipulates the instruments inserted through the secondary sites and clamps the blood vessels and bronchial tubes going to the sections of lung to be removed. With the clamps in place, the tissue is removed. Any cut portions of the lung tissue are repaired by suturing or clipping with surgical clips. At the conclusion of the procedure, the endoscope and the trocar(s) are removed. A chest tube for drainage and re-expansion of the lung is usually inserted through the wound used for the thoracoscopy. Report 32666 for the initial therapeutic wedge resection and 32667 for each additional resection on the same side.

Coding Tips

Note that 32666 is a unilateral procedure. If performed bilaterally, some payers require that the service be reported twice with modifier 50 appended to the second code while others require identification of the service only once with modifier 50 appended. Check with individual payers. Modifier 50 identifies a procedure performed identically on the opposite side of the body (mirror image). When a diagnostic wedge resection is performed and followed by a more complex procedure on the same anatomic location, report 32507 or 32668 with the more complex procedure. When a therapeutic wedge resection is performed on a different lobe than a more complex lung resection, append modifier 59 or an X{EPSU} modifier. Do not report these codes with 32440, 32442, 32445, 32488, or 32671.

ICD-10-CM Diagnostic Codes

A15.0	Tuberculosis of lung
B44.0	Invasive pulmonary aspergillosis
B44.1	Other pulmonary aspergillosis
C34.11	Malignant neoplasm of upper lobe, right bronchus or lung ☑
C34.12	Malignant neoplasm of upper lobe, left bronchus or lung ☑
C34.2	Malignant neoplasm of middle lobe, bronchus or lung
C34.31	Malignant neoplasm of lower lobe, right bronchus or lung ☑
C34.32	Malignant neoplasm of lower lobe, left bronchus or lung ☑
C34.81	Malignant neoplasm of overlapping sites of right bronchus and lung ☑
C34.82	Malignant neoplasm of overlapping sites of left bronchus and lung ☑
C46.51	Kaposi's sarcoma of right lung ☑
C46.52	Kaposi's sarcoma of left lung ☑
C78.01	Secondary malignant neoplasm of right lung ☑
C78.02	Secondary malignant neoplasm of left lung ☑
C7A.090	Malignant carcinoid tumor of the bronchus and lung
D02.21	Carcinoma in situ of right bronchus and lung ☑
D02.22	Carcinoma in situ of left bronchus and lung ☑
D14.31	Benign neoplasm of right bronchus and lung ☑
D14.32	Benign neoplasm of left bronchus and lung ☑
D38.1	Neoplasm of uncertain behavior of trachea, bronchus and lung
D3A.090	Benign carcinoid tumor of the bronchus and lung
D86.0	Sarcoidosis of lung
J43.0	Unilateral pulmonary emphysema [MacLeod's syndrome]
J43.1	Panlobular emphysema
J43.2	Centrilobular emphysema
J43.8	Other emphysema
J47.0	Bronchiectasis with acute lower respiratory infection
J47.1	Bronchiectasis with (acute) exacerbation
J85.0	Gangrene and necrosis of lung
J85.1	Abscess of lung with pneumonia
J85.2	Abscess of lung without pneumonia
J98.4	Other disorders of lung
Q33.2	Sequestration of lung

AMA: **32666** 2018,Jan,8; 2017,Jan,8; 2016,Jan,13; 2015,Jan,16; 2014,Jan,11; 2013,Aug,13 **32667** 2018,Jan,8; 2017,Jan,8; 2016,Jan,13; 2015,Jan,16; 2014,Jan,11; 2013,Aug,13

Relative Value Units/Medicare Edits

Non-Facility RVU	Work	PE	MP	Total
32666	14.5	7.25	3.36	25.11
32667	3.0	0.85	0.69	4.54
Facility RVU	**Work**	**PE**	**MP**	**Total**
32666	14.5	7.25	3.36	25.11
32667	3.0	0.85	0.69	4.54

	FUD	Status	MUE	Modifiers				IOM Reference
32666	90	A	1(3)	51	50	62*	80	None
32667	N/A	A	3(3)	N/A	N/A	62*	80	

* with documentation

32668

\+ **32668** Thoracoscopy, surgical; with diagnostic wedge resection followed by anatomic lung resection (List separately in addition to code for primary procedure)

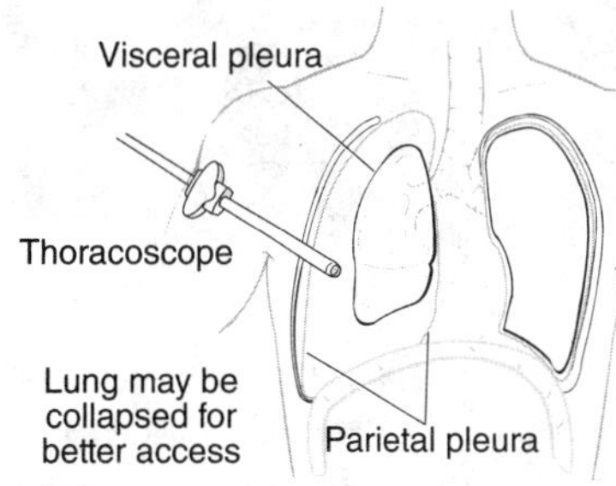

Explanation

The physician performs a wedge resection followed by a lung resection through a rigid or flexible fiberoptic endoscope. The physician makes a small incision between two ribs and by blunt dissection and the use of a trocar enters the thoracic cavity. The endoscope is passed through the trocar and into the chest cavity. The lung is usually partially collapsed by instilling air into the chest through the trocar or the lung may be collapsed through a double lumen endotracheal tube inserted through the mouth into the trachea. The contents of the chest cavity are examined by direct visualization and/or by the use of a video camera. Still photographs may be taken as part of the procedure. Additional instruments may be inserted into the chest cavity through a second and/or third wound in the chest. Under direct visualization through the endoscope, the physician manipulates the instruments inserted through the secondary sites and clamps the blood vessels and bronchial tubes going to the sections of lung to be removed. With the clamps in place, the tissue is removed. Any cut portions of the lung tissue are repaired by suturing or clipping with surgical clips. At the conclusion of the procedure, the endoscope and the trocar(s) are removed. A chest tube for drainage and re-expansion of the lung is usually inserted through the wound used for the thoracoscopy.

Coding Tips

Report 32668 in addition to 32440, 32442, 32445, 32480, 32482, 32484, 32486, 32488, 32503, 32504, 32663, 32669, 32670, or 32671. When a diagnostic wedge resection is performed and followed by a more complex procedure on the same anatomic location, report 32507 or 32668 with the more complex procedure. When a therapeutic wedge resection is performed on a different lobe than a more complex lung resection, append modifier 59 or an X{EPSU} modifier.

ICD-10-CM Diagnostic Codes

This/these CPT code(s) are add on code(s). See the primary procedure code that this code is performed with for your ICD-10-CM code selections. Diagnostic code(s) would be the same as the actual procedure performed.

AMA: **32668** 2018,Jan,8; 2017,Jan,8; 2016,Jan,13; 2015,Jan,16; 2014,Jan,11; 2013,Aug,13

Relative Value Units/Medicare Edits

Non-Facility RVU	Work	PE	MP	Total
32668	3.0	0.85	0.69	4.54
Facility RVU	**Work**	**PE**	**MP**	**Total**
32668	3.0	0.85	0.69	4.54

	FUD	Status	MUE	Modifiers				IOM Reference
32668	N/A	A	2(3)	N/A	N/A	62*	80	None

* with documentation

Terms To Know

diagnostic services. Examination or procedure performed on a patient to obtain information to assess the medical condition of the patient or to identify a disease and to determine the nature and severity of an illness or injury.

malignant. Any condition tending to progress toward death, specifically an invasive tumor with a loss of cellular differentiation that has the ability to spread or metastasize to other body areas.

pleura. One of the two membranes that surround the lungs. The visceral pleura encases the lung and the parietal pleura lines the inner chest walls.

resection. Surgical removal of a part or all of an organ or body part.

trachea. Tube descending from the larynx and branching into the right and left main bronchi.

trocar. Cannula or a sharp pointed instrument used to puncture and aspirate fluid from cavities.

32669-32671

32669 Thoracoscopy, surgical; with removal of a single lung segment (segmentectomy)

32670 with removal of two lobes (bilobectomy)

32671 with removal of lung (pneumonectomy)

Lung segments are defined by bronchopulmonary branches and the tissues they serve. The schematic below shows just some of the main segments within the larger lobes

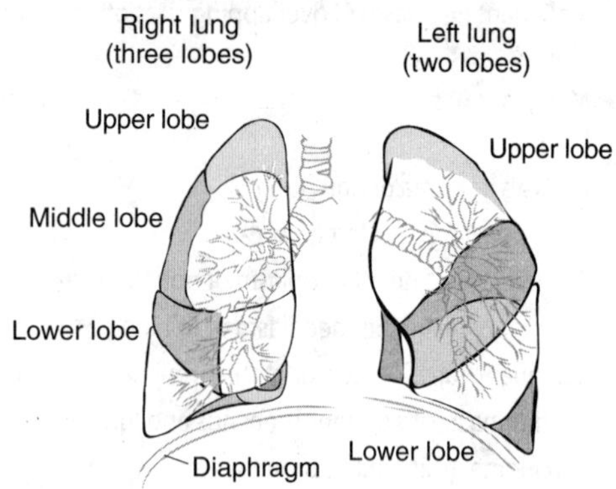

The major lobes of the lung differ from right to left. The right lung has three lobes and the left two, due to the space given over to the heart and pericardium

Explanation

The physician removes a segment of the lung or an entire lung through a rigid or flexible fiberoptic endoscope. The physician makes a small incision between two ribs and by blunt dissection and the use of a trocar enters the thoracic cavity. The endoscope is passed through the trocar and into the chest cavity. The lung is usually partially collapsed by instilling air into the chest through the trocar or the lung may be collapsed through a double lumen endotracheal tube inserted through the mouth into the trachea. The contents of the chest cavity are examined by direct visualization and/or by the use of a video camera. Still photographs may be taken as part of the procedure. Additional instruments may be inserted into the chest cavity through a second and/or third wound in the chest. Under direct visualization through the endoscope, the physician manipulates the instruments inserted through the secondary sites and clamps the blood vessels and bronchial tubes going to the sections of lung to be removed. With the clamps in place, the tissue is removed. Any cut portions of the lung tissue are repaired by suturing or clipping with surgical clips. At the conclusion of the procedure, the endoscope and the trocar(s) are removed. A chest tube for drainage and re-expansion of the lung is usually inserted through the wound used for the thoracoscopy. Report 32669 when the physician removes a single lung segment, 32670 when the physician removes two lobes of a lung, and 32671 when an entire lung is removed.

Coding Tips

Surgical thoracoscopy always includes a diagnostic thoracoscopy. Diagnostic lung biopsies with an intraoperative pathology that determines the need for resection or another definitive procedure should be reported using only the most complex service performed.

ICD-10-CM Diagnostic Codes

A15.0	Tuberculosis of lung
B44.0	Invasive pulmonary aspergillosis
B44.1	Other pulmonary aspergillosis
C34.01	Malignant neoplasm of right main bronchus ☑

C34.02 Malignant neoplasm of left main bronchus ☑
C34.11 Malignant neoplasm of upper lobe, right bronchus or lung ☑
C34.12 Malignant neoplasm of upper lobe, left bronchus or lung ☑
C34.2 Malignant neoplasm of middle lobe, bronchus or lung
C34.31 Malignant neoplasm of lower lobe, right bronchus or lung ☑
C34.32 Malignant neoplasm of lower lobe, left bronchus or lung ☑
C34.81 Malignant neoplasm of overlapping sites of right bronchus and lung ☑
C34.82 Malignant neoplasm of overlapping sites of left bronchus and lung ☑
C46.51 Kaposi's sarcoma of right lung ☑
C46.52 Kaposi's sarcoma of left lung ☑
C78.01 Secondary malignant neoplasm of right lung ☑
C78.02 Secondary malignant neoplasm of left lung ☑
C7A.090 Malignant carcinoid tumor of the bronchus and lung
D02.21 Carcinoma in situ of right bronchus and lung ☑
D02.22 Carcinoma in situ of left bronchus and lung ☑
D14.31 Benign neoplasm of right bronchus and lung ☑
D14.32 Benign neoplasm of left bronchus and lung ☑
D38.1 Neoplasm of uncertain behavior of trachea, bronchus and lung
D3A.090 Benign carcinoid tumor of the bronchus and lung
D86.0 Sarcoidosis of lung
J85.0 Gangrene and necrosis of lung
J85.1 Abscess of lung with pneumonia
J85.2 Abscess of lung without pneumonia
J98.4 Other disorders of lung
Q33.2 Sequestration of lung

AMA: 32669 2018,Jan,8; 2017,Jan,8; 2016,Jan,13; 2015,Jan,16; 2014,Jan,11; 2013,Aug,13 **32670** 2018,Jan,8; 2017,Jan,8; 2016,Jan,13; 2015,Jan,16; 2014,Jan,11; 2013,Aug,13 **32671** 2018,Jan,8; 2017,Jan,8; 2016,Jan,13; 2015,Jan,16; 2014,Jan,11; 2013,Aug,13

Relative Value Units/Medicare Edits

Non-Facility RVU	Work	PE	MP	Total
32669	23.53	9.81	5.45	38.79
32670	28.52	11.28	6.48	46.28
32671	31.92	11.99	7.59	51.5
Facility RVU	**Work**	**PE**	**MP**	**Total**
32669	23.53	9.81	5.45	38.79
32670	28.52	11.28	6.48	46.28
32671	31.92	11.99	7.59	51.5

	FUD	Status	MUE	Modifiers				IOM Reference
32669	90	A	2(3)	51	N/A	62*	80	None
32670	90	A	1(2)	51	N/A	62*	80	
32671	90	A	1(2)	51	N/A	62*	80	

* with documentation

32672

32672 Thoracoscopy, surgical; with resection-plication for emphysematous lung (bullous or non-bullous) for lung volume reduction (LVRS), unilateral includes any pleural procedure, when performed

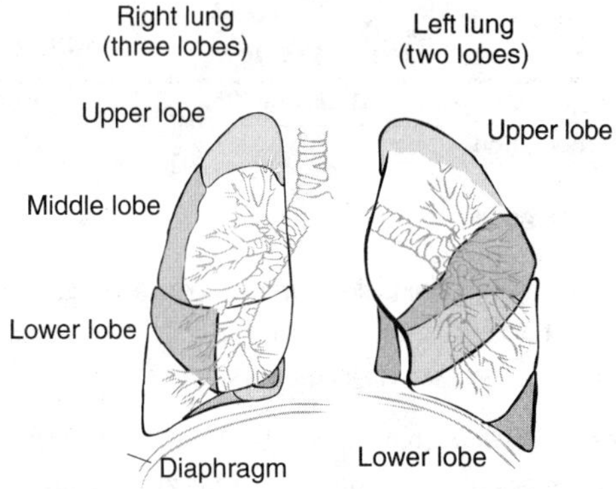

Explanation

The physician removes part of an emphysematous lung. A small incision is made between two ribs and by blunt dissection and the use of a trocar the thoracic cavity is entered. The endoscope is passed through the trocar and into the chest cavity. The lung is usually partially collapsed by instilling air into the chest through the trocar or the lung may be collapsed through a double lumen endotracheal tube inserted through the mouth into the trachea. The contents of the chest cavity are examined by direct visualization and/or by the use of a video camera. Still photographs may be taken as part of the procedure. Additional instruments may be inserted into the chest cavity through a second and/or third wound in the chest. Under direct visualization through the endoscope, the physician manipulates the instruments inserted through the secondary sites and clamps the blood vessels and bronchial tubes going to the section(s) of lung to be removed. With the clamps in place, the emphysematous lung tissue is removed by sharp and blunt dissection and often by folding and suturing of the tissues (plication). Any cut portions of the lung tissue are repaired by suturing or clipping with surgical clips. At the conclusion of the procedure, the endoscope and the trocar(s) are removed. A chest tube for drainage and re-expansion of the lung is usually inserted through the wound used for the thoracoscopy.

Coding Tips

Surgical thoracoscopy always includes a diagnostic thoracoscopy. For an open resection-plication of emphysematous lung(s), see 32491.

ICD-10-CM Diagnostic Codes

J43.0 Unilateral pulmonary emphysema [MacLeod's syndrome]
J43.1 Panlobular emphysema
J43.2 Centrilobular emphysema
J43.8 Other emphysema
J43.9 Emphysema, unspecified

AMA: 32672 2018,Jan,8; 2017,Jan,8; 2016,Jan,13; 2015,Jan,16; 2014,Jan,11; 2013,Aug,13

Relative Value Units/Medicare Edits

Non-Facility RVU	Work	PE	MP	Total
32672	27.0	10.79	6.3	44.09
Facility RVU	**Work**	**PE**	**MP**	**Total**
32672	27.0	10.79	6.3	44.09

	FUD	Status	MUE	Modifiers				IOM Reference
32672	90	A	1(3)	51	N/A	62*	80	None

* with documentation

Terms To Know

emphysema. Pathological condition in which there is destructive enlargement of the air sacs in the lungs resulting in damage and lack of elasticity to the alveolar walls, commonly seen in long-term smokers.

emphysematous bleb. Formation of blisters or vesicles greater than 1.0 mm within an emphysematous lung, containing serum or blood.

LVRS. Lung volume reduction surgery. Treatment for patients with severe or end-stage emphysema. LVRS allows the remaining compressed lung to expand and thus improve respiratory function.

plication. Surgical technique involving folding, tucking, or pleating to reduce the size of a hollow structure or organ.

resection. Surgical removal of a part or all of an organ or body part.

trocar. Cannula or a sharp pointed instrument used to puncture and aspirate fluid from cavities.

Lungs and Pleura

32673

32673 Thoracoscopy, surgical; with resection of thymus, unilateral or bilateral

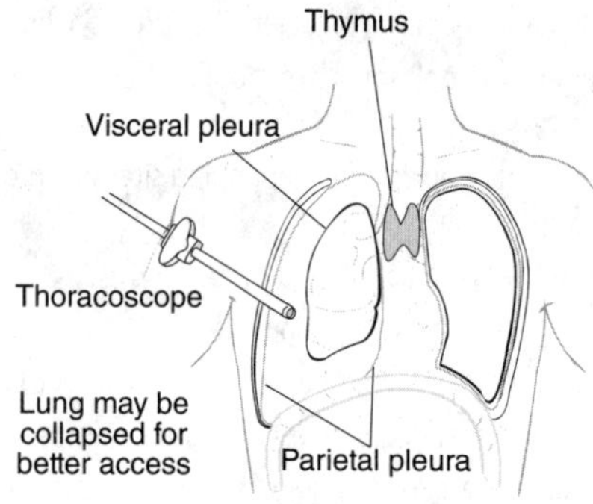

Thymus is resected

Explanation

The physician removes one or both lobes of the thymus gland via thoracoscopic approach. A small incision is made between two ribs and by blunt dissection and the use of a trocar the thoracic cavity is entered. The endoscope is passed through the trocar and into the chest cavity. Additional instruments may be inserted into the chest cavity through a second and/or third wound in the chest. Under direct visualization through the endoscope, the physician manipulates the instruments inserted through the secondary sites and the superior lobe of the thymus is separated from the inferior aspect of the thyroid. The blood supply to the thymus is divided and the thymus is dissected free from the pericardium and removed. A chest tube for drainage is usually inserted through the wound used for the thoracoscopy.

Coding Tips

Surgical thoracoscopy always includes a diagnostic thoracoscopy. For exploratory thoracoscopy with or without biopsy, see 32601–32609. For an open thymectomy, see 60520, 60521, or 60522. For open excision of a mediastinal cyst, see 39200. For open excision of a mediastinal tumor, see 39220.

ICD-10-CM Diagnostic Codes

C37	Malignant neoplasm of thymus
C7A.091	Malignant carcinoid tumor of the thymus
D15.0	Benign neoplasm of thymus
D38.4	Neoplasm of uncertain behavior of thymus
D3A.091	Benign carcinoid tumor of the thymus
G70.00	Myasthenia gravis without (acute) exacerbation
G70.01	Myasthenia gravis with (acute) exacerbation
K51.00	Ulcerative (chronic) pancolitis without complications
K51.011	Ulcerative (chronic) pancolitis with rectal bleeding
K51.012	Ulcerative (chronic) pancolitis with intestinal obstruction
K51.013	Ulcerative (chronic) pancolitis with fistula
K51.014	Ulcerative (chronic) pancolitis with abscess
K51.018	Ulcerative (chronic) pancolitis with other complication
K51.811	Other ulcerative colitis with rectal bleeding
K51.812	Other ulcerative colitis with intestinal obstruction
K51.813	Other ulcerative colitis with fistula
K51.814	Other ulcerative colitis with abscess
K51.818	Other ulcerative colitis with other complication

AMA: 32673 2018,Jan,8; 2017,Jan,8; 2016,Jan,13; 2015,Jan,16; 2014,Jan,11; 2013,Aug,13

Relative Value Units/Medicare Edits

Non-Facility RVU	Work	PE	MP	Total
32673	21.13	9.07	4.82	35.02
Facility RVU	**Work**	**PE**	**MP**	**Total**
32673	21.13	9.07	4.82	35.02

	FUD	Status	MUE	Modifiers				IOM Reference
32673	90	A	1(2)	51	N/A	62*	80	None

* with documentation

Terms To Know

lupus erythematosus. Inflammatory, autoimmune skin condition in which the body's autoimmune system attacks healthy tissue of the integumentary system.

myasthenia gravis. Autoimmune neuromuscular disorder caused by antibodies to the acetylcholine receptors at the neuromuscular junction, interfering with proper binding of the neurotransmitter from the neuron to the target muscle, causing muscle weakness, fatigue, and exhaustion, without pain or atrophy.

thymus. Lymphoid organ located in the front of the upper mediastinum, composed of two symmetrical pyramid-shaped lobes, that is the site where T-lymphocytes are produced.

thyrotoxicosis. Excessive quantities of hormones from the thyroid gland caused by overproduction or loss of storage ability.

32674

\+ **32674** Thoracoscopy, surgical; with mediastinal and regional lymphadenectomy (List separately in addition to code for primary procedure)

Lymph nodes within the mediastinal space are removed in a thoracoscopic surgical procedure

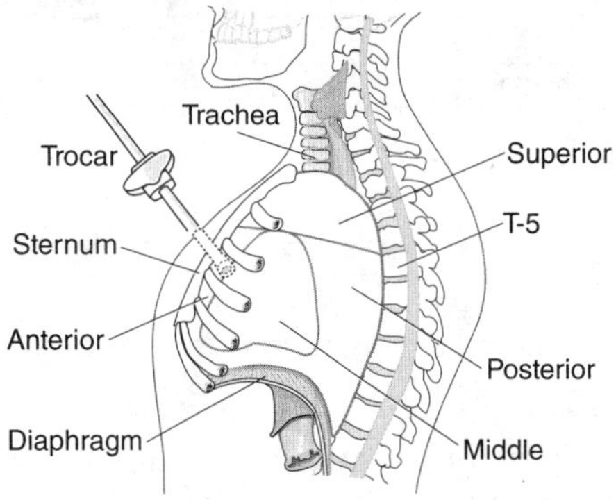

The mediastinal space is the general region between the left and right lungs

Explanation

A regional and mediastinal lymphadenectomy is performed via a thoracoscopic approach. A small incision is made between two ribs and by blunt dissection and the use of a trocar the thoracic cavity is entered. The endoscope is passed through the trocar and into the chest cavity. Additional instruments may be inserted into the chest cavity through a second and/or third wound in the chest. Under direct visualization through the endoscope, the physician manipulates the instruments inserted through the secondary sites and removes the lymph nodes near the lungs, around the heart, and behind the trachea. The area is irrigated, and the operative incision is closed with sutures. A chest tube for drainage is usually inserted through the wound used for the thoracoscopy.

Coding Tips

Surgical thoracoscopy always includes a diagnostic thoracoscopy. Report 32674 in addition to 21601, 31760, 31766, 31786, 32096-32200, 32220-32320, 32440-32491, 32503-32505, 32601-32663, 32666, 32669-32673, 32815, 33025, 33030, 33050-33130, 39200-39220, 39560-39561, 43101, 43112, 43117-43118, 43122-43123, 43287, 43288, 43351, 60270, and 60505. For mediastinal and regional lymphadenectomy by thoracotomy, see 38746.

ICD-10-CM Diagnostic Codes

This/these CPT code(s) are add on code(s). See the primary procedure code that this code is performed with for your ICD-10-CM code selections. Diagnostic code(s) would be the same as the actual procedure performed.

AMA: 32674 2018,Jan,8; 2017,Jan,8; 2016,Jan,13; 2015,Jan,16; 2014,May,3; 2014,Jan,11; 2013,Aug,13

Lungs and Pleura

Relative Value Units/Medicare Edits

Non-Facility RVU	Work	PE	MP	Total
32674	4.12	1.17	0.95	6.24
Facility RVU	**Work**	**PE**	**MP**	**Total**
32674	4.12	1.17	0.95	6.24

	FUD	Status	MUE	Modifiers				IOM Reference
32674	N/A	A	1(2)	N/A	N/A	62*	80	None

* with documentation

Terms To Know

dissection. Separating by cutting tissue or body structures apart.

lymph nodes. Bean-shaped structures along the lymphatic vessels that intercept and destroy foreign materials in the tissue and bloodstream.

lymphadenectomy. Dissection of lymph nodes free from the vessels and removal for examination by frozen section in a separate procedure to detect early-stage metastases.

mediastinum. Collection of organs and tissues that separate the pleural sacs. Located between the sternum and spine above the diaphragm, it contains the heart and great vessels, trachea and bronchi, esophagus, thymus, lymph nodes, and nerves.

trocar. Cannula or a sharp pointed instrument used to puncture and aspirate fluid from cavities.

32800

32800 Repair lung hernia through chest wall

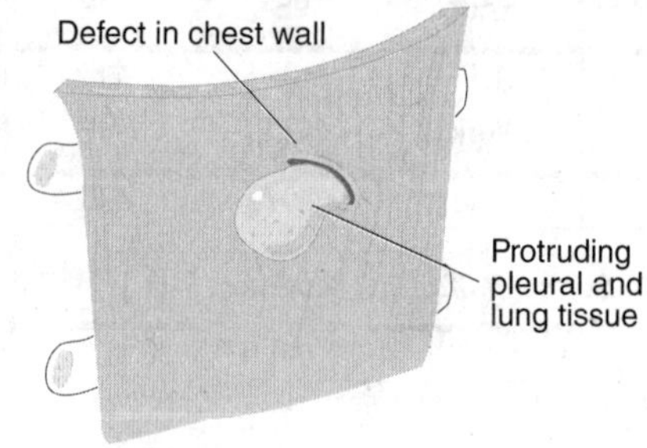

A hernia is a protrusion, usually through a wall containment, and the defect may be congenital

Explanation

The physician repairs a hernia of the chest wall that allows the bulging of the lung through a defect in the chest wall. The physician makes an incision through the skin overlying the defect and carries the incision down to the inside lining of the chest cavity. The defect is repaired by the folding and suturing of tissues or the rotation of muscle and/or thick fibrous tissue flaps over the area and suturing of the flap over the defect. Alternately, the defect can be covered by a synthetic mesh material which is sutured in place. The incision is then closed in layers of sutures.

Coding Tips

Lung hernias may be congenital or acquired and result from a defect in the chest wall causing the lung to protrude through the defect.

ICD-10-CM Diagnostic Codes

J98.4	Other disorders of lung
S21.311A	Laceration without foreign body of right front wall of thorax with penetration into thoracic cavity, initial encounter ☑
S21.312A	Laceration without foreign body of left front wall of thorax with penetration into thoracic cavity, initial encounter ☑
S21.321A	Laceration with foreign body of right front wall of thorax with penetration into thoracic cavity, initial encounter ☑
S21.322A	Laceration with foreign body of left front wall of thorax with penetration into thoracic cavity, initial encounter ☑
S21.331A	Puncture wound without foreign body of right front wall of thorax with penetration into thoracic cavity, initial encounter ☑
S21.332A	Puncture wound without foreign body of left front wall of thorax with penetration into thoracic cavity, initial encounter ☑
S21.341A	Puncture wound with foreign body of right front wall of thorax with penetration into thoracic cavity, initial encounter ☑
S21.342A	Puncture wound with foreign body of left front wall of thorax with penetration into thoracic cavity, initial encounter ☑
S21.351A	Open bite of right front wall of thorax with penetration into thoracic cavity, initial encounter ☑
S21.352A	Open bite of left front wall of thorax with penetration into thoracic cavity, initial encounter ☑
S21.411A	Laceration without foreign body of right back wall of thorax with penetration into thoracic cavity, initial encounter ☑
S21.412A	Laceration without foreign body of left back wall of thorax with penetration into thoracic cavity, initial encounter ☑

S21.421A	Laceration with foreign body of right back wall of thorax with penetration into thoracic cavity, initial encounter ☑
S21.422A	Laceration with foreign body of left back wall of thorax with penetration into thoracic cavity, initial encounter ☑
S21.431A	Puncture wound without foreign body of right back wall of thorax with penetration into thoracic cavity, initial encounter ☑
S21.432A	Puncture wound without foreign body of left back wall of thorax with penetration into thoracic cavity, initial encounter ☑
S21.441A	Puncture wound with foreign body of right back wall of thorax with penetration into thoracic cavity, initial encounter ☑
S21.442A	Puncture wound with foreign body of left back wall of thorax with penetration into thoracic cavity, initial encounter ☑
S21.451A	Open bite of right back wall of thorax with penetration into thoracic cavity, initial encounter ☑
S21.452A	Open bite of left back wall of thorax with penetration into thoracic cavity, initial encounter ☑
S27.893A	Laceration of other specified intrathoracic organs, initial encounter
T81.530A	Perforation due to foreign body accidentally left in body following surgical operation, initial encounter
T81.590A	Other complications of foreign body accidentally left in body following surgical operation, initial encounter

Relative Value Units/Medicare Edits

Non-Facility RVU	Work	PE	MP	Total
32800	15.71	7.83	3.51	27.05
Facility RVU	**Work**	**PE**	**MP**	**Total**
32800	15.71	7.83	3.51	27.05

	FUD	Status	MUE	Modifiers				IOM Reference
32800	90	A	1(3)	51	N/A	62*	80	None

* with documentation

Terms To Know

acquired. Produced by outside influences and not by genetics or birth defect.

anomaly. Irregularity in the structure or position of an organ or tissue.

congenital. Present at birth, occurring through heredity or an influence during gestation up to the moment of birth.

hernia. Protrusion of a body structure through tissue.

incision. Act of cutting into tissue or an organ.

suture. Numerous stitching techniques employed in wound closure.

32810

32810 Closure of chest wall following open flap drainage for empyema (Clagett type procedure)

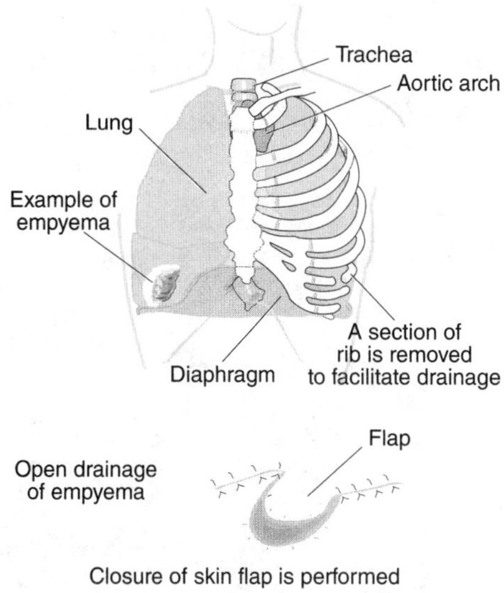

Explanation

The physician treats a draining empyema (accumulation of pus in the chest cavity) by resecting a rib, irrigating the empyema space with an antibiotic solution intermittently over an extended period of time, and closing of the empyema space in six to eight weeks. This code reports the closure portion only.

Coding Tips

Treatment of empyema, an accumulation of pus in the pleural cavity, by open flap drainage requires a second procedure for closure of the flap. This procedure reports the closure portion only. Modifier 58 should be appended to indicate that this is a staged or related procedure performed by the same physician. For thoracostomy with initial creation of an open flap drainage for empyema, see 32036.

ICD-10-CM Diagnostic Codes

A15.6	Tuberculous pleurisy
J86.0	Pyothorax with fistula
J86.9	Pyothorax without fistula

Relative Value Units/Medicare Edits

Non-Facility RVU	Work	PE	MP	Total
32810	14.95	7.54	3.55	26.04
Facility RVU	**Work**	**PE**	**MP**	**Total**
32810	14.95	7.54	3.55	26.04

	FUD	Status	MUE	Modifiers				IOM Reference
32810	90	A	1(3)	51	N/A	N/A	80	None

* with documentation

32815

32815 Open closure of major bronchial fistula

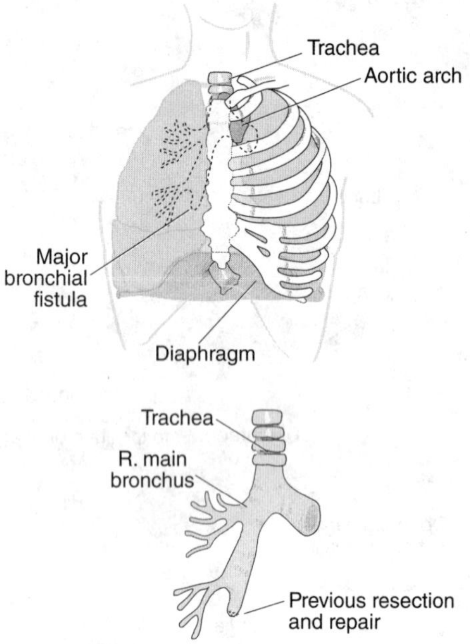

In some instances, the site of a previous bronchial surgery develops into a fistula between the stub and surrounding tissues or pleura

Explanation

The physician repairs a major bronchial fistula (an abnormal passageway between the remaining end of a bronchial tube and the chest that occurs sometimes after the removal of a lung or portion of a lung). The physician enters the chest cavity through a vertical incision made in the middle of the front of the chest. The incision is carried down to the sternum which is split in order to enter the chest cavity at the root of the lung near the center of the chest. The fistula exposure often requires the resection of one or two of the upper ribs. The end of the bronchial tube is located and the stump of the bronchial tube is reamputated and the inside lining of the bronchial tube is treated with silver nitrate to destroy the mucus forming cells lining the bronchus. The stump is sutured or stapled. The chest defect created is repaired and the sternum closed using wire sutures and the skin closed in layers of sutures. A chest tube may be inserted into the chest cavity for drainage.

Coding Tips

For thoracoplasty, Schede type or extrapleural, all stages, with closure of bronchopleural fistula, see 32906.

ICD-10-CM Diagnostic Codes

J86.0 Pyothorax with fistula

Relative Value Units/Medicare Edits

Non-Facility RVU	Work	PE	MP	Total
32815	50.03	19.35	11.67	81.05
Facility RVU	**Work**	**PE**	**MP**	**Total**
32815	50.03	19.35	11.67	81.05

	FUD	Status	MUE	Modifiers				IOM Reference
32815	90	A	1(3)	51	N/A	62*	80	None

* with documentation

32820

32820 Major reconstruction, chest wall (posttraumatic)

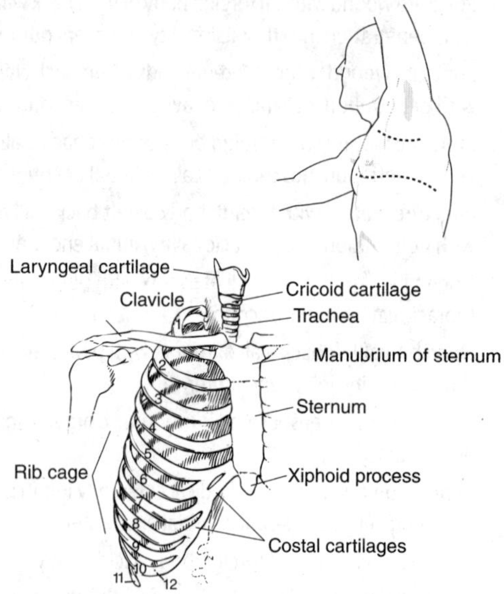

The ribs are the framework of the thoracic cage. Ten pairs connect anteriorly to the sternum and two pairs (11 and 12) float. Ribs numbered 7 to 10 fuse to form the costal margin before attaching to the sternum

Explanation

The physician repairs and reconstructs the chest wall following a major disfiguring injury to the chest (e.g. a shotgun blast). The purpose of the repair is to restore structure and coverage of the chest wall as well as fill any vacant spaces within the chest to prevent infection. The chest wall consists of three layers: the soft tissue layer, including the skin, subcutaneous tissue and muscle; the skeletal layer, consisting of the ribs, cartilage and sometimes the sternum; and the pleural space (parietal cavity). During the procedure, the parietal cavity is checked for air leaks and repaired if necessary. Any empty pleural space may be filled with muscle flap, omentum, or prosthetic material. Bone grafts, muscle or omental flaps or methyl methacrylate reinforced mesh is used to reconstruct the ribs and/or sternum damaged in the trauma. Repair of the soft tissue layer using skin flaps is included in the reconstruction. Skin autograft or substitutes required to close the defect may be reported separately.

Coding Tips

Report 32820 only for reconstruction following trauma. Reconstruction following excision or resection of chest wall tumors should be reported with 21602–21603. For an excision of a chest wall tumor involving the ribs, with plastic reconstruction, without mediastinal lymphadenectomy, see 21602; with mediastinal lymphadenectomy, see 21603. For removal of lung, see 32480–32491.

ICD-10-CM Diagnostic Codes

S21.151A Open bite of right front wall of thorax without penetration into thoracic cavity, initial encounter ☑

S21.152A Open bite of left front wall of thorax without penetration into thoracic cavity, initial encounter ☑

S21.211A Laceration without foreign body of right back wall of thorax without penetration into thoracic cavity, initial encounter ☑

S21.212A Laceration without foreign body of left back wall of thorax without penetration into thoracic cavity, initial encounter ☑

S21.221A Laceration with foreign body of right back wall of thorax without penetration into thoracic cavity, initial encounter ☑

S21.222A Laceration with foreign body of left back wall of thorax without penetration into thoracic cavity, initial encounter ☑

S21.231A Puncture wound without foreign body of right back wall of thorax without penetration into thoracic cavity, initial encounter ☑

S21.232A Puncture wound without foreign body of left back wall of thorax without penetration into thoracic cavity, initial encounter ☑

S21.241A Puncture wound with foreign body of right back wall of thorax without penetration into thoracic cavity, initial encounter ☑

S21.242A Puncture wound with foreign body of left back wall of thorax without penetration into thoracic cavity, initial encounter ☑

S21.251A Open bite of right back wall of thorax without penetration into thoracic cavity, initial encounter ☑

S21.252A Open bite of left back wall of thorax without penetration into thoracic cavity, initial encounter ☑

S21.311A Laceration without foreign body of right front wall of thorax with penetration into thoracic cavity, initial encounter ☑

S21.312A Laceration without foreign body of left front wall of thorax with penetration into thoracic cavity, initial encounter ☑

S21.321A Laceration with foreign body of right front wall of thorax with penetration into thoracic cavity, initial encounter ☑

S21.322A Laceration with foreign body of left front wall of thorax with penetration into thoracic cavity, initial encounter ☑

S21.331A Puncture wound without foreign body of right front wall of thorax with penetration into thoracic cavity, initial encounter ☑

S21.332A Puncture wound without foreign body of left front wall of thorax with penetration into thoracic cavity, initial encounter ☑

S21.341A Puncture wound with foreign body of right front wall of thorax with penetration into thoracic cavity, initial encounter ☑

S21.342A Puncture wound with foreign body of left front wall of thorax with penetration into thoracic cavity, initial encounter ☑

S21.351A Open bite of right front wall of thorax with penetration into thoracic cavity, initial encounter ☑

S21.352A Open bite of left front wall of thorax with penetration into thoracic cavity, initial encounter ☑

S21.411A Laceration without foreign body of right back wall of thorax with penetration into thoracic cavity, initial encounter ☑

S21.412A Laceration without foreign body of left back wall of thorax with penetration into thoracic cavity, initial encounter ☑

S21.421A Laceration with foreign body of right back wall of thorax with penetration into thoracic cavity, initial encounter ☑

S21.422A Laceration with foreign body of left back wall of thorax with penetration into thoracic cavity, initial encounter ☑

S21.431A Puncture wound without foreign body of right back wall of thorax with penetration into thoracic cavity, initial encounter ☑

S21.432A Puncture wound without foreign body of left back wall of thorax with penetration into thoracic cavity, initial encounter ☑

S21.441A Puncture wound with foreign body of right back wall of thorax with penetration into thoracic cavity, initial encounter ☑

S21.442A Puncture wound with foreign body of left back wall of thorax with penetration into thoracic cavity, initial encounter ☑

S21.451A Open bite of right back wall of thorax with penetration into thoracic cavity, initial encounter ☑

S21.452A Open bite of left back wall of thorax with penetration into thoracic cavity, initial encounter ☑

S22.21XB Fracture of manubrium, initial encounter for open fracture

S22.22XB Fracture of body of sternum, initial encounter for open fracture

S22.23XB Sternal manubrial dissociation, initial encounter for open fracture

S22.24XB Fracture of xiphoid process, initial encounter for open fracture

S22.41XB Multiple fractures of ribs, right side, initial encounter for open fracture ☑

S22.5XXA Flail chest, initial encounter for closed fracture

S22.5XXB Flail chest, initial encounter for open fracture

S27.0XXA Traumatic pneumothorax, initial encounter

S27.1XXA Traumatic hemothorax, initial encounter

S27.2XXA Traumatic hemopneumothorax, initial encounter

S27.893A Laceration of other specified intrathoracic organs, initial encounter

S28.0XXA Crushed chest, initial encounter

S29.091A Other injury of muscle and tendon of front wall of thorax, initial encounter

S29.092A Other injury of muscle and tendon of back wall of thorax, initial encounter

S29.8XXA Other specified injuries of thorax, initial encounter

T21.21XA Burn of second degree of chest wall, initial encounter

T21.31XA Burn of third degree of chest wall, initial encounter

T21.61XA Corrosion of second degree of chest wall, initial encounter

T21.71XA Corrosion of third degree of chest wall, initial encounter

T81.31XA Disruption of external operation (surgical) wound, not elsewhere classified, initial encounter

T81.32XA Disruption of internal operation (surgical) wound, not elsewhere classified, initial encounter

Relative Value Units/Medicare Edits

Non-Facility RVU	Work	PE	MP	Total
32820	22.51	10.61	5.34	38.46
Facility RVU	**Work**	**PE**	**MP**	**Total**
32820	22.51	10.61	5.34	38.46

	FUD	Status	MUE	Modifiers				IOM Reference
32820	90	A	1(2)	51	N/A	62*	80	None

* with documentation

Terms To Know

autograft. Any tissue harvested from one anatomical site of a person and grafted to another anatomical site of the same person. Most commonly, blood vessels, skin, tendons, fascia, and bone are used as autografts.

flap. Mass of flesh and skin partially excised from its location but retaining its blood supply that is moved to another site to repair adjacent or distant defects.

omentum. Fold of peritoneal tissue suspended between the stomach and neighboring visceral organs of the abdominal cavity.

32850

32850 Donor pneumonectomy(s) (including cold preservation), from cadaver donor

Lung tissue from a cadaver is prepared and maintained in anticipation of an allograft

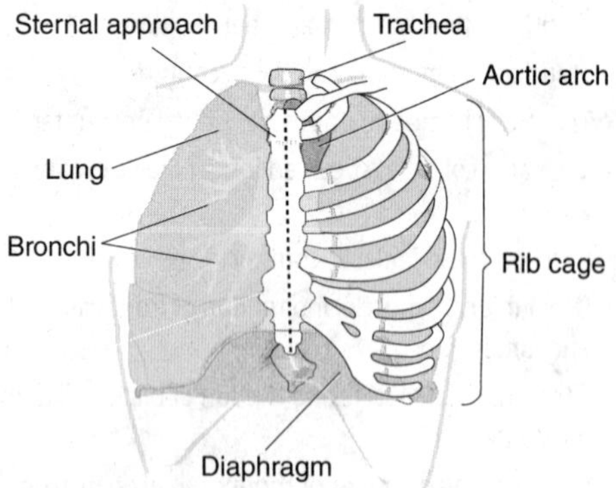

Cardiopulmonary bypass may be initiated during the harvest surgery to keep the tissues viable

Explanation

The physician performs a donor pneumonectomy(ies) for transplant from a cadaver donor. In cases where the donor has been declared brain dead, adequate functioning of the heart, lungs, and circulatory system are maintained prior to removal of the organ. During surgical removal of the lung(s), the donor may be placed on a cardiopulmonary bypass machine to maintain perfusion to the organs. The physician makes a long, mid-line vertical incision through all the layers of the skin down to the sternum bone. The sternum is split and the chest cavity entered. Each lung is removed in one block by dividing the trachea and the major arteries and veins that carry blood to and from the heart. The lung(s) is preserved for transplantation into the recipient. The organ(s) remains under refrigeration, specially packed in a sealable container with some preserving solution and kept on ice in a suitable carrier.

Coding Tips

Lung transplantation involves three distinct components. Code 32850 reports only the cadaver pneumonectomy. Backbench work (32855–32856), which involves preparation of the cadaver donor lung allograft prior to transplant, is reported separately. Transplant of the cadaver lung including recipient pneumonectomy and care of the recipient (32851–32854) is also reported separately. Any additional repair or resection procedures on the donor lung are also reported separately, see 32491, 32505–32507, 35216, and 35276. Donor pneumonectomy and any backbench work, repair, or resection procedures on the donor lung are usually the financial responsibility of the recipient.

ICD-10-CM Diagnostic Codes

Z52.89 Donor of other specified organs or tissues

AMA: **32850** 1993,Win,1

Relative Value Units/Medicare Edits

Non-Facility RVU	Work	PE	MP	Total
32850	0.0	0.0	0.0	0.0
Facility RVU	**Work**	**PE**	**MP**	**Total**
32850	0.0	0.0	0.0	0.0

	FUD	Status	MUE	Modifiers				IOM Reference
32850	N/A	X	1(2)	N/A	N/A	N/A	N/A	None

* with documentation

Terms To Know

allograft. Graft from one individual to another of the same species.

cardiectomy. Excision of the cardiac portion of the stomach.

cardiopulmonary bypass. Venous blood is diverted to a heart-lung machine, which mechanically pumps and oxygenates the blood temporarily so the heart can be bypassed while an open procedure on the heart or coronary arteries is performed. During bypass, the lungs are deflated and immobile.

donor. Person from whom tissues or organs are removed for transplantation.

incision. Act of cutting into tissue or an organ.

pneumonectomy. Surgical removal of a lung or lung tissue.

32851-32854

32851 Lung transplant, single; without cardiopulmonary bypass
32852 with cardiopulmonary bypass
32853 Lung transplant, double (bilateral sequential or en bloc); without cardiopulmonary bypass
32854 with cardiopulmonary bypass

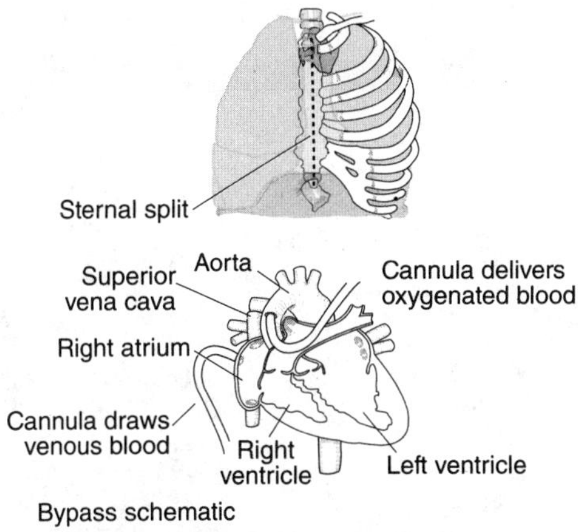

Cardiopulmonary bypass, also known as extracorporeal circulation, is a blood oxygenation technique used in many types of open heart surgeries. A cannula is passed through the right atrium to the vena cava where venous blood is drawn. The blood is oxygenated by machine and returned to arterial circulation, usually through a cannula in the ascending aorta

Explanation

The physician performs a single lung transplantation of the recipient patient. The physician makes a long, mid-line vertical incision through all the layers of the skin down to the sternum bone. The sternum is split and the chest cavity entered. The patient's original lung is deflated and the root of the lung isolated and the major arteries and veins that carry blood to and from the heart are identified and divided. The main bronchial tube to that lung is severed and the lung removed. The donor lung is placed in the chest cavity and its bronchial tube and arteries and veins sutured to the patients where the former lung was attached. Circulation and functioning of the donor lung is assured and the chest is closed. The sternum is closed using wire sutures and the skin closed in layers of sutures. A chest tube(s) is inserted into the chest cavity for drainage. During the procedure the patient's oxygenation and circulation is maintained by the patient's own heart and other lung. In 32852, during the transplantation of the lung, the patient is placed on a cardiopulmonary bypass machine to maintain circulation to the organs. In 32853, the physician performs a double lung transplantation of the recipient patient without cardiopulmonary bypass. In 32854, a double lung transplantation is performed, during which the patient is placed on a cardiopulmonary bypass machine to maintain circulation to the organs.

Coding Tips

Lung transplantation involves three distinct components. Codes 32851–32854 report only the transplant of the cadaver lung including recipient pneumonectomy and care of the recipient. Cadaver pneumonectomy (32850) is reported separately. Backbench work (32855–32856), which involves preparation of the cadaver donor lung allograft prior to transplant, is reported separately. Any additional repair or resection procedures on the donor lung are also reported separately, see 32491, 32505–32507, 35216, and 35276. Donor pneumonectomy and any backbench work, repair, or resection procedures on the donor lung are usually the financial responsibility of the recipient.

ICD-10-CM Diagnostic Codes

D86.0	Sarcoidosis of lung
D86.2	Sarcoidosis of lung with sarcoidosis of lymph nodes
E84.0	Cystic fibrosis with pulmonary manifestations
E88.01	Alpha-1-antitrypsin deficiency
I27.0	Primary pulmonary hypertension
I27.21	Secondary pulmonary arterial hypertension
I27.22	Pulmonary hypertension due to left heart disease
I27.23	Pulmonary hypertension due to lung diseases and hypoxia
I27.24	Chronic thromboembolic pulmonary hypertension
I27.29	Other secondary pulmonary hypertension
I27.81	Cor pulmonale (chronic)
I27.82	Chronic pulmonary embolism
I27.83	Eisenmenger's syndrome
I27.89	Other specified pulmonary heart diseases
J44.1	Chronic obstructive pulmonary disease with (acute) exacerbation
J60	Coalworker's pneumoconiosis
J61	Pneumoconiosis due to asbestos and other mineral fibers
J62.0	Pneumoconiosis due to talc dust
J62.8	Pneumoconiosis due to other dust containing silica
J63.0	Aluminosis (of lung)
J63.1	Bauxite fibrosis (of lung)
J63.2	Berylliosis
J63.3	Graphite fibrosis (of lung)
J63.4	Siderosis
J63.5	Stannosis
J63.6	Pneumoconiosis due to other specified inorganic dusts
J68.4	Chronic respiratory conditions due to chemicals, gases, fumes and vapors
J68.8	Other respiratory conditions due to chemicals, gases, fumes and vapors
J70.1	Chronic and other pulmonary manifestations due to radiation
J84.01	Alveolar proteinosis
J84.112	Idiopathic pulmonary fibrosis
J84.113	Idiopathic non-specific interstitial pneumonitis
J84.114	Acute interstitial pneumonitis
J84.115	Respiratory bronchiolitis interstitial lung disease
J84.117	Desquamative interstitial pneumonia
J84.17	Other interstitial pulmonary diseases with fibrosis in diseases classified elsewhere
J84.2	Lymphoid interstitial pneumonia
J84.81	Lymphangioleiomyomatosis
J84.82	Adult pulmonary Langerhans cell histiocytosis
J84.83	Surfactant mutations of the lung
J84.843	Alveolar capillary dysplasia with vein misalignment
J84.89	Other specified interstitial pulmonary diseases
P26.1	Massive pulmonary hemorrhage originating in the perinatal period
P26.8	Other pulmonary hemorrhages originating in the perinatal period
P27.1	Bronchopulmonary dysplasia originating in the perinatal period
P29.30	Pulmonary hypertension of newborn

P29.38 Other persistent fetal circulation

AMA: **32852** 2017,Dec,3 **32854** 2017,Dec,3

Relative Value Units/Medicare Edits

Non-Facility RVU	Work	PE	MP	Total
32851	59.64	21.55	14.16	95.35
32852	65.5	22.68	15.65	103.83
32853	84.48	28.57	20.47	133.52
32854	90.0	29.85	21.86	141.71
Facility RVU	**Work**	**PE**	**MP**	**Total**
32851	59.64	21.55	14.16	95.35
32852	65.5	22.68	15.65	103.83
32853	84.48	28.57	20.47	133.52
32854	90.0	29.85	21.86	141.71

	FUD	Status	MUE	Modifiers				IOM Reference
32851	90	A	1(2)	51	N/A	62*	80	None
32852	90	A	1(2)	51	N/A	62*	80	
32853	90	A	1(2)	51	N/A	62*	80	
32854	90	A	1(2)	51	N/A	62*	80	

* with documentation

Terms To Know

agenesis. Absence of an organ due to developmental failure in the prenatal period.

asbestosis. Lung disease caused by long-term inhalation of asbestos particles. Asbestos exposure has been linked to lung cancer, most commonly mesothelioma.

dysplasia. Abnormality or alteration in the size, shape, and organization of cells from their normal pattern of development.

fibrosis. Formation of fibrous tissue as part of the restorative process.

hypoplasia. Condition in which there is underdevelopment of an organ or tissue.

meconium. First stool passed by a fetus, sometimes while still in the uterus. In this event, the meconium combines with the maternal amniotic fluid. Complications may occur if meconium is aspirated by the fetus while in utero or at the time of birth.

32855-32856

32855 Backbench standard preparation of cadaver donor lung allograft prior to transplantation, including dissection of allograft from surrounding soft tissues to prepare pulmonary venous/atrial cuff, pulmonary artery, and bronchus; unilateral

32856 bilateral

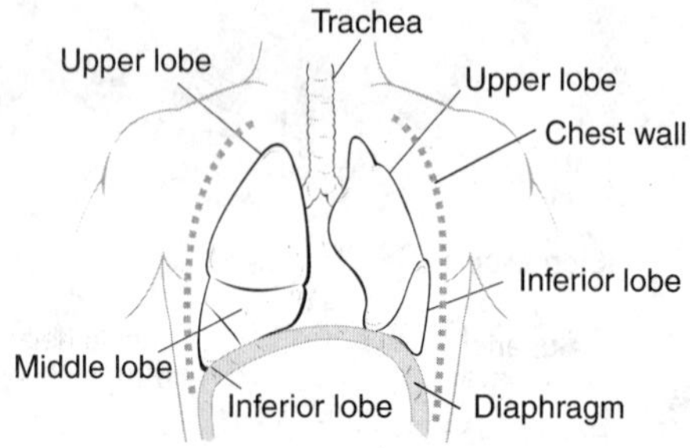

Backbench preparation is performed on one or both lungs from a cadaver in preparation for transplant

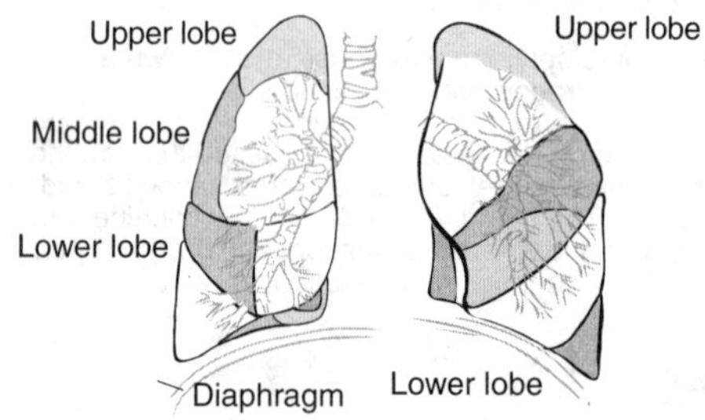

Explanation

The physician performs a standard backbench preparation of one or both lungs following procurement from a cadaver donor. Backbench or back table preparation refers to procedures performed on the donor organs following procurement to prepare the donor organs for transplant. Both lungs are removed or the heart and lungs are removed en bloc. If the heart and lungs are removed en bloc, back table separation of the heart and lungs is performed. The lungs are inspected following procurement to identify any injury or abnormality not noted prior to procurement. The physician prepares the lungs by dissecting free any residual soft tissue. Attention is focused on the pulmonary venous/atrial cuff, pulmonary artery, and bronchus. The pulmonary venous/atrial cuff is inspected and any residual tissue removed. The pulmonary artery, which was divided at its bifurcation, is inspected and any residual tissue removed. The aorta, which was divided distal to the innominate artery, is inspected and residual tissue removed. When all residual soft tissue has been removed and the vessels prepared, the lung(s) is ready for transplant. Report 32855 for backbench preparation of one lung (unilateral). Report 32856 for backbench preparation of both lungs (bilateral).

Coding Tips

Lung transplantation involves three distinct components. Codes 32855–32856 report only the backbench work, which involves preparation of the cadaver donor lung allograft prior to transplant. Cadaver pneumonectomy (32850) is reported separately. Transplant of the cadaver lung including recipient pneumonectomy and care of the recipient (32851–32854) is also reported separately. Any additional repair or resection procedures on the donor lung are also reported separately, see 32491, 32505–32507, 35216, and 35276. Donor pneumonectomy and any backbench work, repair, or resection procedures on the donor lung are usually the financial responsibility of the recipient.

ICD-10-CM Diagnostic Codes

The application of this code is too broad to adequately present ICD-10-CM diagnostic code links here. Refer to your ICD-10-CM book.

Relative Value Units/Medicare Edits

Non-Facility RVU	Work	PE	MP	Total
32855	0.0	0.0	0.0	0.0
32856	0.0	0.0	0.0	0.0
Facility RVU	**Work**	**PE**	**MP**	**Total**
32855	0.0	0.0	0.0	0.0
32856	0.0	0.0	0.0	0.0

	FUD	Status	MUE	Modifiers				IOM Reference
32855	N/A	C	1(2)	51	N/A	62*	80	None
32856	N/A	C	1(2)	51	N/A	62*	80	

* with documentation

Terms To Know

abscess. Circumscribed collection of pus resulting from bacteria, frequently associated with swelling and other signs of inflammation.

allograft. Graft from one individual to another of the same species.

asbestosis. Lung disease caused by long-term inhalation of asbestos particles. Asbestos exposure has been linked to lung cancer, most commonly mesothelioma.

backbench preparation. Procedures performed on a donor organ following procurement to prepare the organ for transplant into the recipient. Excess fat and other tissue may be removed, the organ may be perfused, and vital arteries may be sized, repaired, or modified to fit the patient. These procedures are done on a back table in the operating room before transplantation can begin.

cadaver. Dead body.

empyema. Accumulation of pus within the respiratory or pleural cavity.

32900

32900 Resection of ribs, extrapleural, all stages

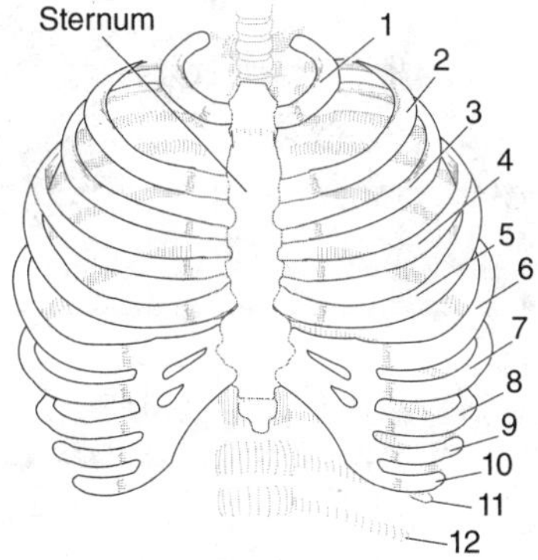

A rib, or a portion of a single rib, is surgically removed without entry into the thoracic cavity

Explanation

The physician resects a rib(s) without entering the chest cavity. The surgeon make an incision in the skin overlying the rib to be removed and carries that incision through the tissues down to the rib. The tissues are dissected away from the rib taking care not to puncture through the pleural membrane on the inside surface of the rib. This avoids the egress of air into the chest cavity. With the tissue removed from the surface of the rib, the rib is cut at two places and the intervening section removed. The resulting defect may be covered by the use of muscle flaps grafted to the area. The remaining tissues and skin are closed by suturing in layers.

Coding Tips

Report this procedure only when performed for the purpose of surgical collapse of the thoracic cavity. For radical resection of the chest wall and rib cage for tumor, see 21601. For partial excision of a rib, see 21600. For excision of the first and/or cervical rib, see 21615. For excision of the first and/or cervical rib with sympathectomy, see 21616. For division of scalenus anticus with resection of the cervical rib, see 21705.

ICD-10-CM Diagnostic Codes

C41.3	Malignant neoplasm of ribs, sternum and clavicle
D16.7	Benign neoplasm of ribs, sternum and clavicle
M41.124	Adolescent idiopathic scoliosis, thoracic region
M41.125	Adolescent idiopathic scoliosis, thoracolumbar region
M41.24	Other idiopathic scoliosis, thoracic region
M41.25	Other idiopathic scoliosis, thoracolumbar region
M41.34	Thoracogenic scoliosis, thoracic region
M41.35	Thoracogenic scoliosis, thoracolumbar region
M41.44	Neuromuscular scoliosis, thoracic region
M41.45	Neuromuscular scoliosis, thoracolumbar region
M41.54	Other secondary scoliosis, thoracic region
M41.55	Other secondary scoliosis, thoracolumbar region
M41.84	Other forms of scoliosis, thoracic region
M41.85	Other forms of scoliosis, thoracolumbar region
M86.38	Chronic multifocal osteomyelitis, other site
M86.48	Chronic osteomyelitis with draining sinus, other site
M86.58	Other chronic hematogenous osteomyelitis, other site
M86.68	Other chronic osteomyelitis, other site

M95.4	Acquired deformity of chest and rib
M99.82	Other biomechanical lesions of thoracic region
M99.88	Other biomechanical lesions of rib cage
Q67.6	Pectus excavatum
Q76.6	Other congenital malformations of ribs

Relative Value Units/Medicare Edits

Non-Facility RVU	Work	PE	MP	Total
32900	23.81	11.75	5.32	40.88
Facility RVU	Work	PE	MP	Total
32900	23.81	11.75	5.32	40.88

	FUD	Status	MUE	Modifiers				IOM Reference
32900	90	A	1(2)	51	N/A	62*	80	None

* with documentation

Terms To Know

benign. Mild or nonmalignant in nature.

deformity. Irregularity or malformation of the body.

dissection. Separating by cutting tissue or body structures apart.

excision. Surgical removal of an organ or tissue.

graft. Tissue implant from another part of the body or another person.

incision. Act of cutting into tissue or an organ.

malignant. Any condition tending to progress toward death, specifically an invasive tumor with a loss of cellular differentiation that has the ability to spread or metastasize to other body areas.

neoplasm. New abnormal growth, tumor.

ostectomy. Excision of bone.

pectus excavatum. Congenital abnormality of the anterior chest wall with depression of the sternum, sinking the appearance of the chest.

resection. Surgical removal of a part or all of an organ or body part.

sympathectomy. Surgical interruption or transection of a sympathetic nervous system pathway.

32905-32906

32905 Thoracoplasty, Schede type or extrapleural (all stages);
32906 with closure of bronchopleural fistula

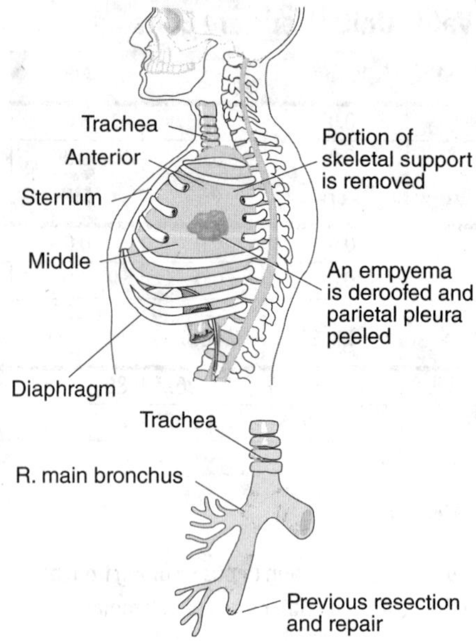

In some instances, the site of a previous bronchial surgery has developed a fistula between the stub and pleura

Explanation

The physician performs a thoracoplasty, which is the removal of the skeletal support of a portion of the chest (32905), and also closes a bronchopleural fistula (32906) to treat chronic thoracic empyema (accumulation of pus in the chest cavity) when there is insufficient lung tissue to fill the chest space. The procedure is carried out primarily on the upper chest. An incision is made through the skin down to the ribs. The Schede operation consists of the extensive unroofing of an empyema space by resecting the overlying ribs and portions of membrane lining the chest cavity (parietal pleural peel). In 32906, the bronchopleural fistula (an abnormal passageway between the remaining end of a bronchial tube that occurs sometimes after the removal of a lung or portion of a lung) is identified and resected, then closed by suturing. Closure of the fistula sometimes requires the use of muscle flap grafts taken from outside the chest cavity. The muscles in the area are partially closed over gauze packing and the skin partially closed by suturing in layers. As the packing is withdrawn in stages a few days later, it is hoped that freshly granulation tissue fills in the space formerly occupied by the empyema. The original Schede type operation is rarely performed but several modifications are currently done.

Coding Tips

For open closure of a major bronchial fistula, see 32815. For resection of the first rib for thoracic outlet syndrome, see 21615–21616.

ICD-10-CM Diagnostic Codes

A15.6	Tuberculous pleurisy
J86.0	Pyothorax with fistula
J86.9	Pyothorax without fistula

Relative Value Units/Medicare Edits

Non-Facility RVU	Work	PE	MP	Total
32905	23.29	9.86	5.52	38.67
32906	29.3	11.53	6.96	47.79
Facility RVU	**Work**	**PE**	**MP**	**Total**
32905	23.29	9.86	5.52	38.67
32906	29.3	11.53	6.96	47.79

	FUD	Status	MUE	Modifiers				IOM Reference
32905	90	A	1(2)	51	N/A	62*	80	None
32906	90	A	1(2)	51	N/A	62*	80	

* with documentation

Terms To Know

closure. Repairing an incision or wound by suture or other means.

empyema. Accumulation of pus within the respiratory or pleural cavity.

fistula. Abnormal tube-like passage between two body cavities or organs or from an organ to the outside surface.

graft. Tissue implant from another part of the body or another person.

granulation tissue. Loose collection of fibroblasts, inflammatory cells, and new vessels in an edematous fleshy projection that forms at the base of open wounds over which new skin forms, unless excessive granulation tissue, or proud flesh, rises above the wound surface.

incision. Act of cutting into tissue or an organ.

open fracture. Exposed break in a bone, always considered compound due to its high risk of infection from the open wound leading to the fracture. Broken bone ends may protrude through the skin and contaminants or foreign bodies are often embedded in the tissues.

resection. Surgical removal of a part or all of an organ or body part.

spontaneous tension pneumothorax. Air leaking from the lung and trapped in the lung lining.

32940

32940 Pneumonolysis, extraperiosteal, including filling or packing procedures

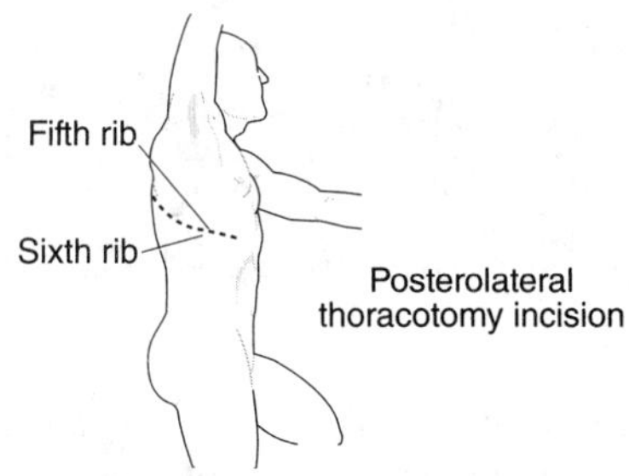

Adhesions between lung tissue and the inside surface of the chest cavity are released in an open surgical procedure

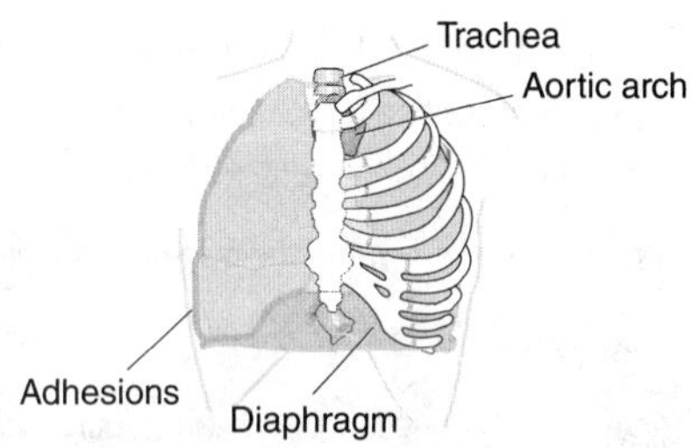

Following lysis, the pleural space may require packing or filling to prevent scar tissue development

Explanation

The physician opens the chest cavity and separates the surface of the lung which has become adherent to the inside surface of the chest cavity. Using a scalpel, the surgeon makes an incision around the side of the chest between two of the ribs. The incision is carried through all the tissue layers down to the tissue lining the chest cavity. Rib spreaders are inserted into the wound and the ribs are spread apart exposing the membrane lining the chest cavity (the parietal pleura). The surgeon separates the tissue between the periosteal membrane adherent to the inside surface of the lung and the parietal pleural membrane. This allows the movement of the lung within the chest cavity. The area or space created is packed or filled and the incision is closed in layers of sutures.

Coding Tips

Pneumolysis procedures are defined by site. Code 32940 reports extraperiosteal lysis of adhesions. For major thoracotomy with open intrapleural pneumonolysis, see 32124. For surgical thoracoscopy with total pulmonary decortication, including intrapleural pneumonolysis, see 32652.

ICD-10-CM Diagnostic Codes

A15.0	Tuberculosis of lung
A15.6	Tuberculous pleurisy
B90.9	Sequelae of respiratory and unspecified tuberculosis

Relative Value Units/Medicare Edits

Non-Facility RVU	Work	PE	MP	Total
32940	21.34	9.31	5.07	35.72
Facility RVU	**Work**	**PE**	**MP**	**Total**
32940	21.34	9.31	5.07	35.72

	FUD	Status	MUE	Modifiers				IOM Reference
32940	90	A	1(3)	51	N/A	62*	80	None

* with documentation

Terms To Know

adhesion. Abnormal fibrous connection between two structures, soft tissue or bony structures, that may occur as the result of surgery, infection, or trauma.

decortication. Removal of the cortical substance, the encapsulating or encasing material, of an organ, such as the kidneys or lungs.

emphysema. Pathological condition in which there is destructive enlargement of the air sacs in the lungs resulting in damage and lack of elasticity to the alveolar walls, commonly seen in long-term smokers.

empyema. Accumulation of pus within the respiratory or pleural cavity.

incision. Act of cutting into tissue or an organ.

late effect. Abnormality, dysfunction, or other residual condition produced after the acute phase of an illness, injury, or disease is over. There is no time limit on when late effects can appear.

lysis. Destruction, breakdown, dissolution, or decomposition of cells or substances by a specific catalyzing agent.

pleurisy. Inflammation of the serous membrane that lines the lungs and the thoracic cavity. Pleurisy may cause effusion within the cavity or have exudate in the pleural space or on the membrane surface.

pneumolysis. Breakdown of tissue attaching the lungs to the wall of the chest cavity, causing lung collapse.

thoracotomy. Surgical procedure for opening the chest wall in order to access the lungs, esophagus, trachea, aorta, heart, and diaphragm.

32960

32960 Pneumothorax, therapeutic, intrapleural injection of air

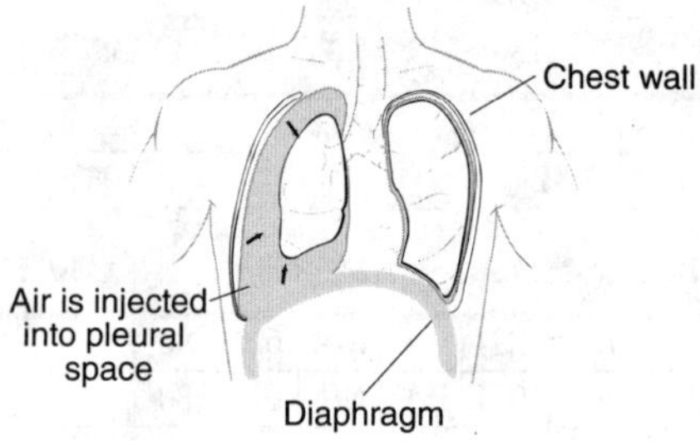

A pleural cavity is normally negatively pressurized and the introduction of atmospheric air causes the lung to begin to collapse

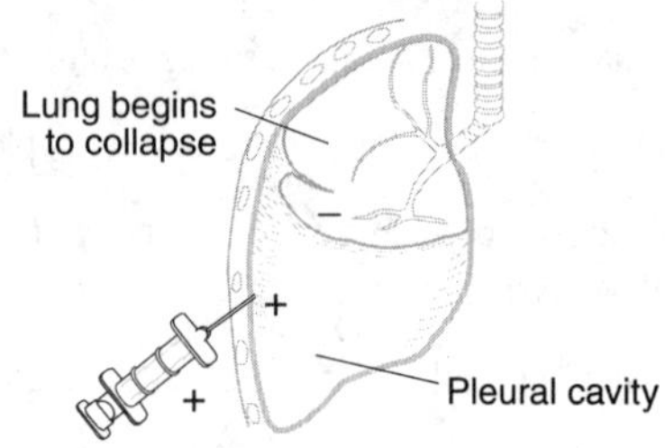

Air is injected into the thoracic cavity for therapeutic purposes

Explanation

The physician partially collapses a lung by injecting air into the chest cavity by puncturing through the space between the ribs. Using a needle attached to a syringe the physician passes the needle over the top of a rib and punctures through the chest tissues and enters the pleural cavity. With the end of the needle in the chest cavity, the physician injects air into the chest cavity to create a partial collapse of one lung, most commonly used to treat tuberculosis. A small plastic tube may be passed through the chest and left in place for repeated injections of air.

Coding Tips

This procedure reports the surgical creation of a pneumothorax used to treat pulmonary effusion, tuberculosis, and other conditions. Do not confuse with procedures performed to correct a spontaneous or traumatic pneumothorax. For thoracentesis for aspiration of the pleural space, see 32554 and 32555. For chemical pleurodesis for recurrent or persistent pneumothorax, see 32560.

ICD-10-CM Diagnostic Codes

A15.0	Tuberculosis of lung
A15.6	Tuberculous pleurisy
A15.7	Primary respiratory tuberculosis
A15.8	Other respiratory tuberculosis
A15.9	Respiratory tuberculosis unspecified
B90.9	Sequelae of respiratory and unspecified tuberculosis

Relative Value Units/Medicare Edits

Non-Facility RVU	Work	PE	MP	Total
32960	1.84	1.63	0.14	3.61
Facility RVU	**Work**	**PE**	**MP**	**Total**
32960	1.84	0.65	0.14	2.63

	FUD	Status	MUE	Modifiers				IOM Reference
32960	0	A	1(2)	51	N/A	N/A	N/A	None

* with documentation

Terms To Know

abscess. Circumscribed collection of pus resulting from bacteria, frequently associated with swelling and other signs of inflammation.

effusion. Escape of fluid from within a body cavity.

hemoptysis. Coughing up or spitting out blood or blood-streaked sputum.

iatrogenic pneumothorax. Air trapped in the lining of the lung following surgery.

pleurisy. Inflammation of the serous membrane that lines the lungs and the thoracic cavity. Pleurisy may cause effusion within the cavity or have exudate in the pleural space or on the membrane surface.

pleurodesis. Injection of a sclerosing agent into the pleural space for creating adhesions between the parietal and the visceral pleura to treat a collapsed lung caused by air trapped in the pleural cavity, or severe cases of pleural effusion.

thoracentesis. Surgical puncture of the chest cavity with a specialized needle or hollow tubing to aspirate fluid from within the pleural space for diagnostic or therapeutic reasons.

32997

32997 Total lung lavage (unilateral)

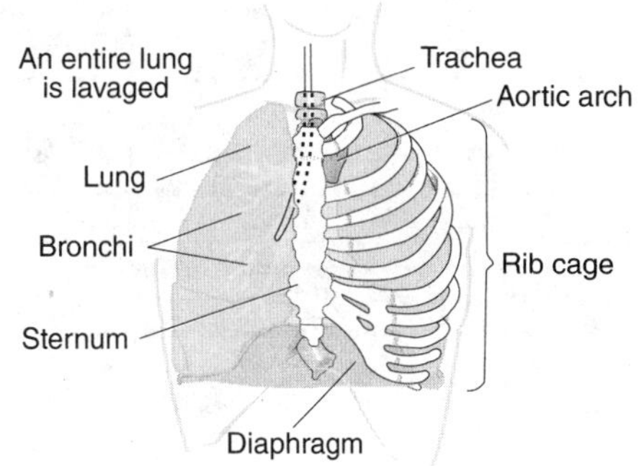

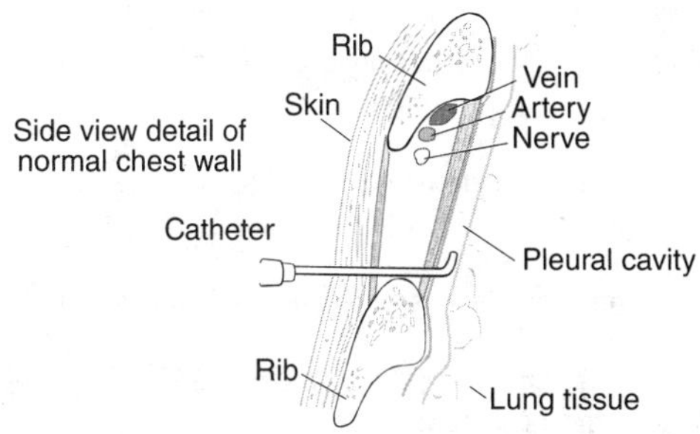

Explanation

The physician performs total lavage on one lung. The physician views the airway using a fiberoptic or rigid bronchoscopy. The airway is anesthetized and the bronchoscope is introduced through the nasal or oral cavity and advanced to the lungs. Saline is introduced through the bronchoscope and the lung tissue is washed or bathed. The saline is removed by suction and the solution containing the cells that have been obtained in the procedure may be sent to pathology to diagnosis certain diseases, such as cancer. The procedure also may be performed to treat specific diseases or injuries.

Coding Tips

This is a unilateral procedure. If performed bilaterally, some payers require that the service be reported twice with modifier 50 appended to the second code, while others require identification of the service only once with modifier 50 appended. Check with individual payers. Modifier 50 identifies a procedure performed identically on the opposite side of the body (mirror image). For bronchial alveolar lavage performed endoscopically, see 31624.

ICD-10-CM Diagnostic Codes

E84.0	Cystic fibrosis with pulmonary manifestations
J44.0	Chronic obstructive pulmonary disease with (acute) lower respiratory infection
J44.1	Chronic obstructive pulmonary disease with (acute) exacerbation
J45.22	Mild intermittent asthma with status asthmaticus
J45.32	Mild persistent asthma with status asthmaticus
J45.42	Moderate persistent asthma with status asthmaticus
J45.52	Severe persistent asthma with status asthmaticus
J68.0	Bronchitis and pneumonitis due to chemicals, gases, fumes and vapors
J69.0	Pneumonitis due to inhalation of food and vomit
J69.1	Pneumonitis due to inhalation of oils and essences
J69.8	Pneumonitis due to inhalation of other solids and liquids

J84.01 Alveolar proteinosis

AMA: **32997** 2018,Jan,8; 2017,Jan,8; 2016,Jan,13; 2015,Jan,16; 2014,Jan,11

Relative Value Units/Medicare Edits

Non-Facility RVU	Work	PE	MP	Total
32997	7.31	1.99	0.54	9.84
Facility RVU	**Work**	**PE**	**MP**	**Total**
32997	7.31	1.99	0.54	9.84

	FUD	Status	MUE	Modifiers				IOM Reference
32997	0	A	1(2)	51	50	N/A	N/A	None

* with documentation

Terms To Know

abscess. Circumscribed collection of pus resulting from bacteria, frequently associated with swelling and other signs of inflammation.

catheter. Flexible tube inserted into an area of the body for introducing or withdrawing fluid.

empyema. Accumulation of pus within the respiratory or pleural cavity.

fistula. Abnormal tube-like passage between two body cavities or organs or from an organ to the outside surface.

instillation. Administering a liquid slowly over time, drop by drop.

intubation. Insertion of a tube into a hollow organ, canal, or cavity within the body.

lavage. Washing.

32998 [32994]

32998 Ablation therapy for reduction or eradication of 1 or more pulmonary tumor(s) including pleura or chest wall when involved by tumor extension, percutaneous, including imaging guidance when performed, unilateral; radiofrequency

32994 Ablation therapy for reduction or eradication of 1 or more pulmonary tumor(s) including pleura or chest wall when involved by tumor extension, percutaneous, including imaging guidance when performed, unilateral; cryoablation

In a percutaneous approach, radiofrequency is used to destroy or reduce a pulmonary tumor

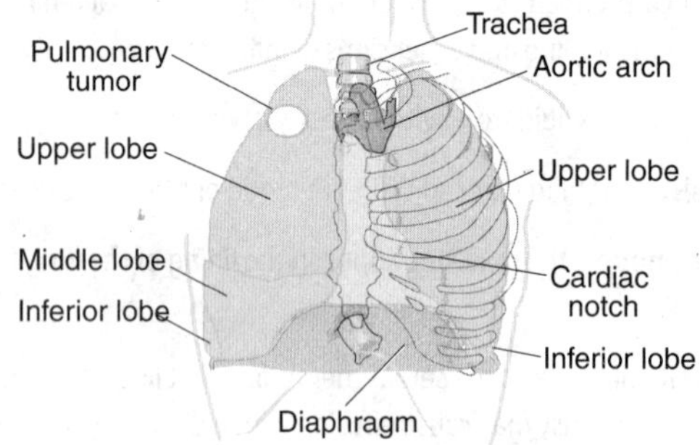

Explanation

In a minimally invasive procedure, the physician uses the heat created from high-frequency radiowaves to destroy one or more tumors in the lung, pleura, or chest wall. A small incision is made in the skin of the chest and the lesion is accessed by inserting an ablation probe connected to a radiofrequency generator between the ribs. Under imaging guidance, the ablation probe is advanced into the lesion of the lung, pleura, or chest wall. Treatment with the heat probe usually takes several minutes and may include repositioning the probe within the lesion so that overlapping ablations treat the entire tumor. The incision is closed with sutures. This process may be repeated for multiple lesions within the same lung. Report 32994 when the procedure is performed using cryoablation. Imaging guidance is included in these procedures, when performed.

Coding Tips

These are unilateral procedures. If performed bilaterally, some payers require that the service be reported twice with modifier 50 appended to the second code, while others require identification of the service only once with modifier 50 appended. Check with individual payers. Modifier 50 identifies a procedure performed identically on the opposite side of the body (mirror image).

ICD-10-CM Diagnostic Codes

C34.11 Malignant neoplasm of upper lobe, right bronchus or lung ☑

C34.12 Malignant neoplasm of upper lobe, left bronchus or lung ☑

C34.2 Malignant neoplasm of middle lobe, bronchus or lung

C34.31 Malignant neoplasm of lower lobe, right bronchus or lung ☑

C34.32 Malignant neoplasm of lower lobe, left bronchus or lung ☑

C34.81 Malignant neoplasm of overlapping sites of right bronchus and lung ☑

C34.82 Malignant neoplasm of overlapping sites of left bronchus and lung ☑

C38.4 Malignant neoplasm of pleura

C38.8 Malignant neoplasm of overlapping sites of heart, mediastinum and pleura

C45.0	Mesothelioma of pleura
C49.3	Malignant neoplasm of connective and soft tissue of thorax
C78.01	Secondary malignant neoplasm of right lung ☑
C78.02	Secondary malignant neoplasm of left lung ☑
C78.2	Secondary malignant neoplasm of pleura
C7A.090	Malignant carcinoid tumor of the bronchus and lung
D02.20	Carcinoma in situ of unspecified bronchus and lung
D02.21	Carcinoma in situ of right bronchus and lung ☑
D02.22	Carcinoma in situ of left bronchus and lung ☑
D14.31	Benign neoplasm of right bronchus and lung ☑
D14.32	Benign neoplasm of left bronchus and lung ☑
D19.0	Benign neoplasm of mesothelial tissue of pleura
D38.1	Neoplasm of uncertain behavior of trachea, bronchus and lung
D38.2	Neoplasm of uncertain behavior of pleura
D3A.090	Benign carcinoid tumor of the bronchus and lung
J91.0	Malignant pleural effusion

AMA: 32994 2018,Jan,8; 2017,Nov,8 **32998** 2018,Jan,8; 2017,Nov,8

Relative Value Units/Medicare Edits

Non-Facility RVU	Work	PE	MP	Total
32998	9.03	90.79	0.8	100.62
32994	9.03	149.65	0.83	159.51
Facility RVU	**Work**	**PE**	**MP**	**Total**
32998	9.03	2.99	0.8	12.82
32994	9.03	3.35	0.83	13.21

	FUD	Status	MUE	Modifiers				IOM Reference
32998	0	A	1(2)	51	50	N/A	80	None
32994	0	A	1(2)	51	50	N/A	80	

* with documentation

Terms To Know

ablation. Removal or destruction of a body part or tissue or its function. Ablation may be performed by surgical means, hormones, drugs, radiofrequency, heat, chemical application, or other methods.

mediastinum. Collection of organs and tissues that separate the pleural sacs. Located between the sternum and spine above the diaphragm, it contains the heart and great vessels, trachea and bronchi, esophagus, thymus, lymph nodes, and nerves.

pleura. One of the two membranes that surround the lungs. The visceral pleura encases the lung and the parietal pleura lines the inner chest walls.

33016

● **33016** Pericardiocentesis, including imaging guidance, when performed

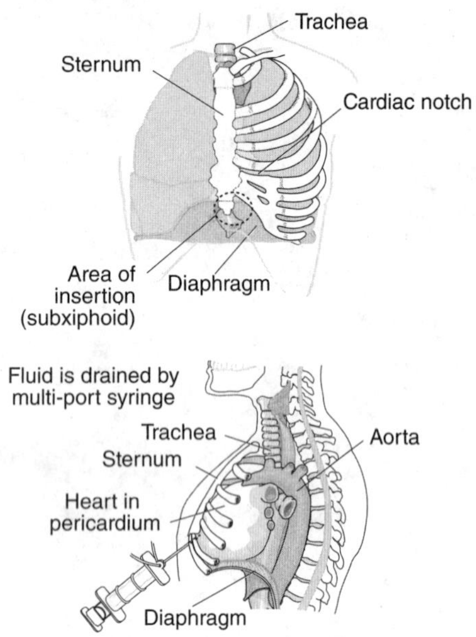

A centesis syringe is inserted into the pericardial sac and excess fluid is aspirated

Explanation

The physician drains fluid from the pericardial space. The physician may perform this procedure using anatomic landmarks or under fluoroscopic or echocardiographic (ultrasound) guidance, which is not separately reportable. The physician places a long needle below the sternum and directs it into the pericardial space. When pericardial fluid is aspirated, the physician may advance a guidewire through the needle into the pericardial space and exchange the needle over the guidewire for a drainage catheter. The physician removes as much pericardial fluid as is required, removes the needle or catheter, and dresses the wound.

Coding Tips

When medically necessary, report moderate (conscious) sedation provided by the performing physician with 99151–99153. When provided by another physician, report 99155–99157. Imaging guidance is included in this procedure and is not reported separately. Do not report 33016 with 76942, 77002, 77012, or 77021. Do not report 33016 with 93303–93325 when echocardiography is performed solely for pericardiocentesis guidance. For pericardial drainage, see 33017–33019.

ICD-10-CM Diagnostic Codes

A18.84	Tuberculosis of heart
A39.53	Meningococcal pericarditis
A43.8	Other forms of nocardiosis
A52.06	Other syphilitic heart involvement
A54.83	Gonococcal heart infection
B33.23	Viral pericarditis
C38.0	Malignant neoplasm of heart
C45.2	Mesothelioma of pericardium
C79.89	Secondary malignant neoplasm of other specified sites
D15.1	Benign neoplasm of heart
D48.7	Neoplasm of uncertain behavior of other specified sites
I01.0	Acute rheumatic pericarditis
I09.2	Chronic rheumatic pericarditis
I23.0	Hemopericardium as current complication following acute myocardial infarction
I24.1	Dressler's syndrome
I30.0	Acute nonspecific idiopathic pericarditis
I30.1	Infective pericarditis
I30.8	Other forms of acute pericarditis
I31.0	Chronic adhesive pericarditis
I31.1	Chronic constrictive pericarditis
I31.2	Hemopericardium, not elsewhere classified
I31.3	Pericardial effusion (noninflammatory)
I31.4	Cardiac tamponade
I31.8	Other specified diseases of pericardium
I32	Pericarditis in diseases classified elsewhere
I97.89	Other postprocedural complications and disorders of the circulatory system, not elsewhere classified
M32.12	Pericarditis in systemic lupus erythematosus
P29.89	Other cardiovascular disorders originating in the perinatal period
P54.8	Other specified neonatal hemorrhages
S26.01XA	Contusion of heart with hemopericardium, initial encounter
S26.09XA	Other injury of heart with hemopericardium, initial encounter
T86.298	Other complications of heart transplant
T86.39	Other complications of heart-lung transplant

Relative Value Units/Medicare Edits

Non-Facility RVU	Work	PE	MP	Total
33016				
Facility RVU	**Work**	**PE**	**MP**	**Total**
33016				

	FUD	Status	MUE	Modifiers				IOM Reference
33016	N/A		-	N/A	N/A	N/A	N/A	None

* with documentation

Terms To Know

percutaneous. Through the skin.

pericardiocentesis. Puncture of a cavity for the purpose of removing fluid from the pericardial sac.

33017-33018

- **33017** Pericardial drainage with insertion of indwelling catheter, percutaneous, including fluoroscopy and/or ultrasound guidance, when performed; 6 years and older without congenital cardiac anomaly
- **33018** birth through 5 years of age or any age with congenital cardiac anomaly

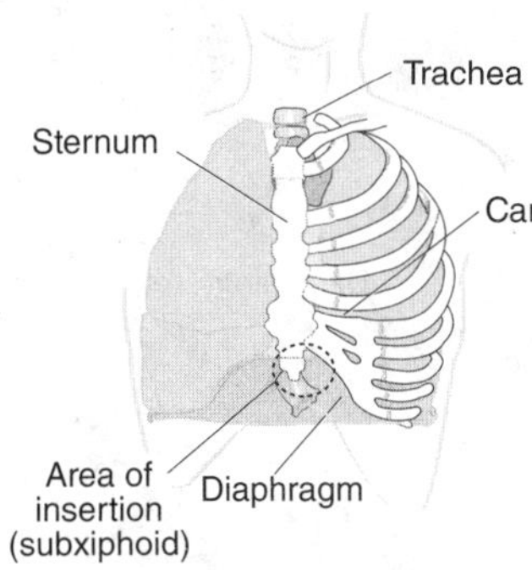

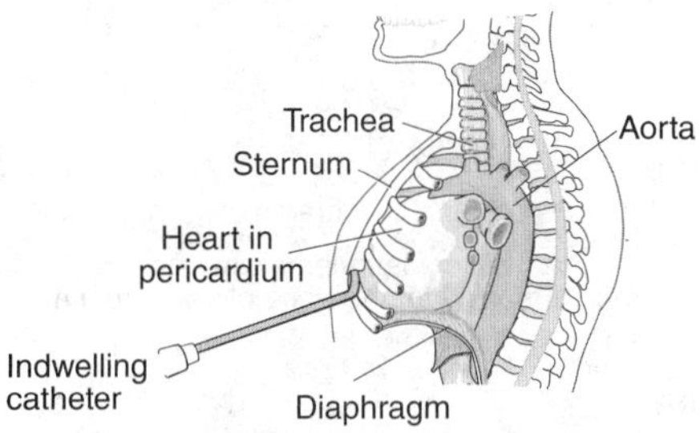

Indwelling catheter is inserted percutaneously for drainage of pericardium

Explanation

The physician drains fluid from the pericardial space. The physician may perform these procedures using anatomic landmarks or under fluoroscopic or echocardiographic (ultrasound) guidance, which is included in these codes and not reported separately. The physician places a long needle percutaneously below the sternum and directs it into the pericardial space. When pericardial fluid flows back through the needle, the physician passes a guidewire through the needle into the pericardial space. The physician exchanges the needle over the wire for an indwelling drainage catheter. The physician attaches the catheter to a drainage bag, sutures the indwelling catheter into place on the chest wall, and dresses the wound. Report 33017 when the procedure is performed on ages 6 years and older without a congenital cardiac anomaly. Report 33018 when the procedure is performed on newborns to 5 years of age with a congenital cardiac anomaly, such as dextrocardia, heterotaxy, mesocardia, or a single ventricle anomaly, or for any age within the first 90-day postop period following surgical repair of a congenital cardiac anomaly.

Coding Tips

When medically necessary, report moderate (conscious) sedation provided by the performing physician with 99151–99153. When provided by another physician, report 99155–99157. Imaging guidance is included in these procedures and is not reported separately. Do not report 33017 or 33018 with 75989, 76942, 77002, 77012, or 77021. Do not report 33017 or 33018 with 93303–93325 when echocardiography is performed solely for pericardiocentesis guidance. Do not report these codes when a catheter is placed to aspirate fluid and then removed at the end of the procedure. For pericardiocentesis, see 33016.

ICD-10-CM Diagnostic Codes

A18.84	Tuberculosis of heart
A39.53	Meningococcal pericarditis
A43.8	Other forms of nocardiosis
A52.06	Other syphilitic heart involvement
A54.83	Gonococcal heart infection
B33.23	Viral pericarditis
C38.0	Malignant neoplasm of heart
C45.2	Mesothelioma of pericardium
C79.89	Secondary malignant neoplasm of other specified sites
D15.1	Benign neoplasm of heart
D48.7	Neoplasm of uncertain behavior of other specified sites
I01.0	Acute rheumatic pericarditis
I09.2	Chronic rheumatic pericarditis
I23.0	Hemopericardium as current complication following acute myocardial infarction
I24.1	Dressler's syndrome
I30.0	Acute nonspecific idiopathic pericarditis
I30.1	Infective pericarditis
I30.8	Other forms of acute pericarditis
I31.0	Chronic adhesive pericarditis
I31.1	Chronic constrictive pericarditis
I31.2	Hemopericardium, not elsewhere classified
I31.3	Pericardial effusion (noninflammatory)
I31.4	Cardiac tamponade
I31.8	Other specified diseases of pericardium
I32	Pericarditis in diseases classified elsewhere
I97.89	Other postprocedural complications and disorders of the circulatory system, not elsewhere classified
M32.12	Pericarditis in systemic lupus erythematosus
P29.89	Other cardiovascular disorders originating in the perinatal period
P54.8	Other specified neonatal hemorrhages
Q20.4	Double inlet ventricle
Q20.6	Isomerism of atrial appendages
Q24.0	Dextrocardia
Q24.8	Other specified congenital malformations of heart
Q89.3	Situs inversus
S26.01XA	Contusion of heart with hemopericardium, initial encounter
S26.09XA	Other injury of heart with hemopericardium, initial encounter
T86.298	Other complications of heart transplant
T86.39	Other complications of heart-lung transplant

Relative Value Units/Medicare Edits

Non-Facility RVU	Work	PE	MP	Total
33017				
33018				
Facility RVU	**Work**	**PE**	**MP**	**Total**
33017				
33018				

	FUD	Status	MUE	Modifiers				IOM Reference
33017	N/A		-	N/A	N/A	N/A	N/A	None
33018	N/A		-	N/A	N/A	N/A	N/A	

* with documentation

Terms To Know

congenital. Present at birth, occurring through heredity or an influence during gestation up to the moment of birth.

fluoroscopy. Radiology technique that allows visual examination of part of the body or a function of an organ using a device that projects an x-ray image on a fluorescent screen.

percutaneous approach. Method used to gain access to a body organ or specific area by puncture or minor incision through the skin or mucous membrane and/or any other body layers necessary to reach the procedure site.

ultrasound. Imaging using ultra-high sound frequency bounced off body structures.

33019

● **33019** Pericardial drainage with insertion of indwelling catheter, percutaneous, including CT guidance

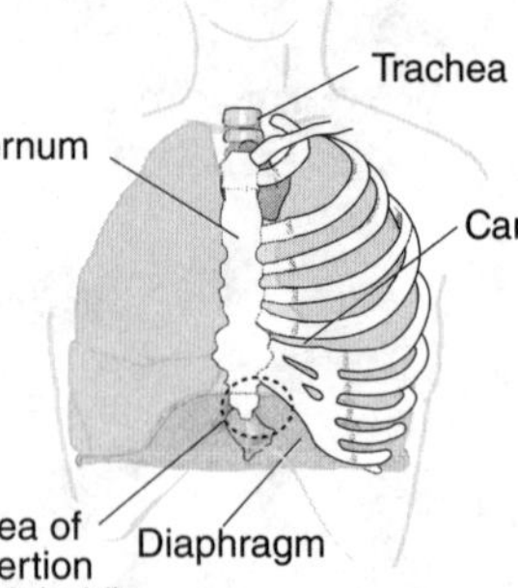

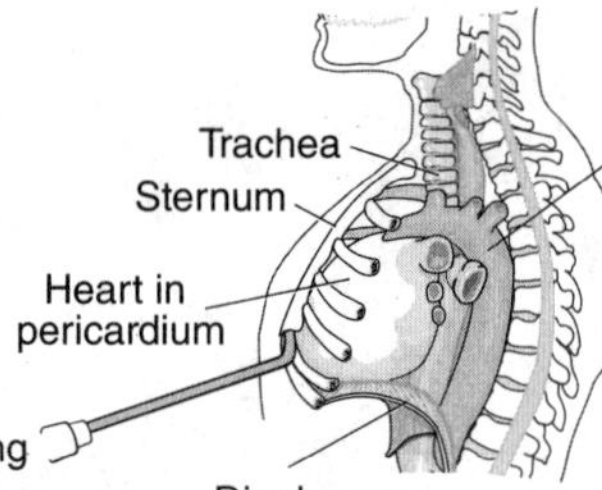

Indwelling catheter is inserted percutaneously for drainage of pericardium

Explanation

The physician drains fluid from the pericardial space. The physician performs this procedure under CT guidance, which is included in this code and not reported separately. The physician places a long needle percutaneously below the sternum and directs it into the pericardial space. When pericardial fluid flows back through the needle, the physician passes a guidewire through the needle into the pericardial space. The physician exchanges the needle over the wire for an indwelling drainage catheter. The physician attaches the catheter to a drainage bag, sutures the indwelling catheter into place on the chest wall, and dresses the wound.

Coding Tips

When medically necessary, report moderate (conscious) sedation provided by the performing physician with 99151–99153. When provided by another physician, report 99155–99157. Imaging (CT) guidance is included in this procedure and is not reported separately. Do not report 33019 with 75989, 76942, 77002, 77012, or 77021. Do not report 33019 when a catheter is placed to aspirate fluid and then removed at the end of the procedure. For pericardial drainage with insertion of an indwelling catheter, percutaneous, using fluoroscopy and/or ultrasound guidance, see 33017–33018.

ICD-10-CM Diagnostic Codes

A18.84	Tuberculosis of heart
A39.53	Meningococcal pericarditis
A43.8	Other forms of nocardiosis
A52.06	Other syphilitic heart involvement
A54.83	Gonococcal heart infection
B33.23	Viral pericarditis
C38.0	Malignant neoplasm of heart
C45.2	Mesothelioma of pericardium
C79.89	Secondary malignant neoplasm of other specified sites

D15.1 Benign neoplasm of heart
D48.7 Neoplasm of uncertain behavior of other specified sites
D49.89 Neoplasm of unspecified behavior of other specified sites
I01.0 Acute rheumatic pericarditis
I09.2 Chronic rheumatic pericarditis
I23.0 Hemopericardium as current complication following acute myocardial infarction
I24.1 Dressler's syndrome
I30.0 Acute nonspecific idiopathic pericarditis
I30.1 Infective pericarditis
I30.8 Other forms of acute pericarditis
I31.0 Chronic adhesive pericarditis
I31.1 Chronic constrictive pericarditis
I31.2 Hemopericardium, not elsewhere classified
I31.3 Pericardial effusion (noninflammatory)
I31.4 Cardiac tamponade
I31.8 Other specified diseases of pericardium
I32 Pericarditis in diseases classified elsewhere
I97.89 Other postprocedural complications and disorders of the circulatory system, not elsewhere classified
M32.12 Pericarditis in systemic lupus erythematosus
P29.89 Other cardiovascular disorders originating in the perinatal period
P54.8 Other specified neonatal hemorrhages
S26.01XA Contusion of heart with hemopericardium, initial encounter
S26.09XA Other injury of heart with hemopericardium, initial encounter
T86.298 Other complications of heart transplant
T86.39 Other complications of heart-lung transplant

Relative Value Units/Medicare Edits

Non-Facility RVU	Work	PE	MP	Total
33019				
Facility RVU	**Work**	**PE**	**MP**	**Total**
33019				

	FUD	Status	MUE	Modifiers				IOM Reference
33019	N/A		-	N/A	N/A	N/A	N/A	None

* with documentation

33020

33020 Pericardiotomy for removal of clot or foreign body (primary procedure)

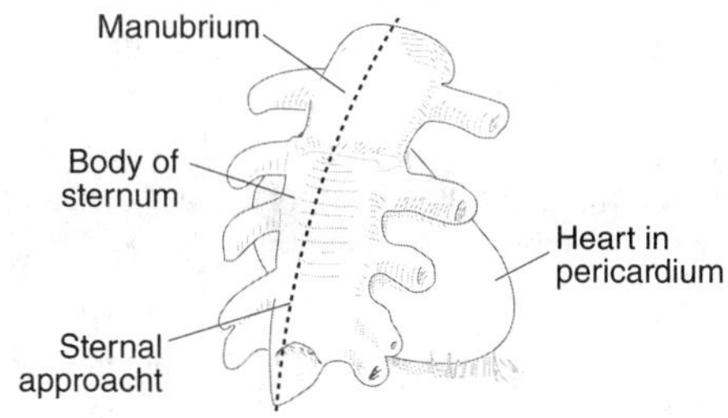

The pericardium is accessed, typically via the sternum, and a clot or foreign body is removed

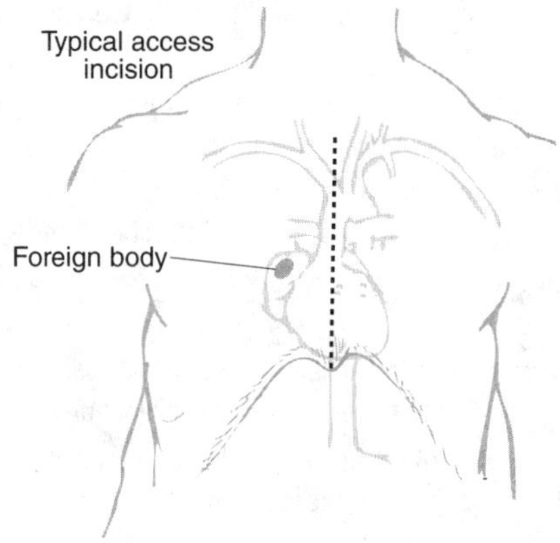

Explanation

The physician removes a clot or foreign body from the pericardial space. The physician performs a midline sternotomy, incising skin, fascia, and the sternum. The pericardium is incised and the clot or foreign body is removed. The pericardium is repaired loosely, leaving gaps for blood and fluid to drain into the pleural space. The sternum is reanastomosed with sternal wires and the skin is sutured in layers. In a less invasive approach for smaller clots or foreign matter, a needle is inserted through the skin under the sternum until it reaches the pericardial sac guided by fluoroscopy or echocardiography. A catheter is inserted to retrieve foreign matter or a catheter with a balloon attachment may also be used. The inflation of the balloon creates an opening within the desired location. The balloon catheter is removed and replaced with another catheter used to retrieve the foreign matter or clot.

Coding Tips

If this procedure is attempted thoracoscopically, but requires thoracotomy for completion, report 33020 for the open portion of the procedure and report a diagnostic thoracoscopy, 32601, as a secondary procedure. Do not report 33020 with 32551 if a pleural drain is placed on the same side. For thoracoscopic removal of a pericardial blood clot or foreign body, see 32658.

ICD-10-CM Diagnostic Codes

I30.0 Acute nonspecific idiopathic pericarditis
I30.8 Other forms of acute pericarditis
I31.1 Chronic constrictive pericarditis
I31.2 Hemopericardium, not elsewhere classified
I31.3 Pericardial effusion (noninflammatory)

S21.311A Laceration without foreign body of right front wall of thorax with penetration into thoracic cavity, initial encounter ☑
S21.312A Laceration without foreign body of left front wall of thorax with penetration into thoracic cavity, initial encounter ☑
S21.321A Laceration with foreign body of right front wall of thorax with penetration into thoracic cavity, initial encounter ☑
S21.322A Laceration with foreign body of left front wall of thorax with penetration into thoracic cavity, initial encounter ☑
S21.331A Puncture wound without foreign body of right front wall of thorax with penetration into thoracic cavity, initial encounter ☑
S21.332A Puncture wound without foreign body of left front wall of thorax with penetration into thoracic cavity, initial encounter ☑
S21.341A Puncture wound with foreign body of right front wall of thorax with penetration into thoracic cavity, initial encounter ☑
S21.342A Puncture wound with foreign body of left front wall of thorax with penetration into thoracic cavity, initial encounter ☑
S21.351A Open bite of right front wall of thorax with penetration into thoracic cavity, initial encounter ☑
S21.352A Open bite of left front wall of thorax with penetration into thoracic cavity, initial encounter ☑
S21.411A Laceration without foreign body of right back wall of thorax with penetration into thoracic cavity, initial encounter ☑
S21.412A Laceration without foreign body of left back wall of thorax with penetration into thoracic cavity, initial encounter ☑
S21.421A Laceration with foreign body of right back wall of thorax with penetration into thoracic cavity, initial encounter ☑
S21.422A Laceration with foreign body of left back wall of thorax with penetration into thoracic cavity, initial encounter ☑
S21.431A Puncture wound without foreign body of right back wall of thorax with penetration into thoracic cavity, initial encounter ☑
S21.432A Puncture wound without foreign body of left back wall of thorax with penetration into thoracic cavity, initial encounter ☑
S21.441A Puncture wound with foreign body of right back wall of thorax with penetration into thoracic cavity, initial encounter ☑
S21.442A Puncture wound with foreign body of left back wall of thorax with penetration into thoracic cavity, initial encounter ☑
S21.451A Open bite of right back wall of thorax with penetration into thoracic cavity, initial encounter ☑
S21.452A Open bite of left back wall of thorax with penetration into thoracic cavity, initial encounter ☑
S26.01XA Contusion of heart with hemopericardium, initial encounter
S26.020A Mild laceration of heart with hemopericardium, initial encounter
S26.021A Moderate laceration of heart with hemopericardium, initial encounter
S26.022A Major laceration of heart with hemopericardium, initial encounter
S26.09XA Other injury of heart with hemopericardium, initial encounter
S26.11XA Contusion of heart without hemopericardium, initial encounter
S26.12XA Laceration of heart without hemopericardium, initial encounter
S26.19XA Other injury of heart without hemopericardium, initial encounter
S28.0XXA Crushed chest, initial encounter
S38.1XXA Crushing injury of abdomen, lower back, and pelvis, initial encounter

AMA: 33020 1997,Nov,1

Relative Value Units/Medicare Edits

Non-Facility RVU	Work	PE	MP	Total
33020	14.95	7.03	3.4	25.38
Facility RVU	**Work**	**PE**	**MP**	**Total**
33020	14.95	7.03	3.4	25.38

	FUD	Status	MUE	Modifiers				IOM Reference
33020	90	A	1(3)	51	N/A	62*	80	None

* with documentation

Terms To Know

fluoroscopy. Radiology technique that allows visual examination of part of the body or a function of an organ using a device that projects an x-ray image on a fluorescent screen.

pericardium. Thin and slippery case in which the heart lies that is lined with fluid so that the heart is free to pulse and move as it beats.

sternotomy. Incision into the sternum, the bone that forms the front of the chest cavity and connects with the ribs.

33025

33025 Creation of pericardial window or partial resection for drainage

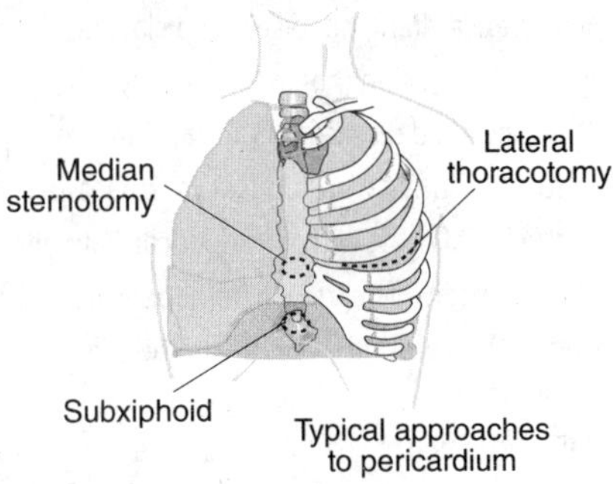

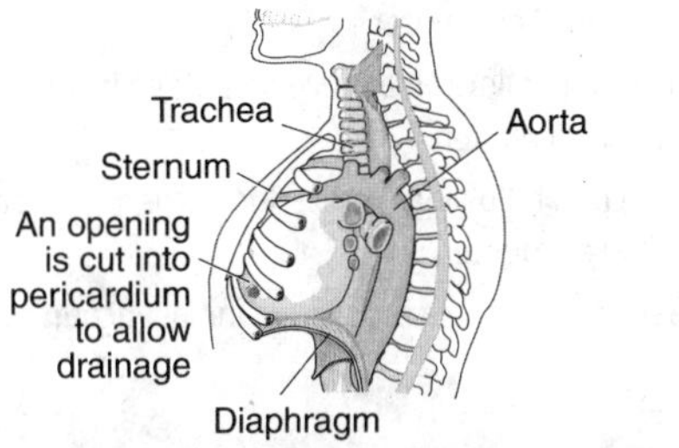

The pericardium is surgically accessed and constricting pericardial matter is removed from around the ventricle (partial) and sometimes from around the atria and cavae (total)

Explanation

The physician gains access to the pericardium in one of three ways: an incision into the subxiphoid space, the chest wall (thoracotomy), or thoracoscopically. The physician may make an incision in the pericardium or use electrocautery to open the pericardium large enough to allow drainage of pericardial fluid into the pleural space. This may require the use of a clamp or forceps to retract the surrounding tissues; however, if the pericardium is distended, a needle aspiration may be utilized under thoracoscopic guidance. The physician closes the sternal or chest wall incision and dresses the wound. The physician may leave chest tubes and/or a mediastinal drainage tube in place following the procedure.

Coding Tips

If this procedure is attempted thoracoscopically, but requires thoracotomy for completion, report 33025 for the open portion of the procedure and report a diagnostic thoracoscopy, 32601, as a secondary procedure. Thoracentesis and thoracostomy are included in this procedure and should not be reported separately. Do not report 33020 with 32551 if pleural drain is placed on the same side. For thoracoscopic creation of a pericardial window or partial resection of the pericardial sac for drainage, see 32659.

ICD-10-CM Diagnostic Codes

A18.84	Tuberculosis of heart
C38.0	Malignant neoplasm of heart
C45.2	Mesothelioma of pericardium
C79.89	Secondary malignant neoplasm of other specified sites
C7B.09	Secondary carcinoid tumors of other sites
C7B.8	Other secondary neuroendocrine tumors
D15.1	Benign neoplasm of heart
I01.0	Acute rheumatic pericarditis
I24.1	Dressler's syndrome
I30.0	Acute nonspecific idiopathic pericarditis
I30.1	Infective pericarditis
I30.8	Other forms of acute pericarditis
I31.0	Chronic adhesive pericarditis
I31.1	Chronic constrictive pericarditis
I31.2	Hemopericardium, not elsewhere classified
I31.3	Pericardial effusion (noninflammatory)
I31.4	Cardiac tamponade
I31.8	Other specified diseases of pericardium
J98.51	Mediastinitis
M32.12	Pericarditis in systemic lupus erythematosus
T81.41XA	Infection following a procedure, superficial incisional surgical site, initial encounter
T81.42XA	Infection following a procedure, deep incisional surgical site, initial encounter
T81.43XA	Infection following a procedure, organ and space surgical site, initial encounter
T81.44XA	Sepsis following a procedure, initial encounter

AMA: 33025 1997,Nov,1

Relative Value Units/Medicare Edits

Non-Facility RVU	Work	PE	MP	Total
33025	13.7	6.2	3.12	23.02
Facility RVU	**Work**	**PE**	**MP**	**Total**
33025	13.7	6.2	3.12	23.02

	FUD	Status	MUE	Modifiers				IOM Reference
33025	90	A	1(2)	51	N/A	62*	80	None

* with documentation

Terms To Know

acute. Sudden, severe.

chronic. Persistent, continuing, or recurring.

neoplasm. New abnormal growth, tumor.

pericarditis. Inflammation affecting the pericardium, the fibroserous membrane that surrounds the heart.

pericardium. Thin and slippery case in which the heart lies that is lined with fluid so that the heart is free to pulse and move as it beats.

resection. Surgical removal of a part or all of an organ or body part.

thoracentesis. Surgical puncture of the chest cavity with a specialized needle or hollow tubing to aspirate fluid from within the pleural space for diagnostic or therapeutic reasons.

thoracotomy. Surgical procedure for opening the chest wall in order to access the lungs, esophagus, trachea, aorta, heart, and diaphragm.

33030-33031

33030 Pericardiectomy, subtotal or complete; without cardiopulmonary bypass

33031 with cardiopulmonary bypass

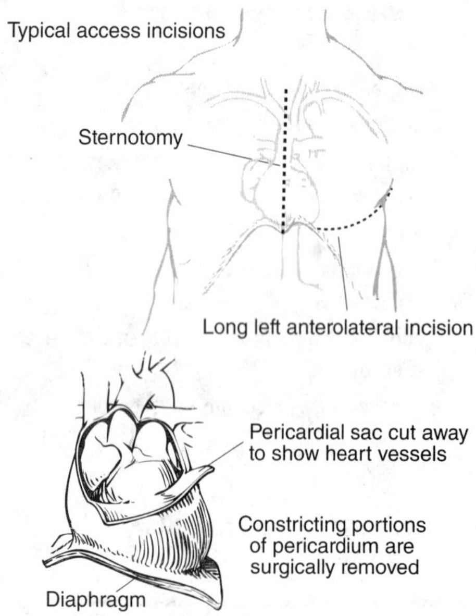

Constricting pericardial matter is removed from around the ventricle (partial) and sometimes also from around the atria and cavae (total)

Explanation

The physician gains access to the pericardium through an incision through the sternum (median sternotomy). The physician cuts away most or all of the pericardial tissue while the heart is still beating (without cardiopulmonary bypass), taking care to leave the phrenic nerves intact. The physician closes the sternal or chest wall incision and dresses the wound. The physician may leave chest tubes and/or a mediastinal drainage tube in place following the procedure. Report 33031 if the procedure is performed with cardiopulmonary bypass.

Coding Tips

If this procedure is attempted thoracoscopically, but requires thoracotomy for completion, report 33030 or 33031 for the open portion of the procedure and report a diagnostic thoracoscopy, 32601, as a secondary procedure. Thoracotomy, thoracentesis, and ECG monitoring are included and should not be reported separately.

ICD-10-CM Diagnostic Codes

A18.84	Tuberculosis of heart
C38.0	Malignant neoplasm of heart
C45.2	Mesothelioma of pericardium
C79.89	Secondary malignant neoplasm of other specified sites
C7B.09	Secondary carcinoid tumors of other sites
C7B.8	Other secondary neuroendocrine tumors
D15.1	Benign neoplasm of heart
D48.7	Neoplasm of uncertain behavior of other specified sites
I01.0	Acute rheumatic pericarditis
I24.1	Dressler's syndrome
I30.0	Acute nonspecific idiopathic pericarditis
I30.1	Infective pericarditis
I30.8	Other forms of acute pericarditis
I31.0	Chronic adhesive pericarditis
I31.1	Chronic constrictive pericarditis
I31.2	Hemopericardium, not elsewhere classified
I31.3	Pericardial effusion (noninflammatory)
I31.8	Other specified diseases of pericardium
M32.12	Pericarditis in systemic lupus erythematosus
S26.01XA	Contusion of heart with hemopericardium, initial encounter
S26.020A	Mild laceration of heart with hemopericardium, initial encounter
S26.021A	Moderate laceration of heart with hemopericardium, initial encounter
S26.022A	Major laceration of heart with hemopericardium, initial encounter
T81.41XA	Infection following a procedure, superficial incisional surgical site, initial encounter
T81.42XA	Infection following a procedure, deep incisional surgical site, initial encounter
T81.43XA	Infection following a procedure, organ and space surgical site, initial encounter
T81.44XA	Sepsis following a procedure, initial encounter

AMA: 33031 2017,Dec,3

Relative Value Units/Medicare Edits

Non-Facility RVU	Work	PE	MP	Total
33030	36.0	13.57	8.28	57.85
33031	45.0	16.23	10.34	71.57
Facility RVU	**Work**	**PE**	**MP**	**Total**
33030	36.0	13.57	8.28	57.85
33031	45.0	16.23	10.34	71.57

	FUD	Status	MUE	Modifiers				IOM Reference
33030	90	A	1(2)	51	N/A	62*	80	None
33031	90	A	1(2)	51	N/A	62*	80	

* with documentation

Terms To Know

cardiopulmonary bypass. Venous blood is diverted to a heart-lung machine, which mechanically pumps and oxygenates the blood temporarily so the heart can be bypassed while an open procedure on the heart or coronary arteries is performed. During bypass, the lungs are deflated and immobile.

late effect. Abnormality, dysfunction, or other residual condition produced after the acute phase of an illness, injury, or disease is over. There is no time limit on when late effects can appear.

thoracotomy. Surgical procedure for opening the chest wall in order to access the lungs, esophagus, trachea, aorta, heart, and diaphragm.

33050

33050 Resection of pericardial cyst or tumor

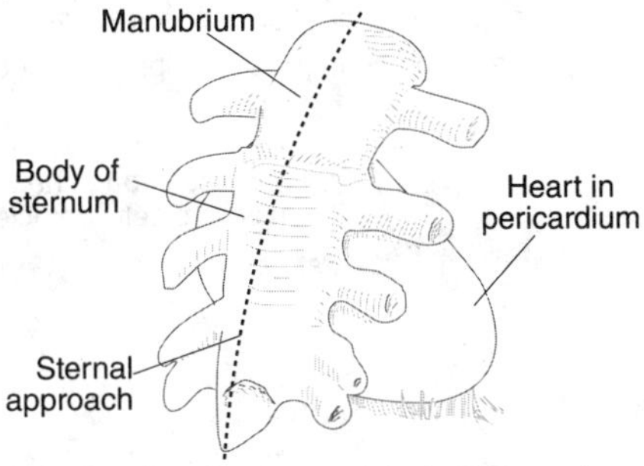

The pericardium is accessed, typically by a sternal split but other accesses may be employed. A pericardial cyst or tumor is removed

Explanation

The physician gains access to the pericardium through an incision through the sternum (median sternotomy) or the chest wall (lateral thoracotomy). If cardiopulmonary bypass is performed, the physician places cardiopulmonary bypass catheters (usually through incisions in the right atrial appendage and aorta or femoral artery). The physician stops the heart by infusing cardioplegia solution into the coronary circulation. The physician cuts away the pericardial cyst or tumor. The physician takes the patient off cardiopulmonary bypass, if used, closes the surgical incisions, and dresses the sternal or chest wall wound. The physician may leave chest tubes and/or a mediastinal drainage tube in place following the procedure.

Coding Tips

If significant additional time and effort are documented, append modifier 22 and submit a cover letter and operative report. For an open pericardial biopsy, see 39010. To report excision of a pericardial cyst, tumor, or mass thoracoscopically, see 32661. For resection of an external cardiac tumor, see 33130.

ICD-10-CM Diagnostic Codes

C45.2	Mesothelioma of pericardium
C79.89	Secondary malignant neoplasm of other specified sites
D15.1	Benign neoplasm of heart
D48.7	Neoplasm of uncertain behavior of other specified sites
D49.89	Neoplasm of unspecified behavior of other specified sites
I31.8	Other specified diseases of pericardium
Q23.8	Other congenital malformations of aortic and mitral valves
Q24.8	Other specified congenital malformations of heart

AMA: **33050** 1997,Nov,1

Relative Value Units/Medicare Edits

Non-Facility RVU	Work	PE	MP	Total
33050	16.97	8.1	4.03	29.1
Facility RVU	**Work**	**PE**	**MP**	**Total**
33050	16.97	8.1	4.03	29.1

	FUD	Status	MUE	Modifiers				IOM Reference
33050	90	A	1(2)	51	N/A	62*	80	None

* with documentation

33120-33130

33120 Excision of intracardiac tumor, resection with cardiopulmonary bypass
33130 Resection of external cardiac tumor

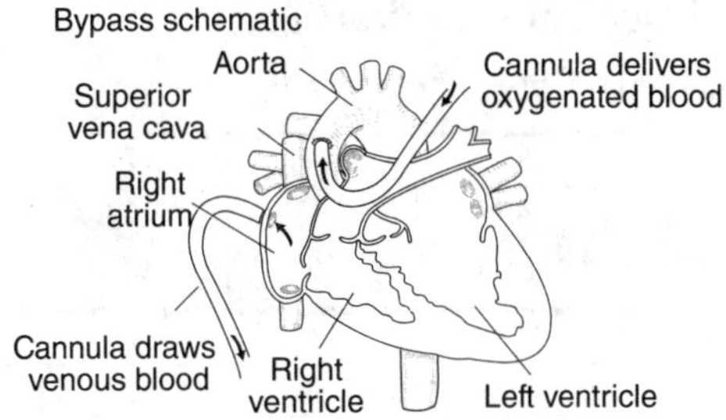

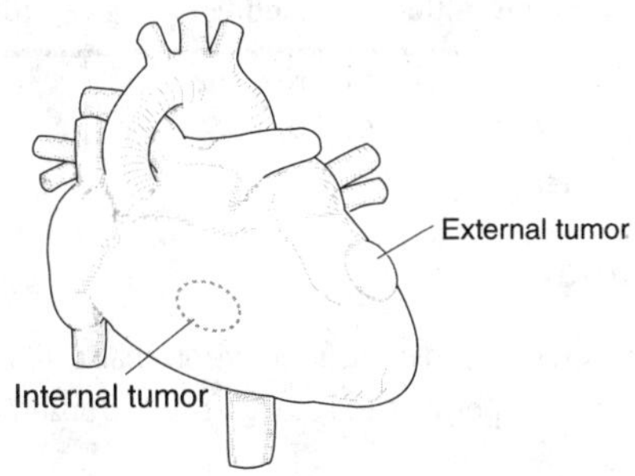

An external or internal cardiac tumor is removed

Explanation

Cardiopulmonary bypass is employed. Venous tubes are placed in both caval veins. The part of the heart which is opened depends on where the tumor is located. Every effort is made to avoid making an incision in any ventricular wall. After the heart is opened, the tumor is resected with a margin of normal heart tissue. Any problems created by this resection (damage to heart valves, holes in the walls between heart chambers or the outside of the heart, injury to coronary arteries) are repaired. All holes in the heart are closed. Cardiopulmonary bypass is stopped when heart function returns. In 33130, cardiopulmonary bypass is only required if a significant portion of the heart or major vessel must be removed with the tumor to get a margin of normal tissue around the tumor. The tumor and surrounding normal tissue are removed. Defects created in the heart, coronary arteries or major vessels are repaired.

Coding Tips

Procedure codes for reporting tumor excision of the heart are classified by site. They may be pericardial, involving only the fibroserous sac surrounding the heart; external, involving the outer portion of the heart; or internal, requiring incision into the heart wall. If significant additional time and effort is documented, append modifier 22 and submit a cover letter and operative report. For excision of a pericardial tumor, see 33050. To report myocardial resection for ventricular aneurysm, see 33542.

ICD-10-CM Diagnostic Codes

C38.0	Malignant neoplasm of heart
C45.2	Mesothelioma of pericardium
C79.89	Secondary malignant neoplasm of other specified sites
C7B.00	Secondary carcinoid tumors, unspecified site
C7B.09	Secondary carcinoid tumors of other sites
D15.1	Benign neoplasm of heart
D48.7	Neoplasm of uncertain behavior of other specified sites

D49.89 Neoplasm of unspecified behavior of other specified sites

AMA: 33120 2018,Jan,8; 2017,Jan,8; 2017,Dec,3; 2016,Jan,13; 2015,Jan,16; 2014,Jan,11 **33130** 2018,Jan,8; 2017,Jan,8; 2016,Jan,13; 2015,Jan,16; 2014,Jan,11

Relative Value Units/Medicare Edits

Non-Facility RVU	Work	PE	MP	Total
33120	38.45	13.44	8.78	60.67
33130	24.17	9.96	5.69	39.82
Facility RVU	**Work**	**PE**	**MP**	**Total**
33120	38.45	13.44	8.78	60.67
33130	24.17	9.96	5.69	39.82

	FUD	Status	MUE	Modifiers				IOM Reference
33120	90	A	1(3)	51	N/A	62*	80	None
33130	90	A	1(3)	51	N/A	62*	80	

* with documentation

Terms To Know

absorbable sutures. Strands used for suture or repair of tissue prepared from collagen or a synthetic polymer and capable of being absorbed by tissue over time.

benign. Mild or nonmalignant in nature.

carcinoma in situ. Malignancy that arises from the cells of the vessel, gland, or organ of origin that remains confined to that site or has not invaded neighboring tissue.

lesion. Area of damaged tissue that has lost continuity or function, due to disease or trauma. Lesions may be located on internal structures such as the brain, nerves, or kidneys, or visible on the skin.

malignant. Any condition tending to progress toward death, specifically an invasive tumor with a loss of cellular differentiation that has the ability to spread or metastasize to other body areas.

neoplasm. New abnormal growth, tumor.

nonabsorbable sutures. Strands of natural or synthetic material that resist absorption into living tissue and are removed once healing is under way. Nonabsorbable sutures are commonly used to close skin wounds and repair tendons or collagenous tissue.

tumor. Pathological swelling or enlargement; a neoplastic growth of uncontrolled, abnormal multiplication of cells.

33140-33141

33140 Transmyocardial laser revascularization, by thoracotomy; (separate procedure)

\+ **33141** performed at the time of other open cardiac procedure(s) (List separately in addition to code for primary procedure)

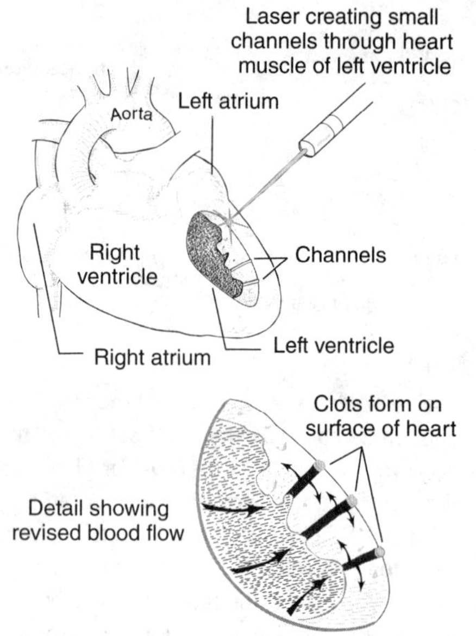

Small holes are burned by laser into the heart tissue to encourage revascularization of diseased muscle

Explanation

The physician performs transmyocardial laser revascularization to restore the flow of blood and oxygen to the heart. Varying approaches may be employed. The procedure is frequently performed on the beating heart, although cardiopulmonary bypass may be initiated. In the beating heart: Using a scalpel the physician makes a 10 centimeters to 15 centimeters incision on the left side of the chest between the ribs and exposes the surface of the heart. The area of ischemia (in still vital tissue) is identified. A laser is inserted through the chest opening and is fired (between heartbeats) through the filled left ventricle. Between 10 channels to 40 channels (small holes) are created to encourage new capillary growth in the area. As the channels are created pressure is applied to each to help close the openings. When the procedure is completed the laser is removed and the wound is closed with layered sutures. If cardiopulmonary bypass was initiated it is discontinued, the patient is rewarmed, and the heartbeat is restored. Report 33140 if the transmyocardial laser revascularization is performed alone. Report 33141 when it is performed at the time of another open cardiac procedure.

Coding Tips

Note that 33140, a separate procedure by definition, is usually a component of a more complex service and is not identified separately. When performed alone or with other unrelated procedures/services, it may be reported. If performed alone, list the code; if performed with other procedures/services, list the code and append modifier 59 or an X{EPSU} modifier. Report 33141 in addition to 33390–33391, 33404–33496, 33510–33536, and 33542.

ICD-10-CM Diagnostic Codes

I20.0 Unstable angina
I20.1 Angina pectoris with documented spasm
I20.8 Other forms of angina pectoris

I21.01	ST elevation (STEMI) myocardial infarction involving left main coronary artery
I21.02	ST elevation (STEMI) myocardial infarction involving left anterior descending coronary artery
I21.09	ST elevation (STEMI) myocardial infarction involving other coronary artery of anterior wall
I21.11	ST elevation (STEMI) myocardial infarction involving right coronary artery
I21.19	ST elevation (STEMI) myocardial infarction involving other coronary artery of inferior wall
I21.21	ST elevation (STEMI) myocardial infarction involving left circumflex coronary artery
I21.29	ST elevation (STEMI) myocardial infarction involving other sites
I21.4	Non-ST elevation (NSTEMI) myocardial infarction
I21.A1	Myocardial infarction type 2
I22.0	Subsequent ST elevation (STEMI) myocardial infarction of anterior wall
I22.1	Subsequent ST elevation (STEMI) myocardial infarction of inferior wall
I22.2	Subsequent non-ST elevation (NSTEMI) myocardial infarction
I22.8	Subsequent ST elevation (STEMI) myocardial infarction of other sites
I24.0	Acute coronary thrombosis not resulting in myocardial infarction
I24.8	Other forms of acute ischemic heart disease
I25.110	Atherosclerotic heart disease of native coronary artery with unstable angina pectoris
I25.111	Atherosclerotic heart disease of native coronary artery with angina pectoris with documented spasm
I25.118	Atherosclerotic heart disease of native coronary artery with other forms of angina pectoris
I25.3	Aneurysm of heart
I25.41	Coronary artery aneurysm
I25.42	Coronary artery dissection
I25.5	Ischemic cardiomyopathy
I25.6	Silent myocardial ischemia
I25.710	Atherosclerosis of autologous vein coronary artery bypass graft(s) with unstable angina pectoris
I25.711	Atherosclerosis of autologous vein coronary artery bypass graft(s) with angina pectoris with documented spasm
I25.718	Atherosclerosis of autologous vein coronary artery bypass graft(s) with other forms of angina pectoris
I25.720	Atherosclerosis of autologous artery coronary artery bypass graft(s) with unstable angina pectoris
I25.721	Atherosclerosis of autologous artery coronary artery bypass graft(s) with angina pectoris with documented spasm
I25.728	Atherosclerosis of autologous artery coronary artery bypass graft(s) with other forms of angina pectoris
I25.730	Atherosclerosis of nonautologous biological coronary artery bypass graft(s) with unstable angina pectoris
I25.731	Atherosclerosis of nonautologous biological coronary artery bypass graft(s) with angina pectoris with documented spasm
I25.738	Atherosclerosis of nonautologous biological coronary artery bypass graft(s) with other forms of angina pectoris
I25.750	Atherosclerosis of native coronary artery of transplanted heart with unstable angina
I25.751	Atherosclerosis of native coronary artery of transplanted heart with angina pectoris with documented spasm
I25.758	Atherosclerosis of native coronary artery of transplanted heart with other forms of angina pectoris
I25.760	Atherosclerosis of bypass graft of coronary artery of transplanted heart with unstable angina
I25.761	Atherosclerosis of bypass graft of coronary artery of transplanted heart with angina pectoris with documented spasm
I25.768	Atherosclerosis of bypass graft of coronary artery of transplanted heart with other forms of angina pectoris
I25.790	Atherosclerosis of other coronary artery bypass graft(s) with unstable angina pectoris
I25.791	Atherosclerosis of other coronary artery bypass graft(s) with angina pectoris with documented spasm
I25.798	Atherosclerosis of other coronary artery bypass graft(s) with other forms of angina pectoris
I25.810	Atherosclerosis of coronary artery bypass graft(s) without angina pectoris
I25.811	Atherosclerosis of native coronary artery of transplanted heart without angina pectoris
I25.812	Atherosclerosis of bypass graft of coronary artery of transplanted heart without angina pectoris
I25.82	Chronic total occlusion of coronary artery
I25.83	Coronary atherosclerosis due to lipid rich plaque
I25.84	Coronary atherosclerosis due to calcified coronary lesion
I25.89	Other forms of chronic ischemic heart disease
Q24.5	Malformation of coronary vessels

AMA: 33140 2018,Jan,8; 2017,Jan,8; 2016,Jan,13; 2015,Jan,16; 2014,Jan,11
33141 2018,Jan,8; 2017,Jan,8; 2016,Jan,13; 2015,Jan,16; 2014,Jan,11

Relative Value Units/Medicare Edits

Non-Facility RVU	Work	PE	MP	Total
33140	28.34	10.48	6.69	45.51
33141	2.54	0.7	0.56	3.8
Facility RVU	**Work**	**PE**	**MP**	**Total**
33140	28.34	10.48	6.69	45.51
33141	2.54	0.7	0.56	3.8

	FUD	Status	MUE	Modifiers				IOM Reference
33140	90	A	1(2)	51	N/A	N/A	80	100-03,20.6
33141	N/A	A	1(2)	N/A	N/A	62*	80	

* with documentation

33202

33202 Insertion of epicardial electrode(s); open incision (eg, thoracotomy, median sternotomy, subxiphoid approach)

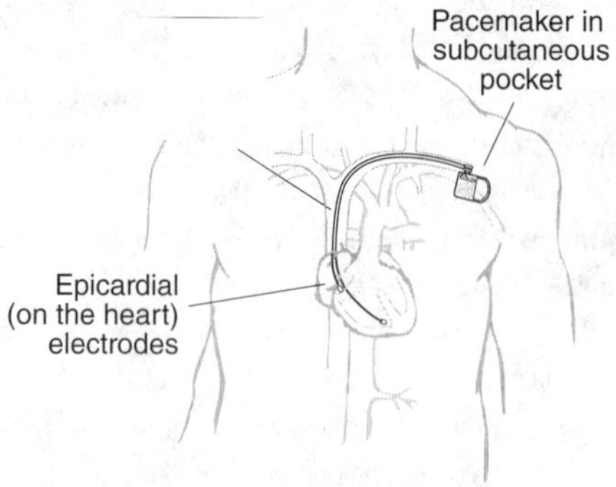

Epicardial electrodes are placed outside the heart in an open procedure

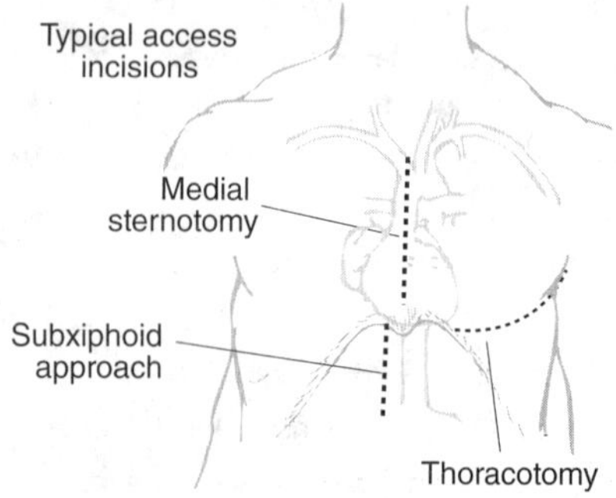

Explanation

The physician places one or more electrical leads on the outside of the heart (epicardial electrodes) by open chest incision. The incision can be in the middle of the chest (midline sternotomy), a vertical incision just below the ribcage (subxiphoid), or between the ribs on the left side of the body (thoracotomy). The chest cavity is opened. After the heart is exposed, electrodes are affixed to the appropriate areas of the heart muscle. The electrodes are tested and then tunneled under the coastal margin to the upper abdomen to a pulse generator or to the infraclavicular area if the generator is in that area. The physician closes the incision with layered sutures.

Coding Tips

Report 33202 when an epicardial lead is placed by the same physician during the same session with the insertion of a pulse generator when performed with 33212, 33213, 33221, 33230, 33231, or 33240. For endoscopic placement of epicardial electrodes by thoracoscopy or pericardioscopy, see 33203.

ICD-10-CM Diagnostic Codes

G90.01	Carotid sinus syncope
I44.0	Atrioventricular block, first degree
I44.1	Atrioventricular block, second degree
I44.2	Atrioventricular block, complete
I45.5	Other specified heart block
I45.6	Pre-excitation syndrome
I45.81	Long QT syndrome
I47.1	Supraventricular tachycardia
I48.0	Paroxysmal atrial fibrillation
I48.11	Longstanding persistent atrial fibrillation
I48.19	Other persistent atrial fibrillation
I48.21	Permanent atrial fibrillation
I49.2	Junctional premature depolarization
I49.5	Sick sinus syndrome
I49.8	Other specified cardiac arrhythmias
Q24.6	Congenital heart block

AMA: 33202 2019,Mar,6; 2018,Jan,8; 2017,Jan,8; 2016,May,5; 2016,Jan,13; 2016,Aug,5; 2015,May,3; 2015,Jan,16; 2014,Nov,5; 2014,Jan,11

Relative Value Units/Medicare Edits

Non-Facility RVU	Work	PE	MP	Total
33202	13.2	6.08	3.1	22.38
Facility RVU	**Work**	**PE**	**MP**	**Total**
33202	13.2	6.08	3.1	22.38

	FUD	Status	MUE	Modifiers				IOM Reference
33202	90	A	1(2)	51	N/A	N/A	N/A	None

* with documentation

Terms To Know

atrioventricular block. Condition in which there is a disturbance of electrical conduction, such as a delay, intermittence, or absence in the transmission of an impulse from the atria to the ventricles and categorized according to degree of severity.

electrode. Electric terminal specialized for a particular electrochemical reaction that acts as a medium between a body surface and another instrument, commonly termed a lead.

epicardial electrode. Stimulation device that is attached to or inserted into the heart muscle and connected to a generator.

ventricular tachycardia. Excessively rapid ventricular rhythm of the heart, usually more than 150 beats per minute, with an origin beat generated in the ventricle, commonly from atrioventricular dissociation.

33203

33203 Insertion of epicardial electrode(s); endoscopic approach (eg, thoracoscopy, pericardioscopy)

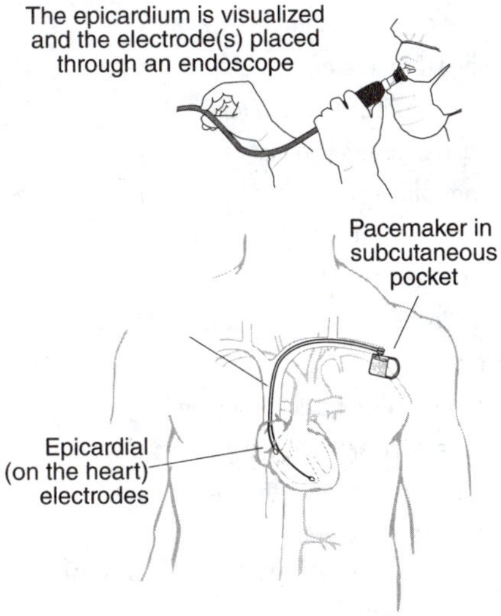

Explanation

The physician places electrical leads on the outside of the heart (epicardial electrodes) using an endoscopic approach. Three trocars are placed in the left anterior chest wall and the left lung is collapsed. A small incision is made in the chest (thoracostomy) and a 12 mm trocar is placed. The thoracoscope (endoscope) is inserted. Two additional trocars are placed under thoracoscopic visualization in the inframammary anterolateral region. Under thoracoscopic guidance, the pericardium is grasped and incised. The lateral trocar is removed and the incision enlarged to allow passage of the epicardial electrode placement device and the electrodes through the intercostal space. The electrodes are placed intrapericardially. The pericardium is approximated with a single stitch to hold the electrodes in place. The electrodes are tested and then tunneled under the costal margin to the upper abdomen to a pulse generator or over the ribs to the infraclavicular area if the generator is in that area. The thoracoscope is removed and a thoracostomy tube is placed at this site. The lung is expanded and the incisions closed with layered sutures.

Coding Tips

Report 33203 when an epicardial lead is placed by the same physician during the same session with the insertion of a pulse generator when performed with 33212, 33213, 33221, 33230, 33231, or 33240. For placement of epicardial electrodes by thoracotomy, see 33202.

ICD-10-CM Diagnostic Codes

G90.01	Carotid sinus syncope
I44.0	Atrioventricular block, first degree
I44.1	Atrioventricular block, second degree
I44.2	Atrioventricular block, complete
I45.5	Other specified heart block
I45.6	Pre-excitation syndrome
I45.81	Long QT syndrome
I47.1	Supraventricular tachycardia
I48.0	Paroxysmal atrial fibrillation
I48.11	Longstanding persistent atrial fibrillation
I48.19	Other persistent atrial fibrillation
I48.21	Permanent atrial fibrillation
I49.2	Junctional premature depolarization
I49.5	Sick sinus syndrome
I49.8	Other specified cardiac arrhythmias
Q24.6	Congenital heart block

AMA: **33203** 2019,Mar,6; 2018,Jan,8; 2017,Jan,8; 2016,May,5; 2016,Jan,13; 2016,Aug,5; 2015,May,3; 2015,Jan,16; 2014,Nov,5; 2014,Jan,11

Relative Value Units/Medicare Edits

Non-Facility RVU	Work	PE	MP	Total
33203	13.97	6.18	3.29	23.44
Facility RVU	**Work**	**PE**	**MP**	**Total**
33203	13.97	6.18	3.29	23.44

	FUD	Status	MUE	Modifiers				IOM Reference
33203	90	A	1(2)	51	N/A	N/A	N/A	None

* with documentation

Terms To Know

atrioventricular block. Condition in which there is a disturbance of electrical conduction, such as a delay, intermittence, or absence in the transmission of an impulse from the atria to the ventricles and categorized according to degree of severity.

ventricular tachycardia. Excessively rapid ventricular rhythm of the heart, usually more than 150 beats per minute, with an origin beat generated in the ventricle, commonly from atrioventricular dissociation.

 ● New ▲ Revised + Add On AMA: CPT Assist [Resequenced] ☑ Laterality

33206-33208

33206 Insertion of new or replacement of permanent pacemaker with transvenous electrode(s); atrial

33207 ventricular

33208 atrial and ventricular

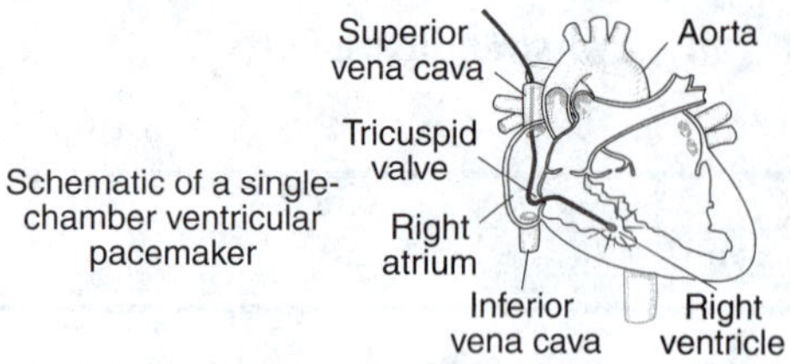

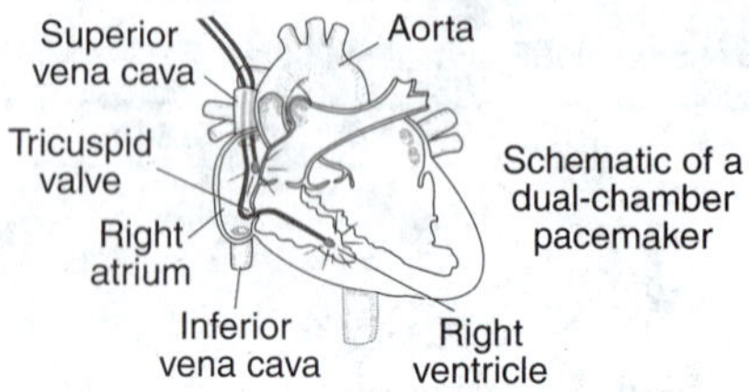

Explanation

Access to the central caval veins is obtained through the subclavian vein or jugular vein. The vein is penetrated with a large needle and a wire is passed through it. A fluoroscope is used to guide the wire into the right atrium. A pocket for the pacemaker generator is created and the wire is tested. The wire is connected to the generator and the generator is closed in its pocket. Report 33206 if the guide and pacemaker wires are placed in the right atrium only; 33207 if the guide and pacemaker wires are placed in the right ventricle only; and 33208 if the elements of 33206 and 33207 are combined.

Coding Tips

When medically necessary, report moderate (conscious) sedation provided by the performing physician with 99151-99153. When provided by another physician, report 99155-99157. Codes 33206–33208 report a global service that includes subcutaneous placement of the pulse generator and transcutaneous placement of the electrode. These procedures include any repositioning or replacement, as well as fluoroscopic guidance. For removal and replacement of a pacemaker pulse generator and transvenous electrodes, report 33233 with 33234 or 33235 and 33206, 33207, or 33208. For removal and replacement of implantable pacing cardioverter-defibrillator, see 33249. For removal and replacement of a subcutaneous implantable defibrillator, see 33270. Removal of subcutaneous leads may be reported separately with 33272. Do not report device evaluation codes (93260, 93261, 93279–93298) in addition to pulse generator and lead insertion/revision codes. Do not report 33206–33208 with 33227–33229. Do not report 33206, 33207, or 33208 with 33216 or 33217.

ICD-10-CM Diagnostic Codes

I44.0	Atrioventricular block, first degree
I44.1	Atrioventricular block, second degree
I44.2	Atrioventricular block, complete
I44.39	Other atrioventricular block
I44.4	Left anterior fascicular block
I44.5	Left posterior fascicular block
I44.69	Other fascicular block
I45.0	Right fascicular block
I45.19	Other right bundle-branch block
I45.2	Bifascicular block
I45.3	Trifascicular block
I45.4	Nonspecific intraventricular block
I45.5	Other specified heart block
I45.6	Pre-excitation syndrome
I45.81	Long QT syndrome
I47.1	Supraventricular tachycardia
I48.0	Paroxysmal atrial fibrillation
I48.11	Longstanding persistent atrial fibrillation
I48.19	Other persistent atrial fibrillation
I48.21	Permanent atrial fibrillation
I49.2	Junctional premature depolarization
I49.5	Sick sinus syndrome
I49.8	Other specified cardiac arrhythmias
I50.1	Left ventricular failure, unspecified
I50.21	Acute systolic (congestive) heart failure
I50.22	Chronic systolic (congestive) heart failure
I50.23	Acute on chronic systolic (congestive) heart failure
I50.31	Acute diastolic (congestive) heart failure
I50.32	Chronic diastolic (congestive) heart failure
I50.33	Acute on chronic diastolic (congestive) heart failure
I50.41	Acute combined systolic (congestive) and diastolic (congestive) heart failure
I50.42	Chronic combined systolic (congestive) and diastolic (congestive) heart failure
I50.43	Acute on chronic combined systolic (congestive) and diastolic (congestive) heart failure
I50.811	Acute right heart failure
I50.812	Chronic right heart failure
I50.813	Acute on chronic right heart failure
I50.814	Right heart failure due to left heart failure
I50.82	Biventricular heart failure
I50.83	High output heart failure
I50.84	End stage heart failure
I51.7	Cardiomegaly
I97.110	Postprocedural cardiac insufficiency following cardiac surgery
I97.111	Postprocedural cardiac insufficiency following other surgery
I97.120	Postprocedural cardiac arrest following cardiac surgery
I97.121	Postprocedural cardiac arrest following other surgery
I97.130	Postprocedural heart failure following cardiac surgery
I97.131	Postprocedural heart failure following other surgery
I97.190	Other postprocedural cardiac functional disturbances following cardiac surgery
I97.191	Other postprocedural cardiac functional disturbances following other surgery
I97.710	Intraoperative cardiac arrest during cardiac surgery
I97.711	Intraoperative cardiac arrest during other surgery
I97.790	Other intraoperative cardiac functional disturbances during cardiac surgery
I97.791	Other intraoperative cardiac functional disturbances during other surgery
I97.88	Other intraoperative complications of the circulatory system, not elsewhere classified

33210-33211

33210 Insertion or replacement of temporary transvenous single chamber cardiac electrode or pacemaker catheter (separate procedure)

33211 Insertion or replacement of temporary transvenous dual chamber pacing electrodes (separate procedure)

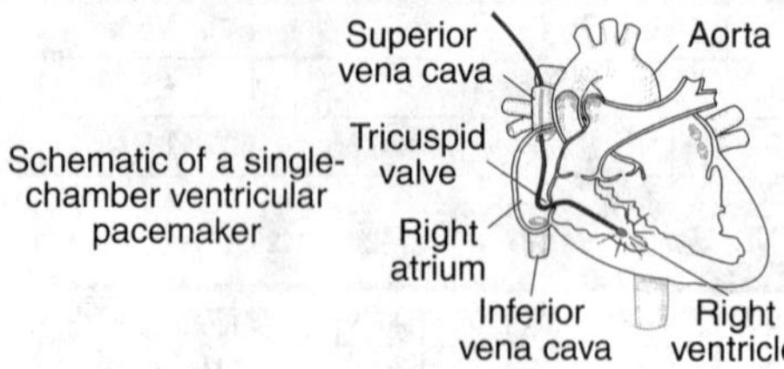

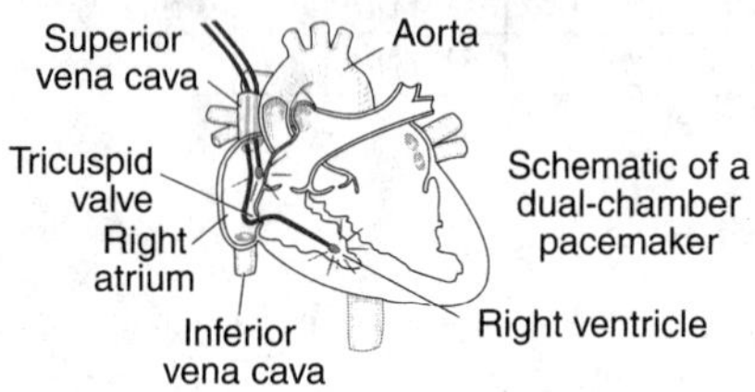

Explanation

Access to the central caval veins is obtained through the subclavian vein or jugular vein. The vein is penetrated with a large needle and a wire is passed through it. A fluoroscope is used to guide the wire into the right atrium. The wire is connected to a generator that is not implanted but temporarily placed outside the body. Report 33210 when a single chamber temporary transvenous electrode or pacemaker catheter is placed and 33211 when a dual chamber electrode(s) is inserted or replaced.

Coding Tips

When medically necessary, report moderate (conscious) sedation provided by the performing physician with 99151-99153. When provided by another physician, report 99155-99157. These separate procedures by definition are usually a component of a more complex service and are not identified separately. When performed alone or with other unrelated procedures/services they may be reported. If performed alone, list the code; if performed with other procedures/services, list the code and append 59 or an X{EPSU} modifier. Fluoroscopy is included in 33210 and 33211 and is not reported separately. Supplies used when providing these procedures may be reported with HCPCS Level II code C1779. Check with the specific payer to determine coverage. Do not report device evaluation codes (93260, 93261, 93279-93298) in addition to pulse generator and lead insertion/revision codes.

ICD-10-CM Diagnostic Codes

I21.01	ST elevation (STEMI) myocardial infarction involving left main coronary artery
I21.02	ST elevation (STEMI) myocardial infarction involving left anterior descending coronary artery
I21.09	ST elevation (STEMI) myocardial infarction involving other coronary artery of anterior wall
I21.11	ST elevation (STEMI) myocardial infarction involving right coronary artery
I21.19	ST elevation (STEMI) myocardial infarction involving other coronary artery of inferior wall
I21.A1	Myocardial infarction type 2
I22.0	Subsequent ST elevation (STEMI) myocardial infarction of anterior wall
I22.1	Subsequent ST elevation (STEMI) myocardial infarction of inferior wall
I44.0	Atrioventricular block, first degree
I44.1	Atrioventricular block, second degree
I44.2	Atrioventricular block, complete
I45.2	Bifascicular block
I45.3	Trifascicular block
I45.5	Other specified heart block
I45.6	Pre-excitation syndrome
I45.81	Long QT syndrome
I46.2	Cardiac arrest due to underlying cardiac condition
I46.8	Cardiac arrest due to other underlying condition
I47.1	Supraventricular tachycardia
I49.2	Junctional premature depolarization
I49.5	Sick sinus syndrome
I49.8	Other specified cardiac arrhythmias
I97.110	Postprocedural cardiac insufficiency following cardiac surgery
I97.111	Postprocedural cardiac insufficiency following other surgery
I97.120	Postprocedural cardiac arrest following cardiac surgery
I97.121	Postprocedural cardiac arrest following other surgery
I97.130	Postprocedural heart failure following cardiac surgery
I97.131	Postprocedural heart failure following other surgery
I97.190	Other postprocedural cardiac functional disturbances following cardiac surgery
I97.191	Other postprocedural cardiac functional disturbances following other surgery
I97.710	Intraoperative cardiac arrest during cardiac surgery
I97.711	Intraoperative cardiac arrest during other surgery
I97.790	Other intraoperative cardiac functional disturbances during cardiac surgery
I97.791	Other intraoperative cardiac functional disturbances during other surgery
I97.88	Other intraoperative complications of the circulatory system, not elsewhere classified
I97.89	Other postprocedural complications and disorders of the circulatory system, not elsewhere classified
Q24.6	Congenital heart block
T82.110A	Breakdown (mechanical) of cardiac electrode, initial encounter
T82.120A	Displacement of cardiac electrode, initial encounter
T82.190A	Other mechanical complication of cardiac electrode, initial encounter
T82.817A	Embolism due to cardiac prosthetic devices, implants and grafts, initial encounter
T82.827A	Fibrosis due to cardiac prosthetic devices, implants and grafts, initial encounter
T82.837A	Hemorrhage due to cardiac prosthetic devices, implants and grafts, initial encounter
T82.847A	Pain due to cardiac prosthetic devices, implants and grafts, initial encounter
T82.857A	Stenosis of other cardiac prosthetic devices, implants and grafts, initial encounter
T82.867A	Thrombosis due to cardiac prosthetic devices, implants and grafts, initial encounter
T82.897A	Other specified complication of cardiac prosthetic devices, implants and grafts, initial encounter

AMA: 33210 2019,Mar,6; 2018,Jan,8; 2017,Jan,8; 2016,May,5; 2016,Jan,13; 2016,Aug,5; 2015,May,3; 2015,Jan,16; 2014,Nov,5; 2014,Jan,11; 2013,Jan,6-8 **33211** 2019,Mar,6; 2018,Jan,8; 2017,Jan,8; 2016,May,5; 2016,Jan,13; 2016,Aug,5; 2015,May,3; 2015,Jan,16; 2014,Nov,5; 2014,Jan,11

Relative Value Units/Medicare Edits

Non-Facility RVU	Work	PE	MP	Total
33210	3.05	1.06	0.65	4.76
33211	3.14	1.12	0.69	4.95
Facility RVU	**Work**	**PE**	**MP**	**Total**
33210	3.05	1.06	0.65	4.76
33211	3.14	1.12	0.69	4.95

	FUD	Status	MUE	Modifiers				IOM Reference
33210	0	A	1(3)	51	N/A	N/A	N/A	None
33211	0	A	1(3)	51	N/A	N/A	N/A	

* with documentation

33212-33214 [33221]

33212 Insertion of pacemaker pulse generator only; with existing single lead

33213 with existing dual leads

33221 Insertion of pacemaker pulse generator only; with existing multiple leads

33214 Upgrade of implanted pacemaker system, conversion of single chamber system to dual chamber system (includes removal of previously placed pulse generator, testing of existing lead, insertion of new lead, insertion of new pulse generator)

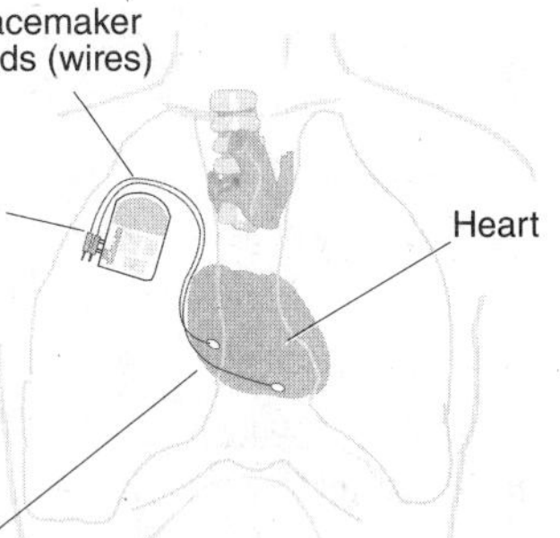

The generator consists of a battery, programmable circuitry, and is attached to the wire leads to the heart

Explanation

A single or dual chamber pacemaker pulse generator is inserted or replaced and connected to previously placed, existing leads. If this is an initial insertion, a pocket for the pacemaker generator is created subcutaneously in the subclavicular region or underneath the abdominal muscles just below the ribcage. The generator is inserted into the pocket. The pocket is closed. Report 33212 if a single chamber (atrial or ventricular) pacemaker pulse generator is inserted, 33213 if a dual chamber (atrial and ventricular) pacemaker pulse generator is inserted, or 33221 for the insertion of the generator with multiple existing leads. In 33214, a single chamber system is converted to a dual chamber system. The existing pacemaker generator pocket is opened and the single chamber generator removed. The dual chamber generator is placed into the existing pocket. The existing pacer wire is tested and connected to the generator. A second lead is placed and tested. The pocket is closed.

Coding Tips

When medically necessary, report moderate (conscious) sedation provided by the performing physician with 99151-99153. When provided by another physician, report 99155-99157. When documentation indicates the replacement of the pulse generator, see 33227–33229, but do not report these codes with 33214. Do not report 33212, 33213, or 33221 with 33233 for removal and replacement of the pacemaker pulse generator. Do not report these codes with 33216 or 33217. When epicardial lead placement is performed with insertion of the generator, see 33202 and/or 33203 in addition to 33212, 33213, and 33221. Revision of skin pocket is included and not reported separately. Fluoroscopy is included in 33212, 33214, and 33221 and is not reported separately. Do not report device evaluation codes (93260, 93261, 93279–93298) in addition to pulse generator and lead insertion/revision codes. Supplies used when providing these procedures may be reported with HCPCS Level II code C1785. Check with the specific payer to determine coverage.

ICD-10-CM Diagnostic Codes

I44.0 Atrioventricular block, first degree

I44.1	Atrioventricular block, second degree
I44.2	Atrioventricular block, complete
I44.4	Left anterior fascicular block
I44.5	Left posterior fascicular block
I45.0	Right fascicular block
I45.2	Bifascicular block
I45.6	Pre-excitation syndrome
I45.81	Long QT syndrome
I47.1	Supraventricular tachycardia
I48.0	Paroxysmal atrial fibrillation
I48.11	Longstanding persistent atrial fibrillation
I48.19	Other persistent atrial fibrillation
I48.21	Permanent atrial fibrillation
I49.2	Junctional premature depolarization
I49.5	Sick sinus syndrome
I50.21	Acute systolic (congestive) heart failure
I50.22	Chronic systolic (congestive) heart failure
I50.23	Acute on chronic systolic (congestive) heart failure
I50.31	Acute diastolic (congestive) heart failure
I50.32	Chronic diastolic (congestive) heart failure
I50.33	Acute on chronic diastolic (congestive) heart failure
I50.41	Acute combined systolic (congestive) and diastolic (congestive) heart failure
I50.42	Chronic combined systolic (congestive) and diastolic (congestive) heart failure
I50.43	Acute on chronic combined systolic (congestive) and diastolic (congestive) heart failure
I50.811	Acute right heart failure
I50.812	Chronic right heart failure
I50.813	Acute on chronic right heart failure
I50.814	Right heart failure due to left heart failure
I50.82	Biventricular heart failure
I50.83	High output heart failure
I50.84	End stage heart failure
Q24.6	Congenital heart block
T82.111A	Breakdown (mechanical) of cardiac pulse generator (battery), initial encounter
T82.121A	Displacement of cardiac pulse generator (battery), initial encounter

AMA: **33212** 2019,Mar,6; 2018,Jan,8; 2017,Jan,8; 2016,May,5; 2016,Jan,13; 2016,Aug,5; 2015,May,3; 2015,Jan,16; 2014,Nov,5; 2014,Jan,11 **33213** 2019,Mar,6; 2018,Jan,8; 2017,Jan,8; 2016,May,5; 2016,Jan,13; 2016,Aug,5; 2015,May,3; 2015,Jan,16; 2014,Nov,5; 2014,Jan,11 **33214** 2019,Mar,6; 2018,Jan,8; 2017,Jan,8; 2016,May,5; 2016,Jan,13; 2016,Aug,5; 2015,May,3; 2015,Jan,16; 2014,Nov,5; 2014,Jan,11 **33221** 2019,Mar,6; 2018,Jan,8; 2017,Jan,8; 2016,May,5; 2016,Jan,13; 2016,Aug,5; 2015,May,3; 2015,Jan,16; 2014,Nov,5; 2014,Jan,11

Relative Value Units/Medicare Edits

Non-Facility RVU	Work	PE	MP	Total
33212	5.01	3.15	1.15	9.31
33213	5.28	3.24	1.22	9.74
33221	5.55	3.62	1.27	10.44
33214	7.59	4.57	1.74	13.9
Facility RVU	**Work**	**PE**	**MP**	**Total**
33212	5.01	3.15	1.15	9.31
33213	5.28	3.24	1.22	9.74
33221	5.55	3.62	1.27	10.44
33214	7.59	4.57	1.74	13.9

	FUD	Status	MUE	Modifiers				IOM Reference
33212	90	A	1(3)	51	N/A	N/A	N/A	None
33213	90	A	1(3)	51	N/A	N/A	N/A	
33221	90	A	1(3)	51	N/A	N/A	N/A	
33214	90	A	1(3)	51	N/A	62	80*	

* with documentation

Terms To Know

fluoroscopy. Radiology technique that allows visual examination of part of the body or a function of an organ using a device that projects an x-ray image on a fluorescent screen.

pacemaker. Implantable cardiac device that controls the heart's rhythm and maintains regular beats by artificial electric discharges. This device consists of the pulse generator with a battery and the electrodes, or leads, which are placed in single or dual chambers of the heart, usually transvenously.

pulse generator. Circuit used to generate pulses. Pulse generators contain the battery, the electronic circuit, and the connector in a hermetically sealed encasement. Pulse generators may be temporary transcutaneous or placed in a subcutaneous pocket.

33215-33217

33215 Repositioning of previously implanted transvenous pacemaker or implantable defibrillator (right atrial or right ventricular) electrode
33216 Insertion of a single transvenous electrode, permanent pacemaker or implantable defibrillator
33217 Insertion of 2 transvenous electrodes, permanent pacemaker or implantable defibrillator

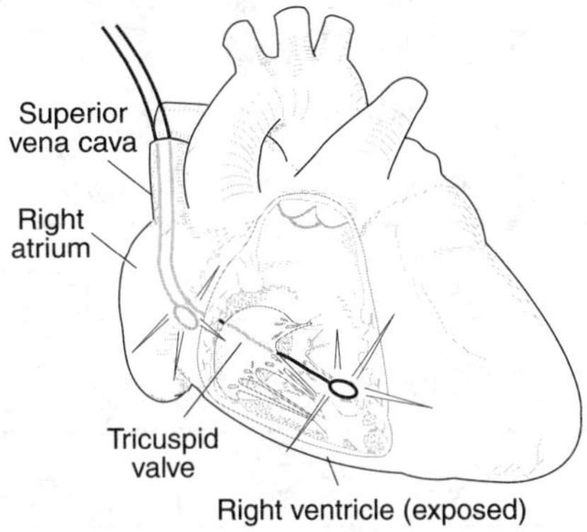

Schematic showing leads and electrodes to both right chambers

Explanation

In 33215, a previously placed transvenous right atrial or right ventricular electrode is repositioned. This is done when the system does not function due to improper placement of the electrode wire itself. The generator is removed and the wire is tested to ensure that the wire is not defective, but simply in the wrong place. It is reattached to the generator in its new position and tested again. In 33216, the physician inserts a single transvenous electrode and in 33217 two transvenous electrodes when there is a malfunction or complication with the electrode wire of a permanent pacemaker or implantable defibrillator. The generator is removed and the wire is tested. When the wire is found defective, another transvenous electrode is inserted. Access to the central caval veins is obtained through the subclavian vein or jugular vein. The vein is penetrated with a large needle and a wire is passed through it. Fluoroscopy is used to guide the wire into position. The wire is connected to the generator and the wound is closed. Various head and body positions are tested again to ensure adequate pacing.

Coding Tips

When medically necessary, report moderate (conscious) sedation provided by the performing physician with 99151-99153. When provided by another physician, report 99155-99157. These codes report insertion or repositioning of electrodes on permanent pacemakers or implantable defibrillators. Do not report 33216–33217 with 33206–33208, 33212–33214, 33221, 33227–33231, 33240, 33249, or 33262–33264. Revision of skin pocket is included and is not reported separately. Imaging guidance is included in these procedures and is not reported separately. For insertion and replacement of a cardiac venous system electrode, see 33224 and 33225. Do not report device evaluation codes (93260, 93261, 93279–93298) in addition to pulse generator and lead insertion/revision codes. Supplies used when providing these procedures may be reported with C1777. Check with the specific payer to determine coverage.

ICD-10-CM Diagnostic Codes

I11.0	Hypertensive heart disease with heart failure
I13.0	Hypertensive heart and chronic kidney disease with heart failure and stage 1 through stage 4 chronic kidney disease, or unspecified chronic kidney disease
I13.2	Hypertensive heart and chronic kidney disease with heart failure and with stage 5 chronic kidney disease, or end stage renal disease
I16.0	Hypertensive urgency
I16.1	Hypertensive emergency
I21.01	ST elevation (STEMI) myocardial infarction involving left main coronary artery
I21.02	ST elevation (STEMI) myocardial infarction involving left anterior descending coronary artery
I21.09	ST elevation (STEMI) myocardial infarction involving other coronary artery of anterior wall
I21.11	ST elevation (STEMI) myocardial infarction involving right coronary artery
I21.19	ST elevation (STEMI) myocardial infarction involving other coronary artery of inferior wall
I21.21	ST elevation (STEMI) myocardial infarction involving left circumflex coronary artery
I21.29	ST elevation (STEMI) myocardial infarction involving other sites
I21.4	Non-ST elevation (NSTEMI) myocardial infarction
I21.A1	Myocardial infarction type 2
I22.0	Subsequent ST elevation (STEMI) myocardial infarction of anterior wall
I22.1	Subsequent ST elevation (STEMI) myocardial infarction of inferior wall
I22.2	Subsequent non-ST elevation (NSTEMI) myocardial infarction
I22.8	Subsequent ST elevation (STEMI) myocardial infarction of other sites
I25.2	Old myocardial infarction
I25.5	Ischemic cardiomyopathy
I25.6	Silent myocardial ischemia
I25.89	Other forms of chronic ischemic heart disease
I42.0	Dilated cardiomyopathy
I42.5	Other restrictive cardiomyopathy
I42.8	Other cardiomyopathies
I44.0	Atrioventricular block, first degree
I44.1	Atrioventricular block, second degree
I44.2	Atrioventricular block, complete
I44.39	Other atrioventricular block
I44.4	Left anterior fascicular block
I44.5	Left posterior fascicular block
I44.69	Other fascicular block
I45.0	Right fascicular block
I45.19	Other right bundle-branch block
I45.2	Bifascicular block
I45.4	Nonspecific intraventricular block
I45.5	Other specified heart block
I45.6	Pre-excitation syndrome
I45.81	Long QT syndrome
I45.89	Other specified conduction disorders
I46.2	Cardiac arrest due to underlying cardiac condition
I46.8	Cardiac arrest due to other underlying condition
I47.0	Re-entry ventricular arrhythmia
I47.1	Supraventricular tachycardia
I47.2	Ventricular tachycardia

I48.0	Paroxysmal atrial fibrillation
I48.11	Longstanding persistent atrial fibrillation
I48.19	Other persistent atrial fibrillation
I48.21	Permanent atrial fibrillation
I48.3	Typical atrial flutter
I48.4	Atypical atrial flutter
I49.01	Ventricular fibrillation
I49.02	Ventricular flutter
I49.2	Junctional premature depolarization
I49.5	Sick sinus syndrome
I49.8	Other specified cardiac arrhythmias
I50.1	Left ventricular failure, unspecified
I50.21	Acute systolic (congestive) heart failure
I50.22	Chronic systolic (congestive) heart failure
I50.23	Acute on chronic systolic (congestive) heart failure
I50.31	Acute diastolic (congestive) heart failure
I50.32	Chronic diastolic (congestive) heart failure
I50.33	Acute on chronic diastolic (congestive) heart failure
I50.41	Acute combined systolic (congestive) and diastolic (congestive) heart failure
I50.42	Chronic combined systolic (congestive) and diastolic (congestive) heart failure
I50.43	Acute on chronic combined systolic (congestive) and diastolic (congestive) heart failure
I50.811	Acute right heart failure
I50.812	Chronic right heart failure
I50.813	Acute on chronic right heart failure
I50.814	Right heart failure due to left heart failure
I50.82	Biventricular heart failure
I50.83	High output heart failure
I50.84	End stage heart failure
Q23.8	Other congenital malformations of aortic and mitral valves
Q24.6	Congenital heart block
Q24.8	Other specified congenital malformations of heart
T82.110A	Breakdown (mechanical) of cardiac electrode, initial encounter
T82.120A	Displacement of cardiac electrode, initial encounter
T82.190A	Other mechanical complication of cardiac electrode, initial encounter
T82.598A	Other mechanical complication of other cardiac and vascular devices and implants, initial encounter
T82.7XXA	Infection and inflammatory reaction due to other cardiac and vascular devices, implants and grafts, initial encounter
T82.817A	Embolism due to cardiac prosthetic devices, implants and grafts, initial encounter
T82.827A	Fibrosis due to cardiac prosthetic devices, implants and grafts, initial encounter
T82.837A	Hemorrhage due to cardiac prosthetic devices, implants and grafts, initial encounter
T82.847A	Pain due to cardiac prosthetic devices, implants and grafts, initial encounter
T82.857A	Stenosis of other cardiac prosthetic devices, implants and grafts, initial encounter
T82.867A	Thrombosis due to cardiac prosthetic devices, implants and grafts, initial encounter
T82.897A	Other specified complication of cardiac prosthetic devices, implants and grafts, initial encounter
Z95.0	Presence of cardiac pacemaker
Z95.810	Presence of automatic (implantable) cardiac defibrillator

AMA: 33215 2019,Mar,6; 2018,Jan,8; 2017,Jan,8; 2016,May,5; 2016,Jan,13; 2016,Aug,5; 2015,May,3; 2015,Jan,16; 2014,Nov,5; 2014,Jan,11 **33216** 2019,Mar,6; 2018,Jan,8; 2017,Jan,8; 2016,May,5; 2016,Jan,13; 2016,Aug,5; 2015,May,3; 2015,Jan,16; 2014,Nov,5; 2014,Jan,11 **33217** 2019,Mar,6; 2018,Jan,8; 2017,Jan,8; 2016,May,5; 2016,Jan,13; 2016,Aug,5; 2015,May,3; 2015,Jan,16; 2014,Nov,5; 2014,Jan,11

Relative Value Units/Medicare Edits

Non-Facility RVU	Work	PE	MP	Total
33215	4.92	2.96	1.14	9.02
33216	5.62	3.85	1.29	10.76
33217	5.59	3.74	1.27	10.6
Facility RVU	**Work**	**PE**	**MP**	**Total**
33215	4.92	2.96	1.14	9.02
33216	5.62	3.85	1.29	10.76
33217	5.59	3.74	1.27	10.6

	FUD	Status	MUE	Modifiers				IOM Reference
33215	90	A	2(3)	51	N/A	N/A	N/A	None
33216	90	A	1(3)	51	N/A	N/A	N/A	
33217	90	A	1(3)	51	N/A	N/A	N/A	

* with documentation

33218-33220

33218 Repair of single transvenous electrode, permanent pacemaker or implantable defibrillator

33220 Repair of 2 transvenous electrodes for permanent pacemaker or implantable defibrillator

Schematic showing leads and electrodes to both right chambers

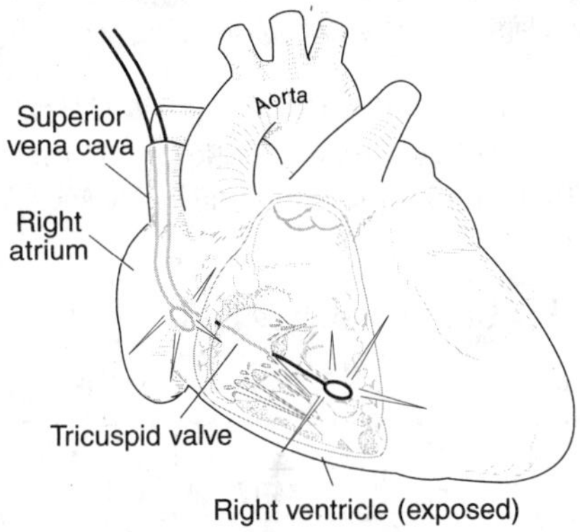

Explanation

A previously placed transvenous electrode is repaired. The permanent pacemaker or implantable defibrillator pocket is opened and the generator is removed. The electrode wire is tested. Repairs are performed on the electrode. The wire is tested again and reconnected to the generator. The generator is placed back in its pocket and the pocket is closed. Report 33218 if a single electrode is repaired and 33220 if two electrodes are repaired.

Coding Tips

When medically necessary, report moderate (conscious) sedation provided by the performing physician with 99151-99153. When provided by another physician, report 99155-99157. These codes report repair of electrodes on permanent pacemakers or implantable defibrillators. For repair of a single permanent pacemaker or implantable defibrillator electrode in addition to the replacement of the pulse generator, report 33218 with 33227–33229 or 33262–33264. For repair of two transvenous electrodes for permanent pacemaker or implantable defibrillator in addition to replacement of the pulse generator, report 33220 with 33228, 33229, 33263, or 33264.

ICD-10-CM Diagnostic Codes

T82.110A	Breakdown (mechanical) of cardiac electrode, initial encounter
T82.120A	Displacement of cardiac electrode, initial encounter
T82.190A	Other mechanical complication of cardiac electrode, initial encounter
T82.7XXA	Infection and inflammatory reaction due to other cardiac and vascular devices, implants and grafts, initial encounter
T82.817A	Embolism due to cardiac prosthetic devices, implants and grafts, initial encounter
T82.827A	Fibrosis due to cardiac prosthetic devices, implants and grafts, initial encounter
T82.837A	Hemorrhage due to cardiac prosthetic devices, implants and grafts, initial encounter
T82.847A	Pain due to cardiac prosthetic devices, implants and grafts, initial encounter
T82.857A	Stenosis of other cardiac prosthetic devices, implants and grafts, initial encounter
T82.867A	Thrombosis due to cardiac prosthetic devices, implants and grafts, initial encounter
T82.897A	Other specified complication of cardiac prosthetic devices, implants and grafts, initial encounter
Z45.09	Encounter for adjustment and management of other cardiac device
Z95.0	Presence of cardiac pacemaker
Z95.810	Presence of automatic (implantable) cardiac defibrillator

AMA: **33218** 2019,Mar,6; 2018,Jan,8; 2017,Jan,8; 2016,May,5; 2016,Jan,13; 2016,Aug,5; 2015,May,3; 2015,Jan,16; 2014,Nov,5; 2014,Jan,11 **33220** 2019,Mar,6; 2018,Jan,8; 2017,Jan,8; 2016,May,5; 2016,Jan,13; 2016,Aug,5; 2015,May,3; 2015,Jan,16; 2014,Nov,5; 2014,Jan,11

Relative Value Units/Medicare Edits

Non-Facility RVU	Work	PE	MP	Total
33218	5.82	4.09	1.34	11.25
33220	5.9	4.09	1.34	11.33
Facility RVU	**Work**	**PE**	**MP**	**Total**
33218	5.82	4.09	1.34	11.25
33220	5.9	4.09	1.34	11.33

	FUD	Status	MUE	Modifiers				IOM Reference
33218	90	A	1(3)	51	N/A	N/A	N/A	None
33220	90	A	1(3)	51	N/A	N/A	N/A	

* with documentation

Terms To Know

cardioverter-defibrillator. Device that uses both low energy cardioversion or defibrillating shocks and antitachycardia pacing to treat ventricular tachycardia or ventricular fibrillation.

complication. Condition arising after the beginning of observation and treatment that modifies the course of the patient's illness or the medical care required, or an undesired result or misadventure in medical care.

heartbeat. Contraction of the heart muscles in a rhythmic pattern, circulating about 70 ml of blood and taking less than a second to complete.

in situ. Located in the natural position or contained within the origin site, not spread into neighboring tissue.

pacemaker. Implantable cardiac device that controls the heart's rhythm and maintains regular beats by artificial electric discharges. This device consists of the pulse generator with a battery and the electrodes, or leads, which are placed in single or dual chambers of the heart, usually transvenously.

transvenous electrode. Electrode placed using a transvenous catheter and wedged into the endocardium of the right ventricle or atrium.

33222-33223

33222 Relocation of skin pocket for pacemaker
33223 Relocation of skin pocket for implantable defibrillator

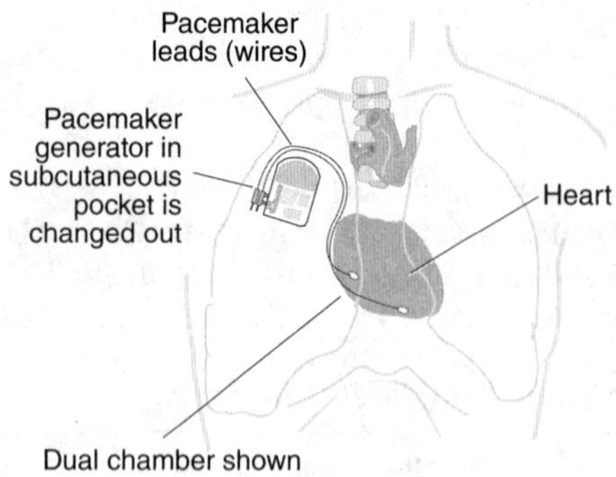

Explanation

The physician relocates a pacemaker or defibrillator pocket due to infection, erosion, or complications from the original generator placement. The pocket is opened and the generator is removed. A new pocket is formed in the subcutaneous tissue within the reach of the already present electrodes. The electrodes are brought through a new subcutaneous tunnel into the new pocket. The old pocket is closed. The existing or new generator is placed in the new pocket and the electrodes are connected. The pocket is closed. Report 33222 when a permanent pacemaker pocket is relocated and 33223 when an implantable defibrillator pocket is relocated.

Coding Tips

When medically necessary, report moderate (conscious) sedation provided by the performing physician with 99151-99153. When provided by another physician, report 99155-99157. Do not report 33222 or 33223 with 10140, 10180, 11042–11047, or 13100–13102.

ICD-10-CM Diagnostic Codes

M79.81	Nontraumatic hematoma of soft tissue
T81.41XA	Infection following a procedure, superficial incisional surgical site, initial encounter
T81.42XA	Infection following a procedure, deep incisional surgical site, initial encounter
T81.43XA	Infection following a procedure, organ and space surgical site, initial encounter
T81.49XA	Infection following a procedure, other surgical site, initial encounter
T81.83XA	Persistent postprocedural fistula, initial encounter
T81.89XA	Other complications of procedures, not elsewhere classified, initial encounter
T82.7XXA	Infection and inflammatory reaction due to other cardiac and vascular devices, implants and grafts, initial encounter
T82.817A	Embolism due to cardiac prosthetic devices, implants and grafts, initial encounter
T82.827A	Fibrosis due to cardiac prosthetic devices, implants and grafts, initial encounter
T82.837A	Hemorrhage due to cardiac prosthetic devices, implants and grafts, initial encounter
T82.847A	Pain due to cardiac prosthetic devices, implants and grafts, initial encounter
T82.855A	Stenosis of coronary artery stent, initial encounter
T82.857A	Stenosis of other cardiac prosthetic devices, implants and grafts, initial encounter
T82.867A	Thrombosis due to cardiac prosthetic devices, implants and grafts, initial encounter
T82.897A	Other specified complication of cardiac prosthetic devices, implants and grafts, initial encounter
Z45.018	Encounter for adjustment and management of other part of cardiac pacemaker
Z45.02	Encounter for adjustment and management of automatic implantable cardiac defibrillator

AMA: **33222** 2019,Mar,6; 2018,Jan,8; 2017,Jan,8; 2016,May,5; 2016,Jan,13; 2016,Aug,5; 2015,May,3; 2015,Jan,16; 2014,Nov,5; 2014,Jan,11 **33223** 2019,Mar,6; 2018,Jan,8; 2017,Jan,8; 2016,Jan,13; 2016,Aug,5; 2015,Jan,16; 2014,Nov,5; 2014,Jan,11

Relative Value Units/Medicare Edits

Non-Facility RVU	Work	PE	MP	Total
33222	4.85	3.84	1.12	9.81
33223	6.3	4.12	1.45	11.87
Facility RVU	**Work**	**PE**	**MP**	**Total**
33222	4.85	3.84	1.12	9.81
33223	6.3	4.12	1.45	11.87

	FUD	Status	MUE	Modifiers				IOM Reference
33222	90	A	1(3)	51	N/A	N/A	N/A	None
33223	90	A	1(3)	51	N/A	N/A	80*	

* with documentation

Terms To Know

cardioverter-defibrillator. Device that uses both low energy cardioversion or defibrillating shocks and antitachycardia pacing to treat ventricular tachycardia or ventricular fibrillation.

hematoma. Tumor-like collection of blood in some part of the body caused by a break in a blood vessel wall, usually as a result of trauma.

pacemaker. Implantable cardiac device that controls the heart's rhythm and maintains regular beats by artificial electric discharges. This device consists of the pulse generator with a battery and the electrodes, or leads, which are placed in single or dual chambers of the heart, usually transvenously.

seroma. Swelling caused by the collection of serum, or clear fluid, in the tissues.

33224

33224 Insertion of pacing electrode, cardiac venous system, for left ventricular pacing, with attachment to previously placed pacemaker or implantable defibrillator pulse generator (including revision of pocket, removal, insertion, and/or replacement of existing generator)

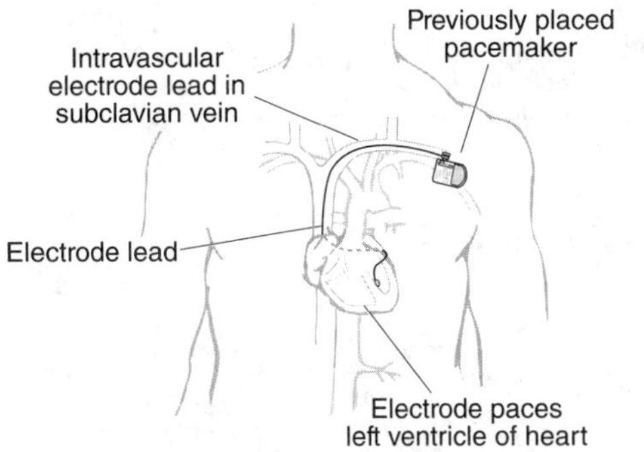

A pacing electrode is placed in the venous system and attached to a previously placed pacemaker or defibrillator generator

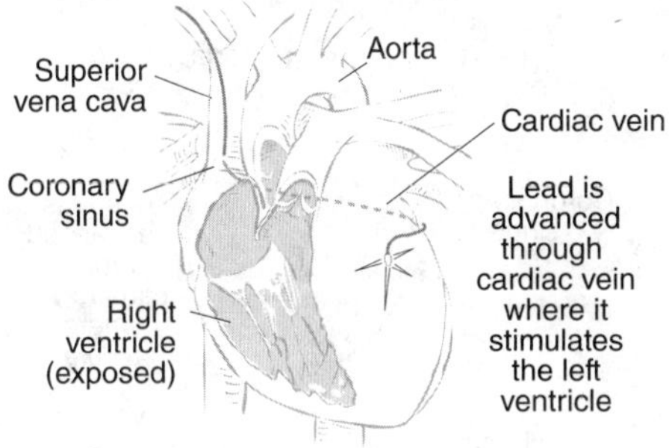

Explanation

If biventricular pacing is required, an additional electrode is placed in the left ventricle. With the pacemaker or implantable defibrillator already in place, the physician gains access transvenously through the subclavian or jugular vein. This procedure is done under local anesthesia. A fluoroscope may be used for guidance and a pacing electrode is inserted in the left ventricular chamber of the heart, usually in the coronary sinus tributary. The electrode is connected to the pulse generator and the pocket is closed. The generator pocket may be revised and/or the existing generator removed, inserted, or replaced. In rare cases, when transvenous approach cannot be used, the device is implanted in the pocket underneath the skin in the lower abdomen (epicardial approach). Implantation using this approach is done under general anesthesia.

Coding Tips

This code reports the insertion of an electrode on a previously placed permanent pacemaker or implantable defibrillator for left ventricular pacing. Fluoroscopy is included in 33224 and is not reported separately. For epicardial electrode placement at the time of insertion of a pacing electrode in the cardiac venous system, report 33202 or 33203 with 33224. For repositioning of an electrode for left ventricular pacing, see 33226. For insertion of a single chamber electrode, see 33216. For insertion of a dual chamber electrode, see 33217. Do not report device evaluation codes (93260, 93261, 93279–93298) in addition to pulse generator and lead insertion/revision codes. Supplies used when providing this procedure may be reported with HCPCS Level II code C1900. Check with the specific payer to determine coverage.

ICD-10-CM Diagnostic Codes

I11.0	Hypertensive heart disease with heart failure
I13.0	Hypertensive heart and chronic kidney disease with heart failure and stage 1 through stage 4 chronic kidney disease, or unspecified chronic kidney disease
I13.2	Hypertensive heart and chronic kidney disease with heart failure and with stage 5 chronic kidney disease, or end stage renal disease
I16.0	Hypertensive urgency
I16.1	Hypertensive emergency
I21.01	ST elevation (STEMI) myocardial infarction involving left main coronary artery
I21.02	ST elevation (STEMI) myocardial infarction involving left anterior descending coronary artery
I21.09	ST elevation (STEMI) myocardial infarction involving other coronary artery of anterior wall
I21.11	ST elevation (STEMI) myocardial infarction involving right coronary artery
I21.19	ST elevation (STEMI) myocardial infarction involving other coronary artery of inferior wall
I21.21	ST elevation (STEMI) myocardial infarction involving left circumflex coronary artery
I21.29	ST elevation (STEMI) myocardial infarction involving other sites
I21.4	Non-ST elevation (NSTEMI) myocardial infarction
I21.A1	Myocardial infarction type 2
I22.0	Subsequent ST elevation (STEMI) myocardial infarction of anterior wall
I22.1	Subsequent ST elevation (STEMI) myocardial infarction of inferior wall
I22.2	Subsequent non-ST elevation (NSTEMI) myocardial infarction
I22.8	Subsequent ST elevation (STEMI) myocardial infarction of other sites
I25.2	Old myocardial infarction
I25.5	Ischemic cardiomyopathy
I25.6	Silent myocardial ischemia
I42.0	Dilated cardiomyopathy
I42.1	Obstructive hypertrophic cardiomyopathy
I42.2	Other hypertrophic cardiomyopathy
I42.3	Endomyocardial (eosinophilic) disease
I42.4	Endocardial fibroelastosis
I42.5	Other restrictive cardiomyopathy
I42.6	Alcoholic cardiomyopathy
I42.7	Cardiomyopathy due to drug and external agent
I43	Cardiomyopathy in diseases classified elsewhere
I44.0	Atrioventricular block, first degree
I44.1	Atrioventricular block, second degree
I44.2	Atrioventricular block, complete
I44.39	Other atrioventricular block
I44.4	Left anterior fascicular block
I44.5	Left posterior fascicular block
I45.0	Right fascicular block
I45.2	Bifascicular block
I45.3	Trifascicular block
I45.4	Nonspecific intraventricular block
I45.5	Other specified heart block
I45.6	Pre-excitation syndrome
I45.81	Long QT syndrome

I46.2	Cardiac arrest due to underlying cardiac condition
I46.8	Cardiac arrest due to other underlying condition
I47.0	Re-entry ventricular arrhythmia
I47.1	Supraventricular tachycardia
I47.2	Ventricular tachycardia
I48.0	Paroxysmal atrial fibrillation
I48.11	Longstanding persistent atrial fibrillation
I48.19	Other persistent atrial fibrillation
I48.21	Permanent atrial fibrillation
I49.01	Ventricular fibrillation
I49.02	Ventricular flutter
I49.2	Junctional premature depolarization
I49.5	Sick sinus syndrome
I49.8	Other specified cardiac arrhythmias
I50.1	Left ventricular failure, unspecified
I50.21	Acute systolic (congestive) heart failure
I50.22	Chronic systolic (congestive) heart failure
I50.23	Acute on chronic systolic (congestive) heart failure
I50.31	Acute diastolic (congestive) heart failure
I50.32	Chronic diastolic (congestive) heart failure
I50.33	Acute on chronic diastolic (congestive) heart failure
I50.41	Acute combined systolic (congestive) and diastolic (congestive) heart failure
I50.42	Chronic combined systolic (congestive) and diastolic (congestive) heart failure
I50.43	Acute on chronic combined systolic (congestive) and diastolic (congestive) heart failure
I50.811	Acute right heart failure
I50.812	Chronic right heart failure
I50.813	Acute on chronic right heart failure
I50.814	Right heart failure due to left heart failure
I50.82	Biventricular heart failure
I50.83	High output heart failure
I50.84	End stage heart failure
I51.7	Cardiomegaly
Q23.8	Other congenital malformations of aortic and mitral valves
Q24.6	Congenital heart block
Q24.8	Other specified congenital malformations of heart
Z95.0	Presence of cardiac pacemaker
Z95.810	Presence of automatic (implantable) cardiac defibrillator

AMA: 33224 2019,Mar,6; 2018,Jan,8; 2017,Jan,8; 2016,May,5; 2016,Jan,13; 2016,Aug,5; 2015,May,3; 2015,Jan,16; 2014,Nov,5; 2014,Jan,11

Relative Value Units/Medicare Edits

Non-Facility RVU	Work	PE	MP	Total
33224	9.04	3.89	2.09	15.02
Facility RVU	**Work**	**PE**	**MP**	**Total**
33224	9.04	3.89	2.09	15.02

	FUD	Status	MUE	Modifiers				IOM Reference
33224	0	A	1(3)	51	N/A	N/A	N/A	None

* with documentation

33225

+ 33225 Insertion of pacing electrode, cardiac venous system, for left ventricular pacing, at time of insertion of implantable defibrillator or pacemaker pulse generator (eg, for upgrade to dual chamber system) (List separately in addition to code for primary procedure)

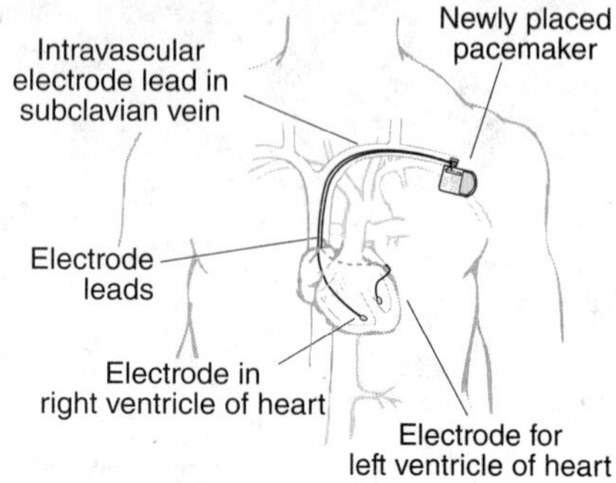

A pacing electrode is placed in the venous system at the time a pacemaker or defibrillator generator is inserted

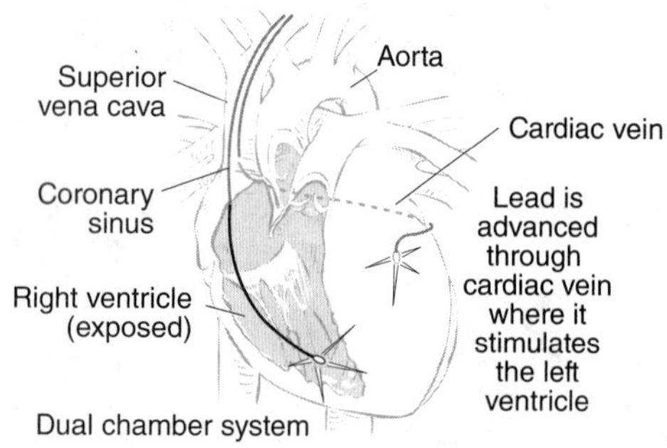

Explanation

If biventricular pacing is required, an additional electrode is placed in the left ventricle. During insertion of an implantable defibrillator or pacemaker pulse generator, the physician gains access transvenously through the subclavian or jugular vein. This procedure is done under local anesthesia. A fluoroscope may be used for guidance and a pacing electrode is inserted in the left ventricular chamber of the heart, usually in the coronary sinus tributary. The generator is upgraded to a dual chamber system. The electrode is connected to the pulse generator and the pocket is closed. In rare cases, when transvenous approach cannot be used, the device is implanted in the pocket underneath the skin in the lower abdomen (epicardial approach). Implantation using this approach is done under general anesthesia.

Coding Tips

Fluoroscopy is included in 33225 and is not reported separately. This code reports the insertion of an electrode at the time of insertion of an implantable defibrillator or pacemaker pulse generator for left ventricular pacing and includes an upgrade to a dual chamber system and pocket revision. Report 33225 in addition to 33206, 33207, 33208, 33212, 33213, 33214, 33216, 33217, 33221, 33223, 33228, 33229, 33230, 33231, 33233, 33234, 33235, 33240, 33249, 33263, and 33264. Use 33225 in addition to 33222 when a pacemaker generator pocket is relocated and 33223 when an implantable defibrillator pocket is relocated. For insertion of an electrode for a previously placed implantable defibrillator or pacemaker pulse generator, see 33224. For repositioning of an electrode for left ventricular pacing, see 33226. Do not report device evaluation codes (93260, 93261, 93279–93298) in addition to pulse generator and lead insertion/revision codes.

ICD-10-CM Diagnostic Codes

This/these CPT code(s) are add on code(s). See the primary procedure code that this code is performed with for your ICD-10-CM code selections. Diagnostic code(s) would be the same as the actual procedure performed.

AMA: **33225** 2019,Mar,6; 2018,Jan,8; 2017,Jan,8; 2016,May,5; 2016,Jan,13; 2016,Aug,5; 2015,May,3; 2015,Jan,16; 2014,Nov,5; 2014,Jan,11

Relative Value Units/Medicare Edits

Non-Facility RVU	Work	PE	MP	Total
33225	8.33	3.42	1.92	13.67
Facility RVU	**Work**	**PE**	**MP**	**Total**
33225	8.33	3.42	1.92	13.67

	FUD	Status	MUE	Modifiers				IOM Reference
33225	N/A	A	1(3)	N/A	N/A	N/A	N/A	100-04,4,10.2.2

* with documentation

Terms To Know

arrhythmia. Irregular heartbeat.

cardioverter-defibrillator. Device that uses both low energy cardioversion or defibrillating shocks and antitachycardia pacing to treat ventricular tachycardia or ventricular fibrillation.

electrode. Electric terminal specialized for a particular electrochemical reaction that acts as a medium between a body surface and another instrument, commonly termed a lead.

fluoroscopy. Radiology technique that allows visual examination of part of the body or a function of an organ using a device that projects an x-ray image on a fluorescent screen.

pacemaker. Implantable cardiac device that controls the heart's rhythm and maintains regular beats by artificial electric discharges. This device consists of the pulse generator with a battery and the electrodes, or leads, which are placed in single or dual chambers of the heart, usually transvenously.

transvenous electrode. Electrode placed using a transvenous catheter and wedged into the endocardium of the right ventricle or atrium.

33226

33226 Repositioning of previously implanted cardiac venous system (left ventricular) electrode (including removal, insertion and/or replacement of existing generator)

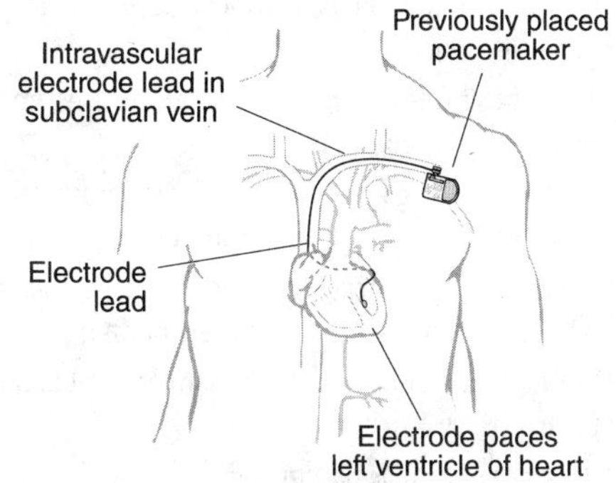

A pacing electrode in the venous system is repositioned

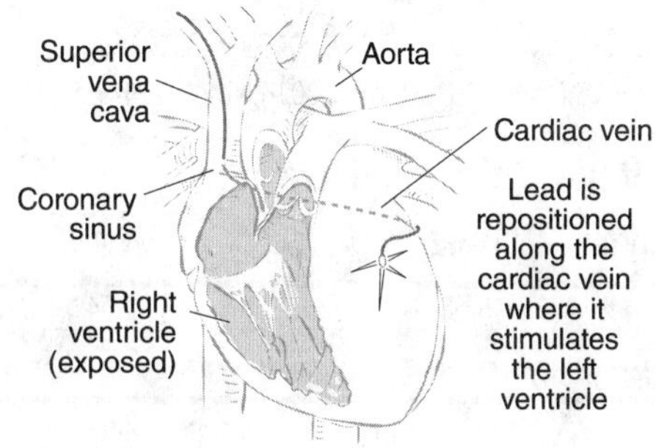

Explanation

The physician gains access transvenously through the subclavian or jugular vein. A fluoroscope may be used for guidance and the pacing electrode that is already in place in the ventricular chamber of the heart, usually in the coronary sinus tributary, is repositioned. The generator pocket may be revised and/or the existing generator removed, inserted, or replaced. The electrode is connected to the generator and the pocket is closed.

Coding Tips

This code reports the repositioning of an electrode in a previously placed pacing cardioverter-defibrillator or pacemaker pulse generator for left ventricular pacing. Fluoroscopy is included in 33226 and is not reported separately. For insertion of an electrode for a previously placed pacing cardioverter-defibrillator or pacemaker pulse generator, see 33224. For insertion of an electrode at the time of insertion of a pacing cardioverter-defibrillator or pacemaker pulse generator for left ventricular pacing, see 33225. For insertion of a single chamber electrode, see 33216. For insertion of a dual chamber electrode, see 33217.

ICD-10-CM Diagnostic Codes

T82.110A	Breakdown (mechanical) of cardiac electrode, initial encounter
T82.120A	Displacement of cardiac electrode, initial encounter
T82.190A	Other mechanical complication of cardiac electrode, initial encounter
T82.7XXA	Infection and inflammatory reaction due to other cardiac and vascular devices, implants and grafts, initial encounter
T82.817A	Embolism due to cardiac prosthetic devices, implants and grafts, initial encounter

T82.827A Fibrosis due to cardiac prosthetic devices, implants and grafts, initial encounter

T82.837A Hemorrhage due to cardiac prosthetic devices, implants and grafts, initial encounter

T82.847A Pain due to cardiac prosthetic devices, implants and grafts, initial encounter

T82.857A Stenosis of other cardiac prosthetic devices, implants and grafts, initial encounter

T82.867A Thrombosis due to cardiac prosthetic devices, implants and grafts, initial encounter

T82.897A Other specified complication of cardiac prosthetic devices, implants and grafts, initial encounter

T82.9XXA Unspecified complication of cardiac and vascular prosthetic device, implant and graft, initial encounter

Z45.09 Encounter for adjustment and management of other cardiac device

Z95.0 Presence of cardiac pacemaker

Z95.810 Presence of automatic (implantable) cardiac defibrillator

AMA: **33226** 2019,Mar,6; 2018,Jan,8; 2017,Jan,8; 2016,May,5; 2016,Jan,13; 2016,Aug,5; 2015,May,3; 2015,Jan,16; 2014,Nov,5; 2014,Jan,11

Relative Value Units/Medicare Edits

Non-Facility RVU	Work	PE	MP	Total
33226	8.68	3.73	2.04	14.45
Facility RVU	**Work**	**PE**	**MP**	**Total**
33226	8.68	3.73	2.04	14.45

	FUD	Status	MUE	Modifiers				IOM Reference
33226	0	A	1(3)	51	N/A	N/A	N/A	None

* with documentation

Terms To Know

electrode. Electric terminal specialized for a particular electrochemical reaction that acts as a medium between a body surface and another instrument, commonly termed a lead.

fluoroscopy. Radiology technique that allows visual examination of part of the body or a function of an organ using a device that projects an x-ray image on a fluorescent screen.

pacemaker. Implantable cardiac device that controls the heart's rhythm and maintains regular beats by artificial electric discharges. This device consists of the pulse generator with a battery and the electrodes, or leads, which are placed in single or dual chambers of the heart, usually transvenously.

33233

33233 Removal of permanent pacemaker pulse generator only

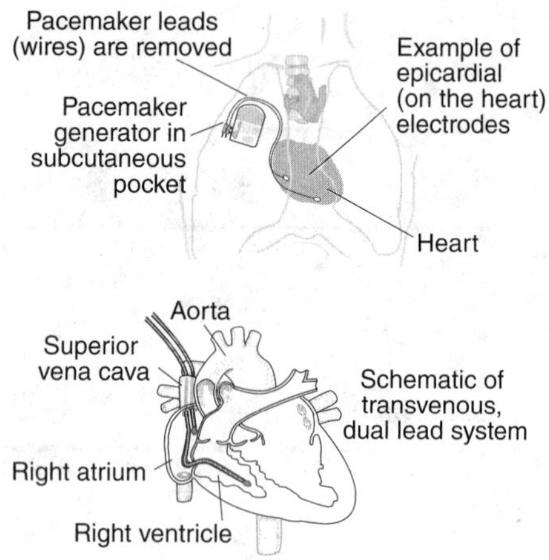

An implanted permanent pacemaker generator is removed

Explanation

In 33233, only the permanent pacemaker pulse generator is removed. The pacemaker generator pocket is opened. The generator is disconnected from the wire(s) and removed. The wire(s) is left in place in the pocket and the pocket is closed.

Coding Tips

When medically necessary, report moderate (conscious) sedation provided by the performing physician with 99151-99153. When provided by another physician, report 99155-99157. An inactive pacemaker does not always require removal. Procedure 33233 reports removal of the pacemaker generator only. For removal with replacement of the pulse generator during the same surgical session, see 33227–33229. For removal of transvenous pacemaker electrodes, see 33234–33235. For removal of a permanent epicardial pacemaker system and/or electrodes by thoracotomy, see 33236–33237. For removal of transvenous electrodes by thoracotomy, see 33238.

ICD-10-CM Diagnostic Codes

T82.111A Breakdown (mechanical) of cardiac pulse generator (battery), initial encounter

T82.121A Displacement of cardiac pulse generator (battery), initial encounter

T82.191A Other mechanical complication of cardiac pulse generator (battery), initial encounter

T82.7XXA Infection and inflammatory reaction due to other cardiac and vascular devices, implants and grafts, initial encounter

T82.817A Embolism due to cardiac prosthetic devices, implants and grafts, initial encounter

T82.827A Fibrosis due to cardiac prosthetic devices, implants and grafts, initial encounter

T82.837A Hemorrhage due to cardiac prosthetic devices, implants and grafts, initial encounter

T82.847A Pain due to cardiac prosthetic devices, implants and grafts, initial encounter

T82.857A Stenosis of other cardiac prosthetic devices, implants and grafts, initial encounter

 ● New ▲ Revised + Add On AMA: CPT Assist [Resequenced] ☑ Laterality

T82.867A	Thrombosis due to cardiac prosthetic devices, implants and grafts, initial encounter
Z45.018	Encounter for adjustment and management of other part of cardiac pacemaker

AMA: **33233** 2019,Mar,6; 2018,Jan,8; 2017,Jan,8; 2016,May,5; 2016,Jan,13; 2016,Aug,5; 2015,Jan,16; 2014,Nov,5; 2014,Jan,11

Relative Value Units/Medicare Edits

Non-Facility RVU	Work	PE	MP	Total
33233	3.14	2.81	0.73	6.68
Facility RVU	**Work**	**PE**	**MP**	**Total**
33233	3.14	2.81	0.73	6.68

	FUD	Status	MUE	Modifiers				IOM Reference
33233	90	A	1(2)	51	N/A	N/A	N/A	100-04,4,10.2.2

* with documentation

Terms To Know

complication. Condition arising after the beginning of observation and treatment that modifies the course of the patient's illness or the medical care required, or an undesired result or misadventure in medical care.

epicardial electrode. Stimulation device that is attached to or inserted into the heart muscle and connected to a generator.

infection. Presence of microorganisms in body tissues that may result in cellular damage.

pacemaker. Implantable cardiac device that controls the heart's rhythm and maintains regular beats by artificial electric discharges. This device consists of the pulse generator with a battery and the electrodes, or leads, which are placed in single or dual chambers of the heart, usually transvenously.

revision. Reordering or rearrangement of tissue to suit a particular need or function.

thoracotomy. Surgical procedure for opening the chest wall in order to access the lungs, esophagus, trachea, aorta, heart, and diaphragm.

transvenous electrode. Electrode placed using a transvenous catheter and wedged into the endocardium of the right ventricle or atrium.

[33227, 33228, 33229]

33227 Removal of permanent pacemaker pulse generator with replacement of pacemaker pulse generator; single lead system

33228 Removal of permanent pacemaker pulse generator with replacement of pacemaker pulse generator; dual lead system

33229 Removal of permanent pacemaker pulse generator with replacement of pacemaker pulse generator; multiple lead system

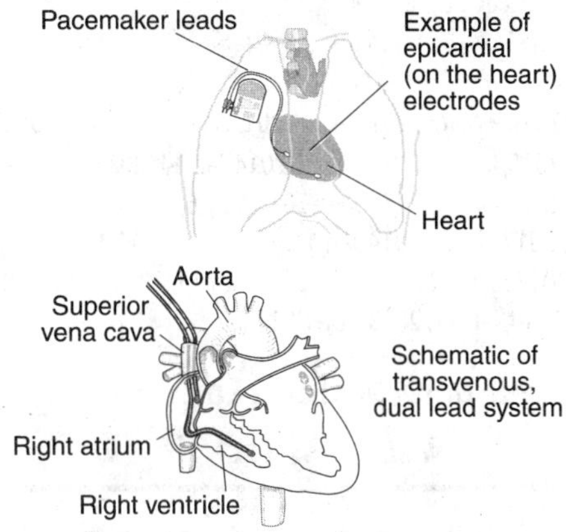

Explanation

A permanent pacemaker pulse generator is removed and replaced. The pacemaker generator pocket is opened. The existing generator is disconnected from the wire(s) and removed. The wire(s) is left in place in the pocket and a new permanent pacemaker pulse generator is inserted. The existing pacer wire(s) is tested and connected to the generator. The pocket is closed. Report 33227 for removal and replacement of a single lead system generator, 33228 for a dual lead system generator, and 33229 for a multiple lead system generator.

Coding Tips

When medically necessary, report moderate (conscious) sedation provided by the performing physician with 99151-99153. When provided by another physician, report 99155-99157. These codes are used when removal and replacement of the permanent pulse generator are performed during the same operative session. For removal and replacement of the pacemaker pulse generator, as well as the transvenous electrodes, see 33233 with 33234 or 33235 and 33206–33208. Do not report 33227–33229 with 33214, 33216, 33217, or 33233.

ICD-10-CM Diagnostic Codes

T82.111A	Breakdown (mechanical) of cardiac pulse generator (battery), initial encounter
T82.121A	Displacement of cardiac pulse generator (battery), initial encounter
T82.191A	Other mechanical complication of cardiac pulse generator (battery), initial encounter
T82.7XXA	Infection and inflammatory reaction due to other cardiac and vascular devices, implants and grafts, initial encounter
T82.817A	Embolism due to cardiac prosthetic devices, implants and grafts, initial encounter
T82.827A	Fibrosis due to cardiac prosthetic devices, implants and grafts, initial encounter
T82.837A	Hemorrhage due to cardiac prosthetic devices, implants and grafts, initial encounter

T82.847A	Pain due to cardiac prosthetic devices, implants and grafts, initial encounter
T82.857A	Stenosis of other cardiac prosthetic devices, implants and grafts, initial encounter
T82.867A	Thrombosis due to cardiac prosthetic devices, implants and grafts, initial encounter
T82.897A	Other specified complication of cardiac prosthetic devices, implants and grafts, initial encounter
Z45.018	Encounter for adjustment and management of other part of cardiac pacemaker
Z95.0	Presence of cardiac pacemaker

AMA: **33227** 2019,Mar,6; 2018,Jan,8; 2017,Jan,8; 2016,May,5; 2016,Jan,13; 2016,Aug,5; 2015,Jan,16; 2014,Nov,5; 2014,Jan,11; 2013,Apr,10-11 **33228** 2019,Mar,6; 2018,Jan,8; 2017,Jan,8; 2016,May,5; 2016,Jan,13; 2016,Aug,5; 2015,Jan,16; 2014,Nov,5; 2014,Jan,11; 2013,Apr,10-11 **33229** 2019,Mar,6; 2018,Jan,8; 2017,Jan,8; 2016,May,5; 2016,Jan,13; 2016,Aug,5; 2015,Jan,16; 2014,Nov,5; 2014,Jan,11; 2013,Apr,10-11

Relative Value Units/Medicare Edits

Non-Facility RVU	Work	PE	MP	Total
33227	5.25	3.35	1.22	9.82
33228	5.52	3.47	1.27	10.26
33229	5.79	3.74	1.34	10.87
Facility RVU	**Work**	**PE**	**MP**	**Total**
33227	5.25	3.35	1.22	9.82
33228	5.52	3.47	1.27	10.26
33229	5.79	3.74	1.34	10.87

	FUD	Status	MUE	Modifiers				IOM Reference
33227	90	A	1(3)	51	N/A	N/A	N/A	None
33228	90	A	1(3)	51	N/A	N/A	N/A	
33229	90	A	1(3)	51	N/A	N/A	N/A	

* with documentation

Terms To Know

dual chamber system. System that includes a pulse generator and one electrode inserted into the right atrium and one into the right ventricle.

multiple-lead device. Implantable cardiac device (pacemaker or implantable cardioverter-defibrillator [ICD]) in which pacing and sensing components are placed in three or more chambers of the heart.

pacemaker. Implantable cardiac device that controls the heart's rhythm and maintains regular beats by artificial electric discharges. This device consists of the pulse generator with a battery and the electrodes, or leads, which are placed in single or dual chambers of the heart, usually transvenously.

pulse generator. Circuit used to generate pulses. Pulse generators contain the battery, the electronic circuit, and the connector in a hermetically sealed encasement. Pulse generators may be temporary transcutaneous or placed in a subcutaneous pocket.

33234-33235

33234 Removal of transvenous pacemaker electrode(s); single lead system, atrial or ventricular

33235 dual lead system

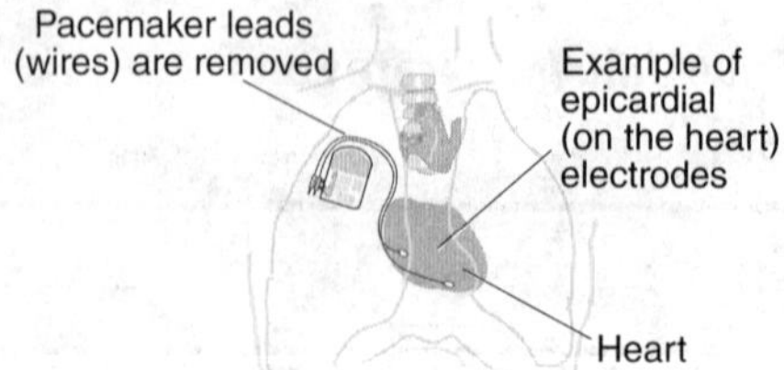

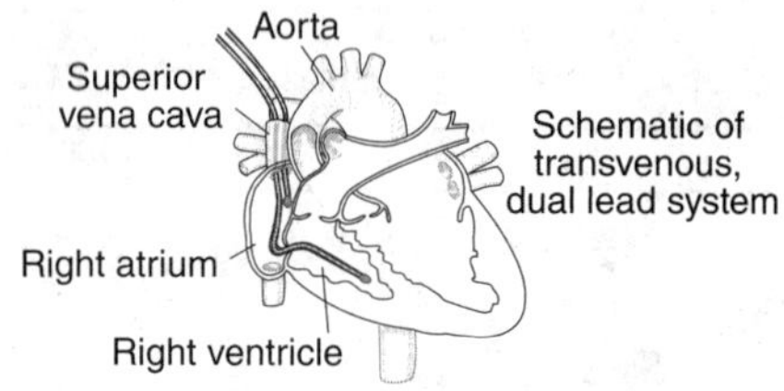

Explanation

In 33234 and 33235, only the transvenous electrode(s) are removed. In 33234, the generator pocket is opened and the wire is disconnected from the generator. The wire is dissected from the scar tissue that has formed around it. Once the wire is completely freed, it is twisted in a direction opposite to that used for insertion (counter clockwise). The wire is withdrawn. Bleeding from the tracts leading to the vein is controlled with sutures. A new wire may be placed, but is reported separately. Report 33235 for a dual lead system (removal of two wires).

Coding Tips

When medically necessary, report moderate (conscious) sedation provided by the performing physician with 99151-99153. When provided by another physician, report 99155-99157. Procedures 33234 and 33235 report removal of pacemaker leads without concurrent replacement. For removal with replacement of generator and leads during the same surgical session, see 33206–33208. For transvenous leads inserted when a pulse generator is in place, see 33216 and 33217. For removal of a permanent pacemaker pulse generator without replacement, see 33233. For removal of a pacemaker system and/or electrodes by thoracotomy, see 33236–33238. Unsuccessful transvenous extraction of electrodes converted to an open procedure should be reported using thoracotomy code 33238 for pacemaker electrodes or 33243 for cardioverter-defibrillator electrodes.

ICD-10-CM Diagnostic Codes

T82.110A	Breakdown (mechanical) of cardiac electrode, initial encounter
T82.120A	Displacement of cardiac electrode, initial encounter
T82.190A	Other mechanical complication of cardiac electrode, initial encounter
T82.7XXA	Infection and inflammatory reaction due to other cardiac and vascular devices, implants and grafts, initial encounter
T82.817A	Embolism due to cardiac prosthetic devices, implants and grafts, initial encounter
T82.827A	Fibrosis due to cardiac prosthetic devices, implants and grafts, initial encounter
T82.837A	Hemorrhage due to cardiac prosthetic devices, implants and grafts, initial encounter

T82.847A Pain due to cardiac prosthetic devices, implants and grafts, initial encounter

T82.857A Stenosis of other cardiac prosthetic devices, implants and grafts, initial encounter

T82.867A Thrombosis due to cardiac prosthetic devices, implants and grafts, initial encounter

Z45.018 Encounter for adjustment and management of other part of cardiac pacemaker

AMA: **33234** 2019,Mar,6; 2018,Jan,8; 2017,Jan,8; 2016,May,5; 2016,Jan,13; 2016,Aug,5; 2015,Jan,16; 2014,Nov,5; 2014,Jan,11 **33235** 2019,Mar,6; 2018,Jan,8; 2017,Jan,8; 2016,May,5; 2016,Jan,13; 2016,Aug,5; 2015,Jan,16; 2014,Nov,5; 2014,Jan,11; 2013,Dec,14

Relative Value Units/Medicare Edits

Non-Facility RVU	Work	PE	MP	Total
33234	7.66	4.67	1.77	14.1
33235	9.9	6.32	2.3	18.52
Facility RVU	**Work**	**PE**	**MP**	**Total**
33234	7.66	4.67	1.77	14.1
33235	9.9	6.32	2.3	18.52

	FUD	Status	MUE	Modifiers				IOM Reference
33234	90	A	1(2)	51	N/A	N/A	N/A	None
33235	90	A	1(2)	51	N/A	N/A	N/A	

* with documentation

Terms To Know

complication. Condition arising after the beginning of observation and treatment that modifies the course of the patient's illness or the medical care required, or an undesired result or misadventure in medical care.

epicardial electrode. Stimulation device that is attached to or inserted into the heart muscle and connected to a generator.

infection. Presence of microorganisms in body tissues that may result in cellular damage.

pacemaker. Implantable cardiac device that controls the heart's rhythm and maintains regular beats by artificial electric discharges. This device consists of the pulse generator with a battery and the electrodes, or leads, which are placed in single or dual chambers of the heart, usually transvenously.

revision. Reordering or rearrangement of tissue to suit a particular need or function.

suture. Numerous stitching techniques employed in wound closure.

thoracotomy. Surgical procedure for opening the chest wall in order to access the lungs, esophagus, trachea, aorta, heart, and diaphragm.

transvenous electrode. Electrode placed using a transvenous catheter and wedged into the endocardium of the right ventricle or atrium.

33236-33237

33236 Removal of permanent epicardial pacemaker and electrodes by thoracotomy; single lead system, atrial or ventricular

33237 dual lead system

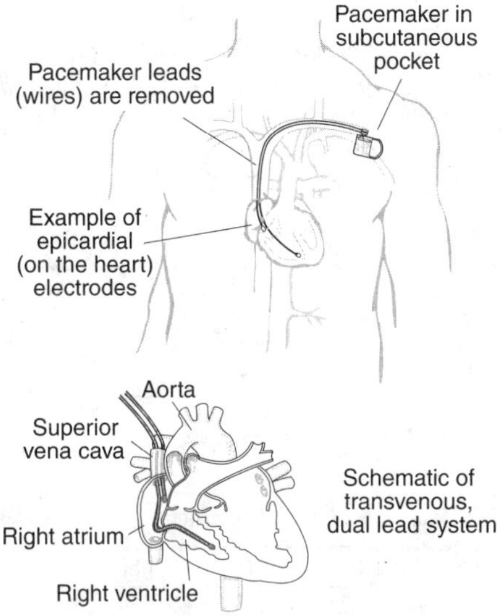

Pacemaker and electrodes are removed

Explanation

Code 33236 reports the removal of a single lead epicardial pacemaker system and electrodes. The old pacemaker pocket is opened and the generator is removed. The old wires are cut and the incision is closed. The old chest incision is opened. The wires are pulled into the chest and they are followed onto the heart surface. The electrodes are detached from the heart. The chest incision is closed. Report 33237 if a dual lead epicardial system is being removed.

Coding Tips

Procedures 33236 and 33237 report removal of the pacemaker system only. For removal of transvenous electrodes not requiring thoracotomy, see 33234–33235. For removal of transvenous electrodes by thoracotomy, see 33238. For insertion of epicardial electrodes, see 33202 and 33203.

ICD-10-CM Diagnostic Codes

T82.110A Breakdown (mechanical) of cardiac electrode, initial encounter

T82.111A Breakdown (mechanical) of cardiac pulse generator (battery), initial encounter

T82.120A Displacement of cardiac electrode, initial encounter

T82.121A Displacement of cardiac pulse generator (battery), initial encounter

T82.190A Other mechanical complication of cardiac electrode, initial encounter

T82.191A Other mechanical complication of cardiac pulse generator (battery), initial encounter

T82.7XXA Infection and inflammatory reaction due to other cardiac and vascular devices, implants and grafts, initial encounter

T82.817A Embolism due to cardiac prosthetic devices, implants and grafts, initial encounter

T82.827A Fibrosis due to cardiac prosthetic devices, implants and grafts, initial encounter

T82.837A	Hemorrhage due to cardiac prosthetic devices, implants and grafts, initial encounter
T82.847A	Pain due to cardiac prosthetic devices, implants and grafts, initial encounter
T82.867A	Thrombosis due to cardiac prosthetic devices, implants and grafts, initial encounter

AMA: 33236 2019,Mar,6; 2018,Jan,8; 2017,Jan,8; 2016,May,5; 2016,Jan,13; 2016,Aug,5; 2015,Jan,16; 2014,Nov,5; 2014,Jan,11 **33237** 2019,Mar,6; 2018,Jan,8; 2017,Jan,8; 2016,May,5; 2016,Jan,13; 2016,Aug,5; 2015,Jan,16; 2014,Nov,5; 2014,Jan,11

Relative Value Units/Medicare Edits

Non-Facility RVU	Work	PE	MP	Total
33236	12.73	6.93	2.99	22.65
33237	13.84	7.24	3.27	24.35
Facility RVU	**Work**	**PE**	**MP**	**Total**
33236	12.73	6.93	2.99	22.65
33237	13.84	7.24	3.27	24.35

	FUD	Status	MUE	Modifiers				IOM Reference
33236	90	A	1(2)	51	N/A	62	80*	None
33237	90	A	1(2)	51	N/A	62	80*	

* with documentation

Terms To Know

complication. Condition arising after the beginning of observation and treatment that modifies the course of the patient's illness or the medical care required, or an undesired result or misadventure in medical care.

dual chamber system. System that includes a pulse generator and one electrode inserted into the right atrium and one into the right ventricle.

epicardial electrode. Stimulation device that is attached to or inserted into the heart muscle and connected to a generator.

infection. Presence of microorganisms in body tissues that may result in cellular damage.

pacemaker. Implantable cardiac device that controls the heart's rhythm and maintains regular beats by artificial electric discharges. This device consists of the pulse generator with a battery and the electrodes, or leads, which are placed in single or dual chambers of the heart, usually transvenously.

pulse generator. Component of a pacemaker or an implantable cardioverter defibrillator that contains the battery and the electronics for producing the electrical discharge sent to the heart to control cardiac rhythm. Insertion or replacement of the pulse generator may be done alone, not in conjunction with insertion or replacement of the entire pacemaker system.

single-lead device. Implantable cardiac device (pacemaker or implantable cardioverter-defibrillator [ICD]) in which pacing and sensing components are placed in only one chamber of the heart.

thoracotomy. Surgical procedure for opening the chest wall in order to access the lungs, esophagus, trachea, aorta, heart, and diaphragm.

33238

33238 Removal of permanent transvenous electrode(s) by thoracotomy

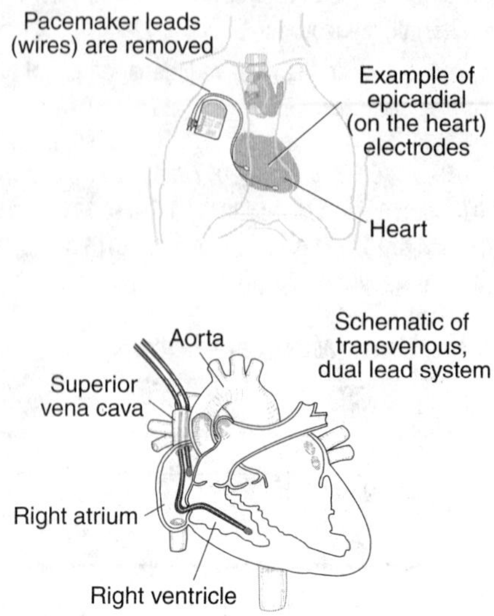

Removal of transvenous electrode(s)

Explanation

The physician removes a transvenous electrode(s) by thoracotomy. Prior to this procedure, the pacemaker pocket was opened, the generator removed, and the wires cut. The right chest is opened and the superior caval vein is dissected out. Tourniquets are placed around the vein above and below the planned site of opening. The tourniquets are tightened and a hole is made in the caval vein. The cut ends of the wires are pulled out through the hole in the caval vein. The ends of the wires that are still in the heart are twisted counterclockwise until they are free and are withdrawn through the caval vein. The hole in the caval vein is closed and the tourniquets released. The chest is closed.

Coding Tips

Procedure 33238 reports removal of pacemaker components only. For removal with replacement of generator and leads during the same surgical session, see 33206–33208. For transvenous leads inserted when a pulse generator is in place, see 33216 and 33217. Note that 33238 may require vein or heart repair with graft; report this separately. For removal of a permanent pacemaker pulse generator, see 33233. For removal of transvenous electrodes not requiring thoracotomy, see 33234–33235. For removal of an epicardial pacemaker system or electrodes by thoracotomy, see 33236–33237.

ICD-10-CM Diagnostic Codes

T82.110A	Breakdown (mechanical) of cardiac electrode, initial encounter
T82.120A	Displacement of cardiac electrode, initial encounter
T82.190A	Other mechanical complication of cardiac electrode, initial encounter
T82.7XXA	Infection and inflammatory reaction due to other cardiac and vascular devices, implants and grafts, initial encounter
T82.817A	Embolism due to cardiac prosthetic devices, implants and grafts, initial encounter
T82.827A	Fibrosis due to cardiac prosthetic devices, implants and grafts, initial encounter
T82.837A	Hemorrhage due to cardiac prosthetic devices, implants and grafts, initial encounter

T82.847A Pain due to cardiac prosthetic devices, implants and grafts, initial encounter

T82.857A Stenosis of other cardiac prosthetic devices, implants and grafts, initial encounter

T82.867A Thrombosis due to cardiac prosthetic devices, implants and grafts, initial encounter

AMA: **33238** 2018,Jan,8; 2017,Jan,8; 2016,May,5; 2016,Jan,13; 2016,Aug,5; 2015,Jan,16; 2014,Nov,5; 2014,Jan,11

Relative Value Units/Medicare Edits

Non-Facility RVU	Work	PE	MP	Total
33238	15.4	8.33	3.36	27.09
Facility RVU	**Work**	**PE**	**MP**	**Total**
33238	15.4	8.33	3.36	27.09

	FUD	Status	MUE	Modifiers				IOM Reference
33238	90	A	1(2)	51	N/A	62	80*	None

* with documentation

Terms To Know

complication. Condition arising after the beginning of observation and treatment that modifies the course of the patient's illness or the medical care required, or an undesired result or misadventure in medical care.

epicardial electrode. Stimulation device that is attached to or inserted into the heart muscle and connected to a generator.

infection. Presence of microorganisms in body tissues that may result in cellular damage.

pacemaker. Implantable cardiac device that controls the heart's rhythm and maintains regular beats by artificial electric discharges. This device consists of the pulse generator with a battery and the electrodes, or leads, which are placed in single or dual chambers of the heart, usually transvenously.

thoracotomy. Surgical procedure for opening the chest wall in order to access the lungs, esophagus, trachea, aorta, heart, and diaphragm.

tourniquet. Device used to apply compressive force to a blood vessel in a limb and slow or prevent blood flow to and from the area.

transvenous electrode. Electrode placed using a transvenous catheter and wedged into the endocardium of the right ventricle or atrium.

33240 [33230, 33231]

33240 Insertion of implantable defibrillator pulse generator only; with existing single lead

33230 Insertion of implantable defibrillator pulse generator only; with existing dual leads

33231 Insertion of implantable defibrillator pulse generator only; with existing multiple leads

+
35266, 59
Axillary
Artery
Graft

Schematic showing epicardial ICD leads and electrodes

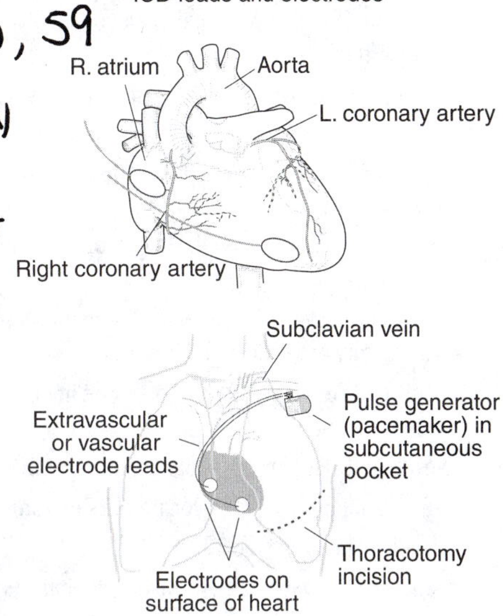

Explanation

This operation is done only when defibrillator electrodes are already in place. The previous pocket is opened or a new pocket is created for the implantable defibrillator pulse generator. The defibrillator pulse generators are implanted subcutaneously usually in an infraclavicular or abdominal pocket with the assistance of fluoroscopy. The electrodes are tested. The electrodes are connected to the defibrillator pulse generator and it is placed in the pocket. The pocket is closed with sutures, adhesive strips, or special glue. Report 33240 when there is an existing single lead (electrode); 33230 when there are existing dual leads (electrodes); and 33231 when there are existing multiple leads (electrodes).

Coding Tips

When medically necessary, report moderate (conscious) sedation provided by the performing physician with 99151-99153. When provided by another physician, report 99155-99157. These codes are appropriate for reporting "battery" change. Epicardial lead placement codes (33202, 33203) can be reported in addition to 33230, 33231, and 33240 when performed by the same physician during the same operative session. For repositioning of a previously implanted electrode, see 33215. For electrode repair, see 33218–33220. Fluoroscopy is included with these procedures and should not be reported separately. For pocket revision, see 33223. Do not report 33230–33231 or 33240 with 33216, 33217, or 33241. Do not report 33240 with 33271, 93260, or 93261. When pulse generator replacement is performed, see 33262–33264. Do not report device evaluation codes (93260, 93261, 93279–93298) in addition to pulse generator and lead insertion/revision codes. Defibrillator threshold testing (DFT) during transvenous implantable defibrillator insertion/replacement is reported separately with 93640 and/or 93641.

ICD-10-CM Diagnostic Codes

I11.0 Hypertensive heart disease with heart failure

I13.0 Hypertensive heart and chronic kidney disease with heart failure and stage 1 through stage 4 chronic kidney disease, or unspecified chronic kidney disease

I13.2 Hypertensive heart and chronic kidney disease with heart failure and with stage 5 chronic kidney disease, or end stage renal disease

I16.0 Hypertensive urgency

I16.1 Hypertensive emergency

I21.01 ST elevation (STEMI) myocardial infarction involving left main coronary artery

I21.02 ST elevation (STEMI) myocardial infarction involving left anterior descending coronary artery

I21.09 ST elevation (STEMI) myocardial infarction involving other coronary artery of anterior wall

I21.11 ST elevation (STEMI) myocardial infarction involving right coronary artery

I21.19 ST elevation (STEMI) myocardial infarction involving other coronary artery of inferior wall

I21.21 ST elevation (STEMI) myocardial infarction involving left circumflex coronary artery

I21.29 ST elevation (STEMI) myocardial infarction involving other sites

I21.4 Non-ST elevation (NSTEMI) myocardial infarction

I21.A1 Myocardial infarction type 2

I22.0 Subsequent ST elevation (STEMI) myocardial infarction of anterior wall

I22.1 Subsequent ST elevation (STEMI) myocardial infarction of inferior wall

I22.2 Subsequent non-ST elevation (NSTEMI) myocardial infarction

I22.8 Subsequent ST elevation (STEMI) myocardial infarction of other sites

I25.2 Old myocardial infarction

I25.5 Ischemic cardiomyopathy

I25.6 Silent myocardial ischemia

I25.89 Other forms of chronic ischemic heart disease

I42.0 Dilated cardiomyopathy

I42.1 Obstructive hypertrophic cardiomyopathy

I42.2 Other hypertrophic cardiomyopathy

I42.5 Other restrictive cardiomyopathy

I42.8 Other cardiomyopathies

I44.0 Atrioventricular block, first degree

I44.1 Atrioventricular block, second degree

I44.2 Atrioventricular block, complete

I44.39 Other atrioventricular block

I44.4 Left anterior fascicular block

I44.5 Left posterior fascicular block

I44.69 Other fascicular block

I45.0 Right fascicular block

I45.19 Other right bundle-branch block

I45.2 Bifascicular block

I45.4 Nonspecific intraventricular block

I45.5 Other specified heart block

I45.6 Pre-excitation syndrome

I45.81 Long QT syndrome

I46.2 Cardiac arrest due to underlying cardiac condition

I46.8 Cardiac arrest due to other underlying condition

I47.0 Re-entry ventricular arrhythmia

I47.1 Supraventricular tachycardia

I47.2 Ventricular tachycardia

I48.0 Paroxysmal atrial fibrillation

I48.11 Longstanding persistent atrial fibrillation

I48.19 Other persistent atrial fibrillation

I48.21 Permanent atrial fibrillation

I49.01 Ventricular fibrillation

I49.02 Ventricular flutter

I49.2 Junctional premature depolarization

I49.5 Sick sinus syndrome

I49.8 Other specified cardiac arrhythmias

I50.1 Left ventricular failure, unspecified

I50.21 Acute systolic (congestive) heart failure

I50.22 Chronic systolic (congestive) heart failure

I50.23 Acute on chronic systolic (congestive) heart failure

I50.31 Acute diastolic (congestive) heart failure

I50.32 Chronic diastolic (congestive) heart failure

I50.33 Acute on chronic diastolic (congestive) heart failure

I50.41 Acute combined systolic (congestive) and diastolic (congestive) heart failure

I50.42 Chronic combined systolic (congestive) and diastolic (congestive) heart failure

I50.43 Acute on chronic combined systolic (congestive) and diastolic (congestive) heart failure

I50.811 Acute right heart failure

I50.812 Chronic right heart failure

I50.813 Acute on chronic right heart failure

I50.814 Right heart failure due to left heart failure

I50.82 Biventricular heart failure

I50.83 High output heart failure

I50.84 End stage heart failure

Q24.6 Congenital heart block

Q24.8 Other specified congenital malformations of heart

T82.110A Breakdown (mechanical) of cardiac electrode, initial encounter

T82.111A Breakdown (mechanical) of cardiac pulse generator (battery), initial encounter

T82.120A Displacement of cardiac electrode, initial encounter

T82.121A Displacement of cardiac pulse generator (battery), initial encounter

T82.190A Other mechanical complication of cardiac electrode, initial encounter

T82.191A Other mechanical complication of cardiac pulse generator (battery), initial encounter

T82.598A Other mechanical complication of other cardiac and vascular devices and implants, initial encounter

T82.7XXA Infection and inflammatory reaction due to other cardiac and vascular devices, implants and grafts, initial encounter

T82.817A Embolism due to cardiac prosthetic devices, implants and grafts, initial encounter

T82.827A	Fibrosis due to cardiac prosthetic devices, implants and grafts, initial encounter
T82.837A	Hemorrhage due to cardiac prosthetic devices, implants and grafts, initial encounter
T82.847A	Pain due to cardiac prosthetic devices, implants and grafts, initial encounter
T82.855A	Stenosis of coronary artery stent, initial encounter
T82.857A	Stenosis of other cardiac prosthetic devices, implants and grafts, initial encounter
T82.867A	Thrombosis due to cardiac prosthetic devices, implants and grafts, initial encounter
T82.897A	Other specified complication of cardiac prosthetic devices, implants and grafts, initial encounter
Z45.02	Encounter for adjustment and management of automatic implantable cardiac defibrillator
Z95.810	Presence of automatic (implantable) cardiac defibrillator

AMA: 33230 2019,Mar,6; 2018,Jan,8; 2017,Jan,8; 2016,Jan,13; 2016,Aug,5; 2015,Jan,16; 2014,Nov,5; 2014,Jan,11 **33231** 2019,Mar,6; 2018,Jan,8; 2017,Jan,8; 2016,Jan,13; 2016,Aug,5; 2015,Jan,16; 2014,Nov,5; 2014,Jan,11 **33240** 2018,Jan,8; 2017,Jan,8; 2016,Jan,13; 2016,Aug,5; 2015,Jan,16; 2014,Nov,5; 2014,Jan,11

Relative Value Units/Medicare Edits

Non-Facility RVU	Work	PE	MP	Total
33240	5.8	3.47	1.34	10.61
33230	6.07	3.64	1.38	11.09
33231	6.34	3.85	1.46	11.65
Facility RVU	**Work**	**PE**	**MP**	**Total**
33240	5.8	3.47	1.34	10.61
33230	6.07	3.64	1.38	11.09
33231	6.34	3.85	1.46	11.65

	FUD	Status	MUE	Modifiers				IOM Reference
33240	90	A	1(3)	51	N/A	N/A	N/A	100-04,4,10.2.2;
33230	90	A	1(3)	51	N/A	N/A	N/A	100-04,32,270;
33231	90	A	1(3)	51	N/A	N/A	N/A	100-04,32,270.1; 100-04,32,270.2

* with documentation

Terms To Know

defibrillation. Arrest of cardiac arrhythmias (atrial or ventricular) with restoration of normal rhythm, usually by applying brief electroshock to the heart.

dual-lead device. Implantable cardiac device (pacemaker or implantable cardioverter-defibrillator [ICD]) in which pacing and sensing components are placed in only two chambers of the heart.

pulse generator. Component of a pacemaker or an implantable cardioverter defibrillator that contains the battery and the electronics for producing the electrical discharge sent to the heart to control cardiac rhythm. Insertion or replacement of the pulse generator may be done alone, not in conjunction with insertion or replacement of the entire pacemaker system.

33241

33241 Removal of implantable defibrillator pulse generator only

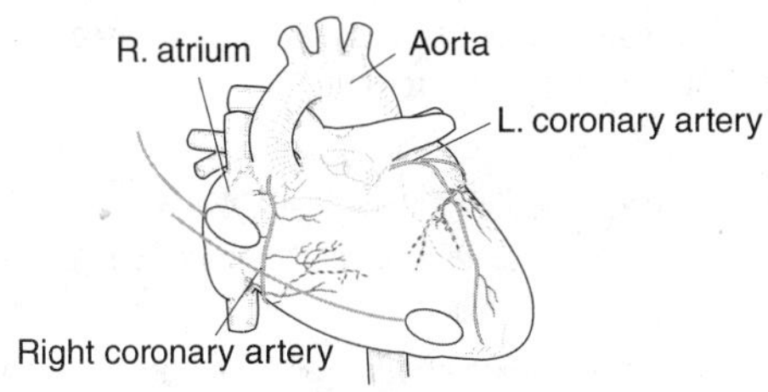

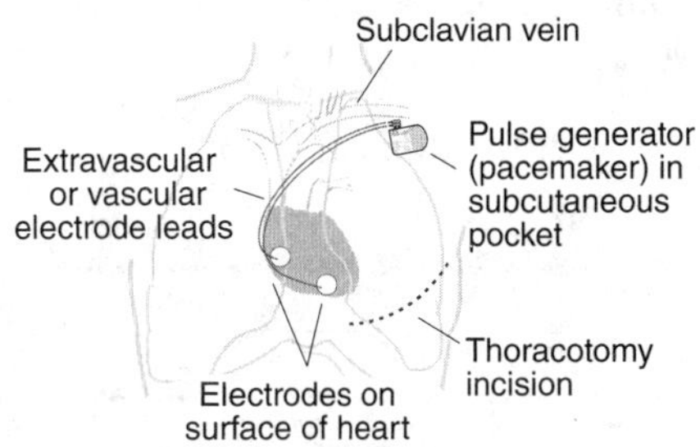

Pulse generator is removed

Explanation

The physician removes only the implantable defibrillator pulse generator. The pulse generator may be removed due to a complication or malfunction. The subcutaneous generator pocket is opened and the generator is removed. The electrodes are detached from the generator and the electrodes are placed in the pocket. The pocket is closed.

Coding Tips

When medically necessary, report moderate (conscious) sedation provided by the performing physician with 99151-99153. When provided by another physician, report 99155-99157. For removal and replacement of an implantable defibrillator pulse generator and electrodes, report 33243 or 33244 and 33249 for transvenous electrodes or 33270 and 33272 for subcutaneous electrodes with 33241. Do not report 33241 with 33230, 33231, or 33240, which includes removal and replacement of an implantable defibrillator pulse generator only. Do not report 33241 in addition to 93260 or 93261. For generator replacement only, see 33262–33264. Fluoroscopy is included and should not be reported separately.

ICD-10-CM Diagnostic Codes

T82.111A	Breakdown (mechanical) of cardiac pulse generator (battery), initial encounter
T82.121A	Displacement of cardiac pulse generator (battery), initial encounter
T82.191A	Other mechanical complication of cardiac pulse generator (battery), initial encounter
T82.598A	Other mechanical complication of other cardiac and vascular devices and implants, initial encounter
T82.7XXA	Infection and inflammatory reaction due to other cardiac and vascular devices, implants and grafts, initial encounter
T82.817A	Embolism due to cardiac prosthetic devices, implants and grafts, initial encounter
T82.827A	Fibrosis due to cardiac prosthetic devices, implants and grafts, initial encounter

T82.837A	Hemorrhage due to cardiac prosthetic devices, implants and grafts, initial encounter
T82.847A	Pain due to cardiac prosthetic devices, implants and grafts, initial encounter
T82.857A	Stenosis of other cardiac prosthetic devices, implants and grafts, initial encounter
T82.867A	Thrombosis due to cardiac prosthetic devices, implants and grafts, initial encounter
T82.897A	Other specified complication of cardiac prosthetic devices, implants and grafts, initial encounter
Z45.02	Encounter for adjustment and management of automatic implantable cardiac defibrillator
Z95.810	Presence of automatic (implantable) cardiac defibrillator

AMA: **33241** 2018,Jan,8; 2017,Jan,8; 2016,Jan,13; 2016,Aug,5; 2015,Jan,16; 2014,Nov,5; 2014,Jan,11

Relative Value Units/Medicare Edits

Non-Facility RVU	Work	PE	MP	Total
33241	3.04	2.49	0.71	6.24
Facility RVU	**Work**	**PE**	**MP**	**Total**
33241	3.04	2.49	0.71	6.24

	FUD	Status	MUE	Modifiers				IOM Reference
33241	90	A	1(2)	51	N/A	N/A	N/A	100-04,32,270; 100-04,32,270.1; 100-04,32,270.2

* with documentation

Terms To Know

atrioventricular block. Condition in which there is a disturbance of electrical conduction, such as a delay, intermittence, or absence in the transmission of an impulse from the atria to the ventricles and categorized according to degree of severity.

cardioverter-defibrillator. Device that uses both low energy cardioversion or defibrillating shocks and antitachycardia pacing to treat ventricular tachycardia or ventricular fibrillation.

electrode. Electric terminal specialized for a particular electrochemical reaction that acts as a medium between a body surface and another instrument, commonly termed a lead.

myocardial infarction. Obstruction of circulation to the heart, resulting in necrosis.

pulse generator. Circuit used to generate pulses. Pulse generators contain the battery, the electronic circuit, and the connector in a hermetically sealed encasement. Pulse generators may be temporary transcutaneous or placed in a subcutaneous pocket.

ventricular tachycardia. Excessively rapid ventricular rhythm of the heart, usually more than 150 beats per minute, with an origin beat generated in the ventricle, commonly from atrioventricular dissociation.

[33262, 33263, 33264]

33262 Removal of implantable defibrillator pulse generator with replacement of implantable defibrillator pulse generator; single lead system

33263 Removal of implantable defibrillator pulse generator with replacement of implantable defibrillator pulse generator; dual lead system

33264 Removal of implantable defibrillator pulse generator with replacement of implantable defibrillator pulse generator; multiple lead system

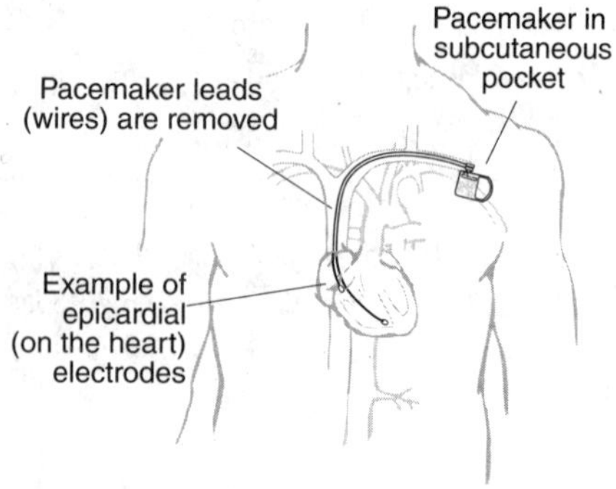

Explanation

An implantable defibrillator pulse generator is removed and replaced. The pulse generator may be removed due to a complication or malfunction. The generator pocket is opened. The existing generator is disconnected from the wire(s) and removed. The wire(s) is left in place in the pocket and a new pulse generator is inserted. The existing wire(s) is tested and connected to the new generator. The pocket is closed. Report 33262 for removal and replacement of a single lead system generator; 33263 for a dual lead system generator; and 33264 for a multiple lead system generator.

Coding Tips

When medically necessary, report moderate (conscious) sedation provided by the performing physician with 99151-99153. When provided by another physician, report 99155-99157. Do not report 33262–33264 with 33216, 33217, or 33241. Do not report 33262 with 33271, 93260, or 93261. For removal of electrodes via thoracotomy and removal/replacement of a pulse generator, use 33243 in addition to 33241 or 33262–33264. For transvenous removal of electrodes and removal/replacement of a pulse generator, use 33244 in addition to 33241 or 33262–33264. For repair of an implantable defibrillator pulse generator and/or leads, see 33218 and/or 33220. For removal of electrodes with removal or replacement of an implantable defibrillator pulse generator, report 33272 in addition to 33241 or 33262. Revision of a skin pocket is included and is not reported separately.

ICD-10-CM Diagnostic Codes

I11.0	Hypertensive heart disease with heart failure
I13.0	Hypertensive heart and chronic kidney disease with heart failure and stage 1 through stage 4 chronic kidney disease, or unspecified chronic kidney disease
I13.2	Hypertensive heart and chronic kidney disease with heart failure and with stage 5 chronic kidney disease, or end stage renal disease
I16.0	Hypertensive urgency
I16.1	Hypertensive emergency
I21.01	ST elevation (STEMI) myocardial infarction involving left main coronary artery

I21.02	ST elevation (STEMI) myocardial infarction involving left anterior descending coronary artery
I21.09	ST elevation (STEMI) myocardial infarction involving other coronary artery of anterior wall
I21.11	ST elevation (STEMI) myocardial infarction involving right coronary artery
I21.19	ST elevation (STEMI) myocardial infarction involving other coronary artery of inferior wall
I21.21	ST elevation (STEMI) myocardial infarction involving left circumflex coronary artery
I21.29	ST elevation (STEMI) myocardial infarction involving other sites
I21.4	Non-ST elevation (NSTEMI) myocardial infarction
I21.A1	Myocardial infarction type 2
I22.0	Subsequent ST elevation (STEMI) myocardial infarction of anterior wall
I22.1	Subsequent ST elevation (STEMI) myocardial infarction of inferior wall
I22.2	Subsequent non-ST elevation (NSTEMI) myocardial infarction
I22.8	Subsequent ST elevation (STEMI) myocardial infarction of other sites
I25.2	Old myocardial infarction
I25.5	Ischemic cardiomyopathy
I25.6	Silent myocardial ischemia
I25.89	Other forms of chronic ischemic heart disease
I42.0	Dilated cardiomyopathy
I42.5	Other restrictive cardiomyopathy
I42.8	Other cardiomyopathies
I44.0	Atrioventricular block, first degree
I44.1	Atrioventricular block, second degree
I44.2	Atrioventricular block, complete
I44.39	Other atrioventricular block
I44.4	Left anterior fascicular block
I44.5	Left posterior fascicular block
I44.69	Other fascicular block
I45.0	Right fascicular block
I45.19	Other right bundle-branch block
I45.2	Bifascicular block
I45.4	Nonspecific intraventricular block
I45.5	Other specified heart block
I45.6	Pre-excitation syndrome
I45.81	Long QT syndrome
I46.2	Cardiac arrest due to underlying cardiac condition
I46.8	Cardiac arrest due to other underlying condition
I47.0	Re-entry ventricular arrhythmia
I47.1	Supraventricular tachycardia
I47.2	Ventricular tachycardia
I48.0	Paroxysmal atrial fibrillation
I48.11	Longstanding persistent atrial fibrillation
I48.19	Other persistent atrial fibrillation
I48.21	Permanent atrial fibrillation
I49.01	Ventricular fibrillation
I49.02	Ventricular flutter
I49.2	Junctional premature depolarization
I49.5	Sick sinus syndrome
I49.8	Other specified cardiac arrhythmias
I50.1	Left ventricular failure, unspecified
I50.21	Acute systolic (congestive) heart failure
I50.22	Chronic systolic (congestive) heart failure
I50.23	Acute on chronic systolic (congestive) heart failure
I50.31	Acute diastolic (congestive) heart failure
I50.32	Chronic diastolic (congestive) heart failure
I50.33	Acute on chronic diastolic (congestive) heart failure
I50.41	Acute combined systolic (congestive) and diastolic (congestive) heart failure
I50.42	Chronic combined systolic (congestive) and diastolic (congestive) heart failure
I50.43	Acute on chronic combined systolic (congestive) and diastolic (congestive) heart failure
I50.811	Acute right heart failure
I50.812	Chronic right heart failure
I50.813	Acute on chronic right heart failure
I50.814	Right heart failure due to left heart failure
I50.82	Biventricular heart failure
I50.83	High output heart failure
I50.84	End stage heart failure
Q23.8	Other congenital malformations of aortic and mitral valves
Q24.6	Congenital heart block
Q24.8	Other specified congenital malformations of heart
T82.111A	Breakdown (mechanical) of cardiac pulse generator (battery), initial encounter
T82.121A	Displacement of cardiac pulse generator (battery), initial encounter
T82.191A	Other mechanical complication of cardiac pulse generator (battery), initial encounter
T82.598A	Other mechanical complication of other cardiac and vascular devices and implants, initial encounter
T82.7XXA	Infection and inflammatory reaction due to other cardiac and vascular devices, implants and grafts, initial encounter
T82.817A	Embolism due to cardiac prosthetic devices, implants and grafts, initial encounter
T82.827A	Fibrosis due to cardiac prosthetic devices, implants and grafts, initial encounter
T82.837A	Hemorrhage due to cardiac prosthetic devices, implants and grafts, initial encounter
T82.847A	Pain due to cardiac prosthetic devices, implants and grafts, initial encounter
T82.855A	Stenosis of coronary artery stent, initial encounter
T82.857A	Stenosis of other cardiac prosthetic devices, implants and grafts, initial encounter
T82.867A	Thrombosis due to cardiac prosthetic devices, implants and grafts, initial encounter
T82.897A	Other specified complication of cardiac prosthetic devices, implants and grafts, initial encounter
Z45.02	Encounter for adjustment and management of automatic implantable cardiac defibrillator
Z95.810	Presence of automatic (implantable) cardiac defibrillator

AMA: **33262** 2018,Jan,8; 2017,Jan,8; 2016,Jan,13; 2016,Aug,5; 2015,Jan,16; 2014,Nov,5; 2014,Jan,11 **33263** 2018,Jan,8; 2017,Jan,8; 2016,Jan,13; 2016,Aug,5; 2015,Jan,16; 2014,Nov,5; 2014,Jan,11; 2013,Dec,16 **33264** 2018,Jan,8;

2017,Jan,8; 2016,Jan,13; 2016,Aug,5; 2015,Jan,16; 2014,Nov,5; 2014,Jan,11; 2013,Dec,16

Relative Value Units/Medicare Edits

Non-Facility RVU	Work	PE	MP	Total
33262	5.81	3.67	1.34	10.82
33263	6.08	3.79	1.4	11.27
33264	6.35	3.94	1.47	11.76
Facility RVU	**Work**	**PE**	**MP**	**Total**
33262	5.81	3.67	1.34	10.82
33263	6.08	3.79	1.4	11.27
33264	6.35	3.94	1.47	11.76

	FUD	Status	MUE	Modifiers				IOM Reference
33262	90	A	1(3)	51	N/A	N/A	N/A	None
33263	90	A	1(3)	51	N/A	N/A	N/A	
33264	90	A	1(3)	51	N/A	N/A	N/A	

* with documentation

Terms To Know

cardioverter-defibrillator. Device that uses both low energy cardioversion or defibrillating shocks and antitachycardia pacing to treat ventricular tachycardia or ventricular fibrillation.

dual-lead device. Implantable cardiac device (pacemaker or implantable cardioverter-defibrillator [ICD]) in which pacing and sensing components are placed in only two chambers of the heart.

hypertension. Abnormally increased pressure, usually referring to arterial pressure, exceeding an acceptable range.

long QT syndrome. Potentially fatal condition precipitated by vigorous exertion, emotional upset, or startling moments due to an imbalance in the electrical timing mechanism that controls the pumping action of the heart's ventricles. This syndrome causes the patient to be susceptible to recurrent episodes of syncope, collapse, and possible ventricular fibrillation that can cause sudden death.

multiple-lead device. Implantable cardiac device (pacemaker or implantable cardioverter-defibrillator [ICD]) in which pacing and sensing components are placed in three or more chambers of the heart.

paroxysmal supraventricular tachycardia. Rapid heartbeat that starts above the ventricles and occurs sporadically.

single-lead device. Implantable cardiac device (pacemaker or implantable cardioverter-defibrillator [ICD]) in which pacing and sensing components are placed in only one chamber of the heart.

thoracotomy. Surgical procedure for opening the chest wall in order to access the lungs, esophagus, trachea, aorta, heart, and diaphragm.

33243-33244

33243 Removal of single or dual chamber implantable defibrillator electrode(s); by thoracotomy

33244 by transvenous extraction

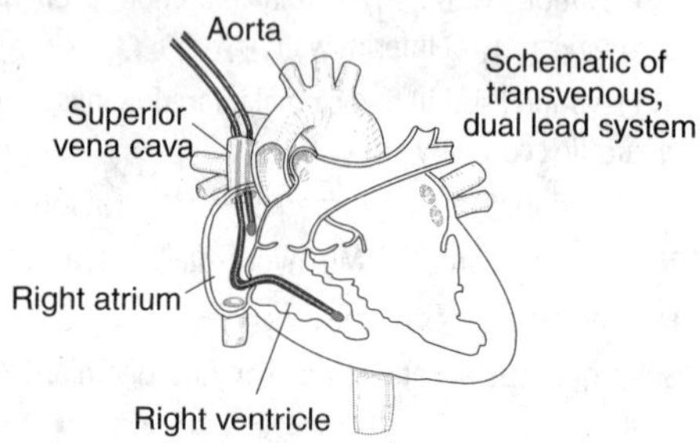

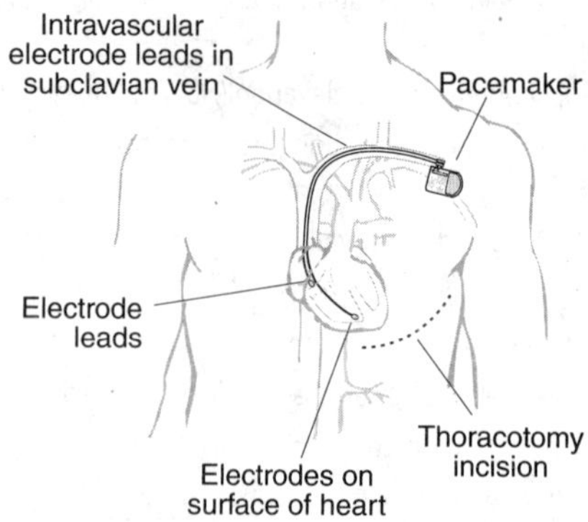

Defibrillator electrodes are removed

Explanation

In 33243, single or dual chamber implantable defibrillator electrodes are removed. Electrodes may be removed due to a complication or malfunction. The generator pocket is opened and the electrode wires are disconnected. The old chest incision is opened and the electrodes are dissected out and removed. The chest incision is closed. In 33244, electrodes only are removed by transvenous extraction, which is currently the most common technique for removing electrodes since most implantable defibrillator electrodes are now placed transvenously. Electrodes may be removed due to a complication or malfunction. The generator pocket is opened and the wire is disconnected from the generator. The wire is dissected from the scar tissue that has formed around it. Once the wire is completely freed, it is twisted in a direction opposite to that used for insertion (counterclockwise). The wire is withdrawn. Bleeding from the tracts leading to the vein is controlled with sutures. A new wire may be placed, but it is reported separately.

Coding Tips

When medically necessary, report moderate (conscious) sedation provided by the performing physician with 99151-99153. When provided by another physician, report 99155-99157. Removal of the pulse generator and electrodes requires reporting of multiple codes. For removal of an electrode by thoracotomy and removal of the pulse generator, report 33243 in addition to 33241. For removal of an electrode by transvenous extraction and removal of the pulse generator, report 33244 in addition to 33241. A transvenous extraction is normally attempted initially, but if it is unsuccessful a thoracotomy is performed. Removal and reinsertion of a new implantable defibrillator system also requires reporting of multiple codes. Report 33241 and 33243 or 33244 for the removal portion of the procedure. Report 33249 for insertion of the new system. For insertion or repositioning of implantable defibrillator electrodes without concurrent insertion of a pulse generator, see 33215–33217.

For repair of implantable defibrillator electrodes, see 33218 or 33220. Unsuccessful transvenous extraction of electrodes converted to an open procedure should be reported using thoracotomy code 33243.

ICD-10-CM Diagnostic Codes

T82.110A	Breakdown (mechanical) of cardiac electrode, initial encounter
T82.120A	Displacement of cardiac electrode, initial encounter
T82.190A	Other mechanical complication of cardiac electrode, initial encounter
T82.7XXA	Infection and inflammatory reaction due to other cardiac and vascular devices, implants and grafts, initial encounter
T82.817A	Embolism due to cardiac prosthetic devices, implants and grafts, initial encounter
T82.827A	Fibrosis due to cardiac prosthetic devices, implants and grafts, initial encounter
T82.837A	Hemorrhage due to cardiac prosthetic devices, implants and grafts, initial encounter
T82.847A	Pain due to cardiac prosthetic devices, implants and grafts, initial encounter
T82.857A	Stenosis of other cardiac prosthetic devices, implants and grafts, initial encounter
T82.867A	Thrombosis due to cardiac prosthetic devices, implants and grafts, initial encounter
T82.897A	Other specified complication of cardiac prosthetic devices, implants and grafts, initial encounter
Z45.02	Encounter for adjustment and management of automatic implantable cardiac defibrillator
Z95.810	Presence of automatic (implantable) cardiac defibrillator

AMA: **33243** 2018,Jan,8; 2017,Jan,8; 2016,Jan,13; 2016,Aug,5; 2015,Jan,16; 2014,Nov,5; 2014,Jan,11 **33244** 2018,Jan,8; 2017,Jan,8; 2016,Jan,13; 2016,Aug,5; 2015,Jan,16; 2014,Nov,5; 2014,Jan,11

Relative Value Units/Medicare Edits

Non-Facility RVU	Work	PE	MP	Total
33243	23.57	10.64	5.48	39.69
33244	13.74	8.14	3.21	25.09
Facility RVU	**Work**	**PE**	**MP**	**Total**
33243	23.57	10.64	5.48	39.69
33244	13.74	8.14	3.21	25.09

	FUD	Status	MUE	Modifiers				IOM Reference
33243	90	A	1(2)	51	N/A	62*	80	100-04,32,270; 100-04,32,270.1; 100-04,32,270.2
33244	90	A	1(2)	51	N/A	62*	N/A	

* with documentation

Terms To Know

cardioverter-defibrillator. Device that uses both low energy cardioversion or defibrillating shocks and antitachycardia pacing to treat ventricular tachycardia or ventricular fibrillation.

33249

33249 Insertion or replacement of permanent implantable defibrillator system, with transvenous lead(s), single or dual chamber

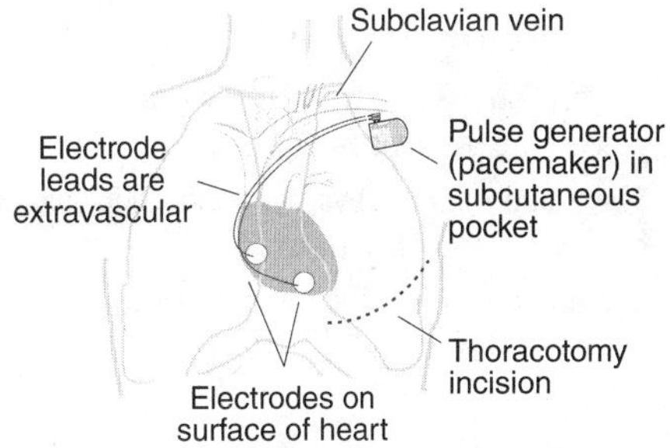

Single or dual chamber electrodes are inserted or repositioned by thoracotomy, with insertion of pulse generator

Explanation

The physician inserts or replaces a permanent implantable defibrillator system, including the pulse generator with transvenous electrode placement. Transvenous placement is currently the most common technique for placing implantable defibrillator electrodes. An implantable defibrillator is a device designed to administer an electric shock to control cardiac arrhythmias and restore a normal heartbeat. Local anesthesia is administered. An incision is made in the infraclavicular area. The subcutaneous tissue is opened and a pocket is created for the pulse generator. The electrode catheter is advanced through the superior vena cava into the heart and placed in the appropriate site in the right ventricle (single chamber system) or in the right ventricle and atrium (dual chamber system). Multiple leads may be required for both single and dual chamber systems. Once all leads are placed, they are tested and connected to the pulse generator that is placed in the previously prepared pocket. All incisions are closed. All radiological supervision and guidance is included.

Coding Tips

When medically necessary, report moderate (conscious) sedation provided by the performing physician with 99151-99153. When provided by another physician, report 99155-99157. For transvenous insertion of electrodes only, see 33216 and 33217; do not report these codes in addition to 33249. For repair of AICD transvenous electrodes, see 33218 or 33220. Removal with reinsertion of an implantable defibrillator system requires reporting of multiple codes. Report 33241 and 33243 or 33244 for the removal portion of the procedure and 33249 for the reinsertion. For insertion of epicardial electrodes by thoracotomy without concurrent pulse generator insertion, see 33202. For insertion of epicardial electrodes by endoscopy (thoracostomy or pericardioscopy) without concurrent pulse generator insertion, see 33203. Revision of a skin pocket is included and is not reported separately. Fluoroscopy is included in this procedure and is not reported separately. Do not report device evaluation codes (93260, 93261, 93279–93298) in addition to pulse generator and lead insertion/revision codes. Defibrillator threshold testing (DFT) during transvenous implantable defibrillator insertion/replacement is reported separately with 93640 or 93641.

ICD-10-CM Diagnostic Codes

I11.0	Hypertensive heart disease with heart failure
I13.0	Hypertensive heart and chronic kidney disease with heart failure and stage 1 through stage 4 chronic kidney disease, or unspecified chronic kidney disease

I13.2 Hypertensive heart and chronic kidney disease with heart failure and with stage 5 chronic kidney disease, or end stage renal disease
I16.0 Hypertensive urgency
I16.1 Hypertensive emergency
I21.01 ST elevation (STEMI) myocardial infarction involving left main coronary artery
I21.02 ST elevation (STEMI) myocardial infarction involving left anterior descending coronary artery
I21.09 ST elevation (STEMI) myocardial infarction involving other coronary artery of anterior wall
I21.11 ST elevation (STEMI) myocardial infarction involving right coronary artery
I21.19 ST elevation (STEMI) myocardial infarction involving other coronary artery of inferior wall
I21.21 ST elevation (STEMI) myocardial infarction involving left circumflex coronary artery
I21.29 ST elevation (STEMI) myocardial infarction involving other sites
I21.4 Non-ST elevation (NSTEMI) myocardial infarction
I21.A1 Myocardial infarction type 2
I22.0 Subsequent ST elevation (STEMI) myocardial infarction of anterior wall
I22.1 Subsequent ST elevation (STEMI) myocardial infarction of inferior wall
I22.2 Subsequent non-ST elevation (NSTEMI) myocardial infarction
I22.8 Subsequent ST elevation (STEMI) myocardial infarction of other sites
I25.2 Old myocardial infarction
I25.5 Ischemic cardiomyopathy
I25.6 Silent myocardial ischemia
I25.89 Other forms of chronic ischemic heart disease
I42.0 Dilated cardiomyopathy
I42.1 Obstructive hypertrophic cardiomyopathy
I42.2 Other hypertrophic cardiomyopathy
I42.5 Other restrictive cardiomyopathy
I42.8 Other cardiomyopathies
I44.0 Atrioventricular block, first degree
I44.1 Atrioventricular block, second degree
I44.2 Atrioventricular block, complete
I44.39 Other atrioventricular block
I44.4 Left anterior fascicular block
I44.5 Left posterior fascicular block
I44.69 Other fascicular block
I45.0 Right fascicular block
I45.19 Other right bundle-branch block
I45.2 Bifascicular block
I45.4 Nonspecific intraventricular block
I45.5 Other specified heart block
I45.6 Pre-excitation syndrome
I45.81 Long QT syndrome
I46.2 Cardiac arrest due to underlying cardiac condition
I46.8 Cardiac arrest due to other underlying condition
I47.0 Re-entry ventricular arrhythmia
I47.1 Supraventricular tachycardia
I47.2 Ventricular tachycardia
I48.0 Paroxysmal atrial fibrillation
I48.21 Permanent atrial fibrillation
I49.01 Ventricular fibrillation
I49.02 Ventricular flutter
I49.2 Junctional premature depolarization
I49.5 Sick sinus syndrome
I49.8 Other specified cardiac arrhythmias
I50.1 Left ventricular failure, unspecified
I50.21 Acute systolic (congestive) heart failure
I50.22 Chronic systolic (congestive) heart failure
I50.23 Acute on chronic systolic (congestive) heart failure
I50.31 Acute diastolic (congestive) heart failure
I50.32 Chronic diastolic (congestive) heart failure
I50.33 Acute on chronic diastolic (congestive) heart failure
I50.41 Acute combined systolic (congestive) and diastolic (congestive) heart failure
I50.42 Chronic combined systolic (congestive) and diastolic (congestive) heart failure
I50.43 Acute on chronic combined systolic (congestive) and diastolic (congestive) heart failure
I50.811 Acute right heart failure
I50.812 Chronic right heart failure
I50.813 Acute on chronic right heart failure
I50.814 Right heart failure due to left heart failure
I50.82 Biventricular heart failure
I50.83 High output heart failure
I50.84 End stage heart failure
T82.110A Breakdown (mechanical) of cardiac electrode, initial encounter
T82.111A Breakdown (mechanical) of cardiac pulse generator (battery), initial encounter
T82.120A Displacement of cardiac electrode, initial encounter
T82.121A Displacement of cardiac pulse generator (battery), initial encounter
T82.190A Other mechanical complication of cardiac electrode, initial encounter
T82.191A Other mechanical complication of cardiac pulse generator (battery), initial encounter
T82.7XXA Infection and inflammatory reaction due to other cardiac and vascular devices, implants and grafts, initial encounter
T82.817A Embolism due to cardiac prosthetic devices, implants and grafts, initial encounter
T82.827A Fibrosis due to cardiac prosthetic devices, implants and grafts, initial encounter
T82.837A Hemorrhage due to cardiac prosthetic devices, implants and grafts, initial encounter
T82.847A Pain due to cardiac prosthetic devices, implants and grafts, initial encounter
T82.857A Stenosis of other cardiac prosthetic devices, implants and grafts, initial encounter
T82.867A Thrombosis due to cardiac prosthetic devices, implants and grafts, initial encounter
T82.897A Other specified complication of cardiac prosthetic devices, implants and grafts, initial encounter

Z45.02 Encounter for adjustment and management of automatic implantable cardiac defibrillator

Z95.810 Presence of automatic (implantable) cardiac defibrillator

AMA: **33249** 2018,Jan,8; 2017,Jan,8; 2016,Jan,13; 2016,Aug,5; 2015,Jan,16; 2014,Nov,5; 2014,Jan,11

Relative Value Units/Medicare Edits

Non-Facility RVU	Work	PE	MP	Total
33249	14.92	8.28	3.47	26.67
Facility RVU	**Work**	**PE**	**MP**	**Total**
33249	14.92	8.28	3.47	26.67

	FUD	Status	MUE	Modifiers				IOM Reference
33249	90	A	1(3)	51	N/A	62*	N/A	100-04,4,10.2.2; 100-04,32,270; 100-04,32,270.1; 100-04,32,270.2

* with documentation

Terms To Know

defibrillator system. System that includes a pulse generator and electrodes, implanted in the same manner as the pacemaker systems.

pulse generator. Component of a pacemaker or an implantable cardioverter defibrillator that contains the battery and the electronics for producing the electrical discharge sent to the heart to control cardiac rhythm. Insertion or replacement of the pulse generator may be done alone, not in conjunction with insertion or replacement of the entire pacemaker system.

[33270, 33271]

33270 Insertion or replacement of permanent subcutaneous implantable defibrillator system, with subcutaneous electrode, including defibrillation threshold evaluation, induction of arrhythmia, evaluation of sensing for arrhythmia termination, and programming or reprogramming of sensing or therapeutic parameters, when performed

33271 Insertion of subcutaneous implantable defibrillator electrode

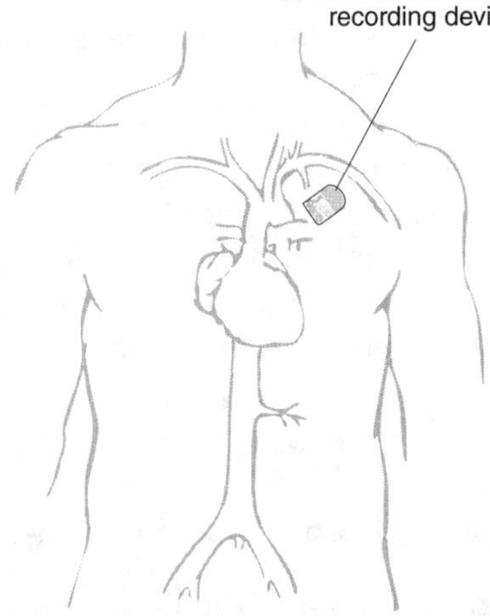

Explanation

In 33270, the physician performs initial insertion or replacement of a permanent subcutaneous implantable defibrillator (S-ICD) system, including the pulse generator and lead. The pulse generator is placed in a subcutaneous pocket on the left side of the chest next to the ribs. Two small incisions are made above the sternum and the lead wire is threaded through and sutured into place. The lead is connected to the pulse generator. The physician records cardiac electrical signals from the leads and paces the heart through the leads to determine pacing threshold. The physician uses the S-ICD pulse generator to pace the heart into an arrhythmia, such as ventricular tachycardia or fibrillation. The S-ICD detects and terminates the arrhythmia using pacing or by shocking the heart through the lead. The physician may reprogram the treatment parameters to optimize the device function to best treat the patient's arrhythmia. The incisions are closed. Report 33271 for insertion of the lead only.

Coding Tips

Do not report 33270 with 33271, 93260, 93261, or 93644. Do not report 33271 with 33240, 33262, 33270, 93260, or 93261. For removal and replacement of an implantable defibrillator generator and subcutaneous electrode, report 33270 and 33272 with 33241. For insertion or replacement of a cardiac venous system electrode, see 33224 and 33225. Revision of a skin pocket is included and is not reported separately. Radiological supervision and interpretation is included and is not reported separately. Device evaluation (93260–93261 and 93279–93298) is included and is not reported separately. For insertion or replacement with a substernal electrode, see 0571T. For insertion of a substernal defibrillator electrode, see 0572T.

ICD-10-CM Diagnostic Codes

I11.0 Hypertensive heart disease with heart failure

I13.0 Hypertensive heart and chronic kidney disease with heart failure and stage 1 through stage 4 chronic kidney disease, or unspecified chronic kidney disease

I13.2	Hypertensive heart and chronic kidney disease with heart failure and with stage 5 chronic kidney disease, or end stage renal disease
I16.0	Hypertensive urgency
I16.1	Hypertensive emergency
I21.01	ST elevation (STEMI) myocardial infarction involving left main coronary artery
I21.02	ST elevation (STEMI) myocardial infarction involving left anterior descending coronary artery
I21.09	ST elevation (STEMI) myocardial infarction involving other coronary artery of anterior wall
I21.11	ST elevation (STEMI) myocardial infarction involving right coronary artery
I21.19	ST elevation (STEMI) myocardial infarction involving other coronary artery of inferior wall
I21.21	ST elevation (STEMI) myocardial infarction involving left circumflex coronary artery
I21.29	ST elevation (STEMI) myocardial infarction involving other sites
I21.4	Non-ST elevation (NSTEMI) myocardial infarction
I21.A1	Myocardial infarction type 2
I22.0	Subsequent ST elevation (STEMI) myocardial infarction of anterior wall
I22.1	Subsequent ST elevation (STEMI) myocardial infarction of inferior wall
I22.2	Subsequent non-ST elevation (NSTEMI) myocardial infarction
I22.8	Subsequent ST elevation (STEMI) myocardial infarction of other sites
I25.2	Old myocardial infarction
I25.5	Ischemic cardiomyopathy
I25.6	Silent myocardial ischemia
I25.89	Other forms of chronic ischemic heart disease
I42.0	Dilated cardiomyopathy
I42.1	Obstructive hypertrophic cardiomyopathy
I42.2	Other hypertrophic cardiomyopathy
I42.5	Other restrictive cardiomyopathy
I42.8	Other cardiomyopathies
I44.0	Atrioventricular block, first degree
I44.1	Atrioventricular block, second degree
I44.2	Atrioventricular block, complete
I44.39	Other atrioventricular block
I44.4	Left anterior fascicular block
I44.5	Left posterior fascicular block
I44.69	Other fascicular block
I45.0	Right fascicular block
I45.19	Other right bundle-branch block
I45.2	Bifascicular block
I45.4	Nonspecific intraventricular block
I45.5	Other specified heart block
I45.6	Pre-excitation syndrome
I45.81	Long QT syndrome
I46.2	Cardiac arrest due to underlying cardiac condition
I46.8	Cardiac arrest due to other underlying condition
I47.0	Re-entry ventricular arrhythmia
I47.1	Supraventricular tachycardia
I47.2	Ventricular tachycardia
I48.0	Paroxysmal atrial fibrillation
I48.11	Longstanding persistent atrial fibrillation
I48.19	Other persistent atrial fibrillation
I48.21	Permanent atrial fibrillation
I49.01	Ventricular fibrillation
I49.02	Ventricular flutter
I49.2	Junctional premature depolarization
I49.5	Sick sinus syndrome
I49.8	Other specified cardiac arrhythmias
I50.1	Left ventricular failure, unspecified
I50.21	Acute systolic (congestive) heart failure
I50.22	Chronic systolic (congestive) heart failure
I50.23	Acute on chronic systolic (congestive) heart failure
I50.31	Acute diastolic (congestive) heart failure
I50.32	Chronic diastolic (congestive) heart failure
I50.33	Acute on chronic diastolic (congestive) heart failure
I50.41	Acute combined systolic (congestive) and diastolic (congestive) heart failure
I50.42	Chronic combined systolic (congestive) and diastolic (congestive) heart failure
I50.43	Acute on chronic combined systolic (congestive) and diastolic (congestive) heart failure
I50.811	Acute right heart failure
I50.812	Chronic right heart failure
I50.813	Acute on chronic right heart failure
I50.814	Right heart failure due to left heart failure
I50.82	Biventricular heart failure
I50.83	High output heart failure
I50.84	End stage heart failure
T82.110A	Breakdown (mechanical) of cardiac electrode, initial encounter
T82.111A	Breakdown (mechanical) of cardiac pulse generator (battery), initial encounter
T82.190A	Other mechanical complication of cardiac electrode, initial encounter
T82.191A	Other mechanical complication of cardiac pulse generator (battery), initial encounter
T82.7XXA	Infection and inflammatory reaction due to other cardiac and vascular devices, implants and grafts, initial encounter
T82.817A	Embolism due to cardiac prosthetic devices, implants and grafts, initial encounter
T82.827A	Fibrosis due to cardiac prosthetic devices, implants and grafts, initial encounter
T82.837A	Hemorrhage due to cardiac prosthetic devices, implants and grafts, initial encounter
T82.847A	Pain due to cardiac prosthetic devices, implants and grafts, initial encounter
T82.857A	Stenosis of other cardiac prosthetic devices, implants and grafts, initial encounter
T82.867A	Thrombosis due to cardiac prosthetic devices, implants and grafts, initial encounter
T82.897A	Other specified complication of cardiac prosthetic devices, implants and grafts, initial encounter
Z45.02	Encounter for adjustment and management of automatic implantable cardiac defibrillator

Z95.810 Presence of automatic (implantable) cardiac defibrillator

AMA: 33270 2018,Jan,8; 2017,Jan,8; 2016,Jan,13; 2016,Aug,5; 2015,Jan,16; 2014,Nov,5 **33271** 2018,Jan,8; 2017,Jan,8; 2016,Jan,13; 2016,Aug,5; 2015,Jan,16; 2014,Nov,5

Relative Value Units/Medicare Edits

Non-Facility RVU	Work	PE	MP	Total
33270	9.1	5.27	2.1	16.47
33271	7.5	3.99	1.76	13.25
Facility RVU	**Work**	**PE**	**MP**	**Total**
33270	9.1	5.27	2.1	16.47
33271	7.5	3.99	1.76	13.25

	FUD	Status	MUE	Modifiers				IOM Reference
33270	90	A	1(3)	51	N/A	N/A	N/A	None
33271	90	A	1(3)	51	N/A	N/A	N/A	

* with documentation

Terms To Know

electrode. Electric terminal specialized for a particular electrochemical reaction that acts as a medium between a body surface and another instrument, commonly termed a lead.

implantable cardioverter-defibrillator. Implantable electronic cardiac device used to control rhythm abnormalities such as tachycardia, fibrillation, or bradycardia by producing high- or low-energy stimulation and pacemaker functions. It may also have the capability to provide the functions of an implantable loop recorder or implantable cardiovascular monitor.

pulse generator. Circuit used to generate pulses. Pulse generators contain the battery, the electronic circuit, and the connector in a hermetically sealed encasement. Pulse generators may be temporary transcutaneous or placed in a subcutaneous pocket.

subcutaneous pocket. Small space created under the skin in a suitable location for holding an implantable device, such as the pulse generator of a pacemaker or cardioverter defibrillator.

[33272]

33272 Removal of subcutaneous implantable defibrillator electrode

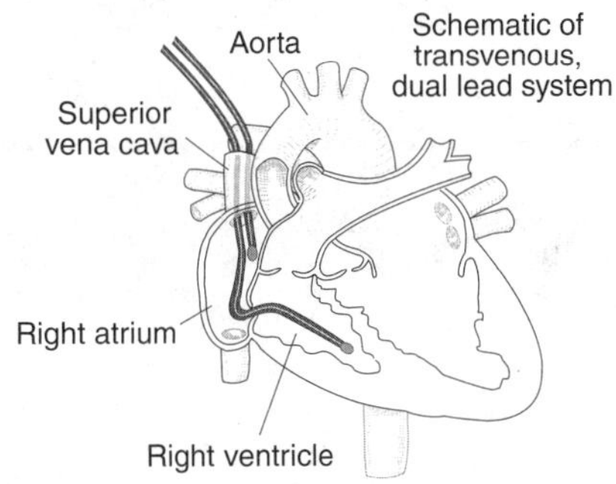

Explanation

The physician performs a procedure to remove the subcutaneous implantable defibrillator lead only. The lead may be removed due to a complication or malfunction. An incision is made in the area above the sternum where the lead is located. The lead is disconnected from the pulse generator, pulled through, and removed. The incision is repaired.

Coding Tips

Insertion or replacement of a pulse generator (33241) may be reported separately, when performed. Radiological supervision and interpretation is included and is not reported separately. Removal and replacement of the pulse generator and electrodes requires reporting of multiple codes: report 33272 in addition to 33241 or 33270. For repositioning of a previously implanted subcutaneous defibrillator electrode, see 33273. Do not report 33272 with 93260 or 93261. For removal of a substernal defibrillator electrode, see 0573T.

ICD-10-CM Diagnostic Codes

T82.110A Breakdown (mechanical) of cardiac electrode, initial encounter

T82.120A Displacement of cardiac electrode, initial encounter

T82.190A Other mechanical complication of cardiac electrode, initial encounter

T82.7XXA Infection and inflammatory reaction due to other cardiac and vascular devices, implants and grafts, initial encounter

T82.817A Embolism due to cardiac prosthetic devices, implants and grafts, initial encounter

T82.827A Fibrosis due to cardiac prosthetic devices, implants and grafts, initial encounter

T82.837A Hemorrhage due to cardiac prosthetic devices, implants and grafts, initial encounter

T82.847A Pain due to cardiac prosthetic devices, implants and grafts, initial encounter

T82.857A Stenosis of other cardiac prosthetic devices, implants and grafts, initial encounter

T82.867A Thrombosis due to cardiac prosthetic devices, implants and grafts, initial encounter

T82.897A Other specified complication of cardiac prosthetic devices, implants and grafts, initial encounter

Z45.02 Encounter for adjustment and management of automatic implantable cardiac defibrillator

Z95.810 Presence of automatic (implantable) cardiac defibrillator

AMA: **33272** 2018,Jan,8; 2017,Jan,8; 2016,Jan,13; 2016,Aug,5; 2015,Jan,16; 2014,Nov,5

Relative Value Units/Medicare Edits

Non-Facility RVU	Work	PE	MP	Total
33272	5.42	3.39	1.27	10.08
Facility RVU	**Work**	**PE**	**MP**	**Total**
33272	5.42	3.39	1.27	10.08

	FUD	Status	MUE	Modifiers				IOM Reference
33272	90	A	1(3)	51	N/A	N/A	N/A	None

* with documentation

Terms To Know

electrode. Electric terminal specialized for a particular electrochemical reaction that acts as a medium between a body surface and another instrument, commonly termed a lead.

pulse generator. Circuit used to generate pulses. Pulse generators contain the battery, the electronic circuit, and the connector in a hermetically sealed encasement. Pulse generators may be temporary transcutaneous or placed in a subcutaneous pocket.

subcutaneous. Below the skin.

supervision and interpretation. Radiology services that usually contain an invasive component and are reported by the radiologist for supervision of the procedure and the personnel involved with performing the examination, reading the film, and preparing the written report.

Heart and Pericardium

[33273]

33273 Repositioning of previously implanted subcutaneous implantable defibrillator electrode

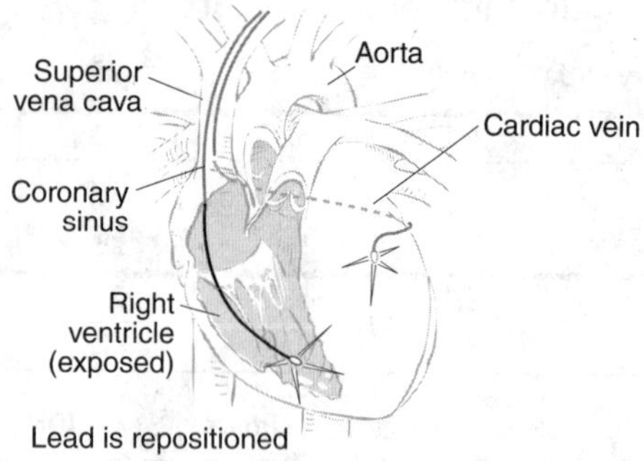

Explanation

A previously placed implanted subcutaneous defibrillator lead (electrode) is repositioned. This procedure is performed when the system does not function due to improper placement of the lead. An incision is made over the previous subcutaneous pocket on the left side of the chest next to the ribs. The lead is disconnected from the pulse generator. The generator is removed and the lead is tested for proper function. It is then reattached to the generator in the new position and retested. The incision is closed.

Coding Tips

Do not report 33273 with 93260 or 93261. Radiological supervision and interpretation is included and is not reported separately. For insertion or replacement of a previously placed subcutaneous defibrillator system, see 33270. For insertion of a subcutaneous implantable defibrillator electrode, see 33271. For removal of a subcutaneous implantable defibrillator electrode, see 33272. For repositioning of a substernal defibrillator electrode, see 0574T.

ICD-10-CM Diagnostic Codes

T82.120A	Displacement of cardiac electrode, initial encounter
T82.897A	Other specified complication of cardiac prosthetic devices, implants and grafts, initial encounter
Z45.02	Encounter for adjustment and management of automatic implantable cardiac defibrillator
Z95.810	Presence of automatic (implantable) cardiac defibrillator

AMA: **33273** 2018,Jan,8; 2017,Jan,8; 2016,Jan,13; 2016,Aug,5; 2015,Jan,16; 2014,Nov,5

Relative Value Units/Medicare Edits

Non-Facility RVU	Work	PE	MP	Total
33273	6.5	3.65	1.53	11.68
Facility RVU	**Work**	**PE**	**MP**	**Total**
33273	6.5	3.65	1.53	11.68

	FUD	Status	MUE	Modifiers				IOM Reference
33273	90	A	1(3)	51	N/A	N/A	N/A	None

* with documentation

[33274, 33275]

33274 Transcatheter insertion or replacement of permanent leadless pacemaker, right ventricular, including imaging guidance (eg, fluoroscopy, venous ultrasound, ventriculography, femoral venography) and device evaluation (eg, interrogation or programming), when performed

▲ **33275** Transcatheter removal of permanent leadless pacemaker, right ventricular, including imaging guidance (eg, fluoroscopy, venous ultrasound, ventriculography, femoral venography), when performed

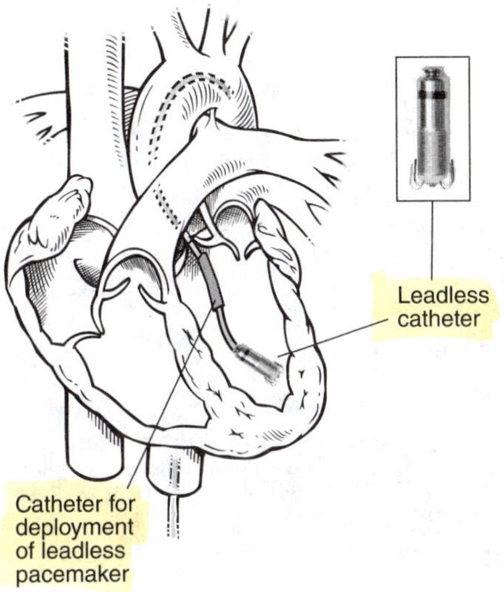

Explanation

The physician performs transcatheter insertion, replacement, or removal of a ventricular permanent leadless pacemaker. This pacemaker is a single-chamber unit without leads that is placed into the right ventricle. The size varies based on manufacturer, but is about 7 mm x 26 mm and weighs 2 grams. The less invasive and shorter implantation procedure of a leadless pacemaker reduces recovery time and eliminates complications related to the transvenous leads and the subcutaneous pulse generator used in traditional pacemaker implantation, specifically infections. The battery typically lasts seven to 15 years, and the pacing, amplitude, and impedance are all relative to the traditional pacemaker. The femoral vein is entered and the device is fed into the right ventricle using a special catheter. Once attached, a continued connection allows for measurements to be taken and to determine positioning. All imaging and device evaluation are included in the procedures and should not be reported separately. For insertion or replacement of the pacemaker, report 33274; for removal of the pacemaker, report 33275.

Coding Tips

Do not report these codes with 75820, 76000, 77002, 76937, or 93566. Do not report 33275 with 33274. Do not report 33274 or 33275 with 93451, 93453, 93456, 93457, 93460, 93461, 93530, 93531, 93532, or 93533 unless complete right heart catheterization is performed for reasons distinct from the leadless pacemaker procedure. For subsequent leadless pacemaker device evaluation, see 93279, 93286, 93288, 93294, or 93296. For insertion, replacement, repositioning, or removal of pacemakers with leads, see 33202-33208, 33212-33221, 33227-33229, and 33233-33237.

ICD-10-CM Diagnostic Codes

I44.0	Atrioventricular block, first degree
I44.1	Atrioventricular block, second degree
I44.2	Atrioventricular block, complete
I44.39	Other atrioventricular block
I44.4	Left anterior fascicular block
I44.5	Left posterior fascicular block
I44.69	Other fascicular block
I45.0	Right fascicular block
I45.19	Other right bundle-branch block
I45.2	Bifascicular block
I45.3	Trifascicular block
I45.4	Nonspecific intraventricular block
I45.5	Other specified heart block
I45.6	Pre-excitation syndrome
I45.81	Long QT syndrome
I47.1	Supraventricular tachycardia
I48.0	Paroxysmal atrial fibrillation
I48.21	Permanent atrial fibrillation
I49.2	Junctional premature depolarization
I49.5	Sick sinus syndrome
I49.8	Other specified cardiac arrhythmias
I50.1	Left ventricular failure, unspecified
I50.21	Acute systolic (congestive) heart failure
I50.22	Chronic systolic (congestive) heart failure
I50.23	Acute on chronic systolic (congestive) heart failure
I50.31	Acute diastolic (congestive) heart failure
I50.32	Chronic diastolic (congestive) heart failure
I50.33	Acute on chronic diastolic (congestive) heart failure
I50.41	Acute combined systolic (congestive) and diastolic (congestive) heart failure
I50.42	Chronic combined systolic (congestive) and diastolic (congestive) heart failure
I50.43	Acute on chronic combined systolic (congestive) and diastolic (congestive) heart failure
I50.810	Right heart failure, unspecified
I50.811	Acute right heart failure
I50.812	Chronic right heart failure
I50.813	Acute on chronic right heart failure
I50.814	Right heart failure due to left heart failure
I50.82	Biventricular heart failure
I50.83	High output heart failure
I50.84	End stage heart failure
I50.89	Other heart failure
I51.7	Cardiomegaly
Q24.6	Congenital heart block
T82.110A	Breakdown (mechanical) of cardiac electrode, initial encounter
T82.111A	Breakdown (mechanical) of cardiac pulse generator (battery), initial encounter
T82.120A	Displacement of cardiac electrode, initial encounter
T82.121A	Displacement of cardiac pulse generator (battery), initial encounter

T82.190A	Other mechanical complication of cardiac electrode, initial encounter
T82.191A	Other mechanical complication of cardiac pulse generator (battery), initial encounter
T82.7XXA	Infection and inflammatory reaction due to other cardiac and vascular devices, implants and grafts, initial encounter
T82.817A	Embolism due to cardiac prosthetic devices, implants and grafts, initial encounter
T82.827A	Fibrosis due to cardiac prosthetic devices, implants and grafts, initial encounter
T82.837A	Hemorrhage due to cardiac prosthetic devices, implants and grafts, initial encounter
T82.847A	Pain due to cardiac prosthetic devices, implants and grafts, initial encounter
T82.857A	Stenosis of other cardiac prosthetic devices, implants and grafts, initial encounter
T82.867A	Thrombosis due to cardiac prosthetic devices, implants and grafts, initial encounter
T82.897A	Other specified complication of cardiac prosthetic devices, implants and grafts, initial encounter
Z45.018	Encounter for adjustment and management of other part of cardiac pacemaker
Z95.0	Presence of cardiac pacemaker

AMA: 33274 2019,Mar,6 **33275** 2019,Mar,6

Relative Value Units/Medicare Edits

Non-Facility RVU	Work	PE	MP	Total
33274	7.8	4.6	1.81	14.21
33275	8.59	4.48	2.03	15.1
Facility RVU	**Work**	**PE**	**MP**	**Total**
33274	7.8	4.6	1.81	14.21
33275	8.59	4.48	2.03	15.1

	FUD	Status	MUE	Modifiers				IOM Reference
33274	90	A	1(3)	51	N/A	62	N/A	None
33275	90	A	1(3)	51	N/A	N/A	N/A	

* with documentation

Terms To Know

catheterization. Use or insertion of a tubular device into a duct, blood vessel, hollow organ, or body cavity for injecting or withdrawing fluids for diagnostic or therapeutic purposes.

fluoroscopy. Radiology technique that allows visual examination of part of the body or a function of an organ using a device that projects an x-ray image on a fluorescent screen.

transcatheter. Procedure or treatment performed via a catheter.

venography. Radiographic study of the veins.

33250-33251

33250 Operative ablation of supraventricular arrhythmogenic focus or pathway (eg, Wolff-Parkinson-White, atrioventricular node re-entry), tract(s) and/or focus (foci); without cardiopulmonary bypass

33251 with cardiopulmonary bypass

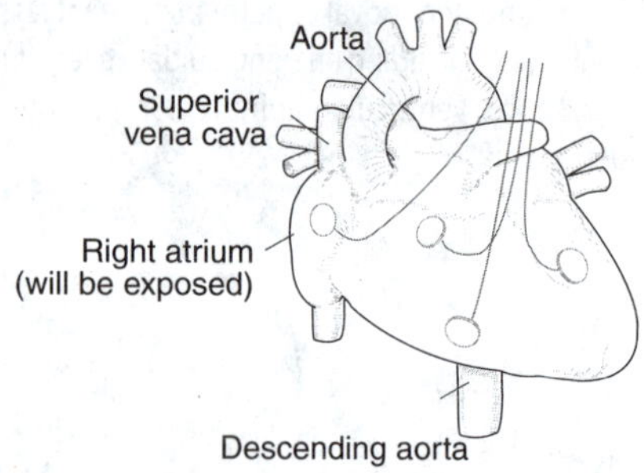

Mapping grid of electrodes is placed on the heart to determine the source of arrhythmia

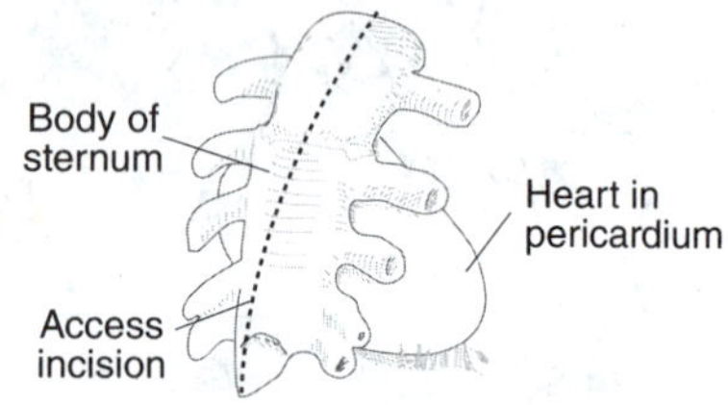

The source of a cardiac arrhythmia is determined in an open surgical procedure and supraventricular tissues are ablated

Explanation

In 33250, the heart is exposed through the sternum. A mapping grid of electrodes is placed over the surface of the beating heart. The location of the arrhythmia source is determined. The source is destroyed using electrical current, freezing, or cutting. Any bleeding is controlled with sutures. The chest is closed. In 33251, cardiopulmonary bypass is required. The heart is exposed through the sternum. A mapping grid of electrodes is placed over the surface of the beating heart. The right atrium is opened and a long cut is made around the tricuspid valve until the cut on the outside of the heart is seen. Any other focuses of the arrhythmia are destroyed with electrical current or freezing. The right atrium is closed. Cardiopulmonary bypass is discontinued when heart function returns. Typically this open approach is reserved for patients requiring surgery for additional conditions being replaced by ablation performed via catheter which is threaded through the femoral vein into the area of the heart requiring treatment.

Coding Tips

When this procedure is performed without cardiopulmonary bypass, report 33250; with cardiopulmonary bypass, report 33251. Report 93631 for intraoperative mapping performed by a separate provider. Note diagnosis when reporting ablation procedures. Ablation of supraventricular focus or pathway (Wolff-Parkinson-White syndrome) is reported with 33250–33251, while ablation of ventricular arrhythmogenic focus is reported with 33261. Open operative tissue ablation and reconstruction of atria is reported with 33254–33256. Endoscopic operative tissue ablation and reconstruction of atria is reported with 33265–33266. Ablation procedures are now frequently performed by intracardiac catheter instead of by thoracotomy. For transvenous intracardiac catheter ablation of supraventricular arrhythmogenic focus, see 93653. Insertion of a permanent pacemaker is reported separately, see 33202, 33203, 33207, or 33208.

ICD-10-CM Diagnostic Codes

I45.6	Pre-excitation syndrome
I45.89	Other specified conduction disorders
I47.0	Re-entry ventricular arrhythmia
I47.1	Supraventricular tachycardia
I47.2	Ventricular tachycardia
I48.0	Paroxysmal atrial fibrillation
I48.11	Longstanding persistent atrial fibrillation
I48.19	Other persistent atrial fibrillation
I48.21	Permanent atrial fibrillation
I48.3	Typical atrial flutter
I48.4	Atypical atrial flutter
I49.01	Ventricular fibrillation
I49.2	Junctional premature depolarization
I49.8	Other specified cardiac arrhythmias

AMA: 33250 2018,Jan,8; 2017,Jan,8; 2016,Jan,13; 2015,Jan,16; 2014,Jan,11
33251 2018,Jan,8; 2017,Jan,8; 2017,Dec,3; 2016,Jan,13; 2015,Jan,16; 2014,Jan,11

Relative Value Units/Medicare Edits

Non-Facility RVU	Work	PE	MP	Total
33250	25.9	10.44	6.11	42.45
33251	28.92	11.42	6.87	47.21
Facility RVU	**Work**	**PE**	**MP**	**Total**
33250	25.9	10.44	6.11	42.45
33251	28.92	11.42	6.87	47.21

	FUD	Status	MUE	Modifiers				IOM Reference
33250	90	A	1(2)	51	N/A	62*	80	None
33251	90	A	1(2)	51	N/A	62*	80	

* with documentation

Terms To Know

ablation. Removal or destruction of tissue by cutting, electrical energy, chemical substances, or excessive heat application.

arrhythmias. Heart disorder of rhythm or rate, due to an electrical conduction system malfunction.

cardiopulmonary bypass. Venous blood is diverted to a heart-lung machine, which mechanically pumps and oxygenates the blood temporarily so the heart can be bypassed while an open procedure on the heart or coronary arteries is performed. During bypass, the lungs are deflated and immobile.

dysrhythmia. Abnormality or disturbance in rhythm.

paroxysmal supraventricular tachycardia. Rapid heartbeat that starts above the ventricles and occurs sporadically.

Wolff-Parkinson-White syndrome. Pre-excitation associated with paroxysmal tachycardia or atrial fibrillation with a short P-R interval on EKG and an early delta wave. The normal conduction pathway is bypassed.

33254-33256

33254 Operative tissue ablation and reconstruction of atria, limited (eg, modified maze procedure)

33255 Operative tissue ablation and reconstruction of atria, extensive (eg, maze procedure); without cardiopulmonary bypass

33256 with cardiopulmonary bypass

Mini maze
Convergent Ablations

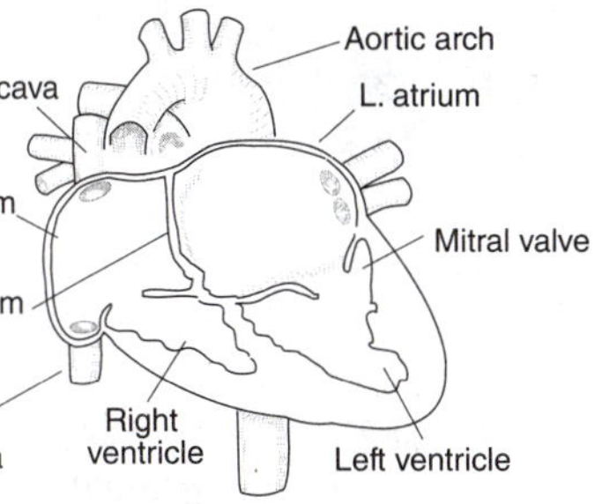

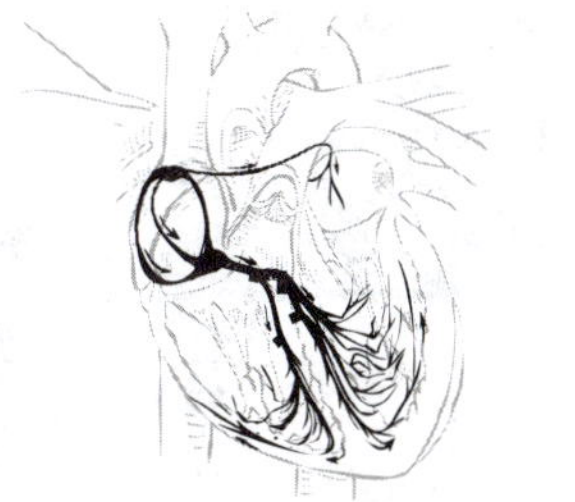

Conduction system of the heart

Explanation

The physician performs operative ablation and reconstruction of the atria to treat atrial fibrillation. Atrial fibrillation is rapid, randomized muscle contraction of the atrial myocardium causing an irregular, rapid heart rate. In a maze procedure, the physician seeks to permanently interrupt aberrant electrical conduction within the atria to restore normal sinus rhythm. The physician performs a midline sternotomy, incising the skin, fascia, muscles, and sternum. The pericardium is incised. For a limited operative ablation and reconstruction (33254), also referred to as a modified maze procedure, an incision is made into the left or right atrium. A combination of surgical incision and/or energy sources such as heat, microwave, laser, ultrasound, or cryoprobe is used to create lesions that will heal into scars that disrupt conduction. In 33255 and 33256, an extensive operative ablation and reconstruction is performed. In an extensive procedure, the right and/or left atrial tissue and/or atrial septum is treated as described in 33254, and additional operative ablation involving the atrioventricular annulus is performed. In any of these procedures, the left atrial appendage may be excised or isolated. In 33256, lines are placed for cardiopulmonary bypass. When cardiopulmonary bypass is achieved, an extensive ablation and reconstruction procedure is performed. The atrial incision lines are reanastomosed. The pericardium is repaired loosely, leaving gaps for blood and fluid to drain into the pleural space. The sternum is reanastomosed with sternal wires and the skin is sutured in layers.

Coding Tips

Excision or isolation of the left atrial appendage by any method, including stapling, oversewing, ligation, or plication, is included in the operative ablation procedure and should not be reported separately. Code 33254–33255 are reported only when there is no concurrently performed procedure requiring median sternotomy or cardiopulmonary bypass. If operative ablation is performed with a concurrent procedure requiring median sternotomy or cardiopulmonary bypass, the operative ablation procedure should be reported with unlisted procedure code 33999. For operative tissue ablation and reconstruction of atria performed endoscopically, see 33265 or 33266. Do not report 33254–33256 with 32100, 32551, 33120, 33130, 33210, 33211, 33390, 33391, 33404–33507, 33510–33523, 33533–33548, 33600–33853, 33858–33864, or 33910–33920.

ICD-10-CM Diagnostic Codes

I47.1	Supraventricular tachycardia
I48.0	Paroxysmal atrial fibrillation
I48.11	Longstanding persistent atrial fibrillation
I48.19	Other persistent atrial fibrillation
I48.21	Permanent atrial fibrillation
I48.3	Typical atrial flutter
I48.4	Atypical atrial flutter
I49.2	Junctional premature depolarization
I49.8	Other specified cardiac arrhythmias

AMA: 33254 2018,Jan,8; 2017,Jan,8; 2016,Jan,13; 2015,Jan,16; 2014,Jan,11 **33255** 2018,Jan,8; 2017,Jan,8; 2016,Jan,13; 2015,Jan,16; 2014,Jan,11 **33256** 2018,Jan,8; 2017,Jan,8; 2017,Dec,3; 2016,Jan,13; 2015,Jan,16; 2014,Jan,11

Relative Value Units/Medicare Edits

Non-Facility RVU	Work	PE	MP	Total
33254	23.71	10.11	5.58	39.4
33255	29.04	11.56	6.85	47.45
33256	34.9	13.32	7.97	56.19
Facility RVU	**Work**	**PE**	**MP**	**Total**
33254	23.71	10.11	5.58	39.4
33255	29.04	11.56	6.85	47.45
33256	34.9	13.32	7.97	56.19

	FUD	Status	MUE	Modifiers				IOM Reference
33254	90	A	1(2)	51	N/A	62*	80	None
33255	90	A	1(2)	51	N/A	62*	80	
33256	90	A	1(2)	51	N/A	62*	80	

* with documentation

Terms To Know

ablation. Removal or destruction of tissue by cutting, electrical energy, chemical substances, or excessive heat application.

arrhythmias. Heart disorder of rhythm or rate, due to an electrical conduction system malfunction.

cardiopulmonary bypass. Venous blood is diverted to a heart-lung machine, which mechanically pumps and oxygenates the blood temporarily so the heart can be bypassed while an open procedure on the heart or coronary arteries is performed. During bypass, the lungs are deflated and immobile.

33257

+ 33257 Operative tissue ablation and reconstruction of atria, performed at the time of other cardiac procedure(s), limited (eg, modified maze procedure) (List separately in addition to code for primary procedure)

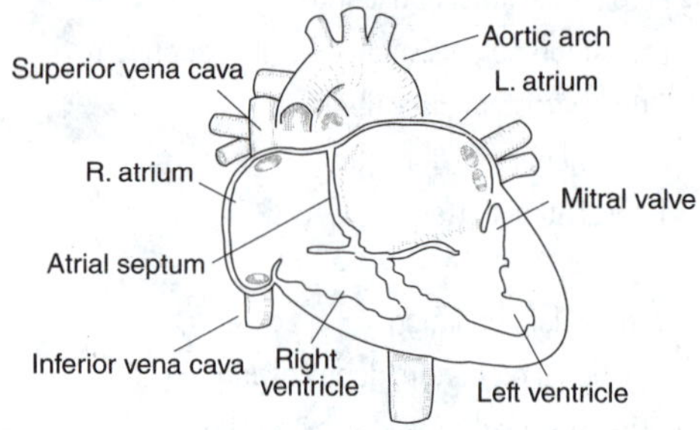

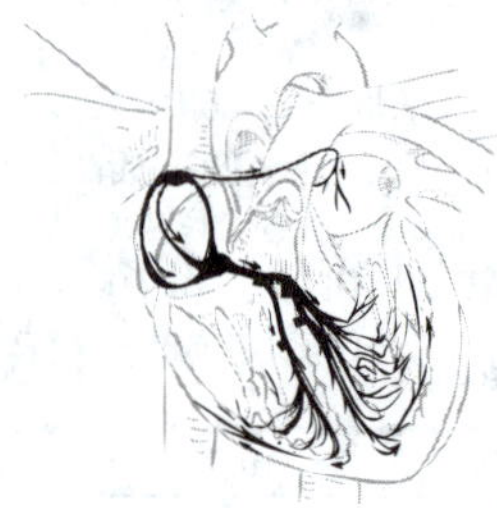

Conduction system of the heart

Aberrant conduction is treated with open heart surgery isolating the pulmonary veins or other anatomically defined triggers in the left or right atrium

Explanation

Concurrently with other cardiac procedures, the physician performs operative tissue ablation and reconstruction of the atria to treat atrial fibrillation. Atrial fibrillation is rapid, randomized muscle contraction of the atrial myocardium causing an irregular, rapid heart rate. In this procedure, the physician seeks to permanently interrupt aberrant electrical conduction within the atria to restore normal sinus rhythm. The physician performs a midline sternotomy, incising the skin, fascia, muscles, and sternum. The pericardium is incised. For a limited operative tissue ablation and reconstruction of atria, also referred to as a modified maze procedure, an incision is made into the left or right atrium. A combination of surgical incision and/or energy sources, such as heat, microwave, laser, ultrasound, or cryoprobe, is used to create lesions that will heal into scars that disrupt conduction. The left atrial appendage may be excised or isolated. The atrial incision lines are reanastomosed. The pericardium is repaired loosely, leaving gaps for blood and fluid to drain into the pleural space. The sternum is reanastomosed with sternal wires and the skin is sutured in layers.

Coding Tips

Report 33257 in addition to 33120–33130, 33250–33251, 33261, 33300–33335, 33390–33391, 33404–33496, 33500–33507, 33510–33516, 33533–33548, 33600–33619, 33641–33697, 33702–33732, 33735–33767, 33770, 33877, 33910–33922, 33925–33926, and 33975–33983. Do not report 33257 with 32551, 33210, 33211, 33254–33256, 33265, or 33266. When performed concurrently, 33257 is reported with open cardiac procedures that require sternotomy.

ICD-10-CM Diagnostic Codes

This/these CPT code(s) are add on code(s). See the primary procedure code that this code is performed with for your ICD-10-CM code selections. Diagnostic code(s) would be the same as the actual procedure performed.

Relative Value Units/Medicare Edits

Non-Facility RVU	Work	PE	MP	Total
33257	9.63	5.0	2.18	16.81
Facility RVU	**Work**	**PE**	**MP**	**Total**
33257	9.63	5.0	2.18	16.81

	FUD	Status	MUE	Modifiers				IOM Reference
33257	N/A	A	1(2)	N/A	N/A	N/A	80	None

* with documentation

Terms To Know

ablation. Removal or destruction of tissue by cutting, electrical energy, chemical substances, or excessive heat application.

reconstruction. Recreating, restoring, or rebuilding a body part or organ.

tissue. Group of similar cells with a similar function that form definite structures and organs. Tissue types include epithelial tissue, muscle tissue, connective tissue, and nervous tissue.

33258

\+ **33258** Operative tissue ablation and reconstruction of atria, performed at the time of other cardiac procedure(s), extensive (eg, maze procedure), without cardiopulmonary bypass (List separately in addition to code for primary procedure)

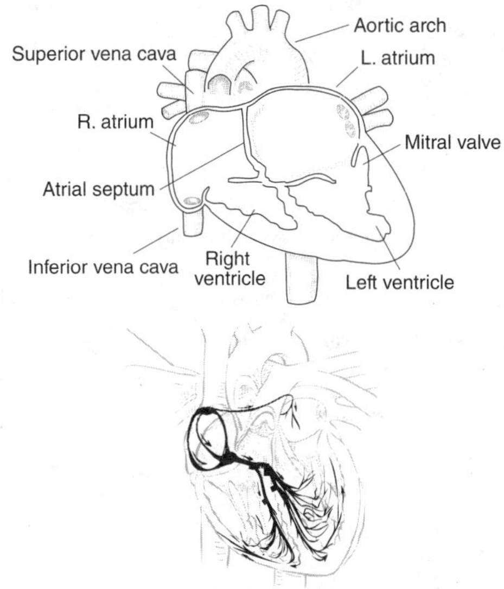

Conduction system of the heart
Aberrant conduction is treated with open heart surgery isolating the pulmonary veins or other anatomically defined triggers in the left or right atrium

Explanation

Concurrently with other cardiac procedures, the physician performs operative tissue ablation and reconstruction of the atria to treat atrial fibrillation. Atrial fibrillation is rapid, randomized muscle contraction of the atrial myocardium causing an irregular, rapid heart rate. In this procedure, the physician seeks to permanently interrupt aberrant electrical conduction within the atria to restore normal sinus rhythm. The physician performs a midline sternotomy, incising the skin, fascia, muscles, and sternum. The pericardium is incised. For an extensive operative tissue ablation and reconstruction of atria, also referred to as a maze procedure, an incision is made into the left or right atrium. A combination of surgical incision and/or energy sources, such as heat, microwave, laser, ultrasound, or cryoprobe, is used to create lesions that will heal into scars that disrupt conduction. Additional operative ablation involving the atrioventricular annulus is also performed. The left atrial appendage may be excised or isolated. The atrial incision lines are reanastomosed. The pericardium is repaired loosely, leaving gaps for blood and fluid to drain into the pleural space. The sternum is reanastomosed with sternal wires and the skin is sutured in layers.

Coding Tips

Report 33258 with the following codes when cardiopulmonary bypass is not performed: 33130, 33250, 33300, 33310, 33320, 33321, 33330, 33365, 33420, 33470–33471, 33501–33503, 33510–33516, 33533–33536, 33690, 33735, 33737, 33750, 33755, 33762-33766, 33820–33824, 33840–33852, 33875, 33877, 33915, 33925, 33981, and 33982. Do not report 33258 with 32551, 33210, 33211, 33254–33256, 33265, or 33266. When performed concurrently, 33258 is reported with open cardiac procedures that require sternotomy.

ICD-10-CM Diagnostic Codes

This/these CPT code(s) are add on code(s). See the primary procedure code that this code is performed with for your ICD-10-CM code selections. Diagnostic code(s) would be the same as the actual procedure performed.

Relative Value Units/Medicare Edits

Non-Facility RVU	Work	PE	MP	Total
33258	11.0	5.41	2.45	18.86
Facility RVU	**Work**	**PE**	**MP**	**Total**
33258	11.0	5.41	2.45	18.86

	FUD	Status	MUE	Modifiers				IOM Reference
33258	N/A	A	1(2)	N/A	N/A	N/A	80	None

* with documentation

Terms To Know

ablation. Removal or destruction of tissue by cutting, electrical energy, chemical substances, or excessive heat application.

reconstruction. Recreating, restoring, or rebuilding a body part or organ.

tissue. Group of similar cells with a similar function that form definite structures and organs. Tissue types include epithelial tissue, muscle tissue, connective tissue, and nervous tissue.

33259

\+ **33259** Operative tissue ablation and reconstruction of atria, performed at the time of other cardiac procedure(s), extensive (eg, maze procedure), with cardiopulmonary bypass (List separately in addition to code for primary procedure)

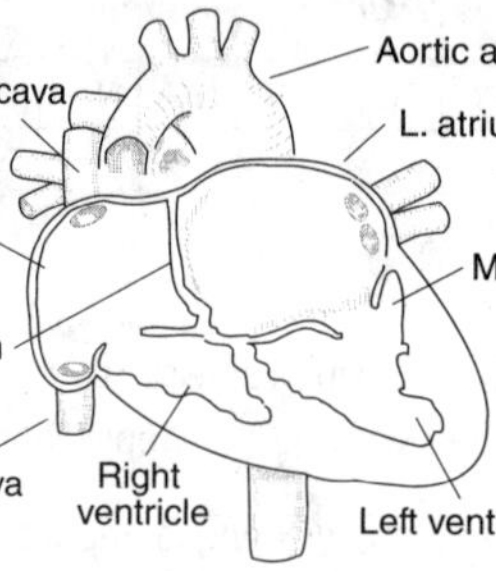

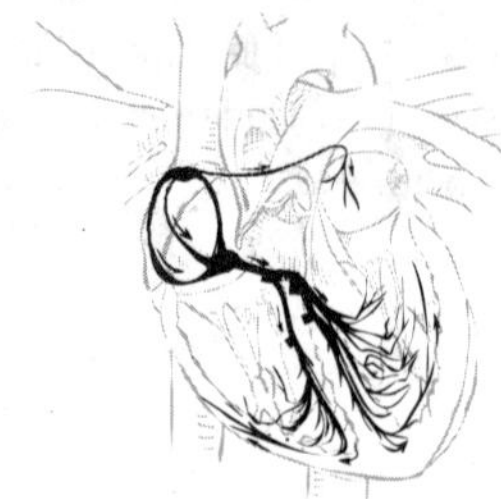

Conduction system of the heart

Aberrant conduction is treated with open heart surgery isolating the pulmonary veins or other anatomically defined triggers in the left or right atrium

Explanation

Concurrently with other cardiac procedures, the physician performs operative tissue ablation and reconstruction of the atria to treat atrial fibrillation. Atrial fibrillation is rapid, randomized muscle contraction of the atrial myocardium causing an irregular, rapid heart rate. In this procedure, the physician seeks to permanently interrupt aberrant electrical conduction within the atria to restore normal sinus rhythm. The physician performs a midline sternotomy, incising the skin, fascia, muscles, and sternum. The pericardium is incised. For an extensive operative tissue ablation and reconstruction of atria with cardiopulmonary bypass, also referred to as a maze procedure, lines are first placed for cardiopulmonary bypass. When cardiopulmonary bypass is achieved, an incision is made into the left or right atrium. A combination of surgical incision and/or energy sources, such as heat, microwave, laser, ultrasound, or cryoprobe, is used to create lesions that will heal into scars that disrupt conduction. Additional operative ablation involving the atrioventricular annulus is also performed. The left atrial appendage may be excised or isolated. The atrial incision lines are reanastomosed. The pericardium is repaired loosely, leaving gaps for blood and fluid to drain into the pleural space. The sternum is reanastomosed with sternal wires and the skin is sutured in layers.

Coding Tips

Report 33259 in addition to the following codes when performed with cardiopulmonary bypass: 33120, 33251, 33261, 33305, 33315, 33322, 33335, 33390–33391, 33404–33417, 33422–33468, 33474–33478, 33496, 33500, 33504–33507, 33510–33516, 33533–33548, 33600–33688, 33692–33726, 33730, 33732, 33736, 33767, 33770, 33783, 33786–33788, 33814, 33853, 33858–33877, 33910, 33916–33922, 33926, 33975–33980, and 33983. Do not report 33259 with 32551, 33210, 33211, 33254–33256, 33265, or 33266. When performed concurrently, 33259 is reported with open cardiac procedures that require sternotomy or cardiopulmonary bypass.

ICD-10-CM Diagnostic Codes

This/these CPT code(s) are add on code(s). See the primary procedure code that this code is performed with for your ICD-10-CM code selections. Diagnostic code(s) would be the same as the actual procedure performed.

AMA: **33259** 2017,Dec,3

Relative Value Units/Medicare Edits

Non-Facility RVU	Work	PE	MP	Total
33259	14.14	7.07	3.2	24.41
Facility RVU	**Work**	**PE**	**MP**	**Total**
33259	14.14	7.07	3.2	24.41

	FUD	Status	MUE	Modifiers				IOM Reference
33259	N/A	A	1(2)	N/A	N/A	N/A	80	None

* with documentation

Terms To Know

ablation. Removal or destruction of tissue by cutting, electrical energy, chemical substances, or excessive heat application.

cardiopulmonary bypass. Venous blood is diverted to a heart-lung machine, which mechanically pumps and oxygenates the blood temporarily so the heart can be bypassed while an open procedure on the heart or coronary arteries is performed. During bypass, the lungs are deflated and immobile.

reconstruction. Recreating, restoring, or rebuilding a body part or organ.

tissue. Group of similar cells with a similar function that form definite structures and organs. Tissue types include epithelial tissue, muscle tissue, connective tissue, and nervous tissue.

33261

33261 Operative ablation of ventricular arrhythmogenic focus with cardiopulmonary bypass

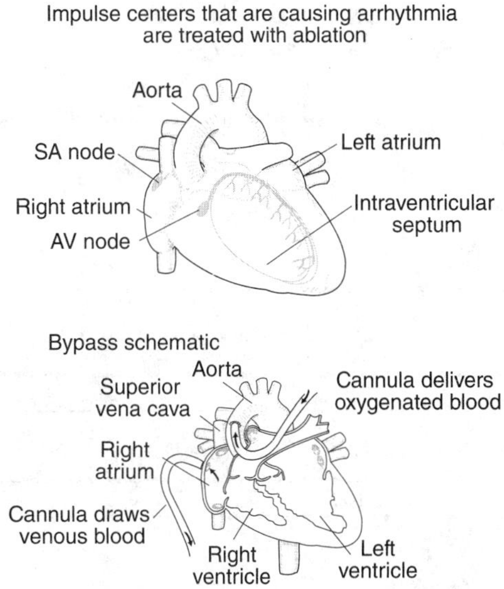

Specialized heart muscle fibers initiate the electrical impulses that contract the atria and the ventricles.The sinoatrial node (SA) is the pacemaker of the heart and initiates the impulse, first contracting the atria. The atrioventricular node (AV) receives the signal from the atria and redistributes it along the intraventricular septum to the muscles that contract the ventricles

Explanation

Following initiation of cardiopulmonary bypass, the physician exposes the heart through the sternum. A mapping grid of electrodes is placed over the surface of the beating heart. The location of the arrhythmia source is determined. The source is destroyed using electrical current, freezing or cutting, though not in the tricuspid valve. Any bleeding is controlled with sutures. The chest is closed.

Coding Tips

To report operative ablation of arrhythmogenic focus by ventricular aneurysmectomy, see 33542. Note diagnosis when reporting ablation procedures. Ablation of ventricular arrhythmogenic focus is reported with 33261, while ablation of supraventricular focus or pathway (Wolff-Parkinson-White syndrome) is reported with 33250–33251. Note also that 33261 involves ventricular ablation below the bundle of His. For open operative tissue ablation and reconstruction of atria, see 33254–33256. For endoscopic operative tissue ablation and reconstruction of atria, see 33265–33266. For transvenous intracardiac catheter ablation of ventricular arrhythmogenic focus, see 93654.

ICD-10-CM Diagnostic Codes

I45.6	Pre-excitation syndrome
I45.89	Other specified conduction disorders
I47.0	Re-entry ventricular arrhythmia
I47.1	Supraventricular tachycardia
I47.2	Ventricular tachycardia
I48.0	Paroxysmal atrial fibrillation
I48.11	Longstanding persistent atrial fibrillation
I48.19	Other persistent atrial fibrillation

I48.21	Permanent atrial fibrillation
I48.3	Typical atrial flutter
I48.4	Atypical atrial flutter
I49.01	Ventricular fibrillation
I49.02	Ventricular flutter
I49.2	Junctional premature depolarization
I49.8	Other specified cardiac arrhythmias

AMA: **33261** 2018,Jan,8; 2017,Jan,8; 2017,Dec,3; 2016,Jan,13; 2015,Jan,16; 2014,Jan,11

Relative Value Units/Medicare Edits

Non-Facility RVU	Work	PE	MP	Total
33261	28.92	11.26	6.82	47.0
Facility RVU	**Work**	**PE**	**MP**	**Total**
33261	28.92	11.26	6.82	47.0

	FUD	Status	MUE	Modifiers				IOM Reference
33261	90	A	1(2)	51	N/A	62*	80	None

* with documentation

Terms To Know

ablation. Removal or destruction of tissue by cutting, electrical energy, chemical substances, or excessive heat application.

arrhythmias. Heart disorder of rhythm or rate, due to an electrical conduction system malfunction.

cardiopulmonary bypass. Venous blood is diverted to a heart-lung machine, which mechanically pumps and oxygenates the blood temporarily so the heart can be bypassed while an open procedure on the heart or coronary arteries is performed. During bypass, the lungs are deflated and immobile.

catheter. Flexible tube inserted into an area of the body for introducing or withdrawing fluid.

dysrhythmia. Abnormality or disturbance in rhythm.

lesion. Area of damaged tissue that has lost continuity or function, due to disease or trauma. Lesions may be located on internal structures such as the brain, nerves, or kidneys, or visible on the skin.

Lown (-Ganong)-Levine syndrome. Electrocardiographic disorder indicated by a short P-R interval with normal duration of the QRS complex.

paroxysmal supraventricular tachycardia. Rapid heartbeat that starts above the ventricles and occurs sporadically.

thoracotomy. Surgical procedure for opening the chest wall in order to access the lungs, esophagus, trachea, aorta, heart, and diaphragm.

Wolff-Parkinson-White syndrome. Pre-excitation associated with paroxysmal tachycardia or atrial fibrillation with a short P-R interval on EKG and an early delta wave. The normal conduction pathway is bypassed.

33265-33266

33265 Endoscopy, surgical; operative tissue ablation and reconstruction of atria, limited (eg, modified maze procedure), without cardiopulmonary bypass

33266 operative tissue ablation and reconstruction of atria, extensive (eg, maze procedure), without cardiopulmonary bypass

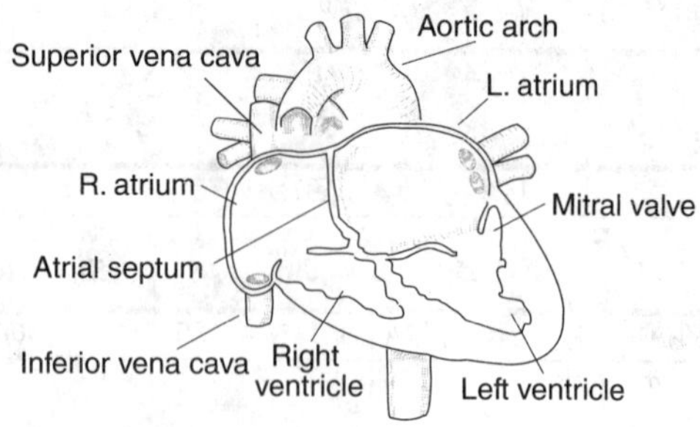

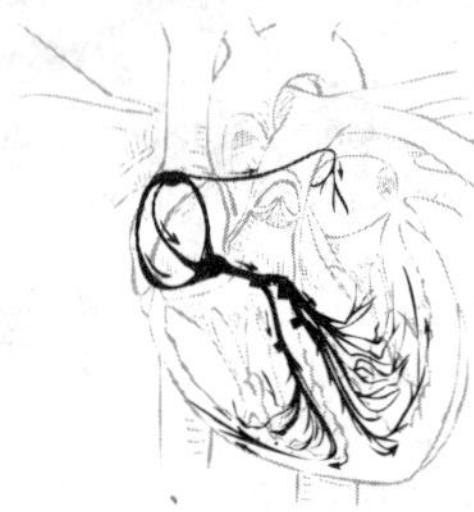

Conduction system of the heart

Aberrant conduction is treated endoscopically through multiple, small chest incisions

Explanation

The physician performs endoscopic operative ablation and reconstruction of the atria to treat atrial fibrillation. Atrial fibrillation is rapid, randomized muscle contraction of the atrial myocardium causing an irregular, rapid heart rate. In a maze procedure, the physician seeks to permanently interrupt aberrant electrical conduction within the atria to restore normal sinus rhythm. Through multiple endoscopic incisions in the chest, the physician accesses and visualizes the outer (epicardial) surface of the heart. For a limited or modified maze procedure performed endoscopically (33265), the pulmonary veins or other anatomically defined triggers are isolated in the left or right atrium and a heat, microwave, laser, ultrasound, or cryoprobe is used to create lesions from the outside of the left atrium that will heal into scars that disrupt conduction. In 33266, the right and/or left atrial tissue and/or atrial septum is treated as described in 33265, and additional operative ablation involving the atrioventricular annulus is performed. In either of these procedures, the left atrial appendage may be excised or isolated. Once sufficient interruption of electrical conduction has been accomplished, the endoscope is removed and access incisions are sutured in layers.

Coding Tips

Excision or isolation of the left atrial appendage by any method, including stapling, oversewing, ligation, or plication, is included in the operative ablation procedure and should not be reported separately. Do not report tube thoracostomy (32551) or temporary pacemaker (33210–33211) separately as these procedures are included in 33265 and 33266. For open operative ablation and reconstruction of atria, see 33254–33256.

ICD-10-CM Diagnostic Codes

I48.0	Paroxysmal atrial fibrillation
I48.11	Longstanding persistent atrial fibrillation

I48.19	Other persistent atrial fibrillation
I48.21	Permanent atrial fibrillation
I48.3	Typical atrial flutter
I48.4	Atypical atrial flutter
I49.2	Junctional premature depolarization
I49.8	Other specified cardiac arrhythmias

AMA: **33265** 2018,Jan,8; 2017,Jan,8; 2016,Jan,13; 2015,Jan,16; 2014,Jan,11
33266 2018,Jan,8; 2017,Jan,8; 2016,Jan,13; 2015,Jan,16; 2014,Jan,11

Relative Value Units/Medicare Edits

Non-Facility RVU	Work	PE	MP	Total
33265	23.71	10.22	5.37	39.3
33266	33.04	12.88	7.55	53.47
Facility RVU	**Work**	**PE**	**MP**	**Total**
33265	23.71	10.22	5.37	39.3
33266	33.04	12.88	7.55	53.47

	FUD	Status	MUE	Modifiers				IOM Reference
33265	90	A	1(2)	51	N/A	62*	80	None
33266	90	A	1(2)	51	N/A	62*	80	

* with documentation

Terms To Know

ablation. Removal or destruction of tissue by cutting, electrical energy, chemical substances, or excessive heat application.

arrhythmias. Heart disorder of rhythm or rate, due to an electrical conduction system malfunction.

cryosurgery. Application of intense cold, usually produced using liquid nitrogen, to locally freeze diseased or unwanted tissue and induce tissue necrosis without causing harm to adjacent tissue.

endoscopy. Visual inspection of the body using a fiberoptic scope.

laser surgery. Use of concentrated, sharply defined light beams to cut, cauterize, coagulate, seal, or vaporize tissue.

ICM Implant Cardiac Monitor

33285-33286

33285 Insertion, subcutaneous cardiac rhythm monitor, including programming
33286 Removal, subcutaneous cardiac rhythm monitor

Insert + Implant

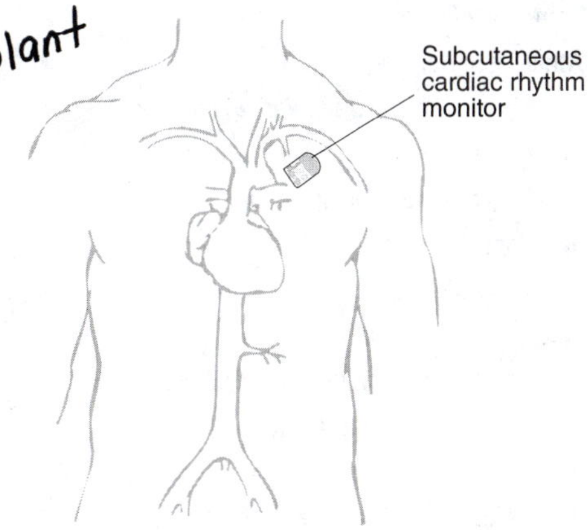

Explanation

The physician implants or removes an electronic device that is capable of recording heartrates and rhythms for over one year (subcutaneous cardiac rhythm monitor, cardiac event recorder, implantable loop recorder or ILR). In 33285, the physician uses a scalpel to make a small parasternal incision and dissects down to the level of subcutaneous tissue located over the left pectoral or mammary area. The monitor is implanted into the subcutaneous tissue. Electrodes that sense heart activity are located on the surface of the monitor, making it unnecessary to place transvenous leads. The device continuously and automatically monitors the heart's electrical activity when sensing the patient's rapid, irregular, or slow heartrate or can also be prompted by the patient in the course of experiencing symptoms. Programming of the device is included in this service. In 33286, the physician removes the monitor when sufficient information regarding the heart's activities has been obtained or when the batteries run out by incising down to the level of the recorder and removing it. In either surgery, the incision is closed with sutures. This type of recorder is capable of storing many separate events. When appropriate, a "programmer" is used by the physician to retrieve the information that can be displayed, stored, or printed.

Coding Tips

Code 33285 includes programming. For subsequent analysis and/or reprogramming, see 93285, 93291, and 93298.

ICD-10-CM Diagnostic Codes

G90.09	Other idiopathic peripheral autonomic neuropathy
I25.2	Old myocardial infarction
I44.0	Atrioventricular block, first degree
I44.1	Atrioventricular block, second degree
I44.2	Atrioventricular block, complete
I45.5	Other specified heart block
I45.6	Pre-excitation syndrome
I47.0	Re-entry ventricular arrhythmia
I47.1	Supraventricular tachycardia
I47.2	Ventricular tachycardia

I48.0	Paroxysmal atrial fibrillation
I48.11	Longstanding persistent atrial fibrillation
I48.19	Other persistent atrial fibrillation
I48.21	Permanent atrial fibrillation
I48.3	Typical atrial flutter
I48.4	Atypical atrial flutter
I49.01	Ventricular fibrillation
I49.02	Ventricular flutter
I49.1	Atrial premature depolarization
I49.2	Junctional premature depolarization
I49.3	Ventricular premature depolarization
I49.49	Other premature depolarization
I49.5	Sick sinus syndrome
I49.8	Other specified cardiac arrhythmias
I50.1	Left ventricular failure, unspecified
I50.21	Acute systolic (congestive) heart failure
I50.22	Chronic systolic (congestive) heart failure
I50.23	Acute on chronic systolic (congestive) heart failure
I50.31	Acute diastolic (congestive) heart failure
I50.32	Chronic diastolic (congestive) heart failure
I50.33	Acute on chronic diastolic (congestive) heart failure
I50.41	Acute combined systolic (congestive) and diastolic (congestive) heart failure
I50.42	Chronic combined systolic (congestive) and diastolic (congestive) heart failure
I50.43	Acute on chronic combined systolic (congestive) and diastolic (congestive) heart failure
I50.811	Acute right heart failure
I50.812	Chronic right heart failure
I50.813	Acute on chronic right heart failure
I50.814	Right heart failure due to left heart failure
I50.82	Biventricular heart failure
I50.83	High output heart failure
I50.84	End stage heart failure
I50.89	Other heart failure
I97.110	Postprocedural cardiac insufficiency following cardiac surgery
I97.111	Postprocedural cardiac insufficiency following other surgery
I97.130	Postprocedural heart failure following cardiac surgery
I97.131	Postprocedural heart failure following other surgery
I97.190	Other postprocedural cardiac functional disturbances following cardiac surgery
I97.191	Other postprocedural cardiac functional disturbances following other surgery
I97.790	Other intraoperative cardiac functional disturbances during cardiac surgery
I97.791	Other intraoperative cardiac functional disturbances during other surgery
Q24.6	Congenital heart block
R00.2	Palpitations
R42	Dizziness and giddiness
R55	Syncope and collapse
R94.31	Abnormal electrocardiogram [ECG] [EKG]
T82.518A	Breakdown (mechanical) of other cardiac and vascular devices and implants, initial encounter
T82.528A	Displacement of other cardiac and vascular devices and implants, initial encounter
T82.538A	Leakage of other cardiac and vascular devices and implants, initial encounter
T82.598A	Other mechanical complication of other cardiac and vascular devices and implants, initial encounter
T82.7XXA	Infection and inflammatory reaction due to other cardiac and vascular devices, implants and grafts, initial encounter
T82.827A	Fibrosis due to cardiac prosthetic devices, implants and grafts, initial encounter
T82.837A	Hemorrhage due to cardiac prosthetic devices, implants and grafts, initial encounter
T82.847A	Pain due to cardiac prosthetic devices, implants and grafts, initial encounter
T82.867A	Thrombosis due to cardiac prosthetic devices, implants and grafts, initial encounter
T82.897A	Other specified complication of cardiac prosthetic devices, implants and grafts, initial encounter
Z45.09	Encounter for adjustment and management of other cardiac device

Associated HCPCS Codes

C1764	Event recorder, cardiac (implantable)
E0616	Implantable cardiac event recorder with memory, activator, and programmer

AMA: 33285 2019,Apr,3 **33286** 2019,Apr,3

Relative Value Units/Medicare Edits

Non-Facility RVU	Work	PE	MP	Total
33285	1.53	144.18	0.36	146.07
33286	1.5	1.95	0.35	3.8
Facility RVU	**Work**	**PE**	**MP**	**Total**
33285	1.53	0.7	0.36	2.59
33286	1.5	0.69	0.35	2.54

	FUD	Status	MUE	Modifiers				IOM Reference
33285	0	A	1(3)	51	N/A	N/A	N/A	None
33286	0	A	1(3)	51	N/A	N/A	N/A	

* with documentation

Terms To Know

event recorder. Portable, ambulatory heart monitor worn by the patient that makes electrocardiographic recordings of the length and frequency of aberrant cardiac rhythm to help diagnose heart conditions and to assess pacemaker functioning or programming.

implantable cardiovascular monitor. Implantable electronic device that stores cardiovascular physiologic data such as intracardiac pressure waveforms collected from internal sensors or data such as weight and blood pressure collected from external sensors. The information stored in these devices is used as an aid in managing patients with heart failure and other cardiac conditions that are non-rhythm related. The data may be transmitted via local telemetry or remotely to a surveillance technician or an internet-based file server.

33289

33289 Transcatheter implantation of wireless pulmonary artery pressure sensor for long-term hemodynamic monitoring, including deployment and calibration of the sensor, right heart catheterization, selective pulmonary catheterization, radiological supervision and interpretation, and pulmonary artery angiography, when performed

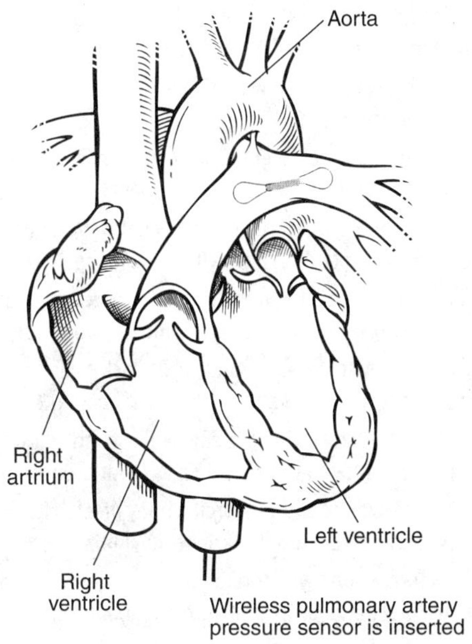

Explanation

The physician places a pulmonary pressure monitoring system. A proprietary device comprised of a battery-free sensor is placed directly in a distal portion of the pulmonary artery of a patient with heart failure to permit ongoing monitoring and measurement of the patient's heartrate, as well as systolic, diastolic, and mean pressures. The system is placed via a corresponding catheter. Pulmonary arterial pressure (PAP) readings transmitted from the sensor to a wireless electronic unit are subsequently transmitted to an online portal that can be accessed by the patient's treating health care provider. Through accurate monitoring of patients diagnosed with heart failure (HF) for exacerbations, it is possible to minimize the need for additional hospitalizations and the associated complications and allow for early pharmacological intervention. Deployment and calibration of the sensor, as well as any associated catheterizations, angiography, and radiological supervision and interpretation, are included in this service, when performed.

Coding Tips

Imaging guidance is included in this procedure and is not reported separately. For remote monitoring of an implantable wireless pulmonary artery pressure sensor, see 93264. Do not report 33289 with 36013-36015, 75741, 75743, 75746, 76000, 93451, 93453, 93456, 93457, 93460, 93461, 93530, 93531, 93532, 93533, or 93568.

ICD-10-CM Diagnostic Codes

I50.1	Left ventricular failure, unspecified
I50.21	Acute systolic (congestive) heart failure
I50.22	Chronic systolic (congestive) heart failure
I50.23	Acute on chronic systolic (congestive) heart failure
I50.31	Acute diastolic (congestive) heart failure
I50.32	Chronic diastolic (congestive) heart failure
I50.33	Acute on chronic diastolic (congestive) heart failure
I50.41	Acute combined systolic (congestive) and diastolic (congestive) heart failure
I50.42	Chronic combined systolic (congestive) and diastolic (congestive) heart failure
I50.43	Acute on chronic combined systolic (congestive) and diastolic (congestive) heart failure
I50.810	Right heart failure, unspecified
I50.811	Acute right heart failure
I50.812	Chronic right heart failure
I50.813	Acute on chronic right heart failure
I50.814	Right heart failure due to left heart failure
I50.82	Biventricular heart failure
I50.83	High output heart failure
I50.84	End stage heart failure
I50.89	Other heart failure

AMA: **33289** 2019,Jun,3

Relative Value Units/Medicare Edits

Non-Facility RVU	Work	PE	MP	Total
33289	6.0	2.23	1.28	9.51
Facility RVU	**Work**	**PE**	**MP**	**Total**
33289	6.0	2.23	1.28	9.51

	FUD	Status	MUE	Modifiers				IOM Reference
33289	0	A	1(3)	51	N/A	N/A	80*	None

* with documentation

Terms To Know

angiography. Radiographic imaging of the arteries. Imaging may be performed to study the vasculature of any given organ, body system, or area of circulation such as the brain, heart, chest, kidneys, limbs, gastrointestinal tract, aorta, and pulmonary circulation to visualize the formation and the function of the blood vessels to detect problems such as a blockage or stricture. A catheter is inserted through an accessible blood vessel and the artery is injected with a radiopaque contrast material after which x-rays are taken.

calibration. Action or process that involves adjusting, checking, or comparing using a standard of accuracy of an instrument in order to ensure consistent and accurate readings.

distal. Located farther away from a specified reference point or the trunk.

hemodynamic monitoring. Measurement of the blood pressure inside the veins, heart, and arteries as well as blood flow and the amount of oxygen in the blood as a way to see how well the heart is functioning.

transcatheter. Procedure or treatment performed via a catheter.

33300-33305

33300 Repair of cardiac wound; without bypass
33305 with cardiopulmonary bypass

A wound to the heart is repaired

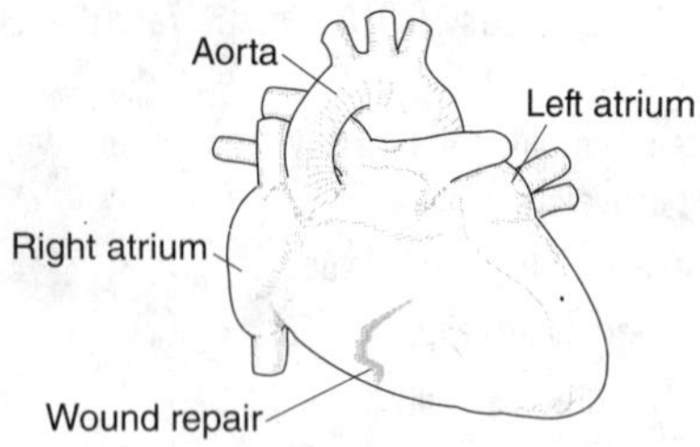

Bypass schematic

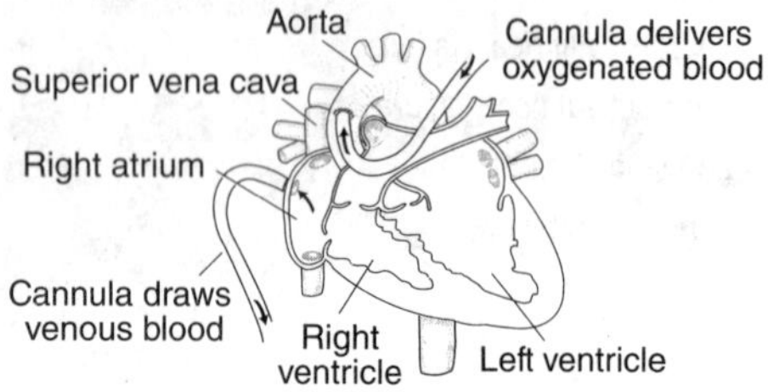

Explanation

The physician gains access to the heart using an incision through the sternum (median sternotomy) or the left anterior chest wall (thoracotomy). A pericardial window may be created if the diagnosis of penetrating cardiac trauma is not confirmed. Once penetrating trauma has been confirmed, the pericardial sac is incised and clotted blood and fluid removed. The entire heart is inspected and wound site(s) identified. Small lacerations are repaired with sutures and reinforced with Teflon felt pledges to anchor the sutures. Lacerations to small coronary vessels are ligated. Lacerations to larger coronary vessels are repaired. Large myocardial wounds may require synthetic grafting to cover the wound. The surgical incision is closed. Chest tubes and/or a mediastinal drainage tube may be left in place following the procedure. Report 33300 when the procedure is performed without cardiopulmonary bypass; report 33305 when cardiopulmonary bypass is required.

Coding Tips

Codes 33300 and 33305 report repair of traumatic wounds, not surgically created wounds. If significant additional time and effort are documented, append modifier 22 and submit a cover letter and operative report. When 33300 or 33305 is performed with another separately identifiable procedure, the highest dollar value code is listed as the primary procedure and subsequent procedures are appended with modifier 51.

ICD-10-CM Diagnostic Codes

I97.51 Accidental puncture and laceration of a circulatory system organ or structure during a circulatory system procedure
I97.52 Accidental puncture and laceration of a circulatory system organ or structure during other procedure
S21.311A Laceration without foreign body of right front wall of thorax with penetration into thoracic cavity, initial encounter ☑
S21.312A Laceration without foreign body of left front wall of thorax with penetration into thoracic cavity, initial encounter ☑
S21.321A Laceration with foreign body of right front wall of thorax with penetration into thoracic cavity, initial encounter ☑
S21.322A Laceration with foreign body of left front wall of thorax with penetration into thoracic cavity, initial encounter ☑
S21.331A Puncture wound without foreign body of right front wall of thorax with penetration into thoracic cavity, initial encounter ☑
S21.332A Puncture wound without foreign body of left front wall of thorax with penetration into thoracic cavity, initial encounter ☑
S21.341A Puncture wound with foreign body of right front wall of thorax with penetration into thoracic cavity, initial encounter ☑
S21.342A Puncture wound with foreign body of left front wall of thorax with penetration into thoracic cavity, initial encounter ☑
S21.351A Open bite of right front wall of thorax with penetration into thoracic cavity, initial encounter ☑
S21.352A Open bite of left front wall of thorax with penetration into thoracic cavity, initial encounter ☑
S21.411A Laceration without foreign body of right back wall of thorax with penetration into thoracic cavity, initial encounter ☑
S21.412A Laceration without foreign body of left back wall of thorax with penetration into thoracic cavity, initial encounter ☑
S21.421A Laceration with foreign body of right back wall of thorax with penetration into thoracic cavity, initial encounter ☑
S21.422A Laceration with foreign body of left back wall of thorax with penetration into thoracic cavity, initial encounter ☑
S21.431A Puncture wound without foreign body of right back wall of thorax with penetration into thoracic cavity, initial encounter ☑
S21.432A Puncture wound without foreign body of left back wall of thorax with penetration into thoracic cavity, initial encounter ☑
S21.441A Puncture wound with foreign body of right back wall of thorax with penetration into thoracic cavity, initial encounter ☑
S21.442A Puncture wound with foreign body of left back wall of thorax with penetration into thoracic cavity, initial encounter ☑
S21.451A Open bite of right back wall of thorax with penetration into thoracic cavity, initial encounter ☑
S21.452A Open bite of left back wall of thorax with penetration into thoracic cavity, initial encounter ☑
S26.01XA Contusion of heart with hemopericardium, initial encounter
S26.020A Mild laceration of heart with hemopericardium, initial encounter
S26.021A Moderate laceration of heart with hemopericardium, initial encounter
S26.022A Major laceration of heart with hemopericardium, initial encounter
S26.09XA Other injury of heart with hemopericardium, initial encounter
S26.11XA Contusion of heart without hemopericardium, initial encounter
S26.12XA Laceration of heart without hemopericardium, initial encounter
S26.19XA Other injury of heart without hemopericardium, initial encounter
T88.8XXA Other specified complications of surgical and medical care, not elsewhere classified, initial encounter

AMA: 33305 2017,Dec,3

Relative Value Units/Medicare Edits

Non-Facility RVU	Work	PE	MP	Total
33300	44.97	15.72	10.33	71.02
33305	76.93	24.29	17.85	119.07
Facility RVU	**Work**	**PE**	**MP**	**Total**
33300	44.97	15.72	10.33	71.02
33305	76.93	24.29	17.85	119.07

	FUD	Status	MUE	Modifiers				IOM Reference
33300	90	A	1(3)	51	N/A	62*	80	None
33305	90	A	1(3)	51	N/A	62*	80	

* with documentation

Terms To Know

cannula. Tube inserted into a blood vessel, duct, or body cavity to facilitate passage.

cardiopulmonary bypass. Venous blood is diverted to a heart-lung machine, which mechanically pumps and oxygenates the blood temporarily so the heart can be bypassed while an open procedure on the heart or coronary arteries is performed. During bypass, the lungs are deflated and immobile.

contusion. Superficial injury (bruising) produced by impact without a break in the skin.

laceration. Tearing injury; a torn, ragged-edged wound.

manubrium. Sternum.

mediastinum. Collection of organs and tissues that separate the pleural sacs. Located between the sternum and spine above the diaphragm, it contains the heart and great vessels, trachea and bronchi, esophagus, thymus, lymph nodes, and nerves.

open wound. Opening or break of the skin.

pericardial window. Incision made in the pericardium to create an opening large enough to allow drainage of pericardial fluid into the pleural space.

pericardium. Thin and slippery case in which the heart lies that is lined with fluid so that the heart is free to pulse and move as it beats.

puncture. Creating a hole.

thoracotomy. Surgical procedure for opening the chest wall in order to access the lungs, esophagus, trachea, aorta, heart, and diaphragm.

33310-33315

33310 Cardiotomy, exploratory (includes removal of foreign body, atrial or ventricular thrombus); without bypass

33315 with cardiopulmonary bypass

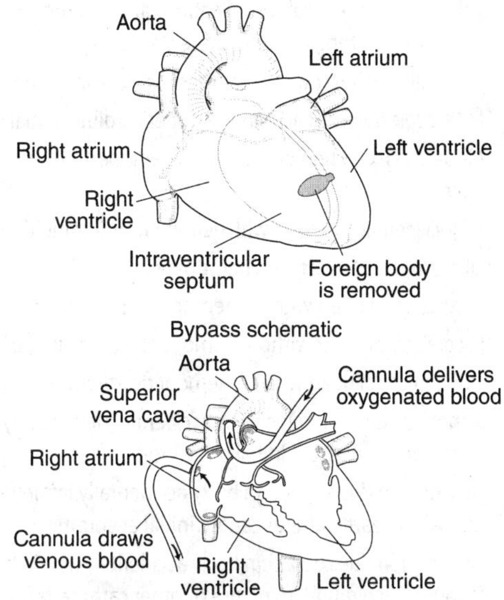

Surgical exploration of the heart is performed, requiring cardiotomy, or incision into heart tissues. A foreign body is removed in the course of the procedure

Explanation

The physician exposes the heart via the sternum. The foreign body is located by feeling the heart. If possible, the object is removed from the surface of the heart. If necessary, a hole is made in one of the ventricles or atria to remove the object or thrombus lodged there. The holes are closed with sutures and small reinforcing patches of Teflon felt. Report 33310 if cardiopulmonary bypass is not initiated; report 33315 if cardiopulmonary bypass is initiated.

Coding Tips

Codes 33310 and 33315 report exploration following trauma to the heart. Removal of foreign body includes objects resulting from penetrating trauma (missiles) or surgical complications (pacing electrodes, catheters, stents). Removal of thrombus includes thrombus due to trauma or complications of surgical procedures. These codes should not be reported for exploration related to congenital anomalies or disease of heart structures. Do not report 33310 or 33315 for removal of thrombus in addition to other cardiac codes unless a separate incision in the heart is required to remove the atrial or ventricular thrombus. When 33515 is performed with other cardiac procedures and requires a separate heart incision, append modifier 59 or an X{EPSU} modifier to 33515. If significant additional time and effort is documented, append modifier 22 and submit a cover letter and operative report. Report any free grafts or flaps separately.

ICD-10-CM Diagnostic Codes

I97.110	Postprocedural cardiac insufficiency following cardiac surgery
I97.111	Postprocedural cardiac insufficiency following other surgery
I97.120	Postprocedural cardiac arrest following cardiac surgery
I97.121	Postprocedural cardiac arrest following other surgery
I97.130	Postprocedural heart failure following cardiac surgery
I97.131	Postprocedural heart failure following other surgery

I97.51	Accidental puncture and laceration of a circulatory system organ or structure during a circulatory system procedure
I97.52	Accidental puncture and laceration of a circulatory system organ or structure during other procedure
I97.710	Intraoperative cardiac arrest during cardiac surgery
I97.711	Intraoperative cardiac arrest during other surgery
I97.89	Other postprocedural complications and disorders of the circulatory system, not elsewhere classified
S26.01XA	Contusion of heart with hemopericardium, initial encounter
S26.020A	Mild laceration of heart with hemopericardium, initial encounter
S26.021A	Moderate laceration of heart with hemopericardium, initial encounter
S26.022A	Major laceration of heart with hemopericardium, initial encounter
S26.09XA	Other injury of heart with hemopericardium, initial encounter
S26.11XA	Contusion of heart without hemopericardium, initial encounter
S26.12XA	Laceration of heart without hemopericardium, initial encounter
S26.19XA	Other injury of heart without hemopericardium, initial encounter
T81.515A	Adhesions due to foreign body accidentally left in body following heart catheterization, initial encounter
T81.525A	Obstruction due to foreign body accidentally left in body following heart catheterization, initial encounter
T81.526A	Obstruction due to foreign body accidentally left in body following aspiration, puncture or other catheterization, initial encounter
T81.535A	Perforation due to foreign body accidentally left in body following heart catheterization, initial encounter
T81.536A	Perforation due to foreign body accidentally left in body following aspiration, puncture or other catheterization, initial encounter
T81.595A	Other complications of foreign body accidentally left in body following heart catheterization, initial encounter
T82.110A	Breakdown (mechanical) of cardiac electrode, initial encounter
T82.120A	Displacement of cardiac electrode, initial encounter
T82.190A	Other mechanical complication of cardiac electrode, initial encounter
T82.513A	Breakdown (mechanical) of balloon (counterpulsation) device, initial encounter
T82.514A	Breakdown (mechanical) of infusion catheter, initial encounter
T82.515A	Breakdown (mechanical) of umbrella device, initial encounter
T82.518A	Breakdown (mechanical) of other cardiac and vascular devices and implants, initial encounter
T82.523A	Displacement of balloon (counterpulsation) device, initial encounter
T82.524A	Displacement of infusion catheter, initial encounter
T82.525A	Displacement of umbrella device, initial encounter
T82.528A	Displacement of other cardiac and vascular devices and implants, initial encounter
T82.533A	Leakage of balloon (counterpulsation) device, initial encounter
T82.534A	Leakage of infusion catheter, initial encounter
T82.535A	Leakage of umbrella device, initial encounter
T82.538A	Leakage of other cardiac and vascular devices and implants, initial encounter
T82.593A	Other mechanical complication of balloon (counterpulsation) device, initial encounter
T82.594A	Other mechanical complication of infusion catheter, initial encounter
T82.595A	Other mechanical complication of umbrella device, initial encounter
T82.598A	Other mechanical complication of other cardiac and vascular devices and implants, initial encounter
T82.898A	Other specified complication of vascular prosthetic devices, implants and grafts, initial encounter

AMA: 33315 2018,Jan,8; 2017,Jan,8; 2017,Dec,3; 2016,Jan,13; 2015,Jan,16; 2014,Jan,11

Relative Value Units/Medicare Edits

Non-Facility RVU	Work	PE	MP	Total
33310	20.34	8.92	4.78	34.04
33315	35.0	12.4	7.96	55.36
Facility RVU	**Work**	**PE**	**MP**	**Total**
33310	20.34	8.92	4.78	34.04
33315	35.0	12.4	7.96	55.36

	FUD	Status	MUE	Modifiers				IOM Reference
33310	90	A	1(2)	51	N/A	62*	80	None
33315	90	A	1(2)	51	N/A	62*	80	

* with documentation

Terms To Know

atria. Two upper chambers of the heart. The left and right atria are divided by the septum, a muscular wall.

cannula. Tube inserted into a blood vessel, duct, or body cavity to facilitate passage.

cardiopulmonary bypass. Venous blood is diverted to a heart-lung machine, which mechanically pumps and oxygenates the blood temporarily so the heart can be bypassed while an open procedure on the heart or coronary arteries is performed. During bypass, the lungs are deflated and immobile.

cardiotomy. Incision of the heart, the cardiac orifice, or the cardiac end of the stomach.

thrombus. Stationary blood clot inside a blood vessel.

33320-33322

33320 Suture repair of aorta or great vessels; without shunt or cardiopulmonary bypass
33321 with shunt bypass
33322 with cardiopulmonary bypass

Schematic of great vessels showing one type of wound repair

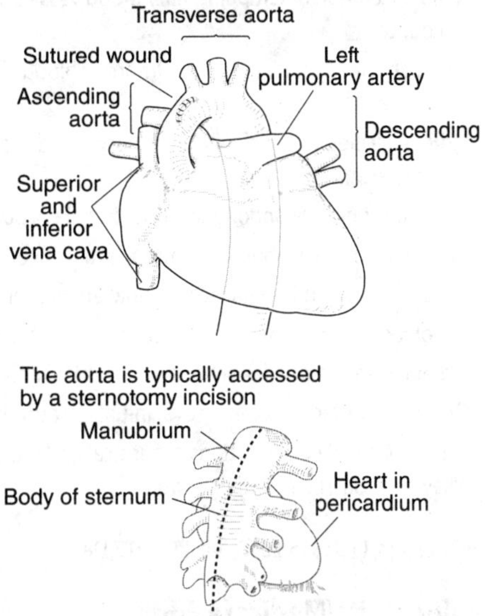

A wound to the aorta or to a great vessel is accessed and repaired using sutures

Explanation

The physician gains access to the mediastinum through an incision through the sternum (median sternotomy) or the chest wall (lateral thoracotomy). The physician repairs the aorta or great vessels while the heart is still beating. The physician closes the surgical incisions and dresses the sternal or chest wall wound. The physician may leave chest tubes and/or a mediastinal drainage tube in place following the procedure. Report 33321 if performed with a shunt bypass; report 33322 if performed with a cardiopulmonary bypass.

Coding Tips

These procedures report repair following trauma to the aorta or great vessels. Repairs related to congenital anomalies or disease should be reported with the appropriate codes for those procedures. If significant additional time and effort are documented, append modifier 22 and submit a cover letter and operative report. When 33320, 33321, or 33322 is performed with another separately identifiable procedure, the highest dollar value code is listed as the primary procedure and subsequent procedures are appended with modifier 51.

ICD-10-CM Diagnostic Codes

I97.51 Accidental puncture and laceration of a circulatory system organ or structure during a circulatory system procedure
I97.52 Accidental puncture and laceration of a circulatory system organ or structure during other procedure
S25.01XA Minor laceration of thoracic aorta, initial encounter
S25.02XA Major laceration of thoracic aorta, initial encounter
S25.09XA Other specified injury of thoracic aorta, initial encounter
S25.21XA Minor laceration of superior vena cava, initial encounter
S25.22XA Major laceration of superior vena cava, initial encounter
S25.29XA Other specified injury of superior vena cava, initial encounter
S25.411A Minor laceration of right pulmonary blood vessels, initial encounter ☑
S25.412A Minor laceration of left pulmonary blood vessels, initial encounter ☑
S25.421A Major laceration of right pulmonary blood vessels, initial encounter ☑
S25.422A Major laceration of left pulmonary blood vessels, initial encounter ☑
S25.491A Other specified injury of right pulmonary blood vessels, initial encounter ☑
S25.492A Other specified injury of left pulmonary blood vessels, initial encounter ☑
S35.01XA Minor laceration of abdominal aorta, initial encounter
S35.02XA Major laceration of abdominal aorta, initial encounter
S35.09XA Other injury of abdominal aorta, initial encounter
S35.11XA Minor laceration of inferior vena cava, initial encounter
S35.12XA Major laceration of inferior vena cava, initial encounter
S35.19XA Other injury of inferior vena cava, initial encounter
T88.8XXA Other specified complications of surgical and medical care, not elsewhere classified, initial encounter

AMA: 33320 2018,Jun,11; 2018,Jan,8; 2017,Jan,8; 2016,Jan,13; 2015,Jan,16; 2014,Jan,11 **33321** 2018,Jun,11 **33322** 2018,Jun,11; 2018,Jan,8; 2017,Jan,8; 2017,Dec,3; 2016,Jan,13; 2015,Jan,16; 2014,Jan,11

Relative Value Units/Medicare Edits

Non-Facility RVU	Work	PE	MP	Total
33320	18.54	7.81	4.19	30.54
33321	20.81	8.89	4.9	34.6
33322	24.42	10.19	5.41	40.02
Facility RVU	**Work**	**PE**	**MP**	**Total**
33320	18.54	7.81	4.19	30.54
33321	20.81	8.89	4.9	34.6
33322	24.42	10.19	5.41	40.02

	FUD	Status	MUE	Modifiers				IOM Reference
33320	90	A	1(3)	51	N/A	62*	80	None
33321	90	A	1(3)	51	N/A	62*	80	
33322	90	A	1(3)	51	N/A	62*	80	

* with documentation

Terms To Know

anomaly. Irregularity in the structure or position of an organ or tissue.

cardiopulmonary bypass. Venous blood is diverted to a heart-lung machine, which mechanically pumps and oxygenates the blood temporarily so the heart can be bypassed while an open procedure on the heart or coronary arteries is performed. During bypass, the lungs are deflated and immobile.

mediastinum. Collection of organs and tissues that separate the pleural sacs. Located between the sternum and spine above the diaphragm, it contains the heart and great vessels, trachea and bronchi, esophagus, thymus, lymph nodes, and nerves.

33330-33335

33330 Insertion of graft, aorta or great vessels; without shunt, or cardiopulmonary bypass

33335 with cardiopulmonary bypass

A graft is inserted on any of the great vessels

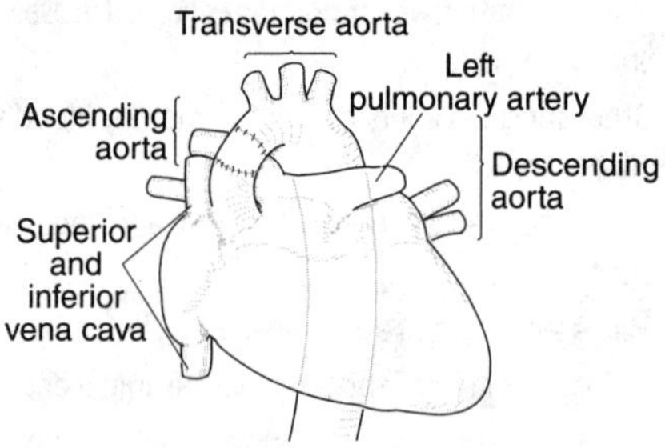

Cardiopulmonary bypass schematic

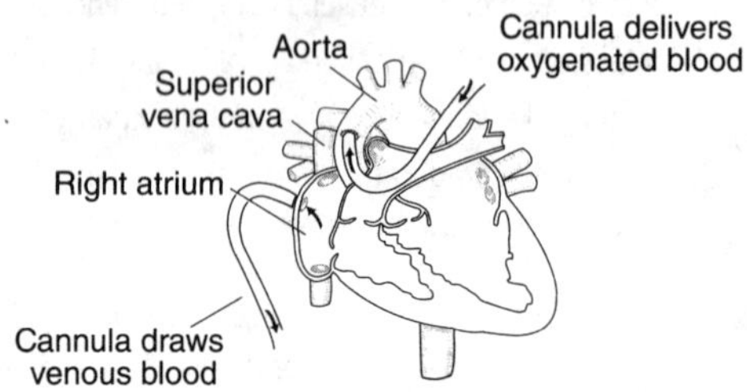

Explanation

In 33330, the physician gains access to the mediastinum through an incision through the sternum (median sternotomy) or the chest wall (lateral thoracotomy). The physician sews in the aortic or great vessel graft while the heart is still beating. In 33335, the physician places cardiopulmonary bypass catheters usually through incisions in the right atrial appendage and aorta or femoral artery. The physician stops the heart by infusing cardioplegia solution into the coronary circulation. The physician sews in the aortic or great vessel graft while the heart is still. The physician takes the patient off cardiopulmonary bypass, closes the surgical incisions and dresses the sternal or chest wall wound. The physician may leave chest tubes and/or a mediastinal drainage tube in place following the procedure.

Coding Tips

These procedures report graft insertion to repair traumatic wounds of the aorta or great vessels. Repairs related to congenital anomalies or disease should be reported with appropriate codes for those procedures. If significant additional time and effort is documented, append modifier 22 and submit a cover letter and operative report. When 33330 or 33335 is performed with another separately identifiable procedure, the highest dollar value code is listed as the primary procedure and subsequent procedures are appended with modifier 51.

ICD-10-CM Diagnostic Codes

I97.51 Accidental puncture and laceration of a circulatory system organ or structure during a circulatory system procedure

I97.52 Accidental puncture and laceration of a circulatory system organ or structure during other procedure

S25.01XA Minor laceration of thoracic aorta, initial encounter

S25.02XA Major laceration of thoracic aorta, initial encounter

S25.09XA Other specified injury of thoracic aorta, initial encounter

S25.21XA Minor laceration of superior vena cava, initial encounter

S25.22XA Major laceration of superior vena cava, initial encounter

S25.29XA Other specified injury of superior vena cava, initial encounter

S25.411A Minor laceration of right pulmonary blood vessels, initial encounter ☑

S25.412A Minor laceration of left pulmonary blood vessels, initial encounter ☑

S25.421A Major laceration of right pulmonary blood vessels, initial encounter ☑

S25.422A Major laceration of left pulmonary blood vessels, initial encounter ☑

S25.491A Other specified injury of right pulmonary blood vessels, initial encounter ☑

S25.492A Other specified injury of left pulmonary blood vessels, initial encounter ☑

S35.01XA Minor laceration of abdominal aorta, initial encounter

S35.02XA Major laceration of abdominal aorta, initial encounter

S35.09XA Other injury of abdominal aorta, initial encounter

S35.11XA Minor laceration of inferior vena cava, initial encounter

S35.12XA Major laceration of inferior vena cava, initial encounter

S35.19XA Other injury of inferior vena cava, initial encounter

T88.8XXA Other specified complications of surgical and medical care, not elsewhere classified, initial encounter

AMA: **33330** 2018,Jun,11 **33335** 2018,Jun,11; 2017,Dec,3

Relative Value Units/Medicare Edits

Non-Facility RVU	Work	PE	MP	Total
33330	25.29	10.27	5.96	41.52
33335	33.91	12.89	7.81	54.61
Facility RVU	**Work**	**PE**	**MP**	**Total**
33330	25.29	10.27	5.96	41.52
33335	33.91	12.89	7.81	54.61

	FUD	Status	MUE	Modifiers				IOM Reference
33330	90	A	1(3)	51	N/A	62*	80	None
33335	90	A	1(3)	51	N/A	62*	80	

* with documentation

33340

33340 Percutaneous transcatheter closure of the left atrial appendage with endocardial implant, including fluoroscopy, transseptal puncture, catheter placement(s), left atrial angiography, left atrial appendage angiography, when performed, and radiological supervision and interpretation

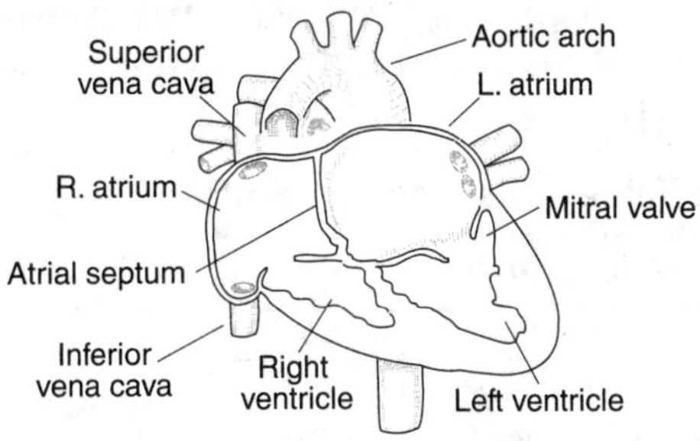

Left atrial appendage is closed with a percutaneously placed endocardial implant

Explanation

A left atrial appendage is closed or occluded using an endocardial implant delivered via catheter. The physician places an introducer sheath in a vein (typically, the femoral vein) using percutaneous puncture. The physician places a lumen catheter through the introducer sheath into the femoral vein and advances it, under fluoroscopic guidance, to the right atrium. The physician exchanges this catheter over a wire for a transseptal puncture needle, dilator, and sheath. The physician advances the transseptal puncture apparatus to the right atrium and punctures the intraatrial septum (in some cases, the physician may use a patent foramen ovale if present rather than performing a septal puncture). The physician advances the needle, dilator, and transseptal sheath into the left atrium. The occlusive device is positioned over the left atrial appendage and deployed blocking the opening completely. The physician removes the catheters and sheaths from the femoral vessels. Pressure is placed on the wound for 20 to 30 minutes to stem bleeding. This code includes fluoroscopy, transseptal puncture, catheter placement, left atrial and left atrial appendage angiography, and radiological supervision and interpretation.

Coding Tips

Do not report this code with 93462. This code should not be reported with 93452–93453, 93458–93461, or 93531–93533 unless left ventricle catheterization is completed via non-transseptal approach for symptoms separate from left atrial appendage closure procedure. This code should not be reported with 93451, 93453, 93456, 93460–93461, or 93530–93533 unless right heart catheterization is completed for symptoms separate from left atrial appendage closure procedure.

ICD-10-CM Diagnostic Codes

I48.0	Paroxysmal atrial fibrillation
I48.11	Longstanding persistent atrial fibrillation
I48.19	Other persistent atrial fibrillation
I48.21	Permanent atrial fibrillation
I48.3	Typical atrial flutter
I48.4	Atypical atrial flutter

AMA: 33340 2018,Jan,8; 2017,Jul,3

Relative Value Units/Medicare Edits

Non-Facility RVU	Work	PE	MP	Total
33340	14.0	5.8	3.21	23.01
Facility RVU	**Work**	**PE**	**MP**	**Total**
33340	14.0	5.8	3.21	23.01

	FUD	Status	MUE	Modifiers				IOM Reference
33340	0	A	1(2)	51	N/A	62	80*	None

* with documentation

Terms To Know

angiography. Radiographic imaging of the arteries. Imaging may be performed to study the vasculature of any given organ, body system, or area of circulation such as the brain, heart, chest, kidneys, limbs, gastrointestinal tract, aorta, and pulmonary circulation to visualize the formation and the function of the blood vessels to detect problems such as a blockage or stricture. A catheter is inserted through an accessible blood vessel and the artery is injected with a radiopaque contrast material after which x-rays are taken.

atrial appendage. Also known as an auricular appendage, a pouch connected to the left and right atria of the heart. The left atrial appendage (LAA) is frequently the source of clots causing embolic strokes in patients with atrial fibrillation.

fibrillation. Spontaneous contraction of individual muscle fibers.

implant. Material or device inserted or placed within the body for therapeutic, reconstructive, or diagnostic purposes.

lumen. Space inside an intestine, artery, vein, duct, or tube.

 ● New ▲ Revised + Add On AMA: CPT Assist [Resequenced] ☑ Laterality

33361-33362

33361 Transcatheter aortic valve replacement (TAVR/TAVI) with prosthetic valve; percutaneous femoral artery approach

33362 open femoral artery approach

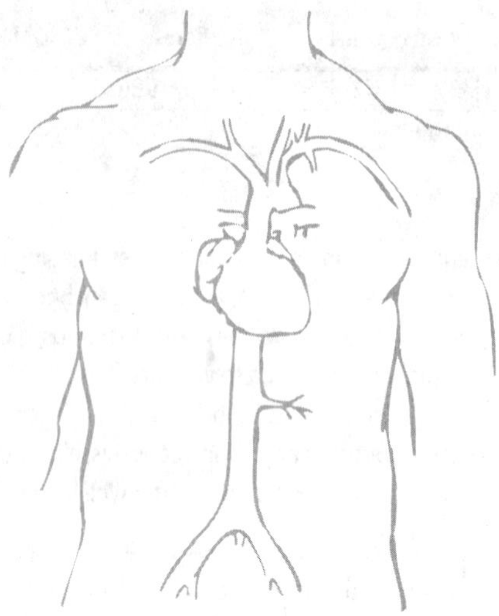

Transcatheter aortic valve is replaced utilizing femoral artery approach

Explanation

Transcatheter aortic valve replacement or implantation (TAVR/TAVI) is performed on patients with symptomatic aortic stenosis that are high risk or not eligible for traditional open chest surgery. A guidewire is placed in the femoral artery in the groin and manipulated into the left ventricle. A catheter is inserted following the guidewire to the aortic valve. A balloon is inflated to compress the native valve. A porcine valve attached to an expandable stent is deployed over the compressed native valve. The catheter and guidewire are removed. Report 33361 if the catheter access is percutaneous and 33362 when access to the femoral artery is open.

Coding Tips

These procedures are typically performed by two surgeons performing their own components of the procedure. In these instances, append modifier 62. Angiography and radiological supervision to guide the procedure are included in the codes and are not separately reported. Diagnostic coronary angiography performed at the time of the procedure may be reported in certain instances, such as when no prior catheter-based angiography study has been performed or a significant change in the patient's condition has occurred since the time of a prior study. Diagnostic coronary angiography services reported at the same surgical session as TAVR/TAVI services must have modifier 59 appended and must meet specific coverage requirements. Check with local payers for requirements. Percutaneous coronary interventional procedures are reported separately when performed with these codes. For cardiopulmonary bypass with TAVR/TAVI procedures, see 33367–33369. For transcatheter ventricular support with TAVR/TAVI, see the ventricular assist device (VAD) procedure codes (33990–33993, 33975–33976, 33999) and the balloon pump insertion codes (33967, 33970, 33973). For a transapical approach, see 33366.

ICD-10-CM Diagnostic Codes

I06.0	Rheumatic aortic stenosis
I06.2	Rheumatic aortic stenosis with insufficiency
I08.0	Rheumatic disorders of both mitral and aortic valves
I08.8	Other rheumatic multiple valve diseases
I35.0	Nonrheumatic aortic (valve) stenosis
I35.1	Nonrheumatic aortic (valve) insufficiency
I35.2	Nonrheumatic aortic (valve) stenosis with insufficiency
I35.8	Other nonrheumatic aortic valve disorders
I35.9	Nonrheumatic aortic valve disorder, unspecified
Q23.0	Congenital stenosis of aortic valve

AMA: 33361 2018,Jan,8; 2017,Jan,8; 2016,Jan,13; 2015,Mar,9; 2015,Jan,16; 2014,Jul,8; 2014,Jan,5; 2014,Jan,11; 2013,Jan,6-8 **33362** 2018,Jan,8; 2017,Jan,8; 2017,Dec,3; 2016,Jan,13; 2015,Mar,9; 2015,Jan,16; 2014,Jul,8; 2014,Jan,11; 2014,Jan,5; 2013,Jan,6-8

Relative Value Units/Medicare Edits

Non-Facility RVU	Work	PE	MP	Total
33361	25.13	8.51	5.84	39.48
33362	27.52	9.17	6.41	43.1
Facility RVU	**Work**	**PE**	**MP**	**Total**
33361	25.13	8.51	5.84	39.48
33362	27.52	9.17	6.41	43.1

	FUD	Status	MUE	Modifiers				IOM Reference
33361	0	A	1(2)	51	N/A	62	80*	100-03,20.32;
33362	0	A	1(2)	51	N/A	62	80*	100-04,32,290.1.1;
								100-04,32,290.2;
								100-04,32,290.3;
								100-04,32,290.4

* with documentation

Terms To Know

aortic stenosis. Narrowing of the aortic valve resulting in backflow of blood into the ventricle.

aortic valve. Heart valve, comprising three cusps, that divides the left ventricle and the aorta.

congenital. Present at birth, occurring through heredity or an influence during gestation up to the moment of birth.

percutaneous. Through the skin.

prosthetic. Device that replaces all or part of an internal body organ or body part, or that replaces part of the function of a permanently inoperable or malfunctioning internal body organ or body part.

 ● New ▲ Revised + Add On AMA: CPT Assist [Resequenced] ☑ Laterality

33363-33364

33363 Transcatheter aortic valve replacement (TAVR/TAVI) with prosthetic valve; open axillary artery approach

33364 open iliac artery approach

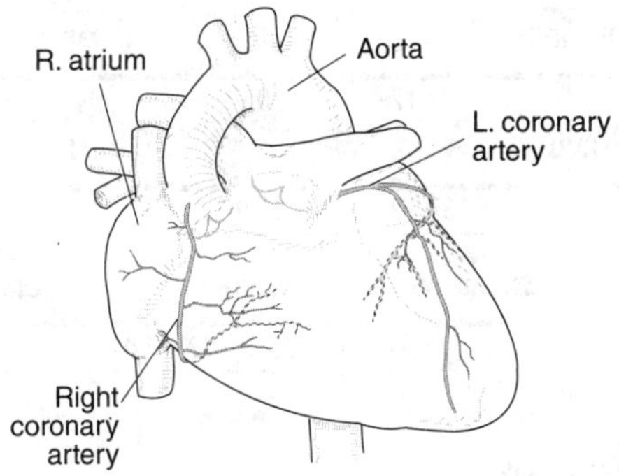

Aortic valves are replaced using a transcather

Explanation

Transcatheter aortic valve replacement or implantation (TAVR/TAVI) is performed on patients with symptomatic aortic stenosis that are high risk or not eligible for traditional open chest surgery. A guidewire is placed in a peripheral or other artery and manipulated into the left ventricle. A catheter is inserted following the guidewire to the aortic valve. A balloon is inflated to compress the native valve. A porcine valve attached to an expandable stent is deployed over the compressed native valve. The catheter and guidewire are removed. Report 33363 if the catheter access is via an open axillary artery approach and 33364 when access is via an open iliac artery approach.

Coding Tips

These procedures are typically performed by two surgeons performing their own components of the procedure. In these instances, append modifier 62. Angiography and radiological supervision to guide the procedure are included in the codes and are not separately reported. Diagnostic coronary angiography performed at the time of the procedure may be reported in certain instances, such as when no prior catheter-based angiography study has been performed or a significant change in the patient's condition has occurred since the time of a prior study. Diagnostic coronary angiography services reported at the same surgical session as TAVR/TAVI services must have modifier 59 appended and must meet specific coverage requirements. Check with local payers for requirements. Percutaneous coronary interventional procedures are reported separately when performed with these codes. For cardiopulmonary bypass with TAVR/TAVI procedures, see 33367–33369. For transcatheter ventricular support with TAVR/TAVI, see the ventricular assist device (VAD) procedure codes (33990–33993, 33975–33976, 33999) and the balloon pump insertion codes (33967, 33970, and 33973). For a transapical approach, see 33366.

ICD-10-CM Diagnostic Codes

I06.0	Rheumatic aortic stenosis
I06.2	Rheumatic aortic stenosis with insufficiency
I08.0	Rheumatic disorders of both mitral and aortic valves
I08.8	Other rheumatic multiple valve diseases
I35.0	Nonrheumatic aortic (valve) stenosis
I35.1	Nonrheumatic aortic (valve) insufficiency
I35.2	Nonrheumatic aortic (valve) stenosis with insufficiency
I35.8	Other nonrheumatic aortic valve disorders
I35.9	Nonrheumatic aortic valve disorder, unspecified
Q23.0	Congenital stenosis of aortic valve

AMA: **33363** 2018,Jan,8; 2017,Jan,8; 2017,Dec,3; 2016,Jan,13; 2015,Mar,9; 2015,Jan,16; 2014,Jul,8; 2014,Jan,5; 2014,Jan,11; 2013,Jan,6-8 **33364** 2018,Jan,8; 2017,Jan,8; 2017,Dec,3; 2016,Jan,13; 2015,Mar,9; 2015,Jan,16; 2014,Jul,8; 2014,Jan,5; 2014,Jan,11; 2013,Jan,6-8

Relative Value Units/Medicare Edits

Non-Facility RVU	Work	PE	MP	Total
33363	28.5	9.46	6.68	44.64
33364	30.0	9.06	7.08	46.14
Facility RVU	**Work**	**PE**	**MP**	**Total**
33363	28.5	9.46	6.68	44.64
33364	30.0	9.06	7.08	46.14

	FUD	Status	MUE	Modifiers				IOM Reference
33363	0	A	1(2)	51	N/A	62	80*	None
33364	0	A	1(2)	51	N/A	62	80*	

* with documentation

Terms To Know

angiography. Radiographic imaging of the arteries.

aortic stenosis. Narrowing of the aortic valve resulting in backflow of blood into the ventricle.

aortic valve. Heart valve, comprising three cusps, that divides the left ventricle and the aorta.

prosthetic. Device that replaces all or part of an internal body organ or body part, or that replaces part of the function of a permanently inoperable or malfunctioning internal body organ or body part.

transcatheter. Procedure or treatment performed via a catheter.

33365

33365 Transcatheter aortic valve replacement (TAVR/TAVI) with prosthetic valve; transaortic approach (eg, median sternotomy, mediastinotomy)

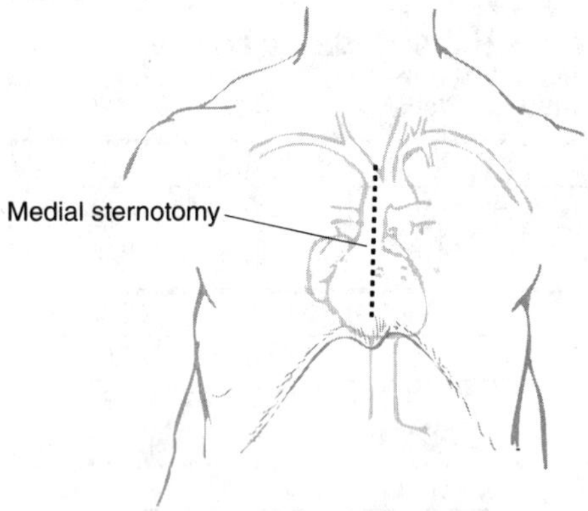

Medial sternotomy approach is utilized for transcatheter aortic value replacement

Explanation

Transcatheter aortic valve replacement or implantation (TAVR/TAVI) is performed on patients with symptomatic aortic stenosis that are high risk or not eligible for traditional open chest surgery. A median sternotomy or mediastinotomy is performed for direct access to the aorta. The aorta is incised and a guidewire is inserted and manipulated into the left ventricle. A catheter is inserted following the guidewire to the aortic valve. A balloon is inflated to compress the native valve. A porcine valve attached to an expandable stent is deployed over the compressed native valve. The catheter and guidewire are removed.

Coding Tips

This procedure is typically performed by two surgeons performing their own components of the procedure. In these instances, append modifier 62. Angiography and radiological supervision to guide the procedure is included in the code and is not reported separately. Diagnostic coronary angiography performed at the time of the procedure may be reported in certain instances, such as when no prior catheter-based angiography study has been performed or a significant change in the patient's condition has occurred since the time of a prior study. Diagnostic coronary angiography services reported at the same surgical session as TAVR/TAVI services must have modifier 59 appended and must meet specific coverage requirements. Check with local payers for requirements. Percutaneous coronary interventional procedures are reported separately when performed with these codes. For cardiopulmonary bypass with TAVR/TAVI procedures, see 33367–33369. For transcatheter ventricular support with TAVR/TAVI, see the ventricular assist device (VAD) procedure codes (33990–33993, 33975–33976, 33999) and the balloon pump insertion codes (33967, 33970, 33973). For a transapical approach, see 33366.

ICD-10-CM Diagnostic Codes

I06.0	Rheumatic aortic stenosis
I06.2	Rheumatic aortic stenosis with insufficiency
I08.0	Rheumatic disorders of both mitral and aortic valves
I08.8	Other rheumatic multiple valve diseases
I35.0	Nonrheumatic aortic (valve) stenosis
I35.1	Nonrheumatic aortic (valve) insufficiency
I35.2	Nonrheumatic aortic (valve) stenosis with insufficiency
I35.8	Other nonrheumatic aortic valve disorders
I35.9	Nonrheumatic aortic valve disorder, unspecified
Q23.0	Congenital stenosis of aortic valve

AMA: 33365 2018,Jan,8; 2017,Jan,8; 2016,Jan,13; 2015,Mar,9; 2015,Jan,16; 2014,Jul,8; 2014,Jan,5; 2014,Jan,11; 2013,Jan,6-8

Relative Value Units/Medicare Edits

Non-Facility RVU	Work	PE	MP	Total
33365	33.12	10.95	7.76	51.83
Facility RVU	**Work**	**PE**	**MP**	**Total**
33365	33.12	10.95	7.76	51.83

	FUD	Status	MUE	Modifiers				IOM Reference
33365	0	A	1(2)	51	N/A	62	80*	None

* with documentation

Terms To Know

aortic valve. Heart valve, comprising three cusps, that divides the left ventricle and the aorta.

median sternotomy. Standard incision for open chest cardiac surgeries, from above the bellybutton to just under the chin, down the center of the chest through the sternum into the thoracic cavity.

mediastinotomy. Incision into the mediastinum for purposes of exploration, foreign body removal, drainage, or biopsy.

prosthetic. Device that replaces all or part of an internal body organ or body part, or that replaces part of the function of a permanently inoperable or malfunctioning internal body organ or body part.

rheumatic heart disease. Manifestation of and sequel to rheumatic fever; any cardiac involvement in rheumatic fever.

33366

33366 Transcatheter aortic valve replacement (TAVR/TAVI) with prosthetic valve; transapical exposure (eg, left thoracotomy)

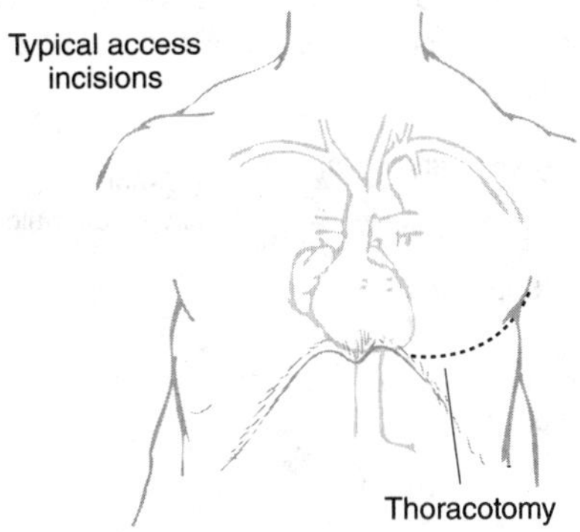

Left thoracotomy approach is used for aortic valve replacement

Explanation

Transcatheter aortic valve replacement or implantation (TAVR/TAVI) is performed on patients with symptomatic aortic stenosis that are high risk or not eligible for traditional open chest surgery. A small incision is made between ribs (usually the fifth or sixth intercostal space) on the lower left side of the patient's chest to achieve direct access to the heart. The pericardium is incised and opened near the left ventricular apex. A guidewire is advanced through the opening into the left ventricle, through the septum, and into the right ventricle. A catheter is inserted following the guidewire to the aortic valve. A balloon is inflated to compress the native valve. A porcine valve attached to an expandable stent is deployed over the compressed native valve. The catheter and guidewire are removed and the pericardium is closed using sutures. A chest tube may be placed. The wound is closed in layers.

Coding Tips

Two surgeons typically perform separate components of this procedure. In this instance, append modifier 62. Angiography and radiological supervision to guide the procedure is included in the procedure and is not reported separately. Diagnostic coronary angiography performed at the time of the procedure may only be reported in certain instances, such as when no prior catheter-based angiography study has been performed or a significant change in the patient's condition has occurred since the time of a prior study. Diagnostic coronary angiography services reported at the same surgical session as TAVR/TAVI services must have modifier 59 appended and must meet specific coverage requirements. Check with local payers for requirements. Percutaneous coronary interventional procedures are reported separately when performed with this procedure. For cardiopulmonary bypass with TAVR/TAVI procedures, see 33367–33369. For transcatheter ventricular support with TAVR/TAVI, see the ventricular assist device (VAD) procedure codes (33990–33993, 33975–33976, 33999) and the balloon pump insertion codes (33967, 33970, 33973).

ICD-10-CM Diagnostic Codes

I06.0	Rheumatic aortic stenosis
I06.2	Rheumatic aortic stenosis with insufficiency
I08.0	Rheumatic disorders of both mitral and aortic valves
I08.8	Other rheumatic multiple valve diseases
I35.0	Nonrheumatic aortic (valve) stenosis
I35.1	Nonrheumatic aortic (valve) insufficiency
I35.2	Nonrheumatic aortic (valve) stenosis with insufficiency
I35.8	Other nonrheumatic aortic valve disorders
I35.9	Nonrheumatic aortic valve disorder, unspecified
Q23.0	Congenital stenosis of aortic valve

AMA: **33366** 2018,Jan,8; 2017,Jan,8; 2016,Jan,13; 2015,Mar,9; 2015,Jan,16; 2014,Jul,8; 2014,Jan,5

Relative Value Units/Medicare Edits

Non-Facility RVU	Work	PE	MP	Total
33366	35.88	11.76	8.39	56.03
Facility RVU	**Work**	**PE**	**MP**	**Total**
33366	35.88	11.76	8.39	56.03

	FUD	Status	MUE	Modifiers				IOM Reference
33366	0	A	1(3)	51	N/A	62	80*	None

* with documentation

Terms To Know

aortic valve. Heart valve, comprising three cusps, that divides the left ventricle and the aorta.

apical. At the top, tip or end of a structure; the opposite of basal.

congenital. Present at birth, occurring through heredity or an influence during gestation up to the moment of birth.

guidewire. Flexible metal instrument designed to lead another instrument in its proper course.

pericardium. Thin and slippery case in which the heart lies that is lined with fluid so that the heart is free to pulse and move as it beats.

stenosis. Narrowing or constriction of a passage.

thoracotomy. Surgical procedure for opening the chest wall in order to access the lungs, esophagus, trachea, aorta, heart, and diaphragm.

33367-33368

+ 33367 Transcatheter aortic valve replacement (TAVR/TAVI) with prosthetic valve; cardiopulmonary bypass support with percutaneous peripheral arterial and venous cannulation (eg, femoral vessels) (List separately in addition to code for primary procedure)

+ 33368 cardiopulmonary bypass support with open peripheral arterial and venous cannulation (eg, femoral, iliac, axillary vessels) (List separately in addition to code for primary procedure)

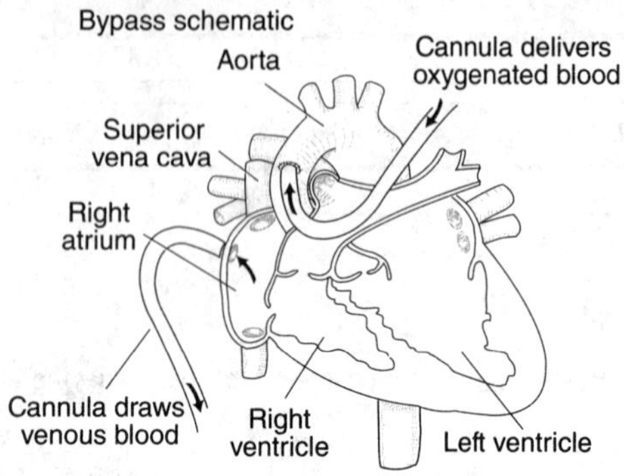

Explanation

The patient's blood is pumped to a bypass machine, oxygenated, and returned to the patient during a transcatheter aortic valve replacement or implantation (TAVR/TAVI). Its purpose is to provide mechanical support for the heart and lungs during the procedure. In 33367, the access for the intake and output of the patient's blood is via percutaneous cannulations of a peripheral artery and vein, typically the femoral vessels. Report 33368 for open peripheral arterial and venous cannulation.

Coding Tips

Report 33367 and 33368 in addition to 33361–33366, 33418, 33477, 0483T, 0484T, 0544T-0545T, and 0569T-0570T. Do not report 33367 or 33368 with one another or with 33369.

ICD-10-CM Diagnostic Codes

This/these CPT code(s) are add on code(s). See the primary procedure code that this code is performed with for your ICD-10-CM code selections. Diagnostic code(s) would be the same as the actual procedure performed.

AMA: **33367** 2018,Jan,8; 2017,Jan,8; 2016,Mar,5; 2016,Jan,13; 2015,Sep,3; 2015,Jan,16; 2013,Jan,6-8 **33368** 2018,Jan,8; 2017,Jan,8; 2016,Mar,5; 2016,Jan,13; 2015,Sep,3; 2015,Jan,16; 2013,Jan,6-8

Relative Value Units/Medicare Edits

Non-Facility RVU	Work	PE	MP	Total
33367	11.88	3.61	2.8	18.29
33368	14.39	3.93	3.4	21.72
Facility RVU	**Work**	**PE**	**MP**	**Total**
33367	11.88	3.61	2.8	18.29
33368	14.39	3.93	3.4	21.72

	FUD	Status	MUE	Modifiers				IOM Reference
33367	N/A	A	1(2)	N/A	N/A	N/A	80*	None
33368	N/A	A	1(2)	N/A	N/A	N/A	80*	

* with documentation

33369

+ 33369 Transcatheter aortic valve replacement (TAVR/TAVI) with prosthetic valve; cardiopulmonary bypass support with central arterial and venous cannulation (eg, aorta, right atrium, pulmonary artery) (List separately in addition to code for primary procedure)

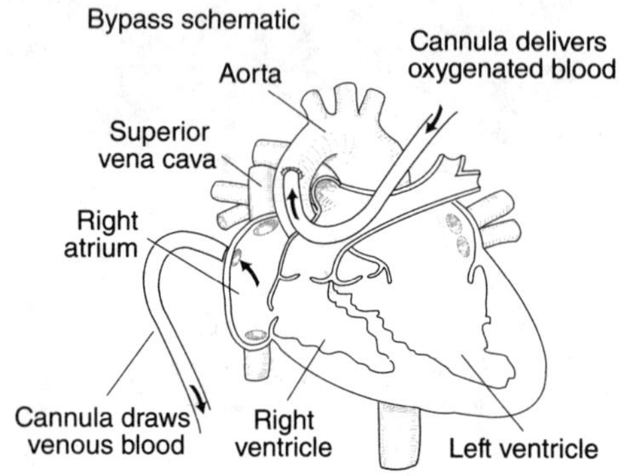

Explanation

The patient's blood is pumped to a bypass machine, oxygenated, and returned to the patient during a transcatheter aortic valve replacement or implantation (TAVR/TAVI). Its purpose is to provide mechanical support for the heart and lungs during the procedure. Access for the intake and output of the patient's blood is via cannulations of a central artery (i.e., aorta, pulmonary artery) and vein.

Coding Tips

Report 33369 in addition to 33361–33366, 33418, 33477, 0483T, 0484T, 0544T-0545T, and 0569T-0570T. Do not report 33369 with 33367–33368.

ICD-10-CM Diagnostic Codes

This/these CPT code(s) are add on code(s). See the primary procedure code that this code is performed with for your ICD-10-CM code selections. Diagnostic code(s) would be the same as the actual procedure performed.

AMA: **33369** 2018,Jan,8; 2017,Jan,8; 2016,Mar,5; 2016,Jan,13; 2015,Sep,3; 2015,Jan,16; 2013,Jan,6-8

Relative Value Units/Medicare Edits

Non-Facility RVU	Work	PE	MP	Total
33369	19.0	5.19	4.48	28.67
Facility RVU	**Work**	**PE**	**MP**	**Total**
33369	19.0	5.19	4.48	28.67

	FUD	Status	MUE	Modifiers				IOM Reference
33369	N/A	A	1(2)	N/A	N/A	N/A	80*	None

* with documentation

33390-33391

33390 Valvuloplasty, aortic valve, open, with cardiopulmonary bypass; simple (ie, valvotomy, debridement, debulking, and/or simple commissural resuspension)

33391 complex (eg, leaflet extension, leaflet resection, leaflet reconstruction, or annuloplasty)

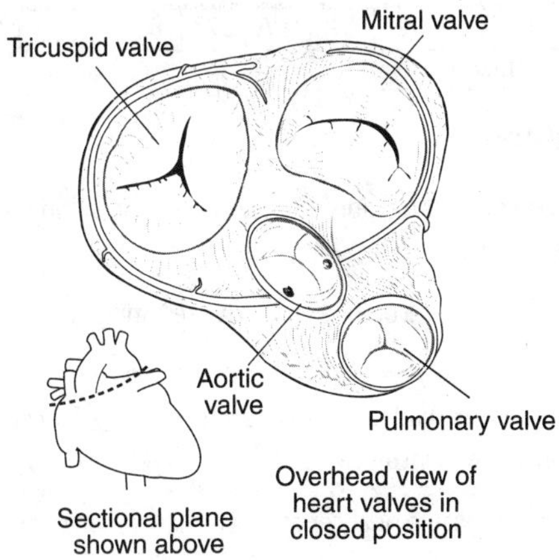

Valvuloplasty of the aortic valve is performed to restore function

Explanation

The physician initiates cardiopulmonary bypass. The aorta is clamped from above the heart and a cold preserving solution is pumped through the heart. The aorta is opened near the valve. The spaces where the heart valve leaflets meet have been fused by inflammation and scarring in diseases requiring this operation. Blunt dilators are passed through the hole and across the aortic valve. Progressively larger dilators are inserted until the valve is wide open. The dilators break the scar tissues that are cut in an open aortic valvoplasty. After the valve is fully dilated, the purse string is tied off. In the simple procedure (33390), cutting into the aortic valve leaflets, debridement utilizing scalpel blades and/or forceps to remove calcium deposits or tumors, and/or simple commissural resuspension may be performed. Commissurotomy requires the physician to stretch or cut the aortic valve due to rigid or fused leaflets. In the complex procedure (33391), extensive repairs to the leaflets may be necessary and/or annuloplasty may also be performed. Annuloplasty requires the physician to attach fibrous tissue to the base of the valve or utilize an implantable ring that prevents blood from accumulating within the left atrium, essentially resizing the valve opening. This procedure assists in maintaining the shape and flexibility of the annulus. The aorta is closed and the clamp is removed. Cardiopulmonary bypass is discontinued when heart function returns.

Coding Tips

These codes should not be reported with each other. Report 33530 in addition to the code for the primary procedure for reoperation on the aortic valve more than one month after the original procedure. For construction of an apical aortic conduit, see 33404. For replacement of an aortic valve, see 33405.

ICD-10-CM Diagnostic Codes

I06.0	Rheumatic aortic stenosis
I06.2	Rheumatic aortic stenosis with insufficiency
I08.0	Rheumatic disorders of both mitral and aortic valves
I08.8	Other rheumatic multiple valve diseases
I35.0	Nonrheumatic aortic (valve) stenosis
I35.1	Nonrheumatic aortic (valve) insufficiency
I35.2	Nonrheumatic aortic (valve) stenosis with insufficiency
I35.8	Other nonrheumatic aortic valve disorders
Q23.0	Congenital stenosis of aortic valve

AMA: 33390 2018,Jan,8; 2017,Dec,3 **33391** 2018,Jan,8; 2017,Dec,3

Relative Value Units/Medicare Edits

Non-Facility RVU	Work	PE	MP	Total
33390	35.0	13.01	7.87	55.88
33391	41.5	15.23	9.4	66.13
Facility RVU	**Work**	**PE**	**MP**	**Total**
33390	35.0	13.01	7.87	55.88
33391	41.5	15.23	9.4	66.13

	FUD	Status	MUE	Modifiers				IOM Reference
33390	90	A	1(2)	51	N/A	62*	80	None
33391	90	A	1(2)	51	N/A	62*	80	

* with documentation

Terms To Know

annuloplasty. Surgical plicaton of weakened tissue of the heart, to improve its muscular function. Annuli are thick, fibrous rings and one is found surrounding each of the cardiac chambers. The atrial and ventricular muscle fibers attach to the annuli. In annuloplasty, weakened annuli may be surgically plicated, or tucked, to improve muscular functions.

aortic stenosis. Narrowing of the aortic valve resulting in backflow of blood into the ventricle.

cardiopulmonary bypass. Venous blood is diverted to a heart-lung machine, which mechanically pumps and oxygenates the blood temporarily so the heart can be bypassed while an open procedure on the heart or coronary arteries is performed. During bypass, the lungs are deflated and immobile.

commissurotomy. Surgical division or disruption of any two parts that are joined to form a commissure in order to increase the opening. The procedure most often refers to opening the adherent leaflet bands of fibrous tissue in a stenosed mitral valve.

valvuloplasty. Surgical repair of a valve.

33404

33404 Construction of apical-aortic conduit

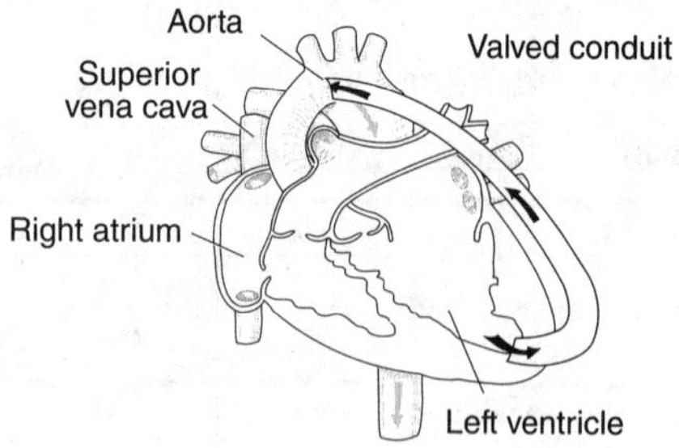

A conduit between the apical tip of the left ventricle and the aorta is established

Explanation

Cardiopulmonary bypass is required. Access to the heart may be achieved by median sternotomy or left thoracotomy. A hole is made in the tip of the left ventricle and another is made in the aorta above the coronary arteries. The conduit is oriented so that the valve in it will only let blood flow out of the heart, but not back in. One end of the conduit is sewn to the hole in the tip of the heart. The other end is sewn to the hole in the aorta. Air is removed from the heart and from the conduit. Cardiopulmonary bypass is discontinued when heart function returns.

Coding Tips

For reoperation on the aortic valve more than one month after the original procedure, report 33530 in addition to the code for the primary procedure. When more than one valve (aortic, mitral, tricuspid, pulmonary) is being repaired or replaced, report each procedure separately and append modifier 51 to the secondary valve procedures. For other valvuloplasty procedures, see 33390–33391. For aortic valve replacement, see 33405–33413. For percutaneous balloon valvuloplasty of the aortic valve, see 92986.

ICD-10-CM Diagnostic Codes

I06.0	Rheumatic aortic stenosis
I06.1	Rheumatic aortic insufficiency
I06.2	Rheumatic aortic stenosis with insufficiency
I06.8	Other rheumatic aortic valve diseases
I35.0	Nonrheumatic aortic (valve) stenosis
I35.1	Nonrheumatic aortic (valve) insufficiency
I35.2	Nonrheumatic aortic (valve) stenosis with insufficiency
I35.8	Other nonrheumatic aortic valve disorders
M31.4	Aortic arch syndrome [Takayasu]
Q23.0	Congenital stenosis of aortic valve
Q25.21	Interruption of aortic arch
Q25.29	Other atresia of aorta
Q25.3	Supravalvular aortic stenosis

AMA: 33404 2018,Jan,8; 2017,Jan,8; 2017,Dec,3; 2016,Jan,13; 2015,Jan,16; 2014,Jan,11

Relative Value Units/Medicare Edits

Non-Facility RVU	Work	PE	MP	Total
33404	31.37	12.24	7.39	51.0
Facility RVU	**Work**	**PE**	**MP**	**Total**
33404	31.37	12.24	7.39	51.0

	FUD	Status	MUE	Modifiers				IOM Reference
33404	90	A	1(2)	51	N/A	62*	80	None

* with documentation

Terms To Know

aortic insufficiency. Malfunction of the aortic valve resulting in backflow of blood into the ventricle.

aortic stenosis. Narrowing of the aortic valve resulting in backflow of blood into the ventricle.

aortic valve disorders. Various types of aortic valve dysfunction, two main types being stenosis and insufficiency.

atresia. Congenital closure or absence of a tubular organ or an opening to the body surface.

cardiopulmonary bypass. Venous blood is diverted to a heart-lung machine, which mechanically pumps and oxygenates the blood temporarily so the heart can be bypassed while an open procedure on the heart or coronary arteries is performed. During bypass, the lungs are deflated and immobile.

congenital. Present at birth, occurring through heredity or an influence during gestation up to the moment of birth.

hypothermia with cardiac bypass. Reduction of the body temperature using a bypass system to reduce the oxygen demands of tissue and to protect the myocardium during a procedure.

scar tissue. Fibrous connective tissue that forms around a wounded area or injury, composed mainly of fibroblasts or collagenous fibers.

stenosis. Narrowing or constriction of a passage.

Takayasu's disease. Rare inflammatory disease of the large arteries, especially affecting the aorta, that is usually fatal.

33405-33410

33405 Replacement, aortic valve, open, with cardiopulmonary bypass; with prosthetic valve other than homograft or stentless valve
33406 with allograft valve (freehand)
33410 with stentless tissue valve

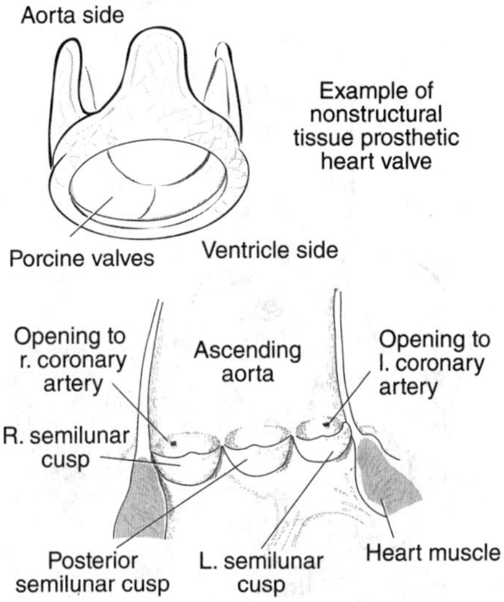

Explanation

Cardiopulmonary bypass is initiated. A clamp is placed on the aorta well above the heart. A cold preserving solution is pumped into the coronary arteries to stop the heart. In 33405, the aorta is opened just above the aortic valve. The valve leaflets are cut out and the annulus of the valve (ring of tissue where the valve leaflets normally attach to the aorta) is cleaned of calcium. The valve annulus size is measured and an appropriate artificial valve is selected. The artificial valve is sewn to the valve annulus. In 33406, an allograft is selected. The tissue valve is trimmed so that it can be sewn to the valve annulus. The aorta above the graft valve is trimmed so that the valve cusps can be suspended when the graft is in place. By doing so, the coronary arteries are not obstructed by the graft. The new valve is sewn in place. The valve annulus size is measured and an appropriate artificial valve is selected. The artificial valve is sewn to the valve annulus. In 33410, the valve annulus size is measured and an appropriate stentless tissue valve is selected, (the stentless valve is unique because unlike other valves it has no rigid external frame or sewing ring) and sutured directly into the aortic wall. The aorta is closed and the clamp is taken off. Cardiopulmonary bypass is discontinued when heart function returns. The wound is closed with layered sutures.

Coding Tips

Report 33530 in addition to the code for the primary procedure for reoperation on the aortic valve more than one month after the original procedure. When more than one valve (aortic, mitral, tricuspid, pulmonary) is being repaired or replaced, report each procedure separately and append modifier 51 to the secondary valve procedures. Do not report these codes with 33440. For valvuloplasty of the aortic valve, see 33390–33391. For construction of an apical aortic conduit, see 33404.

ICD-10-CM Diagnostic Codes

I06.0	Rheumatic aortic stenosis
I06.1	Rheumatic aortic insufficiency
I06.2	Rheumatic aortic stenosis with insufficiency
I06.8	Other rheumatic aortic valve diseases
I08.0	Rheumatic disorders of both mitral and aortic valves
I08.8	Other rheumatic multiple valve diseases
I33.0	Acute and subacute infective endocarditis
I35.0	Nonrheumatic aortic (valve) stenosis
I35.1	Nonrheumatic aortic (valve) insufficiency
I35.2	Nonrheumatic aortic (valve) stenosis with insufficiency
I35.8	Other nonrheumatic aortic valve disorders
Q23.0	Congenital stenosis of aortic valve
Q25.21	Interruption of aortic arch
Q25.29	Other atresia of aorta
Q25.3	Supravalvular aortic stenosis
T82.01XA	Breakdown (mechanical) of heart valve prosthesis, initial encounter
T82.02XA	Displacement of heart valve prosthesis, initial encounter
T82.03XA	Leakage of heart valve prosthesis, initial encounter
T82.09XA	Other mechanical complication of heart valve prosthesis, initial encounter
T82.6XXA	Infection and inflammatory reaction due to cardiac valve prosthesis, initial encounter
T82.817A	Embolism due to cardiac prosthetic devices, implants and grafts, initial encounter
T82.827A	Fibrosis due to cardiac prosthetic devices, implants and grafts, initial encounter
T82.837A	Hemorrhage due to cardiac prosthetic devices, implants and grafts, initial encounter
T82.847A	Pain due to cardiac prosthetic devices, implants and grafts, initial encounter
T82.855A	Stenosis of coronary artery stent, initial encounter
T82.857A	Stenosis of other cardiac prosthetic devices, implants and grafts, initial encounter
T82.867A	Thrombosis due to cardiac prosthetic devices, implants and grafts, initial encounter
T82.897A	Other specified complication of cardiac prosthetic devices, implants and grafts, initial encounter

AMA: 33405 2019,Apr,6; 2018,Jan,8; 2017,Jan,8; 2017,Dec,3; 2016,Jan,13; 2015,Jan,16; 2014,Jan,11; 2013,Jan,6-8 **33406** 2019,Apr,6; 2018,Jan,8; 2017,Jan,8; 2017,Dec,3; 2016,Jan,13; 2015,Jan,16; 2014,Jan,11 **33410** 2019,Apr,6; 2018,Jan,8; 2017,Jan,8; 2017,Dec,3; 2016,Jan,13; 2015,Jan,16; 2014,Jan,11

Relative Value Units/Medicare Edits

Non-Facility RVU	Work	PE	MP	Total
33405	41.32	15.01	9.36	65.69
33406	52.68	18.6	11.92	83.2
33410	46.41	16.71	10.53	73.65
Facility RVU	**Work**	**PE**	**MP**	**Total**
33405	41.32	15.01	9.36	65.69
33406	52.68	18.6	11.92	83.2
33410	46.41	16.71	10.53	73.65

	FUD	Status	MUE	Modifiers				IOM Reference
33405	90	A	1(2)	51	N/A	62*	80	None
33406	90	A	1(2)	51	N/A	62*	80	
33410	90	A	1(2)	51	N/A	62*	80	

* with documentation

Terms To Know

annulus. Ring-shaped object, structure, or region.

cardiopulmonary bypass. Venous blood is diverted to a heart-lung machine, which mechanically pumps and oxygenates the blood temporarily so the heart can be bypassed while an open procedure on the heart or coronary arteries is performed. During bypass, the lungs are deflated and immobile.

homograft. Graft from one individual to another of the same species.

[33440]

33440 Replacement, aortic valve; by translocation of autologous pulmonary valve and transventricular aortic annulus enlargement of the left ventricular outflow tract with valved conduit replacement of pulmonary valve (Ross-Konno procedure)

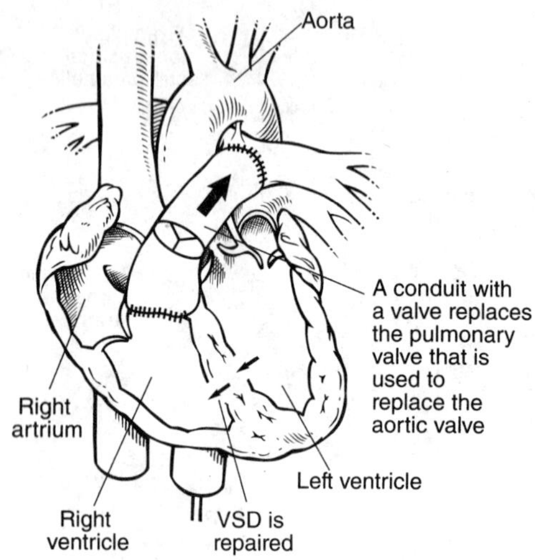

Explanation

Aortoventriculoplasty with pulmonary autograft (Ross-Konno procedure) is a treatment option geared toward younger patients diagnosed with left ventricular outflow tract obstructions who typically require aortic valve replacement reoperation. Cardiopulmonary bypass is initiated. The physician opens the patient using a median sternotomy approach and cold preserving solution is pumped into the coronary arteries to stop the heart. After aortic cross-clamping, the aorta and pulmonary artery are extensively excised and mobilized. Removal of the aortic valve and sinuses of Valsalva are performed. A pulmonary autograft is excised with a muscular tongue of the right ventricular front wall. A Konno technique incision is made in the interventricular septum beginning where the left and right coronary leaflets abut and toward the ventricular septal defect (VSD), if present, resecting the outflow septum. The incision length is based on the morphology of the obstruction and is made as far as needed in order to provide full relief of the left ventricular outflow tract obstruction (LVOTO). The pulmonary autograft is placed into aortic position using great care to precisely position the right ventricular front tongue and avoid injury to the left coronary artery, the pulmonary artery valves, and septal perforator of the left coronary artery. The right and left coronary buttons are implanted back into the autograft avoiding rotation, tension, or kinking. Anastomosis with the ascending aorta is made. Right ventricular (RV) and pulmonary artery (PA) connections are restored via the use of a homograft or bovine jugular vein conduit. Running sutures, including sutures at the base of the root and may include a thin strip of pericardium for reinforcement, are used. An echocardiogram should be performed once the patient has been weaned from bypass.

Coding Tips

For reoperation on the aortic valve more than one month after the original procedure, report 33530 in addition to the code for the primary procedure. Do not report 33440 with 33405-33414, 33416, 33417, 33475, 33608, or 33920. Cardiopulmonary bypass is included in 33440 and should not be reported separately. This code may be reported with codes for mitral valve and atrial septal defect repairs, when performed. For a Ross procedure, see 33413. For a Konno procedure, see 33412.

ICD-10-CM Diagnostic Codes

I06.0	Rheumatic aortic stenosis
I06.1	Rheumatic aortic insufficiency
I06.2	Rheumatic aortic stenosis with insufficiency
I06.8	Other rheumatic aortic valve diseases
I08.0	Rheumatic disorders of both mitral and aortic valves
I08.8	Other rheumatic multiple valve diseases
I35.0	Nonrheumatic aortic (valve) stenosis
I35.1	Nonrheumatic aortic (valve) insufficiency
I35.2	Nonrheumatic aortic (valve) stenosis with insufficiency
I35.8	Other nonrheumatic aortic valve disorders
Q23.0	Congenital stenosis of aortic valve
Q25.21	Interruption of aortic arch
Q25.29	Other atresia of aorta
Q25.3	Supravalvular aortic stenosis
T82.01XA	Breakdown (mechanical) of heart valve prosthesis, initial encounter
T82.02XA	Displacement of heart valve prosthesis, initial encounter
T82.03XA	Leakage of heart valve prosthesis, initial encounter
T82.09XA	Other mechanical complication of heart valve prosthesis, initial encounter
T82.6XXA	Infection and inflammatory reaction due to cardiac valve prosthesis, initial encounter
T82.817A	Embolism due to cardiac prosthetic devices, implants and grafts, initial encounter
T82.827A	Fibrosis due to cardiac prosthetic devices, implants and grafts, initial encounter
T82.837A	Hemorrhage due to cardiac prosthetic devices, implants and grafts, initial encounter
T82.847A	Pain due to cardiac prosthetic devices, implants and grafts, initial encounter
T82.855A	Stenosis of coronary artery stent, initial encounter
T82.857A	Stenosis of other cardiac prosthetic devices, implants and grafts, initial encounter
T82.867A	Thrombosis due to cardiac prosthetic devices, implants and grafts, initial encounter
T82.897A	Other specified complication of cardiac prosthetic devices, implants and grafts, initial encounter

AMA: **33440** 2019,Apr,6

Relative Value Units/Medicare Edits

Non-Facility RVU	Work	PE	MP	Total
33440	64.0	20.02	15.32	99.34
Facility RVU	**Work**	**PE**	**MP**	**Total**
33440	64.0	20.02	15.32	99.34

	FUD	Status	MUE	Modifiers				IOM Reference
33440	90	A	1(2)	51	N/A	62*	80	None

* with documentation

33411-33412

33411 Replacement, aortic valve; with aortic annulus enlargement, noncoronary sinus

33412 with transventricular aortic annulus enlargement (Konno procedure)

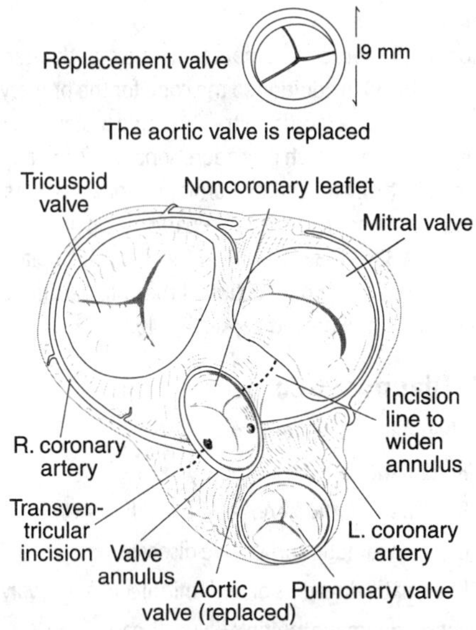

Overhead schematic of major heart valves

Explanation

Cardiopulmonary bypass is initiated. A clamp is placed on the aorta well above the heart. A cold preserving solution is pumped into the coronary arteries to stop the heart. The aorta is opened just above the aortic valve. The valve leaflets (cusps) are cut out and the annulus of the valve (ring of tissue where the valve leaflets normally attach to the aorta) is cleaned of calcium. At this point, a homograft or a xenograft is selected. The tissue valve is trimmed so that it can be sewn to the valve annulus. The aorta above the graft valve is trimmed so that the valve cusps can be suspended when the graft is in place and so the coronary arteries are not obstructed by the graft. When the valve is sized, it must be greater than or equal to 19 mm on a normal sized adult. If a smaller valve is inserted, the heart will slowly fail. Aortic annulus enlargement may be performed utilizing the noncoronary sinus, located just below the aortic valve (Nick's technique). Incision is carried downward posteriorly through the noncoronary aortic sinus across the aortic ring to the origin of the mitral valve. Dacron or other appropriate material is sutured to the fibrous origin of the mitral ring with mattress sutures, which are continued along the anterior and posterior margins of the aortic incision. The valve is sutured to the aortic ring and tied into position. Alternately, the aortic annular enlargement may be performed using the Manougian technique (through the commissure between the left coronary leaflet and the noncoronary leaflet). The aorta is cut longitudinally toward the heart and through the commissure (connecting point where two valve leaflets meet on the aortic wall) between the noncoronary leaflet (no coronary is near this leaflet) and the left coronary leaflet (leaflet near the left coronary artery) and across the valve annulus for a variable distance. The cut may need to extend onto the roof of the left atrium and onto the anterior leaflet of the mitral valve. The end of the cut is determined by the point at which the aortic root accommodates at least a 19 mm valve. The anterior mitral leaflet, left atrial roof, and the aorta are repaired with patches. The new valve is sewn in place. The aorta is closed and the clamp is taken off. Cardiopulmonary bypass is discontinued when heart function returns. In 33412, he physician replaces the aortic valve with transventricular aortic annulus enlargement, also referred to as the Konno procedure. The aorta is incised longitudinally toward a point just to the left of the right coronary artery. The cut is carried across the annulus and for a variable distance onto the right ventricular infundibulum. A triangular patch of pericardium or Dacron (e.g., a gusset) is used to close the incision in the right ventricle and aorta and to enlarge the aortic annulus. The new valve is sewn in place. The aorta is closed and the clamp is taken off. Cardiopulmonary bypass is discontinued when heart function returns.

Coding Tips

For reoperation on the aortic valve more than one month after the original procedure, report 33530 in addition to the code for the primary procedure. When more than one valve (aortic, mitral, tricuspid, pulmonary) is being repaired or replaced, report each procedure separately and append modifier 51 to the secondary valve procedures. Cardiopulmonary bypass is included in these codes and should not be reported separately. Do not report 33412 with 33413. Do not report 33411–33412 with 33440. For valvuloplasty of the aortic valve, see 33390–33391. For construction of the apical aortic conduit, see 33404. For the Ross-Konno procedure, see 33440.

ICD-10-CM Diagnostic Codes

I06.0	Rheumatic aortic stenosis
I06.1	Rheumatic aortic insufficiency
I06.2	Rheumatic aortic stenosis with insufficiency
I06.8	Other rheumatic aortic valve diseases
I08.0	Rheumatic disorders of both mitral and aortic valves
I08.8	Other rheumatic multiple valve diseases
I35.0	Nonrheumatic aortic (valve) stenosis
I35.1	Nonrheumatic aortic (valve) insufficiency
I35.2	Nonrheumatic aortic (valve) stenosis with insufficiency
I35.8	Other nonrheumatic aortic valve disorders
Q23.0	Congenital stenosis of aortic valve
Q25.21	Interruption of aortic arch
Q25.29	Other atresia of aorta
Q25.3	Supravalvular aortic stenosis
T82.01XA	Breakdown (mechanical) of heart valve prosthesis, initial encounter
T82.02XA	Displacement of heart valve prosthesis, initial encounter
T82.03XA	Leakage of heart valve prosthesis, initial encounter
T82.09XA	Other mechanical complication of heart valve prosthesis, initial encounter
T82.6XXA	Infection and inflammatory reaction due to cardiac valve prosthesis, initial encounter
T82.817A	Embolism due to cardiac prosthetic devices, implants and grafts, initial encounter
T82.827A	Fibrosis due to cardiac prosthetic devices, implants and grafts, initial encounter
T82.837A	Hemorrhage due to cardiac prosthetic devices, implants and grafts, initial encounter
T82.847A	Pain due to cardiac prosthetic devices, implants and grafts, initial encounter
T82.855A	Stenosis of coronary artery stent, initial encounter
T82.857A	Stenosis of other cardiac prosthetic devices, implants and grafts, initial encounter
T82.867A	Thrombosis due to cardiac prosthetic devices, implants and grafts, initial encounter
T82.897A	Other specified complication of cardiac prosthetic devices, implants and grafts, initial encounter

AMA: 33411 2019,Apr,6; 2018,Jan,8; 2017,Jan,8; 2017,Dec,3; 2016,Jan,13; 2015,Jan,16; 2014,Jan,11 **33412** 2019,Apr,6; 2018,Jan,8; 2017,Jan,8; 2017,Dec,3; 2016,Jan,13; 2015,Jan,16; 2014,Jan,11

Relative Value Units/Medicare Edits

Non-Facility RVU	Work	PE	MP	Total
33411	62.07	21.05	14.22	97.34
33412	59.0	19.17	14.02	92.19
Facility RVU	**Work**	**PE**	**MP**	**Total**
33411	62.07	21.05	14.22	97.34
33412	59.0	19.17	14.02	92.19

	FUD	Status	MUE	Modifiers				IOM Reference
33411	90	A	1(2)	51	N/A	N/A	80	None
33412	90	A	1(2)	51	N/A	62*	80	

* with documentation

Terms To Know

aortic insufficiency. Malfunction of the aortic valve resulting in backflow of blood into the ventricle.

aortic stenosis. Narrowing of the aortic valve resulting in backflow of blood into the ventricle.

aortic valve. Heart valve, comprising three cusps, that divides the left ventricle and the aorta.

cardiopulmonary bypass. Venous blood is diverted to a heart-lung machine, which mechanically pumps and oxygenates the blood temporarily so the heart can be bypassed while an open procedure on the heart or coronary arteries is performed. During bypass, the lungs are deflated and immobile.

commissure. Juncture where two corresponding parts come together, especially referring to the union site of adjacent heart valve cusps.

congenital. Present at birth, occurring through heredity or an influence during gestation up to the moment of birth.

33413

33413 Replacement, aortic valve; by translocation of autologous pulmonary valve with allograft replacement of pulmonary valve (Ross procedure)

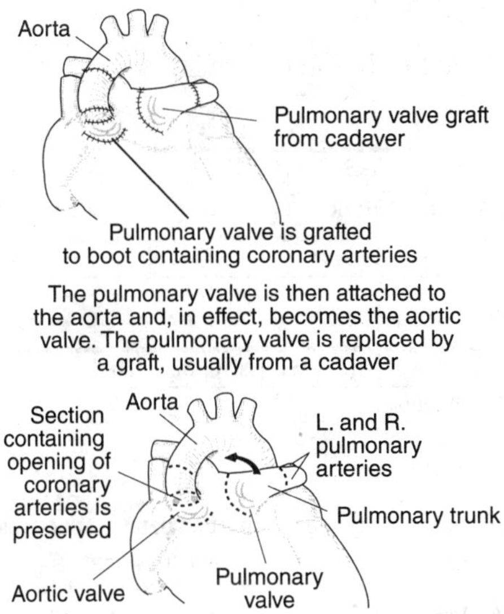

Explanation

Cardiopulmonary bypass is initiated. The aorta and pulmonary artery are separated and the main pulmonary trunk is completely cleaned off. After the heart is stopped, the pulmonary trunk is detached from the branching point of the left and right pulmonary arteries. It is taken off the heart with a small lip of heart muscle. Care is taken when the muscle of interventricular septum is cut. It is possible to damage a large branch of the left anterior descending coronary artery when this muscle is cut. The aorta is opened above the valve. The coronary arteries are detached from the aorta with a surrounding "button" of aortic wall. Next, the aortic valve and its annulus are removed from the heart. A length of the ascending aorta is also removed. The pulmonary artery is sewn to the heart in the aortic position. The commissures and cusps of the pulmonary valve are lined up to be in the same positions as their aortic counterparts were before the aortic valve was removed. The open end of the pulmonary artery is sewn to the ascending aorta. The coronary arteries are re-implanted on the pulmonary artery in positions similar to their positions on the aorta. The pulmonary valve and artery from an organ donor are sewn into the pulmonary position.

Coding Tips

For reoperation on the aortic valve more than one month after the original procedure, report 33530 in addition to the code for the primary procedure. When more than one valve (aortic, mitral, tricuspid, pulmonary) is being repaired or replaced, report each procedure separately and append modifier 51 to the secondary valve procedures. Do not report 33413 with 33412 or 33440. For valvuloplasty of the aortic valve, see 33390–33391. For construction of the apical aortic conduit, see 33404. For the Ross-Konno procedure, see 33440.

ICD-10-CM Diagnostic Codes

I06.0	Rheumatic aortic stenosis
I06.1	Rheumatic aortic insufficiency
I06.2	Rheumatic aortic stenosis with insufficiency
I06.8	Other rheumatic aortic valve diseases
I08.0	Rheumatic disorders of both mitral and aortic valves
I08.8	Other rheumatic multiple valve diseases
I35.0	Nonrheumatic aortic (valve) stenosis
I35.1	Nonrheumatic aortic (valve) insufficiency
I35.2	Nonrheumatic aortic (valve) stenosis with insufficiency
I35.8	Other nonrheumatic aortic valve disorders
Q23.0	Congenital stenosis of aortic valve
Q25.21	Interruption of aortic arch
Q25.29	Other atresia of aorta
Q25.3	Supravalvular aortic stenosis
T82.01XA	Breakdown (mechanical) of heart valve prosthesis, initial encounter
T82.02XA	Displacement of heart valve prosthesis, initial encounter
T82.03XA	Leakage of heart valve prosthesis, initial encounter
T82.09XA	Other mechanical complication of heart valve prosthesis, initial encounter
T82.6XXA	Infection and inflammatory reaction due to cardiac valve prosthesis, initial encounter
T82.817A	Embolism due to cardiac prosthetic devices, implants and grafts, initial encounter
T82.827A	Fibrosis due to cardiac prosthetic devices, implants and grafts, initial encounter
T82.837A	Hemorrhage due to cardiac prosthetic devices, implants and grafts, initial encounter
T82.847A	Pain due to cardiac prosthetic devices, implants and grafts, initial encounter
T82.855A	Stenosis of coronary artery stent, initial encounter
T82.857A	Stenosis of other cardiac prosthetic devices, implants and grafts, initial encounter
T82.867A	Thrombosis due to cardiac prosthetic devices, implants and grafts, initial encounter
T82.897A	Other specified complication of cardiac prosthetic devices, implants and grafts, initial encounter

AMA: **33413** 2019,Apr,6; 2018,Jan,8; 2017,Jan,8; 2017,Dec,3; 2016,Jan,13; 2015,Jan,16; 2014,Jan,11

Relative Value Units/Medicare Edits

Non-Facility RVU	Work	PE	MP	Total
33413	59.87	20.21	14.25	94.33
Facility RVU	**Work**	**PE**	**MP**	**Total**
33413	59.87	20.21	14.25	94.33

	FUD	Status	MUE	Modifiers				IOM Reference
33413	90	A	1(2)	51	N/A	62*	80	None

* with documentation

Heart and Pericardium

33414

33414 Repair of left ventricular outflow tract obstruction by patch enlargement of the outflow tract

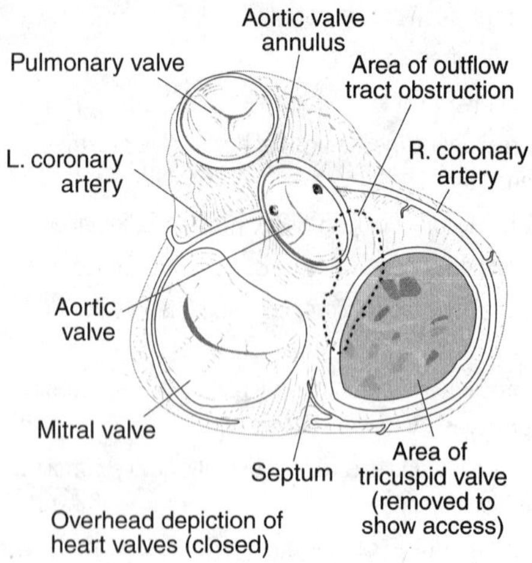

An outflow tract obstruction of the left ventricle is surgically approached

Explanation

The physician enlarges the left ventricular outflow track by patch due to obstruction. The physician performs a midline sternotomy, incising the skin, fascia, muscles, and sternum. The pericardium is incised and lines are placed for cardiopulmonary bypass. Dissection of the aorta is performed within the aorta, right ventricle, and pulmonary artery reaching the aortic annulus. An incision is made in the aorta and the right ventricular outflow tract is opened through the septum. The cusps of the aortic valve are removed. Reconstruction of the left ventricular outflow tract is achieved using a patch of Dacron cut into a diamond shape and the septum is closed to the area of patch placement. The aortic annulus is measured with replacement of aortic valve. An additional patch is attached to broaden the right ventricular outflow tract connecting it to the left ventricular outflow tract patch. The aortic valve prosthesis is connected to the outflow tract patches. The right ventricular outflow tract patch is attached to the right ventriculotomy. The pericardium is repaired loosely, leaving gaps for blood and fluid to drain into the pleural space. The sternum is reanastomosed with sternal wires and the skin is sutured in layers.

Coding Tips

For reoperation on the aortic valve more than one month after the original procedure, report 33530 in addition to the code for the primary procedure. When more than one valve (aortic, mitral, tricuspid, pulmonary) is being repaired or replaced, report each procedure separately and append modifier 51 to the secondary valve procedures. Do not report 33414 with 33440.

ICD-10-CM Diagnostic Codes

I06.0	Rheumatic aortic stenosis
I06.1	Rheumatic aortic insufficiency
I06.2	Rheumatic aortic stenosis with insufficiency
I06.8	Other rheumatic aortic valve diseases
I35.0	Nonrheumatic aortic (valve) stenosis
I35.1	Nonrheumatic aortic (valve) insufficiency
I35.2	Nonrheumatic aortic (valve) stenosis with insufficiency
I35.8	Other nonrheumatic aortic valve disorders
Q23.0	Congenital stenosis of aortic valve
Q25.21	Interruption of aortic arch
Q25.29	Other atresia of aorta
Q25.3	Supravalvular aortic stenosis

AMA: 33414 2019,Apr,6; 2018,Jan,8; 2017,Jan,8; 2017,Dec,3; 2016,Jan,13; 2015,Jan,16; 2014,Jan,11

Relative Value Units/Medicare Edits

Non-Facility RVU	Work	PE	MP	Total
33414	39.37	13.74	8.91	62.02
Facility RVU	**Work**	**PE**	**MP**	**Total**
33414	39.37	13.74	8.91	62.02

	FUD	Status	MUE	Modifiers				IOM Reference
33414	90	A	1(2)	51	N/A	62*	80	None

* with documentation

Terms To Know

anastomosis. Surgically created connection between ducts, blood vessels, or bowel segments to allow flow from one to the other.

aortic insufficiency. Malfunction of the aortic valve resulting in backflow of blood into the ventricle.

aortic stenosis. Narrowing of the aortic valve resulting in backflow of blood into the ventricle.

aortic valve disorders. Various types of aortic valve dysfunction, two main types being stenosis and insufficiency.

atresia. Congenital closure or absence of a tubular organ or an opening to the body surface.

cardiopulmonary bypass. Venous blood is diverted to a heart-lung machine, which mechanically pumps and oxygenates the blood temporarily so the heart can be bypassed while an open procedure on the heart or coronary arteries is performed. During bypass, the lungs are deflated and immobile.

congenital. Present at birth, occurring through heredity or an influence during gestation up to the moment of birth.

pericardium. Thin and slippery case in which the heart lies that is lined with fluid so that the heart is free to pulse and move as it beats.

stenosis. Narrowing or constriction of a passage.

sternotomy. Incision into the sternum, the bone that forms the front of the chest cavity and connects with the ribs.

33415-33416

33415 Resection or incision of subvalvular tissue for discrete subvalvular aortic stenosis

33416 Ventriculomyotomy (-myectomy) for idiopathic hypertrophic subaortic stenosis (eg, asymmetric septal hypertrophy)

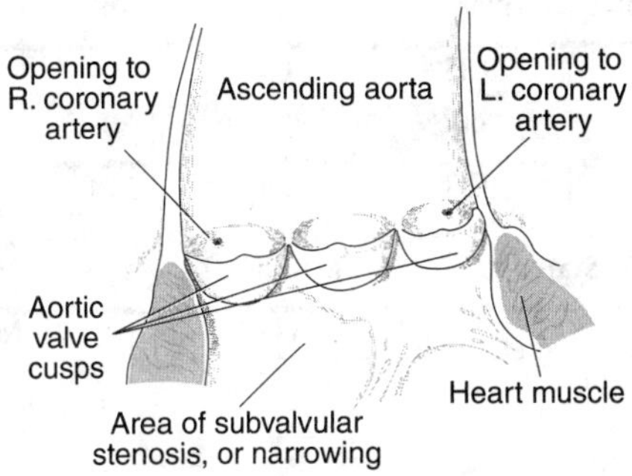

Cutaway schematic of the aortic valve and subvalvular tissues of the septum

Explanation

Cardiopulmonary bypass is initiated. The aorta is opened and the left ventricular outflow tract is assessed below the valve. There is usually a clearly definable ring or shelf below the valve. This is taken off with a tool designed for the purpose. Usually, the left ventricular septal muscle is thickened. A trough of muscle tissue is cut out of the left ventricular septal muscle. The aorta is closed. Cardiopulmonary bypass is discontinued when heart function returns. Report 33416 if there is no ring of subvalvular tissue to remove.

Coding Tips

Note the stenosis site when selecting the code. Subvalvular stenosis, also referred to as subaortic stenosis, is caused by an obstructive lesion in the left ventricle below the aortic valve. Report 33530 in addition to the code for the primary procedure for reoperation on the aortic valve more than one month after the original procedure. For percutaneous transcatheter septal reduction therapy, see 93583. When more than one valve (aortic, mitral, tricuspid, pulmonary) is being repaired or replaced, report each procedure separately and append modifier 51 to the secondary valve procedures. Do not report 33416 with 33440.

ICD-10-CM Diagnostic Codes

I06.0	Rheumatic aortic stenosis
I06.1	Rheumatic aortic insufficiency
I06.2	Rheumatic aortic stenosis with insufficiency
I08.0	Rheumatic disorders of both mitral and aortic valves
I08.2	Rheumatic disorders of both aortic and tricuspid valves
I35.0	Nonrheumatic aortic (valve) stenosis
I35.1	Nonrheumatic aortic (valve) insufficiency
I35.2	Nonrheumatic aortic (valve) stenosis with insufficiency
I35.8	Other nonrheumatic aortic valve disorders
I42.1	Obstructive hypertrophic cardiomyopathy
Q23.0	Congenital stenosis of aortic valve
Q23.1	Congenital insufficiency of aortic valve
Q24.4	Congenital subaortic stenosis
Q25.3	Supravalvular aortic stenosis

AMA: 33415 2018,Jan,8; 2017,Jan,8; 2017,Dec,3; 2016,Jan,13; 2015,Jan,16; 2014,Jan,11 **33416** 2019,Apr,6; 2018,Jan,8; 2017,Jan,8; 2017,Dec,3; 2016,Jan,13; 2015,Jan,16; 2014,Jan,11

Relative Value Units/Medicare Edits

Non-Facility RVU	Work	PE	MP	Total
33415	37.27	13.43	8.08	58.78
33416	36.56	13.7	8.34	58.6
Facility RVU	**Work**	**PE**	**MP**	**Total**
33415	37.27	13.43	8.08	58.78
33416	36.56	13.7	8.34	58.6

	FUD	Status	MUE	Modifiers				IOM Reference
33415	90	A	1(2)	51	N/A	62*	80	None
33416	90	A	1(2)	51	N/A	62*	80	

* with documentation

Terms To Know

aortic insufficiency. Malfunction of the aortic valve resulting in backflow of blood into the ventricle.

aortic stenosis. Narrowing of the aortic valve resulting in backflow of blood into the ventricle.

aortic valve disorders. Various types of aortic valve dysfunction, two main types being stenosis and insufficiency.

atresia. Congenital closure or absence of a tubular organ or an opening to the body surface.

cardiopulmonary bypass. Venous blood is diverted to a heart-lung machine, which mechanically pumps and oxygenates the blood temporarily so the heart can be bypassed while an open procedure on the heart or coronary arteries is performed. During bypass, the lungs are deflated and immobile.

cardiotomy. Incision of the heart, the cardiac orifice, or the cardiac end of the stomach.

congenital. Present at birth, occurring through heredity or an influence during gestation up to the moment of birth.

hypertrophic. Enlarged or overgrown from an increase in cell size of the affected tissue.

incision. Act of cutting into tissue or an organ.

resection. Surgical removal of a part or all of an organ or body part.

stenosis. Narrowing or constriction of a passage.

trabeculae carneae cordis. Bands of muscular tissue that line the walls of the ventricles in the heart.

33417

33417 Aortoplasty (gusset) for supravalvular stenosis

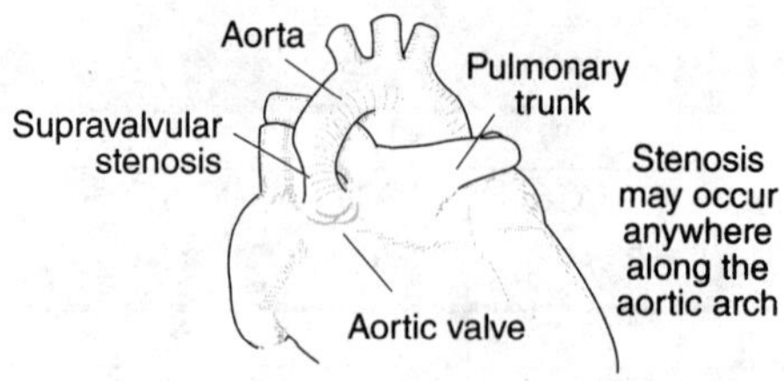

Stenosis, or narrowing, occurs above the aortic valve. Patch graft shown

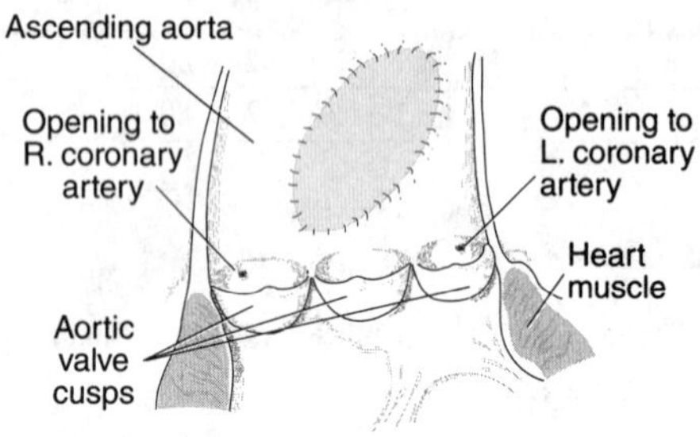

Cutaway schematic of the aortic valve and supravalvular tissues

Explanation

Aortoplasty for supravalvular stenosis is performed with a median sternotomy to gain access. Cardiopulmonary bypass is required. A piece of pericardium or Dacron is prepared. The aorta is clamped beyond the area of narrowing. The heart is stopped with a cold preserving solution. An incision is made into the narrowest point of the ascending aorta and three additional incisions are made that extend into the sinuses of Valsalva. Using patches of pericardium, the sinuses are enlarged. A patch from the noncoronary sinus is extended into the ascending aorta in order to assure symmetrical enlargement. The clamp is released. Cardiopulmonary bypass is discontinued when heart function returns.

Coding Tips

Note the stenosis site when selecting the code. Supravalvular aortic stenosis is a rare condition, occurring above the aortic valve usually caused by a constricting ring of the fibrous tissue at the level of the sinus of Valsalva. Report 33530 in addition to the code for the primary procedure for reoperation on the aortic valve more than one month after the original procedure. When more than one valve (aortic, mitral, tricuspid, pulmonary) is being repaired or replaced, report each procedure separately and append modifier 51 to the secondary valve procedures. Do not report 33417 with 33440.

ICD-10-CM Diagnostic Codes

I06.0	Rheumatic aortic stenosis
I06.1	Rheumatic aortic insufficiency
I06.2	Rheumatic aortic stenosis with insufficiency
I06.8	Other rheumatic aortic valve diseases
I35.0	Nonrheumatic aortic (valve) stenosis
I35.1	Nonrheumatic aortic (valve) insufficiency
I35.2	Nonrheumatic aortic (valve) stenosis with insufficiency
I35.8	Other nonrheumatic aortic valve disorders
Q23.0	Congenital stenosis of aortic valve
Q25.21	Interruption of aortic arch
Q25.29	Other atresia of aorta
Q25.3	Supravalvular aortic stenosis

AMA: 33417 2019,Apr,6; 2018,Jan,8; 2017,Jan,8; 2017,Dec,3; 2016,Jan,13; 2015,Jan,16; 2014,Jan,11

Relative Value Units/Medicare Edits

Non-Facility RVU	Work	PE	MP	Total
33417	29.33	12.09	6.74	48.16
Facility RVU	**Work**	**PE**	**MP**	**Total**
33417	29.33	12.09	6.74	48.16

	FUD	Status	MUE	Modifiers				IOM Reference
33417	90	A	1(2)	51	N/A	62*	80	None

* with documentation

Terms To Know

aortic insufficiency. Malfunction of the aortic valve resulting in backflow of blood into the ventricle.

aortic stenosis. Narrowing of the aortic valve resulting in backflow of blood into the ventricle.

aortic valve disorders. Various types of aortic valve dysfunction, two main types being stenosis and insufficiency.

atresia. Congenital closure or absence of a tubular organ or an opening to the body surface.

cardiopulmonary bypass. Venous blood is diverted to a heart-lung machine, which mechanically pumps and oxygenates the blood temporarily so the heart can be bypassed while an open procedure on the heart or coronary arteries is performed. During bypass, the lungs are deflated and immobile.

gusset. Triangular or diamond shaped patch that is placed for reinforcement or expansion.

incision. Act of cutting into tissue or an organ.

pericardium. Thin and slippery case in which the heart lies that is lined with fluid so that the heart is free to pulse and move as it beats.

stenosis. Narrowing or constriction of a passage.

valvuloplasty. Surgical repair of a valve.

33418-33419

33418 Transcatheter mitral valve repair, percutaneous approach, including transseptal puncture when performed; initial prosthesis

\+ **33419** additional prosthesis(es) during same session (List separately in addition to code for primary procedure)

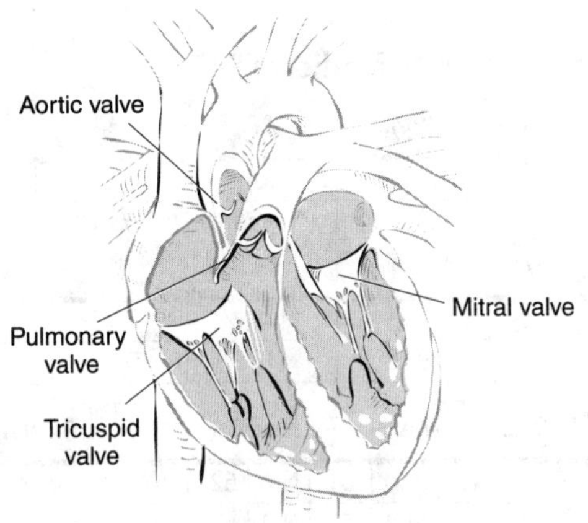

The mitral valve is repaired percutaneously

Explanation

A mitral valve is repaired percutaneously. The procedure is performed under general anesthesia. The physician makes an incision over a lower extremity vessel, usually the femoral vein. A catheter with a specially designed prosthesis or stent is maneuvered through the vessels to the heart under fluoroscopic imaging guidance. Depending on the approach and the device being used, the catheter may be threaded through the inferior vena cava to the right atrium where a septal puncture to access the left atrium and mitral valve is created. Once the device is positioned above the diseased valve, it is secured into place with precautions taken to ensure proper positioning and anchoring. The physician removes the catheter and the surgical wound is closed. Report 33418 for insertion of the initial device and 33419 for any additional devices used during the same operative session.

Coding Tips

Codes 33367 percutaneous bypass, 33368 open peripheral bypass, and 33369 central bypass may be reported in addition to 33418 and 33419 when cardiopulmonary bypass is performed. These codes include percutaneous access, placing sheath, transseptal puncture, advancement of repair device delivery system, repositioning, and deployment of the device, when performed. Report 33419 in addition to 33418 and report only once per encounter. Do not report 33418 with 93462 unless transapical puncture is performed. For transcatheter mitral valve percutaneous approach via coronary sinus, see 0345T. Radiological supervision and interpretation for guidance, including documentation of completion, is included and is not reported separately. Do not report diagnostic heart catheterization with 33418 or 33419 for contrast administration, angiography, road mapping or guidance, to assess regurgitation for guidance, or for hemodynamic measurements occurring before, during, and after the procedure. Other diagnostic cardiac catheterizations may be reported separately when performed for purposes unrelated to TMVR procedures. Percutaneous coronary procedures may be reported separately, when performed. Codes 33990–33993 for ventricular assist devices and 33967, 33970, and 33973 for balloon pump insertion may be reported separately, when performed.

ICD-10-CM Diagnostic Codes

I05.0	Rheumatic mitral stenosis
I05.1	Rheumatic mitral insufficiency
I05.2	Rheumatic mitral stenosis with insufficiency
I05.8	Other rheumatic mitral valve diseases
I08.0	Rheumatic disorders of both mitral and aortic valves
I08.1	Rheumatic disorders of both mitral and tricuspid valves
I08.3	Combined rheumatic disorders of mitral, aortic and tricuspid valves
I08.8	Other rheumatic multiple valve diseases
I34.0	Nonrheumatic mitral (valve) insufficiency
I34.1	Nonrheumatic mitral (valve) prolapse
I34.2	Nonrheumatic mitral (valve) stenosis
I34.8	Other nonrheumatic mitral valve disorders
Q23.2	Congenital mitral stenosis
Q23.3	Congenital mitral insufficiency
Q23.8	Other congenital malformations of aortic and mitral valves

AMA: **33418** 2018,Jan,8; 2017,Jan,8; 2016,Jan,13; 2015,Sep,3 **33419** 2018,Jan,8; 2017,Jan,8; 2016,Jan,13; 2015,Sep,3

Relative Value Units/Medicare Edits

Non-Facility RVU	Work	PE	MP	Total
33418	32.25	12.86	7.28	52.39
33419	7.93	2.68	1.76	12.37
Facility RVU	**Work**	**PE**	**MP**	**Total**
33418	32.25	12.86	7.28	52.39
33419	7.93	2.68	1.76	12.37

	FUD	Status	MUE	Modifiers				IOM Reference
33418	90	A	1(3)	51	N/A	62*	80	None
33419	N/A	A	1(2)	N/A	N/A	62*	80	

* with documentation

Terms To Know

angiography. Radiographic imaging of the arteries.

cardiopulmonary bypass. Venous blood is diverted to a heart-lung machine, which mechanically pumps and oxygenates the blood temporarily so the heart can be bypassed while an open procedure on the heart or coronary arteries is performed. During bypass, the lungs are deflated and immobile.

congenital. Present at birth, occurring through heredity or an influence during gestation up to the moment of birth.

insufficiency. Inadequate closure of the valve that allows abnormal backward blood flow.

mitral valve. Valve with two cusps that is between the left atrium and left ventricle of the heart.

percutaneous. Through the skin.

stenosis. Narrowing or constriction of a passage.

transcatheter. Procedure or treatment performed via a catheter.

33420-33422

33420 Valvotomy, mitral valve; closed heart
33422 open heart, with cardiopulmonary bypass

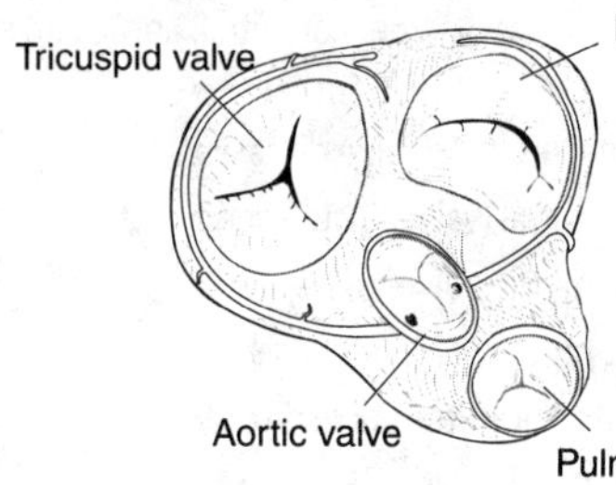

Cutaway view of heart showing left-side valves

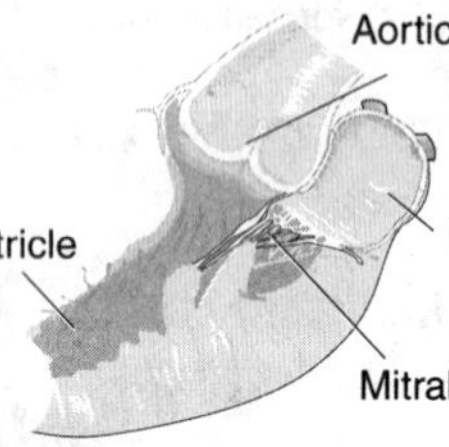

Explanation

In 33420, the chest is opened by median sternotomy or left thoracotomy. The pericardium is opened. An incision is performed within the left atrial appendage where a Tubbs dilator (or gloved physician's finger) is introduced into the left ventricle by way of the apex and opened in the valve. Calcium deposits may be removed from the annulus and leaflets with a bone nibbler. Upon completion of valvotomy, the dilator (or finger) is removed and the incisions are sutured closed. In 33422, the skin and muscle are incised from the sternum to the xiphoid process. The sternum is split and a retractor is utilized to open the chest. An incision is made in the pericardium and cardiopulmonary bypass is initiated. The left atrium is opened from the right side. The mitral valve is exposed. The scar tissue between the lateral ends of the valve leaflets is divided sharply. Cardiopulmonary bypass is discontinued when heart function returns. The pericardium and left atrium are closed. Chest tubes may be inserted to allow drainage.

Coding Tips

For reoperation on the aortic valve more than one month after the original procedure, report 33530 in addition to the code for the primary procedure. When more than one valve (aortic, mitral, tricuspid, pulmonary) is being repaired or replaced, report each procedure separately and append modifier 51 to the secondary valve procedures. For valvuloplasty of the mitral valve with cardiopulmonary bypass, see 33425; with prosthetic ring, see 33426; with radical reconstruction, see 33427. For replacement of the mitral valve with cardiopulmonary bypass, see 33430.

ICD-10-CM Diagnostic Codes

I05.0	Rheumatic mitral stenosis
I05.1	Rheumatic mitral insufficiency
I05.2	Rheumatic mitral stenosis with insufficiency
I05.8	Other rheumatic mitral valve diseases
I08.0	Rheumatic disorders of both mitral and aortic valves
I08.8	Other rheumatic multiple valve diseases
I34.0	Nonrheumatic mitral (valve) insufficiency
I34.1	Nonrheumatic mitral (valve) prolapse
I34.2	Nonrheumatic mitral (valve) stenosis
I34.8	Other nonrheumatic mitral valve disorders
Q23.2	Congenital mitral stenosis
Q23.3	Congenital mitral insufficiency

AMA: **33420** 2018,Jan,8; 2017,Jan,8; 2016,Jan,13; 2015,Sep,3; 2015,Jan,16; 2014,Jan,11 **33422** 2018,Jan,8; 2017,Jan,8; 2017,Dec,3; 2016,Jan,13; 2015,Sep,3; 2015,Jan,16; 2014,Jan,11

Relative Value Units/Medicare Edits

Non-Facility RVU	Work	PE	MP	Total
33420	25.79	10.42	6.09	42.3
33422	29.73	11.79	7.01	48.53
Facility RVU	**Work**	**PE**	**MP**	**Total**
33420	25.79	10.42	6.09	42.3
33422	29.73	11.79	7.01	48.53

	FUD	Status	MUE	Modifiers				IOM Reference
33420	90	A	1(2)	51	N/A	62*	N/A	None
33422	90	A	1(2)	51	N/A	62*	80	

* with documentation

Terms To Know

cardiopulmonary bypass. Venous blood is diverted to a heart-lung machine, which mechanically pumps and oxygenates the blood temporarily so the heart can be bypassed while an open procedure on the heart or coronary arteries is performed. During bypass, the lungs are deflated and immobile.

congenital. Present at birth, occurring through heredity or an influence during gestation up to the moment of birth.

mitral valve. Valve with two cusps that is between the left atrium and left ventricle of the heart.

pericardium. Thin and slippery case in which the heart lies that is lined with fluid so that the heart is free to pulse and move as it beats.

prosthesis. Man-made substitute for a missing body part.

scar tissue. Fibrous connective tissue that forms around a wounded area or injury, composed mainly of fibroblasts or collagenous fibers.

stenosis. Narrowing or constriction of a passage.

valvotomy. Cutting through stenosed cardiac valve leaflets or cusp to relieve or repair the obstruction caused by scar tissue and inflammation.

valvuloplasty. Surgical repair of a valve.

33425-33427

33425 Valvuloplasty, mitral valve, with cardiopulmonary bypass;
33426 with prosthetic ring
33427 radical reconstruction, with or without ring

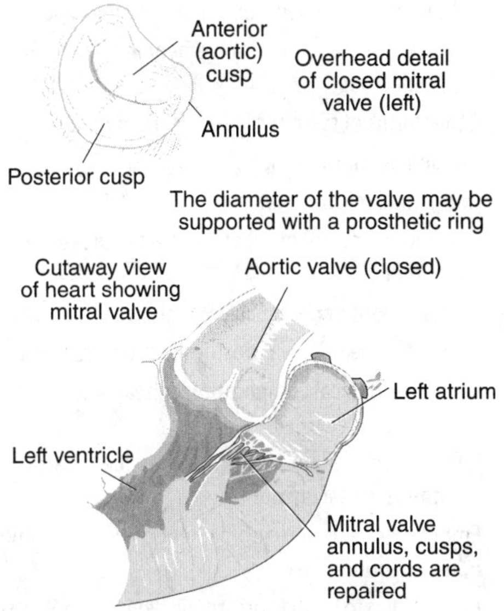

The mitral valve is accessed and surgically repaired

Explanation

This operation is done to improve the ability of the mitral valve to close completely when the ventricle contracts. It is done in patients whose mitral valve has lost the ability to close normally. In almost all cases, this is the result of a mitral valve prolapse in which the mitral leaflets and the cords that tether them on the ventricle have become elongated. Cardiopulmonary bypass is initiated. The left atrium is opened and the mitral valve is exposed. Redundant leaflet tissue is excised and defects in the valve leaflets are closed with sutures. The cords are also shortened with sutures. Valve closure is assessed after the repair. The left atrium is closed and cardiopulmonary bypass is discontinued when heart function returns. Report 33426 if the mitral valve diameter is enlarged requiring placement of a prosthetic ring. Report 33427 if a more extensive repair, including transfer of cords from the posterior leaflet to the anterior leaflet, is performed. A prosthetic ring may be required with extensive reconstruction.

Coding Tips

For reoperation on the mitral valve more than one month after the original procedure, report 33530 in addition to the code for the primary procedure. When more than one valve (aortic, mitral, tricuspid, pulmonary) is being repaired or replaced, report each procedure separately and append modifier 51 to the secondary valve procedures. For valvotomy of the mitral valve, see 33420–33422. For replacement of the mitral valve, see 33430. For percutaneous balloon valvuloplasty of the mitral valve, see 92987.

ICD-10-CM Diagnostic Codes

I05.0	Rheumatic mitral stenosis
I05.1	Rheumatic mitral insufficiency
I05.2	Rheumatic mitral stenosis with insufficiency
I05.8	Other rheumatic mitral valve diseases
I08.0	Rheumatic disorders of both mitral and aortic valves
I08.8	Other rheumatic multiple valve diseases
I34.0	Nonrheumatic mitral (valve) insufficiency
I34.1	Nonrheumatic mitral (valve) prolapse
I34.2	Nonrheumatic mitral (valve) stenosis
I34.8	Other nonrheumatic mitral valve disorders
Q23.2	Congenital mitral stenosis
Q23.3	Congenital mitral insufficiency

AMA: **33425** 2018,Jan,8; 2017,Jan,8; 2017,Dec,3; 2016,Jan,13; 2015,Sep,3; 2015,Jan,16; 2014,Jan,11 **33426** 2018,Jan,8; 2017,Jan,8; 2017,Dec,3; 2016,Jan,13; 2015,Sep,3; 2015,Jan,16; 2014,Jan,11 **33427** 2018,Jan,8; 2017,Jan,8; 2017,Dec,3; 2016,Jan,13; 2015,Sep,3; 2015,Jan,16; 2014,Jan,11

Relative Value Units/Medicare Edits

Non-Facility RVU	Work	PE	MP	Total
33425	49.96	17.75	11.33	79.04
33426	43.28	15.91	9.78	68.97
33427	44.83	15.84	10.13	70.8
Facility RVU	**Work**	**PE**	**MP**	**Total**
33425	49.96	17.75	11.33	79.04
33426	43.28	15.91	9.78	68.97
33427	44.83	15.84	10.13	70.8

	FUD	Status	MUE	Modifiers				IOM Reference
33425	90	A	1(2)	51	N/A	62*	80	None
33426	90	A	1(2)	51	N/A	62*	80	
33427	90	A	1(2)	51	N/A	62*	80	

* with documentation

Terms To Know

cardiopulmonary bypass. Venous blood is diverted to a heart-lung machine, which mechanically pumps and oxygenates the blood temporarily so the heart can be bypassed while an open procedure on the heart or coronary arteries is performed. During bypass, the lungs are deflated and immobile.

congenital. Present at birth, occurring through heredity or an influence during gestation up to the moment of birth.

hypothermia with cardiac bypass. Reduction of the body temperature using a bypass system to reduce the oxygen demands of tissue and to protect the myocardium during a procedure.

mitral valve. Valve with two cusps that is between the left atrium and left ventricle of the heart.

prolapse. Falling, sliding, or sinking of an organ from its normal location in the body.

reconstruction. Recreating, restoring, or rebuilding a body part or organ.

stenosis. Narrowing or constriction of a passage.

33430

33430 Replacement, mitral valve, with cardiopulmonary bypass

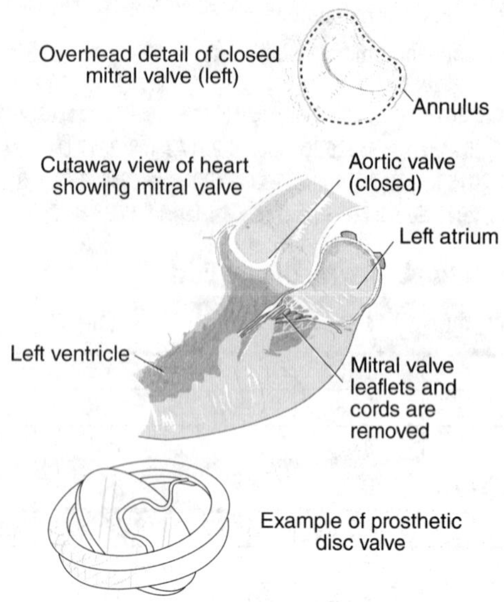

The mitral valve is accessed and surgically removed along with attachment cords. Any of a variety of replacement valves is selected and sutured to the annulus of the former valve

Explanation

The physician performs a sternotomy to gain access to the heart. Cardiopulmonary bypass is initiated. The mitral valve may be accessed by opening the right atrium followed by opening the atrial septum or the left atrium directly, exposing the mitral valve. All leaflet tissue and its attached cords are cut out. Sutures are placed in the mitral annulus. The annulus is sized and an appropriate artificial valve is selected (a totally mechanical valve or a valve with plastic supports and tissue leaflets). The sutures are passed through the sewing ring of the annulus and the sutures are tied down so the sewing ring is adherent to the annulus. The atrial septum (or left atrium) may be sutured closed or left to heal on its own. Cardiopulmonary bypass is discontinued when heart function returns. The sternotomy is closed with wires and the skin is sutured closed.

Coding Tips

For reoperation on the aortic valve more than one month after the original procedure, report 33530 in addition to the code for the primary procedure. When more than one valve (aortic, mitral, tricuspid, pulmonary) is being repaired or replaced, report each procedure separately and append modifier 51 to the secondary valve procedures. For valvuloplasty of the mitral valve, see 33425–33427.

ICD-10-CM Diagnostic Codes

I05.0 Rheumatic mitral stenosis
I05.1 Rheumatic mitral insufficiency
I05.2 Rheumatic mitral stenosis with insufficiency
I05.8 Other rheumatic mitral valve diseases
I08.0 Rheumatic disorders of both mitral and aortic valves
I08.8 Other rheumatic multiple valve diseases
I34.0 Nonrheumatic mitral (valve) insufficiency
I34.1 Nonrheumatic mitral (valve) prolapse
I34.2 Nonrheumatic mitral (valve) stenosis
I34.8 Other nonrheumatic mitral valve disorders
M32.0 Drug-induced systemic lupus erythematosus
M32.11 Endocarditis in systemic lupus erythematosus
M32.12 Pericarditis in systemic lupus erythematosus
M32.13 Lung involvement in systemic lupus erythematosus
M32.14 Glomerular disease in systemic lupus erythematosus
M32.15 Tubulo-interstitial nephropathy in systemic lupus erythematosus
M32.19 Other organ or system involvement in systemic lupus erythematosus
M32.8 Other forms of systemic lupus erythematosus
Q23.2 Congenital mitral stenosis
Q23.3 Congenital mitral insufficiency
T82.01XA Breakdown (mechanical) of heart valve prosthesis, initial encounter
T82.02XA Displacement of heart valve prosthesis, initial encounter
T82.03XA Leakage of heart valve prosthesis, initial encounter
T82.09XA Other mechanical complication of heart valve prosthesis, initial encounter
T82.6XXA Infection and inflammatory reaction due to cardiac valve prosthesis, initial encounter
T82.817A Embolism due to cardiac prosthetic devices, implants and grafts, initial encounter
T82.827A Fibrosis due to cardiac prosthetic devices, implants and grafts, initial encounter
T82.837A Hemorrhage due to cardiac prosthetic devices, implants and grafts, initial encounter
T82.847A Pain due to cardiac prosthetic devices, implants and grafts, initial encounter
T82.855A Stenosis of coronary artery stent, initial encounter
T82.857A Stenosis of other cardiac prosthetic devices, implants and grafts, initial encounter
T82.867A Thrombosis due to cardiac prosthetic devices, implants and grafts, initial encounter
T82.897A Other specified complication of cardiac prosthetic devices, implants and grafts, initial encounter

AMA: 33430 2018,Jan,8; 2017,Jan,8; 2017,Dec,3; 2016,Jan,13; 2015,Sep,3; 2015,Jan,16; 2014,Jan,11

Relative Value Units/Medicare Edits

Non-Facility RVU	Work	PE	MP	Total
33430	50.93	18.56	11.57	81.06
Facility RVU	**Work**	**PE**	**MP**	**Total**
33430	50.93	18.56	11.57	81.06

	FUD	Status	MUE	Modifiers				IOM Reference
33430	90	A	1(2)	51	N/A	62*	80	None

* with documentation

33460-33464

33460 Valvectomy, tricuspid valve, with cardiopulmonary bypass
33463 Valvuloplasty, tricuspid valve; without ring insertion
33464 with ring insertion

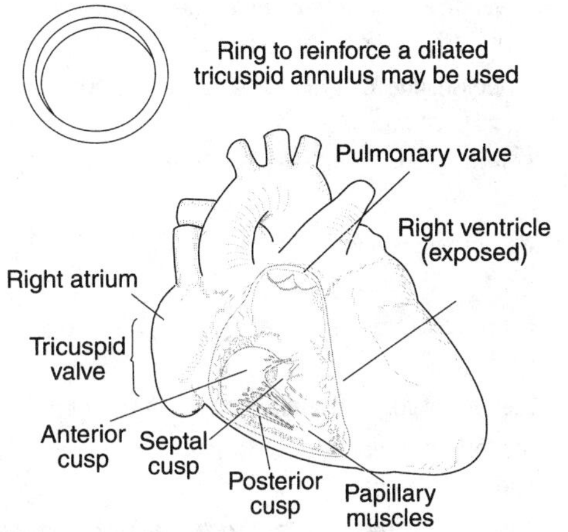

Cutaway view of the heart showing right side valves

Explanation

In 33460, cardiopulmonary bypass is initiated. The right atrium is opened and the tricuspid valve is exposed. The valve tissue and its cords are completely excised. The right atrium is closed. Cardiopulmonary bypass is discontinued when heart function returns. In 33463, cardiopulmonary bypass is initiated with venous uptake tubes in both of the caval veins. The right atrium is opened. Valvuloplasty of the tricuspid valve almost always requires nothing more than reducing the diameter of the tricuspid valve. To accomplish this, a double purse string of sutures is placed around the circumference of the valve and tightened to reduce the valve diameter. The right atrium is closed. Report 33464 if a stiff ring is used to reduce the valve's diameter rather than purse strings.

Coding Tips

For reoperation on the aortic valve more than one month after the original procedure, report 33530 in addition to the code for the primary procedure. When more than one valve (aortic, mitral, tricuspid, pulmonary) is being repaired or replaced, report each procedure separately and append modifier 51 to the secondary valve procedures. For replacement of the tricuspid valve, see 33465.

ICD-10-CM Diagnostic Codes

I07.0	Rheumatic tricuspid stenosis
I07.1	Rheumatic tricuspid insufficiency
I07.2	Rheumatic tricuspid stenosis and insufficiency
I07.8	Other rheumatic tricuspid valve diseases
I36.0	Nonrheumatic tricuspid (valve) stenosis
I36.1	Nonrheumatic tricuspid (valve) insufficiency
I36.2	Nonrheumatic tricuspid (valve) stenosis with insufficiency
I36.8	Other nonrheumatic tricuspid valve disorders
Q22.4	Congenital tricuspid stenosis
Q22.6	Hypoplastic right heart syndrome
Q22.8	Other congenital malformations of tricuspid valve
T82.01XA	Breakdown (mechanical) of heart valve prosthesis, initial encounter
T82.02XA	Displacement of heart valve prosthesis, initial encounter
T82.03XA	Leakage of heart valve prosthesis, initial encounter
T82.09XA	Other mechanical complication of heart valve prosthesis, initial encounter
T82.6XXA	Infection and inflammatory reaction due to cardiac valve prosthesis, initial encounter
T82.7XXA	Infection and inflammatory reaction due to other cardiac and vascular devices, implants and grafts, initial encounter
T82.817A	Embolism due to cardiac prosthetic devices, implants and grafts, initial encounter
T82.827A	Fibrosis due to cardiac prosthetic devices, implants and grafts, initial encounter
T82.837A	Hemorrhage due to cardiac prosthetic devices, implants and grafts, initial encounter
T82.847A	Pain due to cardiac prosthetic devices, implants and grafts, initial encounter
T82.855A	Stenosis of coronary artery stent, initial encounter
T82.857A	Stenosis of other cardiac prosthetic devices, implants and grafts, initial encounter
T82.867A	Thrombosis due to cardiac prosthetic devices, implants and grafts, initial encounter
T82.897A	Other specified complication of cardiac prosthetic devices, implants and grafts, initial encounter

AMA: 33460 2018,Jan,8; 2017,Jan,8; 2017,Dec,3; 2016,Jan,13; 2015,Jan,16; 2014,Jan,11 **33463** 2018,Jan,8; 2017,Jan,8; 2017,Dec,3; 2016,Jan,13; 2015,Jan,16; 2014,Jan,11 **33464** 2018,Jan,8; 2017,Jan,8; 2017,Dec,3; 2016,Jan,13; 2015,Jan,16; 2014,Jan,11

Relative Value Units/Medicare Edits

Non-Facility RVU	Work	PE	MP	Total
33460	44.7	14.96	10.58	70.24
33463	57.08	19.56	12.87	89.51
33464	44.62	16.05	10.04	70.71
Facility RVU	**Work**	**PE**	**MP**	**Total**
33460	44.7	14.96	10.58	70.24
33463	57.08	19.56	12.87	89.51
33464	44.62	16.05	10.04	70.71

	FUD	Status	MUE	Modifiers				IOM Reference
33460	90	A	1(2)	51	N/A	62*	80	None
33463	90	A	1(2)	51	N/A	62*	80	
33464	90	A	1(2)	51	N/A	62*	80	

* with documentation

Terms To Know

endocarditis. Inflammatory disease of the interior lining of the heart chamber and heart valves.

tricuspid valve. Valve with three cusps between the right atrium and the right ventricle.

valvectomy. Excision of a valve.

valvuloplasty. Surgical repair of a valve.

33465

33465 Replacement, tricuspid valve, with cardiopulmonary bypass

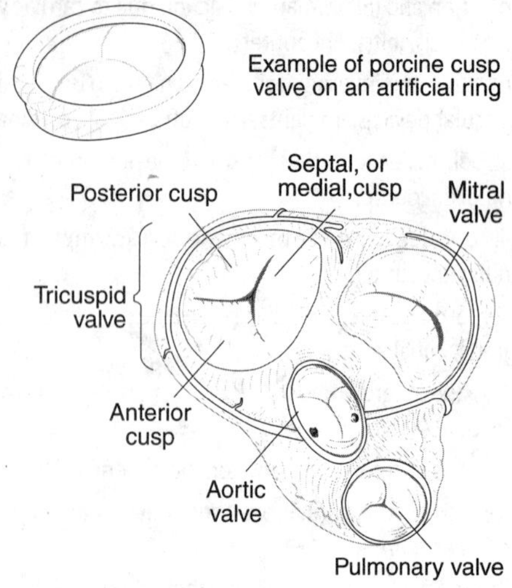

Overhead schematic of heart valves

Explanation

The physician incises the sternum with a cut of about 7 to 9 inches to expose the heart. A minimally invasive procedure could entail a sternal incision of 2 to 4 inches or an incision between the ribs. Cardiopulmonary bypass is initiated with venous uptake tubes in both caval veins. The right atrium is opened and clamps are placed on the aorta. Typically, the tricuspid valve leaflets are left intact; however, when excessive thickening is present, several incisions into the leaflets may be necessary allowing for the best possible fit of the prosthetic. A valve of an appropriate diameter is selected (usually it is a tissue/plastic valve, although a metal valve can also be used). Sutures are placed around the circumference of the tricuspid valve annulus. They are brought through the sewing ring of the valve. The valve is seated so that the sewing ring is resting on the annulus. The sutures are tied tightly. The right atrium is closed. Cardiopulmonary bypass is discontinued when heart function returns.

Coding Tips

For reoperation on the aortic valve more than one month after the original procedure, report 33530 in addition to the code for the primary procedure. When more than one valve (aortic, mitral, tricuspid, pulmonary) is being repaired or replaced, report each procedure separately and append modifier 51 to the secondary valve procedures. For valvectomy of the tricuspid valve, see 33460. For valvuloplasty of the tricuspid valve, see 33463–33464.

ICD-10-CM Diagnostic Codes

I07.0	Rheumatic tricuspid stenosis
I07.1	Rheumatic tricuspid insufficiency
I07.2	Rheumatic tricuspid stenosis and insufficiency
I07.8	Other rheumatic tricuspid valve diseases
I36.0	Nonrheumatic tricuspid (valve) stenosis
I36.1	Nonrheumatic tricuspid (valve) insufficiency
I36.2	Nonrheumatic tricuspid (valve) stenosis with insufficiency
I36.8	Other nonrheumatic tricuspid valve disorders
Q22.4	Congenital tricuspid stenosis
Q22.6	Hypoplastic right heart syndrome
Q22.8	Other congenital malformations of tricuspid valve
T82.01XA	Breakdown (mechanical) of heart valve prosthesis, initial encounter
T82.02XA	Displacement of heart valve prosthesis, initial encounter
T82.03XA	Leakage of heart valve prosthesis, initial encounter
T82.09XA	Other mechanical complication of heart valve prosthesis, initial encounter
T82.6XXA	Infection and inflammatory reaction due to cardiac valve prosthesis, initial encounter
T82.817A	Embolism due to cardiac prosthetic devices, implants and grafts, initial encounter
T82.827A	Fibrosis due to cardiac prosthetic devices, implants and grafts, initial encounter
T82.837A	Hemorrhage due to cardiac prosthetic devices, implants and grafts, initial encounter
T82.847A	Pain due to cardiac prosthetic devices, implants and grafts, initial encounter
T82.855A	Stenosis of coronary artery stent, initial encounter
T82.857A	Stenosis of other cardiac prosthetic devices, implants and grafts, initial encounter
T82.867A	Thrombosis due to cardiac prosthetic devices, implants and grafts, initial encounter
T82.897A	Other specified complication of cardiac prosthetic devices, implants and grafts, initial encounter

AMA: 33465 2018,Jan,8; 2017,Jan,8; 2017,Dec,3; 2016,Jan,13; 2015,Jan,16; 2014,Jan,11

Relative Value Units/Medicare Edits

Non-Facility RVU	Work	PE	MP	Total
33465	50.72	17.57	11.62	79.91
Facility RVU	**Work**	**PE**	**MP**	**Total**
33465	50.72	17.57	11.62	79.91

	FUD	Status	MUE	Modifiers				IOM Reference
33465	90	A	1(2)	51	N/A	62*	80	None

* with documentation

Terms To Know

atresia. Congenital closure or absence of a tubular organ or an opening to the body surface.

atria. Two upper chambers of the heart. The left and right atria are divided by the septum, a muscular wall.

cardiopulmonary bypass. Venous blood is diverted to a heart-lung machine, which mechanically pumps and oxygenates the blood temporarily so the heart can be bypassed while an open procedure on the heart or coronary arteries is performed. During bypass, the lungs are deflated and immobile.

tricuspid valve. Valve with three cusps between the right atrium and the right ventricle.

33468

33468 Tricuspid valve repositioning and plication for Ebstein anomaly

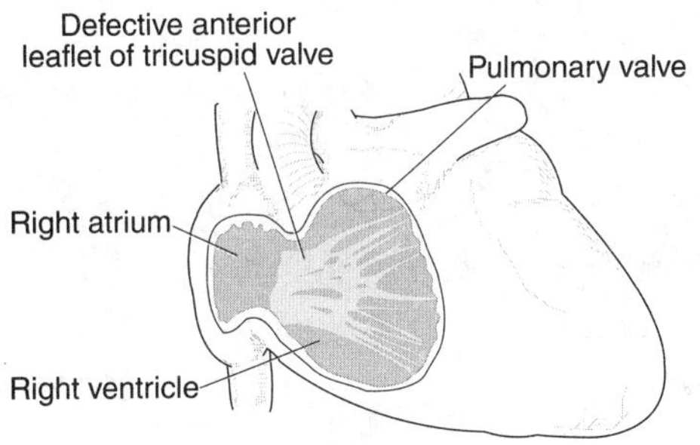

Explanation

In this anomaly, the tricuspid valve annulus is displaced onto the right ventricle, the right ventricle becomes atrophied and the valve leaflets become tethered to the wall of the ventricle. Cardiopulmonary bypass is initiated with venous uptake tubes in both caval veins. The right atrium is opened. The valve is detached from the ventricular wall around its circumference. The edge of the cut valve is sewn circumferentially around the lone port by the true junction of the right atrium and right ventricle. The right atrium is closed. Cardiopulmonary bypass is discontinued when heart function returns.

Coding Tips

For reoperation on the aortic valve more than one month after the original procedure, report 33530 in addition to the code for the primary procedure. When more than one valve (aortic, mitral, tricuspid, pulmonary) is being repaired or replaced, report each procedure separately and append modifier 51 to the secondary valve procedures. For valvuloplasty of the tricuspid valve without ring insertion, see 33463; with ring insertion, see 33464. For replacement of tricuspid valve, see 33465.

ICD-10-CM Diagnostic Codes

Q22.5 Ebstein's anomaly

AMA: 33468 2018,Jan,8; 2017,Jan,8; 2017,Dec,3; 2016,Jan,13; 2015,Jan,16; 2014,Jan,11

Relative Value Units/Medicare Edits

Non-Facility RVU	Work	PE	MP	Total
33468	45.13	15.39	10.76	71.28
Facility RVU	**Work**	**PE**	**MP**	**Total**
33468	45.13	15.39	10.76	71.28

	FUD	Status	MUE	Modifiers				IOM Reference
33468	90	A	1(2)	51	N/A	62*	80	None

* with documentation

33470-33471

33470 Valvotomy, pulmonary valve, closed heart; transventricular
33471 via pulmonary artery

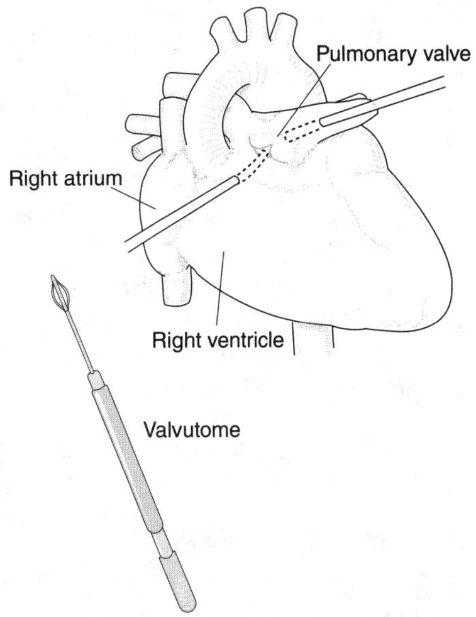

A valvotomy is performed on the pulmonary valve in a closed heart procedure

Explanation

Cardiopulmonary bypass is not required. The heart is exposed through the sternum. A U-stitch reinforced with small patches of Teflon felt is placed in the right ventricular outflow tract muscle. A hole is made in the center of this U-stitch. Dilators are passed through the hole and across the valve. Gradually larger dilators are passed until the valve opening is large enough. The last dilator is removed and the U-stitch is tied to stop any bleeding. The chest is closed. In this operation, the valve is dilated from below. Report 33471 if the U-stitch is placed in the pulmonary artery and the valve is dilated from above.

Coding Tips

For reoperation on the aortic valve more than one month after the original procedure, report 33530 in addition to the code for the primary procedure. When more than one valve (aortic, mitral, tricuspid, pulmonary) is being repaired or replaced, report each procedure separately and append modifier 51 to the secondary valve procedures. For valvotomy of the pulmonary valve, open heart, with cardiopulmonary bypass, see 33474. For percutaneous balloon valvuloplasty of the pulmonary valve, see 92990.

ICD-10-CM Diagnostic Codes

I37.0 Nonrheumatic pulmonary valve stenosis
I37.1 Nonrheumatic pulmonary valve insufficiency
I37.2 Nonrheumatic pulmonary valve stenosis with insufficiency
I37.8 Other nonrheumatic pulmonary valve disorders
Q22.1 Congenital pulmonary valve stenosis
T82.01XA Breakdown (mechanical) of heart valve prosthesis, initial encounter
T82.02XA Displacement of heart valve prosthesis, initial encounter
T82.03XA Leakage of heart valve prosthesis, initial encounter
T82.09XA Other mechanical complication of heart valve prosthesis, initial encounter

T82.6XXA	Infection and inflammatory reaction due to cardiac valve prosthesis, initial encounter
T82.817A	Embolism due to cardiac prosthetic devices, implants and grafts, initial encounter
T82.827A	Fibrosis due to cardiac prosthetic devices, implants and grafts, initial encounter
T82.837A	Hemorrhage due to cardiac prosthetic devices, implants and grafts, initial encounter
T82.847A	Pain due to cardiac prosthetic devices, implants and grafts, initial encounter
T82.855A	Stenosis of coronary artery stent, initial encounter
T82.857A	Stenosis of other cardiac prosthetic devices, implants and grafts, initial encounter
T82.867A	Thrombosis due to cardiac prosthetic devices, implants and grafts, initial encounter
T82.897A	Other specified complication of cardiac prosthetic devices, implants and grafts, initial encounter

AMA: 33470 2018,Jan,8; 2017,Jan,8; 2016,Jan,13; 2015,Jan,16; 2014,Jan,11
33471 2018,Jan,8; 2017,Jan,8; 2016,Jan,13; 2015,Jan,16; 2014,Jan,11

Relative Value Units/Medicare Edits

Non-Facility RVU	Work	PE	MP	Total
33470	21.54	9.24	5.12	35.9
33471	22.96	9.98	5.45	38.39
Facility RVU	**Work**	**PE**	**MP**	**Total**
33470	21.54	9.24	5.12	35.9
33471	22.96	9.98	5.45	38.39

	FUD	Status	MUE	Modifiers				IOM Reference
33470	90	A	1(2)	51	N/A	N/A	80	None
33471	90	A	1(2)	51	N/A	62*	80	

* with documentation

Terms To Know

cardiopulmonary bypass. Venous blood is diverted to a heart-lung machine, which mechanically pumps and oxygenates the blood temporarily so the heart can be bypassed while an open procedure on the heart or coronary arteries is performed. During bypass, the lungs are deflated and immobile.

stenosis. Narrowing or constriction of a passage.

U-stitch. Surgical closure that has a "U" shape.

valvotomy. Cutting through stenosed cardiac valve leaflets or cusp to relieve or repair the obstruction caused by scar tissue and inflammation.

valvuloplasty. Surgical repair of a valve.

33474

33474 Valvotomy, pulmonary valve, open heart, with cardiopulmonary bypass

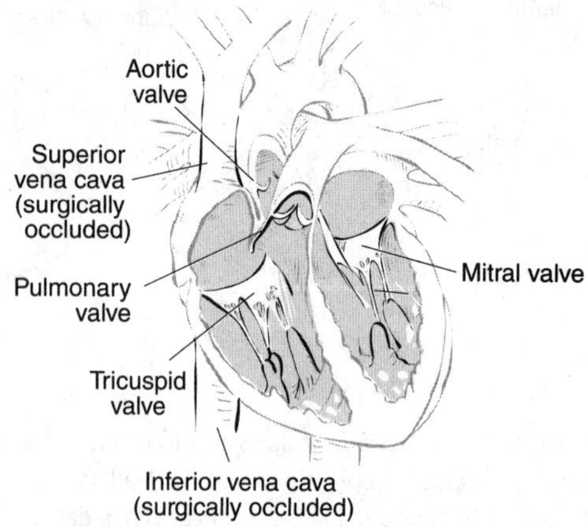

The pulmonary valve is dilated in an open heart surgical session

Explanation

The heart is exposed through the sternum. Tourniquets are placed around the superior and inferior caval veins. These are tightened. A hole is made in the pulmonary artery and the pulmonary valve is cut opened through this hole. The hole in the pulmonary artery is closed and the tourniquets are released. This code includes cardiopulmonary bypass.

Coding Tips

For reoperation on the aortic valve more than one month after the original procedure, report 33530 in addition to the code for the primary procedure. When more than one valve (aortic, mitral, tricuspid, pulmonary) is being repaired or replaced, report each procedure separately and append modifier 51 to the secondary valve procedures. For valvotomy of the pulmonary valve, closed heart, transventricular, see 33470; via pulmonary artery, see 33471. For percutaneous balloon valvuloplasty of the pulmonary valve, see 92990.

ICD-10-CM Diagnostic Codes

I37.1	Nonrheumatic pulmonary valve insufficiency
I37.2	Nonrheumatic pulmonary valve stenosis with insufficiency
I37.8	Other nonrheumatic pulmonary valve disorders
Q22.1	Congenital pulmonary valve stenosis
T82.01XA	Breakdown (mechanical) of heart valve prosthesis, initial encounter
T82.02XA	Displacement of heart valve prosthesis, initial encounter
T82.03XA	Leakage of heart valve prosthesis, initial encounter
T82.09XA	Other mechanical complication of heart valve prosthesis, initial encounter
T82.6XXA	Infection and inflammatory reaction due to cardiac valve prosthesis, initial encounter
T82.817A	Embolism due to cardiac prosthetic devices, implants and grafts, initial encounter
T82.827A	Fibrosis due to cardiac prosthetic devices, implants and grafts, initial encounter
T82.837A	Hemorrhage due to cardiac prosthetic devices, implants and grafts, initial encounter

T82.847A Pain due to cardiac prosthetic devices, implants and grafts, initial encounter

T82.855A Stenosis of coronary artery stent, initial encounter

T82.857A Stenosis of other cardiac prosthetic devices, implants and grafts, initial encounter

T82.867A Thrombosis due to cardiac prosthetic devices, implants and grafts, initial encounter

T82.897A Other specified complication of cardiac prosthetic devices, implants and grafts, initial encounter

AMA: 33474 2017,Dec,3

Relative Value Units/Medicare Edits

Non-Facility RVU	Work	PE	MP	Total
33474	39.4	14.51	9.38	63.29
Facility RVU	**Work**	**PE**	**MP**	**Total**
33474	39.4	14.51	9.38	63.29

	FUD	Status	MUE	Modifiers				IOM Reference
33474	90	A	1(2)	51	N/A	62*	80	None

* with documentation

Terms To Know

cardiopulmonary bypass. Venous blood is diverted to a heart-lung machine, which mechanically pumps and oxygenates the blood temporarily so the heart can be bypassed while an open procedure on the heart or coronary arteries is performed. During bypass, the lungs are deflated and immobile.

complication. Condition arising after the beginning of observation and treatment that modifies the course of the patient's illness or the medical care required, or an undesired result or misadventure in medical care.

congenital. Present at birth, occurring through heredity or an influence during gestation up to the moment of birth.

endocarditis. Inflammatory disease of the interior lining of the heart chamber and heart valves.

infection. Presence of microorganisms in body tissues that may result in cellular damage.

occlusion. Constriction, closure, or blockage of a passage.

percutaneous. Through the skin.

stenosis. Narrowing or constriction of a passage.

tourniquet. Device used to apply compressive force to a blood vessel in a limb and slow or prevent blood flow to and from the area.

valvotomy. Cutting through stenosed cardiac valve leaflets or cusp to relieve or repair the obstruction caused by scar tissue and inflammation.

valvuloplasty. Surgical repair of a valve.

33475

33475 Replacement, pulmonary valve

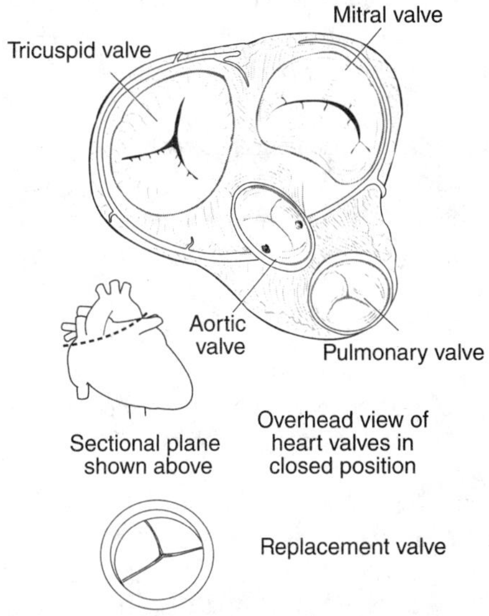

The pulmonary valve is accessed in an open heart surgical session. The valve leaflets are cut out and a replacement valve is secured

Explanation

Cardiopulmonary bypass is initiated with venous uptake tubes in both caval veins. The pulmonary artery is opened and the pulmonary valve leaflets are cut out. Stitches are placed around the circumference of the pulmonary annulus and the valve is sized. An appropriate artificial valve is selected. The stitches are passed through the sewing ring of the valve. The sewing ring is seated against the valve annulus and the stitches are tied. The hole in the pulmonary artery is closed. Cardiopulmonary bypass is discontinued when heart function returns.

Coding Tips

For reoperation on the aortic valve more than one month after the original procedure, report 33530 in addition to the code for the primary procedure. When more than one valve (aortic, mitral, tricuspid, pulmonary) is being repaired or replaced, report each procedure separately and append modifier 51 to the secondary valve procedures. Do not report 33475 with 33440. For valvotomy of the pulmonary valve, closed heart, transventricular, see 33470; via the pulmonary artery, see 33471. For valvotomy of the pulmonary valve, open heart, with cardiopulmonary bypass, see 33474. For percutaneous balloon valvuloplasty of the pulmonary valve, see 92990.

ICD-10-CM Diagnostic Codes

I37.0 Nonrheumatic pulmonary valve stenosis

I37.1 Nonrheumatic pulmonary valve insufficiency

I37.2 Nonrheumatic pulmonary valve stenosis with insufficiency

I37.8 Other nonrheumatic pulmonary valve disorders

Q22.1 Congenital pulmonary valve stenosis

T82.01XA Breakdown (mechanical) of heart valve prosthesis, initial encounter

T82.02XA Displacement of heart valve prosthesis, initial encounter

T82.03XA Leakage of heart valve prosthesis, initial encounter

T82.09XA Other mechanical complication of heart valve prosthesis, initial encounter

T82.6XXA	Infection and inflammatory reaction due to cardiac valve prosthesis, initial encounter
T82.817A	Embolism due to cardiac prosthetic devices, implants and grafts, initial encounter
T82.827A	Fibrosis due to cardiac prosthetic devices, implants and grafts, initial encounter
T82.837A	Hemorrhage due to cardiac prosthetic devices, implants and grafts, initial encounter
T82.847A	Pain due to cardiac prosthetic devices, implants and grafts, initial encounter
T82.855A	Stenosis of coronary artery stent, initial encounter
T82.857A	Stenosis of other cardiac prosthetic devices, implants and grafts, initial encounter
T82.867A	Thrombosis due to cardiac prosthetic devices, implants and grafts, initial encounter
T82.897A	Other specified complication of cardiac prosthetic devices, implants and grafts, initial encounter

AMA: 33475 2019,Apr,6; 2018,Jan,8; 2017,Jan,8; 2017,Dec,3; 2016,Jan,13; 2015,Jan,16; 2014,Jan,11

Relative Value Units/Medicare Edits

Non-Facility RVU	Work	PE	MP	Total
33475	42.4	15.52	9.68	67.6
Facility RVU	**Work**	**PE**	**MP**	**Total**
33475	42.4	15.52	9.68	67.6

	FUD	Status	MUE	Modifiers				IOM Reference
33475	90	A	1(2)	51	N/A	62*	80	None

* with documentation

Terms To Know

cardiopulmonary bypass. Venous blood is diverted to a heart-lung machine, which mechanically pumps and oxygenates the blood temporarily so the heart can be bypassed while an open procedure on the heart or coronary arteries is performed. During bypass, the lungs are deflated and immobile.

complication. Condition arising after the beginning of observation and treatment that modifies the course of the patient's illness or the medical care required, or an undesired result or misadventure in medical care.

congenital. Present at birth, occurring through heredity or an influence during gestation up to the moment of birth.

endocarditis. Inflammatory disease of the interior lining of the heart chamber and heart valves.

infection. Presence of microorganisms in body tissues that may result in cellular damage.

percutaneous. Through the skin.

stenosis. Narrowing or constriction of a passage.

valvotomy. Cutting through stenosed cardiac valve leaflets or cusp to relieve or repair the obstruction caused by scar tissue and inflammation.

valvuloplasty. Surgical repair of a valve.

33476, 33478

33476 Right ventricular resection for infundibular stenosis, with or without commissurotomy

33478 Outflow tract augmentation (gusset), with or without commissurotomy or infundibular resection

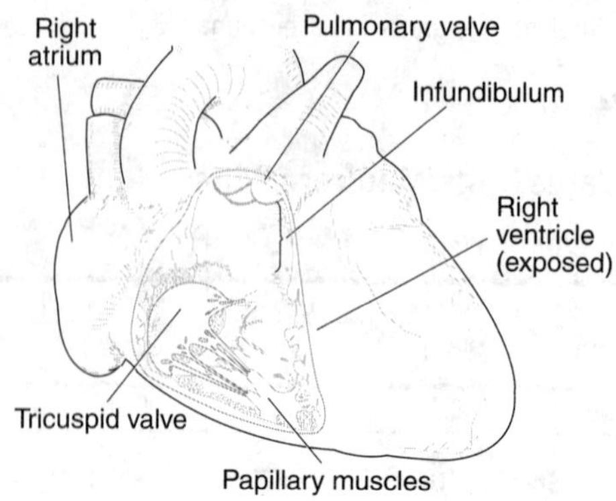

Explanation

Cardiopulmonary bypass is initiated. The right ventricular infundibular muscle is opened and the obstructing muscle bands are cut out. The valve may also need to be opened. If so, the valve is cut open. The hole in the right ventricle is closed with a patch of pericardium. Cardiopulmonary bypass is discontinued when heart function returns. Report 33478 if the operation is performed with a gusset, with or without commissurotomy or infundibular resection.

Coding Tips

For reoperation on the aortic valve more than one month after the original procedure, report 33530 in addition to the code for the primary procedure. When more than one valve (aortic, mitral, tricuspid, pulmonary) is being repaired or replaced, report each procedure separately and append modifier 51 to the secondary valve procedures. For valvotomy of the pulmonary valve, closed heart, transventricular, see 33470; via pulmonary artery, see 33471. For valvotomy of the pulmonary valve, open heart, with cardiopulmonary bypass, see 33474. For replacement of the pulmonary valve, see 33475. For percutaneous balloon valvuloplasty of the pulmonary valve, see 92990. Report 33478 with 33768 when a cavopulmonary anastomosis to a second superior vena cava is performed.

ICD-10-CM Diagnostic Codes

Q22.1	Congenital pulmonary valve stenosis
Q24.3	Pulmonary infundibular stenosis

AMA: 33476 2018,Jan,8; 2017,Jan,8; 2017,Dec,3; 2016,Jan,13; 2015,Jan,16; 2014,Jan,11 **33478** 2018,Jan,8; 2017,Jan,8; 2017,Dec,3; 2016,Jan,13; 2015,Jan,16; 2014,Jan,11

Relative Value Units/Medicare Edits

Non-Facility RVU	Work	PE	MP	Total
33476	26.57	11.28	6.3	44.15
33478	27.54	11.55	6.53	45.62
Facility RVU	**Work**	**PE**	**MP**	**Total**
33476	26.57	11.28	6.3	44.15
33478	27.54	11.55	6.53	45.62

	FUD	Status	MUE	Modifiers				IOM Reference
33476	90	A	1(2)	51	N/A	62*	80	None
33478	90	A	1(2)	51	N/A	62*	80	

* with documentation

Terms To Know

anomaly. Irregularity in the structure or position of an organ or tissue.

augmentation. Add to or increase the substance of a body site, usually performed as plastic reconstructive measures. Augmentation may involve the use of an implant or prosthesis, especially within soft tissue or grafting procedures, such as bone tissue.

cardiopulmonary bypass. Venous blood is diverted to a heart-lung machine, which mechanically pumps and oxygenates the blood temporarily so the heart can be bypassed while an open procedure on the heart or coronary arteries is performed. During bypass, the lungs are deflated and immobile.

commissurotomy. Surgical division or disruption of any two parts that are joined to form a commissure in order to increase the opening. The procedure most often refers to opening the adherent leaflet bands of fibrous tissue in a stenosed mitral valve.

congenital. Present at birth, occurring through heredity or an influence during gestation up to the moment of birth.

gusset. Triangular or diamond shaped patch that is placed for reinforcement or expansion.

infundibulectomy. Excision of the anterosuperior portion of the right ventricle of the heart.

percutaneous. Through the skin.

resection. Surgical removal of a part or all of an organ or body part.

stenosis. Narrowing or constriction of a passage.

valvuloplasty. Surgical repair of a valve.

33477

33477 Transcatheter pulmonary valve implantation, percutaneous approach, including pre-stenting of the valve delivery site, when performed

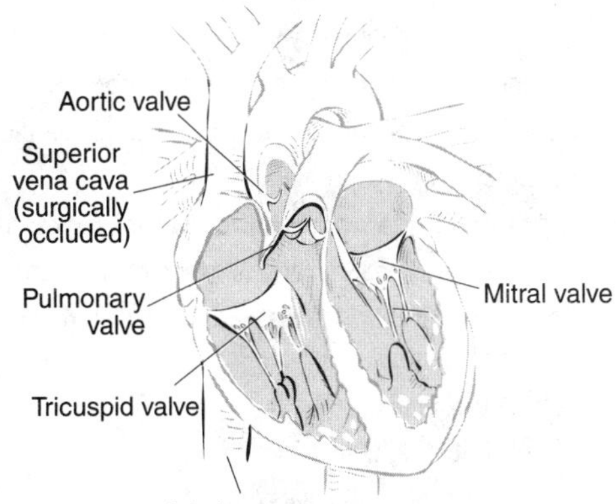

Transcatheter implantation of pulmonary valve

Explanation

Percutaneous placement of a prosthetic pulmonary valve is used primarily to treat patients with stenosis or regurgitation of a previously repaired right ventricular outflow tract (RVOT). The patient is prepped with general anesthesia in addition to endotracheal intubation. The provider inserts a needle through the skin and into an underlying vein, usually a lower extremity vein, although jugular access is also utilized. Angiography and hemodynamic studies are performed and a guidewire is threaded through the needle and advanced into the pulmonary artery. A balloon is inflated in the RVOT conduit to evaluate for coronary compression and an aortogram is performed to visualize the coronary arteries. Pre-stenting is commonly performed with a covered bare metal stent to decrease the risk of fractured stents and more than one stent may be required. The needle is removed and a catheter carrying the prosthetic valve is inserted. The prosthesis is positioned over the diseased pulmonary valve and a balloon is inflated, deploying the prosthetic valve in place. Angiography and hemodynamic evaluations are repeated. The catheter is removed and pressure is applied to stop bleeding at the access site. A single suture may provide hemostasis at the venous access.

Coding Tips

This code should be reported only once per encounter. This procedure includes angiography, cardiac catheterization, contrast injection, imaging guidance, and radiological supervision and interpretation necessary to perform the service. Diagnostic catheterization, diagnostic coronary angiography, and diagnostic pulmonary angiography codes may be reported separately in cases where a previous examination is not available or the anatomic visualization is poor quality, there has been a clinical change in the patient's condition since the previous examination, or complications arise during the course of the procedure requiring the additional study. Cardiopulmonary bypass may be necessary in addition to this procedure. For percutaneous peripheral bypass, see 33367; for open peripheral bypass, see 33368; and for central bypass, see 33369. Do not report 33477 in addition to 76000, 93451, 93453–93461, 93530–93533, 93563, or 93566–93568 for angiography necessary to accomplish the procedure. Do not report this code in addition to 37236–37237 or 92997–92998 for angioplasty, valvuloplasty, or stenting within the treatment site. For transcatheter ventricular assist during this procedure, see 33990–33993 for VAD; see 33946–33989 for ECMO/ECLS; and see 33967, 33970, or 33973 for balloon pump insertion.

ICD-10-CM Diagnostic Codes

A52.03	Syphilitic endocarditis
I33.9	Acute and subacute endocarditis, unspecified
I37.0	Nonrheumatic pulmonary valve stenosis
I37.1	Nonrheumatic pulmonary valve insufficiency
I37.2	Nonrheumatic pulmonary valve stenosis with insufficiency
I37.8	Other nonrheumatic pulmonary valve disorders
I37.9	Nonrheumatic pulmonary valve disorder, unspecified
I97.0	Postcardiotomy syndrome
I97.110	Postprocedural cardiac insufficiency following cardiac surgery
I97.130	Postprocedural heart failure following cardiac surgery
I97.190	Other postprocedural cardiac functional disturbances following cardiac surgery
Q20.0	Common arterial trunk
Q20.1	Double outlet right ventricle
Q20.5	Discordant atrioventricular connection
Q21.3	Tetralogy of Fallot
Q22.0	Pulmonary valve atresia
Q22.1	Congenital pulmonary valve stenosis
Q22.2	Congenital pulmonary valve insufficiency
Q22.3	Other congenital malformations of pulmonary valve
Q24.3	Pulmonary infundibular stenosis

AMA: **33477** 2018,Jan,8; 2017,Jan,8; 2016,Mar,5; 2016,Aug,9

Relative Value Units/Medicare Edits

Non-Facility RVU	Work	PE	MP	Total
33477	25.0	8.82	5.9	39.72
Facility RVU	**Work**	**PE**	**MP**	**Total**
33477	25.0	8.82	5.9	39.72

	FUD	Status	MUE	Modifiers				IOM Reference
33477	0	A	1(2)	51	N/A	62*	80*	None

* with documentation

Terms To Know

angiography. Radiographic imaging of the arteries. Imaging may be performed to study the vasculature of any given organ, body system, or area of circulation such as the brain, heart, chest, kidneys, limbs, gastrointestinal tract, aorta, and pulmonary circulation to visualize the formation and the function of the blood vessels to detect problems such as a blockage or stricture. A catheter is inserted through an accessible blood vessel and the artery is injected with a radiopaque contrast material after which x-rays are taken.

catheterization. Use or insertion of a tubular device into a duct, blood vessel, hollow organ, or body cavity for injecting or withdrawing fluids for diagnostic or therapeutic purposes.

intubation. Insertion of a tube into a hollow organ, canal, or cavity within the body.

regurgitation. Abnormal backward flow.

33496

33496 Repair of non-structural prosthetic valve dysfunction with cardiopulmonary bypass (separate procedure)

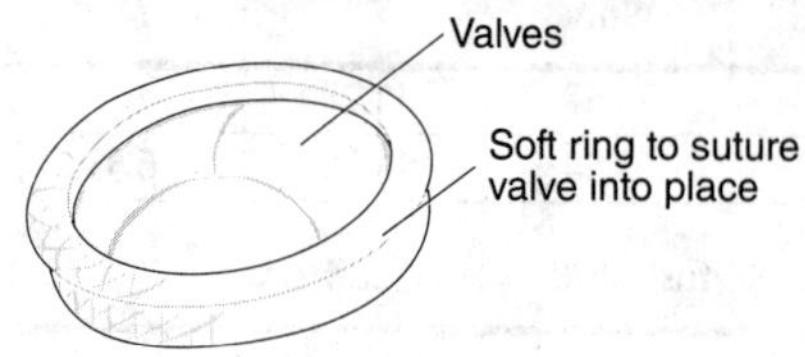

Example of nonstructural prosthetic heart valve

Explanation

This procedure is typically performed to repair an artificial prosthetic valve that is malfunctioning due to leakage around the valve sewing ring or the valve is impeded by blood clot or growth of surrounding tissue (pannus) into the functioning part of the valve. The surgeon exposes the heart through the sternum. Cardiopulmonary bypass is initiated. The prosthetic valve is exposed and the valve is repaired. Cardiopulmonary bypass is discontinued when heart function returns. The sternum is closed with wires or sutures and the soft tissues are closed with sutures.

Coding Tips

This separate procedure by definition is usually a component of a more complex service and is not identified separately. When performed alone or with other unrelated procedures/services, it may be reported. If performed alone, list the code; if performed with other procedures/services, list the code and append modifier 59 or an X{EPSU} modifier. This code is reported for mitral or aortic prosthetic valve repair (e.g., suture of perivalvular prosthetic valve leak, declotting of a prosthetic heart valve). Report 33530 in addition to the code for the primary reoperation procedure on the affected valve more than one month after the original procedure.

ICD-10-CM Diagnostic Codes

T82.02XA	Displacement of heart valve prosthesis, initial encounter
T82.03XA	Leakage of heart valve prosthesis, initial encounter
T82.818A	Embolism due to vascular prosthetic devices, implants and grafts, initial encounter
T82.828A	Fibrosis due to vascular prosthetic devices, implants and grafts, initial encounter
T82.838A	Hemorrhage due to vascular prosthetic devices, implants and grafts, initial encounter
T82.848A	Pain due to vascular prosthetic devices, implants and grafts, initial encounter
T82.856A	Stenosis of peripheral vascular stent, initial encounter
T82.858A	Stenosis of other vascular prosthetic devices, implants and grafts, initial encounter
T82.868A	Thrombosis due to vascular prosthetic devices, implants and grafts, initial encounter
T82.898A	Other specified complication of vascular prosthetic devices, implants and grafts, initial encounter
T82.9XXA	Unspecified complication of cardiac and vascular prosthetic device, implant and graft, initial encounter
Z95.2	Presence of prosthetic heart valve

AMA: **33496** 2018,Jan,8; 2017,Jan,8; 2017,Dec,3; 2016,Jan,13; 2015,Jan,16; 2014,Jan,11

Relative Value Units/Medicare Edits

Non-Facility RVU	Work	PE	MP	Total
33496	29.84	11.69	7.04	48.57
Facility RVU	**Work**	**PE**	**MP**	**Total**
33496	29.84	11.69	7.04	48.57

	FUD	Status	MUE	Modifiers				IOM Reference
33496	90	A	1(3)	51	N/A	62*	80	None

* with documentation

Terms To Know

cardiopulmonary bypass. Venous blood is diverted to a heart-lung machine, which mechanically pumps and oxygenates the blood temporarily so the heart can be bypassed while an open procedure on the heart or coronary arteries is performed. During bypass, the lungs are deflated and immobile.

complication. Condition arising after the beginning of observation and treatment that modifies the course of the patient's illness or the medical care required, or an undesired result or misadventure in medical care.

hypothermia with cardiac bypass. Reduction of the body temperature using a bypass system to reduce the oxygen demands of tissue and to protect the myocardium during a procedure.

prosthesis. Man-made substitute for a missing body part.

suture. Numerous stitching techniques employed in wound closure.

33500-33501

33500 Repair of coronary arteriovenous or arteriocardiac chamber fistula; with cardiopulmonary bypass

33501 without cardiopulmonary bypass

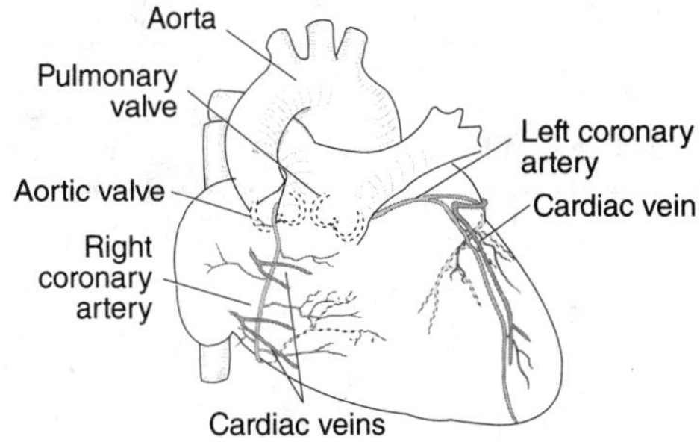

Anatomical variations in coronary vessels are normal; however, a communication between an artery and a vein is a fistula

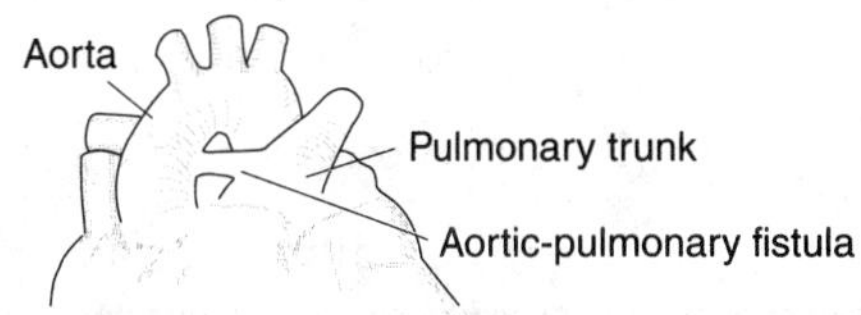

Explanation

Cardiopulmonary bypass is initiated. The site of the fistula has been previously determined by cardiac catheterization. The venous end of the fistula is ligated with sutures. Cardiopulmonary bypass is often discontinued. If the fistula is to a cardiac chamber, that chamber is opened and the chamber end of the fistula is closed with a stitch. Report 33501 if cardiopulmonary bypass is not used.

Coding Tips

If significant additional time and effort are documented, append modifier 22 and submit a cover letter and operative report. When 33500 or 33501 is performed with another separately identifiable procedure, the highest dollar value code is listed as the primary procedure and subsequent procedures are appended with modifier 51. Do not report endarterectomy or angioplasty separately as they are included in the fistula repair.

ICD-10-CM Diagnostic Codes

I25.41	Coronary artery aneurysm
Q24.5	Malformation of coronary vessels

AMA: 33500 2017,Dec,3

Relative Value Units/Medicare Edits

Non-Facility RVU	Work	PE	MP	Total
33500	27.94	10.99	6.58	45.51
33501	19.51	8.4	4.6	32.51
Facility RVU	**Work**	**PE**	**MP**	**Total**
33500	27.94	10.99	6.58	45.51
33501	19.51	8.4	4.6	32.51

	FUD	Status	MUE	Modifiers				IOM Reference
33500	90	A	1(3)	51	N/A	62*	80	None
33501	90	A	1(3)	51	N/A	62	80	

* with documentation

Terms To Know

aneurysm. Circumscribed dilation or outpouching of an artery wall, often containing blood clots and connecting directly with the lumen of the artery.

angioplasty. Reconstruction or repair of a diseased or damaged blood vessel.

anomaly. Irregularity in the structure or position of an organ or tissue.

cardiopulmonary bypass. Venous blood is diverted to a heart-lung machine, which mechanically pumps and oxygenates the blood temporarily so the heart can be bypassed while an open procedure on the heart or coronary arteries is performed. During bypass, the lungs are deflated and immobile.

catheter. Flexible tube inserted into an area of the body for introducing or withdrawing fluid.

congenital. Present at birth, occurring through heredity or an influence during gestation up to the moment of birth.

endarterectomy. Removal of the thickened, endothelial lining of a diseased or damaged artery.

fistula. Abnormal tube-like passage between two body cavities or organs or from an organ to the outside surface.

ligate. To tie off a blood vessel or duct with a suture or a soft, thin wire (ligature wire).

33502-33504

33502 Repair of anomalous coronary artery from pulmonary artery origin; by ligation
33503 by graft, without cardiopulmonary bypass
33504 by graft, with cardiopulmonary bypass

Schematic showing coronary arteries. Normal configuration is for the left and right branches to originate just above the aortic valve

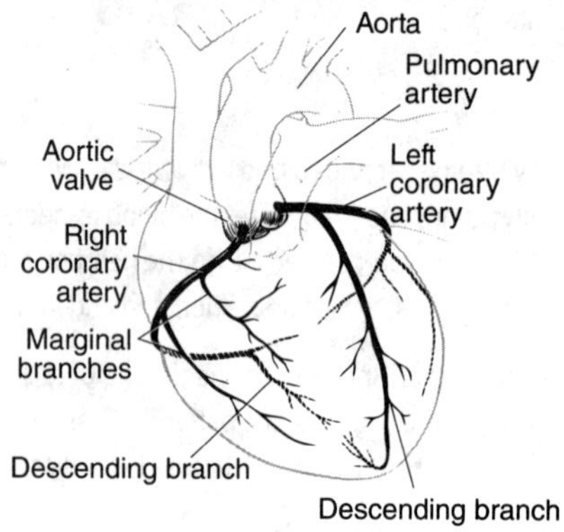

Explanation

In 33502, the physician ligates an anomalous coronary artery arising from the pulmonary artery. Ligation of the anomalous coronary artery has a poor prognosis and may be performed as a temporary measure prior to creation of a double coronary artery system during a subsequent surgical intervention. The anomalous coronary artery is exposed at the site of origin in the pulmonary artery. A suture is placed around the artery and it is ligated. In 33503, the physician repairs an anomalous coronary artery arising from the pulmonary artery using a graft. The anomalous coronary artery is identified and detached. The subsequent hole in the pulmonary artery is sutured closed. An opening is made in the side of the aorta and the free end of the coronary artery is anastomosed to the aorta. Report 33504 if cardiopulmonary bypass is required. This procedure will most always require the cardiopulmonary bypass.

Coding Tips

If significant additional time and effort are documented, append modifier 22 and submit a cover letter and operative report. When 33502, 33503, or 33504 is performed with another separately identifiable procedure, the highest dollar value code is listed as the primary procedure and subsequent procedures are appended with modifier 51. Do not report endarterectomy or angioplasty separately as they are included in the repair of the anomalous artery. Do not append modifier 63 to 33502–33503 as the description of the procedure includes infants up to 4 kg.

ICD-10-CM Diagnostic Codes

Q24.5 Malformation of coronary vessels

AMA: 33502 2017,Dec,3 **33504** 2017,Dec,3

Relative Value Units/Medicare Edits

Non-Facility RVU	Work	PE	MP	Total
33502	21.85	9.97	5.18	37.0
33503	22.51	10.59	5.34	38.44
33504	25.46	11.01	6.04	42.51
Facility RVU	**Work**	**PE**	**MP**	**Total**
33502	21.85	9.97	5.18	37.0
33503	22.51	10.59	5.34	38.44
33504	25.46	11.01	6.04	42.51

	FUD	Status	MUE	Modifiers				IOM Reference
33502	90	A	1(3)	51	N/A	62*	80	None
33503	90	A	1(3)	51	N/A	62*	80*	
33504	90	A	1(3)	51	N/A	62*	80	

* with documentation

Terms To Know

angioplasty. Reconstruction or repair of a diseased or damaged blood vessel.

anomaly. Irregularity in the structure or position of an organ or tissue.

cardiopulmonary bypass. Venous blood is diverted to a heart-lung machine, which mechanically pumps and oxygenates the blood temporarily so the heart can be bypassed while an open procedure on the heart or coronary arteries is performed. During bypass, the lungs are deflated and immobile.

congenital. Present at birth, occurring through heredity or an influence during gestation up to the moment of birth.

endarterectomy. Removal of the thickened, endothelial lining of a diseased or damaged artery.

graft. Tissue implant from another part of the body or another person.

33505-33506

33505 Repair of anomalous coronary artery from pulmonary artery origin; with construction of intrapulmonary artery tunnel (Takeuchi procedure)

33506 by translocation from pulmonary artery to aorta

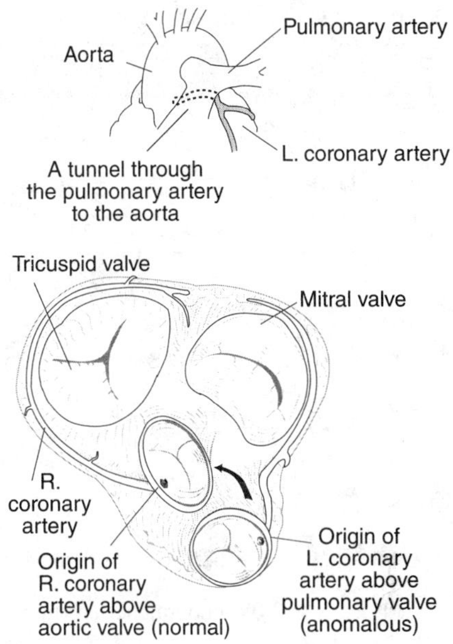

Explanation

In 33505, the physician repairs an anomalous coronary artery arising from the pulmonary artery by construction of an intrapulmonary artery tunnel. Cardiopulmonary bypass is required. This operation is done in cases where the anomalous coronary artery is located far from the aorta on the left lateral side of the pulmonary artery. Openings are made in the aorta and the pulmonary artery at the level of the anomalous coronary artery where the vessels touch each other. The two open areas are sewn together to create a direct aortopulmonary opening. A flap of pulmonary artery wall is created with the anomalous coronary artery at one end. The flap is fashioned into a tunnel with the flap as one side of the tunnel, the back wall of the pulmonary artery as the other side of the tunnel, the hole between the aorta and pulmonary artery as one end, and the anomalous coronary artery as the other end. In this way, blood from the aorta is diverted into the anomalous coronary artery. The hole in the pulmonary artery is closed. Cardiopulmonary bypass is discontinued when heart function returns. This procedure is less common today; surgeons typically repair the defect by direct transfer of the anomalous coronary artery from the pulmonary artery. In 33506, the physician repairs an anomalous coronary artery arising from the pulmonary artery by translocation from the pulmonary artery to the aorta. The anomalous coronary artery arising from the pulmonary artery is detached. The subsequent hole in the pulmonary artery is patched with autologous pericardium. An opening is created in the side of the aorta and the coronary artery is anastomosed into the opening. Cardiopulmonary bypass is almost always required for this operation.

Coding Tips

If significant additional time and effort are documented, append modifier 22 and submit a cover letter and operative report. When 33505 or 33506 is performed with another separately identifiable procedure, the highest dollar value code is listed as the primary procedure and subsequent procedures are appended with modifier 51. Do not report endarterectomy or angioplasty separately as they are included in the repair of the anomalous artery. Do not append modifier 63 to 33505–33506 as the description of the procedure includes infants up to 4 kg.

ICD-10-CM Diagnostic Codes

Q24.5 Malformation of coronary vessels

AMA: **33505** 2017,Dec,3 **33506** 2017,Dec,3

Relative Value Units/Medicare Edits

Non-Facility RVU	Work	PE	MP	Total
33505	38.4	12.46	9.14	60.0
33506	37.85	12.86	9.0	59.71
Facility RVU	**Work**	**PE**	**MP**	**Total**
33505	38.4	12.46	9.14	60.0
33506	37.85	12.86	9.0	59.71

	FUD	Status	MUE	Modifiers				IOM Reference
33505	90	A	1(3)	51	N/A	62*	80	None
33506	90	A	1(3)	51	N/A	62*	80	

* with documentation

Terms To Know

angioplasty. Reconstruction or repair of a diseased or damaged blood vessel.

anomaly. Irregularity in the structure or position of an organ or tissue.

cardiopulmonary bypass. Venous blood is diverted to a heart-lung machine, which mechanically pumps and oxygenates the blood temporarily so the heart can be bypassed while an open procedure on the heart or coronary arteries is performed. During bypass, the lungs are deflated and immobile.

congenital. Present at birth, occurring through heredity or an influence during gestation up to the moment of birth.

endarterectomy. Removal of the thickened, endothelial lining of a diseased or damaged artery.

33507

33507 Repair of anomalous (eg, intramural) aortic origin of coronary artery by unroofing or translocation

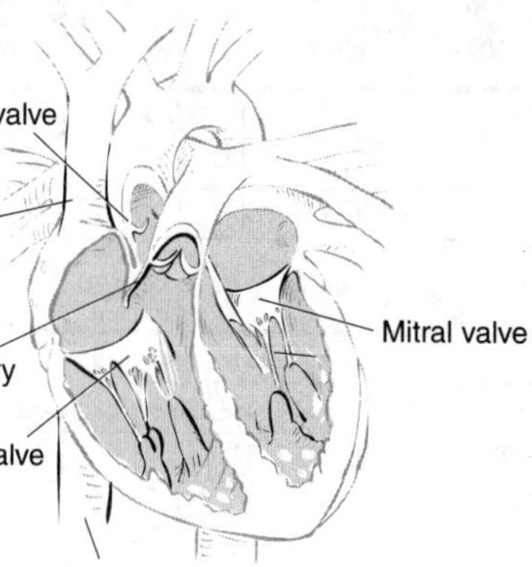

Explanation

The physician repairs an anomalous coronary artery by unroofing or translocation. Common anomalies repaired using this technique include anomalous right coronary artery arising from the left coronary sinus, anomalous left coronary artery arising from the right coronary sinus, and anomalous coronary artery arising from a single ostia. Cardiopulmonary bypass is almost always required. The physician detaches the posterior commissure of the aortic valve. Unroofing of the intramural segment of the coronary artery is accomplished by excision of a triangular portion of the internal aortic wall. The coronary arteries are excised as a single disc and divided into two cuffs. An arterial switch is performed. The posterior commissure of the aortic valve is resuspended to a pericardial patch used to reconstruct the pulmonary artery sinus.

Coding Tips

Endarterectomy and angioplasty are included in the basic procedure and should not be reported separately. For repair of an anomalous coronary artery from pulmonary artery origin, see 33502–33506.

ICD-10-CM Diagnostic Codes

Q24.5 Malformation of coronary vessels

AMA: **33507** 2018,Jan,8; 2017,Jan,8; 2017,Dec,3; 2016,Jan,13; 2015,Jan,16; 2014,Jan,11

Relative Value Units/Medicare Edits

Non-Facility RVU	Work	PE	MP	Total
33507	31.4	11.21	7.45	50.06
Facility RVU	**Work**	**PE**	**MP**	**Total**
33507	31.4	11.21	7.45	50.06

	FUD	Status	MUE	Modifiers				IOM Reference
33507	90	A	1(3)	51	N/A	62*	80	None

* with documentation

Heart and Pericardium

33508

+ 33508 Endoscopy, surgical, including video-assisted harvest of vein(s) for coronary artery bypass procedure (List separately in addition to code for primary procedure)

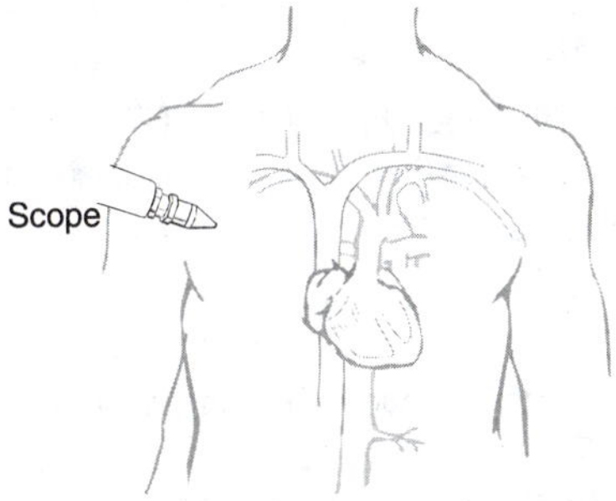

Surgical endoscopy is performed to harvest a suitable vein for coronary artery bypass surgery

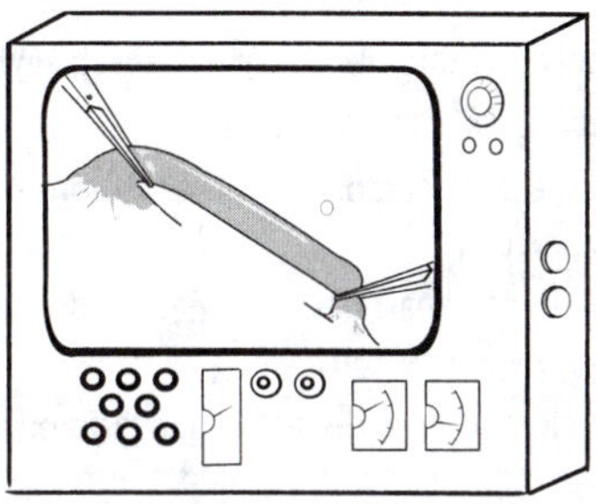

Monitor

Explanation

A surgical vascular endoscopy is done that includes video-assisted harvesting of a vein for a coronary artery bypass. The physician makes a portal incision above the saphenous vein. The endoscope is inserted into the incision and visualization occurs on a video monitor. CO2 gas is insufflated through the endoscope and dissection is made to the vein. A cannula is inserted and a portion of the vein to be removed is released from the surrounding structures. The vein is tied off above and below the portion of the vein to be removed. The vein is removed through the harvesting cannula. The endoscope is removed and the incision is closed with sutures and Steri-strips. The portion of the vein removed is prepared for use in cardiac bypass surgery.

Coding Tips

Report 33508 in addition to 33510–33523. For open harvest of an upper extremity vein, see 35500. For harvest of a femoropopliteal vein not using surgical endoscopy, see 35572.

ICD-10-CM Diagnostic Codes

This/these CPT code(s) are add on code(s). See the primary procedure code that this code is performed with for your ICD-10-CM code selections. Diagnostic code(s) would be the same as the actual procedure performed.

AMA: **33508** 1997,Nov,1

Relative Value Units/Medicare Edits

Non-Facility RVU	Work	PE	MP	Total
33508	0.31	0.09	0.07	0.47
Facility RVU	**Work**	**PE**	**MP**	**Total**
33508	0.31	0.09	0.07	0.47

	FUD	Status	MUE	Modifiers				IOM Reference
33508	N/A	A	1(2)	N/A	N/A	62*	80	None

* with documentation

Terms To Know

bypass graft. Surgically created alternative blood vessel used to reroute blood flow around an area of obstruction or disease.

cannula. Tube inserted into a blood vessel, duct, or body cavity to facilitate passage.

congestive heart failure. Condition caused by the heart's inability to adequately pump and circulate blood, resulting in fluid accumulation in the lungs and other tissues.

dissection. Separating by cutting tissue or body structures apart.

endoscopy. Visual inspection of the body using a fiberoptic scope.

graft. Tissue implant from another part of the body or another person.

harvest. Removal of cells or tissue from their native site to be used as a graft or transplant to another part of the donor's body or placed into another person.

incision. Act of cutting into tissue or an organ.

33510-33513

33510 Coronary artery bypass, vein only; single coronary venous graft
33511 2 coronary venous grafts
33512 3 coronary venous grafts
33513 4 coronary venous grafts

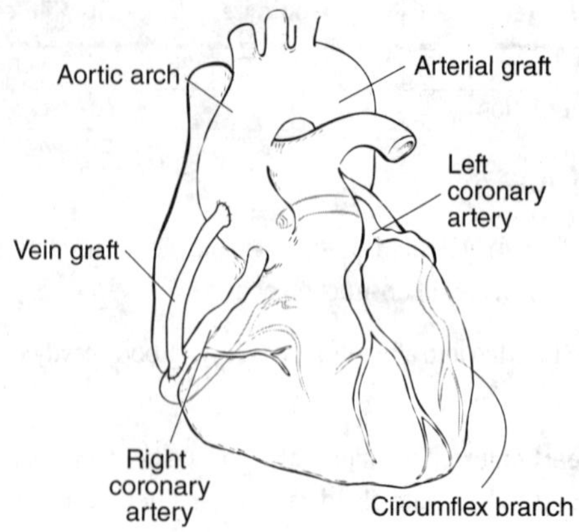

Schematic of a single vein graft bypass

Explanation

Cardiopulmonary bypass is initiated with a single, two-stage venous uptake tube. Saphenous vein is harvested from either leg. Vein may also be taken from the arm, the back of the leg, or from a cadaver. A clamp is placed on the aorta above the heart. Cold preserving solution is pumped through the coronary arteries to stop the heart. A point is chosen on the diseased coronary (arteries) beyond the area of disease and a longitudinal incision is cut in it. The proximal part (the part nearest the thigh) of the vein is trimmed to the same length as the cut in the coronary artery and is cleaned off. The end of the vein is sewn to the side of the coronary artery. A 3 mm to 6 mm hole is punched in the ascending aorta and the other end of the vein graft is sewn to this hole. The clamp on the aorta is released. Cardiopulmonary bypass is discontinued when heart function returns. Report 33511 if two coronary venous grafts are needed; report 33512 if three are needed; report 33513 if four are performed.

Coding Tips

These codes are not to be used to report coronary artery bypass graft (CABG) procedures with arterial grafts and venous grafts during the same procedure. See 33517–33523 and 33533–33536 for reporting combined arterial-venous grafts. Procurement of the saphenous vein graft is included in 33510–33513. When saphenous vein graft procurement is performed by a surgical assistant, add modifier 80 to 33510–33513. Procurement of arm vein is reported separately, see 35500. When coronary endarterectomy of the left anterior descending, circumflex, or right coronary artery is confirmed by the operative report, report 33572 in addition to 33510–33513. For reoperation more than one month after the original procedure, report 33530 in addition to the code for CABG procedure.

ICD-10-CM Diagnostic Codes

I20.0	Unstable angina
I20.1	Angina pectoris with documented spasm
I20.8	Other forms of angina pectoris
I21.01	ST elevation (STEMI) myocardial infarction involving left main coronary artery
I21.02	ST elevation (STEMI) myocardial infarction involving left anterior descending coronary artery
I21.09	ST elevation (STEMI) myocardial infarction involving other coronary artery of anterior wall
I21.11	ST elevation (STEMI) myocardial infarction involving right coronary artery
I21.19	ST elevation (STEMI) myocardial infarction involving other coronary artery of inferior wall
I21.21	ST elevation (STEMI) myocardial infarction involving left circumflex coronary artery
I21.29	ST elevation (STEMI) myocardial infarction involving other sites
I21.4	Non-ST elevation (NSTEMI) myocardial infarction
I21.A1	Myocardial infarction type 2
I22.0	Subsequent ST elevation (STEMI) myocardial infarction of anterior wall
I22.1	Subsequent ST elevation (STEMI) myocardial infarction of inferior wall
I22.2	Subsequent non-ST elevation (NSTEMI) myocardial infarction
I22.8	Subsequent ST elevation (STEMI) myocardial infarction of other sites
I24.0	Acute coronary thrombosis not resulting in myocardial infarction
I24.8	Other forms of acute ischemic heart disease
I25.10	Atherosclerotic heart disease of native coronary artery without angina pectoris
I25.110	Atherosclerotic heart disease of native coronary artery with unstable angina pectoris
I25.111	Atherosclerotic heart disease of native coronary artery with angina pectoris with documented spasm
I25.118	Atherosclerotic heart disease of native coronary artery with other forms of angina pectoris
I25.3	Aneurysm of heart
I25.41	Coronary artery aneurysm
I25.42	Coronary artery dissection
I25.5	Ischemic cardiomyopathy
I25.6	Silent myocardial ischemia
I25.710	Atherosclerosis of autologous vein coronary artery bypass graft(s) with unstable angina pectoris
I25.711	Atherosclerosis of autologous vein coronary artery bypass graft(s) with angina pectoris with documented spasm
I25.718	Atherosclerosis of autologous vein coronary artery bypass graft(s) with other forms of angina pectoris
I25.720	Atherosclerosis of autologous artery coronary artery bypass graft(s) with unstable angina pectoris
I25.721	Atherosclerosis of autologous artery coronary artery bypass graft(s) with angina pectoris with documented spasm
I25.728	Atherosclerosis of autologous artery coronary artery bypass graft(s) with other forms of angina pectoris
I25.730	Atherosclerosis of nonautologous biological coronary artery bypass graft(s) with unstable angina pectoris
I25.731	Atherosclerosis of nonautologous biological coronary artery bypass graft(s) with angina pectoris with documented spasm
I25.738	Atherosclerosis of nonautologous biological coronary artery bypass graft(s) with other forms of angina pectoris
I25.750	Atherosclerosis of native coronary artery of transplanted heart with unstable angina
I25.751	Atherosclerosis of native coronary artery of transplanted heart with angina pectoris with documented spasm

I25.758 Atherosclerosis of native coronary artery of transplanted heart with other forms of angina pectoris
I25.760 Atherosclerosis of bypass graft of coronary artery of transplanted heart with unstable angina
I25.761 Atherosclerosis of bypass graft of coronary artery of transplanted heart with angina pectoris with documented spasm
I25.768 Atherosclerosis of bypass graft of coronary artery of transplanted heart with other forms of angina pectoris
I25.790 Atherosclerosis of other coronary artery bypass graft(s) with unstable angina pectoris
I25.791 Atherosclerosis of other coronary artery bypass graft(s) with angina pectoris with documented spasm
I25.798 Atherosclerosis of other coronary artery bypass graft(s) with other forms of angina pectoris
I25.810 Atherosclerosis of coronary artery bypass graft(s) without angina pectoris
I25.811 Atherosclerosis of native coronary artery of transplanted heart without angina pectoris
I25.812 Atherosclerosis of bypass graft of coronary artery of transplanted heart without angina pectoris
I25.82 Chronic total occlusion of coronary artery
I25.83 Coronary atherosclerosis due to lipid rich plaque
I25.84 Coronary atherosclerosis due to calcified coronary lesion
I25.89 Other forms of chronic ischemic heart disease
I45.6 Pre-excitation syndrome
I50.1 Left ventricular failure, unspecified
I50.21 Acute systolic (congestive) heart failure
I50.22 Chronic systolic (congestive) heart failure
I50.23 Acute on chronic systolic (congestive) heart failure
I50.31 Acute diastolic (congestive) heart failure
I50.32 Chronic diastolic (congestive) heart failure
I50.33 Acute on chronic diastolic (congestive) heart failure
I50.41 Acute combined systolic (congestive) and diastolic (congestive) heart failure
I50.42 Chronic combined systolic (congestive) and diastolic (congestive) heart failure
I50.43 Acute on chronic combined systolic (congestive) and diastolic (congestive) heart failure
I50.811 Acute right heart failure
I50.812 Chronic right heart failure
I50.813 Acute on chronic right heart failure
I50.814 Right heart failure due to left heart failure
I50.82 Biventricular heart failure
I50.83 High output heart failure
I50.84 End stage heart failure
Q24.5 Malformation of coronary vessels
Q26.2 Total anomalous pulmonary venous connection

AMA: 33510 2018,Jan,8; 2017,Jan,8; 2017,Dec,3; 2016,Jan,13; 2015,Jan,16; 2014,Jan,11; 2014,Aug,14 **33511** 2018,Jan,8; 2017,Jan,8; 2017,Dec,3; 2016,Jan,13; 2015,Jan,16; 2014,Jan,11; 2014,Aug,14 **33512** 2018,Jan,8; 2017,Jan,8; 2017,Dec,3; 2016,Jan,13; 2015,Jan,16; 2014,Jan,11; 2014,Aug,14 **33513** 2018,Jan,8; 2017,Jan,8; 2017,Dec,3; 2016,Jan,13; 2015,Jan,16; 2014,Jan,11; 2014,Aug,14

Relative Value Units/Medicare Edits

Non-Facility RVU	Work	PE	MP	Total
33510	34.98	13.07	7.9	55.95
33511	38.45	14.3	8.7	61.45
33512	43.98	16.0	9.99	69.97
33513	45.37	16.28	10.41	72.06
Facility RVU	**Work**	**PE**	**MP**	**Total**
33510	34.98	13.07	7.9	55.95
33511	38.45	14.3	8.7	61.45
33512	43.98	16.0	9.99	69.97
33513	45.37	16.28	10.41	72.06

	FUD	Status	MUE	Modifiers				IOM Reference
33510	90	A	1(2)	51	N/A	N/A	80	None
33511	90	A	1(2)	51	N/A	N/A	80	
33512	90	A	1(2)	51	N/A	N/A	80	
33513	90	A	1(2)	51	N/A	N/A	80	

* with documentation

Terms To Know

atherosclerosis. Buildup of yellowish plaques composed of cholesterol and lipoid material within the arteries.

bypass graft. Surgically created alternative blood vessel used to reroute blood flow around an area of obstruction or disease.

cardiopulmonary bypass. Venous blood is diverted to a heart-lung machine, which mechanically pumps and oxygenates the blood temporarily so the heart can be bypassed while an open procedure on the heart or coronary arteries is performed. During bypass, the lungs are deflated and immobile.

harvest. Removal of cells or tissue from their native site to be used as a graft or transplant to another part of the donor's body or placed into another person.

33514-33516

33514 Coronary artery bypass, vein only; 5 coronary venous grafts
33516 6 or more coronary venous grafts

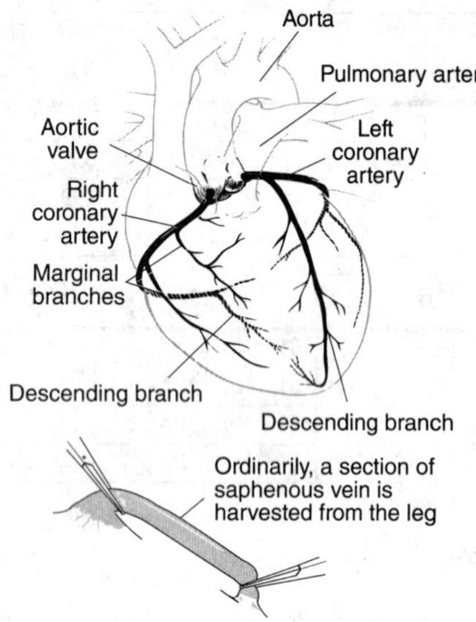

Explanation

Cardiopulmonary bypass is initiated with a single, two-stage venous uptake tube. Saphenous vein is harvested from either leg. Vein may also be taken from the arm, the back of the leg, or from a cadaver. A clamp is placed on the aorta above the heart. Cold preserving solution is pumped through the coronary arteries to stop the heart. A point is chosen on the diseased coronary (arteries) beyond the area of disease and a longitudinal incision is cut in it. The proximal part (the part nearest the thigh) of the vein is trimmed to the same length as the cut in the coronary artery and is cleaned off. The end of the vein is sewn to the side of the coronary artery. A 3 mm to 6 mm hole is punched in the ascending aorta and the other end of the vein graft is sewn to this hole. The clamp on the aorta is released. Cardiopulmonary bypass is discontinued when heart function returns. Report 33514 if five are performed; report 33516 if six or more are performed.

Coding Tips

To report coronary venous grafts, single and up to four, see 33510–33513. These codes are not to be used to report coronary artery bypass graft (CABG) procedures with arterial grafts and venous grafts during the same procedure. See 33517–33523 and 33533–33536 for reporting combined arterial-venous grafts. Procurement of the saphenous vein graft is included in 33514–33516. When saphenous vein graft procurement is performed by a surgical assistant, add modifier 80 to 33514–33516. Procurement of arm vein is reported separately, see 35500. When coronary endarterectomy of the left anterior descending, circumflex, or right coronary artery is confirmed by the operative report, report 33572 in addition to 33514–33516. For reoperation more than one month after the original procedure, report 33530 in addition to the code for CABG procedure.

ICD-10-CM Diagnostic Codes

I20.0	Unstable angina
I20.1	Angina pectoris with documented spasm
I20.8	Other forms of angina pectoris
I21.01	ST elevation (STEMI) myocardial infarction involving left main coronary artery
I21.02	ST elevation (STEMI) myocardial infarction involving left anterior descending coronary artery
I21.09	ST elevation (STEMI) myocardial infarction involving other coronary artery of anterior wall
I21.11	ST elevation (STEMI) myocardial infarction involving right coronary artery
I21.19	ST elevation (STEMI) myocardial infarction involving other coronary artery of inferior wall
I21.21	ST elevation (STEMI) myocardial infarction involving left circumflex coronary artery
I21.29	ST elevation (STEMI) myocardial infarction involving other sites
I21.4	Non-ST elevation (NSTEMI) myocardial infarction
I21.A1	Myocardial infarction type 2
I22.0	Subsequent ST elevation (STEMI) myocardial infarction of anterior wall
I22.1	Subsequent ST elevation (STEMI) myocardial infarction of inferior wall
I22.2	Subsequent non-ST elevation (NSTEMI) myocardial infarction
I22.8	Subsequent ST elevation (STEMI) myocardial infarction of other sites
I24.0	Acute coronary thrombosis not resulting in myocardial infarction
I24.8	Other forms of acute ischemic heart disease
I25.110	Atherosclerotic heart disease of native coronary artery with unstable angina pectoris
I25.111	Atherosclerotic heart disease of native coronary artery with angina pectoris with documented spasm
I25.118	Atherosclerotic heart disease of native coronary artery with other forms of angina pectoris
I25.3	Aneurysm of heart
I25.41	Coronary artery aneurysm
I25.42	Coronary artery dissection
I25.5	Ischemic cardiomyopathy
I25.6	Silent myocardial ischemia
I25.710	Atherosclerosis of autologous vein coronary artery bypass graft(s) with unstable angina pectoris
I25.711	Atherosclerosis of autologous vein coronary artery bypass graft(s) with angina pectoris with documented spasm
I25.718	Atherosclerosis of autologous vein coronary artery bypass graft(s) with other forms of angina pectoris
I25.720	Atherosclerosis of autologous artery coronary artery bypass graft(s) with unstable angina pectoris
I25.721	Atherosclerosis of autologous artery coronary artery bypass graft(s) with angina pectoris with documented spasm
I25.728	Atherosclerosis of autologous artery coronary artery bypass graft(s) with other forms of angina pectoris
I25.730	Atherosclerosis of nonautologous biological coronary artery bypass graft(s) with unstable angina pectoris
I25.731	Atherosclerosis of nonautologous biological coronary artery bypass graft(s) with angina pectoris with documented spasm
I25.738	Atherosclerosis of nonautologous biological coronary artery bypass graft(s) with other forms of angina pectoris
I25.750	Atherosclerosis of native coronary artery of transplanted heart with unstable angina
I25.751	Atherosclerosis of native coronary artery of transplanted heart with angina pectoris with documented spasm

I25.758	Atherosclerosis of native coronary artery of transplanted heart with other forms of angina pectoris
I25.760	Atherosclerosis of bypass graft of coronary artery of transplanted heart with unstable angina
I25.761	Atherosclerosis of bypass graft of coronary artery of transplanted heart with angina pectoris with documented spasm
I25.768	Atherosclerosis of bypass graft of coronary artery of transplanted heart with other forms of angina pectoris
I25.790	Atherosclerosis of other coronary artery bypass graft(s) with unstable angina pectoris
I25.791	Atherosclerosis of other coronary artery bypass graft(s) with angina pectoris with documented spasm
I25.798	Atherosclerosis of other coronary artery bypass graft(s) with other forms of angina pectoris
I25.810	Atherosclerosis of coronary artery bypass graft(s) without angina pectoris
I25.811	Atherosclerosis of native coronary artery of transplanted heart without angina pectoris
I25.812	Atherosclerosis of bypass graft of coronary artery of transplanted heart without angina pectoris
I25.82	Chronic total occlusion of coronary artery
I25.83	Coronary atherosclerosis due to lipid rich plaque
I25.84	Coronary atherosclerosis due to calcified coronary lesion
I25.89	Other forms of chronic ischemic heart disease
I45.6	Pre-excitation syndrome
I50.1	Left ventricular failure, unspecified
I50.21	Acute systolic (congestive) heart failure
I50.22	Chronic systolic (congestive) heart failure
I50.23	Acute on chronic systolic (congestive) heart failure
I50.31	Acute diastolic (congestive) heart failure
I50.32	Chronic diastolic (congestive) heart failure
I50.33	Acute on chronic diastolic (congestive) heart failure
I50.41	Acute combined systolic (congestive) and diastolic (congestive) heart failure
I50.42	Chronic combined systolic (congestive) and diastolic (congestive) heart failure
I50.43	Acute on chronic combined systolic (congestive) and diastolic (congestive) heart failure
I50.811	Acute right heart failure
I50.812	Chronic right heart failure
I50.813	Acute on chronic right heart failure
I50.814	Right heart failure due to left heart failure
I50.82	Biventricular heart failure
I50.83	High output heart failure
I50.84	End stage heart failure
Q24.5	Malformation of coronary vessels
Q26.2	Total anomalous pulmonary venous connection

AMA: **33514** 2018,Jan,8; 2017,Jan,8; 2017,Dec,3; 2016,Jan,13; 2015,Jan,16; 2014,Jan,11; 2014,Aug,14 **33516** 2018,Jan,8; 2017,Jan,8; 2017,Dec,3; 2016,Jan,13; 2015,Jan,16; 2014,Jan,11; 2014,Aug,14

Relative Value Units/Medicare Edits

Non-Facility RVU	Work	PE	MP	Total
33514	48.08	16.87	10.82	75.77
33516	49.76	17.46	11.77	78.99
Facility RVU	**Work**	**PE**	**MP**	**Total**
33514	48.08	16.87	10.82	75.77
33516	49.76	17.46	11.77	78.99

	FUD	Status	MUE	Modifiers				IOM Reference
33514	90	A	1(2)	51	N/A	N/A	80	None
33516	90	A	1(2)	51	N/A	N/A	80	

* with documentation

Terms To Know

cadaver. Dead body.

cardiopulmonary bypass. Venous blood is diverted to a heart-lung machine, which mechanically pumps and oxygenates the blood temporarily so the heart can be bypassed while an open procedure on the heart or coronary arteries is performed. During bypass, the lungs are deflated and immobile.

graft. Tissue implant from another part of the body or another person.

harvest. Removal of cells or tissue from their native site to be used as a graft or transplant to another part of the donor's body or placed into another person.

33517-33519

+ 33517 Coronary artery bypass, using venous graft(s) and arterial graft(s); single vein graft (List separately in addition to code for primary procedure)

+ 33518 2 venous grafts (List separately in addition to code for primary procedure)

+ 33519 3 venous grafts (List separately in addition to code for primary procedure)

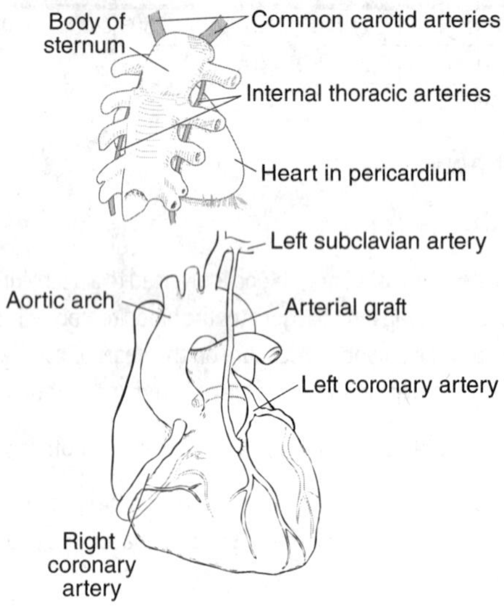

Explanation

The physician initiates cardiopulmonary bypass with a single, two-stage venous uptake tube. The physician harvests saphenous vein from the legs. Other vein grafts may be obtained from the arms, backs of the legs, or cadavers (organ donors). These sources are inferior to the saphenous vein. Arterial grafts may be obtained from the internal mammary artery (along the lateral side of the breastbone), the gastroepiploic artery (from the abdomen), the inferior epigastric artery (from the abdominal wall), or the radial artery (from the nondominant hand). The most commonly used vessel is the internal mammary artery. It is left connected at one end to the subclavian artery from which it arises. Report 33517 for a single vein graft, 33518 if two venous grafts are performed, and 33519 if three venous grafts are performed.

Coding Tips

These codes report combined arterial-venous grafting for coronary bypass and should be reported in addition to the code(s) for the primary procedure(s). To report combined arterial-venous grafts, it is necessary to report two codes: 1) the appropriate combined arterial-venous graft code (33517–33523); and 2) the appropriate arterial graft code (33533–33536). If venous grafting only is performed, see 33510–33516. If arterial grafting only is performed, see 33533–33536. Procurement of saphenous vein graft is included in 33517–33519. When a surgical assistant performs graft procurement, append modifier 80 to 33517–33519. Report procurement of upper extremity vein separately, see 35500. When coronary endarterectomy of the left anterior descending, circumflex, or right coronary artery is confirmed by the operative report, report 33572 in addition to 33513–33516. For reoperation more than one month after the original procedure, report 33530 in addition to the code for CABG procedure.

ICD-10-CM Diagnostic Codes

This/these CPT code(s) are add on code(s). See the primary procedure code that this code is performed with for your ICD-10-CM code selections. Diagnostic code(s) would be the same as the actual procedure performed.

AMA: **33517** 2018,Jan,8; 2017,Jan,8; 2016,Jan,13; 2015,Jan,16; 2014,Jan,11 **33518** 2018,Jan,8; 2017,Jan,8; 2016,Jan,13; 2015,Jan,16; 2014,Jan,11 **33519** 2018,Jan,8; 2017,Jan,8; 2016,Jan,13; 2015,Jan,16; 2014,Jan,11

Relative Value Units/Medicare Edits

Non-Facility RVU	Work	PE	MP	Total
33517	3.61	1.0	0.8	5.41
33518	7.93	2.21	1.79	11.93
33519	10.49	2.92	2.37	15.78
Facility RVU	**Work**	**PE**	**MP**	**Total**
33517	3.61	1.0	0.8	5.41
33518	7.93	2.21	1.79	11.93
33519	10.49	2.92	2.37	15.78

	FUD	Status	MUE	Modifiers				IOM Reference
33517	N/A	A	1(2)	N/A	N/A	N/A	80	None
33518	N/A	A	1(2)	N/A	N/A	N/A	80	
33519	N/A	A	1(2)	N/A	N/A	N/A	80	

* with documentation

Terms To Know

cardiopulmonary bypass. Venous blood is diverted to a heart-lung machine, which mechanically pumps and oxygenates the blood temporarily so the heart can be bypassed while an open procedure on the heart or coronary arteries is performed. During bypass, the lungs are deflated and immobile.

myocardial infarction. Obstruction of circulation to the heart, resulting in necrosis.

occlusion. Constriction, closure, or blockage of a passage.

Heart and Pericardium

33521-33523

\+ **33521** Coronary artery bypass, using venous graft(s) and arterial graft(s); 4 venous grafts (List separately in addition to code for primary procedure)

\+ **33522** 5 venous grafts (List separately in addition to code for primary procedure)

\+ **33523** 6 or more venous grafts (List separately in addition to code for primary procedure)

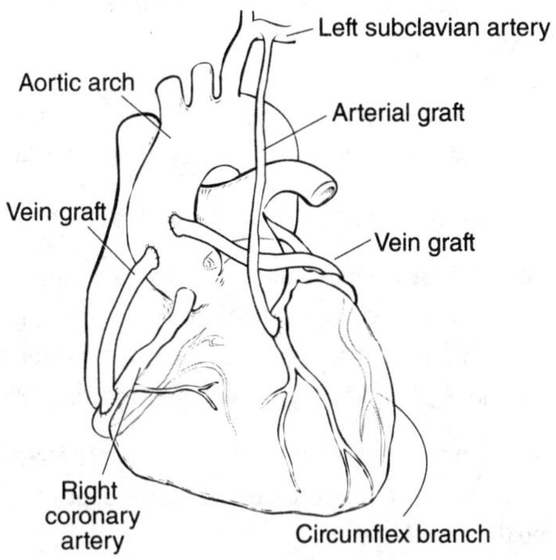

Explanation

The physician initiates cardiopulmonary bypass with a single, two-stage venous uptake tube. The physician harvests saphenous vein from the legs. Other vein grafts may be obtained from the arms, backs of the legs, or cadavers (organ donors). These sources are inferior to the saphenous vein. Arterial grafts may be obtained from the internal mammary artery (along the lateral side of the breastbone), the gastroepiploic artery (from the abdomen), the inferior epigastric artery (from the abdominal wall), or the radial artery (from the nondominant hand). The most commonly used vessel is the internal mammary artery. It is left connected at one end to the subclavian artery from which it arises. Report 33521 if four venous grafts are performed, 33522 if five venous grafts are performed, and 33523 if six or more venous grafts are performed.

Coding Tips

These codes report combined arterial-venous grafting for coronary bypass and should be reported in addition to the code(s) for the primary procedure(s). To report combined arterial-venous grafts, it is necessary to report two codes: 1) the appropriate combined arterial-venous graft code (33517–33523); and 2) the appropriate arterial graft code (33533–33536). If venous grafting only is performed, see 33510–33516. If arterial grafting only is performed, see 33533–33536. Procurement of saphenous vein graft is included in 33521–33523. When a surgical assistant performs graft procurement, append modifier 80 to 33521–33523. Report procurement of upper extremity vein separately, see 35500. When coronary endarterectomy of the left anterior descending, circumflex, or right coronary artery is confirmed by the operative report, report 33572 in addition to 33513–33516. For reoperation more than one month after the original procedure, report 33530 in addition to the code for CABG procedure.

ICD-10-CM Diagnostic Codes

This/these CPT code(s) are add on code(s). See the primary procedure code that this code is performed with for your ICD-10-CM code selections. Diagnostic code(s) would be the same as the actual procedure performed.

AMA: **33521** 2018,Jan,8; 2017,Jan,8; 2016,Jan,13; 2015,Jan,16; 2014,Jan,11 **33522** 2018,Jan,8; 2017,Jan,8; 2016,Jan,13; 2015,Jan,16; 2014,Jan,11 **33523** 2018,Jan,8; 2017,Jan,8; 2016,Jan,13; 2015,Jan,16; 2014,Jan,11

Relative Value Units/Medicare Edits

Non-Facility RVU	Work	PE	MP	Total
33521	12.59	3.49	2.85	18.93
33522	14.14	3.91	3.21	21.26
33523	16.08	4.34	3.58	24.0
Facility RVU	**Work**	**PE**	**MP**	**Total**
33521	12.59	3.49	2.85	18.93
33522	14.14	3.91	3.21	21.26
33523	16.08	4.34	3.58	24.0

	FUD	Status	MUE	Modifiers				IOM Reference
33521	N/A	A	1(2)	N/A	N/A	N/A	80	None
33522	N/A	A	1(2)	N/A	N/A	N/A	80	
33523	N/A	A	1(2)	N/A	N/A	N/A	80	

* with documentation

Terms To Know

cardiopulmonary bypass. Venous blood is diverted to a heart-lung machine, which mechanically pumps and oxygenates the blood temporarily so the heart can be bypassed while an open procedure on the heart or coronary arteries is performed. During bypass, the lungs are deflated and immobile.

graft. Tissue implant from another part of the body or another person.

insufficiency. Inadequate closure of the valve that allows abnormal backward blood flow.

occlusion. Constriction, closure, or blockage of a passage.

venous. Relating to the veins.

33530

\+ **33530** Reoperation, coronary artery bypass procedure or valve procedure, more than 1 month after original operation (List separately in addition to code for primary procedure)

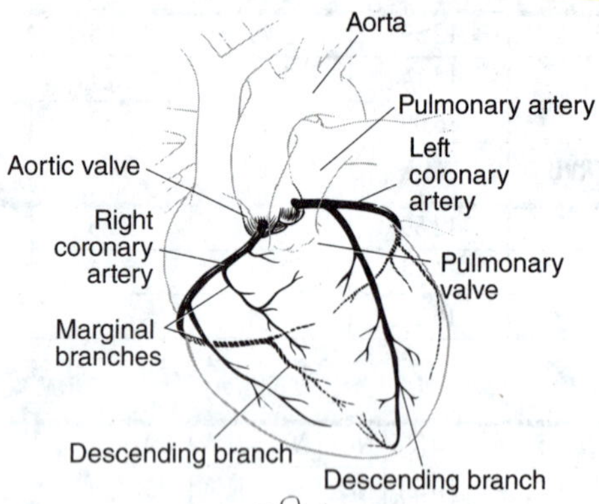

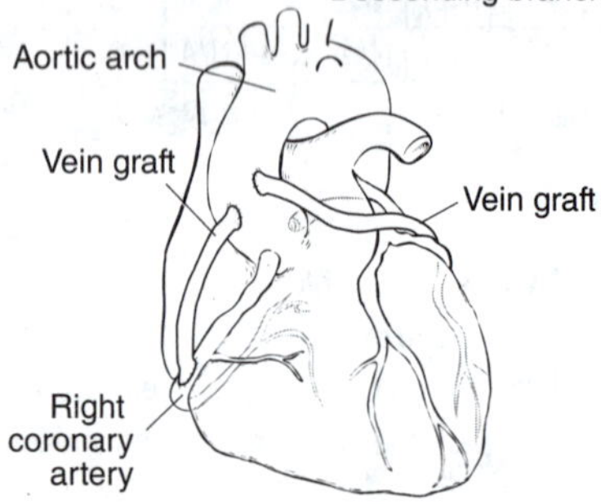

Explanation

For descriptions of the actual therapeutic procedure to be performed, please see the description of that procedure. The breast bone must be split again. Because the heart is invariably tightly adherent to the underside of the sternum in a redo operation, a vibrating saw is used to cut through it. After the sternum is cut, its halves are gently retracted while the tissues that have adhered to its undersurface are carefully cut down. Once the sternum can be opened, the heart is exposed by cutting any chest tissues that have adhered to it since the last operation. It is usually necessary to initiate cardiopulmonary bypass before the heart is completely cleaned off.

Coding Tips

Report 33530 in addition to 33390–33391, 33404–33496, 33510–33536, and 33863.

ICD-10-CM Diagnostic Codes

This/these CPT code(s) are add on code(s). See the primary procedure code that this code is performed with for your ICD-10-CM code selections. Diagnostic code(s) would be the same as the actual procedure performed.

AMA: 33530 2018,Jan,8; 2017,Jan,8; 2016,Jan,13; 2015,Jan,16; 2014,Jan,11

Relative Value Units/Medicare Edits

Non-Facility RVU	Work	PE	MP	Total
33530	10.13	2.82	2.3	15.25
Facility RVU	**Work**	**PE**	**MP**	**Total**
33530	10.13	2.82	2.3	15.25

	FUD	Status	MUE	Modifiers				IOM Reference
33530	N/A	A	1(2)	N/A	N/A	N/A	80	None

* with documentation

Terms To Know

adhesion. Abnormal fibrous connection between two structures, soft tissue or bony structures, that may occur as the result of surgery, infection, or trauma.

bypass. Auxiliary or diverted route to maintain continuous flow.

cardiopulmonary bypass. Venous blood is diverted to a heart-lung machine, which mechanically pumps and oxygenates the blood temporarily so the heart can be bypassed while an open procedure on the heart or coronary arteries is performed. During bypass, the lungs are deflated and immobile.

coronary atherosclerosis. Chronic condition marked by thickening and loss of elasticity of the coronary artery, caused by deposits of plaque containing cholesterol, lipoid material, and lipophages.

manubrium. Sternum.

occlusion. Constriction, closure, or blockage of a passage.

retraction. Act of holding tissue or a structure back away from its normal position or the field of interest.

CABG

33533-33536

33533 Coronary artery bypass, using arterial graft(s); single arterial graft
33534 2 coronary arterial grafts
33535 3 coronary arterial grafts
33536 4 or more coronary arterial grafts

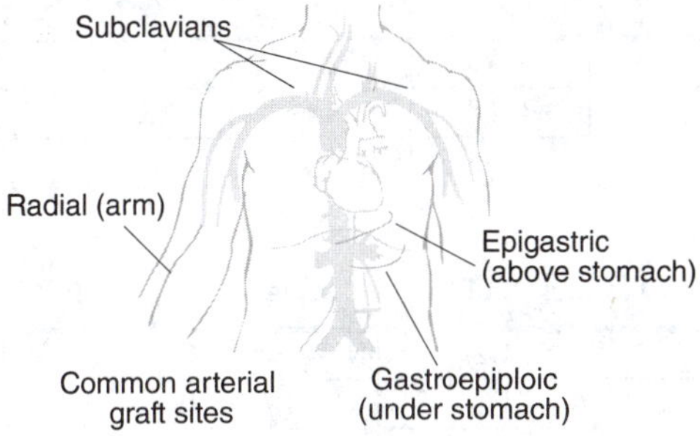

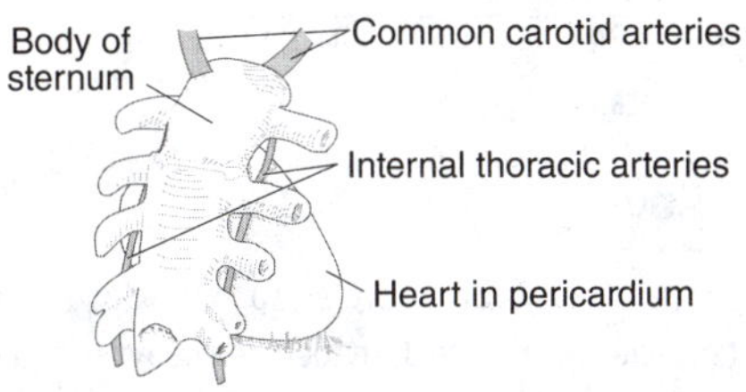

Explanation

Cardiopulmonary bypass is initiated with a single, two-stage venous uptake tube. Arterial grafts may be obtained from the internal mammary artery (along the lateral side of the breastbone), the gastroepiploic artery (from the abdomen), the inferior epigastric artery (from the abdominal wall), or the radial artery (from the non-dominant hand). The most commonly used vessel is the internal mammary artery. It is left connected at one end to the arm artery from which it arises. Report 33534 if two arterial grafts are placed; report 33535 if three are placed; report 33536 if four or more are placed.

Coding Tips

These codes are used to report coronary artery bypass graft (CABG) procedures using either arterial grafts only or combined arterial-venous grafts. To report combined arterial-venous grafts, it is necessary to use two codes: 1) the appropriate arterial graft (33533–33536); and 2) the appropriate combined arterial-venous graft code (33517–33523). Note that 33533–33536 includes the use of the internal mammary artery, gastroepiploic artery, epigastric artery, and arterial conduits procured from other sites except the upper extremity. If a surgical assistant performs arterial graft procurement from these sites, report 33533–33536 and append modifier 80 as appropriate. Procurement of an upper extremity artery graft, including the radial artery or other upper extremity artery, is reported separately, see 35600. Report 33572 with 33533–33536 when coronary endarterectomy of the left anterior descending, circumflex, or right coronary artery is confirmed by the operative report. For reoperation more than one month after the original procedure, report 33530 in addition to the code for CABG procedure.

ICD-10-CM Diagnostic Codes

I20.0	Unstable angina
I20.1	Angina pectoris with documented spasm
I20.8	Other forms of angina pectoris
I21.01	ST elevation (STEMI) myocardial infarction involving left main coronary artery
I21.02	ST elevation (STEMI) myocardial infarction involving left anterior descending coronary artery
I21.09	ST elevation (STEMI) myocardial infarction involving other coronary artery of anterior wall
I21.11	ST elevation (STEMI) myocardial infarction involving right coronary artery
I21.19	ST elevation (STEMI) myocardial infarction involving other coronary artery of inferior wall
I21.21	ST elevation (STEMI) myocardial infarction involving left circumflex coronary artery
I21.29	ST elevation (STEMI) myocardial infarction involving other sites
I21.4	Non-ST elevation (NSTEMI) myocardial infarction
I21.A1	Myocardial infarction type 2
I22.0	Subsequent ST elevation (STEMI) myocardial infarction of anterior wall
I22.1	Subsequent ST elevation (STEMI) myocardial infarction of inferior wall
I22.2	Subsequent non-ST elevation (NSTEMI) myocardial infarction
I22.8	Subsequent ST elevation (STEMI) myocardial infarction of other sites
I24.0	Acute coronary thrombosis not resulting in myocardial infarction
I24.8	Other forms of acute ischemic heart disease
I25.110	Atherosclerotic heart disease of native coronary artery with unstable angina pectoris
I25.111	Atherosclerotic heart disease of native coronary artery with angina pectoris with documented spasm
I25.118	Atherosclerotic heart disease of native coronary artery with other forms of angina pectoris
I25.3	Aneurysm of heart
I25.41	Coronary artery aneurysm
I25.42	Coronary artery dissection
I25.5	Ischemic cardiomyopathy
I25.6	Silent myocardial ischemia
I25.710	Atherosclerosis of autologous vein coronary artery bypass graft(s) with unstable angina pectoris
I25.711	Atherosclerosis of autologous vein coronary artery bypass graft(s) with angina pectoris with documented spasm
I25.718	Atherosclerosis of autologous vein coronary artery bypass graft(s) with other forms of angina pectoris
I25.720	Atherosclerosis of autologous artery coronary artery bypass graft(s) with unstable angina pectoris
I25.721	Atherosclerosis of autologous artery coronary artery bypass graft(s) with angina pectoris with documented spasm
I25.728	Atherosclerosis of autologous artery coronary artery bypass graft(s) with other forms of angina pectoris
I25.730	Atherosclerosis of nonautologous biological coronary artery bypass graft(s) with unstable angina pectoris
I25.731	Atherosclerosis of nonautologous biological coronary artery bypass graft(s) with angina pectoris with documented spasm
I25.738	Atherosclerosis of nonautologous biological coronary artery bypass graft(s) with other forms of angina pectoris
I25.750	Atherosclerosis of native coronary artery of transplanted heart with unstable angina
I25.751	Atherosclerosis of native coronary artery of transplanted heart with angina pectoris with documented spasm

I25.758	Atherosclerosis of native coronary artery of transplanted heart with other forms of angina pectoris
I25.760	Atherosclerosis of bypass graft of coronary artery of transplanted heart with unstable angina
I25.761	Atherosclerosis of bypass graft of coronary artery of transplanted heart with angina pectoris with documented spasm
I25.768	Atherosclerosis of bypass graft of coronary artery of transplanted heart with other forms of angina pectoris
I25.790	Atherosclerosis of other coronary artery bypass graft(s) with unstable angina pectoris
I25.791	Atherosclerosis of other coronary artery bypass graft(s) with angina pectoris with documented spasm
I25.798	Atherosclerosis of other coronary artery bypass graft(s) with other forms of angina pectoris
I25.810	Atherosclerosis of coronary artery bypass graft(s) without angina pectoris
I25.811	Atherosclerosis of native coronary artery of transplanted heart without angina pectoris
I25.812	Atherosclerosis of bypass graft of coronary artery of transplanted heart without angina pectoris
I25.82	Chronic total occlusion of coronary artery
I25.83	Coronary atherosclerosis due to lipid rich plaque
I25.84	Coronary atherosclerosis due to calcified coronary lesion
I25.89	Other forms of chronic ischemic heart disease
I50.1	Left ventricular failure, unspecified
I50.21	Acute systolic (congestive) heart failure
I50.22	Chronic systolic (congestive) heart failure
I50.23	Acute on chronic systolic (congestive) heart failure
I50.31	Acute diastolic (congestive) heart failure
I50.32	Chronic diastolic (congestive) heart failure
I50.33	Acute on chronic diastolic (congestive) heart failure
I50.41	Acute combined systolic (congestive) and diastolic (congestive) heart failure
I50.42	Chronic combined systolic (congestive) and diastolic (congestive) heart failure
I50.43	Acute on chronic combined systolic (congestive) and diastolic (congestive) heart failure
I50.811	Acute right heart failure
I50.812	Chronic right heart failure
I50.813	Acute on chronic right heart failure
I50.814	Right heart failure due to left heart failure
I50.82	Biventricular heart failure
I50.83	High output heart failure
I50.84	End stage heart failure
Q24.5	Malformation of coronary vessels
Q26.2	Total anomalous pulmonary venous connection

AMA: **33533** 2018,Jan,8; 2017,Jan,8; 2017,Dec,3; 2016,Jan,13; 2015,Jan,16; 2014,Nov,14; 2014,Jan,11 **33534** 2018,Jan,8; 2017,Jan,8; 2017,Dec,3; 2016,Jan,13; 2015,Jan,16; 2014,Jan,11 **33535** 2018,Jan,8; 2017,Jan,8; 2017,Dec,3; 2016,Jan,13; 2015,Jan,16; 2014,Jan,11 **33536** 2018,Jan,8; 2017,Jan,8; 2017,Dec,3; 2016,Jan,13; 2015,Jan,16; 2014,Nov,14; 2014,Jan,11

Relative Value Units/Medicare Edits

Non-Facility RVU	Work	PE	MP	Total
33533	33.75	12.72	7.62	54.09
33534	39.88	14.69	9.05	63.62
33535	44.75	16.07	10.16	70.98
33536	48.43	17.06	10.62	76.11
Facility RVU	**Work**	**PE**	**MP**	**Total**
33533	33.75	12.72	7.62	54.09
33534	39.88	14.69	9.05	63.62
33535	44.75	16.07	10.16	70.98
33536	48.43	17.06	10.62	76.11

	FUD	Status	MUE	Modifiers				IOM Reference
33533	90	A	1(2)	51	N/A	N/A	80	None
33534	90	A	1(2)	51	N/A	N/A	80	
33535	90	A	1(2)	51	N/A	N/A	80	
33536	90	A	1(2)	51	N/A	N/A	80	

* with documentation

Terms To Know

angina. Chest pain that occurs secondary to the inadequate delivery of oxygen to the heart muscle and may be described as a heavy or squeezing pain in the midsternal area of the chest.

bypass. Auxiliary or diverted route to maintain continuous flow.

dissection. (dis. apart; -section, act of cutting) Separating by cutting tissue or body structures apart.

myocardial infarction. Obstruction of circulation to the heart, resulting in necrosis.

33542

33542 Myocardial resection (eg, ventricular aneurysmectomy)

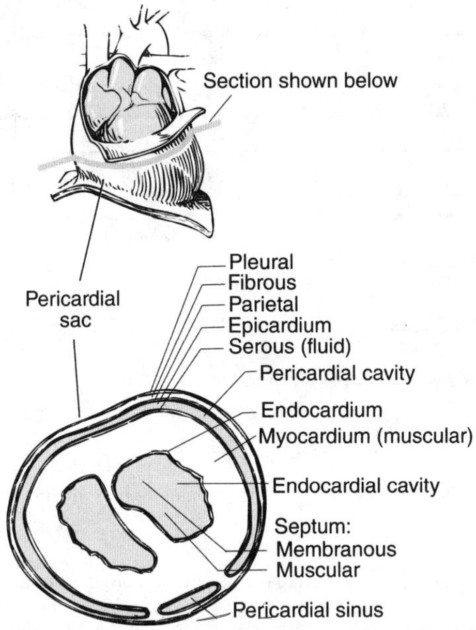

The myocardium is the muscle tissue of the heart

Explanation

This operation is almost always done in conjunction with coronary artery bypass grafting. Prior to placing the bypass grafts, the aneurysm is opened and any clot is removed from the ventricle. The aneurysm is opened widely and damaged tissue is removed from the ventricular wall. The ventricle is repaired by suturing the walls of the ventricle back together directly or with a patch of Gortex, Dacron, or other appropriate material sewn into the defect. All stitches are placed in healthy (not aneurysm) heart tissue and care is taken to avoid the coronary arteries.

Coding Tips

Ventricular aneurysms are usually a complication of myocardial infarction, but may also be caused by bacterial endocarditis or trauma. For ablation of ventricular arrhythmogenic focus to control a ventricular arrhythmia, see 33261. For ventriculomyotomy (-myectomy) for idiopathic hypertrophic subaortic stenosis, see 33416. For excision of an intracardiac tumor without myocardial resection, see 33120. For excision of an external cardiac tumor without myocardial resection, see 33130.

ICD-10-CM Diagnostic Codes

I25.3 Aneurysm of heart

AMA: 33542 2018,Jan,8; 2017,Jan,8; 2017,Dec,3; 2016,Jan,13; 2015,Jan,16; 2014,Jan,11

Relative Value Units/Medicare Edits

Non-Facility RVU	Work	PE	MP	Total
33542	48.21	16.85	11.14	76.2
Facility RVU	**Work**	**PE**	**MP**	**Total**
33542	48.21	16.85	11.14	76.2

	FUD	Status	MUE	Modifiers				IOM Reference
33542	90	A	1(2)	51	N/A	62*	80	None

* with documentation

Terms To Know

aneurysm. Circumscribed dilation or outpouching of an artery wall, often containing blood clots and connecting directly with the lumen of the artery.

bypass graft. Surgically created alternative blood vessel used to reroute blood flow around an area of obstruction or disease.

cardiomegaly. Enlargement of the heart due to a thickened heart muscle or an enlarged heart chamber. Cardiomegaly is a result of the heart having to work harder than normal.

endocarditis. Inflammatory disease of the interior lining of the heart chamber and heart valves.

excision. Surgical removal of an organ or tissue.

hypertrophic. Enlarged or overgrown from an increase in cell size of the affected tissue.

lesion. Area of damaged tissue that has lost continuity or function, due to disease or trauma. Lesions may be located on internal structures such as the brain, nerves, or kidneys, or visible on the skin.

myocardial infarction. Obstruction of circulation to the heart, resulting in necrosis.

resection. Surgical removal of a part or all of an organ or body part.

stenosis. Narrowing or constriction of a passage.

tumor. Pathological swelling or enlargement; a neoplastic growth of uncontrolled, abnormal multiplication of cells.

33545

33545 Repair of postinfarction ventricular septal defect, with or without myocardial resection

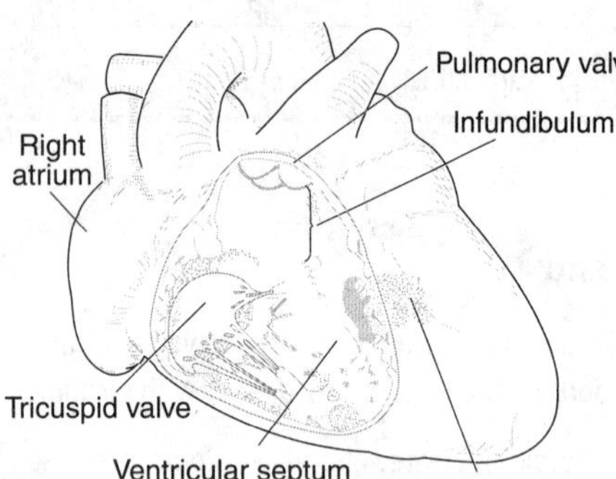

A defect in the ventricular septum caused by myocardial infarction is repaired

Explanation

This operation is always done in conjunction with coronary artery bypass grafting. The heart muscle involved in the infarction extends from the septum onto the surface of the heart. The heart is opened through this dead muscle and all dead muscle on the surface of the heart is cut out as is all the dead muscle in the septum. The septum is reconstructed by sewing in a patch of Gortex, for example, or Dacron. The surface of the heart is closed directly with sutures or with a patch sewn over the hole.

Coding Tips

When 33545 is performed with another separately identifiable procedure, the highest dollar value code is listed as the primary procedure and subsequent procedures are appended with modifier 51. Excision of a ventricular aneurysm is included in 33545. For coronary artery bypass grafting, report 33510–33536 in addition to 33545.

ICD-10-CM Diagnostic Codes

I21.01 ST elevation (STEMI) myocardial infarction involving left main coronary artery
I21.02 ST elevation (STEMI) myocardial infarction involving left anterior descending coronary artery
I21.09 ST elevation (STEMI) myocardial infarction involving other coronary artery of anterior wall
I21.11 ST elevation (STEMI) myocardial infarction involving right coronary artery
I21.19 ST elevation (STEMI) myocardial infarction involving other coronary artery of inferior wall
I21.21 ST elevation (STEMI) myocardial infarction involving left circumflex coronary artery
I21.4 Non-ST elevation (NSTEMI) myocardial infarction
I21.A1 Myocardial infarction type 2
I22.0 Subsequent ST elevation (STEMI) myocardial infarction of anterior wall
I22.1 Subsequent ST elevation (STEMI) myocardial infarction of inferior wall

AMA: 33545 2018,Jan,8; 2017,Jan,8; 2017,Dec,3; 2016,Jan,13; 2015,Jan,16; 2014,Jan,11

Relative Value Units/Medicare Edits

Non-Facility RVU	Work	PE	MP	Total
33545	57.06	19.13	13.54	89.73
Facility RVU	**Work**	**PE**	**MP**	**Total**
33545	57.06	19.13	13.54	89.73

	FUD	Status	MUE	Modifiers				IOM Reference
33545	90	A	1(2)	51	N/A	62*	80	None

* with documentation

Terms To Know

coronary atherosclerosis. Chronic condition marked by thickening and loss of elasticity of the coronary artery, caused by deposits of plaque containing cholesterol, lipoid material, and lipophages.

myocardial infarction. Obstruction of circulation to the heart, resulting in necrosis.

resection. Surgical removal of a part or all of an organ or body part.

tricuspid valve. Valve with three cusps between the right atrium and the right ventricle.

 ● New ▲ Revised + Add On AMA: CPT Assist [Resequenced] ☑ Laterality

33548

33548 Surgical ventricular restoration procedure, includes prosthetic patch, when performed (eg, ventricular remodeling, SVR, SAVER, Dor procedures)

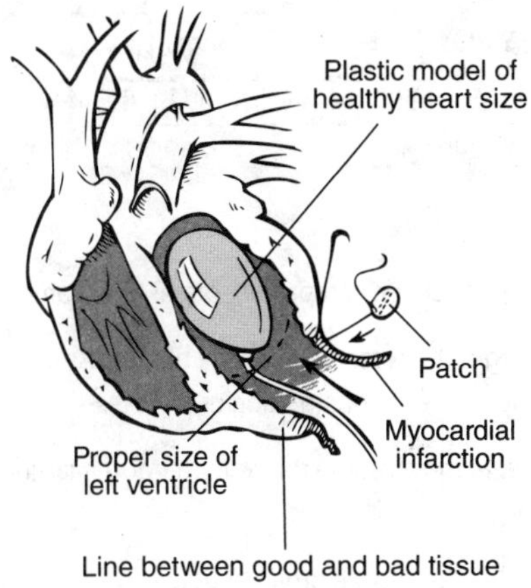

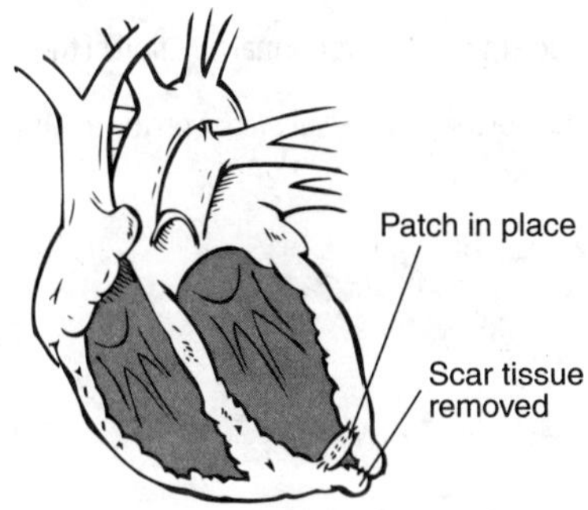

Explanation

The physician performs a surgical ventricular restoration (SVR) procedure to treat congestive heart failure subsequent to a myocardial infarction that has caused scarring or aneurysm of the left ventricle resulting in an enlarged rounded heart. SVR restores the heart to a more normal size and shape thereby improving function. Cardiopulmonary bypass is initiated. The ventricle is collapsed. A small incision is made in the bottom of the left ventricle through the scar tissue. The heart is opened and the area between the scar and the good heart muscle is identified. Using a plastic model of the heart selected based on the body surface area of the patient, the physician reshapes the heart. Rather than closing the defect, the physician sutures a patch over the defect to restore the normal spherical shape of the heart.

Coding Tips

Do not report 33548 with 32551, 33210, 33211, 33310, or 33315. For a Batista procedure or pachopexy, use unlisted code 33999.

ICD-10-CM Diagnostic Codes

I25.3	Aneurysm of heart
I25.41	Coronary artery aneurysm
I25.42	Coronary artery dissection
I25.5	Ischemic cardiomyopathy
I50.1	Left ventricular failure, unspecified
I50.21	Acute systolic (congestive) heart failure
I50.22	Chronic systolic (congestive) heart failure
I50.23	Acute on chronic systolic (congestive) heart failure
I50.31	Acute diastolic (congestive) heart failure
I50.32	Chronic diastolic (congestive) heart failure
I50.33	Acute on chronic diastolic (congestive) heart failure
I50.41	Acute combined systolic (congestive) and diastolic (congestive) heart failure
I50.42	Chronic combined systolic (congestive) and diastolic (congestive) heart failure
I50.43	Acute on chronic combined systolic (congestive) and diastolic (congestive) heart failure
I50.811	Acute right heart failure
I50.812	Chronic right heart failure
I50.813	Acute on chronic right heart failure
I50.814	Right heart failure due to left heart failure
I50.82	Biventricular heart failure
I50.83	High output heart failure
I50.84	End stage heart failure

AMA: 33548 2018,Jan,8; 2017,Jan,8; 2017,Dec,3; 2016,Jan,13; 2015,Jan,16; 2014,Jan,11

Relative Value Units/Medicare Edits

Non-Facility RVU	Work	PE	MP	Total
33548	54.14	19.51	12.09	85.74
Facility RVU	Work	PE	MP	Total
33548	54.14	19.51	12.09	85.74

	FUD	Status	MUE	Modifiers				IOM Reference
33548	90	A	1(2)	51	N/A	62*	80	100-03,20.26

* with documentation

Terms To Know

aneurysm. Circumscribed dilation or outpouching of an artery wall, often containing blood clots and connecting directly with the lumen of the artery.

atherosclerosis. Buildup of yellowish plaques composed of cholesterol and lipoid material within the arteries.

cardiopulmonary bypass. Venous blood is diverted to a heart-lung machine, which mechanically pumps and oxygenates the blood temporarily so the heart can be bypassed while an open procedure on the heart or coronary arteries is performed. During bypass, the lungs are deflated and immobile.

congestive heart failure. Condition caused by the heart's inability to adequately pump and circulate blood, resulting in fluid accumulation in the lungs and other tissues.

ischemia. Deficiency in blood supply causing tissues to be deprived of oxygen, resulting from trauma, mechanical or functional constriction of blood vessels, or a physical obstruction.

myocardial infarction. Obstruction of circulation to the heart, resulting in necrosis.

occlusion. Constriction, closure, or blockage of a passage.

33572

+ **33572** Coronary endarterectomy, open, any method, of left anterior descending, circumflex, or right coronary artery performed in conjunction with coronary artery bypass graft procedure, each vessel (List separately in addition to primary procedure)

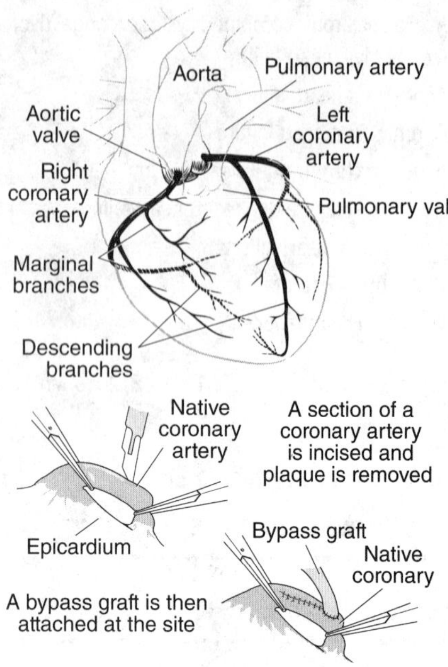

Explanation

This operation is only done when a coronary artery is so full of disease along its length that a good site for sewing on the bypass graft cannot be found. Coronary artery bypass grafts are almost always done along with an endarterectomy. The coronary artery to be cleaned out is opened along its length for a distance greater than that usually opened for a bypass alone, sometimes along its length. The plaque within the artery is separated from the outer layer of the arterial wall with a tool designed for this purpose. The plaque is removed from as much of the artery as is possible. A bypass graft is usually sewn to part of the hole left in the coronary. The rest of the hole is closed directly with suture or a patch of opened vein graft is laid over the open artery and sewn to the coronary artery wall to close the hole.

Coding Tips

Report 33572 in addition to 33510–33516 and 33533–33536. Note that 33572 reports only endarterectomy of the left anterior descending, circumflex, or right coronary artery. Endarterectomy of other coronary arteries is not reported separately. For pulmonary endarterectomy, see 33916. For coronary artery angiography, see 93454–93461.

ICD-10-CM Diagnostic Codes

This/these CPT code(s) are add on code(s). See the primary procedure code that this code is performed with for your ICD-10-CM code selections. Diagnostic code(s) would be the same as the actual procedure performed.

AMA: 33572 1997,Nov,1

Relative Value Units/Medicare Edits

Non-Facility RVU	Work	PE	MP	Total
33572	4.44	1.23	1.0	6.67
Facility RVU	**Work**	**PE**	**MP**	**Total**
33572	4.44	1.23	1.0	6.67

	FUD	Status	MUE	Modifiers				IOM Reference
33572	N/A	A	3(2)	N/A	N/A	N/A	80	None

* with documentation

Terms To Know

angioplasty. Reconstruction or repair of a diseased or damaged blood vessel.

bypass graft. Surgically created alternative blood vessel used to reroute blood flow around an area of obstruction or disease.

endarterectomy. Removal of the thickened, endothelial lining of a diseased or damaged artery.

excision. Surgical removal of an organ or tissue.

obstruction. Blockage that prevents normal function of the valve or structure.

plaque. Accumulation of a soft sticky substance on the teeth largely composed of bacteria and its byproducts.

33600-33602

33600 Closure of atrioventricular valve (mitral or tricuspid) by suture or patch
33602 Closure of semilunar valve (aortic or pulmonary) by suture or patch

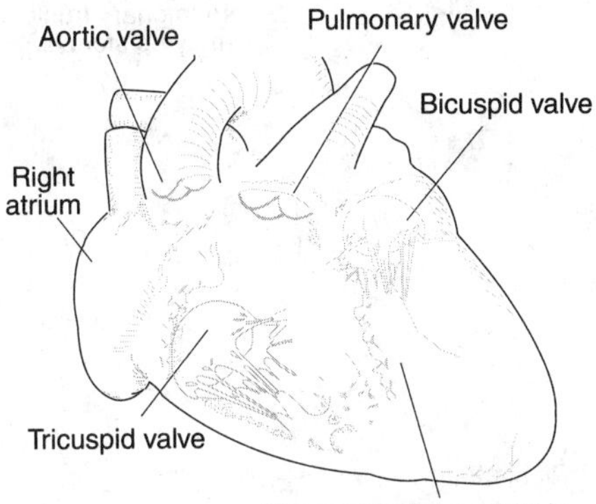

Explanation

Cardiopulmonary bypass is initiated. The appropriate heart chamber (right atrium for the tricuspid valve; left atrium for the mitral valve) is opened and the valve is assessed. The hole in the leaflet is cleaned of any infection. If it can be closed directly without distorting the valve significantly, suture alone is used. If the hole is large, it is closed with a patch made of pericardium. The open heart chamber is closed and cardiopulmonary bypass is discontinued when heart function returns. Report 33602 if the pulmonary artery or aorta are opened to gain access to the valve.

Coding Tips

If significant additional time and effort are documented, append modifier 22 and submit a cover letter and operative report. When 33600 or 33602 is performed with another separately identified procedure, the highest dollar value code is listed as the primary procedure and subsequent procedures are appended with modifier 51. When ligation and takedown of a systemic-to-pulmonary shunt is performed in addition to this procedure, it should be reported separately, see 33924.

ICD-10-CM Diagnostic Codes

I34.0	Nonrheumatic mitral (valve) insufficiency
I34.1	Nonrheumatic mitral (valve) prolapse
I34.2	Nonrheumatic mitral (valve) stenosis
I34.8	Other nonrheumatic mitral valve disorders
I35.0	Nonrheumatic aortic (valve) stenosis
I35.1	Nonrheumatic aortic (valve) insufficiency
I35.2	Nonrheumatic aortic (valve) stenosis with insufficiency
I35.8	Other nonrheumatic aortic valve disorders
I36.0	Nonrheumatic tricuspid (valve) stenosis
I36.1	Nonrheumatic tricuspid (valve) insufficiency
I36.2	Nonrheumatic tricuspid (valve) stenosis with insufficiency
I36.8	Other nonrheumatic tricuspid valve disorders
I37.0	Nonrheumatic pulmonary valve stenosis
I37.1	Nonrheumatic pulmonary valve insufficiency
I37.2	Nonrheumatic pulmonary valve stenosis with insufficiency
I37.8	Other nonrheumatic pulmonary valve disorders
Q20.8	Other congenital malformations of cardiac chambers and connections
Q21.2	Atrioventricular septal defect
Q21.8	Other congenital malformations of cardiac septa
Q22.0	Pulmonary valve atresia
Q22.2	Congenital pulmonary valve insufficiency
Q22.3	Other congenital malformations of pulmonary valve
Q22.4	Congenital tricuspid stenosis
Q22.5	Ebstein's anomaly
Q22.6	Hypoplastic right heart syndrome
Q22.8	Other congenital malformations of tricuspid valve
Q23.1	Congenital insufficiency of aortic valve
Q23.3	Congenital mitral insufficiency

AMA: **33600** 2018,Jan,8; 2017,Jan,8; 2017,Dec,3; 2016,Jan,13; 2015,Jan,16; 2014,Jan,11 **33602** 2017,Dec,3

Relative Value Units/Medicare Edits

Non-Facility RVU	Work	PE	MP	Total
33600	30.31	12.36	7.2	49.87
33602	29.34	12.09	6.97	48.4
Facility RVU	**Work**	**PE**	**MP**	**Total**
33600	30.31	12.36	7.2	49.87
33602	29.34	12.09	6.97	48.4

	FUD	Status	MUE	Modifiers				IOM Reference
33600	90	A	1(3)	51	N/A	62*	80	None
33602	90	A	1(3)	51	N/A	62*	80	

* with documentation

Terms To Know

cardiopulmonary bypass. Venous blood is diverted to a heart-lung machine, which mechanically pumps and oxygenates the blood temporarily so the heart can be bypassed while an open procedure on the heart or coronary arteries is performed. During bypass, the lungs are deflated and immobile.

shunt. Surgically created passage between blood vessels or other natural passages, such as an arteriovenous anastomosis, to divert or bypass blood flow from the normal channel.

33606

33606 Anastomosis of pulmonary artery to aorta (Damus-Kaye-Stansel procedure)

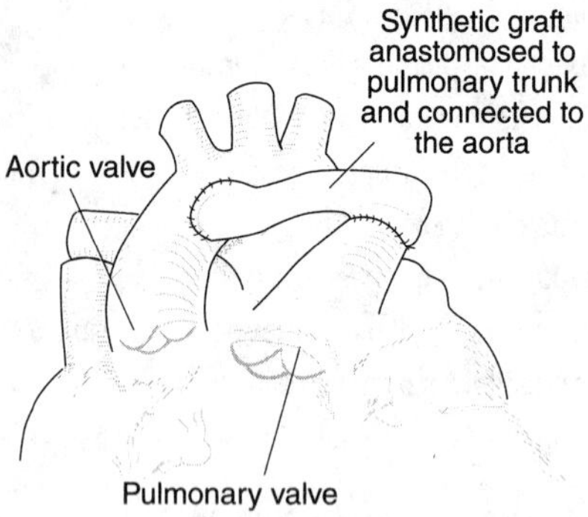

Explanation

The heart is exposed by dividing the breastbone longitudinally. Mechanical, extracorporeal circulation is established and the heart is stopped (cardiopulmonary bypass). The pulmonary artery is cut just before it divides into right and left branches. The pulmonary artery end is connected to the side of the ascending aorta. A piece of Dacron graft is used to construct this connection. This allows the single ventricle to pump blood to the body.

Coding Tips

If significant additional time and effort are documented, append modifier 22 and submit a cover letter and operative report. When 33606 is performed with another separately identifiable procedure, the highest dollar value code is listed as the primary procedure and subsequent procedures are appended with modifier 51. When ligation and takedown of a systemic-to-pulmonary shunt is performed in addition to this procedure, it should be reported separately, see 33924.

ICD-10-CM Diagnostic Codes

Q20.1	Double outlet right ventricle
Q20.3	Discordant ventriculoarterial connection
Q21.3	Tetralogy of Fallot
Q22.0	Pulmonary valve atresia
Q23.4	Hypoplastic left heart syndrome

AMA: 33606 2017,Dec,3

Relative Value Units/Medicare Edits

Non-Facility RVU	Work	PE	MP	Total
33606	31.53	12.58	7.49	51.6
Facility RVU	**Work**	**PE**	**MP**	**Total**
33606	31.53	12.58	7.49	51.6

	FUD	Status	MUE	Modifiers				IOM Reference
33606	90	A	1(2)	51	N/A	62*	80	None

* with documentation

33608

33608 Repair of complex cardiac anomaly other than pulmonary atresia with ventricular septal defect by construction or replacement of conduit from right or left ventricle to pulmonary artery

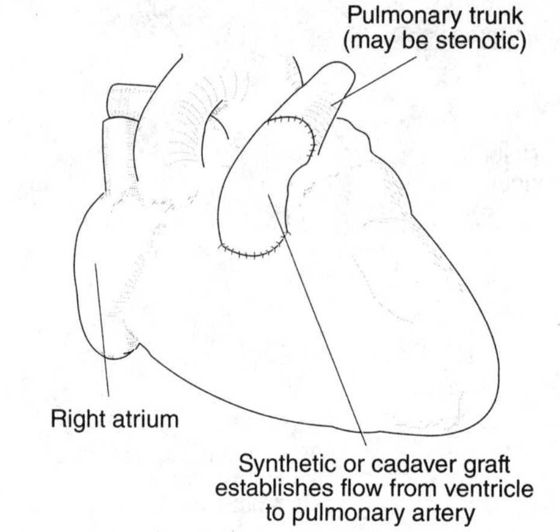

Any of a variety of congenital cardiac malformations may be addressed by creating a shunt from a ventricle to the pulmonary artery

Explanation

Mechanical, extracorporeal circulation is established and the heart is stopped (cardiopulmonary bypass). A hole is made in the pulmonary artery and is enlarged to cross any areas of narrowing. A cadaver ascending aorta is trimmed to the right length. A tube of artery or Dacron is sewn to the valve end of the cadaver aorta. The cadaver artery is connected to the hole in the pulmonary artery. The tube of aorta or Dacron is sewn to the hole in the ventricle to close the hole and allow blood to flow through the new valved tube that now connects the ventricle to the pulmonary artery.

Coding Tips

If significant additional time and effort are documented, append modifier 22 and submit a cover letter and operative report. When 33608 is performed with another separately identifiable procedure, the highest dollar value code is listed as the primary procedure and subsequent procedures are appended with modifier 51. Do not report 33608 with 33440. When ligation and takedown of a systemic-to-pulmonary shunt is performed in addition to this procedure, it should be reported separately, see 33924. For repair of pulmonary atresia with a ventricular septal defect, see 33920. For repair of pulmonary artery arborization anomalies by unifocalization, see 33925–33926.

ICD-10-CM Diagnostic Codes

Q20.1	Double outlet right ventricle
Q20.3	Discordant ventriculoarterial connection
Q21.3	Tetralogy of Fallot

AMA: 33608 2019,Apr,6; 2017,Dec,3

Relative Value Units/Medicare Edits

Non-Facility RVU	Work	PE	MP	Total
33608	31.88	12.8	7.58	52.26
Facility RVU	**Work**	**PE**	**MP**	**Total**
33608	31.88	12.8	7.58	52.26

	FUD	Status	MUE	Modifiers				IOM Reference
33608	90	A	1(2)	51	N/A	62*	80	None

* with documentation

Terms To Know

anomaly. Irregularity in the structure or position of an organ or tissue.

atresia. Congenital closure or absence of a tubular organ or an opening to the body surface.

cadaver. Dead body.

cardiopulmonary bypass. Venous blood is diverted to a heart-lung machine, which mechanically pumps and oxygenates the blood temporarily so the heart can be bypassed while an open procedure on the heart or coronary arteries is performed. During bypass, the lungs are deflated and immobile.

conduit. Surgically created channel for the passage of fluids.

ligation. Tying off a blood vessel or duct with a suture or a soft, thin wire.

tetralogy of Fallot. Specific combination of congenital cardiac defects: obstruction of the right ventricular outflow tract with pulmonary stenosis, interventricular septal defect, malposition of the aorta, overriding the interventricular septum and receiving blood from both the venous and arterial systems, and enlargement of the right ventricle.

ventricular septal defect. Congenital cardiac anomaly resulting in a continual opening in the septum between the ventricles that, in severe cases, causes oxygenated blood to flow back into the lungs, resulting in pulmonary hypertension.

33610

33610 Repair of complex cardiac anomalies (eg, single ventricle with subaortic obstruction) by surgical enlargement of ventricular septal defect

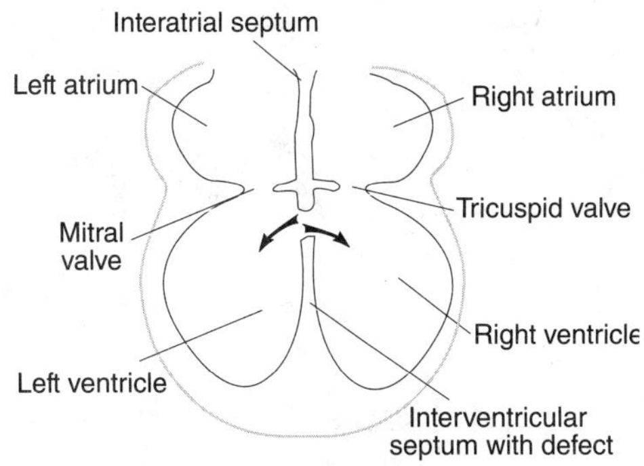

Posterior schematic showing septal defect

In some instances, an interventricular septal defect is desirable, due to anomalies occuring elsewhere in the heart

Explanation

The heart is exposed by dividing the breast bone longitudinally. Mechanical, extra corporeal circulation is established and the heart is stopped (cardiopulmonary bypass). The heart is opened and the hole in the wall between the two ventricles is enlarged so that blood will flow freely across it. A baffle is placed to direct blood that flows across the enlarged ventricular septal defect out the aorta.

Coding Tips

If significant additional time and effort are documented, append modifier 22 and submit a cover letter and operative report. When 33610 is performed with another separately identifiable procedure, the highest dollar value code is listed as the primary procedure and subsequent procedures are appended with modifier 51. Do not append modifier 63 to 33610 as the description or nature of the procedure includes infants up to 4 kg. When ligation and takedown of a systemic-to-pulmonary shunt is performed in addition to this procedure, it should be reported separately, see 33924.

ICD-10-CM Diagnostic Codes

Q20.1 Double outlet right ventricle
Q20.4 Double inlet ventricle

AMA: 33610 2017,Dec,3

Relative Value Units/Medicare Edits

Non-Facility RVU	Work	PE	MP	Total
33610	31.4	12.67	7.46	51.53
Facility RVU	**Work**	**PE**	**MP**	**Total**
33610	31.4	12.67	7.46	51.53

	FUD	Status	MUE	Modifiers				IOM Reference
33610	90	A	1(2)	51	N/A	62*	80	None

* with documentation

33611-33612

33611 Repair of double outlet right ventricle with intraventricular tunnel repair;

33612 with repair of right ventricular outflow tract obstruction

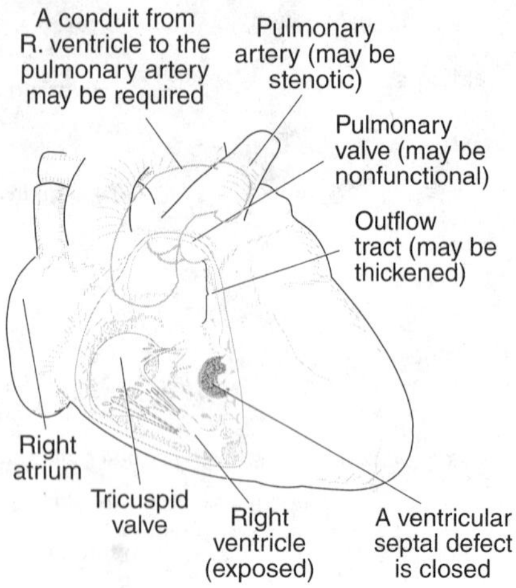

Explanation

Cardiopulmonary bypass is initiated. A hole is made in the right ventricle free wall. This exposes the hole between the right and left ventricles. A patch of pericardium or Dacron is sewn in place to block the hole and directs blood ejected from the left ventricle (i.e. blood coming from the lungs) out the aorta. If the pulmonary artery is of adequate size, blood will flow from the right ventricle to the lungs. If it is inadequate or if the valve does not open, a conduit containing a valve (natural or artificial) is sewn to the hole in the right ventricle free wall. The far end of the conduit is attached to the pulmonary artery. This will allow blood to be pumped from the right ventricle to the lungs. Report 33612 if the obstructing muscles bundles in the outflow part of the right ventricle are excised when the heart is open.

Coding Tips

If significant additional time and effort are documented, append modifier 22 and submit a cover letter and operative report. When 33611 or 33612 is performed with another separately identifiable procedure, the highest dollar value code is listed as the primary procedure and subsequent procedures are appended with modifier 51. Do not append modifier 63 to 33611 as the description or nature of the procedure includes infants up to 4 kg. When ligation and takedown of a systemic-to-pulmonary shunt is performed in addition to this procedure, it should be reported separately, see 33924.

ICD-10-CM Diagnostic Codes

Q20.1 Double outlet right ventricle

Q24.8 Other specified congenital malformations of heart

AMA: 33611 2017,Dec,3 **33612** 2017,Dec,3

Relative Value Units/Medicare Edits

Non-Facility RVU	Work	PE	MP	Total
33611	35.57	12.68	8.46	56.71
33612	36.57	12.96	8.7	58.23
Facility RVU	**Work**	**PE**	**MP**	**Total**
33611	35.57	12.68	8.46	56.71
33612	36.57	12.96	8.7	58.23

	FUD	Status	MUE	Modifiers				IOM Reference
33611	90	A	1(2)	51	N/A	62*	80	None
33612	90	A	1(2)	51	N/A	62*	80	

* with documentation

Terms To Know

anomaly. Irregularity in the structure or position of an organ or tissue.

conduit. Surgically created channel for the passage of fluids.

congenital. Present at birth, occurring through heredity or an influence during gestation up to the moment of birth.

ligation. Tying off a blood vessel or duct with a suture or a soft, thin wire.

obstruction. Blockage that prevents normal function of the valve or structure.

pericardium. Thin and slippery case in which the heart lies that is lined with fluid so that the heart is free to pulse and move as it beats.

septum. Anatomical partition or dividing wall.

suture. Numerous stitching techniques employed in wound closure.

ventricular septal defect. Congenital cardiac anomaly resulting in a continual opening in the septum between the ventricles that, in severe cases, causes oxygenated blood to flow back into the lungs, resulting in pulmonary hypertension.

33615

33615 Repair of complex cardiac anomalies (eg, tricuspid atresia) by closure of atrial septal defect and anastomosis of atria or vena cava to pulmonary artery (simple Fontan procedure)

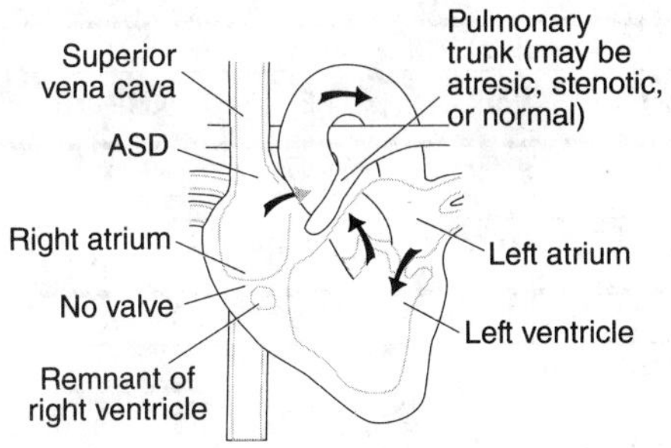

Example of tricuspid atresia with pulmonary atresia (single ventricle)

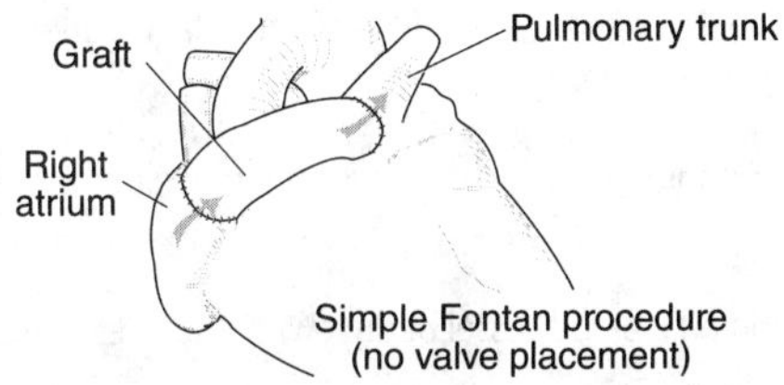

Simple Fontan procedure (no valve placement)

Explanation

The right pulmonary artery (or left in situs inverses) is exposed from the main pulmonary trunk to the hilum of the lung. The superior vena cava is detached from the right atrium. The atrial hole is closed. A hole is made in the top part of the pulmonary artery and the cut end of the superior vena cava is connected to the hole in the pulmonary artery. Pulmonary blood flow comes directly from the venous system and bypasses the heart. Later the process is completed by performing a Fontan operation. This procedure may also be referred to as a simple Fontan or Bidirectional Glenn Shunt (BDG).

Coding Tips

If significant additional time and effort are documented, append modifier 22 and submit a cover letter and operative report. When 33615 is performed with another separately identifiable procedure, the highest dollar value code is listed as the primary procedure and subsequent procedures are appended with modifier 51. For repair of pulmonary atresia with a ventricular septal defect, see 33920. When ligation and takedown of a systemic-to-pulmonary shunt is performed in addition to this procedure, it should be reported separately, see 33924.

ICD-10-CM Diagnostic Codes

Q20.4	Double inlet ventricle
Q21.1	Atrial septal defect
Q21.2	Atrioventricular septal defect
Q22.0	Pulmonary valve atresia
Q22.4	Congenital tricuspid stenosis
Q22.5	Ebstein's anomaly
Q22.6	Hypoplastic right heart syndrome
Q22.8	Other congenital malformations of tricuspid valve
Q26.2	Total anomalous pulmonary venous connection
Q26.3	Partial anomalous pulmonary venous connection

AMA: **33615** 2017,Dec,3

Relative Value Units/Medicare Edits

Non-Facility RVU	Work	PE	MP	Total
33615	35.89	13.57	8.54	58.0
Facility RVU	**Work**	**PE**	**MP**	**Total**
33615	35.89	13.57	8.54	58.0

	FUD	Status	MUE	Modifiers				IOM Reference
33615	90	A	1(2)	51	N/A	62*	80	None

* with documentation

Terms To Know

anastomosis. Surgically created connection between ducts, blood vessels, or bowel segments to allow flow from one to the other.

anomaly. Irregularity in the structure or position of an organ or tissue.

atresia. Congenital closure or absence of a tubular organ or an opening to the body surface.

atrial septal defect. Cardiac anomaly consisting of a patent opening in the atrial septum due to a fusion failure, classified as ostium secundum type, ostium primum defect, or endocardial cushion defect.

bypass. Auxiliary or diverted route to maintain continuous flow.

congenital. Present at birth, occurring through heredity or an influence during gestation up to the moment of birth.

Fontan procedure. Surgical bypass procedure that corrects tricuspid atresia and other selected congenital conditions by connecting the right atrium directly to the pulmonary artery by anastomosis or by inserting a closed prosthesis between the right atrium and the pulmonary artery and closing the interatrial communication.

ligation. Tying off a blood vessel or duct with a suture or a soft, thin wire.

shunt. Surgically created passage between blood vessels or other natural passages, such as an arteriovenous anastomosis, to divert or bypass blood flow from the normal channel.

stenosis. Narrowing or constriction of a passage.

tricuspid atresia. Congenital absence of the valve that may occur with other defects, such as atrial septal defect, pulmonary atresia, and transposition of great vessels.

33617

33617 Repair of complex cardiac anomalies (eg, single ventricle) by modified Fontan procedure

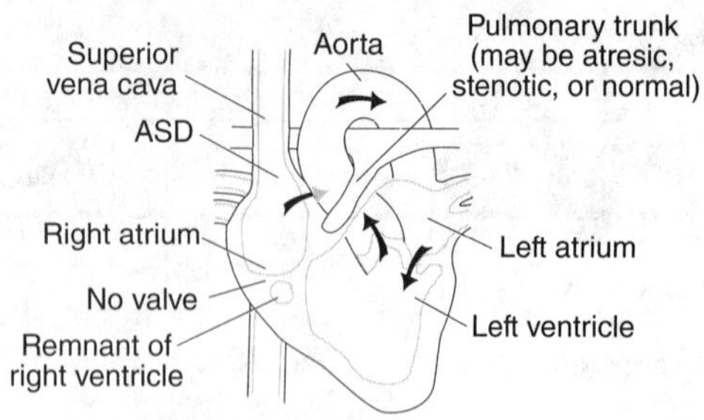

Example of tricuspid atresia with pulmonary atresia (single ventricle)

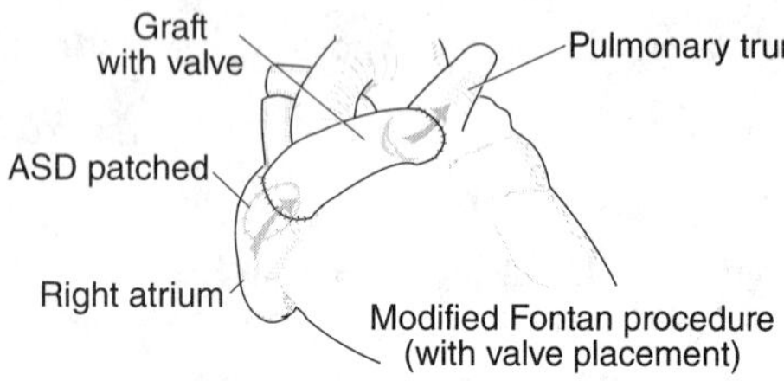

Modified Fontan procedure (with valve placement)

Explanation

This operation is usually considered to be the second stage of a Glen repair. Cardiopulmonary bypass with or without circulatory arrest is required. In this operation, blood flow is directed from the inferior caval vein, through a tunnel created inside the right atrium to the pulmonary artery. All systemic venous return is diverted away from the heart and directly into the pulmonary circulation. The right atrium is widely opened. A large patch of pericardium or Dacron is used for one wall of the tunnel. The lateral wall of the right atrium forms the other half of the tunnel. The tunnel leads from the inferior caval vein, where it joins the right atrium, to the undersurface of the pulmonary artery. The mouth of the tunnel is connected to a hole on the undersurface of the pulmonary artery. Previously, or at the same time, the superior caval vein will already have been directly connected to the upper surface of the pulmonary artery.

Coding Tips

If significant additional time and effort are documented, append modifier 22 and submit a cover letter and operative report. When 33617 is performed with another separately identifiable procedure, the highest dollar value code is listed as the primary procedure and subsequent procedures are appended with modifier 51. When ligation and takedown of a systemic-to-pulmonary shunt is performed with this procedure, it should be reported separately, see 33924. For repair of complex cardiac anomalies (e.g., single ventricle with subaortic obstruction) by surgical enlargement of the interventricular septal defect, see 33610. For repair of a single ventricle with aortic outflow obstruction and aortic arch hypoplasia (hypoplastic left heart syndrome) (e.g., Norwood procedure), see 33619. Report 33617 with 33768 when a cavopulmonary anastomosis to a second superior vena cava is performed.

ICD-10-CM Diagnostic Codes

Q20.4	Double inlet ventricle
Q20.8	Other congenital malformations of cardiac chambers and connections
Q21.4	Aortopulmonary septal defect
Q21.8	Other congenital malformations of cardiac septa
Q21.9	Congenital malformation of cardiac septum, unspecified
Q23.4	Hypoplastic left heart syndrome

AMA: **33617** 2017,Dec,3

Relative Value Units/Medicare Edits

Non-Facility RVU	Work	PE	MP	Total
33617	39.09	14.47	9.31	62.87
Facility RVU	**Work**	**PE**	**MP**	**Total**
33617	39.09	14.47	9.31	62.87

	FUD	Status	MUE	Modifiers				IOM Reference
33617	90	A	1(2)	51	N/A	62*	80	None

* with documentation

Terms To Know

anomaly. Irregularity in the structure or position of an organ or tissue.

atresia. Congenital closure or absence of a tubular organ or an opening to the body surface.

hypoplasia. Condition in which there is underdevelopment of an organ or tissue.

ligation. Tying off a blood vessel or duct with a suture or a soft, thin wire.

obstruction. Blockage that prevents normal function of the valve or structure.

pericardium. Thin and slippery case in which the heart lies that is lined with fluid so that the heart is free to pulse and move as it beats.

suture. Numerous stitching techniques employed in wound closure.

33619

33619 Repair of single ventricle with aortic outflow obstruction and aortic arch hypoplasia (hypoplastic left heart syndrome) (eg, Norwood procedure)

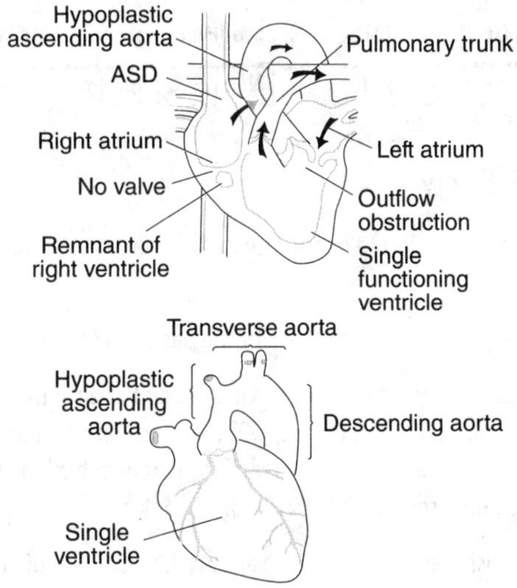

Explanation

Cardiopulmonary bypass and circulatory arrest are required. The small aorta is opened on the inner surface of its arch up to the point where the aortic diameter becomes normal. The pulmonary artery is removed and its connection to the branched pulmonary artery is closed with a patch. A large, rectangular patch of pericardium is used to enlarge the small aorta. The pulmonary valve becomes the systemic arterial valve of the heart and is encircled by the large patch that becomes shaped like a tube as it is sewn along either side of the small ascending aorta and arch that have been opened longitudinally. The coronary arteries are small and still originate in the root of the abnormal aorta.

Coding Tips

If significant additional time and effort are documented, append modifier 22 and submit a cover letter and operative report. When 33619 is performed with another separately identifiable procedure, the highest dollar value code is listed as the primary procedure and subsequent procedures are appended with modifier 51. Do not append modifier 63 to 33619 as the description or nature of the procedure includes infants up to 4 kg. When ligation and takedown of a systemic-to-pulmonary shunt is performed in addition to this procedure, it should be reported separately, see 33924. For repair of complex cardiac anomalies (e.g., single ventricle with subaortic obstruction) by surgical enlargement of the interventricular septal defect, see 33610. For repair of a single ventricle by modified Fontan procedure, see 33617.

ICD-10-CM Diagnostic Codes

Q20.4	Double inlet ventricle
Q20.8	Other congenital malformations of cardiac chambers and connections
Q21.4	Aortopulmonary septal defect
Q21.8	Other congenital malformations of cardiac septa
Q21.9	Congenital malformation of cardiac septum, unspecified
Q23.4	Hypoplastic left heart syndrome

AMA: 33619 2018,Jan,8; 2017,Jan,8; 2017,Dec,3; 2016,Jul,3; 2016,Jan,13; 2015,Jan,16; 2014,Jan,11

Relative Value Units/Medicare Edits

Non-Facility RVU	Work	PE	MP	Total
33619	48.76	18.98	11.63	79.37
Facility RVU	**Work**	**PE**	**MP**	**Total**
33619	48.76	18.98	11.63	79.37

	FUD	Status	MUE	Modifiers				IOM Reference
33619	90	A	1(2)	51	N/A	62*	80	None

* with documentation

Terms To Know

anomaly. Irregularity in the structure or position of an organ or tissue.

cardiopulmonary bypass. Venous blood is diverted to a heart-lung machine, which mechanically pumps and oxygenates the blood temporarily so the heart can be bypassed while an open procedure on the heart or coronary arteries is performed. During bypass, the lungs are deflated and immobile.

hypoplasia. Condition in which there is underdevelopment of an organ or tissue.

ligation. Tying off a blood vessel or duct with a suture or a soft, thin wire.

obstruction. Blockage that prevents normal function of the valve or structure.

pericardium. Thin and slippery case in which the heart lies that is lined with fluid so that the heart is free to pulse and move as it beats.

● New ▲ Revised + Add On AMA: CPT Assist [Resequenced] ☑ Laterality

33620

33620 Application of right and left pulmonary artery bands (eg, hybrid approach stage 1)

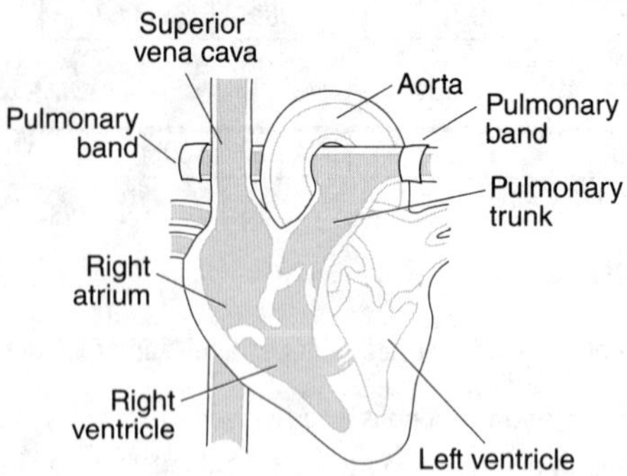

Explanation

The cardiovascular surgeon performs bilateral pulmonary artery banding (bPAB) using a hybrid stage 1 approach, which does not require open heart surgery or circulatory arrest. Hybrid procedures utilize the services of both a cardiovascular surgeon and an interventional cardiologist. This procedure is typically performed on high-risk neonates with hypoplastic left heart syndrome or related congenital anomalies for short-term palliation as part of a staged approach to more definitive surgical repair. Following a median sternotomy, the pulmonary arteries are banded individually in order to restrict some of the pulmonary blood flow. In a separately reportable procedure, the interventional cardiologist may place a stent in the ductus arteriosus under fluoroscopic guidance. Incisions are closed.

Coding Tips

For banding of the main pulmonary artery in connection with a septal defect, see 33690.

ICD-10-CM Diagnostic Codes

Q20.1	Double outlet right ventricle
Q20.2	Double outlet left ventricle
Q20.3	Discordant ventriculoarterial connection
Q20.4	Double inlet ventricle
Q20.5	Discordant atrioventricular connection
Q20.8	Other congenital malformations of cardiac chambers and connections
Q21.0	Ventricular septal defect
Q21.2	Atrioventricular septal defect
Q21.4	Aortopulmonary septal defect
Q21.8	Other congenital malformations of cardiac septa
Q23.4	Hypoplastic left heart syndrome
Q25.1	Coarctation of aorta
Q25.21	Interruption of aortic arch
Q25.29	Other atresia of aorta

AMA: 33620 2018,Jan,8; 2017,Jan,8; 2017,Dec,3; 2016,Jul,3; 2016,Jan,13; 2015,Jan,16; 2014,Jan,11

Relative Value Units/Medicare Edits

Non-Facility RVU	Work	PE	MP	Total
33620	30.0	10.81	7.13	47.94
Facility RVU	**Work**	**PE**	**MP**	**Total**
33620	30.0	10.81	7.13	47.94

	FUD	Status	MUE	Modifiers				IOM Reference
33620	90	A	1(2)	51	N/A	62*	80	None

* with documentation

Terms To Know

atresia. Congenital closure or absence of a tubular organ or an opening to the body surface.

conduit. Surgically created channel for the passage of fluids.

congenital anomaly. Abnormality that is present at birth that may be the result of genetic factors, teratogens, or other conditions that affect the fetus in utero. The abnormalities may be readily apparent at birth or may remain undiscovered until some point after birth.

cyanosis. Bluish discoloration due to an excessive amount of deoxygenated hemoglobin in the blood.

fluoroscopy. Radiology technique that allows visual examination of part of the body or a function of an organ using a device that projects an x-ray image on a fluorescent screen.

hypoplasia. Condition in which there is underdevelopment of an organ or tissue.

hypoplastic left heart syndrome. Hypoplasia or atresia of the left ventricle and aorta or mitral valve with respiratory distress and extreme cyanosis. Cardiac failure and death often result in early infancy.

palliative. Alleviating care or medicine that is intended to provide relief from symptoms, but not cure the disease. Palliative care is employed in cases of terminal illness or severe chronic diseases.

pulmonary artery banding. Surgical constriction of the pulmonary artery to prevent irreversible pulmonary vascular obstructive changes and overflow into the left ventricle.

 ● New ▲ Revised + Add On AMA: CPT Assist [Resequenced] ☑ Laterality

33621

33621 Transthoracic insertion of catheter for stent placement with catheter removal and closure (eg, hybrid approach stage 1)

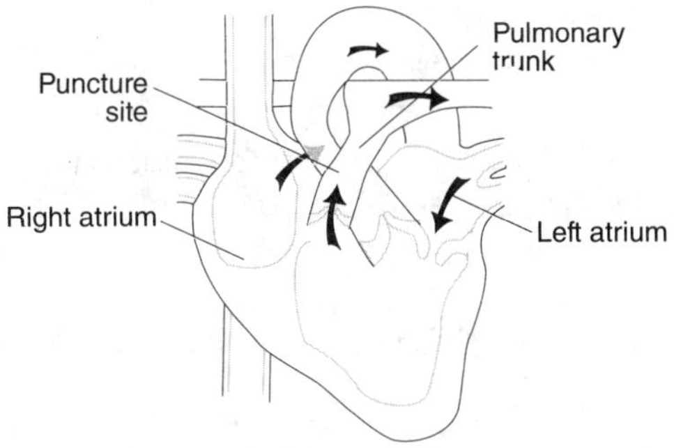

Explanation

The interventional cardiologist performs a transthoracic insertion of a catheter for stent placement using a hybrid stage 1 approach, which does not require open heart surgery or circulatory arrest. Hybrid procedures utilize the services of both an interventional cardiologist and a cardiovascular surgeon. This procedure is typically performed on high-risk neonates with hypoplastic left heart syndrome or related congenital anomalies for short-term palliation as part of a staged approach to more definitive surgical repair. Because pulmonary arteries in a newborn are difficult to access for catheter interventions, access is obtained by direct puncture of the right ventricular outflow tract, typically in the same operative episode as another, separately reportable procedure performed by the cardiovascular surgeon (i.e., pulmonary artery banding, which requires sternotomy). Upon completion of the separately reportable stent placement, the catheter is removed and the incisions are closed.

Coding Tips

Report 33620 in addition to 33621 if both procedures are performed during the same encounter. For stent placement, see 37236.

ICD-10-CM Diagnostic Codes

Q20.1	Double outlet right ventricle
Q20.2	Double outlet left ventricle
Q20.3	Discordant ventriculoarterial connection
Q20.4	Double inlet ventricle
Q20.5	Discordant atrioventricular connection
Q20.8	Other congenital malformations of cardiac chambers and connections
Q21.0	Ventricular septal defect
Q21.2	Atrioventricular septal defect
Q21.4	Aortopulmonary septal defect
Q21.8	Other congenital malformations of cardiac septa
Q23.4	Hypoplastic left heart syndrome
Q25.1	Coarctation of aorta
Q25.21	Interruption of aortic arch
Q25.29	Other atresia of aorta

AMA: 33621 2018,Jan,8; 2017,Jan,8; 2017,Dec,3; 2016,Jul,3; 2016,Jan,13; 2015,Jan,16; 2014,Jan,11

Relative Value Units/Medicare Edits

Non-Facility RVU	Work	PE	MP	Total
33621	16.18	6.98	3.84	27.0
Facility RVU	**Work**	**PE**	**MP**	**Total**
33621	16.18	6.98	3.84	27.0

	FUD	Status	MUE	Modifiers				IOM Reference
33621	90	A	1(3)	51	N/A	62*	80	None

* with documentation

Terms To Know

approach. Method or anatomical location used to gain access to a body organ or specific area for procedures. The approach is not coded separately although it may be a specified component of the procedure, such as laparoscopic versus incisional, or spinal procedures in which the amount of dissection required to expose the spine significantly alters with the site of approach.

atresia. Congenital closure or absence of a tubular organ or an opening to the body surface.

catheter. Flexible tube inserted into an area of the body for introducing or withdrawing fluid.

conduit. Surgically created channel for the passage of fluids.

congenital anomaly. Abnormality that is present at birth that may be the result of genetic factors, teratogens, or other conditions that affect the fetus in utero. The abnormalities may be readily apparent at birth or may remain undiscovered until some point after birth.

extracorporeal. Located or taking place outside the body.

hypoplastic left heart syndrome. Hypoplasia or atresia of the left ventricle and aorta or mitral valve with respiratory distress and extreme cyanosis. Cardiac failure and death often result in early infancy.

palliative. Alleviating care or medicine that is intended to provide relief from symptoms, but not cure the disease. Palliative care is employed in cases of terminal illness or severe chronic diseases.

stent. Tube to provide support in a body cavity or lumen.

33622

33622 Reconstruction of complex cardiac anomaly (eg, single ventricle or hypoplastic left heart) with palliation of single ventricle with aortic outflow obstruction and aortic arch hypoplasia, creation of cavopulmonary anastomosis, and removal of right and left pulmonary bands (eg, hybrid approach stage 2, Norwood, bidirectional Glenn, pulmonary artery debanding)

Hypoplastic left heart with single right ventricle

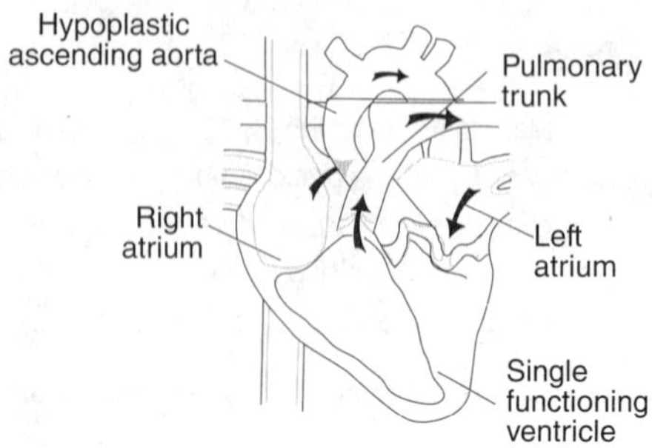

Explanation

While a "hybrid procedure" is one that combines both surgical and transcatheter interventional approaches, a "hybrid approach" may be any of a group of staged procedures that follow (not all procedures classified as hybrid approach are true hybrid procedures). The hybrid approach stage 2 reported by 33622 is part of a planned staged approach that typically follows a hybrid procedure; it is not a hybrid procedure in and of itself. The physician performs a hybrid stage 2 reconstruction of a congenital cardiac abnormality, such as left heart hypoplasia or a single ventricle. The physician gains access to the mediastinum through a sternal incision (median sternotomy). Cardiopulmonary bypass and circulatory arrest are required. For palliation of a single ventricle with aortic outflow obstruction and aortic arch hypoplasia, the physician performs a Norwood procedure. After the bypass pump is turned off, the small aorta is opened on the inner surface of its arch up to the point where the aortic diameter becomes "normal." The physician removes the pulmonary artery bands (placed during a previous surgery). The pulmonary artery is removed and its connection to the branched pulmonary artery is closed with a patch. A large, rectangular patch of pericardium is used to enlarge the small aorta. The pulmonary valve becomes the systemic arterial valve of the heart and is encircled by the large patch that becomes shaped like a tube as it is sewn along either side of the small ascending aorta and arch that have been opened longitudinally. The coronary arteries are small and still originate in the root of the abnormal aorta. The physician creates a cavopulmonary anastomosis. The left superior vena cava is dissected free. The left superior vena cava is divided and anastomosed in end-to-side fashion to the left pulmonary artery. The physician closes the cardiac incisions, takes the patient off cardiopulmonary bypass, closes the remaining surgical incisions, and dresses the sternal or chest wall wound. The physician may leave chest tubes and/or a mediastinal drainage tube in place following the procedure.

Coding Tips

Do not report 33622 with 33619, 33767, 33822, 33840, 33845, 33851, 33853, or 33917. For a bilateral, bidirectional Glenn procedure, report 33768 in addition to 33622.

ICD-10-CM Diagnostic Codes

Q20.1	Double outlet right ventricle
Q20.2	Double outlet left ventricle
Q20.3	Discordant ventriculoarterial connection
Q20.4	Double inlet ventricle
Q20.5	Discordant atrioventricular connection
Q20.6	Isomerism of atrial appendages
Q20.8	Other congenital malformations of cardiac chambers and connections
Q21.0	Ventricular septal defect
Q21.2	Atrioventricular septal defect
Q21.4	Aortopulmonary septal defect
Q21.8	Other congenital malformations of cardiac septa
Q23.4	Hypoplastic left heart syndrome
Q25.1	Coarctation of aorta

AMA: **33622** 2018,Jan,8; 2017,Jan,8; 2017,Dec,3; 2016,Jul,3; 2016,Jan,13; 2015,Jan,16; 2014,Jan,11

Relative Value Units/Medicare Edits

Non-Facility RVU	Work	PE	MP	Total
33622	64.0	20.62	15.39	100.01
Facility RVU	**Work**	**PE**	**MP**	**Total**
33622	64.0	20.62	15.39	100.01

	FUD	Status	MUE	Modifiers				IOM Reference
33622	90	A	1(2)	51	N/A	62*	80	None

* with documentation

Terms To Know

Glenn procedure. Creation of a shunt by anastomosing the superior vena cava to the pulmonary artery to increase perfusion to both lungs.

hypoplastic left heart syndrome. Hypoplasia or atresia of the left ventricle and aorta or mitral valve with respiratory distress and extreme cyanosis. Cardiac failure and death often result in early infancy.

pericardium. Thin and slippery case in which the heart lies that is lined with fluid so that the heart is free to pulse and move as it beats.

ASD

33641

33641 Repair atrial septal defect, secundum, with cardiopulmonary bypass, with or without patch

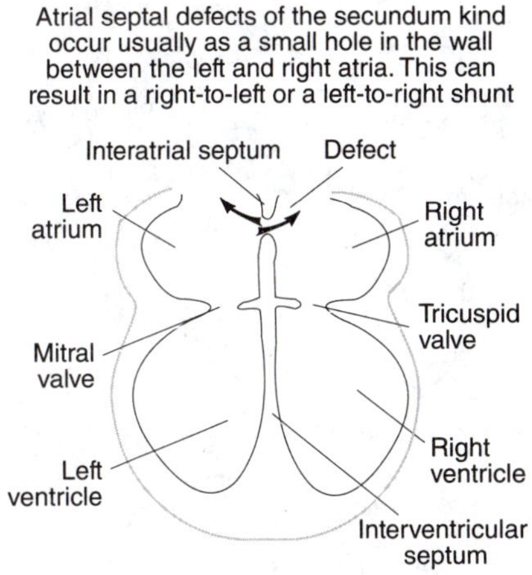

Posterior schematic showing atrial septal defect

Explanation

Cardiopulmonary bypass is necessary. Two venous tubes are placed for the bypass machine–one draining the superior caval vein and one draining the inferior caval vein. The right atrium is isolated by putting tourniquets around the superior vena cava and inferior vena cava and their corresponding tubes. The right atrium is opened and the size and location of the atrial septal defect is assessed. If it is small enough or if the atrial septal tissue is sufficiently redundant, the defect is closed primarily with suture. If not, a patch of pericardium or Dacron is sewn to the edge of the defect to close it.

Coding Tips

Atrial septal defects are normally congenital anomalies; however, they may also be the result of myocardial infarction. Note the diagnosis when selecting codes for repair of atrial septal defects as the code selected is dependent on the exact nature of the defect. For repair of atrial septal defect with repair of ventricular septal defect, see 33647. For repair of ostium primum atrial septal defect, see 33660.

ICD-10-CM Diagnostic Codes

I23.1	Atrial septal defect as current complication following acute myocardial infarction
I51.0	Cardiac septal defect, acquired
Q21.1	Atrial septal defect

AMA: 33641 2018,Jan,8; 2017,Jan,8; 2017,Dec,3; 2016,Jan,13; 2015,Jan,16; 2014,Jan,11

Relative Value Units/Medicare Edits

Non-Facility RVU	Work	PE	MP	Total
33641	29.58	11.02	6.78	47.38
Facility RVU	**Work**	**PE**	**MP**	**Total**
33641	29.58	11.02	6.78	47.38

	FUD	Status	MUE	Modifiers				IOM Reference
33641	90	A	1(2)	51	N/A	62*	80	None

* with documentation

Terms To Know

atrial septal defect. Cardiac anomaly consisting of a patent opening in the atrial septum due to a fusion failure, classified as ostium secundum type, ostium primum defect, or endocardial cushion defect.

cardiopulmonary bypass. Venous blood is diverted to a heart-lung machine, which mechanically pumps and oxygenates the blood temporarily so the heart can be bypassed while an open procedure on the heart or coronary arteries is performed. During bypass, the lungs are deflated and immobile.

ischemia. Deficiency in blood supply causing tissues to be deprived of oxygen, resulting from trauma, mechanical or functional constriction of blood vessels, or a physical obstruction.

ostium primum. Temporary opening between the right and left atrium between the lower margin of the septum primum and the atrioventricular canal in a fetal heart. In an adult heart, this condition results in an endocardial cushion defect of a cleft in the basal portion of the atrial septum with abnormal passage of blood through the congenital opening, usually associated with a cleft mitral valve.

33645

33645 Direct or patch closure, sinus venosus, with or without anomalous pulmonary venous drainage

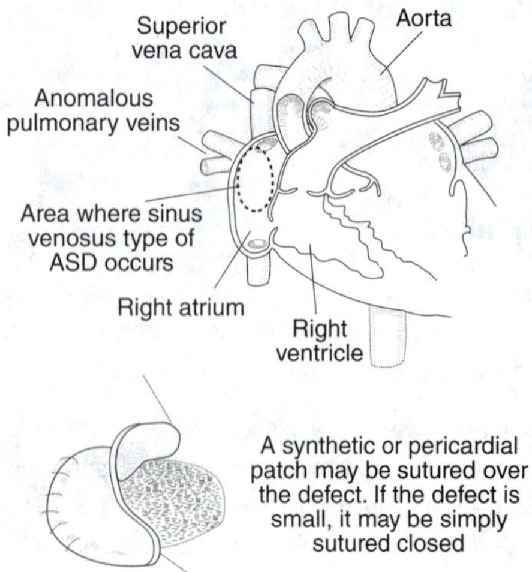

The sinus venosus is the area of the right atrium where the superior vena cava enters the chamber

Explanation

The right atrium is opened and the size and location of the congenital sinus venosus defect is assessed. If it is small enough or if the atrial septal tissue is sufficiently redundant, the defect is closed primarily with suture. If not, a patch of pericardium or Dacron is sewn to the edge of the defect to close it. Care is taken to place the patch so that all pulmonary veins remain patent and there is no obstruction of the superior vena cava, right ventricle, or pulmonary veins by the patch.

Coding Tips

Any repair of pulmonary venous drainage is included in 33645. Do not report 33645 with repair of isolated partial anomalous pulmonary venous return (33724) or repair of pulmonary venous stenosis (33726). Note the diagnosis when selecting codes for repair of septal defects as the code selected is dependent on the exact nature of the defect.

ICD-10-CM Diagnostic Codes

I23.1	Atrial septal defect as current complication following acute myocardial infarction
I51.0	Cardiac septal defect, acquired
Q21.1	Atrial septal defect

AMA: **33645** 2017,Dec,3

Relative Value Units/Medicare Edits

Non-Facility RVU	Work	PE	MP	Total
33645	31.3	11.55	7.43	50.28
Facility RVU	**Work**	**PE**	**MP**	**Total**
33645	31.3	11.55	7.43	50.28

	FUD	Status	MUE	Modifiers				IOM Reference
33645	90	A	1(2)	51	N/A	62*	80	None

* with documentation

33647

33647 Repair of atrial septal defect and ventricular septal defect, with direct or patch closure

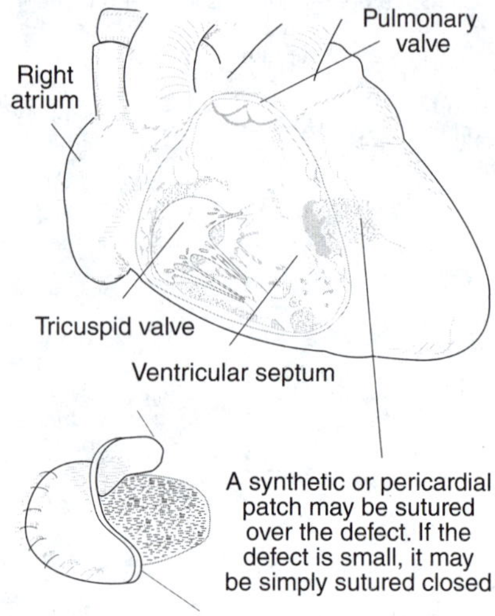

Repair of a ventricular septal defect is accomplished during the same session as a repair of an atrial septal defect

Explanation

Cardiopulmonary bypass is established with the venous uptake tubes in the superior and inferior caval veins. A hole in the right atrium or, if needed, a hole in one of the ventricles is made. The hole in the ventricle is made in the area of scar (if the ventricular septal defect is due to ischemia) or in the anterior part of the right ventricle (if the ventricular septal defect is congenital). All dead heart muscles are cut out (in ischemic ventricular septal defect) and the ventricular septal defect is closed with a patch of Dacron or pericardium. The hole in the atrium or ventricle is closed. Cardiopulmonary bypass is discontinued when heart function is restored.

Coding Tips

Note the diagnosis when selecting codes for repair of septal defects as the code selected is dependent on the exact nature of the defect. Ventricular septal defects are often associated with other cardiac anomalies. Many cardiac procedures include repair of ventricular septal defect in the code description. Code 33647 should not be reported additionally when the procedure specifically includes repair of ventricular septal defect. Do not append modifier 63 to 33647 as the description or nature of the procedure includes infants up to 4 kg. For repair of tricuspid atresia, see 33615. For closure of ventricular septal defect with or without patch, see 33681. For repair of transposition of great arteries, atrial baffle procedure (e.g., Mustard or Senning type) with cardiopulmonary bypass, with closure of ventricular septal defect, see 33776. For repair of transposition of the great arteries, aortic pulmonary artery reconstruction (e.g., Jatene type), with closure of ventricular septal defect, see 33780.

ICD-10-CM Diagnostic Codes

I23.1	Atrial septal defect as current complication following acute myocardial infarction
I23.2	Ventricular septal defect as current complication following acute myocardial infarction

I27.89	Other specified pulmonary heart diseases
I51.0	Cardiac septal defect, acquired
Q20.9	Congenital malformation of cardiac chambers and connections, unspecified
Q21.1	Atrial septal defect
Q21.2	Atrioventricular septal defect
Q21.9	Congenital malformation of cardiac septum, unspecified
Q24.9	Congenital malformation of heart, unspecified

AMA: 33647 2017,Dec,3

Relative Value Units/Medicare Edits

Non-Facility RVU	Work	PE	MP	Total
33647	33.0	11.97	7.86	52.83

Facility RVU	Work	PE	MP	Total
33647	33.0	11.97	7.86	52.83

	FUD	Status	MUE	Modifiers				IOM Reference
33647	90	A	1(2)	51	N/A	62*	80	None

* with documentation

Terms To Know

atrial septal defect. Cardiac anomaly consisting of a patent opening in the atrial septum due to a fusion failure, classified as ostium secundum type, ostium primum defect, or endocardial cushion defect.

cardiopulmonary bypass. Venous blood is diverted to a heart-lung machine, which mechanically pumps and oxygenates the blood temporarily so the heart can be bypassed while an open procedure on the heart or coronary arteries is performed. During bypass, the lungs are deflated and immobile.

myocardial infarction. Obstruction of circulation to the heart, resulting in necrosis.

ostium primum. Temporary opening between the right and left atrium between the lower margin of the septum primum and the atrioventricular canal in a fetal heart. In an adult heart, this condition results in an endocardial cushion defect of a cleft in the basal portion of the atrial septum with abnormal passage of blood through the congenital opening, usually associated with a cleft mitral valve.

ventricular septal defect. Congenital cardiac anomaly resulting in a continual opening in the septum between the ventricles that, in severe cases, causes oxygenated blood to flow back into the lungs, resulting in pulmonary hypertension.

33660-33665

33660 Repair of incomplete or partial atrioventricular canal (ostium primum atrial septal defect), with or without atrioventricular valve repair

33665 Repair of intermediate or transitional atrioventricular canal, with or without atrioventricular valve repair

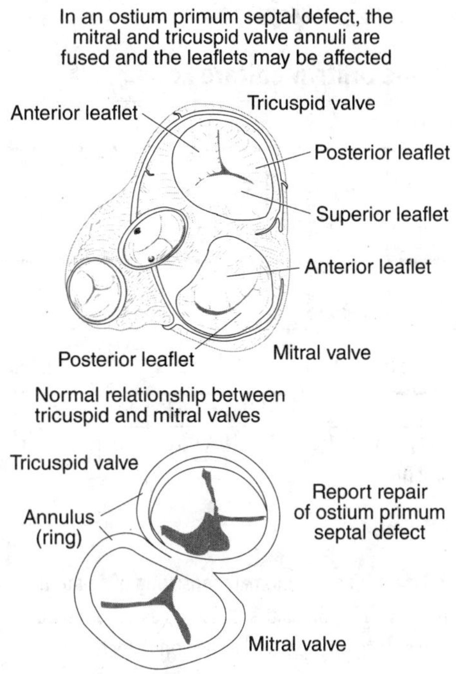

Explanation

Cardiopulmonary bypass is established using venous uptake tubes in both the superior and inferior caval veins. In 33660, the right atrium is opened. A radially oriented cleft or division in the anterior leaflet of the mitral valve is closed with interrupted sutures. Care is taken to assure that the valve closes properly after it is repaired. There is a line of denser valve tissue marking the anatomic line between the two AV valves. The ventricular septal defect is obliterated by sewing this line to the top of the septal muscle. The arterial septal defect is closed with a patch of Dacron or pericardium. The right atrium is closed and cardiopulmonary bypass is discontinued after heart function is restored. In 33665, a hole in the right atrium or, if needed, a hole in one of the ventricles is made. The hole in the ventricle is made in the area of scar tissue (if the ventricular septal defect is due to ischemia) or in the anterior part of the right ventricle (if the ventricular septal defect is congenital). The AV valve anatomy can be highly variable, ranging from normal mitral and tricuspid anatomy with a subvalvular ventricular septal defect to grossly abnormal AV valve leaflet with two separate valves present separated by a line of tissue. The AV valves are repaired. Repair is all that is done if valvular competence can be restored to the left AV valve. If not, the valve is replaced with a mechanical valve on a tissue valve.

Coding Tips

Note the diagnosis when selecting codes for repair of septal defects as the code selected is dependent on the exact nature of the defect. For closure of an atrioventricular valve, see 33600. For repair of an atrial septal defect, secundum, see 33641. For repair of an atrial septal defect and a ventricular septal defect, see 33647. For repair of complete atrioventricular canal, with or without prosthetic valve, see 33670.

Heart and Pericardium

 ● New ▲ Revised + Add On AMA: CPT Assist [Resequenced] ☑ Laterality

ICD-10-CM Diagnostic Codes

Q20.9	Congenital malformation of cardiac chambers and connections, unspecified
Q21.2	Atrioventricular septal defect
Q21.9	Congenital malformation of cardiac septum, unspecified
Q24.9	Congenital malformation of heart, unspecified

AMA: 33660 2017,Dec,3 **33665** 2017,Dec,3

Relative Value Units/Medicare Edits

Non-Facility RVU	Work	PE	MP	Total
33660	31.83	11.65	7.57	51.05
33665	34.85	12.48	8.29	55.62
Facility RVU	**Work**	**PE**	**MP**	**Total**
33660	31.83	11.65	7.57	51.05
33665	34.85	12.48	8.29	55.62

	FUD	Status	MUE	Modifiers				IOM Reference
33660	90	A	1(2)	51	N/A	62*	80	None
33665	90	A	1(2)	51	N/A	62*	80	

* with documentation

Terms To Know

atrial septal defect. Cardiac anomaly consisting of a patent opening in the atrial septum due to a fusion failure, classified as ostium secundum type, ostium primum defect, or endocardial cushion defect.

cardiopulmonary bypass. Venous blood is diverted to a heart-lung machine, which mechanically pumps and oxygenates the blood temporarily so the heart can be bypassed while an open procedure on the heart or coronary arteries is performed. During bypass, the lungs are deflated and immobile.

congenital. Present at birth, occurring through heredity or an influence during gestation up to the moment of birth.

ischemia. Deficiency in blood supply causing tissues to be deprived of oxygen, resulting from trauma, mechanical or functional constriction of blood vessels, or a physical obstruction.

ventricular septal defect. Congenital cardiac anomaly resulting in a continual opening in the septum between the ventricles that, in severe cases, causes oxygenated blood to flow back into the lungs, resulting in pulmonary hypertension.

33670

33670 Repair of complete atrioventricular canal, with or without prosthetic valve

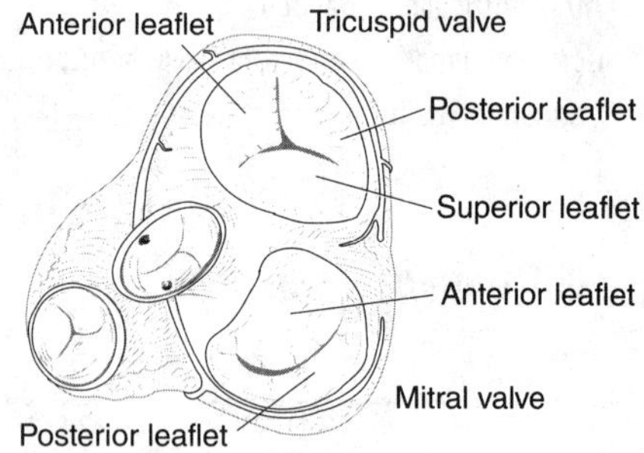

Normal relationship between tricuspid and mitral valves

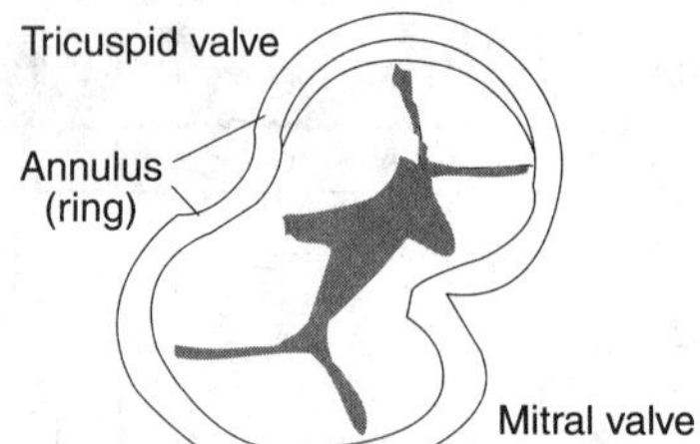

In a complete atrioventricular septal defect, the valves have merged into a single valve. Repair involves closing the VSD and sometimes installing a prosthetic valve

Explanation

Cardiopulmonary bypass is established using venous uptake tubes in the superior and inferior caval veins. The right atrium is opened. A radially oriented cleft or division in the anterior leaflet of the mitral value is closed with the interrupted sutures. Care is taken to assure that the valve closes properly after it is repaired. There is a raphe or line of denser value tissue marking the anatomic line between the two AV valves. The ventricular septal defect is obliterated by sewing this line to the top of the septal muscle. The atrial septal defect is closed with a patch of Dacron or pericardium. The competency of the single AV valve is assessed as is the imaginary line where the plane extending upward from the ventricular septal defect intersects the AV valve. The AV valve leaflets are divided along this line. The ventricular septal defect patch is placed. The valve leaflets are resuspended by sewing them to the ventricular septal defect patch. The competency of the valves is assessed. The atrial septal defect is closed with a patch sewn to the top of the ventricular septal defect patch or an extension of the ventricular septal defect patch is used to close the atrial septal defect (single patch technique). The hole in the right atrium is closed. Cardiopulmonary bypass is discontinued when cardiac function has returned.

Coding Tips

Do not append modifier 63 to 33670 as the description or nature of the procedure includes infants up to 4 kg. For repair of an incomplete or partial atrioventricular canal (ostium primum atrial septal defect), with or without atrial ventricular valve repair, see 33660. For repair of an intermediate or transitional atrioventricular canal, with or without atrioventricular valve repair, see 33665. For repair of an atrial septal defect, secundum, with cardiopulmonary bypass, with or without patch, see 33641. For closure of a ventricular septal defect, with or without patch, see 33681. For repair of transposition of great arteries, atrial baffle procedure (e.g., Mustard or Senning type) with cardiopulmonary bypass, with closure of ventricular septal defect, see 33776. For repair of transposition of the great arteries, aortic pulmonary artery reconstruction (e.g., Jatene type), with closure of ventricular septal defect, see 33780.

ICD-10-CM Diagnostic Codes

Q21.2	Atrioventricular septal defect

AMA: 33670 2017,Dec,3

Relative Value Units/Medicare Edits

Non-Facility RVU	Work	PE	MP	Total
33670	36.63	12.05	8.72	57.4
Facility RVU	**Work**	**PE**	**MP**	**Total**
33670	36.63	12.05	8.72	57.4

	FUD	Status	MUE	Modifiers				IOM Reference
33670	90	A	1(2)	51	N/A	62*	80	None

* with documentation

Terms To Know

anomaly. Irregularity in the structure or position of an organ or tissue.

atrial septal defect. Cardiac anomaly consisting of a patent opening in the atrial septum due to a fusion failure, classified as ostium secundum type, ostium primum defect, or endocardial cushion defect.

cardiopulmonary bypass. Venous blood is diverted to a heart-lung machine, which mechanically pumps and oxygenates the blood temporarily so the heart can be bypassed while an open procedure on the heart or coronary arteries is performed. During bypass, the lungs are deflated and immobile.

congenital. Present at birth, occurring through heredity or an influence during gestation up to the moment of birth.

ventricular septal defect. Congenital cardiac anomaly resulting in a continual opening in the septum between the ventricles that, in severe cases, causes oxygenated blood to flow back into the lungs, resulting in pulmonary hypertension.

33675

33675 Closure of multiple ventricular septal defects;

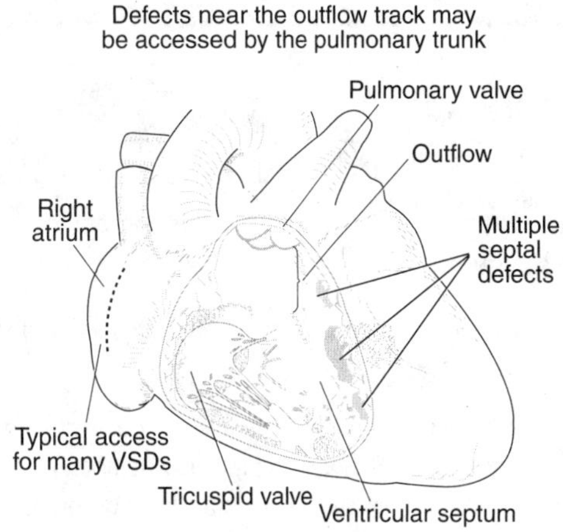

Depiction is of a cutaway view of the right ventricle

Explanation

The physician repairs multiple defects in the tissue separating the right and left ventricles of the heart in an open heart procedure. Cardiopulmonary bypass is established with tubes in both the caval veins. The ventricular septal defects can almost always be accessed and repaired through an incision in the right atrium. Each ventricular septal defect is usually repaired with a patch of Dacron or pericardium, but may be closed using only sutures. The septal defects may be repaired with a pair of patches, one in each ventricle. After the ventricular septal defects are repaired, the access incision in the right atrium is closed with sutures. Cardiopulmonary bypass is discontinued when heart function returns. The chest incision is repaired.

Coding Tips

Aspiration of the pleural space via thoracentesis (32554, 32555), as well as tube thoracostomy (32551), is included and should not be reported separately. Do not report thoracotomy (32100) separately. Temporary transvenous pacemaker placement (33210) is also included and should not be reported separately. Do not report closure of a single ventricular septal defect (33681–33688) separately. For closure of multiple ventricular septal defects with pulmonary valvotomy or infundibular resection, see 33676; with removal of pulmonary artery band, with or without gusset, see 33677. For percutaneous closure, see 93581.

ICD-10-CM Diagnostic Codes

I51.0	Cardiac septal defect, acquired
Q20.8	Other congenital malformations of cardiac chambers and connections
Q20.9	Congenital malformation of cardiac chambers and connections, unspecified
Q21.0	Ventricular septal defect
Q21.4	Aortopulmonary septal defect
Q21.8	Other congenital malformations of cardiac septa
Q21.9	Congenital malformation of cardiac septum, unspecified
Q24.9	Congenital malformation of heart, unspecified

AMA: 33675 2018,Jan,8; 2017,Jan,8; 2017,Dec,3; 2016,Jan,13; 2015,Jan,16; 2014,Jan,11

Relative Value Units/Medicare Edits

Non-Facility RVU	Work	PE	MP	Total
33675	35.95	12.82	8.55	57.32
Facility RVU	Work	PE	MP	Total
33675	35.95	12.82	8.55	57.32

	FUD	Status	MUE	Modifiers				IOM Reference
33675	90	A	1(2)	51	N/A	62*	80	None

* with documentation

Terms To Know

atresia. Congenital closure or absence of a tubular organ or an opening to the body surface.

cardiopulmonary bypass. Venous blood is diverted to a heart-lung machine, which mechanically pumps and oxygenates the blood temporarily so the heart can be bypassed while an open procedure on the heart or coronary arteries is performed. During bypass, the lungs are deflated and immobile.

cor biloculare. Congenital anomaly in which the heart is two-chambered, lacking both an atrial and a ventricular septum. Few newborns with this condition live to the first year.

myocardial infarction. Obstruction of circulation to the heart, resulting in necrosis.

ventricular septal defect. Congenital cardiac anomaly resulting in a continual opening in the septum between the ventricles that, in severe cases, causes oxygenated blood to flow back into the lungs, resulting in pulmonary hypertension.

33676

33676 Closure of multiple ventricular septal defects; with pulmonary valvotomy or infundibular resection (acyanotic)

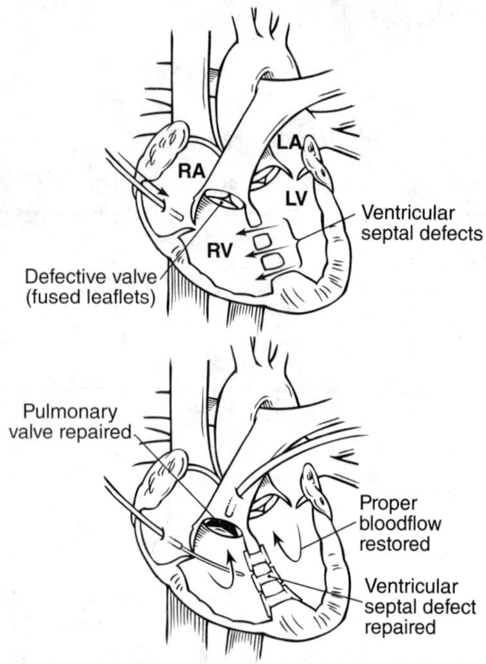

Explanation

The physician repairs multiple defects in the tissue separating the right and left ventricles of the heart, and surgically releases fused leaflets within the pulmonary valve or resects the anterosuperior portion of the right ventricle (infundibulum). The heart is accessed through a midline sternal incision. Cardiopulmonary bypass is established with tubes in both the caval veins. The septal and ventricular defects can almost always be accessed and repaired through an incision in the right atrium, and the pulmonary valve is usually accessed through an incision in the pulmonary artery. Each ventricular septal defect is usually repaired with a patch of Dacron or pericardium, but may be closed using only sutures. The septal defects alternately may be repaired with a pair of patches, applied on each side of the septum. Fused pulmonary valve leaflets are incised and any abnormal tethering of the leaflets to the arterial wall is released. For infundibular resection, obstructions within the right ventricle are excised and the ventricle repaired. After repairs are complete, the access incision in the right atrium is closed with sutures. Cardiopulmonary bypass is discontinued when heart function returns. The chest incision is repaired.

Coding Tips

Aspiration of the pleural space via thoracentesis (32554, 32555), as well as tube thoracostomy (32551), is included and should not be reported separately. Do not report thoracotomy (32100) separately. Temporary transvenous pacemaker placement (33210) is also included and should not be reported separately. Do not report closure of a single ventricular septal defect (33681–33688) separately. For closure of multiple ventricular septal defects only, see 33675; with removal of pulmonary artery band, with or without gusset, see 33677. For percutaneous closure, see 93581.

ICD-10-CM Diagnostic Codes

I23.2	Ventricular septal defect as current complication following acute myocardial infarction

I51.0	Cardiac septal defect, acquired
Q20.8	Other congenital malformations of cardiac chambers and connections
Q20.9	Congenital malformation of cardiac chambers and connections, unspecified
Q21.0	Ventricular septal defect
Q21.8	Other congenital malformations of cardiac septa
Q21.9	Congenital malformation of cardiac septum, unspecified
Q22.0	Pulmonary valve atresia
Q22.1	Congenital pulmonary valve stenosis
Q22.2	Congenital pulmonary valve insufficiency
Q22.3	Other congenital malformations of pulmonary valve
Q24.9	Congenital malformation of heart, unspecified

AMA: 33676 2018,Jan,8; 2017,Jan,8; 2017,Dec,3; 2016,Jan,13; 2015,Jan,16; 2014,Jan,11

Relative Value Units/Medicare Edits

Non-Facility RVU	Work	PE	MP	Total
33676	36.95	13.1	8.79	58.84
Facility RVU	**Work**	**PE**	**MP**	**Total**
33676	36.95	13.1	8.79	58.84

	FUD	Status	MUE	Modifiers				IOM Reference
33676	90	A	1(2)	51	N/A	62*	80	None

* with documentation

Terms To Know

anomaly. Irregularity in the structure or position of an organ or tissue.

congenital. Present at birth, occurring through heredity or an influence during gestation up to the moment of birth.

infundibulectomy. Excision of the anterosuperior portion of the right ventricle of the heart.

valvotomy. Cutting through stenosed cardiac valve leaflets or cusp to relieve or repair the obstruction caused by scar tissue and inflammation.

ventricular septal defect. Congenital cardiac anomaly resulting in a continual opening in the septum between the ventricles that, in severe cases, causes oxygenated blood to flow back into the lungs, resulting in pulmonary hypertension.

33677

33677 Closure of multiple ventricular septal defects; with removal of pulmonary artery band, with or without gusset

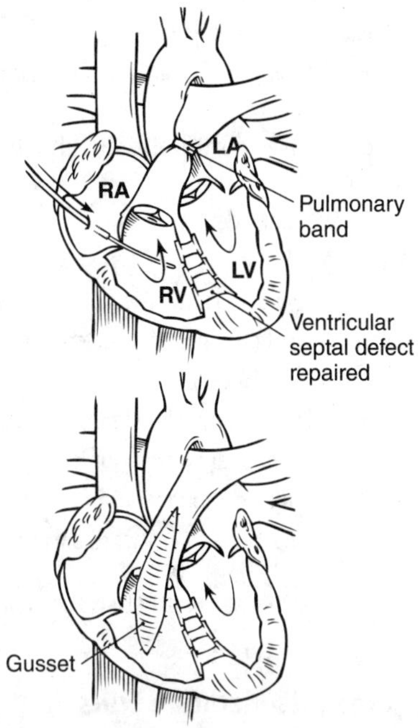

Multiple ventricular septal defects are repaired and a pulmonary artery band is removed, and normal blood flow returns to the heart

Explanation

The physician repairs multiple defects in the tissue separating the right and left ventricles of the heart, removes a previously placed band from the pulmonary artery, and may place a gusset. The heart is accessed through a midline sternal incision. The physician gains access to the mediastinum through an incision through the sternum (median sternotomy). The physician places cardiopulmonary bypass catheters through incisions in the low inferior vena cava, the superior vena cava, and aorta or femoral artery. The physician stops the heart by infusing cardioplegia solution into the coronary circulation. The septal defects can almost always be accessed and repaired through an incision in the right atrium, and the pulmonary valve is usually accessed through an incision in the pulmonary artery. Each ventricular septal defect is usually repaired with a patch of Dacron or pericardium, but may be closed using only sutures. The septal defects alternately may be repaired with a pair of patches applied on each side of the septum. The physician removes the pulmonary artery band (placed during a previous surgery) and dilates the pulmonary artery to normal size. A triangular patch (gusset) may be sutured into the incised pulmonary artery to enlarge its circumference. The physician closes the cardiac incisions, takes the patient off cardiopulmonary bypass, closes the remaining surgical incisions, and dresses the sternal or chest wall wound. The physician may leave chest tubes and/or a mediastinal drainage tube in place following the procedure.

Coding Tips

Aspiration of the pleural space via thoracentesis (32554, 32555), as well as tube thoracostomy (32551), is included and should not be reported separately. Do not report thoracotomy (32100) separately. Temporary transvenous pacemaker placement (33210) is also included and should not be reported separately. Do not report closure of a single ventricular septal defect (33681–33688) separately. For closure of multiple ventricular septal defects only, see 33675; with pulmonary valvotomy or infundibular resection, see 33676. For percutaneous closure, see 93581.

ICD-10-CM Diagnostic Codes

I23.2	Ventricular septal defect as current complication following acute myocardial infarction
I51.0	Cardiac septal defect, acquired
Q20.8	Other congenital malformations of cardiac chambers and connections
Q20.9	Congenital malformation of cardiac chambers and connections, unspecified
Q21.0	Ventricular septal defect
Q21.3	Tetralogy of Fallot
Q21.8	Other congenital malformations of cardiac septa
Q21.9	Congenital malformation of cardiac septum, unspecified
Q22.0	Pulmonary valve atresia
Q22.1	Congenital pulmonary valve stenosis
Q22.2	Congenital pulmonary valve insufficiency
Q22.3	Other congenital malformations of pulmonary valve
Q24.9	Congenital malformation of heart, unspecified

AMA: **33677** 2018,Jan,8; 2017,Jan,8; 2017,Dec,3; 2016,Jan,13; 2015,Jan,16; 2014,Jan,11

Relative Value Units/Medicare Edits

Non-Facility RVU	Work	PE	MP	Total
33677	38.45	13.51	9.15	61.11
Facility RVU	**Work**	**PE**	**MP**	**Total**
33677	38.45	13.51	9.15	61.11

	FUD	Status	MUE	Modifiers				IOM Reference
33677	90	A	1(2)	51	N/A	62*	80	None

* with documentation

Terms To Know

anomaly. Irregularity in the structure or position of an organ or tissue.

congenital. Present at birth, occurring through heredity or an influence during gestation up to the moment of birth.

pulmonary artery banding. Surgical constriction of the pulmonary artery to prevent irreversible pulmonary vascular obstructive changes and overflow into the left ventricle.

ventricular septal defect. Congenital cardiac anomaly resulting in a continual opening in the septum between the ventricles that, in severe cases, causes oxygenated blood to flow back into the lungs, resulting in pulmonary hypertension.

33681

33681 Closure of single ventricular septal defect, with or without patch;

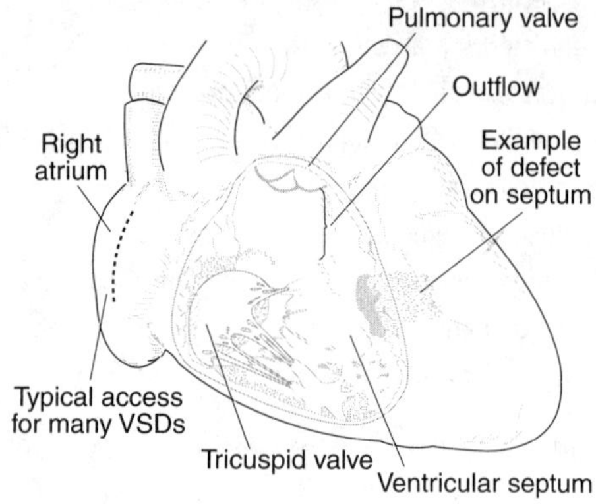

Depiction is of a cutaway view of the right ventricle

A single defect in the ventricular septum is repaired

Explanation

The physician repairs a solitary defect in the tissue separating the right and left ventricles of the heart in an open heart procedure. Cardiopulmonary bypass is established with tubes in both the caval veins. The ventricular septal defect can almost always be accessed and repaired through an incision in the right atrium, except in the case of a supracristal ventricular septal defect, in which the ventricle is higher in the outflow part of the right ventricle. This type of ventricular septal defect is most often accessed and repaired through an incision in the pulmonary artery. All types of ventricular septal defects can be accessed and repaired through an incision in the muscle of the right ventricle, but this causes more damage and is avoided if possible. The ventricular septal defect is usually repaired with a patch of Dacron or pericardium, but may be closed using only sutures. After the ventricular septal defect is closed, the hole that has been created in the right atrium, right ventricle, or pulmonary artery is closed. The chest incision is repaired. Cardiopulmonary bypass is discontinued when heart function returns.

Coding Tips

Ventricular septal defects are often associated with other cardiac anomalies. Many cardiac procedures include repair of a ventricular septal defect in the code description. Code 33681 should not be reported additionally when the procedure description specifically includes repair of ventricular septal defect. For repair of atrial septal defect and ventricular septal defect, with or without direct or patch closure, see 33647.

ICD-10-CM Diagnostic Codes

I23.2	Ventricular septal defect as current complication following acute myocardial infarction
I51.0	Cardiac septal defect, acquired
Q20.8	Other congenital malformations of cardiac chambers and connections
Q20.9	Congenital malformation of cardiac chambers and connections, unspecified
Q21.0	Ventricular septal defect
Q21.8	Other congenital malformations of cardiac septa
Q21.9	Congenital malformation of cardiac septum, unspecified
Q22.3	Other congenital malformations of pulmonary valve
Q24.9	Congenital malformation of heart, unspecified

AMA: **33681** 2018,Jan,8; 2017,Jan,8; 2017,Dec,3; 2016,Jan,13; 2015,Jan,16; 2014,Jan,11

Relative Value Units/Medicare Edits

Non-Facility RVU	Work	PE	MP	Total
33681	32.34	13.38	7.31	53.03
Facility RVU	**Work**	**PE**	**MP**	**Total**
33681	32.34	13.38	7.31	53.03

	FUD	Status	MUE	Modifiers				IOM Reference
33681	90	A	1(2)	51	N/A	62*	80	None

* with documentation

Terms To Know

cardiopulmonary bypass. Venous blood is diverted to a heart-lung machine, which mechanically pumps and oxygenates the blood temporarily so the heart can be bypassed while an open procedure on the heart or coronary arteries is performed. During bypass, the lungs are deflated and immobile.

cor biloculare. Congenital anomaly in which the heart is two-chambered, lacking both an atrial and a ventricular septum. Few newborns with this condition live to the first year.

myocardial infarction. Obstruction of circulation to the heart, resulting in necrosis.

ventricular septal defect. Congenital cardiac anomaly resulting in a continual opening in the septum between the ventricles that, in severe cases, causes oxygenated blood to flow back into the lungs, resulting in pulmonary hypertension.

33684

33684 Closure of single ventricular septal defect, with or without patch; with pulmonary valvotomy or infundibular resection (acyanotic)

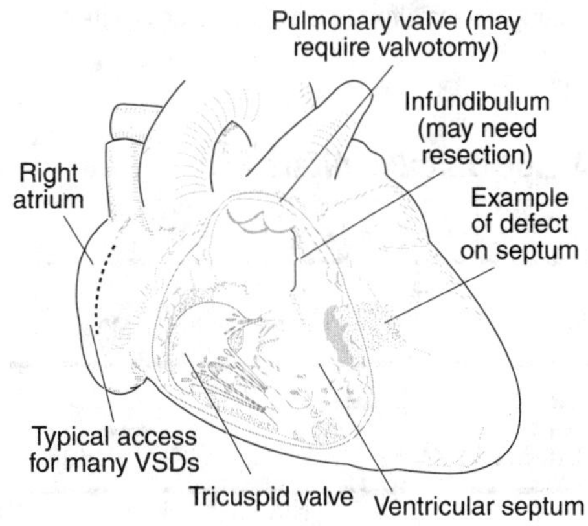

Depiction is of a cutaway view of the right ventricle

Explanation

The physician repairs a solitary defect in the tissue separating the right and left ventricles of the heart in an open heart procedure in conjunction with a pulmonary valvotomy or infundibular resection. Cardiopulmonary bypass is established with venous uptake tubes in both the caval veins. Prior to surgery, it is established by echocardiography, cardiac catheterization, or both that the diameter of the tricuspid valve is large enough to permit a normal cardiac output. If not, the operation is combined with a modified Blalock-Taussig shunt. The right ventricle or pulmonary artery is opened. Through either opening, the infundibular muscle blocking blood flow to the pulmonary artery can be cut out and cuts can be made in the pulmonary valve to reduce the restriction to blood flow that it presents. A singular ventricular septal defect is closed through either of these incisions, if possible. If it is not possible to close the ventricular septal defect with the exposure thus provided, the right atrium is opened and the ventricular septal defect closed. A patch is almost always used. All holes in the heart are closed. Cardiopulmonary bypass is discontinued when heart function is restored.

Coding Tips

When 33684 is performed with another separately identifiable procedure, the highest dollar value code is listed as the primary procedure and subsequent procedures are appended with modifier 51. When ligation and takedown of systemic-to-pulmonary artery shunt is performed in addition to this procedure, it should be reported separately, see 33924. For shunt, subclavian to pulmonary artery (Blalock-Taussig type operation), see 33750. For closure of a ventricular septal defect only, with or without a patch, see 33681.

ICD-10-CM Diagnostic Codes

I23.2	Ventricular septal defect as current complication following acute myocardial infarction
I51.0	Cardiac septal defect, acquired
Q20.8	Other congenital malformations of cardiac chambers and connections
Q20.9	Congenital malformation of cardiac chambers and connections, unspecified
Q21.0	Ventricular septal defect
Q21.8	Other congenital malformations of cardiac septa

Q21.9 Congenital malformation of cardiac septum, unspecified
Q22.0 Pulmonary valve atresia
Q22.1 Congenital pulmonary valve stenosis
Q22.2 Congenital pulmonary valve insufficiency
Q22.3 Other congenital malformations of pulmonary valve
Q24.9 Congenital malformation of heart, unspecified

AMA: 33684 2017,Dec,3

Relative Value Units/Medicare Edits

Non-Facility RVU	Work	PE	MP	Total
33684	34.37	12.35	8.17	54.89
Facility RVU	**Work**	**PE**	**MP**	**Total**
33684	34.37	12.35	8.17	54.89

	FUD	Status	MUE	Modifiers				IOM Reference
33684	90	A	1(2)	51	N/A	62*	80	None

* with documentation

Terms To Know

atresia. Congenital closure or absence of a tubular organ or an opening to the body surface.

infundibulectomy. Excision of the anterosuperior portion of the right ventricle of the heart.

myocardial infarction. Obstruction of circulation to the heart, resulting in necrosis.

valvuloplasty. Surgical repair of a valve.

ventricular septal defect. Congenital cardiac anomaly resulting in a continual opening in the septum between the ventricles that, in severe cases, causes oxygenated blood to flow back into the lungs, resulting in pulmonary hypertension.

33688

33688 Closure of single ventricular septal defect, with or without patch; with removal of pulmonary artery band, with or without gusset

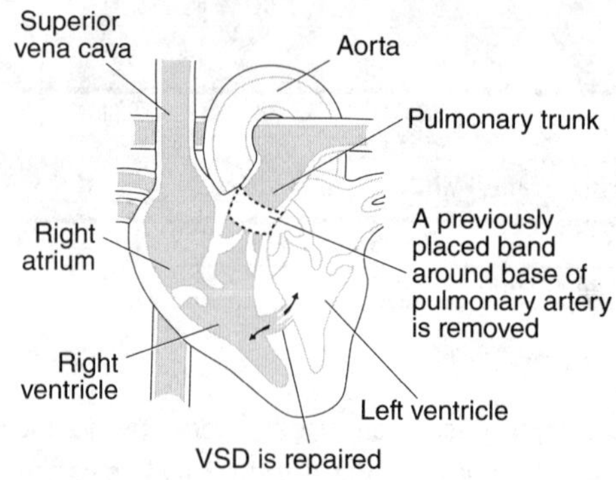

Schematic showing pulmonary band removal and VSD repair

Explanation

The physician repairs a solitary defect in the tissue separating the right and left ventricles of the heart in an open heart procedure in conjunction with removal of a previously placed pulmonary artery (PA) band. The patient is prepared for cardiopulmonary bypass, but it is not established yet. The previously placed pulmonary artery band is dissected out and removed. Stenosis at the site of the pulmonary artery band is assessed before and after band removal with a pressure transducer connected to a needle probe that measures any pressure drop across the area of narrowing. Cardiopulmonary bypass is then established and the ventricular septal defect is repaired. If pulmonary artery pressures proximal to the band site remain high after band removal and ventricular septal defect closure or if the surgeon feels the residual stenosis is too tight, cardiopulmonary bypass is restarted. The surgeon then removes the stenosed segment of pulmonary artery followed by a primary repair or the surgeon makes an incision in the pulmonary artery across the area of narrowing and closes the defect with a patch graft. Heart function is restored and cardiopulmonary bypass is discontinued.

Coding Tips

When ligation and takedown of systemic-to-pulmonary artery shunt is performed in addition to this procedure, it should be reported separately, see 33924. For pulmonary vein repair requiring creation of an atrial septal defect, see 33724. For repair of transposition of great arteries, atrial baffle procedure (e.g., Mustard or Senning type) with cardiopulmonary bypass, with removal of pulmonary band, see 33775. For repair of transposition of the great arteries, aortic pulmonary artery reconstruction (e.g., Jatene type), with removal of pulmonary band, see 33779.

ICD-10-CM Diagnostic Codes

I23.2 Ventricular septal defect as current complication following acute myocardial infarction
I51.0 Cardiac septal defect, acquired
Q20.8 Other congenital malformations of cardiac chambers and connections
Q20.9 Congenital malformation of cardiac chambers and connections, unspecified
Q21.0 Ventricular septal defect
Q21.8 Other congenital malformations of cardiac septa
Q21.9 Congenital malformation of cardiac septum, unspecified

Q22.0	Pulmonary valve atresia
Q22.1	Congenital pulmonary valve stenosis
Q22.2	Congenital pulmonary valve insufficiency
Q22.3	Other congenital malformations of pulmonary valve
Q24.9	Congenital malformation of heart, unspecified

AMA: **33688** 2017,Dec,3

Relative Value Units/Medicare Edits

Non-Facility RVU	Work	PE	MP	Total
33688	34.75	11.78	8.27	54.8
Facility RVU	**Work**	**PE**	**MP**	**Total**
33688	34.75	11.78	8.27	54.8

	FUD	Status	MUE	Modifiers				IOM Reference
33688	90	A	1(2)	51	N/A	62*	80	None

* with documentation

Terms To Know

cardiopulmonary bypass. Venous blood is diverted to a heart-lung machine, which mechanically pumps and oxygenates the blood temporarily so the heart can be bypassed while an open procedure on the heart or coronary arteries is performed. During bypass, the lungs are deflated and immobile.

stenosis. Narrowing or constriction of a passage.

transposition. Removal or exchange from one side to another; change of position from one place to another.

vena cava. Main venous trunk that empties into the right atrium from both the lower and upper regions, beginning at the junction of the common iliac veins inferiorly and the two brachiocephalic veins superiorly.

ventricular septal defect. Congenital cardiac anomaly resulting in a continual opening in the septum between the ventricles that, in severe cases, causes oxygenated blood to flow back into the lungs, resulting in pulmonary hypertension.

33690

33690 Banding of pulmonary artery

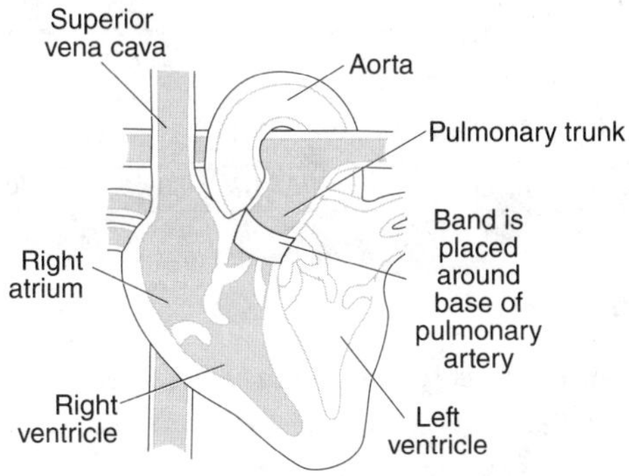

A synthetic band is placed around the base of the pulmonary artery

Explanation

Cardiopulmonary bypass is not required. The pulmonary artery is exposed through a median sternotomy or left thoracotomy. A band of heavy Dacron suture or tape is place around the base of the pulmonary artery. Once the PA pressure distal to the band is less than half of the systemic pressure and the patients arterial saturation is greater than 70 percent, the band is tight enough, but not too tight. The incision is closed.

Coding Tips

Placement of the pulmonary band (banding) is sometimes performed with other procedures on the heart and should be reported separately unless specifically included in the procedure description. When 33690 is performed with another separately identifiable procedure, the highest dollar value code is listed as the primary procedure and subsequent procedures are appended with modifier 51. Do not append modifier 63 to 33690 as the description or nature of the procedure includes infants up to 4 kg. For right and left pulmonary banding within one ventricle, see 33620. For repair of a ventricular septal defect, with or without patch, with removal of pulmonary artery band, with or without gusset, see 33688. For repair of transposition of the great arteries, atrial baffle procedure (e.g., Mustard or Senning type), with cardiopulmonary bypass, with removal of pulmonary band, see 33775. For repair of transposition of the great arteries, aortic pulmonary artery reconstruction (e.g., Jatene type), with removal of pulmonary band, see 33779.

ICD-10-CM Diagnostic Codes

Q20.1	Double outlet right ventricle
Q20.3	Discordant ventriculoarterial connection
Q21.0	Ventricular septal defect
Q21.2	Atrioventricular septal defect
Q21.9	Congenital malformation of cardiac septum, unspecified
Q22.4	Congenital tricuspid stenosis
Q22.6	Hypoplastic right heart syndrome
Q22.8	Other congenital malformations of tricuspid valve
Q22.9	Congenital malformation of tricuspid valve, unspecified

AMA: **33690** 2018,Jan,8; 2017,Jan,8; 2016,Jan,13; 2015,Jan,16; 2014,Jan,11

Relative Value Units/Medicare Edits

Non-Facility RVU	Work	PE	MP	Total
33690	20.36	9.6	4.82	34.78
Facility RVU	**Work**	**PE**	**MP**	**Total**
33690	20.36	9.6	4.82	34.78

	FUD	Status	MUE	Modifiers				IOM Reference
33690	90	A	1(2)	51	N/A	62*	80	None

* with documentation

Terms To Know

atresia. Congenital closure or absence of a tubular organ or an opening to the body surface.

cardiopulmonary bypass. Venous blood is diverted to a heart-lung machine, which mechanically pumps and oxygenates the blood temporarily so the heart can be bypassed while an open procedure on the heart or coronary arteries is performed. During bypass, the lungs are deflated and immobile.

congenital. Present at birth, occurring through heredity or an influence during gestation up to the moment of birth.

gusset. Triangular or diamond shaped patch that is placed for reinforcement or expansion.

incision. Act of cutting into tissue or an organ.

occlusion. Constriction, closure, or blockage of a passage.

stenosis. Narrowing or constriction of a passage.

sternotomy. Incision into the sternum, the bone that forms the front of the chest cavity and connects with the ribs.

thoracotomy. Surgical procedure for opening the chest wall in order to access the lungs, esophagus, trachea, aorta, heart, and diaphragm.

ventricular septal defect. Congenital cardiac anomaly resulting in a continual opening in the septum between the ventricles that, in severe cases, causes oxygenated blood to flow back into the lungs, resulting in pulmonary hypertension.

33692-33694

33692 Complete repair tetralogy of Fallot without pulmonary atresia;
33694 with transannular patch

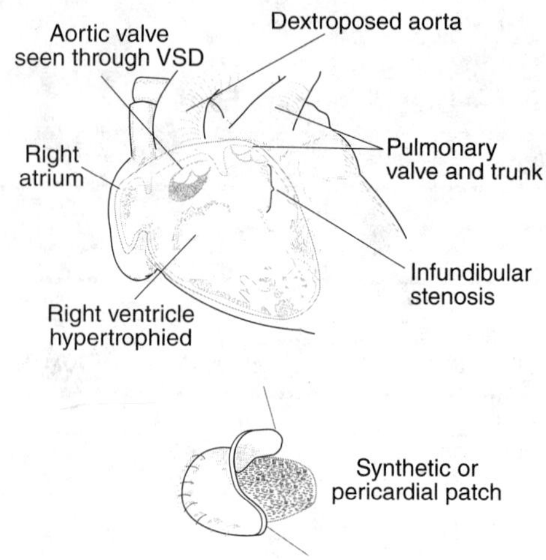

Explanation

In this defect, there are four cardiac anomalies: narrowing of the pulmonary valve annulus and/or the right ventricular infundibulum that restricts normal pulmonary blood flow, a ventricular septal defect, hypertrophy of the right ventricle, and an overriding aorta. In 33692, repair of this defect assumes that the pulmonary valve and right ventricular outflow tract are of adequate size to permit normal pulmonary blood flow. Cardiopulmonary bypass is required. The surgical approach relies on the anatomical location of the VSD, by way of atrial incision or ventriculotomy. The ventricular septal defect is closed with a patch of Dacron allowing normal blood flow from the left ventricle to the aorta. The physician enlarges the pulmonary artery from the right ventricle in order to increase blood flow to the lungs allowing the proper amount of oxygen distribution to the body. Upon completion of the repair, the pericardium is closed and drainage tubes are placed. In 33694, surgical approach may be by right arteriotomy or right ventriculotomy based on the extent of obstruction within the right ventricular outflow tract. Cardiopulmonary bypass is required. Resection of the infundibular muscle is performed first. The ventricular septal defect is sutured closed. A longitudinal incision is made in the pulmonary artery and carried proximally across the pulmonary valve annulus and onto the muscles of the right ventricular outflow tract. The defect is closed with a patch placed across the pulmonary valve annulus. Cardiopulmonary bypass is discontinued when heart function returns.

Coding Tips

When ligation and takedown of systemic-to-pulmonary artery shunt is performed in addition to this procedure, it should be reported separately, see 33924. Do not append modifier 63 to 33694 as the description or nature of the procedure includes infants up to 4 kg. For repair of a complex cardiac anomaly other than pulmonary atresia with ventricular septal defect by construction or replacement of conduit from right to left ventricle to pulmonary artery, see 33608. For complete repair tetralogy of Fallot with pulmonary atresia, including construction of conduit from right ventricle to pulmonary artery and closure of ventricular septal defect, see 33697.

ICD-10-CM Diagnostic Codes

Q21.3 Tetralogy of Fallot

AMA: 33692 2017,Dec,3 **33694** 2017,Dec,3

Relative Value Units/Medicare Edits

Non-Facility RVU	Work	PE	MP	Total
33692	36.15	12.16	8.6	56.91
33694	35.57	12.68	8.46	56.71
Facility RVU	**Work**	**PE**	**MP**	**Total**
33692	36.15	12.16	8.6	56.91
33694	35.57	12.68	8.46	56.71

	FUD	Status	MUE	Modifiers				IOM Reference
33692	90	A	1(2)	51	N/A	62*	80	None
33694	90	A	1(2)	51	N/A	62*	80	

* with documentation

Terms To Know

atresia. Congenital closure or absence of a tubular organ or an opening to the body surface.

Blalock-Taussig procedure. Anastomosis of the left subclavian artery to the left pulmonary artery or the right subclavian artery to the right pulmonary artery in order to shunt some of the blood flow from the systemic to the pulmonary circulation.

ligation. Tying off a blood vessel or duct with a suture or a soft, thin wire.

pericardium. Thin and slippery case in which the heart lies that is lined with fluid so that the heart is free to pulse and move as it beats.

Potts-Smith-Gibson procedure. Side-to-side anastomosis of the aorta and left pulmonary artery creating a shunt that enlarges as the child grows.

tetralogy of Fallot. Specific combination of congenital cardiac defects: obstruction of the right ventricular outflow tract with pulmonary stenosis, interventricular septal defect, malposition of the aorta, overriding the interventricular septum and receiving blood from both the venous and arterial systems, and enlargement of the right ventricle.

ventricular septal defect. Congenital cardiac anomaly resulting in a continual opening in the septum between the ventricles that, in severe cases, causes oxygenated blood to flow back into the lungs, resulting in pulmonary hypertension.

Waterston procedure. Type of aortopulmonary shunting done to increase pulmonary blood flow. The ascending aorta is anastomosed to the right pulmonary artery.

33697

33697 Complete repair tetralogy of Fallot with pulmonary atresia including construction of conduit from right ventricle to pulmonary artery and closure of ventricular septal defect

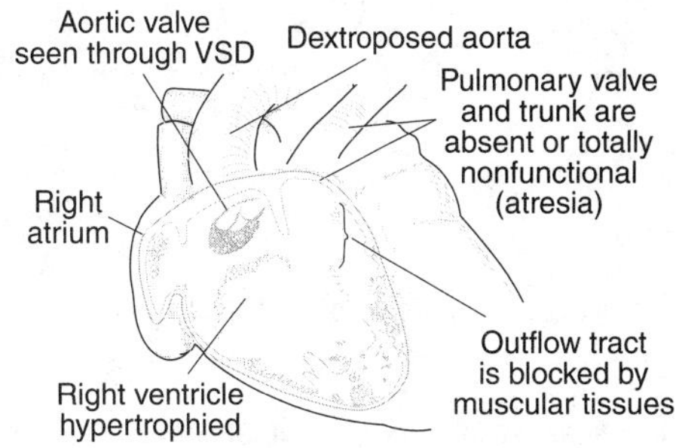

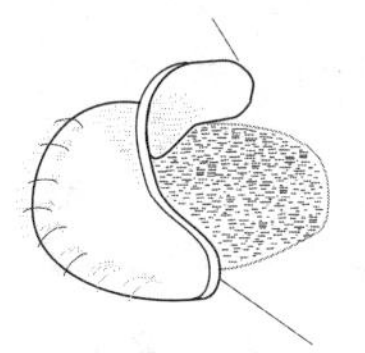

Explanation

The physician completely repairs tetralogy of Fallot with pulmonary atresia, including construction of a conduit from the right ventricle to the pulmonary artery and closure of the ventricular septal defect. Cardiopulmonary bypass is required. A hole is made in the right ventricle and any muscular obstruction in the outflow tract of the right ventricle is removed. The pulmonary artery or its branches are opened longitudinally until normal-sized vessels are encountered. The ventricular septal defect is closed. An aortic graft from a donor is trimmed to form a patch over the opened pulmonary artery. Any excess artery from the donor graft or a patch of pericardium or Dacron is sewn to the graft below the valve to use as a secondary patch for closing the hole in the right ventricle. The graft valve becomes the new pulmonary valve. After the patches and graft are sewn in place and heart function returns, cardiopulmonary bypass is stopped.

Coding Tips

When ligation and takedown of systemic-to-pulmonary artery shunt is performed in addition to this procedure, it should be reported separately, see 33924. For complete repair of tetralogy of Fallot without pulmonary atresia, see 33692; with transannular patch, see 33694. For repair of pulmonary atresia with a ventricular septal defect, see 33920. For closure of a ventricular septal defect, with or without patch, see 33681; with pulmonary valvotomy or infundibular resection (acyanotic), see 33684; with removal of a pulmonary artery band, with or without gusset, see 33688.

ICD-10-CM Diagnostic Codes

Q21.3 Tetralogy of Fallot

AMA: 33697 2018,Jan,8; 2017,Jan,8; 2017,Dec,3; 2016,Jan,13; 2015,Jan,16; 2014,Jan,11

Relative Value Units/Medicare Edits

Non-Facility RVU	Work	PE	MP	Total
33697	37.57	13.23	8.93	59.73
Facility RVU	**Work**	**PE**	**MP**	**Total**
33697	37.57	13.23	8.93	59.73

	FUD	Status	MUE	Modifiers				IOM Reference
33697	90	A	1(2)	51	N/A	62*	80	None

* with documentation

Terms To Know

atresia. Congenital closure or absence of a tubular organ or an opening to the body surface.

blue baby. Infant born with bluish discoloration due to cyanosis.

cardiopulmonary bypass. Venous blood is diverted to a heart-lung machine, which mechanically pumps and oxygenates the blood temporarily so the heart can be bypassed while an open procedure on the heart or coronary arteries is performed. During bypass, the lungs are deflated and immobile.

congenital. Present at birth, occurring through heredity or an influence during gestation up to the moment of birth.

graft. Tissue implant from another part of the body or another person.

gusset. Triangular or diamond shaped patch that is placed for reinforcement or expansion.

ligation. Tying off a blood vessel or duct with a suture or a soft, thin wire.

obstruction. Blockage that prevents normal function of the valve or structure.

pericardium. Thin and slippery case in which the heart lies that is lined with fluid so that the heart is free to pulse and move as it beats.

tetralogy of Fallot. Specific combination of congenital cardiac defects: obstruction of the right ventricular outflow tract with pulmonary stenosis, interventricular septal defect, malposition of the aorta, overriding the interventricular septum and receiving blood from both the venous and arterial systems, and enlargement of the right ventricle.

ventricular septal defect. Congenital cardiac anomaly resulting in a continual opening in the septum between the ventricles that, in severe cases, causes oxygenated blood to flow back into the lungs, resulting in pulmonary hypertension.

33702-33710

33702 Repair sinus of Valsalva fistula, with cardiopulmonary bypass;

33710 with repair of ventricular septal defect

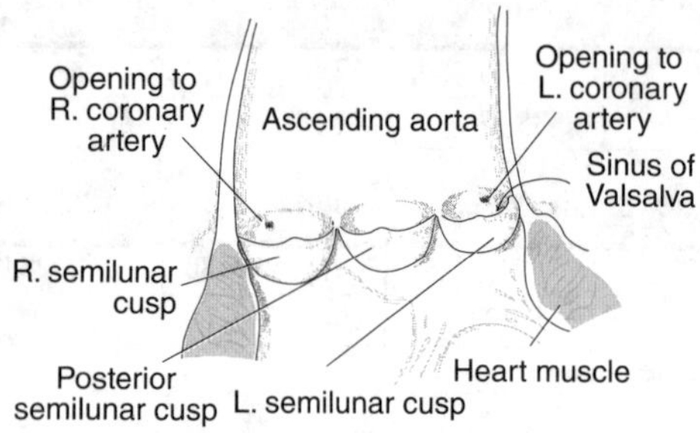

Cutaway depiction of the three cusps of the aortic valve showing location of sinus of Valsalva

Explanation

The physician repairs a sinus of Valsalva fistula. Cardiopulmonary bypass is required. After the heart is stopped, the aorta is opened and the fistula is identified. It is closed with a patch of pericardium. Any aorta valve incompetence is repaired by shortening the redundant valve leaflet diameter with stitches that reef in its free edge. The hole in the aorta is closed. Report 33710 if the sinus of Valsalva fistula is closed through the right atrium or through an incision in the aorta.

Coding Tips

When 33702 or 33710 is performed with another separately identifiable procedure, the highest dollar value code is listed as the primary procedure and subsequent procedures are appended with modifier 51. The patch of the pericardium used for the repair of the fistula is not reported separately. For repair of sinus of Valsalva aneurysm, see 33720. For closure of aortico-left ventricular tunnel, see 33722. For aortic valve replacement, see 33405–33413. For repair of ventricular septal defect alone, see 33681–33688.

ICD-10-CM Diagnostic Codes

Q21.0	Ventricular septal defect
Q25.41	Absence and aplasia of aorta
Q25.42	Hypoplasia of aorta
Q25.44	Congenital dilation of aorta
Q25.45	Double aortic arch
Q25.46	Tortuous aortic arch
Q25.47	Right aortic arch
Q25.48	Anomalous origin of subclavian artery
Q25.49	Other congenital malformations of aorta

AMA: 33702 2018,Jan,8; 2017,Jan,8; 2017,Dec,3; 2016,Jan,13; 2015,Jan,16; 2014,Jan,11 **33710** 2017,Dec,3

Relative Value Units/Medicare Edits

Non-Facility RVU	Work	PE	MP	Total
33702	27.24	11.17	6.46	44.87
33710	37.5	13.23	8.92	59.65
Facility RVU	**Work**	**PE**	**MP**	**Total**
33702	27.24	11.17	6.46	44.87
33710	37.5	13.23	8.92	59.65

	FUD	Status	MUE	Modifiers				IOM Reference
33702	90	A	1(2)	51	N/A	62*	80	None
33710	90	A	1(2)	51	N/A	N/A	80	

* with documentation

Terms To Know

aneurysm. Circumscribed dilation or outpouching of an artery wall, often containing blood clots and connecting directly with the lumen of the artery.

anomaly. Irregularity in the structure or position of an organ or tissue.

cardiopulmonary bypass. Venous blood is diverted to a heart-lung machine, which mechanically pumps and oxygenates the blood temporarily so the heart can be bypassed while an open procedure on the heart or coronary arteries is performed. During bypass, the lungs are deflated and immobile.

congenital. Present at birth, occurring through heredity or an influence during gestation up to the moment of birth.

fistula. Abnormal tube-like passage between two body cavities or organs or from an organ to the outside surface.

graft. Tissue implant from another part of the body or another person.

incision. Act of cutting into tissue or an organ.

pericardium. Thin and slippery case in which the heart lies that is lined with fluid so that the heart is free to pulse and move as it beats.

prosthesis. Man-made substitute for a missing body part.

sinus of Valsalva. Any of three sinuses corresponding to the individual cusps of the aortic valve, located in the most proximal part of the aorta just above the cusps. These structures are contained within the pericardium and appear as distinct but subtle outpouchings or dilations of the aortic wall between each of the semilunar cusps of the valve.

ventricular septal defect. Congenital cardiac anomaly resulting in a continual opening in the septum between the ventricles that, in severe cases, causes oxygenated blood to flow back into the lungs, resulting in pulmonary hypertension.

33720

33720 Repair sinus of Valsalva aneurysm, with cardiopulmonary bypass

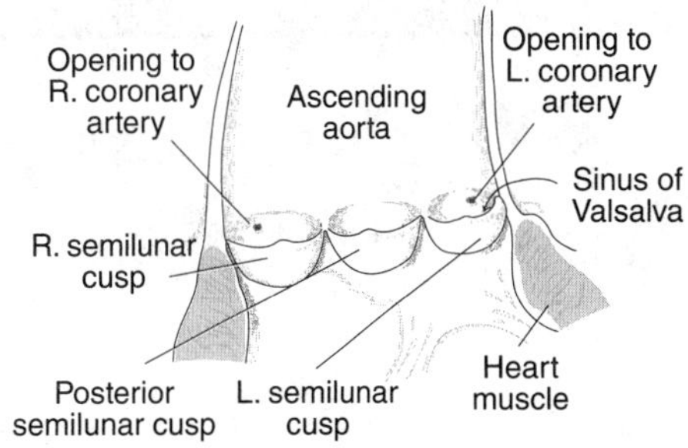

Cutaway depiction of the three cusps of the aortic valve showing location of sinus of Valsalva

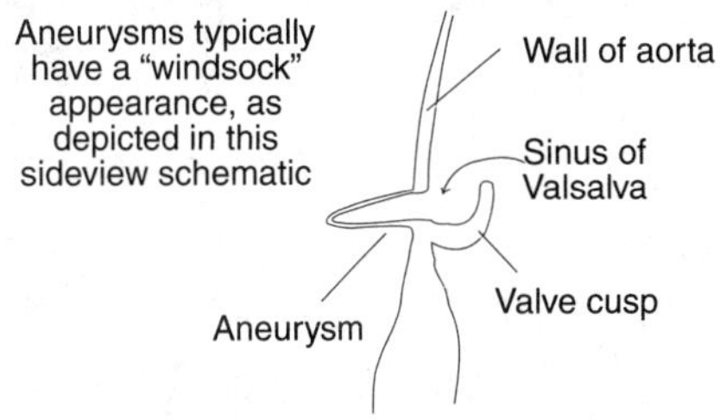

Explanation

Cardiopulmonary bypass is required. The aorta is opened after the heart has stopped. Thrombus (clot) in the aneurysm is removed. The neck of the aneurysm is closed with stitches. The aortic valve is usually incompetent. If the aortic annulus is sufficiently dilated by the aneurysm the aortic valve may need to be replaced with a mechanical aortic valve, a biomechanical valve or a tissue valve from an organ donor. After the valve is repaired or replaced, the aorta is closed. Cardiopulmonary bypass is discontinued after heart function returns.

Coding Tips

When 33720 is performed with another separately identifiable procedure, the highest dollar value code is listed as the primary procedure and subsequent procedures are appended with modifier 51. For aortic valve replacement, see 33405–33413. For closure of aortico-left ventricular tunnel, see 33722. For repair of ventricular septal defect, see 33681–33688.

ICD-10-CM Diagnostic Codes

Q25.41	Absence and aplasia of aorta
Q25.42	Hypoplasia of aorta
Q25.43	Congenital aneurysm of aorta
Q25.44	Congenital dilation of aorta
Q25.45	Double aortic arch
Q25.46	Tortuous aortic arch
Q25.47	Right aortic arch
Q25.48	Anomalous origin of subclavian artery
Q25.49	Other congenital malformations of aorta

AMA: 33720 2017,Dec,3

Relative Value Units/Medicare Edits

Non-Facility RVU	Work	PE	MP	Total
33720	27.26	11.18	6.46	44.9
Facility RVU	**Work**	**PE**	**MP**	**Total**
33720	27.26	11.18	6.46	44.9

	FUD	Status	MUE	Modifiers				IOM Reference
33720	90	A	1(2)	51	N/A	62*	80	None

* with documentation

Terms To Know

aneurysm. Circumscribed dilation or outpouching of an artery wall, often containing blood clots and connecting directly with the lumen of the artery.

anomaly. Irregularity in the structure or position of an organ or tissue.

aortic annulus. Aortic valve.

aortic valve. Heart valve, comprising three cusps, that divides the left ventricle and the aorta.

ascending aorta. Thoracic aorta, ascending/arch.

cardiopulmonary bypass. Venous blood is diverted to a heart-lung machine, which mechanically pumps and oxygenates the blood temporarily so the heart can be bypassed while an open procedure on the heart or coronary arteries is performed. During bypass, the lungs are deflated and immobile.

congenital. Present at birth, occurring through heredity or an influence during gestation up to the moment of birth.

dilation. Artificial increase in the diameter of an opening or lumen made by medication or by instrumentation.

extracorporeal. Located or taking place outside the body.

hypothermia with cardiac bypass. Reduction of the body temperature using a bypass system to reduce the oxygen demands of tissue and to protect the myocardium during a procedure.

sinus of Valsalva. Any of three sinuses corresponding to the individual cusps of the aortic valve, located in the most proximal part of the aorta just above the cusps. These structures are contained within the pericardium and appear as distinct but subtle outpouchings or dilations of the aortic wall between each of the semilunar cusps of the valve.

thrombus. Stationary blood clot inside a blood vessel.

ventricular septal defect. Congenital cardiac anomaly resulting in a continual opening in the septum between the ventricles that, in severe cases, causes oxygenated blood to flow back into the lungs, resulting in pulmonary hypertension.

33722

33722 Closure of aortico-left ventricular tunnel

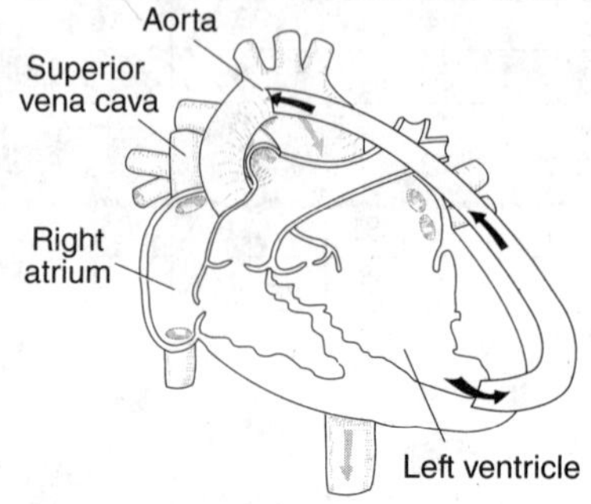

Depiction of an aortico-left ventricular tunnel

Explanation

The physician closes an aortic-left ventricular tunnel. The physician performs a midline sternotomy, incising the skin, fascia, muscles, and sternum. The pericardium is incised and lines are placed for cardiopulmonary bypass. An aortotomy is performed and the aortic hole is patched at the ascending aorta distal to the sinus of Valsalva. The ventricular hole is sealed with another patch which is attached to the ventricular myocardium, the wall of the aortic sinus, and the bottom of the first patch. The incision in the aorta is sutured closed. The sternum is reanastomosed with sternal wires and the skin is sutured in layers.

Coding Tips

When 33722 is performed with another separately identifiable procedure, the highest dollar value code is listed as the primary procedure and subsequent procedures are appended with modifier 51. For repair of sinus of Valsalva fistula, with cardiopulmonary bypass, see 33702 or 33710. For repair of sinus of Valsalva aneurysm, with cardiopulmonary bypass, see 33720.

ICD-10-CM Diagnostic Codes

Q20.8	Other congenital malformations of cardiac chambers and connections
Q21.0	Ventricular septal defect
Q21.4	Aortopulmonary septal defect
Q21.8	Other congenital malformations of cardiac septa
Q21.9	Congenital malformation of cardiac septum, unspecified

AMA: **33722** 2018,Jan,8; 2017,Jan,8; 2017,Dec,3; 2016,Jan,13; 2015,Jan,16; 2014,Jan,11

Relative Value Units/Medicare Edits

Non-Facility RVU	Work	PE	MP	Total
33722	29.21	11.09	6.94	47.24
Facility RVU	**Work**	**PE**	**MP**	**Total**
33722	29.21	11.09	6.94	47.24

	FUD	Status	MUE	Modifiers				IOM Reference
33722	90	A	1(3)	51	N/A	62*	80	None

* with documentation

33724

33724 Repair of isolated partial anomalous pulmonary venous return (eg, Scimitar Syndrome)

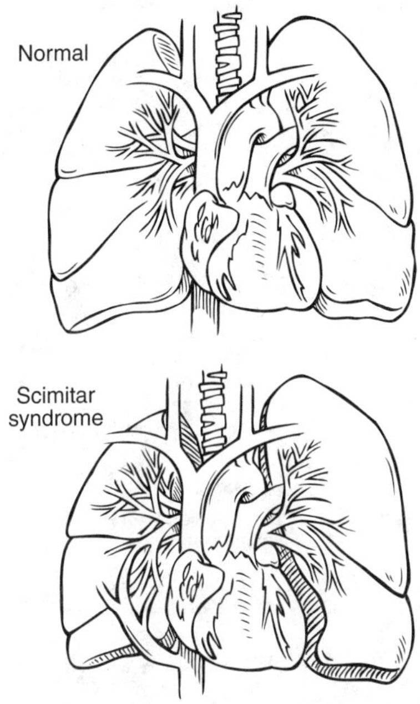

Scimitar syndrome is so named because the aberrant vein casts a shadow shaped like a curved Turkishsword, a scimitar, upon x-ray

Explanation

The physician repairs an isolated partial anomalous venous return (scimitar syndrome) using one of two open techniques. Scimitar syndrome describes a congenital condition in which an aberrant vessel connects the pulmonary vein in the right lung to the inferior vena cava. It can be diagnosed in infancy through adulthood, and symptoms occurring in infancy suggest a more severe form of the disease. Scimitar syndrome is so named because the aberrant vein casts a shadow shaped like a curved Turkish sword, a scimitar, upon x-ray. A midline sternotomy is performed. In one technique, a long pericardial patch graft is used to divert the anomalous pulmonary venous drainage from the inferior vena cava into the left atrium. In the second technique, the anomalous pulmonary vein is divided off the inferior vena cava and reimplanted into the posterior wall of the right atrium. A short pericardial baffle is used to divert flow to the left atrium through an atrial septal defect. Grafts may be required to enlarge remaining vessels. In some cases, a separately reported right pneumonectomy is performed.

Coding Tips

Insertion of a chest tube (32551) is included and should not be reported separately. Temporary transvenous pacemaker placement (33210, 33211) is also included and should not be reported separately. Scimitar syndrome can also be repaired by transcatheter occlusion or embolization. For repair of pulmonary venous stenosis, see 33726. For complete repair of anomalous pulmonary venous return, see 33730.

ICD-10-CM Diagnostic Codes

Q26.3	Partial anomalous pulmonary venous connection
Q26.4	Anomalous pulmonary venous connection, unspecified
Q26.8	Other congenital malformations of great veins
Q26.9	Congenital malformation of great vein, unspecified

AMA: **33724** 2018,Jan,8; 2017,Jan,8; 2017,Dec,3; 2016,Jan,13; 2015,Jan,16; 2014,Jan,11

Relative Value Units/Medicare Edits

Non-Facility RVU	Work	PE	MP	Total
33724	27.63	10.5	6.55	44.68
Facility RVU	**Work**	**PE**	**MP**	**Total**
33724	27.63	10.5	6.55	44.68

	FUD	Status	MUE	Modifiers				IOM Reference
33724	90	A	1(2)	51	N/A	62*	80	None

* with documentation

Terms To Know

anomaly. Irregularity in the structure or position of an organ or tissue.

embolization. Placement of a clotting agent, such as a coil, plastic particles, gel, foam, etc., into an area of hemorrhage to stop the bleeding or to block blood flow to a problem area, such as an aneurysm or a tumor.

graft. Tissue implant from another part of the body or another person.

pericardium. Thin and slippery case in which the heart lies that is lined with fluid so that the heart is free to pulse and move as it beats.

sternotomy. Incision into the sternum, the bone that forms the front of the chest cavity and connects with the ribs.

transcatheter. Procedure or treatment performed via a catheter.

33726

33726 Repair of pulmonary venous stenosis

Stenosis is a narrowing or blockage of a passage

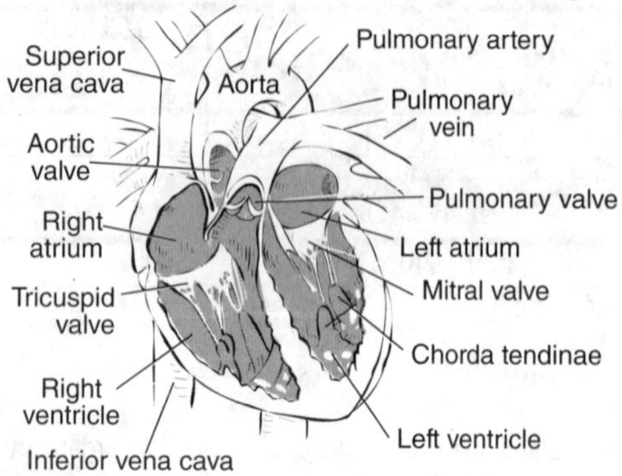

Explanation

The physician gains access to the heart through a midline sternotomy. The physician places cardiopulmonary bypass catheters usually through incisions in the right atrial appendage and aorta or femoral artery. The physician stops the heart by infusing cardioplegia solution into the coronary circulation. Either atria may be incised for exploration to locate and better visualize the defect. The blocked pulmonary vein is opened along its length. The inner layer of the artery is removed. The outer layer of the artery is closed with suture directly or with a patch of pericardium, saphenous vein, or Dacron.

Coding Tips

Insertion of a chest tube (32551) is included and should not be reported separately. Temporary transvenous pacemaker placement (33210, 33211) is also included and should not be reported separately. For partial repair of anomalous pulmonary venous return, see 33724; complete repair, see 33730.

ICD-10-CM Diagnostic Codes

I28.8	Other diseases of pulmonary vessels
Q26.0	Congenital stenosis of vena cava
Q26.1	Persistent left superior vena cava
Q26.2	Total anomalous pulmonary venous connection
Q26.3	Partial anomalous pulmonary venous connection
Q26.4	Anomalous pulmonary venous connection, unspecified
Q26.8	Other congenital malformations of great veins
Q26.9	Congenital malformation of great vein, unspecified

AMA: **33726** 2018,Jan,8; 2017,Jan,8; 2017,Dec,3; 2016,Jan,13; 2015,Jan,16; 2014,Jan,11

Relative Value Units/Medicare Edits

Non-Facility RVU	Work	PE	MP	Total
33726	37.12	13.15	8.83	59.1
Facility RVU	**Work**	**PE**	**MP**	**Total**
33726	37.12	13.15	8.83	59.1

	FUD	Status	MUE	Modifiers				IOM Reference
33726	90	A	1(2)	51	N/A	62*	80	None

* with documentation

33730

33730 Complete repair of anomalous pulmonary venous return (supracardiac, intracardiac, or infracardiac types)

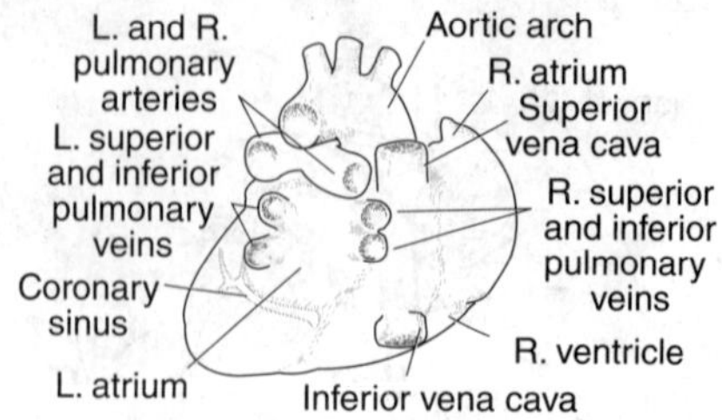

Posterior depiction of normal heart and its major venous returns

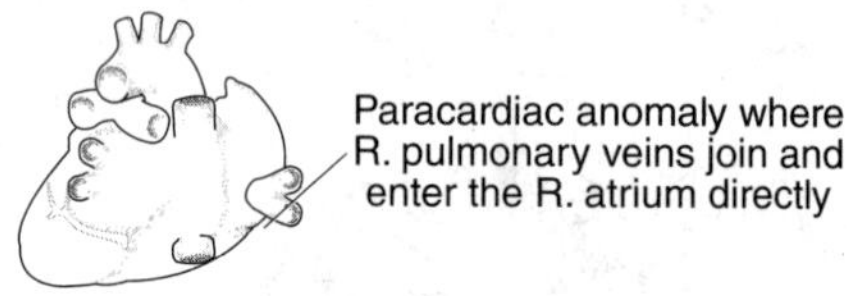

The anomaly typically involves the R. pulmonary veins and a VSD is usually also present

Numerous configurations of anomalous venous drainage occur

Explanation

The physician performs a complete repair of total anomalous pulmonary venous return (TAPVR), a rare congenital defect in which all four pulmonary veins do not connect normally to the left atrium, but rather drain to the right atrium by way of an abnormal connection. Via a midline sternotomy, the physician exposes the heart. Cardiopulmonary bypass is initiated. The abnormal veins are rerouted to the left atrium, most often by connecting them directly to the back wall of the atrium. Any abnormal routes for pulmonary venous drainage are tied off, and any existing atrial septal defect is closed. The heart is restarted, cardiopulmonary bypass is discontinued, and the sternotomy is closed.

Coding Tips

This procedure is performed for total anomalous pulmonary venous return (TAPVR). Do not append modifier 63 to 33730 as the description or nature of the procedure includes infants up to 4 kg. For repair of atrial septal defect, secundum, with cardiopulmonary bypass, with or without patch, see 33641. For direct or patch closure, sinus venosus, with or without anomalous pulmonary venous drainage, see 33645. For repair of an incomplete or partial atrioventricular canal (ostium primum atrial septal defect), with or without atrioventricular valve repair, see 33660. For repair of partial anomalous pulmonary venous return, see 33724. For repair of pulmonary venous stenosis, see 33726.

ICD-10-CM Diagnostic Codes

Q26.2	Total anomalous pulmonary venous connection
Q26.3	Partial anomalous pulmonary venous connection
Q26.4	Anomalous pulmonary venous connection, unspecified
Q26.8	Other congenital malformations of great veins
Q26.9	Congenital malformation of great vein, unspecified

AMA: **33730** 2018,Jan,8; 2017,Jan,8; 2017,Dec,3; 2016,Jan,13; 2015,Jan,16; 2014,Jan,11

Relative Value Units/Medicare Edits

Non-Facility RVU	Work	PE	MP	Total
33730	36.14	13.52	8.6	58.26
Facility RVU	Work	PE	MP	Total
33730	36.14	13.52	8.6	58.26

	FUD	Status	MUE	Modifiers				IOM Reference
33730	90	A	1(2)	51	N/A	62*	80	None

* with documentation

Terms To Know

anomaly. Irregularity in the structure or position of an organ or tissue.

atrial septal defect. Cardiac anomaly consisting of a patent opening in the atrial septum due to a fusion failure, classified as ostium secundum type, ostium primum defect, or endocardial cushion defect.

cardiopulmonary bypass. Venous blood is diverted to a heart-lung machine, which mechanically pumps and oxygenates the blood temporarily so the heart can be bypassed while an open procedure on the heart or coronary arteries is performed. During bypass, the lungs are deflated and immobile.

congenital. Present at birth, occurring through heredity or an influence during gestation up to the moment of birth.

extracorporeal. Located or taking place outside the body.

para-. Indicates near, similar, beside, or past.

sternotomy. Incision into the sternum, the bone that forms the front of the chest cavity and connects with the ribs.

supra. Above.

ventricular septal defect. Congenital cardiac anomaly resulting in a continual opening in the septum between the ventricles that, in severe cases, causes oxygenated blood to flow back into the lungs, resulting in pulmonary hypertension.

33732

33732 Repair of cor triatriatum or supravalvular mitral ring by resection of left atrial membrane

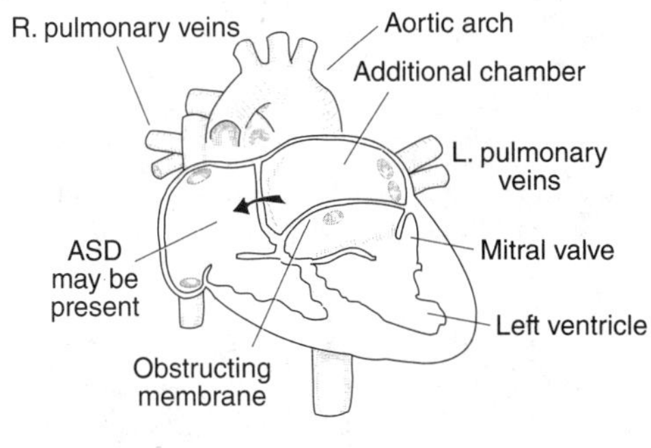

Cardiac anomalies are repaired

Explanation

This lesion is frequently considered to be related to TAPVR, but it is distinctly different. In this anomaly, there is a wall subdividing the left atrium between the pulmonary veins and the mitral valve. This restricts blood flow to the left ventricle and therefore to the rest of the body. Cardiopulmonary bypass is readied. The left atrium is opened and the membrane is cut out. The left atrium is closed. Cardiopulmonary bypass is discontinued when heart function returns.

Coding Tips

When 33732 is performed with another separately identifiable procedure, the highest dollar value code is listed as the primary procedure and subsequent procedures are appended with modifier 51. Do not append modifier 63 to 33732 as the description or nature of the procedure includes infants up to 4 kg. For repair of complex cardiac anomalies (e.g., tricuspid atresia) by closure of atrial septal defect and anastomosis of atria or vena cava (simple Fontan procedures), see 33615. For repair of atrial septal defect, secundum, with cardiopulmonary bypass, with or without patch, see 33641.

ICD-10-CM Diagnostic Codes

Q23.2	Congenital mitral stenosis
Q24.2	Cor triatriatum

AMA: **33732** 2018,Jan,8; 2017,Jan,8; 2017,Dec,3; 2016,Jan,13; 2015,Jan,16; 2014,Jan,11

Relative Value Units/Medicare Edits

Non-Facility RVU	Work	PE	MP	Total
33732	28.96	11.98	6.88	47.82
Facility RVU	Work	PE	MP	Total
33732	28.96	11.98	6.88	47.82

	FUD	Status	MUE	Modifiers				IOM Reference
33732	90	A	1(2)	51	N/A	62*	80	None

* with documentation

Terms To Know

anomaly. Irregularity in the structure or position of an organ or tissue.

congenital. Present at birth, occurring through heredity or an influence during gestation up to the moment of birth.

Heart and Pericardium

33735-33737

33735 Atrial septectomy or septostomy; closed heart (Blalock-Hanlon type operation)
33736 open heart with cardiopulmonary bypass
33737 open heart, with inflow occlusion

The usual goal of this series of procedures is to surgically create a left-to-right mixing of atrial blood by removal of tissues from the atrial septum (septectomy) or by creation of a hole in the septum

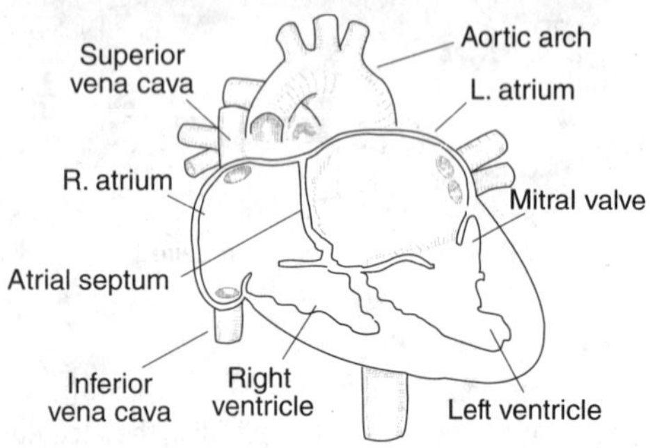

Explanation

These procedures are largely of historical interest only. Code 33735 requires access by lateral thoracotomy. An incision is made in the pericardium with the right pulmonary artery and pulmonary veins tied off. A clamp is utilized at the anterior position of the right atrium and the posterior position of the left atrium. Incisions are made within the right atrium and right pulmonary vein. The atrial septum is removed and incisions are closed. The clamps are removed and ligatures previously placed in the pulmonary veins and right pulmonary artery are released. Alternatively, a purse string may be placed in the right atrial appendage and the appendage is opened in the middle of the purse string. A finger or a dilating tool is passed through the hole in the atrium and the wall between the right and left atria is torn open. The dilating instrument is removed and the purse string is tied to stop the bleeding. The thoracotomy is closed in standard fashion. In 33736, in most pediatric cardiac surgery centers, it has been supplanted by balloon dilation of a naturally occurring hole in the wall between the atrial chambers. No incision is needed for balloon dilation. Operative septostomy/septectomy requires cardiopulmonary bypass with venous uptake tubes in both caval veins. The right atrium is opened and the thin part of the wall between the right and left atria is cut out or opened widely. The goal is to allow free mixing of the blood from the right and left atria. Cardiopulmonary bypass is discontinued when heart function returns. Report 33737 if tourniquets are placed around the caval veins and the patient is placed head down so no air entering the right atrium crosses the wall between the right and left atria.

Coding Tips

Code these procedures with caution as they are used quite infrequently. Open chest atrial septectomy or septostomy has largely been replaced with balloon dilation of a naturally occurring hole in the wall between the atrial chambers. When ligation and takedown of systemic-to-pulmonary artery shunt is performed in addition to this procedure, it should be reported separately, see 33924. Do not append modifier 63 to 33735–33736 as the description or nature of the procedure includes infants up to 4 kg. For atrial septectomy or septostomy, transvenous method, balloon (Rashkind type), see 92992. For atrial septectomy or septostomy, blade method (Sang-Park septostomy), see 92993.

ICD-10-CM Diagnostic Codes

Q20.3	Discordant ventriculoarterial connection
Q22.6	Hypoplastic right heart syndrome
Q22.8	Other congenital malformations of tricuspid valve
Q22.9	Congenital malformation of tricuspid valve, unspecified
Q23.8	Other congenital malformations of aortic and mitral valves
Q23.9	Congenital malformation of aortic and mitral valves, unspecified
Q24.8	Other specified congenital malformations of heart
Q26.2	Total anomalous pulmonary venous connection

AMA: **33735** 2018,Jan,8; 2017,Jan,8; 2016,Jan,13; 2015,Jan,16; 2014,Jan,11 **33736** 2017,Dec,3

Relative Value Units/Medicare Edits

Non-Facility RVU	Work	PE	MP	Total
33735	22.2	10.11	5.26	37.57
33736	24.32	10.69	5.76	40.77
33737	22.47	9.84	5.33	37.64
Facility RVU	**Work**	**PE**	**MP**	**Total**
33735	22.2	10.11	5.26	37.57
33736	24.32	10.69	5.76	40.77
33737	22.47	9.84	5.33	37.64

	FUD	Status	MUE	Modifiers				IOM Reference
33735	90	A	1(2)	51	N/A	N/A	80	None
33736	90	A	1(2)	51	N/A	62*	80	
33737	90	A	1(2)	51	N/A	62*	80	

* with documentation

Terms To Know

Blalock-Hanlon procedure. Atrial septectomy procedure to allow free mixing of the blood from the right and left atria.

occlusion. Constriction, closure, or blockage of a passage.

pulmonary artery banding. Surgical constriction of the pulmonary artery to prevent irreversible pulmonary vascular obstructive changes and overflow into the left ventricle.

Rashkind procedure. Transvenous balloon atrial septectomy or septostomy performed by cardiac catheterization. A balloon catheter is inserted into the heart either to create or enlarge an opening in the interatrial septal wall.

stenosis. Narrowing or constriction of a passage.

tricuspid atresia. Congenital absence of the valve that may occur with other defects, such as atrial septal defect, pulmonary atresia, and transposition of great vessels.

33750

33750 Shunt; subclavian to pulmonary artery (Blalock-Taussig type operation)

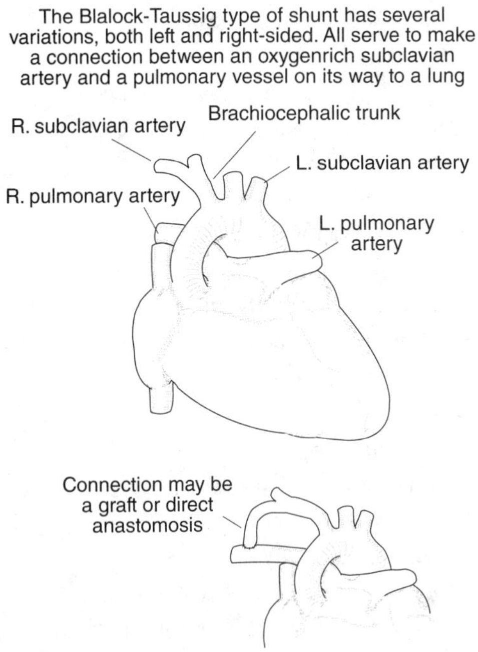

Explanation

In its unmodified form, this operation involves dividing the left subclavian artery, tying off the end of the artery going to the arm, and creating a connection between the end of this artery coming from the heart and the side of the pulmonary artery. The difficulty with this operation is making the connection to the pulmonary artery exactly the right size to supply adequate, but not excessive blood flow to the lungs. Instead, a modified version of the operation is usually performed. The artery to the arm is not divided. Instead, one end of a 3 mm to 5 mm diameter tube of Gortex is sewn to the side of the artery to the arm and the other end is sewn to the side of the pulmonary artery. The size of the tube determines the amount of blood flow to the lungs. Cardiopulmonary bypass is not required. The ductus arteriosus (a connection between the aorta and pulmonary artery that has been supplying blood to the lungs, but usually closes at birth) is tied off.

Coding Tips

This procedure is sometimes performed in addition to 33684. When ligation and takedown of systemic-to-pulmonary artery shunt is performed in addition to this procedure, it should be reported separately, see 33924. Do not append modifier 63 to 33750 as the description or nature of the procedure includes infants up to 4 kg. For shunt, ascending aorta to pulmonary artery (Waterston type operation), see 33755. For descending aorta to pulmonary artery (Potts-Smith type operation), see 33762, and for flow to one lung (classical Glenn procedure), see 33766. For superior vena cava to pulmonary artery for flow to both lungs (bidirectional Glenn procedure), see 33767.

ICD-10-CM Diagnostic Codes

I24.8	Other forms of acute ischemic heart disease
I37.0	Nonrheumatic pulmonary valve stenosis
I37.1	Nonrheumatic pulmonary valve insufficiency
I37.2	Nonrheumatic pulmonary valve stenosis with insufficiency
I37.8	Other nonrheumatic pulmonary valve disorders
Q20.4	Double inlet ventricle
Q20.8	Other congenital malformations of cardiac chambers and connections
Q21.0	Ventricular septal defect
Q21.3	Tetralogy of Fallot
Q21.8	Other congenital malformations of cardiac septa
Q22.0	Pulmonary valve atresia
Q22.1	Congenital pulmonary valve stenosis
Q22.2	Congenital pulmonary valve insufficiency
Q22.3	Other congenital malformations of pulmonary valve
Q22.4	Congenital tricuspid stenosis
Q22.5	Ebstein's anomaly
Q22.6	Hypoplastic right heart syndrome
Q22.8	Other congenital malformations of tricuspid valve
Q24.3	Pulmonary infundibular stenosis
Q24.8	Other specified congenital malformations of heart
Q25.5	Atresia of pulmonary artery
Q25.6	Stenosis of pulmonary artery
Q25.71	Coarctation of pulmonary artery
Q25.72	Congenital pulmonary arteriovenous malformation
Q25.79	Other congenital malformations of pulmonary artery
Q25.8	Other congenital malformations of other great arteries

AMA: 33750 2017,Dec,3

Relative Value Units/Medicare Edits

Non-Facility RVU	Work	PE	MP	Total
33750	22.22	9.14	5.27	36.63
Facility RVU	**Work**	**PE**	**MP**	**Total**
33750	22.22	9.14	5.27	36.63

	FUD	Status	MUE	Modifiers				IOM Reference
33750	90	A	1(3)	51	N/A	62*	80	None

* with documentation

Terms To Know

atresia. Congenital closure or absence of a tubular organ or an opening to the body surface.

Blalock-Taussig procedure. Anastomosis of the left subclavian artery to the left pulmonary artery or the right subclavian artery to the right pulmonary artery in order to shunt some of the blood flow from the systemic to the pulmonary circulation.

cardiopulmonary bypass. Venous blood is diverted to a heart-lung machine, which mechanically pumps and oxygenates the blood temporarily so the heart can be bypassed while an open procedure on the heart or coronary arteries is performed. During bypass, the lungs are deflated and immobile.

shunt. Surgically created passage between blood vessels or other natural passages, such as an arteriovenous anastomosis, to divert or bypass blood flow from the normal channel.

33755

33755 Shunt; ascending aorta to pulmonary artery (Waterston type operation)

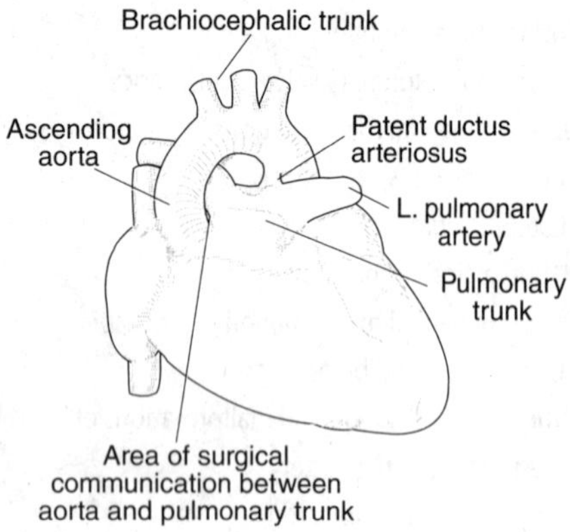

A surgical shunt is created between the ascending aorta and the pulmonary artery

Explanation

This procedure is largely of historic interest. This procedure requires cardiopulmonary bypass. It is designed to allow adequate blood flow to the lungs. After cardiopulmonary bypass is initiated, the aorta is occluded above the heart. A hole may be cut in the aorta with the shunt closed from within by sutures. A more common method utilizes the pulmonary artery detached from the aorta and consequently reattached to the defect of the ascending aorta by sutures. The remaining defect in the pulmonary artery may be closed with sutures, but typically is patched with pericardium or pulmonary homograft. It is difficult to accurately control the diameter of the resulting connection and the resulting flow of blood into the lungs. Cardiopulmonary bypass is discontinued when heart function returns.

Coding Tips

When ligation and takedown of systemic-to-pulmonary artery shunt is performed with this procedure, it should be reported separately, see 33924. Do not append modifier 63 to 33755 as the description or nature of the procedure includes infants up to 4 kg. For shunt, subclavian to pulmonary artery (Blalock-Taussig type operation), see 33750. For descending aorta to pulmonary artery (Potts-Smith type operation), see 33762. For central shunt, with prosthetic graft, see 33764. For superior vena cava to pulmonary artery for flow to one lung (classical Glenn procedure), see 33766. For superior vena cava to pulmonary artery for flow to both lungs (bidirectional Glenn procedure), see 33767.

ICD-10-CM Diagnostic Codes

I24.8	Other forms of acute ischemic heart disease
I37.0	Nonrheumatic pulmonary valve stenosis
I37.1	Nonrheumatic pulmonary valve insufficiency
I37.2	Nonrheumatic pulmonary valve stenosis with insufficiency
I37.8	Other nonrheumatic pulmonary valve disorders
Q20.4	Double inlet ventricle
Q20.8	Other congenital malformations of cardiac chambers and connections
Q21.0	Ventricular septal defect
Q21.3	Tetralogy of Fallot
Q21.8	Other congenital malformations of cardiac septa
Q22.0	Pulmonary valve atresia
Q22.1	Congenital pulmonary valve stenosis
Q22.2	Congenital pulmonary valve insufficiency
Q22.3	Other congenital malformations of pulmonary valve
Q22.4	Congenital tricuspid stenosis
Q22.5	Ebstein's anomaly
Q22.6	Hypoplastic right heart syndrome
Q24.3	Pulmonary infundibular stenosis
Q24.4	Congenital subaortic stenosis
Q24.8	Other specified congenital malformations of heart
Q25.21	Interruption of aortic arch
Q25.3	Supravalvular aortic stenosis
Q25.41	Absence and aplasia of aorta
Q25.42	Hypoplasia of aorta
Q25.43	Congenital aneurysm of aorta
Q25.44	Congenital dilation of aorta
Q25.45	Double aortic arch
Q25.46	Tortuous aortic arch
Q25.47	Right aortic arch
Q25.48	Anomalous origin of subclavian artery
Q25.5	Atresia of pulmonary artery
Q25.6	Stenosis of pulmonary artery
Q25.71	Coarctation of pulmonary artery
Q25.72	Congenital pulmonary arteriovenous malformation
Q25.79	Other congenital malformations of pulmonary artery
Q25.8	Other congenital malformations of other great arteries

AMA: **33755** 2017,Dec,3

Relative Value Units/Medicare Edits

Non-Facility RVU	Work	PE	MP	Total
33755	22.6	10.22	5.36	38.18
Facility RVU	**Work**	**PE**	**MP**	**Total**
33755	22.6	10.22	5.36	38.18

	FUD	Status	MUE	Modifiers				IOM Reference
33755	90	A	1(2)	51	N/A	62*	80	None

* with documentation

Terms To Know

atresia. Congenital closure or absence of a tubular organ or an opening to the body surface.

patent ductus arteriosus. Condition in which the normal channel between the pulmonary artery and the aorta fails to close at birth, causing arterial blood to recirculate in the lungs and inhibiting the blood supply to the aorta.

33762

33762 Shunt; descending aorta to pulmonary artery (Potts-Smith type operation)

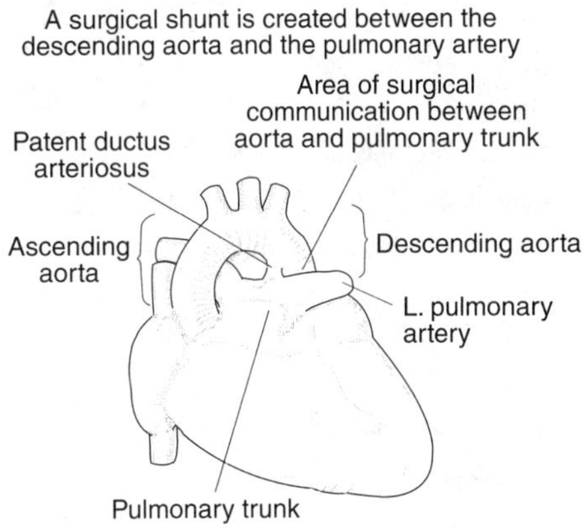

Explanation

This procedure is performed through the left side of the chest. Cardiopulmonary bypass is not required. The pulmonary artery is dissected from its original position to the branches and the aorta is visualized. Occlusion of the pulmonary artery is conducted and incisions are made into both arteries. One end of a 3 mm to 5 mm diameter tube made of polytetrafluoroethylene (PTFE) (e.g., Gortex) is sewn to the side of the descending aorta and the other end is sewn to the pulmonary artery. The ductus arteriosus (a connection between the aorta and pulmonary artery that has been supplying blood to the lungs, but usually closes at birth) is tied off.

Coding Tips

When ligation and takedown of systemic-to-pulmonary artery shunt is performed with this procedure, it should be reported separately, see 33924. Do not append modifier 63 to 33762 as the description or the nature of the procedure includes infants up to 4 kg. For shunt, subclavian to pulmonary artery (Blalock-Taussig type operation), see 33750. For ascending aorta to pulmonary artery (Waterston type operation), see 33755. For central shunt, with prosthetic graft, see 33764. For superior vena cava to pulmonary artery for flow to one lung (classical Glenn procedure), see 33766. For superior vena cava to pulmonary artery for flow to both lungs (bidirectional Glenn procedure), see 33767.

ICD-10-CM Diagnostic Codes

I24.8	Other forms of acute ischemic heart disease
I37.0	Nonrheumatic pulmonary valve stenosis
I37.1	Nonrheumatic pulmonary valve insufficiency
I37.2	Nonrheumatic pulmonary valve stenosis with insufficiency
I37.8	Other nonrheumatic pulmonary valve disorders
Q20.4	Double inlet ventricle
Q20.8	Other congenital malformations of cardiac chambers and connections
Q21.0	Ventricular septal defect
Q21.3	Tetralogy of Fallot
Q21.4	Aortopulmonary septal defect
Q21.8	Other congenital malformations of cardiac septa
Q22.0	Pulmonary valve atresia
Q22.1	Congenital pulmonary valve stenosis
Q22.2	Congenital pulmonary valve insufficiency
Q22.3	Other congenital malformations of pulmonary valve
Q22.4	Congenital tricuspid stenosis
Q22.5	Ebstein's anomaly
Q22.6	Hypoplastic right heart syndrome
Q22.8	Other congenital malformations of tricuspid valve
Q24.3	Pulmonary infundibular stenosis
Q24.4	Congenital subaortic stenosis
Q24.8	Other specified congenital malformations of heart
Q25.3	Supravalvular aortic stenosis
Q25.41	Absence and aplasia of aorta
Q25.42	Hypoplasia of aorta
Q25.43	Congenital aneurysm of aorta
Q25.44	Congenital dilation of aorta
Q25.45	Double aortic arch
Q25.46	Tortuous aortic arch
Q25.47	Right aortic arch
Q25.48	Anomalous origin of subclavian artery
Q25.49	Other congenital malformations of aorta
Q25.5	Atresia of pulmonary artery
Q25.6	Stenosis of pulmonary artery
Q25.71	Coarctation of pulmonary artery
Q25.72	Congenital pulmonary arteriovenous malformation
Q25.79	Other congenital malformations of pulmonary artery
Q25.8	Other congenital malformations of other great arteries

AMA: 33762 2017,Dec,3

Relative Value Units/Medicare Edits

Non-Facility RVU	Work	PE	MP	Total
33762	22.6	9.25	5.36	37.21
Facility RVU	**Work**	**PE**	**MP**	**Total**
33762	22.6	9.25	5.36	37.21

	FUD	Status	MUE	Modifiers				IOM Reference
33762	90	A	1(2)	51	N/A	62*	80	None

* with documentation

Terms To Know

anastomosis. Surgically created connection between ducts, blood vessels, or bowel segments to allow flow from one to the other.

atresia. Congenital closure or absence of a tubular organ or an opening to the body surface.

patent ductus arteriosus. Condition in which the normal channel between the pulmonary artery and the aorta fails to close at birth, causing arterial blood to recirculate in the lungs and inhibiting the blood supply to the aorta.

33764

33764 Shunt; central, with prosthetic graft

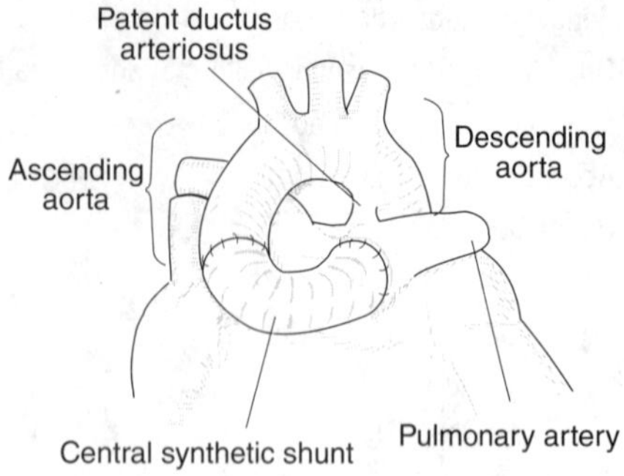

A central prosthetic shunt is installed between the ascending aorta and the pulmonary artery

Explanation

The operation is done through an incision in the middle of the breast bone or through an incision in the left chest. Cardiopulmonary bypass is usually not required. One end of a 3 mm to 5 mm diameter tube made of Gortex is sewn to the side of the ascending aorta and the other end is sewn to some part of the pulmonary artery. The ductus arteriosus (a connection between the aorta and pulmonary artery that has been supplying blood to the lungs, but usually closes at birth) is tied off.

Coding Tips

When ligation and takedown of systemic-to-pulmonary artery shunt is performed in addition to this procedure, it should be reported separately, see 33924. For shunt, subclavian to pulmonary artery (Blalock-Taussig type operation), see 33750. For ascending aorta to pulmonary artery (Waterston type operation), see 33755. For descending aorta to pulmonary artery (Potts-Smith type operation), see 33762. For superior vena cava to pulmonary artery for flow to one lung (classical Glenn procedure), see 33766. For superior vena cava to pulmonary artery for flow to both lungs (bidirectional Glenn procedure), see 33767.

ICD-10-CM Diagnostic Codes

I24.8	Other forms of acute ischemic heart disease
I37.0	Nonrheumatic pulmonary valve stenosis
I37.1	Nonrheumatic pulmonary valve insufficiency
I37.2	Nonrheumatic pulmonary valve stenosis with insufficiency
I37.8	Other nonrheumatic pulmonary valve disorders
Q20.4	Double inlet ventricle
Q20.8	Other congenital malformations of cardiac chambers and connections
Q21.0	Ventricular septal defect
Q21.2	Atrioventricular septal defect
Q21.3	Tetralogy of Fallot
Q21.4	Aortopulmonary septal defect
Q21.8	Other congenital malformations of cardiac septa
Q22.0	Pulmonary valve atresia
Q22.1	Congenital pulmonary valve stenosis
Q22.2	Congenital pulmonary valve insufficiency
Q22.3	Other congenital malformations of pulmonary valve
Q22.4	Congenital tricuspid stenosis
Q22.5	Ebstein's anomaly
Q22.6	Hypoplastic right heart syndrome
Q22.8	Other congenital malformations of tricuspid valve
Q24.3	Pulmonary infundibular stenosis
Q24.8	Other specified congenital malformations of heart
Q25.21	Interruption of aortic arch
Q25.29	Other atresia of aorta
Q25.3	Supravalvular aortic stenosis
Q25.41	Absence and aplasia of aorta
Q25.42	Hypoplasia of aorta
Q25.43	Congenital aneurysm of aorta
Q25.44	Congenital dilation of aorta
Q25.45	Double aortic arch
Q25.46	Tortuous aortic arch
Q25.47	Right aortic arch
Q25.48	Anomalous origin of subclavian artery
Q25.49	Other congenital malformations of aorta
Q25.5	Atresia of pulmonary artery
Q25.6	Stenosis of pulmonary artery
Q25.71	Coarctation of pulmonary artery
Q25.72	Congenital pulmonary arteriovenous malformation
Q25.79	Other congenital malformations of pulmonary artery
Q25.8	Other congenital malformations of other great arteries

AMA: 33764 2017,Dec,3

Relative Value Units/Medicare Edits

Non-Facility RVU	Work	PE	MP	Total
33764	22.6	10.22	5.36	38.18
Facility RVU	**Work**	**PE**	**MP**	**Total**
33764	22.6	10.22	5.36	38.18

	FUD	Status	MUE	Modifiers				IOM Reference
33764	90	A	1(3)	51	N/A	62*	80	None

* with documentation

Terms To Know

atresia. Congenital closure or absence of a tubular organ or an opening to the body surface.

congenital. Present at birth, occurring through heredity or an influence during gestation up to the moment of birth.

ligation. Tying off a blood vessel or duct with a suture or a soft, thin wire.

patent ductus arteriosus. Condition in which the normal channel between the pulmonary artery and the aorta fails to close at birth, causing arterial blood to recirculate in the lungs and inhibiting the blood supply to the aorta.

33766-33767

33766 Shunt; superior vena cava to pulmonary artery for flow to 1 lung (classical Glenn procedure)

33767 superior vena cava to pulmonary artery for flow to both lungs (bidirectional Glenn procedure)

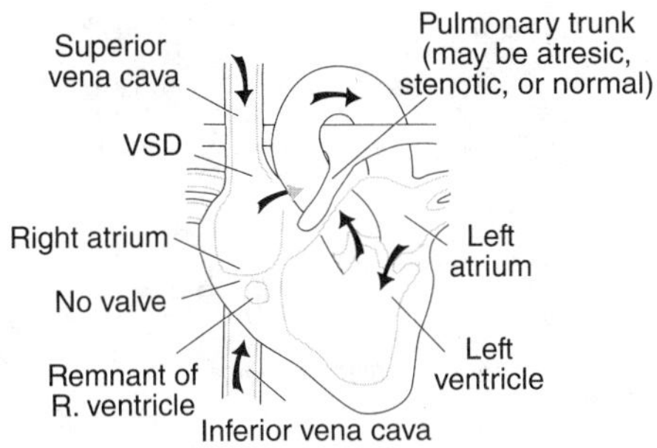

Example of tricuspid atresia with pulmonary atresia (single ventricle)

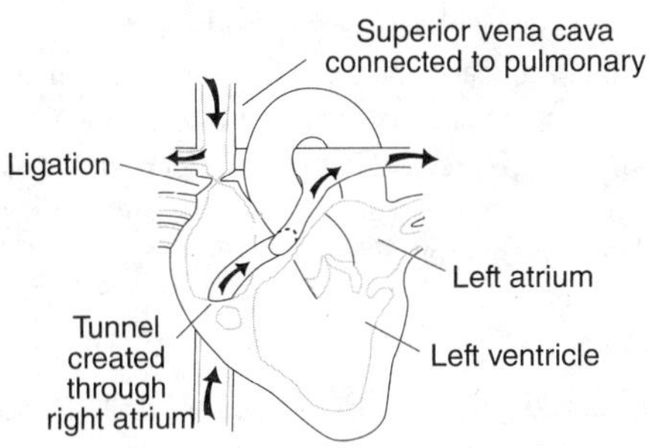

Explanation

In 33766, the operation is performed when there is an irreparable obstruction to blood flow through the right side of the heart. It is usually done as a prelude to a bidirectional or bilateral Glenn procedure, which is usually a prelude to a Fontan procedure. Cardiopulmonary bypass is usually required. The right (or the persistent left) superior caval vein is occluded and its connection with the heart is divided. The heart end of the superior caval vein is closed. The free end of the superior caval vein is sewn to the side of the corresponding pulmonary artery. It is assumed that the corresponding pulmonary artery is isolated from the opposite lung congenitally or surgically. The goal is to permit blood to flow directly from the superior caval vein to the lungs, thereby bypassing the right side of the heart. In 33767, it is assumed that all the pulmonary arteries from both lungs communicate freely. Cardiopulmonary bypass is required. Circulatory arrest and deep cooling of the body are usually employed. The main pulmonary artery is often tied off. The superior caval vein is detached from its connection to the right atrium. The hole left in the right atrium is closed with sutures. The free end of the superior caval vein is sewn to a hole in the side of the pulmonary artery. In this way, blood can flow to the lungs without passing through the right side of the heart. This operation is usually done as a prelude to a Fontan procedure.

Coding Tips

When ligation and takedown of systemic-to-pulmonary artery shunt is performed with this procedure, it should be reported separately, see 33924. For shunt, subclavian to pulmonary artery (Blalock-Taussig type operation), see 33750. For ascending aorta to pulmonary artery (Waterston type operation), see 33755. For descending aorta to pulmonary artery (Potts-Smith type operation), see 33762. For central shunt, with prosthetic graft, see 33764.

ICD-10-CM Diagnostic Codes

I24.8	Other forms of acute ischemic heart disease
I37.0	Nonrheumatic pulmonary valve stenosis
I37.1	Nonrheumatic pulmonary valve insufficiency
I37.2	Nonrheumatic pulmonary valve stenosis with insufficiency
I37.8	Other nonrheumatic pulmonary valve disorders
Q20.4	Double inlet ventricle
Q20.8	Other congenital malformations of cardiac chambers and connections
Q21.0	Ventricular septal defect
Q21.2	Atrioventricular septal defect
Q21.3	Tetralogy of Fallot
Q21.4	Aortopulmonary septal defect
Q21.8	Other congenital malformations of cardiac septa
Q22.0	Pulmonary valve atresia
Q22.1	Congenital pulmonary valve stenosis
Q22.2	Congenital pulmonary valve insufficiency
Q22.3	Other congenital malformations of pulmonary valve
Q22.4	Congenital tricuspid stenosis
Q22.5	Ebstein's anomaly
Q22.6	Hypoplastic right heart syndrome
Q22.8	Other congenital malformations of tricuspid valve
Q24.3	Pulmonary infundibular stenosis
Q24.8	Other specified congenital malformations of heart
Q25.3	Supravalvular aortic stenosis
Q25.41	Absence and aplasia of aorta
Q25.42	Hypoplasia of aorta
Q25.43	Congenital aneurysm of aorta
Q25.44	Congenital dilation of aorta
Q25.45	Double aortic arch
Q25.46	Tortuous aortic arch
Q25.47	Right aortic arch
Q25.48	Anomalous origin of subclavian artery
Q25.49	Other congenital malformations of aorta
Q25.5	Atresia of pulmonary artery
Q25.6	Stenosis of pulmonary artery
Q25.71	Coarctation of pulmonary artery
Q25.72	Congenital pulmonary arteriovenous malformation
Q25.79	Other congenital malformations of pulmonary artery
Q25.8	Other congenital malformations of other great arteries
Q26.0	Congenital stenosis of vena cava
Q26.3	Partial anomalous pulmonary venous connection
Q26.8	Other congenital malformations of great veins
R23.0	Cyanosis

AMA: 33766 2017,Dec,3 **33767** 2018,Jan,8; 2017,Jan,8; 2017,Dec,3; 2016,Jul,3

Relative Value Units/Medicare Edits

Non-Facility RVU	Work	PE	MP	Total
33766	23.57	9.52	5.59	38.68
33767	25.3	10.0	6.01	41.31
Facility RVU	**Work**	**PE**	**MP**	**Total**
33766	23.57	9.52	5.59	38.68
33767	25.3	10.0	6.01	41.31

	FUD	Status	MUE	Modifiers				IOM Reference
33766	90	A	1(2)	51	N/A	62*	80	None
33767	90	A	1(2)	51	N/A	62*	80	

* with documentation

Terms To Know

atresia. Congenital closure or absence of a tubular organ or an opening to the body surface.

cardiopulmonary bypass. Venous blood is diverted to a heart-lung machine, which mechanically pumps and oxygenates the blood temporarily so the heart can be bypassed while an open procedure on the heart or coronary arteries is performed. During bypass, the lungs are deflated and immobile.

cyanosis. Bluish discoloration due to an excessive amount of deoxygenated hemoglobin in the blood.

Ebstein's anomaly. Malformation of the tricuspid valve characterized by septal and posterior leaflets attaching to the wall of the right ventricle. Ebstein's anomaly causes the right ventricle to fuse with the atrium into a large right atrium and a small ventricle and leads to heart failure and abnormal cardiac rhythm.

shunt. Surgically created passage between blood vessels or other natural passages, such as an arteriovenous anastomosis, to divert or bypass blood flow from the normal channel.

stenosis. Narrowing or constriction of a passage.

tetralogy of Fallot. Specific combination of congenital cardiac defects: obstruction of the right ventricular outflow tract with pulmonary stenosis, interventricular septal defect, malposition of the aorta, overriding the interventricular septum and receiving blood from both the venous and arterial systems, and enlargement of the right ventricle.

Waterston procedure. Type of aortopulmonary shunting done to increase pulmonary blood flow. The ascending aorta is anastomosed to the right pulmonary artery.

33768

\+ **33768** Anastomosis, cavopulmonary, second superior vena cava (List separately in addition to primary procedure)

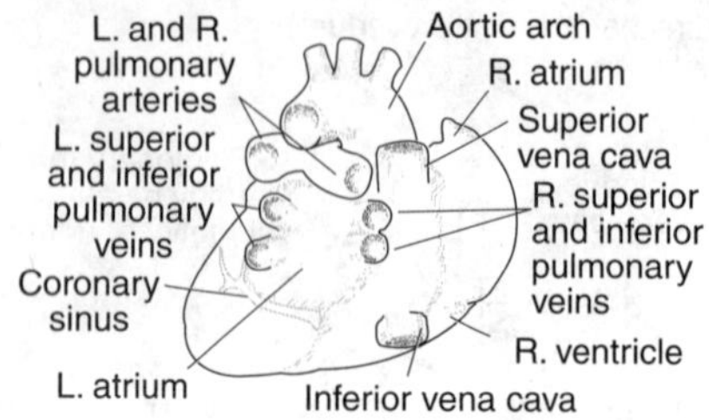

Posterior depiction of normal heart and its major venous returns

An anomalous left superior vena cava is repaired using anastomosis

Explanation

A cavopulmonary anastomosis of an anomalous left superior vena cava is performed in conjunction with separately reportable repair of other cardiac anomalies (e.g., bidirectional Glenn procedure, modified Fontan procedure, outflow tract augmentation). Cavopulmonary anastomosis is required when a left superior vena cava is present. The left superior vena cava is dissected free. The left superior vena cava is divided and anastomosed in end-to-side fashion to the left pulmonary artery.

Coding Tips

Report 33768 in addition to 33478, 33617, 33622, and 33767. Insertion of a chest tube (32551) is included and should not be reported separately. Temporary transvenous pacemaker placement (33210, 33211) is also included and should not be reported separately.

ICD-10-CM Diagnostic Codes

This/these CPT code(s) are add on code(s). See the primary procedure code that this code is performed with for your ICD-10-CM code selections. Diagnostic code(s) would be the same as the actual procedure performed.

AMA: **33768** 2018,Jan,8; 2017,Jan,8; 2016,Jul,3; 2016,Jan,13; 2015,Jan,16; 2014,Jan,11

Relative Value Units/Medicare Edits

Non-Facility RVU	Work	PE	MP	Total
33768	8.0	2.22	1.88	12.1
Facility RVU	**Work**	**PE**	**MP**	**Total**
33768	8.0	2.22	1.88	12.1

	FUD	Status	MUE	Modifiers				IOM Reference
33768	N/A	A	1(2)	N/A	N/A	62	80	None

* with documentation

Terms To Know

anastomosis. Surgically created connection between ducts, blood vessels, or bowel segments to allow flow from one to the other.

33770-33771

33770 Repair of transposition of the great arteries with ventricular septal defect and subpulmonary stenosis; without surgical enlargement of ventricular septal defect

33771 with surgical enlargement of ventricular septal defect

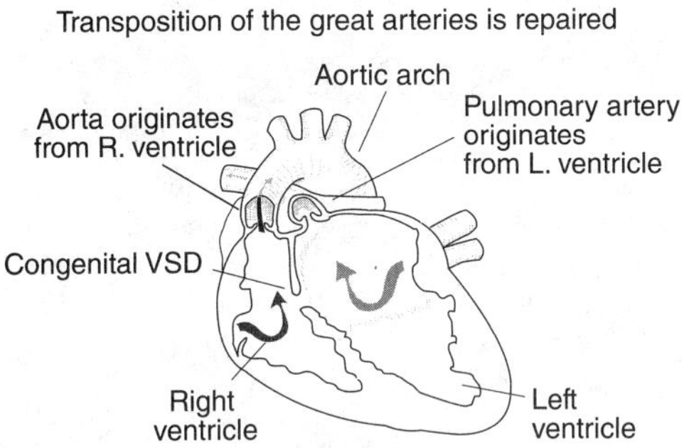

Explanation

In 33770, the physician gains access to the mediastinum through the sternum (median sternotomy). Cardiopulmonary bypass catheters are usually placed through an incision in the right atrial appendage and aorta or femoral artery and the heart is stopped by infusion of cardioplegia solution into the coronary circulation. A large Dacron patch is applied to direct oxygenated blood from the left ventricle through the large ventricular septal defect into the aortic valve and ascending aorta. The physician ligates the proximal main pulmonary artery or oversews the pulmonic valve. A fabric conduit or human cadaveric homograft is placed to direct unoxygenated blood from the right ventricle to the branch pulmonary arteries. The physician may place a bioprosthetic valve in the pulmonary outflow conduit if the pulmonary vascular resistance is elevated. In 33771, the physician gains access to the mediastinum through the sternum (median sternotomy). Cardiopulmonary bypass catheters are usually placed through incision in the right atrial appendage and aorta or femoral artery and the heart is stopped by infusion of cardioplegia solution into the coronary circulation. The physician enlarges the ventricular septal defect anteriorly to avoid damage to the conduction bundles. A large Dacron patch is applied to direct oxygenated blood from the left ventricle through the large ventricular septal defect into the aortic valve and ascending aorta. The physician ligates the proximal main pulmonary artery or oversews the pulmonic valve. A fabric conduit is placed to direct right ventricular flow to the pulmonary artery. The physician may place a bioprosthetic valve in the pulmonary outflow conduit if the pulmonary vascular resistance is elevated. The cardiac incisions are closed, the patient is removed from cardiopulmonary bypass, and the remaining surgical incisions are closed. Chest tubes and/or a mediastinal drainage tube may be inserted for drainage following the procedure.

Coding Tips

Congenital anomalies involving transposition of the great vessels may occur with other anomalies of the heart that also require repair. In addition, repair may be accomplished by a variety of techniques. Review all procedure descriptions in CPT for repair of transposition of the great vessels (33770–33781) prior to selecting a code. When ligation and takedown of systemic-to-pulmonary artery shunt is performed in addition to this procedure, it should be reported separately, see 33924. For repair of transposition of the great arteries, atrial baffle procedure (e.g., Mustard or Senning type), see 33774; with removal of pulmonary artery band, see 33775; with closure of ventricular septal defect, see 33776; and with repair of subpulmonic obstruction, see 33777. For repair of transposition of the great arteries, aortic pulmonary artery reconstruction (e.g., Jatene type), see 33778; with removal of pulmonary artery band, see 33779; with closure of ventricular septal defect, see 33780; and with repair of subpulmonic obstruction, see 33781.

ICD-10-CM Diagnostic Codes

I24.8	Other forms of acute ischemic heart disease
I37.0	Nonrheumatic pulmonary valve stenosis
I37.1	Nonrheumatic pulmonary valve insufficiency
I37.2	Nonrheumatic pulmonary valve stenosis with insufficiency
I37.8	Other nonrheumatic pulmonary valve disorders
Q20.1	Double outlet right ventricle
Q20.2	Double outlet left ventricle
Q20.3	Discordant ventriculoarterial connection
Q20.4	Double inlet ventricle
Q20.5	Discordant atrioventricular connection
Q20.8	Other congenital malformations of cardiac chambers and connections
Q21.8	Other congenital malformations of cardiac septa
Q22.0	Pulmonary valve atresia
Q22.1	Congenital pulmonary valve stenosis
Q22.2	Congenital pulmonary valve insufficiency
Q22.3	Other congenital malformations of pulmonary valve
Q22.4	Congenital tricuspid stenosis
Q22.5	Ebstein's anomaly
Q22.6	Hypoplastic right heart syndrome
Q22.8	Other congenital malformations of tricuspid valve
Q24.8	Other specified congenital malformations of heart
Q25.41	Absence and aplasia of aorta
Q25.42	Hypoplasia of aorta
Q25.43	Congenital aneurysm of aorta
Q25.44	Congenital dilation of aorta
Q25.45	Double aortic arch
Q25.46	Tortuous aortic arch
Q25.47	Right aortic arch
Q25.48	Anomalous origin of subclavian artery
Q25.49	Other congenital malformations of aorta
Q25.72	Congenital pulmonary arteriovenous malformation
Q25.79	Other congenital malformations of pulmonary artery
Q25.8	Other congenital malformations of other great arteries
R23.0	Cyanosis

AMA: 33770 2018,Jan,8; 2017,Jan,8; 2017,Dec,3; 2016,Jan,13; 2015,Jan,16; 2014,Jan,11 **33771** 2017,Dec,3

Relative Value Units/Medicare Edits

Non-Facility RVU	Work	PE	MP	Total
33770	39.07	13.2	9.3	61.57
33771	40.63	13.08	9.67	63.38
Facility RVU	**Work**	**PE**	**MP**	**Total**
33770	39.07	13.2	9.3	61.57
33771	40.63	13.08	9.67	63.38

	FUD	Status	MUE	Modifiers				IOM Reference
33770	90	A	1(2)	51	N/A	62*	80	None
33771	90	A	1(2)	51	N/A	62*	80	

* with documentation

Terms To Know

homograft. Graft from one individual to another of the same species.

Rashkind procedure. Transvenous balloon atrial septectomy or septostomy performed by cardiac catheterization. A balloon catheter is inserted into the heart either to create or enlarge an opening in the interatrial septal wall.

transposition of great vessels. Life-threatening congenital malformation of the two main vessels of the cardiovascular system in which the pulmonary artery branches from the left ventricle and the aorta branches from the right ventricle. This condition causes the blood being returned from the extremities to be shunted back into the systemic circulation without being oxygenated. This condition may appear in differing forms: complete or classical transposition; double outlet right ventricle in which there is incomplete transposition of the vessels or both vessels arise from the right ventricle; and corrected transposition of the great vessels in which a developmental cardiac anomaly inverts the ventricles and valves to compensate for the transposed vessels by producing mirror-image blood flow through the heart.

ventricular septal defect. Congenital cardiac anomaly resulting in a continual opening in the septum between the ventricles that, in severe cases, causes oxygenated blood to flow back into the lungs, resulting in pulmonary hypertension.

33774-33777

33774 Repair of transposition of the great arteries, atrial baffle procedure (eg, Mustard or Senning type) with cardiopulmonary bypass;
33775 with removal of pulmonary band
33776 with closure of ventricular septal defect
33777 with repair of subpulmonic obstruction

Transposition of the great arteries and other anomalies are repaired

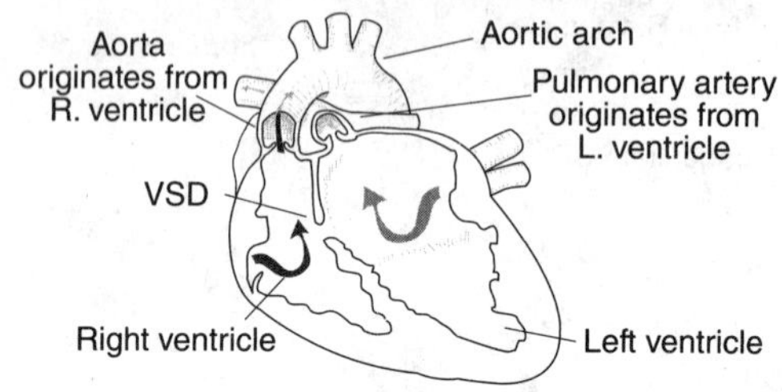

Explanation

The physician gains access to the mediastinum through an incision through the sternum (median sternotomy). Cardiopulmonary bypass catheters are placed through incisions in the low inferior vena cava, the superior vena cava, and aorta or femoral artery and the heart is stopped by infusion of cardioplegia solution into the coronary circulation. In 33774, the physician excises the interatrial septum and sews baffle material (pericardium or Dacron) to direct blood from the pulmonary veins to the right ventricle and the systemic venous drainage to the left ventricle. The pulmonary venous chamber may be enlarged with a woven Dacron or pericardial patch. In 33775, the physician removes the pulmonary artery band (placed during a previous surgery) and dilates the pulmonary artery to normal size. If this is not possible, the pulmonary band and the constricted area of pulmonary artery are removed, and a woven Dacron patch is applied over the hole. The physician excises the interatrial septum and sews baffle material (pericardium or Dacron) to direct blood from the pulmonary veins to the right ventricle and the systemic venous drainage to the left ventricle. The pulmonary venous chamber may be enlarged with a woven Dacron or pericardial patch. In 33776, the ventricular septal defect is closed, usually with a Dacron patch and the interatrial septum is excised. The physician sews baffle material (pericardium or Dacron) to direct blood from the pulmonary veins to the right ventricle and the systemic venous drainage to the left ventricle. The pulmonary venous chamber may be enlarged with a woven Dacron or pericardial patch. In 33777, the physician makes an incision in the right ventricular outflow tract, resects the fibrous muscular tissue causing the subpulmonic obstruction, and sews the ventriculotomy closed. The interatrial septum is excised and baffle material (pericardium or Dacron) is sewn in to direct blood from the pulmonary veins to the right ventricle and the systemic venous drainage to the left ventricle. The pulmonary venous chamber may be enlarged with a woven Dacron or pericardial patch. The cardiac incisions are closed and the patient is taken off cardiopulmonary bypass. The remaining surgical incisions are closed and the sternal or chest wall wounds are dressed. Chest tubes and/or mediastinal drainage tubes may be inserted for drainage following the procedure.

Coding Tips

Congenital anomalies involving transposition of the great vessels may occur with other anomalies of the heart that also require repair. In addition, repair may be accomplished by a variety of techniques. Review all procedure descriptions in CPT for repair of transposition of the great vessels (33770–33781) prior to selecting a code. When ligation and takedown of systemic-to-pulmonary artery shunt is performed in addition to this procedure, it should be reported separately, see 33924. For repair of transposition of the great arteries with ventricular septal defect and subpulmonary stenosis, see 33770–33771.

ICD-10-CM Diagnostic Codes

I24.8	Other forms of acute ischemic heart disease
I37.0	Nonrheumatic pulmonary valve stenosis
I37.1	Nonrheumatic pulmonary valve insufficiency
I37.2	Nonrheumatic pulmonary valve stenosis with insufficiency
I37.8	Other nonrheumatic pulmonary valve disorders
Q20.1	Double outlet right ventricle
Q20.2	Double outlet left ventricle
Q20.3	Discordant ventriculoarterial connection
Q20.4	Double inlet ventricle
Q20.5	Discordant atrioventricular connection
Q20.8	Other congenital malformations of cardiac chambers and connections
Q21.0	Ventricular septal defect
Q21.1	Atrial septal defect
Q21.2	Atrioventricular septal defect
Q21.3	Tetralogy of Fallot
Q21.4	Aortopulmonary septal defect
Q21.8	Other congenital malformations of cardiac septa
Q22.0	Pulmonary valve atresia
Q22.1	Congenital pulmonary valve stenosis
Q22.2	Congenital pulmonary valve insufficiency
Q22.3	Other congenital malformations of pulmonary valve
Q22.4	Congenital tricuspid stenosis
Q22.5	Ebstein's anomaly
Q22.6	Hypoplastic right heart syndrome
Q22.8	Other congenital malformations of tricuspid valve
Q24.8	Other specified congenital malformations of heart
Q25.41	Absence and aplasia of aorta
Q25.42	Hypoplasia of aorta
Q25.43	Congenital aneurysm of aorta
Q25.44	Congenital dilation of aorta
Q25.45	Double aortic arch
Q25.46	Tortuous aortic arch
Q25.47	Right aortic arch
Q25.48	Anomalous origin of subclavian artery
Q25.49	Other congenital malformations of aorta
Q25.72	Congenital pulmonary arteriovenous malformation
Q25.79	Other congenital malformations of pulmonary artery
Q25.8	Other congenital malformations of other great arteries
R23.0	Cyanosis

AMA: 33774 2017,Dec,3 **33775** 2017,Dec,3 **33776** 2017,Dec,3 **33777** 2017,Dec,3

Relative Value Units/Medicare Edits

Non-Facility RVU	Work	PE	MP	Total
33774	31.73	12.96	7.54	52.23
33775	32.99	12.99	7.86	53.84
33776	34.75	13.88	8.27	56.9
33777	34.17	12.67	8.12	54.96
Facility RVU	**Work**	**PE**	**MP**	**Total**
33774	31.73	12.96	7.54	52.23
33775	32.99	12.99	7.86	53.84
33776	34.75	13.88	8.27	56.9
33777	34.17	12.67	8.12	54.96

	FUD	Status	MUE	Modifiers				IOM Reference
33774	90	A	1(2)	51	N/A	62*	80	None
33775	90	A	1(2)	51	N/A	N/A	80	
33776	90	A	1(2)	51	N/A	62*	80	
33777	90	A	1(2)	51	N/A	N/A	80	

* with documentation

Terms To Know

congenital. Present at birth, occurring through heredity or an influence during gestation up to the moment of birth.

transposition of great vessels. Life-threatening congenital malformation of the two main vessels of the cardiovascular system in which the pulmonary artery branches from the left ventricle and the aorta branches from the right ventricle. This condition causes the blood being returned from the extremities to be shunted back into the systemic circulation without being oxygenated. This condition may appear in differing forms: complete or classical transposition; double outlet right ventricle in which there is incomplete transposition of the vessels or both vessels arise from the right ventricle; and corrected transposition of the great vessels in which a developmental cardiac anomaly inverts the ventricles and valves to compensate for the transposed vessels by producing mirror-image blood flow through the heart.

ventricular septal defect. Congenital cardiac anomaly resulting in a continual opening in the septum between the ventricles that, in severe cases, causes oxygenated blood to flow back into the lungs, resulting in pulmonary hypertension.

33778-33781

33778 Repair of transposition of the great arteries, aortic pulmonary artery reconstruction (eg, Jatene type);
33779 with removal of pulmonary band
33780 with closure of ventricular septal defect
33781 with repair of subpulmonic obstruction

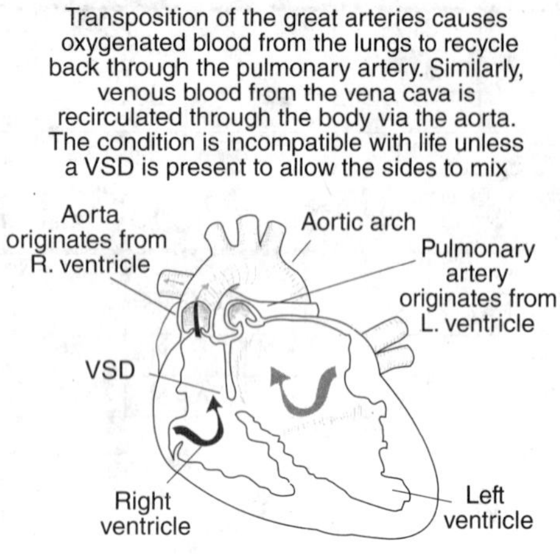

Explanation

The physician gains access to the mediastinum through an incision of the sternum (median sternotomy). Cardiopulmonary bypass catheters are placed through incisions in the low inferior vena cava, the superior vena cava, and aorta or femoral artery and the heart is stopped by infusion of cardioplegia solution into the coronary circulation. In 33778, the physician performs an arterial switch (or Jatene type procedure) for transposition of the great arteries, aortic pulmonary artery reconstruction. The physician removes the coronary ostia from the aortic root and sews them into the root of the pulmonary trunk. The pulmonary trunk and aortic root are each transected and interchanged to direct blood from the pulmonary veins through the left ventricle to the aorta, and the systemic venous drainage to the pulmonary trunk via the right ventricle. In 33779, the physician removes the pulmonary artery band placed during a previous surgery and dilates the pulmonary artery to normal size. If this is not possible, the pulmonary band and constricted area of pulmonary artery are removed and a woven Dacron patch is applied over the hole. The physician removes the coronary ostia from the aortic root and sews into the root of the pulmonary trunk. The pulmonary trunk and aortic root are each transected and interchanged to direct blood from the pulmonary veins through the left ventricle to the aorta, and the systemic venous drainage to the pulmonary trunk via the right ventricle. In 33780, the physician removes the coronary ostia from the aortic root and sews into the root of the pulmonary trunk. The pulmonary trunk and aortic root are each transected and interchanged to direct blood from the pulmonary veins through the left ventricle to the aorta, and the systemic venous drainage to the pulmonary trunk via the right ventricle. The ventricular septal defect is closed, usually with a Dacron patch. In 33781, the physician removes the coronary ostia from the aortic root and sews them into the root of the pulmonary trunk. The pulmonary trunk and aortic root are each transected and interchanged to direct blood from the pulmonary veins through the left ventricle to the aorta, and the systemic venous drainage to the pulmonary trunk via the right ventricle. An incision is made in the right ventricular outflow tract, resection of the fibrous muscular tissue causing the subpulmonic obstruction is performed, and the ventriculotomy is closed. Cardiac incisions are closed and patient is taken off cardiopulmonary bypass. The remaining surgical incisions are closed and the sternal or chest wall wounds are dressed. Chest tubes and/or mediastinal drainage tubes may be inserted following the procedure.

Coding Tips

When ligation and takedown of systemic-to-pulmonary artery shunt is performed in addition to this procedure, it should be reported separately, see 33924. Do not append modifier 63 to 33778 as the description or nature of the procedure includes infants up to 4 kg. For repair of transposition of the great arteries with ventricular septal defect and subpulmonary stenosis, see 33770–33771. For repair of transposition of the great arteries, atrial baffle procedure (e.g., Mustard or Senning type), see 33774; with removal of pulmonary artery band, see 33775; with closure of ventricular septal defect, see 33776; and with repair of subpulmonic obstruction, see 33777.

ICD-10-CM Diagnostic Codes

I37.0	Nonrheumatic pulmonary valve stenosis
I37.1	Nonrheumatic pulmonary valve insufficiency
I37.2	Nonrheumatic pulmonary valve stenosis with insufficiency
I37.8	Other nonrheumatic pulmonary valve disorders
Q20.1	Double outlet right ventricle
Q20.2	Double outlet left ventricle
Q20.3	Discordant ventriculoarterial connection
Q20.4	Double inlet ventricle
Q20.5	Discordant atrioventricular connection
Q20.8	Other congenital malformations of cardiac chambers and connections
Q21.0	Ventricular septal defect
Q21.4	Aortopulmonary septal defect
Q21.8	Other congenital malformations of cardiac septa
Q22.0	Pulmonary valve atresia
Q22.1	Congenital pulmonary valve stenosis
Q22.2	Congenital pulmonary valve insufficiency
Q22.3	Other congenital malformations of pulmonary valve
Q22.4	Congenital tricuspid stenosis
Q22.5	Ebstein's anomaly
Q22.6	Hypoplastic right heart syndrome
Q22.8	Other congenital malformations of tricuspid valve
Q24.8	Other specified congenital malformations of heart
Q25.41	Absence and aplasia of aorta
Q25.42	Hypoplasia of aorta
Q25.43	Congenital aneurysm of aorta
Q25.44	Congenital dilation of aorta
Q25.45	Double aortic arch
Q25.46	Tortuous aortic arch
Q25.47	Right aortic arch
Q25.48	Anomalous origin of subclavian artery
Q25.49	Other congenital malformations of aorta
Q25.72	Congenital pulmonary arteriovenous malformation
Q25.79	Other congenital malformations of pulmonary artery
Q25.8	Other congenital malformations of other great arteries
R23.0	Cyanosis

AMA: **33778** 2017,Dec,3 **33779** 2017,Dec,3 **33780** 2017,Dec,3 **33781** 2018,Jan,8; 2017,Jan,8; 2017,Dec,3; 2016,Jan,13; 2015,Jan,16; 2014,Jan,11

Relative Value Units/Medicare Edits

Non-Facility RVU	Work	PE	MP	Total
33778	42.75	15.36	10.19	68.3
33779	43.23	14.14	10.31	67.68
33780	43.9	14.55	10.47	68.92
33781	43.21	13.79	10.3	67.3
Facility RVU	**Work**	**PE**	**MP**	**Total**
33778	42.75	15.36	10.19	68.3
33779	43.23	14.14	10.31	67.68
33780	43.9	14.55	10.47	68.92
33781	43.21	13.79	10.3	67.3

	FUD	Status	MUE	Modifiers				IOM Reference
33778	90	A	1(2)	51	N/A	62*	80	None
33779	90	A	1(2)	51	N/A	62*	80	
33780	90	A	1(2)	51	N/A	62*	80	
33781	90	A	1(2)	51	N/A	N/A	80	

* with documentation

Terms To Know

coronary ostia. One or both of the two openings in the aortic sinuses that mark the origins of the left and right coronary arteries.

hypoplastic left heart syndrome. Hypoplasia or atresia of the left ventricle and aorta or mitral valve with respiratory distress and extreme cyanosis. Cardiac failure and death often result in early infancy.

transposition of great vessels. Life-threatening congenital malformation of the two main vessels of the cardiovascular system in which the pulmonary artery branches from the left ventricle and the aorta branches from the right ventricle. This condition causes the blood being returned from the extremities to be shunted back into the systemic circulation without being oxygenated. This condition may appear in differing forms: complete or classical transposition; double outlet right ventricle in which there is incomplete transposition of the vessels or both vessels arise from the right ventricle; and corrected transposition of the great vessels in which a developmental cardiac anomaly inverts the ventricles and valves to compensate for the transposed vessels by producing mirror-image blood flow through the heart.

ventricular septal defect. Congenital cardiac anomaly resulting in a continual opening in the septum between the ventricles that, in severe cases, causes oxygenated blood to flow back into the lungs, resulting in pulmonary hypertension.

33782-33783

33782 Aortic root translocation with ventricular septal defect and pulmonary stenosis repair (ie, Nikaidoh procedure); without coronary ostium reimplantation

33783 with reimplantation of 1 or both coronary ostia

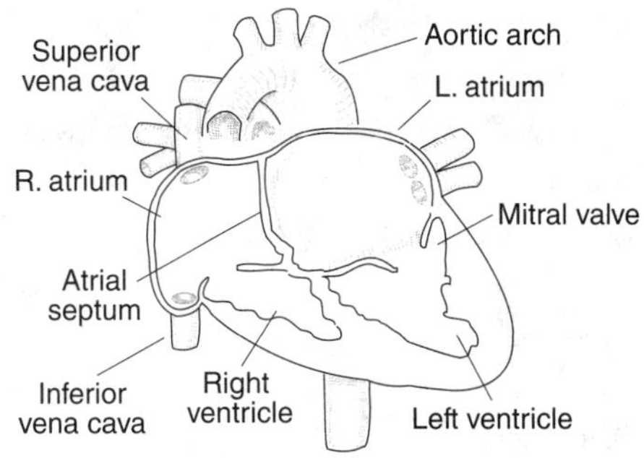

Explanation

The physician repairs anomalies of ventriculoarterial connection, ventricular septal defect (VSD), and pulmonary outflow tract obstruction (stenosis) in the Nikaidoh procedure. A median sternotomy incision is made and cardiopulmonary bypass is initiated. The physician may harvest a piece of pericardium to be used in the reconstruction of the right ventricular outflow tract, and mobilizes the branch pulmonary arteries. The physician harvests the aortic root from the right ventricle, with coronary arteries attached. The outlet septum is divided and the physician excises the pulmonary valve. The left ventricular outflow tract is reconstructed with the posteriorly translocated aortic root and the VSD patch. Using the pericardial patch, the physician reconstructs the right ventricular outflow tract. Report 33782 if no reimplantation of the coronary ostium is performed and 33783 if the physician reimplants one or both coronary ostia.

Coding Tips

For 33782, codes 33412, 33413, 33608, 33681, 33770, 33771, 33778, 33780, and 33920 are not reported separately.

ICD-10-CM Diagnostic Codes

I24.8	Other forms of acute ischemic heart disease
I28.8	Other diseases of pulmonary vessels
I37.0	Nonrheumatic pulmonary valve stenosis
I37.1	Nonrheumatic pulmonary valve insufficiency
I37.2	Nonrheumatic pulmonary valve stenosis with insufficiency
I37.8	Other nonrheumatic pulmonary valve disorders
Q20.0	Common arterial trunk
Q20.1	Double outlet right ventricle
Q20.2	Double outlet left ventricle
Q20.3	Discordant ventriculoarterial connection
Q20.4	Double inlet ventricle
Q20.5	Discordant atrioventricular connection
Q20.8	Other congenital malformations of cardiac chambers and connections
Q21.0	Ventricular septal defect
Q21.2	Atrioventricular septal defect
Q21.3	Tetralogy of Fallot
Q21.4	Aortopulmonary septal defect
Q21.8	Other congenital malformations of cardiac septa

Q22.0	Pulmonary valve atresia
Q22.1	Congenital pulmonary valve stenosis
Q22.2	Congenital pulmonary valve insufficiency
Q22.3	Other congenital malformations of pulmonary valve
Q22.4	Congenital tricuspid stenosis
Q22.5	Ebstein's anomaly
Q22.6	Hypoplastic right heart syndrome
Q22.8	Other congenital malformations of tricuspid valve
Q24.3	Pulmonary infundibular stenosis
Q24.8	Other specified congenital malformations of heart
Q25.3	Supravalvular aortic stenosis
Q25.41	Absence and aplasia of aorta
Q25.42	Hypoplasia of aorta
Q25.43	Congenital aneurysm of aorta
Q25.44	Congenital dilation of aorta
Q25.45	Double aortic arch
Q25.46	Tortuous aortic arch
Q25.47	Right aortic arch
Q25.48	Anomalous origin of subclavian artery
Q25.49	Other congenital malformations of aorta
Q25.5	Atresia of pulmonary artery
Q25.6	Stenosis of pulmonary artery
Q25.71	Coarctation of pulmonary artery
Q25.72	Congenital pulmonary arteriovenous malformation
Q25.79	Other congenital malformations of pulmonary artery
Q25.8	Other congenital malformations of other great arteries

AMA: **33782** 2017,Dec,3 **33783** 2017,Dec,3

Relative Value Units/Medicare Edits

Non-Facility RVU	Work	PE	MP	Total
33782	60.08	19.53	14.41	94.02
33783	65.08	20.92	15.66	101.66
Facility RVU	**Work**	**PE**	**MP**	**Total**
33782	60.08	19.53	14.41	94.02
33783	65.08	20.92	15.66	101.66

	FUD	Status	MUE	Modifiers				IOM Reference
33782	90	A	1(2)	51	N/A	62*	80	None
33783	90	A	1(2)	51	N/A	62*	80	

* with documentation

Terms To Know

congenital. Present at birth, occurring through heredity or an influence during gestation up to the moment of birth.

coronary ostia. One or both of the two openings in the aortic sinuses that mark the origins of the left and right coronary arteries.

ventricular septal defect. Congenital cardiac anomaly resulting in a continual opening in the septum between the ventricles that, in severe cases, causes oxygenated blood to flow back into the lungs, resulting in pulmonary hypertension.

33786

33786 Total repair, truncus arteriosus (Rastelli type operation)

Two types of truncus arteriosus

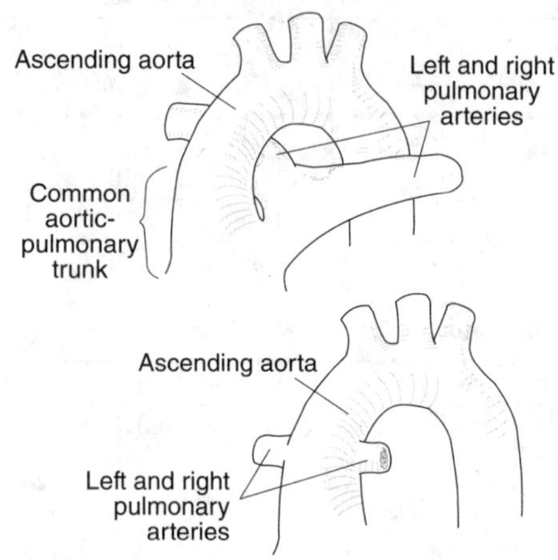

Truncus arteriosus is an anomaly in which the aortic and pulmonary systems are fused into a common trunk. A VSD is always present. Surgical intervention is almost always early in life

Explanation

Total repair, truncus arteriosus (Rastelli type operation) is performed by access to the mediastinum through an incision in the sternum (median sternotomy). Cardiopulmonary bypass catheters are placed usually through incisions in the right atrial appendage and the aorta or femoral artery. The heart is stopped by infusion of cardioplegia solution into the coronary circulation. A large Dacron patch is placed to direct oxygenated blood from the left ventricle through the large ventricular septal defect into the aortic valve and ascending aorta. The proximal main pulmonary artery is ligated or the pulmonic valve is oversewn. A fabric conduit or a human cadaveric homograft is placed to direct unoxygenated blood from the right ventricle to the branch pulmonary arteries after removing them from their origin(s) at the truncal vessel. A pericardial patch is sewn in place to close the defect(s) in the truncal vessel. A bioprosthetic valve may be placed in the pulmonary outflow conduit if the pulmonary vascular resistance is elevated. The cardiac incisions are closed and the patient is taken off cardiopulmonary bypass. The remaining surgical incisions are closed and the sternal or chest wall wounds are dressed. Chest tubes and/or mediastinal drainage tubes may be placed following the procedure.

Coding Tips

When ligation and takedown of systemic-to-pulmonary artery shunt is performed in addition to this procedure, it should be reported separately, see 33924. Do not append modifier 63 to 33786 as the description or nature of the procedure includes infants up to 4 kg. For closure of a ventricular septal defect only, with or without patch, see 33681; with pulmonary valvotomy or infundibular resection (acyanotic), see 33684.

ICD-10-CM Diagnostic Codes

Q20.0	Common arterial trunk
Q20.3	Discordant ventriculoarterial connection
Q20.5	Discordant atrioventricular connection
Q20.8	Other congenital malformations of cardiac chambers and connections
Q22.0	Pulmonary valve atresia
Q22.1	Congenital pulmonary valve stenosis

Q22.2 Congenital pulmonary valve insufficiency
Q22.3 Other congenital malformations of pulmonary valve
Q24.3 Pulmonary infundibular stenosis
Q24.8 Other specified congenital malformations of heart
Q25.21 Interruption of aortic arch
Q25.29 Other atresia of aorta
Q25.41 Absence and aplasia of aorta
Q25.42 Hypoplasia of aorta
Q25.43 Congenital aneurysm of aorta
Q25.44 Congenital dilation of aorta
Q25.45 Double aortic arch
Q25.46 Tortuous aortic arch
Q25.47 Right aortic arch
Q25.48 Anomalous origin of subclavian artery
Q25.49 Other congenital malformations of aorta
Q25.5 Atresia of pulmonary artery
Q25.6 Stenosis of pulmonary artery
Q25.71 Coarctation of pulmonary artery
Q25.72 Congenital pulmonary arteriovenous malformation
Q25.79 Other congenital malformations of pulmonary artery
Q25.8 Other congenital malformations of other great arteries

AMA: 33786 2018,Jan,8; 2017,Jan,8; 2017,Dec,3; 2016,Jan,13; 2015,Jan,16; 2014,Jan,11

Relative Value Units/Medicare Edits

Non-Facility RVU	Work	PE	MP	Total
33786	41.87	14.36	9.98	66.21
Facility RVU	**Work**	**PE**	**MP**	**Total**
33786	41.87	14.36	9.98	66.21

	FUD	Status	MUE	Modifiers				IOM Reference
33786	90	A	1(2)	51	N/A	62*	80	None

* with documentation

Terms To Know

anomaly. Irregularity in the structure or position of an organ or tissue.

conduit. Surgically created channel for the passage of fluids.

congenital. Present at birth, occurring through heredity or an influence during gestation up to the moment of birth.

homograft. Graft from one individual to another of the same species.

incision. Act of cutting into tissue or an organ.

suture. Numerous stitching techniques employed in wound closure.

valve. Fold or membrane within a body canal or passageway that prevents backflow of fluids running through it.

33788

33788 Reimplantation of an anomalous pulmonary artery

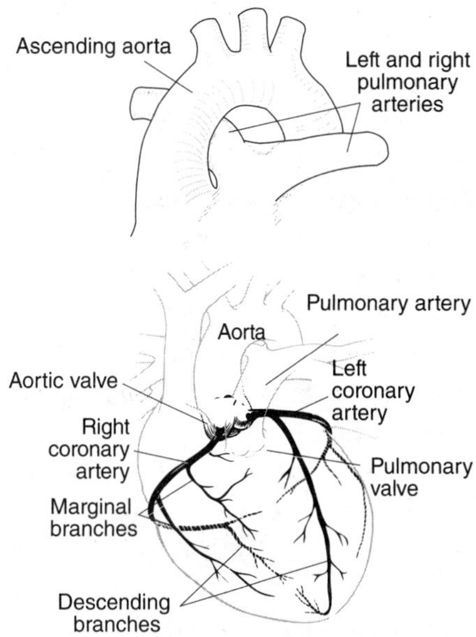

Explanation

Reimplantation of an anomalous pulmonary artery is performed with access to the mediastinum through an incision in the sternum (median sternotomy). Cardiopulmonary bypass catheters are placed usually through incisions in the right atrial appendage and aorta or femoral artery and the heart is stopped by infusion of cardioplegia solution into the coronary circulation. The physician identifies the coronary artery anomaly and reattaches the unperfused pulmonary artery to the pulmonic outflow tract, directly or using a Dacron graft, and ligates the patent ductus arteriosus, if present. The cardiac incisions are closed and the patient is taken off cardiopulmonary bypass. The remaining surgical incisions are closed and the sternal or chest wall wounds are dressed. Chest tubes and/or mediastinal drainage tubes may be inserted following the procedure.

Coding Tips

For pulmonary artery band, see 33690. For complete repair of anomalous venous return (supracardiac, intracardiac, or infracardiac types), see 33730. For partial anomalous returns, see atrial septal defect. For repair of pulmonary artery stenosis by reconstruction with patch or graft, see 33917. For repair of pulmonary atresia with ventricular septal defect, see 33920. For transection of pulmonary artery with cardiopulmonary bypass, see 33922.

ICD-10-CM Diagnostic Codes

Q20.0 Common arterial trunk
Q20.3 Discordant ventriculoarterial connection
Q20.5 Discordant atrioventricular connection
Q20.8 Other congenital malformations of cardiac chambers and connections
Q22.0 Pulmonary valve atresia
Q22.1 Congenital pulmonary valve stenosis
Q22.2 Congenital pulmonary valve insufficiency
Q22.3 Other congenital malformations of pulmonary valve
Q24.3 Pulmonary infundibular stenosis
Q24.8 Other specified congenital malformations of heart

Q25.21 Interruption of aortic arch
Q25.29 Other atresia of aorta
Q25.41 Absence and aplasia of aorta
Q25.42 Hypoplasia of aorta
Q25.43 Congenital aneurysm of aorta
Q25.44 Congenital dilation of aorta
Q25.45 Double aortic arch
Q25.46 Tortuous aortic arch
Q25.47 Right aortic arch
Q25.48 Anomalous origin of subclavian artery
Q25.49 Other congenital malformations of aorta
Q25.5 Atresia of pulmonary artery
Q25.6 Stenosis of pulmonary artery
Q25.71 Coarctation of pulmonary artery
Q25.72 Congenital pulmonary arteriovenous malformation
Q25.79 Other congenital malformations of pulmonary artery
Q25.8 Other congenital malformations of other great arteries

AMA: 33788 2018,Jan,8; 2017,Jan,8; 2017,Dec,3; 2016,Jan,13; 2015,Jan,16; 2014,Jan,11

Relative Value Units/Medicare Edits

Non-Facility RVU	Work	PE	MP	Total
33788	27.42	10.59	6.5	44.51
Facility RVU	**Work**	**PE**	**MP**	**Total**
33788	27.42	10.59	6.5	44.51

	FUD	Status	MUE	Modifiers				IOM Reference
33788	90	A	1(2)	51	N/A	62*	80	None

* with documentation

Terms To Know

anomaly. Irregularity in the structure or position of an organ or tissue.

atresia. Congenital closure or absence of a tubular organ or an opening to the body surface.

atrial septal defect. Cardiac anomaly consisting of a patent opening in the atrial septum due to a fusion failure, classified as ostium secundum type, ostium primum defect, or endocardial cushion defect.

ventricular septal defect. Congenital cardiac anomaly resulting in a continual opening in the septum between the ventricles that, in severe cases, causes oxygenated blood to flow back into the lungs, resulting in pulmonary hypertension.

33800

33800 Aortic suspension (aortopexy) for tracheal decompression (eg, for tracheomalacia) (separate procedure)

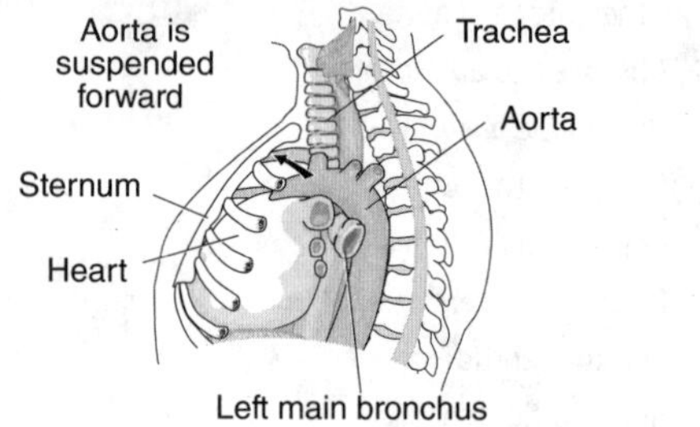

Tissues surrounding an anomalous aortic arch are sutured to those of the sternum to prevent the aorta from pressuring the trachea and causing respiratory compromise. The thymus gland may be removed to allow mobilization of the aorta

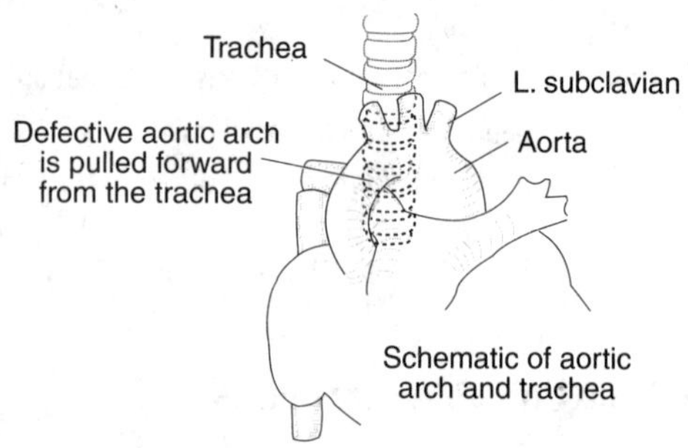

Schematic of aortic arch and trachea

Explanation

Aortopexy for tracheal decompression is performed to open the tracheal lumen thereby preventing collapse. A right lateral thoracotomy or, sometimes, a midline sternotomy is performed to identify the ascending aorta. The thymus is isolated with partial removal performed to allow the ascending aorta to be mobilized and pulled forward. The physician sutures the adventitia of the ascending aorta and base of the innominate artery to the periosteum of the posterior aspect of the sternum or anterior rib. A similar operation may be performed on the descending aorta, depending upon the site of tracheomalacia. The thoracotomy or sternotomy is closed, leaving chest or mediastinal tubes in place.

Coding Tips

Thymectomy is included in this procedure. When 33800 is performed with another separately identifiable procedure, the highest dollar value code is listed as the primary procedure and subsequent procedures are appended with modifier 51. For tracheoplasty, intrathoracic, see 31760.

ICD-10-CM Diagnostic Codes

J39.8 Other specified diseases of upper respiratory tract
Q32.0 Congenital tracheomalacia
Q32.1 Other congenital malformations of trachea
Q34.8 Other specified congenital malformations of respiratory system

AMA: 33800 2018,Jan,8; 2017,Jan,8; 2016,Jan,13; 2015,Jan,16; 2014,Jan,11

Relative Value Units/Medicare Edits

Non-Facility RVU	Work	PE	MP	Total
33800	17.28	7.26	4.1	28.64
Facility RVU	**Work**	**PE**	**MP**	**Total**
33800	17.28	7.26	4.1	28.64

	FUD	Status	MUE	Modifiers				IOM Reference
33800	90	A	1(2)	51	N/A	62	80	None

* with documentation

Terms To Know

anomaly. Irregularity in the structure or position of an organ or tissue.

anterior. Situated in the front area or toward the belly surface of the body; an anatomical reference point used to show the position and relationship of one body structure to another.

congenital. Present at birth, occurring through heredity or an influence during gestation up to the moment of birth.

excision. Surgical removal of an organ or tissue.

incision. Act of cutting into tissue or an organ.

ligate. To tie off a blood vessel or duct with a suture or a soft, thin wire (ligature wire).

mediastinum. Collection of organs and tissues that separate the pleural sacs. Located between the sternum and spine above the diaphragm, it contains the heart and great vessels, trachea and bronchi, esophagus, thymus, lymph nodes, and nerves.

posterior. Located in the back part or caudal end of the body.

sternotomy. Incision into the sternum, the bone that forms the front of the chest cavity and connects with the ribs.

thoracotomy. Surgical procedure for opening the chest wall in order to access the lungs, esophagus, trachea, aorta, heart, and diaphragm.

thymectomy. Excision of the thymus gland, situated in the anterior superior mediastinum.

tracheoplasty. Plastic repair of the trachea, the tube descending from the larynx that branches into the right and left main bronchi.

33802-33803

33802 Division of aberrant vessel (vascular ring);
33803 with reanastomosis

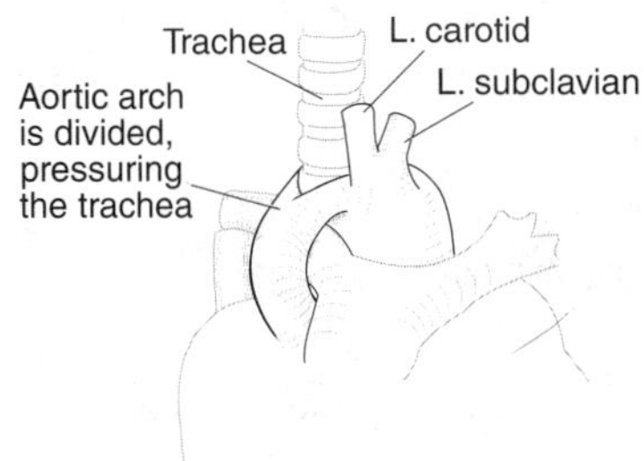

Schematic of aortic arch vascular ring

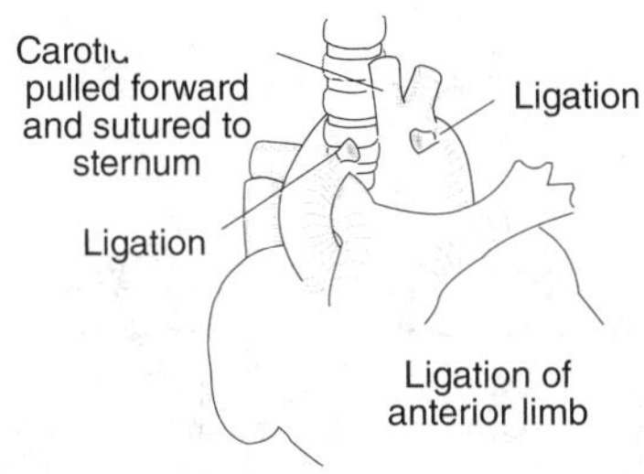

A divided aortic arch is surgically accessed

Explanation

The physician gains access to the mediastinum through an incision through the left chest (posterolateral thoracotomy). The physician identifies the two aortic arches and occludes the smaller left arch with vascular clamps. The physician divides the arch and oversews and possibly ligates the divided ends. The physician dissects away the stumps of the divided left arch and frees them from their mediastinal attachments. The physician attaches traction sutures to the ligated stumps and to the endothoracic fascia anteriorly and posteriorly to minimize obstruction to the esophagus and trachea. The physician closes the remaining surgical incisions and dresses the chest wall wound. The physician may leave a chest tube and/or a mediastinal drainage tube in place following the procedure. Report 33803 if the procedure includes reanastomosis.

Coding Tips

When 33802 or 33803 is performed with another separately identifiable procedure, the highest dollar value code is listed as the primary procedure and subsequent procedures are appended with modifier 51. For repair of transposition of the great arteries, see 33770–33781. For repair of patent ductus arteriosus, see 33820–33824. For excision of coarctation of aorta, see 33840–33851.

ICD-10-CM Diagnostic Codes

I28.8	Other diseases of pulmonary vessels
I77.89	Other specified disorders of arteries and arterioles
Q25.1	Coarctation of aorta
Q25.41	Absence and aplasia of aorta
Q25.42	Hypoplasia of aorta
Q25.43	Congenital aneurysm of aorta
Q25.44	Congenital dilation of aorta
Q25.45	Double aortic arch
Q25.46	Tortuous aortic arch
Q25.47	Right aortic arch

Q25.48	Anomalous origin of subclavian artery
Q25.49	Other congenital malformations of aorta
Q25.6	Stenosis of pulmonary artery
Q25.71	Coarctation of pulmonary artery
Q25.72	Congenital pulmonary arteriovenous malformation
Q25.79	Other congenital malformations of pulmonary artery
Q25.8	Other congenital malformations of other great arteries

AMA: **33802** 2017,Dec,3 **33803** 2017,Dec,3

Relative Value Units/Medicare Edits

Non-Facility RVU	Work	PE	MP	Total
33802	18.37	8.71	4.37	31.45
33803	20.31	8.28	4.81	33.4
Facility RVU	**Work**	**PE**	**MP**	**Total**
33802	18.37	8.71	4.37	31.45
33803	20.31	8.28	4.81	33.4

	FUD	Status	MUE	Modifiers				IOM Reference
33802	90	A	1(3)	51	N/A	62*	80	None
33803	90	A	1(3)	51	N/A	62*	80	

* with documentation

Terms To Know

anastomosis. Surgically created connection between ducts, blood vessels, or bowel segments to allow flow from one to the other.

anomaly. Irregularity in the structure or position of an organ or tissue.

anterior. Situated in the front area or toward the belly surface of the body; an anatomical reference point used to show the position and relationship of one body structure to another.

congenital. Present at birth, occurring through heredity or an influence during gestation up to the moment of birth.

fascia. Fibrous sheet or band of tissue that envelops organs, muscles, and groupings of muscles.

ligate. To tie off a blood vessel or duct with a suture or a soft, thin wire (ligature wire).

mediastinum. Collection of organs and tissues that separate the pleural sacs. Located between the sternum and spine above the diaphragm, it contains the heart and great vessels, trachea and bronchi, esophagus, thymus, lymph nodes, and nerves.

obstruction. Blockage that prevents normal function of the valve or structure.

occlusion. Constriction, closure, or blockage of a passage.

posterior. Located in the back part or caudal end of the body.

33813-33814

33813 Obliteration of aortopulmonary septal defect; without cardiopulmonary bypass

33814 with cardiopulmonary bypass

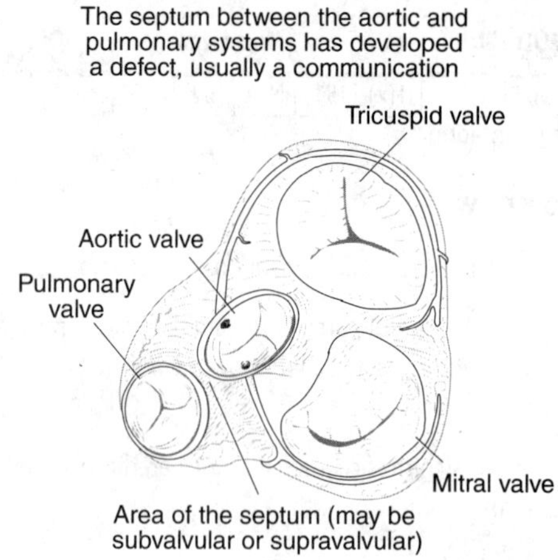

Explanation

The physician performs obliteration of an aortopulmonary septal defect. In 33813, the physician gains access to the mediastinum through an incision through the sternum (median sternotomy). The physician exposes the aortopulmonary septal defect by cutting through the ascending aorta or main pulmonary artery. The physician closes the defect with a Dacron fabric patch, closes the aortic or pulmonary arterial incision, closes the remaining surgical incisions, and dresses the sternal wound. The physician may leave chest tubes and/or a mediastinal drainage tube in place following the procedure. In 33814, the physician places cardiopulmonary bypass catheters through incisions in the low inferior vena cava, the superior vena cava, and high aorta or femoral artery. The physician stops the heart by infusing cardioplegia solution into the coronary circulation. The physician cross-clamps the aorta and places sump suction in the left atrium to obtain a bloodless surgical field. Cardiopulmonary bypass is almost always required if the defect is in the wall between the right and left ventricle. If the hole is above the aortic and pulmonary valves, it may be possible to avoid cardiopulmonary bypass if the connection can be isolated and controlled with side-biting clamps on both the aorta and pulmonary artery.

Coding Tips

When 33813 or 33814 is performed with another separately identifiable procedure, the highest dollar value code is listed as the primary procedure and subsequent procedures are appended with modifier 51. For repair of an atrial septal defect, secundum, with cardiopulmonary bypass, with or without patch, see 33641. For direct or patch closure, sinus venosus, with or without anomalous pulmonary venous drainage, see 33645. For repair of an atrial septal defect and ventricular septal defect, with direct or patch closure, see 33647. For repair of an incomplete or partial atrioventricular canal (ostium primum atrial septal defect), with or without atrioventricular valve repair, see 33660. For closure of a ventricular septal defect, with or without patch graft, see 33681–33688.

ICD-10-CM Diagnostic Codes

Q21.4	Aortopulmonary septal defect
Q21.8	Other congenital malformations of cardiac septa

AMA: **33814** 2017,Dec,3

Relative Value Units/Medicare Edits

Non-Facility RVU	Work	PE	MP	Total
33813	21.36	9.53	5.07	35.96
33814	26.57	11.32	6.3	44.19
Facility RVU	**Work**	**PE**	**MP**	**Total**
33813	21.36	9.53	5.07	35.96
33814	26.57	11.32	6.3	44.19

	FUD	Status	MUE	Modifiers				IOM Reference
33813	90	A	1(2)	51	N/A	62*	80	None
33814	90	A	1(2)	51	N/A	62*	80	

* with documentation

Terms To Know

atrial septal defect. Cardiac anomaly consisting of a patent opening in the atrial septum due to a fusion failure, classified as ostium secundum type, ostium primum defect, or endocardial cushion defect.

cardiopulmonary bypass. Venous blood is diverted to a heart-lung machine, which mechanically pumps and oxygenates the blood temporarily so the heart can be bypassed while an open procedure on the heart or coronary arteries is performed. During bypass, the lungs are deflated and immobile.

obliterate. Get rid or do away with completely.

ventricular septal defect. Congenital cardiac anomaly resulting in a continual opening in the septum between the ventricles that, in severe cases, causes oxygenated blood to flow back into the lungs, resulting in pulmonary hypertension.

33820-33824

33820 Repair of patent ductus arteriosus; by ligation
33822 by division, younger than 18 years
33824 by division, 18 years and older

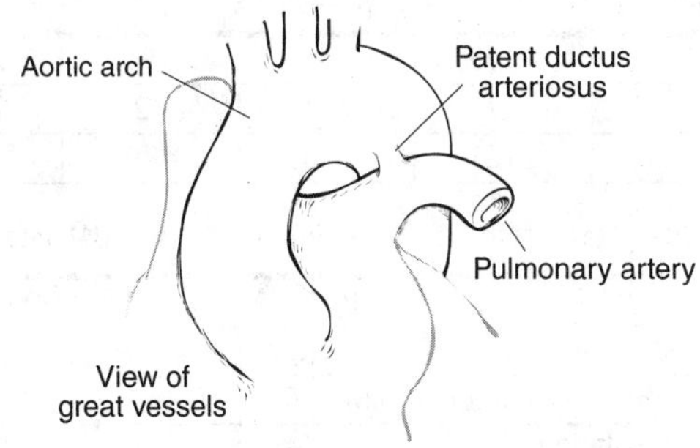

The ductus arteriosus is the natural shunt that bypasses lung circulation in the prenatal phase

Explanation

In 33820, the physician repairs patent ductus arteriosus (PDA) by ligation with access to the mediastinum through an incision of the posterolateral left chest wall (posterolateral thoracotomy). Dissection is performed through the posterior chest wall musculature to expose the superior mediastinum with continued dissection of the tissues surrounding the ductus. Several heavy ligatures are passed around the ductus followed by ligation. The surgical incisions are closed and the chest wall wound is dressed. Chest tubes and/or mediastinal drainage tubes may be inserted following the procedure. In 33822, the repair is performed by division in a patient younger than 18 years of age. The physician dissects away the tissues surrounding the ductus and passes several heavy ligatures around the ductus and ties it off (ligation) at each end. The physician occludes the ductus with vascular clamps and divides the ductus with scissors. The physician closes the aortic end with suture then closes the pulmonary stump. The physician removes the vascular clamps, sutures the pleura closed, closes the remaining surgical incisions, and dresses the chest wall wound. The physician may leave chest tubes and/or a mediastinal drainage tube in place following the procedure. Report 33824 if the patient is 18 years and older.

Coding Tips

When 33820, 33822, or 33824 is performed with another separately identifiable procedure, the highest dollar value code is listed as the primary procedure and subsequent procedures are appended with modifier 51. For excision of coarctation of the aorta, with or without associated patent ductus arteriosus, see 33840–33851. For closure of a ventricular septal defect, see 33681–33688. Use 93582 when closure of patent ductus areteriosus is performed via percutaneous transcatheter.

ICD-10-CM Diagnostic Codes

Q24.8	Other specified congenital malformations of heart
Q25.0	Patent ductus arteriosus
Q25.8	Other congenital malformations of other great arteries
Q28.8	Other specified congenital malformations of circulatory system

AMA: 33820 2018,Jan,8; 2017,Jan,8; 2017,Dec,3; 2016,Jan,13; 2015,Jan,16; 2014,Jan,11 **33822** 2018,Jan,8; 2017,Jan,8; 2017,Dec,3; 2016,Jul,3; 2016,Jan,13; 2015,Jan,16; 2014,Jan,11 **33824** 2017,Dec,3

Relative Value Units/Medicare Edits

Non-Facility RVU	Work	PE	MP	Total
33820	16.69	7.44	3.96	28.09
33822	17.71	7.71	4.2	29.62
33824	20.23	9.18	4.79	34.2
Facility RVU	**Work**	**PE**	**MP**	**Total**
33820	16.69	7.44	3.96	28.09
33822	17.71	7.71	4.2	29.62
33824	20.23	9.18	4.79	34.2

	FUD	Status	MUE	Modifiers				IOM Reference
33820	90	A	1(2)	51	N/A	N/A	80	None
33822	90	A	1(2)	51	N/A	62*	80	
33824	90	A	1(2)	51	N/A	62*	80	

* with documentation

Terms To Know

ligation. Tying off a blood vessel or duct with a suture or a soft, thin wire.

mediastinum. Collection of organs and tissues that separate the pleural sacs. Located between the sternum and spine above the diaphragm, it contains the heart and great vessels, trachea and bronchi, esophagus, thymus, lymph nodes, and nerves.

musculature. Entire muscle tissue apparatus of the body or a specific part of the body.

occlusion. Constriction, closure, or blockage of a passage.

patent ductus arteriosus. Condition in which the normal channel between the pulmonary artery and the aorta fails to close at birth, causing arterial blood to recirculate in the lungs and inhibiting the blood supply to the aorta.

posterior. Located in the back part or caudal end of the body.

ventricular septal defect. Congenital cardiac anomaly resulting in a continual opening in the septum between the ventricles that, in severe cases, causes oxygenated blood to flow back into the lungs, resulting in pulmonary hypertension.

Heart and Pericardium

33840-33851

33840 Excision of coarctation of aorta, with or without associated patent ductus arteriosus; with direct anastomosis

33845 with graft

33851 repair using either left subclavian artery or prosthetic material as gusset for enlargement

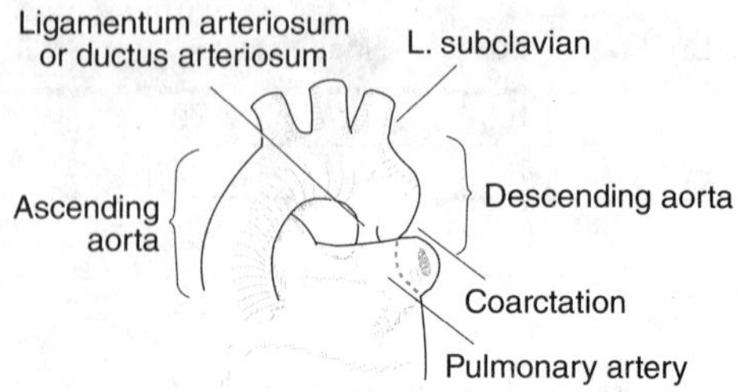

Coarctation is a stenotic narrowing of the descending aorta that is associated with the ductus arteriosum as it turns into the ligamentum arteriosum. This ligament is attached to the heart side of the localized stenosis

Explanation

In 33840–33845, the physician gains access to the mediastinum through an incision through the posterolateral left chest wall (posterolateral thoracotomy). The physician dissects through the posterior chest wall musculature to expose the superior mediastinum, clamping and ligating large collateral vessels as they are encountered. The physician dissects away the tissues surrounding the aorta. The physician clamps the aorta on either side of the coarctation and ties off and divides the ligamentum arteriosum (or patent ductus arteriosus, if present). The physician excises the stricture and sutures the two ends of the aorta to each other. Report 33845 if a graft is placed. In 33851, the physician gains access to the mediastinum through an incision through the posterolateral left chest wall (posterolateral thoracotomy). Dissection through the posterior chest wall musculature to expose the superior mediastinum is performed with clamping and ligating of large collateral vessels as they are encountered. The tissues surrounding the aorta are dissected away and clamps are placed on the aorta at either side of the coarctation and tied off with division of the ligamentum arteriosum (or patent ductus arteriosus, if present). The aorta is opened with a longitudinal incision that extends along the subclavian artery above and for a distance distally. Any extra tissue at the stricture site is excised. The physician sews in the left subclavian artery or a Dacron patch graft to attach and enlarge the aorta at the longitudinal incision. The mediastinal pleura and chest wounds are closed and dressing is applied to the chest wall wound. Chest tubes and/or a mediastinal drainage tube may be placed following the procedure.

Coding Tips

When 33840, 33845, or 33851 is performed with another separately identifiable procedure, the highest dollar value code is listed as the primary procedure and subsequent procedures are appended with modifier 51. For repair of patent ductus arteriosus without excision of coarctation of the aorta, see 33820–33824. For closure of a ventricular septal defect, see 33681–33688.

ICD-10-CM Diagnostic Codes

Q25.0	Patent ductus arteriosus
Q25.1	Coarctation of aorta
Q25.41	Absence and aplasia of aorta
Q25.42	Hypoplasia of aorta

Q25.43	Congenital aneurysm of aorta
Q25.44	Congenital dilation of aorta
Q25.45	Double aortic arch
Q25.46	Tortuous aortic arch
Q25.47	Right aortic arch
Q25.48	Anomalous origin of subclavian artery
Q25.49	Other congenital malformations of aorta

AMA: 33840 2018,Jan,8; 2017,Jan,8; 2017,Dec,3; 2016,Jul,3 **33845** 2018,Jan,8; 2017,Jan,8; 2017,Dec,3; 2016,Jul,3 **33851** 2018,Jan,8; 2017,Jan,8; 2017,Dec,3; 2016,Jul,3

Relative Value Units/Medicare Edits

Non-Facility RVU	Work	PE	MP	Total
33840	21.34	9.53	5.07	35.94
33845	22.93	10.32	5.44	38.69
33851	21.98	9.71	5.21	36.9
Facility RVU	**Work**	**PE**	**MP**	**Total**
33840	21.34	9.53	5.07	35.94
33845	22.93	10.32	5.44	38.69
33851	21.98	9.71	5.21	36.9

	FUD	Status	MUE	Modifiers				IOM Reference
33840	90	A	1(2)	51	N/A	62*	80	None
33845	90	A	1(2)	51	N/A	62*	80	
33851	90	A	1(2)	51	N/A	62*	80	

* with documentation

Terms To Know

anastomosis. Surgically created connection between ducts, blood vessels, or bowel segments to allow flow from one to the other.

graft. Tissue implant from another part of the body or another person.

posterior. Located in the back part or caudal end of the body.

stenosis. Narrowing or constriction of a passage.

stricture. Narrowing of an anatomical structure.

ventricular septal defect. Congenital cardiac anomaly resulting in a continual opening in the septum between the ventricles that, in severe cases, causes oxygenated blood to flow back into the lungs, resulting in pulmonary hypertension.

33852-33853

33852 Repair of hypoplastic or interrupted aortic arch using autogenous or prosthetic material; without cardiopulmonary bypass

33853 with cardiopulmonary bypass

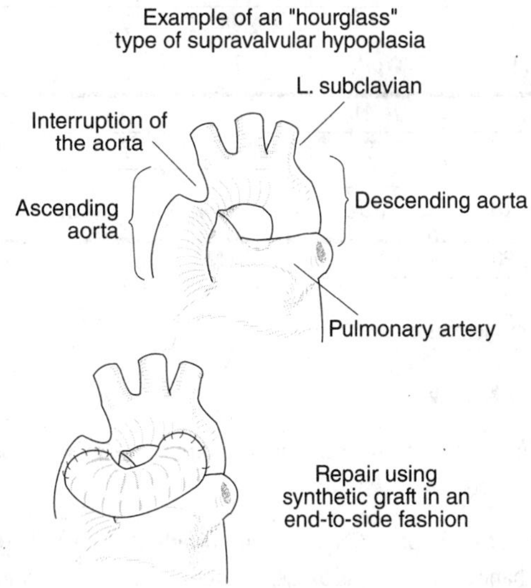

Explanation

The physician surgically attaches the ascending and descending parts of the aorta, where normal connection is too small or interrupted entirely. Access to the mediastinum is achieved through an incision in the sternum (midline sternotomy). The aorta and left carotid artery are clamped to allow completion of the end-to-side attachment of a Dacron mesh graft to the ascending aorta. The physician cross-clamps the graft and releases the proximal clamp and the left carotid artery clamp. End-to-side attachment is performed to secure the distal graft to the descending aorta. The mediastinal pleura and chest are closed with dressing applied to the chest wall wound. Chest tubes and/or a mediastinal drainage tube may be placed following the procedure. Report 33853 when cardiopulmonary bypass is utilized.

Coding Tips

For repair of hypoplastic left heart syndrome (e.g., Norwood type), via excision of coarctation of aorta, see 33619. For excision of coarctation of the aorta with or without associated patent ductus arteriosus, see 33840–33845.

ICD-10-CM Diagnostic Codes

Q25.1	Coarctation of aorta
Q25.21	Interruption of aortic arch
Q25.29	Other atresia of aorta
Q25.3	Supravalvular aortic stenosis
Q25.41	Absence and aplasia of aorta
Q25.42	Hypoplasia of aorta
Q25.43	Congenital aneurysm of aorta
Q25.44	Congenital dilation of aorta
Q25.45	Double aortic arch
Q25.46	Tortuous aortic arch
Q25.47	Right aortic arch
Q25.48	Anomalous origin of subclavian artery
Q25.49	Other congenital malformations of aorta

AMA: 33853 2018,Jan,8; 2017,Jan,8; 2017,Dec,3; 2016,Jul,3; 2016,Jan,13; 2015,Jan,16; 2014,Jan,11

Relative Value Units/Medicare Edits

Non-Facility RVU	Work	PE	MP	Total
33852	24.41	10.39	5.78	40.58
33853	32.51	12.98	7.73	53.22
Facility RVU	**Work**	**PE**	**MP**	**Total**
33852	24.41	10.39	5.78	40.58
33853	32.51	12.98	7.73	53.22

	FUD	Status	MUE	Modifiers				IOM Reference
33852	90	A	1(2)	51	N/A	N/A	80	None
33853	90	A	1(2)	51	N/A	62*	80	

* with documentation

Terms To Know

atresia. Congenital closure or absence of a tubular organ or an opening to the body surface.

cardiopulmonary bypass. Venous blood is diverted to a heart-lung machine, which mechanically pumps and oxygenates the blood temporarily so the heart can be bypassed while an open procedure on the heart or coronary arteries is performed. During bypass, the lungs are deflated and immobile.

catheter. Flexible tube inserted into an area of the body for introducing or withdrawing fluid.

congenital. Present at birth, occurring through heredity or an influence during gestation up to the moment of birth.

excision. Surgical removal of an organ or tissue.

graft. Tissue implant from another part of the body or another person.

hypoplasia. Condition in which there is underdevelopment of an organ or tissue.

stenosis. Narrowing or constriction of a passage.

33858-33859

- **33858** Ascending aorta graft, with cardiopulmonary bypass, includes valve suspension, when performed; for aortic dissection
- **33859** for aortic disease other than dissection (eg, aneurysm)

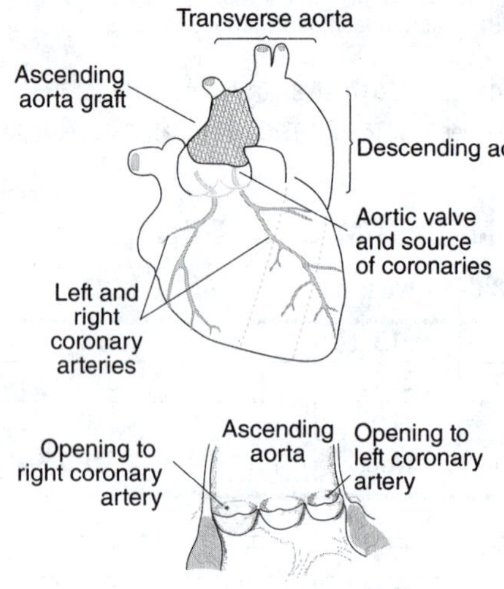

Aortic valve may be suspended with ascending aortic graft

Explanation

In 33858, the surgeon places an ascending aortic graft for aortic dissection and in 33859, for aortic disease other than dissection, such as aneurysm. Following induction of general anesthesia, a median sternotomy is performed. The physician places appropriate arterial and venous cannulation and initiates cardiopulmonary bypass. Following cross-clamp of the distal ascending aorta at the base of the innominate artery, the physician opens the proximal ascending aorta. The affected section of the ascending aorta is removed, the inside and outside of the aortic wall is lined with strips of felt for reinforcement, and a piece of synthetic graft material such as Dacron or PTFE is put in place of the missing piece of the aorta. The patient's aortic valve is preserved, although valve suspension may be performed. The physician closes the sternal incision and dresses the wound. If the patient's ascending aortic disease process includes the aortic arch and requires an aortic hemiarch graft, it is reported separately.

Coding Tips

Thoracic aortic aneurysm repair codes are dependent on aneurysm site: ascending, transverse arch, descending, or thoracoabdominal. Do not report an ascending aortic repair with a beveled anastomosis into the arch with a cross-clamp as a hemiarch graft using 33866. For a transverse arch graft, see 33871. For a descending thoracic aorta graft, see 33875. For repair of a thoracoabdominal aneurysm, see 33877. For direct repair of an aneurysm, a false aneurysm, or excision (partial or total) and graft insertion, with or without patch graft, of the abdominal aorta, see 35081 and 35091; for ruptured aneurysm, abdominal aorta, see 35082.

ICD-10-CM Diagnostic Codes

A52.01	Syphilitic aneurysm of aorta
I71.01	Dissection of thoracic aorta
I71.03	Dissection of thoracoabdominal aorta
I71.1	Thoracic aortic aneurysm, ruptured
I71.2	Thoracic aortic aneurysm, without rupture
I71.5	Thoracoabdominal aortic aneurysm, ruptured

I71.6 Thoracoabdominal aortic aneurysm, without rupture
I79.0 Aneurysm of aorta in diseases classified elsewhere
Q25.43 Congenital aneurysm of aorta

Relative Value Units/Medicare Edits

Non-Facility RVU	Work	PE	MP	Total
33858				
33859				
Facility RVU	**Work**	**PE**	**MP**	**Total**
33858				
33859				

	FUD	Status	MUE	Modifiers				IOM Reference
33858	N/A		-	N/A	N/A	N/A	N/A	None
33859	N/A		-	N/A	N/A	N/A	N/A	

* with documentation

33863-33866

33863 Ascending aorta graft, with cardiopulmonary bypass, with aortic root replacement using valved conduit and coronary reconstruction (eg, Bentall)

33864 Ascending aorta graft, with cardiopulmonary bypass with valve suspension, with coronary reconstruction and valve-sparing aortic root remodeling (eg, David Procedure, Yacoub Procedure)

\+ **33866** Aortic hemiarch graft including isolation and control of the arch vessels, beveled open distal aortic anastomosis extending under one or more of the arch vessels, and total circulatory arrest or isolated cerebral perfusion (List separately in addition to code for primary procedure)

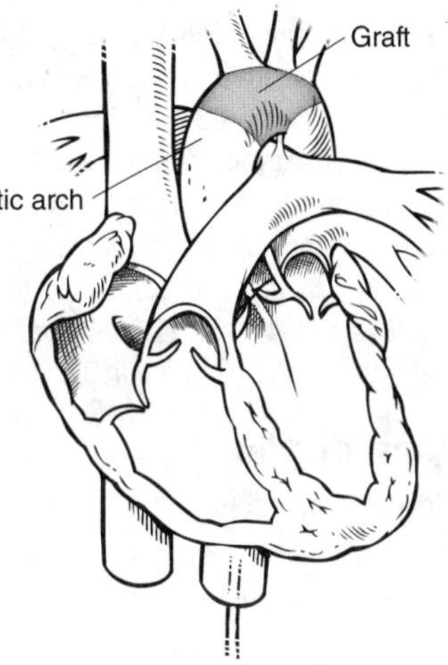

Graft of the aortic hemiarch isolates the arch vessels

Explanation

In 33863, the surgeon places an ascending aortic graft. The aorta is the largest artery in the body, extending from the heart through the chest and down into the abdomen. Cardiopulmonary bypass is required. Deep cooling of the body and circulatory arrest are often required, especially if the transverse arch of the aorta must be replaced. After circulatory arrest or if a cross-clamp can be placed on the aorta before its first branch, the aneurysm (an abnormally widened or weakened section of an artery) is opened. The hole in the aneurysm is lengthened along the aorta until the end of the aneurysm is reached. The aorta is divided at this point. A double layer of felt strips is placed circumferentially around the inner and outer circumference of the normal aorta with the aortic wall sandwiched in between. A Dacron tube graft is sewn to this end of the aorta and its felt layers. The aortic root is also replaced using a valved conduit and coronary reconstruction (e.g., Bentall procedure). In 33864, following induction of general anesthesia, the surgeon accesses the operative field via median sternotomy. Cardiopulmonary bypass is initiated. The coronary ostia are identified, detached from the aorta using dissecting scissors, and mobilized. After exposing the aneurysm site and clamping the artery above and below the aneurysm, the physician makes an incision into the aneurysm and removes any plaque deposits or clotted blood. The arterial section that is affected by the aneurysm is replaced with a synthetic graft. One end of the graft is attached to the arterial wall just above the beginning point of the aneurysm, while the other continues down through the artery to a point below the end of the aneurysm. The proximal coronary arteries are implanted into the aortic vascular graft. The physician performs a valve-sparing aortic root remodeling in which the dilated aortic root is replaced with a Dacron tube (graft) and the native aortic valve is integrated within the graft. The patient is taken off cardiopulmonary bypass and incisions are repaired. This procedure may be referred to as a David or Yacoub procedure in the operative note. When the patient's ascending aortic disease process includes the aortic arch requiring an aortic hemiarch graft, 33866 may be reported in addition to one of the procedures described above. This code describes three distinct elements: complete circulatory arrest or isolated cerebral retro- or antegrade perfusion, transverse arch incision performed under a single or multiple arch vessel(s) such as the left common carotid or innominate, and extending the ascending aortic graft beneath the aortic arch using a slanted or sloped (beveled) anastomosis. All three elements must be performed in order to use this code.

Coding Tips

Thoracic aortic aneurysm repair codes are dependent on aneurysm site: ascending, transverse arch, descending, or thoracoabdominal. Do not report an ascending aortic repair with a beveled anastomosis into the arch with a cross-clamp as a hemiarch graft using 33866. Report 33866 for aortic hemiarch graft when performed with ascending aortic graft codes 33858, 33859, 33863, or 33864. For a transverse arch graft, see 33871. For a descending thoracic aorta graft, see 33875. For repair of a thoracoabdominal aneurysm, see 33877. For direct repair of an aneurysm, a false aneurysm, or excision (partial or total) and graft insertion, with or without patch graft, of the abdominal aorta, see 35081 and 35091; for ruptured aneurysm, abdominal aorta, see 35082. Do not report 33863 with 33405, 33406, 33410–33413, 33858, or 33859. Do not report 33864 with 33858, 33859, or 33863. Do not report 33866 with 33871.

ICD-10-CM Diagnostic Codes

A52.01	Syphilitic aneurysm of aorta
A52.02	Syphilitic aortitis
I06.0	Rheumatic aortic stenosis
I06.1	Rheumatic aortic insufficiency
I06.2	Rheumatic aortic stenosis with insufficiency
I06.8	Other rheumatic aortic valve diseases
I08.0	Rheumatic disorders of both mitral and aortic valves
I08.2	Rheumatic disorders of both aortic and tricuspid valves
I08.3	Combined rheumatic disorders of mitral, aortic and tricuspid valves
I08.8	Other rheumatic multiple valve diseases
I35.0	Nonrheumatic aortic (valve) stenosis
I35.1	Nonrheumatic aortic (valve) insufficiency
I35.2	Nonrheumatic aortic (valve) stenosis with insufficiency
I35.8	Other nonrheumatic aortic valve disorders
I71.01	Dissection of thoracic aorta
I71.1	Thoracic aortic aneurysm, ruptured
I71.2	Thoracic aortic aneurysm, without rupture
I79.0	Aneurysm of aorta in diseases classified elsewhere
Q23.0	Congenital stenosis of aortic valve
Q23.1	Congenital insufficiency of aortic valve
Q23.8	Other congenital malformations of aortic and mitral valves
Q25.1	Coarctation of aorta
Q25.3	Supravalvular aortic stenosis
Q25.41	Absence and aplasia of aorta
Q25.42	Hypoplasia of aorta
Q25.43	Congenital aneurysm of aorta
Q25.44	Congenital dilation of aorta
Q25.45	Double aortic arch
Q25.46	Tortuous aortic arch
Q25.47	Right aortic arch
Q25.48	Anomalous origin of subclavian artery
Q25.49	Other congenital malformations of aorta
Q25.8	Other congenital malformations of other great arteries
Q87.410	Marfan's syndrome with aortic dilation

AMA: 33863 2018,Jan,8; 2017,Jan,8; 2017,Dec,3; 2016,Jan,13; 2015,Jan,16; 2014,Jan,11 **33864** 2018,Jan,8; 2017,Jan,8; 2017,Dec,3; 2016,Jan,13; 2015,Jan,16; 2014,Jan,11

Relative Value Units/Medicare Edits

Non-Facility RVU	Work	PE	MP	Total
33863	58.79	19.13	13.46	91.38
33864	60.08	19.69	13.84	93.61
33866	19.74	6.05	4.06	29.85
Facility RVU	**Work**	**PE**	**MP**	**Total**
33863	58.79	19.13	13.46	91.38
33864	60.08	19.69	13.84	93.61
33866	19.74	6.05	4.06	29.85

	FUD	Status	MUE	Modifiers				IOM Reference
33863	90	A	1(2)	51	N/A	62*	80	None
33864	90	A	1(2)	51	N/A	62*	80	
33866	N/A	A	1(2)	N/A	N/A	N/A	80*	

* with documentation

Heart and Pericardium

33871

● **33871** Transverse aortic arch graft, with cardiopulmonary bypass, with profound hypothermia, total circulatory arrest and isolated cerebral perfusion with reimplantation of arch vessel(s) (eg, island pedicle or individual arch vessel reimplantation)

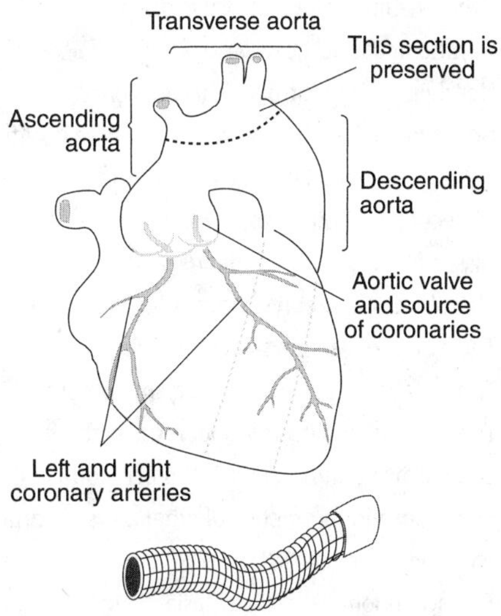

An aortic graft is placed and the transverse section containing the great arteries is sutured to it

Explanation

The physician performs a transverse aortic arch graft in which the entire aortic arch is replaced. This operation requires cardiopulmonary bypass, profound hypothermia, total circulatory arrest, and isolated cerebral perfusion. The patient's body temperature is lowered to 18 to 21 degrees centigrade and the bypass pump is stopped. The aneurysm is opened along its length and a patch of aortic wall containing the openings of the arteries to the head and arms is cut out. Each of these vessels will have been surrounded by tourniquets that were tightened before the bypass pump was stopped. The hole in the aneurysm is lengthened along the aorta until the end of the aneurysm is reached. The aorta is divided at this point. A double layer of felt strips is placed circumferentially around the inner and outer circumference of the normal aorta with the aortic wall sandwiched between. A Dacron tube graft is sewn to this end of the aorta and its felt layers. The aortic root where the aorta emerges from the heart is assessed. This area is where the aortic valve is located. If the valve closes normally, the aortic root size is reduced using stitches that also sew a double layer of felt to the aorta as previously described. Arch vessels are reimplanted individually or using an island pedicle. The physician closes the sternal incision and dresses the wound.

Coding Tips

Thoracic aortic aneurysm repair codes are dependent on aneurysm site: ascending, transverse arch, descending, or thoracoabdominal. For ascending aorta graft, see 33858, 33859, 33863, or 33864. For aortic hemiarch graft performed with ascending aortic graft, see 33866. For descending thoracic aorta graft, see 33875. For repair of a thoracoabdominal aneurysm, see 33877. For direct repair of an aneurysm, false aneurysm, or excision (partial or total) and graft insertion, with or without patch graft, of the abdominal aorta, see 35081–35103. Do not report 33871 with 33866.

ICD-10-CM Diagnostic Codes

A52.01	Syphilitic aneurysm of aorta
I71.01	Dissection of thoracic aorta
I71.03	Dissection of thoracoabdominal aorta
I71.1	Thoracic aortic aneurysm, ruptured
I71.2	Thoracic aortic aneurysm, without rupture
I71.5	Thoracoabdominal aortic aneurysm, ruptured
I71.6	Thoracoabdominal aortic aneurysm, without rupture
I79.0	Aneurysm of aorta in diseases classified elsewhere
Q25.43	Congenital aneurysm of aorta

Relative Value Units/Medicare Edits

Non-Facility RVU	Work	PE	MP	Total
33871				

Facility RVU	Work	PE	MP	Total
33871				

	FUD	Status	MUE	Modifiers				IOM Reference
33871	N/A		-	N/A	N/A	N/A	N/A	None

* with documentation

33875-33877

33875 Descending thoracic aorta graft, with or without bypass
33877 Repair of thoracoabdominal aortic aneurysm with graft, with or without cardiopulmonary bypass

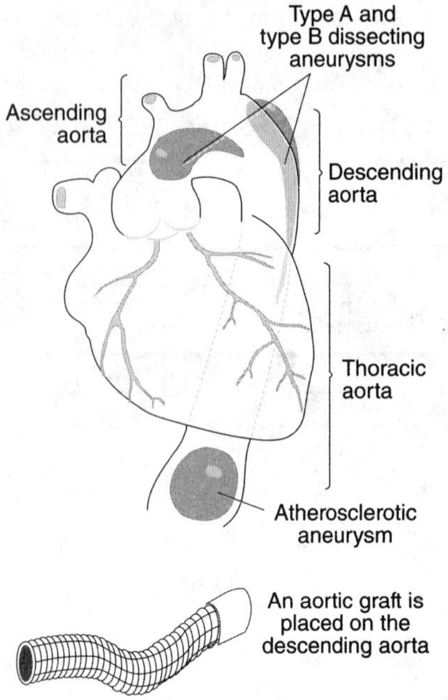

Explanation

A segment of the intrathoracic descending aorta is replaced with a tube of Dacron. This is done through an incision in the left chest cavity. The great concern in performing this operation is possible damage to the spinal cord. Preserving the spinal cord can be accomplished using a cardiopulmonary bypass circuit from above the aneurysm to below it, using deep cooling of the body and stopping the bypass machine, using perfusion of one or more spinal artery branches with blood pumped through it or using the "clamp and go" method in which no effort, except a speedy operation, is used to preserve the spinal cord. No matter what spinal cord preservation method is chosen, clamps are placed across the aorta above and below the aneurysm. The aneurysm is cut out and the ends of any small branches are closed with sutures. One end of a Dacron tube graft is sewn to the end of the aorta above the aneurysm and the other end of the graft is sewn to the aorta below the aneurysm. The clamps on the aorta are released. Report 33877 if aorta is exposed through the left chest.

Coding Tips

Thoracic aortic aneurysm repair codes are dependent on aneurysm site: ascending, transverse arch, descending, or thoracoabdominal. For ascending aorta graft, see 33858–33864. For transverse arch graft, see 33871. For direct repair of aneurysm, false aneurysm, or excision (partial or total) and graft insertion, with or without patch graft, of the abdominal aorta, see 35081–35103. Aneurysms of the thoracic aorta can also be performed endoscopically. For endoscopic repair of the descending thoracic aorta, see 33880–33891. For endoscopic repair of abdominal aortic aneurysm, see 34701–34848.

ICD-10-CM Diagnostic Codes

A52.01	Syphilitic aneurysm of aorta
A52.02	Syphilitic aortitis
I06.0	Rheumatic aortic stenosis
I06.1	Rheumatic aortic insufficiency
I06.2	Rheumatic aortic stenosis with insufficiency
I08.0	Rheumatic disorders of both mitral and aortic valves
I08.2	Rheumatic disorders of both aortic and tricuspid valves
I08.3	Combined rheumatic disorders of mitral, aortic and tricuspid valves
I08.8	Other rheumatic multiple valve diseases
I35.0	Nonrheumatic aortic (valve) stenosis
I35.1	Nonrheumatic aortic (valve) insufficiency
I35.2	Nonrheumatic aortic (valve) stenosis with insufficiency
I35.8	Other nonrheumatic aortic valve disorders
I71.01	Dissection of thoracic aorta
I71.03	Dissection of thoracoabdominal aorta
I71.1	Thoracic aortic aneurysm, ruptured
I71.2	Thoracic aortic aneurysm, without rupture
I71.5	Thoracoabdominal aortic aneurysm, ruptured
I71.6	Thoracoabdominal aortic aneurysm, without rupture
I74.11	Embolism and thrombosis of thoracic aorta
I74.19	Embolism and thrombosis of other parts of aorta
I77.810	Thoracic aortic ectasia
I77.812	Thoracoabdominal aortic ectasia
I77.89	Other specified disorders of arteries and arterioles
I79.0	Aneurysm of aorta in diseases classified elsewhere
Q23.0	Congenital stenosis of aortic valve
Q23.1	Congenital insufficiency of aortic valve
Q23.8	Other congenital malformations of aortic and mitral valves
Q25.1	Coarctation of aorta
Q25.3	Supravalvular aortic stenosis
Q25.41	Absence and aplasia of aorta
Q25.42	Hypoplasia of aorta
Q25.43	Congenital aneurysm of aorta
Q25.44	Congenital dilation of aorta
Q25.45	Double aortic arch
Q25.46	Tortuous aortic arch
Q25.47	Right aortic arch
Q25.48	Anomalous origin of subclavian artery
Q25.49	Other congenital malformations of aorta
Q25.8	Other congenital malformations of other great arteries
Q87.410	Marfan's syndrome with aortic dilation
Q87.418	Marfan's syndrome with other cardiovascular manifestations
S25.01XA	Minor laceration of thoracic aorta, initial encounter
S25.02XA	Major laceration of thoracic aorta, initial encounter
S25.09XA	Other specified injury of thoracic aorta, initial encounter
S26.01XA	Contusion of heart with hemopericardium, initial encounter
S26.020A	Mild laceration of heart with hemopericardium, initial encounter
S26.021A	Moderate laceration of heart with hemopericardium, initial encounter
S26.022A	Major laceration of heart with hemopericardium, initial encounter
S26.09XA	Other injury of heart with hemopericardium, initial encounter
S26.11XA	Contusion of heart without hemopericardium, initial encounter
S26.12XA	Laceration of heart without hemopericardium, initial encounter
S26.19XA	Other injury of heart without hemopericardium, initial encounter

Heart and Pericardium

AMA: **33875** 2017,Dec,3 **33877** 2017,Dec,3

Relative Value Units/Medicare Edits

Non-Facility RVU	Work	PE	MP	Total
33875	50.72	17.09	11.91	79.72
33877	69.03	19.78	16.34	105.15
Facility RVU	**Work**	**PE**	**MP**	**Total**
33875	50.72	17.09	11.91	79.72
33877	69.03	19.78	16.34	105.15

	FUD	Status	MUE	Modifiers				IOM Reference
33875	90	A	1(2)	51	N/A	62	80	None
33877	90	A	1(2)	51	N/A	62	80	

* with documentation

Terms To Know

aneurysm. Circumscribed dilation or outpouching of an artery wall, often containing blood clots and connecting directly with the lumen of the artery.

cardiopulmonary bypass. Venous blood is diverted to a heart-lung machine, which mechanically pumps and oxygenates the blood temporarily so the heart can be bypassed while an open procedure on the heart or coronary arteries is performed. During bypass, the lungs are deflated and immobile.

33880-33881

cutdown

+34812

33880 Endovascular repair of descending thoracic aorta (eg, aneurysm, pseudoaneurysm, dissection, penetrating ulcer, intramural hematoma, or traumatic disruption); involving coverage of left subclavian artery origin, initial endoprosthesis plus descending thoracic aortic extension(s), if required, to level of celiac artery origin

33881 not involving coverage of left subclavian artery origin, initial endoprosthesis plus descending thoracic aortic extension(s), if required, to level of celiac artery origin

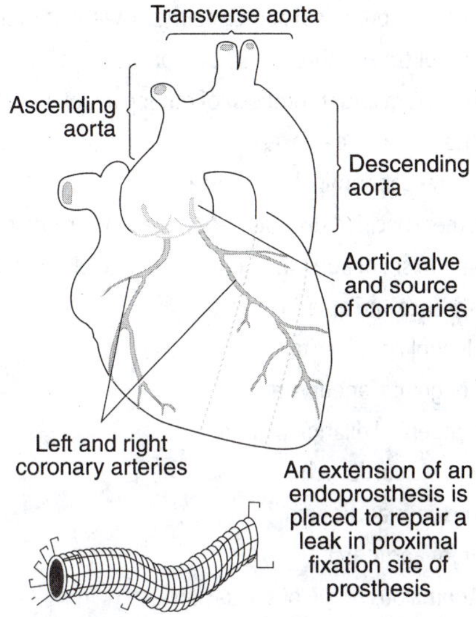

This procedure is performed by threading the prosthesis through the patient's vessels rather than through an open approach

Explanation

The physician repairs the descending thoracic aorta by placing an endoprosthesis from within the artery. Endovascular repair may be performed for an aneurysm, pseudoaneurysm, dissection, penetrating ulcer, intramural hematoma, or traumatic disruption. The defect in the descending thoracic aorta is identified using aortography. The endoprosthesis, contained inside a holding device, is introduced into the artery under fluoroscopy and positioned at the target zone area of repair. Extension prostheses may be required to the level of the celiac artery origin. When the endoprosthesis is in position, it is deployed within the artery at the target site in the descending thoracic aorta, covering the origin of the left subclavian artery in 33880. A balloon angioplasty may be necessary to achieve proper positioning and functioning of the endoprosthesis. The placement position is confirmed, the catheter is removed, and the arteriotomy site is closed. Report 33880 when the repair covers the left subclavian artery origin and 33881 when the repair does not cover the left subclavian artery origin.

Coding Tips

These codes include all device introduction, manipulation, positioning, and deployment. Balloon angioplasty and/or stent deployment is not reported separately. Open arterial exposure, introduction of guidewires and catheters, and extensive repair or replacement of an artery should be reported separately. Report transposition of subclavian to carotid (33889) and carotid-carotid bypass (33891) separately. These codes include distal extensions in the distal thoracic aorta, but proximal extensions (33883–33884) are reported separately. For radiological supervision and interpretation, see 75956–75957.

ICD-10-CM Diagnostic Codes

A52.01	Syphilitic aneurysm of aorta
A52.02	Syphilitic aortitis
I71.01	Dissection of thoracic aorta
I71.03	Dissection of thoracoabdominal aorta
I71.1	Thoracic aortic aneurysm, ruptured
I71.2	Thoracic aortic aneurysm, without rupture
I71.3	Abdominal aortic aneurysm, ruptured
I71.4	Abdominal aortic aneurysm, without rupture
I71.5	Thoracoabdominal aortic aneurysm, ruptured
I71.6	Thoracoabdominal aortic aneurysm, without rupture
I74.11	Embolism and thrombosis of thoracic aorta
I74.19	Embolism and thrombosis of other parts of aorta
I77.810	Thoracic aortic ectasia
I77.812	Thoracoabdominal aortic ectasia
I77.89	Other specified disorders of arteries and arterioles
I79.0	Aneurysm of aorta in diseases classified elsewhere
Q25.41	Absence and aplasia of aorta
Q25.42	Hypoplasia of aorta
Q25.43	Congenital aneurysm of aorta
Q25.44	Congenital dilation of aorta
Q25.45	Double aortic arch
Q25.46	Tortuous aortic arch
Q25.47	Right aortic arch
Q25.48	Anomalous origin of subclavian artery
Q25.49	Other congenital malformations of aorta
Q25.8	Other congenital malformations of other great arteries
S25.01XA	Minor laceration of thoracic aorta, initial encounter
S25.02XA	Major laceration of thoracic aorta, initial encounter
S25.09XA	Other specified injury of thoracic aorta, initial encounter
S25.112A	Minor laceration of left innominate or subclavian artery, initial encounter ☑
S25.122A	Major laceration of left innominate or subclavian artery, initial encounter ☑
S25.192A	Other specified injury of left innominate or subclavian artery, initial encounter ☑
S26.01XA	Contusion of heart with hemopericardium, initial encounter
S26.020A	Mild laceration of heart with hemopericardium, initial encounter
S26.021A	Moderate laceration of heart with hemopericardium, initial encounter
S26.022A	Major laceration of heart with hemopericardium, initial encounter
S26.09XA	Other injury of heart with hemopericardium, initial encounter
S26.11XA	Contusion of heart without hemopericardium, initial encounter
S26.12XA	Laceration of heart without hemopericardium, initial encounter
S26.19XA	Other injury of heart without hemopericardium, initial encounter
S35.211A	Minor laceration of celiac artery, initial encounter
S35.212A	Major laceration of celiac artery, initial encounter
S35.218A	Other injury of celiac artery, initial encounter

AMA: 33880 2018,Jan,8; 2017,Jan,8; 2017,Dec,3; 2016,Jan,13; 2015,Jan,16; 2014,Jan,11 **33881** 2018,Jan,8; 2017,Jan,8; 2017,Dec,3; 2016,Jan,13; 2015,Jan,16; 2014,Jan,11

Relative Value Units/Medicare Edits

Non-Facility RVU	Work	PE	MP	Total
33880	34.58	9.65	7.78	52.01
33881	29.58	8.39	6.67	44.64
Facility RVU	**Work**	**PE**	**MP**	**Total**
33880	34.58	9.65	7.78	52.01
33881	29.58	8.39	6.67	44.64

	FUD	Status	MUE	Modifiers				IOM Reference
33880	90	A	1(2)	51	N/A	62	80	None
33881	90	A	1(2)	51	N/A	62	80	

* with documentation

Terms To Know

aneurysm. Circumscribed dilation or outpouching of an artery wall, often containing blood clots and connecting directly with the lumen of the artery.

angioplasty. Reconstruction or repair of a diseased or damaged blood vessel.

angioplasty balloon. Balloon-tipped medical device used to clear the blockage of an artery. After insertion into the clogged artery, the balloon is inflated to expand a narrowing arterial section.

balloon catheter. Any catheter equipped with an inflatable balloon at the end to hold it in place in a body cavity or to be used for dilation of a vessel lumen.

embolism. Obstruction of a blood vessel resulting from a clot or foreign substance.

thrombosis. Condition arising from the presence or formation of blood clots within a blood vessel that may cause vascular obstruction and insufficient oxygenation.

33883-33884

33883 Placement of proximal extension prosthesis for endovascular repair of descending thoracic aorta (eg, aneurysm, pseudoaneurysm, dissection, penetrating ulcer, intramural hematoma, or traumatic disruption); initial extension

+ 33884 each additional proximal extension (List separately in addition to code for primary procedure)

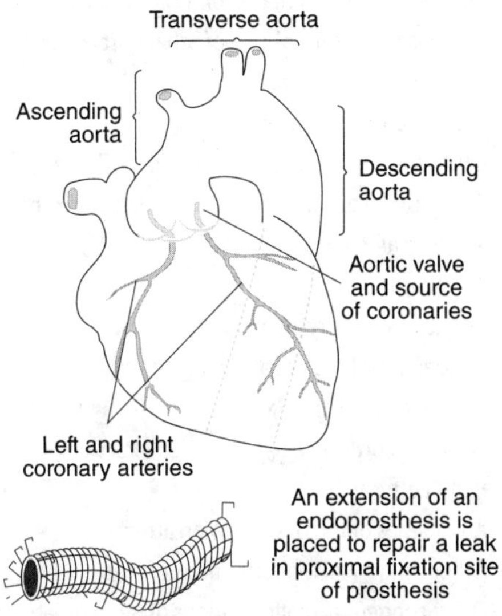

This procedure is performed by threading the prosthesis through the patient's vessels rather than through an open approach

Explanation

A leak, called an endoleak, may occur at the proximal fixation sites of a grafted descending thoracic aorta defect through the body of the graft or from patent arteries within the defect and may require endovascular repair. A proximal extension prosthesis is placed endovascularly to repair an endoleak in a grafted descending thoracic aortic aneurysm, pseudoaneurysm, dissection, penetrating ulcer, intramural hematoma, or traumatic disruption. The target site is identified by aortography and the proper extension prosthesis is selected. Under fluoroscopy, the extension prosthesis, contained inside a long plastic holding capsule, is threaded through the arteries to the site of the leak. Once the extension prosthesis is in place, the holding capsule is removed. The extension prosthesis, activated by heat, expands like a spring and becomes anchored to the artery wall at the site of the endoleak. If full expansion of the prosthesis does not occur automatically, a balloon catheter is threaded to the graft site and inflated within the endovascular prosthesis until full expansion is achieved. The placement position is confirmed, the catheter is removed, and the arteriotomy site is closed. Report 33883 for an initial proximal extension and 33884 for each additional proximal extension.

Coding Tips

Report 33884 in addition to 33883. These codes include all device introduction, manipulation, positioning, and deployment. Balloon angioplasty and/or stent deployment is not reported separately. Open arterial exposure, introduction of guidewires and catheters, and extensive repair or replacement of an artery should be reported separately. For radiological supervision and interpretation, see 75958.

ICD-10-CM Diagnostic Codes

A52.01	Syphilitic aneurysm of aorta
A52.02	Syphilitic aortitis
I71.01	Dissection of thoracic aorta
I71.03	Dissection of thoracoabdominal aorta
I71.1	Thoracic aortic aneurysm, ruptured
I71.2	Thoracic aortic aneurysm, without rupture
I71.3	Abdominal aortic aneurysm, ruptured
I71.4	Abdominal aortic aneurysm, without rupture
I71.5	Thoracoabdominal aortic aneurysm, ruptured
I71.6	Thoracoabdominal aortic aneurysm, without rupture
I74.11	Embolism and thrombosis of thoracic aorta
I74.19	Embolism and thrombosis of other parts of aorta
I77.810	Thoracic aortic ectasia
I77.812	Thoracoabdominal aortic ectasia
I77.89	Other specified disorders of arteries and arterioles
I79.0	Aneurysm of aorta in diseases classified elsewhere
Q25.41	Absence and aplasia of aorta
Q25.42	Hypoplasia of aorta
Q25.43	Congenital aneurysm of aorta
Q25.44	Congenital dilation of aorta
Q25.45	Double aortic arch
Q25.46	Tortuous aortic arch
Q25.47	Right aortic arch
Q25.48	Anomalous origin of subclavian artery
Q25.49	Other congenital malformations of aorta
Q25.8	Other congenital malformations of other great arteries
S25.01XA	Minor laceration of thoracic aorta, initial encounter
S25.02XA	Major laceration of thoracic aorta, initial encounter
S25.09XA	Other specified injury of thoracic aorta, initial encounter
S26.01XA	Contusion of heart with hemopericardium, initial encounter
S26.020A	Mild laceration of heart with hemopericardium, initial encounter
S26.021A	Moderate laceration of heart with hemopericardium, initial encounter
S26.022A	Major laceration of heart with hemopericardium, initial encounter
S26.09XA	Other injury of heart with hemopericardium, initial encounter
S26.11XA	Contusion of heart without hemopericardium, initial encounter
S26.12XA	Laceration of heart without hemopericardium, initial encounter
S26.19XA	Other injury of heart without hemopericardium, initial encounter

AMA: **33883** 2018,Jan,8; 2017,Jan,8; 2017,Dec,3; 2016,Jan,13; 2015,Jan,16; 2014,Jan,11 **33884** 2018,Jan,8; 2017,Jan,8; 2017,Dec,3; 2016,Jan,13; 2015,Jan,16; 2014,Jan,11

Relative Value Units/Medicare Edits

Non-Facility RVU	Work	PE	MP	Total
33883	21.09	6.57	4.66	32.32
33884	8.2	1.34	1.89	11.43
Facility RVU	**Work**	**PE**	**MP**	**Total**
33883	21.09	6.57	4.66	32.32
33884	8.2	1.34	1.89	11.43

	FUD	Status	MUE	Modifiers				IOM Reference
33883	90	A	1(2)	51	N/A	62	80	None
33884	N/A	A	2(3)	N/A	N/A	62	80	

* with documentation

33886

33886 Placement of distal extension prosthesis(s) delayed after endovascular repair of descending thoracic aorta

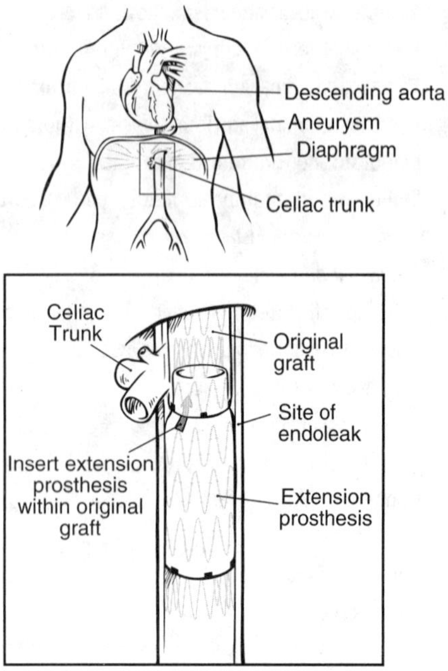

Repair of endoleak in descending thoracic aorta

Explanation

A leak, called an endoleak, may occur at the distal fixation sites of a previously grafted descending thoracic aorta defect through the body of the graft or from patent arteries within the defect and may require endovascular repair. One or more distal extension prosthesis modules are placed endovascularly to the level of the celiac artery to repair an endoleak in a previously grafted descending thoracic aortic aneurysm, pseudoaneurysm, dissection, penetrating ulcer, intramural hematoma, or traumatic disruption. The target site is identified by aortography and the proper extension prosthesis is selected. Under fluoroscopy, the extension prosthesis, contained inside a long plastic holding capsule, is threaded through the arteries to the site of the leak. Once the extension prosthesis is in place, the holding capsule is removed. The extension prosthesis, activated by heat, expands like a spring and becomes anchored to the artery wall at the site of the endoleak. If full expansion of the prosthesis does not occur automatically, a balloon catheter is threaded to the graft site and inflated within the endovascular prosthesis until full expansion is achieved. The placement position is confirmed, the catheter is removed, and the arteriotomy site is closed. This code is reported only once regardless of the number of extension modules deployed.

Coding Tips

This code includes all device introduction, manipulation, positioning, and deployment. Balloon angioplasty and/or stent deployment is not reported separately. Do not report 33886 with 33880 or 33881. Report 33886 once, regardless of the number of modules deployed. Open arterial exposure, introduction of guidewires and catheters, and extensive repair or replacement of an artery should be reported separately. For radiological supervision and interpretation, see 75959.

ICD-10-CM Diagnostic Codes

A52.01	Syphilitic aneurysm of aorta
A52.02	Syphilitic aortitis
I71.01	Dissection of thoracic aorta
I71.03	Dissection of thoracoabdominal aorta
I71.1	Thoracic aortic aneurysm, ruptured
I71.2	Thoracic aortic aneurysm, without rupture
I71.3	Abdominal aortic aneurysm, ruptured
I71.4	Abdominal aortic aneurysm, without rupture
I71.5	Thoracoabdominal aortic aneurysm, ruptured
I71.6	Thoracoabdominal aortic aneurysm, without rupture
I74.11	Embolism and thrombosis of thoracic aorta
I74.19	Embolism and thrombosis of other parts of aorta
I77.810	Thoracic aortic ectasia
I77.812	Thoracoabdominal aortic ectasia
I77.89	Other specified disorders of arteries and arterioles
I79.0	Aneurysm of aorta in diseases classified elsewhere
Q25.41	Absence and aplasia of aorta
Q25.42	Hypoplasia of aorta
Q25.43	Congenital aneurysm of aorta
Q25.44	Congenital dilation of aorta
Q25.45	Double aortic arch
Q25.46	Tortuous aortic arch
Q25.47	Right aortic arch
Q25.48	Anomalous origin of subclavian artery
Q25.49	Other congenital malformations of aorta
Q25.8	Other congenital malformations of other great arteries
S25.01XA	Minor laceration of thoracic aorta, initial encounter
S25.02XA	Major laceration of thoracic aorta, initial encounter
S25.09XA	Other specified injury of thoracic aorta, initial encounter
S26.01XA	Contusion of heart with hemopericardium, initial encounter
S26.020A	Mild laceration of heart with hemopericardium, initial encounter
S26.021A	Moderate laceration of heart with hemopericardium, initial encounter
S26.022A	Major laceration of heart with hemopericardium, initial encounter
S26.09XA	Other injury of heart with hemopericardium, initial encounter
S26.11XA	Contusion of heart without hemopericardium, initial encounter
S26.12XA	Laceration of heart without hemopericardium, initial encounter
S26.19XA	Other injury of heart without hemopericardium, initial encounter

AMA: 33886 2018,Jan,8; 2017,Jan,8; 2017,Dec,3; 2016,Jan,13; 2015,Jan,16; 2014,Jan,11

Relative Value Units/Medicare Edits

Non-Facility RVU	Work	PE	MP	Total
33886	18.09	5.62	3.99	27.7
Facility RVU	**Work**	**PE**	**MP**	**Total**
33886	18.09	5.62	3.99	27.7

	FUD	Status	MUE	Modifiers				IOM Reference
33886	90	A	1(2)	51	N/A	62	80	None

* with documentation

33889

33889 Open subclavian to carotid artery transposition performed in conjunction with endovascular repair of descending thoracic aorta, by neck incision, unilateral

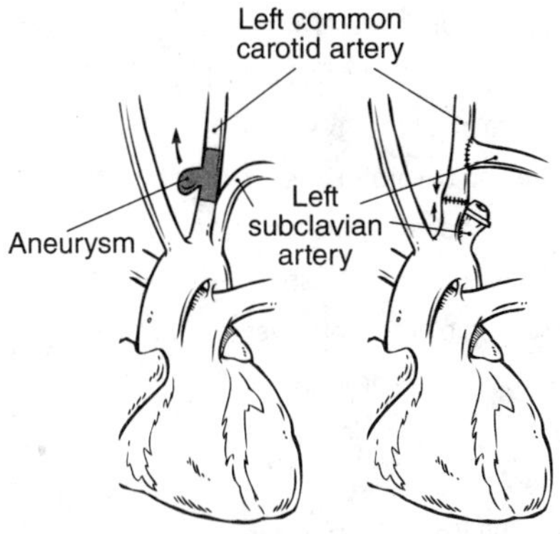

The left subclavian artery is anastomosed to the side of the left common carotid artery

Explanation

The physician performs a unilateral open subclavian to carotid artery transposition in conjunction with endovascular repair of the descending aorta. The physician performs a 2 to 3 cm supraclavicular incision to gain access to the carotid and subclavian arteries. The clavicular section of the sternocleidomastoid muscle is partially divided exposing the phrenic nerve, which is identified and avoided. The physician clears the adventitia of the chosen translocation site in the wall of the common carotid artery. The section of artery where the aneurysm occurs is isolated and dissected from adjacent structures. Vessel clamps are affixed above and below the defect. The repair is accomplished by excising the segment containing the aneurysm. The vessel ends are sutured in an end-to-end fashion. Next, the subclavian artery is transposed and anastomosed to the common carotid artery in an end-to-side fashion. Vessel clamps are removed and the incision is closed with layered sutures.

Coding Tips

Report 33889 in addition to 33880 or 33881 when an open subclavian-to-carotid artery transposition is performed during the same surgical session as the endovascular repair of the descending thoracic aorta. Do not report 33889 with 35694.

ICD-10-CM Diagnostic Codes

G45.1	Carotid artery syndrome (hemispheric)
I63.031	Cerebral infarction due to thrombosis of right carotid artery ☑
I63.131	Cerebral infarction due to embolism of right carotid artery ☑
I63.81	Other cerebral infarction due to occlusion or stenosis of small artery
I63.89	Other cerebral infarction
I65.21	Occlusion and stenosis of right carotid artery ☑
I70.0	Atherosclerosis of aorta
I70.8	Atherosclerosis of other arteries
I72.0	Aneurysm of carotid artery
I72.6	Aneurysm of vertebral artery
I77.1	Stricture of artery
I77.71	Dissection of carotid artery
I77.76	Dissection of artery of upper extremity
Q25.21	Interruption of aortic arch
Q25.3	Supravalvular aortic stenosis
Q25.41	Absence and aplasia of aorta
Q25.42	Hypoplasia of aorta
Q25.43	Congenital aneurysm of aorta
Q25.44	Congenital dilation of aorta
Q25.45	Double aortic arch
Q25.46	Tortuous aortic arch
Q25.47	Right aortic arch
Q25.48	Anomalous origin of subclavian artery
Q25.49	Other congenital malformations of aorta
Q25.8	Other congenital malformations of other great arteries
S15.011A	Minor laceration of right carotid artery, initial encounter ☑
S15.012A	Minor laceration of left carotid artery, initial encounter ☑
S15.021A	Major laceration of right carotid artery, initial encounter ☑
S15.022A	Major laceration of left carotid artery, initial encounter ☑
S15.091A	Other specified injury of right carotid artery, initial encounter ☑
S15.092A	Other specified injury of left carotid artery, initial encounter ☑
S25.111A	Minor laceration of right innominate or subclavian artery, initial encounter ☑
S25.112A	Minor laceration of left innominate or subclavian artery, initial encounter ☑
S25.121A	Major laceration of right innominate or subclavian artery, initial encounter ☑
S25.122A	Major laceration of left innominate or subclavian artery, initial encounter ☑
S25.191A	Other specified injury of right innominate or subclavian artery, initial encounter ☑
S25.192A	Other specified injury of left innominate or subclavian artery, initial encounter ☑

AMA: **33889** 2018,Jan,8; 2017,Jan,8; 2016,Jan,13; 2015,Jan,16; 2014,Jan,11

Relative Value Units/Medicare Edits

Non-Facility RVU	Work	PE	MP	Total
33889	15.92	3.31	3.62	22.85
Facility RVU	**Work**	**PE**	**MP**	**Total**
33889	15.92	3.31	3.62	22.85

	FUD	Status	MUE	Modifiers				IOM Reference
33889	0	A	1(2)	51	50	62	80	None

* with documentation

Terms To Know

aneurysm. Circumscribed dilation or outpouching of an artery wall, often containing blood clots and connecting directly with the lumen of the artery.

stenosis. Narrowing or constriction of a passage.

stricture. Narrowing of an anatomical structure.

33891

33891 Bypass graft, with other than vein, transcervical retropharyngeal carotid-carotid, performed in conjunction with endovascular repair of descending thoracic aorta, by neck incision

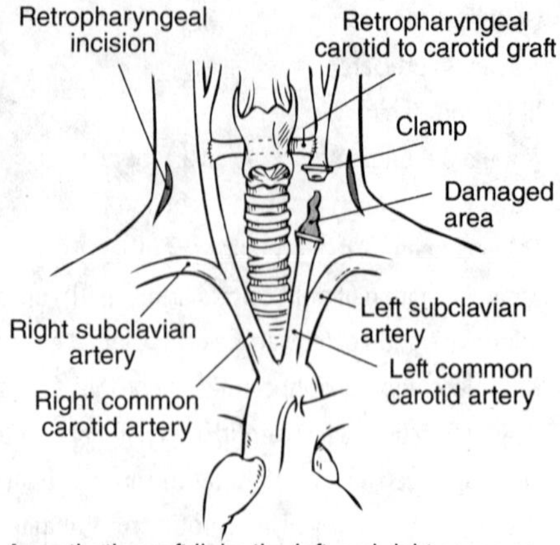

A synthetic graft links the left and right common carotid arteries as an adjunct to an endovascular repair of the descending thoracic aorta

Explanation

The physician performs a transcervical retropharyngeal carotid-to-carotid bypass graft with other than vein in conjunction with endovascular repair of the descending thoracic aorta. Through incisions in the neck, the physician isolates and dissects the common carotid arteries, separating them from adjacent critical structures. The physician creates a bypass around a section of carotid artery that is damaged or blocked using a synthetic vein graft and one of two methods of repair. After vessel clamps have been affixed above and below the damaged area, the ends of the synthetic vein graft are sutured into the side of the carotid arterial wall (end-to-side). In the second method, the carotid artery may be cut above the damaged area and sutured to one end of a synthetic vein graft, which is sutured to the side of the carotid artery on the opposite side of the neck (end-to-end). In either case, the blocked or damaged section of artery is not removed. When the clamps are removed, the synthetic vein graft forms a new path through which blood can easily bypass the blocked or damaged area. After the graft procedure is completed, the skin incisions are repaired with layered sutures.

Coding Tips

Report 33891 in addition to 33880 and 33881 when an open carotid-to-carotid artery bypass graft with other than vein is performed during the same surgical session as the endovascular repair of the descending thoracic aorta. Do not report 33891 with 35509 or 35601.

ICD-10-CM Diagnostic Codes

G45.1	Carotid artery syndrome (hemispheric)
G45.8	Other transient cerebral ischemic attacks and related syndromes
I63.031	Cerebral infarction due to thrombosis of right carotid artery ☑
I63.032	Cerebral infarction due to thrombosis of left carotid artery ☑
I63.131	Cerebral infarction due to embolism of right carotid artery ☑
I63.132	Cerebral infarction due to embolism of left carotid artery ☑
I63.19	Cerebral infarction due to embolism of other precerebral artery
I63.81	Other cerebral infarction due to occlusion or stenosis of small artery
I63.89	Other cerebral infarction
I65.21	Occlusion and stenosis of right carotid artery ☑
I65.22	Occlusion and stenosis of left carotid artery ☑
I65.23	Occlusion and stenosis of bilateral carotid arteries ☑
I70.0	Atherosclerosis of aorta
I70.8	Atherosclerosis of other arteries
I72.0	Aneurysm of carotid artery
I72.5	Aneurysm of other precerebral arteries
I72.6	Aneurysm of vertebral artery
I72.8	Aneurysm of other specified arteries
I77.1	Stricture of artery
I77.71	Dissection of carotid artery
I77.75	Dissection of other precerebral arteries
I77.76	Dissection of artery of upper extremity
I77.77	Dissection of artery of lower extremity
Q25.21	Interruption of aortic arch
Q25.41	Absence and aplasia of aorta
Q25.42	Hypoplasia of aorta
Q25.43	Congenital aneurysm of aorta
Q25.44	Congenital dilation of aorta
Q25.45	Double aortic arch
Q25.46	Tortuous aortic arch
Q25.47	Right aortic arch
Q25.48	Anomalous origin of subclavian artery
Q25.8	Other congenital malformations of other great arteries
S15.011A	Minor laceration of right carotid artery, initial encounter ☑
S15.012A	Minor laceration of left carotid artery, initial encounter ☑
S15.021A	Major laceration of right carotid artery, initial encounter ☑
S15.022A	Major laceration of left carotid artery, initial encounter ☑
S15.091A	Other specified injury of right carotid artery, initial encounter ☑
S15.092A	Other specified injury of left carotid artery, initial encounter ☑

AMA: 33891 2018,Jan,8; 2017,Jan,8; 2016,Jan,13; 2015,Jan,16; 2014,Jan,11

Relative Value Units/Medicare Edits

Non-Facility RVU	Work	PE	MP	Total
33891	20.0	3.28	4.62	27.9
Facility RVU	**Work**	**PE**	**MP**	**Total**
33891	20.0	3.28	4.62	27.9

	FUD	Status	MUE	Modifiers				IOM Reference
33891	0	A	1(2)	51	50	62	80	None

* with documentation

33910-33915

33910 Pulmonary artery embolectomy; with cardiopulmonary bypass
33915 without cardiopulmonary bypass

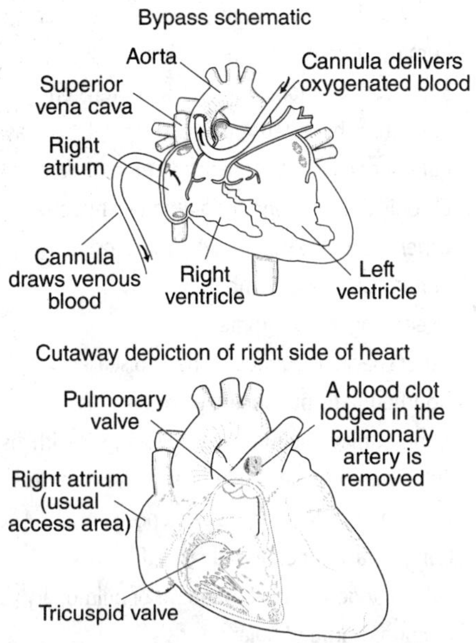

A blood clot (embolism) has broken free and traveled the venous route to the right side of the heart where it has lodged in the pulmonary artery

Explanation

This operation is only done for patients who are in extremis following a pulmonary artery embolism (i.e., a blood clot originating in one of the large veins in the leg breaks loose and travels into the heart via the caval vein where it obstructs blood flow to the lungs). Survival is low. If cardiopulmonary bypass is used, the physician opens the right atrium widely. If cardiopulmonary bypass is not used, the right atrium is opened through a hole in the middle of a purse string. The clot is "milked" out of the pulmonary artery into the right atrium and out the hole. Report 33910 if cardiopulmonary bypass is required and the right atrium is opened widely. Report 33910 if cardiopulmonary bypass is initiated. Report 33915 if cardiopulmonary bypass is not initiated.

Coding Tips

If significant additional time and effort are documented, append modifier 22 and submit a cover letter and operative report. When 33910 or 33915 is performed with another separately identifiable procedure, the highest dollar value code is listed as the primary procedure and subsequent procedures are appended with modifier 51. For embolectomy of other arteries, see 34001–34203.

ICD-10-CM Diagnostic Codes

I26.01	Septic pulmonary embolism with acute cor pulmonale
I26.02	Saddle embolus of pulmonary artery with acute cor pulmonale
I26.09	Other pulmonary embolism with acute cor pulmonale
I26.90	Septic pulmonary embolism without acute cor pulmonale
I26.92	Saddle embolus of pulmonary artery without acute cor pulmonale
I26.99	Other pulmonary embolism without acute cor pulmonale
I27.82	Chronic pulmonary embolism
I27.89	Other specified pulmonary heart diseases
T81.718A	Complication of other artery following a procedure, not elsewhere classified, initial encounter
T82.817A	Embolism due to cardiac prosthetic devices, implants and grafts, initial encounter
T82.818A	Embolism due to vascular prosthetic devices, implants and grafts, initial encounter

AMA: 33910 2018,Jan,8; 2017,Jan,8; 2017,Dec,3; 2016,Jan,13; 2015,Jan,16; 2014,Jan,11 **33915** 2018,Jan,8; 2017,Jan,8; 2016,Jan,13; 2015,Jan,16; 2014,Jan,11

Relative Value Units/Medicare Edits

Non-Facility RVU	Work	PE	MP	Total
33910	48.21	17.14	10.87	76.22
33915	24.95	9.35	5.87	40.17
Facility RVU	**Work**	**PE**	**MP**	**Total**
33910	48.21	17.14	10.87	76.22
33915	24.95	9.35	5.87	40.17

	FUD	Status	MUE	Modifiers				IOM Reference
33910	90	A	1(3)	51	N/A	62*	80	None
33915	90	A	1(3)	51	N/A	62*	80	

* with documentation

Terms To Know

cardiopulmonary bypass. Venous blood is diverted to a heart-lung machine, which mechanically pumps and oxygenates the blood temporarily so the heart can be bypassed while an open procedure on the heart or coronary arteries is performed. During bypass, the lungs are deflated and immobile.

embolectomy. Surgical excision of a blood clot or other foreign material that broke away from its original source and traveled in the blood stream, becoming lodged in a blood vessel and blocking circulation.

embolism. Obstruction of a blood vessel resulting from a clot or foreign substance.

iatrogenic. Adversely induced in the patient; caused by medical treatment.

incision. Act of cutting into tissue or an organ.

infarction. Area of necrosis in tissue, due to ischemia from lack of circulation, usually from a thrombus or an embolus.

33916-33917

33916 Pulmonary endarterectomy, with or without embolectomy, with cardiopulmonary bypass

33917 Repair of pulmonary artery stenosis by reconstruction with patch or graft

The inner tissues of the lumen are removed and the artery is repaired directly or with a patch

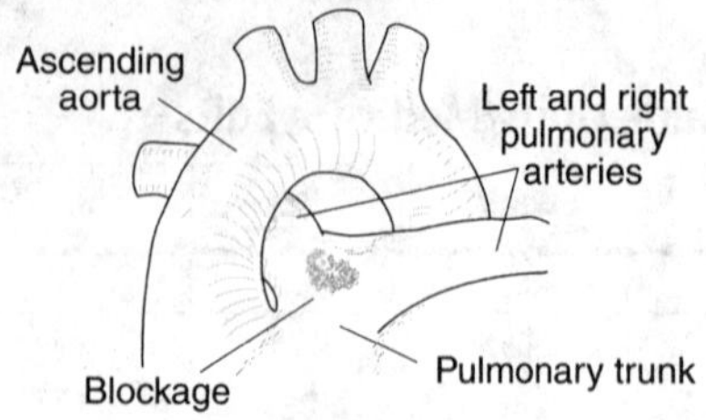

A stenotic (narrowed) pulmonary artery is repaired using a patch or graft

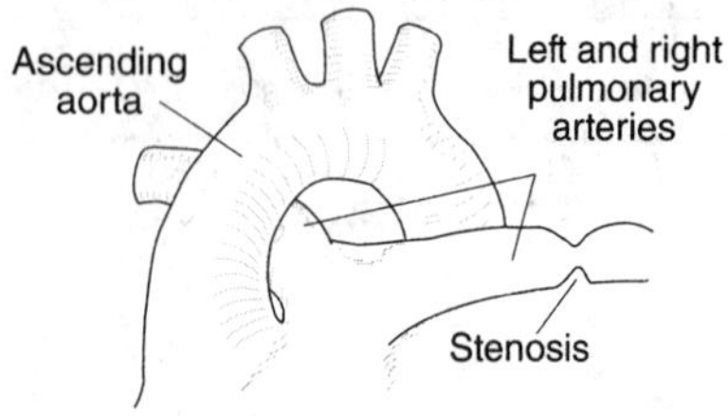

Repair of a blockage in the greater pulmonary arteries is accomplished by opening the artery along its length overlying the blockage. If an embolism is present it is removed

Explanation

In 33916, a pulmonary endarterectomy is performed to treat patients diagnosed with chronic thromboembolic pulmonary hypertension. Cardiopulmonary bypass and hypothermia is required in order to perform this procedure. Only the main and branch pulmonary arteries can be treated. Via a median sternotomy, the pulmonary arteries are opened along their lengths. If present, any thrombotic or embolic material is extracted. The inner layer of each artery is removed. Once the endarterectomies are complete, the arteries are closed with suture directly or with a patch of pericardium, saphenous vein or Dacron. Homeostasis is achieved and the chest is closed in layers using standard techniques. In 33917, the physician reconstructs the pulmonary artery to correct any outflow tract obstruction caused by stenosis. Cardiopulmonary bypass is required. Via a median sternotomy, the stenotic pulmonary artery is opened longitudinally until healthy artery is encountered. The diseased vessel is removed. A patch is trimmed to reconstruct the defect in the artery or grafting may be performed if the defect is too complex or large for a patch. After the patch or graft is placed, homeostasis is achieved and the chest is closed in layers using standard techniques.

Coding Tips

The insertion of grafts or implanted materials is considered part of this procedure and is not reported separately. If significant additional time and effort are documented, append modifier 22 and submit a cover letter and operative report. When 33916 or 33917 is performed with another separately identifiable procedure, the highest dollar value code is listed as the primary procedure and subsequent procedures are appended with modifier 51. For coronary endarterectomy, see 33572.

ICD-10-CM Diagnostic Codes

I26.01	Septic pulmonary embolism with acute cor pulmonale
I26.02	Saddle embolus of pulmonary artery with acute cor pulmonale
I26.09	Other pulmonary embolism with acute cor pulmonale
I26.90	Septic pulmonary embolism without acute cor pulmonale
I26.92	Saddle embolus of pulmonary artery without acute cor pulmonale
I26.99	Other pulmonary embolism without acute cor pulmonale
I27.0	Primary pulmonary hypertension
I27.21	Secondary pulmonary arterial hypertension
I27.22	Pulmonary hypertension due to left heart disease
I27.23	Pulmonary hypertension due to lung diseases and hypoxia
I27.24	Chronic thromboembolic pulmonary hypertension
I27.29	Other secondary pulmonary hypertension
I27.82	Chronic pulmonary embolism
I27.83	Eisenmenger's syndrome
I27.89	Other specified pulmonary heart diseases
I37.0	Nonrheumatic pulmonary valve stenosis
I37.2	Nonrheumatic pulmonary valve stenosis with insufficiency
I37.8	Other nonrheumatic pulmonary valve disorders
Q22.1	Congenital pulmonary valve stenosis
Q22.2	Congenital pulmonary valve insufficiency
Q22.3	Other congenital malformations of pulmonary valve
Q24.3	Pulmonary infundibular stenosis
Q25.6	Stenosis of pulmonary artery
Q25.72	Congenital pulmonary arteriovenous malformation
Q25.79	Other congenital malformations of pulmonary artery
S25.411A	Minor laceration of right pulmonary blood vessels, initial encounter ☑
S25.412A	Minor laceration of left pulmonary blood vessels, initial encounter ☑
S25.421A	Major laceration of right pulmonary blood vessels, initial encounter ☑
S25.422A	Major laceration of left pulmonary blood vessels, initial encounter ☑
S25.491A	Other specified injury of right pulmonary blood vessels, initial encounter ☑
S25.492A	Other specified injury of left pulmonary blood vessels, initial encounter ☑
T81.718A	Complication of other artery following a procedure, not elsewhere classified, initial encounter
T82.817A	Embolism due to cardiac prosthetic devices, implants and grafts, initial encounter
T82.818A	Embolism due to vascular prosthetic devices, implants and grafts, initial encounter

AMA: 33916 2018,Jan,8; 2017,Jan,8; 2017,Dec,3; 2016,Jan,13; 2015,Jan,16; 2014,Jan,11 **33917** 2018,Jan,8; 2017,Jan,8; 2017,Dec,3; 2016,Jul,3; 2016,Jan,13; 2015,Jan,16; 2014,Jan,11

Relative Value Units/Medicare Edits

Non-Facility RVU	Work	PE	MP	Total
33916	78.0	26.74	18.43	123.17
33917	25.3	10.97	6.01	42.28
Facility RVU	**Work**	**PE**	**MP**	**Total**
33916	78.0	26.74	18.43	123.17
33917	25.3	10.97	6.01	42.28

	FUD	Status	MUE	Modifiers				IOM Reference
33916	90	A	1(3)	51	N/A	62*	80	None
33917	90	A	1(2)	51	N/A	62*	80	

* with documentation

Terms To Know

cardiopulmonary bypass. Venous blood is diverted to a heart-lung machine, which mechanically pumps and oxygenates the blood temporarily so the heart can be bypassed while an open procedure on the heart or coronary arteries is performed. During bypass, the lungs are deflated and immobile.

embolectomy. Surgical excision of a blood clot or other foreign material that broke away from its original source and traveled in the blood stream, becoming lodged in a blood vessel and blocking circulation.

endarterectomy. Removal of the thickened, endothelial lining of a diseased or damaged artery.

hypothermia with cardiac bypass. Reduction of the body temperature using a bypass system to reduce the oxygen demands of tissue and to protect the myocardium during a procedure.

stenosis. Narrowing or constriction of a passage.

sternotomy. Incision into the sternum, the bone that forms the front of the chest cavity and connects with the ribs.

33920

33920 Repair of pulmonary atresia with ventricular septal defect, by construction or replacement of conduit from right or left ventricle to pulmonary artery

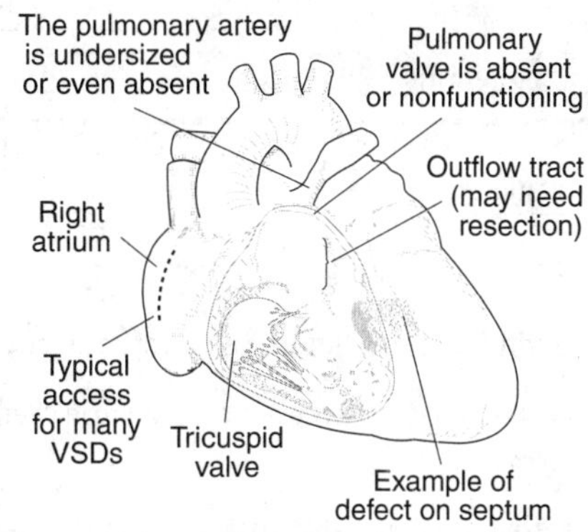

Pulmonary atresia (the absence of an outlet) is surgically treated by constructing a connection from a ventricle (usually the right) to a point on the pulmonary artery that is of normal

Explanation

Cardiopulmonary bypass is required. A hole is made in the right ventricle and any muscular obstruction in the outflow tract of the right ventricle is removed. The pulmonary artery or its branches are opened longitudinally until normal-sized vessels are encountered. The ventricular septal defect is closed. An aortic graft from an organ donor is trimmed to form a patch over the opened pulmonary artery. Any excess artery from the donor graft or a patch of pericardium or Dacron is sewn to the graft below the valve to use as a secondary patch for closing the hole in the right ventricle. The graft valve becomes the new pulmonary valve. After the patches and graft are sewn in place, cardiopulmonary bypass is stopped when heart function returns.

Coding Tips

The insertion of grafts or implanted materials is considered part of this procedure and is not reported separately. If significant additional time and effort are documented, append modifier 22 and submit a cover letter and operative report. When 33920 is performed with another separately identifiable procedure, the highest dollar value code is listed as the primary procedure and subsequent procedures are appended with modifier 51. When ligation and takedown of systemic-to-pulmonary artery shunt is performed in addition to this procedure, it should be reported separately, see 33924. Do not report 33920 with 33440. For repair of other complex cardiac anomalies by construction or replacement of right or left ventricle to pulmonary artery conduit, see 33608. For closure of a ventricular septal defect only, with or without patch, see 33681–33688.

ICD-10-CM Diagnostic Codes

Q21.0	Ventricular septal defect
Q21.8	Other congenital malformations of cardiac septa
Q22.0	Pulmonary valve atresia
Q22.3	Other congenital malformations of pulmonary valve
Q25.5	Atresia of pulmonary artery
Q25.79	Other congenital malformations of pulmonary artery

Heart and Pericardium

AMA: **33920** 2019,Apr,6; 2018,Jan,8; 2017,Jan,8; 2017,Dec,3; 2016,Jan,13; 2015,Jan,16; 2014,Jan,11

Relative Value Units/Medicare Edits

Non-Facility RVU	Work	PE	MP	Total
33920	32.74	12.07	7.8	52.61
Facility RVU	**Work**	**PE**	**MP**	**Total**
33920	32.74	12.07	7.8	52.61

	FUD	Status	MUE	Modifiers				IOM Reference
33920	90	A	1(2)	51	N/A	62*	80	None

* with documentation

Terms To Know

anomaly. Irregularity in the structure or position of an organ or tissue.

atresia. Congenital closure or absence of a tubular organ or an opening to the body surface.

cardiopulmonary bypass. Venous blood is diverted to a heart-lung machine, which mechanically pumps and oxygenates the blood temporarily so the heart can be bypassed while an open procedure on the heart or coronary arteries is performed. During bypass, the lungs are deflated and immobile.

conduit. Surgically created channel for the passage of fluids.

congenital. Present at birth, occurring through heredity or an influence during gestation up to the moment of birth.

graft. Tissue implant from another part of the body or another person.

ligation. Tying off a blood vessel or duct with a suture or a soft, thin wire.

obstruction. Blockage that prevents normal function of the valve or structure.

shunt. Surgically created passage between blood vessels or other natural passages, such as an arteriovenous anastomosis, to divert or bypass blood flow from the normal channel.

stenosis. Narrowing or constriction of a passage.

ventricular septal defect. Congenital cardiac anomaly resulting in a continual opening in the septum between the ventricles that, in severe cases, causes oxygenated blood to flow back into the lungs, resulting in pulmonary hypertension.

33922

33922 Transection of pulmonary artery with cardiopulmonary bypass

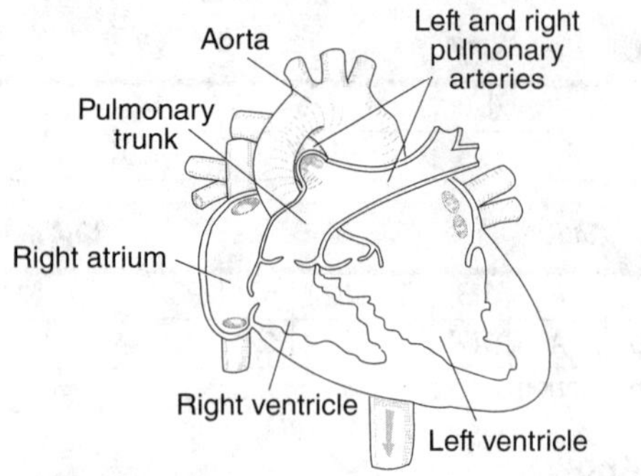

A pulmonary artery is transected and a diseased portion removed. The ends are then anastomosed together. Cardiopulmonary bypass is employed

Explanation

Cardiopulmonary bypass is required. After it is started, cuts are made all the way across the pulmonary artery just above and just below the part of the artery containing the disease. The pulmonary artery is closed directly or is closed using a piece of the pulmonary artery or a piece of the aorta from an organ donor that is placed as an interposition graft.

Coding Tips

The insertion of grafts or implanted materials is considered part of this procedure and is not reported separately. If significant additional time and effort are documented, append modifier 22 and submit a cover letter and operative report. When 33922 is performed with another separately identifiable procedure, the highest dollar value code is listed as the primary procedure and subsequent procedures are appended with modifier 51. Do not append modifier 63 to 33922 as the description or nature of the procedure includes infants up to 4 kg. When ligation and takedown of systemic-to-pulmonary artery shunt is performed in addition to this procedure, it should be reported separately, see 33924.

ICD-10-CM Diagnostic Codes

I28.1	Aneurysm of pulmonary artery
I28.8	Other diseases of pulmonary vessels
Q22.0	Pulmonary valve atresia
Q22.3	Other congenital malformations of pulmonary valve
Q25.5	Atresia of pulmonary artery
Q25.6	Stenosis of pulmonary artery
Q25.71	Coarctation of pulmonary artery
Q25.72	Congenital pulmonary arteriovenous malformation
Q25.79	Other congenital malformations of pulmonary artery
Q25.8	Other congenital malformations of other great arteries
S25.411A	Minor laceration of right pulmonary blood vessels, initial encounter ☑
S25.412A	Minor laceration of left pulmonary blood vessels, initial encounter ☑
S25.421A	Major laceration of right pulmonary blood vessels, initial encounter ☑
S25.422A	Major laceration of left pulmonary blood vessels, initial encounter ☑

S25.491A Other specified injury of right pulmonary blood vessels, initial encounter ☑

S25.492A Other specified injury of left pulmonary blood vessels, initial encounter ☑

AMA: **33922** 2017,Dec,3

Relative Value Units/Medicare Edits

Non-Facility RVU	Work	PE	MP	Total
33922	24.22	10.33	5.74	40.29
Facility RVU	Work	PE	MP	Total
33922	24.22	10.33	5.74	40.29

	FUD	Status	MUE	Modifiers				IOM Reference
33922	90	A	1(2)	51	N/A	62*	80	None

* with documentation

Terms To Know

anastomosis. Surgically created connection between ducts, blood vessels, or bowel segments to allow flow from one to the other.

anomaly. Irregularity in the structure or position of an organ or tissue.

cardiopulmonary bypass. Venous blood is diverted to a heart-lung machine, which mechanically pumps and oxygenates the blood temporarily so the heart can be bypassed while an open procedure on the heart or coronary arteries is performed. During bypass, the lungs are deflated and immobile.

congenital. Present at birth, occurring through heredity or an influence during gestation up to the moment of birth.

graft. Tissue implant from another part of the body or another person.

hypothermia with cardiac bypass. Reduction of the body temperature using a bypass system to reduce the oxygen demands of tissue and to protect the myocardium during a procedure.

ligation. Tying off a blood vessel or duct with a suture or a soft, thin wire.

transection. Transverse dissection; to cut across a long axis; cross section.

33924

+ 33924 Ligation and takedown of a systemic-to-pulmonary artery shunt, performed in conjunction with a congenital heart procedure (List separately in addition to code for primary procedure)

Surgery to correct a congenital heart defect, a systemic-to-pulmonary artery shunt is ligated and removed

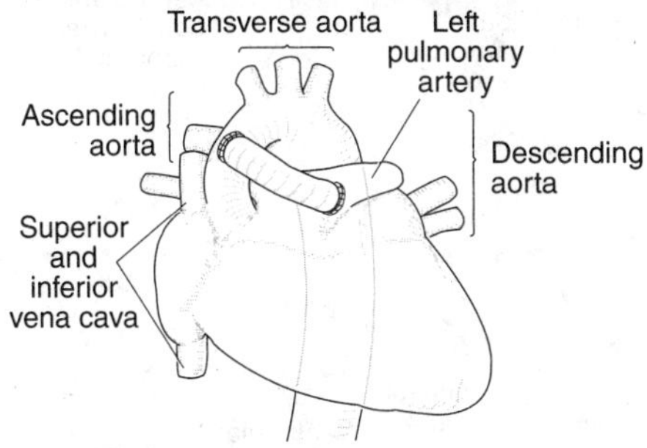

Explanation

During a separately reportable congenital heart procedure, the physician ligates and takes down a previously formed systemic-to-pulmonary artery shunt. The shunt is ligated and the systemic arteries are returned to their correct anatomic position.

Coding Tips

Report 33924 with 33470–33478, 33600–33617, 33622, 33684–33688, 33692–33697, 33735–33767, 33770–33783, 33786, 33917, 33920, 33922, 33925, 33926, 33935, or 33945.

ICD-10-CM Diagnostic Codes

This/these CPT code(s) are add on code(s). See the primary procedure code that this code is performed with for your ICD-10-CM code selections. Diagnostic code(s) would be the same as the actual procedure performed.

AMA: **33924** 1997,Nov,1

Relative Value Units/Medicare Edits

Non-Facility RVU	Work	PE	MP	Total
33924	5.49	1.53	1.29	8.31
Facility RVU	Work	PE	MP	Total
33924	5.49	1.53	1.29	8.31

	FUD	Status	MUE	Modifiers				IOM Reference
33924	N/A	A	1(2)	N/A	N/A	62*	80	None

* with documentation

Terms To Know

congenital. Present at birth, occurring through heredity or an influence during gestation up to the moment of birth.

ligation. Tying off a blood vessel or duct with a suture or a soft, thin wire.

33925-33926

33925 Repair of pulmonary artery arborization anomalies by unifocalization; without cardiopulmonary bypass

33926 with cardiopulmonary bypass

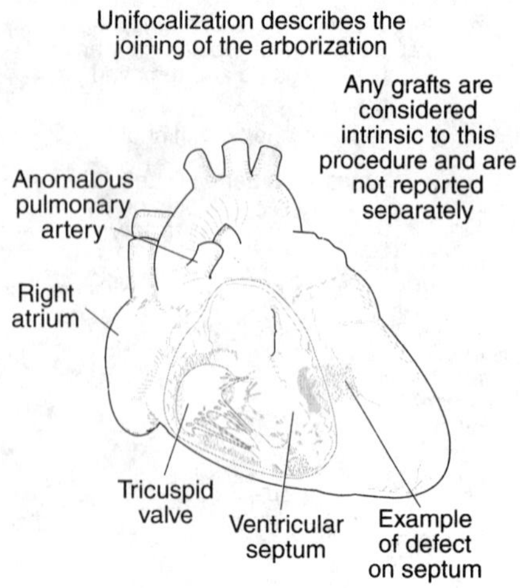

Explanation

The physician repairs pulmonary artery arborization anomalies (i.e., stenosis of unbranched and intrapulmonary arteries) by unifocalization, a surgical technique in which the various sources of pulmonary blood supply can be perfused from a single source. In patients with pulmonary atresia or with a ventricular septal defect (VSD), the pulmonary blood supply often comes from multiple sources, particularly major aortopulmonary collateral arteries (MAPCA), which often arise from the aorta and its direct branches. Unifocalization, which may be performed as a single operation or as a staged procedure, interrupts the extracardiac sources of pulmonary arterial blood flow; restores segmental, lobar, and pulmonary arterial confluence; replaces missing central pulmonary arterial branches; and creates a central, accessible source of pulmonary arterial blood flow. The physician accesses the mediastinum through an extended median sternotomy or a bilateral transsternal thoracotomy. The major aortopulmonary collateral arteries are identified, mobilized, and dissected, using a variety of techniques, from the upper descending aorta, the aortic arch, brachiocephalic vessels, or coronary arteries, and anastomosed to the native pulmonary artery. Ligation of the collateral arteries at their origin is performed to achieve controlled perfusion. As each artery is ligated, desaturation is assessed by pulse oximetry. If desaturation approaches a compromising level, the surgeon may proceed with cardiopulmonary bypass at this point. Report 33925 when the procedure is performed without cardiopulmonary bypass and 33926 when it is performed with cardiopulmonary bypass.

Coding Tips

If significant additional time and effort is documented, append modifier 22 and submit a cover letter and operative report. For repair of other complex cardiac anomalies by construction or replacement of right or left ventricle to pulmonary artery conduit, see 33608.

ICD-10-CM Diagnostic Codes

I28.8	Other diseases of pulmonary vessels
I28.9	Disease of pulmonary vessels, unspecified
I77.1	Stricture of artery
Q21.0	Ventricular septal defect
Q21.2	Atrioventricular septal defect
Q21.3	Tetralogy of Fallot
Q21.4	Aortopulmonary septal defect
Q21.8	Other congenital malformations of cardiac septa
Q25.5	Atresia of pulmonary artery
Q25.6	Stenosis of pulmonary artery
Q25.71	Coarctation of pulmonary artery
Q25.72	Congenital pulmonary arteriovenous malformation
Q25.79	Other congenital malformations of pulmonary artery
Q25.8	Other congenital malformations of other great arteries

AMA: **33926** 2017,Dec,3

Relative Value Units/Medicare Edits

Non-Facility RVU	Work	PE	MP	Total
33925	31.3	11.18	7.43	49.91
33926	44.73	14.91	10.66	70.3
Facility RVU	**Work**	**PE**	**MP**	**Total**
33925	31.3	11.18	7.43	49.91
33926	44.73	14.91	10.66	70.3

	FUD	Status	MUE	Modifiers				IOM Reference
33925	90	A	1(2)	51	N/A	62*	80	None
33926	90	A	1(2)	51	N/A	62*	80	

* with documentation

Terms To Know

anomaly. Irregularity in the structure or position of an organ or tissue.

cardiopulmonary bypass. Venous blood is diverted to a heart-lung machine, which mechanically pumps and oxygenates the blood temporarily so the heart can be bypassed while an open procedure on the heart or coronary arteries is performed. During bypass, the lungs are deflated and immobile.

tetralogy of Fallot. Specific combination of congenital cardiac defects: obstruction of the right ventricular outflow tract with pulmonary stenosis, interventricular septal defect, malposition of the aorta, overriding the interventricular septum and receiving blood from both the venous and arterial systems, and enlargement of the right ventricle.

ventricular septal defect. Congenital cardiac anomaly resulting in a continual opening in the septum between the ventricles that, in severe cases, causes oxygenated blood to flow back into the lungs, resulting in pulmonary hypertension.

33927-33929

33927 Implantation of a total replacement heart system (artificial heart) with recipient cardiectomy

33928 Removal and replacement of total replacement heart system (artificial heart)

+ **33929** Removal of a total replacement heart system (artificial heart) for heart transplantation (List separately in addition to code for primary procedure)

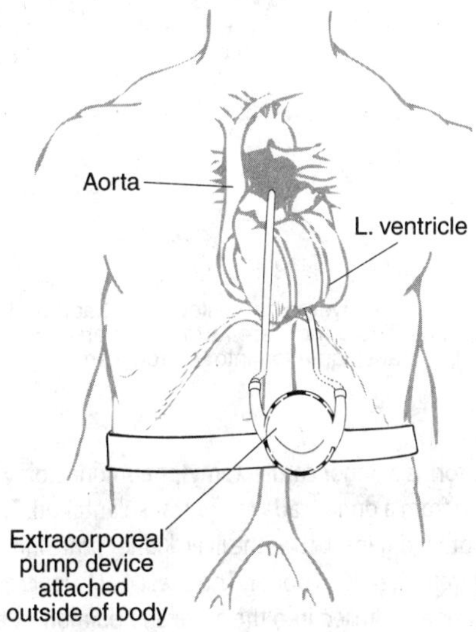

Implantable replacement heart system with removal of native heart

Explanation

In 33927, the physician implants a total replacement heart system, or artificial heart, as a temporary measure until transplantation or to prolong life for patients not eligible for transplant. One artificial heart system, described here, is a self-contained, electrohydraulic action heart, charged from a battery source through the skin. Once attached, the natural atria pump blood into the artificial ventricles of the replacement heart and the hydraulic pump moves the blood into circulation. The patient is prepared for open heart surgery, and an extended median sternotomy is made. A subcutaneous/submuscular pocket is created in the patient's abdominal area for the internal battery and the heart's pumping controller unit, and these internal components are placed between muscle layers. A separate incision is made over the chest wall for placement of the internal transcutaneous energy transmission coil, which is sutured into an appropriate position where the external coil may lie flat over it without much interposing tissue. Cardiopulmonary bypass is initiated, the aorta is cross-clamped, and cardiectomy is undertaken to remove the native ventricles and transect the great vessels. Outflow grafts are anastomosed to the pulmonary artery and the aorta. The artificial ventricles are anastomosed to the native atrial cuffs and all air is removed from the system. The aortic cross-clamp is released and cardiopulmonary bypass weaned onto the artificial heart support. The internal components are connected to the artificial heart and energy is transferred through the transcutaneous coils, where external battery packs transmit power across the skin to keep the internal battery charged. In 33928, the physician removes and replaces a total replacement heart system or artificial heart. The thoracic unit is the pump that consists of the artificial ventricles, which are attached to the natural atria, containing their corresponding valves, and the motor-driven hydraulic pumping system, or the pneumatic air pressure valves, depending on the system. Removal and replacement of this component requires open chest access in a procedure following the same kind of steps for implantation (see 33927). Internal components include the implanted rechargeable battery, which is continually charged by external battery packs, the internal transcutaneous coil for receiving the battery charge across the skin, or the control unit, which monitors and controls the pumping speed of the artificial heart. These components are removed and replaced back in their prepared subcutaneous/submuscular pockets and tunneled back to their connection with the thoracic unit. Report 33929 for removal of a total replacement heart system or artificial heart for heart transplantation.

Coding Tips

Report 33929 in addition to 33945. For implantation with replacement of a total heart system with recipient cardiectomy, see 33927. For implant of a ventricular assist device, see 33975, 33976, 33979, 33990, and 33991. For revision or replacement of components only, see 33999.

ICD-10-CM Diagnostic Codes

I50.1	Left ventricular failure, unspecified
I50.21	Acute systolic (congestive) heart failure
I50.22	Chronic systolic (congestive) heart failure
I50.23	Acute on chronic systolic (congestive) heart failure
I50.31	Acute diastolic (congestive) heart failure
I50.32	Chronic diastolic (congestive) heart failure
I50.33	Acute on chronic diastolic (congestive) heart failure
I50.41	Acute combined systolic (congestive) and diastolic (congestive) heart failure
I50.42	Chronic combined systolic (congestive) and diastolic (congestive) heart failure
I50.43	Acute on chronic combined systolic (congestive) and diastolic (congestive) heart failure
I50.810	Right heart failure, unspecified
I50.811	Acute right heart failure
I50.812	Chronic right heart failure
I50.813	Acute on chronic right heart failure
I50.814	Right heart failure due to left heart failure
I50.82	Biventricular heart failure
I50.83	High output heart failure
I50.84	End stage heart failure
I50.89	Other heart failure
T82.512A	Breakdown (mechanical) of artificial heart, initial encounter
T82.522A	Displacement of artificial heart, initial encounter
T82.532A	Leakage of artificial heart, initial encounter
T82.592A	Other mechanical complication of artificial heart, initial encounter
T86.20	Unspecified complication of heart transplant
T86.21	Heart transplant rejection
T86.22	Heart transplant failure
T86.23	Heart transplant infection
Z76.82	Awaiting organ transplant status
Z95.812	Presence of fully implantable artificial heart

AMA: 33927 2018,Jun,3 **33928** 2018,Jun,3 **33929** 2018,Jun,3

Heart and Pericardium

Relative Value Units/Medicare Edits

Non-Facility RVU	Work	PE	MP	Total
33927	49.0	13.59	11.68	74.27
33928	0.0	0.0	0.0	0.0
33929	0.0	0.0	0.0	0.0
Facility RVU	**Work**	**PE**	**MP**	**Total**
33927	49.0	13.59	11.68	74.27
33928	0.0	0.0	0.0	0.0
33929	0.0	0.0	0.0	0.0

	FUD	Status	MUE	Modifiers				IOM Reference
33927	N/A	A	1(3)	51	N/A	N/A	80	None
33928	N/A	C	1(3)	51	N/A	N/A	80	
33929	N/A	C	1(3)	N/A	N/A	N/A	80	

* with documentation

Terms To Know

cardiectomy. Excision of the cardiac portion of the stomach.

ventricular assist device. Temporary measure used to support the heart by substituting for left and/or right heart function. The device replaces the work of the left and/or right ventricle when a patient has a damaged or weakened heart. A left ventricular assist device (VAD) helps the heart pump blood through the rest of the body. A right VAD helps the heart pump blood to the lungs to become oxygenated again. Catheters are inserted to circulate the blood through external tubing to a pump machine located outside of the body and back to the correct artery.

33930

33930 Donor cardiectomy-pneumonectomy (including cold preservation)

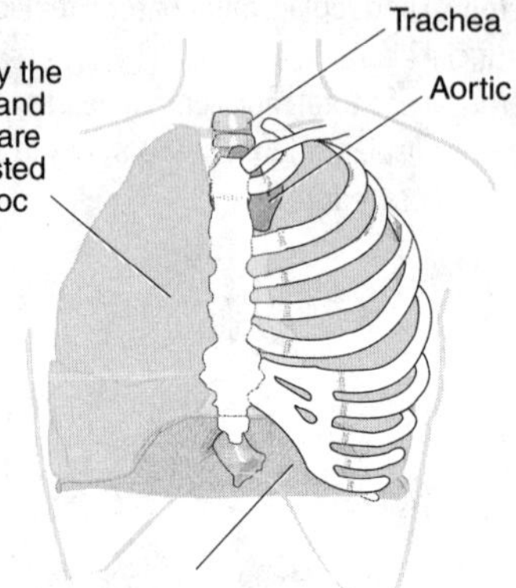

A donor cadaver is harvested of its heart and lungs. The organs are further prepared for transplantation into the recipient

Explanation

The physician performs a donor cardiectomy-pneumonectomy by removing the heart and lung from a donor cadaver for transplantation. This is usually performed when other organs such as the liver, kidneys, intestines, or pancreas are also acquired from the organ donor. The chest cavity is accessed and cold preserving solutions are infused into the aorta and pulmonary arteries. After enough solution has been given, the heart and lungs are removed by transection, en bloc. This includes the aorta well above the heart, the right atrium, the atrial septum, and the left atrium—completely and as close to the patient's spine (or as posteriorly) as possible. The heart/lung block is preserved for transplantation into the recipient. The organ remains under refrigeration, specially packed in a sealable container with some preserving solution and kept on ice in a suitable carrier.

Coding Tips

Combined heart and lung transplantation involves three distinct components. Code 33930 reports only the cadaver cardiectomy-pneumonectomy. Backbench work (33933), which involves preparation of the cadaver donor heart and lung allograft prior to transplant, is reported separately. Transplant of the cadaver donor heart and lung including recipient cardiectomy-pneumonectomy and care of the recipient (33935) is also reported separately. Any additional repair or resection procedures on the donor heart or lung are also reported separately, see 33300, 33310, 33320, 33390, 33463, 33464, 33510, 33641, 35216, 35276, or 35685. Donor cardiectomy-pneumonectomy and any backbench work, repair, or resection procedures on the donor heart are usually the financial responsibility of the recipient.

ICD-10-CM Diagnostic Codes

Z52.89 Donor of other specified organs or tissues

AMA: 33930 1997,Nov,1

Relative Value Units/Medicare Edits

Non-Facility RVU	Work	PE	MP	Total
33930	0.0	0.0	0.0	0.0
Facility RVU	**Work**	**PE**	**MP**	**Total**
33930	0.0	0.0	0.0	0.0

	FUD	Status	MUE	Modifiers				IOM Reference
33930	N/A	X	1(2)	N/A	N/A	N/A	N/A	100-03,260.9

* with documentation

Terms To Know

allograft. Graft from one individual to another of the same species.

backbench preparation. Procedures performed on a donor organ following procurement to prepare the organ for transplant into the recipient. Excess fat and other tissue may be removed, the organ may be perfused, and vital arteries may be sized, repaired, or modified to fit the patient. These procedures are done on a back table in the operating room before transplantation can begin.

cardiectomy. Excision of the cardiac portion of the stomach.

donor. Person from whom tissues or organs are removed for transplantation.

en bloc. In total.

excision. Surgical removal of an organ or tissue.

pneumonectomy. Surgical removal of a lung or lung tissue.

transection. Transverse dissection; to cut across a long axis; cross section.

transplant. Insertion of an organ or tissue from one person or site into another.

33933

33933 Backbench standard preparation of cadaver donor heart/lung allograft prior to transplantation, including dissection of allograft from surrounding soft tissues to prepare aorta, superior vena cava, inferior vena cava, and trachea for implantation

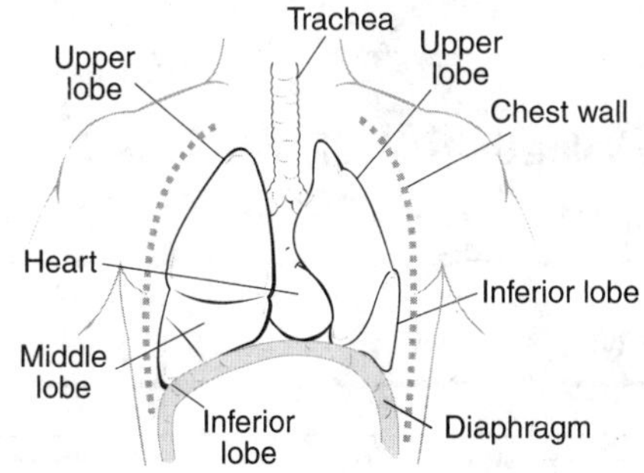

Backbench preparation is performed on the heart and lungs from a cadaver in preparation for transplantation

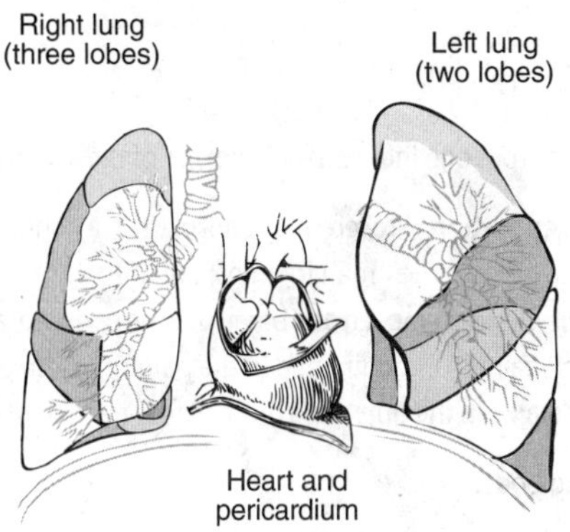

Explanation

The physician performs a standard backbench preparation of the heart and lungs following procurement from a cadaver donor. Backbench or back table preparation refers to procedures performed on the donor organs following procurement to prepare the donor organs for transplant. The heart and lungs are removed en bloc. The heart and lungs are inspected following procurement to identify any injury or abnormality not noted prior to procurement. The physician prepares the heart and lungs by dissecting free any residual soft tissue. Attention is focused on the aorta, superior vena cava, inferior vena cava, and the trachea. The aorta, which was divided at the aortic arch, is inspected and residual tissue removed. The superior vena cava is inspected and residual tissue removed. The inferior vena cava is inspected to assure adequate length has been preserved. Any residual tissue is removed from the inferior vena cava. The trachea, which was divided as far above the carina as possible, is inspected and residual tissue removed. When all residual soft tissue has been removed and the vessels prepared, the heart and lungs are ready for transplant.

Coding Tips

Combined heart and lung transplantation involves three distinct components. Code 33933 includes only backbench work to prepare the cadaver donor heart and lung allograft prior to transplant. Cadaver cardiectomy-pneumonectomy (33930) is reported separately. Transplant of the cadaver donor heart and lung including recipient cardiectomy-pneumonectomy and care of the recipient (33935) is also reported separately. Any additional repair or resection procedures on the donor heart are also reported separately, see 33300, 33310, 33320, 33390, 33463, 33464, 33510, 33641, 35216, 35276, or 35685. Donor cardiectomy-pneumonectomy and any backbench work, repair, or resection procedures on the donor heart are usually the financial responsibility of the recipient.

ICD-10-CM Diagnostic Codes

This code is not identified as an add-on code by CPT® but is performed at the same time as another primary procedure. Refer to the corresponding primary procedure code for ICD-10-CM diagnosis code links.

AMA: **33933** 1997,Nov,1

Relative Value Units/Medicare Edits

Non-Facility RVU	Work	PE	MP	Total
33933	0.0	0.0	0.0	0.0
Facility RVU	**Work**	**PE**	**MP**	**Total**
33933	0.0	0.0	0.0	0.0

	FUD	Status	MUE	Modifiers				IOM Reference
33933	N/A	C	1(2)	51	N/A	62*	80	None

* with documentation

Terms To Know

allograft. Graft from one individual to another of the same species.

backbench preparation. Procedures performed on a donor organ following procurement to prepare the organ for transplant into the recipient. Excess fat and other tissue may be removed, the organ may be perfused, and vital arteries may be sized, repaired, or modified to fit the patient. These procedures are done on a back table in the operating room before transplantation can begin.

cadaver. Dead body.

carina. Ridge at the junction of the trachea and the bronchi formed by a projection of the lowest tracheal cartilage separating the openings of the two bronchi.

en bloc. In total.

resection. Surgical removal of a part or all of an organ or body part.

vena cava. Main venous trunk that empties into the right atrium from both the lower and upper regions, beginning at the junction of the common iliac veins inferiorly and the two brachiocephalic veins superiorly.

Heart and Pericardium

33935

33935 Heart-lung transplant with recipient cardiectomy-pneumonectomy

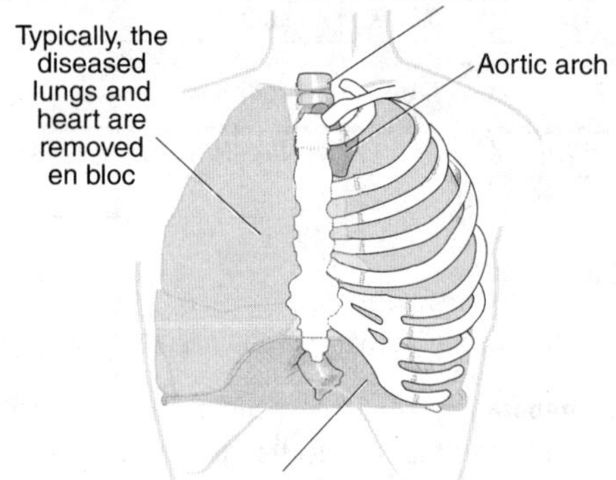

The diseased heart and lung are removed from the patient and the donor organs are placed and surgically connected

Explanation

The patient is placed on cardiopulmonary bypass and the heart and lungs are removed. The donor's organs are placed by sewing the left atrium of the donor to the left atrium of the recipient's first, and then sewing together the atrial septums and the right atrium. The donor aorta is trimmed to an appropriate length and sewn to the ascending aorta of the recipient. Immunosuppressive drugs may be given to the patient before, during, and after surgery. Cardiopulmonary bypass is discontinued when function returns to the donor heart.

Coding Tips

Combined heart and lung transplantation involves three distinct components. Code 33935 includes only transplant of the cadaver donor heart and lung including recipient cardiectomy-pneumonectomy and care of the recipient. Cadaver cardiectomy-pneumonectomy (33930) is reported separately. Backbench work (33933), which involves preparation of the cadaver donor heart and lung allograft prior to transplant, is also reported separately. Any additional repair or resection procedures on the donor heart are also reported separately, see 33300, 33310, 33320, 33390, 33463, 33464, 33510, 33641, 35216, 35276, or 35685. Donor cardiectomy-pneumonectomy and any backbench work, repair, or resection procedures on the donor heart are usually the financial responsibility of the recipient.

ICD-10-CM Diagnostic Codes

C34.01	Malignant neoplasm of right main bronchus ☑
C34.02	Malignant neoplasm of left main bronchus ☑
C34.11	Malignant neoplasm of upper lobe, right bronchus or lung ☑
C34.12	Malignant neoplasm of upper lobe, left bronchus or lung ☑
C34.2	Malignant neoplasm of middle lobe, bronchus or lung
C34.31	Malignant neoplasm of lower lobe, right bronchus or lung ☑
C34.32	Malignant neoplasm of lower lobe, left bronchus or lung ☑
C38.0	Malignant neoplasm of heart
C38.4	Malignant neoplasm of pleura
C45.2	Mesothelioma of pericardium
E84.0	Cystic fibrosis with pulmonary manifestations
I11.0	Hypertensive heart disease with heart failure
I16.0	Hypertensive urgency

I16.1 Hypertensive emergency
I20.0 Unstable angina
I20.1 Angina pectoris with documented spasm
I20.8 Other forms of angina pectoris
I25.110 Atherosclerotic heart disease of native coronary artery with unstable angina pectoris
I25.111 Atherosclerotic heart disease of native coronary artery with angina pectoris with documented spasm
I25.118 Atherosclerotic heart disease of native coronary artery with other forms of angina pectoris
I25.2 Old myocardial infarction
I25.3 Aneurysm of heart
I25.41 Coronary artery aneurysm
I25.42 Coronary artery dissection
I25.5 Ischemic cardiomyopathy
I25.6 Silent myocardial ischemia
I25.82 Chronic total occlusion of coronary artery
I25.83 Coronary atherosclerosis due to lipid rich plaque
I25.84 Coronary atherosclerosis due to calcified coronary lesion
I27.0 Primary pulmonary hypertension
I27.21 Secondary pulmonary arterial hypertension
I27.22 Pulmonary hypertension due to left heart disease
I27.23 Pulmonary hypertension due to lung diseases and hypoxia
I27.24 Chronic thromboembolic pulmonary hypertension
I27.83 Eisenmenger's syndrome
I40.0 Infective myocarditis
I40.1 Isolated myocarditis
I42.0 Dilated cardiomyopathy
I42.1 Obstructive hypertrophic cardiomyopathy
I42.3 Endomyocardial (eosinophilic) disease
I42.4 Endocardial fibroelastosis
I50.1 Left ventricular failure, unspecified
I50.21 Acute systolic (congestive) heart failure
I50.22 Chronic systolic (congestive) heart failure
I50.23 Acute on chronic systolic (congestive) heart failure
I50.31 Acute diastolic (congestive) heart failure
I50.32 Chronic diastolic (congestive) heart failure
I50.33 Acute on chronic diastolic (congestive) heart failure
I50.41 Acute combined systolic (congestive) and diastolic (congestive) heart failure
I50.42 Chronic combined systolic (congestive) and diastolic (congestive) heart failure
I50.43 Acute on chronic combined systolic (congestive) and diastolic (congestive) heart failure
I50.811 Acute right heart failure
I50.812 Chronic right heart failure
I50.813 Acute on chronic right heart failure
I50.814 Right heart failure due to left heart failure
I50.82 Biventricular heart failure
I50.83 High output heart failure
I50.84 End stage heart failure
I51.5 Myocardial degeneration
I51.7 Cardiomegaly
J43.0 Unilateral pulmonary emphysema [MacLeod's syndrome]
J44.0 Chronic obstructive pulmonary disease with (acute) lower respiratory infection
J44.1 Chronic obstructive pulmonary disease with (acute) exacerbation
J47.0 Bronchiectasis with acute lower respiratory infection
J47.1 Bronchiectasis with (acute) exacerbation
J70.1 Chronic and other pulmonary manifestations due to radiation
J70.3 Chronic drug-induced interstitial lung disorders
J81.1 Chronic pulmonary edema
J84.112 Idiopathic pulmonary fibrosis
J84.113 Idiopathic non-specific interstitial pneumonitis
J84.114 Acute interstitial pneumonitis
J84.115 Respiratory bronchiolitis interstitial lung disease
J84.116 Cryptogenic organizing pneumonia
J84.117 Desquamative interstitial pneumonia
J84.2 Lymphoid interstitial pneumonia
J96.11 Chronic respiratory failure with hypoxia
J96.12 Chronic respiratory failure with hypercapnia
J96.21 Acute and chronic respiratory failure with hypoxia
J96.22 Acute and chronic respiratory failure with hypercapnia
J98.11 Atelectasis
J98.2 Interstitial emphysema
Q20.6 Isomerism of atrial appendages
Q24.4 Congenital subaortic stenosis
Q24.5 Malformation of coronary vessels
Q24.6 Congenital heart block
Q33.0 Congenital cystic lung
Q33.3 Agenesis of lung
Q33.4 Congenital bronchiectasis
Q33.6 Congenital hypoplasia and dysplasia of lung

AMA: **33935** 2017,Dec,3

Relative Value Units/Medicare Edits

Non-Facility RVU	Work	PE	MP	Total
33935	91.78	29.67	22.45	143.9
Facility RVU	**Work**	**PE**	**MP**	**Total**
33935	91.78	29.67	22.45	143.9

	FUD	Status	MUE	Modifiers				IOM Reference
33935	90	R	1(2)	51	N/A	62*	80	None

* with documentation

Heart and Pericardium

33940

33940 Donor cardiectomy (including cold preservation)

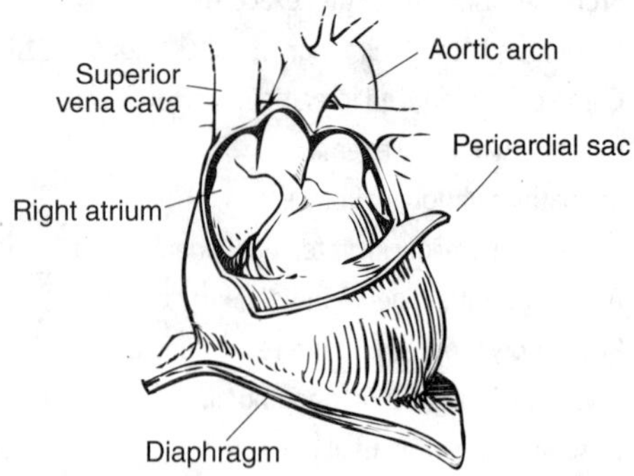

A cadaver donor heart is removed and additional work is performed to prepare and maintain the harvested heart in anticipation of a transplant

Explanation

The physician performs a donor cardiectomy by removing the heart from a donor cadaver for transplantation. This is usually performed when other organs such as the liver, kidneys, intestines, or pancreas are also acquired from the organ donor. The chest cavity is accessed and cold preserving solutions are infused into the aorta. After enough solution has been given, the heart is removed by transection, en bloc. This includes the aorta well above the heart, the right atrium, the atrial septum, and the left atrium, completely and as close to the patient's spine (or as posteriorly) as possible. The heart is preserved for transplantation into the recipient. The organ remains under refrigeration, specially packed in a sealable container with some preserving solution and kept on ice in a suitable carrier to maintain hypothermia.

Coding Tips

Heart transplantation involves three distinct components. Code 33940 reports only the cadaver cardiectomy. Backbench work (33944), which involves preparation of the cadaver donor heart allograft prior to transplant, is reported separately. Transplant of the cadaver donor heart with or without recipient cardiectomy and care of the recipient (33945) is also reported separately. Any additional repair or resection procedures on the donor heart are also reported separately, see 33300, 33310, 33320, 33390, 33463, 33464, 33510, 33641, 35216, 35276, or 35685. Donor cardiectomy and any backbench work, repair, or resection procedures on the donor heart are usually the financial responsibility of the recipient.

ICD-10-CM Diagnostic Codes

Z52.89 Donor of other specified organs or tissues

AMA: 33940 2018,Jan,8; 2017,Jan,8; 2016,Jan,13; 2015,Jan,16; 2014,Jan,11

Relative Value Units/Medicare Edits

Non-Facility RVU	Work	PE	MP	Total
33940	0.0	0.0	0.0	0.0
Facility RVU	**Work**	**PE**	**MP**	**Total**
33940	0.0	0.0	0.0	0.0

	FUD	Status	MUE	Modifiers				IOM Reference
33940	N/A	X	1(2)	N/A	N/A	N/A	N/A	None

* with documentation

33944

33944 Backbench standard preparation of cadaver donor heart allograft prior to transplantation, including dissection of allograft from surrounding soft tissues to prepare aorta, superior vena cava, inferior vena cava, pulmonary artery, and left atrium for implantation

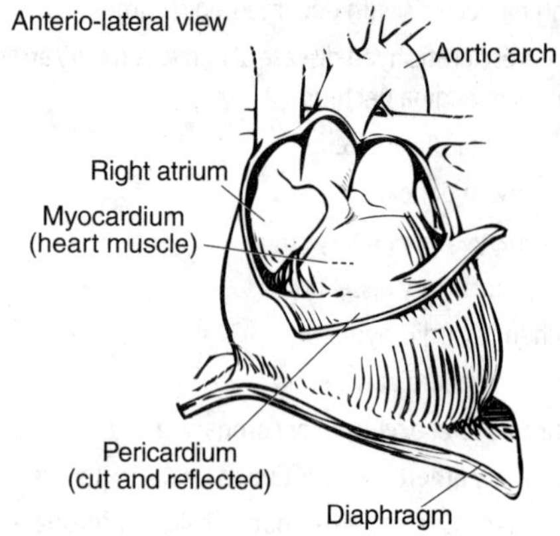

Backbench preparation is performed on the heart from a cadaver in preparation for transplantation

Explanation

The physician performs a standard backbench preparation of the heart following procurement from a cadaver donor. Backbench or back table preparation refers to procedures performed on the donor organs following procurement to prepare the donor organs for transplant. The heart is removed or the heart and lungs are removed en bloc. If the heart and lungs are removed en bloc, back table separation of the heart and lungs is performed. The heart is inspected following procurement to identify any injury or abnormality not noted prior to procurement. The physician prepares the heart by dissecting free any residual soft tissue. Attention is focused on the aorta, superior vena cava, inferior vena cava, and the left atrium. The aorta, which was divided at the aortic arch, is inspected and residual tissue removed. The superior vena cava is inspected and residual tissue removed. The inferior vena cava is inspected to assure adequate length has been preserved. Any residual tissue is removed. The left atrium is inspected and residual tissue removed. When all residual soft tissue has been removed and the vessels prepared, the heart is ready for transplant.

Coding Tips

Heart transplantation involves three distinct components. Code 33944 includes only backbench work to prepare the cadaver donor heart allograft prior to transplant. Cadaver cardiectomy (33940) is reported separately. Transplant of the cadaver donor heart with or without recipient cardiectomy and care of the recipient (33945) is also reported separately. Any additional repair or resection procedures on the donor heart are also reported separately, see 33300, 33310, 33320, 33390, 33463, 33464, 33510, 33641, 35216, 35276, or 35685. Donor cardiectomy and any backbench work, repair, or resection procedures on the donor heart are usually the financial responsibility of the recipient.

ICD-10-CM Diagnostic Codes

This code is not identified as an add-on code by CPT® but is performed at the same time as another primary procedure. Refer to the corresponding primary procedure code for ICD-10-CM diagnosis code links.

AMA: 33944 1997,Nov,1

Relative Value Units/Medicare Edits

Non-Facility RVU	Work	PE	MP	Total
33944	0.0	0.0	0.0	0.0
Facility RVU	**Work**	**PE**	**MP**	**Total**
33944	0.0	0.0	0.0	0.0

	FUD	Status	MUE	Modifiers				IOM Reference
33944	N/A	C	1(2)	51	N/A	62*	80	None

* with documentation

Terms To Know

allograft. Graft from one individual to another of the same species.

backbench preparation. Procedures performed on a donor organ following procurement to prepare the organ for transplant into the recipient. Excess fat and other tissue may be removed, the organ may be perfused, and vital arteries may be sized, repaired, or modified to fit the patient. These procedures are done on a back table in the operating room before transplantation can begin.

cadaver. Dead body.

dissection. (dis. apart; -section, act of cutting) Separating by cutting tissue or body structures apart.

en bloc. In total.

pericardium. Thin and slippery case in which the heart lies that is lined with fluid so that the heart is free to pulse and move as it beats.

vena cava. Main venous trunk that empties into the right atrium from both the lower and upper regions, beginning at the junction of the common iliac veins inferiorly and the two brachiocephalic veins superiorly.

33945

33945 Heart transplant, with or without recipient cardiectomy

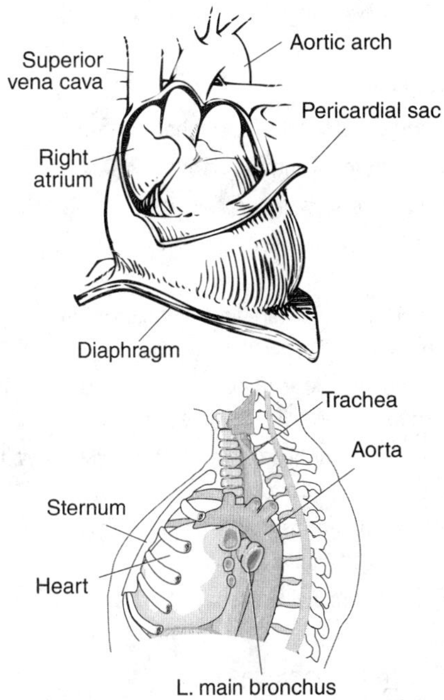

A cadaver donor heart has been prepared and maintained. The recipient's diseased heart may or may not be removed as part of the transplant procedure

Explanation

The patient is placed on cardiopulmonary bypass. Cardiac transplantation may be performed by one of two techniques: total orthotopic heart replacement or heterotropic implantation. A total orthotopic heart replacement involves excising the ventricles, atrial appendages, and most of the coronary sinus from the donor heart. The recipient heart is then opened. The atria, aorta, and pulmonary artery of the recipient heart are anastomosed to the donor heart. The sinoatrial nodes of both the donor and recipient heart are left intact. In a heterotropic implantation, the donor's organs are placed by sewing the left atrium of the donor heart to the left atrium of the recipient, and then sewing together the atrial septums and the right atrium. The donor aorta is then trimmed to an appropriate length and sewn to the ascending aorta of the recipient. Immunosuppressive drugs may be given to the patient before, during, and after the operation. Cardiopulmonary bypass is discontinued when the donor heart begins functioning in the recipient.

Coding Tips

Heart transplantation involves three distinct components. Code 33945 includes only transplant of the cadaver donor heart with or without recipient cardiectomy and care of the recipient. Cadaver cardiectomy (33940) is reported separately. Backbench work (33944), which involves preparation of the cadaver donor heart allograft prior to transplant, is also reported separately. Any additional repair or resection procedures on the donor heart are also reported separately, see 33300, 33310, 33320, 33390, 33463, 33464, 33510, 33641, 35216, 35276, or 35685. Donor cardiectomy and any backbench work, repair, or resection procedures on the donor heart are usually the financial responsibility of the recipient.

ICD-10-CM Diagnostic Codes

C38.0 Malignant neoplasm of heart

C38.8	Malignant neoplasm of overlapping sites of heart, mediastinum and pleura
C45.2	Mesothelioma of pericardium
I11.0	Hypertensive heart disease with heart failure
I16.0	Hypertensive urgency
I16.1	Hypertensive emergency
I20.0	Unstable angina
I20.1	Angina pectoris with documented spasm
I20.8	Other forms of angina pectoris
I20.9	Angina pectoris, unspecified
I25.10	Atherosclerotic heart disease of native coronary artery without angina pectoris
I25.110	Atherosclerotic heart disease of native coronary artery with unstable angina pectoris
I25.111	Atherosclerotic heart disease of native coronary artery with angina pectoris with documented spasm
I25.118	Atherosclerotic heart disease of native coronary artery with other forms of angina pectoris
I25.119	Atherosclerotic heart disease of native coronary artery with unspecified angina pectoris
I25.2	Old myocardial infarction
I25.3	Aneurysm of heart
I25.41	Coronary artery aneurysm
I25.42	Coronary artery dissection
I25.5	Ischemic cardiomyopathy
I25.6	Silent myocardial ischemia
I25.700	Atherosclerosis of coronary artery bypass graft(s), unspecified, with unstable angina pectoris
I25.701	Atherosclerosis of coronary artery bypass graft(s), unspecified, with angina pectoris with documented spasm
I25.708	Atherosclerosis of coronary artery bypass graft(s), unspecified, with other forms of angina pectoris
I25.710	Atherosclerosis of autologous vein coronary artery bypass graft(s) with unstable angina pectoris
I25.711	Atherosclerosis of autologous vein coronary artery bypass graft(s) with angina pectoris with documented spasm
I25.718	Atherosclerosis of autologous vein coronary artery bypass graft(s) with other forms of angina pectoris
I25.720	Atherosclerosis of autologous artery coronary artery bypass graft(s) with unstable angina pectoris
I25.721	Atherosclerosis of autologous artery coronary artery bypass graft(s) with angina pectoris with documented spasm
I25.728	Atherosclerosis of autologous artery coronary artery bypass graft(s) with other forms of angina pectoris
I25.730	Atherosclerosis of nonautologous biological coronary artery bypass graft(s) with unstable angina pectoris
I25.731	Atherosclerosis of nonautologous biological coronary artery bypass graft(s) with angina pectoris with documented spasm
I25.738	Atherosclerosis of nonautologous biological coronary artery bypass graft(s) with other forms of angina pectoris
I25.790	Atherosclerosis of other coronary artery bypass graft(s) with unstable angina pectoris
I25.791	Atherosclerosis of other coronary artery bypass graft(s) with angina pectoris with documented spasm
I25.798	Atherosclerosis of other coronary artery bypass graft(s) with other forms of angina pectoris
I25.810	Atherosclerosis of coronary artery bypass graft(s) without angina pectoris
I25.82	Chronic total occlusion of coronary artery
I25.83	Coronary atherosclerosis due to lipid rich plaque
I25.84	Coronary atherosclerosis due to calcified coronary lesion
I25.89	Other forms of chronic ischemic heart disease
I25.9	Chronic ischemic heart disease, unspecified
I27.0	Primary pulmonary hypertension
I27.21	Secondary pulmonary arterial hypertension
I27.22	Pulmonary hypertension due to left heart disease
I27.23	Pulmonary hypertension due to lung diseases and hypoxia
I27.24	Chronic thromboembolic pulmonary hypertension
I27.29	Other secondary pulmonary hypertension
I27.83	Eisenmenger's syndrome
I27.89	Other specified pulmonary heart diseases
I27.9	Pulmonary heart disease, unspecified
I40.0	Infective myocarditis
I40.1	Isolated myocarditis
I40.8	Other acute myocarditis
I42.0	Dilated cardiomyopathy
I42.1	Obstructive hypertrophic cardiomyopathy
I42.3	Endomyocardial (eosinophilic) disease
I42.4	Endocardial fibroelastosis
I42.5	Other restrictive cardiomyopathy
I42.8	Other cardiomyopathies
I43	Cardiomyopathy in diseases classified elsewhere
I50.1	Left ventricular failure, unspecified
I50.21	Acute systolic (congestive) heart failure
I50.22	Chronic systolic (congestive) heart failure
I50.23	Acute on chronic systolic (congestive) heart failure
I50.31	Acute diastolic (congestive) heart failure
I50.32	Chronic diastolic (congestive) heart failure
I50.33	Acute on chronic diastolic (congestive) heart failure
I50.41	Acute combined systolic (congestive) and diastolic (congestive) heart failure
I50.42	Chronic combined systolic (congestive) and diastolic (congestive) heart failure
I50.43	Acute on chronic combined systolic (congestive) and diastolic (congestive) heart failure
I50.811	Acute right heart failure
I50.812	Chronic right heart failure
I50.813	Acute on chronic right heart failure
I50.814	Right heart failure due to left heart failure
I50.82	Biventricular heart failure
I50.83	High output heart failure
I50.84	End stage heart failure
I50.9	Heart failure, unspecified
I51.5	Myocardial degeneration
I51.7	Cardiomegaly
I51.89	Other ill-defined heart diseases
Q20.6	Isomerism of atrial appendages
Q20.8	Other congenital malformations of cardiac chambers and connections

Q21.8	Other congenital malformations of cardiac septa
Q24.4	Congenital subaortic stenosis
Q24.5	Malformation of coronary vessels
Q24.6	Congenital heart block
Q24.8	Other specified congenital malformations of heart
Q24.9	Congenital malformation of heart, unspecified

AMA: 33945 2018,Jun,3; 2017,Dec,3

Relative Value Units/Medicare Edits

Non-Facility RVU	Work	PE	MP	Total
33945	89.5	30.58	21.26	141.34
Facility RVU	**Work**	**PE**	**MP**	**Total**
33945	89.5	30.58	21.26	141.34

	FUD	Status	MUE	Modifiers				IOM Reference
33945	90	R	1(2)	51	N/A	62*	80	None

* with documentation

Terms To Know

atherosclerosis. Buildup of yellowish plaques composed of cholesterol and lipoid material within the arteries.

cadaver. Dead body.

cardiectomy. Excision of the cardiac portion of the stomach.

cardiomyopathy. General term used to describe a number of conditions of the heart muscle.

cardiopulmonary bypass. Venous blood is diverted to a heart-lung machine, which mechanically pumps and oxygenates the blood temporarily so the heart can be bypassed while an open procedure on the heart or coronary arteries is performed. During bypass, the lungs are deflated and immobile.

congestive heart failure. Condition caused by the heart's inability to adequately pump and circulate blood, resulting in fluid accumulation in the lungs and other tissues.

rheumatic heart disease. Manifestation of and sequel to rheumatic fever; any cardiac involvement in rheumatic fever.

transplant. Insertion of an organ or tissue from one person or site into another.

33946-33947

33946 Extracorporeal membrane oxygenation (ECMO)/extracorporeal life support (ECLS) provided by physician; initiation, veno-venous

33947 initiation, veno-arterial

Any of several variations of extracorporeal circulation may be employed. The configurations vary according to the type of surgery that has taken place or the type of heart/lung insufficiency

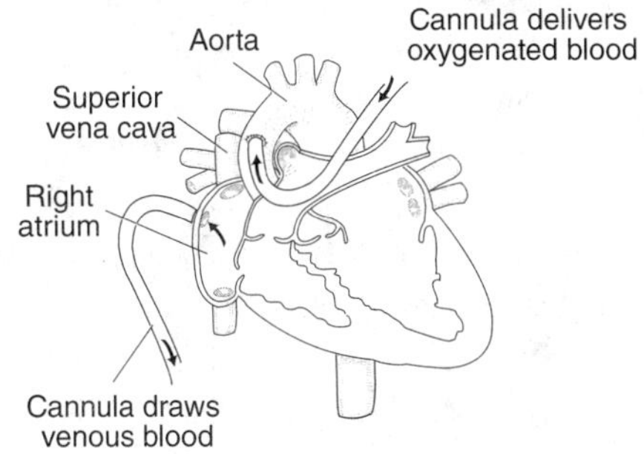

Explanation

The physician initiates veno-venous or veno-arterial extracorporeal membrane oxygenation (ECMO)/extracorporeal life support (ECLS). In ECMO/ECLS, the patient's blood is pumped to a machine, oxygenated, and returned to the patient, similar to a cardiopulmonary bypass but modified for prolonged use (days to weeks) at the bedside. Its purpose is to provide mechanical support for the heart and lungs in order to allow time for recovery. Report 33946 for initiation of veno-venous ECMO/ECLS, which exchanges blood between large veins through a single double-lumen cannula. Report 33947 for initiation of veno-arterial ECMO/ECLS, which exchanges oxygen poor blood from a central vein or right atrium with oxygen rich blood pumped back into the patient within the arterial circulation through two cannulae: one into a vein and the other into an artery.

Coding Tips

These services are reported separately in addition to daily management, hospital observation, inpatient, or critical care codes. The physician providing all components of ECMO/ECLS should report all codes for services provided. When performed by different providers, each should bill for the service performed. If extensive repair or replacement of an artery is required and performed, report 35266, 35286, 35371, or 35665 in addition to 33946 and 33947. Do not report 33946 or 33947 with daily management codes 33948 and 33949 or repositioning codes 33957–33959 and 33962–33964. Do not append modifier 63 to 33946 and 33947 as the description or nature of the procedure includes infants up to 4 kg. For cannula insertion, see 33951–33956.

ICD-10-CM Diagnostic Codes

I40.0	Infective myocarditis
I40.1	Isolated myocarditis
I50.21	Acute systolic (congestive) heart failure
I50.22	Chronic systolic (congestive) heart failure
I50.23	Acute on chronic systolic (congestive) heart failure
I50.31	Acute diastolic (congestive) heart failure
I50.32	Chronic diastolic (congestive) heart failure
I50.33	Acute on chronic diastolic (congestive) heart failure
I50.41	Acute combined systolic (congestive) and diastolic (congestive) heart failure

I50.42	Chronic combined systolic (congestive) and diastolic (congestive) heart failure
I50.43	Acute on chronic combined systolic (congestive) and diastolic (congestive) heart failure
I50.811	Acute right heart failure
I50.812	Chronic right heart failure
I50.813	Acute on chronic right heart failure
I50.814	Right heart failure due to left heart failure
I50.82	Biventricular heart failure
I50.83	High output heart failure
I50.84	End stage heart failure
I97.0	Postcardiotomy syndrome
I97.110	Postprocedural cardiac insufficiency following cardiac surgery
I97.120	Postprocedural cardiac arrest following cardiac surgery
I97.130	Postprocedural heart failure following cardiac surgery
J80	Acute respiratory distress syndrome
J93.0	Spontaneous tension pneumothorax
J93.11	Primary spontaneous pneumothorax
J93.12	Secondary spontaneous pneumothorax
J93.81	Chronic pneumothorax
J95.1	Acute pulmonary insufficiency following thoracic surgery
J95.3	Chronic pulmonary insufficiency following surgery
J95.822	Acute and chronic postprocedural respiratory failure
J95.851	Ventilator associated pneumonia
J96.01	Acute respiratory failure with hypoxia
J96.02	Acute respiratory failure with hypercapnia
J96.11	Chronic respiratory failure with hypoxia
J96.12	Chronic respiratory failure with hypercapnia
J96.21	Acute and chronic respiratory failure with hypoxia
J96.22	Acute and chronic respiratory failure with hypercapnia
P22.0	Respiratory distress syndrome of newborn
P25.0	Interstitial emphysema originating in the perinatal period
P25.1	Pneumothorax originating in the perinatal period
P28.5	Respiratory failure of newborn
P28.81	Respiratory arrest of newborn
P29.0	Neonatal cardiac failure
P29.2	Neonatal hypertension
P29.30	Pulmonary hypertension of newborn
P29.4	Transient myocardial ischemia in newborn
P29.81	Cardiac arrest of newborn
Q22.2	Congenital pulmonary valve insufficiency
R06.03	Acute respiratory distress
R09.2	Respiratory arrest
R57.0	Cardiogenic shock
S27.0XXA	Traumatic pneumothorax, initial encounter
S27.1XXA	Traumatic hemothorax, initial encounter
S27.2XXA	Traumatic hemopneumothorax, initial encounter
T81.11XA	Postprocedural cardiogenic shock, initial encounter

AMA: 33946 2018,Jan,8; 2017,Jan,8; 2016,Mar,5; 2016,Jan,13; 2015,Jul,3
33947 2018,Jan,8; 2017,Jan,8; 2016,Mar,5; 2016,Jan,13; 2015,Jul,3

Relative Value Units/Medicare Edits

Non-Facility RVU	Work	PE	MP	Total
33946	6.0	1.76	1.23	8.99
33947	6.63	1.93	1.41	9.97
Facility RVU	**Work**	**PE**	**MP**	**Total**
33946	6.0	1.76	1.23	8.99
33947	6.63	1.93	1.41	9.97

	FUD	Status	MUE	Modifiers				IOM Reference
33946	N/A	A	1(2)	N/A	N/A	N/A	N/A	None
33947	N/A	A	1(2)	N/A	N/A	N/A	N/A	

* with documentation

Terms To Know

anomaly. Irregularity in the structure or position of an organ or tissue.

cardiogenic shock. Shock caused by an inadequate supply of oxygen to the body's tissues due to a malfunction of the pumping action of the heart.

congenital anomaly. Abnormality that is present at birth that may be the result of genetic factors, teratogens, or other conditions that affect the fetus in utero. The abnormalities may be readily apparent at birth or may remain undiscovered until some point after birth.

extracorporeal. Located or taking place outside the body.

meconium aspiration syndrome. Newborn respiratory complications resulting from the passage and subsequent aspiration of meconium (fetal intestinal waste material) prior to or during delivery.

respiratory distress syndrome. Premature neonates with respiratory distress and associated with reduced amounts of lung surfactant. Frequently fatal.

33948-33949

33948 Extracorporeal membrane oxygenation (ECMO)/extracorporeal life support (ECLS) provided by physician; daily management, each day, veno-venous

33949 daily management, each day, veno-arterial

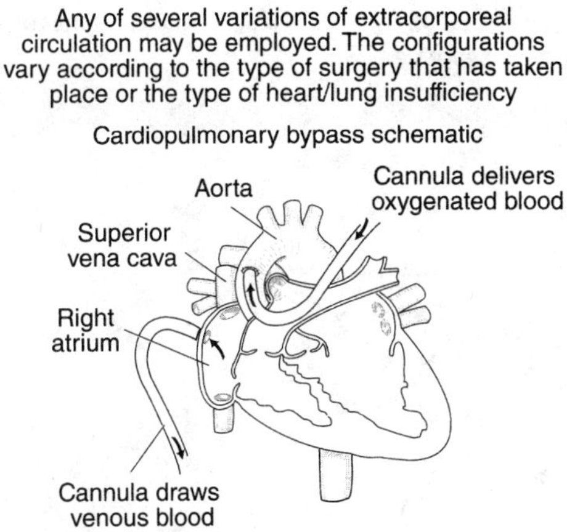

Explanation

The physician performs daily management of extracorporeal membrane oxygenation (ECMO)/extracorporeal life support (ECLS). In ECMO/ECLS, the patient's blood is pumped to a machine, oxygenated, and returned to the patient, similar to a cardiopulmonary bypass but modified for prolonged use (days to weeks) at the bedside. Its purpose is to provide mechanical support for the heart and lungs in order to allow time for recovery. Patients receiving ECMO/ECLS require daily management to monitor for infections of the skin along cannulas and to identify any evidence of clotting in the legs or any deposits visualized within the pump. Report 33948 for daily management of veno-venous ECMO/ECLS, which exchanges blood between large veins through a single double-lumen cannula. Report 33949 for daily management of veno-arterial ECMO/ECLS, which exchanges oxygen poor blood from a central vein or right atrium with oxygen rich blood pumped back into the patient within the arterial circulation through two cannulae: one into a vein and the other into an artery.

Coding Tips

These services are separately reported in addition to daily overall management reported with hospital observation, inpatient, or critical care codes. Do not append modifier 63 to 33948 and 33949 as the description or nature of the procedure includes infants up to 4 kg. Do not report 33948 and 33949 with 33946 or 33947.

ICD-10-CM Diagnostic Codes

I40.0	Infective myocarditis
I40.1	Isolated myocarditis
I50.21	Acute systolic (congestive) heart failure
I50.22	Chronic systolic (congestive) heart failure
I50.23	Acute on chronic systolic (congestive) heart failure
I50.31	Acute diastolic (congestive) heart failure
I50.32	Chronic diastolic (congestive) heart failure
I50.33	Acute on chronic diastolic (congestive) heart failure
I50.41	Acute combined systolic (congestive) and diastolic (congestive) heart failure
I50.42	Chronic combined systolic (congestive) and diastolic (congestive) heart failure
I50.43	Acute on chronic combined systolic (congestive) and diastolic (congestive) heart failure
I50.811	Acute right heart failure
I50.812	Chronic right heart failure
I50.813	Acute on chronic right heart failure
I50.814	Right heart failure due to left heart failure
I50.82	Biventricular heart failure
I50.83	High output heart failure
I50.84	End stage heart failure
I97.0	Postcardiotomy syndrome
I97.110	Postprocedural cardiac insufficiency following cardiac surgery
I97.120	Postprocedural cardiac arrest following cardiac surgery
I97.130	Postprocedural heart failure following cardiac surgery
J80	Acute respiratory distress syndrome
J93.0	Spontaneous tension pneumothorax
J93.11	Primary spontaneous pneumothorax
J93.12	Secondary spontaneous pneumothorax
J93.81	Chronic pneumothorax
J95.1	Acute pulmonary insufficiency following thoracic surgery
J95.3	Chronic pulmonary insufficiency following surgery
J95.822	Acute and chronic postprocedural respiratory failure
J95.851	Ventilator associated pneumonia
J96.01	Acute respiratory failure with hypoxia
J96.02	Acute respiratory failure with hypercapnia
J96.11	Chronic respiratory failure with hypoxia
J96.12	Chronic respiratory failure with hypercapnia
J96.21	Acute and chronic respiratory failure with hypoxia
J96.22	Acute and chronic respiratory failure with hypercapnia
P22.0	Respiratory distress syndrome of newborn
P25.0	Interstitial emphysema originating in the perinatal period
P25.1	Pneumothorax originating in the perinatal period
P28.5	Respiratory failure of newborn
P28.81	Respiratory arrest of newborn
P29.0	Neonatal cardiac failure
P29.2	Neonatal hypertension
P29.30	Pulmonary hypertension of newborn
P29.4	Transient myocardial ischemia in newborn
P29.81	Cardiac arrest of newborn
Q22.2	Congenital pulmonary valve insufficiency
R06.03	Acute respiratory distress
R09.2	Respiratory arrest
R57.0	Cardiogenic shock
S27.0XXA	Traumatic pneumothorax, initial encounter
S27.1XXA	Traumatic hemothorax, initial encounter
S27.2XXA	Traumatic hemopneumothorax, initial encounter
T81.11XA	Postprocedural cardiogenic shock, initial encounter

AMA: 33948 2018,Jan,8; 2017,Jan,8; 2016,Mar,5; 2016,Jan,13; 2015,Jul,3
33949 2018,Jan,8; 2017,Jan,8; 2016,Mar,5; 2016,Jan,13; 2015,Jul,3

Relative Value Units/Medicare Edits

Non-Facility RVU	Work	PE	MP	Total
33948	4.73	1.44	0.74	6.91
33949	4.6	1.34	0.78	6.72
Facility RVU	**Work**	**PE**	**MP**	**Total**
33948	4.73	1.44	0.74	6.91
33949	4.6	1.34	0.78	6.72

	FUD	Status	MUE	Modifiers				IOM Reference
33948	N/A	A	1(2)	N/A	N/A	N/A	N/A	None
33949	N/A	A	1(2)	N/A	N/A	N/A	N/A	

* with documentation

Terms To Know

hypercapnia. Excess carbon dioxide in the blood.

hypoxia. Organ or tissue receiving an oxygen supply that is below the necessary oxygen levels, even when there is adequate blood perfusion.

myocarditis. Inflammation of the middle layer of the heart, which is composed of muscle tissue.

pneumothorax. Collapsed lung due to air or gas trapped in the pleural space formed by the membrane that encloses the lungs and lines the thoracic cavity.

33951-33952

33951 Extracorporeal membrane oxygenation (ECMO)/extracorporeal life support (ECLS) provided by physician; insertion of peripheral (arterial and/or venous) cannula(e), percutaneous, birth through 5 years of age (includes fluoroscopic guidance, when performed)

33952 insertion of peripheral (arterial and/or venous) cannula(e), percutaneous, 6 years and older (includes fluoroscopic guidance, when performed)

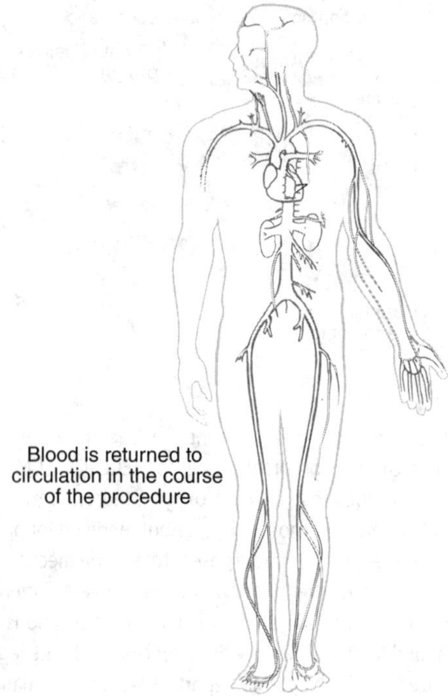

Explanation

The physician inserts a peripheral cannula for extracorporeal membrane oxygenation (ECMO)/extracorporeal life support (ECLS) percutaneously. When veno-arterial ECMO/ECLS is performed, a cannula is typically placed in the inferior vena cava or right atrium allowing for drainage. This cannula is introduced at the internal jugular or femoral vein. The blood is pumped back into the patient through a cannula placed within the femoral artery. When veno-venous ECMO/ECLS is performed, two or more cannulae are used within the large veins (jugular, femoral, or both) to assist with draining and oxygenated blood flow. A relatively new dual-chamber cannula is being utilized in some facilities for improved drainage, to reduce the risk of complications, and to improve the ability to move the patient. Report 33951 for peripheral insertion of a cannula performed percutaneously on patients from birth through age 5 and 33952 for patients age 6 years and older. Fluoroscopic guidance is included in these procedures when performed.

Coding Tips

For initiation and daily management/maintenance of extracorporeal circulation, see 33946, 33947, 33948, and 33949. The physician providing all components of ECMO/ECLS should report all codes for services provided. When performed by different providers, each should bill for the service performed. If cannula is taken from one vessel and inserted into another, report the removal (33965–33969, 33984–33986, and 33955–33956) and insertion (33951–33955) codes. However, if cannula(e) is removed and reinserted into the same vessel, report only the insertion codes. If extensive repair or replacement of an artery is required and performed, report 35266, 35286, 35371, or 35665 in addition to 33951 and 33952. Do not report repositioning of cannula (33957–33959 and 33962–33964) with 33951 and 33952.

ICD-10-CM Diagnostic Codes

I40.0	Infective myocarditis
I40.1	Isolated myocarditis
I50.21	Acute systolic (congestive) heart failure
I50.22	Chronic systolic (congestive) heart failure
I50.23	Acute on chronic systolic (congestive) heart failure
I50.31	Acute diastolic (congestive) heart failure
I50.32	Chronic diastolic (congestive) heart failure
I50.33	Acute on chronic diastolic (congestive) heart failure
I50.41	Acute combined systolic (congestive) and diastolic (congestive) heart failure
I50.42	Chronic combined systolic (congestive) and diastolic (congestive) heart failure
I50.43	Acute on chronic combined systolic (congestive) and diastolic (congestive) heart failure
I50.811	Acute right heart failure
I50.812	Chronic right heart failure
I50.813	Acute on chronic right heart failure
I50.814	Right heart failure due to left heart failure
I50.82	Biventricular heart failure
I50.83	High output heart failure
I50.84	End stage heart failure
I97.0	Postcardiotomy syndrome
I97.110	Postprocedural cardiac insufficiency following cardiac surgery
I97.120	Postprocedural cardiac arrest following cardiac surgery
I97.130	Postprocedural heart failure following cardiac surgery
J80	Acute respiratory distress syndrome
J93.0	Spontaneous tension pneumothorax
J93.11	Primary spontaneous pneumothorax
J93.12	Secondary spontaneous pneumothorax
J93.81	Chronic pneumothorax
J95.1	Acute pulmonary insufficiency following thoracic surgery
J95.3	Chronic pulmonary insufficiency following surgery
J95.822	Acute and chronic postprocedural respiratory failure
J95.851	Ventilator associated pneumonia
J96.01	Acute respiratory failure with hypoxia
J96.02	Acute respiratory failure with hypercapnia
J96.11	Chronic respiratory failure with hypoxia
J96.12	Chronic respiratory failure with hypercapnia
J96.21	Acute and chronic respiratory failure with hypoxia
J96.22	Acute and chronic respiratory failure with hypercapnia
P22.0	Respiratory distress syndrome of newborn
P25.0	Interstitial emphysema originating in the perinatal period
P25.1	Pneumothorax originating in the perinatal period
P28.5	Respiratory failure of newborn
P28.81	Respiratory arrest of newborn
P29.0	Neonatal cardiac failure
P29.2	Neonatal hypertension
P29.30	Pulmonary hypertension of newborn
P29.4	Transient myocardial ischemia in newborn
P29.81	Cardiac arrest of newborn
Q22.2	Congenital pulmonary valve insufficiency
R06.03	Acute respiratory distress
R09.2	Respiratory arrest
R57.0	Cardiogenic shock
S27.0XXA	Traumatic pneumothorax, initial encounter
S27.1XXA	Traumatic hemothorax, initial encounter
S27.2XXA	Traumatic hemopneumothorax, initial encounter
T81.11XA	Postprocedural cardiogenic shock, initial encounter

AMA: 33951 2018,Jan,8; 2017,Jan,8; 2016,Mar,5; 2016,Jan,13; 2015,Jul,3
33952 2018,Jan,8; 2017,Jan,8; 2016,Mar,5; 2016,Jan,13; 2015,Jul,3

Relative Value Units/Medicare Edits

Non-Facility RVU	Work	PE	MP	Total
33951	8.15	2.32	1.91	12.38
33952	8.15	2.46	1.82	12.43
Facility RVU	**Work**	**PE**	**MP**	**Total**
33951	8.15	2.32	1.91	12.38
33952	8.15	2.46	1.82	12.43

	FUD	Status	MUE	Modifiers				IOM Reference
33951	0	A	1(3)	51	N/A	N/A	80*	None
33952	0	A	1(3)	51	N/A	N/A	80*	

* with documentation

Terms To Know

asphyxia. Insufficient intake of oxygen, resulting in pathological changes brought on by a lack of oxygen perfusion to the tissues or excessive carbon dioxide in the blood.

cannula. Tube inserted into a blood vessel, duct, or body cavity to facilitate passage.

extracorporeal. Located or taking place outside the body.

fluoroscopy. Radiology technique that allows visual examination of part of the body or a function of an organ using a device that projects an x-ray image on a fluorescent screen.

meconium aspiration syndrome. Newborn respiratory complications resulting from the passage and subsequent aspiration of meconium (fetal intestinal waste material) prior to or during delivery.

33953-33954

33953 Extracorporeal membrane oxygenation (ECMO)/extracorporeal life support (ECLS) provided by physician; insertion of peripheral (arterial and/or venous) cannula(e), open, birth through 5 years of age

33954 insertion of peripheral (arterial and/or venous) cannula(e), open, 6 years and older

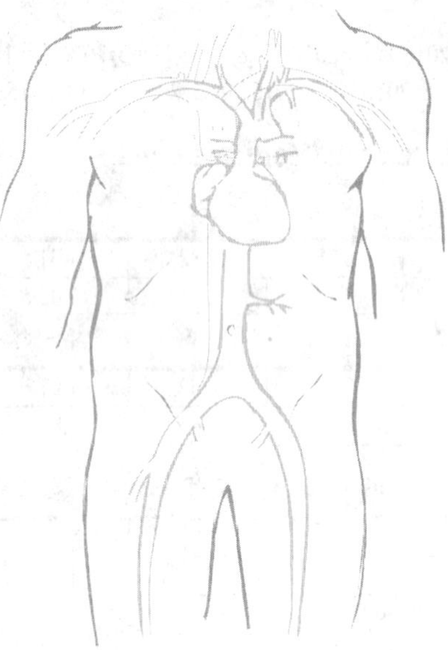

Open insertion of a cannula into a peripheral artery or vein, such as the femoral artery

Explanation

The physician inserts a peripheral cannula for extracorporeal membrane oxygenation (ECMO)/extracorporeal life support (ECLS) using an open approach. When veno-arterial ECMO/ECLS is performed, a cannula is typically placed in the inferior vena cava or right atrium allowing for drainage. This cannula is introduced at the internal jugular or femoral vein. The blood is pumped back into the patient through a cannula placed within the femoral artery. When veno-venous ECMO/ECLS is performed, two or more cannulae are used within the large veins (jugular, femoral, or both) to assist with draining and oxygenated blood flow. A relatively new dual-chamber cannula is being utilized in some facilities for improved drainage, to reduce the risk of complications, and to improve the ability to move the patient. Report 33953 for peripheral insertion of a cannula using an open approach on patients from birth through age 5 and 33954 for patients age 6 years and older.

Coding Tips

For initiation and daily management/maintenance of extracorporeal circulation, see 33946, 33947, 33948, and 33949. The physician providing all components of ECMO/ECLS should report all codes for services provided. When performed by different providers, each should bill for the service performed. If cannula is taken from one vessel and inserted into another, report the removal (33965–33969, 33984–33986, and 33955–33956) and insertion (33951–33955) codes. However, if cannula(e) is removed and reinserted into the same vessel, report only the insertion codes. If extensive repair or replacement of an artery is required and performed, report 35266, 35286, 35371, or 35665 in addition to 33953 and 33954. Do not report 33953 or 33954 with 34714-34716, 34812, 34820, 34833, and 34834.

ICD-10-CM Diagnostic Codes

I40.0	Infective myocarditis
I40.1	Isolated myocarditis
I50.21	Acute systolic (congestive) heart failure
I50.22	Chronic systolic (congestive) heart failure
I50.23	Acute on chronic systolic (congestive) heart failure
I50.31	Acute diastolic (congestive) heart failure
I50.32	Chronic diastolic (congestive) heart failure
I50.33	Acute on chronic diastolic (congestive) heart failure
I50.41	Acute combined systolic (congestive) and diastolic (congestive) heart failure
I50.42	Chronic combined systolic (congestive) and diastolic (congestive) heart failure
I50.43	Acute on chronic combined systolic (congestive) and diastolic (congestive) heart failure
I50.811	Acute right heart failure
I50.812	Chronic right heart failure
I50.813	Acute on chronic right heart failure
I50.814	Right heart failure due to left heart failure
I50.82	Biventricular heart failure
I50.83	High output heart failure
I50.84	End stage heart failure
I97.0	Postcardiotomy syndrome
I97.110	Postprocedural cardiac insufficiency following cardiac surgery
I97.120	Postprocedural cardiac arrest following cardiac surgery
I97.130	Postprocedural heart failure following cardiac surgery
J80	Acute respiratory distress syndrome
J93.0	Spontaneous tension pneumothorax
J93.11	Primary spontaneous pneumothorax
J93.12	Secondary spontaneous pneumothorax
J93.81	Chronic pneumothorax
J95.1	Acute pulmonary insufficiency following thoracic surgery
J95.3	Chronic pulmonary insufficiency following surgery
J95.822	Acute and chronic postprocedural respiratory failure
J95.851	Ventilator associated pneumonia
J96.01	Acute respiratory failure with hypoxia
J96.02	Acute respiratory failure with hypercapnia
J96.11	Chronic respiratory failure with hypoxia
J96.12	Chronic respiratory failure with hypercapnia
J96.21	Acute and chronic respiratory failure with hypoxia
J96.22	Acute and chronic respiratory failure with hypercapnia
P22.0	Respiratory distress syndrome of newborn
P25.0	Interstitial emphysema originating in the perinatal period
P25.1	Pneumothorax originating in the perinatal period
P28.5	Respiratory failure of newborn
P28.81	Respiratory arrest of newborn
P29.0	Neonatal cardiac failure
P29.2	Neonatal hypertension
P29.30	Pulmonary hypertension of newborn
P29.4	Transient myocardial ischemia in newborn
P29.81	Cardiac arrest of newborn
Q22.2	Congenital pulmonary valve insufficiency
R06.03	Acute respiratory distress
R09.2	Respiratory arrest
R57.0	Cardiogenic shock
S27.0XXA	Traumatic pneumothorax, initial encounter

S27.1XXA Traumatic hemothorax, initial encounter
S27.2XXA Traumatic hemopneumothorax, initial encounter
T81.11XA Postprocedural cardiogenic shock, initial encounter

AMA: **33953** 2018,Jan,8; 2017,Jan,8; 2017,Dec,3; 2016,Mar,5; 2016,Jan,13; 2015,Jul,3 **33954** 2018,Jan,8; 2017,Jan,8; 2017,Dec,3; 2016,Mar,5; 2016,Jan,13; 2015,Jul,3

Relative Value Units/Medicare Edits

Non-Facility RVU	Work	PE	MP	Total
33953	9.11	2.59	2.14	13.84
33954	9.11	2.68	2.09	13.88
Facility RVU	**Work**	**PE**	**MP**	**Total**
33953	9.11	2.59	2.14	13.84
33954	9.11	2.68	2.09	13.88

	FUD	Status	MUE	Modifiers				IOM Reference
33953	0	A	1(3)	51	N/A	N/A	80*	None
33954	0	A	1(3)	51	N/A	N/A	80*	

* with documentation

Terms To Know

asphyxia. Insufficient intake of oxygen, resulting in pathological changes brought on by a lack of oxygen perfusion to the tissues or excessive carbon dioxide in the blood.

cannula. Tube inserted into a blood vessel, duct, or body cavity to facilitate passage.

cardiogenic shock. Shock caused by an inadequate supply of oxygen to the body's tissues due to a malfunction of the pumping action of the heart.

congenital. Present at birth, occurring through heredity or an influence during gestation up to the moment of birth.

extracorporeal. Located or taking place outside the body.

meconium aspiration syndrome. Newborn respiratory complications resulting from the passage and subsequent aspiration of meconium (fetal intestinal waste material) prior to or during delivery.

vena cava. Main venous trunk that empties into the right atrium from both the lower and upper regions, beginning at the junction of the common iliac veins inferiorly and the two brachiocephalic veins superiorly.

33955-33956

33955 Extracorporeal membrane oxygenation (ECMO)/extracorporeal life support (ECLS) provided by physician; insertion of central cannula(e) by sternotomy or thoracotomy, birth through 5 years of age

33956 insertion of central cannula(e) by sternotomy or thoracotomy, 6 years and older

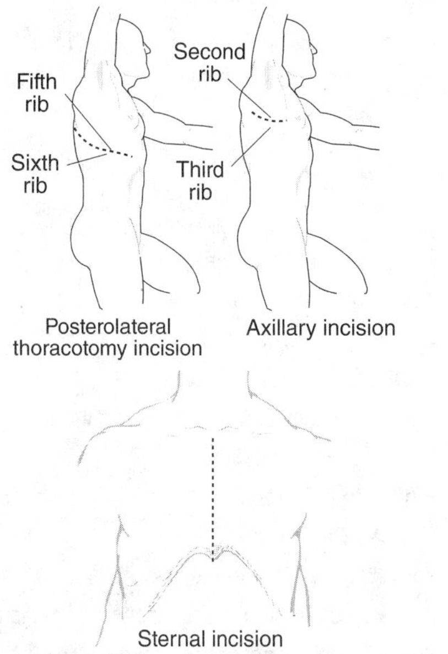

Any of a number of access incisions may be used

Explanation

The physician inserts central cannulae for extracorporeal membrane oxygenation (ECMO)/extracorporeal life support (ECLS) via sternotomy or thoracotomy. A cannula is placed in the inferior vena cava or right atrium allowing for drainage. This cannula is introduced at the internal jugular or femoral vein accomplished by sternotomy or thoracotomy. The blood is pumped back into the patient through a cannula surgically placed within the ascending aorta, referred to as central ECMO/ECLS. This form of introduction is typically utilized following cardiopulmonary bypass since the location of cannulae placement would be the same as location during surgery. When veno-venous ECMO/ECLS is performed, two or more cannulae are used within the large veins (jugular, femoral, or both) to assist with draining and oxygenated blood flow. A relatively new dual-chamber cannula is being utilized in some facilities for improved drainage, to reduce the risk of complications, and to improve the ability to move the patient. Report 33955 for centrally inserted cannulae by sternotomy or thoracotomy performed on patients from birth through age 5 and 33956 for patients age 6 years and older.

Coding Tips

For initiation and daily management/maintenance of extracorporeal circulation, see 33946, 33947, 33948, and 33949. The physician providing all components of ECMO/ECLS should report all codes for services provided. When performed by different providers, each should bill for the service performed. If cannula is taken from one vessel and inserted into another, report the removal (33965–33969, 33984–33986), and insertion (33951–33955) codes. However, if cannula(e) is removed and reinserted into the same vessel, report only the insertion codes. If extensive repair or replacement of an artery is required and performed, report 35266, 35286, 35371, or 35665 in addition to 33955 and 33956. Do not report 33955 or 33956 with 32100 or 39010.

ICD-10-CM Diagnostic Codes

I40.0	Infective myocarditis
I40.1	Isolated myocarditis
I50.21	Acute systolic (congestive) heart failure
I50.22	Chronic systolic (congestive) heart failure
I50.23	Acute on chronic systolic (congestive) heart failure
I50.31	Acute diastolic (congestive) heart failure
I50.32	Chronic diastolic (congestive) heart failure
I50.33	Acute on chronic diastolic (congestive) heart failure
I50.41	Acute combined systolic (congestive) and diastolic (congestive) heart failure
I50.42	Chronic combined systolic (congestive) and diastolic (congestive) heart failure
I50.43	Acute on chronic combined systolic (congestive) and diastolic (congestive) heart failure
I50.811	Acute right heart failure
I50.812	Chronic right heart failure
I50.813	Acute on chronic right heart failure
I50.814	Right heart failure due to left heart failure
I50.82	Biventricular heart failure
I50.83	High output heart failure
I50.84	End stage heart failure
I97.0	Postcardiotomy syndrome
I97.110	Postprocedural cardiac insufficiency following cardiac surgery
I97.120	Postprocedural cardiac arrest following cardiac surgery
I97.130	Postprocedural heart failure following cardiac surgery
J80	Acute respiratory distress syndrome
J93.0	Spontaneous tension pneumothorax
J93.11	Primary spontaneous pneumothorax
J93.12	Secondary spontaneous pneumothorax
J93.81	Chronic pneumothorax
J95.1	Acute pulmonary insufficiency following thoracic surgery
J95.3	Chronic pulmonary insufficiency following surgery
J95.822	Acute and chronic postprocedural respiratory failure
J95.851	Ventilator associated pneumonia
J96.01	Acute respiratory failure with hypoxia
J96.02	Acute respiratory failure with hypercapnia
J96.11	Chronic respiratory failure with hypoxia
J96.12	Chronic respiratory failure with hypercapnia
J96.21	Acute and chronic respiratory failure with hypoxia
J96.22	Acute and chronic respiratory failure with hypercapnia
P22.0	Respiratory distress syndrome of newborn
P25.0	Interstitial emphysema originating in the perinatal period
P25.1	Pneumothorax originating in the perinatal period
P28.5	Respiratory failure of newborn
P28.81	Respiratory arrest of newborn
P29.0	Neonatal cardiac failure
P29.2	Neonatal hypertension
P29.30	Pulmonary hypertension of newborn
P29.4	Transient myocardial ischemia in newborn
P29.81	Cardiac arrest of newborn
Q22.2	Congenital pulmonary valve insufficiency
R06.03	Acute respiratory distress
R09.2	Respiratory arrest
R57.0	Cardiogenic shock
S27.0XXA	Traumatic pneumothorax, initial encounter
S27.1XXA	Traumatic hemothorax, initial encounter
S27.2XXA	Traumatic hemopneumothorax, initial encounter
T81.11XA	Postprocedural cardiogenic shock, initial encounter

AMA: 33955 2018,Jan,8; 2017,Jan,8; 2016,Mar,5; 2016,Jan,13; 2015,Jul,3 **33956** 2018,Jan,8; 2017,Jan,8; 2016,Mar,5; 2016,Jan,13; 2015,Jul,3

Relative Value Units/Medicare Edits

Non-Facility RVU	Work	PE	MP	Total
33955	16.0	4.48	3.78	24.26
33956	16.0	4.6	3.62	24.22
Facility RVU	**Work**	**PE**	**MP**	**Total**
33955	16.0	4.48	3.78	24.26
33956	16.0	4.6	3.62	24.22

	FUD	Status	MUE	Modifiers				IOM Reference
33955	0	A	1(3)	51	N/A	62*	80*	None
33956	0	A	1(3)	51	N/A	62*	80*	

* with documentation

Terms To Know

asphyxia. Insufficient intake of oxygen, resulting in pathological changes brought on by a lack of oxygen perfusion to the tissues or excessive carbon dioxide in the blood.

cannula. Tube inserted into a blood vessel, duct, or body cavity to facilitate passage.

cardiogenic shock. Shock caused by an inadequate supply of oxygen to the body's tissues due to a malfunction of the pumping action of the heart.

congenital. Present at birth, occurring through heredity or an influence during gestation up to the moment of birth.

extracorporeal. Located or taking place outside the body.

meconium aspiration syndrome. Newborn respiratory complications resulting from the passage and subsequent aspiration of meconium (fetal intestinal waste material) prior to or during delivery.

vena cava. Main venous trunk that empties into the right atrium from both the lower and upper regions, beginning at the junction of the common iliac veins inferiorly and the two brachiocephalic veins superiorly.

33957-33958

33957 Extracorporeal membrane oxygenation (ECMO)/extracorporeal life support (ECLS) provided by physician; reposition peripheral (arterial and/or venous) cannula(e), percutaneous, birth through 5 years of age (includes fluoroscopic guidance, when performed)

33958 reposition peripheral (arterial and/or venous) cannula(e), percutaneous, 6 years and older (includes fluoroscopic guidance, when performed)

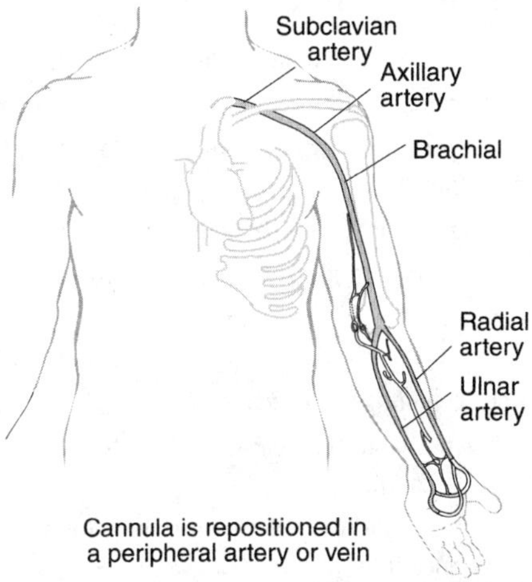

Explanation

The physician repositions a peripheral cannula used for extracorporeal membrane oxygenation (ECMO)/extracorporeal life support (ECLS) percutaneously. Repositioning of the cannula may be necessary in the event of technical and/or vascular complications, such as blood flow obstruction, movement of the cannula from the original position, and/or bleeding issues resulting from the use of heparin during ECMO/ECLS. Oftentimes this requires a pull back of the cannula until it is back in an optimal position; however, in some cases, repositioning may require another procedure to achieve an appropriate position based on the specific location of the cannula and the complication. Report 33957 for percutaneous repositioning performed on a peripheral vessel for patients from birth through age 5 and 33958 for patients age 6 years and older. These codes include fluoroscopic guidance when performed.

Coding Tips

Do not report daily management codes 33948 and 33949 or repositioning codes 33957–33959 and 33962–33964 with 33946 or 33947. Repositioning of the cannula is not reported separately during the same encounter as insertion (33951–33955). Fluoroscopic guidance is included and is not reported separately. Do not report 33957 or 33958 with 34713, 34812, 34820, or 34834.

ICD-10-CM Diagnostic Codes

T82.310A Breakdown (mechanical) of aortic (bifurcation) graft (replacement), initial encounter
T82.311A Breakdown (mechanical) of carotid arterial graft (bypass), initial encounter
T82.312A Breakdown (mechanical) of femoral arterial graft (bypass), initial encounter
T82.318A Breakdown (mechanical) of other vascular grafts, initial encounter
T82.320A Displacement of aortic (bifurcation) graft (replacement), initial encounter
T82.321A Displacement of carotid arterial graft (bypass), initial encounter
T82.322A Displacement of femoral arterial graft (bypass), initial encounter
T82.328A Displacement of other vascular grafts, initial encounter
T82.330A Leakage of aortic (bifurcation) graft (replacement), initial encounter
T82.331A Leakage of carotid arterial graft (bypass), initial encounter
T82.332A Leakage of femoral arterial graft (bypass), initial encounter
T82.338A Leakage of other vascular grafts, initial encounter
T82.390A Other mechanical complication of aortic (bifurcation) graft (replacement), initial encounter
T82.391A Other mechanical complication of carotid arterial graft (bypass), initial encounter
T82.392A Other mechanical complication of femoral arterial graft (bypass), initial encounter
T82.398A Other mechanical complication of other vascular grafts, initial encounter
T82.528A Displacement of other cardiac and vascular devices and implants, initial encounter
T82.538A Leakage of other cardiac and vascular devices and implants, initial encounter
T82.598A Other mechanical complication of other cardiac and vascular devices and implants, initial encounter
T82.818A Embolism due to vascular prosthetic devices, implants and grafts, initial encounter
T82.828A Fibrosis due to vascular prosthetic devices, implants and grafts, initial encounter
T82.838A Hemorrhage due to vascular prosthetic devices, implants and grafts, initial encounter
T82.848A Pain due to vascular prosthetic devices, implants and grafts, initial encounter
T82.856A Stenosis of peripheral vascular stent, initial encounter
T82.858A Stenosis of other vascular prosthetic devices, implants and grafts, initial encounter
T82.868A Thrombosis due to vascular prosthetic devices, implants and grafts, initial encounter
T82.898A Other specified complication of vascular prosthetic devices, implants and grafts, initial encounter
T88.8XXA Other specified complications of surgical and medical care, not elsewhere classified, initial encounter

AMA: **33957** 2018,Jan,8; 2017,Jan,8; 2016,Mar,5; 2016,Jan,13; 2015,Jul,3
33958 2018,Jan,8; 2017,Jan,8; 2016,Mar,5; 2016,Jan,13; 2015,Jul,3

Relative Value Units/Medicare Edits

Non-Facility RVU	Work	PE	MP	Total
33957	3.51	1.06	0.81	5.38
33958	3.51	1.06	0.81	5.38
Facility RVU	**Work**	**PE**	**MP**	**Total**
33957	3.51	1.06	0.81	5.38
33958	3.51	1.06	0.81	5.38

	FUD	Status	MUE	Modifiers				IOM Reference
33957	0	A	1(3)	51	N/A	N/A	80*	None
33958	0	A	1(3)	51	N/A	N/A	80*	

* with documentation

Heart and Pericardium

33959 [33962]

33959 Extracorporeal membrane oxygenation (ECMO)/extracorporeal life support (ECLS) provided by physician; reposition peripheral (arterial and/or venous) cannula(e), open, birth through 5 years of age (includes fluoroscopic guidance, when performed)

33962 Extracorporeal membrane oxygenation (ECMO)/extracorporeal life support (ECLS) provided by physician; reposition peripheral (arterial and/or venous) cannula(e), open, 6 years and older (includes fluoroscopic guidance, when performed)

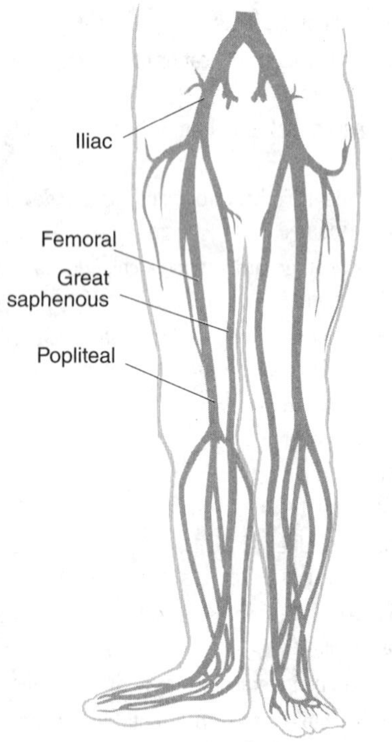

A single segment of femoropopliteal vein is harvested for a vascular reconstruction

Explanation

The physician repositions a peripheral cannula used for extracorporeal membrane oxygenation (ECMO)/extracorporeal life support (ECLS) via an open approach. Repositioning of the cannula may be necessary in the event of technical and/or vascular complications, such as blood flow obstruction, movement of the cannula from the original position, and/or bleeding issues resulting from the use of heparin during ECMO/ECLS. Oftentimes this requires a pull back of the cannula until it is back in an optimal position; however, in some cases, repositioning may require another procedure to achieve an appropriate position based on the specific location of the cannula and the complication. Report 33959 if the reposition is performed by open approach on a peripheral vessel for patients from birth through age 5 and 33962 for patients age 6 years and older. These codes include fluoroscopic guidance when performed.

Coding Tips

Do not report daily management codes 33948 and 33949 or repositioning codes 33957–33959 and 33962–33964 with 33946 and 33947. Repositioning of cannula is not reported separately during the same encounter as insertion (33951–33955). Fluoroscopic guidance is included and is not reported separately. Do not report 33959 or 33962 with 34714-34716, 34812, 34820, or 34834.

ICD-10-CM Diagnostic Codes

T82.310A	Breakdown (mechanical) of aortic (bifurcation) graft (replacement), initial encounter
T82.311A	Breakdown (mechanical) of carotid arterial graft (bypass), initial encounter
T82.312A	Breakdown (mechanical) of femoral arterial graft (bypass), initial encounter
T82.318A	Breakdown (mechanical) of other vascular grafts, initial encounter
T82.320A	Displacement of aortic (bifurcation) graft (replacement), initial encounter
T82.321A	Displacement of carotid arterial graft (bypass), initial encounter
T82.322A	Displacement of femoral arterial graft (bypass), initial encounter
T82.328A	Displacement of other vascular grafts, initial encounter
T82.330A	Leakage of aortic (bifurcation) graft (replacement), initial encounter
T82.331A	Leakage of carotid arterial graft (bypass), initial encounter
T82.332A	Leakage of femoral arterial graft (bypass), initial encounter
T82.338A	Leakage of other vascular grafts, initial encounter
T82.390A	Other mechanical complication of aortic (bifurcation) graft (replacement), initial encounter
T82.391A	Other mechanical complication of carotid arterial graft (bypass), initial encounter
T82.392A	Other mechanical complication of femoral arterial graft (bypass), initial encounter
T82.398A	Other mechanical complication of other vascular grafts, initial encounter
T82.518A	Breakdown (mechanical) of other cardiac and vascular devices and implants, initial encounter
T82.528A	Displacement of other cardiac and vascular devices and implants, initial encounter
T82.538A	Leakage of other cardiac and vascular devices and implants, initial encounter
T82.598A	Other mechanical complication of other cardiac and vascular devices and implants, initial encounter
T82.818A	Embolism due to vascular prosthetic devices, implants and grafts, initial encounter
T82.828A	Fibrosis due to vascular prosthetic devices, implants and grafts, initial encounter
T82.838A	Hemorrhage due to vascular prosthetic devices, implants and grafts, initial encounter
T82.848A	Pain due to vascular prosthetic devices, implants and grafts, initial encounter
T82.858A	Stenosis of other vascular prosthetic devices, implants and grafts, initial encounter
T82.868A	Thrombosis due to vascular prosthetic devices, implants and grafts, initial encounter
T82.898A	Other specified complication of vascular prosthetic devices, implants and grafts, initial encounter
T88.8XXA	Other specified complications of surgical and medical care, not elsewhere classified, initial encounter

AMA: 33959 2018,Jan,8; 2017,Jan,8; 2017,Dec,3; 2016,Mar,5; 2016,Jan,13; 2015,Jul,3 **33962** 2018,Jan,8; 2017,Jan,8; 2017,Dec,3; 2016,Mar,5; 2016,Jan,13; 2015,Jul,3

Heart and Pericardium

Relative Value Units/Medicare Edits

Non-Facility RVU	Work	PE	MP	Total
33959	4.47	1.32	1.05	6.84
33962	4.47	1.32	1.05	6.84
Facility RVU	**Work**	**PE**	**MP**	**Total**
33959	4.47	1.32	1.05	6.84
33962	4.47	1.32	1.05	6.84

	FUD	Status	MUE	Modifiers				IOM Reference
33959	0	A	1(3)	51	N/A	N/A	80*	None
33962	0	A	1(3)	51	N/A	N/A	80*	

* with documentation

Terms To Know

cannula. Tube inserted into a blood vessel, duct, or body cavity to facilitate passage.

extracorporeal membrane oxygenation. Procedure done for cardiopulmonary insufficiency that shunts the circulating venous blood through catheters inserted into the right atrium to the outside of the body where it is oxygenated, bypassing the lungs, then returned to the body through another cannula inserted in the femoral artery.

fluoroscopy. Radiology technique that allows visual examination of part of the body or a function of an organ using a device that projects an x-ray image on a fluorescent screen.

graft. Tissue implant from another part of the body or another person.

implant. Material or device inserted or placed within the body for therapeutic, reconstructive, or diagnostic purposes.

reposition. Placement of an organ or structure into another position or return of an organ or structure to its original position.

vascular. Pertaining to blood vessels.

[33963, 33964]

33963 Extracorporeal membrane oxygenation (ECMO)/extracorporeal life support (ECLS) provided by physician; reposition of central cannula(e) by sternotomy or thoracotomy, birth through 5 years of age (includes fluoroscopic guidance, when performed)

33964 Extracorporeal membrane oxygenation (ECMO)/extracorporeal life support (ECLS) provided by physician; reposition central cannula(e) by sternotomy or thoracotomy, 6 years and older (includes fluoroscopic guidance, when performed)

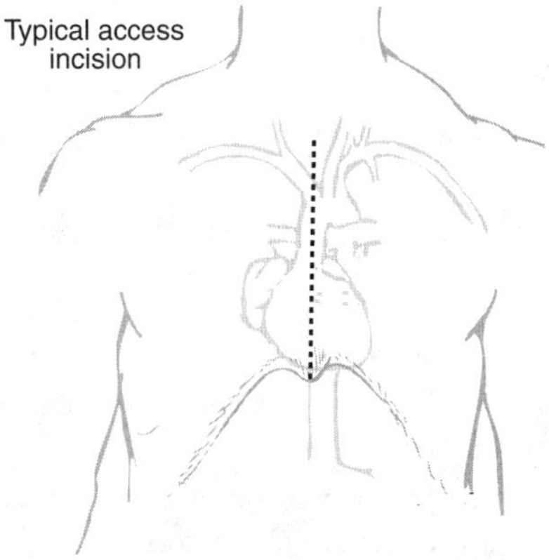

Central cannula is repositioned by sternotomy or thoracotomy

Explanation

The physician repositions a central cannula used for extracorporeal membrane oxygenation (ECMO)/extracorporeal life support (ECLS) via a sternotomy or thoracotomy. Repositioning of the cannula may be necessary in the event of technical and/or vascular complications, such as blood flow obstruction, movement of the cannula from the original position, and/or bleeding issues resulting from the use of heparin during ECMO/ECLS. Oftentimes this requires a pull back of the cannula until it is back in an optimal position; however, in some cases, repositioning may require another procedure to achieve an appropriate position based on the specific location of the cannula and the complication. Report 33963 for repositioning of a central cannula by sternotomy or thoracotomy performed on patients from birth through age 5 and 33964 for patients age 6 years and older. These codes include fluoroscopic guidance when performed.

Coding Tips

Do not report daily management codes 33948 and 33949 or repositioning codes 33957–33959 and 33962–33964 with 33946 and 33947. Repositioning of cannula in not reported separately during the same encounter as insertion (33951–33955). Fluoroscopic guidance is included and is not reported separately. Do not report 33963 or 33964 with 32100 or 39010.

ICD-10-CM Diagnostic Codes

T82.310A	Breakdown (mechanical) of aortic (bifurcation) graft (replacement), initial encounter
T82.311A	Breakdown (mechanical) of carotid arterial graft (bypass), initial encounter
T82.312A	Breakdown (mechanical) of femoral arterial graft (bypass), initial encounter
T82.318A	Breakdown (mechanical) of other vascular grafts, initial encounter
T82.320A	Displacement of aortic (bifurcation) graft (replacement), initial encounter
T82.321A	Displacement of carotid arterial graft (bypass), initial encounter

T82.322A Displacement of femoral arterial graft (bypass), initial encounter
T82.328A Displacement of other vascular grafts, initial encounter
T82.330A Leakage of aortic (bifurcation) graft (replacement), initial encounter
T82.331A Leakage of carotid arterial graft (bypass), initial encounter
T82.332A Leakage of femoral arterial graft (bypass), initial encounter
T82.338A Leakage of other vascular grafts, initial encounter
T82.390A Other mechanical complication of aortic (bifurcation) graft (replacement), initial encounter
T82.391A Other mechanical complication of carotid arterial graft (bypass), initial encounter
T82.392A Other mechanical complication of femoral arterial graft (bypass), initial encounter
T82.398A Other mechanical complication of other vascular grafts, initial encounter
T82.518A Breakdown (mechanical) of other cardiac and vascular devices and implants, initial encounter
T82.528A Displacement of other cardiac and vascular devices and implants, initial encounter
T82.538A Leakage of other cardiac and vascular devices and implants, initial encounter
T82.598A Other mechanical complication of other cardiac and vascular devices and implants, initial encounter
T82.818A Embolism due to vascular prosthetic devices, implants and grafts, initial encounter
T82.828A Fibrosis due to vascular prosthetic devices, implants and grafts, initial encounter
T82.838A Hemorrhage due to vascular prosthetic devices, implants and grafts, initial encounter
T82.848A Pain due to vascular prosthetic devices, implants and grafts, initial encounter
T82.856A Stenosis of peripheral vascular stent, initial encounter
T82.858A Stenosis of other vascular prosthetic devices, implants and grafts, initial encounter
T82.868A Thrombosis due to vascular prosthetic devices, implants and grafts, initial encounter
T82.898A Other specified complication of vascular prosthetic devices, implants and grafts, initial encounter
T88.8XXA Other specified complications of surgical and medical care, not elsewhere classified, initial encounter

AMA: **33963** 2018,Jan,8; 2017,Jan,8; 2016,Mar,5; 2016,Jan,13; 2015,Jul,3
33964 2018,Jan,8; 2017,Jan,8; 2016,Mar,5; 2016,Jan,13; 2015,Jul,3

Relative Value Units/Medicare Edits

Non-Facility RVU	Work	PE	MP	Total
33963	9.0	2.56	2.12	13.68
33964	9.5	2.7	2.24	14.44
Facility RVU	**Work**	**PE**	**MP**	**Total**
33963	9.0	2.56	2.12	13.68
33964	9.5	2.7	2.24	14.44

	FUD	Status	MUE	Modifiers				IOM Reference
33963	0	A	1(3)	51	N/A	62*	80*	None
33964	0	A	1(3)	51	N/A	62*	80*	

* with documentation

[33965, 33966]

33965 Extracorporeal membrane oxygenation (ECMO)/extracorporeal life support (ECLS) provided by physician; removal of peripheral (arterial and/or venous) cannula(e), percutaneous, birth through 5 years of age

33966 Extracorporeal membrane oxygenation (ECMO)/extracorporeal life support (ECLS) provided by physician; removal of peripheral (arterial and/or venous) cannula(e), percutaneous, 6 years and older

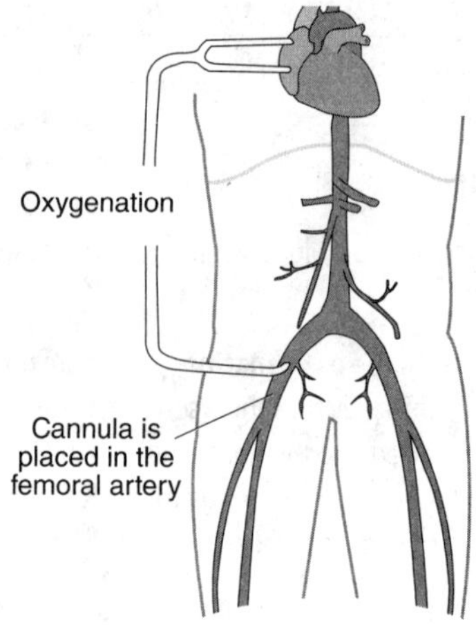

Percutaneous removal of a cannula from a peripheral artery or vein

Explanation

When extracorporeal membrane oxygenation (ECMO)/extracorporeal life support (ECLS) therapy is complete, the physician removes the cannula. Cannulae introduced percutaneously are simply pulled out like any other percutaneous placed catheter. Pressure is applied to the site for a limited time to stop bleeding. Report 33965 for removal of a peripheral percutaneous cannula for patients from birth through age 5 and 33966 for patients age 6 and older.

Coding Tips

If cannula is taken from one vessel and inserted into another, report the removal (33965–33969, 33984–33986, and 33955–33956) and insertion (33951–33955) codes. However, if cannula(e) is removed and reinserted into the same vessel, report only the insertion codes. If extensive repair or replacement of an artery is required and performed, report 35266, 35286, 35371, or 35665 in addition to 33965 and 33966.

ICD-10-CM Diagnostic Codes

T80.1XXA Vascular complications following infusion, transfusion and therapeutic injection, initial encounter
T80.211A Bloodstream infection due to central venous catheter, initial encounter
T80.212A Local infection due to central venous catheter, initial encounter
T80.29XA Infection following other infusion, transfusion and therapeutic injection, initial encounter
T82.310A Breakdown (mechanical) of aortic (bifurcation) graft (replacement), initial encounter
T82.311A Breakdown (mechanical) of carotid arterial graft (bypass), initial encounter

Heart and Pericardium

T82.312A	Breakdown (mechanical) of femoral arterial graft (bypass), initial encounter
T82.318A	Breakdown (mechanical) of other vascular grafts, initial encounter
T82.320A	Displacement of aortic (bifurcation) graft (replacement), initial encounter
T82.321A	Displacement of carotid arterial graft (bypass), initial encounter
T82.322A	Displacement of femoral arterial graft (bypass), initial encounter
T82.328A	Displacement of other vascular grafts, initial encounter
T82.330A	Leakage of aortic (bifurcation) graft (replacement), initial encounter
T82.331A	Leakage of carotid arterial graft (bypass), initial encounter
T82.332A	Leakage of femoral arterial graft (bypass), initial encounter
T82.338A	Leakage of other vascular grafts, initial encounter
T82.390A	Other mechanical complication of aortic (bifurcation) graft (replacement), initial encounter
T82.391A	Other mechanical complication of carotid arterial graft (bypass), initial encounter
T82.392A	Other mechanical complication of femoral arterial graft (bypass), initial encounter
T82.398A	Other mechanical complication of other vascular grafts, initial encounter
T82.518A	Breakdown (mechanical) of other cardiac and vascular devices and implants, initial encounter
T82.528A	Displacement of other cardiac and vascular devices and implants, initial encounter
T82.538A	Leakage of other cardiac and vascular devices and implants, initial encounter
T82.598A	Other mechanical complication of other cardiac and vascular devices and implants, initial encounter
T82.7XXA	Infection and inflammatory reaction due to other cardiac and vascular devices, implants and grafts, initial encounter
T82.818A	Embolism due to vascular prosthetic devices, implants and grafts, initial encounter
T82.828A	Fibrosis due to vascular prosthetic devices, implants and grafts, initial encounter
T82.838A	Hemorrhage due to vascular prosthetic devices, implants and grafts, initial encounter
T82.848A	Pain due to vascular prosthetic devices, implants and grafts, initial encounter
T82.856A	Stenosis of peripheral vascular stent, initial encounter
T82.858A	Stenosis of other vascular prosthetic devices, implants and grafts, initial encounter
T82.868A	Thrombosis due to vascular prosthetic devices, implants and grafts, initial encounter
T82.898A	Other specified complication of vascular prosthetic devices, implants and grafts, initial encounter
T88.8XXA	Other specified complications of surgical and medical care, not elsewhere classified, initial encounter

AMA: 33965 2018,Jan,8; 2017,Jan,8; 2016,Mar,5; 2016,Jan,13; 2015,Jul,3
33966 2018,Jan,8; 2017,Jan,8; 2016,Mar,5; 2016,Jan,13; 2015,Jul,3

Relative Value Units/Medicare Edits

Non-Facility RVU	Work	PE	MP	Total
33965	3.51	1.06	0.81	5.38
33966	4.5	1.4	1.01	6.91
Facility RVU	**Work**	**PE**	**MP**	**Total**
33965	3.51	1.06	0.81	5.38
33966	4.5	1.4	1.01	6.91

	FUD	Status	MUE	Modifiers				IOM Reference
33965	0	A	1(3)	51	N/A	N/A	80*	None
33966	0	A	1(3)	51	N/A	N/A	80*	

* with documentation

Terms To Know

central venous catheter. Catheter positioned in the superior vena cava or right atrium and introduced through a large vein, such as the jugular or subclavian, and used to measure venous pressure or administer fluids or medication.

inflammatory. Pertaining to, characterized by, causing, or resulting from or affected by inflammation.

percutaneous. Through the skin.

peripheral. Outside of a structure or organ.

transfusion. Process of transferring whole blood or blood components from one person, the donor, to another person, the recipient, or the process of taking liquid from one vessel and putting it into another.

[33969, 33984]

33969 Extracorporeal membrane oxygenation (ECMO)/extracorporeal life support (ECLS) provided by physician; removal of peripheral (arterial and/or venous) cannula(e), open, birth through 5 years of age

33984 Extracorporeal membrane oxygenation (ECMO)/extracorporeal life support (ECLS) provided by physician; removal of peripheral (arterial and/or venous) cannula(e), open, 6 years and older

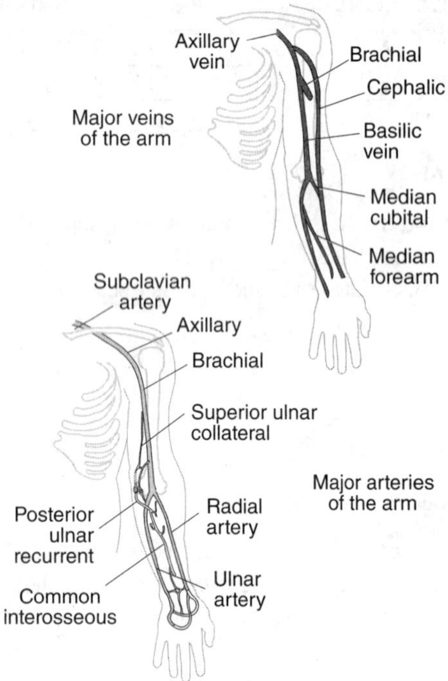

Explanation

When extracorporeal membrane oxygenation (ECMO)/extracorporeal life support (ECLS) therapy is complete, the physician removes the cannula. Cannulae placed via an open procedure require surgical intervention, sometimes performed bedside. The vessels cannulated are repaired and the skin is closed with stitches. Some patients require continued ventilation upon discontinuation of ECMO/ECLS therapy. Report 33969 for removal of a peripheral cannula performed by open approach for patients from birth through age 5 and 33984 for patients age 6 and older.

Coding Tips

If cannula is taken from one vessel and inserted into another, report the removal (33965–33969, 33984–33986, and 33955–33956) and insertion (33951–33955) codes. However, if cannula(e) is removed and reinserted into the same vessel, report only the insertion codes. If extensive repair or replacement of an artery is required and performed, report 35266, 35286, 35371, or 35665 in addition to 33965 and 33966. Do not report 33969 or 33984 with 34714-34716, 34812, 34820, 34834, 35201, 35206, 35211, or 35226.

ICD-10-CM Diagnostic Codes

T80.1XXA	Vascular complications following infusion, transfusion and therapeutic injection, initial encounter
T80.211A	Bloodstream infection due to central venous catheter, initial encounter
T80.212A	Local infection due to central venous catheter, initial encounter
T80.29XA	Infection following other infusion, transfusion and therapeutic injection, initial encounter
T82.310A	Breakdown (mechanical) of aortic (bifurcation) graft (replacement), initial encounter
T82.311A	Breakdown (mechanical) of carotid arterial graft (bypass), initial encounter
T82.312A	Breakdown (mechanical) of femoral arterial graft (bypass), initial encounter
T82.318A	Breakdown (mechanical) of other vascular grafts, initial encounter
T82.320A	Displacement of aortic (bifurcation) graft (replacement), initial encounter
T82.321A	Displacement of carotid arterial graft (bypass), initial encounter
T82.322A	Displacement of femoral arterial graft (bypass), initial encounter
T82.328A	Displacement of other vascular grafts, initial encounter
T82.330A	Leakage of aortic (bifurcation) graft (replacement), initial encounter
T82.331A	Leakage of carotid arterial graft (bypass), initial encounter
T82.332A	Leakage of femoral arterial graft (bypass), initial encounter
T82.338A	Leakage of other vascular grafts, initial encounter
T82.390A	Other mechanical complication of aortic (bifurcation) graft (replacement), initial encounter
T82.391A	Other mechanical complication of carotid arterial graft (bypass), initial encounter
T82.392A	Other mechanical complication of femoral arterial graft (bypass), initial encounter
T82.398A	Other mechanical complication of other vascular grafts, initial encounter
T82.518A	Breakdown (mechanical) of other cardiac and vascular devices and implants, initial encounter
T82.528A	Displacement of other cardiac and vascular devices and implants, initial encounter
T82.538A	Leakage of other cardiac and vascular devices and implants, initial encounter
T82.598A	Other mechanical complication of other cardiac and vascular devices and implants, initial encounter
T82.7XXA	Infection and inflammatory reaction due to other cardiac and vascular devices, implants and grafts, initial encounter
T82.818A	Embolism due to vascular prosthetic devices, implants and grafts, initial encounter
T82.828A	Fibrosis due to vascular prosthetic devices, implants and grafts, initial encounter
T82.838A	Hemorrhage due to vascular prosthetic devices, implants and grafts, initial encounter
T82.848A	Pain due to vascular prosthetic devices, implants and grafts, initial encounter
T82.856A	Stenosis of peripheral vascular stent, initial encounter
T82.858A	Stenosis of other vascular prosthetic devices, implants and grafts, initial encounter
T82.868A	Thrombosis due to vascular prosthetic devices, implants and grafts, initial encounter
T82.898A	Other specified complication of vascular prosthetic devices, implants and grafts, initial encounter
T88.8XXA	Other specified complications of surgical and medical care, not elsewhere classified, initial encounter

AMA: 33969 2018,Jan,8; 2017,Jan,8; 2017,Dec,3; 2016,Mar,5; 2016,Jan,13; 2015,Jul,3 **33984** 2018,Jan,8; 2017,Jan,8; 2017,Dec,3; 2016,Mar,5; 2016,Jan,13; 2015,Jul,3

Relative Value Units/Medicare Edits

Non-Facility RVU	Work	PE	MP	Total
33969	5.22	1.53	1.23	7.98
33984	5.46	1.57	1.22	8.25
Facility RVU	**Work**	**PE**	**MP**	**Total**
33969	5.22	1.53	1.23	7.98
33984	5.46	1.57	1.22	8.25

	FUD	Status	MUE	Modifiers				IOM Reference
33969	0	A	1(3)	51	N/A	N/A	80*	None
33984	0	A	1(3)	51	N/A	N/A	80*	

* with documentation

Terms To Know

acute. Sudden, severe.

infusion. Introduction of a therapeutic fluid, other than blood, into the bloodstream.

intervention. Purposeful interaction of the physical therapist with the patient and, when appropriate, with other individuals involved in patient care, using various physical therapy procedures and techniques to produce changes in the condition.

vascular. Pertaining to blood vessels.

[33985, 33986]

33985 Extracorporeal membrane oxygenation (ECMO)/extracorporeal life support (ECLS) provided by physician; removal of central cannula(e) by sternotomy or thoracotomy, birth through 5 years of age

33986 Extracorporeal membrane oxygenation (ECMO)/extracorporeal life support (ECLS) provided by physician; removal of central cannula(e) by sternotomy or thoracotomy, 6 years and older

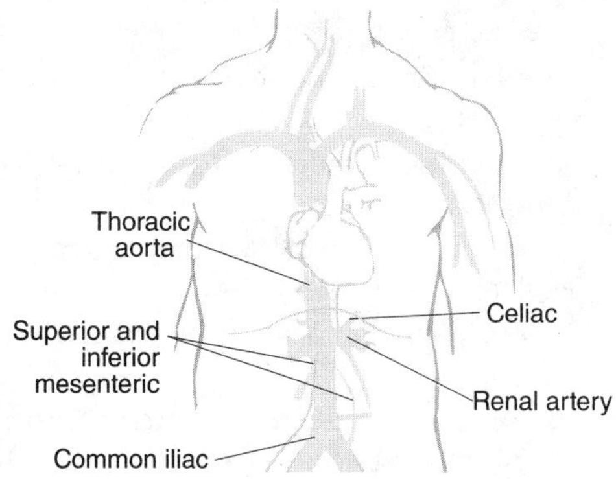

Removal of central cannula through sternotomy or thoracotomy

Explanation

When extracorporeal membrane oxygenation (ECMO)/extracorporeal life support (ECLS) therapy is complete, the physician removes the cannula. Cannulae placed via sternotomy or thoracotomy requires surgical intervention. The vessels cannulated are repaired and the skin is closed with stitches. Some patients require continued ventilation upon discontinuation of ECMO therapy. Report 33985 for removal of a central cannula performed by sternotomy or thoracotomy for patients from birth through age 5 and 33986 for patients age 6 and older.

Coding Tips

If cannula is taken from one vessel and inserted into another, report the removal (33965–33969, 33984–33986, and 33955–33956) and insertion (33951–33955) codes. However, if cannula(e) is removed and reinserted into the same vessel, report only the insertion codes. If extensive repair or replacement of an artery is required and performed, report 35266, 35286, 35371, or 35665 in addition to 33965 and 33966. Do not report 33985 or 33986 with 35211.

ICD-10-CM Diagnostic Codes

T80.1XXA Vascular complications following infusion, transfusion and therapeutic injection, initial encounter

T80.211A Bloodstream infection due to central venous catheter, initial encounter

T80.212A Local infection due to central venous catheter, initial encounter

T80.29XA Infection following other infusion, transfusion and therapeutic injection, initial encounter

T82.310A Breakdown (mechanical) of aortic (bifurcation) graft (replacement), initial encounter

T82.311A Breakdown (mechanical) of carotid arterial graft (bypass), initial encounter

T82.312A Breakdown (mechanical) of femoral arterial graft (bypass), initial encounter

T82.318A Breakdown (mechanical) of other vascular grafts, initial encounter

Heart and Pericardium

T82.320A Displacement of aortic (bifurcation) graft (replacement), initial encounter
T82.321A Displacement of carotid arterial graft (bypass), initial encounter
T82.322A Displacement of femoral arterial graft (bypass), initial encounter
T82.328A Displacement of other vascular grafts, initial encounter
T82.330A Leakage of aortic (bifurcation) graft (replacement), initial encounter
T82.331A Leakage of carotid arterial graft (bypass), initial encounter
T82.332A Leakage of femoral arterial graft (bypass), initial encounter
T82.338A Leakage of other vascular grafts, initial encounter
T82.390A Other mechanical complication of aortic (bifurcation) graft (replacement), initial encounter
T82.391A Other mechanical complication of carotid arterial graft (bypass), initial encounter
T82.392A Other mechanical complication of femoral arterial graft (bypass), initial encounter
T82.398A Other mechanical complication of other vascular grafts, initial encounter
T82.510A Breakdown (mechanical) of surgically created arteriovenous fistula, initial encounter
T82.511A Breakdown (mechanical) of surgically created arteriovenous shunt, initial encounter
T82.513A Breakdown (mechanical) of balloon (counterpulsation) device, initial encounter
T82.518A Breakdown (mechanical) of other cardiac and vascular devices and implants, initial encounter
T82.528A Displacement of other cardiac and vascular devices and implants, initial encounter
T82.538A Leakage of other cardiac and vascular devices and implants, initial encounter
T82.598A Other mechanical complication of other cardiac and vascular devices and implants, initial encounter
T82.7XXA Infection and inflammatory reaction due to other cardiac and vascular devices, implants and grafts, initial encounter
T82.818A Embolism due to vascular prosthetic devices, implants and grafts, initial encounter
T82.828A Fibrosis due to vascular prosthetic devices, implants and grafts, initial encounter
T82.838A Hemorrhage due to vascular prosthetic devices, implants and grafts, initial encounter
T82.848A Pain due to vascular prosthetic devices, implants and grafts, initial encounter
T82.856A Stenosis of peripheral vascular stent, initial encounter
T82.858A Stenosis of other vascular prosthetic devices, implants and grafts, initial encounter
T82.868A Thrombosis due to vascular prosthetic devices, implants and grafts, initial encounter
T82.898A Other specified complication of vascular prosthetic devices, implants and grafts, initial encounter
T88.8XXA Other specified complications of surgical and medical care, not elsewhere classified, initial encounter

AMA: 33985 2018,Jan,8; 2017,Jan,8; 2016,Mar,5; 2016,Jan,13; 2015,Jul,3
33986 2018,Jan,8; 2017,Jan,8; 2016,Mar,5; 2016,Jan,13; 2015,Jul,3

Relative Value Units/Medicare Edits

Non-Facility RVU	Work	PE	MP	Total
33985	9.89	2.8	2.33	15.02
33986	10.0	2.9	2.25	15.15
Facility RVU	**Work**	**PE**	**MP**	**Total**
33985	9.89	2.8	2.33	15.02
33986	10.0	2.9	2.25	15.15

	FUD	Status	MUE	Modifiers				IOM Reference
33985	0	A	1(3)	51	N/A	62*	80*	None
33986	0	A	1(3)	51	N/A	62*	80*	

* with documentation

Terms To Know

cannula. Tube inserted into a blood vessel, duct, or body cavity to facilitate passage.

central venous catheter. Catheter positioned in the superior vena cava or right atrium and introduced through a large vein, such as the jugular or subclavian, and used to measure venous pressure or administer fluids or medication.

injection. Forcing a liquid substance into a body part such as a joint or muscle.

sternotomy. Incision into the sternum, the bone that forms the front of the chest cavity and connects with the ribs.

thoracotomy. Surgical procedure for opening the chest wall in order to access the lungs, esophagus, trachea, aorta, heart, and diaphragm.

[33987]

\+ **33987** Arterial exposure with creation of graft conduit (eg, chimney graft) to facilitate arterial perfusion for ECMO/ECLS (List separately in addition to code for primary procedure)

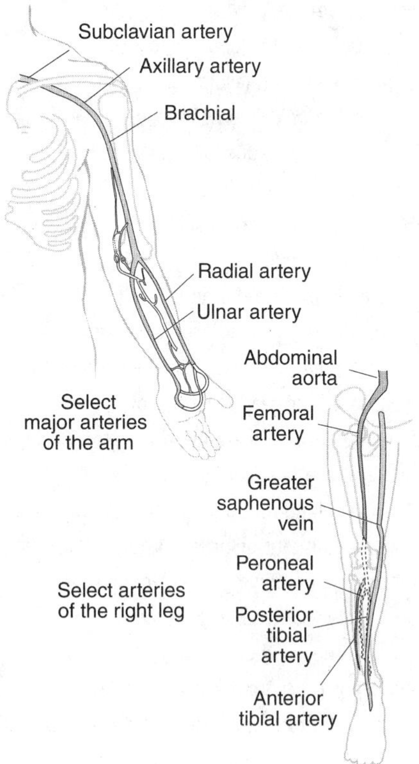

Explanation

The physician inserts a cannula(e) to provide prolonged extracorporeal circulation for cardiopulmonary insufficiency. The artery is exposed to create a graft that will broaden the vessel upwards (similar to a chimney) from the main artery being utilized. The graft is placed next to the artery often allowing for improved blood flow to smaller branches. Creating this type of graft requires special attention to the length needed to effectively use this technique. This cannula carries blood that is low in oxygen and high in carbon dioxide into the extracorporeal membrane oxygenation (ECMO) circuit. In veno-venous ECMO, if a double lumen cannula was inserted, blood that has passed through the membrane oxygenator that is now high in oxygen and low in carbon dioxide (oxygenated blood) is rewarmed to body temperature and returned via the same cannula. If a single lumen cannula is used, a second cannula is inserted into a second vein (venovenous ECMO) or a main artery (venoarterial ECMO), usually the femoral but in children the carotid may be used. This second cannula passes from the ECMO circuit carrying oxygenated, rewarmed blood back to the vein or artery.

Coding Tips

Report 33987 in addition to 33953–33956. Do not report 33987 with 34714, 34716, or 34833.

ICD-10-CM Diagnostic Codes

This/these CPT code(s) are add on code(s). See the primary procedure code that this code is performed with for your ICD-10-CM code selections. Diagnostic code(s) would be the same as the actual procedure performed.

AMA: **33987** 2018,Jan,8; 2017,Jan,8; 2017,Dec,3; 2016,Mar,5; 2016,Jan,13; 2015,Jul,3

Relative Value Units/Medicare Edits

Non-Facility RVU	Work	PE	MP	Total
33987	4.04	1.1	0.95	6.09
Facility RVU	**Work**	**PE**	**MP**	**Total**
33987	4.04	1.1	0.95	6.09

	FUD	Status	MUE	Modifiers				IOM Reference
33987	N/A	A	1(3)	N/A	N/A	62*	80*	None

* with documentation

Terms To Know

conduit. Surgically created channel for the passage of fluids.

extracorporeal membrane oxygenation. Procedure done for cardiopulmonary insufficiency that shunts the circulating venous blood through catheters inserted into the right atrium to the outside of the body where it is oxygenated, bypassing the lungs, then returned to the body through another cannula inserted in the femoral artery.

graft. Tissue implant from another part of the body or another person.

perfusion. Act of pouring over or through, especially the passage of a fluid through the vessels of a specific organ.

[33988, 33989]

33988 Insertion of left heart vent by thoracic incision (eg, sternotomy, thoracotomy) for ECMO/ECLS

33989 Removal of left heart vent by thoracic incision (eg, sternotomy, thoracotomy) for ECMO/ECLS

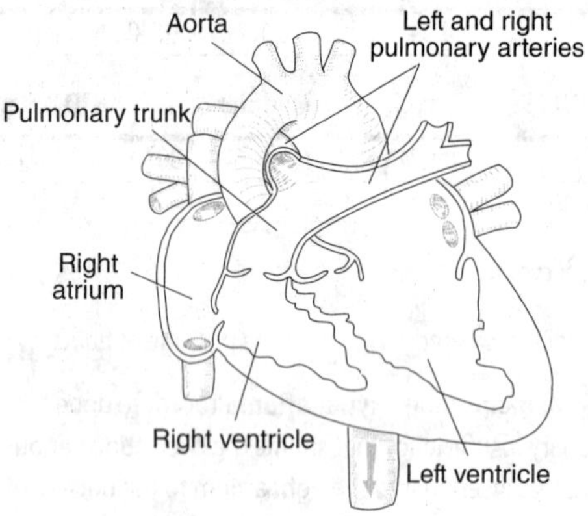

A vent cannula is inserted into the left ventricle of the heart

Explanation

The physician inserts a cannula(e) to provide extracorporeal membrane oxygenation (ECMO) or extracorporeal life support services (ECLS). A small incision is made to access the vessel. A single or double lumen cannula is inserted and passed into the inferior vena cava or right atrium. This cannula carries blood that is low in oxygen and high in carbon dioxide into the ECMO circuit. If a single lumen cannula is used, a second cannula is inserted into a main artery (venoarterial ECMO), usually the femoral but in children the carotid may be used. This second cannula passes from the ECMO circuit carrying oxygenated, rewarmed blood back to the vein or artery. This process reduces the amount of work the cardiac muscle must provide and if recovery is anticipated, ventricle expansion should be minimal and is often achieved by placing a catheter (to vent) in the left ventricle for draining. ECMO with ventricular decompression can be attained by insertion of a vent catheter directly into the left ventricle. Through an open incision into the thorax, the vent cannula is most commonly inserted into the pulmonary artery and positioned in the left ventricle. Report 33988 for insertion of the left heart vent and 33989 for removal of the left heart vent.

Coding Tips

The physician providing all components of ECMO/ECLS should report all codes for services provided. When performed by different providers, each should bill for the service performed. All services pertaining to cannulation, initiation, management, and discontinuation of the ECMO/ECLS circuit and parameters are separate from the daily overall management of the patient. Daily overall management is reported with hospital observation, inpatient, or critical care codes.

ICD-10-CM Diagnostic Codes

I40.0	Infective myocarditis
I40.1	Isolated myocarditis
I50.21	Acute systolic (congestive) heart failure
I50.22	Chronic systolic (congestive) heart failure
I50.23	Acute on chronic systolic (congestive) heart failure
I50.31	Acute diastolic (congestive) heart failure
I50.32	Chronic diastolic (congestive) heart failure
I50.33	Acute on chronic diastolic (congestive) heart failure
I50.41	Acute combined systolic (congestive) and diastolic (congestive) heart failure
I50.42	Chronic combined systolic (congestive) and diastolic (congestive) heart failure
I50.43	Acute on chronic combined systolic (congestive) and diastolic (congestive) heart failure
I50.811	Acute right heart failure
I50.812	Chronic right heart failure
I50.813	Acute on chronic right heart failure
I50.814	Right heart failure due to left heart failure
I50.82	Biventricular heart failure
I50.83	High output heart failure
I50.84	End stage heart failure
I97.0	Postcardiotomy syndrome
I97.110	Postprocedural cardiac insufficiency following cardiac surgery
I97.120	Postprocedural cardiac arrest following cardiac surgery
I97.130	Postprocedural heart failure following cardiac surgery
I97.710	Intraoperative cardiac arrest during cardiac surgery
J80	Acute respiratory distress syndrome
J85.1	Abscess of lung with pneumonia
J93.0	Spontaneous tension pneumothorax
J93.11	Primary spontaneous pneumothorax
J93.12	Secondary spontaneous pneumothorax
J93.81	Chronic pneumothorax
J95.821	Acute postprocedural respiratory failure
J95.822	Acute and chronic postprocedural respiratory failure
J96.01	Acute respiratory failure with hypoxia
J96.02	Acute respiratory failure with hypercapnia
J96.11	Chronic respiratory failure with hypoxia
J96.12	Chronic respiratory failure with hypercapnia
J96.21	Acute and chronic respiratory failure with hypoxia
J96.22	Acute and chronic respiratory failure with hypercapnia
P22.0	Respiratory distress syndrome of newborn
P24.01	Meconium aspiration with respiratory symptoms
P24.11	Neonatal aspiration of (clear) amniotic fluid and mucus with respiratory symptoms
P24.21	Neonatal aspiration of blood with respiratory symptoms
P25.1	Pneumothorax originating in the perinatal period
P25.2	Pneumomediastinum originating in the perinatal period
P25.3	Pneumopericardium originating in the perinatal period
P28.5	Respiratory failure of newborn
P28.81	Respiratory arrest of newborn
P29.0	Neonatal cardiac failure
P29.30	Pulmonary hypertension of newborn
P29.4	Transient myocardial ischemia in newborn
P29.81	Cardiac arrest of newborn
R06.03	Acute respiratory distress
R09.2	Respiratory arrest
R57.0	Cardiogenic shock
S27.0XXA	Traumatic pneumothorax, initial encounter
S27.1XXA	Traumatic hemothorax, initial encounter
S27.2XXA	Traumatic hemopneumothorax, initial encounter

T79.4XXA	Traumatic shock, initial encounter
T81.11XA	Postprocedural cardiogenic shock, initial encounter

AMA: 33988 2018,Jan,8; 2017,Jan,8; 2016,Mar,5; 2016,Jan,13; 2015,Jul,3 **33989** 2018,Jan,8; 2017,Jan,8; 2016,Mar,5; 2016,Jan,13; 2015,Jul,3

Relative Value Units/Medicare Edits

Non-Facility RVU	Work	PE	MP	Total
33988	15.0	4.2	3.54	22.74
33989	9.5	2.7	2.24	14.44
Facility RVU	**Work**	**PE**	**MP**	**Total**
33988	15.0	4.2	3.54	22.74
33989	9.5	2.7	2.24	14.44

	FUD	Status	MUE	Modifiers				IOM Reference
33988	0	A	1(3)	51	N/A	62*	80*	None
33989	0	A	1(3)	51	N/A	62*	80*	

* with documentation

Terms To Know

cannula. Tube inserted into a blood vessel, duct, or body cavity to facilitate passage.

catheter. Flexible tube inserted into an area of the body for introducing or withdrawing fluid.

critical care. Treatment of critically ill patients in a variety of medical emergencies that requires the constant attendance of the physician (e.g., cardiac arrest, shock, bleeding, respiratory failure, postoperative complications, critically ill neonate).

lumen. Space inside an intestine, artery, vein, duct, or tube.

thoracentesis. Surgical puncture of the chest cavity with a specialized needle or hollow tubing to aspirate fluid from within the pleural space for diagnostic or therapeutic reasons.

vena cava. Main venous trunk that empties into the right atrium from both the lower and upper regions, beginning at the junction of the common iliac veins inferiorly and the two brachiocephalic veins superiorly.

33967

33967 Insertion of intra-aortic balloon assist device, percutaneous

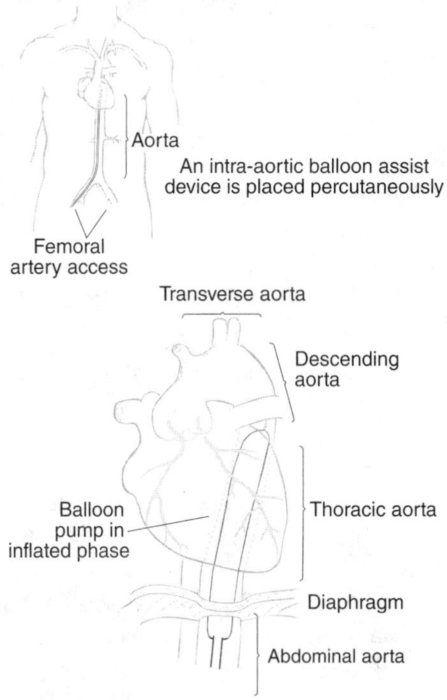

Explanation

An intra-aortic balloon catheter, usually with a 40 cc volume capacity, is inserted into the femoral artery and advanced under fluoroscopy to the distal portion of the aortic arch. After correct placement of the intra-aortic balloon assist device (IAB) in the descending aorta with its tip at the distal aortic arch, the balloon is connected to a drive console. The console consists of a pressurized gas reservoir, a monitor for ECG and pressure wave recording, adjustments for inflation/deflation timing, triggering selection switches, and battery back-up power sources. Helium or carbon dioxide is used for inflation. Inflation and deflation are synchronized to the patient's cardiac cycle. Inflation at the onset of diastole results in proximal and distal displacement of blood volume in the aorta. Deflation occurs just prior to the onset of systole. Once the patient's cardiac performance improves, weaning from the intra-aortic balloon catheter pump (IABP) begins by gradually decreasing the balloon augmentation ratio under control of hemodynamic stability.

Coding Tips

When 33967 is performed with another separately identifiable procedure, the highest dollar value code is listed as the primary procedure and subsequent procedures are appended with modifier 51. If the approach is open through the femoral artery, see 33970. For insertion through the ascending aorta, see 33973. For removal of an intra-aortic balloon assist device, percutaneous, see 33968.

ICD-10-CM Diagnostic Codes

I11.0	Hypertensive heart disease with heart failure
I16.0	Hypertensive urgency
I16.1	Hypertensive emergency
I20.0	Unstable angina
I20.1	Angina pectoris with documented spasm
I20.8	Other forms of angina pectoris

I21.01	ST elevation (STEMI) myocardial infarction involving left main coronary artery
I21.02	ST elevation (STEMI) myocardial infarction involving left anterior descending coronary artery
I21.09	ST elevation (STEMI) myocardial infarction involving other coronary artery of anterior wall
I21.11	ST elevation (STEMI) myocardial infarction involving right coronary artery
I21.19	ST elevation (STEMI) myocardial infarction involving other coronary artery of inferior wall
I21.21	ST elevation (STEMI) myocardial infarction involving left circumflex coronary artery
I21.29	ST elevation (STEMI) myocardial infarction involving other sites
I21.4	Non-ST elevation (NSTEMI) myocardial infarction
I21.A1	Myocardial infarction type 2
I22.0	Subsequent ST elevation (STEMI) myocardial infarction of anterior wall
I22.1	Subsequent ST elevation (STEMI) myocardial infarction of inferior wall
I22.2	Subsequent non-ST elevation (NSTEMI) myocardial infarction
I22.8	Subsequent ST elevation (STEMI) myocardial infarction of other sites
I24.8	Other forms of acute ischemic heart disease
I25.10	Atherosclerotic heart disease of native coronary artery without angina pectoris
I25.2	Old myocardial infarction
I25.3	Aneurysm of heart
I25.41	Coronary artery aneurysm
I25.42	Coronary artery dissection
I25.5	Ischemic cardiomyopathy
I25.6	Silent myocardial ischemia
I34.0	Nonrheumatic mitral (valve) insufficiency
I34.1	Nonrheumatic mitral (valve) prolapse
I34.2	Nonrheumatic mitral (valve) stenosis
I34.8	Other nonrheumatic mitral valve disorders
I35.0	Nonrheumatic aortic (valve) stenosis
I35.1	Nonrheumatic aortic (valve) insufficiency
I35.2	Nonrheumatic aortic (valve) stenosis with insufficiency
I35.8	Other nonrheumatic aortic valve disorders
I42.0	Dilated cardiomyopathy
I42.5	Other restrictive cardiomyopathy
I42.8	Other cardiomyopathies
I46.2	Cardiac arrest due to underlying cardiac condition
I46.8	Cardiac arrest due to other underlying condition
I47.0	Re-entry ventricular arrhythmia
I47.1	Supraventricular tachycardia
I47.2	Ventricular tachycardia
I50.1	Left ventricular failure, unspecified
I50.21	Acute systolic (congestive) heart failure
I50.22	Chronic systolic (congestive) heart failure
I50.23	Acute on chronic systolic (congestive) heart failure
I50.31	Acute diastolic (congestive) heart failure
I50.32	Chronic diastolic (congestive) heart failure
I50.33	Acute on chronic diastolic (congestive) heart failure
I50.41	Acute combined systolic (congestive) and diastolic (congestive) heart failure
I50.42	Chronic combined systolic (congestive) and diastolic (congestive) heart failure
I50.43	Acute on chronic combined systolic (congestive) and diastolic (congestive) heart failure
I50.811	Acute right heart failure
I50.812	Chronic right heart failure
I50.813	Acute on chronic right heart failure
I50.814	Right heart failure due to left heart failure
I50.82	Biventricular heart failure
I50.83	High output heart failure
I50.84	End stage heart failure
I51.5	Myocardial degeneration
I97.0	Postcardiotomy syndrome
I97.110	Postprocedural cardiac insufficiency following cardiac surgery
I97.111	Postprocedural cardiac insufficiency following other surgery
I97.120	Postprocedural cardiac arrest following cardiac surgery
I97.121	Postprocedural cardiac arrest following other surgery
I97.130	Postprocedural heart failure following cardiac surgery
I97.131	Postprocedural heart failure following other surgery
I97.190	Other postprocedural cardiac functional disturbances following cardiac surgery
I97.191	Other postprocedural cardiac functional disturbances following other surgery
I97.710	Intraoperative cardiac arrest during cardiac surgery
I97.711	Intraoperative cardiac arrest during other surgery
I97.790	Other intraoperative cardiac functional disturbances during cardiac surgery
I97.791	Other intraoperative cardiac functional disturbances during other surgery
I97.88	Other intraoperative complications of the circulatory system, not elsewhere classified
I97.89	Other postprocedural complications and disorders of the circulatory system, not elsewhere classified
Q21.0	Ventricular septal defect
Q21.1	Atrial septal defect
Q21.2	Atrioventricular septal defect
Q21.3	Tetralogy of Fallot
Q21.4	Aortopulmonary septal defect
Q21.8	Other congenital malformations of cardiac septa
Q23.0	Congenital stenosis of aortic valve
Q23.1	Congenital insufficiency of aortic valve
Q23.2	Congenital mitral stenosis
Q23.3	Congenital mitral insufficiency
Q23.8	Other congenital malformations of aortic and mitral valves
Q24.4	Congenital subaortic stenosis
Q24.5	Malformation of coronary vessels
Q24.6	Congenital heart block
Q24.8	Other specified congenital malformations of heart
R09.2	Respiratory arrest
R09.89	Other specified symptoms and signs involving the circulatory and respiratory systems
R57.0	Cardiogenic shock

AMA: **33967** 2018,Jan,8; 2017,Jan,8; 2016,Mar,5; 2016,Jan,13; 2015,Sep,3; 2015,Jul,3; 2015,Jan,16; 2014,Jan,11; 2013,Mar,10-11

Relative Value Units/Medicare Edits

Non-Facility RVU	Work	PE	MP	Total
33967	4.84	1.62	1.1	7.56
Facility RVU	**Work**	**PE**	**MP**	**Total**
33967	4.84	1.62	1.1	7.56

	FUD	Status	MUE	Modifiers				IOM Reference
33967	0	A	1(3)	51	N/A	N/A	80*	None

* with documentation

Terms To Know

augmentation. Add to or increase the substance of a body site, usually performed as plastic reconstructive measures. Augmentation may involve the use of an implant or prosthesis, especially within soft tissue or grafting procedures, such as bone tissue.

balloon assist device. Circulation assist device consisting of a balloon placed in the thoracic aorta that inflates and deflates in coordination with the beating of the heart.

distal. Located farther away from a specified reference point or the trunk.

percutaneous. Through the skin.

reservoir. Space or body cavity for storage of liquid.

transverse. Crosswise at right angles to the long axis of a structure or part.

33968

33968 Removal of intra-aortic balloon assist device, percutaneous

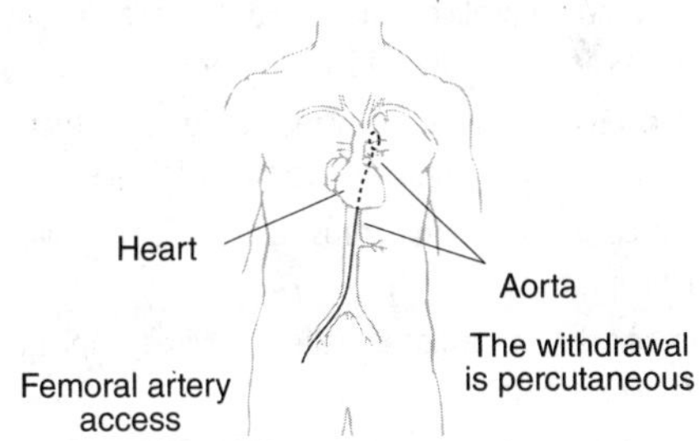

A balloon assist device in the aortic region is removed percutaneously

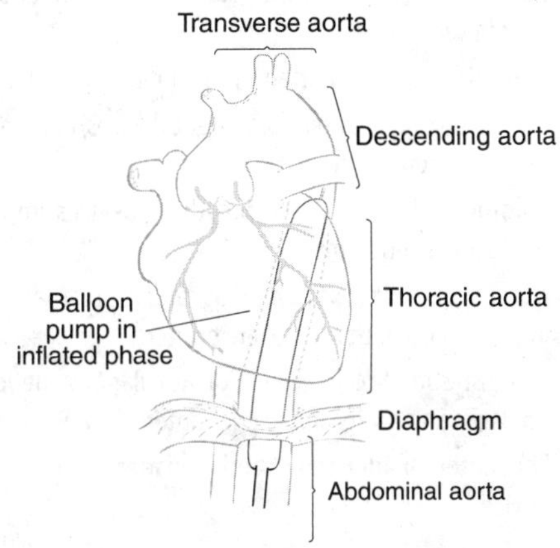

Explanation

The physician removes an intra-aortic balloon assist device (IABP). In a previous separately reportable procedure an IABP was inserted. When the patient is stabilized they are weaned off of the IAPB. The pump is turned off and the IABP catheter with the attached balloon is withdrawn from the femoral artery. Pressure is placed over the wound in the groin for a specified period of time. A light dressing is applied. The patient may be placed at bed rest and observed for several hours to avoid problems that could arise from bleeding or a hematoma at the puncture site.

Coding Tips

The approach may be either percutaneous, open through the femoral artery, or open through the ascending aorta and the approach is key to correct coding of insertion and removal of intra-aortic balloon assist device. For insertion and removal through the femoral artery, open approach, see 33970–33971. For insertion and removal through the ascending aorta, see 33973–33974. For percutaneous insertion, see 33967. For removal of implantable aortic counterpulsation ventricular assist system, see 0455T–0458T.

ICD-10-CM Diagnostic Codes

T82.513A	Breakdown (mechanical) of balloon (counterpulsation) device, initial encounter
T82.518A	Breakdown (mechanical) of other cardiac and vascular devices and implants, initial encounter
T82.523A	Displacement of balloon (counterpulsation) device, initial encounter
T82.528A	Displacement of other cardiac and vascular devices and implants, initial encounter
T82.533A	Leakage of balloon (counterpulsation) device, initial encounter

T82.538A	Leakage of other cardiac and vascular devices and implants, initial encounter
T82.593A	Other mechanical complication of balloon (counterpulsation) device, initial encounter
T82.598A	Other mechanical complication of other cardiac and vascular devices and implants, initial encounter
T82.7XXA	Infection and inflammatory reaction due to other cardiac and vascular devices, implants and grafts, initial encounter
T82.817A	Embolism due to cardiac prosthetic devices, implants and grafts, initial encounter
T82.827A	Fibrosis due to cardiac prosthetic devices, implants and grafts, initial encounter
T82.837A	Hemorrhage due to cardiac prosthetic devices, implants and grafts, initial encounter
T82.847A	Pain due to cardiac prosthetic devices, implants and grafts, initial encounter
T82.855A	Stenosis of coronary artery stent, initial encounter
T82.857A	Stenosis of other cardiac prosthetic devices, implants and grafts, initial encounter
T82.867A	Thrombosis due to cardiac prosthetic devices, implants and grafts, initial encounter
T82.897A	Other specified complication of cardiac prosthetic devices, implants and grafts, initial encounter
T82.898A	Other specified complication of vascular prosthetic devices, implants and grafts, initial encounter
Z45.09	Encounter for adjustment and management of other cardiac device

AMA: **33968** 2018,Jan,8; 2017,Jan,8; 2016,Mar,5; 2016,Jan,13; 2015,Jul,3; 2015,Jan,16; 2014,Jan,11

Relative Value Units/Medicare Edits

Non-Facility RVU	Work	PE	MP	Total
33968	0.64	0.21	0.13	0.98
Facility RVU	**Work**	**PE**	**MP**	**Total**
33968	0.64	0.21	0.13	0.98

	FUD	Status	MUE	Modifiers				IOM Reference
33968	0	A	1(3)	N/A	N/A	N/A	N/A	None

* with documentation

Terms To Know

ascending aorta. Thoracic aorta, ascending/arch.

graft. Tissue implant from another part of the body or another person.

hematoma. Tumor-like collection of blood in some part of the body caused by a break in a blood vessel wall, usually as a result of trauma.

intra-aortic balloon pump. Internal cardiac assist device usually inserted through the femoral artery into the descending aorta, either percutaneously or by open approach, and connected to a drive console that monitors the patient's condition as the balloon is synchronously inflated and deflated to improve cardiac performance.

33970-33971

33970 Insertion of intra-aortic balloon assist device through the femoral artery, open approach

33971 Removal of intra-aortic balloon assist device including repair of femoral artery, with or without graft

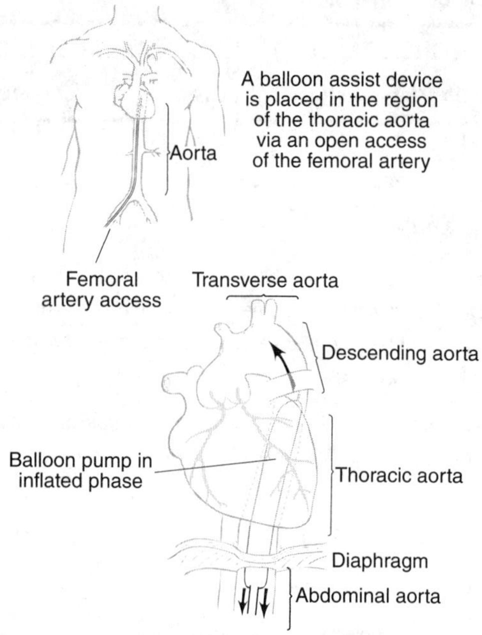

Removal of the device with repair to the artery

Explanation

This operation is done to help support the function of the left ventricle of the heart. In 33970, the left or right femoral artery is exposed in the groin. After the vessel is occluded above and below the proposed insertion site, the artery is opened transversely. In some cases, the end of a small tube of Gortex may be sewn to the side of the artery. The tip of the balloon catheter is inserted into the artery (or Gortex tube). The clamp occluding the artery upstream is released and the balloon catheter is advanced through the femoral artery and into the aorta above the level of the kidney arteries, but not beyond the left arm artery. It is connected to a pump and the pump is turned on. The pump inflates and deflates the balloon during each heartbeat cycle. In 33971, the previously placed balloon pump is withdrawn and the artery is occluded above and below the hole. If a Gortex sleeve has been used, it is simply tied off and no other repair is needed. If the balloon was directly introduced into the artery, the hole is sewn shut. If sewing the hole shut narrows the artery significantly, the hole can be patched with a piece of saphenous vein or Dacron. If the arterial diameter has been damaged, the segment of artery containing the hole can be removed and the artery replaced with an interposition graft of saphenous vein or Dacron tube.

Coding Tips

The approach may be percutaneous, open through the femoral artery, or open through the ascending aorta; the approach is key to correct coding of insertion and removal of the intra-aortic balloon assist device. For insertion and removal through the ascending aorta, see 33973–33974. For percutaneous insertion, see 33967. For removal of an intra-aortic balloon assist device, percutaneous, see 33968. For insertion or replacement of implantable aortic counterpulsation ventricular assist system, see 0451T–0454T. For removal of implantable aortic counterpulsation ventricular system, see 0455T–0458T.

ICD-10-CM Diagnostic Codes

I11.0	Hypertensive heart disease with heart failure
I16.0	Hypertensive urgency
I16.1	Hypertensive emergency
I20.0	Unstable angina
I20.1	Angina pectoris with documented spasm
I20.8	Other forms of angina pectoris
I21.01	ST elevation (STEMI) myocardial infarction involving left main coronary artery
I21.02	ST elevation (STEMI) myocardial infarction involving left anterior descending coronary artery
I21.09	ST elevation (STEMI) myocardial infarction involving other coronary artery of anterior wall
I21.11	ST elevation (STEMI) myocardial infarction involving right coronary artery
I21.19	ST elevation (STEMI) myocardial infarction involving other coronary artery of inferior wall
I21.21	ST elevation (STEMI) myocardial infarction involving left circumflex coronary artery
I21.29	ST elevation (STEMI) myocardial infarction involving other sites
I21.4	Non-ST elevation (NSTEMI) myocardial infarction
I21.A1	Myocardial infarction type 2
I22.0	Subsequent ST elevation (STEMI) myocardial infarction of anterior wall
I22.1	Subsequent ST elevation (STEMI) myocardial infarction of inferior wall
I22.2	Subsequent non-ST elevation (NSTEMI) myocardial infarction
I22.8	Subsequent ST elevation (STEMI) myocardial infarction of other sites
I24.8	Other forms of acute ischemic heart disease
I25.10	Atherosclerotic heart disease of native coronary artery without angina pectoris
I25.2	Old myocardial infarction
I25.3	Aneurysm of heart
I25.41	Coronary artery aneurysm
I25.42	Coronary artery dissection
I25.5	Ischemic cardiomyopathy
I25.6	Silent myocardial ischemia
I34.0	Nonrheumatic mitral (valve) insufficiency
I34.1	Nonrheumatic mitral (valve) prolapse
I34.2	Nonrheumatic mitral (valve) stenosis
I34.8	Other nonrheumatic mitral valve disorders
I35.0	Nonrheumatic aortic (valve) stenosis
I35.1	Nonrheumatic aortic (valve) insufficiency
I35.2	Nonrheumatic aortic (valve) stenosis with insufficiency
I35.8	Other nonrheumatic aortic valve disorders
I42.0	Dilated cardiomyopathy
I42.5	Other restrictive cardiomyopathy
I42.8	Other cardiomyopathies
I46.2	Cardiac arrest due to underlying cardiac condition
I46.8	Cardiac arrest due to other underlying condition
I47.0	Re-entry ventricular arrhythmia
I47.1	Supraventricular tachycardia
I47.2	Ventricular tachycardia
I50.1	Left ventricular failure, unspecified
I50.21	Acute systolic (congestive) heart failure
I50.22	Chronic systolic (congestive) heart failure
I50.23	Acute on chronic systolic (congestive) heart failure
I50.31	Acute diastolic (congestive) heart failure
I50.32	Chronic diastolic (congestive) heart failure
I50.33	Acute on chronic diastolic (congestive) heart failure
I50.41	Acute combined systolic (congestive) and diastolic (congestive) heart failure
I50.42	Chronic combined systolic (congestive) and diastolic (congestive) heart failure
I50.43	Acute on chronic combined systolic (congestive) and diastolic (congestive) heart failure
I50.811	Acute right heart failure
I50.812	Chronic right heart failure
I50.813	Acute on chronic right heart failure
I50.814	Right heart failure due to left heart failure
I50.82	Biventricular heart failure
I50.83	High output heart failure
I50.84	End stage heart failure
I51.5	Myocardial degeneration
I97.0	Postcardiotomy syndrome
I97.110	Postprocedural cardiac insufficiency following cardiac surgery
I97.111	Postprocedural cardiac insufficiency following other surgery
I97.120	Postprocedural cardiac arrest following cardiac surgery
I97.121	Postprocedural cardiac arrest following other surgery
I97.130	Postprocedural heart failure following cardiac surgery
I97.131	Postprocedural heart failure following other surgery
I97.190	Other postprocedural cardiac functional disturbances following cardiac surgery
I97.191	Other postprocedural cardiac functional disturbances following other surgery
I97.710	Intraoperative cardiac arrest during cardiac surgery
I97.711	Intraoperative cardiac arrest during other surgery
I97.790	Other intraoperative cardiac functional disturbances during cardiac surgery
I97.791	Other intraoperative cardiac functional disturbances during other surgery
I97.88	Other intraoperative complications of the circulatory system, not elsewhere classified
I97.89	Other postprocedural complications and disorders of the circulatory system, not elsewhere classified
Q21.0	Ventricular septal defect
Q21.1	Atrial septal defect
Q21.2	Atrioventricular septal defect
Q21.3	Tetralogy of Fallot
Q21.4	Aortopulmonary septal defect
Q21.8	Other congenital malformations of cardiac septa
Q23.0	Congenital stenosis of aortic valve
Q23.1	Congenital insufficiency of aortic valve
Q23.2	Congenital mitral stenosis
Q23.3	Congenital mitral insufficiency
Q23.8	Other congenital malformations of aortic and mitral valves
Q24.4	Congenital subaortic stenosis

Q24.5	Malformation of coronary vessels
Q24.6	Congenital heart block
Q24.8	Other specified congenital malformations of heart
R09.2	Respiratory arrest
R57.0	Cardiogenic shock
T82.513A	Breakdown (mechanical) of balloon (counterpulsation) device, initial encounter
T82.518A	Breakdown (mechanical) of other cardiac and vascular devices and implants, initial encounter
T82.523A	Displacement of balloon (counterpulsation) device, initial encounter
T82.528A	Displacement of other cardiac and vascular devices and implants, initial encounter
T82.533A	Leakage of balloon (counterpulsation) device, initial encounter
T82.538A	Leakage of other cardiac and vascular devices and implants, initial encounter
T82.593A	Other mechanical complication of balloon (counterpulsation) device, initial encounter
T82.598A	Other mechanical complication of other cardiac and vascular devices and implants, initial encounter
T82.7XXA	Infection and inflammatory reaction due to other cardiac and vascular devices, implants and grafts, initial encounter
T82.817A	Embolism due to cardiac prosthetic devices, implants and grafts, initial encounter
T82.827A	Fibrosis due to cardiac prosthetic devices, implants and grafts, initial encounter
T82.837A	Hemorrhage due to cardiac prosthetic devices, implants and grafts, initial encounter
T82.847A	Pain due to cardiac prosthetic devices, implants and grafts, initial encounter
T82.855A	Stenosis of coronary artery stent, initial encounter
T82.857A	Stenosis of other cardiac prosthetic devices, implants and grafts, initial encounter
T82.867A	Thrombosis due to cardiac prosthetic devices, implants and grafts, initial encounter

AMA: 33970 2018,Jan,8; 2017,Jan,8; 2016,Mar,5; 2016,Jan,13; 2015,Sep,3; 2015,Jul,3; 2015,Jan,16; 2014,Jan,11; 2013,Mar,10-11 **33971** 2018,Jan,8; 2017,Jan,8; 2016,Mar,5; 2016,Jan,13; 2015,Jul,3; 2015,Jan,16; 2014,Jan,11

Relative Value Units/Medicare Edits

Non-Facility RVU	Work	PE	MP	Total
33970	6.74	2.03	1.51	10.28
33971	11.99	5.78	2.74	20.51
Facility RVU	**Work**	**PE**	**MP**	**Total**
33970	6.74	2.03	1.51	10.28
33971	11.99	5.78	2.74	20.51

	FUD	Status	MUE	Modifiers				IOM Reference
33970	0	A	1(3)	51	N/A	62*	80	None
33971	90	A	1(3)	51	N/A	N/A	N/A	

* with documentation

Heart and Pericardium

33973-33974

33973 Insertion of intra-aortic balloon assist device through the ascending aorta

33974 Removal of intra-aortic balloon assist device from the ascending aorta, including repair of the ascending aorta, with or without graft

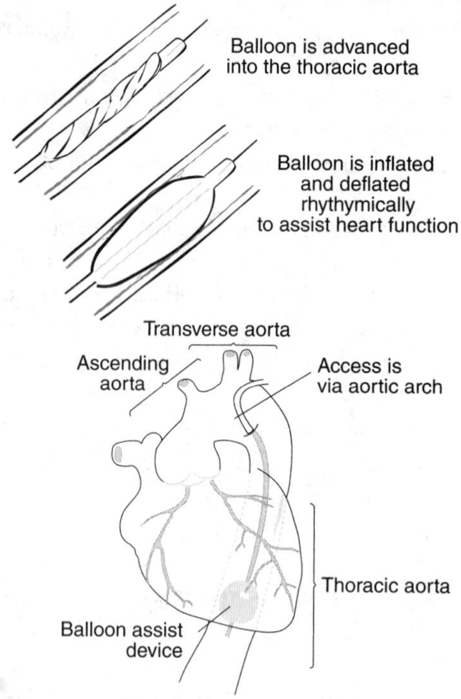

Explanation

The procedure is done when 1) the femoral arteries cannot be readily exposed in the operating room because of patient positioning; 2) the arteries are occluded by atherosclerosis or trauma; 3) there will be a need to reopen the patient's chest soon. In 33973, a balloon placed in this fashion must be removed in the operating room and the chest must be reopened. A purse string is placed in the aorta. A hole is made in the aorta in the middle of the purse string. The balloon is inserted through this hole until it lies beyond the left arm artery but above the kidney arteries. The purse string is tightened with a tourniquet. The chest incision is not closed. The balloon is driven by a pump outside the patient. In 33974, the physician removes an ascending aortic intra-aortic balloon assist device during performance of a primary procedure. If the sternum is open, the physician removes the aortic balloon while tightening purse-string sutures around the hole. When hemostasis is assured, the pericardium is repaired loosely with or without graft, leaving gaps for blood and fluid to drain into the pleural space. The sternum is reanastomosed with sternal wires and the skin is sutured in layers. If the sternum is closed, a Dacron-tube graft (reported separately) is used as a vehicle for balloon removal. As the balloon is removed, the Dacron-tube graft tightens around the aortic incision to create aortic hemostasis.

Coding Tips

The approach may be percutaneous, open through the femoral artery, or open through the ascending aorta. The approach is key to correct coding of insertion and removal of the intra-aortic balloon assist device. For open approach through the femoral artery, see 33970–33971. For percutaneous insertion, see 33967. For percutaneous removal, see 33968. For insertion or replacement of implantable aortic counterpulsation ventricular assist system, see

0451T-0454T. For removal of implantable aortic counterpulsation ventricular assist system, see 0455T-0458T.

ICD-10-CM Diagnostic Codes

I11.0	Hypertensive heart disease with heart failure
I20.0	Unstable angina
I20.1	Angina pectoris with documented spasm
I20.8	Other forms of angina pectoris
I21.01	ST elevation (STEMI) myocardial infarction involving left main coronary artery
I21.02	ST elevation (STEMI) myocardial infarction involving left anterior descending coronary artery
I21.09	ST elevation (STEMI) myocardial infarction involving other coronary artery of anterior wall
I21.11	ST elevation (STEMI) myocardial infarction involving right coronary artery
I21.19	ST elevation (STEMI) myocardial infarction involving other coronary artery of inferior wall
I21.21	ST elevation (STEMI) myocardial infarction involving left circumflex coronary artery
I21.29	ST elevation (STEMI) myocardial infarction involving other sites
I21.4	Non-ST elevation (NSTEMI) myocardial infarction
I22.0	Subsequent ST elevation (STEMI) myocardial infarction of anterior wall
I22.1	Subsequent ST elevation (STEMI) myocardial infarction of inferior wall
I22.2	Subsequent non-ST elevation (NSTEMI) myocardial infarction
I22.8	Subsequent ST elevation (STEMI) myocardial infarction of other sites
I24.8	Other forms of acute ischemic heart disease
I25.2	Old myocardial infarction
I25.3	Aneurysm of heart
I25.41	Coronary artery aneurysm
I25.42	Coronary artery dissection
I25.5	Ischemic cardiomyopathy
I25.6	Silent myocardial ischemia
I34.0	Nonrheumatic mitral (valve) insufficiency
I34.1	Nonrheumatic mitral (valve) prolapse
I34.2	Nonrheumatic mitral (valve) stenosis
I34.8	Other nonrheumatic mitral valve disorders
I35.0	Nonrheumatic aortic (valve) stenosis
I35.1	Nonrheumatic aortic (valve) insufficiency
I35.2	Nonrheumatic aortic (valve) stenosis with insufficiency
I35.8	Other nonrheumatic aortic valve disorders
I42.0	Dilated cardiomyopathy
I42.5	Other restrictive cardiomyopathy
I42.8	Other cardiomyopathies
I46.2	Cardiac arrest due to underlying cardiac condition
I46.8	Cardiac arrest due to other underlying condition
I47.0	Re-entry ventricular arrhythmia
I47.1	Supraventricular tachycardia
I47.2	Ventricular tachycardia
I50.1	Left ventricular failure, unspecified
I50.21	Acute systolic (congestive) heart failure
I50.22	Chronic systolic (congestive) heart failure
I50.23	Acute on chronic systolic (congestive) heart failure
I50.31	Acute diastolic (congestive) heart failure
I50.32	Chronic diastolic (congestive) heart failure
I50.33	Acute on chronic diastolic (congestive) heart failure
I50.41	Acute combined systolic (congestive) and diastolic (congestive) heart failure
I50.42	Chronic combined systolic (congestive) and diastolic (congestive) heart failure
I50.43	Acute on chronic combined systolic (congestive) and diastolic (congestive) heart failure
I51.5	Myocardial degeneration
I97.0	Postcardiotomy syndrome
I97.110	Postprocedural cardiac insufficiency following cardiac surgery
I97.111	Postprocedural cardiac insufficiency following other surgery
I97.120	Postprocedural cardiac arrest following cardiac surgery
I97.121	Postprocedural cardiac arrest following other surgery
I97.130	Postprocedural heart failure following cardiac surgery
I97.131	Postprocedural heart failure following other surgery
I97.190	Other postprocedural cardiac functional disturbances following cardiac surgery
I97.191	Other postprocedural cardiac functional disturbances following other surgery
I97.710	Intraoperative cardiac arrest during cardiac surgery
I97.711	Intraoperative cardiac arrest during other surgery
I97.790	Other intraoperative cardiac functional disturbances during cardiac surgery
I97.791	Other intraoperative cardiac functional disturbances during other surgery
I97.88	Other intraoperative complications of the circulatory system, not elsewhere classified
I97.89	Other postprocedural complications and disorders of the circulatory system, not elsewhere classified
Q21.0	Ventricular septal defect
Q21.1	Atrial septal defect
Q21.2	Atrioventricular septal defect
Q21.3	Tetralogy of Fallot
Q21.4	Aortopulmonary septal defect
Q21.8	Other congenital malformations of cardiac septa
Q23.0	Congenital stenosis of aortic valve
Q23.1	Congenital insufficiency of aortic valve
Q23.2	Congenital mitral stenosis
Q23.3	Congenital mitral insufficiency
Q23.8	Other congenital malformations of aortic and mitral valves
Q24.4	Congenital subaortic stenosis
Q24.5	Malformation of coronary vessels
Q24.6	Congenital heart block
Q24.8	Other specified congenital malformations of heart
R09.2	Respiratory arrest
R57.0	Cardiogenic shock
T82.513A	Breakdown (mechanical) of balloon (counterpulsation) device, initial encounter
T82.518A	Breakdown (mechanical) of other cardiac and vascular devices and implants, initial encounter

T82.523A	Displacement of balloon (counterpulsation) device, initial encounter
T82.528A	Displacement of other cardiac and vascular devices and implants, initial encounter
T82.533A	Leakage of balloon (counterpulsation) device, initial encounter
T82.538A	Leakage of other cardiac and vascular devices and implants, initial encounter
T82.593A	Other mechanical complication of balloon (counterpulsation) device, initial encounter
T82.598A	Other mechanical complication of other cardiac and vascular devices and implants, initial encounter
T82.7XXA	Infection and inflammatory reaction due to other cardiac and vascular devices, implants and grafts, initial encounter
T82.817A	Embolism due to cardiac prosthetic devices, implants and grafts, initial encounter
T82.827A	Fibrosis due to cardiac prosthetic devices, implants and grafts, initial encounter
T82.837A	Hemorrhage due to cardiac prosthetic devices, implants and grafts, initial encounter
T82.847A	Pain due to cardiac prosthetic devices, implants and grafts, initial encounter
T82.857A	Stenosis of other cardiac prosthetic devices, implants and grafts, initial encounter
T82.867A	Thrombosis due to cardiac prosthetic devices, implants and grafts, initial encounter
T82.897A	Other specified complication of cardiac prosthetic devices, implants and grafts, initial encounter
T82.898A	Other specified complication of vascular prosthetic devices, implants and grafts, initial encounter
Z45.09	Encounter for adjustment and management of other cardiac device

AMA: **33973** 2018,Jan,8; 2017,Jan,8; 2016,Mar,5; 2016,Jan,13; 2015,Sep,3; 2015,Jul,3; 2015,Jan,16; 2014,Jan,11; 2013,Mar,10-11 **33974** 2018,Jan,8; 2017,Jan,8; 2016,Mar,5; 2016,Jan,13; 2015,Jul,3; 2015,Jan,16; 2014,Jan,11

Relative Value Units/Medicare Edits

Non-Facility RVU	Work	PE	MP	Total
33973	9.75	3.0	2.28	15.03
33974	15.03	7.3	3.54	25.87
Facility RVU	**Work**	**PE**	**MP**	**Total**
33973	9.75	3.0	2.28	15.03
33974	15.03	7.3	3.54	25.87

	FUD	Status	MUE	Modifiers				IOM Reference
33973	0	A	1(3)	51	N/A	62*	80	None
33974	90	A	1(3)	51	N/A	N/A	N/A	

* with documentation

33975-33976

33975 Insertion of ventricular assist device; extracorporeal, single ventricle
33976 extracorporeal, biventricular

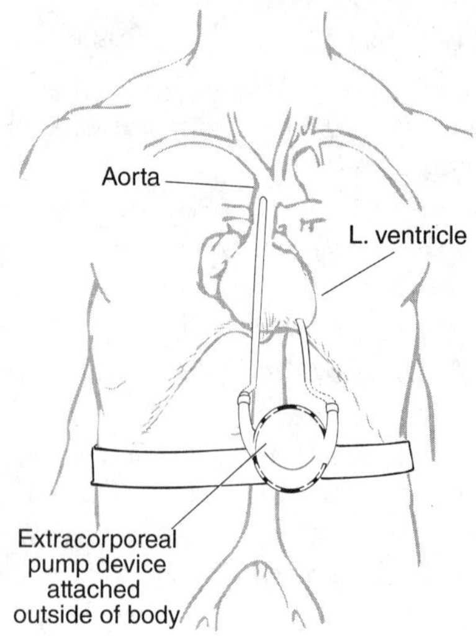

A single ventricle assist device is located outside of the body and its lines attached to the heart and aorta

The configurations vary according to which side of the heart is failing

Explanation

Cardiopulmonary bypass is required. For right ventricular failure, a pump uptake tube is placed in the right ventricular apex. A pump delivery tube is placed in the pulmonary artery. The pump is turned on and the patient is weaned off cardiopulmonary bypass. For left ventricular failure, the pump uptake tube is placed in one of the pulmonary veins or in the left ventricle apex. The arterial delivery tube is placed in the aorta. The pump is turned on and the patient is removed from cardiopulmonary bypass. The implanted pump is placed in a pocket formed in the upper abdominal wall, but outside the abdominal cavity. Tubes for the pump drive are brought out through separate incisions in the skin. The pump is started and the patient is weaned off cardiopulmonary bypass. The device is removed when the patient's ventricle recovers, a total artificial heart is placed or the patient undergoes heart transplantation. Report 33976 if biventricular support is needed.

Coding Tips

These codes are used to report initial insertion or replacement of the entire ventricular assist device. Removal of the device being replaced is included and should not be reported separately. For percutaneous implantation of a ventricular assist device, see 33990–33991; for the removal of the device, see 33992. For heart transplant, with or without recipient cardiectomy, see 33945.

ICD-10-CM Diagnostic Codes

I09.81	Rheumatic heart failure
I11.0	Hypertensive heart disease with heart failure
I16.0	Hypertensive urgency
I16.1	Hypertensive emergency
I20.0	Unstable angina
I20.1	Angina pectoris with documented spasm
I20.8	Other forms of angina pectoris

I21.01	ST elevation (STEMI) myocardial infarction involving left main coronary artery
I21.02	ST elevation (STEMI) myocardial infarction involving left anterior descending coronary artery
I21.09	ST elevation (STEMI) myocardial infarction involving other coronary artery of anterior wall
I21.11	ST elevation (STEMI) myocardial infarction involving right coronary artery
I21.19	ST elevation (STEMI) myocardial infarction involving other coronary artery of inferior wall
I21.21	ST elevation (STEMI) myocardial infarction involving left circumflex coronary artery
I21.29	ST elevation (STEMI) myocardial infarction involving other sites
I21.4	Non-ST elevation (NSTEMI) myocardial infarction
I21.A1	Myocardial infarction type 2
I22.0	Subsequent ST elevation (STEMI) myocardial infarction of anterior wall
I22.1	Subsequent ST elevation (STEMI) myocardial infarction of inferior wall
I22.2	Subsequent non-ST elevation (NSTEMI) myocardial infarction
I22.8	Subsequent ST elevation (STEMI) myocardial infarction of other sites
I24.8	Other forms of acute ischemic heart disease
I25.2	Old myocardial infarction
I25.3	Aneurysm of heart
I25.41	Coronary artery aneurysm
I25.42	Coronary artery dissection
I25.5	Ischemic cardiomyopathy
I25.6	Silent myocardial ischemia
I25.89	Other forms of chronic ischemic heart disease
I34.0	Nonrheumatic mitral (valve) insufficiency
I34.1	Nonrheumatic mitral (valve) prolapse
I34.2	Nonrheumatic mitral (valve) stenosis
I34.8	Other nonrheumatic mitral valve disorders
I35.0	Nonrheumatic aortic (valve) stenosis
I35.1	Nonrheumatic aortic (valve) insufficiency
I35.2	Nonrheumatic aortic (valve) stenosis with insufficiency
I35.8	Other nonrheumatic aortic valve disorders
I40.0	Infective myocarditis
I40.1	Isolated myocarditis
I41	Myocarditis in diseases classified elsewhere
I42.0	Dilated cardiomyopathy
I42.1	Obstructive hypertrophic cardiomyopathy
I42.2	Other hypertrophic cardiomyopathy
I42.5	Other restrictive cardiomyopathy
I42.7	Cardiomyopathy due to drug and external agent
I42.8	Other cardiomyopathies
I43	Cardiomyopathy in diseases classified elsewhere
I46.2	Cardiac arrest due to underlying cardiac condition
I46.8	Cardiac arrest due to other underlying condition
I47.0	Re-entry ventricular arrhythmia
I47.1	Supraventricular tachycardia
I47.2	Ventricular tachycardia
I50.1	Left ventricular failure, unspecified
I50.21	Acute systolic (congestive) heart failure
I50.22	Chronic systolic (congestive) heart failure
I50.23	Acute on chronic systolic (congestive) heart failure
I50.31	Acute diastolic (congestive) heart failure
I50.32	Chronic diastolic (congestive) heart failure
I50.33	Acute on chronic diastolic (congestive) heart failure
I50.41	Acute combined systolic (congestive) and diastolic (congestive) heart failure
I50.42	Chronic combined systolic (congestive) and diastolic (congestive) heart failure
I50.43	Acute on chronic combined systolic (congestive) and diastolic (congestive) heart failure
I50.811	Acute right heart failure
I50.812	Chronic right heart failure
I50.813	Acute on chronic right heart failure
I50.814	Right heart failure due to left heart failure
I50.82	Biventricular heart failure
I50.83	High output heart failure
I50.84	End stage heart failure
I51.5	Myocardial degeneration
I97.110	Postprocedural cardiac insufficiency following cardiac surgery
I97.111	Postprocedural cardiac insufficiency following other surgery
I97.120	Postprocedural cardiac arrest following cardiac surgery
I97.121	Postprocedural cardiac arrest following other surgery
I97.130	Postprocedural heart failure following cardiac surgery
I97.131	Postprocedural heart failure following other surgery
I97.190	Other postprocedural cardiac functional disturbances following cardiac surgery
I97.191	Other postprocedural cardiac functional disturbances following other surgery
I97.710	Intraoperative cardiac arrest during cardiac surgery
I97.711	Intraoperative cardiac arrest during other surgery
I97.790	Other intraoperative cardiac functional disturbances during cardiac surgery
I97.791	Other intraoperative cardiac functional disturbances during other surgery
I97.88	Other intraoperative complications of the circulatory system, not elsewhere classified
I97.89	Other postprocedural complications and disorders of the circulatory system, not elsewhere classified
Q21.0	Ventricular septal defect
Q21.1	Atrial septal defect
Q21.2	Atrioventricular septal defect
Q21.3	Tetralogy of Fallot
Q21.4	Aortopulmonary septal defect
Q21.8	Other congenital malformations of cardiac septa
Q23.0	Congenital stenosis of aortic valve
Q23.1	Congenital insufficiency of aortic valve
Q23.2	Congenital mitral stenosis
Q23.3	Congenital mitral insufficiency
Q23.8	Other congenital malformations of aortic and mitral valves
Q24.4	Congenital subaortic stenosis
Q24.5	Malformation of coronary vessels
Q24.6	Congenital heart block

Q24.8	Other specified congenital malformations of heart
R09.2	Respiratory arrest
R09.89	Other specified symptoms and signs involving the circulatory and respiratory systems
R57.0	Cardiogenic shock

AMA: 33975 2018,Jun,3; 2018,Jan,8; 2017,Jan,8; 2017,Dec,3; 2016,Mar,5; 2016,Jan,13; 2015,Jul,3; 2015,Jan,16; 2014,Jan,11; 2013,Mar,10-11 **33976** 2018,Jun,3; 2018,Jan,8; 2017,Jan,8; 2017,Dec,3; 2016,Mar,5; 2016,Jan,13; 2015,Jul,3; 2015,Jan,16; 2014,Jan,11; 2013,Mar,10-11

Relative Value Units/Medicare Edits

Non-Facility RVU	Work	PE	MP	Total
33975	25.0	7.24	5.71	37.95
33976	30.75	8.41	7.25	46.41
Facility RVU	**Work**	**PE**	**MP**	**Total**
33975	25.0	7.24	5.71	37.95
33976	30.75	8.41	7.25	46.41

	FUD	Status	MUE	Modifiers				IOM Reference
33975	N/A	A	1(3)	51	N/A	N/A	80	100-03,20.9; 100-03,20.9.1; 100-04,32,320.3.1; 100-04,32,320.3.2
33976	N/A	A	1(3)	51	N/A	N/A	80	

* with documentation

Terms To Know

cardiogenic shock. Shock caused by an inadequate supply of oxygen to the body's tissues due to a malfunction of the pumping action of the heart.

cardiopulmonary bypass. Venous blood is diverted to a heart-lung machine, which mechanically pumps and oxygenates the blood temporarily so the heart can be bypassed while an open procedure on the heart or coronary arteries is performed. During bypass, the lungs are deflated and immobile.

ventricular assist device. Temporary measure used to support the heart by substituting for left and/or right heart function. The device replaces the work of the left and/or right ventricle when a patient has a damaged or weakened heart. A left ventricular assist device (VAD) helps the heart pump blood through the rest of the body. A right VAD helps the heart pump blood to the lungs to become oxygenated again. Catheters are inserted to circulate the blood through external tubing to a pump machine located outside of the body and back to the correct artery.

33977-33978

33977 Removal of ventricular assist device; extracorporeal, single ventricle
33978 extracorporeal, biventricular

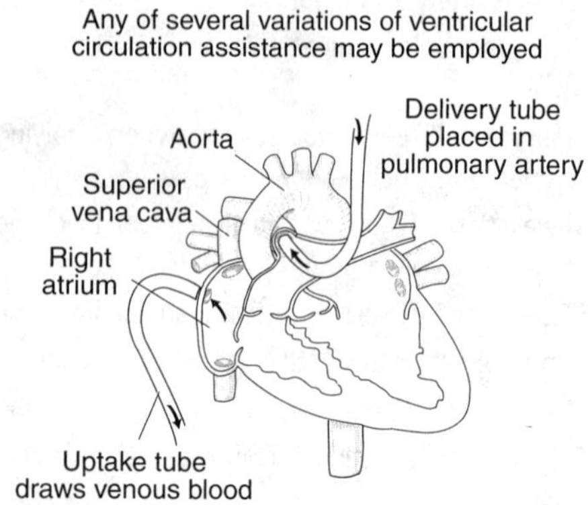

Depiction of right ventricular circulation support

Explanation

Cardiopulmonary bypass is required. The pump is stopped. All the tubes are removed and any holes in the heart or vessels are closed. The device is removed from the patient's body. Cardiopulmonary bypass is discontinued when the patient's heart function returns. An intra-aortic balloon pump is often required to allow discontinuation of bypass. All wounds are closed. Report 33978 if biventricular support is needed.

Coding Tips

These codes are used to report removal of the entire ventricular assist device. Removal of the device is included when the entire ventricular assist device is replaced and should not be reported separately. For percutaneous implantation of a ventricular assist device, see 33990–33991; for removal of the device, see 33992. For heart transplant, with or without recipient cardiectomy, see 33945.

ICD-10-CM Diagnostic Codes

T82.518A	Breakdown (mechanical) of other cardiac and vascular devices and implants, initial encounter
T82.528A	Displacement of other cardiac and vascular devices and implants, initial encounter
T82.538A	Leakage of other cardiac and vascular devices and implants, initial encounter
T82.598A	Other mechanical complication of other cardiac and vascular devices and implants, initial encounter
T82.7XXA	Infection and inflammatory reaction due to other cardiac and vascular devices, implants and grafts, initial encounter
T82.817A	Embolism due to cardiac prosthetic devices, implants and grafts, initial encounter
T82.827A	Fibrosis due to cardiac prosthetic devices, implants and grafts, initial encounter
T82.837A	Hemorrhage due to cardiac prosthetic devices, implants and grafts, initial encounter
T82.847A	Pain due to cardiac prosthetic devices, implants and grafts, initial encounter
T82.855A	Stenosis of coronary artery stent, initial encounter
T82.857A	Stenosis of other cardiac prosthetic devices, implants and grafts, initial encounter
T82.867A	Thrombosis due to cardiac prosthetic devices, implants and grafts, initial encounter

T82.897A	Other specified complication of cardiac prosthetic devices, implants and grafts, initial encounter
T82.898A	Other specified complication of vascular prosthetic devices, implants and grafts, initial encounter
Z45.09	Encounter for adjustment and management of other cardiac device
Z95.811	Presence of heart assist device

AMA: 33977 2018,Jan,8; 2017,Jan,8; 2017,Dec,3; 2016,Mar,5; 2016,Jan,13; 2015,Jul,3; 2015,Jan,16; 2014,Jan,11; 2013,Mar,10-11 **33978** 2018,Jan,8; 2017,Jan,8; 2017,Dec,3; 2016,Mar,5; 2016,Jan,13; 2015,Jul,3; 2015,Jan,16; 2014,Jan,11; 2013,Mar,10-11

Relative Value Units/Medicare Edits

Non-Facility RVU	Work	PE	MP	Total
33977	20.86	7.07	4.72	32.65
33978	25.0	8.01	5.88	38.89
Facility RVU	**Work**	**PE**	**MP**	**Total**
33977	20.86	7.07	4.72	32.65
33978	25.0	8.01	5.88	38.89

	FUD	Status	MUE	Modifiers				IOM Reference
33977	N/A	A	1(3)	51	N/A	N/A	80	None
33978	N/A	A	1(3)	51	N/A	N/A	80	

* with documentation

Terms To Know

cardiopulmonary bypass. Venous blood is diverted to a heart-lung machine, which mechanically pumps and oxygenates the blood temporarily so the heart can be bypassed while an open procedure on the heart or coronary arteries is performed. During bypass, the lungs are deflated and immobile.

complication. Condition arising after the beginning of observation and treatment that modifies the course of the patient's illness or the medical care required, or an undesired result or misadventure in medical care.

extracorporeal. Located or taking place outside the body.

graft. Tissue implant from another part of the body or another person.

implant. Material or device inserted or placed within the body for therapeutic, reconstructive, or diagnostic purposes.

infection. Presence of microorganisms in body tissues that may result in cellular damage.

intra-aortic balloon pump. Internal cardiac assist device usually inserted through the femoral artery into the descending aorta, either percutaneously or by open approach, and connected to a drive console that monitors the patient's condition as the balloon is synchronously inflated and deflated to improve cardiac performance.

percutaneous. Through the skin.

33979-33980

33979 Insertion of ventricular assist device, implantable intracorporeal, single ventricle

33980 Removal of ventricular assist device, implantable intracorporeal, single ventricle

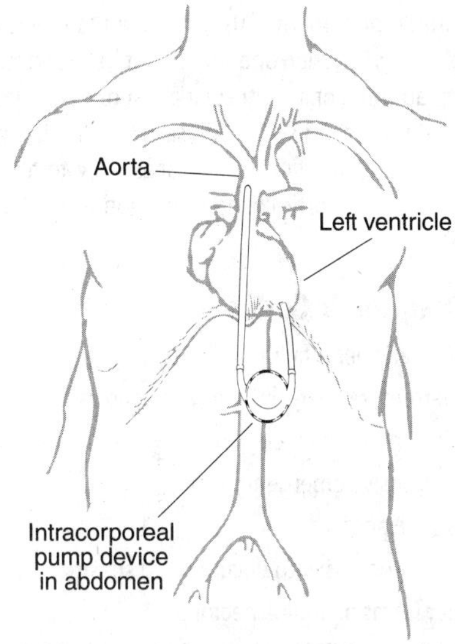

A single ventricular assist device

Explanation

The physician makes a midline incision extending from the sternal notch to the umbilicus. Sternotomy is performed prior to creation of the pocket. The preperitoneal fat is dissected from the undersurface of the rectus sheath using low-power cautery. Superiorly the dissection is carried to the undersurface of the diaphragm until the apex of the heart can be palpated just lateral to the inferior phrenic artery and vein and carried well back into the retroperitoneum. The preperitoneal space is opened to allow room for the device outflow valve and graft conduit. The muscular attachment of the right hemidiaphragm to the medial edge of the sternum is divided to allow room for the graft. A small incision is made and a tunneling device is passed subcutaneously inferiorly around the umbilicus, and into the pocket through the rectus sheath at its most inferior aspect. The tunneler is screwed onto the end of the drive line, which is pulled back through the tunnel to the skin. The drive line is not attached to the skin. Cardiopulmonary bypass is instituted using standard aortic and dual stage venous cannulae. The apex of the left ventricle is elevated. The physician cores out a piece of ventricle and places the apical cuff sutures. An apical vent is passed into the left ventricle. Pledgeted 2-0 Ethibond sutures are placed circumferentially partial thickness into the myocardium and passed through the sewing ring of the apical cuff. Once the apical cuff is secure, a cruciate incision in the diaphragm opposite the ventricular apex is made just lateral to the inferior phrenic vessels, and the inflow cannula is brought into the chest. The inflow cannula is inserted through the apical cuff until the sintered titanium surface is within the cuff. The Dacron tie of the inflow cuff is secured and an additional plastic band and Dacron tie are used to reinforce the connection and flatten out the silicone cuff. Blood is allowed to passively fill the device and exit via the outflow valve. A partial occluding clamp is placed on the right lateral aspect of the ascending aorta and a longitudinal aortotomy is performed. The periaortic adventitia is left in place and a strip of pericardium is incorporated into the anastomosis. The apex and heel of the anastomosis are reinforced with interrupted 4-0 Prolene pledgeted horizontal mattress stitches. Inotropic support is started before separating from bypass and activating the LVAD. The device is switched to automatic mode after the cessation of cardiopulmonary bypass. Transesophageal echocardiography is used to ensure adequate ventricular decompression and a bubble study is performed to rule out a patent foramen ovale. A thermodilution cardiac output is performed and compared to the output from the LVAD. In the presence of severe coagulopathy, the chest may need to be packed open. The device is removed (33980) when the patient's ventricle recovers, an artificial heart is placed, or the patient undergoes heart transplantation.

Coding Tips

Code 33979 includes replacement of the pump and cannulas. Removal of the device being replaced is included and should not be reported separately. For percutaneous implantation of a ventricular assist device, see 33990–33991; for removal of the device, see 33992. For insertion or replacement of implantable aortic counterpulsation ventricular assist system, see 0451T-0454T. For removal of implantable aortic counterpulsation ventricluar assist system, see 0455T-0458T.

ICD-10-CM Diagnostic Codes

I09.81	Rheumatic heart failure
I11.0	Hypertensive heart disease with heart failure
I16.0	Hypertensive urgency
I16.1	Hypertensive emergency
I20.0	Unstable angina
I20.1	Angina pectoris with documented spasm
I20.8	Other forms of angina pectoris
I21.01	ST elevation (STEMI) myocardial infarction involving left main coronary artery
I21.02	ST elevation (STEMI) myocardial infarction involving left anterior descending coronary artery
I21.09	ST elevation (STEMI) myocardial infarction involving other coronary artery of anterior wall
I21.11	ST elevation (STEMI) myocardial infarction involving right coronary artery
I21.19	ST elevation (STEMI) myocardial infarction involving other coronary artery of inferior wall
I21.21	ST elevation (STEMI) myocardial infarction involving left circumflex coronary artery
I21.29	ST elevation (STEMI) myocardial infarction involving other sites
I21.4	Non-ST elevation (NSTEMI) myocardial infarction
I21.A1	Myocardial infarction type 2
I22.0	Subsequent ST elevation (STEMI) myocardial infarction of anterior wall
I22.1	Subsequent ST elevation (STEMI) myocardial infarction of inferior wall
I22.2	Subsequent non-ST elevation (NSTEMI) myocardial infarction
I22.8	Subsequent ST elevation (STEMI) myocardial infarction of other sites
I24.8	Other forms of acute ischemic heart disease
I25.2	Old myocardial infarction
I25.3	Aneurysm of heart
I25.41	Coronary artery aneurysm
I25.42	Coronary artery dissection
I25.5	Ischemic cardiomyopathy
I25.6	Silent myocardial ischemia
I25.89	Other forms of chronic ischemic heart disease
I34.0	Nonrheumatic mitral (valve) insufficiency
I34.1	Nonrheumatic mitral (valve) prolapse
I34.2	Nonrheumatic mitral (valve) stenosis
I34.8	Other nonrheumatic mitral valve disorders
I35.0	Nonrheumatic aortic (valve) stenosis
I35.1	Nonrheumatic aortic (valve) insufficiency
I35.2	Nonrheumatic aortic (valve) stenosis with insufficiency
I35.8	Other nonrheumatic aortic valve disorders
I40.0	Infective myocarditis
I40.1	Isolated myocarditis
I41	Myocarditis in diseases classified elsewhere
I42.0	Dilated cardiomyopathy
I42.1	Obstructive hypertrophic cardiomyopathy
I42.2	Other hypertrophic cardiomyopathy
I42.5	Other restrictive cardiomyopathy
I42.7	Cardiomyopathy due to drug and external agent
I42.8	Other cardiomyopathies
I43	Cardiomyopathy in diseases classified elsewhere
I46.2	Cardiac arrest due to underlying cardiac condition
I46.8	Cardiac arrest due to other underlying condition
I47.0	Re-entry ventricular arrhythmia
I47.1	Supraventricular tachycardia
I47.2	Ventricular tachycardia
I50.1	Left ventricular failure, unspecified
I50.21	Acute systolic (congestive) heart failure
I50.22	Chronic systolic (congestive) heart failure
I50.23	Acute on chronic systolic (congestive) heart failure
I50.31	Acute diastolic (congestive) heart failure
I50.32	Chronic diastolic (congestive) heart failure
I50.33	Acute on chronic diastolic (congestive) heart failure
I50.41	Acute combined systolic (congestive) and diastolic (congestive) heart failure
I50.42	Chronic combined systolic (congestive) and diastolic (congestive) heart failure
I50.43	Acute on chronic combined systolic (congestive) and diastolic (congestive) heart failure
I50.811	Acute right heart failure
I50.812	Chronic right heart failure
I50.813	Acute on chronic right heart failure
I50.814	Right heart failure due to left heart failure
I50.82	Biventricular heart failure
I50.83	High output heart failure
I50.84	End stage heart failure
I51.5	Myocardial degeneration
I97.110	Postprocedural cardiac insufficiency following cardiac surgery
I97.111	Postprocedural cardiac insufficiency following other surgery
I97.120	Postprocedural cardiac arrest following cardiac surgery
I97.121	Postprocedural cardiac arrest following other surgery
I97.130	Postprocedural heart failure following cardiac surgery
I97.131	Postprocedural heart failure following other surgery
I97.190	Other postprocedural cardiac functional disturbances following cardiac surgery
I97.191	Other postprocedural cardiac functional disturbances following other surgery
I97.710	Intraoperative cardiac arrest during cardiac surgery

I97.711 Intraoperative cardiac arrest during other surgery
I97.790 Other intraoperative cardiac functional disturbances during cardiac surgery
I97.791 Other intraoperative cardiac functional disturbances during other surgery
I97.88 Other intraoperative complications of the circulatory system, not elsewhere classified
I97.89 Other postprocedural complications and disorders of the circulatory system, not elsewhere classified
Q21.0 Ventricular septal defect
Q21.1 Atrial septal defect
Q21.2 Atrioventricular septal defect
Q21.3 Tetralogy of Fallot
Q21.4 Aortopulmonary septal defect
Q23.0 Congenital stenosis of aortic valve
Q23.1 Congenital insufficiency of aortic valve
Q23.2 Congenital mitral stenosis
Q23.3 Congenital mitral insufficiency
Q24.4 Congenital subaortic stenosis
Q24.5 Malformation of coronary vessels
Q24.6 Congenital heart block
R57.0 Cardiogenic shock

AMA: **33979** 2018,Jun,3; 2018,Jan,8; 2017,Jan,8; 2017,Dec,3; 2016,Mar,5; 2016,Jan,13; 2015,Jul,3; 2015,Jan,16; 2014,Jan,11; 2013,Mar,10-11 **33980** 2018,Jan,8; 2017,Jan,8; 2017,Dec,3; 2016,Mar,5; 2016,Jan,13; 2015,Jul,3; 2015,Jan,16; 2014,Jan,11; 2013,Mar,10-11

Relative Value Units/Medicare Edits

Non-Facility RVU	Work	PE	MP	Total
33979	37.5	10.54	8.63	56.67
33980	33.5	10.52	7.8	51.82
Facility RVU	**Work**	**PE**	**MP**	**Total**
33979	37.5	10.54	8.63	56.67
33980	33.5	10.52	7.8	51.82

	FUD	Status	MUE	Modifiers				IOM Reference
33979	N/A	A	1(3)	51	N/A	N/A	80	None
33980	N/A	A	1(3)	51	N/A	N/A	80	

* with documentation

33981

33981 Replacement of extracorporeal ventricular assist device, single or biventricular, pump(s), single or each pump

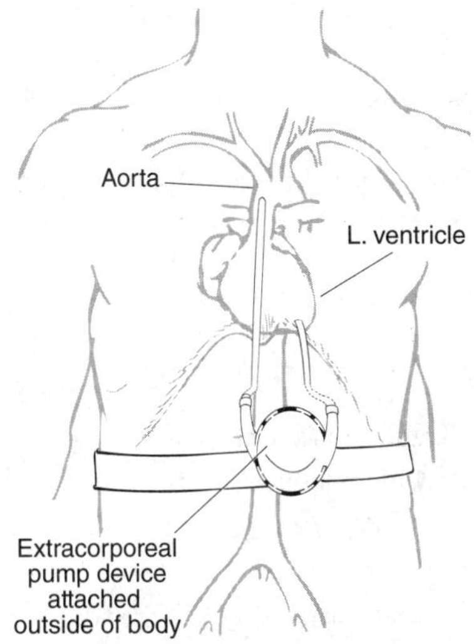

A single ventricle assist device is located outside of the body and its lines attached to the heart and aorta

Explanation

The physician replaces the blood pump component of an extracorporeal ventricular assist device (VAD). The previously implanted pump, which was placed in a pocket formed in the upper abdominal wall (but outside the abdominal cavity), is removed. Pump replacement includes removal of the existing pump, insertion of a new pump, connection, de-airing, and new pump initiation. Report 33981 for one or more pumps; this code reports pump replacement of single or biventricular VAD systems.

Coding Tips

Replacement of the pump includes removal of the previous pump, insertion of a new pump, and connection, de-airing, and initiation of the pump. For replacement of a ventricular assist device, extracorporeal, using percutaneous transseptal access, see 33999.

ICD-10-CM Diagnostic Codes

I11.0 Hypertensive heart disease with heart failure
I16.0 Hypertensive urgency
I16.1 Hypertensive emergency
I20.0 Unstable angina
I20.1 Angina pectoris with documented spasm
I20.8 Other forms of angina pectoris
I21.01 ST elevation (STEMI) myocardial infarction involving left main coronary artery
I21.02 ST elevation (STEMI) myocardial infarction involving left anterior descending coronary artery
I21.09 ST elevation (STEMI) myocardial infarction involving other coronary artery of anterior wall
I21.11 ST elevation (STEMI) myocardial infarction involving right coronary artery
I21.19 ST elevation (STEMI) myocardial infarction involving other coronary artery of inferior wall

I21.21	ST elevation (STEMI) myocardial infarction involving left circumflex coronary artery
I21.29	ST elevation (STEMI) myocardial infarction involving other sites
I21.4	Non-ST elevation (NSTEMI) myocardial infarction
I21.A1	Myocardial infarction type 2
I22.0	Subsequent ST elevation (STEMI) myocardial infarction of anterior wall
I22.1	Subsequent ST elevation (STEMI) myocardial infarction of inferior wall
I22.2	Subsequent non-ST elevation (NSTEMI) myocardial infarction
I22.8	Subsequent ST elevation (STEMI) myocardial infarction of other sites
I24.8	Other forms of acute ischemic heart disease
I25.2	Old myocardial infarction
I25.3	Aneurysm of heart
I25.41	Coronary artery aneurysm
I25.42	Coronary artery dissection
I25.5	Ischemic cardiomyopathy
I25.6	Silent myocardial ischemia
I34.0	Nonrheumatic mitral (valve) insufficiency
I34.1	Nonrheumatic mitral (valve) prolapse
I34.2	Nonrheumatic mitral (valve) stenosis
I34.8	Other nonrheumatic mitral valve disorders
I35.0	Nonrheumatic aortic (valve) stenosis
I35.1	Nonrheumatic aortic (valve) insufficiency
I35.2	Nonrheumatic aortic (valve) stenosis with insufficiency
I35.8	Other nonrheumatic aortic valve disorders
I42.0	Dilated cardiomyopathy
I42.5	Other restrictive cardiomyopathy
I42.8	Other cardiomyopathies
I46.2	Cardiac arrest due to underlying cardiac condition
I46.8	Cardiac arrest due to other underlying condition
I47.0	Re-entry ventricular arrhythmia
I47.1	Supraventricular tachycardia
I47.2	Ventricular tachycardia
I50.1	Left ventricular failure, unspecified
I50.21	Acute systolic (congestive) heart failure
I50.22	Chronic systolic (congestive) heart failure
I50.23	Acute on chronic systolic (congestive) heart failure
I50.31	Acute diastolic (congestive) heart failure
I50.32	Chronic diastolic (congestive) heart failure
I50.33	Acute on chronic diastolic (congestive) heart failure
I50.41	Acute combined systolic (congestive) and diastolic (congestive) heart failure
I50.42	Chronic combined systolic (congestive) and diastolic (congestive) heart failure
I50.43	Acute on chronic combined systolic (congestive) and diastolic (congestive) heart failure
I50.811	Acute right heart failure
I50.812	Chronic right heart failure
I50.813	Acute on chronic right heart failure
I50.814	Right heart failure due to left heart failure
I50.82	Biventricular heart failure
I50.83	High output heart failure
I50.84	End stage heart failure
I51.5	Myocardial degeneration
I97.0	Postcardiotomy syndrome
I97.110	Postprocedural cardiac insufficiency following cardiac surgery
I97.111	Postprocedural cardiac insufficiency following other surgery
I97.120	Postprocedural cardiac arrest following cardiac surgery
I97.121	Postprocedural cardiac arrest following other surgery
I97.130	Postprocedural heart failure following cardiac surgery
I97.131	Postprocedural heart failure following other surgery
I97.190	Other postprocedural cardiac functional disturbances following cardiac surgery
I97.191	Other postprocedural cardiac functional disturbances following other surgery
I97.710	Intraoperative cardiac arrest during cardiac surgery
I97.711	Intraoperative cardiac arrest during other surgery
I97.790	Other intraoperative cardiac functional disturbances during cardiac surgery
I97.791	Other intraoperative cardiac functional disturbances during other surgery
I97.88	Other intraoperative complications of the circulatory system, not elsewhere classified
I97.89	Other postprocedural complications and disorders of the circulatory system, not elsewhere classified
Q21.0	Ventricular septal defect
Q21.1	Atrial septal defect
Q21.2	Atrioventricular septal defect
Q21.3	Tetralogy of Fallot
Q21.4	Aortopulmonary septal defect
Q21.8	Other congenital malformations of cardiac septa
Q23.0	Congenital stenosis of aortic valve
Q23.1	Congenital insufficiency of aortic valve
Q23.2	Congenital mitral stenosis
Q23.3	Congenital mitral insufficiency
Q23.8	Other congenital malformations of aortic and mitral valves
Q24.4	Congenital subaortic stenosis
Q24.5	Malformation of coronary vessels
Q24.6	Congenital heart block
Q24.8	Other specified congenital malformations of heart
R09.2	Respiratory arrest
R09.89	Other specified symptoms and signs involving the circulatory and respiratory systems
R57.0	Cardiogenic shock
T82.518A	Breakdown (mechanical) of other cardiac and vascular devices and implants, initial encounter
T82.528A	Displacement of other cardiac and vascular devices and implants, initial encounter
T82.538A	Leakage of other cardiac and vascular devices and implants, initial encounter
T82.598A	Other mechanical complication of other cardiac and vascular devices and implants, initial encounter
T82.7XXA	Infection and inflammatory reaction due to other cardiac and vascular devices, implants and grafts, initial encounter
T82.817A	Embolism due to cardiac prosthetic devices, implants and grafts, initial encounter

T82.827A	Fibrosis due to cardiac prosthetic devices, implants and grafts, initial encounter
T82.837A	Hemorrhage due to cardiac prosthetic devices, implants and grafts, initial encounter
T82.847A	Pain due to cardiac prosthetic devices, implants and grafts, initial encounter
T82.857A	Stenosis of other cardiac prosthetic devices, implants and grafts, initial encounter
T82.867A	Thrombosis due to cardiac prosthetic devices, implants and grafts, initial encounter
T82.897A	Other specified complication of cardiac prosthetic devices, implants and grafts, initial encounter
T82.898A	Other specified complication of vascular prosthetic devices, implants and grafts, initial encounter
Z45.09	Encounter for adjustment and management of other cardiac device
Z95.811	Presence of heart assist device

AMA: 33981 2018,Jan,8; 2017,Jan,8; 2016,Mar,5; 2016,Jan,13; 2015,Jul,3; 2015,Jan,16; 2014,Jan,11

Relative Value Units/Medicare Edits

Non-Facility RVU	Work	PE	MP	Total
33981	16.11	4.41	3.8	24.32
Facility RVU	**Work**	**PE**	**MP**	**Total**
33981	16.11	4.41	3.8	24.32

	FUD	Status	MUE	Modifiers				IOM Reference
33981	N/A	A	1(3)	51	N/A	N/A	80	100-04,32,320.3.2

* with documentation

33982-33983

33982 Replacement of ventricular assist device pump(s); implantable intracorporeal, single ventricle, without cardiopulmonary bypass

33983 implantable intracorporeal, single ventricle, with cardiopulmonary bypass

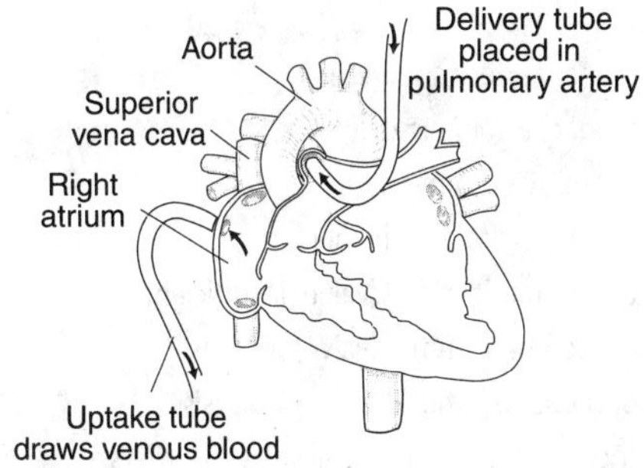

Depiction of right ventricular circulation support

Explanation

The physician replaces the blood pump component of an implantable, intracorporeal, single ventricle VAD (ventricular assist device). This may be accomplished without cardiopulmonary bypass (33982) or with cardiopulmonary bypass (33983). Pump replacement includes removal of the existing pump, insertion of a new pump, connection, de-airing, and new pump initiation.

Coding Tips

Replacement of the new pump includes removal of the previous pump, insertion of the new pump, and connection, de-airing, and initiation of the pump. For replacement of a ventricular assist device, extracorporeal, using percutaneous transseptal access, see 33999. For insertion or replacement of implantable aortic counterpulsation ventricular assist system, see 0451T-0454T.

ICD-10-CM Diagnostic Codes

I11.0	Hypertensive heart disease with heart failure
I16.0	Hypertensive urgency
I16.1	Hypertensive emergency
I20.0	Unstable angina
I20.1	Angina pectoris with documented spasm
I20.8	Other forms of angina pectoris
I21.01	ST elevation (STEMI) myocardial infarction involving left main coronary artery
I21.02	ST elevation (STEMI) myocardial infarction involving left anterior descending coronary artery
I21.09	ST elevation (STEMI) myocardial infarction involving other coronary artery of anterior wall
I21.11	ST elevation (STEMI) myocardial infarction involving right coronary artery
I21.19	ST elevation (STEMI) myocardial infarction involving other coronary artery of inferior wall
I21.21	ST elevation (STEMI) myocardial infarction involving left circumflex coronary artery
I21.29	ST elevation (STEMI) myocardial infarction involving other sites
I21.4	Non-ST elevation (NSTEMI) myocardial infarction
I21.A1	Myocardial infarction type 2
I22.0	Subsequent ST elevation (STEMI) myocardial infarction of anterior wall

I22.1	Subsequent ST elevation (STEMI) myocardial infarction of inferior wall
I22.2	Subsequent non-ST elevation (NSTEMI) myocardial infarction
I22.8	Subsequent ST elevation (STEMI) myocardial infarction of other sites
I24.8	Other forms of acute ischemic heart disease
I25.2	Old myocardial infarction
I25.3	Aneurysm of heart
I25.41	Coronary artery aneurysm
I25.42	Coronary artery dissection
I25.5	Ischemic cardiomyopathy
I25.6	Silent myocardial ischemia
I34.0	Nonrheumatic mitral (valve) insufficiency
I34.1	Nonrheumatic mitral (valve) prolapse
I34.2	Nonrheumatic mitral (valve) stenosis
I34.8	Other nonrheumatic mitral valve disorders
I35.0	Nonrheumatic aortic (valve) stenosis
I35.1	Nonrheumatic aortic (valve) insufficiency
I35.2	Nonrheumatic aortic (valve) stenosis with insufficiency
I35.8	Other nonrheumatic aortic valve disorders
I42.0	Dilated cardiomyopathy
I42.5	Other restrictive cardiomyopathy
I42.8	Other cardiomyopathies
I46.2	Cardiac arrest due to underlying cardiac condition
I46.8	Cardiac arrest due to other underlying condition
I47.0	Re-entry ventricular arrhythmia
I47.1	Supraventricular tachycardia
I47.2	Ventricular tachycardia
I50.1	Left ventricular failure, unspecified
I50.21	Acute systolic (congestive) heart failure
I50.22	Chronic systolic (congestive) heart failure
I50.23	Acute on chronic systolic (congestive) heart failure
I50.31	Acute diastolic (congestive) heart failure
I50.32	Chronic diastolic (congestive) heart failure
I50.33	Acute on chronic diastolic (congestive) heart failure
I50.41	Acute combined systolic (congestive) and diastolic (congestive) heart failure
I50.42	Chronic combined systolic (congestive) and diastolic (congestive) heart failure
I50.43	Acute on chronic combined systolic (congestive) and diastolic (congestive) heart failure
I50.811	Acute right heart failure
I50.812	Chronic right heart failure
I50.813	Acute on chronic right heart failure
I50.814	Right heart failure due to left heart failure
I50.82	Biventricular heart failure
I50.83	High output heart failure
I50.84	End stage heart failure
I51.5	Myocardial degeneration
I97.0	Postcardiotomy syndrome
I97.110	Postprocedural cardiac insufficiency following cardiac surgery
I97.111	Postprocedural cardiac insufficiency following other surgery
I97.120	Postprocedural cardiac arrest following cardiac surgery
I97.121	Postprocedural cardiac arrest following other surgery
I97.130	Postprocedural heart failure following cardiac surgery
I97.131	Postprocedural heart failure following other surgery
I97.190	Other postprocedural cardiac functional disturbances following cardiac surgery
I97.191	Other postprocedural cardiac functional disturbances following other surgery
I97.710	Intraoperative cardiac arrest during cardiac surgery
I97.711	Intraoperative cardiac arrest during other surgery
I97.790	Other intraoperative cardiac functional disturbances during cardiac surgery
I97.791	Other intraoperative cardiac functional disturbances during other surgery
I97.88	Other intraoperative complications of the circulatory system, not elsewhere classified
I97.89	Other postprocedural complications and disorders of the circulatory system, not elsewhere classified
Q21.0	Ventricular septal defect
Q21.1	Atrial septal defect
Q21.2	Atrioventricular septal defect
Q21.3	Tetralogy of Fallot
Q21.4	Aortopulmonary septal defect
Q21.8	Other congenital malformations of cardiac septa
Q23.0	Congenital stenosis of aortic valve
Q23.1	Congenital insufficiency of aortic valve
Q23.2	Congenital mitral stenosis
Q23.3	Congenital mitral insufficiency
Q23.8	Other congenital malformations of aortic and mitral valves
Q24.4	Congenital subaortic stenosis
Q24.5	Malformation of coronary vessels
Q24.6	Congenital heart block
Q24.8	Other specified congenital malformations of heart
R09.2	Respiratory arrest
R09.89	Other specified symptoms and signs involving the circulatory and respiratory systems
R57.0	Cardiogenic shock
T82.518A	Breakdown (mechanical) of other cardiac and vascular devices and implants, initial encounter
T82.528A	Displacement of other cardiac and vascular devices and implants, initial encounter
T82.538A	Leakage of other cardiac and vascular devices and implants, initial encounter
T82.598A	Other mechanical complication of other cardiac and vascular devices and implants, initial encounter
T82.7XXA	Infection and inflammatory reaction due to other cardiac and vascular devices, implants and grafts, initial encounter
T82.817A	Embolism due to cardiac prosthetic devices, implants and grafts, initial encounter
T82.827A	Fibrosis due to cardiac prosthetic devices, implants and grafts, initial encounter
T82.837A	Hemorrhage due to cardiac prosthetic devices, implants and grafts, initial encounter
T82.847A	Pain due to cardiac prosthetic devices, implants and grafts, initial encounter

T82.857A Stenosis of other cardiac prosthetic devices, implants and grafts, initial encounter

T82.867A Thrombosis due to cardiac prosthetic devices, implants and grafts, initial encounter

T82.897A Other specified complication of cardiac prosthetic devices, implants and grafts, initial encounter

T82.898A Other specified complication of vascular prosthetic devices, implants and grafts, initial encounter

Z45.09 Encounter for adjustment and management of other cardiac device

Z95.811 Presence of heart assist device

AMA: 33982 2018,Jan,8; 2017,Jan,8; 2016,Mar,5; 2016,Jan,13; 2015,Jul,3; 2015,Jan,16; 2014,Jan,11 **33983** 2018,Jan,8; 2017,Jan,8; 2017,Dec,3; 2016,Mar,5; 2016,Jan,13; 2015,Jul,3; 2015,Jan,16; 2014,Jan,11

Relative Value Units/Medicare Edits

Non-Facility RVU	Work	PE	MP	Total
33982	37.86	10.36	8.94	57.16
33983	44.54	12.33	10.26	67.13
Facility RVU	**Work**	**PE**	**MP**	**Total**
33982	37.86	10.36	8.94	57.16
33983	44.54	12.33	10.26	67.13

	FUD	Status	MUE	Modifiers				IOM Reference
33982	N/A	A	1(3)	51	N/A	N/A	80	None
33983	N/A	A	1(3)	51	N/A	N/A	80	

* with documentation

33990-33991

33990 Insertion of ventricular assist device, percutaneous including radiological supervision and interpretation; arterial access only

33991 both arterial and venous access, with transseptal puncture

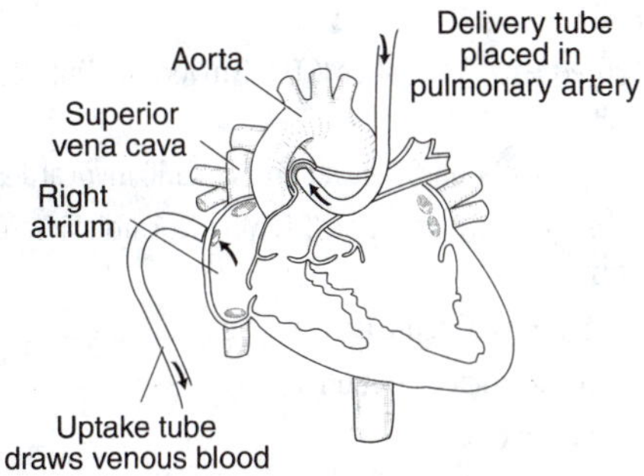

Depiction of right ventricular circulation support

Explanation

A ventricular assist device (VAD) bypasses the left ventricle during the blood oxygenation cycle making the ventricle work less during the systolic phase. In percutaneous placement of a VAD, a catheter is inserted in the patient's femoral vein and maneuvered to the left atrium. A centrifugal assist device is placed outside the body, usually on the patient's thigh. The catheter is attached to the device. Oxygenated blood is pumped from the left atrium to the device and distributed to one or both femoral arteries via catheter. Report 33990 when the VAD is inserted with a single arterial access. Report 33991 if the septum is punctured for left atrial access and the procedure includes both arterial and venous access.

Coding Tips

When medically necessary, report moderate (conscious) sedation provided by the performing physician with 99151-99153. When provided by another physician, report 99155-99157. For repositioning of the percutaneous ventricular assist device, see 33993. For removal of the percutaneous ventricular assist device, see 33992. For insertion of implantable intracorporeal ventricular assist devices, see 33979. For insertion or replacement of implantable aortic counterpulsation ventricular assist system, see 0451T-0454T.

ICD-10-CM Diagnostic Codes

I09.81 Rheumatic heart failure

I11.0 Hypertensive heart disease with heart failure

I16.0 Hypertensive urgency

I16.1 Hypertensive emergency

I20.0 Unstable angina

I20.1 Angina pectoris with documented spasm

I20.8 Other forms of angina pectoris

I21.01 ST elevation (STEMI) myocardial infarction involving left main coronary artery

I21.02 ST elevation (STEMI) myocardial infarction involving left anterior descending coronary artery

I21.09 ST elevation (STEMI) myocardial infarction involving other coronary artery of anterior wall

I21.11 ST elevation (STEMI) myocardial infarction involving right coronary artery

I21.19 ST elevation (STEMI) myocardial infarction involving other coronary artery of inferior wall

I21.21	ST elevation (STEMI) myocardial infarction involving left circumflex coronary artery
I21.29	ST elevation (STEMI) myocardial infarction involving other sites
I21.4	Non-ST elevation (NSTEMI) myocardial infarction
I21.A1	Myocardial infarction type 2
I22.0	Subsequent ST elevation (STEMI) myocardial infarction of anterior wall
I22.1	Subsequent ST elevation (STEMI) myocardial infarction of inferior wall
I22.2	Subsequent non-ST elevation (NSTEMI) myocardial infarction
I22.8	Subsequent ST elevation (STEMI) myocardial infarction of other sites
I24.8	Other forms of acute ischemic heart disease
I25.2	Old myocardial infarction
I25.3	Aneurysm of heart
I25.41	Coronary artery aneurysm
I25.42	Coronary artery dissection
I25.5	Ischemic cardiomyopathy
I25.6	Silent myocardial ischemia
I25.89	Other forms of chronic ischemic heart disease
I34.0	Nonrheumatic mitral (valve) insufficiency
I34.1	Nonrheumatic mitral (valve) prolapse
I34.2	Nonrheumatic mitral (valve) stenosis
I34.8	Other nonrheumatic mitral valve disorders
I35.0	Nonrheumatic aortic (valve) stenosis
I35.1	Nonrheumatic aortic (valve) insufficiency
I35.2	Nonrheumatic aortic (valve) stenosis with insufficiency
I35.8	Other nonrheumatic aortic valve disorders
I40.0	Infective myocarditis
I40.1	Isolated myocarditis
I41	Myocarditis in diseases classified elsewhere
I42.0	Dilated cardiomyopathy
I42.1	Obstructive hypertrophic cardiomyopathy
I42.2	Other hypertrophic cardiomyopathy
I42.5	Other restrictive cardiomyopathy
I42.7	Cardiomyopathy due to drug and external agent
I42.8	Other cardiomyopathies
I43	Cardiomyopathy in diseases classified elsewhere
I46.2	Cardiac arrest due to underlying cardiac condition
I46.8	Cardiac arrest due to other underlying condition
I47.0	Re-entry ventricular arrhythmia
I47.1	Supraventricular tachycardia
I47.2	Ventricular tachycardia
I50.1	Left ventricular failure, unspecified
I50.21	Acute systolic (congestive) heart failure
I50.22	Chronic systolic (congestive) heart failure
I50.23	Acute on chronic systolic (congestive) heart failure
I50.31	Acute diastolic (congestive) heart failure
I50.32	Chronic diastolic (congestive) heart failure
I50.33	Acute on chronic diastolic (congestive) heart failure
I50.41	Acute combined systolic (congestive) and diastolic (congestive) heart failure
I50.42	Chronic combined systolic (congestive) and diastolic (congestive) heart failure
I50.43	Acute on chronic combined systolic (congestive) and diastolic (congestive) heart failure
I50.811	Acute right heart failure
I50.812	Chronic right heart failure
I50.813	Acute on chronic right heart failure
I50.814	Right heart failure due to left heart failure
I50.82	Biventricular heart failure
I50.83	High output heart failure
I50.84	End stage heart failure
I51.5	Myocardial degeneration
I97.110	Postprocedural cardiac insufficiency following cardiac surgery
I97.111	Postprocedural cardiac insufficiency following other surgery
I97.120	Postprocedural cardiac arrest following cardiac surgery
I97.121	Postprocedural cardiac arrest following other surgery
I97.130	Postprocedural heart failure following cardiac surgery
I97.131	Postprocedural heart failure following other surgery
I97.190	Other postprocedural cardiac functional disturbances following cardiac surgery
I97.191	Other postprocedural cardiac functional disturbances following other surgery
I97.710	Intraoperative cardiac arrest during cardiac surgery
I97.711	Intraoperative cardiac arrest during other surgery
I97.790	Other intraoperative cardiac functional disturbances during cardiac surgery
I97.791	Other intraoperative cardiac functional disturbances during other surgery
I97.88	Other intraoperative complications of the circulatory system, not elsewhere classified
I97.89	Other postprocedural complications and disorders of the circulatory system, not elsewhere classified
Q21.0	Ventricular septal defect
Q21.1	Atrial septal defect
Q21.2	Atrioventricular septal defect
Q21.3	Tetralogy of Fallot
Q21.4	Aortopulmonary septal defect
Q21.8	Other congenital malformations of cardiac septa
Q23.0	Congenital stenosis of aortic valve
Q23.1	Congenital insufficiency of aortic valve
Q23.2	Congenital mitral stenosis
Q23.3	Congenital mitral insufficiency
Q23.8	Other congenital malformations of aortic and mitral valves
Q24.4	Congenital subaortic stenosis
Q24.5	Malformation of coronary vessels
Q24.6	Congenital heart block
Q24.8	Other specified congenital malformations of heart
R57.0	Cardiogenic shock

AMA: 33990 2018,Jun,3; 2018,Jan,8; 2017,Jan,8; 2017,Dec,3; 2016,Mar,5; 2016,Jan,13; 2015,Sep,3; 2015,Jan,16; 2014,Oct,14; 2014,Jan,11; 2013,Mar,10-11 **33991** 2018,Jun,3; 2018,Jan,8; 2017,Jan,8; 2017,Dec,3; 2016,Mar,5; 2016,Jan,13; 2015,Sep,3; 2015,Jan,16; 2014,Jan,11; 2013,Mar,10-11

Relative Value Units/Medicare Edits

Non-Facility RVU	Work	PE	MP	Total
33990	7.9	2.69	1.81	12.4
33991	11.63	3.92	2.64	18.19
Facility RVU	**Work**	**PE**	**MP**	**Total**
33990	7.9	2.69	1.81	12.4
33991	11.63	3.92	2.64	18.19

	FUD	Status	MUE	Modifiers				IOM Reference
33990	N/A	A	1(3)	51	N/A	N/A	80	100-03,20.9; 100-03,20.9.1; 100-04,32,320.3.1; 100-04,32,320.3.2
33991	N/A	A	1(3)	51	N/A	N/A	80	

* with documentation

Terms To Know

cardiogenic shock. Shock caused by an inadequate supply of oxygen to the body's tissues due to a malfunction of the pumping action of the heart.

hypertrophic. Enlarged or overgrown from an increase in cell size of the affected tissue.

idiopathic. Having no known cause.

percutaneous. Through the skin.

rheumatic heart disease. Manifestation of and sequel to rheumatic fever; any cardiac involvement in rheumatic fever.

ventricular assist device. Temporary measure used to support the heart by substituting for left and/or right heart function. The device replaces the work of the left and/or right ventricle when a patient has a damaged or weakened heart. A left ventricular assist device (VAD) helps the heart pump blood through the rest of the body. A right VAD helps the heart pump blood to the lungs to become oxygenated again. Catheters are inserted to circulate the blood through external tubing to a pump machine located outside of the body and back to the correct artery.

33992

33992 Removal of percutaneous ventricular assist device at separate and distinct session from insertion

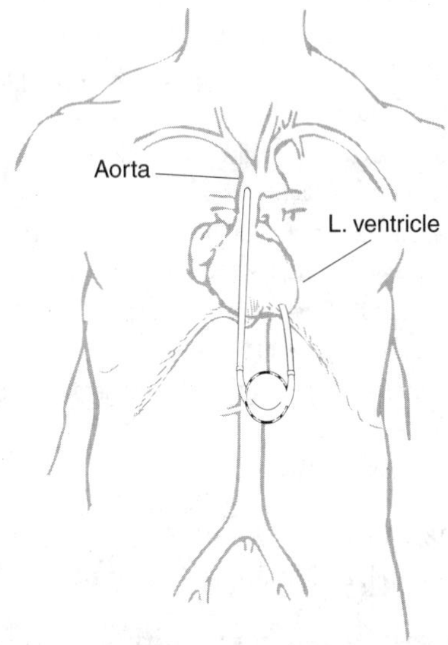

Ventricular assist device is removed percutaneously

Explanation

A ventricular assist device (VAD) bypasses the left ventricle during the blood oxygenation cycle making the ventricle work less during the systolic phase. The device is removed when the patient's ventricle recovers, an artificial heart is placed, or the patient undergoes heart transplantation. The catheters are removed from the left atrium and one or more femoral vessels and the external centrifugal assist device is discontinued and removed. This code can only be reported for the removal of a VAD during a different operative encounter than the insertion, and is only used for a percutaneous VAD, not an implantable VAD.

Coding Tips

When medically necessary, report moderate (conscious) sedation provided by the performing physician with 99151-99153. When provided by another physician, report 99155-99157. For insertion of a percutaneous ventricular assist device, see 33990–33991. For repositioning of a percutaneous ventricular assist device, see 33993. For removal of implantable intracorporeal ventricular assist devices, see 33980. For removal of extracorporeal ventricular assist devices, see 33977–33978. For removal of an implantable aortic counterpulsation ventricular assist system, see 0455T-0458T.

ICD-10-CM Diagnostic Codes

T82.518A	Breakdown (mechanical) of other cardiac and vascular devices and implants, initial encounter
T82.528A	Displacement of other cardiac and vascular devices and implants, initial encounter
T82.538A	Leakage of other cardiac and vascular devices and implants, initial encounter
T82.598A	Other mechanical complication of other cardiac and vascular devices and implants, initial encounter
T82.7XXA	Infection and inflammatory reaction due to other cardiac and vascular devices, implants and grafts, initial encounter
T82.817A	Embolism due to cardiac prosthetic devices, implants and grafts, initial encounter

T82.827A Fibrosis due to cardiac prosthetic devices, implants and grafts, initial encounter

T82.837A Hemorrhage due to cardiac prosthetic devices, implants and grafts, initial encounter

T82.847A Pain due to cardiac prosthetic devices, implants and grafts, initial encounter

T82.855A Stenosis of coronary artery stent, initial encounter

T82.857A Stenosis of other cardiac prosthetic devices, implants and grafts, initial encounter

T82.867A Thrombosis due to cardiac prosthetic devices, implants and grafts, initial encounter

T82.897A Other specified complication of cardiac prosthetic devices, implants and grafts, initial encounter

T82.898A Other specified complication of vascular prosthetic devices, implants and grafts, initial encounter

Z45.09 Encounter for adjustment and management of other cardiac device

Z95.811 Presence of heart assist device

AMA: 33992 2018,Jan,8; 2017,Jan,8; 2016,Mar,5; 2016,Jan,13; 2015,Sep,3; 2015,Jan,16; 2014,Jan,11; 2013,Mar,10-11

Relative Value Units/Medicare Edits

Non-Facility RVU	Work	PE	MP	Total
33992	3.75	1.21	0.84	5.8
Facility RVU	**Work**	**PE**	**MP**	**Total**
33992	3.75	1.21	0.84	5.8

	FUD	Status	MUE	Modifiers				IOM Reference
33992	N/A	A	1(2)	51	N/A	N/A	80	None

* with documentation

Terms To Know

extracorporeal. Located or taking place outside the body.

moderate sedation. Medically controlled state of depressed consciousness, with or without analgesia, while maintaining the patient's airway, protective reflexes, and ability to respond to stimulation or verbal commands.

percutaneous. Through the skin.

ventricular assist device. Temporary measure used to support the heart by substituting for left and/or right heart function. The device replaces the work of the left and/or right ventricle when a patient has a damaged or weakened heart. A left ventricular assist device (VAD) helps the heart pump blood through the rest of the body. A right VAD helps the heart pump blood to the lungs to become oxygenated again. Catheters are inserted to circulate the blood through external tubing to a pump machine located outside of the body and back to the correct artery.

33993

33993 Repositioning of percutaneous ventricular assist device with imaging guidance at separate and distinct session from insertion

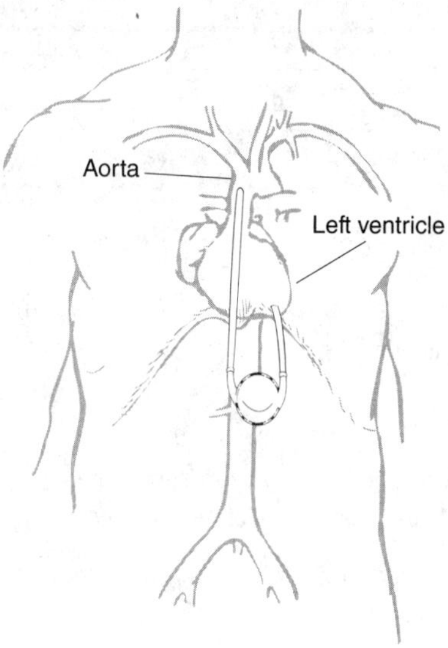

Ventricular assist device is repositioned percutaneously

Explanation

A ventricular assist device (VAD) bypasses the left ventricle during the blood oxygenation cycle making the ventricle work less during the systolic phase. A catheter is inserted in the patient's femoral vein and maneuvered to the left atrium. A centrifugal assist device is placed outside the body, usually on the patient's thigh. The catheter is attached to the device. Oxygenated blood is pumped from the left atrium to the device and distributed to one or both femoral arteries via catheter. Report 33993 when the components of a percutaneously placed VAD need to be repositioned any time other than during the surgical encounter for insertion.

Coding Tips

When medically necessary, report moderate (conscious) sedation provided by the performing physician with 99151-99153. When provided by another physician, report 99155-99157. Imaging guidance is considered part of this procedure and is not reported separately. For insertion of the percutaneous ventricular assist device, see 33990–33991. For removal of the percutaneous ventricular assist device, see 33992. For relocating and repositioning of an implantable aortic counterpulsation ventricular assist system, see 0459T-0461T.

ICD-10-CM Diagnostic Codes

I11.0 Hypertensive heart disease with heart failure

I16.0 Hypertensive urgency

I16.1 Hypertensive emergency

I20.0 Unstable angina

I20.1 Angina pectoris with documented spasm

I20.8 Other forms of angina pectoris

I21.01 ST elevation (STEMI) myocardial infarction involving left main coronary artery

I21.02 ST elevation (STEMI) myocardial infarction involving left anterior descending coronary artery

I21.09 ST elevation (STEMI) myocardial infarction involving other coronary artery of anterior wall

I21.11	ST elevation (STEMI) myocardial infarction involving right coronary artery
I21.19	ST elevation (STEMI) myocardial infarction involving other coronary artery of inferior wall
I21.21	ST elevation (STEMI) myocardial infarction involving left circumflex coronary artery
I21.29	ST elevation (STEMI) myocardial infarction involving other sites
I21.4	Non-ST elevation (NSTEMI) myocardial infarction
I21.A1	Myocardial infarction type 2
I22.0	Subsequent ST elevation (STEMI) myocardial infarction of anterior wall
I22.1	Subsequent ST elevation (STEMI) myocardial infarction of inferior wall
I22.2	Subsequent non-ST elevation (NSTEMI) myocardial infarction
I22.8	Subsequent ST elevation (STEMI) myocardial infarction of other sites
I24.8	Other forms of acute ischemic heart disease
I25.2	Old myocardial infarction
I25.3	Aneurysm of heart
I25.41	Coronary artery aneurysm
I25.42	Coronary artery dissection
I25.5	Ischemic cardiomyopathy
I25.6	Silent myocardial ischemia
I34.0	Nonrheumatic mitral (valve) insufficiency
I34.1	Nonrheumatic mitral (valve) prolapse
I34.2	Nonrheumatic mitral (valve) stenosis
I34.8	Other nonrheumatic mitral valve disorders
I35.0	Nonrheumatic aortic (valve) stenosis
I35.1	Nonrheumatic aortic (valve) insufficiency
I35.2	Nonrheumatic aortic (valve) stenosis with insufficiency
I35.8	Other nonrheumatic aortic valve disorders
I42.0	Dilated cardiomyopathy
I42.5	Other restrictive cardiomyopathy
I42.8	Other cardiomyopathies
I46.2	Cardiac arrest due to underlying cardiac condition
I46.8	Cardiac arrest due to other underlying condition
I47.0	Re-entry ventricular arrhythmia
I47.1	Supraventricular tachycardia
I47.2	Ventricular tachycardia
I50.1	Left ventricular failure, unspecified
I50.21	Acute systolic (congestive) heart failure
I50.22	Chronic systolic (congestive) heart failure
I50.23	Acute on chronic systolic (congestive) heart failure
I50.31	Acute diastolic (congestive) heart failure
I50.32	Chronic diastolic (congestive) heart failure
I50.33	Acute on chronic diastolic (congestive) heart failure
I50.41	Acute combined systolic (congestive) and diastolic (congestive) heart failure
I50.42	Chronic combined systolic (congestive) and diastolic (congestive) heart failure
I50.43	Acute on chronic combined systolic (congestive) and diastolic (congestive) heart failure
I50.811	Acute right heart failure
I50.812	Chronic right heart failure
I50.813	Acute on chronic right heart failure
I50.814	Right heart failure due to left heart failure
I50.82	Biventricular heart failure
I50.83	High output heart failure
I50.84	End stage heart failure
I51.5	Myocardial degeneration
I97.0	Postcardiotomy syndrome
I97.110	Postprocedural cardiac insufficiency following cardiac surgery
I97.111	Postprocedural cardiac insufficiency following other surgery
I97.120	Postprocedural cardiac arrest following cardiac surgery
I97.121	Postprocedural cardiac arrest following other surgery
I97.130	Postprocedural heart failure following cardiac surgery
I97.131	Postprocedural heart failure following other surgery
I97.190	Other postprocedural cardiac functional disturbances following cardiac surgery
I97.191	Other postprocedural cardiac functional disturbances following other surgery
I97.710	Intraoperative cardiac arrest during cardiac surgery
I97.711	Intraoperative cardiac arrest during other surgery
I97.790	Other intraoperative cardiac functional disturbances during cardiac surgery
I97.791	Other intraoperative cardiac functional disturbances during other surgery
I97.88	Other intraoperative complications of the circulatory system, not elsewhere classified
I97.89	Other postprocedural complications and disorders of the circulatory system, not elsewhere classified
Q21.0	Ventricular septal defect
Q21.1	Atrial septal defect
Q21.2	Atrioventricular septal defect
Q21.3	Tetralogy of Fallot
Q21.4	Aortopulmonary septal defect
Q21.8	Other congenital malformations of cardiac septa
Q23.0	Congenital stenosis of aortic valve
Q23.1	Congenital insufficiency of aortic valve
Q23.2	Congenital mitral stenosis
Q23.3	Congenital mitral insufficiency
Q23.8	Other congenital malformations of aortic and mitral valves
Q24.4	Congenital subaortic stenosis
Q24.5	Malformation of coronary vessels
Q24.6	Congenital heart block
Q24.8	Other specified congenital malformations of heart
R09.2	Respiratory arrest
R09.89	Other specified symptoms and signs involving the circulatory and respiratory systems
R57.0	Cardiogenic shock
T82.518A	Breakdown (mechanical) of other cardiac and vascular devices and implants, initial encounter
T82.528A	Displacement of other cardiac and vascular devices and implants, initial encounter
T82.538A	Leakage of other cardiac and vascular devices and implants, initial encounter
T82.598A	Other mechanical complication of other cardiac and vascular devices and implants, initial encounter

T82.7XXA	Infection and inflammatory reaction due to other cardiac and vascular devices, implants and grafts, initial encounter
T82.817A	Embolism due to cardiac prosthetic devices, implants and grafts, initial encounter
T82.827A	Fibrosis due to cardiac prosthetic devices, implants and grafts, initial encounter
T82.837A	Hemorrhage due to cardiac prosthetic devices, implants and grafts, initial encounter
T82.847A	Pain due to cardiac prosthetic devices, implants and grafts, initial encounter
T82.857A	Stenosis of other cardiac prosthetic devices, implants and grafts, initial encounter
T82.867A	Thrombosis due to cardiac prosthetic devices, implants and grafts, initial encounter
T82.897A	Other specified complication of cardiac prosthetic devices, implants and grafts, initial encounter
T82.898A	Other specified complication of vascular prosthetic devices, implants and grafts, initial encounter
Z45.09	Encounter for adjustment and management of other cardiac device
Z95.811	Presence of heart assist device

AMA: **33993** 2018,Jan,8; 2017,Jan,8; 2016,Mar,5; 2016,Jan,13; 2015,Sep,3; 2015,Jan,16; 2014,Jan,11; 2013,Mar,10-11

Relative Value Units/Medicare Edits

Non-Facility RVU	Work	PE	MP	Total
33993	3.26	1.13	0.7	5.09
Facility RVU	**Work**	**PE**	**MP**	**Total**
33993	3.26	1.13	0.7	5.09

	FUD	Status	MUE	Modifiers				IOM Reference
33993	N/A	A	1(3)	51	N/A	N/A	80	None

* with documentation

34001

34001 Embolectomy or thrombectomy, with or without catheter; carotid, subclavian or innominate artery, by neck incision

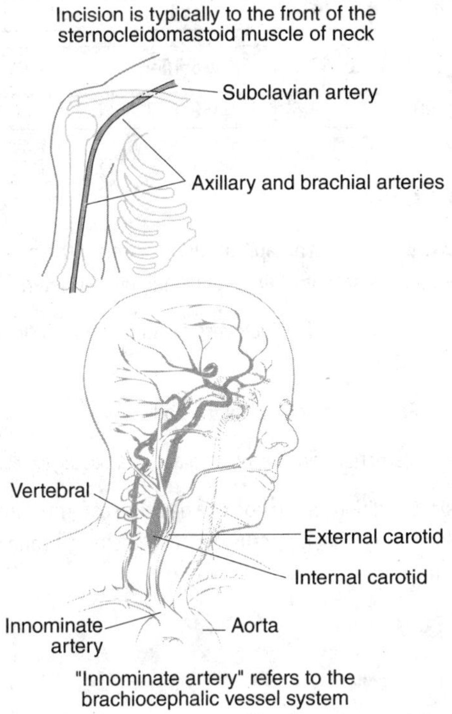

Explanation

To remove a blood clot in the carotid, subclavian, or innominate artery, the physician makes an incision in the skin of the neck usually in front of the sternocleidomastoid muscle over the site of the clot or immediately above it. The artery is isolated and dissected from critical structures. The artery may be clamped above and below the clot and incised. The physician removes the blood clot and sutures the artery. The clamps are removed. If a catheter is required, it is threaded past the clot and a small balloon at its tip is inflated. The catheter is withdrawn, capturing and retrieving the clot. The physician may make several passes to remove the entire clot. The blood vessel is repaired with sutures and the skin incision is repaired with layered closure.

Coding Tips

Establishing both inflow and outflow by any method is included. That portion of the operative arteriogram performed by the surgeon is also included. Angioscopy performed during therapeutic intervention should be reported in addition to the code for the primary procedure; see 35400. For arterial embolectomy or thrombectomy, innominate, subclavian, by thoracic incision, see 34051; by arm incision, see 34101. For venous thrombectomy subclavian by neck incision, see 34471; by arm incision, see 34490. For thrombectomy of an arterial graft, see 35875–35876.

ICD-10-CM Diagnostic Codes

G45.0	Vertebro-basilar artery syndrome
G45.1	Carotid artery syndrome (hemispheric)
G45.2	Multiple and bilateral precerebral artery syndromes
G45.3	Amaurosis fugax
G45.8	Other transient cerebral ischemic attacks and related syndromes
G45.9	Transient cerebral ischemic attack, unspecified
I63.031	Cerebral infarction due to thrombosis of right carotid artery ☑
I63.032	Cerebral infarction due to thrombosis of left carotid artery ☑
I63.033	Cerebral infarction due to thrombosis of bilateral carotid arteries ☑
I63.09	Cerebral infarction due to thrombosis of other precerebral artery
I63.131	Cerebral infarction due to embolism of right carotid artery ☑
I63.132	Cerebral infarction due to embolism of left carotid artery ☑
I63.133	Cerebral infarction due to embolism of bilateral carotid arteries ☑
I63.231	Cerebral infarction due to unspecified occlusion or stenosis of right carotid arteries ☑
I63.232	Cerebral infarction due to unspecified occlusion or stenosis of left carotid arteries ☑
I63.29	Cerebral infarction due to unspecified occlusion or stenosis of other precerebral arteries
I65.21	Occlusion and stenosis of right carotid artery ☑
I65.22	Occlusion and stenosis of left carotid artery ☑
I65.23	Occlusion and stenosis of bilateral carotid arteries ☑
I65.8	Occlusion and stenosis of other precerebral arteries
I67.2	Cerebral atherosclerosis
I67.81	Acute cerebrovascular insufficiency
I67.841	Reversible cerebrovascular vasoconstriction syndrome
I67.848	Other cerebrovascular vasospasm and vasoconstriction
I67.89	Other cerebrovascular disease
I76	Septic arterial embolism

AMA: **34001** 1997,Nov,1

Relative Value Units/Medicare Edits

Non-Facility RVU	Work	PE	MP	Total
34001	17.88	5.92	4.07	27.87
Facility RVU	**Work**	**PE**	**MP**	**Total**
34001	17.88	5.92	4.07	27.87

	FUD	Status	MUE	Modifiers				IOM Reference
34001	90	A	1(3)	51	50	62*	80	100-03,160.8

* with documentation

Terms To Know

embolism. Obstruction of a blood vessel resulting from a clot or foreign substance.

thrombosis. Condition arising from the presence or formation of blood clots within a blood vessel that may cause vascular obstruction and insufficient oxygenation.

34051

34051 Embolectomy or thrombectomy, with or without catheter; innominate, subclavian artery, by thoracic incision

"Innominate artery" refers to the brachiocephalic trunk, i.e., between the aorta and the bifurcation to the right subclavian and the right common carotid arteries

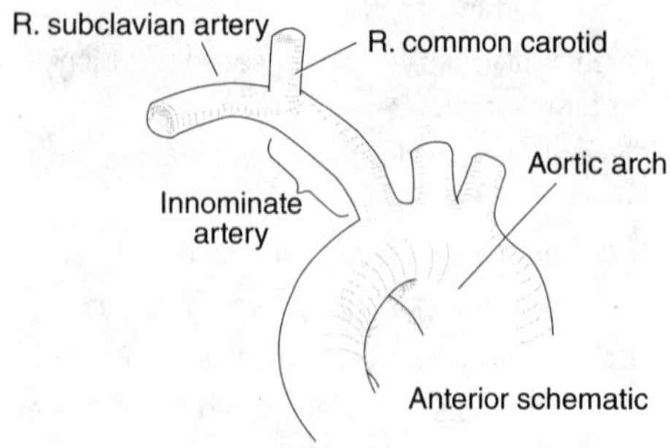

Access is via a thoracic incision

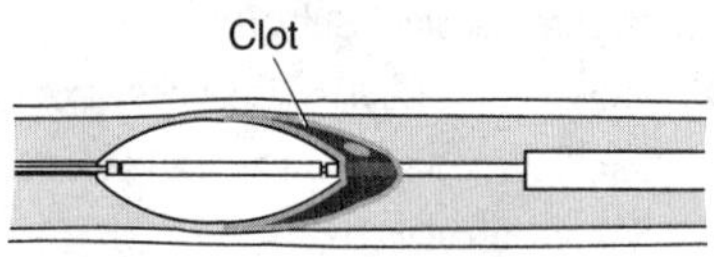

Balloon catheter may be inserted beyond clot and withdrawn through structure, removing the clot

Explanation

The physician exposes the innominate or subclavian artery by making an incision in the anterior chest (midline sternotomy or lateral thoracotomy). The physician identifies the embolus or thrombus and occludes the artery proximal to the clot. The physician makes a small incision in the artery proximal to the clot and withdraws it using ring forceps, or by passing a Fogarty balloon catheter beyond the clot, inflating and withdrawing the balloon. The physician establishes proof of patency by injecting contrast in the artery under fluoroscope. The physician sutures the arteriotomy closed, removes the vascular clamp or tie, and closes the chest wall. The physician may leave chest tubes and/or a mediastinal drainage tube in place following the procedure.

Coding Tips

Establishing both inflow and outflow by any method is included. That portion of the operative arteriogram performed by the surgeon is also included. Angioscopy performed during therapeutic intervention should be reported in addition to the code for the primary procedure; see 35400.

ICD-10-CM Diagnostic Codes

G45.0	Vertebro-basilar artery syndrome
G45.2	Multiple and bilateral precerebral artery syndromes
G45.8	Other transient cerebral ischemic attacks and related syndromes
G45.9	Transient cerebral ischemic attack, unspecified
I63.09	Cerebral infarction due to thrombosis of other precerebral artery
I63.19	Cerebral infarction due to embolism of other precerebral artery
I63.29	Cerebral infarction due to unspecified occlusion or stenosis of other precerebral arteries
I63.9	Cerebral infarction, unspecified
I76	Septic arterial embolism

AMA: 34051 1997,Nov,1

Relative Value Units/Medicare Edits

Non-Facility RVU	Work	PE	MP	Total
34051	16.99	7.83	4.01	28.83
Facility RVU	**Work**	**PE**	**MP**	**Total**
34051	16.99	7.83	4.01	28.83

	FUD	Status	MUE	Modifiers				IOM Reference
34051	90	A	1(3)	51	50	62*	80	None

* with documentation

Terms To Know

angioscopy. Visualization of capillary blood vessels with a microscope, or the inside of a blood vessel with a fiberoptic-equipped catheter.

embolism. Obstruction of a blood vessel resulting from a clot or foreign substance.

hemiplegia. Paralysis of one side of the body.

occlusion. Constriction, closure, or blockage of a passage.

thrombosis. Condition arising from the presence or formation of blood clots within a blood vessel that may cause vascular obstruction and insufficient oxygenation.

34101-34111

34101 Embolectomy or thrombectomy, with or without catheter; axillary, brachial, innominate, subclavian artery, by arm incision

34111 radial or ulnar artery, by arm incision

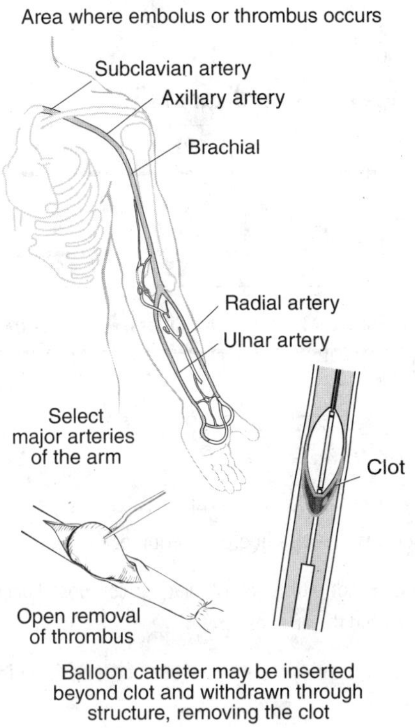

Explanation

In 34101, to remove a blood clot in the axillary, brachial, innominate, or subclavian artery, the physician makes an incision in the skin of the arm at the site of the blood clot or above it. In 34111, to remove a blood clot in the radial or ulnar artery, the physician makes an incision in the skin of the arm, over the site of the clot or immediately above it. The artery is isolated and dissected from adjacent critical structures. The artery may be clamped above and below the clot, and incised. The physician removes the blood clot and repairs the artery. The clamps are removed. If a catheter is required, it is threaded past the clot and a small balloon at its tip is inflated. The catheter is withdrawn, capturing and retrieving the clot. The physician may make several passes to remove all of the clot. The blood vessel is repaired with sutures and the skin incision is repaired with a layered closure.

Coding Tips

Establishing both inflow and outflow by any method is included. The portion of the operative arteriogram performed by the surgeon is also included. Angioscopy performed during therapeutic intervention should be reported in addition to the code for the primary procedure; see 35400. For arterial embolectomy or thrombectomy, carotid, innominate, subclavian, by thoracic incision, see 34001; innominate, subclavian, by thoracic incision, see 34051. For venous thrombectomy, subclavian, by neck incision, see 34471; axillary and subclavian by arm incision, see 34490. For thrombectomy of an arterial graft, see 35875–35876.

ICD-10-CM Diagnostic Codes

G45.2	Multiple and bilateral precerebral artery syndromes
I63.09	Cerebral infarction due to thrombosis of other precerebral artery
I63.29	Cerebral infarction due to unspecified occlusion or stenosis of other precerebral arteries
I65.8	Occlusion and stenosis of other precerebral arteries
I72.8	Aneurysm of other specified arteries
I73.89	Other specified peripheral vascular diseases
I73.9	Peripheral vascular disease, unspecified
I74.2	Embolism and thrombosis of arteries of the upper extremities
I75.011	Atheroembolism of right upper extremity ☑
I75.012	Atheroembolism of left upper extremity ☑
I75.013	Atheroembolism of bilateral upper extremities ☑
I75.019	Atheroembolism of unspecified upper extremity
I76	Septic arterial embolism

AMA: 34101 1997,Nov,1 **34111** 1997,Nov,1

Relative Value Units/Medicare Edits

Non-Facility RVU	Work	PE	MP	Total
34101	10.93	3.88	2.51	17.32
34111	10.93	3.99	2.47	17.39
Facility RVU	**Work**	**PE**	**MP**	**Total**
34101	10.93	3.88	2.51	17.32
34111	10.93	3.99	2.47	17.39

	FUD	Status	MUE	Modifiers				IOM Reference
34101	90	A	1(3)	51	50	62*	80	None
34111	90	A	2(3)	51	50	62*	80	

* with documentation

Terms To Know

angioscopy. Visualization of capillary blood vessels with a microscope, or the inside of a blood vessel with a fiberoptic-equipped catheter.

catheter. Flexible tube inserted into an area of the body for introducing or withdrawing fluid.

dissect. Cut apart or separate tissue for surgical purposes or for visual or microscopic study.

embolism. Obstruction of a blood vessel resulting from a clot or foreign substance.

thrombosis. Condition arising from the presence or formation of blood clots within a blood vessel that may cause vascular obstruction and insufficient oxygenation.

Arteries and Veins

34151

34151 Embolectomy or thrombectomy, with or without catheter; renal, celiac, mesentery, aortoiliac artery, by abdominal incision

Access is via an abdominal incision

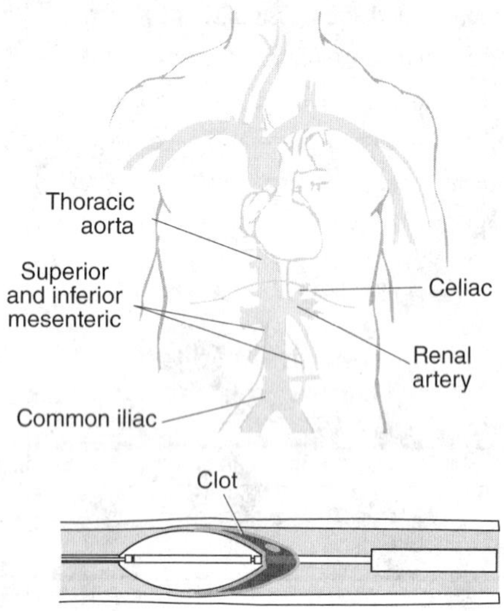

Balloon catheter may be inserted beyond clot and withdrawn through structure, removing the clot

Explanation

To remove a blood clot in the renal, celiac, mesentery, aortoiliac artery, the physician makes an incision in the skin of the abdomen over the site of the clot or immediately above or below it. The vein is isolated and dissected from adjacent critical structures. The artery may be clamped above and below the clot and incised. The physician removes the blood clot. The clamps are removed. If a catheter is required, it is threaded past the clot and a small balloon at its tip is inflated. The catheter is withdrawn, capturing and retrieving the clot. The physician may make several passes to remove all of the clot. The blood vessel is repaired with sutures and the skin incision is repaired with a layered closure.

Coding Tips

Establishing both inflow and outflow by any method is included. The portion of the operative arteriogram performed by the surgeon is also included. Angioscopy performed during therapeutic intervention should be reported in addition to the code for the primary procedure; see 35400. For thrombectomy of an arterial or venous graft, see 35875–35876.

ICD-10-CM Diagnostic Codes

I70.1	Atherosclerosis of renal artery
I74.01	Saddle embolus of abdominal aorta
I74.09	Other arterial embolism and thrombosis of abdominal aorta
I74.19	Embolism and thrombosis of other parts of aorta
I74.5	Embolism and thrombosis of iliac artery
I75.81	Atheroembolism of kidney
I76	Septic arterial embolism
K55.011	Focal (segmental) acute (reversible) ischemia of small intestine
K55.012	Diffuse acute (reversible) ischemia of small intestine
K55.021	Focal (segmental) acute infarction of small intestine
K55.022	Diffuse acute infarction of small intestine
K55.031	Focal (segmental) acute (reversible) ischemia of large intestine
K55.032	Diffuse acute (reversible) ischemia of large intestine
K55.041	Focal (segmental) acute infarction of large intestine
K55.042	Diffuse acute infarction of large intestine
K55.1	Chronic vascular disorders of intestine
K55.8	Other vascular disorders of intestine
N28.0	Ischemia and infarction of kidney

AMA: **34151** 1997,Nov,1

Relative Value Units/Medicare Edits

Non-Facility RVU	Work	PE	MP	Total
34151	26.52	7.95	5.93	40.4
Facility RVU	**Work**	**PE**	**MP**	**Total**
34151	26.52	7.95	5.93	40.4

	FUD	Status	MUE	Modifiers				IOM Reference
34151	90	A	1(3)	51	50	62*	80	None

* with documentation

Terms To Know

angioscopy. Visualization of capillary blood vessels with a microscope, or the inside of a blood vessel with a fiberoptic-equipped catheter.

atherosclerosis. Buildup of yellowish plaques composed of cholesterol and lipoid material within the arteries.

catheter. Flexible tube inserted into an area of the body for introducing or withdrawing fluid.

complication. Condition arising after the beginning of observation and treatment that modifies the course of the patient's illness or the medical care required, or an undesired result or misadventure in medical care.

embolism. Obstruction of a blood vessel resulting from a clot or foreign substance.

34201

34201 Embolectomy or thrombectomy, with or without catheter; femoropopliteal, aortoiliac artery, by leg incision

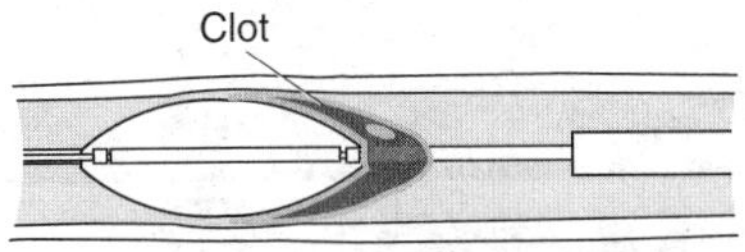

Balloon catheter may be inserted beyond clot and withdrawn through structure, removing the clot

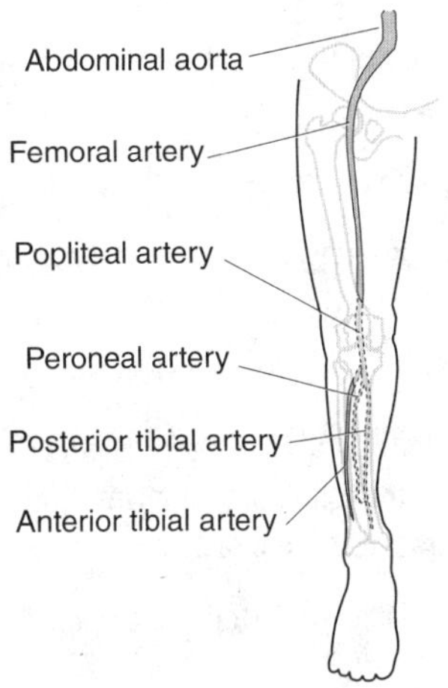

Explanation

To remove a blood clot in the femoropopliteal or aortoiliac artery, the physician makes an incision in the skin of the leg over the femoral artery. The artery is isolated and dissected from adjacent critical structures. The artery may be clamped above and below the clot and incised. The physician removes the blood clot and repairs the vessel. The clamps are removed. If a catheter is required, it is threaded past the clot and a small balloon at its tip is inflated. The catheter is withdrawn, capturing and retrieving the clot. The physician may make several passes to remove all of the clot. The blood vessel is repaired with sutures and the skin incision is repaired with a layered closure.

Coding Tips

Establishing both inflow and outflow by any method is included. The portion of the operative arteriogram performed by the surgeon is also included. Angioscopy performed during therapeutic intervention should be reported in addition to the code for the primary procedure; see 35400. For venous thrombectomy of the vena cava, iliac, or femoropopliteal vein by leg incision, see 34421. For thrombectomy of an arterial or venous graft, see 35875–35876.

ICD-10-CM Diagnostic Codes

I74.01	Saddle embolus of abdominal aorta
I74.09	Other arterial embolism and thrombosis of abdominal aorta
I74.19	Embolism and thrombosis of other parts of aorta
I74.3	Embolism and thrombosis of arteries of the lower extremities
I74.5	Embolism and thrombosis of iliac artery
I75.021	Atheroembolism of right lower extremity ☑
I75.022	Atheroembolism of left lower extremity ☑
I75.023	Atheroembolism of bilateral lower extremities ☑
I75.029	Atheroembolism of unspecified lower extremity

AMA: 34201 2018,Jan,8; 2017,Jan,8; 2016,Jan,13; 2015,Jan,16; 2014,Jan,11

Relative Value Units/Medicare Edits

Non-Facility RVU	Work	PE	MP	Total
34201	19.48	5.8	4.5	29.78
Facility RVU	**Work**	**PE**	**MP**	**Total**
34201	19.48	5.8	4.5	29.78

	FUD	Status	MUE	Modifiers				IOM Reference
34201	90	A	1(3)	51	50	62*	80	None

* with documentation

Terms To Know

angioscopy. Visualization of capillary blood vessels with a microscope, or the inside of a blood vessel with a fiberoptic-equipped catheter.

catheter. Flexible tube inserted into an area of the body for introducing or withdrawing fluid.

embolism. Obstruction of a blood vessel resulting from a clot or foreign substance.

graft. Tissue implant from another part of the body or another person.

incision. Act of cutting into tissue or an organ.

thrombectomy. Removal of a clot (thrombus) from a blood vessel utilizing various methods.

34203

34203 Embolectomy or thrombectomy, with or without catheter; popliteal-tibio-peroneal artery, by leg incision

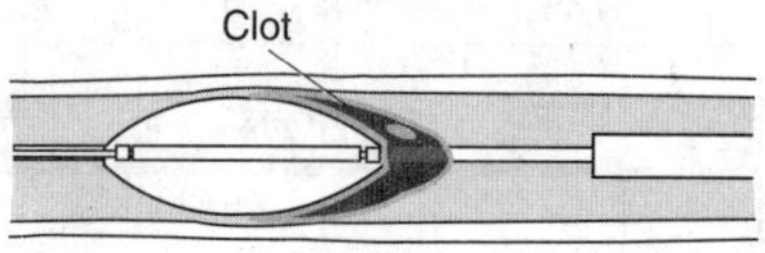

Balloon catheter may be inserted beyond clot and withdrawn through structure, removing the clot

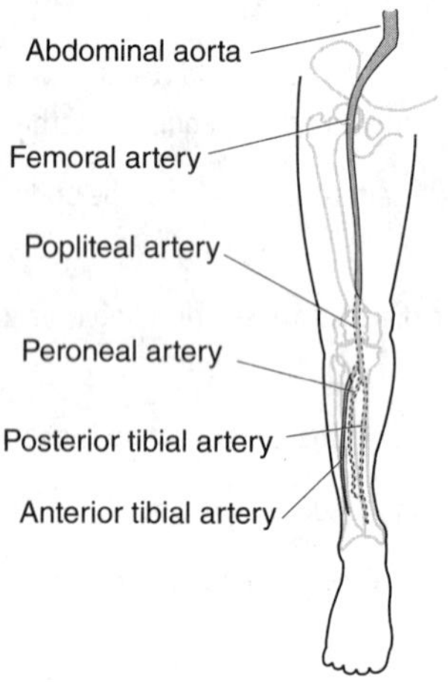

Explanation

To remove a blood clot in the popliteal-tibio-peroneal artery, the physician makes an incision in the skin of the leg over the femoral or popliteal artery. The artery is isolated and dissected from adjacent critical structures. The artery may be clamped above and below the clot and incised. The physician removes the blood clot. The clamps are removed. If a catheter is required, it is threaded past the clot and a small balloon at its tip is inflated. The catheter is withdrawn, capturing and retrieving the clot. The physician may make several passes to remove all of the clot. The blood vessel is repaired with sutures and the skin incision is repaired with a layered closure.

Coding Tips

Establishing both inflow and outflow by any method is included. The portion of the operative arteriogram performed by the surgeon is also included. Angioscopy performed during therapeutic intervention should be reported in addition to the code for the primary procedure; see 35400. For thrombectomy of an arterial or venous graft, see 35875–35876.

ICD-10-CM Diagnostic Codes

I74.3	Embolism and thrombosis of arteries of the lower extremities
I75.021	Atheroembolism of right lower extremity ☑
I75.022	Atheroembolism of left lower extremity ☑
I75.023	Atheroembolism of bilateral lower extremities ☑
I75.029	Atheroembolism of unspecified lower extremity

AMA: 34203 1997,Nov,1

Relative Value Units/Medicare Edits

Non-Facility RVU	Work	PE	MP	Total
34203	17.86	5.58	4.09	27.53
Facility RVU	**Work**	**PE**	**MP**	**Total**
34203	17.86	5.58	4.09	27.53

	FUD	Status	MUE	Modifiers				IOM Reference
34203	90	A	1(2)	51	50	62*	80	None

* with documentation

Terms To Know

angioscopy. Visualization of capillary blood vessels with a microscope, or the inside of a blood vessel with a fiberoptic-equipped catheter.

arteriogram. Radiograph of arteries.

catheter. Flexible tube inserted into an area of the body for introducing or withdrawing fluid.

closed fracture. Break in a bone without a concomitant opening in the skin.

complication. Condition arising after the beginning of observation and treatment that modifies the course of the patient's illness or the medical care required, or an undesired result or misadventure in medical care.

dissect. Cut apart or separate tissue for surgical purposes or for visual or microscopic study.

embolism. Obstruction of a blood vessel resulting from a clot or foreign substance.

graft. Tissue implant from another part of the body or another person.

incision. Act of cutting into tissue or an organ.

thrombectomy. Removal of a clot (thrombus) from a blood vessel utilizing various methods.

thrombosis. Condition arising from the presence or formation of blood clots within a blood vessel that may cause vascular obstruction and insufficient oxygenation.

34401

34401 Thrombectomy, direct or with catheter; vena cava, iliac vein, by abdominal incision

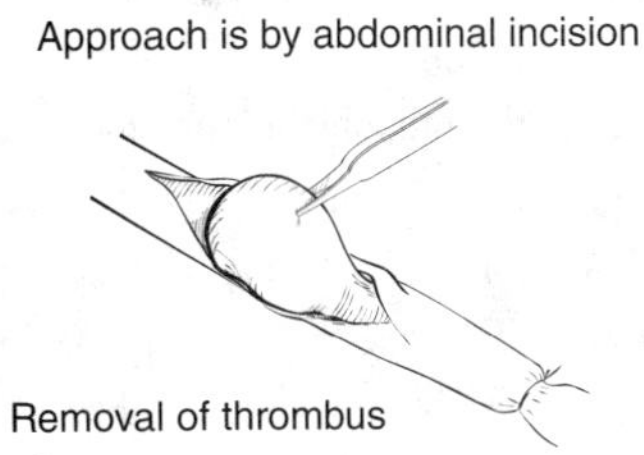

A thrombus in the vena cava and/or iliac vein is removed by an abdominal incision

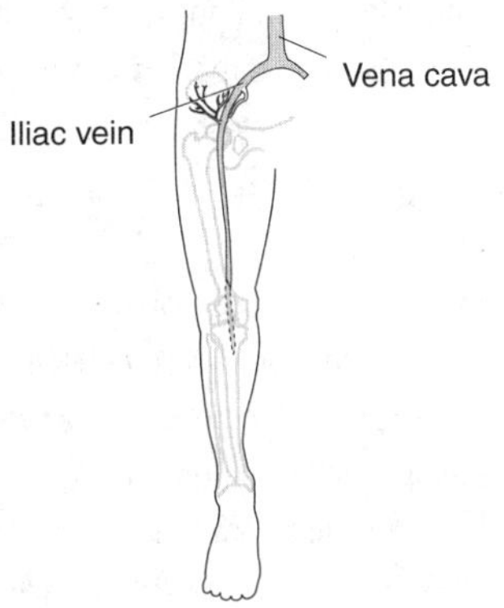

Explanation

The physician exposes the vena cava or iliac vein by making an abdominal incision. The physician identifies the thrombus by venogram and may perform a contralateral femoral venogram to rule out inferior vena caval involvement. The physician makes an incision in the vena cava or iliac vein. The physician withdraws the clot by passing a Fogarty balloon catheter beyond the clot, inflating and withdrawing the balloon. The physician may attempt to reduce the risk of pulmonary embolism by increasing intrathoracic pressure in a ventilated patient. The physician may establish proof of patency by repeat venography. The physician sutures the venotomy closed and closes the wound.

Coding Tips

Establishing both inflow and outflow by any method is included. The portion of the operative arteriogram performed by the surgeon is also included. Angioscopy performed during therapeutic intervention should be reported in addition to the code for the primary procedure; see 35400. For arterial thrombectomy aortoiliac by abdominal incision, see 34151; by leg incision, see 34201. For venous thrombectomy of the vena cava or the iliac or femoropopliteal vein by leg incision, see 34421; by abdominal and leg incision, see 34451. For thrombectomy of an arterial or venous graft, see 35875–35876.

ICD-10-CM Diagnostic Codes

I80.211	Phlebitis and thrombophlebitis of right iliac vein ☑
I80.212	Phlebitis and thrombophlebitis of left iliac vein ☑
I80.213	Phlebitis and thrombophlebitis of iliac vein, bilateral ☑
I82.220	Acute embolism and thrombosis of inferior vena cava
I82.221	Chronic embolism and thrombosis of inferior vena cava
I82.421	Acute embolism and thrombosis of right iliac vein ☑
I82.422	Acute embolism and thrombosis of left iliac vein ☑
I82.423	Acute embolism and thrombosis of iliac vein, bilateral ☑
I82.521	Chronic embolism and thrombosis of right iliac vein ☑
I82.522	Chronic embolism and thrombosis of left iliac vein ☑
I82.523	Chronic embolism and thrombosis of iliac vein, bilateral ☑
T81.72XA	Complication of vein following a procedure, not elsewhere classified, initial encounter

AMA: **34401** 1997,Nov,1

Relative Value Units/Medicare Edits

Non-Facility RVU	Work	PE	MP	Total
34401	26.52	10.21	5.67	42.4
Facility RVU	**Work**	**PE**	**MP**	**Total**
34401	26.52	10.21	5.67	42.4

	FUD	Status	MUE	Modifiers				IOM Reference
34401	90	A	1(3)	51	50	62*	80	None

* with documentation

Terms To Know

embolism. Obstruction of a blood vessel resulting from a clot or foreign substance.

thrombectomy. Removal of a clot (thrombus) from a blood vessel utilizing various methods.

thrombosis. Condition arising from the presence or formation of blood clots within a blood vessel that may cause vascular obstruction and insufficient oxygenation.

vena cava. Main venous trunk that empties into the right atrium from both the lower and upper regions, beginning at the junction of the common iliac veins inferiorly and the two brachiocephalic veins superiorly.

34421-34451

34421 Thrombectomy, direct or with catheter; vena cava, iliac, femoropopliteal vein, by leg incision

34451 vena cava, iliac, femoropopliteal vein, by abdominal and leg incision

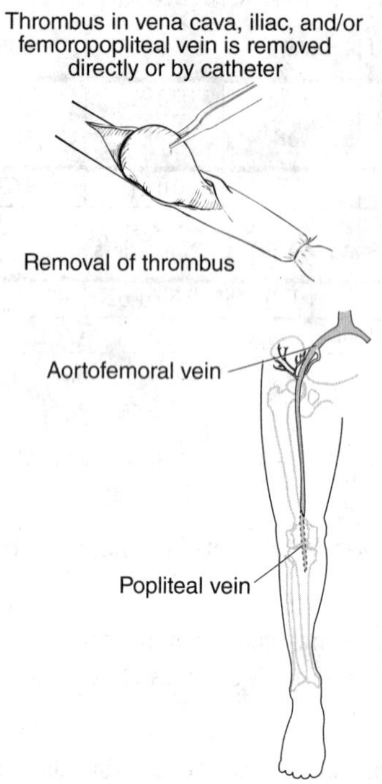

Explanation

In 34421, to remove a blood clot in the vena cava, iliac, or femoropopliteal vein, the physician makes an incision in the skin of the upper leg over the site of the clot or immediately above or below it. The vein is isolated and dissected from adjacent critical structures. The vein may be clamped above and below the clot and incised. The physician removes the blood clot. The clamps are removed. If a catheter is required, it is threaded past the clot and a small balloon at its tip is inflated. The catheter is withdrawn, capturing and retrieving the clot. The physician may make several passes to remove all of the clot. The blood vessel is repaired with sutures and the skin incision is repaired with a layered closure. In 34451, the physician exposes the vena cava, iliac, or femoropopliteal veins by making abdominal and leg incisions. The physician identifies the thrombus by venogram and may perform a contralateral femoral venogram to rule out inferior vena caval involvement. An incision is made over the site of the clot or immediately above or below it. The vein is isolated and dissected from adjacent critical structures. The vein may be clamped above and below the clot and incised. The physician removes the blood clot. The clamps are removed. The physician may cut down and introduce a Fogarty catheter via the popliteal vein, advancing the catheter toward the femoral vein while extruding thrombus through the femoral venotomy. The physician withdraws the clot by passing a Fogarty balloon catheter beyond the clot, inflating, and withdrawing the balloon. The physician may establish proof of patency by repeat venography. The physician sutures the venotomy closed and closes the wound.

Coding Tips

Establishing both inflow and outflow by any method is included. The portion of the operative arteriogram performed by the surgeon is also included. Angioscopy performed during therapeutic intervention should be reported in addition to the code for the primary procedure; see 35400. For arterial thrombectomy of the aortoiliac artery by abdominal incision, see 34151; aortoiliac, femoropopliteal by leg incision, see 34201.

ICD-10-CM Diagnostic Codes

I80.11	Phlebitis and thrombophlebitis of right femoral vein ☑
I80.12	Phlebitis and thrombophlebitis of left femoral vein ☑
I80.13	Phlebitis and thrombophlebitis of femoral vein, bilateral ☑
I80.211	Phlebitis and thrombophlebitis of right iliac vein ☑
I80.212	Phlebitis and thrombophlebitis of left iliac vein ☑
I80.213	Phlebitis and thrombophlebitis of iliac vein, bilateral ☑
I80.221	Phlebitis and thrombophlebitis of right popliteal vein ☑
I80.222	Phlebitis and thrombophlebitis of left popliteal vein ☑
I80.223	Phlebitis and thrombophlebitis of popliteal vein, bilateral ☑
I82.220	Acute embolism and thrombosis of inferior vena cava
I82.221	Chronic embolism and thrombosis of inferior vena cava
I82.411	Acute embolism and thrombosis of right femoral vein ☑
I82.412	Acute embolism and thrombosis of left femoral vein ☑
I82.413	Acute embolism and thrombosis of femoral vein, bilateral ☑
I82.421	Acute embolism and thrombosis of right iliac vein ☑
I82.422	Acute embolism and thrombosis of left iliac vein ☑
I82.423	Acute embolism and thrombosis of iliac vein, bilateral ☑
I82.431	Acute embolism and thrombosis of right popliteal vein ☑
I82.432	Acute embolism and thrombosis of left popliteal vein ☑
I82.433	Acute embolism and thrombosis of popliteal vein, bilateral ☑
I82.491	Acute embolism and thrombosis of other specified deep vein of right lower extremity ☑
I82.492	Acute embolism and thrombosis of other specified deep vein of left lower extremity ☑
I82.493	Acute embolism and thrombosis of other specified deep vein of lower extremity, bilateral ☑
I82.511	Chronic embolism and thrombosis of right femoral vein ☑
I82.512	Chronic embolism and thrombosis of left femoral vein ☑
I82.513	Chronic embolism and thrombosis of femoral vein, bilateral ☑
I82.521	Chronic embolism and thrombosis of right iliac vein ☑
I82.522	Chronic embolism and thrombosis of left iliac vein ☑
I82.523	Chronic embolism and thrombosis of iliac vein, bilateral ☑
I82.531	Chronic embolism and thrombosis of right popliteal vein ☑
I82.532	Chronic embolism and thrombosis of left popliteal vein ☑
I82.533	Chronic embolism and thrombosis of popliteal vein, bilateral ☑
I82.591	Chronic embolism and thrombosis of other specified deep vein of right lower extremity ☑
I82.592	Chronic embolism and thrombosis of other specified deep vein of left lower extremity ☑
I82.593	Chronic embolism and thrombosis of other specified deep vein of lower extremity, bilateral ☑
T81.72XA	Complication of vein following a procedure, not elsewhere classified, initial encounter

AMA: 34421 2018,Jan,8; 2017,Jan,8; 2016,Jan,13; 2015,Jan,16; 2014,Jan,11

Relative Value Units/Medicare Edits

Non-Facility RVU	Work	PE	MP	Total
34421	13.37	4.87	3.1	21.34
34451	28.52	6.34	6.59	41.45
Facility RVU	**Work**	**PE**	**MP**	**Total**
34421	13.37	4.87	3.1	21.34
34451	28.52	6.34	6.59	41.45

	FUD	Status	MUE	Modifiers				IOM Reference
34421	90	A	1(3)	51	50	62*	80	None
34451	90	A	1(3)	51	50	62*	80	

* with documentation

Terms To Know

angioscopy. Visualization of capillary blood vessels with a microscope, or the inside of a blood vessel with a fiberoptic-equipped catheter.

contralateral. Located on, or affecting, the opposite side of the body, usually as it relates to a bilateral body part.

embolism. Obstruction of a blood vessel resulting from a clot or foreign substance.

thrombosis. Condition arising from the presence or formation of blood clots within a blood vessel that may cause vascular obstruction and insufficient oxygenation.

vena cava. Main venous trunk that empties into the right atrium from both the lower and upper regions, beginning at the junction of the common iliac veins inferiorly and the two brachiocephalic veins superiorly.

34471-34490

34471 Thrombectomy, direct or with catheter; subclavian vein, by neck incision

34490 axillary and subclavian vein, by arm incision

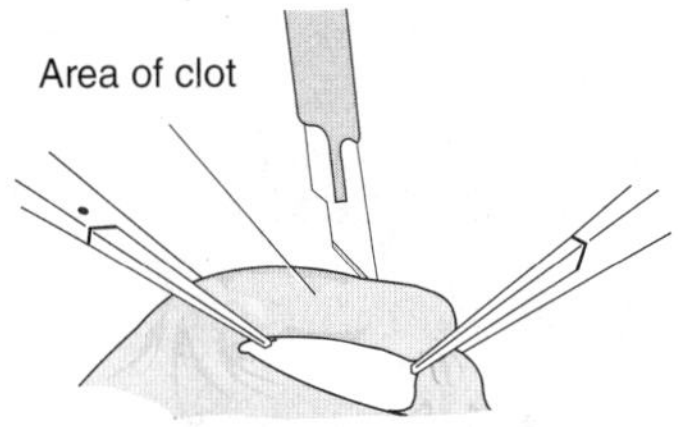

A thrombus may be approached directly by incision

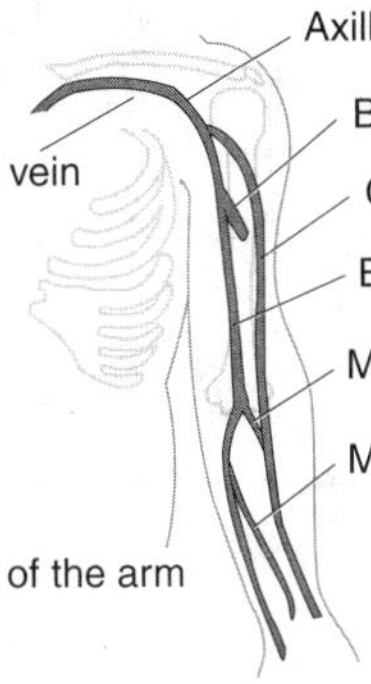

Major veins of the arm

Explanation

In 34471, to remove a blood clot in the subclavian vein, the physician makes an incision in the skin of the neck over the site of the clot or immediately above or below it. In 34490, to remove a blood clot in the axillary and subclavian vein, the physician makes an incision in the skin of the arm over the site of the clot or immediately above or below it. The vein is isolated and dissected from adjacent critical structures. The vein may be clamped above and below the clot and incised. The physician removes the blood clot. The clamps are removed. If a catheter is required, it is threaded past the clot and a small balloon at its tip is inflated. The catheter is withdrawn, capturing and retrieving the clot. The physician may make several passes to remove the entire clot. The blood vessel is repaired with sutures and the skin incision is repaired with a layered closure.

Coding Tips

Establishing both inflow and outflow by any method is included. The portion of the operative arteriogram performed by the surgeon is also included. Angioscopy performed during therapeutic intervention should be reported in addition to the code for the primary procedure; see 35400. For arterial embolectomy/thrombectomy of the subclavian vein, by neck incision, see 34001; by thoracic incision, see 34051. For arterial embolectomy/thrombectomy of the axillary or subclavian artery by arm incision, see 34101. For thrombectomy of an arterial or venous graft, see 35875–35876.

ICD-10-CM Diagnostic Codes

I82.A11 Acute embolism and thrombosis of right axillary vein ☑
I82.A12 Acute embolism and thrombosis of left axillary vein ☑
I82.A13 Acute embolism and thrombosis of axillary vein, bilateral ☑
I82.A21 Chronic embolism and thrombosis of right axillary vein ☑
I82.A22 Chronic embolism and thrombosis of left axillary vein ☑
I82.A23 Chronic embolism and thrombosis of axillary vein, bilateral ☑

I82.B11	Acute embolism and thrombosis of right subclavian vein ☑
I82.B12	Acute embolism and thrombosis of left subclavian vein ☑
I82.B13	Acute embolism and thrombosis of subclavian vein, bilateral ☑
I82.B21	Chronic embolism and thrombosis of right subclavian vein ☑
I82.B22	Chronic embolism and thrombosis of left subclavian vein ☑
I82.B23	Chronic embolism and thrombosis of subclavian vein, bilateral ☑
T81.72XA	Complication of vein following a procedure, not elsewhere classified, initial encounter

AMA: **34471** 1997,Nov,1 **34490** 1997,Nov,1

Relative Value Units/Medicare Edits

Non-Facility RVU	Work	PE	MP	Total
34471	21.11	5.13	4.87	31.11
34490	10.91	5.09	2.56	18.56
Facility RVU	**Work**	**PE**	**MP**	**Total**
34471	21.11	5.13	4.87	31.11
34490	10.91	5.09	2.56	18.56

	FUD	Status	MUE	Modifiers				IOM Reference
34471	90	A	1(2)	51	50	62*	N/A	None
34490	90	A	1(2)	51	50	N/A	N/A	

* with documentation

Terms To Know

angioscopy. Visualization of capillary blood vessels with a microscope, or the inside of a blood vessel with a fiberoptic-equipped catheter.

arteriogram. Radiograph of arteries.

embolism. Obstruction of a blood vessel resulting from a clot or foreign substance.

thrombosis. Condition arising from the presence or formation of blood clots within a blood vessel that may cause vascular obstruction and insufficient oxygenation.

34501

34501 Valvuloplasty, femoral vein

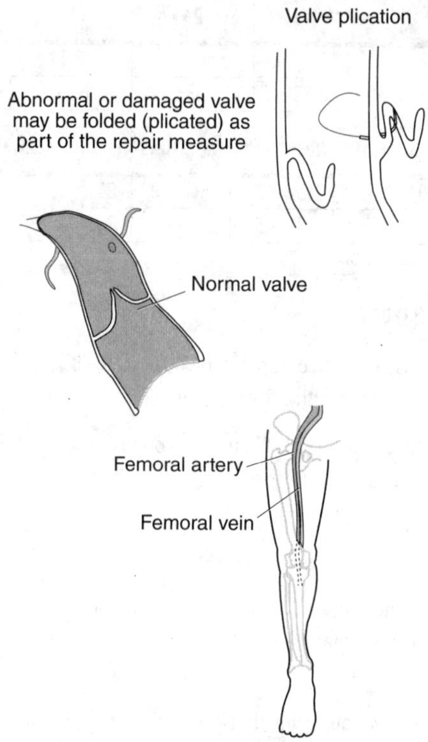

Explanation

The physician makes an incision in the skin overlying the site of the incompetent valve. The femoral vein is isolated and dissected from adjacent critical structures. The physician affixes vessel clamps above and below the malfunctioning valve. The physician opens the vein and repairs the valve leaflets by suture plication (tacking the excess valve material). The vein is repaired with sutures. The clamps are removed and the skin incision is repaired with a layered closure.

Coding Tips

Establishing both inflow and outflow by any method is included. The portion of the operative arteriogram performed by the surgeon is also included. Angioscopy performed during therapeutic intervention should be reported in addition to the code for the primary procedure; see 35400. For venous valve transposition, any vein donor, see 34510.

ICD-10-CM Diagnostic Codes

I80.11	Phlebitis and thrombophlebitis of right femoral vein ☑
I80.12	Phlebitis and thrombophlebitis of left femoral vein ☑
I80.13	Phlebitis and thrombophlebitis of femoral vein, bilateral ☑
I82.411	Acute embolism and thrombosis of right femoral vein ☑
I82.412	Acute embolism and thrombosis of left femoral vein ☑
I82.413	Acute embolism and thrombosis of femoral vein, bilateral ☑
I82.511	Chronic embolism and thrombosis of right femoral vein ☑
I82.512	Chronic embolism and thrombosis of left femoral vein ☑
I82.513	Chronic embolism and thrombosis of femoral vein, bilateral ☑
I83.011	Varicose veins of right lower extremity with ulcer of thigh ☑
I83.012	Varicose veins of right lower extremity with ulcer of calf ☑
I83.013	Varicose veins of right lower extremity with ulcer of ankle ☑

I83.014 Varicose veins of right lower extremity with ulcer of heel and midfoot ☑

I83.015 Varicose veins of right lower extremity with ulcer other part of foot ☑

I83.018 Varicose veins of right lower extremity with ulcer other part of lower leg ☑

I83.021 Varicose veins of left lower extremity with ulcer of thigh ☑

I83.022 Varicose veins of left lower extremity with ulcer of calf ☑

I83.023 Varicose veins of left lower extremity with ulcer of ankle ☑

I83.024 Varicose veins of left lower extremity with ulcer of heel and midfoot ☑

I83.025 Varicose veins of left lower extremity with ulcer other part of foot ☑

I83.028 Varicose veins of left lower extremity with ulcer other part of lower leg ☑

I83.11 Varicose veins of right lower extremity with inflammation ☑

I83.12 Varicose veins of left lower extremity with inflammation ☑

I83.211 Varicose veins of right lower extremity with both ulcer of thigh and inflammation ☑

I83.212 Varicose veins of right lower extremity with both ulcer of calf and inflammation ☑

I83.213 Varicose veins of right lower extremity with both ulcer of ankle and inflammation ☑

I83.214 Varicose veins of right lower extremity with both ulcer of heel and midfoot and inflammation ☑

I83.215 Varicose veins of right lower extremity with both ulcer other part of foot and inflammation ☑

I83.218 Varicose veins of right lower extremity with both ulcer of other part of lower extremity and inflammation ☑

I83.221 Varicose veins of left lower extremity with both ulcer of thigh and inflammation ☑

I83.222 Varicose veins of left lower extremity with both ulcer of calf and inflammation ☑

I83.223 Varicose veins of left lower extremity with both ulcer of ankle and inflammation ☑

I83.224 Varicose veins of left lower extremity with both ulcer of heel and midfoot and inflammation ☑

I83.225 Varicose veins of left lower extremity with both ulcer other part of foot and inflammation ☑

I83.228 Varicose veins of left lower extremity with both ulcer of other part of lower extremity and inflammation ☑

I83.811 Varicose veins of right lower extremity with pain ☑

I83.812 Varicose veins of left lower extremity with pain ☑

I83.813 Varicose veins of bilateral lower extremities with pain ☑

I83.891 Varicose veins of right lower extremity with other complications ☑

I83.892 Varicose veins of left lower extremity with other complications ☑

I83.893 Varicose veins of bilateral lower extremities with other complications ☑

I83.91 Asymptomatic varicose veins of right lower extremity ☑

I83.92 Asymptomatic varicose veins of left lower extremity ☑

I83.93 Asymptomatic varicose veins of bilateral lower extremities ☑

I87.001 Postthrombotic syndrome without complications of right lower extremity ☑

I87.002 Postthrombotic syndrome without complications of left lower extremity ☑

I87.003 Postthrombotic syndrome without complications of bilateral lower extremity ☑

I87.011 Postthrombotic syndrome with ulcer of right lower extremity ☑

I87.012 Postthrombotic syndrome with ulcer of left lower extremity ☑

I87.013 Postthrombotic syndrome with ulcer of bilateral lower extremity ☑

I87.021 Postthrombotic syndrome with inflammation of right lower extremity ☑

I87.022 Postthrombotic syndrome with inflammation of left lower extremity ☑

I87.023 Postthrombotic syndrome with inflammation of bilateral lower extremity ☑

I87.031 Postthrombotic syndrome with ulcer and inflammation of right lower extremity ☑

I87.032 Postthrombotic syndrome with ulcer and inflammation of left lower extremity ☑

I87.033 Postthrombotic syndrome with ulcer and inflammation of bilateral lower extremity ☑

I87.091 Postthrombotic syndrome with other complications of right lower extremity ☑

I87.092 Postthrombotic syndrome with other complications of left lower extremity ☑

I87.093 Postthrombotic syndrome with other complications of bilateral lower extremity ☑

I87.2 Venous insufficiency (chronic) (peripheral)

Q27.32 Arteriovenous malformation of vessel of lower limb

S75.111A Minor laceration of femoral vein at hip and thigh level, right leg, initial encounter ☑

S75.112A Minor laceration of femoral vein at hip and thigh level, left leg, initial encounter ☑

S75.121A Major laceration of femoral vein at hip and thigh level, right leg, initial encounter ☑

S75.122A Major laceration of femoral vein at hip and thigh level, left leg, initial encounter ☑

S75.191A Other specified injury of femoral vein at hip and thigh level, right leg, initial encounter ☑

S75.192A Other specified injury of femoral vein at hip and thigh level, left leg, initial encounter ☑

AMA: 34501 1997,Nov,1

Relative Value Units/Medicare Edits

Non-Facility RVU	Work	PE	MP	Total
34501	16.85	4.97	3.9	25.72
Facility RVU	**Work**	**PE**	**MP**	**Total**
34501	16.85	4.97	3.9	25.72

	FUD	Status	MUE	Modifiers				IOM Reference
34501	90	A	1(2)	51	50	62*	80	None

* with documentation

34502

34502 Reconstruction of vena cava, any method

The vena cava is the largest of the venous return vessels and are the lengths closest to, with attachments upon, the right atrium of the heart

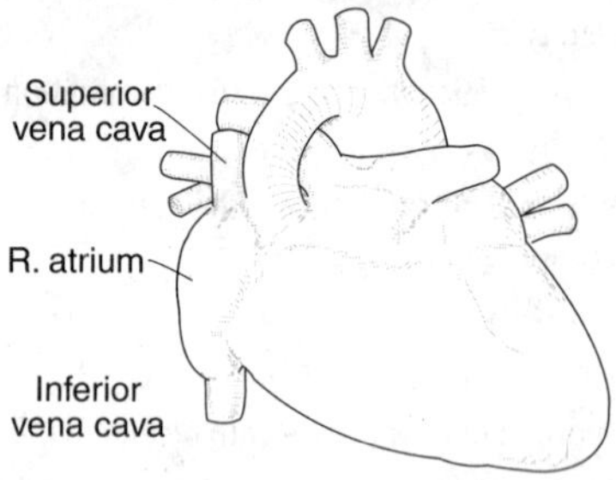

Explanation

The physician exposes the inferior vena cava by making an incision in the anterior abdomen. Clamps are placed on the vena cava proximally and any defects are sutured closed. Abnormal vena caval tissue may be replaced or bypassed with synthetic graft material. An injection of intravenous contrast may be administered under fluoroscopy to demonstrate appropriate flow. The clamps are removed and the abdominal wall incision is closed. A surgical drain may be left in place at the conclusion of the procedure.

Coding Tips

Establishing both inflow and outflow by any method is included. The portion of the operative arteriogram performed by the surgeon is also included. Angioscopy performed during therapeutic intervention should be reported in addition to the code for the primary procedure; see 35400. For resection with reconstruction of the vena cava, see 37799.

ICD-10-CM Diagnostic Codes

I82.210	Acute embolism and thrombosis of superior vena cava
I82.211	Chronic embolism and thrombosis of superior vena cava
I82.220	Acute embolism and thrombosis of inferior vena cava
I82.221	Chronic embolism and thrombosis of inferior vena cava
I87.1	Compression of vein
I87.2	Venous insufficiency (chronic) (peripheral)
Q26.0	Congenital stenosis of vena cava
Q26.1	Persistent left superior vena cava
Q26.8	Other congenital malformations of great veins
S25.21XA	Minor laceration of superior vena cava, initial encounter
S25.22XA	Major laceration of superior vena cava, initial encounter
S25.29XA	Other specified injury of superior vena cava, initial encounter
S35.11XA	Minor laceration of inferior vena cava, initial encounter
S35.12XA	Major laceration of inferior vena cava, initial encounter
S35.19XA	Other injury of inferior vena cava, initial encounter
T81.72XA	Complication of vein following a procedure, not elsewhere classified, initial encounter

AMA: 34502 1997,Nov,1

Relative Value Units/Medicare Edits

Non-Facility RVU	Work	PE	MP	Total
34502	28.07	10.59	6.02	44.68
Facility RVU	**Work**	**PE**	**MP**	**Total**
34502	28.07	10.59	6.02	44.68

	FUD	Status	MUE	Modifiers				IOM Reference
34502	90	A	1(2)	51	N/A	N/A	80	None

* with documentation

Terms To Know

angioscopy. Visualization of capillary blood vessels with a microscope, or the inside of a blood vessel with a fiberoptic-equipped catheter.

arteriogram. Radiograph of arteries.

embolism. Obstruction of a blood vessel resulting from a clot or foreign substance.

fluoroscopy. Radiology technique that allows visual examination of part of the body or a function of an organ using a device that projects an x-ray image on a fluorescent screen.

graft. Tissue implant from another part of the body or another person.

thrombosis. Condition arising from the presence or formation of blood clots within a blood vessel that may cause vascular obstruction and insufficient oxygenation.

34510

34510 Venous valve transposition, any vein donor

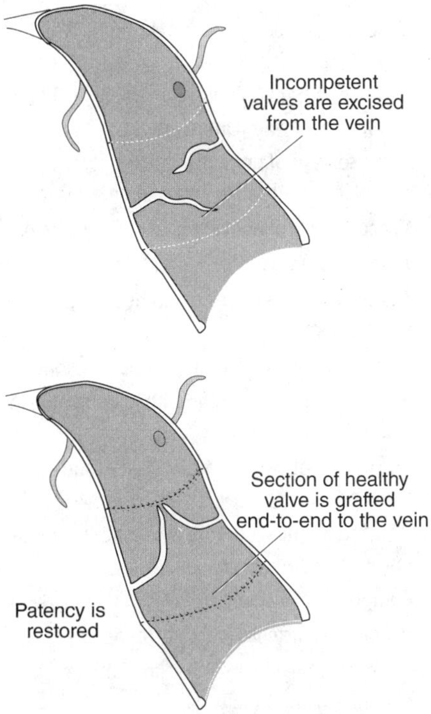

Explanation

The physician makes an incision in the skin overlying the site of the malfunctioning valve. The vein is isolated and dissected from adjacent critical structures. The physician affixes vessel clamps above and below the vein and excises the section of vein containing the malfunctioning valve. A section of harvested vein containing functional valves is sutured end-to-end to the vein. The clamps are removed and the skin incision is repaired with a layered closure.

Coding Tips

Establishing both inflow and outflow by any method is included. The portion of the operative arteriogram performed by the surgeon is also included. Angioscopy performed during therapeutic intervention should be reported in addition to the code for the primary procedure; see 35400. For crossover vein graft to venous system, see 34520.

ICD-10-CM Diagnostic Codes

I80.291 Phlebitis and thrombophlebitis of other deep vessels of right lower extremity ☑
I82.491 Acute embolism and thrombosis of other specified deep vein of right lower extremity ☑
I82.591 Chronic embolism and thrombosis of other specified deep vein of right lower extremity ☑
I83.011 Varicose veins of right lower extremity with ulcer of thigh ☑
I83.012 Varicose veins of right lower extremity with ulcer of calf ☑
I83.013 Varicose veins of right lower extremity with ulcer of ankle ☑
I83.014 Varicose veins of right lower extremity with ulcer of heel and midfoot ☑
I83.015 Varicose veins of right lower extremity with ulcer other part of foot ☑
I83.018 Varicose veins of right lower extremity with ulcer other part of lower leg ☑
I83.11 Varicose veins of right lower extremity with inflammation ☑
I83.211 Varicose veins of right lower extremity with both ulcer of thigh and inflammation ☑
I83.212 Varicose veins of right lower extremity with both ulcer of calf and inflammation ☑
I83.213 Varicose veins of right lower extremity with both ulcer of ankle and inflammation ☑
I83.214 Varicose veins of right lower extremity with both ulcer of heel and midfoot and inflammation ☑
I83.215 Varicose veins of right lower extremity with both ulcer other part of foot and inflammation ☑
I83.218 Varicose veins of right lower extremity with both ulcer of other part of lower extremity and inflammation ☑
I83.811 Varicose veins of right lower extremity with pain ☑
I83.891 Varicose veins of right lower extremity with other complications ☑
I83.91 Asymptomatic varicose veins of right lower extremity ☑
I87.001 Postthrombotic syndrome without complications of right lower extremity ☑
I87.011 Postthrombotic syndrome with ulcer of right lower extremity ☑
I87.021 Postthrombotic syndrome with inflammation of right lower extremity ☑
I87.031 Postthrombotic syndrome with ulcer and inflammation of right lower extremity ☑
I87.091 Postthrombotic syndrome with other complications of right lower extremity ☑
I87.1 Compression of vein
I87.2 Venous insufficiency (chronic) (peripheral)
I87.301 Chronic venous hypertension (idiopathic) without complications of right lower extremity ☑
I87.311 Chronic venous hypertension (idiopathic) with ulcer of right lower extremity ☑
I87.321 Chronic venous hypertension (idiopathic) with inflammation of right lower extremity ☑
I87.331 Chronic venous hypertension (idiopathic) with ulcer and inflammation of right lower extremity ☑
I87.391 Chronic venous hypertension (idiopathic) with other complications of right lower extremity ☑
Q27.32 Arteriovenous malformation of vessel of lower limb

AMA: **34510** 1997,Nov,1

Relative Value Units/Medicare Edits

Non-Facility RVU	Work	PE	MP	Total
34510	19.91	4.94	4.6	29.45
Facility RVU	**Work**	**PE**	**MP**	**Total**
34510	19.91	4.94	4.6	29.45

	FUD	Status	MUE	Modifiers				IOM Reference
34510	90	A	2(3)	51	50	62*	80	None

* with documentation

34520

34520 Cross-over vein graft to venous system

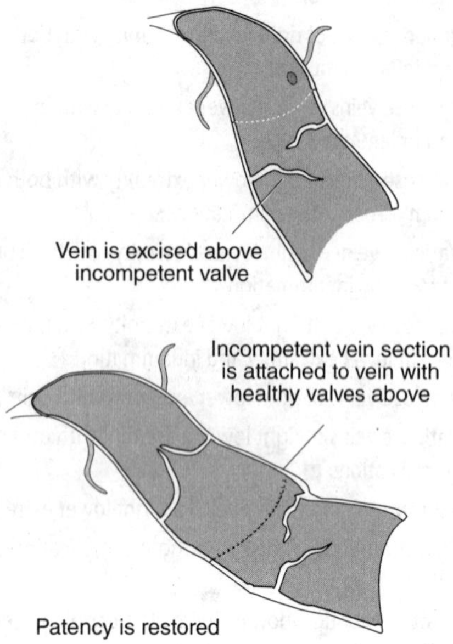

Explanation

The physician makes an incision in the skin overlying the site of the incompetent valve. The incompetent vein is isolated and dissected from adjacent critical structures. The physician affixes vessel clamps above and below the vein. The divided section of incompetent vein is connected to a nearby vein with functioning valves, placing competent values above the incompetent vein. Both the vein and the skin incision are closed with sutures.

Coding Tips

Establishing both inflow and outflow by any method is included. The portion of the operative arteriogram performed by the surgeon is also included. Angioscopy performed during therapeutic intervention should be reported in addition to the code for the primary procedure; see 35400. For venous valve transposition, any vein donor, see 34510.

ICD-10-CM Diagnostic Codes

I80.11	Phlebitis and thrombophlebitis of right femoral vein ☑
I80.211	Phlebitis and thrombophlebitis of right iliac vein ☑
I80.291	Phlebitis and thrombophlebitis of other deep vessels of right lower extremity ☑
I82.411	Acute embolism and thrombosis of right femoral vein ☑
I82.421	Acute embolism and thrombosis of right iliac vein ☑
I82.511	Chronic embolism and thrombosis of right femoral vein ☑
I82.521	Chronic embolism and thrombosis of right iliac vein ☑
I82.591	Chronic embolism and thrombosis of other specified deep vein of right lower extremity ☑
I83.011	Varicose veins of right lower extremity with ulcer of thigh ☑
I83.012	Varicose veins of right lower extremity with ulcer of calf ☑
I83.013	Varicose veins of right lower extremity with ulcer of ankle ☑
I83.014	Varicose veins of right lower extremity with ulcer of heel and midfoot ☑
I83.015	Varicose veins of right lower extremity with ulcer other part of foot ☑
I83.11	Varicose veins of right lower extremity with inflammation ☑
I83.211	Varicose veins of right lower extremity with both ulcer of thigh and inflammation ☑
I83.212	Varicose veins of right lower extremity with both ulcer of calf and inflammation ☑
I83.213	Varicose veins of right lower extremity with both ulcer of ankle and inflammation ☑
I83.214	Varicose veins of right lower extremity with both ulcer of heel and midfoot and inflammation ☑
I83.218	Varicose veins of right lower extremity with both ulcer of other part of lower extremity and inflammation ☑
I83.811	Varicose veins of right lower extremity with pain ☑
I83.91	Asymptomatic varicose veins of right lower extremity ☑
I87.001	Postthrombotic syndrome without complications of right lower extremity ☑
I87.011	Postthrombotic syndrome with ulcer of right lower extremity ☑
I87.021	Postthrombotic syndrome with inflammation of right lower extremity ☑
I87.031	Postthrombotic syndrome with ulcer and inflammation of right lower extremity ☑
I87.091	Postthrombotic syndrome with other complications of right lower extremity ☑
I87.1	Compression of vein
I87.2	Venous insufficiency (chronic) (peripheral)
I87.301	Chronic venous hypertension (idiopathic) without complications of right lower extremity ☑
I87.311	Chronic venous hypertension (idiopathic) with ulcer of right lower extremity ☑
I87.321	Chronic venous hypertension (idiopathic) with inflammation of right lower extremity ☑
I87.331	Chronic venous hypertension (idiopathic) with ulcer and inflammation of right lower extremity ☑
Q26.0	Congenital stenosis of vena cava
Q26.1	Persistent left superior vena cava
Q27.32	Arteriovenous malformation of vessel of lower limb
S35.514A	Injury of right iliac vein, initial encounter ☑
S75.121A	Major laceration of femoral vein at hip and thigh level, right leg, initial encounter ☑

AMA: 34520 1997,Nov,1

Relative Value Units/Medicare Edits

Non-Facility RVU	Work	PE	MP	Total
34520	19.18	4.91	4.44	28.53
Facility RVU	**Work**	**PE**	**MP**	**Total**
34520	19.18	4.91	4.44	28.53

	FUD	Status	MUE	Modifiers				IOM Reference
34520	90	A	1(3)	51	50	62*	80	None

* with documentation

34530

34530 Saphenopopliteal vein anastomosis

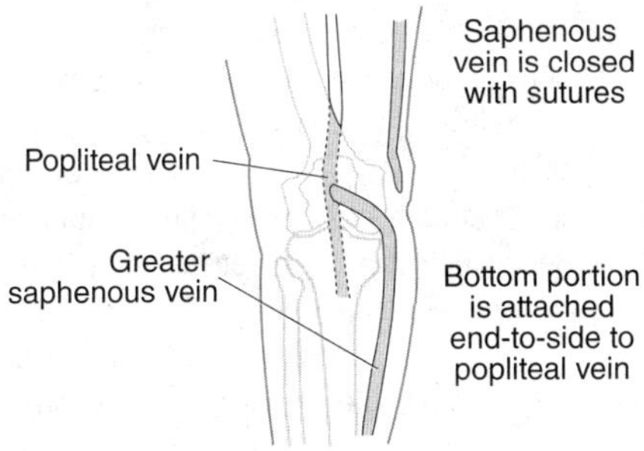

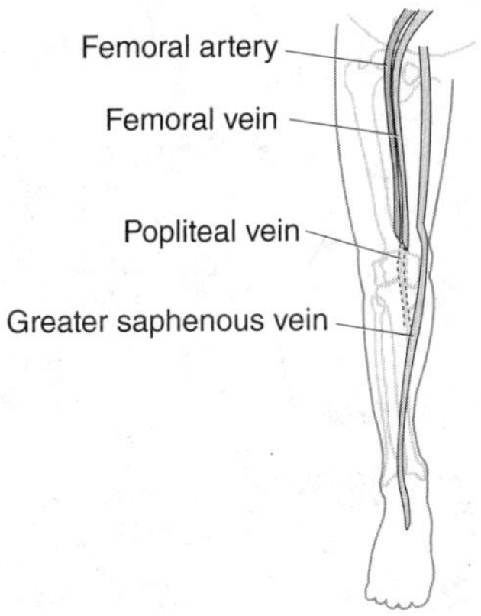

Explanation

The physician makes an incision in the skin overlying the site of the greater saphenous vein just below the knee. The vein is isolated and dissected from adjacent critical structures. The physician affixes vessel clamps above and below the incision site. The dissected section of saphenous vein is connected to the popliteal vein in an end-to-side anastomosis. The other end of the saphenous vein is closed with sutures. Once the saphenous vein and the popliteal vein are connected, the clamps are removed and the skin incision is repaired with layered closure.

Coding Tips

Establishing both inflow and outflow by any method is included. The portion of the operative arteriogram performed by the surgeon is also included. Angioscopy performed during therapeutic intervention should be reported in addition to the code for the primary procedure; see 35400. For venous valve transposition, any vein donor, see 34510. For crossover vein graft, see 34520. For direct repair of a blood vessel other than for fistula, see 35226, 35256, and 35286.

ICD-10-CM Diagnostic Codes

I80.221	Phlebitis and thrombophlebitis of right popliteal vein ☑
I82.431	Acute embolism and thrombosis of right popliteal vein ☑
I82.491	Acute embolism and thrombosis of other specified deep vein of right lower extremity ☑
I82.591	Chronic embolism and thrombosis of other specified deep vein of right lower extremity ☑
I83.011	Varicose veins of right lower extremity with ulcer of thigh ☑
I83.012	Varicose veins of right lower extremity with ulcer of calf ☑
I83.013	Varicose veins of right lower extremity with ulcer of ankle ☑
I83.014	Varicose veins of right lower extremity with ulcer of heel and midfoot ☑
I83.015	Varicose veins of right lower extremity with ulcer other part of foot ☑
I83.018	Varicose veins of right lower extremity with ulcer other part of lower leg ☑
I83.11	Varicose veins of right lower extremity with inflammation ☑
I83.211	Varicose veins of right lower extremity with both ulcer of thigh and inflammation ☑
I83.212	Varicose veins of right lower extremity with both ulcer of calf and inflammation ☑
I83.213	Varicose veins of right lower extremity with both ulcer of ankle and inflammation ☑
I83.214	Varicose veins of right lower extremity with both ulcer of heel and midfoot and inflammation ☑
I83.215	Varicose veins of right lower extremity with both ulcer other part of foot and inflammation ☑
I83.218	Varicose veins of right lower extremity with both ulcer of other part of lower extremity and inflammation ☑
I83.811	Varicose veins of right lower extremity with pain ☑
I83.891	Varicose veins of right lower extremity with other complications ☑
I87.011	Postthrombotic syndrome with ulcer of right lower extremity ☑
I87.021	Postthrombotic syndrome with inflammation of right lower extremity ☑
I87.031	Postthrombotic syndrome with ulcer and inflammation of right lower extremity ☑
I87.091	Postthrombotic syndrome with other complications of right lower extremity ☑
I87.1	Compression of vein
I87.2	Venous insufficiency (chronic) (peripheral)
I87.311	Chronic venous hypertension (idiopathic) with ulcer of right lower extremity ☑
I87.321	Chronic venous hypertension (idiopathic) with inflammation of right lower extremity ☑
I87.331	Chronic venous hypertension (idiopathic) with ulcer and inflammation of right lower extremity ☑
I87.391	Chronic venous hypertension (idiopathic) with other complications of right lower extremity ☑
Q27.32	Arteriovenous malformation of vessel of lower limb
S75.221A	Major laceration of greater saphenous vein at hip and thigh level, right leg, initial encounter ☑
S85.311A	Laceration of greater saphenous vein at lower leg level, right leg, initial encounter ☑
S85.411A	Laceration of lesser saphenous vein at lower leg level, right leg, initial encounter ☑
S85.511A	Laceration of popliteal vein, right leg, initial encounter ☑

AMA: 34530 1997,Nov,1

Arteries and Veins

Relative Value Units/Medicare Edits

Non-Facility RVU	Work	PE	MP	Total
34530	17.93	4.99	4.14	27.06
Facility RVU	Work	PE	MP	Total
34530	17.93	4.99	4.14	27.06

	FUD	Status	MUE	Modifiers				IOM Reference
34530	90	A	1(2)	51	50	62*	80	None

* with documentation

Terms To Know

anastomosis. Surgically created connection between ducts, blood vessels, or bowel segments to allow flow from one to the other.

angioscopy. Visualization of capillary blood vessels with a microscope, or the inside of a blood vessel with a fiberoptic-equipped catheter.

arteriogram. Radiograph of arteries.

dissect. Cut apart or separate tissue for surgical purposes or for visual or microscopic study.

fistula. Abnormal tube-like passage between two body cavities or organs or from an organ to the outside surface.

incision. Act of cutting into tissue or an organ.

laceration. Tearing injury; a torn, ragged-edged wound.

resection. Surgical removal of a part or all of an organ or body part.

transposition. Removal or exchange from one side to another; change of position from one place to another.

ulcer. Open sore or excavating lesion of skin or the tissue on the surface of an organ from the sloughing of chronically inflamed and necrosing tissue.

varicose vein. Abnormal, permanently distended or stretched vein.

34701-34702

34701 Endovascular repair of infrarenal aorta by deployment of an aorto-aortic tube endograft including pre-procedure sizing and device selection, all nonselective catheterization(s), all associated radiological supervision and interpretation, all endograft extension(s) placed in the aorta from the level of the renal arteries to the aortic bifurcation, and all angioplasty/stenting performed from the level of the renal arteries to the aortic bifurcation; for other than rupture (eg, for aneurysm, pseudoaneurysm, dissection, penetrating ulcer)

34702 for rupture including temporary aortic and/or iliac balloon occlusion, when performed (eg, for aneurysm, pseudoaneurysm, dissection, penetrating ulcer, traumatic disruption)

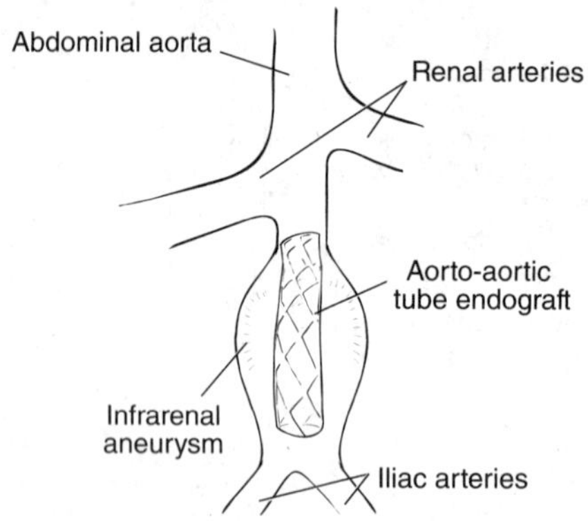

Explanation

The physician introduces, positions, and deploys an endograft to treat abdominal aortic conditions, with or without rupture, such as an aneurysm, pseudoaneurysm, dissection, penetrating ulcer, or traumatic disruption located in the infrarenal abdominal aorta that may or may not extend into the iliac arteries. A covered stent may be referred to using terms such as endovascular graft, endoprosthesis, endograft, or stent graft. The infrarenal aortic endograft may be an aortic tube device, a bifurcated unibody device, a modular bifurcated docking system with docking limbs, or an aorto-uni-iliac device. The abdominal aortic treatment zone is defined as the infrarenal aorta. This procedure requires a vascular surgeon and a radiologist. In 34701, an incision is made over the femoral artery, which is normally used for access, and a guidewire is threaded into the blood vessel. A catheter with a stent-transporting tip is advanced over the guidewire into the vessel. The catheter carries the aortic tube prosthesis, approximately 6 inches long and contained inside a holding capsule, through the arterial tree to the site of the aortic infrarenal aneurysm. Once the stent is in proper position, the holding capsule is removed and the stent is deployed, expanding like a spring to anchor itself to normal walls of the aorta above and below the aneurysm. The device serves as a substitute channel for blood flow. If full expansion of the prosthesis does not occur, or leaks are present, a balloon catheter is threaded to the graft site and inflated within the prosthesis until full expansion is achieved and leaking is stopped. The catheter/guidewire is removed and the arteriotomy site is closed. The aneurysm, excluded from the blood flow, typically shrinks over time. The treatment zone for endograft procedures is defined by those vessels that contain an endograft (main body, docking limbs, and/or extensions) deployed during that operative session. Report 34702 when endovascular repair is performed on a ruptured aneurysm in the aorta. Rupture is defined as clinical and/or radiographic evidence of acute hemorrhage. A chronic, contained rupture is considered a pseudoaneurysm and its endovascular treatment is reported with 34701. Nonselective catheterization is included in these codes. Balloon angioplasty and/or stenting at the sealing zone of an endograft is an integral part of the procedure. Fluoroscopic guidance and radiological supervision and interpretation in conjunction with endograft repair is not reported separately, and includes all intraprocedural imaging (e.g., angiography, rotational CT) of the aorta and its branches prior to deployment of the endovascular device, fluoroscopic guidance, and roadmapping used in the delivery of the endovascular components, and intraprocedural and completion angiography (e.g., confirm position, detect endoleak, evaluate runoff) performed at the time of the endovascular infrarenal aorta repair.

Coding Tips

Preprocedure sizing and device selection, all nonselective catheterizations, radiological supervision and interpretation, endograft extensions, and angioplasty stenting are included in these procedures and should not be reported separately. For repair requiring a decompressive laparotomy for abdominal compartment syndrome, report 49000 in addition to 34702. Report 34709 in addition to 34701 or 34702 for placement of an extension prosthesis that terminates in the abdominal aorta proximal to the renal arteries. For covered stent placements for atherosclerotic occlusive disease of the abdominal aorta, see 37236 and 37237. For repair of infrarenal aorta and/or iliac arteries by deployment of an aorto-uni-iliac endograft, see 34703 and 34704. For repair of infrarenal aorta and/or iliac arteries by deployment of an aorto-bi-iliac endograft, see 34705 and 34706.

ICD-10-CM Diagnostic Codes

A52.01	Syphilitic aneurysm of aorta
I71.02	Dissection of abdominal aorta
I71.3	Abdominal aortic aneurysm, ruptured
I71.4	Abdominal aortic aneurysm, without rupture
I77.811	Abdominal aortic ectasia
I77.89	Other specified disorders of arteries and arterioles
Q25.43	Congenital aneurysm of aorta
Q25.44	Congenital dilation of aorta
Q25.49	Other congenital malformations of aorta
Q79.61	Classical Ehlers-Danlos syndrome
Q79.62	Hypermobile Ehlers-Danlos syndrome
Q79.63	Vascular Ehlers-Danlos syndrome
Q79.69	Other Ehlers-Danlos syndromes
Q87.410	Marfan's syndrome with aortic dilation
S35.02XA	Major laceration of abdominal aorta, initial encounter
S35.09XA	Other injury of abdominal aorta, initial encounter

AMA: 34701 2018,Jan,8; 2017,Dec,3 **34702** 2018,Jan,8; 2017,Dec,3

Relative Value Units/Medicare Edits

Non-Facility RVU	Work	PE	MP	Total
34701	23.71	6.88	5.26	35.85
34702	36.0	9.8	7.95	53.75
Facility RVU	**Work**	**PE**	**MP**	**Total**
34701	23.71	6.88	5.26	35.85
34702	36.0	9.8	7.95	53.75

	FUD	Status	MUE	Modifiers				IOM Reference
34701	90	A	1(2)	51	N/A	62	80	None
34702	90	A	1(2)	51	N/A	62	80	

* with documentation

34703-34706

34703 Endovascular repair of infrarenal aorta and/or iliac artery(ies) by deployment of an aorto-uni-iliac endograft including pre-procedure sizing and device selection, all nonselective catheterization(s), all associated radiological supervision and interpretation, all endograft extension(s) placed in the aorta from the level of the renal arteries to the iliac bifurcation, and all angioplasty/stenting performed from the level of the renal arteries to the iliac bifurcation; for other than rupture (eg, for aneurysm, pseudoaneurysm, dissection, penetrating ulcer)

34704 for rupture including temporary aortic and/or iliac balloon occlusion, when performed (eg, for aneurysm, pseudoaneurysm, dissection, penetrating ulcer, traumatic disruption)

34705 Endovascular repair of infrarenal aorta and/or iliac artery(ies) by deployment of an aorto-bi-iliac endograft including pre-procedure sizing and device selection, all nonselective catheterization(s), all associated radiological supervision and interpretation, all endograft extension(s) placed in the aorta from the level of the renal arteries to the iliac bifurcation, and all angioplasty/stenting performed from the level of the renal arteries to the iliac bifurcation; for other than rupture (eg, for aneurysm, pseudoaneurysm, dissection, penetrating ulcer)

34706 for rupture including temporary aortic and/or iliac balloon occlusion, when performed (eg, for aneurysm, pseudoaneurysm, dissection, penetrating ulcer, traumatic disruption)

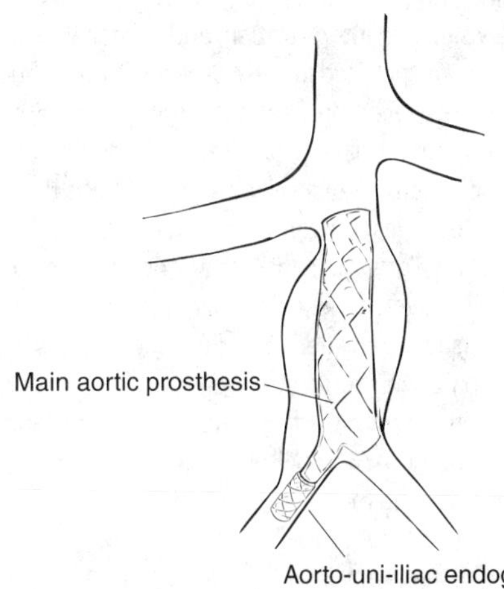

Explanation

The physician introduces, positions, and deploys an endograft to treat abdominal aortic conditions, with or without rupture, such as an aneurysm, pseudoaneurysm, dissection, penetrating ulcer, or traumatic disruption located in the infrarenal abdominal aorta that may or may not extend into the iliac arteries. A covered stent may be referred to as an endovascular graft, endoprosthesis, endograft, or stent graft. The infrarenal aortic endograft may be an aortic tube device, a bifurcated unibody device, a modular bifurcated docking system with docking limbs, or an aorto-uni-iliac device. In 34703 and 34704, the abdominal aortic treatment zone is typically defined as the infrarenal aorta and ipsilateral common iliac artery. In 34705 and 34706, the abdominal aortic treatment zone is typically defined as the infrarenal aorta and both common iliac arteries. These procedures require a vascular surgeon and a radiologist. In 34703, under general anesthesia, a small incision is made in the groin over one femoral artery or both femoral arteries through which the endovascular devices are inserted. If contralateral femoral access is necessary, a percutaneous sheath may be placed. An aorta-uni-iliac prosthetic graft device contained inside a plastic holding capsule is threaded through the arteries to the site of the infrarenal aneurysm. The endograft is deployed by slowly removing the holding capsule away from the endograft, with continual monitoring of exact positioning. Once the prosthesis is in place, the holding capsule is removed. Balloon angioplasty is performed at the ends of the prosthesis to expand and seat the graft. Stents are deployed within the body of the endograft to maintain expansion forces. The aorta-uni-iliac prosthetic endograft is supported along its length by a series of metal rings sutured to the graft and is held in place by the radial force applied by the rings to the patient's aorta. Once in place, the arteriotomy site is closed. Report 34705 for simultaneous bilateral iliac artery aneurysm repairs with aorto-bi-iliac endograft. Report 34704 and 34706 when endovascular repair is performed on a ruptured aneurysm in the aorta or iliac arteries. Rupture is defined as clinical and/or radiographic evidence of acute hemorrhage. A chronic, contained rupture is considered a pseudoaneurysm and its endovascular treatment is reported with 34703 and 34705. Nonselective catheterization is included in 34703, 34704, 34705, and 34706. Balloon angioplasty and/or stenting at the sealing zone of an endograft is an integral part of the procedure. Fluoroscopic guidance and radiological supervision and interpretation in conjunction with endograft repair is not separately reported, and includes all intraprocedural imaging (e.g., angiography, rotational CT) of the aorta and its branches prior to deployment of the endovascular device, fluoroscopic guidance and roadmapping used in the delivery of the endovascular components, and intraprocedural and completion angiography (e.g., confirm position, detect endoleak, evaluate runoff) performed at the time of the endovascular infrarenal aorta and/or iliac repair.

Coding Tips

Preprocedure sizing and device selection, all nonselective catheterizations, radiological supervision and interpretation, endograft extensions, and angioplasty stenting are included in these procedures and should not be reported separately. For decompressive laparotomy, report 49000 in addition to 34704 or 34706, as appropriate. Report 34709 in addition to 34703, 34704, 34705, or 34706 for placement of an extension prosthesis that terminates in the internal iliac, external iliac, or common femoral arteries. For treatment of atherosclerotic occlusive disease in the iliac arteries with covered stents, see 37221 and 37223. For covered stent placement for atherosclerotic occlusive disease in the aorta, see 37236 and 37237. For simultaneous bilateral iliac artery aneurysm repairs with aorto-bi-iliac endograft, see 34705 and 34706. For repair of an infrarenal aorta by deployment of an aorto-aortic tube endograft, see 34701 and 34702. For isolated bilateral iliac artery repair, see 34707 or 34708 and append modifier 50.

ICD-10-CM Diagnostic Codes

A52.01	Syphilitic aneurysm of aorta
I71.02	Dissection of abdominal aorta
I71.3	Abdominal aortic aneurysm, ruptured
I71.4	Abdominal aortic aneurysm, without rupture
I72.3	Aneurysm of iliac artery
I77.72	Dissection of iliac artery
I77.811	Abdominal aortic ectasia
I77.89	Other specified disorders of arteries and arterioles
Q25.43	Congenital aneurysm of aorta
Q25.44	Congenital dilation of aorta
Q25.49	Other congenital malformations of aorta
Q25.8	Other congenital malformations of other great arteries
Q79.61	Classical Ehlers-Danlos syndrome
Q79.63	Vascular Ehlers-Danlos syndrome
Q87.410	Marfan's syndrome with aortic dilation
Q87.418	Marfan's syndrome with other cardiovascular manifestations
S35.02XA	Major laceration of abdominal aorta, initial encounter
S35.09XA	Other injury of abdominal aorta, initial encounter
S35.511A	Injury of right iliac artery, initial encounter ☑
S35.512A	Injury of left iliac artery, initial encounter ☑
S35.59XA	Injury of other iliac blood vessels, initial encounter

AMA: **34703** 2018,Jan,8; 2017,Dec,3 **34704** 2018,Jan,8; 2017,Dec,3 **34705** 2018,Jan,8; 2017,Dec,3 **34706** 2018,Jan,8; 2017,Dec,3

Relative Value Units/Medicare Edits

Non-Facility RVU	Work	PE	MP	Total
34703	26.52	7.54	6.3	40.36
34704	45.0	11.84	10.42	67.26
34705	29.58	8.21	6.6	44.39
34706	45.0	11.83	10.05	66.88
Facility RVU	**Work**	**PE**	**MP**	**Total**
34703	26.52	7.54	6.3	40.36
34704	45.0	11.84	10.42	67.26
34705	29.58	8.21	6.6	44.39
34706	45.0	11.83	10.05	66.88

	FUD	Status	MUE	Modifiers				IOM Reference
34703	90	A	1(2)	51	N/A	62	80	None
34704	90	A	1(2)	51	N/A	62	80	
34705	90	A	1(2)	51	N/A	62	80	
34706	90	A	1(2)	51	N/A	62	80	

* with documentation

Terms To Know

aneurysm. Circumscribed dilation or outpouching of an artery wall, often containing blood clots and connecting directly with the lumen of the artery.

dissection. (dis. apart; -section, act of cutting) Separating by cutting tissue or body structures apart.

endometriosis interna. Abnormal presence of endometrial glands and tissue within the myometrium, the smooth muscle walls of the uterus, causing hypertrophy of the myometrium. At menses, blood is trapped within the muscle of the uterus, causing pain and cramping.

endoprosthesis. Intravascular device in the form of a hollow stent placed within a duct or artery to provide passage through an obstructed area, such as in a bile duct, or to act as a replacement for damaged arterial walls, as in treating an aneurysm.

fluoroscopy. Radiology technique that allows visual examination of part of the body or a function of an organ using a device that projects an x-ray image on a fluorescent screen.

34707-34708

34707 Endovascular repair of iliac artery by deployment of an ilio-iliac tube endograft including pre-procedure sizing and device selection, all nonselective catheterization(s), all associated radiological supervision and interpretation, and all endograft extension(s) proximally to the aortic bifurcation and distally to the iliac bifurcation, and treatment zone angioplasty/stenting, when performed, unilateral; for other than rupture (eg, for aneurysm, pseudoaneurysm, dissection, arteriovenous malformation)

34708 for rupture including temporary aortic and/or iliac balloon occlusion, when performed (eg, for aneurysm, pseudoaneurysm, dissection, arteriovenous malformation, traumatic disruption)

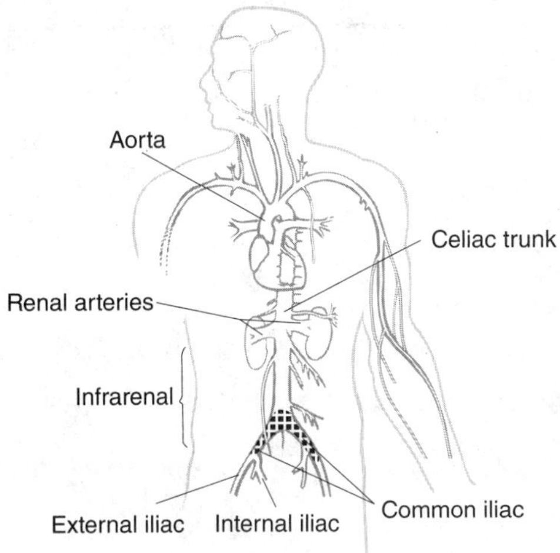

Ilio-iliac tube endograft

Explanation

The physician introduces, positions, and deploys an ilio-iliac endograft for treatment of isolated arterial pathology (with or without rupture), such as an aneurysm, pseudoaneurysm, dissection, arteriovenous malformation, or trauma involving the iliac artery. The treatment zone is defined as the portion of the iliac artery (e.g., common, internal, external iliac arteries) involved. The procedure requires a vascular surgeon and a radiologist. The patient receives medication (Heparin) to help prevent blood clots prior to the procedure. In 34707, under general anesthesia, the physician makes a small incision near the patient's hipbone area to enter the iliac artery. A proprietary device is used, such as the GORE® EXCLUDER® Iliac Branch Endoprosthesis. The device is comprised of two main components: a trunk component and a contralateral leg component. The endoprosthesis, contained inside a holding device, is introduced into the artery under fluoroscopy and positioned at the target zone area of repair by threading guidewires and catheters. Nonselective catheterization is included. Report 34708 when endovascular repair is performed on a ruptured aneurysm in the iliac artery. Rupture is defined as clinical and/or radiographic evidence of acute hemorrhage. A chronic, contained rupture is considered a pseudoaneurysm, and its endovascular treatment is reported with 34707. Balloon angioplasty and/or stenting at the treatment zone of an endograft is an integral part of the procedure. Fluoroscopic guidance and radiological supervision and interpretation, in conjunction with endograft repair, are not reported separately. Included are all intraprocedural imaging (e.g., angiography, rotational CT) of the iliac artery prior to deployment of the endovascular device, fluoroscopic guidance and roadmapping used in the delivery of the endovascular components, and intraprocedural and completion angiography (e.g., confirm position, detect endoleak, evaluate runoff) performed at the time of the endovascular iliac repair.

Coding Tips

Preprocedure sizing and device selection, all nonselective catheterizations, radiological supervision and interpretation, endograft extensions, and angioplasty stenting are included in the procedure and should not be reported separately. Report 34709 in addition to 34707 or 34708 for placement of an extension prosthesis that terminates in the internal iliac, external iliac, or common femoral arteries. For isolated bilateral iliac artery repair, append modifier 50. For decompressive laparotomy, report 49000 in addition to 34708. For covered stent placements for atherosclerotic occlusive disease of the abdominal aorta, see 37236 and 37237; iliac artery, see 37221 and 37223. For simultaneous bilateral iliac artery aneurysm repairs with aorto-bi-iliac endograft, see 34705 and 34706. For repair of an infrarenal aorta by deployment of an aorto-aortic tube endograft, see 34701 and 34702.

ICD-10-CM Diagnostic Codes

I72.3	Aneurysm of iliac artery
I77.72	Dissection of iliac artery
I77.89	Other specified disorders of arteries and arterioles
Q25.8	Other congenital malformations of other great arteries
Q25.9	Congenital malformation of great arteries, unspecified
S35.50XA	Injury of unspecified iliac blood vessel(s), initial encounter
S35.511A	Injury of right iliac artery, initial encounter ☑
S35.512A	Injury of left iliac artery, initial encounter ☑
S35.513A	Injury of unspecified iliac artery, initial encounter
S35.59XA	Injury of other iliac blood vessels, initial encounter

AMA: **34707** 2018,Jan,8; 2017,Dec,3 **34708** 2018,Jan,8; 2017,Dec,3

Relative Value Units/Medicare Edits

Non-Facility RVU	Work	PE	MP	Total
34707	22.28	6.35	4.81	33.44
34708	36.5	9.59	7.59	53.68
Facility RVU	**Work**	**PE**	**MP**	**Total**
34707	22.28	6.35	4.81	33.44
34708	36.5	9.59	7.59	53.68

	FUD	Status	MUE	Modifiers				IOM Reference
34707	90	A	1(2)	51	50	62	80	None
34708	90	A	1(2)	51	50	62	80	

* with documentation

Terms To Know

aneurysm. Circumscribed dilation or outpouching of an artery wall, often containing blood clots and connecting directly with the lumen of the artery.

arteriovenous malformation. Connecting passage between an artery and a vein.

endoprosthesis. Intravascular device in the form of a hollow stent placed within a duct or artery to provide passage through an obstructed area, such as in a bile duct, or to act as a replacement for damaged arterial walls, as in treating an aneurysm.

[34717]

+ ● 34717 Endovascular repair of iliac artery at the time of aorto-iliac artery endograft placement by deployment of an iliac branched endograft including pre-procedure sizing and device selection, all ipsilateral selective iliac artery catheterization(s), all associated radiological supervision and interpretation, and all endograft extension(s) proximally to the aortic bifurcation and distally in the internal iliac, external iliac, and common femoral artery(ies), and treatment zone angioplasty/stenting, when performed, for rupture or other than rupture (eg, for aneurysm, pseudoaneurysm, dissection, arteriovenous malformation, penetrating ulcer, traumatic disruption), unilateral (List separately in addition to code for primary procedure)

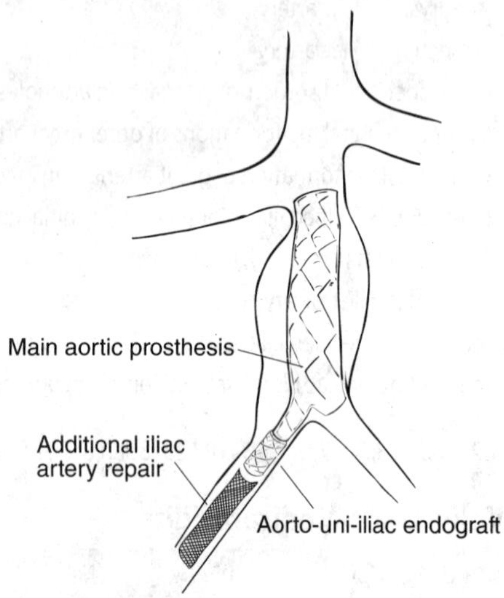

Explanation

At the time of aorto-iliac artery endograft placement, the physician repairs a unilateral iliac artery rupture, aneurysm, pseudoaneurysm, arteriovenous (AV) malformation, dissection, penetrating ulcer, or traumatic disruption by placing an iliac branched endograft. The endograft, contained inside a holding device, is introduced into the artery under fluoroscopy and positioned at the target zone area of repair. This may require open access exposure of the artery or may be accomplished by threading guidewires and catheters through to the site. Once the endoprosthesis is in place, it is deployed within the artery at the targeted site. The position of the endoprosthesis is confirmed, any endoleaks are identified, and the status of runoff vessels is evaluated for any related stenosis, dissection, thrombosis, or embolism. All selective ipsilateral catheterization(s) necessary for device placement, device selection and preprocedural sizing, endograft extension(s), angioplasty or stenting within the treatment zone, as well as radiological supervision and interpretation are included in this procedure. Report 34717, once per side, in addition to the code for the primary procedure.

Coding Tips

Report 34717 in addition to 34703–34706. Code 34717 should be reported twice when performed bilaterally. Do not report with modifier 50. Do not report 34717 with 34709 on the same side. Do not report 34717 with 34710 or 34711. Selective arterial catheterization of the internal and external iliac arteries on the same side as the iliac branched endograft should not be reported separately. Selective catheterization of the renal artery, opposite hypogastric artery, and other artery families outside of the treatment area of the graft may be reported separately. For placement of an iliac branched endograft at a setting separate from the aorto-iliac endograft placement, see 34718.

ICD-10-CM Diagnostic Codes

This/these CPT code(s) are add on code(s). See the primary procedure code that this code is performed with for your ICD-10-CM code selections.

Relative Value Units/Medicare Edits

Non-Facility RVU	Work	PE	MP	Total
34717				
Facility RVU	**Work**	**PE**	**MP**	**Total**
34717				

	FUD	Status	MUE	Modifiers				IOM Reference
34717	N/A		-	N/A	N/A	N/A	N/A	None

* with documentation

34709

\+ **34709** Placement of extension prosthesis(es) distal to the common iliac artery(ies) or proximal to the renal artery(ies) for endovascular repair of infrarenal abdominal aortic or iliac aneurysm, false aneurysm, dissection, penetrating ulcer, including pre-procedure sizing and device selection, all nonselective catheterization(s), all associated radiological supervision and interpretation, and treatment zone angioplasty/stenting, when performed, per vessel treated (List separately in addition to code for primary procedure)

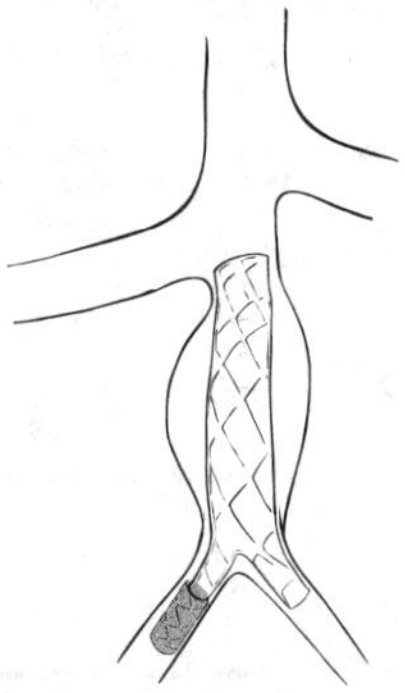

Extension prosthesis

Explanation

The physician places an extension prosthesis distal to the common iliac artery or proximal to the renal artery for endovascular repair of an infrarenal abdominal aortic or iliac aneurysm, pseudoaneurysm, dissection or penetrating ulcer that terminates in the internal iliac, external iliac, or common femoral arteries or in the abdominal aorta proximal to the renal arteries. Using separately reportable aortography, the target site is identified. The proper extension prosthesis is selected. Under separately reportable fluoroscopy, the extension prosthesis, contained inside a long plastic holding capsule, is threaded through the arteries to the leak site. Once the extension prosthesis is in place, the holding capsule is removed. The extension prosthesis, activated by heat, expands like a spring and becomes anchored to the artery wall at the site of the endoleak. If full expansion of the prosthesis does not occur automatically, a balloon catheter is threaded to the graft site and inflated within the endovascular prosthesis until full expansion is achieved. The catheter is removed and the arteriotomy site is closed. Report 34709 once per vessel treated.

Coding Tips

Report 34709 in addition to 34701-34708. Report 34709 only once per vessel treated. Do not report 34709 for placement of a docking limb extending into the external iliac artery. Selective catheterization of the renal arteries, hypogastric arteries, and/or arterial families outside of the treatment area may be reported separately. For endograft placement into a renal artery covered by a proximal extension, see 37236 and 37237.

ICD-10-CM Diagnostic Codes

This/these CPT code(s) are add on code(s). See the primary procedure code that this code is performed with for your ICD-10-CM code selections. Diagnostic code(s) would be the same as the actual procedure performed.

AMA: 34709 2018,Jan,8; 2017,Dec,3

Relative Value Units/Medicare Edits

Non-Facility RVU	Work	PE	MP	Total
34709	6.5	1.43	1.45	9.38
Facility RVU	**Work**	**PE**	**MP**	**Total**
34709	6.5	1.43	1.45	9.38

	FUD	Status	MUE	Modifiers				IOM Reference
34709	N/A	A	3(3)	N/A	N/A	62	80	None

* with documentation

Terms To Know

aneurysm. Circumscribed dilation or outpouching of an artery wall, often containing blood clots and connecting directly with the lumen of the artery.

dissection. Separating by cutting tissue or body structures apart.

nonselective placement. Insertion of a large needle with passage of a guidewire via the needle into the punctured vein or artery. The needle is removed leaving the guidewire and catheter in place. In direct punctures to peripheral veins or arteries, the catheter is not manipulated further after the initial stick is secured. Regardless of the site of the puncture, catheterization of the aorta or of the vena cava is considered nonselective placement.

[34718]

- **34718** Endovascular repair of iliac artery, not associated with placement of an aorto-iliac artery endograft at the same session, by deployment of an iliac branched endograft, including pre-procedure sizing and device selection, all ipsilateral selective iliac artery catheterization(s), all associated radiological supervision and interpretation, and all endograft extension(s) proximally to the aortic bifurcation and distally in the internal iliac, external iliac, and common femoral artery(ies), and treatment zone angioplasty/stenting, when performed, for other than rupture (eg, for aneurysm, pseudoaneurysm, dissection, arteriovenous malformation, penetrating ulcer), unilateral

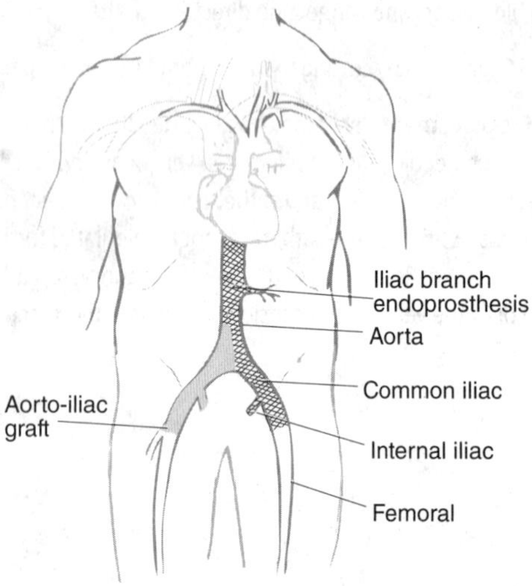

Iliac Vessels

Explanation

The physician repairs a unilateral iliac artery aneurysm, pseudoaneurysm, arteriovenous (AV) malformation, dissection, or penetrating ulcer by placing an iliac branched endograft. The endograft, contained inside a holding device, is introduced into the artery under fluoroscopy and positioned at the target zone area of repair. This may require open access exposure of the artery or may be accomplished by threading guidewires and catheters through to the site. Once the endoprosthesis is in place, it is deployed within the artery at the targeted site. The position of the endoprosthesis is confirmed, any endoleaks are identified, and the status of runoff vessels is evaluated for any related stenosis, dissection, thrombosis, or embolism. All selective ipsilateral catheterization(s) necessary for device placement, device selection and preprocedural sizing, endograft extension(s), angioplasty or stenting within the treatment zone, as well as radiological supervision and interpretation is included in this procedure. Placement of an aorto-iliac artery endograft is not performed during this session.

Coding Tips

These are unilateral procedures. If performed bilaterally, some payers require that the service be reported twice with modifier 50 appended to the second code while others require identification of the service only once with modifier 50 appended. Check with individual payers. Modifier 50 identifies a procedure performed identically on the opposite side of the body (mirror image). Do not report 34718 with 34701–34709 or 34717. Do not report 34718 with 34710 or 34711 on the same side. Selective arterial catheterization of the internal and external iliac arteries on the same side as the iliac branched endograft should not be reported separately. Selective catheterization of the renal artery, opposite hypogastric artery, and other artery families outside of the treatment area of the graft may be reported separately. For placement of an iliac branched endograft in the same setting as an aorto-iliac endograft placement, see 34717. For placement of an isolated iliac branched endograft for rupture, see 37799.

ICD-10-CM Diagnostic Codes

I72.3	Aneurysm of iliac artery
I77.2	Rupture of artery
I77.72	Dissection of iliac artery
Q27.32	Arteriovenous malformation of vessel of lower limb
S35.511A	Injury of right iliac artery, initial encounter ☑
S35.512A	Injury of left iliac artery, initial encounter ☑
S35.513A	Injury of unspecified iliac artery, initial encounter

Relative Value Units/Medicare Edits

Non-Facility RVU	Work	PE	MP	Total
34718				
Facility RVU	**Work**	**PE**	**MP**	**Total**
34718				

	FUD	Status	MUE	Modifiers				IOM Reference
34718	N/A		-	N/A	N/A	N/A	N/A	None

* with documentation

Terms To Know

angioplasty. Reconstruction or repair of a diseased or damaged blood vessel.

bifurcated. Having two branches or divisions, such as the left pulmonary veins that split off from the left atrium to carry oxygenated blood away from the heart.

distal. Located farther away from a specified reference point or the trunk.

ipsilateral. Located on, or affecting, the same side of the body, usually as it relates to a bilateral body part.

selective placement. Introduction and manipulation of a catheter or guidewire within a vascular tree or family into a specified target area that is identified and monitored by radiographic imaging in order to carry out a diagnostic or therapeutic procedure.

34710-34711

34710 Delayed placement of distal or proximal extension prosthesis for endovascular repair of infrarenal abdominal aortic or iliac aneurysm, false aneurysm, dissection, endoleak, or endograft migration, including pre-procedure sizing and device selection, all nonselective catheterization(s), all associated radiological supervision and interpretation, and treatment zone angioplasty/stenting, when performed; initial vessel treated

\+ **34711** each additional vessel treated (List separately in addition to code for primary procedure)

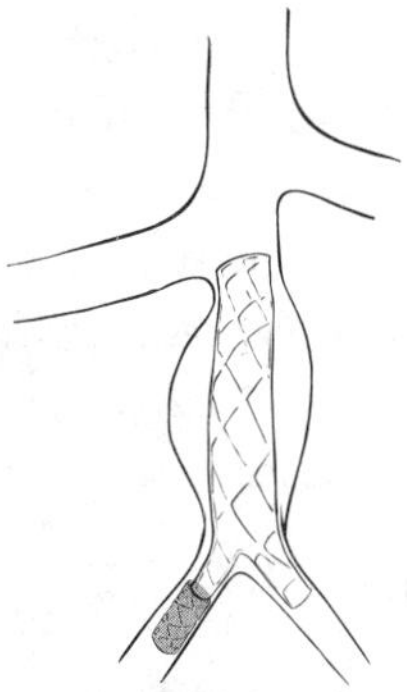

Extension prosthesis

Explanation

The physician performs delayed endovascular placement of a distal or proximal extension prosthesis to repair an infrarenal abdominal aortic or iliac aneurysm, pseudoaneurysm, dissection, endoleak, or endograft migration. A leak may occur at fixation sites of a grafted aneurysm through the body of the graft or from patent arteries within the aneurysm sac and may require endovascular reparation. Using separately reportable aortography, the target site is identified. The proper extension prosthesis is selected. Under separately reportable fluoroscopy, the extension prosthesis, contained inside a long plastic holding capsule, is threaded through the arteries to the leak site. Once the extension prosthesis is in place, the holding capsule is removed. The extension prosthesis, activated by heat, expands like a spring and becomes anchored to the artery wall at the site of the endoleak. If full expansion of the prosthesis does not occur automatically, a balloon catheter is threaded to the graft site and inflated within the endovascular prosthesis until full expansion is achieved. The catheter is removed and the arteriotomy site is closed. These procedures include all nonselective catheterizations, sizing, and device selection prior to the procedure; radiological supervision and interpretation; and treatment zone angioplasty or stenting, when performed. These codes may only be reported once per vessel treated (e.g., multiple endograft extensions placed in a single vessel may only be reported once). Report 34710 for placement of an extension prosthesis in the initial vessel and 34711 for placement of an extension prosthesis in each additional vessel.

Coding Tips

These are unilateral procedures. If performed bilaterally, some payers require that the service be reported twice with modifier 50 appended to the second code while others require identification of the service only once with modifier 50 appended. Check with individual payers. Modifier 50 identifies a procedure performed identically on the opposite side of the body (mirror image). Report 34711 in addition to 34710. These codes may only be reported once per operative session. For decompressive laparotomy, report 49000 in addition to 34710. For delayed revision using a transcatheter enhanced fixation device, see 34712. Do not report 34710 or 34711 with 34701-34709 or 34841-34848. Do not report these codes in addition to 34718 for the same side. For endovascular repair of an iliac artery bifurcation, see 34717-34718. For intravascular ultrasound performed during an endovascular aneurysm repair, see 37252 and 37253. For isolated bilateral iliac artery repair, see 34707 and 34708 and append modifier 50. For open artery exposure, use 34714-34716, 34812, 34820, 34833, or 34834 in addition to 34701-34708, 34710, 34712, or 34718, when applicable. For percutaneous arterial closure, use 34713 in addition to 34701-34708, 34710, 34712, or 34718, when applicable. For simultaneous bilateral iliac artery aneurysm repairs with an aorto-bi-iliac endograft, report 34705 or 34706, when applicable.

ICD-10-CM Diagnostic Codes

A52.01	Syphilitic aneurysm of aorta
I71.02	Dissection of abdominal aorta
I71.3	Abdominal aortic aneurysm, ruptured
I71.4	Abdominal aortic aneurysm, without rupture
I72.3	Aneurysm of iliac artery
I77.72	Dissection of iliac artery
I77.811	Abdominal aortic ectasia
I77.89	Other specified disorders of arteries and arterioles
Q25.43	Congenital aneurysm of aorta
Q25.44	Congenital dilation of aorta
Q25.49	Other congenital malformations of aorta
Q25.8	Other congenital malformations of other great arteries
Q25.9	Congenital malformation of great arteries, unspecified
Q79.61	Classical Ehlers-Danlos syndrome
Q79.62	Hypermobile Ehlers-Danlos syndrome
Q79.63	Vascular Ehlers-Danlos syndrome
Q79.69	Other Ehlers-Danlos syndromes
Q87.410	Marfan's syndrome with aortic dilation
Q87.418	Marfan's syndrome with other cardiovascular manifestations
S35.01XA	Minor laceration of abdominal aorta, initial encounter
S35.02XA	Major laceration of abdominal aorta, initial encounter
S35.09XA	Other injury of abdominal aorta, initial encounter
S35.511A	Injury of right iliac artery, initial encounter ☑
S35.512A	Injury of left iliac artery, initial encounter ☑
S35.59XA	Injury of other iliac blood vessels, initial encounter

AMA: 34710 2018,Jan,8; 2017,Dec,3 **34711** 2018,Jan,8; 2017,Dec,3

Relative Value Units/Medicare Edits

Non-Facility RVU	Work	PE	MP	Total
34710	15.0	4.98	3.26	23.24
34711	6.0	1.32	1.34	8.66
Facility RVU	**Work**	**PE**	**MP**	**Total**
34710	15.0	4.98	3.26	23.24
34711	6.0	1.32	1.34	8.66

	FUD	Status	MUE	Modifiers				IOM Reference
34710	90	A	1(2)	51	N/A	62	80	None
34711	N/A	A	2(3)	N/A	N/A	62	80	

* with documentation

34712

34712 Transcatheter delivery of enhanced fixation device(s) to the endograft (eg, anchor, screw, tack) and all associated radiological supervision and interpretation

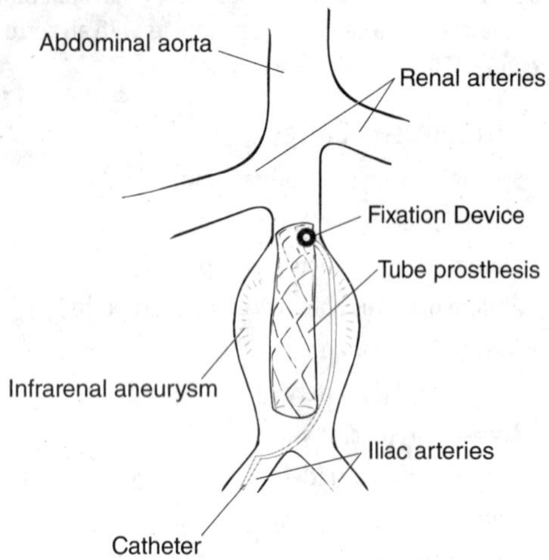

Explanation

The physician performs transcatheter delivery of accessory-enhanced fixation devices, such as an anchor, screw, or tack, to the endograft. Commonly referred to as a bioprosthesis, this procedure is used for patients with abdominal aortic and/or iliac artery conditions, such as an aneurysm with complex anatomies, or for patients who are experiencing an endoleak. Proprietary devices such as the Aptus™ Heli-FX™ EndoAnchor™ system and the Aptus™ Heli-FX™ Thoracic EndoAnchor™ system ensure a safe and effective treatment solution for these types of repairs. They enhance durability to the level of a surgical anastomosis and address concerns for future complications. They are used to improve fixation and sealing of an endovascular graft, either in primary cases or to fix endoleaks and stent migration. The devices lock the endograft to the abdominal aorta and/or iliac artery to secure the patient's future and maximize outcomes in challenging patients. The fixation devices quickly identify, aim, and activate a sealing mechanism to close up endoleaks. Endoanchors are used to repair an endovascular graft in cases where the original graft has moved away from the implant site and developed endoleaks. In such cases, augmented fixation and/or sealing is required to regain or maintain effective aneurysm exclusion. These devices can be placed during the initial endoprosthesis placement procedure or for a subsequent repair procedure. Radiologic supervision and interpretation are included in this procedure.

Coding Tips

Report this code only once per operative session. Radiological supervision and interpretation is included and should not be reported separately. For vascular access requiring the use of closure devices for sheaths of 12 French or larger, or access requiring open surgical arterial exposure, see 34713-34716, 34812, 34820, 34833, and 34834. Percutaneous access using a sheath smaller than 12 French is included in 34712 and should not be reported separately.

ICD-10-CM Diagnostic Codes

A52.01	Syphilitic aneurysm of aorta
I71.02	Dissection of abdominal aorta
I71.3	Abdominal aortic aneurysm, ruptured
I71.4	Abdominal aortic aneurysm, without rupture
I72.3	Aneurysm of iliac artery
I77.72	Dissection of iliac artery
I77.811	Abdominal aortic ectasia
I77.89	Other specified disorders of arteries and arterioles
Q25.43	Congenital aneurysm of aorta
Q25.44	Congenital dilation of aorta
Q25.49	Other congenital malformations of aorta
Q25.8	Other congenital malformations of other great arteries
Q25.9	Congenital malformation of great arteries, unspecified
Q79.61	Classical Ehlers-Danlos syndrome
Q79.62	Hypermobile Ehlers-Danlos syndrome
Q79.63	Vascular Ehlers-Danlos syndrome
Q87.410	Marfan's syndrome with aortic dilation
Q87.418	Marfan's syndrome with other cardiovascular manifestations
S35.01XA	Minor laceration of abdominal aorta, initial encounter
S35.02XA	Major laceration of abdominal aorta, initial encounter
S35.09XA	Other injury of abdominal aorta, initial encounter
S35.511A	Injury of right iliac artery, initial encounter ☑
S35.512A	Injury of left iliac artery, initial encounter ☑
S35.59XA	Injury of other iliac blood vessels, initial encounter

AMA: 34712 2018,Jan,8; 2017,Dec,3

Relative Value Units/Medicare Edits

Non-Facility RVU	Work	PE	MP	Total
34712	12.0	5.42	2.43	19.85
Facility RVU	**Work**	**PE**	**MP**	**Total**
34712	12.0	5.42	2.43	19.85

	FUD	Status	MUE	Modifiers				IOM Reference
34712	90	A	1(2)	51	N/A	62	80	None

* with documentation

Terms To Know

fixation. Act or condition of being attached, secured, fastened, or held in position.

transcatheter. Procedure or treatment performed via a catheter.

34713-34714 [34812]

+ **34713** Percutaneous access and closure of femoral artery for delivery of endograft through a large sheath (12 French or larger), including ultrasound guidance, when performed, unilateral (List separately in addition to code for primary procedure)
+ **34812** Open femoral artery exposure for delivery of endovascular prosthesis, by groin incision, unilateral (List separately in addition to code for primary procedure)
+ **34714** Open femoral artery exposure with creation of conduit for delivery of endovascular prosthesis or for establishment of cardiopulmonary bypass, by groin incision, unilateral (List separately in addition to code for primary procedure)

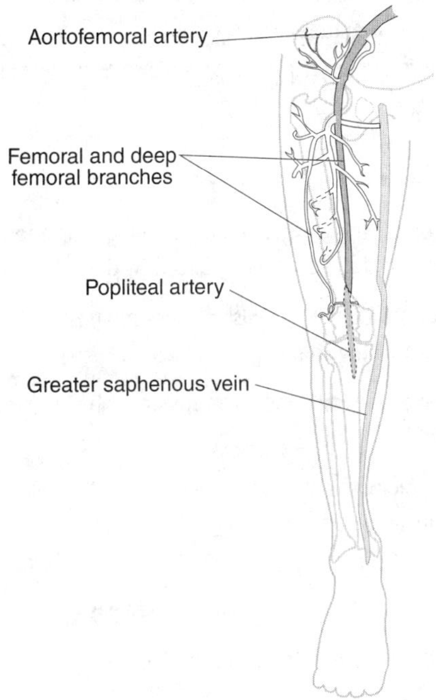

Explanation

The femoral artery may be accessed percutaneously or by open incision. For percutaneous access the femoral artery is identified using ultrasound guidance and the guide catheter is percutaneously inserted with subsequent insertion of a large arterial sheath (i.e., 12 French or larger). Closure may involve the use of an arterial closure device (ACD). Several types of ACDs may be used for closure including a small balloon that ensures sealant coverage of the arteriotomy, four needles that anchor and close suture material upon removal, or a collagen sponge with polymer that forms a self-tightening suture seal. Alternately, the femoral artery may be examined via an open technique. With the patient in the supine position, the physician exposes the femoral artery through an incision in the groin area revealing the femoral artery on one side while underlying subcutaneous layers and muscles incised to reach the artery are placed out of the way as hemostasis is achieved in preparation for delivery of the endograft, endovascular prosthesis, or creation of a conduit. Closure may be by direct suture. Report 34713 for percutaneous access and closure of a femoral arteriotomy for delivery of an endovascular prosthesis. Ultrasound guidance is included. Report 34812 for open femoral artery exposure with delivery of an endovascular prosthesis and repair and closure of the femoral artery. Report 34714 for open femoral artery exposure with endovascular device delivery or establishment of cardiopulmonary bypass that requires creation of a prosthetic conduit utilizing a femoral artery.

Coding Tips

These codes should only be reported once per side and should be reported twice when performed bilaterally. Do not report with modifier 50. Report 34713 and 34812 in addition to 33880, 33881, 33883, 33884, 33886, 34701-34708, 34710, 34712, 34718, and 34841-34848. Do not report 34812 with 33990 or 33991. Do not report 34713 with the prior list of codes if a sheath smaller than 12 French was used or for percutaneous access and closure of the femoral artery in addition to 37221, 37223, 37236, or 37237. Do not report 34812 with 33953, 33954, 33959, 33962, 33969, 33984, or 33987. Code 34714 may be reported with an extensive number of primary procedures ranging from 32852-34848. Refer to the CPT manual for details. Do not report 34714 with 33362, 33953, 33954, 33959, 33962, 33969, 33984, or 34812 when performed on the same side.

ICD-10-CM Diagnostic Codes

This/these CPT code(s) are add on code(s). See the primary procedure code that this code is performed with for your ICD-10-CM code selections. Diagnostic code(s) would be the same as the actual procedure performed.

AMA: **34713** 2018,Jan,8; 2017,Dec,3 **34714** 2018,Jan,8; 2017,Dec,3 **34812** 2018,Jan,8; 2017,Jan,8; 2017,Dec,3; 2016,Jan,13; 2015,Jul,3; 2015,Jan,16; 2014,Jan,11; 2013,Mar,10-11; 2013,Dec,8

Relative Value Units/Medicare Edits

Non-Facility RVU	Work	PE	MP	Total
34713	2.5	0.72	0.51	3.73
34812	4.13	0.92	0.95	6.0
34714	5.25	1.54	1.05	7.84
Facility RVU	**Work**	**PE**	**MP**	**Total**
34713	2.5	0.72	0.51	3.73
34812	4.13	0.92	0.95	6.0
34714	5.25	1.54	1.05	7.84

	FUD	Status	MUE	Modifiers				IOM Reference
34713	N/A	A	1(2)	N/A	50	62	80	None
34812	N/A	A	1(2)	N/A	50	62	80	
34714	N/A	A	1(2)	N/A	50	62	80	

* with documentation

[34820]

+ **34820** Open iliac artery exposure for delivery of endovascular prosthesis or iliac occlusion during endovascular therapy, by abdominal or retroperitoneal incision, unilateral (List separately in addition to code for primary procedure)

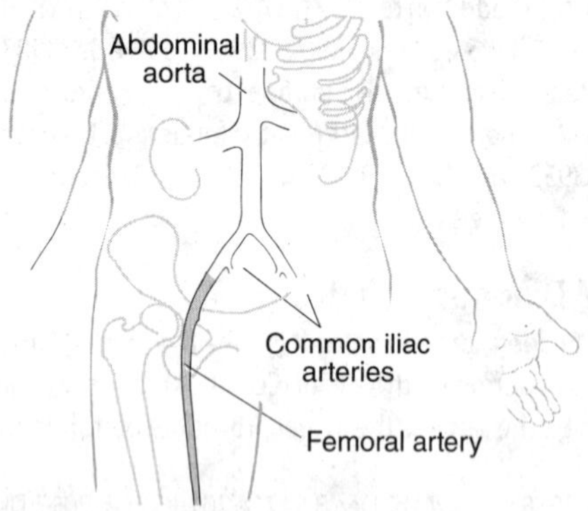

An iliac artery is surgically exposed to deliver an endovascular prosthesis or to occlude an iliac artery. The procedure occurs during endovascular therapy and access is abdominal or retroperitoneal

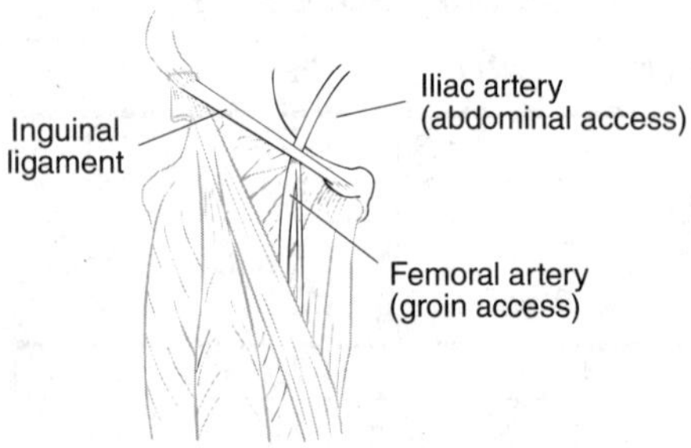

Explanation

The physician makes an abdominal or retroperitoneal incision to expose the iliac artery on one side to facilitate the delivery of an endovascular prosthesis or to perform temporary iliac artery occlusion during a procedure for endovascular therapy. The patient is placed supine and the buttocks are elevated. An incision is made parallel with and just above the inguinal ligament. The incision is in the middle third of a proximally curved line extending from the anterior superior iliac spine to the pubic symphysis. Hemostasis of vessels is achieved and the aponeuroses of the external and internal oblique and the transversus muscles are incised parallel to the inguinal ligament. The structures are reflected upward and medially, the transversalis fascia is opened, and the retroperitoneal space is entered. The iliac artery is exposed in preparation for delivering an endovascular prosthesis and its sheath is opened with tape placed about it. If the artery has been exposed for the purpose of placing a temporary occlusion device, the clamp is placed.

Coding Tips

Depending on the type of exposure required, this service may be performed by a surgeon other than the one performing the endovascular repair. Code 34820 should only be reported once per side and should be reported twice when performed bilaterally. Do not report with modifier 50. Report 34820 in addition to 33880, 33881, 33883, 33884, 33886, 33990, 33991, 34701-34708, 34710, 34712, 34718, or 34841-34848. Do not report 34820 with 33953, 33954, 33959, 33962, 33969, or 33984.

ICD-10-CM Diagnostic Codes

This/these CPT code(s) are add on code(s). See the primary procedure code that this code is performed with for your ICD-10-CM code selections. Diagnostic code(s) would be the same as the actual procedure performed.

AMA: 34820 2018,Jan,8; 2017,Jan,8; 2017,Dec,3; 2016,Jan,13; 2015,Jul,3; 2015,Jan,16; 2014,Jan,11

Relative Value Units/Medicare Edits

Non-Facility RVU	Work	PE	MP	Total
34820	7.0	1.51	1.58	10.09
Facility RVU	**Work**	**PE**	**MP**	**Total**
34820	7.0	1.51	1.58	10.09

	FUD	Status	MUE	Modifiers				IOM Reference
34820	N/A	A	1(2)	N/A	50	62	80	None

* with documentation

Terms To Know

aneurysm. Circumscribed dilation or outpouching of an artery wall, often containing blood clots and connecting directly with the lumen of the artery.

atherosclerosis. Buildup of yellowish plaques composed of cholesterol and lipoid material within the arteries.

catheter. Flexible tube inserted into an area of the body for introducing or withdrawing fluid.

fluoroscopy. Radiology technique that allows visual examination of part of the body or a function of an organ using a device that projects an x-ray image on a fluorescent screen.

occlusion. Constriction, closure, or blockage of a passage.

sheath. Covering enclosing an organ or part.

stent. Tube to provide support in a body cavity or lumen.

[34833, 34834]

- \+ **34833** Open iliac artery exposure with creation of conduit for delivery of endovascular prosthesis or for establishment of cardiopulmonary bypass, by abdominal or retroperitoneal incision, unilateral (List separately in addition to code for primary procedure)
- \+ **34834** Open brachial artery exposure for delivery of endovascular prosthesis, unilateral (List separately in addition to code for primary procedure)

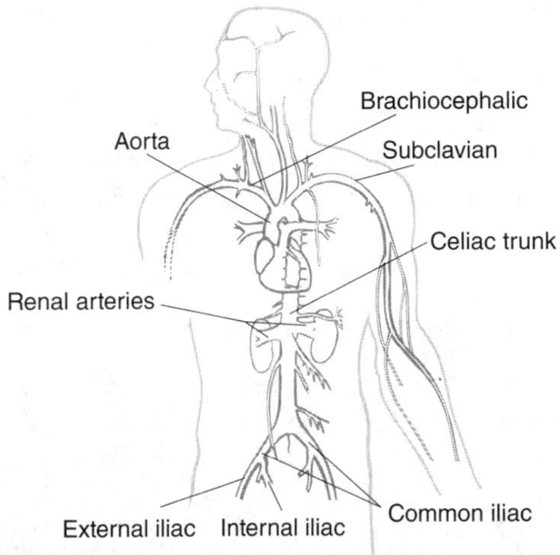

Explanation

In 34833, a conduit is created for the delivery of an endovascular prosthesis or for the establishment of cardiopulmonary bypass via transabdominal or retroperitoneal incision. A skin incision is made parallel with and just above the inguinal ligament. The skin is incised and the retroperitoneal space is entered to access the iliac artery. Bowels, blood vessels, and other soft tissue are mobilized from the area to give clear access to the iliac artery. With adequate exposure, loops are passed around the vessel proximally and distally. Anticoagulation is achieved and vascular clamps are applied. An arteriotomy is made for creation of the conduit, which is formed by placing a tubular piece of bypass graft material that has been fashioned into the right size onto the iliac artery and suturing it together. The conduit is clamped and the vascular clamps are removed from the iliac artery. Additional sutures are placed as needed. Through the newly created conduit, endovascular repair by deployment of a prosthesis may be undertaken. After the repair is complete, the conduit may be closed in one of two ways. The open end of the conduit may be sewn to the distal external iliac artery, and thereby left in place as a channel for external iliac bypass graft, or it may be cut close to the iliac artery and simply oversewn with sutures. This code reports the creation of the conduit, not the endovascular repair. In 34834, open brachial artery exposure is done for delivery of an endovascular prosthesis. An incision is made in the skin of the upper arm and nerves, blood vessels, and other soft tissues are mobilized from the area to give clear access to the brachial artery. With adequate exposure, loops are passed around the vessel proximally and distally. Anticoagulation is achieved and vascular clamps are alternately applied and removed as needed for introduction of guidewires, sheaths, and catheters through the brachial artery for accomplishing deployment of an aortic or iliac endovascular prosthesis. After the endovascular repair is complete, the opening remaining in the brachial artery is closed with fine sutures after irrigation and trimming of the edges has been done. Hemostasis is achieved and the wound is irrigated and closed. This code reports the open brachial artery exposure, not the endovascular repair.

Coding Tips

Depending on the type of exposure required, this service may be performed by a surgeon other than the one performing the endovascular repair. These codes should only be reported once per side and should be reported twice when performed bilaterally. Do not report with modifier 50. Code 34833 may be reported with an extensive number of primary procedures ranging from 32852-34848. Refer to the CPT manual for details. Do not report 34833 with 33364, 33953, 33954, 33959, 33962, 33969, 33984, or 34820 when performed on the same side. Report 34834 in addition to 33880-33884, 33886, 33990, 33991, 34701-34708, 34710, 34712, 34718, or 34841-34848. Do not report 34834 with 33953, 33954, 33959, 33962, 33969, or 33984.

ICD-10-CM Diagnostic Codes

This/these CPT code(s) are add on code(s). See the primary procedure code that this code is performed with for your ICD-10-CM code selections. Diagnostic code(s) would be the same as the actual procedure performed.

AMA: **34833** 2018,Jan,8; 2017,Jan,8; 2017,Dec,3; 2016,Jan,13; 2015,Jul,3; 2015,Jan,16; 2014,Jan,11 **34834** 2018,Jan,8; 2017,Jan,8; 2017,Dec,3; 2016,Jan,13; 2015,Jul,3; 2015,Jan,16; 2014,Jan,11

Relative Value Units/Medicare Edits

Non-Facility RVU	Work	PE	MP	Total
34833	8.16	1.7	1.86	11.72
34834	2.65	0.5	0.6	3.75
Facility RVU	**Work**	**PE**	**MP**	**Total**
34833	8.16	1.7	1.86	11.72
34834	2.65	0.5	0.6	3.75

	FUD	Status	MUE	Modifiers				IOM Reference
34833	N/A	A	1(2)	N/A	50	62	80	None
34834	N/A	A	1(2)	N/A	50	62	80	

* with documentation

34715-34716

\+ **34715** Open axillary/subclavian artery exposure for delivery of endovascular prosthesis by infraclavicular or supraclavicular incision, unilateral (List separately in addition to code for primary procedure)

\+ **34716** Open axillary/subclavian artery exposure with creation of conduit for delivery of endovascular prosthesis or for establishment of cardiopulmonary bypass, by infraclavicular or supraclavicular incision, unilateral (List separately in addition to code for primary procedure)

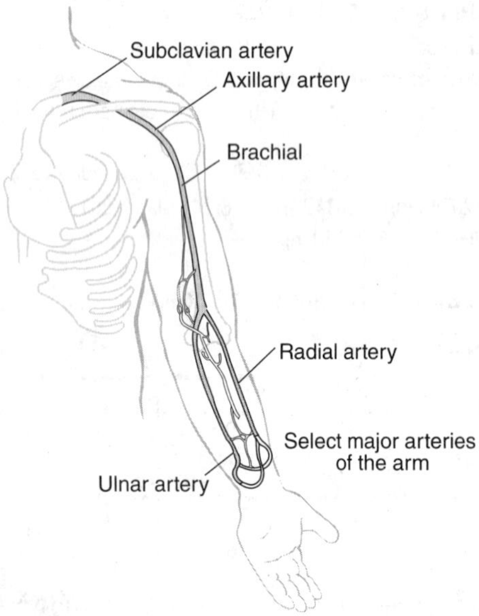

Explanation

The physician exposes the axillary or subclavian artery for delivery of an endovascular prosthesis and performs closure of the artery with an arterial closure device (ACD). The Mynx Vascular Closure Device® is an ACD that is inserted through the existing procedural sheath. A small balloon is inflated within the artery and pulled back to the arterial wall, serving as an anchor to ensure proper placement, and is inflated. The balloon is deflated and removed through the tract, leaving behind only the expanded sealant, which seals the arteriotomy. The Prostar® system is an ACD that uses four needles (two sutures) directed outward from within the arterial lumen. It is advanced over a guidewire until blood return indicates proper placement. When the physician pulls the device handle, the needles are deployed and pulled through the arterial wall. The needles remain contained within the device shaft and are removed by pulling them up through the device shaft, leaving behind the suture ends, which are then tied and the device is removed. The Angio-Seal STS Plus ACD is composed of collagen sponge and polymer anchor joined together with a self-tightening suture that seals and sandwiches the arteriotomy for a more complete closure. The device stops the flow of blood mechanically, which is supported by the platelet-inducing properties of the collagen. Report 34715 for delivery of an endovascular prosthesis by axillary or subclavian exposure through an infraclavicular or supraclavicular or sternotomy incision during endovascular aneurysm repair. The patient is placed in supine position and open incision is made. Hemostasis of vessels is achieved. The underlying subcutaneous layers and muscles are incised to reach the artery and reflected out of the way. The axillary or subclavian artery is exposed in preparation for delivery of the endovascular prosthesis and its sheath is opened with tape placed about it. Report 34716 for endovascular device delivery or establishment of cardiopulmonary bypass that requires creation of a prosthetic conduit utilizing axillary or subclavian artery exposure through an infraclavicular or supraclavicular or sternotomy incision during endovascular aneurysm repair or cardiac procedures requiring cardiopulmonary bypass.

Coding Tips

These codes should only be reported once per side and should be reported twice when performed bilaterally. Do not report with modifier 50. Report 34715 in addition to 33880-33884, 33886, 33990, 33991, 34701-34708, 34710, 34712, 34718, or 34841-34848. Do not report 34715 with 33363, 33953, 33954, 33959, 33962, 33969, 33984, 0451T, 0452T, 0455T, or 0456T. Code 34716 may be reported with an extensive number of primary procedures ranging from 32852-34848. Refer to the CPT manual for details. Do not report 34716 with 33953, 33954, 33959, 33962, 33969, 33984, 0451T, 0452T, 0455T, or 0456T.

ICD-10-CM Diagnostic Codes

This/these CPT code(s) are add on code(s). See the primary procedure code that this code is performed with for your ICD-10-CM code selections. Diagnostic code(s) would be the same as the actual procedure performed.

AMA: **34715** 2018,Jan,8; 2017,Dec,3 **34716** 2018,Jan,8; 2017,Dec,3

Relative Value Units/Medicare Edits

Non-Facility RVU	Work	PE	MP	Total
34715	6.0	1.64	1.15	8.79
34716	7.19	2.26	1.6	11.05
Facility RVU	**Work**	**PE**	**MP**	**Total**
34715	6.0	1.64	1.15	8.79
34716	7.19	2.26	1.6	11.05

	FUD	Status	MUE	Modifiers				IOM Reference
34715	N/A	A	1(2)	N/A	50	62	80	None
34716	N/A	A	1(2)	N/A	50	62	80	

* with documentation

Terms To Know

arteriotomy. Incision into an artery.

endovascular therapy. Intravascular catheters, scopes, stents, balloons, and other devices or methods used to treat vascular disease.

Arteries and Veins

34808

+ **34808** Endovascular placement of iliac artery occlusion device (List separately in addition to code for primary procedure)

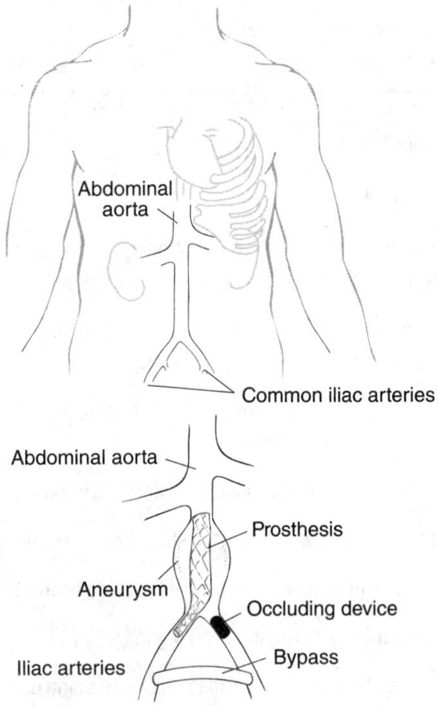

A device is placed endovascularly into an iliac artery in order to occlude blood flow

Explanation

Endovascular placement of an iliac artery occlusion device is performed during separately reportable repair of an abdominal aortic aneurysm and/or endovascular graft procedure. As part of the repair, the iliac artery is occluded. Under separately reportable fluoroscopy, an iliac artery occlusion device is threaded through the arteries and placed distal to the aneurysm. When the aneurysmal repair is complete, the endovascular occlusion device may be left in the artery. Catheters and devices used for access and to deploy the occlusion device are removed and any bleeding controlled.

Coding Tips

Report 34808 in addition to 34701-34704, 34707-34710, 34813, or 34841-34844. When an open approach is required, report the appropriate arterial exposure code (34714, 34812, 34820, 34833) in addition to the endovascular placement of the occlusion device.

ICD-10-CM Diagnostic Codes

This/these CPT code(s) are add on code(s). See the primary procedure code that this code is performed with for your ICD-10-CM code selections. Diagnostic code(s) would be the same as the actual procedure performed.

AMA: 34808 2018,Jan,8; 2017,Jan,8; 2016,Jan,13; 2015,Jan,16; 2014,Jan,11

Relative Value Units/Medicare Edits

Non-Facility RVU	Work	PE	MP	Total
34808	4.12	0.97	1.02	6.11
Facility RVU	**Work**	**PE**	**MP**	**Total**
34808	4.12	0.97	1.02	6.11

	FUD	Status	MUE	Modifiers				IOM Reference
34808	N/A	A	1(3)	N/A	N/A	62	80	None

* with documentation

Terms To Know

aneurysm. Circumscribed dilation or outpouching of an artery wall, often containing blood clots and connecting directly with the lumen of the artery.

fluoroscopy. Radiology technique that allows visual examination of part of the body or a function of an organ using a device that projects an x-ray image on a fluorescent screen.

graft. Tissue implant from another part of the body or another person.

occlusion. Constriction, closure, or blockage of a passage.

suture. Numerous stitching techniques employed in wound closure.

buried suture. Continuous or interrupted suture placed under the skin for a layered closure.

continuous suture. Running stitch with tension evenly distributed across a single strand to provide a leakproof closure line.

interrupted suture. Series of single stitches with tension isolated at each stitch, in which all stitches are not affected if one becomes loose, and the isolated sutures cannot act as a wick to transport an infection.

purse-string suture. Continuous suture placed around a tubular structure and tightened, to reduce or close the lumen.

retention suture. Secondary stitching that bridges the primary suture, providing support for the primary repair; a plastic or rubber bolster may be placed over the primary repair and under the retention sutures.

34813

+ 34813 Placement of femoral-femoral prosthetic graft during endovascular aortic aneurysm repair (List separately in addition to code for primary procedure)

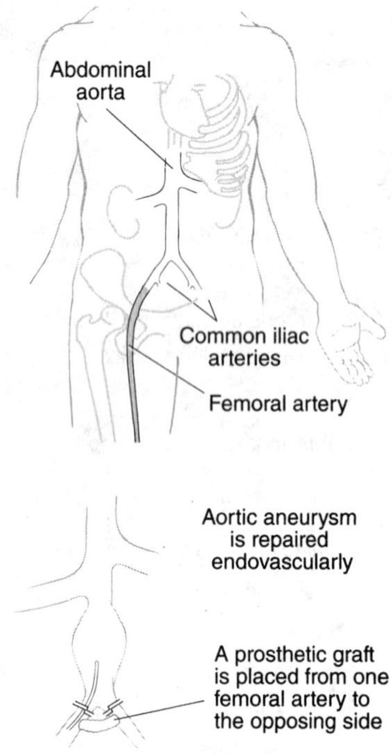

Explanation

During separately reportable endovascular repair of an aortic aneurysm, a diseased or damaged femoral artery is repaired by placing a prosthetic femoral-femoral graft. Through incisions in the skin of the upper thighs, the physician isolates and dissects a section of the affected femoral artery. Once vessel clamps have been affixed above and below the area of damaged vessel to be anastomosed, the femoral artery is cut above and below the diseased or damaged area and the new distal and proximal ends are sutured to the ends of the prosthetic graft, which now replaces the section of diseased or damaged artery. When the clamps are removed, the blood flows unobstructed through the femoral artery. After the graft is complete, the skin incisions are repaired with layered closures.

Coding Tips

Report 34813 in addition to 34812 as appropriate. For femoral artery grafting, see 35521, 35533, 35539, 35540, 35556, 35558, 35566, 35621, 35646, 35654–35661, 35666, and 35700.

ICD-10-CM Diagnostic Codes

This/these CPT code(s) are add on code(s). See the primary procedure code that this code is performed with for your ICD-10-CM code selections. Diagnostic code(s) would be the same as the actual procedure performed.

AMA: 34813 2018,Jan,8; 2017,Jan,8; 2016,Jan,13; 2015,Jan,16; 2014,Jan,11

Relative Value Units/Medicare Edits

Non-Facility RVU	Work	PE	MP	Total
34813	4.79	0.96	1.1	6.85
Facility RVU	**Work**	**PE**	**MP**	**Total**
34813	4.79	0.96	1.1	6.85

	FUD	Status	MUE	Modifiers				IOM Reference
34813	N/A	A	1(2)	N/A	N/A	62	80	None

* with documentation

Terms To Know

anastomosis. Surgically created connection between ducts, blood vessels, or bowel segments to allow flow from one to the other.

aneurysm. Circumscribed dilation or outpouching of an artery wall, often containing blood clots and connecting directly with the lumen of the artery.

atherosclerosis. Buildup of yellowish plaques composed of cholesterol and lipoid material within the arteries.

bypass. Auxiliary or diverted route to maintain continuous flow.

distal. Located farther away from a specified reference point or the trunk.

graft. Tissue implant from another part of the body or another person.

incision. Act of cutting into tissue or an organ.

proximal. Located closest to a specified reference point, usually the midline or trunk.

stricture. Narrowing of an anatomical structure.

34830-34832

34830 Open repair of infrarenal aortic aneurysm or dissection, plus repair of associated arterial trauma, following unsuccessful endovascular repair; tube prosthesis

34831 aorto-bi-iliac prosthesis

34832 aorto-bifemoral prosthesis

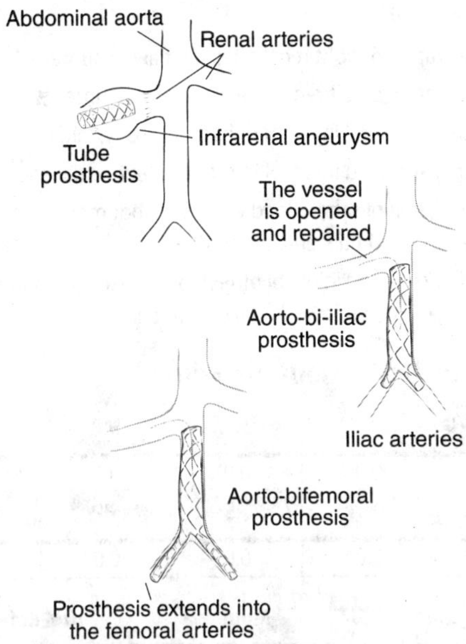

An infrarenal aortic aneurysm or dissection is treated in an open surgical session following an unsuccessful endovascular treatment attempt. A tube prosthesis is placed and any associated arterial trauma is repaired

Explanation

An attempted endovascular repair of an aortic aneurysm originating below the renal arteries (infrarenal) fails necessitating open repair of the aneurysm as well as repair of any trauma associated with the endovascular attempt. An incision is made in the abdomen from just below the diaphragm to the umbilicus. The aorta is exposed, the aneurysm identified, and the aorta and other arteries inspected for injury resulting from the failed endovascular procedure. Repair of the aneurysm is accomplished by temporarily clamping the aorta both above and below the aneurysm. It is usually possible to place the upper clamp just below the origins of the renal arteries so that the kidneys continue to receive blood flow throughout the operation. Blood flow to the legs is interrupted while the aorta is clamped. The aneurysm is opened lengthwise and any thrombi (blood clots) removed. The aneurysm wall is not removed. The aorta is cut above and below the aneurysm and a prosthetic graft made of synthetic material is sutured in place between the two ends. The aneurysm wall is wrapped around the synthetic graft. The clamps are removed allowing blood to flow through the graft and into the vessels of the lower extremities. The surgical wound is closed. Repair using a tube prosthesis is reported with 34830; repair with an aorto-bi-iliac prosthesis is reported with 34831; and repair with an aorto-bifemoral prosthesis is reported with 34832.

Coding Tips

These codes should be used only when an endovascular repair has been attempted but has been unsuccessful. To report direct repair of an abdominal aortic aneurysm not preceded by attempted endovascular repair, see 35081–35103.

ICD-10-CM Diagnostic Codes

A52.01	Syphilitic aneurysm of aorta
I71.02	Dissection of abdominal aorta
I71.3	Abdominal aortic aneurysm, ruptured
I71.4	Abdominal aortic aneurysm, without rupture
Q25.43	Congenital aneurysm of aorta
Q25.44	Congenital dilation of aorta
Q25.47	Right aortic arch
Q25.48	Anomalous origin of subclavian artery
Q25.49	Other congenital malformations of aorta
Q25.8	Other congenital malformations of other great arteries
Q79.61	Classical Ehlers-Danlos syndrome
Q79.62	Hypermobile Ehlers-Danlos syndrome
Q79.63	Vascular Ehlers-Danlos syndrome
Q87.410	Marfan's syndrome with aortic dilation
Q87.418	Marfan's syndrome with other cardiovascular manifestations
S35.01XA	Minor laceration of abdominal aorta, initial encounter
S35.02XA	Major laceration of abdominal aorta, initial encounter
S35.09XA	Other injury of abdominal aorta, initial encounter

AMA: 34830 2018,Jan,8; 2017,Jan,8; 2016,Jan,13; 2015,Jan,16; 2014,Jan,11 **34831** 2018,Jan,8; 2017,Jan,8; 2016,Jan,13; 2015,Jan,16; 2014,Jan,11 **34832** 2018,Jan,8; 2017,Jan,8; 2016,Jan,13; 2015,Jan,16; 2014,Jan,11

Relative Value Units/Medicare Edits

Non-Facility RVU	Work	PE	MP	Total
34830	35.23	7.53	8.15	50.91
34831	37.98	9.44	8.57	55.99
34832	37.98	7.97	8.8	54.75
Facility RVU	**Work**	**PE**	**MP**	**Total**
34830	35.23	7.53	8.15	50.91
34831	37.98	9.44	8.57	55.99
34832	37.98	7.97	8.8	54.75

	FUD	Status	MUE	Modifiers				IOM Reference
34830	90	A	1(2)	51	N/A	62	80	None
34831	90	A	1(2)	51	N/A	62	80	
34832	90	A	1(2)	51	N/A	62	80	

* with documentation

Terms To Know

aneurysm. Circumscribed dilation or outpouching of an artery wall, often containing blood clots and connecting directly with the lumen of the artery.

34839

34839 Physician planning of a patient-specific fenestrated visceral aortic endograft requiring a minimum of 90 minutes of physician time

Explanation

The physician spends at least 90 minutes planning for the placement of a fenestrated visceral aortic endograft, which requires detailed preparation prior to implantation. The planning includes review of radiological imaging enhanced by computer software to assist in the production of the device. Before placement, the physician needs to determine the size parameters of the graft that will conform to the branches of the aorta. These dimensions allow the physician to cut holes (fenestrations) in the device at each visceral artery orifice to allow side branch perfusion of these vessels. Precise planning must allow for adequate blood flow upon completion of placement. The physician must document at least 90 minutes of planning in the medical record.

Coding Tips

This code is reported the date the planning is completed. Do not report 34839 with 76376 or 76377. Do not report 34839 with 34841–34848 when performed the day before or the day of the fenestrated endovascular repair.

ICD-10-CM Diagnostic Codes

A52.01	Syphilitic aneurysm of aorta
I71.01	Dissection of thoracic aorta
I71.02	Dissection of abdominal aorta
I71.03	Dissection of thoracoabdominal aorta
I71.1	Thoracic aortic aneurysm, ruptured
I71.2	Thoracic aortic aneurysm, without rupture
I71.3	Abdominal aortic aneurysm, ruptured
I71.4	Abdominal aortic aneurysm, without rupture
I71.5	Thoracoabdominal aortic aneurysm, ruptured
I71.6	Thoracoabdominal aortic aneurysm, without rupture
I72.2	Aneurysm of renal artery
I72.8	Aneurysm of other specified arteries
I77.73	Dissection of renal artery
I77.79	Dissection of other specified artery
I79.0	Aneurysm of aorta in diseases classified elsewhere
Q25.41	Absence and aplasia of aorta
Q25.42	Hypoplasia of aorta
Q25.43	Congenital aneurysm of aorta
Q25.44	Congenital dilation of aorta
Q25.45	Double aortic arch
Q25.46	Tortuous aortic arch
Q25.47	Right aortic arch
Q25.48	Anomalous origin of subclavian artery
Q25.49	Other congenital malformations of aorta
Q25.8	Other congenital malformations of other great arteries
S35.01XA	Minor laceration of abdominal aorta, initial encounter
S35.02XA	Major laceration of abdominal aorta, initial encounter
S35.09XA	Other injury of abdominal aorta, initial encounter
S35.211A	Minor laceration of celiac artery, initial encounter
S35.212A	Major laceration of celiac artery, initial encounter
S35.218A	Other injury of celiac artery, initial encounter
S35.221A	Minor laceration of superior mesenteric artery, initial encounter
S35.222A	Major laceration of superior mesenteric artery, initial encounter
S35.228A	Other injury of superior mesenteric artery, initial encounter
S35.291A	Minor laceration of branches of celiac and mesenteric artery, initial encounter
S35.292A	Major laceration of branches of celiac and mesenteric artery, initial encounter
S35.298A	Other injury of branches of celiac and mesenteric artery, initial encounter
S35.411A	Laceration of right renal artery, initial encounter ☑
S35.412A	Laceration of left renal artery, initial encounter ☑
S35.491A	Other specified injury of right renal artery, initial encounter ☑
S35.492A	Other specified injury of left renal artery, initial encounter ☑
S35.8X1A	Laceration of other blood vessels at abdomen, lower back and pelvis level, initial encounter
S35.8X8A	Other specified injury of other blood vessels at abdomen, lower back and pelvis level, initial encounter

Relative Value Units/Medicare Edits

Non-Facility RVU	Work	PE	MP	Total
34839	0.0	0.0	0.0	0.0
Facility RVU	**Work**	**PE**	**MP**	**Total**
34839	0.0	0.0	0.0	0.0

	FUD	Status	MUE	Modifiers				IOM Reference
34839	N/A	B	1(2)	N/A	N/A	N/A	80*	None

* with documentation

Terms To Know

aneurysm. Circumscribed dilation or outpouching of an artery wall, often containing blood clots and connecting directly with the lumen of the artery.

dissection. (dis. apart; -section, act of cutting) Separating by cutting tissue or body structures apart.

fenestration. Presence of small openings from piercing or perforations.

graft. Tissue implant from another part of the body or another person.

vascular. Pertaining to blood vessels.

34841-34844

34841 Endovascular repair of visceral aorta (eg, aneurysm, pseudoaneurysm, dissection, penetrating ulcer, intramural hematoma, or traumatic disruption) by deployment of a fenestrated visceral aortic endograft and all associated radiological supervision and interpretation, including target zone angioplasty, when performed; including one visceral artery endoprosthesis (superior mesenteric, celiac or renal artery)

34842 including two visceral artery endoprostheses (superior mesenteric, celiac and/or renal artery[s])

34843 including three visceral artery endoprostheses (superior mesenteric, celiac and/or renal artery[s])

34844 including four or more visceral artery endoprostheses (superior mesenteric, celiac and/or renal artery[s])

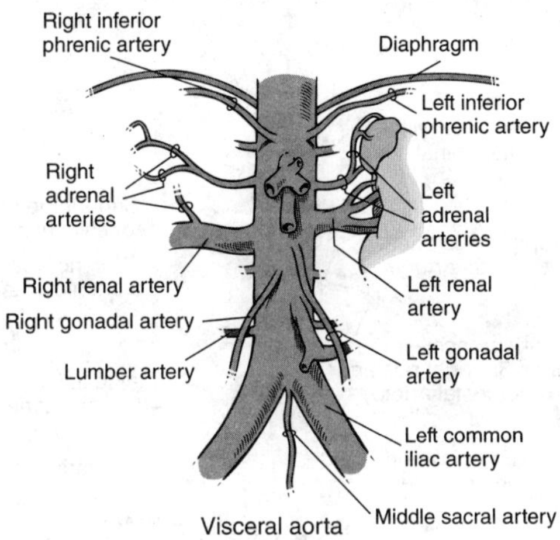

Visceral aorta

Explanation

Endovascular repair of an abdominal aortic aneurysm, pseudoaneurysm, or dissection, using a prosthesis, and involving visceral branches (superior mesenteric, celiac, and/or renal artery) requires the skills of a vascular surgeon and a radiologist. A small incision is made in the groin over both femoral arteries. Under fluoroscopic guidance, the physician inserts an aortic component through one femoral artery. These are contained inside a plastic holding capsule that is threaded through the arteries to the site of the aneurysm. The physician places the necessary extension prostheses and cuts fenestrations (holes) at each visceral artery orifice to allow side branch perfusion of these vessels. Next, catheters are used to place overlapping stents at each fenestration and vessel orifice to secure the junction. Once the graft components and stents are in place, the holding capsule and catheters are removed and the arteriotomy site is closed. Report 34841 when one visceral artery is included, 34842 for two, 34843 for three, and 34844 for four or more arteries.

Coding Tips

Do not report introduction of catheters and guidewires into the aorta and visceral and/or renal arteries separately in addition to these procedures. Balloon angioplasty within the target zone of the endograft is also not reported separately, whether prior to or after graft deployment. Fluoroscopic guidance is included in these procedures and not reported separately. Catheterization of the hypogastric arteries, arterial families outside of the treatment zone of the graft, exposure of the access vessels, extensive repair of the access vessels, and other separate interventional procedures outside of the target treatment zone performed at the time of this service may be reported separately. For endovascular treatment of the descending thoracic aorta, see 33880–33886 and 75956–75959. For endovascular infrarenal abdominal aortic aneurysm repair without the use of a graft, see 34701–34706. Do not report these codes with 34701–34706 or 34845–34848. Do not report these codes in addition to 34839 when planning is performed the day before or the day of the fenestrated repair. These codes should not be reported with 37236 or 37237 when covered or bare metal stents are placed into the visceral branches of the endoprosthesis target zone.

ICD-10-CM Diagnostic Codes

A52.01	Syphilitic aneurysm of aorta
I71.02	Dissection of abdominal aorta
I71.03	Dissection of thoracoabdominal aorta
I71.3	Abdominal aortic aneurysm, ruptured
I71.4	Abdominal aortic aneurysm, without rupture
I71.5	Thoracoabdominal aortic aneurysm, ruptured
I79.0	Aneurysm of aorta in diseases classified elsewhere
Q25.41	Absence and aplasia of aorta
Q25.42	Hypoplasia of aorta
Q25.43	Congenital aneurysm of aorta
Q25.44	Congenital dilation of aorta
Q25.48	Anomalous origin of subclavian artery
Q25.49	Other congenital malformations of aorta
S35.01XA	Minor laceration of abdominal aorta, initial encounter
S35.02XA	Major laceration of abdominal aorta, initial encounter
S35.09XA	Other injury of abdominal aorta, initial encounter
T82.818A	Embolism due to vascular prosthetic devices, implants and grafts, initial encounter
T82.858A	Stenosis of other vascular prosthetic devices, implants and grafts, initial encounter
T82.868A	Thrombosis due to vascular prosthetic devices, implants and grafts, initial encounter

AMA: 34841 2018,Jan,8; 2017,Jul,3; 2017,Jan,8; 2017,Dec,3; 2016,Jan,13; 2015,Jan,16; 2014,Jan,11; 2013,Dec,8 **34842** 2018,Jan,8; 2017,Jul,3; 2017,Jan,8; 2017,Dec,3; 2016,Jan,13; 2015,Jan,16; 2014,Jan,11; 2013,Dec,8 **34843** 2018,Jan,8; 2017,Jul,3; 2017,Jan,8; 2017,Dec,3; 2016,Jan,13; 2015,Jan,16; 2014,Jan,11; 2013,Dec,8 **34844** 2018,Jan,8; 2017,Jul,3; 2017,Jan,8; 2017,Dec,3; 2016,Jan,13; 2015,Jan,16; 2014,Jan,11; 2013,Dec,8

Relative Value Units/Medicare Edits

Non-Facility RVU	Work	PE	MP	Total
34841	0.0	0.0	0.0	0.0
34842	0.0	0.0	0.0	0.0
34843	0.0	0.0	0.0	0.0
34844	0.0	0.0	0.0	0.0
Facility RVU	**Work**	**PE**	**MP**	**Total**
34841	0.0	0.0	0.0	0.0
34842	0.0	0.0	0.0	0.0
34843	0.0	0.0	0.0	0.0
34844	0.0	0.0	0.0	0.0

	FUD	Status	MUE	Modifiers				IOM Reference
34841	N/A	C	1(2)	51	N/A	62	80	None
34842	N/A	C	1(2)	51	N/A	62	80	
34843	N/A	C	1(2)	51	N/A	62	80	
34844	N/A	C	1(2)	51	N/A	62	80	

* with documentation

Terms To Know

aneurysm. Circumscribed dilation or outpouching of an artery wall, often containing blood clots and connecting directly with the lumen of the artery.

angioplasty. Reconstruction or repair of a diseased or damaged blood vessel.

endovascular therapy. Intravascular catheters, scopes, stents, balloons, and other devices or methods used to treat vascular disease.

fenestrate. Pierce or perforate with one or more openings.

intramural. Within the wall of an organ.

34845-34848

34845 Endovascular repair of visceral aorta and infrarenal abdominal aorta (eg, aneurysm, pseudoaneurysm, dissection, penetrating ulcer, intramural hematoma, or traumatic disruption) with a fenestrated visceral aortic endograft and concomitant unibody or modular infrarenal aortic endograft and all associated radiological supervision and interpretation, including target zone angioplasty, when performed; including one visceral artery endoprosthesis (superior mesenteric, celiac or renal artery)

34846 including two visceral artery endoprostheses (superior mesenteric, celiac and/or renal artery[s])

34847 including three visceral artery endoprostheses (superior mesenteric, celiac and/or renal artery[s])

34848 including four or more visceral artery endoprostheses (superior mesenteric, celiac and/or renal artery[s])

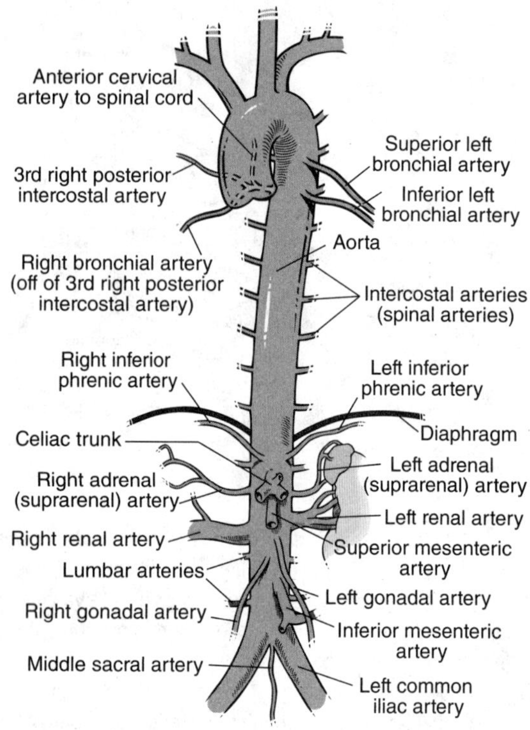

Explanation

Endovascular repair of an abdominal aortic aneurysm, pseudoaneurysm, or dissection, using a prosthesis, and involving visceral branches (superior mesenteric, celiac, and/or renal artery) requires the skills of a vascular surgeon and a radiologist. A small incision is made in the groin over both femoral arteries through which the endovascular devices are inserted. Under fluoroscopic guidance, the physician inserts the aortic component and one iliac limb through one femoral artery. These are contained inside a plastic holding capsule that is threaded through the arteries to the site of the aneurysm. Next, the physician inserts the opposite iliac limb by contralateral femoral artery access. The physician mates the aortic and iliac limb inserted into the first femoral artery to the opposite iliac limb inserted by contralateral femoral artery access. Since this repair extends above the visceral vessels, a visceral extension prosthesis is required. The physician places the extension prosthesis and cuts fenestrations (holes) at each visceral artery orifice to allow side branch perfusion of these vessels. Catheters are used to place overlapping stents at each fenestration and vessel orifice to secure the junction. Once the graft components and stents are in place, the holding capsule and catheters are removed and the arteriotomy site is closed. Report 34845 when one visceral artery is included, 34846 for two, 34847 for three, and 34848 for four or more arteries.

Coding Tips

Do not report introduction of catheters and guidewires into the aorta and visceral and/or renal arteries separately with these procedures. Balloon angioplasty within the target zone of the endograft is also not reported separately, whether prior to or after graft deployment. Fluoroscopic guidance with these procedures is included and is not reported separately. Catheterization of the hypogastric arteries, arterial families outside of the treatment zone of the graft, exposure of the access vessels, extensive repair of the access vessels, and other separate interventional procedures outside of the target treatment zone performed at the time of this service may be reported separately. For endovascular treatment of the descending thoracic aorta, see 33880–33886 and 75956–75959. For endovascular infrarenal abdominal aortic aneurysm repair without the use of a graft, see 34701–34706. Do not report these codes with 34701–34706, 34841–34844, 35081, or 35102. Do not report these codes with 37220–37223 for endovascular revascularization except when performed outside of the area treated with the endoprosthesis. Do not report these codes with 34839 when planning occurs the day before or the day of repair. For placement of distal extension prosthesis terminating in the internal or external iliac or common femoral artery, see 34709-34711 or 34718. These codes should not be reported with 37236 or 37237 when covered or bare metal stents are placed into the visceral branches of the endoprosthesis target zone.

ICD-10-CM Diagnostic Codes

A52.01	Syphilitic aneurysm of aorta
I71.02	Dissection of abdominal aorta
I71.03	Dissection of thoracoabdominal aorta
I71.3	Abdominal aortic aneurysm, ruptured
I71.4	Abdominal aortic aneurysm, without rupture
I71.5	Thoracoabdominal aortic aneurysm, ruptured
I79.0	Aneurysm of aorta in diseases classified elsewhere
Q25.41	Absence and aplasia of aorta
Q25.42	Hypoplasia of aorta
Q25.43	Congenital aneurysm of aorta
Q25.44	Congenital dilation of aorta
Q25.48	Anomalous origin of subclavian artery
Q25.49	Other congenital malformations of aorta
S35.01XA	Minor laceration of abdominal aorta, initial encounter
S35.02XA	Major laceration of abdominal aorta, initial encounter
S35.09XA	Other injury of abdominal aorta, initial encounter

AMA: **34845** 2018,Jan,8; 2017,Jul,3; 2017,Jan,8; 2017,Dec,3; 2016,Jan,13; 2015,Jan,16; 2014,Jan,11; 2013,Dec,8 **34846** 2018,Jan,8; 2017,Jul,3; 2017,Jan,8; 2017,Dec,3; 2016,Jan,13; 2015,Jan,16; 2014,Jan,11; 2013,Dec,8 **34847** 2018,Jan,8; 2017,Jul,3; 2017,Jan,8; 2017,Dec,3; 2016,Jan,13; 2015,Jan,16; 2014,Jan,11; 2013,Dec,8 **34848** 2018,Jan,8; 2017,Jul,3; 2017,Jan,8; 2017,Dec,3; 2017,Aug,9; 2016,Jul,6; 2016,Jan,13; 2015,Jan,16; 2014,Jan,11; 2013,Dec,8

Relative Value Units/Medicare Edits

Non-Facility RVU	Work	PE	MP	Total
34845	0.0	0.0	0.0	0.0
34846	0.0	0.0	0.0	0.0
34847	0.0	0.0	0.0	0.0
34848	0.0	0.0	0.0	0.0
Facility RVU	**Work**	**PE**	**MP**	**Total**
34845	0.0	0.0	0.0	0.0
34846	0.0	0.0	0.0	0.0
34847	0.0	0.0	0.0	0.0
34848	0.0	0.0	0.0	0.0

	FUD	Status	MUE	Modifiers				IOM Reference
34845	N/A	C	1(2)	51	N/A	62	80	None
34846	N/A	C	1(2)	51	N/A	62	80	
34847	N/A	C	1(2)	51	N/A	62	80	
34848	N/A	C	1(2)	51	N/A	62	80	

* with documentation

Terms To Know

aneurysm. Circumscribed dilation or outpouching of an artery wall, often containing blood clots and connecting directly with the lumen of the artery.

angioplasty. Reconstruction or repair of a diseased or damaged blood vessel.

dissection. (dis. apart; -section, act of cutting) Separating by cutting tissue or body structures apart.

endoprosthesis. Intravascular device in the form of a hollow stent placed within a duct or artery to provide passage through an obstructed area, such as in a bile duct, or to act as a replacement for damaged arterial walls, as in treating an aneurysm.

pseudoaneurysm. False aneurysm produced by a dilated vessel wall, or a ruptured blood vessel that has formed a clot that pulsates, mimicking a true aneurysm.

vascular. Pertaining to blood vessels.

35001-35002

35001 Direct repair of aneurysm, pseudoaneurysm, or excision (partial or total) and graft insertion, with or without patch graft; for aneurysm and associated occlusive disease, carotid, subclavian artery, by neck incision

35002 for ruptured aneurysm, carotid, subclavian artery, by neck incision

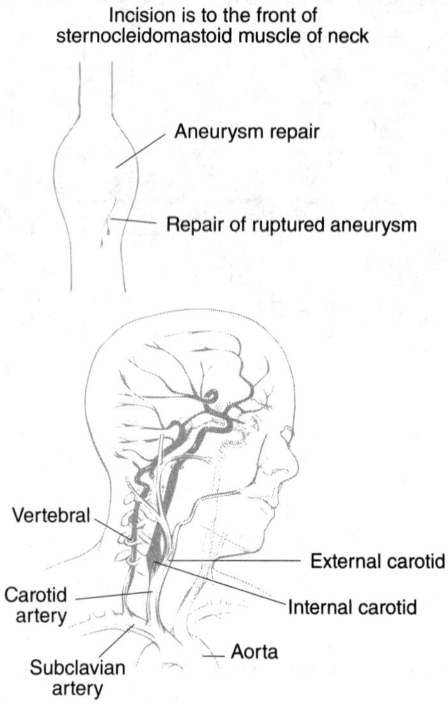

Explanation

The physician makes an incision in the neck in front of the sternocleidomastoid muscle. The section of the carotid or subclavian artery (35001) or the ruptured section (35002) is isolated and dissected from adjacent critical structures. Vessel clamps are affixed above and below the defect. The repair may be accomplished by removing the segment of artery containing the aneurysm and suturing the exposed ends of the vessel in an end-to-end fashion or the aneurysm may be bypassed with a venous or synthetic graft. If a large section is removed, a harvested or synthetic graft is inserted into the defect, or a patch may be sutured into place to open up the diameter of the vessel. The skin incision is repaired with a layered closure.

Coding Tips

Preparation of the artery for anastomosis, including endarterectomy, is integral to the procedure and should not be reported separately. Establishing inflow and outflow by any method is included. The portion of the operative arteriogram performed by the surgeon is also included. Angioscopy performed during therapeutic intervention should be reported in addition to the code for the primary procedure; see 35400. Harvested vein or synthetic material may be used for the graft. Any graft harvest is not reported separately. For direct repairs associated with occlusive disease only, see 35201, 35231, and 35261.

ICD-10-CM Diagnostic Codes

G45.1 Carotid artery syndrome (hemispheric)
G45.2 Multiple and bilateral precerebral artery syndromes
G45.3 Amaurosis fugax
G45.8 Other transient cerebral ischemic attacks and related syndromes
G45.9 Transient cerebral ischemic attack, unspecified
I63.031 Cerebral infarction due to thrombosis of right carotid artery ☑
I63.032 Cerebral infarction due to thrombosis of left carotid artery ☑
I63.09 Cerebral infarction due to thrombosis of other precerebral artery
I63.131 Cerebral infarction due to embolism of right carotid artery ☑
I63.132 Cerebral infarction due to embolism of left carotid artery ☑
I63.19 Cerebral infarction due to embolism of other precerebral artery
I63.231 Cerebral infarction due to unspecified occlusion or stenosis of right carotid arteries ☑
I63.232 Cerebral infarction due to unspecified occlusion or stenosis of left carotid arteries ☑
I63.29 Cerebral infarction due to unspecified occlusion or stenosis of other precerebral arteries
I63.81 Other cerebral infarction due to occlusion or stenosis of small artery
I63.89 Other cerebral infarction
I65.21 Occlusion and stenosis of right carotid artery ☑
I65.22 Occlusion and stenosis of left carotid artery ☑
I65.23 Occlusion and stenosis of bilateral carotid arteries ☑
I65.8 Occlusion and stenosis of other precerebral arteries
I72.0 Aneurysm of carotid artery
I72.6 Aneurysm of vertebral artery
I72.8 Aneurysm of other specified arteries
I77.1 Stricture of artery
I77.2 Rupture of artery
I77.71 Dissection of carotid artery
I77.76 Dissection of artery of upper extremity
I77.77 Dissection of artery of lower extremity
I77.79 Dissection of other specified artery
I77.89 Other specified disorders of arteries and arterioles
Q28.1 Other malformations of precerebral vessels
Q28.8 Other specified congenital malformations of circulatory system

AMA: **35001** 2002,May,7 **35002** 2002,May,7

Relative Value Units/Medicare Edits

Non-Facility RVU	Work	PE	MP	Total
35001	20.81	6.7	4.69	32.2
35002	22.23	5.41	5.14	32.78
Facility RVU	**Work**	**PE**	**MP**	**Total**
35001	20.81	6.7	4.69	32.2
35002	22.23	5.41	5.14	32.78

	FUD	Status	MUE	Modifiers				IOM Reference
35001	90	A	1(2)	51	50	62*	80	None
35002	90	A	1(2)	51	50	62*	80	

* with documentation

Terms To Know

anastomosis. Surgically created connection between ducts, blood vessels, or bowel segments to allow flow from one to the other.

35005

35005 Direct repair of aneurysm, pseudoaneurysm, or excision (partial or total) and graft insertion, with or without patch graft; for aneurysm, pseudoaneurysm, and associated occlusive disease, vertebral artery

Incision is made in the back of the neck to repair or remove the aneurysm or occlusion in this area

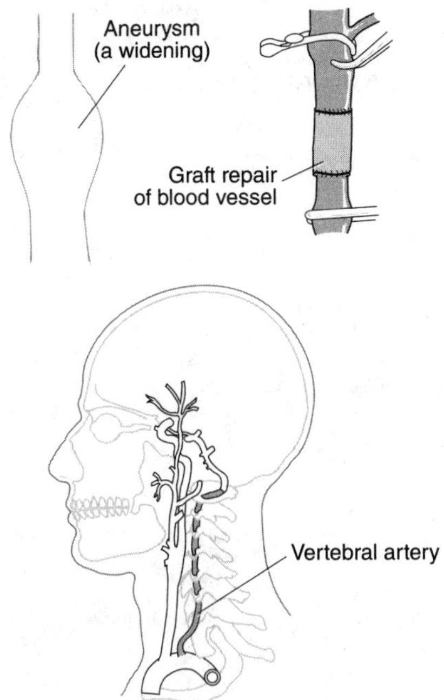

Explanation

The physician makes an incision in the skin overlying the neck. The enlarged or blocked section of the vertebral artery is isolated and dissected from muscles and adjacent critical structures. A portion of a cervical vertebra may be removed to access the defect. Vessel clamps are affixed above and below the defect, which may be repaired or removed. The repair may be accomplished by removing the segment of artery containing the aneurysm and suturing the exposed ends of the vessel in an end-to-end fashion or the aneurysm may be bypassed with a venous or synthetic graft. If a large section is removed, a harvested or synthetic graft is inserted into the defect. Instead of a complete graft, a patch may be sutured into place to open up the diameter of the vessel. Once the vessel is repaired, the clamps are removed. The skin incision is repaired with a layered closure.

Coding Tips

Preparation of the artery for anastomosis, including endarterectomy, is integral to the procedure and should not be reported separately. Establishing both inflow and outflow by any method is included. The portion of the operative arteriogram performed by the surgeon is also included. Angioscopy performed during therapeutic intervention should be reported in addition to the code for the primary procedure, see 35400. Harvested vein or synthetic material may be used for the graft. Any graft harvest is not reported separately. For direct repairs associated with occlusive disease only, see 35201, 35231, and 35261.

ICD-10-CM Diagnostic Codes

G45.8	Other transient cerebral ischemic attacks and related syndromes
I63.011	Cerebral infarction due to thrombosis of right vertebral artery ☑
I63.012	Cerebral infarction due to thrombosis of left vertebral artery ☑
I63.013	Cerebral infarction due to thrombosis of bilateral vertebral arteries ☑
I63.033	Cerebral infarction due to thrombosis of bilateral carotid arteries ☑
I63.09	Cerebral infarction due to thrombosis of other precerebral artery
I63.111	Cerebral infarction due to embolism of right vertebral artery ☑
I63.112	Cerebral infarction due to embolism of left vertebral artery ☑
I63.113	Cerebral infarction due to embolism of bilateral vertebral arteries ☑
I63.133	Cerebral infarction due to embolism of bilateral carotid arteries ☑
I63.19	Cerebral infarction due to embolism of other precerebral artery
I63.211	Cerebral infarction due to unspecified occlusion or stenosis of right vertebral artery ☑
I63.212	Cerebral infarction due to unspecified occlusion or stenosis of left vertebral artery ☑
I63.233	Cerebral infarction due to unspecified occlusion or stenosis of bilateral carotid arteries ☑
I63.29	Cerebral infarction due to unspecified occlusion or stenosis of other precerebral arteries
I63.313	Cerebral infarction due to thrombosis of bilateral middle cerebral arteries ☑
I63.323	Cerebral infarction due to thrombosis of bilateral anterior cerebral arteries ☑
I63.333	Cerebral infarction due to thrombosis of bilateral posterior cerebral arteries ☑
I63.343	Cerebral infarction due to thrombosis of bilateral cerebellar arteries ☑
I63.413	Cerebral infarction due to embolism of bilateral middle cerebral arteries ☑
I63.423	Cerebral infarction due to embolism of bilateral anterior cerebral arteries ☑
I63.433	Cerebral infarction due to embolism of bilateral posterior cerebral arteries ☑
I63.443	Cerebral infarction due to embolism of bilateral cerebellar arteries ☑
I63.81	Other cerebral infarction due to occlusion or stenosis of small artery
I63.89	Other cerebral infarction
I65.01	Occlusion and stenosis of right vertebral artery ☑
I65.02	Occlusion and stenosis of left vertebral artery ☑
I65.03	Occlusion and stenosis of bilateral vertebral arteries ☑
I67.850	Cerebral autosomal dominant arteriopathy with subcortical infarcts and leukoencephalopathy
I67.858	Other hereditary cerebrovascular disease
I77.2	Rupture of artery
I77.74	Dissection of vertebral artery
I77.89	Other specified disorders of arteries and arterioles

AMA: 35005 2002,May,7

Relative Value Units/Medicare Edits

Non-Facility RVU	Work	PE	MP	Total
35005	19.29	4.92	4.47	28.68
Facility RVU	**Work**	**PE**	**MP**	**Total**
35005	19.29	4.92	4.47	28.68

	FUD	Status	MUE	Modifiers				IOM Reference
35005	90	A	1(2)	51	50	62*	80	None

* with documentation

Terms To Know

aneurysm. Circumscribed dilation or outpouching of an artery wall, often containing blood clots and connecting directly with the lumen of the artery.

dissection. Separating by cutting tissue or body structures apart.

embolism. Obstruction of a blood vessel resulting from a clot or foreign substance.

pseudoaneurysm. False aneurysm produced by a dilated vessel wall, or a ruptured blood vessel that has formed a clot that pulsates, mimicking a true aneurysm.

stenosis. Narrowing or constriction of a passage.

35011-35013

35011 Direct repair of aneurysm, pseudoaneurysm, or excision (partial or total) and graft insertion, with or without patch graft; for aneurysm and associated occlusive disease, axillary-brachial artery, by arm incision

35013 for ruptured aneurysm, axillary-brachial artery, by arm incision

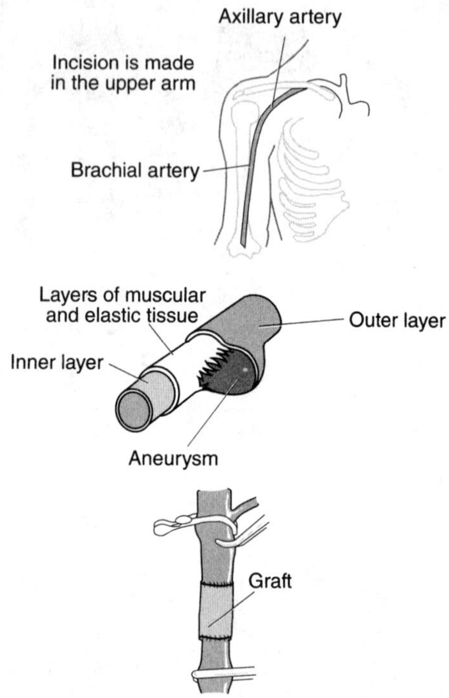

Explanation

The physician makes an incision in the skin of the arm or axilla. The enlarged or blocked section of the axillary or brachial artery (35011) or the ruptured section (35013) is isolated and dissected from adjacent critical structures. Vessel clamps are affixed above and below the defect, which may be repaired or removed. The repair may be accomplished by removing the segment of artery containing the aneurysm and suturing the exposed ends of the vessel in an end-to-end fashion or the aneurysm may be bypassed with a venous or synthetic graft. If a large section is removed, a harvested or synthetic graft is inserted into the defect. Instead of a complete graft, a patch may be sutured into place to open up the diameter of the vessel. Once the vessel is repaired, the clamps are removed. The skin incision is repaired with a layered closure.

Coding Tips

Preparation of the artery for anastomosis, including endarterectomy, is integral to the procedure and should not be reported separately. Establishing both inflow and outflow by any method is included. The portion of the operative arteriogram performed by the surgeon is also included. Angioscopy performed during therapeutic intervention should be reported in addition to the code for the primary procedure; see 35400. Harvested vein or synthetic material may be used for the graft. Any graft harvest is not reported separately. For direct repairs associated with occlusive disease only, see 35206, 35236, and 35266.

ICD-10-CM Diagnostic Codes

I70.8	Atherosclerosis of other arteries
I70.92	Chronic total occlusion of artery of the extremities

I72.1 Aneurysm of artery of upper extremity
I72.8 Aneurysm of other specified arteries
I74.2 Embolism and thrombosis of arteries of the upper extremities
I75.011 Atheroembolism of right upper extremity ☑
I75.012 Atheroembolism of left upper extremity ☑
I75.013 Atheroembolism of bilateral upper extremities ☑
I77.1 Stricture of artery
I77.2 Rupture of artery
I77.79 Dissection of other specified artery

AMA: **35011** 2002,May,7 **35013** 2002,May,7

Relative Value Units/Medicare Edits

Non-Facility RVU	Work	PE	MP	Total
35011	18.58	6.19	4.28	29.05
35013	23.23	7.77	5.35	36.35
Facility RVU	**Work**	**PE**	**MP**	**Total**
35011	18.58	6.19	4.28	29.05
35013	23.23	7.77	5.35	36.35

	FUD	Status	MUE	Modifiers				IOM Reference
35011	90	A	1(2)	51	50	62*	80	None
35013	90	A	1(2)	51	50	62*	80	

* with documentation

Terms To Know

anastomosis. Surgically created connection between ducts, blood vessels, or bowel segments to allow flow from one to the other.

aneurysm. Circumscribed dilation or outpouching of an artery wall, often containing blood clots and connecting directly with the lumen of the artery.

angioscopy. Visualization of capillary blood vessels with a microscope, or the inside of a blood vessel with a fiberoptic-equipped catheter.

atherosclerosis. Buildup of yellowish plaques composed of cholesterol and lipoid material within the arteries.

claudication. Lameness, pain, and weakness occurring in the arms or legs during exercise due to muscles not receiving the needed oxygen and nutrients.

embolism. Obstruction of a blood vessel resulting from a clot or foreign substance.

pseudoaneurysm. False aneurysm produced by a dilated vessel wall, or a ruptured blood vessel that has formed a clot that pulsates, mimicking a true aneurysm.

stricture. Narrowing of an anatomical structure.

35021-35022

35021 Direct repair of aneurysm, pseudoaneurysm, or excision (partial or total) and graft insertion, with or without patch graft; for aneurysm, pseudoaneurysm, and associated occlusive disease, innominate, subclavian artery, by thoracic incision

35022 for ruptured aneurysm, innominate, subclavian artery, by thoracic incision

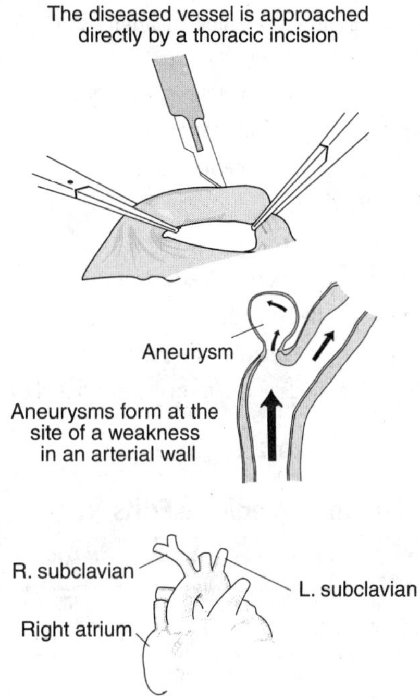

Explanation

The physician exposes the innominate or subclavian artery by median sternotomy or lateral thoracotomy. In 35021, the physician anticoagulates the patient with heparin, clamps the aortic arch widely around the origin of the innominate artery, and clamps the right common carotid and right subclavian arteries. The physician excises the aneurysmal tissue. In 35022, the physician clamps the aortic arch widely around the origin of the innominate artery, and clamps the right common carotid and right subclavian arteries. The physician excises the ruptured aneurysmal tissue. In both procedures, the physician may use a woven Dacron patch graft or harvested vein to repair the aneurysmal artery. The physician unclamps the aorta, as well as the right common carotid and right subclavian arteries. The physician closes the sternotomy or thoracotomy, leaving a chest tube in place.

Coding Tips

Preparation of the artery for anastomosis, including endarterectomy, is integral to the procedure and should not be reported separately. Establishing both inflow and outflow by any method is included. The portion of the operative arteriogram performed by the surgeon is also included. Angioscopy performed during therapeutic intervention should be reported in addition to the code for the primary procedure; see 35400. Harvested vein or synthetic material may be used for the graft. Any graft harvest is not reported separately. For direct repairs associated with occlusive disease only, see 35211, 35216, 35241, 35246, 35271, and 35276.

ICD-10-CM Diagnostic Codes

G45.2 Multiple and bilateral precerebral artery syndromes

G45.3	Amaurosis fugax
G45.8	Other transient cerebral ischemic attacks and related syndromes
I63.09	Cerebral infarction due to thrombosis of other precerebral artery
I63.19	Cerebral infarction due to embolism of other precerebral artery
I63.29	Cerebral infarction due to unspecified occlusion or stenosis of other precerebral arteries
I63.81	Other cerebral infarction due to occlusion or stenosis of small artery
I63.89	Other cerebral infarction
I67.850	Cerebral autosomal dominant arteriopathy with subcortical infarcts and leukoencephalopathy
I67.858	Other hereditary cerebrovascular disease
I70.8	Atherosclerosis of other arteries
I72.8	Aneurysm of other specified arteries
I77.1	Stricture of artery
I77.2	Rupture of artery
I77.79	Dissection of other specified artery
I77.89	Other specified disorders of arteries and arterioles
Q28.1	Other malformations of precerebral vessels
Q28.8	Other specified congenital malformations of circulatory system

AMA: 35021 2002,May,7 **35022** 2002,May,7

Relative Value Units/Medicare Edits

Non-Facility RVU	Work	PE	MP	Total
35021	22.17	9.25	5.22	36.64
35022	25.7	10.22	6.06	41.98
Facility RVU	**Work**	**PE**	**MP**	**Total**
35021	22.17	9.25	5.22	36.64
35022	25.7	10.22	6.06	41.98

	FUD	Status	MUE	Modifiers				IOM Reference
35021	90	A	1(2)	51	50	62*	80	None
35022	90	A	1(2)	51	50	62*	80	

* with documentation

Terms To Know

anastomosis. Surgically created connection between ducts, blood vessels, or bowel segments to allow flow from one to the other.

aneurysm. Circumscribed dilation or outpouching of an artery wall, often containing blood clots and connecting directly with the lumen of the artery.

atherosclerosis. Buildup of yellowish plaques composed of cholesterol and lipoid material within the arteries.

median sternotomy. Standard incision for open chest cardiac surgeries, from above the bellybutton to just under the chin, down the center of the chest through the sternum into the thoracic cavity.

pseudoaneurysm. False aneurysm produced by a dilated vessel wall, or a ruptured blood vessel that has formed a clot that pulsates, mimicking a true aneurysm.

rupture. Tearing or breaking open of tissue.

thoracotomy. Surgical procedure for opening the chest wall in order to access the lungs, esophagus, trachea, aorta, heart, and diaphragm.

35045

35045 Direct repair of aneurysm, pseudoaneurysm, or excision (partial or total) and graft insertion, with or without patch graft; for aneurysm, pseudoaneurysm, and associated occlusive disease, radial or ulnar artery

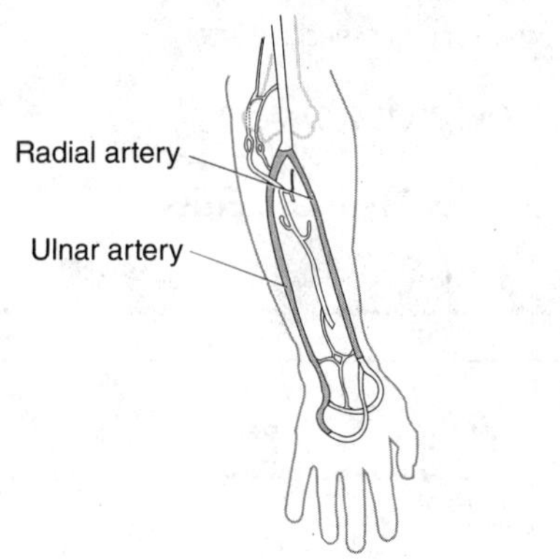

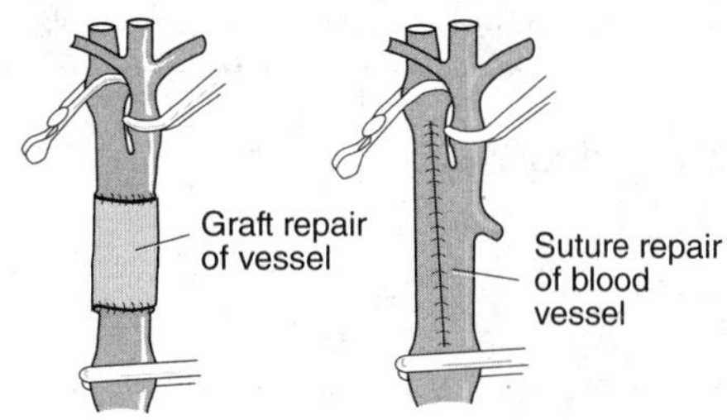

Explanation

The physician makes an incision in the skin overlying the arm. The enlarged or blocked section of the radial or ulnar artery is isolated and dissected from adjacent critical structures. Vessel clamps are affixed above and below the defect, which may be repaired or removed. The repair may be accomplished by removing the segment of artery containing the aneurysm and suturing the exposed ends of the vessel in an end-to-end fashion or the aneurysm may be bypassed with a venous or synthetic graft. If a large section is removed, a harvested or synthetic graft is inserted into the defect. Instead of a complete graft, a patch may be sutured into place to open up the diameter of the vessel. Once the vessel is repaired, the clamps are removed. The skin incision is repaired with a layered closure.

Coding Tips

Preparation of the artery for anastomosis, including endarterectomy, is integral to the procedure and should not be reported separately. Establishing both inflow and outflow by any method is included. The portion of the operative arteriogram performed by the surgeon is also included. Angioscopy performed during therapeutic intervention should be reported in addition to the code for the primary procedure; see 35400. Harvested vein or synthetic material may be used for the graft. Any graft harvest is not reported separately. For direct repairs associated with occlusive disease only, see 35206, 35236, and 35266.

ICD-10-CM Diagnostic Codes

I70.8	Atherosclerosis of other arteries
I70.92	Chronic total occlusion of artery of the extremities
I72.1	Aneurysm of artery of upper extremity

I72.8 Aneurysm of other specified arteries
I74.2 Embolism and thrombosis of arteries of the upper extremities
I75.011 Atheroembolism of right upper extremity ☑
I75.012 Atheroembolism of left upper extremity ☑
I75.013 Atheroembolism of bilateral upper extremities ☑
I77.1 Stricture of artery
I77.2 Rupture of artery
I77.79 Dissection of other specified artery
I77.89 Other specified disorders of arteries and arterioles

AMA: 35045 2002,May,7

Relative Value Units/Medicare Edits

Non-Facility RVU	Work	PE	MP	Total
35045	18.01	6.41	4.03	28.45
Facility RVU	**Work**	**PE**	**MP**	**Total**
35045	18.01	6.41	4.03	28.45

	FUD	Status	MUE	Modifiers				IOM Reference
35045	90	A	1(3)	51	50	62*	80	None

* with documentation

Terms To Know

anastomosis. Surgically created connection between ducts, blood vessels, or bowel segments to allow flow from one to the other.

aneurysm. Circumscribed dilation or outpouching of an artery wall, often containing blood clots and connecting directly with the lumen of the artery.

atherosclerosis. Buildup of yellowish plaques composed of cholesterol and lipoid material within the arteries.

suture. Numerous stitching techniques employed in wound closure.

buried suture. Continuous or interrupted suture placed under the skin for a layered closure.

continuous suture. Running stitch with tension evenly distributed across a single strand to provide a leakproof closure line.

interrupted suture. Series of single stitches with tension isolated at each stitch, in which all stitches are not affected if one becomes loose, and the isolated sutures cannot act as a wick to transport an infection.

purse-string suture. Continuous suture placed around a tubular structure and tightened, to reduce or close the lumen.

retention suture. Secondary stitching that bridges the primary suture, providing support for the primary repair; a plastic or rubber bolster may be placed over the primary repair and under the retention sutures.

35081

35081 Direct repair of aneurysm, pseudoaneurysm, or excision (partial or total) and graft insertion, with or without patch graft; for aneurysm, pseudoaneurysm, and associated occlusive disease, abdominal aorta

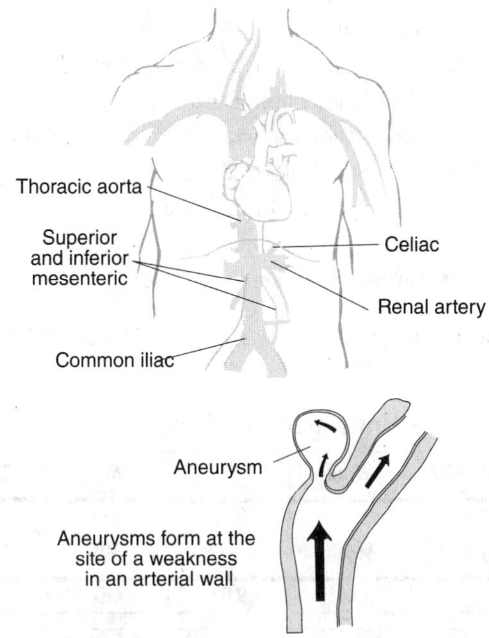

The aneurysm or occlusion of the abdominal aorta is repaired with a graft insertion. A patch graft may be required

Explanation

The physician exposes the abdominal aorta using a transperitoneal approach, placing a long incision in the mid abdomen. The physician retracts the transverse colon and small bowel to allow dissection and exposure of the aorta. The physician places an umbilical tape or rubber catheter around the aorta proximal to the aneurysm. The physician exposes the iliac arteries and achieves control of blood flow with umbilical tape or rubber catheters. The physician anticoagulates the patient and cross-clamps the iliac arteries and proximal aorta. The physician opens and clears the aneurysm, controls collateral bleeding from the lumbar arteries with suture, and sutures a Y-shaped knitted Dacron graft to the proximal aorta. The physician sutures the distal ends of the graft to the iliac arteries. The physician may anastomose the inferior mesenteric arteries and any aberrant or accessory renal arteries to the Dacron graft. The physician sutures the remaining aneurysmal shell around the graft and closes the retroperitoneum. The physician closes the abdominal wound, leaving drains in place.

Coding Tips

Preparation of the artery for anastomosis, including endarterectomy, is integral to the procedure and should not be reported separately. Establishing both inflow and outflow by any method is included. The portion of the operative arteriogram performed by the surgeon is also included. Angioscopy performed during therapeutic intervention should be reported in addition to the code for the primary procedure; see 35400. Harvested vein or synthetic material may be used for the graft. Any graft harvest is not reported separately. For thoracic aortic aneurysm, see 33858–33875. For direct repairs associated with occlusive disease only, see 35221, 35251, and 35281.

ICD-10-CM Diagnostic Codes

I70.0 Atherosclerosis of aorta

I71.02	Dissection of abdominal aorta
I71.4	Abdominal aortic aneurysm, without rupture
I71.6	Thoracoabdominal aortic aneurysm, without rupture
I74.01	Saddle embolus of abdominal aorta
I74.09	Other arterial embolism and thrombosis of abdominal aorta
I76	Septic arterial embolism
I77.1	Stricture of artery
I77.89	Other specified disorders of arteries and arterioles
Q25.43	Congenital aneurysm of aorta
Q25.44	Congenital dilation of aorta
Q79.61	Classical Ehlers-Danlos syndrome
Q79.62	Hypermobile Ehlers-Danlos syndrome
Q79.63	Vascular Ehlers-Danlos syndrome
Q87.410	Marfan's syndrome with aortic dilation

AMA: 35081 2018,Jan,8; 2017,Jan,8; 2016,Jan,13; 2015,Jan,16; 2014,Jan,11; 2013,Dec,8

Relative Value Units/Medicare Edits

Non-Facility RVU	Work	PE	MP	Total
35081	33.53	9.02	7.67	50.22
Facility RVU	**Work**	**PE**	**MP**	**Total**
35081	33.53	9.02	7.67	50.22

	FUD	Status	MUE	Modifiers				IOM Reference
35081	90	A	1(2)	51	N/A	62*	80	100-03,20.23

* with documentation

Terms To Know

aneurysm. Circumscribed dilation or outpouching of an artery wall, often containing blood clots and connecting directly with the lumen of the artery.

atherosclerosis. Buildup of yellowish plaques composed of cholesterol and lipoid material within the arteries.

embolism. Obstruction of a blood vessel resulting from a clot or foreign substance.

pseudoaneurysm. False aneurysm produced by a dilated vessel wall, or a ruptured blood vessel that has formed a clot that pulsates, mimicking a true aneurysm.

35082

35082 Direct repair of aneurysm, pseudoaneurysm, or excision (partial or total) and graft insertion, with or without patch graft; for ruptured aneurysm, abdominal aorta

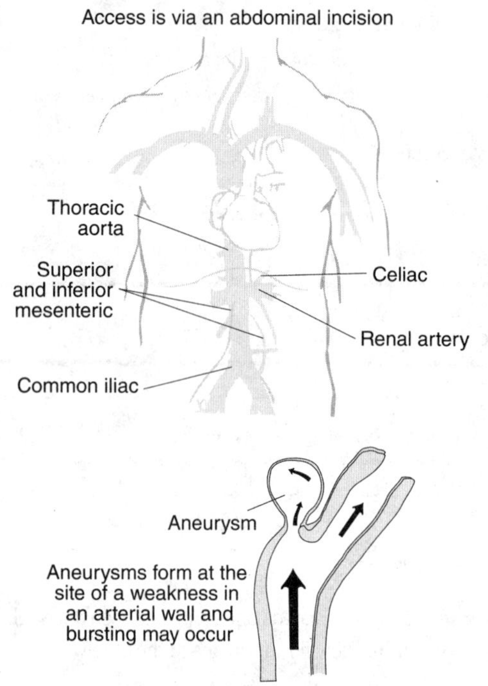

A burst aneurysm or occlusion of the abdominal aorta is repaired with a graft insertion. A patch graft may be required

Explanation

The physician quickly exposes the abdominal aorta using a transperitoneal approach, placing a long incision in the midabdomen, and retracts the transverse colon and small bowel to allow dissection and exposure of the aorta. Bleeding control is achieved by pushing the liver aside and compressing the aorta manually against the spine. The aorta is cross-clamped proximal to the dissection. The physician exposes the iliac arteries and achieves control of blood flow with umbilical tape or rubber catheters. If bleeding is controlled, the patient receives anticoagulation while the iliac arteries and proximal aorta are cross-clamped. The physician opens and clears the aneurysm, controls collateral bleeding from the lumbar arteries with suture, and sutures a Y-shaped knitted Dacron graft to the proximal aorta. The distal ends of the graft are sutured to the iliac arteries with the remaining aneurysmal shell around the graft. The retroperitoneum and abdominal wounds are closed, leaving drains in place.

Coding Tips

Preparation of the artery for anastomosis, including endarterectomy, is integral to the procedure and should not be reported separately. Establishing both inflow and outflow by any method is included. The portion of the operative arteriogram performed by the surgeon is also included. Angioscopy performed during therapeutic intervention should be reported in addition to the code for the primary procedure; see 35400. Harvested vein or synthetic material may be used for the graft. Any graft harvest is not reported separately. For thoracic aortic aneurysm, see 33858–33875. For direct repairs associated with occlusive disease only, see 35221, 35251, and 35281.

ICD-10-CM Diagnostic Codes

I71.3	Abdominal aortic aneurysm, ruptured
I71.5	Thoracoabdominal aortic aneurysm, ruptured
I74.01	Saddle embolus of abdominal aorta
I74.19	Embolism and thrombosis of other parts of aorta
S35.02XA	Major laceration of abdominal aorta, initial encounter

AMA: 35082 2002,May,7

Relative Value Units/Medicare Edits

Non-Facility RVU	Work	PE	MP	Total
35082	42.09	11.61	9.67	63.37
Facility RVU	**Work**	**PE**	**MP**	**Total**
35082	42.09	11.61	9.67	63.37

	FUD	Status	MUE	Modifiers				IOM Reference
35082	90	A	1(2)	51	N/A	62*	80	100-03,20.23

* with documentation

Terms To Know

anastomosis. Surgically created connection between ducts, blood vessels, or bowel segments to allow flow from one to the other.

aneurysm. Circumscribed dilation or outpouching of an artery wall, often containing blood clots and connecting directly with the lumen of the artery.

angioscopy. Visualization of capillary blood vessels with a microscope, or the inside of a blood vessel with a fiberoptic-equipped catheter.

arteriogram. Radiograph of arteries.

atherosclerosis. Buildup of yellowish plaques composed of cholesterol and lipoid material within the arteries.

35091

35091 Direct repair of aneurysm, pseudoaneurysm, or excision (partial or total) and graft insertion, with or without patch graft; for aneurysm, pseudoaneurysm, and associated occlusive disease, abdominal aorta involving visceral vessels (mesenteric, celiac, renal)

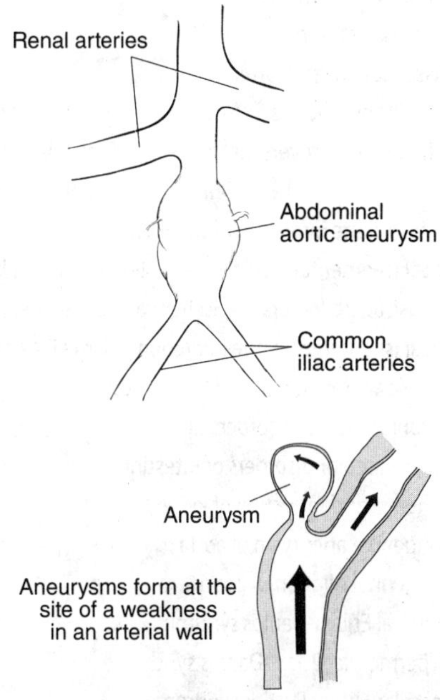

An aneurysm or occlusion of the abdominal aorta is repaired with a graft insertion. Mesenteric, celiac, or renal vessels may be involved and a patch graft may be required

Explanation

The physician exposes the abdominal aorta using a transperitoneal approach, placing a long incision in the midabdomen. The physician retracts the transverse colon and small bowel to allow dissection and exposure of the aorta. The physician places an umbilical tape or rubber catheter around the aorta proximal to the aneurysm. The physician exposes the iliac arteries and achieves control of blood flow with umbilical tape or rubber catheters. The physician anticoagulates the patient and cross-clamps the iliac arteries and proximal aorta. The physician opens and clears the aneurysm, controls collateral bleeding from the lumbar arteries with suture, and sutures a Y-shaped knitted Dacron graft to the proximal aorta. The physician sutures the distal ends of the graft to the iliac arteries. The physician will anastomose the inferior mesenteric arteries and any aberrant or accessory renal arteries to the Dacron graft, when applicable. The physician sutures the remaining aneurysmal shell around the graft and closes the retroperitoneum. The physician closes the abdominal wound, leaving drains in place.

Coding Tips

Preparation of the artery for anastomosis, including endarterectomy, is integral to the procedure and should not be reported separately. Establishing both inflow and outflow by any method is included. The portion of the operative arteriogram performed by the surgeon is also included. Angioscopy performed during therapeutic intervention should be reported in addition to the code for the primary procedure; see 35400. Harvested vein or synthetic material may be used for the graft. Any graft harvest is not reported separately. For thoracic aortic aneurysm, see 33858–33875. For direct repairs associated with occlusive disease only, see 35221, 35251, and 35281.

ICD-10-CM Diagnostic Codes

I70.0	Atherosclerosis of aorta
I70.1	Atherosclerosis of renal artery
I71.02	Dissection of abdominal aorta
I71.4	Abdominal aortic aneurysm, without rupture
I71.6	Thoracoabdominal aortic aneurysm, without rupture
I72.2	Aneurysm of renal artery
I77.1	Stricture of artery
I77.73	Dissection of renal artery
K55.011	Focal (segmental) acute (reversible) ischemia of small intestine
K55.012	Diffuse acute (reversible) ischemia of small intestine
K55.021	Focal (segmental) acute infarction of small intestine
K55.022	Diffuse acute infarction of small intestine
K55.031	Focal (segmental) acute (reversible) ischemia of large intestine
K55.032	Diffuse acute (reversible) ischemia of large intestine
K55.041	Focal (segmental) acute infarction of large intestine
K55.042	Diffuse acute infarction of large intestine
K55.1	Chronic vascular disorders of intestine
K55.8	Other vascular disorders of intestine
N28.0	Ischemia and infarction of kidney
Q25.43	Congenital aneurysm of aorta
Q25.44	Congenital dilation of aorta
Q79.61	Classical Ehlers-Danlos syndrome
Q79.62	Hypermobile Ehlers-Danlos syndrome
Q79.63	Vascular Ehlers-Danlos syndrome
Q87.410	Marfan's syndrome with aortic dilation

AMA: **35091** 2018,Jan,8; 2017,Jan,8; 2016,Jan,13; 2015,Jan,16; 2014,Jan,11

Relative Value Units/Medicare Edits

Non-Facility RVU	Work	PE	MP	Total
35091	35.35	8.31	8.16	51.82
Facility RVU	**Work**	**PE**	**MP**	**Total**
35091	35.35	8.31	8.16	51.82

	FUD	Status	MUE	Modifiers				IOM Reference
35091	90	A	1(2)	51	50	62*	80	100-03,20.23

* with documentation

Terms To Know

anastomosis. Surgically created connection between ducts, blood vessels, or bowel segments to allow flow from one to the other.

aneurysm. Circumscribed dilation or outpouching of an artery wall, often containing blood clots and connecting directly with the lumen of the artery.

atherosclerosis. Buildup of yellowish plaques composed of cholesterol and lipoid material within the arteries.

pseudoaneurysm. False aneurysm produced by a dilated vessel wall, or a ruptured blood vessel that has formed a clot that pulsates, mimicking a true aneurysm.

35092

35092 Direct repair of aneurysm, pseudoaneurysm, or excision (partial or total) and graft insertion, with or without patch graft; for ruptured aneurysm, abdominal aorta involving visceral vessels (mesenteric, celiac, renal)

Report direct repair of a ruptured aneurysm of the abdominal aorta involving visceral vessels, such as celiac, renal, and/or mesenteric

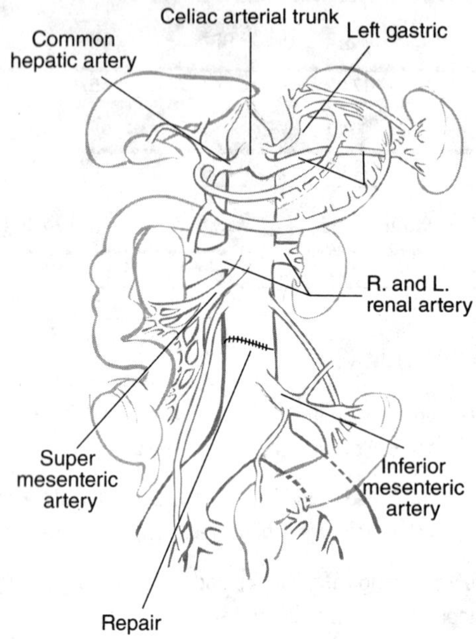

Explanation

The physician quickly exposes the abdominal aorta using a transperitoneal approach, placing a long incision in the midabdomen and retracting the transverse colon and small bowel to allow dissection and exposure of the aorta. Control of bleeding is achieved by pushing the liver aside and compressing the aorta manually against the spine. The aorta is cross-clamped proximal to the dissection and the iliac arteries are exposed. Control of blood flow is done with umbilical tape or rubber catheters. If bleeding is controlled, the iliac arteries and proximal aorta are cross-clamped. The physician opens and clears the aneurysm, controls collateral bleeding from the lumbar arteries with suture, then sutures a Y-shaped knitted Dacron graft to the proximal aorta. The distal ends of the graft are sutured to the iliac arteries. The physician may anastomose the celiac, inferior mesenteric, and/or renal arteries to the Dacron graft. The remaining aneurysmal shell is sutured around the graft. The retroperitoneum and abdominal wounds are closed, leaving drains in place.

Coding Tips

Preparation of the artery for anastomosis, including endarterectomy, is integral to the procedure and should not be reported separately. Establishing both inflow and outflow by any method is included. The portion of the operative arteriogram performed by the surgeon is also included. Angioscopy performed during therapeutic intervention should be reported in addition to the code for the primary procedure; see 35400. Harvested vein or synthetic material may be used for the graft. Any graft harvest is not reported separately. For thoracic aortic aneurysm, see 33858–33875. For direct repairs associated with occlusive disease only, see 35221, 35251, and 35281.

ICD-10-CM Diagnostic Codes

I71.3	Abdominal aortic aneurysm, ruptured

I71.5	Thoracoabdominal aortic aneurysm, ruptured
I72.2	Aneurysm of renal artery
I72.8	Aneurysm of other specified arteries

AMA: **35092** 2002,May,7

Relative Value Units/Medicare Edits

Non-Facility RVU	Work	PE	MP	Total
35092	50.97	12.7	11.87	75.54
Facility RVU	**Work**	**PE**	**MP**	**Total**
35092	50.97	12.7	11.87	75.54

	FUD	Status	MUE	Modifiers				IOM Reference
35092	90	A	1(2)	51	50	62*	80	None

* with documentation

Terms To Know

aneurysm. Circumscribed dilation or outpouching of an artery wall, often containing blood clots and connecting directly with the lumen of the artery.

endarterectomy. Removal of the thickened, endothelial lining of a diseased or damaged artery.

pseudoaneurysm. False aneurysm produced by a dilated vessel wall, or a ruptured blood vessel that has formed a clot that pulsates, mimicking a true aneurysm.

35102

35102 Direct repair of aneurysm, pseudoaneurysm, or excision (partial or total) and graft insertion, with or without patch graft; for aneurysm, pseudoaneurysm, and associated occlusive disease, abdominal aorta involving iliac vessels (common, hypogastric, external)

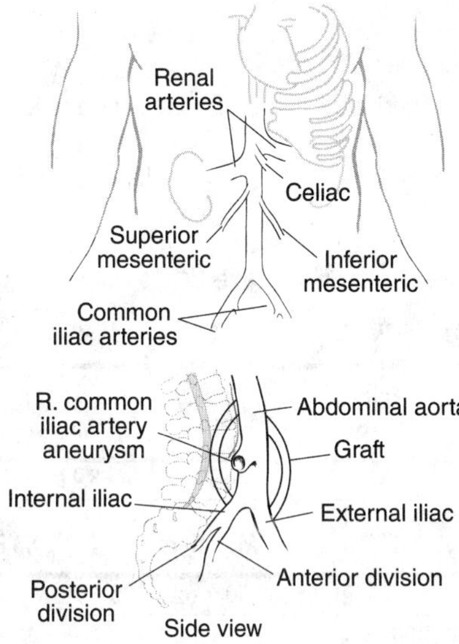

Explanation

The physician exposes the abdominal aorta using a transperitoneal approach, placing a long incision in the midabdomen, and retracting the transverse colon and small bowel to allow dissection and exposure of the aorta. Umbilical tape or a rubber catheter is placed around the aorta proximal to the aneurysm. The iliac arteries are exposed and control of blood flow is achieved with umbilical tape or rubber catheters. The physician anticoagulates the patient and cross-clamps the iliac arteries and proximal aorta. The physician opens and clears the aneurysm, controls collateral bleeding from the lumbar arteries with suture, then sutures a Y-shaped knitted Dacron graft to the proximal aorta. The distal ends of the graft are sutured to the iliac arteries. The physician may anastomose grafts from other involved iliac vessels (common, hypogastric, external) to the Dacron graft. The remaining aneurysmal shell is sutured around the graft. The retroperitoneal and abdominal wounds are closed, leaving drains in place.

Coding Tips

Preparation of the artery for anastomosis, including endarterectomy, is integral to the procedure and should not be reported separately. Establishing both inflow and outflow by any method is included. The portion of the operative arteriogram performed by the surgeon is also included. Angioscopy performed during therapeutic intervention should be reported in addition to the code for the primary procedure; see 35400. Harvested vein or synthetic material may be used for the graft. Any graft harvest is not reported separately. For thoracic aortic aneurysm, see 33858–33875. For direct repairs associated with occlusive disease only, see 35221, 35251, and 35281.

ICD-10-CM Diagnostic Codes

I70.0	Atherosclerosis of aorta
I71.3	Abdominal aortic aneurysm, ruptured
I71.4	Abdominal aortic aneurysm, without rupture
I71.5	Thoracoabdominal aortic aneurysm, ruptured
I71.6	Thoracoabdominal aortic aneurysm, without rupture

I72.3	Aneurysm of iliac artery
I73.89	Other specified peripheral vascular diseases
I74.01	Saddle embolus of abdominal aorta
I74.09	Other arterial embolism and thrombosis of abdominal aorta
I74.19	Embolism and thrombosis of other parts of aorta
I74.5	Embolism and thrombosis of iliac artery
I76	Septic arterial embolism
I77.1	Stricture of artery
I77.72	Dissection of iliac artery
I77.89	Other specified disorders of arteries and arterioles

AMA: **35102** 2018,Jan,8; 2017,Jan,8; 2016,Jan,13; 2015,Jan,16; 2014,Jan,11; 2013,Dec,8

Relative Value Units/Medicare Edits

Non-Facility RVU	Work	PE	MP	Total
35102	36.53	9.56	8.42	54.51
Facility RVU	**Work**	**PE**	**MP**	**Total**
35102	36.53	9.56	8.42	54.51

	FUD	Status	MUE	Modifiers				IOM Reference
35102	90	A	1(2)	51	50	62*	80	None

* with documentation

Terms To Know

anastomosis. Surgically created connection between ducts, blood vessels, or bowel segments to allow flow from one to the other.

atherosclerosis. Buildup of yellowish plaques composed of cholesterol and lipoid material within the arteries.

35103

35103 Direct repair of aneurysm, pseudoaneurysm, or excision (partial or total) and graft insertion, with or without patch graft; for ruptured aneurysm, abdominal aorta involving iliac vessels (common, hypogastric, external)

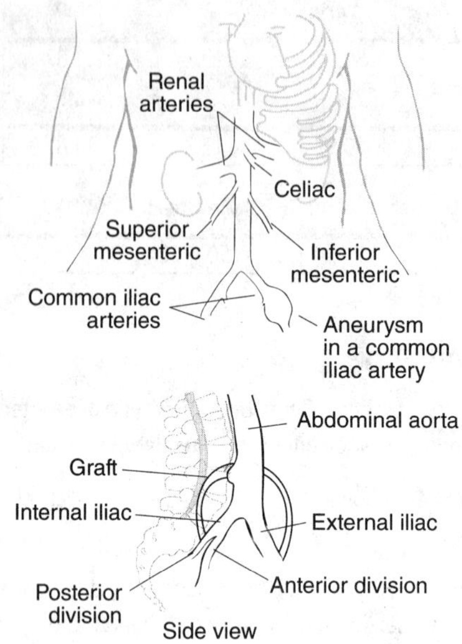

Explanation

The physician quickly exposes the abdominal aorta using a transperitoneal approach, placing a long incision in the midabdomen. The transverse colon and small bowel are retracted to allow dissection and exposure of the aorta. The physician quickly achieves control of bleeding by pushing the liver aside and compressing the aorta manually against the spine. The aorta is cross-clamped proximal to the dissection and the iliac arteries are exposed. Control of blood flow is achieved with umbilical tape or rubber catheters. Anticoagulation is provided (if bleeding is controlled) and the iliac arteries and proximal aorta are cross-clamped. The physician opens and clears the aneurysm, controls collateral bleeding from the lumbar arteries with suture, and sutures a Y-shaped knitted Dacron graft to the proximal aorta. The distal ends of the graft are sutured to the iliac arteries. The physician may anastomose grafts from other involved iliac vessels (common, hypogastric, external) to the Dacron graft. The remaining aneurysmal shell is sutured around the graft. The retroperitoneal and abdominal wounds are closed, leaving drains in place.

Coding Tips

Preparation of the artery for anastomosis, including endarterectomy, is integral to the procedure and should not be reported separately. Establishing both inflow and outflow by any method is included. The portion of the operative arteriogram performed by the surgeon is also included. Angioscopy performed during therapeutic intervention should be reported in addition to the code for the primary procedure; see 35400. Harvested vein or synthetic material may be used for the graft. Any graft harvest is not reported separately. For thoracic aortic aneurysm, see 33858–33875. For direct repairs associated with occlusive disease only, see 35221, 35251, and 35281.

ICD-10-CM Diagnostic Codes

I70.0	Atherosclerosis of aorta
I71.02	Dissection of abdominal aorta
I71.3	Abdominal aortic aneurysm, ruptured

I71.5	Thoracoabdominal aortic aneurysm, ruptured
I72.3	Aneurysm of iliac artery
I73.89	Other specified peripheral vascular diseases
I74.01	Saddle embolus of abdominal aorta
I74.09	Other arterial embolism and thrombosis of abdominal aorta
I74.19	Embolism and thrombosis of other parts of aorta
I74.5	Embolism and thrombosis of iliac artery
I76	Septic arterial embolism
I77.1	Stricture of artery
I77.72	Dissection of iliac artery

AMA: 35103 2002,May,7

Relative Value Units/Medicare Edits

Non-Facility RVU	Work	PE	MP	Total
35103	43.62	11.27	10.1	64.99
Facility RVU	**Work**	**PE**	**MP**	**Total**
35103	43.62	11.27	10.1	64.99

	FUD	Status	MUE	Modifiers				IOM Reference
35103	90	A	1(2)	51	50	62*	80	None

* with documentation

Terms To Know

anastomosis. Surgically created connection between ducts, blood vessels, or bowel segments to allow flow from one to the other.

arteriogram. Radiograph of arteries.

atherosclerosis. Buildup of yellowish plaques composed of cholesterol and lipoid material within the arteries.

complication. Condition arising after the beginning of observation and treatment that modifies the course of the patient's illness or the medical care required, or an undesired result or misadventure in medical care.

pseudoaneurysm. False aneurysm produced by a dilated vessel wall, or a ruptured blood vessel that has formed a clot that pulsates, mimicking a true aneurysm.

35111-35112

35111 Direct repair of aneurysm, pseudoaneurysm, or excision (partial or total) and graft insertion, with or without patch graft; for aneurysm, pseudoaneurysm, and associated occlusive disease, splenic artery

35112 for ruptured aneurysm, splenic artery

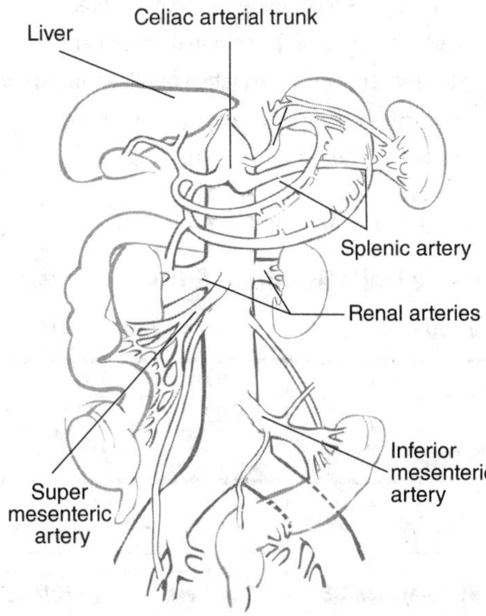

Explanation

The physician exposes the splenic artery using an abdominal incision. If the aneurysm involves the proximal or distal (hilar) splenic artery, in 35111, the physician may repair the aneurysm using harvested venous material or synthetic graft material or simply tie off the diseased artery and vein. In 35112, the physician may repair the aneurysm using harvested venous material or synthetic graft material or simply tie off the diseased artery and vein. If the aneurysm involves the middle splenic artery, which is surrounded by pancreatic tissue, the artery may be tied off to avoid dissection of the pancreas. The abdominal wound is closed, leaving drains in place.

Coding Tips

Preparation of the artery for anastomosis, including endarterectomy, is integral to the procedure and should not be reported separately. Establishing both inflow and outflow by any method is included. That portion of the operative arteriogram performed by the surgeon is also included. Angioscopy performed during therapeutic intervention should be reported in addition to the code for the primary procedure; see 35400. Harvested vein or synthetic material may be used for the graft. Any graft harvest is not reported separately. For direct repairs associated with occlusive disease only, see 35221, 35251, and 35281.

ICD-10-CM Diagnostic Codes

D73.5	Infarction of spleen
I72.8	Aneurysm of other specified arteries
I73.89	Other specified peripheral vascular diseases
I74.19	Embolism and thrombosis of other parts of aorta
I74.8	Embolism and thrombosis of other arteries
I76	Septic arterial embolism
I77.1	Stricture of artery
I77.79	Dissection of other specified artery

I77.89	Other specified disorders of arteries and arterioles
S35.291A	Minor laceration of branches of celiac and mesenteric artery, initial encounter
S35.292A	Major laceration of branches of celiac and mesenteric artery, initial encounter
S35.298A	Other injury of branches of celiac and mesenteric artery, initial encounter
S36.020A	Minor contusion of spleen, initial encounter
S36.021A	Major contusion of spleen, initial encounter
S36.030A	Superficial (capsular) laceration of spleen, initial encounter
S36.031A	Moderate laceration of spleen, initial encounter
S36.032A	Major laceration of spleen, initial encounter

AMA: 35111 2002,May,7 **35112** 2002,May,7

Relative Value Units/Medicare Edits

Non-Facility RVU	Work	PE	MP	Total
35111	26.28	5.99	6.09	38.36
35112	32.57	7.09	7.54	47.2
Facility RVU	**Work**	**PE**	**MP**	**Total**
35111	26.28	5.99	6.09	38.36
35112	32.57	7.09	7.54	47.2

	FUD	Status	MUE	Modifiers				IOM Reference
35111	90	A	1(2)	51	50	62*	80	None
35112	90	A	1(2)	51	50	62*	80	

* with documentation

Terms To Know

aneurysm. Circumscribed dilation or outpouching of an artery wall, often containing blood clots and connecting directly with the lumen of the artery.

late effect. Abnormality, dysfunction, or other residual condition produced after the acute phase of an illness, injury, or disease is over. There is no time limit on when late effects can appear.

pseudoaneurysm. False aneurysm produced by a dilated vessel wall, or a ruptured blood vessel that has formed a clot that pulsates, mimicking a true aneurysm.

35121-35122

35121 Direct repair of aneurysm, pseudoaneurysm, or excision (partial or total) and graft insertion, with or without patch graft; for aneurysm, pseudoaneurysm, and associated occlusive disease, hepatic, celiac, renal, or mesenteric artery

35122 for ruptured aneurysm, hepatic, celiac, renal, or mesenteric artery

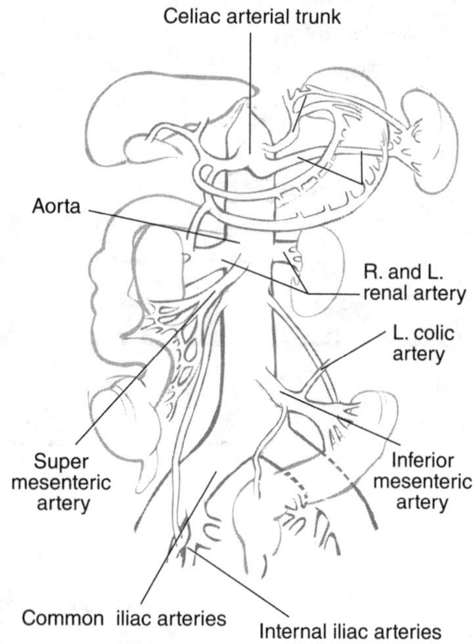

Explanation

In 35121, the physician exposes the involved hepatic, celiac, renal, or mesenteric artery using an abdominal incision, retracting and dissecting past large and small bowel. If the aneurysm involves an artery whose vascular distribution has adequate collaterals (the common hepatic artery, for example), the physician may simply tie off the diseased artery. Otherwise, the physician repairs the aneurysm, often using harvested vein graft, harvested internal iliac artery graft, or synthetic graft material. The physician closes the abdominal wound, leaving drains in place. In 35122, the physician quickly exposes the involved hepatic, celiac, renal, or mesenteric artery using an abdominal incision, retracting and dissecting past large and small bowel. Bleeding is controlled by clamping or compressing the involved artery proximal to the rupture. If the aneurysm involves an artery whose vascular distribution has adequate collaterals (e.g., the common hepatic artery), the physician may simply tie off the diseased artery. Otherwise, the aneurysm is repaired, often using harvested vein graft, harvested internal iliac artery graft, or synthetic graft material. The abdominal wound is closed, leaving drains in place.

Coding Tips

Preparation of the artery for anastomosis, including endarterectomy, is integral to the procedure and should not be reported separately. Establishing both inflow and outflow by any method is included. That portion of the operative arteriogram performed by the surgeon is also included. Angioscopy performed during therapeutic intervention should be reported in addition to the code for the primary procedure; see 35400. Harvested vein or synthetic material may be used for the graft. Any graft harvest is not reported separately. For direct repairs associated with occlusive disease only, see 35221, 35251, and 35281.

ICD-10-CM Diagnostic Codes

I70.1	Atherosclerosis of renal artery
I70.8	Atherosclerosis of other arteries
I72.2	Aneurysm of renal artery
I72.8	Aneurysm of other specified arteries
I77.1	Stricture of artery
I77.73	Dissection of renal artery
I77.79	Dissection of other specified artery
K55.011	Focal (segmental) acute (reversible) ischemia of small intestine
K55.012	Diffuse acute (reversible) ischemia of small intestine
K55.021	Focal (segmental) acute infarction of small intestine
K55.022	Diffuse acute infarction of small intestine
K55.031	Focal (segmental) acute (reversible) ischemia of large intestine
K55.032	Diffuse acute (reversible) ischemia of large intestine
K55.041	Focal (segmental) acute infarction of large intestine
K55.042	Diffuse acute infarction of large intestine
K55.1	Chronic vascular disorders of intestine
K55.8	Other vascular disorders of intestine
N28.0	Ischemia and infarction of kidney

AMA: **35121** 2002,May,7 **35122** 2002,May,7

Relative Value Units/Medicare Edits

Non-Facility RVU	Work	PE	MP	Total
35121	31.52	9.59	7.19	48.3
35122	37.89	7.96	8.78	54.63
Facility RVU	**Work**	**PE**	**MP**	**Total**
35121	31.52	9.59	7.19	48.3
35122	37.89	7.96	8.78	54.63

	FUD	Status	MUE	Modifiers				IOM Reference
35121	90	A	1(3)	51	50	N/A	80	None
35122	90	A	1(3)	51	50	62*	80	

* with documentation

Terms To Know

anastomosis. Surgically created connection between ducts, blood vessels, or bowel segments to allow flow from one to the other.

aneurysm. Circumscribed dilation or outpouching of an artery wall, often containing blood clots and connecting directly with the lumen of the artery.

pseudoaneurysm. False aneurysm produced by a dilated vessel wall, or a ruptured blood vessel that has formed a clot that pulsates, mimicking a true aneurysm.

35131-35132

35131 Direct repair of aneurysm, pseudoaneurysm, or excision (partial or total) and graft insertion, with or without patch graft; for aneurysm, pseudoaneurysm, and associated occlusive disease, iliac artery (common, hypogastric, external)

35132 for ruptured aneurysm, iliac artery (common, hypogastric, external)

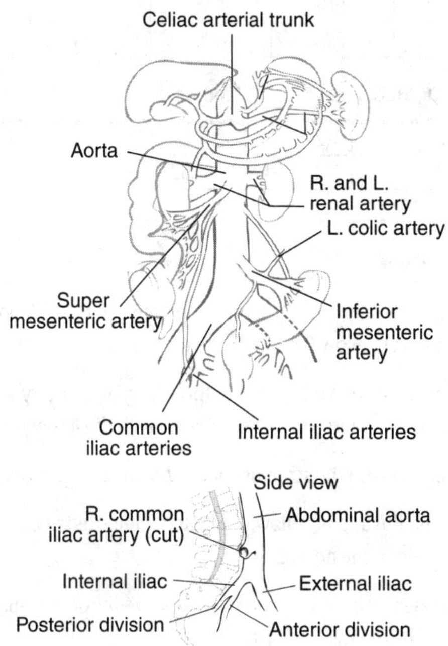

Explanation

The physician exposes the involved iliac arterial branch(es) (common, hypogastric, external) using a low abdominal incision. In 35131, the aneurysm is repaired by clamping off the affected artery proximally and distally and replacing the affected arterial segment with harvested venous material or synthetic graft material such as Dacron mesh. In 35132, bleeding is controlled by clamping or compressing the proximal segment of the affected artery. The ruptured aneurysm is repaired by clamping off the affected artery proximally and distally and replacing the affected arterial segment with harvested venous material or synthetic graft material such as Dacron mesh. The arterial patency is confirmed with a Doppler probe or by angiography. The abdominal wound is closed, leaving drains in place.

Coding Tips

Preparation of the artery for anastomosis, including endarterectomy, is integral to the procedure and should not be reported separately. Establishing both inflow and outflow by any method is included. That portion of the operative arteriogram performed by the surgeon is also included. Angioscopy performed during therapeutic intervention should be reported in addition to the code for the primary procedure; see 35400. Harvested vein or synthetic material may be used for the graft. Any graft harvest is not reported separately. For direct repairs associated with occlusive disease only, see 35221, 35251, and 35281.

ICD-10-CM Diagnostic Codes

I72.3	Aneurysm of iliac artery
I74.5	Embolism and thrombosis of iliac artery
I77.1	Stricture of artery
I77.72	Dissection of iliac artery

AMA: 35131 2018,Jan,8; 2017,Jan,8; 2016,Jan,13; 2015,Jan,16; 2014,Jan,11

Relative Value Units/Medicare Edits

Non-Facility RVU	Work	PE	MP	Total
35131	26.4	7.76	6.06	40.22
35132	32.57	7.09	7.54	47.2
Facility RVU	**Work**	**PE**	**MP**	**Total**
35131	26.4	7.76	6.06	40.22
35132	32.57	7.09	7.54	47.2

	FUD	Status	MUE	Modifiers				IOM Reference
35131	90	A	1(2)	51	50	62*	80	None
35132	90	A	1(2)	51	50	62*	80	

* with documentation

Terms To Know

anastomosis. Surgically created connection between ducts, blood vessels, or bowel segments to allow flow from one to the other.

aneurysm. Circumscribed dilation or outpouching of an artery wall, often containing blood clots and connecting directly with the lumen of the artery.

anomaly. Irregularity in the structure or position of an organ or tissue.

atherosclerosis. Buildup of yellowish plaques composed of cholesterol and lipoid material within the arteries.

congenital. Present at birth, occurring through heredity or an influence during gestation up to the moment of birth.

digital subtraction angiography. Diagnostic imaging technique that applies computer technology to fluoroscopy for the purpose of visualizing the same vascular structures observable with conventional angiography.

excision. Surgical removal of an organ or tissue.

graft. Tissue implant from another part of the body or another person.

late effect. Abnormality, dysfunction, or other residual condition produced after the acute phase of an illness, injury, or disease is over. There is no time limit on when late effects can appear.

pseudoaneurysm. False aneurysm produced by a dilated vessel wall, or a ruptured blood vessel that has formed a clot that pulsates, mimicking a true aneurysm.

35141-35142

35141 Direct repair of aneurysm, pseudoaneurysm, or excision (partial or total) and graft insertion, with or without patch graft; for aneurysm, pseudoaneurysm, and associated occlusive disease, common femoral artery (profunda femoris, superficial femoral)

35142 for ruptured aneurysm, common femoral artery (profunda femoris, superficial femoral)

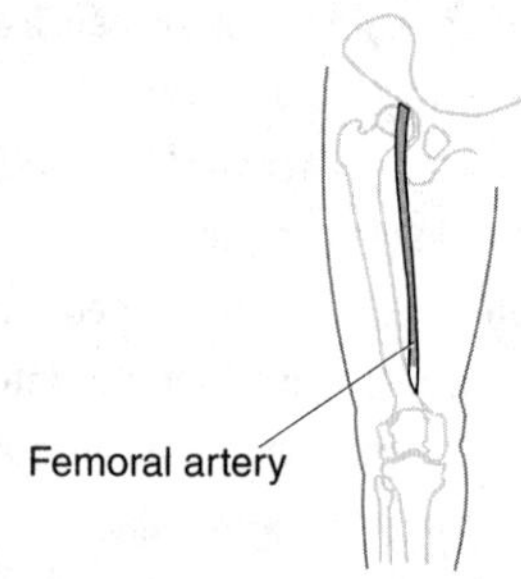

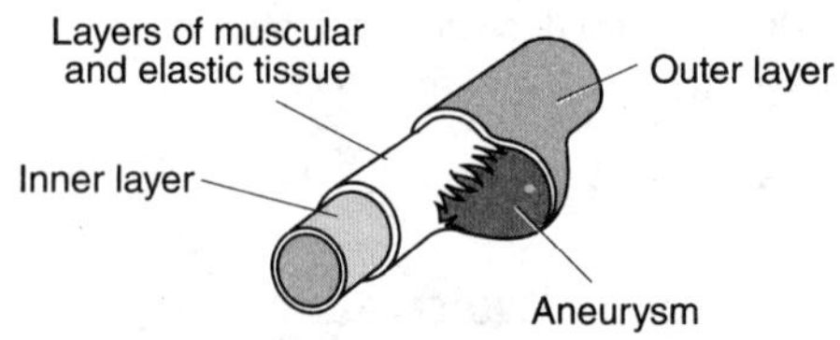

Area of aneurysm or occlusion

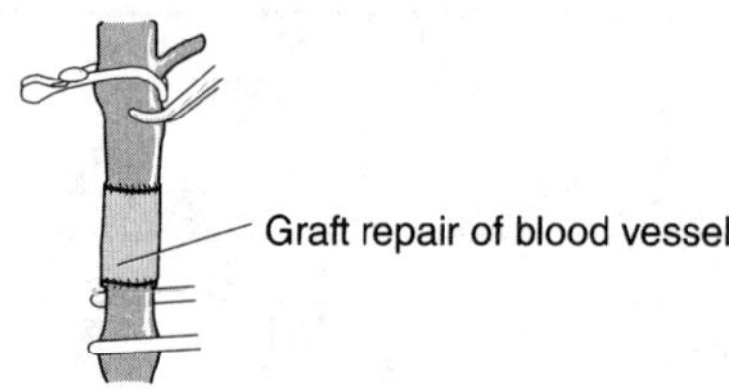

Explanation

The physician makes an incision in the skin of the leg. The enlarged or blocked section of the femoral artery (35141) or ruptured section (35142) is isolated and dissected from adjacent critical structures. Vessel clamps are affixed above and below the defect, which may be repaired or removed. The repair may be accomplished by removing the segment of artery containing the aneurysm and suturing the exposed ends of the vessel in an end-to-end fashion or the aneurysm may be bypassed with a venous or synthetic graft. If a large section is removed, a harvested or synthetic graft is inserted into the defect. Instead of a complete graft, a patch may be sutured into place to open up the diameter of the vessel. Once the vessel is repaired, the clamps are removed. The skin incision is repaired with a layered closure.

Coding Tips

Preparation of the artery for anastomosis, including endarterectomy, is integral to the procedure and should not be reported separately. Establishing both inflow and outflow by any method is included. That portion of the operative arteriogram performed by the surgeon is also included. Angioscopy performed during therapeutic intervention should be reported in addition to the code for the primary procedure; see 35400. Harvested vein or synthetic material may be used for the graft. Any graft harvest is not reported separately. For direct repairs associated with occlusive disease only, see 35226, 35256, and 35286.

ICD-10-CM Diagnostic Codes

I70.211	Atherosclerosis of native arteries of extremities with intermittent claudication, right leg ☑
I70.212	Atherosclerosis of native arteries of extremities with intermittent claudication, left leg ☑
I70.213	Atherosclerosis of native arteries of extremities with intermittent claudication, bilateral legs ☑
I70.221	Atherosclerosis of native arteries of extremities with rest pain, right leg ☑
I70.222	Atherosclerosis of native arteries of extremities with rest pain, left leg ☑
I70.223	Atherosclerosis of native arteries of extremities with rest pain, bilateral legs ☑
I72.4	Aneurysm of artery of lower extremity
I74.3	Embolism and thrombosis of arteries of the lower extremities
I75.021	Atheroembolism of right lower extremity ☑
I75.022	Atheroembolism of left lower extremity ☑
I75.023	Atheroembolism of bilateral lower extremities ☑
I76	Septic arterial embolism

AMA: **35141** 2002,May,7 **35142** 2002,May,7

Relative Value Units/Medicare Edits

Non-Facility RVU	Work	PE	MP	Total
35141	20.91	6.26	4.8	31.97
35142	25.16	7.58	5.77	38.51
Facility RVU	**Work**	**PE**	**MP**	**Total**
35141	20.91	6.26	4.8	31.97
35142	25.16	7.58	5.77	38.51

	FUD	Status	MUE	Modifiers				IOM Reference
35141	90	A	1(2)	51	50	62*	80	None
35142	90	A	1(2)	51	50	62*	80	

* with documentation

Terms To Know

anastomosis. Surgically created connection between ducts, blood vessels, or bowel segments to allow flow from one to the other.

aneurysm. Circumscribed dilation or outpouching of an artery wall, often containing blood clots and connecting directly with the lumen of the artery.

pseudoaneurysm. False aneurysm produced by a dilated vessel wall, or a ruptured blood vessel that has formed a clot that pulsates, mimicking a true aneurysm.

35151-35152

35151 Direct repair of aneurysm, pseudoaneurysm, or excision (partial or total) and graft insertion, with or without patch graft; for aneurysm, pseudoaneurysm, and associated occlusive disease, popliteal artery

35152 for ruptured aneurysm, popliteal artery

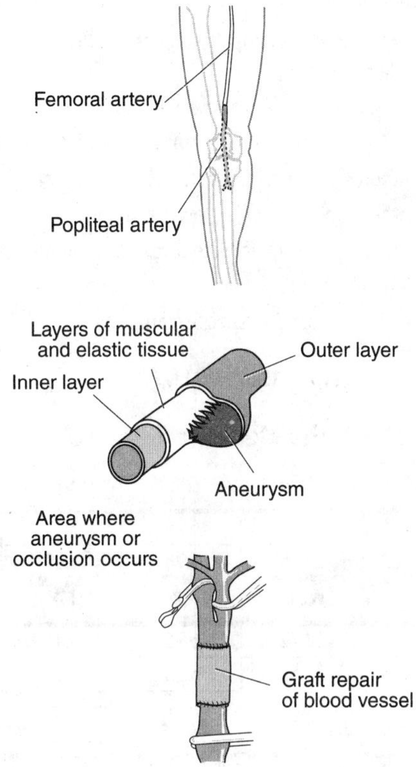

Explanation

The physician makes an incision in the skin over the leg. The enlarged or blocked section of the popliteal artery (35151) or the ruptured section (35152) is isolated and dissected from adjacent critical structures. Vessel clamps are affixed above and below the defect, which may be repaired or removed. The repair may be accomplished by removing the segment of artery containing the aneurysm and suturing the exposed ends of the vessel in an end-to-end fashion or the aneurysm may be bypassed with a venous or synthetic graft. If a large section is removed, a harvested or synthetic graft is inserted into the defect. Instead of a complete graft, a patch may be sutured into place to open up the diameter of the vessel. Once the vessel is repaired, the clamps are removed. The skin incision is repaired with a layered closure.

Coding Tips

Preparation of the artery for anastomosis, including endarterectomy, is integral to the procedure and should not be reported separately. Establishing both inflow and outflow by any method is included. That portion of the operative arteriogram performed by the surgeon is also included. Angioscopy performed during therapeutic intervention should be reported in addition to the code for the primary procedure; see 35400. Harvested vein or synthetic material may be used for the graft. Any graft harvest is not reported separately. For direct repairs associated with occlusive disease only, see 35226, 35256, and 35286.

ICD-10-CM Diagnostic Codes

I70.211	Atherosclerosis of native arteries of extremities with intermittent claudication, right leg ☑

I70.212 Atherosclerosis of native arteries of extremities with intermittent claudication, left leg ☑
I70.213 Atherosclerosis of native arteries of extremities with intermittent claudication, bilateral legs ☑
I70.221 Atherosclerosis of native arteries of extremities with rest pain, right leg ☑
I70.222 Atherosclerosis of native arteries of extremities with rest pain, left leg ☑
I70.223 Atherosclerosis of native arteries of extremities with rest pain, bilateral legs ☑
I72.4 Aneurysm of artery of lower extremity
I74.3 Embolism and thrombosis of arteries of the lower extremities
I75.021 Atheroembolism of right lower extremity ☑
I75.022 Atheroembolism of left lower extremity ☑
I75.023 Atheroembolism of bilateral lower extremities ☑
I77.1 Stricture of artery
I77.79 Dissection of other specified artery

AMA: **35151** 2002,May,7 **35152** 2002,May,7

Relative Value Units/Medicare Edits

Non-Facility RVU	Work	PE	MP	Total
35151	23.72	6.75	5.41	35.88
35152	27.66	6.28	6.39	40.33
Facility RVU	**Work**	**PE**	**MP**	**Total**
35151	23.72	6.75	5.41	35.88
35152	27.66	6.28	6.39	40.33

	FUD	Status	MUE	Modifiers				IOM Reference
35151	90	A	1(2)	51	50	62*	80	None
35152	90	A	1(2)	51	50	62*	80	

* with documentation

Terms To Know

aneurysm. Circumscribed dilation or outpouching of an artery wall, often containing blood clots and connecting directly with the lumen of the artery.

pseudoaneurysm. False aneurysm produced by a dilated vessel wall, or a ruptured blood vessel that has formed a clot that pulsates, mimicking a true aneurysm.

35180

35180 Repair, congenital arteriovenous fistula; head and neck

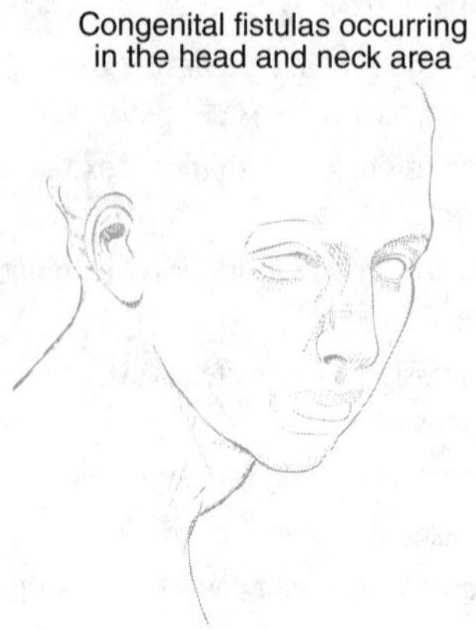

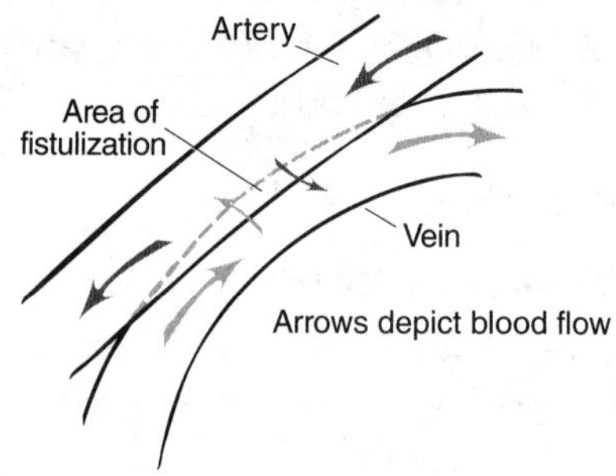

Explanation

The physician makes an incision in the skin of the head or neck over the site of the unnatural opening, a congenital fistula, that exists between an artery and vein. The fistula is isolated and dissected from adjacent critical structures, and vessel clamps are applied to the vein and the artery. The walls of the artery and vein creating the fistula are each sutured closed. A graft or patch graft may be required to complete the repair. The fistula is tied off, or it may be excised. Once the fistula has been eliminated, the clamps are removed and the skin incision is repaired with a layered closure.

Coding Tips

Fistula repair may be performed in stages during multiple operative or invasive radiology sessions. Report each separate session according to the procedure performed. Establishing both inflow and outflow by any method is included. That portion of the operative arteriogram performed by the surgeon is also included. Angioscopy performed during therapeutic intervention should be reported in addition to the code for the primary procedure; see 35400. For repair of an acquired or traumatic arteriovenous fistula, head and neck, see 35188. For repair of blood vessel other than for fistula, neck, see 35201, 35231, and 35261.

ICD-10-CM Diagnostic Codes

I60.01 Nontraumatic subarachnoid hemorrhage from right carotid siphon and bifurcation ☑
I60.02 Nontraumatic subarachnoid hemorrhage from left carotid siphon and bifurcation ☑
I60.11 Nontraumatic subarachnoid hemorrhage from right middle cerebral artery ☑
I60.12 Nontraumatic subarachnoid hemorrhage from left middle cerebral artery ☑

I60.31	Nontraumatic subarachnoid hemorrhage from right posterior communicating artery ☑
I60.32	Nontraumatic subarachnoid hemorrhage from left posterior communicating artery ☑
I60.4	Nontraumatic subarachnoid hemorrhage from basilar artery
I60.51	Nontraumatic subarachnoid hemorrhage from right vertebral artery ☑
I60.52	Nontraumatic subarachnoid hemorrhage from left vertebral artery ☑
I60.6	Nontraumatic subarachnoid hemorrhage from other intracranial arteries
I60.8	Other nontraumatic subarachnoid hemorrhage
I61.0	Nontraumatic intracerebral hemorrhage in hemisphere, subcortical
I61.1	Nontraumatic intracerebral hemorrhage in hemisphere, cortical
I61.3	Nontraumatic intracerebral hemorrhage in brain stem
I61.4	Nontraumatic intracerebral hemorrhage in cerebellum
I61.5	Nontraumatic intracerebral hemorrhage, intraventricular
I61.6	Nontraumatic intracerebral hemorrhage, multiple localized
I61.8	Other nontraumatic intracerebral hemorrhage
I62.01	Nontraumatic acute subdural hemorrhage
I62.02	Nontraumatic subacute subdural hemorrhage
I62.03	Nontraumatic chronic subdural hemorrhage
I62.1	Nontraumatic extradural hemorrhage
I67.0	Dissection of cerebral arteries, nonruptured
I67.1	Cerebral aneurysm, nonruptured
I67.89	Other cerebrovascular disease
Q25.8	Other congenital malformations of other great arteries
Q26.8	Other congenital malformations of great veins
Q27.8	Other specified congenital malformations of peripheral vascular system
Q28.0	Arteriovenous malformation of precerebral vessels
Q28.1	Other malformations of precerebral vessels
Q28.2	Arteriovenous malformation of cerebral vessels
Q28.3	Other malformations of cerebral vessels
Q28.8	Other specified congenital malformations of circulatory system

AMA: 35180 2018,Jan,8; 2017,Jan,8; 2016,Jan,13; 2015,Jan,16; 2014,Jan,11

Relative Value Units/Medicare Edits

Non-Facility RVU	Work	PE	MP	Total
35180	15.1	6.76	3.58	25.44
Facility RVU	**Work**	**PE**	**MP**	**Total**
35180	15.1	6.76	3.58	25.44

	FUD	Status	MUE	Modifiers				IOM Reference
35180	90	A	2(3)	51	N/A	62*	80	None

* with documentation

35182

35182 Repair, congenital arteriovenous fistula; thorax and abdomen

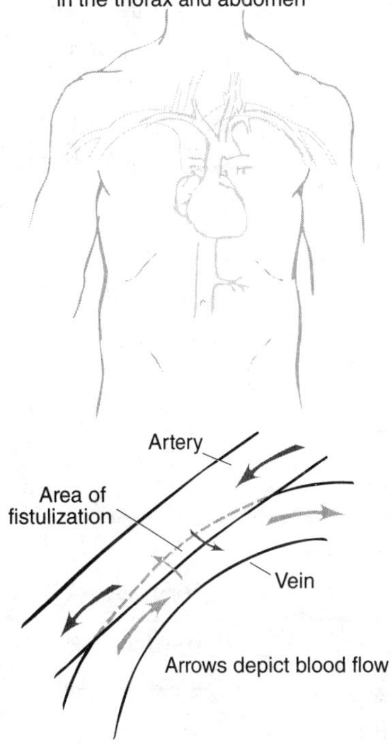

Explanation

The congenital arteriovenous fistula is exposed by choosing an incision appropriate to the fistula site. The physician examines the fistulous connection and repairs it by ligation (tying it off) or may repair the fistula by clamping the connection from both sides, dividing the connection with scissors, and closing each side with suture. A synthetic graft material or vein material harvested from the patient may be sewn in to enlarge the arterial or venous lumen. The vessel patency is confirmed with a Doppler probe or angiography prior to closing the wound. The physician may leave surgical drains in place.

Coding Tips

Fistula repair may be performed in stages during multiple operative or invasive radiology sessions. Report each separate session according to the procedure performed. Establishing both inflow and outflow by any method is included. That portion of the operative arteriogram performed by the surgeon is also included. Angioscopy performed during therapeutic intervention should be reported in addition to the code for the primary procedure; see 35400. For repair of an acquired or traumatic arteriovenous fistula, thorax and abdomen, see 35189. For repair of blood vessel other than for fistula, see 35211–35221, 35241–35251, and 35271–35281.

ICD-10-CM Diagnostic Codes

Q24.5	Malformation of coronary vessels
Q25.41	Absence and aplasia of aorta
Q25.42	Hypoplasia of aorta
Q25.43	Congenital aneurysm of aorta
Q25.44	Congenital dilation of aorta
Q25.45	Double aortic arch
Q25.46	Tortuous aortic arch
Q25.47	Right aortic arch

Q25.48	Anomalous origin of subclavian artery
Q25.49	Other congenital malformations of aorta
Q25.72	Congenital pulmonary arteriovenous malformation
Q25.79	Other congenital malformations of pulmonary artery
Q25.8	Other congenital malformations of other great arteries
Q26.6	Portal vein-hepatic artery fistula
Q26.8	Other congenital malformations of great veins
Q27.2	Other congenital malformations of renal artery
Q27.33	Arteriovenous malformation of digestive system vessel
Q27.34	Arteriovenous malformation of renal vessel
Q27.8	Other specified congenital malformations of peripheral vascular system

AMA: 35182 2018,Jan,8; 2017,Jan,8; 2016,Jan,13; 2015,Jan,16; 2014,Jan,11

Relative Value Units/Medicare Edits

Non-Facility RVU	Work	PE	MP	Total
35182	31.71	12.66	7.54	51.91
Facility RVU	**Work**	**PE**	**MP**	**Total**
35182	31.71	12.66	7.54	51.91

	FUD	Status	MUE	Modifiers				IOM Reference
35182	90	A	2(3)	51	N/A	62*	80	None

* with documentation

Terms To Know

acquired. Produced by outside influences and not by genetics or birth defect.

angioscopy. Visualization of capillary blood vessels with a microscope, or the inside of a blood vessel with a fiberoptic-equipped catheter.

anomaly. Irregularity in the structure or position of an organ or tissue.

arteriogram. Radiograph of arteries.

congenital. Present at birth, occurring through heredity or an influence during gestation up to the moment of birth.

digital subtraction angiography. Diagnostic imaging technique that applies computer technology to fluoroscopy for the purpose of visualizing the same vascular structures observable with conventional angiography.

excision. Surgical removal of an organ or tissue.

fistula. Abnormal tube-like passage between two body cavities or organs or from an organ to the outside surface.

graft. Tissue implant from another part of the body or another person.

incision. Act of cutting into tissue or an organ.

ligation. Tying off a blood vessel or duct with a suture or a soft, thin wire.

35184

35184 Repair, congenital arteriovenous fistula; extremities

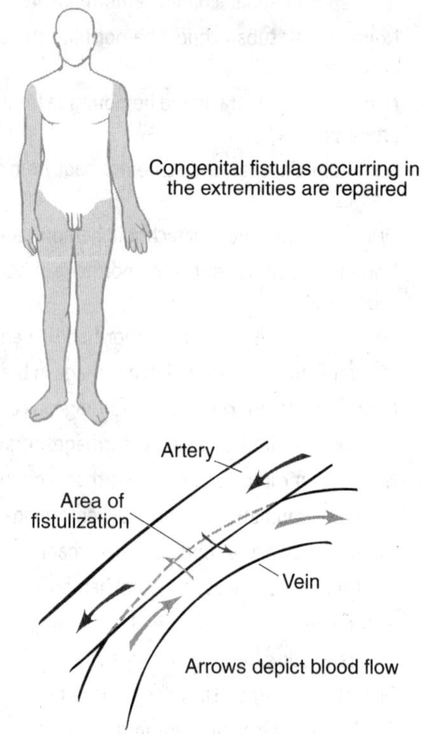

Explanation

The physician makes an incision in the skin of an extremity over the site of the unnatural opening, a congenital fistula, that exists between an artery and vein. The fistula is isolated and dissected from adjacent critical structures, and vessel clamps are applied to the vein and the artery. The walls of the artery and vein creating the fistula are each sutured closed. A graft or patch graft may be required to complete the repair. The fistula is tied off, or it may be excised. Once the fistula has been eliminated, the clamps are removed and the skin incision is repaired with a layered closure.

Coding Tips

Fistula repair may be performed in stages during multiple operative or invasive radiology sessions. Report each separate session according to the procedure performed. Establishing both inflow and outflow by any method is included. That portion of the operative arteriogram performed by the surgeon is also included. Angioscopy performed during therapeutic intervention should be reported in addition to the code for the primary procedure; see 35400. For repair of an acquired or traumatic arteriovenous fistula, extremities, see 35190. For repair of blood vessel other than for fistula, see 35206, 35226, 35236, 35256, 35266, and 35286. For revision of an arteriovenous fistula, with or without thrombectomy, autogenous or nonautogenous graft (separate procedure), see 36832.

ICD-10-CM Diagnostic Codes

Q27.31	Arteriovenous malformation of vessel of upper limb
Q27.32	Arteriovenous malformation of vessel of lower limb

AMA: 35184 2018,Jan,8; 2017,Jan,8; 2016,Jan,13; 2015,Jan,16; 2014,Jan,11

35188-35189

35188 Repair, acquired or traumatic arteriovenous fistula; head and neck
35189 thorax and abdomen

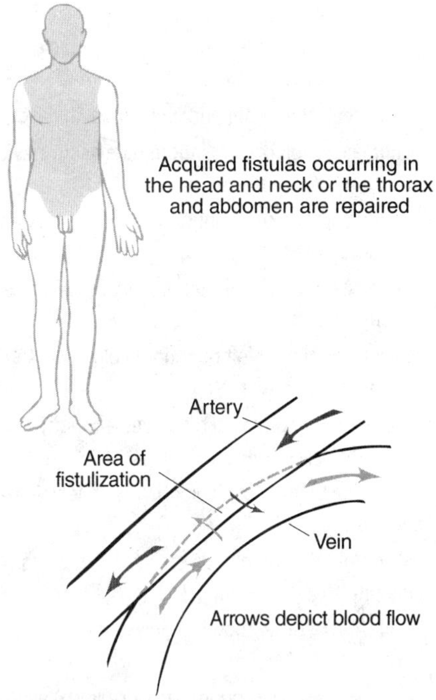

Explanation

The physician makes an incision in the skin over the site of the unnatural opening, a fistula, created through trauma. The fistula connects an artery to a vein. The fistula is isolated and dissected from adjacent critical structures, and vessel clamps are applied to the vein and the artery. The walls of the artery and vein creating the fistula are each repaired and closed. A graft or patch graft may be required to complete the repair. The fistula is tied off or excised. Once the fistula has been eliminated, the clamps are removed and the skin incision is repaired with a layered closure. Report 35189 if fistula is in the thorax or abdomen.

Coding Tips

Fistula repair may be performed in stages during multiple operative or invasive radiology sessions. Report each separate session according to the procedure performed. Establishing inflow and outflow by any method is included. That portion of the operative arteriogram performed by the surgeon is also included. Angioscopy performed during therapeutic intervention should be reported in addition to the code for the primary procedure; see 35400. For repair of a congenital arteriovenous fistula, head and neck, see 35180; thorax and abdomen, see 35182. For repair of a blood vessel other than for fistula, see 35201, 35211–35221, 35231, 35241–35251, 35261, and 35271–35281.

ICD-10-CM Diagnostic Codes

I67.1	Cerebral aneurysm, nonruptured
I77.0	Arteriovenous fistula, acquired
I77.2	Rupture of artery
S15.021A	Major laceration of right carotid artery, initial encounter ☑
S15.022A	Major laceration of left carotid artery, initial encounter ☑
S15.121A	Major laceration of right vertebral artery, initial encounter ☑
S15.122A	Major laceration of left vertebral artery, initial encounter ☑

Relative Value Units/Medicare Edits

Non-Facility RVU	Work	PE	MP	Total
35184	18.82	4.65	4.36	27.83
Facility RVU	**Work**	**PE**	**MP**	**Total**
35184	18.82	4.65	4.36	27.83

	FUD	Status	MUE	Modifiers				IOM Reference
35184	90	A	2(3)	51	N/A	62*	80	None

* with documentation

Terms To Know

acquired. Produced by outside influences and not by genetics or birth defect.

angioscopy. Visualization of capillary blood vessels with a microscope, or the inside of a blood vessel with a fiberoptic-equipped catheter.

anomaly. Irregularity in the structure or position of an organ or tissue.

arteriogram. Radiograph of arteries.

arteriovenous fistula. Connecting passage between an artery and a vein.

autogenous transplant. Tissue, such as bone, that is harvested from the patient and used for transplantation back into the same patient.

congenital. Present at birth, occurring through heredity or an influence during gestation up to the moment of birth.

graft. Tissue implant from another part of the body or another person.

suture. Numerous stitching techniques employed in wound closure.

thrombectomy. Removal of a clot (thrombus) from a blood vessel utilizing various methods.

S15.221A Major laceration of right external jugular vein, initial encounter ☑
S15.222A Major laceration of left external jugular vein, initial encounter ☑
S15.321A Major laceration of right internal jugular vein, initial encounter ☑
S15.322A Major laceration of left internal jugular vein, initial encounter ☑
S25.121A Major laceration of right innominate or subclavian artery, initial encounter ☑
S25.122A Major laceration of left innominate or subclavian artery, initial encounter ☑
S25.22XA Major laceration of superior vena cava, initial encounter
S25.321A Major laceration of right innominate or subclavian vein, initial encounter ☑
S25.322A Major laceration of left innominate or subclavian vein, initial encounter ☑
S25.421A Major laceration of right pulmonary blood vessels, initial encounter ☑
S25.422A Major laceration of left pulmonary blood vessels, initial encounter ☑
S25.511A Laceration of intercostal blood vessels, right side, initial encounter ☑
S25.512A Laceration of intercostal blood vessels, left side, initial encounter ☑
S25.811A Laceration of other blood vessels of thorax, right side, initial encounter ☑
S25.812A Laceration of other blood vessels of thorax, left side, initial encounter ☑
S35.02XA Major laceration of abdominal aorta, initial encounter
S35.12XA Major laceration of inferior vena cava, initial encounter
S35.212A Major laceration of celiac artery, initial encounter
S35.222A Major laceration of superior mesenteric artery, initial encounter
S35.232A Major laceration of inferior mesenteric artery, initial encounter
S35.292A Major laceration of branches of celiac and mesenteric artery, initial encounter
S35.311A Laceration of portal vein, initial encounter
S35.321A Laceration of splenic vein, initial encounter
S35.331A Laceration of superior mesenteric vein, initial encounter
S35.341A Laceration of inferior mesenteric vein, initial encounter
S35.411A Laceration of right renal artery, initial encounter ☑
S35.412A Laceration of left renal artery, initial encounter ☑
S35.414A Laceration of right renal vein, initial encounter ☑
S35.415A Laceration of left renal vein, initial encounter ☑
S35.511A Injury of right iliac artery, initial encounter ☑
S35.512A Injury of left iliac artery, initial encounter ☑
S35.514A Injury of right iliac vein, initial encounter ☑
S35.515A Injury of left iliac vein, initial encounter ☑

AMA: **35188** 2018,Jan,8; 2017,Jan,8; 2016,Jan,13; 2015,Jan,16; 2014,Jan,11
35189 2018,Jan,8; 2017,Jan,8; 2016,Jan,13; 2015,Jan,16; 2014,Jan,11

Relative Value Units/Medicare Edits

Non-Facility RVU	Work	PE	MP	Total
35188	18.0	12.25	7.46	37.71
35189	29.98	6.66	6.94	43.58
Facility RVU	**Work**	**PE**	**MP**	**Total**
35188	18.0	12.25	7.46	37.71
35189	29.98	6.66	6.94	43.58

	FUD	Status	MUE	Modifiers				IOM Reference
35188	90	A	2(3)	51	N/A	62*	80	None
35189	90	A	1(3)	51	N/A	62*	80	

* with documentation

Terms To Know

aneurysm. Circumscribed dilation or outpouching of an artery wall, often containing blood clots and connecting directly with the lumen of the artery.

angioscopy. Visualization of capillary blood vessels with a microscope, or the inside of a blood vessel with a fiberoptic-equipped catheter.

arteriogram. Radiograph of arteries.

embolism. Obstruction of a blood vessel resulting from a clot or foreign substance.

excision. Surgical removal of an organ or tissue.

graft. Tissue implant from another part of the body or another person.

hemorrhage syndrome. Fulminating meningococcal septicemia occurring in children younger than 10 years of age with vomiting, cyanosis, diarrhea, purpura, convulsions, circulatory collapse, meningitis, and hemorrhaging into adrenal glands.

incision. Act of cutting into tissue or an organ.

stricture. Narrowing of an anatomical structure.

35190

35190 Repair, acquired or traumatic arteriovenous fistula; extremities

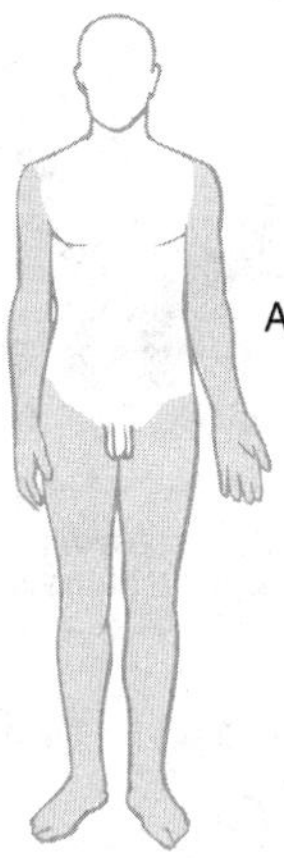

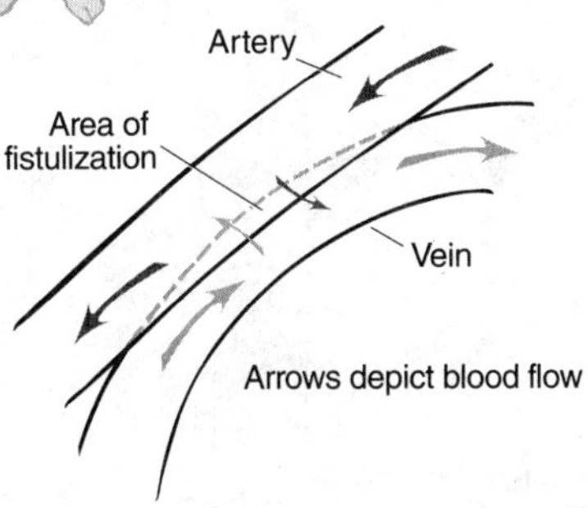

Explanation

The physician makes an incision in the skin of an extremity at the site of the unnatural opening, a fistula, created through trauma. It connects an artery to a vein. The fistula is isolated and dissected from adjacent critical structures, and vessel clamps are applied to the vein and the artery. The walls of the artery and vein creating the fistula are each repaired and closed. A graft or patch graft may be required to complete the repair. The fistula is tied off or excised. Once the fistula has been eliminated, the clamps are removed and the skin incision is repaired with a layered closure.

Coding Tips

Fistula repair may be performed in stages during multiple operative or invasive radiology sessions. Report each separate session according to the procedure performed. Establishing both inflow and outflow by any method is included. That portion of the operative arteriogram performed by the surgeon is also included. Angioscopy performed during therapeutic intervention should be reported in addition to the code for the primary procedure; see 35400. For repair of a congenital arteriovenous fistula, extremities, see 35184. For repair of blood vessel other than for fistula, see 35206, 35236, and 35286. For revision of a surgically created arteriovenous fistula, with or without thrombectomy, autogenous or non-autogenous graft (separate procedure), see 36832.

ICD-10-CM Diagnostic Codes

I77.0	Arteriovenous fistula, acquired
I77.2	Rupture of artery
S45.011A	Laceration of axillary artery, right side, initial encounter ☑
S45.012A	Laceration of axillary artery, left side, initial encounter ☑
S45.111A	Laceration of brachial artery, right side, initial encounter ☑
S45.112A	Laceration of brachial artery, left side, initial encounter ☑
S45.211A	Laceration of axillary or brachial vein, right side, initial encounter ☑
S45.212A	Laceration of axillary or brachial vein, left side, initial encounter ☑
S45.311A	Laceration of superficial vein at shoulder and upper arm level, right arm, initial encounter ☑
S45.312A	Laceration of superficial vein at shoulder and upper arm level, left arm, initial encounter ☑
S55.011A	Laceration of ulnar artery at forearm level, right arm, initial encounter ☑
S55.012A	Laceration of ulnar artery at forearm level, left arm, initial encounter ☑
S55.111A	Laceration of radial artery at forearm level, right arm, initial encounter ☑
S55.112A	Laceration of radial artery at forearm level, left arm, initial encounter ☑
S55.211A	Laceration of vein at forearm level, right arm, initial encounter ☑
S55.212A	Laceration of vein at forearm level, left arm, initial encounter ☑
S65.011A	Laceration of ulnar artery at wrist and hand level of right arm, initial encounter ☑
S65.012A	Laceration of ulnar artery at wrist and hand level of left arm, initial encounter ☑
S65.111A	Laceration of radial artery at wrist and hand level of right arm, initial encounter ☑
S65.112A	Laceration of radial artery at wrist and hand level of left arm, initial encounter ☑
S75.021A	Major laceration of femoral artery, right leg, initial encounter ☑
S75.022A	Major laceration of femoral artery, left leg, initial encounter ☑
S75.121A	Major laceration of femoral vein at hip and thigh level, right leg, initial encounter ☑
S75.122A	Major laceration of femoral vein at hip and thigh level, left leg, initial encounter ☑
S75.221A	Major laceration of greater saphenous vein at hip and thigh level, right leg, initial encounter ☑
S75.222A	Major laceration of greater saphenous vein at hip and thigh level, left leg, initial encounter ☑
S85.011A	Laceration of popliteal artery, right leg, initial encounter ☑
S85.012A	Laceration of popliteal artery, left leg, initial encounter ☑
S85.141A	Laceration of anterior tibial artery, right leg, initial encounter ☑
S85.142A	Laceration of anterior tibial artery, left leg, initial encounter ☑
S85.171A	Laceration of posterior tibial artery, right leg, initial encounter ☑
S85.172A	Laceration of posterior tibial artery, left leg, initial encounter ☑
S85.211A	Laceration of peroneal artery, right leg, initial encounter ☑
S85.212A	Laceration of peroneal artery, left leg, initial encounter ☑
S85.311A	Laceration of greater saphenous vein at lower leg level, right leg, initial encounter ☑
S85.312A	Laceration of greater saphenous vein at lower leg level, left leg, initial encounter ☑
S85.511A	Laceration of popliteal vein, right leg, initial encounter ☑
S85.512A	Laceration of popliteal vein, left leg, initial encounter ☑

AMA: **35190** 2018,Jan,8; 2017,Jan,8; 2016,Jan,13; 2015,Jan,16; 2014,Jan,11

Relative Value Units/Medicare Edits

Non-Facility RVU	Work	PE	MP	Total
35190	13.42	5.51	3.1	22.03
Facility RVU	**Work**	**PE**	**MP**	**Total**
35190	13.42	5.51	3.1	22.03

	FUD	Status	MUE	Modifiers				IOM Reference
35190	90	A	2(3)	51	N/A	62*	80	None

* with documentation

Terms To Know

angioscopy. Visualization of capillary blood vessels with a microscope, or the inside of a blood vessel with a fiberoptic-equipped catheter.

arteriogram. Radiograph of arteries.

embolism. Obstruction of a blood vessel resulting from a clot or foreign substance.

fistula. Abnormal tube-like passage between two body cavities or organs or from an organ to the outside surface.

graft. Tissue implant from another part of the body or another person.

late effect. Abnormality, dysfunction, or other residual condition produced after the acute phase of an illness, injury, or disease is over. There is no time limit on when late effects can appear.

suture. Numerous stitching techniques employed in wound closure.

thrombectomy. Removal of a clot (thrombus) from a blood vessel utilizing various methods.

thrombosis. Condition arising from the presence or formation of blood clots within a blood vessel that may cause vascular obstruction and insufficient oxygenation.

35201

35201 Repair blood vessel, direct; neck

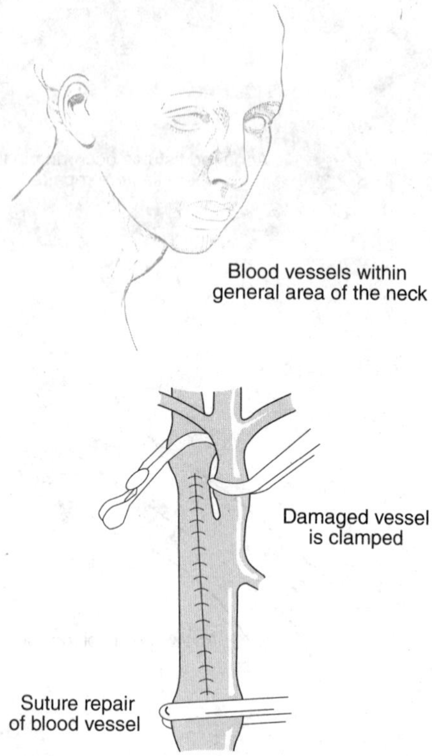

Explanation

The physician makes an incision in the skin of the neck over the site of an injured blood vessel. The vessel is isolated and dissected from adjacent critical structures, and vessel clamps are applied. The edges of the injured vessel may be trimmed to ease repair. A patch graft may be sutured over the defect or the hole in the vessel may be repaired with sutures. The clamps are removed and the skin incision is repaired with a layered closure.

Coding Tips

Establishing both inflow and outflow by any method is included. That portion of the operative arteriogram performed by the surgeon is also included. Angioscopy performed during therapeutic intervention should be reported in addition to the code for the primary procedure; see 35400. Any graft harvest is not reported separately. For repair of aneurysm carotid, subclavian, see 35001–35002. For repair of a blood vessel of the neck with vein graft, see 35231; with synthetic graft, see 35261. For repair of a congenital arteriovenous fistula, see 35180. For repair of an acquired or traumatic arteriovenous fistula, see 35188. Do not report 35201 with 33969, 33984, 33985, 33986.

ICD-10-CM Diagnostic Codes

G45.0	Vertebro-basilar artery syndrome
G45.1	Carotid artery syndrome (hemispheric)
G45.2	Multiple and bilateral precerebral artery syndromes
I65.01	Occlusion and stenosis of right vertebral artery ☑
I65.02	Occlusion and stenosis of left vertebral artery ☑
I65.03	Occlusion and stenosis of bilateral vertebral arteries ☑
I65.21	Occlusion and stenosis of right carotid artery ☑
I65.22	Occlusion and stenosis of left carotid artery ☑

I65.23 Occlusion and stenosis of bilateral carotid arteries ☑
I77.71 Dissection of carotid artery
I77.89 Other specified disorders of arteries and arterioles
S15.011A Minor laceration of right carotid artery, initial encounter ☑
S15.012A Minor laceration of left carotid artery, initial encounter ☑
S15.021A Major laceration of right carotid artery, initial encounter ☑
S15.022A Major laceration of left carotid artery, initial encounter ☑
S15.091A Other specified injury of right carotid artery, initial encounter ☑
S15.092A Other specified injury of left carotid artery, initial encounter ☑
S15.111A Minor laceration of right vertebral artery, initial encounter ☑
S15.112A Minor laceration of left vertebral artery, initial encounter ☑
S15.121A Major laceration of right vertebral artery, initial encounter ☑
S15.122A Major laceration of left vertebral artery, initial encounter ☑
S15.191A Other specified injury of right vertebral artery, initial encounter ☑
S15.192A Other specified injury of left vertebral artery, initial encounter ☑
S15.211A Minor laceration of right external jugular vein, initial encounter ☑
S15.212A Minor laceration of left external jugular vein, initial encounter ☑
S15.221A Major laceration of right external jugular vein, initial encounter ☑
S15.222A Major laceration of left external jugular vein, initial encounter ☑
S15.291A Other specified injury of right external jugular vein, initial encounter ☑
S15.292A Other specified injury of left external jugular vein, initial encounter ☑
S15.311A Minor laceration of right internal jugular vein, initial encounter ☑
S15.312A Minor laceration of left internal jugular vein, initial encounter ☑
S15.321A Major laceration of right internal jugular vein, initial encounter ☑
S15.322A Major laceration of left internal jugular vein, initial encounter ☑
S15.391A Other specified injury of right internal jugular vein, initial encounter ☑
S15.392A Other specified injury of left internal jugular vein, initial encounter ☑
S15.8XXA Injury of other specified blood vessels at neck level, initial encounter
S25.311A Minor laceration of right innominate or subclavian vein, initial encounter ☑
S25.312A Minor laceration of left innominate or subclavian vein, initial encounter ☑
S25.321A Major laceration of right innominate or subclavian vein, initial encounter ☑
S25.322A Major laceration of left innominate or subclavian vein, initial encounter ☑
S25.391A Other specified injury of right innominate or subclavian vein, initial encounter ☑
S25.392A Other specified injury of left innominate or subclavian vein, initial encounter ☑

AMA: 35201 2018,Jan,8; 2017,Jan,8; 2016,Jan,13; 2015,Jul,3; 2015,Jan,16; 2014,Mar,8

Relative Value Units/Medicare Edits

Non-Facility RVU	Work	PE	MP	Total
35201	16.93	6.57	3.78	27.28
Facility RVU	**Work**	**PE**	**MP**	**Total**
35201	16.93	6.57	3.78	27.28

	FUD	Status	MUE	Modifiers				IOM Reference
35201	90	A	2(3)	51	50	62*	80	None

* with documentation

Terms To Know

graft. Tissue implant from another part of the body or another person.

occlusion. Constriction, closure, or blockage of a passage.

stenosis. Narrowing or constriction of a passage.

35206

35206 Repair blood vessel, direct; upper extremity

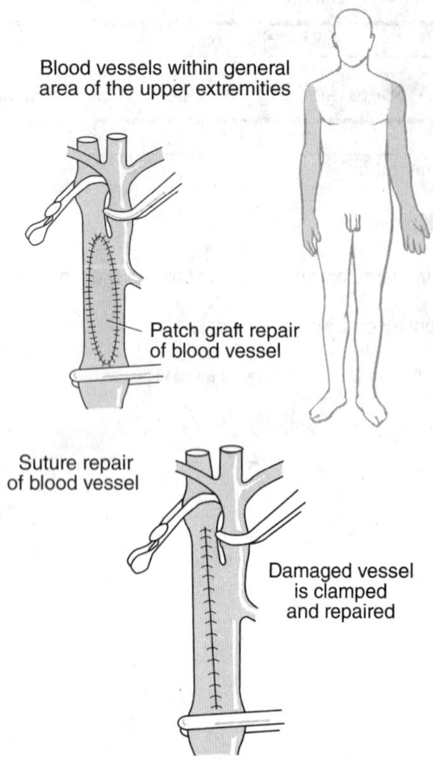

Explanation

The physician makes an incision in the skin of an upper extremity over the site of an injured blood vessel. The vessel is isolated and dissected from adjacent critical structures, and vessel clamps are applied. The edges of the injured vessel may be trimmed to ease repair. A patch graft may be sutured over the defect or the hole in the vessel may be repaired with sutures. The clamps are removed and the skin incision is repaired with a layered closure.

Coding Tips

Establishing both inflow and outflow by any method is included. That portion of the operative arteriogram performed by the surgeon is also included. Angioscopy performed during therapeutic intervention should be reported in addition to the code for the primary procedure; see 35400. Any graft harvest is not reported separately. For repair of an axillary-brachial aneurysm, see 35011–35013; ulnar, radial aneurysm, see 35045. For repair of a blood vessel of an upper extremity with vein graft, see 35236; with synthetic graft, see 35266. For repair of a congenital arteriovenous fistula, see 35184. For repair of an acquired or traumatic arteriovenous fistula, see 35190. Do not report 35206 with 33969, 33984, 33985, 33986.

ICD-10-CM Diagnostic Codes

I77.1	Stricture of artery
I77.2	Rupture of artery
S45.011A	Laceration of axillary artery, right side, initial encounter ☑
S45.012A	Laceration of axillary artery, left side, initial encounter ☑
S45.091A	Other specified injury of axillary artery, right side, initial encounter ☑
S45.092A	Other specified injury of axillary artery, left side, initial encounter ☑
S45.111A	Laceration of brachial artery, right side, initial encounter ☑
S45.112A	Laceration of brachial artery, left side, initial encounter ☑
S45.191A	Other specified injury of brachial artery, right side, initial encounter ☑
S45.192A	Other specified injury of brachial artery, left side, initial encounter ☑
S45.211A	Laceration of axillary or brachial vein, right side, initial encounter ☑
S45.212A	Laceration of axillary or brachial vein, left side, initial encounter ☑
S45.291A	Other specified injury of axillary or brachial vein, right side, initial encounter ☑
S45.292A	Other specified injury of axillary or brachial vein, left side, initial encounter ☑
S45.311A	Laceration of superficial vein at shoulder and upper arm level, right arm, initial encounter ☑
S45.312A	Laceration of superficial vein at shoulder and upper arm level, left arm, initial encounter ☑
S45.391A	Other specified injury of superficial vein at shoulder and upper arm level, right arm, initial encounter ☑
S45.392A	Other specified injury of superficial vein at shoulder and upper arm level, left arm, initial encounter ☑
S45.811A	Laceration of other specified blood vessels at shoulder and upper arm level, right arm, initial encounter ☑
S45.812A	Laceration of other specified blood vessels at shoulder and upper arm level, left arm, initial encounter ☑
S45.891A	Other specified injury of other specified blood vessels at shoulder and upper arm level, right arm, initial encounter ☑
S45.892A	Other specified injury of other specified blood vessels at shoulder and upper arm level, left arm, initial encounter ☑
S55.011A	Laceration of ulnar artery at forearm level, right arm, initial encounter ☑
S55.012A	Laceration of ulnar artery at forearm level, left arm, initial encounter ☑
S55.091A	Other specified injury of ulnar artery at forearm level, right arm, initial encounter ☑
S55.092A	Other specified injury of ulnar artery at forearm level, left arm, initial encounter ☑
S55.111A	Laceration of radial artery at forearm level, right arm, initial encounter ☑
S55.112A	Laceration of radial artery at forearm level, left arm, initial encounter ☑
S55.191A	Other specified injury of radial artery at forearm level, right arm, initial encounter ☑
S55.192A	Other specified injury of radial artery at forearm level, left arm, initial encounter ☑
S55.211A	Laceration of vein at forearm level, right arm, initial encounter ☑
S55.212A	Laceration of vein at forearm level, left arm, initial encounter ☑
S55.291A	Other specified injury of vein at forearm level, right arm, initial encounter ☑
S55.292A	Other specified injury of vein at forearm level, left arm, initial encounter ☑
S55.811A	Laceration of other blood vessels at forearm level, right arm, initial encounter ☑
S55.812A	Laceration of other blood vessels at forearm level, left arm, initial encounter ☑

S55.891A Other specified injury of other blood vessels at forearm level, right arm, initial encounter ☑

S55.892A Other specified injury of other blood vessels at forearm level, left arm, initial encounter ☑

S65.011A Laceration of ulnar artery at wrist and hand level of right arm, initial encounter ☑

S65.012A Laceration of ulnar artery at wrist and hand level of left arm, initial encounter ☑

S65.091A Other specified injury of ulnar artery at wrist and hand level of right arm, initial encounter ☑

S65.092A Other specified injury of ulnar artery at wrist and hand level of left arm, initial encounter ☑

S65.111A Laceration of radial artery at wrist and hand level of right arm, initial encounter ☑

S65.112A Laceration of radial artery at wrist and hand level of left arm, initial encounter ☑

S65.191A Other specified injury of radial artery at wrist and hand level of right arm, initial encounter ☑

S65.192A Other specified injury of radial artery at wrist and hand level of left arm, initial encounter ☑

S65.811A Laceration of other blood vessels at wrist and hand level of right arm, initial encounter ☑

S65.812A Laceration of other blood vessels at wrist and hand level of left arm, initial encounter ☑

S65.891A Other specified injury of other blood vessels at wrist and hand level of right arm, initial encounter ☑

S65.892A Other specified injury of other blood vessels at wrist and hand level of left arm, initial encounter ☑

AMA: 35206 2018,Jan,8; 2017,Jan,8; 2016,Jan,13; 2015,Jul,3; 2015,Jan,16; 2014,Jan,11; 2014,Apr,10

Relative Value Units/Medicare Edits

Non-Facility RVU	Work	PE	MP	Total
35206	13.84	5.76	3.07	22.67
Facility RVU	**Work**	**PE**	**MP**	**Total**
35206	13.84	5.76	3.07	22.67

	FUD	Status	MUE	Modifiers				IOM Reference
35206	90	A	2(3)	51	50	62*	80	None

* with documentation

Terms To Know

aneurysm. Circumscribed dilation or outpouching of an artery wall, often containing blood clots and connecting directly with the lumen of the artery.

angioscopy. Visualization of capillary blood vessels with a microscope, or the inside of a blood vessel with a fiberoptic-equipped catheter.

arteriogram. Radiograph of arteries.

atherosclerosis. Buildup of yellowish plaques composed of cholesterol and lipoid material within the arteries.

claudication. Lameness, pain, and weakness occurring in the arms or legs during exercise due to muscles not receiving the needed oxygen and nutrients.

congenital. Present at birth, occurring through heredity or an influence during gestation up to the moment of birth.

35207

35207 Repair blood vessel, direct; hand, finger

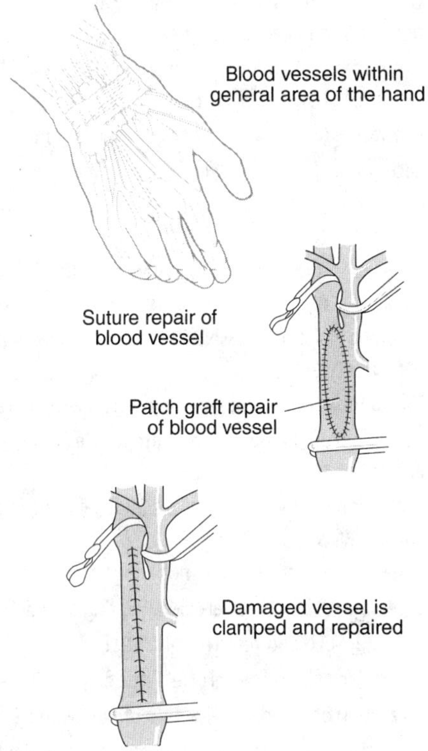

Explanation

The physician makes an incision in the skin of the hand or finger over the site of an injured blood vessel. The vessel is isolated and dissected from adjacent critical structures, and vessel clamps are applied. The edges of the injured vessel may be trimmed to ease repair. A patch graft may be sutured over the defect or the hole in the vessel may be repaired with sutures. The clamps are removed and the skin incision is repaired with a layered closure.

Coding Tips

Establishing both inflow and outflow by any method is included. That portion of the operative arteriogram performed by the surgeon is also included. Angioscopy performed during therapeutic intervention should be reported in addition to the code for the primary procedure; see 35400. Any graft harvest is not reported separately. For repair of a congenital arteriovenous fistula, see 35184. For repair of an acquired or traumatic arteriovenous fistula, see 35190.

ICD-10-CM Diagnostic Codes

I77.1 Stricture of artery

I77.2 Rupture of artery

S65.011A Laceration of ulnar artery at wrist and hand level of right arm, initial encounter ☑

S65.012A Laceration of ulnar artery at wrist and hand level of left arm, initial encounter ☑

S65.091A Other specified injury of ulnar artery at wrist and hand level of right arm, initial encounter ☑

S65.092A Other specified injury of ulnar artery at wrist and hand level of left arm, initial encounter ☑

S65.111A Laceration of radial artery at wrist and hand level of right arm, initial encounter ☑

S65.112A Laceration of radial artery at wrist and hand level of left arm, initial encounter ☑

S65.191A Other specified injury of radial artery at wrist and hand level of right arm, initial encounter ☑

S65.192A Other specified injury of radial artery at wrist and hand level of left arm, initial encounter ☑

S65.411A Laceration of blood vessel of right thumb, initial encounter ☑

S65.412A Laceration of blood vessel of left thumb, initial encounter ☑

S65.491A Other specified injury of blood vessel of right thumb, initial encounter ☑

S65.492A Other specified injury of blood vessel of left thumb, initial encounter ☑

S65.510A Laceration of blood vessel of right index finger, initial encounter ☑

S65.511A Laceration of blood vessel of left index finger, initial encounter ☑

S65.512A Laceration of blood vessel of right middle finger, initial encounter ☑

S65.513A Laceration of blood vessel of left middle finger, initial encounter ☑

S65.514A Laceration of blood vessel of right ring finger, initial encounter ☑

S65.515A Laceration of blood vessel of left ring finger, initial encounter ☑

S65.516A Laceration of blood vessel of right little finger, initial encounter ☑

S65.517A Laceration of blood vessel of left little finger, initial encounter ☑

S65.518A Laceration of blood vessel of other finger, initial encounter

S65.590A Other specified injury of blood vessel of right index finger, initial encounter ☑

S65.591A Other specified injury of blood vessel of left index finger, initial encounter ☑

S65.592A Other specified injury of blood vessel of right middle finger, initial encounter ☑

S65.593A Other specified injury of blood vessel of left middle finger, initial encounter ☑

S65.594A Other specified injury of blood vessel of right ring finger, initial encounter ☑

S65.595A Other specified injury of blood vessel of left ring finger, initial encounter ☑

S65.596A Other specified injury of blood vessel of right little finger, initial encounter ☑

S65.597A Other specified injury of blood vessel of left little finger, initial encounter ☑

S65.598A Other specified injury of blood vessel of other finger, initial encounter

S65.811A Laceration of other blood vessels at wrist and hand level of right arm, initial encounter ☑

S65.812A Laceration of other blood vessels at wrist and hand level of left arm, initial encounter ☑

S65.891A Other specified injury of other blood vessels at wrist and hand level of right arm, initial encounter ☑

S65.892A Other specified injury of other blood vessels at wrist and hand level of left arm, initial encounter ☑

S69.81XA Other specified injuries of right wrist, hand and finger(s), initial encounter ☑

S69.82XA Other specified injuries of left wrist, hand and finger(s), initial encounter ☑

AMA: **35207** 2012,Apr,3-9

Relative Value Units/Medicare Edits

Non-Facility RVU	Work	PE	MP	Total
35207	10.94	8.9	1.92	21.76
Facility RVU	**Work**	**PE**	**MP**	**Total**
35207	10.94	8.9	1.92	21.76

	FUD	Status	MUE	Modifiers				IOM Reference
35207	90	A	3(3)	51	50	62*	N/A	None

* with documentation

Terms To Know

angioscopy. Visualization of capillary blood vessels with a microscope, or the inside of a blood vessel with a fiberoptic-equipped catheter.

arteriogram. Radiograph of arteries.

fistula. Abnormal tube-like passage between two body cavities or organs or from an organ to the outside surface.

graft. Tissue implant from another part of the body or another person.

incision. Act of cutting into tissue or an organ.

laceration. Tearing injury; a torn, ragged-edged wound.

rupture. Tearing or breaking open of tissue.

suture. Numerous stitching techniques employed in wound closure.

35211-35216

35211 Repair blood vessel, direct; intrathoracic, with bypass
35216 intrathoracic, without bypass

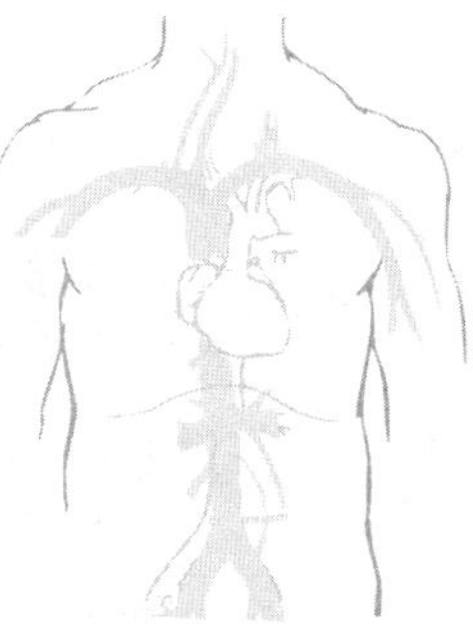

Procedures are within the thorax

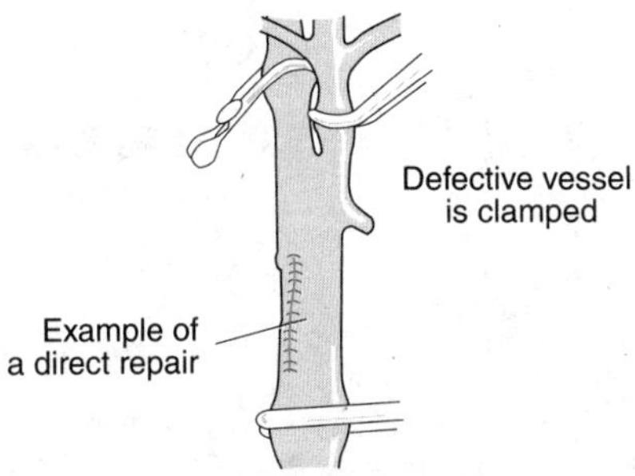

Explanation

The abnormal blood vessel (arterial or venous) is exposed by choosing a thoracic incision appropriate to the involved vessel. In 35211, the physician places cardiopulmonary bypass catheters (through incisions in the low inferior vena cava, the superior vena cava, and high aorta or femoral artery). The heart is stopped by infusing cardioplegia solution into the coronary circulation. The abnormal vessel is examined and repaired by ligation (tying it off) or may be repaired by clamping it proximally and distally to the defect, and suturing the defect closed. The physician may repair the vessel by sewing in synthetic graft material or vein material harvested from the patient in order to enlarge the lumen of the repaired vessel (patch graft). Vessel patency is confirmed with a Doppler probe or angiography prior to taking the patient off cardiopulmonary bypass and closing the wound. The physician leaves chest and, possibly, mediastinal drains in place. Report 35216 when the procedure is performed without the use of cardiopulmonary bypass.

Coding Tips

Establishing both inflow and outflow by any method is included. That portion of the operative arteriogram performed by the surgeon is also included. Angioscopy performed during therapeutic intervention should be reported in addition to the code for the primary procedure; see 35400. Any graft harvest is not reported separately. For repair of a thoracic aortic aneurysm, see 33858–33875. For repair of an innominate, subclavian aneurysm by thoracic incision, see 35021–35022. For vein graft repair of an intrathoracic blood vessel, see 35241–35246; with graft other than vein, see 35271–35276. Do not report these codes with 33969, 33984, 33985, or 33986.

ICD-10-CM Diagnostic Codes

I70.0	Atherosclerosis of aorta
I71.01	Dissection of thoracic aorta
I71.1	Thoracic aortic aneurysm, ruptured
I71.2	Thoracic aortic aneurysm, without rupture
I77.1	Stricture of artery
I77.2	Rupture of artery
I77.5	Necrosis of artery
I77.810	Thoracic aortic ectasia
I77.812	Thoracoabdominal aortic ectasia
I77.89	Other specified disorders of arteries and arterioles
I80.8	Phlebitis and thrombophlebitis of other sites
I87.1	Compression of vein
S21.121A	Laceration with foreign body of right front wall of thorax without penetration into thoracic cavity, initial encounter ☑
S21.122A	Laceration with foreign body of left front wall of thorax without penetration into thoracic cavity, initial encounter ☑
S21.141A	Puncture wound with foreign body of right front wall of thorax without penetration into thoracic cavity, initial encounter ☑
S21.142A	Puncture wound with foreign body of left front wall of thorax without penetration into thoracic cavity, initial encounter ☑
S25.01XA	Minor laceration of thoracic aorta, initial encounter
S25.02XA	Major laceration of thoracic aorta, initial encounter
S25.09XA	Other specified injury of thoracic aorta, initial encounter
S25.111A	Minor laceration of right innominate or subclavian artery, initial encounter ☑
S25.112A	Minor laceration of left innominate or subclavian artery, initial encounter ☑
S25.121A	Major laceration of right innominate or subclavian artery, initial encounter ☑
S25.122A	Major laceration of left innominate or subclavian artery, initial encounter ☑
S25.191A	Other specified injury of right innominate or subclavian artery, initial encounter ☑
S25.192A	Other specified injury of left innominate or subclavian artery, initial encounter ☑
S25.21XA	Minor laceration of superior vena cava, initial encounter
S25.22XA	Major laceration of superior vena cava, initial encounter
S25.29XA	Other specified injury of superior vena cava, initial encounter
S25.311A	Minor laceration of right innominate or subclavian vein, initial encounter ☑
S25.312A	Minor laceration of left innominate or subclavian vein, initial encounter ☑
S25.321A	Major laceration of right innominate or subclavian vein, initial encounter ☑
S25.322A	Major laceration of left innominate or subclavian vein, initial encounter ☑
S25.391A	Other specified injury of right innominate or subclavian vein, initial encounter ☑
S25.392A	Other specified injury of left innominate or subclavian vein, initial encounter ☑
S25.411A	Minor laceration of right pulmonary blood vessels, initial encounter ☑
S25.412A	Minor laceration of left pulmonary blood vessels, initial encounter ☑
S25.421A	Major laceration of right pulmonary blood vessels, initial encounter ☑
S25.422A	Major laceration of left pulmonary blood vessels, initial encounter ☑

S25.491A Other specified injury of right pulmonary blood vessels, initial encounter ☑

S25.492A Other specified injury of left pulmonary blood vessels, initial encounter ☑

S25.511A Laceration of intercostal blood vessels, right side, initial encounter ☑

S25.512A Laceration of intercostal blood vessels, left side, initial encounter ☑

S25.591A Other specified injury of intercostal blood vessels, right side, initial encounter ☑

S25.592A Other specified injury of intercostal blood vessels, left side, initial encounter ☑

S25.811A Laceration of other blood vessels of thorax, right side, initial encounter ☑

S25.812A Laceration of other blood vessels of thorax, left side, initial encounter ☑

S25.891A Other specified injury of other blood vessels of thorax, right side, initial encounter ☑

S25.892A Other specified injury of other blood vessels of thorax, left side, initial encounter ☑

S35.11XA Minor laceration of inferior vena cava, initial encounter

S35.12XA Major laceration of inferior vena cava, initial encounter

S35.19XA Other injury of inferior vena cava, initial encounter

AMA: **35211** 2015,Jul,3 **35216** 2018,Jan,8; 2017,Jan,8; 2016,Jan,13; 2015,Jan,16; 2014,Jan,11

Relative Value Units/Medicare Edits

Non-Facility RVU	Work	PE	MP	Total
35211	24.58	9.88	5.58	40.04
35216	36.61	14.87	8.23	59.71
Facility RVU	**Work**	**PE**	**MP**	**Total**
35211	24.58	9.88	5.58	40.04
35216	36.61	14.87	8.23	59.71

	FUD	Status	MUE	Modifiers				IOM Reference
35211	90	A	3(3)	51	50	62*	80	None
35216	90	A	2(3)	51	50	62*	80	

* with documentation

35221

35221 Repair blood vessel, direct; intra-abdominal

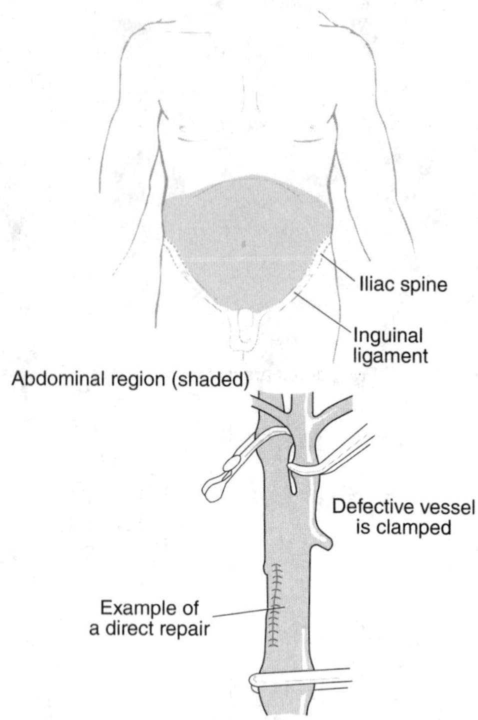

Explanation

The physician exposes the abnormal blood vessel (arterial or venous) by choosing an abdominal incision appropriate to the involved vessel. The abnormal vessel is examined and repaired by ligation (tying it off) or may be repaired by clamping it proximally and distally to the defect. The defect is sutured closed. A patch graft may be sutured over any remaining defect. Vessel patency is confirmed with a Doppler probe or angiography prior to closing the wound, leaving surgical drains in place.

Coding Tips

Establishing both inflow and outflow by any method is included. That portion of the operative arteriogram performed by the surgeon is also included. Angioscopy performed during therapeutic intervention should be reported in addition to the code for the primary procedure; see 35400. Any graft harvest is not reported separately. For repair of an intra-abdominal aneurysm, see 35081–35132. For repair of an intra-abdominal blood vessel with vein graft, see 35251; with graft other than vein, see 35281.

ICD-10-CM Diagnostic Codes

I70.1 Atherosclerosis of renal artery

I77.1 Stricture of artery

I77.811 Abdominal aortic ectasia

I77.812 Thoracoabdominal aortic ectasia

I82.0 Budd-Chiari syndrome

K55.011 Focal (segmental) acute (reversible) ischemia of small intestine

K55.012 Diffuse acute (reversible) ischemia of small intestine

K55.021 Focal (segmental) acute infarction of small intestine

K55.022 Diffuse acute infarction of small intestine

K55.031 Focal (segmental) acute (reversible) ischemia of large intestine

K55.032 Diffuse acute (reversible) ischemia of large intestine

K55.041	Focal (segmental) acute infarction of large intestine
K55.042	Diffuse acute infarction of large intestine
S35.01XA	Minor laceration of abdominal aorta, initial encounter
S35.02XA	Major laceration of abdominal aorta, initial encounter
S35.09XA	Other injury of abdominal aorta, initial encounter
S35.211A	Minor laceration of celiac artery, initial encounter
S35.212A	Major laceration of celiac artery, initial encounter
S35.218A	Other injury of celiac artery, initial encounter
S35.221A	Minor laceration of superior mesenteric artery, initial encounter
S35.222A	Major laceration of superior mesenteric artery, initial encounter
S35.228A	Other injury of superior mesenteric artery, initial encounter
S35.231A	Minor laceration of inferior mesenteric artery, initial encounter
S35.232A	Major laceration of inferior mesenteric artery, initial encounter
S35.238A	Other injury of inferior mesenteric artery, initial encounter
S35.291A	Minor laceration of branches of celiac and mesenteric artery, initial encounter
S35.292A	Major laceration of branches of celiac and mesenteric artery, initial encounter
S35.298A	Other injury of branches of celiac and mesenteric artery, initial encounter
S35.311A	Laceration of portal vein, initial encounter
S35.318A	Other specified injury of portal vein, initial encounter
S35.321A	Laceration of splenic vein, initial encounter
S35.328A	Other specified injury of splenic vein, initial encounter
S35.331A	Laceration of superior mesenteric vein, initial encounter
S35.338A	Other specified injury of superior mesenteric vein, initial encounter
S35.341A	Laceration of inferior mesenteric vein, initial encounter
S35.348A	Other specified injury of inferior mesenteric vein, initial encounter
S35.411A	Laceration of right renal artery, initial encounter ☑
S35.412A	Laceration of left renal artery, initial encounter ☑
S35.414A	Laceration of right renal vein, initial encounter ☑
S35.415A	Laceration of left renal vein, initial encounter ☑
S35.491A	Other specified injury of right renal artery, initial encounter ☑
S35.492A	Other specified injury of left renal artery, initial encounter ☑
S35.494A	Other specified injury of right renal vein, initial encounter ☑
S35.495A	Other specified injury of left renal vein, initial encounter ☑
S35.511A	Injury of right iliac artery, initial encounter ☑
S35.512A	Injury of left iliac artery, initial encounter ☑
S35.514A	Injury of right iliac vein, initial encounter ☑
S35.515A	Injury of left iliac vein, initial encounter ☑
S35.531A	Injury of right uterine artery, initial encounter ☑
S35.532A	Injury of left uterine artery, initial encounter ☑
S35.534A	Injury of right uterine vein, initial encounter ☑
S35.535A	Injury of left uterine vein, initial encounter ☑
S35.59XA	Injury of other iliac blood vessels, initial encounter
S35.8X1A	Laceration of other blood vessels at abdomen, lower back and pelvis level, initial encounter
S35.8X8A	Other specified injury of other blood vessels at abdomen, lower back and pelvis level, initial encounter

AMA: 35221 2012,Apr,3-9

Relative Value Units/Medicare Edits

Non-Facility RVU	Work	PE	MP	Total
35221	26.62	9.69	6.17	42.48
Facility RVU	**Work**	**PE**	**MP**	**Total**
35221	26.62	9.69	6.17	42.48

	FUD	Status	MUE	Modifiers				IOM Reference
35221	90	A	3(3)	51	50	62*	80	None

* with documentation

Terms To Know

arteriography. Radiologic study of an artery upon injection of dye.

Budd-Chiari syndrome. Thrombus or other obstruction of the hepatic vein, with an enlarged liver, intractable ascites, portal hypertension, and the growth of extensive collateral vessels.

ectasia. Pathological expansion, dilation, or distension of a hollow or tubular anatomic organ or structure.

35226

35226 Repair blood vessel, direct; lower extremity

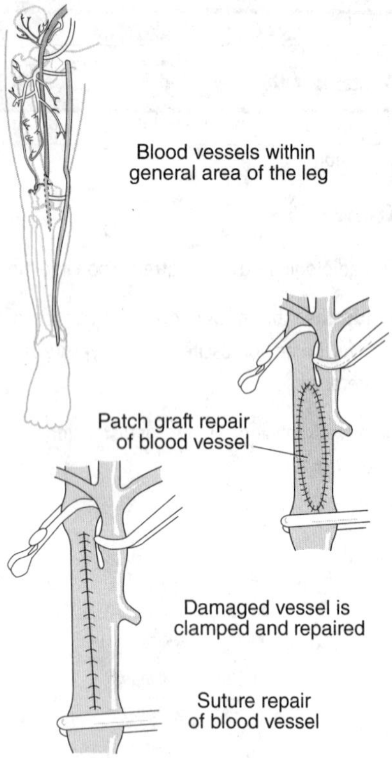

Explanation

The physician makes an incision in the skin of a lower extremity over the site of an injured blood vessel. The vessel is isolated and dissected from adjacent critical structures, and vessel clamps are applied. The edges of the injured vessel may be trimmed to ease repair. A patch graft may be sutured over the defect or the hole in the vessel may be repaired with sutures. The clamps are removed and the skin incision is repaired with a layered closure.

Coding Tips

Establishing both inflow and outflow by any method is included. That portion of the operative arteriogram performed by the surgeon is also included. Simple direct repair of a vessel is included in most primary cardiac procedures. Do not report 35226 separately for direct vessel repair following removal of the cannula during a cardiac procedure. Angioscopy performed during therapeutic intervention should be reported in addition to the code for the primary procedure, see 35400. Any graft harvest is not reported separately. For repair of an aneurysm, lower extremity, see 35141–35152. For repair of a blood vessel of a lower extremity with vein graft, see 35256; with synthetic graft, see 35286. For repair of a congenital arteriovenous fistula, see 35184. For repair of an acquired or traumatic arteriovenous fistula, see 35190. Do not report 35226 with 33969, 33984, 33985, or 33986.

ICD-10-CM Diagnostic Codes

I70.92 Chronic total occlusion of artery of the extremities
I77.2 Rupture of artery
I80.01 Phlebitis and thrombophlebitis of superficial vessels of right lower extremity ☑
I80.02 Phlebitis and thrombophlebitis of superficial vessels of left lower extremity ☑
I80.03 Phlebitis and thrombophlebitis of superficial vessels of lower extremities, bilateral ☑
I80.11 Phlebitis and thrombophlebitis of right femoral vein ☑
I80.12 Phlebitis and thrombophlebitis of left femoral vein ☑
I80.13 Phlebitis and thrombophlebitis of femoral vein, bilateral ☑
I80.221 Phlebitis and thrombophlebitis of right popliteal vein ☑
I80.222 Phlebitis and thrombophlebitis of left popliteal vein ☑
I80.223 Phlebitis and thrombophlebitis of popliteal vein, bilateral ☑
I80.231 Phlebitis and thrombophlebitis of right tibial vein ☑
I80.232 Phlebitis and thrombophlebitis of left tibial vein ☑
I80.233 Phlebitis and thrombophlebitis of tibial vein, bilateral ☑
S75.021A Major laceration of femoral artery, right leg, initial encounter ☑
S75.022A Major laceration of femoral artery, left leg, initial encounter ☑
S75.221A Major laceration of greater saphenous vein at hip and thigh level, right leg, initial encounter ☑
S75.222A Major laceration of greater saphenous vein at hip and thigh level, left leg, initial encounter ☑
S85.011A Laceration of popliteal artery, right leg, initial encounter ☑
S85.012A Laceration of popliteal artery, left leg, initial encounter ☑
S85.141A Laceration of anterior tibial artery, right leg, initial encounter ☑
S85.142A Laceration of anterior tibial artery, left leg, initial encounter ☑
S85.171A Laceration of posterior tibial artery, right leg, initial encounter ☑
S85.172A Laceration of posterior tibial artery, left leg, initial encounter ☑
S85.211A Laceration of peroneal artery, right leg, initial encounter ☑
S85.212A Laceration of peroneal artery, left leg, initial encounter ☑
S85.311A Laceration of greater saphenous vein at lower leg level, right leg, initial encounter ☑
S85.312A Laceration of greater saphenous vein at lower leg level, left leg, initial encounter ☑
S85.411A Laceration of lesser saphenous vein at lower leg level, right leg, initial encounter ☑
S85.412A Laceration of lesser saphenous vein at lower leg level, left leg, initial encounter ☑
S85.511A Laceration of popliteal vein, right leg, initial encounter ☑
S85.512A Laceration of popliteal vein, left leg, initial encounter ☑
S95.011A Laceration of dorsal artery of right foot, initial encounter ☑
S95.012A Laceration of dorsal artery of left foot, initial encounter ☑
S95.211A Laceration of dorsal vein of right foot, initial encounter ☑
S95.212A Laceration of dorsal vein of left foot, initial encounter ☑

AMA: 35226 2019,Jul,10; 2018,Jan,8; 2017,Jul,3; 2017,Jan,8; 2017,Aug,10; 2016,Jul,6; 2016,Jan,13; 2015,Jul,3; 2015,Jan,16; 2014,Jan,11; 2013,Mar,10-11; 2013,Dec,8

Relative Value Units/Medicare Edits

Non-Facility RVU	Work	PE	MP	Total
35226	15.3	5.35	3.5	24.15
Facility RVU	**Work**	**PE**	**MP**	**Total**
35226	15.3	5.35	3.5	24.15

	FUD	Status	MUE	Modifiers				IOM Reference
35226	90	A	3(3)	51	50	62*	80	None

* with documentation

35231

35231 Repair blood vessel with vein graft; neck

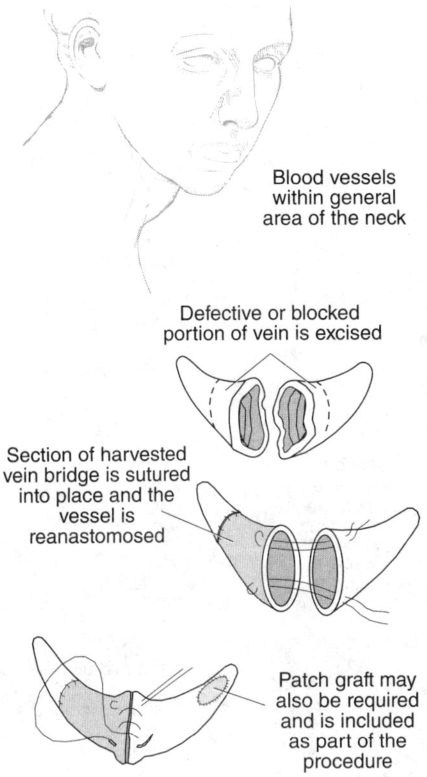

Explanation

The physician makes an incision in the skin in the neck over the site of an injured blood vessel. The vessel is isolated and dissected from adjacent critical structures, and vessel clamps are applied. The defect is too extensive to repair directly, so the physician removes a short length of vein. The physician repairs the injured vessel with a length of vein harvested from another site in the body or with cadaver vein. The vein is sutured end-to-end to the vessel, replacing the excised portion, or is used as a patch to repair a large hole in the side of the vessel. A patch graft may be sutured over any remaining defect. The clamps are removed and the skin incision is repaired with a layered closure.

Coding Tips

Establishing both inflow and outflow by any method is included. That portion of the operative arteriogram performed by the surgeon is also included. Angioscopy performed during therapeutic intervention should be reported in addition to the code for the primary procedure; see 35400. Any graft harvest is not reported separately. For repair of aneurysm carotid, subclavian, see 35001–35002. For direct repair of a blood vessel, neck, see 35201. For repair of a blood vessel of neck with synthetic graft, see 35261. For repair of a congenital arteriovenous fistula, see 35180. For repair of an acquired or traumatic arteriovenous fistula, see 35188.

ICD-10-CM Diagnostic Codes

G45.0	Vertebro-basilar artery syndrome
G45.1	Carotid artery syndrome (hemispheric)
G45.2	Multiple and bilateral precerebral artery syndromes
G45.8	Other transient cerebral ischemic attacks and related syndromes
G45.9	Transient cerebral ischemic attack, unspecified
I65.01	Occlusion and stenosis of right vertebral artery ☑
I65.02	Occlusion and stenosis of left vertebral artery ☑
I65.03	Occlusion and stenosis of bilateral vertebral arteries ☑
I65.1	Occlusion and stenosis of basilar artery
I65.21	Occlusion and stenosis of right carotid artery ☑
I65.22	Occlusion and stenosis of left carotid artery ☑
I65.23	Occlusion and stenosis of bilateral carotid arteries ☑
I65.8	Occlusion and stenosis of other precerebral arteries
I67.0	Dissection of cerebral arteries, nonruptured
I77.1	Stricture of artery
I77.2	Rupture of artery
I77.71	Dissection of carotid artery
I77.79	Dissection of other specified artery
I77.89	Other specified disorders of arteries and arterioles
S15.011A	Minor laceration of right carotid artery, initial encounter ☑
S15.012A	Minor laceration of left carotid artery, initial encounter ☑
S15.021A	Major laceration of right carotid artery, initial encounter ☑
S15.022A	Major laceration of left carotid artery, initial encounter ☑
S15.091A	Other specified injury of right carotid artery, initial encounter ☑
S15.092A	Other specified injury of left carotid artery, initial encounter ☑
S15.111A	Minor laceration of right vertebral artery, initial encounter ☑
S15.112A	Minor laceration of left vertebral artery, initial encounter ☑
S15.121A	Major laceration of right vertebral artery, initial encounter ☑
S15.122A	Major laceration of left vertebral artery, initial encounter ☑
S15.191A	Other specified injury of right vertebral artery, initial encounter ☑
S15.192A	Other specified injury of left vertebral artery, initial encounter ☑
S15.211A	Minor laceration of right external jugular vein, initial encounter ☑
S15.212A	Minor laceration of left external jugular vein, initial encounter ☑
S15.221A	Major laceration of right external jugular vein, initial encounter ☑
S15.222A	Major laceration of left external jugular vein, initial encounter ☑
S15.291A	Other specified injury of right external jugular vein, initial encounter ☑
S15.292A	Other specified injury of left external jugular vein, initial encounter ☑
S15.311A	Minor laceration of right internal jugular vein, initial encounter ☑
S15.312A	Minor laceration of left internal jugular vein, initial encounter ☑
S15.321A	Major laceration of right internal jugular vein, initial encounter ☑
S15.322A	Major laceration of left internal jugular vein, initial encounter ☑
S15.391A	Other specified injury of right internal jugular vein, initial encounter ☑
S15.392A	Other specified injury of left internal jugular vein, initial encounter ☑
S15.8XXA	Injury of other specified blood vessels at neck level, initial encounter
S25.111A	Minor laceration of right innominate or subclavian artery, initial encounter ☑
S25.112A	Minor laceration of left innominate or subclavian artery, initial encounter ☑
S25.121A	Major laceration of right innominate or subclavian artery, initial encounter ☑
S25.122A	Major laceration of left innominate or subclavian artery, initial encounter ☑
S25.191A	Other specified injury of right innominate or subclavian artery, initial encounter ☑

S25.192A Other specified injury of left innominate or subclavian artery, initial encounter ☑
S25.311A Minor laceration of right innominate or subclavian vein, initial encounter ☑
S25.312A Minor laceration of left innominate or subclavian vein, initial encounter ☑
S25.321A Major laceration of right innominate or subclavian vein, initial encounter ☑
S25.322A Major laceration of left innominate or subclavian vein, initial encounter ☑
S25.391A Other specified injury of right innominate or subclavian vein, initial encounter ☑
S25.392A Other specified injury of left innominate or subclavian vein, initial encounter ☑

AMA: 35231 2012,Apr,3-9

Relative Value Units/Medicare Edits

Non-Facility RVU	Work	PE	MP	Total
35231	21.16	10.68	3.92	35.76
Facility RVU	**Work**	**PE**	**MP**	**Total**
35231	21.16	10.68	3.92	35.76

	FUD	Status	MUE	Modifiers				IOM Reference
35231	90	A	2(3)	51	50	62*	80	None

* with documentation

35236

35236 Repair blood vessel with vein graft; upper extremity

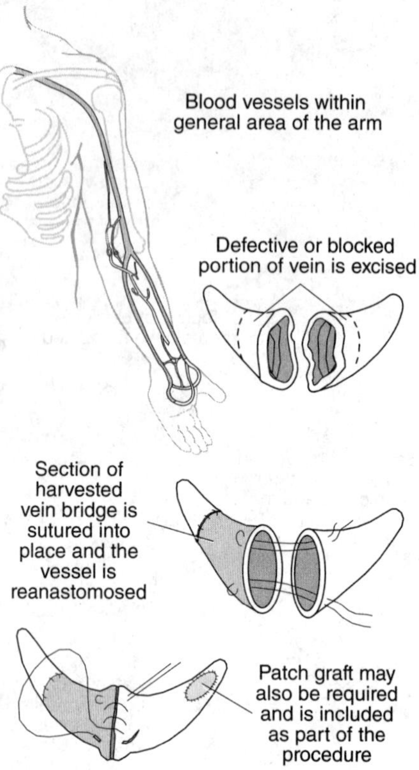

Explanation

The physician makes an incision in the skin of an upper extremity over the site of an injured blood vessel. The vessel is isolated and dissected from adjacent critical structures, and vessel clamps are applied. The defect is too extensive to repair directly, so the physician removes a short length of vein. The physician repairs the injured vessel with a length of vein harvested from another site in the body or with cadaver vein. The vein is sutured end-to-end to the vessel, replacing the excised portion, or is used as a patch to repair a large hole in the side of the vessel. A patch graft may be sutured over any remaining defect. The clamps are removed and the skin incision is repaired with a layered closure.

Coding Tips

Establishing both inflow and outflow by any method is included. That portion of the operative arteriogram performed by the surgeon is also included. Angioscopy performed during therapeutic intervention should be reported in addition to the code for the primary procedure; see 35400. Any graft harvest is not reported separately. For repair of an axillary-brachial aneurysm, see 35011–35013; for repair ulnar, radial aneurysm, see 35045. For direct repair of a blood vessel, upper extremity, see 35206. For repair of a blood vessel of the upper extremity with a synthetic graft, see 35266. For repair of a congenital arteriovenous fistula, see 35184. For repair of an acquired or traumatic arteriovenous fistula, see 35190.

ICD-10-CM Diagnostic Codes

I77.2 Rupture of artery
S45.011A Laceration of axillary artery, right side, initial encounter ☑
S45.091A Other specified injury of axillary artery, right side, initial encounter ☑
S45.111A Laceration of brachial artery, right side, initial encounter ☑

S45.191A Other specified injury of brachial artery, right side, initial encounter ☑

S45.211A Laceration of axillary or brachial vein, right side, initial encounter ☑

S45.291A Other specified injury of axillary or brachial vein, right side, initial encounter ☑

S45.311A Laceration of superficial vein at shoulder and upper arm level, right arm, initial encounter ☑

S45.391A Other specified injury of superficial vein at shoulder and upper arm level, right arm, initial encounter ☑

S45.811A Laceration of other specified blood vessels at shoulder and upper arm level, right arm, initial encounter ☑

S45.891A Other specified injury of other specified blood vessels at shoulder and upper arm level, right arm, initial encounter ☑

S55.011A Laceration of ulnar artery at forearm level, right arm, initial encounter ☑

S55.091A Other specified injury of ulnar artery at forearm level, right arm, initial encounter ☑

S55.111A Laceration of radial artery at forearm level, right arm, initial encounter ☑

S55.191A Other specified injury of radial artery at forearm level, right arm, initial encounter ☑

S55.211A Laceration of vein at forearm level, right arm, initial encounter ☑

S55.291A Other specified injury of vein at forearm level, right arm, initial encounter ☑

S55.811A Laceration of other blood vessels at forearm level, right arm, initial encounter ☑

S55.891A Other specified injury of other blood vessels at forearm level, right arm, initial encounter ☑

S65.011A Laceration of ulnar artery at wrist and hand level of right arm, initial encounter ☑

S65.091A Other specified injury of ulnar artery at wrist and hand level of right arm, initial encounter ☑

S65.111A Laceration of radial artery at wrist and hand level of right arm, initial encounter ☑

S65.191A Other specified injury of radial artery at wrist and hand level of right arm, initial encounter ☑

S65.411A Laceration of blood vessel of right thumb, initial encounter ☑

S65.491A Other specified injury of blood vessel of right thumb, initial encounter ☑

S65.510A Laceration of blood vessel of right index finger, initial encounter ☑

S65.512A Laceration of blood vessel of right middle finger, initial encounter ☑

S65.514A Laceration of blood vessel of right ring finger, initial encounter ☑

S65.516A Laceration of blood vessel of right little finger, initial encounter ☑

S65.590A Other specified injury of blood vessel of right index finger, initial encounter ☑

S65.592A Other specified injury of blood vessel of right middle finger, initial encounter ☑

S65.594A Other specified injury of blood vessel of right ring finger, initial encounter ☑

S65.596A Other specified injury of blood vessel of right little finger, initial encounter ☑

S65.811A Laceration of other blood vessels at wrist and hand level of right arm, initial encounter ☑

S65.891A Other specified injury of other blood vessels at wrist and hand level of right arm, initial encounter ☑

AMA: 35236 2018,Jan,8; 2017,Jan,8; 2016,Jan,13; 2015,Jan,16; 2014,Jan,11

Relative Value Units/Medicare Edits

Non-Facility RVU	Work	PE	MP	Total
35236	18.02	7.01	3.99	29.02
Facility RVU	**Work**	**PE**	**MP**	**Total**
35236	18.02	7.01	3.99	29.02

	FUD	Status	MUE	Modifiers				IOM Reference
35236	90	A	2(3)	51	50	62*	80	None

* with documentation

Terms To Know

anastomosis. Surgically created connection between ducts, blood vessels, or bowel segments to allow flow from one to the other.

graft. Tissue implant from another part of the body or another person.

Arteries and Veins

35241-35246

35241 Repair blood vessel with vein graft; intrathoracic, with bypass
35246 intrathoracic, without bypass

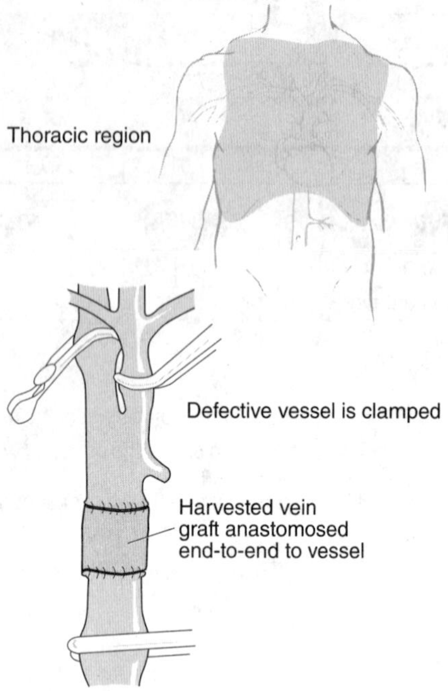

Explanation

The physician exposes the abnormal blood vessel (arterial or venous) by choosing a thoracic incision appropriate to the involved vessel. The physician places cardiopulmonary bypass catheters (in 35241) through incisions in the low inferior vena cava, the superior vena cava, and high aorta or femoral artery. The physician stops the heart by infusing cardioplegia solution into the coronary circulation. For both procedures, the physician examines the abnormal vessel and repairs it by clamping proximally and distally to the defect, and sewing in venous graft material harvested from the patient in order to bypass the abnormal area of the vessel (bypass graft). The physician confirms vessel patency with Doppler probe or angiography prior to taking the patient off cardiopulmonary bypass (in 35241) and closing the wound. The physician leaves chest and, possibly, mediastinal drains in place. Report 35246 when the procedure is performed without cardiopulmonary bypass.

Coding Tips

Establishing both inflow and outflow by any method is included. That portion of the operative arteriogram performed by the surgeon is also included. Angioscopy performed during therapeutic intervention should be reported in addition to the code for the primary procedure; see 35400. Any graft harvest is not reported separately. For repair of a thoracic aortic aneurysm, see 33858–33875. For repair of an innominate, subclavian aneurysm by thoracic incision, see 35021–35022. For a direct repair of an intrathoracic blood vessel, see 35211–35216; with graft other than vein, see 35271–35276.

ICD-10-CM Diagnostic Codes

I70.0	Atherosclerosis of aorta
I71.01	Dissection of thoracic aorta
I71.1	Thoracic aortic aneurysm, ruptured
I71.2	Thoracic aortic aneurysm, without rupture
I77.1	Stricture of artery
I77.2	Rupture of artery
I77.5	Necrosis of artery
I77.810	Thoracic aortic ectasia
I77.812	Thoracoabdominal aortic ectasia
I77.89	Other specified disorders of arteries and arterioles
I80.8	Phlebitis and thrombophlebitis of other sites
I87.1	Compression of vein
S25.01XA	Minor laceration of thoracic aorta, initial encounter
S25.02XA	Major laceration of thoracic aorta, initial encounter
S25.09XA	Other specified injury of thoracic aorta, initial encounter
S25.111A	Minor laceration of right innominate or subclavian artery, initial encounter ☑
S25.112A	Minor laceration of left innominate or subclavian artery, initial encounter ☑
S25.121A	Major laceration of right innominate or subclavian artery, initial encounter ☑
S25.122A	Major laceration of left innominate or subclavian artery, initial encounter ☑
S25.191A	Other specified injury of right innominate or subclavian artery, initial encounter ☑
S25.192A	Other specified injury of left innominate or subclavian artery, initial encounter ☑
S25.21XA	Minor laceration of superior vena cava, initial encounter
S25.22XA	Major laceration of superior vena cava, initial encounter
S25.29XA	Other specified injury of superior vena cava, initial encounter
S25.311A	Minor laceration of right innominate or subclavian vein, initial encounter ☑
S25.312A	Minor laceration of left innominate or subclavian vein, initial encounter ☑
S25.321A	Major laceration of right innominate or subclavian vein, initial encounter ☑
S25.322A	Major laceration of left innominate or subclavian vein, initial encounter ☑
S25.391A	Other specified injury of right innominate or subclavian vein, initial encounter ☑
S25.392A	Other specified injury of left innominate or subclavian vein, initial encounter ☑
S25.411A	Minor laceration of right pulmonary blood vessels, initial encounter ☑
S25.412A	Minor laceration of left pulmonary blood vessels, initial encounter ☑
S25.421A	Major laceration of right pulmonary blood vessels, initial encounter ☑
S25.422A	Major laceration of left pulmonary blood vessels, initial encounter ☑
S25.491A	Other specified injury of right pulmonary blood vessels, initial encounter ☑
S25.492A	Other specified injury of left pulmonary blood vessels, initial encounter ☑
S25.511A	Laceration of intercostal blood vessels, right side, initial encounter ☑
S25.512A	Laceration of intercostal blood vessels, left side, initial encounter ☑
S25.591A	Other specified injury of intercostal blood vessels, right side, initial encounter ☑

S25.592A Other specified injury of intercostal blood vessels, left side, initial encounter ☑
S25.811A Laceration of other blood vessels of thorax, right side, initial encounter ☑
S25.812A Laceration of other blood vessels of thorax, left side, initial encounter ☑
S25.891A Other specified injury of other blood vessels of thorax, right side, initial encounter ☑
S25.892A Other specified injury of other blood vessels of thorax, left side, initial encounter ☑
S35.11XA Minor laceration of inferior vena cava, initial encounter
S35.12XA Major laceration of inferior vena cava, initial encounter
S35.19XA Other injury of inferior vena cava, initial encounter

AMA: 35241 2012,Apr,3-9 **35246** 2012,Apr,3-9

Relative Value Units/Medicare Edits

Non-Facility RVU	Work	PE	MP	Total
35241	25.58	10.19	6.03	41.8
35246	28.23	10.73	6.66	45.62
Facility RVU	**Work**	**PE**	**MP**	**Total**
35241	25.58	10.19	6.03	41.8
35246	28.23	10.73	6.66	45.62

	FUD	Status	MUE	Modifiers				IOM Reference
35241	90	A	2(3)	51	50	62*	80	None
35246	90	A	2(3)	51	50	62*	80	

* with documentation

Terms To Know

aneurysm. Circumscribed dilation or outpouching of an artery wall, often containing blood clots and connecting directly with the lumen of the artery.

angioscopy. Visualization of capillary blood vessels with a microscope, or the inside of a blood vessel with a fiberoptic-equipped catheter.

arteriogram. Radiograph of arteries.

atherosclerosis. Buildup of yellowish plaques composed of cholesterol and lipoid material within the arteries.

bypass. Auxiliary or diverted route to maintain continuous flow.

catheter. Flexible tube inserted into an area of the body for introducing or withdrawing fluid.

graft. Tissue implant from another part of the body or another person.

necrosis. Death of cells or tissue within a living organ or structure.

35251

35251 Repair blood vessel with vein graft; intra-abdominal

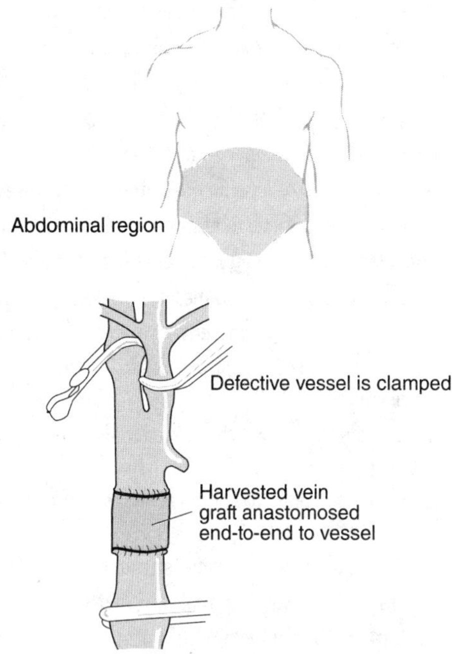

Explanation

The physician exposes the abnormal blood vessel (arterial or venous) by choosing an abdominal incision appropriate to the involved vessel. The physician examines the abnormal vessel and repairs it by clamping proximally and distally to the defect, and sewing in vein material harvested from the patient in order to bypass the abnormal area of the diseased vessel (bypass graft). The physician confirms vessel patency with Doppler probe or angiography prior to closing the wound. The physician leaves surgical drains in place.

Coding Tips

Establishing both inflow and outflow by any method is included. That portion of the operative arteriogram performed by the surgeon is also included. Angioscopy performed during therapeutic intervention should be reported in addition to the code for the primary procedure; see 35400. Any graft harvest is not reported separately. For repair of an intra-abdominal aneurysm, see 35081–35132. For direct repair of an intra-abdominal blood vessel, see 35221. For repair of an intra-abdominal blood vessel with graft other than vein, see 35281.

ICD-10-CM Diagnostic Codes

I70.1 Atherosclerosis of renal artery
I77.1 Stricture of artery
I77.811 Abdominal aortic ectasia
I77.812 Thoracoabdominal aortic ectasia
I82.0 Budd-Chiari syndrome
K55.011 Focal (segmental) acute (reversible) ischemia of small intestine
K55.012 Diffuse acute (reversible) ischemia of small intestine
K55.021 Focal (segmental) acute infarction of small intestine
K55.022 Diffuse acute infarction of small intestine
K55.031 Focal (segmental) acute (reversible) ischemia of large intestine
K55.032 Diffuse acute (reversible) ischemia of large intestine

K55.041	Focal (segmental) acute infarction of large intestine
K55.042	Diffuse acute infarction of large intestine
S35.01XA	Minor laceration of abdominal aorta, initial encounter
S35.02XA	Major laceration of abdominal aorta, initial encounter
S35.09XA	Other injury of abdominal aorta, initial encounter
S35.211A	Minor laceration of celiac artery, initial encounter
S35.212A	Major laceration of celiac artery, initial encounter
S35.218A	Other injury of celiac artery, initial encounter
S35.221A	Minor laceration of superior mesenteric artery, initial encounter
S35.222A	Major laceration of superior mesenteric artery, initial encounter
S35.228A	Other injury of superior mesenteric artery, initial encounter
S35.231A	Minor laceration of inferior mesenteric artery, initial encounter
S35.232A	Major laceration of inferior mesenteric artery, initial encounter
S35.238A	Other injury of inferior mesenteric artery, initial encounter
S35.291A	Minor laceration of branches of celiac and mesenteric artery, initial encounter
S35.292A	Major laceration of branches of celiac and mesenteric artery, initial encounter
S35.298A	Other injury of branches of celiac and mesenteric artery, initial encounter
S35.311A	Laceration of portal vein, initial encounter
S35.318A	Other specified injury of portal vein, initial encounter
S35.321A	Laceration of splenic vein, initial encounter
S35.328A	Other specified injury of splenic vein, initial encounter
S35.331A	Laceration of superior mesenteric vein, initial encounter
S35.338A	Other specified injury of superior mesenteric vein, initial encounter
S35.341A	Laceration of inferior mesenteric vein, initial encounter
S35.348A	Other specified injury of inferior mesenteric vein, initial encounter
S35.411A	Laceration of right renal artery, initial encounter ☑
S35.412A	Laceration of left renal artery, initial encounter ☑
S35.414A	Laceration of right renal vein, initial encounter ☑
S35.415A	Laceration of left renal vein, initial encounter ☑
S35.491A	Other specified injury of right renal artery, initial encounter ☑
S35.492A	Other specified injury of left renal artery, initial encounter ☑
S35.494A	Other specified injury of right renal vein, initial encounter ☑
S35.495A	Other specified injury of left renal vein, initial encounter ☑
S35.511A	Injury of right iliac artery, initial encounter ☑
S35.512A	Injury of left iliac artery, initial encounter ☑
S35.514A	Injury of right iliac vein, initial encounter ☑
S35.515A	Injury of left iliac vein, initial encounter ☑
S35.531A	Injury of right uterine artery, initial encounter ☑
S35.532A	Injury of left uterine artery, initial encounter ☑
S35.534A	Injury of right uterine vein, initial encounter ☑
S35.535A	Injury of left uterine vein, initial encounter ☑
S35.59XA	Injury of other iliac blood vessels, initial encounter
S35.8X1A	Laceration of other blood vessels at abdomen, lower back and pelvis level, initial encounter
S35.8X8A	Other specified injury of other blood vessels at abdomen, lower back and pelvis level, initial encounter

AMA: **35251** 2012,Apr,3-9

Relative Value Units/Medicare Edits

Non-Facility RVU	Work	PE	MP	Total
35251	31.91	11.19	7.3	50.4
Facility RVU	**Work**	**PE**	**MP**	**Total**
35251	31.91	11.19	7.3	50.4

	FUD	Status	MUE	Modifiers				IOM Reference
35251	90	A	2(3)	51	50	62*	80	None

* with documentation

Terms To Know

angioscopy. Visualization of capillary blood vessels with a microscope, or the inside of a blood vessel with a fiberoptic-equipped catheter.

arteriogram. Radiograph of arteries.

atherosclerosis. Buildup of yellowish plaques composed of cholesterol and lipoid material within the arteries.

Budd-Chiari syndrome. Thrombus or other obstruction of the hepatic vein, with an enlarged liver, intractable ascites, portal hypertension, and the growth of extensive collateral vessels.

bypass. Auxiliary or diverted route to maintain continuous flow.

digital subtraction angiography. Diagnostic imaging technique that applies computer technology to fluoroscopy for the purpose of visualizing the same vascular structures observable with conventional angiography.

graft. Tissue implant from another part of the body or another person.

harvest. Removal of cells or tissue from their native site to be used as a graft or transplant to another part of the donor's body or placed into another person.

stricture. Narrowing of an anatomical structure.

35256

35256 Repair blood vessel with vein graft; lower extremity

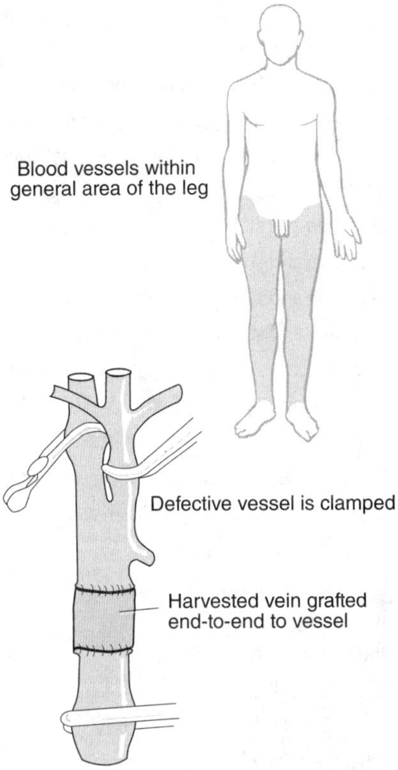

Explanation

The physician makes an incision in the skin of a lower extremity over the site of an injured blood vessel. The vessel is isolated and dissected from adjacent critical structures, and vessel clamps are applied. The defect is too extensive to repair directly, so the physician removes a short length of vein. The physician repairs the injured vessel with a length of vein harvested from another site in the body or with cadaver vein. The vein is sutured end-to-end to the vessel, replacing the excised portion, or is used as a patch to repair a large hole in the side of the vessel. A patch graft may be sutured over any remaining defect. The clamps are removed and the skin incision is repaired with a layered closure.

Coding Tips

Establishing both inflow and outflow by any method is included. That portion of the operative arteriogram performed by the surgeon is also included. Angioscopy performed during therapeutic intervention should be reported in addition to the code for the primary procedure; see 35400. Any graft harvest is not reported separately. For repair of an aneurysm, lower extremity, see 35141–35152. For direct repair of a blood vessel, lower extremity, see 35226. For repair of a lower extremity blood vessel with graft other than vein, see 35286. For repair of a congenital arteriovenous fistula, see 35184. For repair of an acquired or traumatic arteriovenous fistula, see 35190.

ICD-10-CM Diagnostic Codes

I70.92	Chronic total occlusion of artery of the extremities
I77.2	Rupture of artery
I80.01	Phlebitis and thrombophlebitis of superficial vessels of right lower extremity ☑
I80.02	Phlebitis and thrombophlebitis of superficial vessels of left lower extremity ☑
I80.03	Phlebitis and thrombophlebitis of superficial vessels of lower extremities, bilateral ☑
I80.11	Phlebitis and thrombophlebitis of right femoral vein ☑
I80.12	Phlebitis and thrombophlebitis of left femoral vein ☑
I80.13	Phlebitis and thrombophlebitis of femoral vein, bilateral ☑
I80.221	Phlebitis and thrombophlebitis of right popliteal vein ☑
I80.222	Phlebitis and thrombophlebitis of left popliteal vein ☑
I80.223	Phlebitis and thrombophlebitis of popliteal vein, bilateral ☑
I80.231	Phlebitis and thrombophlebitis of right tibial vein ☑
I80.232	Phlebitis and thrombophlebitis of left tibial vein ☑
I80.233	Phlebitis and thrombophlebitis of tibial vein, bilateral ☑
S75.021A	Major laceration of femoral artery, right leg, initial encounter ☑
S75.022A	Major laceration of femoral artery, left leg, initial encounter ☑
S75.221A	Major laceration of greater saphenous vein at hip and thigh level, right leg, initial encounter ☑
S75.222A	Major laceration of greater saphenous vein at hip and thigh level, left leg, initial encounter ☑
S85.011A	Laceration of popliteal artery, right leg, initial encounter ☑
S85.012A	Laceration of popliteal artery, left leg, initial encounter ☑
S85.141A	Laceration of anterior tibial artery, right leg, initial encounter ☑
S85.142A	Laceration of anterior tibial artery, left leg, initial encounter ☑
S85.171A	Laceration of posterior tibial artery, right leg, initial encounter ☑
S85.172A	Laceration of posterior tibial artery, left leg, initial encounter ☑
S85.211A	Laceration of peroneal artery, right leg, initial encounter ☑
S85.212A	Laceration of peroneal artery, left leg, initial encounter ☑
S85.311A	Laceration of greater saphenous vein at lower leg level, right leg, initial encounter ☑
S85.312A	Laceration of greater saphenous vein at lower leg level, left leg, initial encounter ☑
S85.411A	Laceration of lesser saphenous vein at lower leg level, right leg, initial encounter ☑
S85.412A	Laceration of lesser saphenous vein at lower leg level, left leg, initial encounter ☑
S85.511A	Laceration of popliteal vein, right leg, initial encounter ☑
S85.512A	Laceration of popliteal vein, left leg, initial encounter ☑
S95.011A	Laceration of dorsal artery of right foot, initial encounter ☑
S95.012A	Laceration of dorsal artery of left foot, initial encounter ☑
S95.211A	Laceration of dorsal vein of right foot, initial encounter ☑
S95.212A	Laceration of dorsal vein of left foot, initial encounter ☑

AMA: 35256 2012,Apr,3-9

Relative Value Units/Medicare Edits

Non-Facility RVU	Work	PE	MP	Total
35256	19.06	6.29	4.34	29.69
Facility RVU	**Work**	**PE**	**MP**	**Total**
35256	19.06	6.29	4.34	29.69

	FUD	Status	MUE	Modifiers				IOM Reference
35256	90	A	2(3)	51	50	62*	80	None

* with documentation

35261

35261 Repair blood vessel with graft other than vein; neck

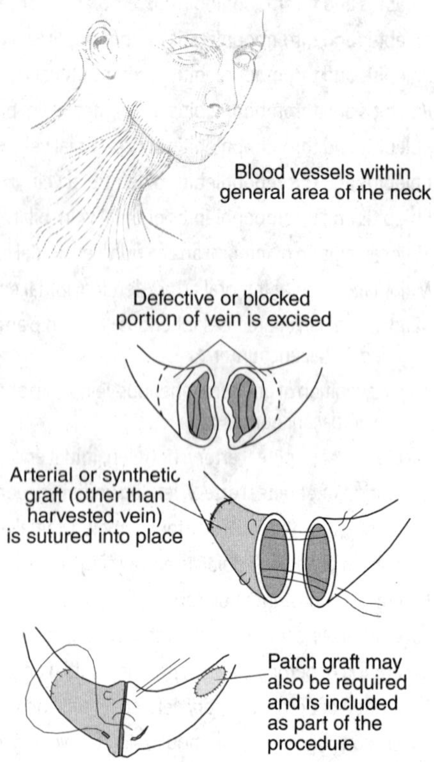

Explanation

The physician makes an incision in the skin of the neck over the site of an injured blood vessel. The vessel is isolated and dissected from adjacent critical structures and vessel clamps are applied. If the defect is too extensive to repair directly, the physician repairs the injured vessel with a length of synthetic graft material. The synthetic graft is sutured end-to-end to the vessel, replacing the excised portion. A patch graft may be sutured over any remaining defect. The clamps are removed and the skin incision is repaired with a layered closure.

Coding Tips

Establishing both inflow and outflow by any method is included. That portion of the operative arteriogram performed by the surgeon is also included. Angioscopy performed during therapeutic intervention should be reported in addition to the code for the primary procedure; see 35400. Any graft harvest is not reported separately. For repair of an aneurysm, carotid, subclavian, see 35001–35002. For direct repair of a blood vessel, neck, see 35201. For repair of a blood vessel of neck with vein graft, see 35231. For repair of a congenital arteriovenous fistula, see 35180. For repair of an acquired or traumatic arteriovenous fistula, see 35188.

ICD-10-CM Diagnostic Codes

G45.0	Vertebro-basilar artery syndrome
G45.1	Carotid artery syndrome (hemispheric)
G45.2	Multiple and bilateral precerebral artery syndromes
G45.3	Amaurosis fugax
G45.8	Other transient cerebral ischemic attacks and related syndromes
G45.9	Transient cerebral ischemic attack, unspecified
I63.011	Cerebral infarction due to thrombosis of right vertebral artery ☑
I63.012	Cerebral infarction due to thrombosis of left vertebral artery ☑
I63.02	Cerebral infarction due to thrombosis of basilar artery
I63.031	Cerebral infarction due to thrombosis of right carotid artery ☑
I63.032	Cerebral infarction due to thrombosis of left carotid artery ☑
I63.111	Cerebral infarction due to embolism of right vertebral artery ☑
I63.112	Cerebral infarction due to embolism of left vertebral artery ☑
I63.12	Cerebral infarction due to embolism of basilar artery
I63.131	Cerebral infarction due to embolism of right carotid artery ☑
I63.132	Cerebral infarction due to embolism of left carotid artery ☑
I65.01	Occlusion and stenosis of right vertebral artery ☑
I65.02	Occlusion and stenosis of left vertebral artery ☑
I65.03	Occlusion and stenosis of bilateral vertebral arteries ☑
I65.1	Occlusion and stenosis of basilar artery
I65.21	Occlusion and stenosis of right carotid artery ☑
I65.22	Occlusion and stenosis of left carotid artery ☑
I65.23	Occlusion and stenosis of bilateral carotid arteries ☑
I65.8	Occlusion and stenosis of other precerebral arteries
I67.81	Acute cerebrovascular insufficiency
I67.841	Reversible cerebrovascular vasoconstriction syndrome
I67.848	Other cerebrovascular vasospasm and vasoconstriction
I67.89	Other cerebrovascular disease
I72.0	Aneurysm of carotid artery
I77.1	Stricture of artery
I77.2	Rupture of artery
I77.71	Dissection of carotid artery
I77.79	Dissection of other specified artery
I77.89	Other specified disorders of arteries and arterioles
S15.011A	Minor laceration of right carotid artery, initial encounter ☑
S15.012A	Minor laceration of left carotid artery, initial encounter ☑
S15.021A	Major laceration of right carotid artery, initial encounter ☑
S15.022A	Major laceration of left carotid artery, initial encounter ☑
S15.091A	Other specified injury of right carotid artery, initial encounter ☑
S15.092A	Other specified injury of left carotid artery, initial encounter ☑
S15.111A	Minor laceration of right vertebral artery, initial encounter ☑
S15.112A	Minor laceration of left vertebral artery, initial encounter ☑
S15.121A	Major laceration of right vertebral artery, initial encounter ☑
S15.122A	Major laceration of left vertebral artery, initial encounter ☑
S15.191A	Other specified injury of right vertebral artery, initial encounter ☑
S15.192A	Other specified injury of left vertebral artery, initial encounter ☑
S15.211A	Minor laceration of right external jugular vein, initial encounter ☑
S15.212A	Minor laceration of left external jugular vein, initial encounter ☑
S15.221A	Major laceration of right external jugular vein, initial encounter ☑
S15.222A	Major laceration of left external jugular vein, initial encounter ☑
S15.291A	Other specified injury of right external jugular vein, initial encounter ☑
S15.292A	Other specified injury of left external jugular vein, initial encounter ☑
S15.311A	Minor laceration of right internal jugular vein, initial encounter ☑
S15.312A	Minor laceration of left internal jugular vein, initial encounter ☑
S15.321A	Major laceration of right internal jugular vein, initial encounter ☑
S15.322A	Major laceration of left internal jugular vein, initial encounter ☑
S15.391A	Other specified injury of right internal jugular vein, initial encounter ☑

S15.392A Other specified injury of left internal jugular vein, initial encounter ☑

S15.8XXA Injury of other specified blood vessels at neck level, initial encounter

AMA: 35261 2012,Apr,3-9

Relative Value Units/Medicare Edits

Non-Facility RVU	Work	PE	MP	Total
35261	18.96	4.93	4.39	28.28
Facility RVU	**Work**	**PE**	**MP**	**Total**
35261	18.96	4.93	4.39	28.28

	FUD	Status	MUE	Modifiers				IOM Reference
35261	90	A	1(3)	51	50	62*	80	None

* with documentation

Terms To Know

aneurysm. Circumscribed dilation or outpouching of an artery wall, often containing blood clots and connecting directly with the lumen of the artery.

angioscopy. Visualization of capillary blood vessels with a microscope, or the inside of a blood vessel with a fiberoptic-equipped catheter.

arteriogram. Radiograph of arteries.

fistula. Abnormal tube-like passage between two body cavities or organs or from an organ to the outside surface.

graft. Tissue implant from another part of the body or another person.

harvest. Removal of cells or tissue from their native site to be used as a graft or transplant to another part of the donor's body or placed into another person.

occlusion. Constriction, closure, or blockage of a passage.

stenosis. Narrowing or constriction of a passage.

35266

35266 Repair blood vessel with graft other than vein; upper extremity

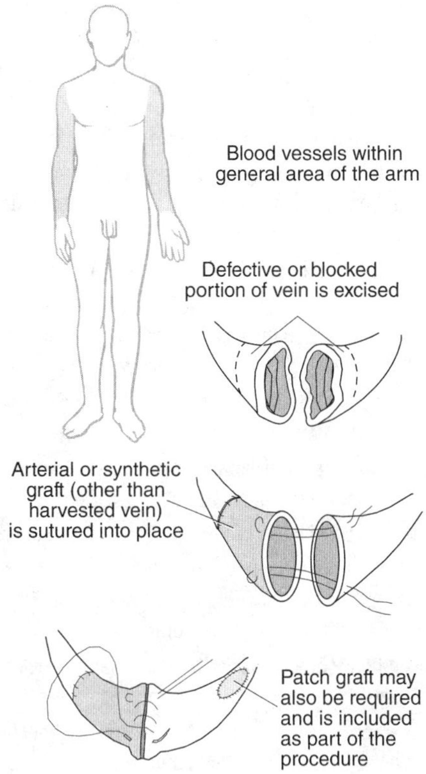

Explanation

The physician makes an incision in the skin of an upper extremity over the site of an injured blood vessel. The vessel is isolated and dissected from adjacent critical structures and vessel clamps are applied. If the defect is too extensive to repair directly, the physician repairs the injured vessel with a length of synthetic graft material. The synthetic graft is sutured end-to-end to the vessel, replacing the excised portion. A patch graft may be sutured over any remaining defect. The clamps are removed and the skin incision is repaired with layered closure.

Coding Tips

Establishing both inflow and outflow by any method is included. That portion of the operative arteriogram performed by the surgeon is also included. Angioscopy performed during therapeutic intervention should be reported in addition to the code for the primary procedure; see 35400. Any graft harvest is not reported separately. For repair of an axillary-brachial aneurysm, see 35011–35013; for repair ulnar, radial aneurysm, see 35045. For direct repair of a blood vessel, upper extremity, see 35206. For repair of a blood vessel, upper extremity, with vein graft, see 35236. For repair of a congenital arteriovenous fistula, see 35184. For repair of an acquired or traumatic arteriovenous fistula, see 35190.

ICD-10-CM Diagnostic Codes

I70.92 Chronic total occlusion of artery of the extremities

I77.2 Rupture of artery

S45.011A Laceration of axillary artery, right side, initial encounter ☑

S45.012A Laceration of axillary artery, left side, initial encounter ☑

S45.091A Other specified injury of axillary artery, right side, initial encounter ☑

S45.092A Other specified injury of axillary artery, left side, initial encounter ☑

S45.111A Laceration of brachial artery, right side, initial encounter ☑

S45.112A Laceration of brachial artery, left side, initial encounter ☑

S45.191A Other specified injury of brachial artery, right side, initial encounter ☑

S45.192A Other specified injury of brachial artery, left side, initial encounter ☑

S45.211A Laceration of axillary or brachial vein, right side, initial encounter ☑

S45.212A Laceration of axillary or brachial vein, left side, initial encounter ☑

S45.291A Other specified injury of axillary or brachial vein, right side, initial encounter ☑

S45.292A Other specified injury of axillary or brachial vein, left side, initial encounter ☑

S45.311A Laceration of superficial vein at shoulder and upper arm level, right arm, initial encounter ☑

S45.312A Laceration of superficial vein at shoulder and upper arm level, left arm, initial encounter ☑

S45.391A Other specified injury of superficial vein at shoulder and upper arm level, right arm, initial encounter ☑

S45.392A Other specified injury of superficial vein at shoulder and upper arm level, left arm, initial encounter ☑

S45.811A Laceration of other specified blood vessels at shoulder and upper arm level, right arm, initial encounter ☑

S45.812A Laceration of other specified blood vessels at shoulder and upper arm level, left arm, initial encounter ☑

S45.891A Other specified injury of other specified blood vessels at shoulder and upper arm level, right arm, initial encounter ☑

S45.892A Other specified injury of other specified blood vessels at shoulder and upper arm level, left arm, initial encounter ☑

S55.011A Laceration of ulnar artery at forearm level, right arm, initial encounter ☑

S55.012A Laceration of ulnar artery at forearm level, left arm, initial encounter ☑

S55.091A Other specified injury of ulnar artery at forearm level, right arm, initial encounter ☑

S55.092A Other specified injury of ulnar artery at forearm level, left arm, initial encounter ☑

S55.111A Laceration of radial artery at forearm level, right arm, initial encounter ☑

S55.112A Laceration of radial artery at forearm level, left arm, initial encounter ☑

S55.191A Other specified injury of radial artery at forearm level, right arm, initial encounter ☑

S55.192A Other specified injury of radial artery at forearm level, left arm, initial encounter ☑

S55.211A Laceration of vein at forearm level, right arm, initial encounter ☑

S55.212A Laceration of vein at forearm level, left arm, initial encounter ☑

S55.291A Other specified injury of vein at forearm level, right arm, initial encounter ☑

S55.292A Other specified injury of vein at forearm level, left arm, initial encounter ☑

S55.811A Laceration of other blood vessels at forearm level, right arm, initial encounter ☑

S55.812A Laceration of other blood vessels at forearm level, left arm, initial encounter ☑

S55.891A Other specified injury of other blood vessels at forearm level, right arm, initial encounter ☑

S55.892A Other specified injury of other blood vessels at forearm level, left arm, initial encounter ☑

S65.011A Laceration of ulnar artery at wrist and hand level of right arm, initial encounter ☑

S65.012A Laceration of ulnar artery at wrist and hand level of left arm, initial encounter ☑

S65.091A Other specified injury of ulnar artery at wrist and hand level of right arm, initial encounter ☑

S65.092A Other specified injury of ulnar artery at wrist and hand level of left arm, initial encounter ☑

S65.111A Laceration of radial artery at wrist and hand level of right arm, initial encounter ☑

S65.112A Laceration of radial artery at wrist and hand level of left arm, initial encounter ☑

S65.191A Other specified injury of radial artery at wrist and hand level of right arm, initial encounter ☑

S65.192A Other specified injury of radial artery at wrist and hand level of left arm, initial encounter ☑

S65.411A Laceration of blood vessel of right thumb, initial encounter ☑

S65.412A Laceration of blood vessel of left thumb, initial encounter ☑

S65.510A Laceration of blood vessel of right index finger, initial encounter ☑

S65.511A Laceration of blood vessel of left index finger, initial encounter ☑

S65.512A Laceration of blood vessel of right middle finger, initial encounter ☑

S65.513A Laceration of blood vessel of left middle finger, initial encounter ☑

S65.514A Laceration of blood vessel of right ring finger, initial encounter ☑

S65.515A Laceration of blood vessel of left ring finger, initial encounter ☑

S65.516A Laceration of blood vessel of right little finger, initial encounter ☑

S65.517A Laceration of blood vessel of left little finger, initial encounter ☑

S65.811A Laceration of other blood vessels at wrist and hand level of right arm, initial encounter ☑

S65.812A Laceration of other blood vessels at wrist and hand level of left arm, initial encounter ☑

S65.891A Other specified injury of other blood vessels at wrist and hand level of right arm, initial encounter ☑

S65.892A Other specified injury of other blood vessels at wrist and hand level of left arm, initial encounter ☑

AMA: 35266 2018,Jan,8; 2017,Jan,8; 2016,Jan,13; 2015,Jan,16; 2014,Jan,11

Relative Value Units/Medicare Edits

Non-Facility RVU	Work	PE	MP	Total
35266	15.83	5.68	3.63	25.14
Facility RVU	**Work**	**PE**	**MP**	**Total**
35266	15.83	5.68	3.63	25.14

	FUD	Status	MUE	Modifiers				IOM Reference
35266	90	A	2(3)	51	50	62*	80	None

* with documentation

35271-35276

35271 Repair blood vessel with graft other than vein; intrathoracic, with bypass

35276 intrathoracic, without bypass

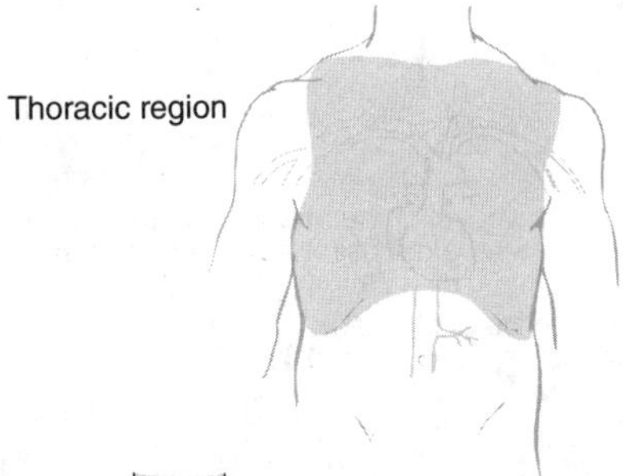

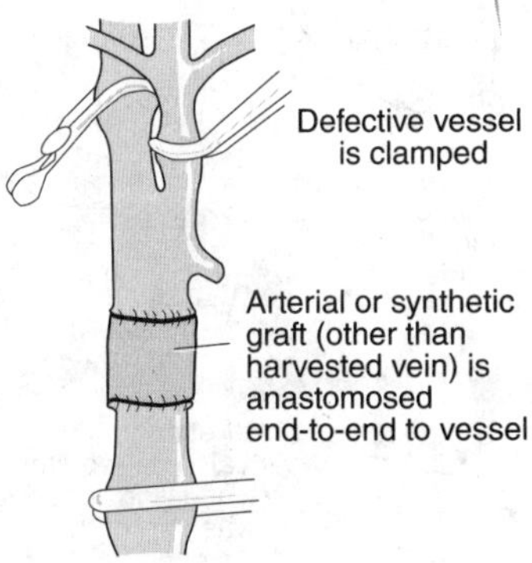

Explanation

In 35271, the physician exposes the abnormal blood vessel (arterial or venous) by choosing a thoracic incision appropriate to the involved vessel. The physician places cardiopulmonary bypass catheters (through incisions in the low inferior vena cava, the superior vena cava, and high aorta or femoral artery). The physician stops the heart by infusing cardioplegia solution into the coronary circulation. The physician examines the abnormal vessel and repairs it by clamping proximally and distally to the defect, and sewing in synthetic graft material in order to bypass the abnormal area of the vessel (bypass graft). The physician confirms vessel patency with Doppler probe or angiography prior to taking the patient off cardiopulmonary bypass and closing the wound. The physician leaves chest and, possibly, mediastinal drains in place. In 35276, the physician exposes the abnormal blood vessel (arterial or venous) by choosing a thoracic incision appropriate to the involved vessel. The physician examines the abnormal vessel and repairs it by clamping proximally and distally to the defect, and sewing in synthetic graft material in order to bypass the abnormal portion of the repaired vessel (bypass graft). The physician confirms vessel patency with Doppler probe or angiography prior to closing the wound. The physician leaves chest and, possibly, mediastinal drains in place.

Coding Tips

Establishing both inflow and outflow by any method is included. That portion of the operative arteriogram performed by the surgeon is also included. Angioscopy performed during therapeutic intervention should be reported in addition to the code for the primary procedure; see 35400. Any graft harvest is not reported separately. For repair of a thoracic aortic aneurysm, see 33858-33875. For repair of an innominate, subclavian aneurysm by thoracic incision, see 35021-35022. For direct repair of an intrathoracic blood vessel, see 35211-35216. For repair of an intrathoracic blood vessel with vein graft, see 35241-35246.

ICD-10-CM Diagnostic Codes

I70.0	Atherosclerosis of aorta
I71.01	Dissection of thoracic aorta
I71.1	Thoracic aortic aneurysm, ruptured
I71.2	Thoracic aortic aneurysm, without rupture
I77.1	Stricture of artery
I77.2	Rupture of artery
I77.5	Necrosis of artery
I77.810	Thoracic aortic ectasia
I77.812	Thoracoabdominal aortic ectasia
I77.89	Other specified disorders of arteries and arterioles
I80.8	Phlebitis and thrombophlebitis of other sites
I87.1	Compression of vein
S25.01XA	Minor laceration of thoracic aorta, initial encounter
S25.02XA	Major laceration of thoracic aorta, initial encounter
S25.09XA	Other specified injury of thoracic aorta, initial encounter
S25.111A	Minor laceration of right innominate or subclavian artery, initial encounter ☑
S25.112A	Minor laceration of left innominate or subclavian artery, initial encounter ☑
S25.121A	Major laceration of right innominate or subclavian artery, initial encounter ☑
S25.122A	Major laceration of left innominate or subclavian artery, initial encounter ☑
S25.191A	Other specified injury of right innominate or subclavian artery, initial encounter ☑
S25.192A	Other specified injury of left innominate or subclavian artery, initial encounter ☑
S25.21XA	Minor laceration of superior vena cava, initial encounter
S25.22XA	Major laceration of superior vena cava, initial encounter
S25.29XA	Other specified injury of superior vena cava, initial encounter
S25.311A	Minor laceration of right innominate or subclavian vein, initial encounter ☑
S25.312A	Minor laceration of left innominate or subclavian vein, initial encounter ☑
S25.321A	Major laceration of right innominate or subclavian vein, initial encounter ☑
S25.322A	Major laceration of left innominate or subclavian vein, initial encounter ☑
S25.391A	Other specified injury of right innominate or subclavian vein, initial encounter ☑
S25.392A	Other specified injury of left innominate or subclavian vein, initial encounter ☑
S25.411A	Minor laceration of right pulmonary blood vessels, initial encounter ☑
S25.412A	Minor laceration of left pulmonary blood vessels, initial encounter ☑
S25.421A	Major laceration of right pulmonary blood vessels, initial encounter ☑
S25.422A	Major laceration of left pulmonary blood vessels, initial encounter ☑
S25.491A	Other specified injury of right pulmonary blood vessels, initial encounter ☑
S25.492A	Other specified injury of left pulmonary blood vessels, initial encounter ☑

S25.511A Laceration of intercostal blood vessels, right side, initial encounter ☑

S25.512A Laceration of intercostal blood vessels, left side, initial encounter ☑

S25.591A Other specified injury of intercostal blood vessels, right side, initial encounter ☑

S25.592A Other specified injury of intercostal blood vessels, left side, initial encounter ☑

S25.811A Laceration of other blood vessels of thorax, right side, initial encounter ☑

S25.812A Laceration of other blood vessels of thorax, left side, initial encounter ☑

S25.891A Other specified injury of other blood vessels of thorax, right side, initial encounter ☑

S25.892A Other specified injury of other blood vessels of thorax, left side, initial encounter ☑

S35.11XA Minor laceration of inferior vena cava, initial encounter

S35.12XA Major laceration of inferior vena cava, initial encounter

S35.19XA Other injury of inferior vena cava, initial encounter

AMA: 35271 2012,Apr,3-9 **35276** 2012,Apr,3-9

Relative Value Units/Medicare Edits

Non-Facility RVU	Work	PE	MP	Total
35271	24.58	9.88	5.56	40.02
35276	25.83	10.51	6.09	42.43
Facility RVU	**Work**	**PE**	**MP**	**Total**
35271	24.58	9.88	5.56	40.02
35276	25.83	10.51	6.09	42.43

	FUD	Status	MUE	Modifiers				IOM Reference
35271	90	A	2(3)	51	50	62*	80	None
35276	90	A	2(3)	51	50	62*	80	

* with documentation

35281

35281 Repair blood vessel with graft other than vein; intra-abdominal

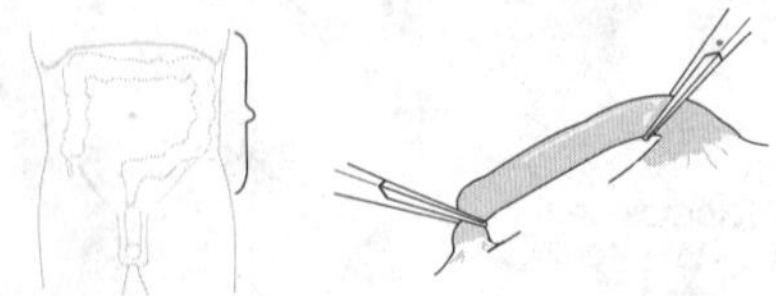

A defective vessel of the abdominal area, venous or arterial, is repaired using a graft other than vein

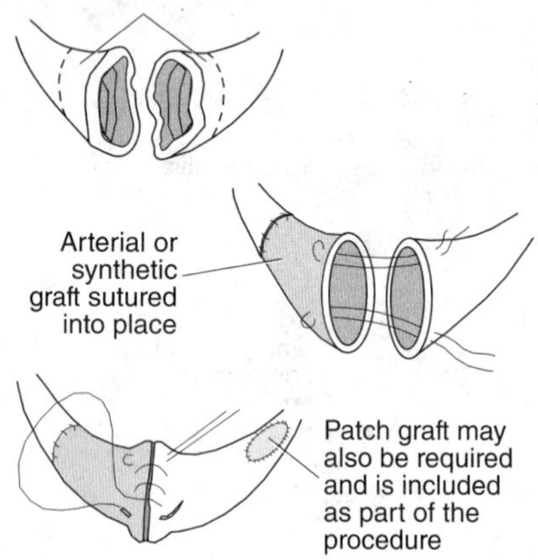

Explanation

The physician exposes the abnormal blood vessel (arterial or venous) by choosing an abdominal incision appropriate to the involved vessel. The physician examines the abnormal vessel and repairs it by clamping proximally and distally to the defect, and sewing in synthetic graft material in order to bypass the abnormal area of the diseased vessel (bypass graft). The physician confirms vessel patency with Doppler probe or angiography prior to closing the wound. The physician leaves surgical drains in place.

Coding Tips

Establishing both inflow and outflow by any method is included. That portion of the operative arteriogram performed by the surgeon is also included. Angioscopy performed during therapeutic intervention should be reported in addition to the code for the primary procedure; see 35400. Any graft harvest is not reported separately. For repair of an intra-abdominal aneurysm, see 35081–35132. For direct repair of an intra-abdominal blood vessel, see 35221. For repair of an intra-abdominal blood vessel with vein graft, see 35251.

ICD-10-CM Diagnostic Codes

I70.1 Atherosclerosis of renal artery

I77.1 Stricture of artery

I77.2 Rupture of artery

I77.811 Abdominal aortic ectasia

I77.812 Thoracoabdominal aortic ectasia

I82.0 Budd-Chiari syndrome

K55.011 Focal (segmental) acute (reversible) ischemia of small intestine

K55.012 Diffuse acute (reversible) ischemia of small intestine

K55.021 Focal (segmental) acute infarction of small intestine

K55.022 Diffuse acute infarction of small intestine

K55.031 Focal (segmental) acute (reversible) ischemia of large intestine

K55.032 Diffuse acute (reversible) ischemia of large intestine
K55.041 Focal (segmental) acute infarction of large intestine
K55.042 Diffuse acute infarction of large intestine
S35.01XA Minor laceration of abdominal aorta, initial encounter
S35.02XA Major laceration of abdominal aorta, initial encounter
S35.09XA Other injury of abdominal aorta, initial encounter
S35.211A Minor laceration of celiac artery, initial encounter
S35.212A Major laceration of celiac artery, initial encounter
S35.218A Other injury of celiac artery, initial encounter
S35.221A Minor laceration of superior mesenteric artery, initial encounter
S35.222A Major laceration of superior mesenteric artery, initial encounter
S35.228A Other injury of superior mesenteric artery, initial encounter
S35.231A Minor laceration of inferior mesenteric artery, initial encounter
S35.232A Major laceration of inferior mesenteric artery, initial encounter
S35.238A Other injury of inferior mesenteric artery, initial encounter
S35.291A Minor laceration of branches of celiac and mesenteric artery, initial encounter
S35.292A Major laceration of branches of celiac and mesenteric artery, initial encounter
S35.298A Other injury of branches of celiac and mesenteric artery, initial encounter
S35.311A Laceration of portal vein, initial encounter
S35.318A Other specified injury of portal vein, initial encounter
S35.321A Laceration of splenic vein, initial encounter
S35.328A Other specified injury of splenic vein, initial encounter
S35.331A Laceration of superior mesenteric vein, initial encounter
S35.338A Other specified injury of superior mesenteric vein, initial encounter
S35.341A Laceration of inferior mesenteric vein, initial encounter
S35.348A Other specified injury of inferior mesenteric vein, initial encounter
S35.411A Laceration of right renal artery, initial encounter ☑
S35.412A Laceration of left renal artery, initial encounter ☑
S35.414A Laceration of right renal vein, initial encounter ☑
S35.415A Laceration of left renal vein, initial encounter ☑
S35.491A Other specified injury of right renal artery, initial encounter ☑
S35.492A Other specified injury of left renal artery, initial encounter ☑
S35.494A Other specified injury of right renal vein, initial encounter ☑
S35.495A Other specified injury of left renal vein, initial encounter ☑
S35.511A Injury of right iliac artery, initial encounter ☑
S35.512A Injury of left iliac artery, initial encounter ☑
S35.514A Injury of right iliac vein, initial encounter ☑
S35.515A Injury of left iliac vein, initial encounter ☑
S35.531A Injury of right uterine artery, initial encounter ☑
S35.532A Injury of left uterine artery, initial encounter ☑
S35.534A Injury of right uterine vein, initial encounter ☑
S35.535A Injury of left uterine vein, initial encounter ☑
S35.59XA Injury of other iliac blood vessels, initial encounter
S35.8X1A Laceration of other blood vessels at abdomen, lower back and pelvis level, initial encounter
S35.8X8A Other specified injury of other blood vessels at abdomen, lower back and pelvis level, initial encounter

AMA: 35281 2012,Apr,3-9

Relative Value Units/Medicare Edits

Non-Facility RVU	Work	PE	MP	Total
35281	30.06	9.84	6.93	46.83
Facility RVU	**Work**	**PE**	**MP**	**Total**
35281	30.06	9.84	6.93	46.83

	FUD	Status	MUE	Modifiers				IOM Reference
35281	90	A	2(3)	51	50	62*	80	None

* with documentation

Terms To Know

atherosclerosis. Buildup of yellowish plaques composed of cholesterol and lipoid material within the arteries.

bypass graft. Surgically created alternative blood vessel used to reroute blood flow around an area of obstruction or disease.

graft. Tissue implant from another part of the body or another person.

35286

35286 Repair blood vessel with graft other than vein; lower extremity

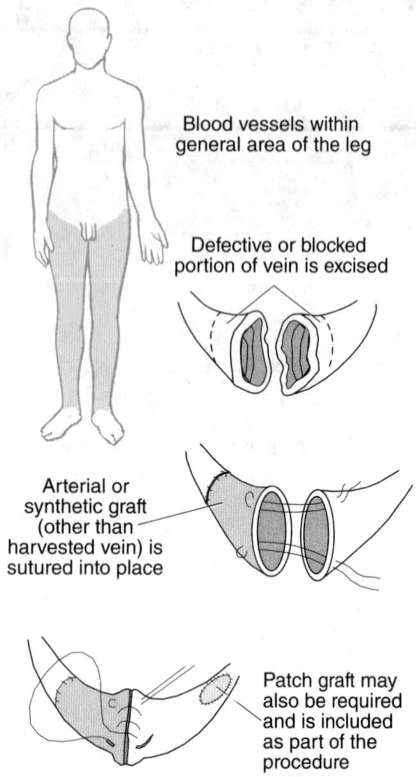

Explanation

The physician makes an incision in the skin of a lower extremity over the site of an injured blood vessel. The vessel is isolated and dissected from adjacent critical structures and vessel clamps are applied. If the defect is too extensive to repair directly, the physician repairs the injured vessel with a length of synthetic graft material. The synthetic graft is sutured end-to-end to the vessel, replacing the excised portion. A patch graft may be sutured over any remaining defect. The clamps are removed and the skin incision is repaired with a layered closure.

Coding Tips

Establishing both inflow and outflow by any method is included. That portion of the operative arteriogram performed by the surgeon is also included. Angioscopy performed during therapeutic intervention should be reported in addition to the code for the primary procedure; see 35400. Any graft harvest is not reported separately. For repair of an aneurysm, lower extremity, see 35141–35152. For direct repair of a blood vessel, lower extremity, see 35226. For repair of a blood vessel of lower extremity with vein graft, see 35256. For repair of a congenital arteriovenous fistula, see 35184. For repair of an acquired or traumatic arteriovenous blood fistula, see 35190.

ICD-10-CM Diagnostic Codes

I70.92	Chronic total occlusion of artery of the extremities
I77.2	Rupture of artery
I80.01	Phlebitis and thrombophlebitis of superficial vessels of right lower extremity ☑
I80.02	Phlebitis and thrombophlebitis of superficial vessels of left lower extremity ☑
I80.11	Phlebitis and thrombophlebitis of right femoral vein ☑
I80.12	Phlebitis and thrombophlebitis of left femoral vein ☑
I80.221	Phlebitis and thrombophlebitis of right popliteal vein ☑
I80.222	Phlebitis and thrombophlebitis of left popliteal vein ☑
I80.231	Phlebitis and thrombophlebitis of right tibial vein ☑
I80.232	Phlebitis and thrombophlebitis of left tibial vein ☑
I80.291	Phlebitis and thrombophlebitis of other deep vessels of right lower extremity ☑
I80.292	Phlebitis and thrombophlebitis of other deep vessels of left lower extremity ☑
S75.021A	Major laceration of femoral artery, right leg, initial encounter ☑
S75.022A	Major laceration of femoral artery, left leg, initial encounter ☑
S75.221A	Major laceration of greater saphenous vein at hip and thigh level, right leg, initial encounter ☑
S75.222A	Major laceration of greater saphenous vein at hip and thigh level, left leg, initial encounter ☑
S85.011A	Laceration of popliteal artery, right leg, initial encounter ☑
S85.012A	Laceration of popliteal artery, left leg, initial encounter ☑
S85.141A	Laceration of anterior tibial artery, right leg, initial encounter ☑
S85.142A	Laceration of anterior tibial artery, left leg, initial encounter ☑
S85.171A	Laceration of posterior tibial artery, right leg, initial encounter ☑
S85.172A	Laceration of posterior tibial artery, left leg, initial encounter ☑
S85.211A	Laceration of peroneal artery, right leg, initial encounter ☑
S85.212A	Laceration of peroneal artery, left leg, initial encounter ☑
S85.311A	Laceration of greater saphenous vein at lower leg level, right leg, initial encounter ☑
S85.312A	Laceration of greater saphenous vein at lower leg level, left leg, initial encounter ☑
S85.411A	Laceration of lesser saphenous vein at lower leg level, right leg, initial encounter ☑
S85.412A	Laceration of lesser saphenous vein at lower leg level, left leg, initial encounter ☑
S85.511A	Laceration of popliteal vein, right leg, initial encounter ☑
S85.512A	Laceration of popliteal vein, left leg, initial encounter ☑
S85.811A	Laceration of other blood vessels at lower leg level, right leg, initial encounter ☑
S85.812A	Laceration of other blood vessels at lower leg level, left leg, initial encounter ☑
S95.011A	Laceration of dorsal artery of right foot, initial encounter ☑
S95.012A	Laceration of dorsal artery of left foot, initial encounter ☑
S95.211A	Laceration of dorsal vein of right foot, initial encounter ☑
S95.212A	Laceration of dorsal vein of left foot, initial encounter ☑
S95.811A	Laceration of other blood vessels at ankle and foot level, right leg, initial encounter ☑
S95.812A	Laceration of other blood vessels at ankle and foot level, left leg, initial encounter ☑

AMA: 35286 2019,Jul,10; 2018,Jan,8; 2017,Jul,3; 2017,Jan,8; 2017,Aug,10; 2016,Jul,6; 2016,Jan,13; 2015,Jan,16; 2014,Jan,11; 2013,Mar,10-11; 2013,Dec,8

Relative Value Units/Medicare Edits

Non-Facility RVU	Work	PE	MP	Total
35286	17.19	5.84	3.95	26.98
Facility RVU	**Work**	**PE**	**MP**	**Total**
35286	17.19	5.84	3.95	26.98

	FUD	Status	MUE	Modifiers				IOM Reference
35286	90	A	2(3)	51	50	62*	80	None

* with documentation

Terms To Know

acquired. Produced by outside influences and not by genetics or birth defect.

aneurysm. Circumscribed dilation or outpouching of an artery wall, often containing blood clots and connecting directly with the lumen of the artery.

atherosclerosis. Buildup of yellowish plaques composed of cholesterol and lipoid material within the arteries.

claudication. Lameness, pain, and weakness occurring in the arms or legs during exercise due to muscles not receiving the needed oxygen and nutrients.

congenital. Present at birth, occurring through heredity or an influence during gestation up to the moment of birth.

dissect. Cut apart or separate tissue for surgical purposes or for visual or microscopic study.

gangrene. Death of tissue, usually resulting from a loss of vascular supply, followed by a bacterial attack or onset of disease.

graft. Tissue implant from another part of the body or another person.

incision. Act of cutting into tissue or an organ.

ulcer. Open sore or excavating lesion of skin or the tissue on the surface of an organ from the sloughing of chronically inflamed and necrosing tissue.

35301

35301 Thromboendarterectomy, including patch graft, if performed; carotid, vertebral, subclavian, by neck incision

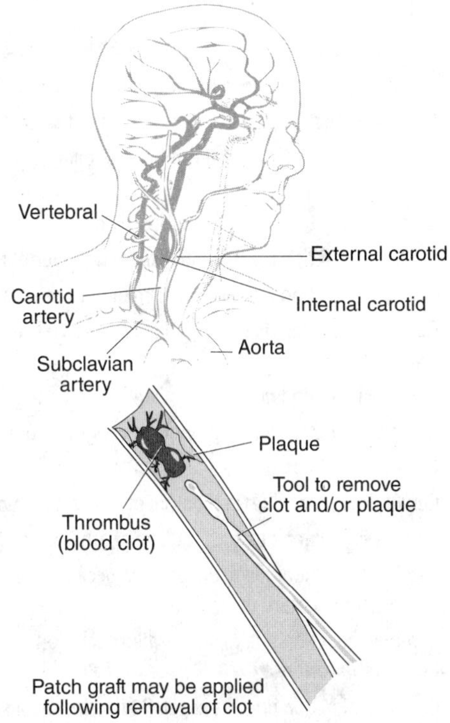

Explanation

The physician makes an incision in the skin of the neck over the site of plaque or abnormal lining of the carotid, vertebral, or subclavian artery. The vessel is isolated and dissected from adjacent critical structures and vessel clamps are applied. A temporary vascular shunt may be placed, bypassing the area and allowing blood supply to continue uninterrupted during the procedure. The vessel is incised. Using a blunt, spatula-like tool, the plaque and the vessel lining are separated from the artery and removed. The edge of the normal artery lining may be sutured to the artery wall to prevent separation when blood flow resumes. After the plaque and lining are removed, a patch graft may be applied and sutured to the vessel. This enlarges the diameter of the artery. The vessel clamps are removed and the skin incision is repaired with layered closure.

Coding Tips

Establishing both inflow and outflow by any method is included. That portion of the operative arteriogram performed by the surgeon is also included. Angioscopy performed during therapeutic intervention should be reported in addition to the code for the primary procedure; see 35400. Report 35390 in addition to 35301 for reoperation on the carotid artery involving repeat thromboendarterectomy more than one month after the original operation. Any graft harvest of saphenous or upper extremity vein is not reported separately. Do not report this procedure with codes for repair of an aneurysm (35001–35152) as aneurysm repair includes endarterectomy and treatment of associated occlusive disease.

ICD-10-CM Diagnostic Codes

G45.0	Vertebro-basilar artery syndrome
G45.1	Carotid artery syndrome (hemispheric)
G45.2	Multiple and bilateral precerebral artery syndromes

G45.3 Amaurosis fugax
G45.8 Other transient cerebral ischemic attacks and related syndromes
I63.011 Cerebral infarction due to thrombosis of right vertebral artery ☑
I63.012 Cerebral infarction due to thrombosis of left vertebral artery ☑
I63.013 Cerebral infarction due to thrombosis of bilateral vertebral arteries ☑
I63.02 Cerebral infarction due to thrombosis of basilar artery
I63.031 Cerebral infarction due to thrombosis of right carotid artery ☑
I63.032 Cerebral infarction due to thrombosis of left carotid artery ☑
I63.033 Cerebral infarction due to thrombosis of bilateral carotid arteries ☑
I63.09 Cerebral infarction due to thrombosis of other precerebral artery
I63.111 Cerebral infarction due to embolism of right vertebral artery ☑
I63.112 Cerebral infarction due to embolism of left vertebral artery ☑
I63.113 Cerebral infarction due to embolism of bilateral vertebral arteries ☑
I63.12 Cerebral infarction due to embolism of basilar artery
I63.131 Cerebral infarction due to embolism of right carotid artery ☑
I63.132 Cerebral infarction due to embolism of left carotid artery ☑
I63.133 Cerebral infarction due to embolism of bilateral carotid arteries ☑
I63.19 Cerebral infarction due to embolism of other precerebral artery
I63.211 Cerebral infarction due to unspecified occlusion or stenosis of right vertebral artery ☑
I63.212 Cerebral infarction due to unspecified occlusion or stenosis of left vertebral artery ☑
I63.213 Cerebral infarction due to unspecified occlusion or stenosis of bilateral vertebral arteries ☑
I63.22 Cerebral infarction due to unspecified occlusion or stenosis of basilar artery
I63.231 Cerebral infarction due to unspecified occlusion or stenosis of right carotid arteries ☑
I63.232 Cerebral infarction due to unspecified occlusion or stenosis of left carotid arteries ☑
I63.233 Cerebral infarction due to unspecified occlusion or stenosis of bilateral carotid arteries ☑
I63.29 Cerebral infarction due to unspecified occlusion or stenosis of other precerebral arteries
I63.313 Cerebral infarction due to thrombosis of bilateral middle cerebral arteries ☑
I63.323 Cerebral infarction due to thrombosis of bilateral anterior cerebral arteries ☑
I63.333 Cerebral infarction due to thrombosis of bilateral posterior cerebral arteries ☑
I63.343 Cerebral infarction due to thrombosis of bilateral cerebellar arteries ☑
I63.413 Cerebral infarction due to embolism of bilateral middle cerebral arteries ☑
I63.423 Cerebral infarction due to embolism of bilateral anterior cerebral arteries ☑
I63.433 Cerebral infarction due to embolism of bilateral posterior cerebral arteries ☑
I63.443 Cerebral infarction due to embolism of bilateral cerebellar arteries ☑
I63.59 Cerebral infarction due to unspecified occlusion or stenosis of other cerebral artery
I65.01 Occlusion and stenosis of right vertebral artery ☑
I65.02 Occlusion and stenosis of left vertebral artery ☑
I65.03 Occlusion and stenosis of bilateral vertebral arteries ☑
I65.1 Occlusion and stenosis of basilar artery
I65.21 Occlusion and stenosis of right carotid artery ☑
I65.22 Occlusion and stenosis of left carotid artery ☑
I65.23 Occlusion and stenosis of bilateral carotid arteries ☑
I65.8 Occlusion and stenosis of other precerebral arteries
I67.81 Acute cerebrovascular insufficiency
I67.841 Reversible cerebrovascular vasoconstriction syndrome
I67.848 Other cerebrovascular vasospasm and vasoconstriction
I67.89 Other cerebrovascular disease
I72.0 Aneurysm of carotid artery
I72.6 Aneurysm of vertebral artery
I72.8 Aneurysm of other specified arteries
I73.89 Other specified peripheral vascular diseases
I76 Septic arterial embolism
I77.74 Dissection of vertebral artery

AMA: **35301** 2018,Jan,8; 2017,Jan,8; 2016,Jan,13; 2015,Jan,16; 2014,Jan,11

Relative Value Units/Medicare Edits

Non-Facility RVU	Work	PE	MP	Total
35301	21.16	6.71	4.92	32.79
Facility RVU	**Work**	**PE**	**MP**	**Total**
35301	21.16	6.71	4.92	32.79

	FUD	Status	MUE	Modifiers				IOM Reference
35301	90	A	2(3)	51	50	62*	80	100-03,160.8

* with documentation

Terms To Know

angioscopy. Visualization of capillary blood vessels with a microscope, or the inside of a blood vessel with a fiberoptic-equipped catheter.

plaque. Accumulation of a soft sticky substance on the teeth largely composed of bacteria and its byproducts.

shunt. Surgically created passage between blood vessels or other natural passages, such as an arteriovenous anastomosis, to divert or bypass blood flow from the normal channel.

thrombo-. Relating to blood clots.

35302-35304

35302 Thromboendarterectomy, including patch graft, if performed; superficial femoral artery
35303 popliteal artery
35304 tibioperoneal trunk artery

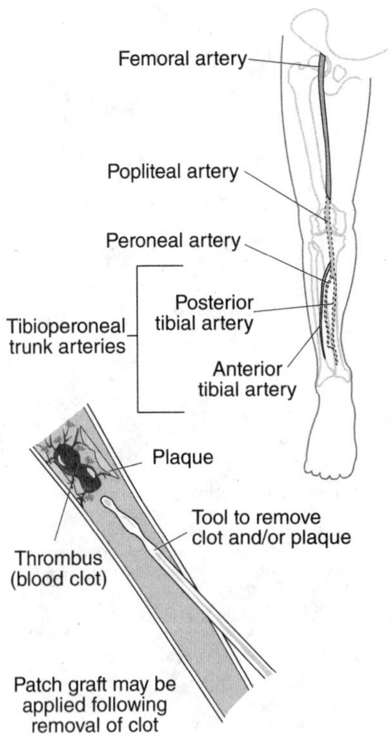

Explanation

The physician makes an incision in the skin of the leg over the site of a blood clot, plaque, or abnormal lining of the superficial femoral (35302), popliteal (35303), or tibioperoneal trunk (35304) arteries. The vessels are isolated and dissected from adjacent critical structures and vessel clamps are applied. The vessels are incised. Using a blunt, spatula-like tool, the plaque and the vessel lining are separated from the arteries and removed. The edge of the normal artery linings may be sutured to the artery walls to prevent separation when blood flow resumes. After the plaque and lining are removed, a patch graft may be applied and sutured to the vessels. This enlarges the diameter of the arteries. The vessel clamps are removed and the skin incision is repaired with layered closure.

Coding Tips

Establishing both inflow and outflow by any method is included. That portion of the operative arteriogram performed by the surgeon is also included. Angioscopy performed during therapeutic intervention should be reported in addition to the code for the primary procedure, see 35400. Any graft harvest of saphenous or upper extremity vein (35500) is not reported separately. Do not report 35302 or 35303 with 37225 or 37227 when the procedures are performed in the same vessel. Do not report 35304 with 37229, 37231, 37233, or 37235 when the procedures are performed in the same vessel.

ICD-10-CM Diagnostic Codes

D68.61 Antiphospholipid syndrome
I70.211 Atherosclerosis of native arteries of extremities with intermittent claudication, right leg ☑
I70.212 Atherosclerosis of native arteries of extremities with intermittent claudication, left leg ☑
I70.213 Atherosclerosis of native arteries of extremities with intermittent claudication, bilateral legs ☑
I70.221 Atherosclerosis of native arteries of extremities with rest pain, right leg ☑
I70.222 Atherosclerosis of native arteries of extremities with rest pain, left leg ☑
I70.223 Atherosclerosis of native arteries of extremities with rest pain, bilateral legs ☑
I70.231 Atherosclerosis of native arteries of right leg with ulceration of thigh ☑
I70.232 Atherosclerosis of native arteries of right leg with ulceration of calf ☑
I70.233 Atherosclerosis of native arteries of right leg with ulceration of ankle ☑
I70.234 Atherosclerosis of native arteries of right leg with ulceration of heel and midfoot ☑
I70.235 Atherosclerosis of native arteries of right leg with ulceration of other part of foot ☑
I70.238 Atherosclerosis of native arteries of right leg with ulceration of other part of lower leg ☑
I70.241 Atherosclerosis of native arteries of left leg with ulceration of thigh ☑
I70.242 Atherosclerosis of native arteries of left leg with ulceration of calf ☑
I70.243 Atherosclerosis of native arteries of left leg with ulceration of ankle ☑
I70.244 Atherosclerosis of native arteries of left leg with ulceration of heel and midfoot ☑
I70.245 Atherosclerosis of native arteries of left leg with ulceration of other part of foot ☑
I70.248 Atherosclerosis of native arteries of left leg with ulceration of other part of lower leg ☑
I70.261 Atherosclerosis of native arteries of extremities with gangrene, right leg ☑
I70.262 Atherosclerosis of native arteries of extremities with gangrene, left leg ☑
I70.263 Atherosclerosis of native arteries of extremities with gangrene, bilateral legs ☑
I70.291 Other atherosclerosis of native arteries of extremities, right leg ☑
I70.292 Other atherosclerosis of native arteries of extremities, left leg ☑
I70.293 Other atherosclerosis of native arteries of extremities, bilateral legs ☑
I70.461 Atherosclerosis of autologous vein bypass graft(s) of the extremities with gangrene, right leg ☑
I70.462 Atherosclerosis of autologous vein bypass graft(s) of the extremities with gangrene, left leg ☑
I70.463 Atherosclerosis of autologous vein bypass graft(s) of the extremities with gangrene, bilateral legs ☑
I70.561 Atherosclerosis of nonautologous biological bypass graft(s) of the extremities with gangrene, right leg ☑
I70.562 Atherosclerosis of nonautologous biological bypass graft(s) of the extremities with gangrene, left leg ☑
I70.563 Atherosclerosis of nonautologous biological bypass graft(s) of the extremities with gangrene, bilateral legs ☑

I70.661	Atherosclerosis of nonbiological bypass graft(s) of the extremities with gangrene, right leg ☑
I70.662	Atherosclerosis of nonbiological bypass graft(s) of the extremities with gangrene, left leg ☑
I70.663	Atherosclerosis of nonbiological bypass graft(s) of the extremities with gangrene, bilateral legs ☑
I70.761	Atherosclerosis of other type of bypass graft(s) of the extremities with gangrene, right leg ☑
I70.762	Atherosclerosis of other type of bypass graft(s) of the extremities with gangrene, left leg ☑
I70.763	Atherosclerosis of other type of bypass graft(s) of the extremities with gangrene, bilateral legs ☑
I72.4	Aneurysm of artery of lower extremity
I74.3	Embolism and thrombosis of arteries of the lower extremities
I75.021	Atheroembolism of right lower extremity ☑
I75.022	Atheroembolism of left lower extremity ☑
I75.023	Atheroembolism of bilateral lower extremities ☑
I76	Septic arterial embolism
I77.1	Stricture of artery
I77.2	Rupture of artery
S75.021A	Major laceration of femoral artery, right leg, initial encounter ☑
S75.022A	Major laceration of femoral artery, left leg, initial encounter ☑
S85.011A	Laceration of popliteal artery, right leg, initial encounter ☑
S85.012A	Laceration of popliteal artery, left leg, initial encounter ☑
S85.141A	Laceration of anterior tibial artery, right leg, initial encounter ☑
S85.142A	Laceration of anterior tibial artery, left leg, initial encounter ☑
S85.171A	Laceration of posterior tibial artery, right leg, initial encounter ☑
S85.172A	Laceration of posterior tibial artery, left leg, initial encounter ☑
S85.181A	Other specified injury of posterior tibial artery, right leg, initial encounter ☑
S85.211A	Laceration of peroneal artery, right leg, initial encounter ☑
S85.212A	Laceration of peroneal artery, left leg, initial encounter ☑

AMA: **35302** 2018,Jan,8; 2017,Jan,8; 2016,Jan,13; 2015,Jan,16; 2014,Jan,11 **35303** 2018,Jan,8; 2017,Jan,8; 2016,Jan,13; 2015,Jan,16; 2014,Jan,11 **35304** 2018,Jan,8; 2017,Jan,8; 2016,Jan,13; 2015,Jan,16; 2014,Jan,11

Relative Value Units/Medicare Edits

Non-Facility RVU	Work	PE	MP	Total
35302	21.35	6.25	4.9	32.5
35303	23.6	6.94	5.41	35.95
35304	24.6	6.81	5.61	37.02
Facility RVU	**Work**	**PE**	**MP**	**Total**
35302	21.35	6.25	4.9	32.5
35303	23.6	6.94	5.41	35.95
35304	24.6	6.81	5.61	37.02

	FUD	Status	MUE	Modifiers				IOM Reference
35302	90	A	1(2)	51	50	62*	80	None
35303	90	A	1(2)	51	50	62*	80	
35304	90	A	1(2)	51	50	62*	80	

* with documentation

35305-35306

35305 Thromboendarterectomy, including patch graft, if performed; tibial or peroneal artery, initial vessel

\+ **35306** each additional tibial or peroneal artery (List separately in addition to code for primary procedure)

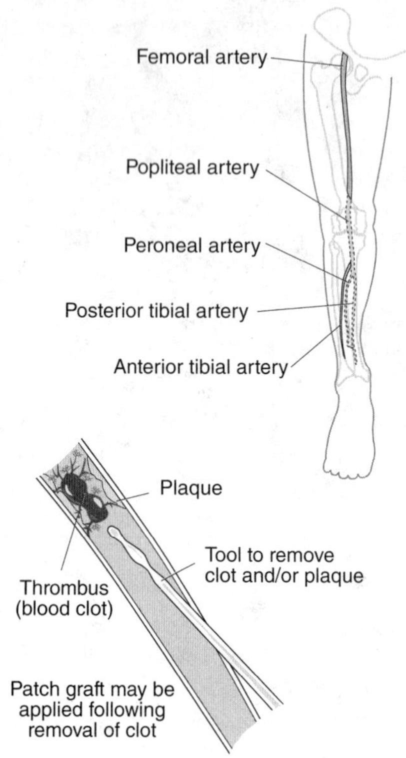

Explanation

A thromboendarterectomy is performed on a tibial or peroneal artery. The physician makes an incision in the skin over the site of plaque or abnormal lining of a tibial or peroneal artery. The vessel is isolated and dissected from adjacent critical structures and vessel clamps are applied. The vessel is incised. Using a blunt, spatula-like tool, the plaque and the vessel lining are separated from the artery and removed. The edge of the normal artery lining may be sutured to the artery wall to prevent separation when blood flow resumes. After the plaque and lining are removed, a patch graft may be applied and sutured to the vessel. This enlarges the diameter of the artery. The vessel clamps are removed and the skin incision is repaired with layered closure. Report 35305 for thromboendarterectomy of the initial tibial or peroneal vessel and 35306 for each additional tibial or peroneal vessel.

Coding Tips

Report 35306 in addition to 35305. Establishing both inflow and outflow by any method is included. That portion of the operative arteriogram performed by the surgeon is also included. Angioscopy performed during therapeutic intervention should be reported in addition to the code for the primary procedure, see 35400. Any graft harvest of saphenous or upper extremity vein (35500) is not reported separately. Do not report 35305 or 35306 with transluminal peripheral atherectomy (37229, 37231, 37233, 37235) when performed in the same vessel.

ICD-10-CM Diagnostic Codes

I70.211	Atherosclerosis of native arteries of extremities with intermittent claudication, right leg ☑

I70.212 Atherosclerosis of native arteries of extremities with intermittent claudication, left leg ☑
I70.213 Atherosclerosis of native arteries of extremities with intermittent claudication, bilateral legs ☑
I70.221 Atherosclerosis of native arteries of extremities with rest pain, right leg ☑
I70.222 Atherosclerosis of native arteries of extremities with rest pain, left leg ☑
I70.223 Atherosclerosis of native arteries of extremities with rest pain, bilateral legs ☑
I70.231 Atherosclerosis of native arteries of right leg with ulceration of thigh ☑
I70.232 Atherosclerosis of native arteries of right leg with ulceration of calf ☑
I70.233 Atherosclerosis of native arteries of right leg with ulceration of ankle ☑
I70.234 Atherosclerosis of native arteries of right leg with ulceration of heel and midfoot ☑
I70.235 Atherosclerosis of native arteries of right leg with ulceration of other part of foot ☑
I70.238 Atherosclerosis of native arteries of right leg with ulceration of other part of lower leg ☑
I70.241 Atherosclerosis of native arteries of left leg with ulceration of thigh ☑
I70.242 Atherosclerosis of native arteries of left leg with ulceration of calf ☑
I70.243 Atherosclerosis of native arteries of left leg with ulceration of ankle ☑
I70.244 Atherosclerosis of native arteries of left leg with ulceration of heel and midfoot ☑
I70.245 Atherosclerosis of native arteries of left leg with ulceration of other part of foot ☑
I70.248 Atherosclerosis of native arteries of left leg with ulceration of other part of lower leg ☑
I70.261 Atherosclerosis of native arteries of extremities with gangrene, right leg ☑
I70.262 Atherosclerosis of native arteries of extremities with gangrene, left leg ☑
I70.263 Atherosclerosis of native arteries of extremities with gangrene, bilateral legs ☑
I70.291 Other atherosclerosis of native arteries of extremities, right leg ☑
I70.292 Other atherosclerosis of native arteries of extremities, left leg ☑
I70.293 Other atherosclerosis of native arteries of extremities, bilateral legs ☑
I70.361 Atherosclerosis of unspecified type of bypass graft(s) of the extremities with gangrene, right leg ☑
I70.362 Atherosclerosis of unspecified type of bypass graft(s) of the extremities with gangrene, left leg ☑
I70.363 Atherosclerosis of unspecified type of bypass graft(s) of the extremities with gangrene, bilateral legs ☑
I70.461 Atherosclerosis of autologous vein bypass graft(s) of the extremities with gangrene, right leg ☑
I70.462 Atherosclerosis of autologous vein bypass graft(s) of the extremities with gangrene, left leg ☑
I70.463 Atherosclerosis of autologous vein bypass graft(s) of the extremities with gangrene, bilateral legs ☑
I70.561 Atherosclerosis of nonautologous biological bypass graft(s) of the extremities with gangrene, right leg ☑
I70.562 Atherosclerosis of nonautologous biological bypass graft(s) of the extremities with gangrene, left leg ☑
I70.563 Atherosclerosis of nonautologous biological bypass graft(s) of the extremities with gangrene, bilateral legs ☑
I70.661 Atherosclerosis of nonbiological bypass graft(s) of the extremities with gangrene, right leg ☑
I70.662 Atherosclerosis of nonbiological bypass graft(s) of the extremities with gangrene, left leg ☑
I70.663 Atherosclerosis of nonbiological bypass graft(s) of the extremities with gangrene, bilateral legs ☑
I70.761 Atherosclerosis of other type of bypass graft(s) of the extremities with gangrene, right leg ☑
I70.762 Atherosclerosis of other type of bypass graft(s) of the extremities with gangrene, left leg ☑
I70.763 Atherosclerosis of other type of bypass graft(s) of the extremities with gangrene, bilateral legs ☑
I72.4 Aneurysm of artery of lower extremity
I74.3 Embolism and thrombosis of arteries of the lower extremities
I75.021 Atheroembolism of right lower extremity ☑
I75.022 Atheroembolism of left lower extremity ☑
I75.023 Atheroembolism of bilateral lower extremities ☑
I77.1 Stricture of artery
I77.2 Rupture of artery
I77.79 Dissection of other specified artery
S85.141A Laceration of anterior tibial artery, right leg, initial encounter ☑
S85.142A Laceration of anterior tibial artery, left leg, initial encounter ☑
S85.171A Laceration of posterior tibial artery, right leg, initial encounter ☑
S85.172A Laceration of posterior tibial artery, left leg, initial encounter ☑
S85.211A Laceration of peroneal artery, right leg, initial encounter ☑
S85.212A Laceration of peroneal artery, left leg, initial encounter ☑

AMA: **35305** 2018,Jan,8; 2017,Jan,8; 2016,Jan,13; 2015,Jan,16; 2014,Jan,11
35306 2018,Jan,8; 2017,Jan,8; 2016,Jan,13; 2015,Jan,16; 2014,Jan,11

Relative Value Units/Medicare Edits

Non-Facility RVU	Work	PE	MP	Total
35305	23.6	6.68	5.33	35.61
35306	9.25	1.51	2.14	12.9
Facility RVU	**Work**	**PE**	**MP**	**Total**
35305	23.6	6.68	5.33	35.61
35306	9.25	1.51	2.14	12.9

	FUD	Status	MUE	Modifiers				IOM Reference
35305	90	A	1(2)	51	50	62*	80	None
35306	N/A	A	2(3)	N/A	N/A	62*	80	

* with documentation

35311

35311 Thromboendarterectomy, including patch graft, if performed; subclavian, innominate, by thoracic incision

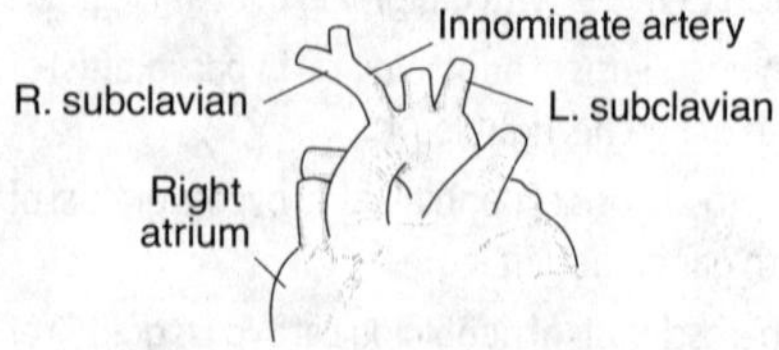

The vessel is accessed by a thoracic incision

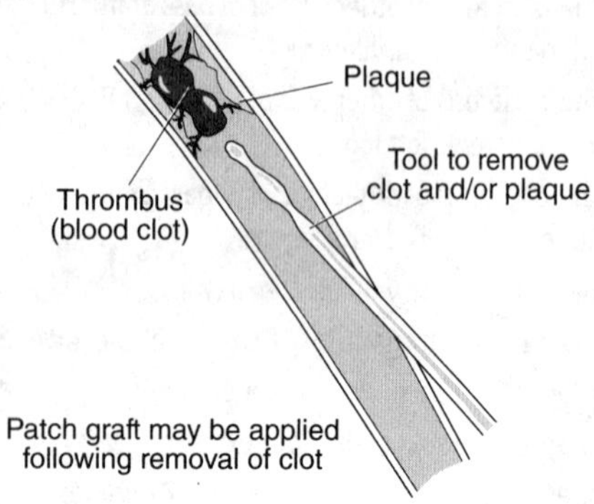

Explanation

The physician exposes the innominate or subclavian artery by median sternotomy or lateral thoracotomy. The physician clamps the aortic arch widely around the origin of the diseased artery and clamps the distal end of the diseased artery. After making a longitudinal incision in the diseased artery, the physician uses a spatula to remove the atherosclerotic material. The physician may tack (suture) down the inner layer of the artery with a few 6-0 sutures before closing the artery with suture. A patch graft may be used to enlarge the arterial lumen. The physician unclamps the aorta, as well as the distal arterial clamp, and closes the sternotomy or thoracotomy, leaving a chest tube in place.

Coding Tips

Establishing both inflow and outflow by any method is included. That portion of the operative arteriogram performed by the surgeon is also included. Angioscopy performed during therapeutic intervention should be reported in addition to the code for the primary procedure; see 35400. Any graft harvest is not reported separately. Do not report this procedure with codes for repair of an aneurysm (35001–35152) as aneurysm repair includes endarterectomy and treatment of associated occlusive disease. For innominate or subclavian embolectomy and/or thrombectomy, see 34051. For repair of a congenital arteriovenous fistula, see 35182. For repair of an acquired or traumatic arteriovenous fistula, see 35189.

ICD-10-CM Diagnostic Codes

G45.2	Multiple and bilateral precerebral artery syndromes
G45.8	Other transient cerebral ischemic attacks and related syndromes
G45.9	Transient cerebral ischemic attack, unspecified
G54.0	Brachial plexus disorders
I63.09	Cerebral infarction due to thrombosis of other precerebral artery
I63.19	Cerebral infarction due to embolism of other precerebral artery
I63.29	Cerebral infarction due to unspecified occlusion or stenosis of other precerebral arteries
I70.8	Atherosclerosis of other arteries
I74.8	Embolism and thrombosis of other arteries
S25.191A	Other specified injury of right innominate or subclavian artery, initial encounter ☑
S25.192A	Other specified injury of left innominate or subclavian artery, initial encounter ☑

AMA: **35311** 1997,Nov,1

Relative Value Units/Medicare Edits

Non-Facility RVU	Work	PE	MP	Total
35311	28.6	10.11	6.75	45.46
Facility RVU	**Work**	**PE**	**MP**	**Total**
35311	28.6	10.11	6.75	45.46

	FUD	Status	MUE	Modifiers				IOM Reference
35311	90	A	1(2)	51	50	62*	80	None

* with documentation

Terms To Know

angioscopy. Visualization of capillary blood vessels with a microscope, or the inside of a blood vessel with a fiberoptic-equipped catheter.

arteriogram. Radiograph of arteries.

atherosclerosis. Buildup of yellowish plaques composed of cholesterol and lipoid material within the arteries.

embolism. Obstruction of a blood vessel resulting from a clot or foreign substance.

fistula. Abnormal tube-like passage between two body cavities or organs or from an organ to the outside surface.

graft. Tissue implant from another part of the body or another person.

thrombosis. Condition arising from the presence or formation of blood clots within a blood vessel that may cause vascular obstruction and insufficient oxygenation.

35321

35321 Thromboendarterectomy, including patch graft, if performed; axillary-brachial

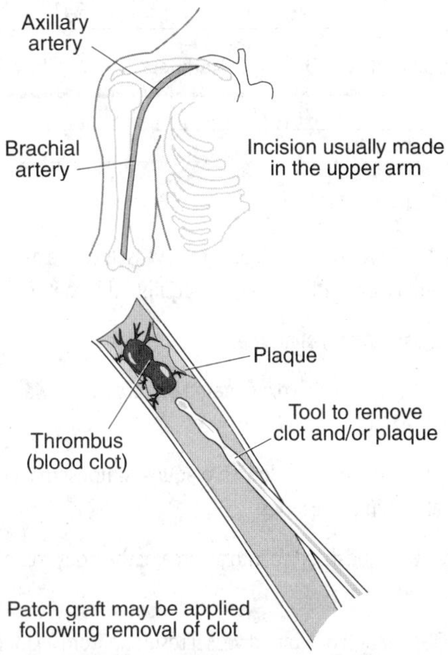

Explanation

The physician makes an incision in the skin of the axilla or arm over the site of a blood clot, plaque, or abnormal lining of the axillary or brachial artery. The vessel is isolated and dissected from adjacent critical structures and vessel clamps are applied. The vessel is incised. Using a blunt, spatula-like tool, the plaque and the vessel lining are separated from the artery and removed. The edge of the normal artery lining may be sutured to the artery wall to prevent separation when blood flow resumes. After the plaque and lining are removed, a patch graft may be applied and sutured to the vessel. This enlarges the diameter of the artery. The vessel clamps are removed and the skin incision is repaired with layered closure.

Coding Tips

Establishing both inflow and outflow by any method is included. That portion of the operative arteriogram performed by the surgeon is also included. Angioscopy performed during therapeutic intervention should be reported in addition to the code for the primary procedure; see 35400. Any graft harvest is not reported separately. Do not report this procedure with codes for repair of an aneurysm (35001–35152) as aneurysm repair includes endarterectomy and treatment of associated occlusive disease. For axillary, brachial embolectomy and/or thrombectomy, see 34101. For repair of a congenital arteriovenous fistula, see 35184. For repair of an acquired or traumatic arteriovenous fistula, see 35190.

ICD-10-CM Diagnostic Codes

I70.92	Chronic total occlusion of artery of the extremities
I74.2	Embolism and thrombosis of arteries of the upper extremities
I75.011	Atheroembolism of right upper extremity ☑
I75.012	Atheroembolism of left upper extremity ☑
I75.013	Atheroembolism of bilateral upper extremities ☑
I77.1	Stricture of artery
I77.2	Rupture of artery

AMA: **35321** 1997,Nov,1

Relative Value Units/Medicare Edits

Non-Facility RVU	Work	PE	MP	Total
35321	16.59	5.47	3.8	25.86
Facility RVU	**Work**	**PE**	**MP**	**Total**
35321	16.59	5.47	3.8	25.86

	FUD	Status	MUE	Modifiers				IOM Reference
35321	90	A	1(2)	51	50	62*	80	None

* with documentation

Terms To Know

angioscopy. Visualization of capillary blood vessels with a microscope, or the inside of a blood vessel with a fiberoptic-equipped catheter.

dissection. Separating by cutting tissue or body structures apart.

graft. Tissue implant from another part of the body or another person.

plaque. Accumulation of a soft sticky substance on the teeth largely composed of bacteria and its byproducts.

35331

35331 Thromboendarterectomy, including patch graft, if performed; abdominal aorta

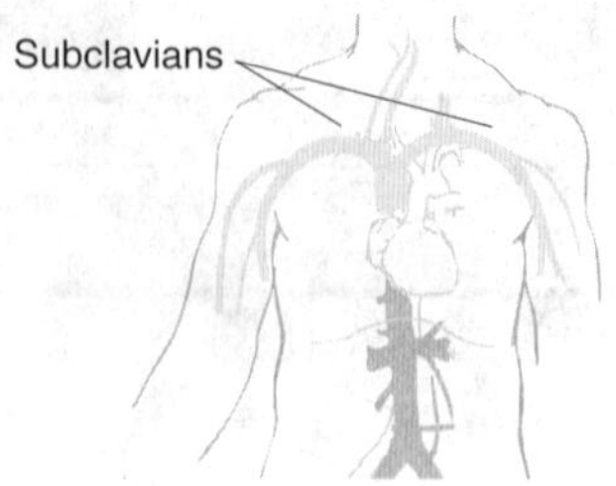

Abdominal aorta and select branches

A thromboendarterectomy is performed on the abdominal aorta

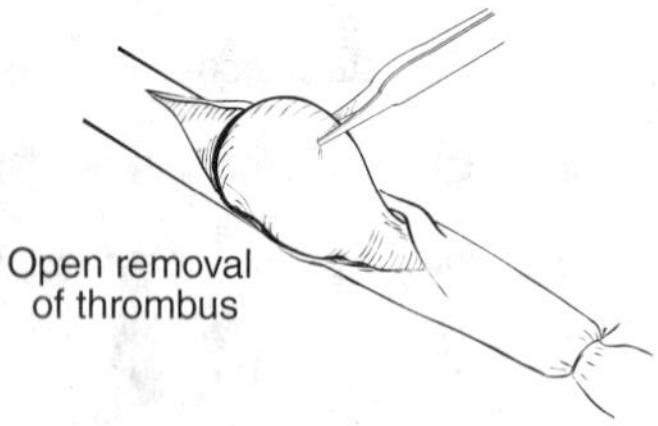

Patch graft may be applied following removal of clot

Explanation

The physician exposes the abdominal aorta using a transperitoneal approach, placing a long incision in the midabdomen. The transverse colon and small bowel are retracted to allow dissection and exposure of the aorta. The iliac arteries are exposed and control of blood flow is achieved with umbilical tape or rubber catheters placed proximal to the diseased area. The physician anticoagulates the patient and cross-clamps the iliac arteries and proximal aorta. A longitudinal incision down the affected portion of abdominal aorta is performed and a spatula is used to remove the atherosclerotic material. The inner layer of the aorta may be tacked down with small sutures. A patch graft may be applied and sutured to the vessel. The physician sutures the aorta closed and closes the retroperitoneum and abdominal wound, leaving drains in place.

Coding Tips

Establishing both inflow and outflow by any method is included. That portion of the operative arteriogram performed by the surgeon is also included. Angioscopy performed during therapeutic intervention should be reported in addition to the code for the primary procedure; see 35400. Any graft harvest is not reported separately. Do not report this procedure with codes for repair of aneurysm (35001–35152) as aneurysm repair includes endarterectomy and treatment of associated occlusive disease. For repair of a congenital arteriovenous fistula, see 35182. For repair of an acquired or traumatic arteriovenous fistula, see 35189.

ICD-10-CM Diagnostic Codes

I70.0	Atherosclerosis of aorta
I74.01	Saddle embolus of abdominal aorta
I74.09	Other arterial embolism and thrombosis of abdominal aorta
I76	Septic arterial embolism
I77.1	Stricture of artery
I77.89	Other specified disorders of arteries and arterioles

AMA: **35331** 1997,Nov,1

Relative Value Units/Medicare Edits

Non-Facility RVU	Work	PE	MP	Total
35331	27.72	8.22	6.41	42.35
Facility RVU	**Work**	**PE**	**MP**	**Total**
35331	27.72	8.22	6.41	42.35

	FUD	Status	MUE	Modifiers				IOM Reference
35331	90	A	1(2)	51	50	62*	80	None

* with documentation

Terms To Know

angioscopy. Visualization of capillary blood vessels with a microscope, or the inside of a blood vessel with a fiberoptic-equipped catheter.

arteriogram. Radiograph of arteries.

artery. Vessel through which oxygenated blood passes away from the heart to any part of the body.

atherosclerosis. Buildup of yellowish plaques composed of cholesterol and lipoid material within the arteries.

catheter. Flexible tube inserted into an area of the body for introducing or withdrawing fluid.

embolism. Obstruction of a blood vessel resulting from a clot or foreign substance.

incision. Act of cutting into tissue or an organ.

suture. Numerous stitching techniques employed in wound closure.

thrombosis. Condition arising from the presence or formation of blood clots within a blood vessel that may cause vascular obstruction and insufficient oxygenation.

35341

35341 Thromboendarterectomy, including patch graft, if performed; mesenteric, celiac, or renal

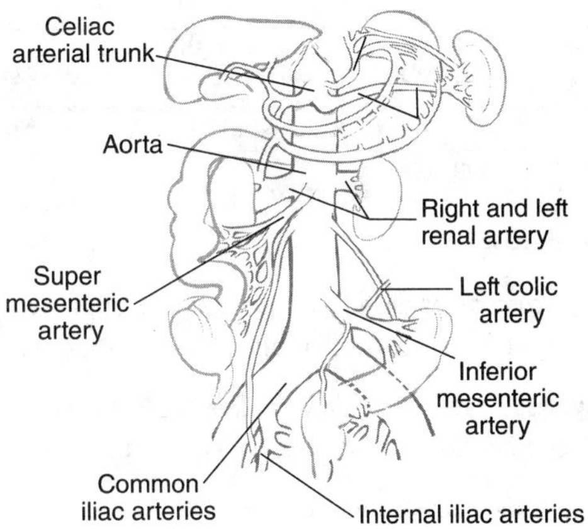

A thromboendarterectomy is performed on the mesenteric, celiac, and renal arteries

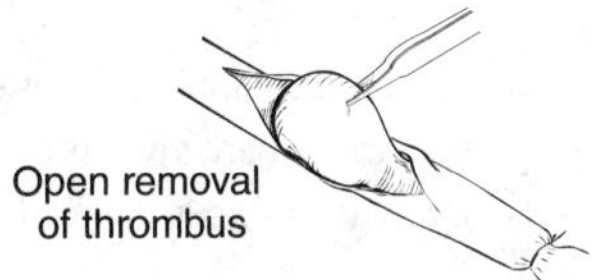

Patch graft may be applied following removal of clot

Explanation

The physician exposes the involved mesenteric, celiac, or renal artery using an abdominal incision, retracting and dissecting past large and small bowel. The aorta is clamped to isolate the involved vessel with a longitudinal incision placed down the affected vessel, and a spatula is used to remove the atherosclerotic material. If there is significant stenosis at the arterial takeoff, the aorta may be opened and the atherosclerotic material removed from within the aorta before suturing the aorta and diseased artery closed. A patch graft may be applied and sutured to the vessel An arteriography may be performed or a Doppler probe may be used to establish patency of the vessel, before closing the abdominal wound, leaving drains in place.

Coding Tips

Establishing both inflow and outflow by any method is included. That portion of the operative arteriogram performed by the surgeon is also included. Angioscopy performed during therapeutic intervention should be reported in addition to the code for the primary procedure; see 35400. Any graft harvest is not reported separately. Do not report this procedure with codes for repair of an aneurysm (35001–35152) as aneurysm repair includes endarterectomy and treatment of associated occlusive disease. For renal, celiac, mesenteric, or aortoiliac embolectomy and/or thrombectomy, by abdominal incision, see 34151. For repair of a congenital arteriovenous fistula, see 35182. For repair of an acquired or traumatic arteriovenous fistula, see 35189.

ICD-10-CM Diagnostic Codes

I70.1	Atherosclerosis of renal artery
I70.8	Atherosclerosis of other arteries
I77.1	Stricture of artery
I77.89	Other specified disorders of arteries and arterioles
Q27.1	Congenital renal artery stenosis
Q27.2	Other congenital malformations of renal artery
Q79.61	Classical Ehlers-Danlos syndrome
Q79.62	Hypermobile Ehlers-Danlos syndrome
Q79.63	Vascular Ehlers-Danlos syndrome

AMA: 35341 1997,Nov,1

Relative Value Units/Medicare Edits

Non-Facility RVU	Work	PE	MP	Total
35341	26.21	7.67	6.06	39.94
Facility RVU	**Work**	**PE**	**MP**	**Total**
35341	26.21	7.67	6.06	39.94

	FUD	Status	MUE	Modifiers				IOM Reference
35341	90	A	3(3)	51	50	62*	80	None

* with documentation

Terms To Know

aneurysm. Circumscribed dilation or outpouching of an artery wall, often containing blood clots and connecting directly with the lumen of the artery.

angioscopy. Visualization of capillary blood vessels with a microscope, or the inside of a blood vessel with a fiberoptic-equipped catheter.

embolism. Obstruction of a blood vessel resulting from a clot or foreign substance.

endarterectomy. Removal of the thickened, endothelial lining of a diseased or damaged artery.

fistula. Abnormal tube-like passage between two body cavities or organs or from an organ to the outside surface.

35351

35351 Thromboendarterectomy, including patch graft, if performed; iliac

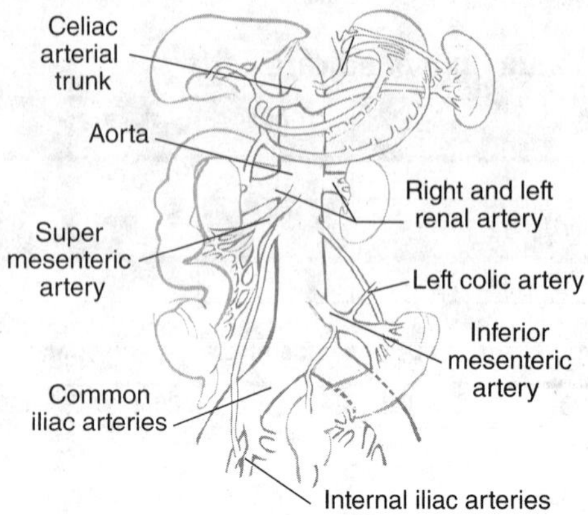

A thromboendarterectomy is performed on the iliac artery

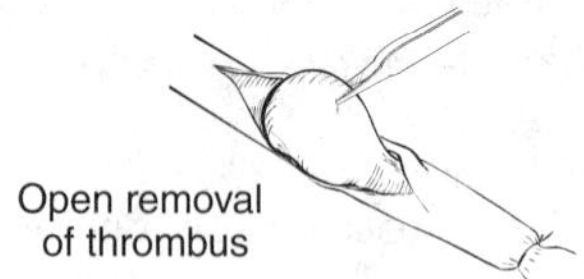

Patch graft may be applied following removal of clot

Explanation

The physician exposes the involved iliac artery using an abdominal incision, retracting and dissecting past large and small bowel. The aorta is clamped to isolate the involved vessel, with a longitudinal incision down the affected vessel, and a spatula is used to remove the atherosclerotic material. If there is significant stenosis at the arterial takeoff, the aorta may be opened and the atherosclerotic material removed before suturing the aorta and diseased artery closed. A patch graft may be applied and sutured to the vessel. The physician may perform arteriography or use a Doppler probe to establish patency of the vessel before closing the abdominal wound, leaving drains in place.

Coding Tips

Establishing both inflow and outflow by any method is included. That portion of the operative arteriogram performed by the surgeon is also included. Angioscopy performed during therapeutic intervention should be reported in addition to the code for the primary procedure, see 35400. Any graft harvest is not reported separately. Do not report this procedure with codes for repair of an aneurysm (35001–35152) as aneurysm repair includes endarterectomy and treatment of associated occlusive disease. For repair of a congenital arteriovenous fistula, see 35182. For repair of an acquired or traumatic arteriovenous fistula, see 35189.

ICD-10-CM Diagnostic Codes

I74.5	Embolism and thrombosis of iliac artery
I76	Septic arterial embolism
I77.1	Stricture of artery
I77.72	Dissection of iliac artery
I77.89	Other specified disorders of arteries and arterioles
S35.511A	Injury of right iliac artery, initial encounter ☑
S35.512A	Injury of left iliac artery, initial encounter ☑
S35.59XA	Injury of other iliac blood vessels, initial encounter

AMA: 35351 1997,Nov,1

Relative Value Units/Medicare Edits

Non-Facility RVU	Work	PE	MP	Total
35351	24.61	6.85	5.63	37.09
Facility RVU	**Work**	**PE**	**MP**	**Total**
35351	24.61	6.85	5.63	37.09

	FUD	Status	MUE	Modifiers				IOM Reference
35351	90	A	1(3)	51	50	62*	80	None

* with documentation

Terms To Know

aneurysm. Circumscribed dilation or outpouching of an artery wall, often containing blood clots and connecting directly with the lumen of the artery.

angioscopy. Visualization of capillary blood vessels with a microscope, or the inside of a blood vessel with a fiberoptic-equipped catheter.

arteriogram. Radiograph of arteries.

atherosclerosis. Buildup of yellowish plaques composed of cholesterol and lipoid material within the arteries.

complication. Condition arising after the beginning of observation and treatment that modifies the course of the patient's illness or the medical care required, or an undesired result or misadventure in medical care.

digital subtraction angiography. Diagnostic imaging technique that applies computer technology to fluoroscopy for the purpose of visualizing the same vascular structures observable with conventional angiography.

embolism. Obstruction of a blood vessel resulting from a clot or foreign substance.

fistula. Abnormal tube-like passage between two body cavities or organs or from an organ to the outside surface.

graft. Tissue implant from another part of the body or another person.

harvest. Removal of cells or tissue from their native site to be used as a graft or transplant to another part of the donor's body or placed into another person.

patency. State of a tube-like structure or conduit being open and unobstructed.

stenosis. Narrowing or constriction of a passage.

● New ▲ Revised + Add On AMA: CPT Assist [Resequenced] ☑ Laterality

35355

35355 Thromboendarterectomy, including patch graft, if performed; iliofemoral

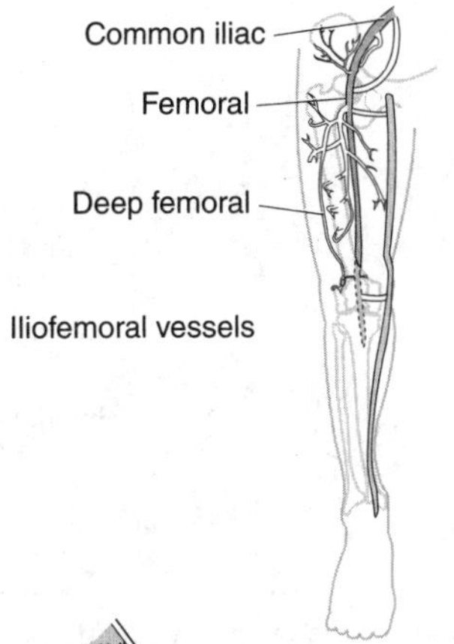

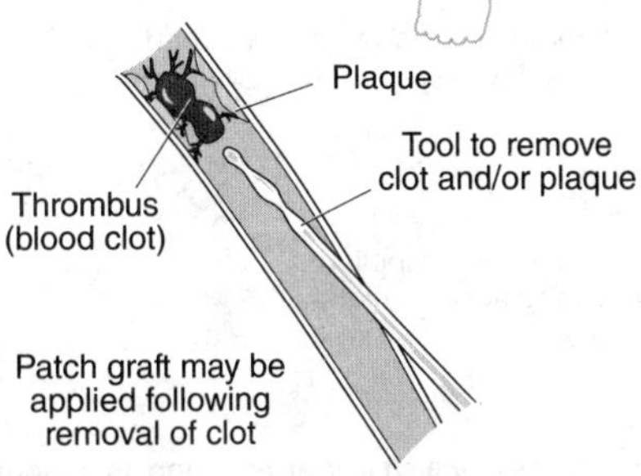

Explanation

The physician exposes the involved iliac artery using abdominal and femoral incisions, retracting and dissecting past large and small bowel. The femoral artery is exposed via a femoral incision. The aorta is clamped to isolate the involved vessel, a longitudinal incision is performed down the involved vessel, and a spatula is used to remove the atherosclerotic material. If there is significant stenosis at the arterial takeoff, the physician may open the aorta and remove the atherosclerotic material from within the aorta before suturing the aorta and diseased artery closed. A patch graft may be applied and sutured to the vessel. An arteriography may be performed or a Doppler probe may be used to establish patency of the vessel before closing the abdominal and femoral wounds, leaving drains in place.

Coding Tips

Establishing both inflow and outflow by any method is included. That portion of the operative arteriogram performed by the surgeon is also included. Angioscopy performed during therapeutic intervention should be reported in addition to the code for the primary procedure; see 35400. Any graft harvest is not reported separately. Do not report this procedure with codes for repair of an aneurysm (35001–35152) as aneurysm repair includes endarterectomy and treatment of associated occlusive disease.

ICD-10-CM Diagnostic Codes

D68.61	Antiphospholipid syndrome
I70.211	Atherosclerosis of native arteries of extremities with intermittent claudication, right leg ☑
I70.212	Atherosclerosis of native arteries of extremities with intermittent claudication, left leg ☑
I70.213	Atherosclerosis of native arteries of extremities with intermittent claudication, bilateral legs ☑
I70.221	Atherosclerosis of native arteries of extremities with rest pain, right leg ☑
I70.222	Atherosclerosis of native arteries of extremities with rest pain, left leg ☑
I70.223	Atherosclerosis of native arteries of extremities with rest pain, bilateral legs ☑
I70.231	Atherosclerosis of native arteries of right leg with ulceration of thigh ☑
I70.232	Atherosclerosis of native arteries of right leg with ulceration of calf ☑
I70.233	Atherosclerosis of native arteries of right leg with ulceration of ankle ☑
I70.234	Atherosclerosis of native arteries of right leg with ulceration of heel and midfoot ☑
I70.235	Atherosclerosis of native arteries of right leg with ulceration of other part of foot ☑
I70.238	Atherosclerosis of native arteries of right leg with ulceration of other part of lower leg ☑
I70.241	Atherosclerosis of native arteries of left leg with ulceration of thigh ☑
I70.242	Atherosclerosis of native arteries of left leg with ulceration of calf ☑
I70.243	Atherosclerosis of native arteries of left leg with ulceration of ankle ☑
I70.244	Atherosclerosis of native arteries of left leg with ulceration of heel and midfoot ☑
I70.245	Atherosclerosis of native arteries of left leg with ulceration of other part of foot ☑
I70.248	Atherosclerosis of native arteries of left leg with ulceration of other part of lower leg ☑
I70.261	Atherosclerosis of native arteries of extremities with gangrene, right leg ☑
I70.262	Atherosclerosis of native arteries of extremities with gangrene, left leg ☑
I70.263	Atherosclerosis of native arteries of extremities with gangrene, bilateral legs ☑
I70.291	Other atherosclerosis of native arteries of extremities, right leg ☑
I70.292	Other atherosclerosis of native arteries of extremities, left leg ☑
I70.293	Other atherosclerosis of native arteries of extremities, bilateral legs ☑
I70.461	Atherosclerosis of autologous vein bypass graft(s) of the extremities with gangrene, right leg ☑
I70.462	Atherosclerosis of autologous vein bypass graft(s) of the extremities with gangrene, left leg ☑
I70.463	Atherosclerosis of autologous vein bypass graft(s) of the extremities with gangrene, bilateral legs ☑
I70.561	Atherosclerosis of nonautologous biological bypass graft(s) of the extremities with gangrene, right leg ☑
I70.562	Atherosclerosis of nonautologous biological bypass graft(s) of the extremities with gangrene, left leg ☑
I70.563	Atherosclerosis of nonautologous biological bypass graft(s) of the extremities with gangrene, bilateral legs ☑
I70.661	Atherosclerosis of nonbiological bypass graft(s) of the extremities with gangrene, right leg ☑
I70.662	Atherosclerosis of nonbiological bypass graft(s) of the extremities with gangrene, left leg ☑

I70.663	Atherosclerosis of nonbiological bypass graft(s) of the extremities with gangrene, bilateral legs ☑
I70.761	Atherosclerosis of other type of bypass graft(s) of the extremities with gangrene, right leg ☑
I70.762	Atherosclerosis of other type of bypass graft(s) of the extremities with gangrene, left leg ☑
I70.763	Atherosclerosis of other type of bypass graft(s) of the extremities with gangrene, bilateral legs ☑
I72.4	Aneurysm of artery of lower extremity
I74.3	Embolism and thrombosis of arteries of the lower extremities
I74.5	Embolism and thrombosis of iliac artery
I75.021	Atheroembolism of right lower extremity ☑
I75.022	Atheroembolism of left lower extremity ☑
I75.023	Atheroembolism of bilateral lower extremities ☑
I76	Septic arterial embolism
I77.1	Stricture of artery
I77.72	Dissection of iliac artery
S35.511A	Injury of right iliac artery, initial encounter ☑
S35.512A	Injury of left iliac artery, initial encounter ☑
S35.59XA	Injury of other iliac blood vessels, initial encounter
S75.091A	Other specified injury of femoral artery, right leg, initial encounter ☑
S75.092A	Other specified injury of femoral artery, left leg, initial encounter ☑

AMA: 35355 1997,Nov,1

Relative Value Units/Medicare Edits

Non-Facility RVU	Work	PE	MP	Total
35355	19.86	5.47	4.55	29.88
Facility RVU	**Work**	**PE**	**MP**	**Total**
35355	19.86	5.47	4.55	29.88

	FUD	Status	MUE	Modifiers				IOM Reference
35355	90	A	1(2)	51	50	62*	80	None

* with documentation

Terms To Know

aneurysm. Circumscribed dilation or outpouching of an artery wall, often containing blood clots and connecting directly with the lumen of the artery.

angioscopy. Visualization of capillary blood vessels with a microscope, or the inside of a blood vessel with a fiberoptic-equipped catheter.

arteriogram. Radiograph of arteries.

atherosclerosis. Buildup of yellowish plaques composed of cholesterol and lipoid material within the arteries.

35361

35361 Thromboendarterectomy, including patch graft, if performed; combined aortoiliac

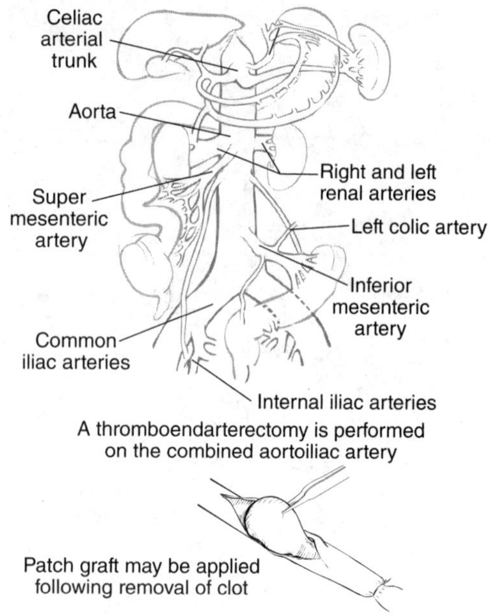

Explanation

The physician exposes the involved iliac artery using an abdominal incision, retracting and dissecting past large and small bowel. The proximal aorta is clamped above the diseased area, a longitudinal incision is performed down the distal aorta and affected iliac artery, and a spatula is utilized to remove the atherosclerotic material before suturing the aorta and iliac artery closed. A patch graft may be applied and sutured to the vessel. Arteriography or use of a Doppler probe may be necessary to establish patency of the vessel before closing the abdominal wound, leaving drains in place.

Coding Tips

Establishing both inflow and outflow by any method is included. That portion of the operative arteriogram performed by the surgeon is also included. Angioscopy performed during therapeutic intervention should be reported in addition to the code for the primary procedure; see 35400. Any graft harvest is not reported separately. Do not report this procedure with codes for repair of an aneurysm (35001–35152) as aneurysm repair includes endarterectomy and treatment of associated occlusive disease. For renal, celiac, mesenteric, or aortoiliac embolectomy and/or thrombectomy, by abdominal incision, see 34151. For repair of a congenital arteriovenous fistula, see 35182. For repair of an acquired or traumatic arteriovenous fistula, see 35189.

ICD-10-CM Diagnostic Codes

I70.0	Atherosclerosis of aorta
I74.01	Saddle embolus of abdominal aorta
I74.09	Other arterial embolism and thrombosis of abdominal aorta
I74.19	Embolism and thrombosis of other parts of aorta
I74.5	Embolism and thrombosis of iliac artery
I76	Septic arterial embolism
I77.1	Stricture of artery
I77.72	Dissection of iliac artery
I77.89	Other specified disorders of arteries and arterioles
S35.02XA	Major laceration of abdominal aorta, initial encounter

S35.511A Injury of right iliac artery, initial encounter ☑

S35.512A Injury of left iliac artery, initial encounter ☑

AMA: **35361** 1997,Nov,1

Relative Value Units/Medicare Edits

Non-Facility RVU	Work	PE	MP	Total
35361	30.24	6.71	7.0	43.95
Facility RVU	**Work**	**PE**	**MP**	**Total**
35361	30.24	6.71	7.0	43.95

	FUD	Status	MUE	Modifiers				IOM Reference
35361	90	A	1(2)	51	50	62*	80	None

* with documentation

Terms To Know

aneurysm. Circumscribed dilation or outpouching of an artery wall, often containing blood clots and connecting directly with the lumen of the artery.

angioscopy. Visualization of capillary blood vessels with a microscope, or the inside of a blood vessel with a fiberoptic-equipped catheter.

arteriogram. Radiograph of arteries.

atherosclerosis. Buildup of yellowish plaques composed of cholesterol and lipoid material within the arteries.

complication. Condition arising after the beginning of observation and treatment that modifies the course of the patient's illness or the medical care required, or an undesired result or misadventure in medical care.

embolism. Obstruction of a blood vessel resulting from a clot or foreign substance.

graft. Tissue implant from another part of the body or another person.

harvest. Removal of cells or tissue from their native site to be used as a graft or transplant to another part of the donor's body or placed into another person.

incision. Act of cutting into tissue or an organ.

patency. State of a tube-like structure or conduit being open and unobstructed.

proximal. Located closest to a specified reference point, usually the midline or trunk.

35363

35363 Thromboendarterectomy, including patch graft, if performed; combined aortoiliofemoral

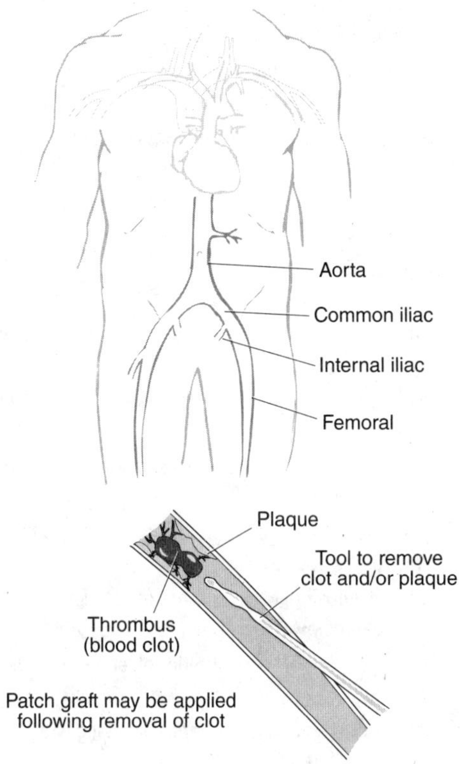

Explanation

The physician exposes the involved abdominal aorta and iliac artery using an abdominal incision, retracting and dissecting past large and small bowel. The involved femoral artery is exposed via a femoral incision and dissection. The proximal aorta is clamped above the diseased area, a longitudinal incision is performed down the distal aorta and affected iliac artery, and a spatula is used to remove the atherosclerotic material before suturing the aorta and iliac artery closed. A longitudinal incision is performed down the femoral artery and a spatula is used to remove any atherosclerotic material before sewing the femoral artery closed. A patch graft may be applied and sutured to the vessel. An arteriography or Doppler imaging may be performed to establish patency of the vessel. The physician closes the femoral and abdominal wounds, leaving drains in place.

Coding Tips

Establishing both inflow and outflow by any method is included. That portion of the operative arteriogram performed by the surgeon is also included. Angioscopy performed during therapeutic intervention should be reported in addition to the code for the primary procedure; see 35400. Any graft harvest is not reported separately. Do not report this procedure with codes for repair of aneurysm (35001–35152) as aneurysm repair includes endarterectomy and treatment of associated occlusive disease. For renal, celiac, mesentery, aortoiliac, embolectomy and/or thrombectomy, by abdominal incision, see 34151. For repair of a congenital arteriovenous fistula, see 35182. For repair of an acquired or traumatic arteriovenous fistula, see 35189.

ICD-10-CM Diagnostic Codes

D68.61 Antiphospholipid syndrome

I70.0 Atherosclerosis of aorta

I70.211 Atherosclerosis of native arteries of extremities with intermittent claudication, right leg ☑

I70.212 Atherosclerosis of native arteries of extremities with intermittent claudication, left leg ☑

I70.213 Atherosclerosis of native arteries of extremities with intermittent claudication, bilateral legs ☑

I70.221 Atherosclerosis of native arteries of extremities with rest pain, right leg ☑

I70.222 Atherosclerosis of native arteries of extremities with rest pain, left leg ☑

I70.223 Atherosclerosis of native arteries of extremities with rest pain, bilateral legs ☑

I70.231 Atherosclerosis of native arteries of right leg with ulceration of thigh ☑

I70.232 Atherosclerosis of native arteries of right leg with ulceration of calf ☑

I70.233 Atherosclerosis of native arteries of right leg with ulceration of ankle ☑

I70.234 Atherosclerosis of native arteries of right leg with ulceration of heel and midfoot ☑

I70.235 Atherosclerosis of native arteries of right leg with ulceration of other part of foot ☑

I70.238 Atherosclerosis of native arteries of right leg with ulceration of other part of lower leg ☑

I70.241 Atherosclerosis of native arteries of left leg with ulceration of thigh ☑

I70.242 Atherosclerosis of native arteries of left leg with ulceration of calf ☑

I70.243 Atherosclerosis of native arteries of left leg with ulceration of ankle ☑

I70.244 Atherosclerosis of native arteries of left leg with ulceration of heel and midfoot ☑

I70.245 Atherosclerosis of native arteries of left leg with ulceration of other part of foot ☑

I70.248 Atherosclerosis of native arteries of left leg with ulceration of other part of lower leg ☑

I70.261 Atherosclerosis of native arteries of extremities with gangrene, right leg ☑

I70.262 Atherosclerosis of native arteries of extremities with gangrene, left leg ☑

I70.263 Atherosclerosis of native arteries of extremities with gangrene, bilateral legs ☑

I70.291 Other atherosclerosis of native arteries of extremities, right leg ☑

I70.292 Other atherosclerosis of native arteries of extremities, left leg ☑

I70.293 Other atherosclerosis of native arteries of extremities, bilateral legs ☑

I70.461 Atherosclerosis of autologous vein bypass graft(s) of the extremities with gangrene, right leg ☑

I70.462 Atherosclerosis of autologous vein bypass graft(s) of the extremities with gangrene, left leg ☑

I70.463 Atherosclerosis of autologous vein bypass graft(s) of the extremities with gangrene, bilateral legs ☑

I70.561 Atherosclerosis of nonautologous biological bypass graft(s) of the extremities with gangrene, right leg ☑

I70.562 Atherosclerosis of nonautologous biological bypass graft(s) of the extremities with gangrene, left leg ☑

I70.563 Atherosclerosis of nonautologous biological bypass graft(s) of the extremities with gangrene, bilateral legs ☑

I70.661 Atherosclerosis of nonbiological bypass graft(s) of the extremities with gangrene, right leg ☑

I70.662 Atherosclerosis of nonbiological bypass graft(s) of the extremities with gangrene, left leg ☑

I70.663 Atherosclerosis of nonbiological bypass graft(s) of the extremities with gangrene, bilateral legs ☑

I70.761 Atherosclerosis of other type of bypass graft(s) of the extremities with gangrene, right leg ☑

I70.762 Atherosclerosis of other type of bypass graft(s) of the extremities with gangrene, left leg ☑

I70.763 Atherosclerosis of other type of bypass graft(s) of the extremities with gangrene, bilateral legs ☑

I74.01 Saddle embolus of abdominal aorta

I74.09 Other arterial embolism and thrombosis of abdominal aorta

I74.19 Embolism and thrombosis of other parts of aorta

I74.3 Embolism and thrombosis of arteries of the lower extremities

I74.5 Embolism and thrombosis of iliac artery

I75.021 Atheroembolism of right lower extremity ☑

I75.022 Atheroembolism of left lower extremity ☑

I75.023 Atheroembolism of bilateral lower extremities ☑

I76 Septic arterial embolism

I77.1 Stricture of artery

I77.72 Dissection of iliac artery

I77.89 Other specified disorders of arteries and arterioles

S35.511A Injury of right iliac artery, initial encounter ☑

S35.512A Injury of left iliac artery, initial encounter ☑

S35.59XA Injury of other iliac blood vessels, initial encounter

S35.8X8A Other specified injury of other blood vessels at abdomen, lower back and pelvis level, initial encounter

S75.091A Other specified injury of femoral artery, right leg, initial encounter ☑

S75.092A Other specified injury of femoral artery, left leg, initial encounter ☑

AMA: 35363 1997,Nov,1

Relative Value Units/Medicare Edits

Non-Facility RVU	Work	PE	MP	Total
35363	32.35	7.06	7.48	46.89
Facility RVU	**Work**	**PE**	**MP**	**Total**
35363	32.35	7.06	7.48	46.89

	FUD	Status	MUE	Modifiers				IOM Reference
35363	90	A	1(2)	51	50	62*	80	None

* with documentation

35371-35372

35371 Thromboendarterectomy, including patch graft, if performed; common femoral

35372 deep (profunda) femoral

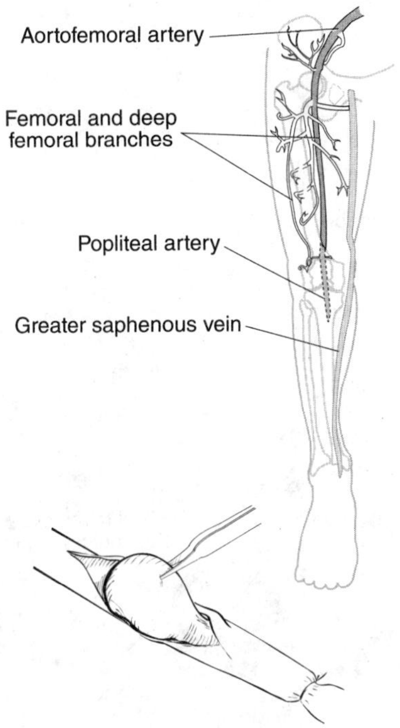

Explanation

The physician makes an incision in the skin over the leg at the site of a blood clot, plaque, or abnormal lining of the common femoral artery (35371) or the deep (profunda) femoral artery (35372). The vessel is isolated and dissected from adjacent critical structures and vessel clamps are applied. The vessel is incised. Using a blunt, spatula-like tool, the plaque and the vessel lining are separated from the artery and removed. The edge of the normal artery lining may be sutured to the artery wall to prevent separation when blood flow resumes. After the plaque and lining are removed, a patch graft may be applied and sutured to the vessel. This enlarges the diameter of the artery. The vessel clamps are removed and the skin incision is repaired with layered closure.

Coding Tips

Unless the procedure involves a significant length of the deep or superficial femoral artery, report only the common femoral procedure (35371). Establishing both inflow and outflow by any method is included. That portion of the operative arteriogram performed by the surgeon is also included. Angioscopy performed during therapeutic intervention should be reported in addition to the code for the primary procedure; see 35400. Any graft harvest is not reported separately. Do not report this procedure with codes for repair of an aneurysm (35001–35152) as aneurysm repair includes endarterectomy and treatment of associated occlusive disease. For femoropopliteal embolectomy and/or thrombectomy, see 34201. For repair of a congenital arteriovenous fistula, see 35184. For repair of an acquired or traumatic arteriovenous fistula, see 35190.

ICD-10-CM Diagnostic Codes

I70.211 Atherosclerosis of native arteries of extremities with intermittent claudication, right leg ☑

I70.212 Atherosclerosis of native arteries of extremities with intermittent claudication, left leg ☑

I70.213 Atherosclerosis of native arteries of extremities with intermittent claudication, bilateral legs ☑

I70.221 Atherosclerosis of native arteries of extremities with rest pain, right leg ☑

I70.222 Atherosclerosis of native arteries of extremities with rest pain, left leg ☑

I70.223 Atherosclerosis of native arteries of extremities with rest pain, bilateral legs ☑

I70.231 Atherosclerosis of native arteries of right leg with ulceration of thigh ☑

I70.232 Atherosclerosis of native arteries of right leg with ulceration of calf ☑

I70.233 Atherosclerosis of native arteries of right leg with ulceration of ankle ☑

I70.234 Atherosclerosis of native arteries of right leg with ulceration of heel and midfoot ☑

I70.235 Atherosclerosis of native arteries of right leg with ulceration of other part of foot ☑

I70.238 Atherosclerosis of native arteries of right leg with ulceration of other part of lower leg ☑

I70.241 Atherosclerosis of native arteries of left leg with ulceration of thigh ☑

I70.242 Atherosclerosis of native arteries of left leg with ulceration of calf ☑

I70.243 Atherosclerosis of native arteries of left leg with ulceration of ankle ☑

I70.244 Atherosclerosis of native arteries of left leg with ulceration of heel and midfoot ☑

I70.245 Atherosclerosis of native arteries of left leg with ulceration of other part of foot ☑

I70.248 Atherosclerosis of native arteries of left leg with ulceration of other part of lower leg ☑

I70.261 Atherosclerosis of native arteries of extremities with gangrene, right leg ☑

I70.262 Atherosclerosis of native arteries of extremities with gangrene, left leg ☑

I70.263 Atherosclerosis of native arteries of extremities with gangrene, bilateral legs ☑

I70.291 Other atherosclerosis of native arteries of extremities, right leg ☑

I70.292 Other atherosclerosis of native arteries of extremities, left leg ☑

I70.293 Other atherosclerosis of native arteries of extremities, bilateral legs ☑

I70.461 Atherosclerosis of autologous vein bypass graft(s) of the extremities with gangrene, right leg ☑

I70.462 Atherosclerosis of autologous vein bypass graft(s) of the extremities with gangrene, left leg ☑

I70.463 Atherosclerosis of autologous vein bypass graft(s) of the extremities with gangrene, bilateral legs ☑

I70.561 Atherosclerosis of nonautologous biological bypass graft(s) of the extremities with gangrene, right leg ☑

I70.562 Atherosclerosis of nonautologous biological bypass graft(s) of the extremities with gangrene, left leg ☑

I70.563 Atherosclerosis of nonautologous biological bypass graft(s) of the extremities with gangrene, bilateral legs ☑

I70.661	Atherosclerosis of nonbiological bypass graft(s) of the extremities with gangrene, right leg ☑
I70.662	Atherosclerosis of nonbiological bypass graft(s) of the extremities with gangrene, left leg ☑
I70.663	Atherosclerosis of nonbiological bypass graft(s) of the extremities with gangrene, bilateral legs ☑
I70.761	Atherosclerosis of other type of bypass graft(s) of the extremities with gangrene, right leg ☑
I70.762	Atherosclerosis of other type of bypass graft(s) of the extremities with gangrene, left leg ☑
I70.763	Atherosclerosis of other type of bypass graft(s) of the extremities with gangrene, bilateral legs ☑
I70.92	Chronic total occlusion of artery of the extremities
I74.3	Embolism and thrombosis of arteries of the lower extremities
I75.021	Atheroembolism of right lower extremity ☑
I75.022	Atheroembolism of left lower extremity ☑
I75.023	Atheroembolism of bilateral lower extremities ☑
I76	Septic arterial embolism
I77.1	Stricture of artery

AMA: 35371 2018,Jan,8; 2017,Jul,3; 2017,Jan,8; 2017,Aug,10; 2016,Jan,13; 2015,Jan,16; 2014,Jan,11 **35372** 2018,Jan,8; 2017,Jan,8; 2016,Jan,13; 2015,Jan,16; 2014,Jan,11

Relative Value Units/Medicare Edits

Non-Facility RVU	Work	PE	MP	Total
35371	15.31	4.87	3.52	23.7
35372	18.58	5.55	4.24	28.37
Facility RVU	**Work**	**PE**	**MP**	**Total**
35371	15.31	4.87	3.52	23.7
35372	18.58	5.55	4.24	28.37

	FUD	Status	MUE	Modifiers				IOM Reference
35371	90	A	1(2)	51	50	62*	80	None
35372	90	A	1(2)	51	50	62*	80	

* with documentation

Terms To Know

embolism. Obstruction of a blood vessel resulting from a clot or foreign substance.

35390

\+ **35390** Reoperation, carotid, thromboendarterectomy, more than 1 month after original operation (List separately in addition to code for primary procedure)

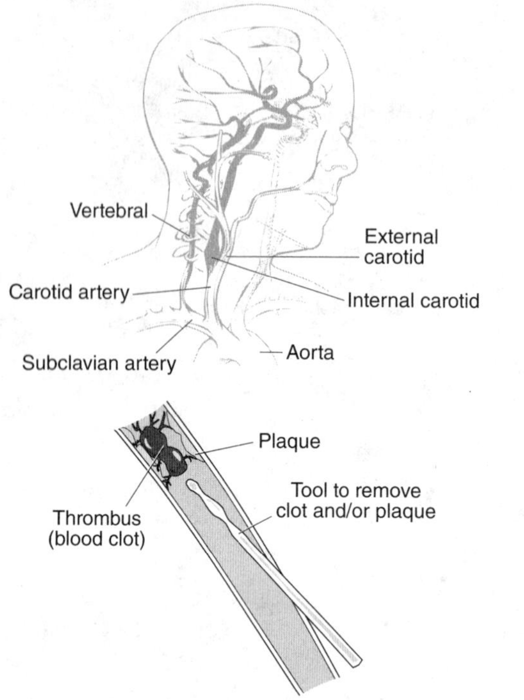

Explanation

The physician makes an incision in the skin of the neck over the site of plaque or abnormal lining of the carotid, vertebral, or subclavian artery. The vessel is isolated and dissected from adjacent critical structures, and vessel clamps are applied. A temporary vascular shunt may be placed, bypassing the area and allowing blood supply to continue uninterrupted during the procedure. The vessel is incised. Using a blunt, spatula-like tool, the plaque and the vessel lining are separated from the artery and removed. The edge of the normal artery lining may be sutured to the artery wall to prevent separation when blood flow resumes. After the plaque and lining are removed, a patch graft taken from another portion of the patient's body, a cadaver, or a synthetic source may be applied and sutured to the vessel. This enlarges the diameter of the artery. The vessel clamps are removed and the skin incision is repaired with a layered closure.

Coding Tips

Report 35390 in addition to 35301 and for a repeat thromboendarterectomy on the carotid artery.

ICD-10-CM Diagnostic Codes

This/these CPT code(s) are add on code(s). See the primary procedure code that this code is performed with for your ICD-10-CM code selections. Diagnostic code(s) would be the same as the actual procedure performed.

AMA: 35390 1997,Nov,1

Relative Value Units/Medicare Edits

Non-Facility RVU	Work	PE	MP	Total
35390	3.19	0.7	0.72	4.61
Facility RVU	**Work**	**PE**	**MP**	**Total**
35390	3.19	0.7	0.72	4.61

	FUD	Status	MUE	Modifiers				IOM Reference
35390	N/A	A	1(3)	N/A	N/A	62*	80	None

* with documentation

Terms To Know

artery. Vessel through which oxygenated blood passes away from the heart to any part of the body.

atherosclerosis. Buildup of yellowish plaques composed of cholesterol and lipoid material within the arteries.

graft. Tissue implant from another part of the body or another person.

plaque. Accumulation of a soft sticky substance on the teeth largely composed of bacteria and its byproducts.

shunt. Surgically created passage between blood vessels or other natural passages, such as an arteriovenous anastomosis, to divert or bypass blood flow from the normal channel.

suture. Numerous stitching techniques employed in wound closure.

buried suture. Continuous or interrupted suture placed under the skin for a layered closure.

continuous suture. Running stitch with tension evenly distributed across a single strand to provide a leakproof closure line.

interrupted suture. Series of single stitches with tension isolated at each stitch, in which all stitches are not affected if one becomes loose, and the isolated sutures cannot act as a wick to transport an infection.

purse-string suture. Continuous suture placed around a tubular structure and tightened, to reduce or close the lumen.

retention suture. Secondary stitching that bridges the primary suture, providing support for the primary repair; a plastic or rubber bolster may be placed over the primary repair and under the retention sutures.

thrombus. Stationary blood clot inside a blood vessel.

35400

\+ **35400** Angioscopy (noncoronary vessels or grafts) during therapeutic intervention (List separately in addition to code for primary procedure)

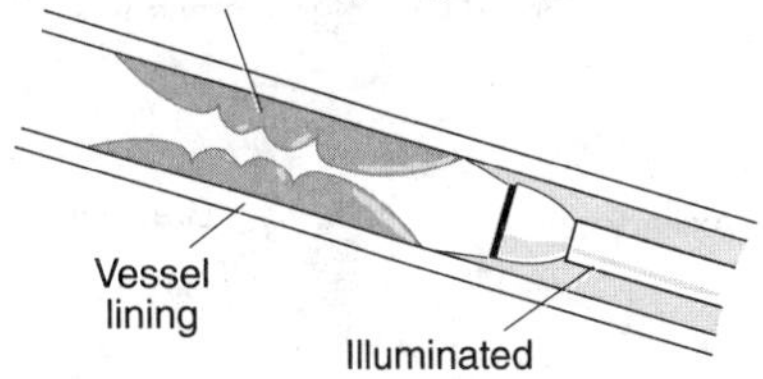

Explanation

The purpose of this procedure is to use an endoscope to look inside a blood vessel. The physician places an introducer sheath in the vessel to be examined, using percutaneous puncture or a cutdown technique. The physician places an angioscopy catheter through the introducer sheath into the vessel to be examined. The physician advances the angioscope through the vessel, clearing the view with injections of saline. Once the inside of the vessel has been examined, the angioscope and sheath are withdrawn. Vessel hemostasis is achieved using sutures or manual pressure.

Coding Tips

Fiberoptic intraoperative angioscopy provides three-dimensional endovascular visualization for assessment of vessels during revascularization procedures, such as endarterectomy and bypass.

ICD-10-CM Diagnostic Codes

This/these CPT code(s) are add on code(s). See the primary procedure code that this code is performed with for your ICD-10-CM code selections.

AMA: **35400** 1997,Nov,1; 1997,Dec,1

Relative Value Units/Medicare Edits

Non-Facility RVU	Work	PE	MP	Total
35400	3.0	0.63	0.69	4.32
Facility RVU	**Work**	**PE**	**MP**	**Total**
35400	3.0	0.63	0.69	4.32

	FUD	Status	MUE	Modifiers				IOM Reference
35400	N/A	A	1(3)	N/A	N/A	62*	80*	None

* with documentation

Terms To Know

angioscopy. Visualization of capillary blood vessels with a microscope, or the inside of a blood vessel with a fiberoptic-equipped catheter.

bypass. Auxiliary or diverted route to maintain continuous flow.

catheter. Flexible tube inserted into an area of the body for introducing or withdrawing fluid.

Arteries and Veins

35500

+ **35500** Harvest of upper extremity vein, 1 segment, for lower extremity or coronary artery bypass procedure (List separately in addition to code for primary procedure)

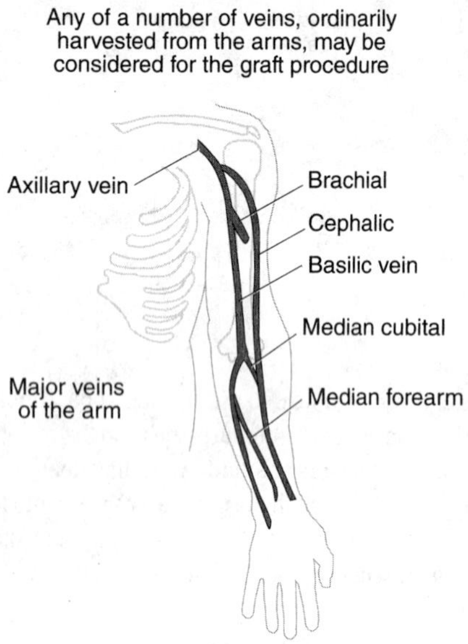

Explanation

The physician harvests a vein from an upper extremity (arm) to use for a planned bypass procedure on a lower extremity vessel (leg) or coronary artery. An incision is made over the site on the arm. Tissue is dissected to the vein. The portion of the vein to be removed is released from the surrounding structures, and is tied off above and below the portion of vein to be removed. The vein is removed. The wound is closed with layered sutures. The portion of vein removed is prepared for use in a separately reportable bypass graft procedure of a leg vessel or coronary artery.

Coding Tips

Report 35500 in addition to 33510–33536, 35556, 35566, 35570, 35571, and 35583–35587. For endoscopic harvest of veins for a coronary artery bypass procedure, see 33508. Note that 35500 reports harvest of a single vein segment. For harvest of more than one vein segment, see 35682 or 35683.

ICD-10-CM Diagnostic Codes

This/these CPT code(s) are add on code(s). See the primary procedure code that this code is performed with for your ICD-10-CM code selections. Diagnostic code(s) would be the same as the actual procedure performed.

AMA: **35500** 2018,Jan,8; 2017,Jan,8; 2016,Jan,13; 2015,Jan,16; 2014,Jan,11

Relative Value Units/Medicare Edits

Non-Facility RVU	Work	PE	MP	Total
35500	6.44	1.37	1.48	9.29
Facility RVU	**Work**	**PE**	**MP**	**Total**
35500	6.44	1.37	1.48	9.29

	FUD	Status	MUE	Modifiers				IOM Reference
35500	N/A	A	2(3)	N/A	N/A	62*	80	None

* with documentation

35501

35501 Bypass graft, with vein; common carotid-ipsilateral internal carotid

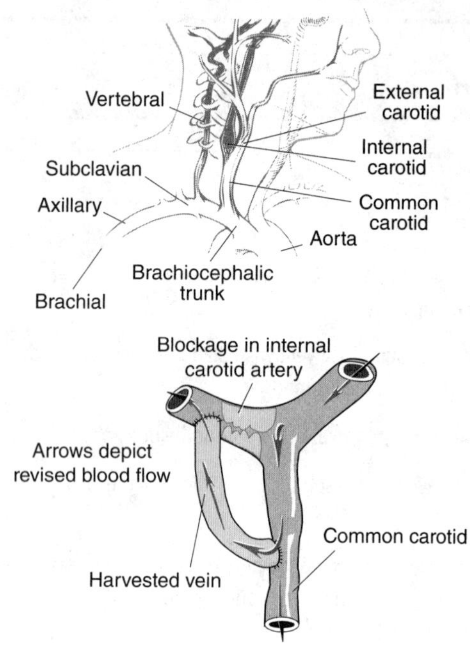

A portion of blocked internal carotid artery is bypassed

Explanation

The physician bypasses a blocked segment of common carotid artery to a segment of internal carotid artery on the same side of the neck. Through an incision in the skin of the neck in front of the sternocleidomastoid muscle, the physician isolates and dissects the common carotid artery, separating it from adjacent structures. After vessel clamps are affixed above and below the defect, the physician creates a bypass around the defective section of common carotid artery. The common carotid artery may be cut through below the damaged area and sutured to one end of the harvest vein (end-to-end), which is then sutured to the internal carotid artery beyond the affected area. As an alternative, the ends of the harvested vein are sutured into the side of the common carotid arterial wall and to the side of the internal carotid arterial wall (end-to-side). Either method results in a bypass of the damaged area. When the clamps are removed, the section of vein graft forms a new path through which blood can easily bypass the blocked area. The defective common carotid artery is not removed. After the graft is complete, the skin incision is repaired with layered closure.

Coding Tips

Establishing both inflow and outflow by any method is included. That portion of the operative arteriogram performed by the surgeon is also included. Angioscopy performed during therapeutic intervention should be reported in addition to the code for the primary procedure, see 35400. Harvesting of the saphenous vein graft is included in the description of the work for 35501 and should not be reported as a separate procedure. For harvesting of a femoropopliteal vein segment, use 35572 in addition to the bypass procedure. If a composite (combination of vein and synthetic graft) is used, report 35681 in addition to the code for the primary procedure.

ICD-10-CM Diagnostic Codes

G45.1 Carotid artery syndrome (hemispheric)

G45.3 Amaurosis fugax

G45.8 Other transient cerebral ischemic attacks and related syndromes
G45.9 Transient cerebral ischemic attack, unspecified
I63.031 Cerebral infarction due to thrombosis of right carotid artery ☑
I63.032 Cerebral infarction due to thrombosis of left carotid artery ☑
I63.131 Cerebral infarction due to embolism of right carotid artery ☑
I63.132 Cerebral infarction due to embolism of left carotid artery ☑
I63.81 Other cerebral infarction due to occlusion or stenosis of small artery
I63.89 Other cerebral infarction
I65.21 Occlusion and stenosis of right carotid artery ☑
I65.22 Occlusion and stenosis of left carotid artery ☑
I65.23 Occlusion and stenosis of bilateral carotid arteries ☑
I67.81 Acute cerebrovascular insufficiency
I67.82 Cerebral ischemia
I67.850 Cerebral autosomal dominant arteriopathy with subcortical infarcts and leukoencephalopathy
I67.858 Other hereditary cerebrovascular disease
I67.89 Other cerebrovascular disease
I72.0 Aneurysm of carotid artery
I77.1 Stricture of artery
I77.2 Rupture of artery
I77.71 Dissection of carotid artery
S15.011A Minor laceration of right carotid artery, initial encounter ☑
S15.012A Minor laceration of left carotid artery, initial encounter ☑
S15.021A Major laceration of right carotid artery, initial encounter ☑
S15.022A Major laceration of left carotid artery, initial encounter ☑
S15.091A Other specified injury of right carotid artery, initial encounter ☑
S15.092A Other specified injury of left carotid artery, initial encounter ☑
S15.8XXA Injury of other specified blood vessels at neck level, initial encounter

AMA: 35501 2018,Jan,8; 2017,Jan,8; 2016,Jan,13; 2015,Jan,16; 2014,Jan,11

Relative Value Units/Medicare Edits

Non-Facility RVU	Work	PE	MP	Total
35501	29.09	7.71	6.54	43.34
Facility RVU	**Work**	**PE**	**MP**	**Total**
35501	29.09	7.71	6.54	43.34

	FUD	Status	MUE	Modifiers				IOM Reference
35501	90	A	1(3)	51	50	62*	80	None

* with documentation

35506

35506 Bypass graft, with vein; carotid-subclavian or subclavian-carotid

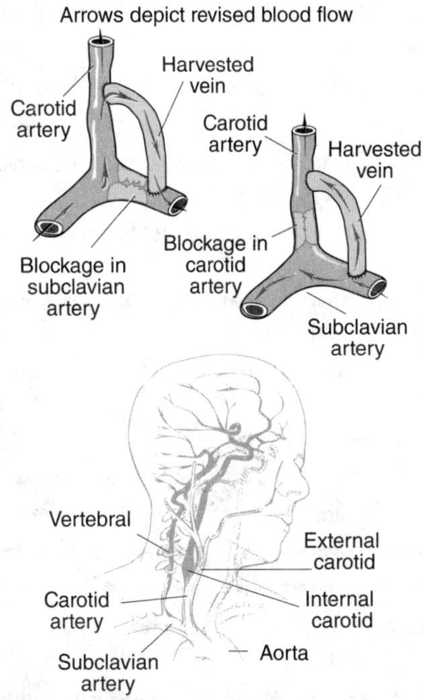

Explanation

The physician bypasses a segment of blocked common carotid or subclavian artery. Through an incision in the skin at the side of the neck, the physician isolates and dissects the subclavian and common carotid arteries, separating them from adjacent critical structures. In this procedure, a blocked common carotid arterial flow may be bypassed to the subclavian artery, or a blocked subclavian arterial flow may be bypassed to the common carotid artery. To create a bypass around a section of artery that is damaged or blocked, the physician uses a harvested vein and one of two methods of repair. After vessel clamps have been affixed above and below the damaged area, the graft is sewn to the side of the two arteries (end-to-side) or cut ends may be sewn (end-to-end). The graft is attached above the portion of blocked artery. The blocked portion of artery is not removed. When the clamps are removed in either case, the section of vein graft forms a new path through which blood can easily bypass the blocked area. After the graft is complete, the skin incision is repaired with layered closure.

Coding Tips

Establishing both inflow and outflow by any method is included. That portion of the operative arteriogram performed by the surgeon is also included. Angioscopy performed during therapeutic intervention should be reported in addition to the code for the primary procedure, see 35400. Harvesting of the saphenous vein graft is included in the description of the work for 35506 and should not be reported as a separate procedure. For harvesting of a femoropopliteal vein segment, use 35572 in addition to the bypass procedure. If a composite (combination of vein and synthetic graft) is used, report 35681 in addition to the code for the primary procedure. If synthetic graft material is used, see 35606.

ICD-10-CM Diagnostic Codes

G45.1 Carotid artery syndrome (hemispheric)
G45.2 Multiple and bilateral precerebral artery syndromes
G45.3 Amaurosis fugax

G45.8	Other transient cerebral ischemic attacks and related syndromes
G45.9	Transient cerebral ischemic attack, unspecified
I63.031	Cerebral infarction due to thrombosis of right carotid artery ☑
I63.032	Cerebral infarction due to thrombosis of left carotid artery ☑
I63.09	Cerebral infarction due to thrombosis of other precerebral artery
I63.131	Cerebral infarction due to embolism of right carotid artery ☑
I63.132	Cerebral infarction due to embolism of left carotid artery ☑
I63.19	Cerebral infarction due to embolism of other precerebral artery
I63.231	Cerebral infarction due to unspecified occlusion or stenosis of right carotid arteries ☑
I63.232	Cerebral infarction due to unspecified occlusion or stenosis of left carotid arteries ☑
I63.29	Cerebral infarction due to unspecified occlusion or stenosis of other precerebral arteries
I63.81	Other cerebral infarction due to occlusion or stenosis of small artery
I63.89	Other cerebral infarction
I65.21	Occlusion and stenosis of right carotid artery ☑
I65.22	Occlusion and stenosis of left carotid artery ☑
I65.23	Occlusion and stenosis of bilateral carotid arteries ☑
I65.8	Occlusion and stenosis of other precerebral arteries
I67.81	Acute cerebrovascular insufficiency
I67.82	Cerebral ischemia
I67.850	Cerebral autosomal dominant arteriopathy with subcortical infarcts and leukoencephalopathy
I67.858	Other hereditary cerebrovascular disease
I67.89	Other cerebrovascular disease
I72.8	Aneurysm of other specified arteries
I77.1	Stricture of artery
I77.2	Rupture of artery
I77.79	Dissection of other specified artery
I77.89	Other specified disorders of arteries and arterioles
Q28.1	Other malformations of precerebral vessels
Q28.8	Other specified congenital malformations of circulatory system
S15.011A	Minor laceration of right carotid artery, initial encounter ☑
S15.012A	Minor laceration of left carotid artery, initial encounter ☑
S15.021A	Major laceration of right carotid artery, initial encounter ☑
S15.022A	Major laceration of left carotid artery, initial encounter ☑
S15.091A	Other specified injury of right carotid artery, initial encounter ☑
S15.092A	Other specified injury of left carotid artery, initial encounter ☑
S15.8XXA	Injury of other specified blood vessels at neck level, initial encounter
S25.191A	Other specified injury of right innominate or subclavian artery, initial encounter ☑
S25.192A	Other specified injury of left innominate or subclavian artery, initial encounter ☑

AMA: 35506 2018,Jan,8; 2017,Jan,8; 2016,Jan,13; 2015,Jan,16; 2014,Jan,11

Relative Value Units/Medicare Edits

Non-Facility RVU	Work	PE	MP	Total
35506	25.33	5.62	5.84	36.79
Facility RVU	**Work**	**PE**	**MP**	**Total**
35506	25.33	5.62	5.84	36.79

	FUD	Status	MUE	Modifiers				IOM Reference
35506	90	A	1(3)	51	50	62*	80	None

* with documentation

Terms To Know

aneurysm. Circumscribed dilation or outpouching of an artery wall, often containing blood clots and connecting directly with the lumen of the artery.

artery. Vessel through which oxygenated blood passes away from the heart to any part of the body.

graft. Tissue implant from another part of the body or another person.

infarction. Area of necrosis in tissue, due to ischemia from lack of circulation, usually from a thrombus or an embolus.

ischemia. Deficiency in blood supply causing tissues to be deprived of oxygen, resulting from trauma, mechanical or functional constriction of blood vessels, or a physical obstruction.

stenosis. Narrowing or constriction of a passage.

35508

35508 Bypass graft, with vein; carotid-vertebral

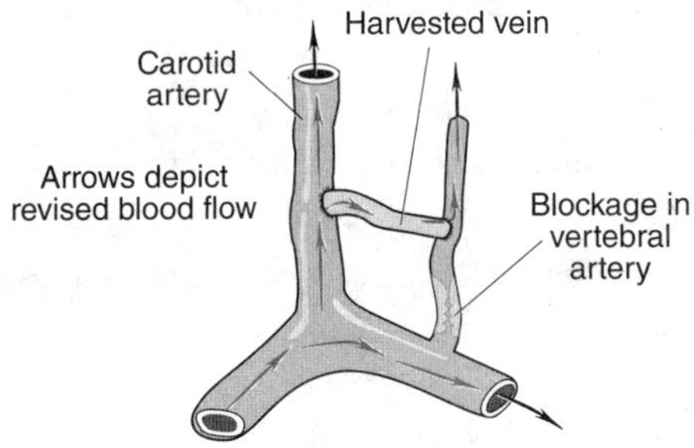

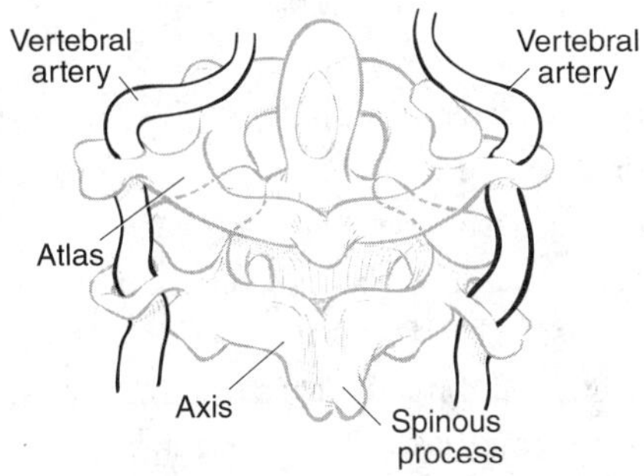

Posterior view of the first two vertebrae showing route of vertebral arteries

Explanation

Through an incision in the skin of the neck, the physician isolates and dissects the vertebral and carotid arteries, separating them from adjacent critical structures. The physician creates a bypass around a section of vertebral artery that is damaged or blocked, using a harvested vein and one of two methods of repair. After vessel clamps have been affixed above and below the damaged area, the graft is sewn to the side of the carotid artery and either sewn to the side of the vertebral artery beyond the affected area (end-to-side) or sewn over the cut end of the vertebral artery after dividing it beyond the affected area (end-to-end). The damaged or blocked section of the vertebral artery is not removed. When the clamps are removed, the section of vein graft forms a new path through which blood can easily bypass the blocked area. After the graft is complete, the skin incision is repaired with a layered closure.

Coding Tips

Establishing both inflow and outflow by any method is included. That portion of the operative arteriogram performed by the surgeon is also included. Angioscopy performed during therapeutic intervention should be reported in addition to the code for the primary procedure; see 35400. Harvesting of the saphenous vein graft is included in the description of the work for 35508 and should not be reported as a separate procedure. For harvesting of a femoropopliteal vein segment, use 35572 in addition to the bypass procedure. If a composite (combination of vein and synthetic graft) is used, report 35681 in addition to the code for the primary procedure. If synthetic graft material is used, see 35642.

ICD-10-CM Diagnostic Codes

G45.0 Vertebro-basilar artery syndrome
I63.011 Cerebral infarction due to thrombosis of right vertebral artery ☑
I63.012 Cerebral infarction due to thrombosis of left vertebral artery ☑
I63.013 Cerebral infarction due to thrombosis of bilateral vertebral arteries ☑
I63.033 Cerebral infarction due to thrombosis of bilateral carotid arteries ☑
I63.111 Cerebral infarction due to embolism of right vertebral artery ☑
I63.112 Cerebral infarction due to embolism of left vertebral artery ☑
I63.113 Cerebral infarction due to embolism of bilateral vertebral arteries ☑
I63.133 Cerebral infarction due to embolism of bilateral carotid arteries ☑
I65.01 Occlusion and stenosis of right vertebral artery ☑
I65.02 Occlusion and stenosis of left vertebral artery ☑
I65.03 Occlusion and stenosis of bilateral vertebral arteries ☑
I76 Septic arterial embolism
I77.1 Stricture of artery
I77.2 Rupture of artery
I77.74 Dissection of vertebral artery
I77.89 Other specified disorders of arteries and arterioles
S15.111A Minor laceration of right vertebral artery, initial encounter ☑
S15.112A Minor laceration of left vertebral artery, initial encounter ☑
S15.121A Major laceration of right vertebral artery, initial encounter ☑
S15.122A Major laceration of left vertebral artery, initial encounter ☑
S15.191A Other specified injury of right vertebral artery, initial encounter ☑
S15.192A Other specified injury of left vertebral artery, initial encounter ☑

AMA: **35508** 1999,Mar,6; 1999,Apr,11

Relative Value Units/Medicare Edits

Non-Facility RVU	Work	PE	MP	Total
35508	26.09	6.22	6.03	38.34
Facility RVU	**Work**	**PE**	**MP**	**Total**
35508	26.09	6.22	6.03	38.34

	FUD	Status	MUE	Modifiers				IOM Reference
35508	90	A	1(3)	51	50	62*	80	None

* with documentation

Terms To Know

arteriogram. Radiograph of arteries.

bypass graft. Surgically created alternative blood vessel used to reroute blood flow around an area of obstruction or disease.

ischemia. Deficiency in blood supply causing tissues to be deprived of oxygen, resulting from trauma, mechanical or functional constriction of blood vessels, or a physical obstruction.

35509

35509 Bypass graft, with vein; carotid-contralateral carotid

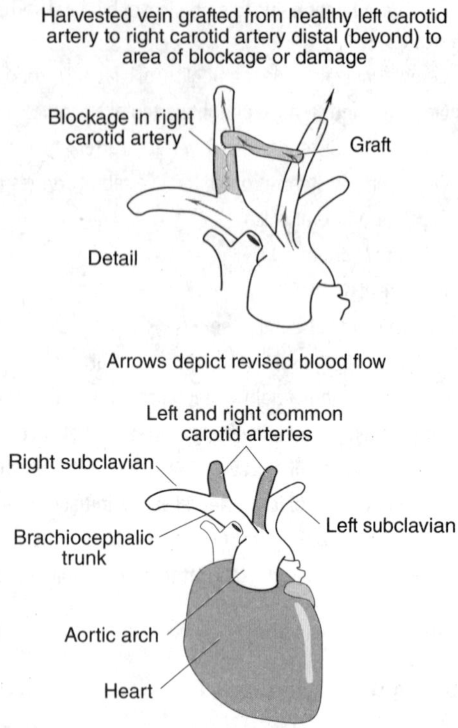

Explanation

The physician performs a vein bypass graft from one carotid to the contralateral carotid. Through incisions in the skin of the neck, the physician isolates and dissects the carotid arteries, separating them from adjacent critical structures. The physician creates a bypass around a section of carotid artery that is damaged or blocked, using a harvested vein and one of two methods of repair. After vessel clamps have been affixed above and below the damaged area, the ends of the vein graft are sutured into the side of the carotid arterial wall (end-to-side). In the second method, the carotid artery may be cut through above the damaged area and sutured to one end of a harvested vein, which is sutured to the side of the carotid artery on the opposite side of the neck (end-to-end). In either case, the blocked or damaged section of artery is not removed. When the clamps are removed, the section of vein graft forms a new path through which blood can easily bypass the blocked or damaged area. After the graft is complete, the skin incisions are repaired with layered closures.

Coding Tips

Establishing both inflow and outflow by any method is included. That portion of the operative arteriogram performed by the surgeon is also included. Angioscopy performed during therapeutic intervention should be reported in addition to the code for the primary procedure; see 35400. Harvesting of the saphenous vein graft is included in the description of the work for 35509 and should not be reported as a separate procedure. For harvesting of a femoropopliteal vein segment, use 35572 in addition to the bypass procedure. If a composite (combination of vein and synthetic graft) is used, report 35681 in addition to the code for the primary procedure.

ICD-10-CM Diagnostic Codes

G45.1	Carotid artery syndrome (hemispheric)
G45.3	Amaurosis fugax
G45.9	Transient cerebral ischemic attack, unspecified
I63.031	Cerebral infarction due to thrombosis of right carotid artery ☑
I63.032	Cerebral infarction due to thrombosis of left carotid artery ☑
I63.131	Cerebral infarction due to embolism of right carotid artery ☑
I63.132	Cerebral infarction due to embolism of left carotid artery ☑
I63.81	Other cerebral infarction due to occlusion or stenosis of small artery
I63.89	Other cerebral infarction
I65.21	Occlusion and stenosis of right carotid artery ☑
I65.22	Occlusion and stenosis of left carotid artery ☑
I65.23	Occlusion and stenosis of bilateral carotid arteries ☑
I67.81	Acute cerebrovascular insufficiency
I67.850	Cerebral autosomal dominant arteriopathy with subcortical infarcts and leukoencephalopathy
I67.858	Other hereditary cerebrovascular disease
I72.0	Aneurysm of carotid artery
I77.71	Dissection of carotid artery
S15.011A	Minor laceration of right carotid artery, initial encounter ☑
S15.012A	Minor laceration of left carotid artery, initial encounter ☑
S15.021A	Major laceration of right carotid artery, initial encounter ☑
S15.022A	Major laceration of left carotid artery, initial encounter ☑
S15.091A	Other specified injury of right carotid artery, initial encounter ☑
S15.092A	Other specified injury of left carotid artery, initial encounter ☑
S15.8XXA	Injury of other specified blood vessels at neck level, initial encounter

AMA: 35509 2018,Jan,8; 2017,Jan,8; 2016,Jan,13; 2015,Jan,16; 2014,Jan,11

Relative Value Units/Medicare Edits

Non-Facility RVU	Work	PE	MP	Total
35509	28.09	6.25	6.49	40.83
Facility RVU	**Work**	**PE**	**MP**	**Total**
35509	28.09	6.25	6.49	40.83

	FUD	Status	MUE	Modifiers				IOM Reference
35509	90	A	1(3)	51	50	62*	80	None

* with documentation

35510

35510 Bypass graft, with vein; carotid-brachial

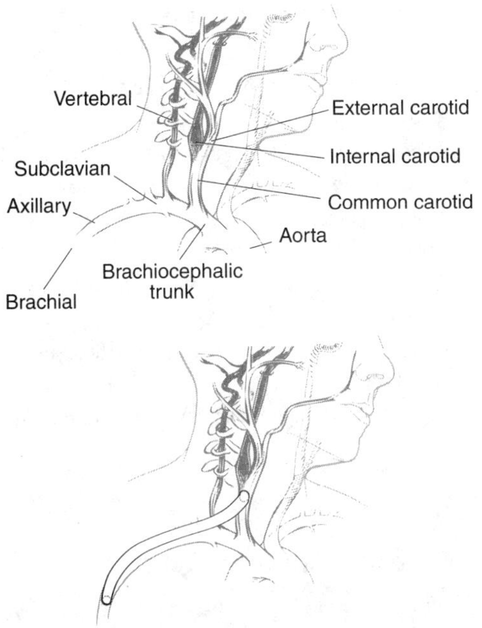

A vein graft from the carotid to the brachial artery is performed

Explanation

Through an incision in the skin at the side of the neck, the physician dissects down to the common carotid artery, separating soft tissue and adjacent critical structures. Soft tissue must be cleared for several centimeters. Dissection through the skin and soft tissue at the distal anastomosis site of this bypass graft is also done over the brachial artery in the arm. Next, a tunnel is made from the carotid through the axilla and down the arm to the brachial artery site. To create a bypass graft around the section of brachial artery that is damaged or blocked, the physician uses a harvested vein, usually the greater saphenous. After vascular clamps have been affixed above and below the anastomosis area on the carotid artery, the proximal arteriotomy is carried out and the harvested vein is sutured to the carotid artery. When this is completed and checked for hemorrhaging, the arterial clamps are removed. The vein graft is tunneled through the prepared space to the brachial artery and the distal arteriotomy and anastomosis are carried out in the same manner. The clamps are removed, additional sutures may be placed for complete hemostasis, and the patency of the graft is checked. The incisions are closed and the appropriate pulses are checked again before dressings are applied.

Coding Tips

Establishing both inflow and outflow by any method is included. That portion of the operative arteriogram performed by the surgeon is also included. Angioscopy performed during therapeutic intervention should be reported in addition to the code for the primary procedure; see 35400. Harvesting of the saphenous vein graft is included in the description of the work for 35510 and should not be reported as a separate procedure. For harvesting of a femoropopliteal vein segment, use 35572 in addition to the bypass procedure. If a composite (combination of vein and synthetic graft) is used, report 35681 in addition to the code for the primary procedure.

ICD-10-CM Diagnostic Codes

I70.92	Chronic total occlusion of artery of the extremities
I74.2	Embolism and thrombosis of arteries of the upper extremities
I74.8	Embolism and thrombosis of other arteries
I75.011	Atheroembolism of right upper extremity ☑
I75.012	Atheroembolism of left upper extremity ☑
I75.013	Atheroembolism of bilateral upper extremities ☑
I77.1	Stricture of artery
I77.2	Rupture of artery
S45.111A	Laceration of brachial artery, right side, initial encounter ☑
S45.112A	Laceration of brachial artery, left side, initial encounter ☑
S45.191A	Other specified injury of brachial artery, right side, initial encounter ☑
S45.192A	Other specified injury of brachial artery, left side, initial encounter ☑

AMA: **35510** 2018,Jan,8; 2017,Jan,8; 2016,Jan,13; 2015,Jan,16; 2014,Jan,11

Relative Value Units/Medicare Edits

Non-Facility RVU	Work	PE	MP	Total
35510	24.39	5.49	5.64	35.52
Facility RVU	**Work**	**PE**	**MP**	**Total**
35510	24.39	5.49	5.64	35.52

	FUD	Status	MUE	Modifiers				IOM Reference
35510	90	A	1(3)	51	50	62*	80	None

* with documentation

Terms To Know

anastomosis. Surgically created connection between ducts, blood vessels, or bowel segments to allow flow from one to the other.

bypass graft. Surgically created alternative blood vessel used to reroute blood flow around an area of obstruction or disease.

dissection. Separating by cutting tissue or body structures apart.

hemostasis. Interruption of blood flow or the cessation or arrest of bleeding.

patency. State of a tube-like structure or conduit being open and unobstructed.

35511

35511 Bypass graft, with vein; subclavian-subclavian

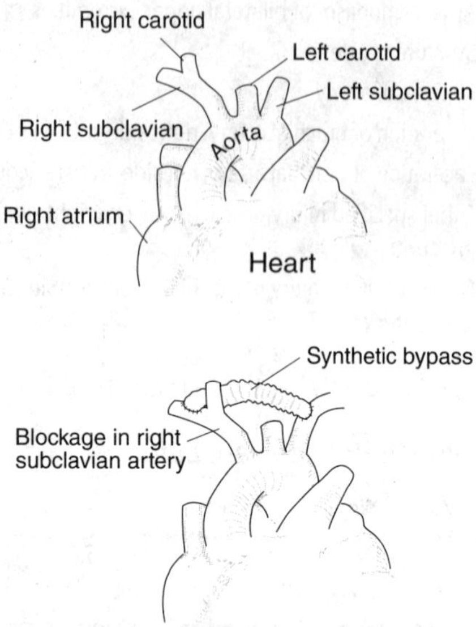

Harvested vein grafted from healthy left subclavian artery to right subclavian artery distal (beyond) area of blockage or damage

Explanation

Through incisions in the skin at the base of the neck, the physician isolates and dissects the subclavian arteries, separating them from adjacent critical structures. The physician creates a bypass around a section of subclavian artery that is damaged or blocked, using a harvested vein and one of two methods of repair after vessel clamps have been affixed above and below the defect. In the first method of repair the ends of the vein graft are sutured into the sides of the walls of the two subclavian arteries, resulting in a bypass of the damaged area. In the second method, the subclavian artery may be cut through beyond the damaged area and sutured to one end of a harvested vein, which is sutured to the subclavian artery on the opposite side of the neck. In either case, the blocked or damaged portion of the artery is not removed. When the clamps are removed, the section of vein graft forms a new path through which blood can easily bypass the blocked area. After the graft is complete, the skin incisions are repaired with a layered closure.

Coding Tips

Establishing both inflow and outflow by any method is included. That portion of the operative arteriogram performed by the surgeon is also included. Angioscopy performed during therapeutic intervention should be reported in addition to the code for the primary procedure; see 35400. Harvesting of the saphenous vein graft is included in the description of the work for 35511 and should not be reported as a separate procedure. For harvesting of a femoropopliteal vein segment, use 35572 in addition to the bypass procedure. If a composite (combination of vein and synthetic graft) is used, report 35681 in addition to the code for the primary procedure. If synthetic graft material is used, see 35612.

ICD-10-CM Diagnostic Codes

I74.2	Embolism and thrombosis of arteries of the upper extremities
I74.8	Embolism and thrombosis of other arteries
I75.011	Atheroembolism of right upper extremity ☑
I75.012	Atheroembolism of left upper extremity ☑
I75.013	Atheroembolism of bilateral upper extremities ☑
I77.1	Stricture of artery
I77.2	Rupture of artery
I77.5	Necrosis of artery
I77.79	Dissection of other specified artery
I77.89	Other specified disorders of arteries and arterioles
S25.111A	Minor laceration of right innominate or subclavian artery, initial encounter ☑
S25.112A	Minor laceration of left innominate or subclavian artery, initial encounter ☑
S25.121A	Major laceration of right innominate or subclavian artery, initial encounter ☑
S25.122A	Major laceration of left innominate or subclavian artery, initial encounter ☑
S25.191A	Other specified injury of right innominate or subclavian artery, initial encounter ☑
S25.192A	Other specified injury of left innominate or subclavian artery, initial encounter ☑

AMA: **35511** 2018,Jan,8; 2017,Jan,8; 2016,Jan,13; 2015,Jan,16; 2014,Jan,11

Relative Value Units/Medicare Edits

Non-Facility RVU	Work	PE	MP	Total
35511	22.2	5.02	5.13	32.35
Facility RVU	**Work**	**PE**	**MP**	**Total**
35511	22.2	5.02	5.13	32.35

	FUD	Status	MUE	Modifiers				IOM Reference
35511	90	A	1(3)	51	50	62*	80	None

* with documentation

Terms To Know

angioscopy. Visualization of capillary blood vessels with a microscope, or the inside of a blood vessel with a fiberoptic-equipped catheter.

ischemia. Deficiency in blood supply causing tissues to be deprived of oxygen, resulting from trauma, mechanical or functional constriction of blood vessels, or a physical obstruction.

35512

35512 Bypass graft, with vein; subclavian-brachial

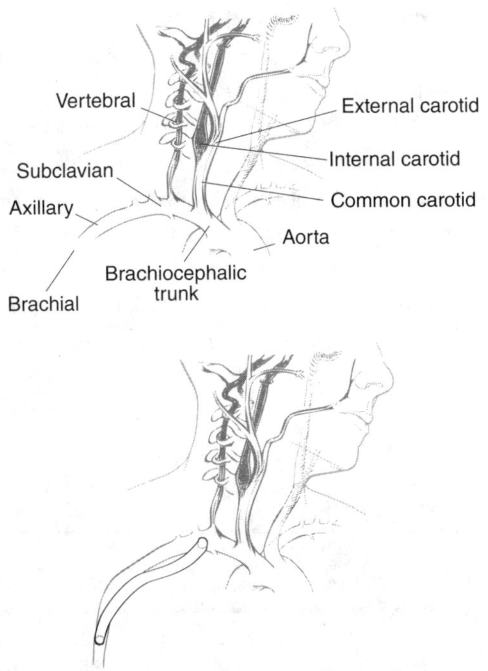

A vein graft from the subclavian to the brachial artery is performed

Explanation

Through an incision in the skin at the base of the neck, the physician dissects down to the subclavian artery just above the clavicle, separating soft tissue and adjacent critical structures. Soft tissue must be cleared for several centimeters. Dissection through the skin and soft tissue at the distal anastomosis site for this bypass graft is also done over the brachial artery in the arm. Next, a tunnel is made from the subclavian, under the clavicle, through the axilla, and down the arm to the brachial artery site. To create a bypass graft around the section of brachial artery that is damaged or blocked, the physician uses a harvested vein, usually the greater saphenous. After vascular clamps have been affixed above and below the anastomosis area on the subclavian artery, the proximal arteriotomy is carried out and the harvested vein is sutured to the subclavian artery. When this is completed and checked for hemorrhaging, the arterial clamps are removed. The vein graft is tunneled through the prepared space to the brachial artery and the distal arteriotomy and anastomosis are carried out in the same manner. The clamps are removed, additional sutures may be placed for complete hemostasis, and the patency of the graft is checked. The incisions are closed and the appropriate pulses are checked again before dressings are applied.

Coding Tips

Establishing both inflow and outflow by any method is included. That portion of the operative arteriogram performed by the surgeon is also included. Angioscopy performed during therapeutic intervention should be reported in addition to the code for the primary procedure; see 35400. Harvesting of the saphenous vein graft is included in the description of the work for 35512 and should not be reported as a separate procedure. For harvesting of a femoropopliteal vein segment, use 35572 in addition to the bypass procedure. If a composite (combination of vein and synthetic graft) is used, report 35681 in addition to the code for the primary procedure.

ICD-10-CM Diagnostic Codes

I72.1	Aneurysm of artery of upper extremity
I74.2	Embolism and thrombosis of arteries of the upper extremities
I74.8	Embolism and thrombosis of other arteries
I75.011	Atheroembolism of right upper extremity ☑
I75.012	Atheroembolism of left upper extremity ☑
I75.013	Atheroembolism of bilateral upper extremities ☑
I77.1	Stricture of artery
I77.2	Rupture of artery
I77.79	Dissection of other specified artery
I77.89	Other specified disorders of arteries and arterioles
S45.111A	Laceration of brachial artery, right side, initial encounter ☑
S45.112A	Laceration of brachial artery, left side, initial encounter ☑
S45.191A	Other specified injury of brachial artery, right side, initial encounter ☑
S45.192A	Other specified injury of brachial artery, left side, initial encounter ☑

AMA: 35512 2018,Jan,8; 2017,Jan,8; 2016,Jan,13; 2015,Jan,16; 2014,Jan,11

Relative Value Units/Medicare Edits

Non-Facility RVU	Work	PE	MP	Total
35512	23.89	5.41	5.52	34.82
Facility RVU	**Work**	**PE**	**MP**	**Total**
35512	23.89	5.41	5.52	34.82

	FUD	Status	MUE	Modifiers				IOM Reference
35512	90	A	1(3)	51	50	62*	80	None

* with documentation

Terms To Know

anastomosis. Surgically created connection between ducts, blood vessels, or bowel segments to allow flow from one to the other.

arteriotomy. Incision into an artery.

axillary region. Area immediately surrounding the armpit.

vascular insufficiency. Inadequate blood flow and oxygenation.

35515

35515 Bypass graft, with vein; subclavian-vertebral

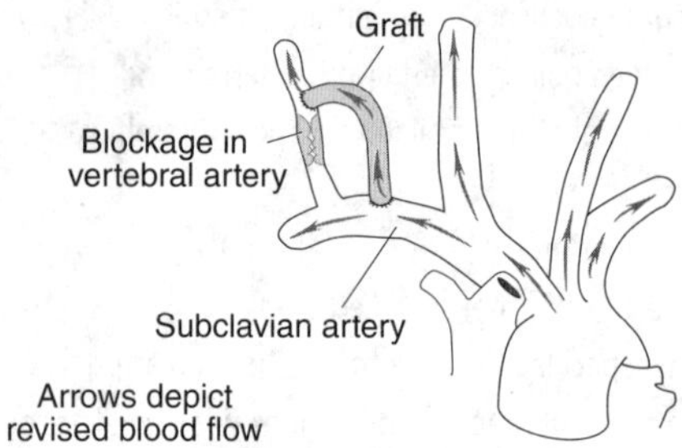

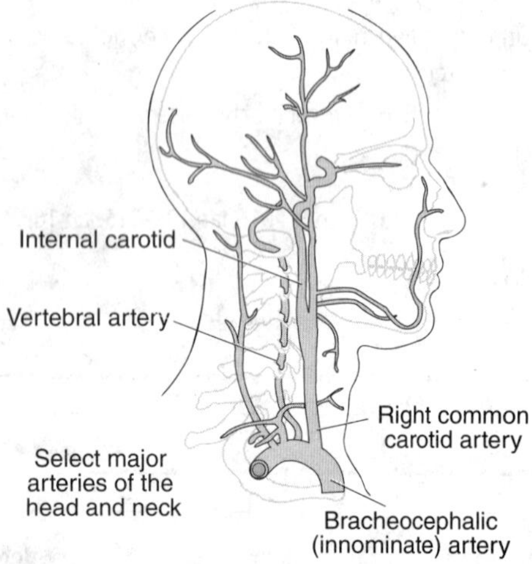

Explanation

Through an incision in the skin of the neck, the physician isolates and dissects the vertebral and subclavian arteries, separating them from adjacent critical structures. The physician creates a bypass around a section of vertebral artery that is damaged or blocked, using a harvested vein and one of two methods of repair. Once vessel clamps are affixed above and below the defect, the ends of the harvested vein are sutured into the sides of the subclavian and vertebral arterial walls resulting in a bypass of the damaged area (end-to-side). In the second method, the vertebral artery can be cut through above the damaged area and sutured to one end of a harvested vein (end-to-end). The remaining end is sutured to the subclavian artery. In either case, the blocked or damaged vertebral artery is not removed. When the clamps are removed, the section of vein graft forms a new path through which blood can easily bypass the blocked area. After the graft is complete, the skin incision is repaired with a layered closure.

Coding Tips

Establishing both inflow and outflow by any method is included. That portion of the operative arteriogram performed by the surgeon is also included. Angioscopy performed during therapeutic intervention should be reported in addition to the code for the primary procedure; see 35400. Harvesting of the saphenous vein graft is included in the description of the work for 35515 and should not be reported as a separate procedure. For harvesting of a femoropopliteal vein segment, use 35572 in addition to the bypass procedure. If a composite (combination of vein and synthetic graft) is used, report 35681 in addition to the code for the primary procedure.

ICD-10-CM Diagnostic Codes

G45.0 Vertebro-basilar artery syndrome
I63.011 Cerebral infarction due to thrombosis of right vertebral artery ☑
I63.012 Cerebral infarction due to thrombosis of left vertebral artery ☑
I63.111 Cerebral infarction due to embolism of right vertebral artery ☑
I63.112 Cerebral infarction due to embolism of left vertebral artery ☑
I65.01 Occlusion and stenosis of right vertebral artery ☑
I65.02 Occlusion and stenosis of left vertebral artery ☑
I65.03 Occlusion and stenosis of bilateral vertebral arteries ☑
I77.74 Dissection of vertebral artery
I77.89 Other specified disorders of arteries and arterioles
S15.111A Minor laceration of right vertebral artery, initial encounter ☑
S15.112A Minor laceration of left vertebral artery, initial encounter ☑
S15.121A Major laceration of right vertebral artery, initial encounter ☑
S15.122A Major laceration of left vertebral artery, initial encounter ☑
S15.191A Other specified injury of right vertebral artery, initial encounter ☑
S15.192A Other specified injury of left vertebral artery, initial encounter ☑

AMA: **35515** 1999,Mar,6; 1999,Apr,11

Relative Value Units/Medicare Edits

Non-Facility RVU	Work	PE	MP	Total
35515	26.09	6.22	6.03	38.34
Facility RVU	**Work**	**PE**	**MP**	**Total**
35515	26.09	6.22	6.03	38.34

	FUD	Status	MUE	Modifiers				IOM Reference
35515	90	A	1(3)	51	50	62*	80	None

* with documentation

Terms To Know

angioscopy. Visualization of capillary blood vessels with a microscope, or the inside of a blood vessel with a fiberoptic-equipped catheter.

graft. Tissue implant from another part of the body or another person.

ischemia. Deficiency in blood supply causing tissues to be deprived of oxygen, resulting from trauma, mechanical or functional constriction of blood vessels, or a physical obstruction.

occlusion. Constriction, closure, or blockage of a passage.

stenosis. Narrowing or constriction of a passage.

stricture. Narrowing of an anatomical structure.

35516

35516 Bypass graft, with vein; subclavian-axillary

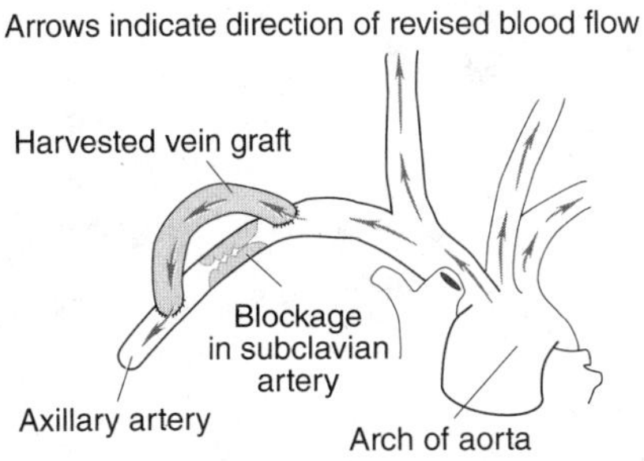

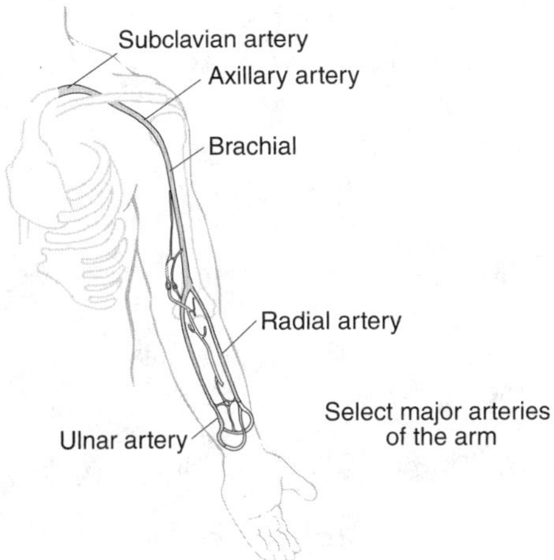

Explanation

Through an incision in the skin at the base of the neck and axilla, the physician isolates and dissects the subclavian and axillary arteries, separating them from adjacent critical structures. The physician creates a bypass around a section of subclavian artery that is damaged or blocked, using a harvested vein and one of two methods of repair. Once vessel clamps have been affixed above and below the defect, the ends of the harvested vein are sutured into the sides of the subclavian and axillary arterial walls resulting in a bypass of the damaged area (end-to-side). In the second method, the subclavian artery may be cut through before the damaged area and sutured to one end of a harvested vein, which is sutured to the axillary artery (end-to-end). The blocked or damaged portion of the subclavian artery is not removed. When the clamps are removed, the section of vein graft forms a new path through which blood can easily bypass the blocked area. After the graft is complete, the skin incisions are repaired with a layered closure.

Coding Tips

Establishing both inflow and outflow by any method is included. That portion of the operative arteriogram performed by the surgeon is also included. Angioscopy performed during therapeutic intervention should be reported in addition to the code for the primary procedure; see 35400. Harvesting of the saphenous vein graft is included in the description of the work for 35516 and should not be reported as a separate procedure. For harvesting of a femoropopliteal vein segment, use 35572 in addition to the bypass procedure. If a composite (combination of vein and synthetic graft) is used, report 35681 in addition to the code for the primary procedure. If synthetic graft material is used, see 35616.

ICD-10-CM Diagnostic Codes

G45.2	Multiple and bilateral precerebral artery syndromes
G45.8	Other transient cerebral ischemic attacks and related syndromes
I63.19	Cerebral infarction due to embolism of other precerebral artery
I63.29	Cerebral infarction due to unspecified occlusion or stenosis of other precerebral arteries
I63.89	Other cerebral infarction
I65.8	Occlusion and stenosis of other precerebral arteries
I67.850	Cerebral autosomal dominant arteriopathy with subcortical infarcts and leukoencephalopathy
I67.858	Other hereditary cerebrovascular disease
I70.92	Chronic total occlusion of artery of the extremities
I74.2	Embolism and thrombosis of arteries of the upper extremities
I74.8	Embolism and thrombosis of other arteries
I75.011	Atheroembolism of right upper extremity ☑
I75.012	Atheroembolism of left upper extremity ☑
I75.013	Atheroembolism of bilateral upper extremities ☑
I77.1	Stricture of artery
I77.2	Rupture of artery
I77.5	Necrosis of artery
I77.79	Dissection of other specified artery
I77.89	Other specified disorders of arteries and arterioles
S15.8XXA	Injury of other specified blood vessels at neck level, initial encounter
S25.111A	Minor laceration of right innominate or subclavian artery, initial encounter ☑
S25.112A	Minor laceration of left innominate or subclavian artery, initial encounter ☑
S25.121A	Major laceration of right innominate or subclavian artery, initial encounter ☑
S25.122A	Major laceration of left innominate or subclavian artery, initial encounter ☑
S25.191A	Other specified injury of right innominate or subclavian artery, initial encounter ☑
S25.192A	Other specified injury of left innominate or subclavian artery, initial encounter ☑

AMA: 35516 1999,Mar,6; 1999,Apr,11

Relative Value Units/Medicare Edits

Non-Facility RVU	Work	PE	MP	Total
35516	24.21	5.43	5.59	35.23
Facility RVU	**Work**	**PE**	**MP**	**Total**
35516	24.21	5.43	5.59	35.23

	FUD	Status	MUE	Modifiers				IOM Reference
35516	90	A	1(3)	51	50	62*	80	None

* with documentation

Terms To Know

bypass graft. Surgically created alternative blood vessel used to reroute blood flow around an area of obstruction or disease.

35518

35518 Bypass graft, with vein; axillary-axillary

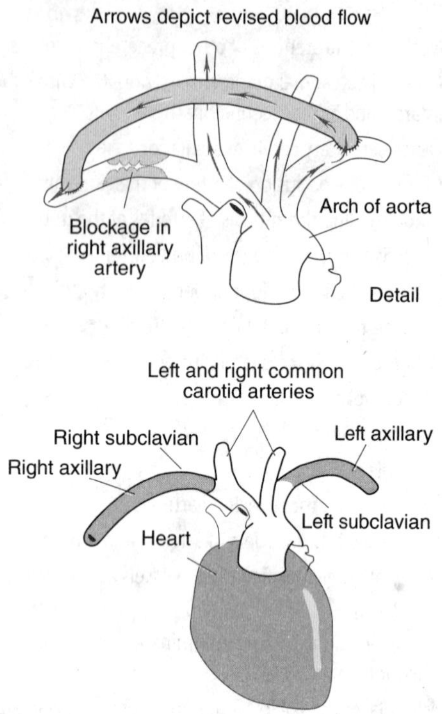

Explanation

The physician makes an incision in the skin of both axillae. The physician creates a bypass around the section of axillary artery that is damaged or blocked, using a harvested vein and one of two methods of repair. Once vessel clamps have been affixed above and below the defect, the ends of the harvested vein are sutured into the sides of the two axillary arterial walls, resulting in a bypass of the damaged area. In the second method, the axillary artery may be cut through beyond the damaged area and sutured to one end of a harvested vein, which is passed across the front of the chest under the skin and sutured to the side of the contralateral axillary artery. The blocked or damaged portion of the axillary artery is not removed. When the clamps are removed, the section of vein graft forms a new path through which blood can easily bypass the blocked area. After the graft is complete, the skin incisions are repaired with layered closures.

Coding Tips

Establishing both inflow and outflow by any method is included. That portion of the operative arteriogram performed by the surgeon is also included. Angioscopy performed during therapeutic intervention should be reported in addition to the code for the primary procedure; see 35400. Harvesting of the saphenous vein graft is included in the description of the work for 35518 and should not be reported as a separate procedure. For harvesting of a femoropopliteal vein segment, use 35572 in addition to the bypass procedure. If a composite (combination of vein and synthetic graft) is used, report 35681 in addition to the code for the primary procedure.

ICD-10-CM Diagnostic Codes

G45.2	Multiple and bilateral precerebral artery syndromes
I63.09	Cerebral infarction due to thrombosis of other precerebral artery
I63.19	Cerebral infarction due to embolism of other precerebral artery
I63.81	Other cerebral infarction due to occlusion or stenosis of small artery
I63.89	Other cerebral infarction
I65.8	Occlusion and stenosis of other precerebral arteries
I67.81	Acute cerebrovascular insufficiency
I67.850	Cerebral autosomal dominant arteriopathy with subcortical infarcts and leukoencephalopathy
I67.858	Other hereditary cerebrovascular disease
I74.8	Embolism and thrombosis of other arteries
I76	Septic arterial embolism
I77.1	Stricture of artery
I77.2	Rupture of artery
I77.5	Necrosis of artery
I77.79	Dissection of other specified artery
I77.89	Other specified disorders of arteries and arterioles
S15.8XXA	Injury of other specified blood vessels at neck level, initial encounter
S45.011A	Laceration of axillary artery, right side, initial encounter ☑
S45.012A	Laceration of axillary artery, left side, initial encounter ☑
S45.091A	Other specified injury of axillary artery, right side, initial encounter ☑
S45.092A	Other specified injury of axillary artery, left side, initial encounter ☑

AMA: 35518 2018,Jan,8; 2017,Jan,8; 2016,Jan,13; 2015,Jan,16; 2014,Jan,11

Relative Value Units/Medicare Edits

Non-Facility RVU	Work	PE	MP	Total
35518	22.65	5.09	5.23	32.97
Facility RVU	**Work**	**PE**	**MP**	**Total**
35518	22.65	5.09	5.23	32.97

	FUD	Status	MUE	Modifiers				IOM Reference
35518	90	A	1(3)	51	50	62*	80	None

* with documentation

Terms To Know

angioscopy. Visualization of capillary blood vessels with a microscope, or the inside of a blood vessel with a fiberoptic-equipped catheter.

arteriogram. Radiograph of arteries.

atherosclerosis. Buildup of yellowish plaques composed of cholesterol and lipoid material within the arteries.

graft. Tissue implant from another part of the body or another person.

35521

35521 Bypass graft, with vein; axillary-femoral

A vein bypass graft from the axillary artery to the femoral artery is accomplished

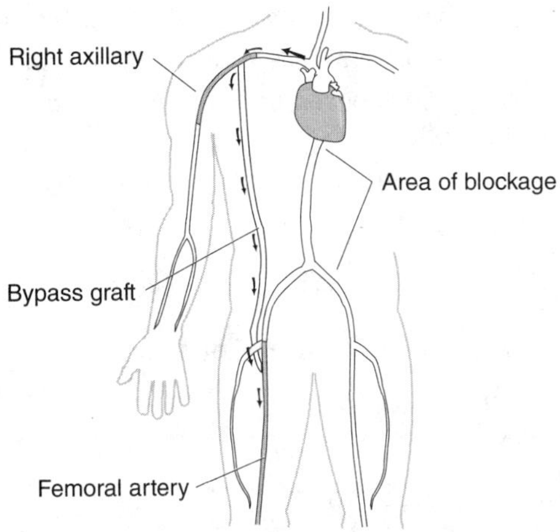

Explanation

The physician makes incisions in the skin of the axilla and upper thigh. The axillary and femoral arteries are isolated and dissected from adjacent critical structures. The physician creates a bypass around the section of damaged or blocked artery using a harvested vein and one of two methods of repair. Once vessel clamps have been affixed above and below the areas of anastomosis, the harvested vein is sutured to an incision in the side of the axillary artery and passed through a subcutaneous tunnel on the side of the body and to the upper thigh. The harvested vein is sutured to the femoral artery (common, deep, or superficial) in an end-to-side or end-to-end fashion. The blocked or damaged portion of artery is not removed. When the clamps are removed, the section of vein graft forms a new path through which blood can easily bypass the blocked area. After the graft is complete, the skin incisions are repaired with layered closures.

Coding Tips

Establishing both inflow and outflow by any method is included. That portion of the operative arteriogram performed by the surgeon is also included. Angioscopy performed during therapeutic intervention should be reported in addition to the code for the primary procedure; see 35400. Harvesting of the saphenous vein graft is included in the description of the work for 35521 and should not be reported as a separate procedure. For harvesting of a femoropopliteal vein segment, use 35572 in addition to the bypass procedure. If a composite (combination of vein and synthetic graft) is used, report 35681 in addition to the code for the primary procedure. If synthetic graft material is used, see 35621.

ICD-10-CM Diagnostic Codes

A52.02	Syphilitic aortitis
I70.0	Atherosclerosis of aorta
I70.8	Atherosclerosis of other arteries
I70.92	Chronic total occlusion of artery of the extremities
I71.01	Dissection of thoracic aorta
I71.02	Dissection of abdominal aorta
I71.03	Dissection of thoracoabdominal aorta
I73.89	Other specified peripheral vascular diseases
I73.9	Peripheral vascular disease, unspecified
I74.01	Saddle embolus of abdominal aorta
I74.09	Other arterial embolism and thrombosis of abdominal aorta
I74.19	Embolism and thrombosis of other parts of aorta
I74.5	Embolism and thrombosis of iliac artery
I76	Septic arterial embolism
I77.1	Stricture of artery
I77.3	Arterial fibromuscular dysplasia
I77.5	Necrosis of artery
I77.72	Dissection of iliac artery
I77.89	Other specified disorders of arteries and arterioles
Q25.21	Interruption of aortic arch
Q25.41	Absence and aplasia of aorta
Q25.42	Hypoplasia of aorta
Q25.43	Congenital aneurysm of aorta
Q25.44	Congenital dilation of aorta
Q25.45	Double aortic arch
Q25.46	Tortuous aortic arch
Q25.47	Right aortic arch
Q25.48	Anomalous origin of subclavian artery
Q25.8	Other congenital malformations of other great arteries
S25.01XA	Minor laceration of thoracic aorta, initial encounter
S25.02XA	Major laceration of thoracic aorta, initial encounter
S25.09XA	Other specified injury of thoracic aorta, initial encounter
S35.01XA	Minor laceration of abdominal aorta, initial encounter
S35.02XA	Major laceration of abdominal aorta, initial encounter
S35.09XA	Other injury of abdominal aorta, initial encounter
S35.511A	Injury of right iliac artery, initial encounter ☑
S35.512A	Injury of left iliac artery, initial encounter ☑
S35.59XA	Injury of other iliac blood vessels, initial encounter

AMA: **35521** 2018,Jan,8; 2017,Jan,8; 2016,Jan,13; 2015,Jan,16; 2014,Jan,11

Relative Value Units/Medicare Edits

Non-Facility RVU	Work	PE	MP	Total
35521	24.13	5.71	5.57	35.41
Facility RVU	**Work**	**PE**	**MP**	**Total**
35521	24.13	5.71	5.57	35.41

	FUD	Status	MUE	Modifiers				IOM Reference
35521	90	A	1(3)	51	50	62*	80	None

* with documentation

Terms To Know

aneurysm. Circumscribed dilation or outpouching of an artery wall, often containing blood clots and connecting directly with the lumen of the artery.

bypass graft. Surgically created alternative blood vessel used to reroute blood flow around an area of obstruction or disease.

35522

35522 Bypass graft, with vein; axillary-brachial

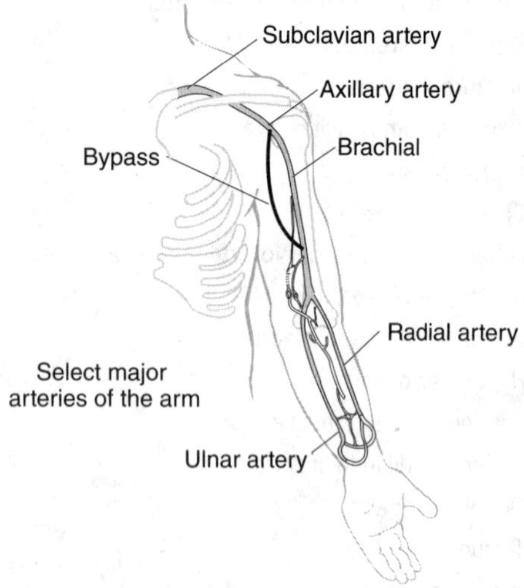

A bypass from the axillary artery to another site along the brachial artery is performed

Explanation

Through an incision in the skin of the chest wall, the physician dissects down to the axillary artery just below the clavicle, separating soft tissue and adjacent critical structures. Soft tissue must be cleared for several centimeters. Dissection through the skin and soft tissue at the distal anastomosis site for this bypass graft is also done over the brachial artery in the arm near the elbow. Next, a tunnel is made from the exposed axillary, through the axilla and down the arm to the brachial artery site. To create a bypass graft around the section of brachial artery that is damaged or blocked, the physician uses a harvested vein, usually the greater saphenous. After vascular clamps have been affixed above and below the anastomosis area on the axillary artery, the proximal arteriotomy is carried out and the harvested vein is sutured to the axillary artery. When this is completed and checked for hemorrhaging, the arterial clamps are removed. The vein graft is tunneled through the prepared space to the brachial artery and the distal arteriotomy and anastomosis are carried out in the same manner. The clamps are removed, additional sutures may be placed for complete hemostasis, and the patency of the graft is checked. The incisions are closed and the appropriate pulses are checked again before dressings are applied.

Coding Tips

Establishing both inflow and outflow by any method is included. That portion of the operative arteriogram performed by the surgeon is also included. Angioscopy performed during therapeutic intervention should be reported in addition to the code for the primary procedure; see 35400. Harvesting of the saphenous vein graft is included in the description of the work for 35522 and should not be reported as a separate procedure. For harvesting of a femoropopliteal vein segment, use 35572 in addition to the bypass procedure.

ICD-10-CM Diagnostic Codes

I70.92	Chronic total occlusion of artery of the extremities
I72.1	Aneurysm of artery of upper extremity
I73.9	Peripheral vascular disease, unspecified
I74.2	Embolism and thrombosis of arteries of the upper extremities
I74.8	Embolism and thrombosis of other arteries
I75.011	Atheroembolism of right upper extremity ☑
I75.012	Atheroembolism of left upper extremity ☑
I75.013	Atheroembolism of bilateral upper extremities ☑
I77.1	Stricture of artery
I77.2	Rupture of artery
I77.5	Necrosis of artery
I77.89	Other specified disorders of arteries and arterioles
S45.111A	Laceration of brachial artery, right side, initial encounter ☑
S45.112A	Laceration of brachial artery, left side, initial encounter ☑
S45.191A	Other specified injury of brachial artery, right side, initial encounter ☑
S45.192A	Other specified injury of brachial artery, left side, initial encounter ☑

AMA: **35522** 2018,Jan,8; 2017,Jan,8; 2016,Jan,13; 2015,Jan,16; 2014,Jan,11

Relative Value Units/Medicare Edits

Non-Facility RVU	Work	PE	MP	Total
35522	23.15	6.56	5.26	34.97
Facility RVU	**Work**	**PE**	**MP**	**Total**
35522	23.15	6.56	5.26	34.97

	FUD	Status	MUE	Modifiers				IOM Reference
35522	90	A	1(3)	51	50	62*	80	None

* with documentation

Terms To Know

anastomosis. Surgically created connection between ducts, blood vessels, or bowel segments to allow flow from one to the other.

bypass graft. Surgically created alternative blood vessel used to reroute blood flow around an area of obstruction or disease.

35523

35523 Bypass graft, with vein; brachial-ulnar or -radial

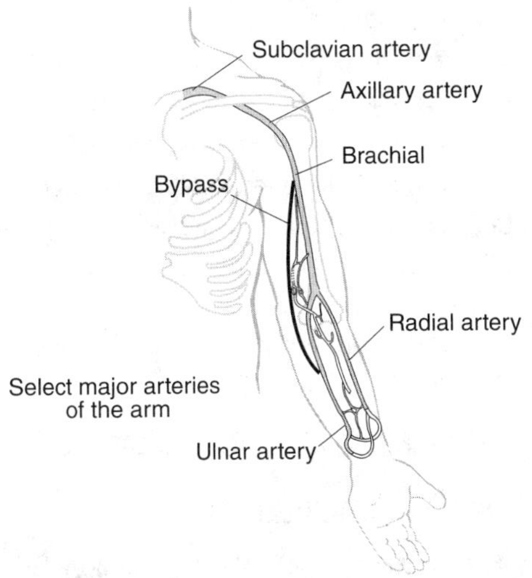

A bypass from the brachial artery to another site along the ulnar or radial artery

Explanation

The physician performs a brachial-ulnar or –radial bypass graft. Through an incision in the skin of the upper arm, the physician dissects down to the brachial artery at a site above the diseased or damaged portion of the artery. Soft tissue and adjacent critical structures are separated. Soft tissue must be cleared for several centimeters. Dissection through the skin and soft tissue at the distal anastomosis site for this bypass graft is also done over the radial or ulnar artery. A tunnel is made from the exposed proximal brachial site down the arm to the radial or ulnar artery site. To create a bypass graft around the section of the artery that is damaged or blocked, the physician uses a harvested vein, usually the greater saphenous. After vascular clamps have been affixed above and below the proximal anastomosis area on the brachial artery, arteriotomy is carried out and the harvested vein is sutured to the artery. When this is completed and checked for hemorrhaging, the arterial clamps are removed. The vein graft is tunneled through the prepared space to the distal site on the radial or ulnar artery and arteriotomy and anastomosis are carried out again in the same manner. The clamps are removed, additional sutures may be placed for complete hemostasis, and the patency of the graft is checked. The incisions are closed and the appropriate pulses are checked again before dressings are applied.

Coding Tips

Establishing both inflow and outflow by any method is included. That portion of the operative arteriogram performed by the surgeon is also included. Angioscopy performed during therapeutic intervention should be reported in addition to the code for the primary procedure, see 35400. Harvesting of the saphenous vein graft is included in the description of the work for 35523 and should not be reported as a separate procedure. For harvesting of a femoropopliteal vein segment, use 35572 in addition to the bypass procedure. If a composite (combination of vein and synthetic graft) is used, report 35681 in addition to the code for the primary procedure. For a bypass graft performed with synthetic conduit, see 37799. Do not report 33523 with 35206, 35500, 35525, or 36838.

ICD-10-CM Diagnostic Codes

I70.92	Chronic total occlusion of artery of the extremities
I73.9	Peripheral vascular disease, unspecified
I74.2	Embolism and thrombosis of arteries of the upper extremities
I74.8	Embolism and thrombosis of other arteries
I75.011	Atheroembolism of right upper extremity ☑
I75.012	Atheroembolism of left upper extremity ☑
I75.013	Atheroembolism of bilateral upper extremities ☑
I77.1	Stricture of artery
I77.2	Rupture of artery
I77.5	Necrosis of artery
I77.89	Other specified disorders of arteries and arterioles
S45.111A	Laceration of brachial artery, right side, initial encounter ☑
S45.112A	Laceration of brachial artery, left side, initial encounter ☑
S45.191A	Other specified injury of brachial artery, right side, initial encounter ☑
S45.192A	Other specified injury of brachial artery, left side, initial encounter ☑
S55.011A	Laceration of ulnar artery at forearm level, right arm, initial encounter ☑
S55.012A	Laceration of ulnar artery at forearm level, left arm, initial encounter ☑
S55.091A	Other specified injury of ulnar artery at forearm level, right arm, initial encounter ☑
S55.092A	Other specified injury of ulnar artery at forearm level, left arm, initial encounter ☑
S55.111A	Laceration of radial artery at forearm level, right arm, initial encounter ☑
S55.112A	Laceration of radial artery at forearm level, left arm, initial encounter ☑
S55.191A	Other specified injury of radial artery at forearm level, right arm, initial encounter ☑
S55.192A	Other specified injury of radial artery at forearm level, left arm, initial encounter ☑

Relative Value Units/Medicare Edits

Non-Facility RVU	Work	PE	MP	Total
35523	24.13	7.55	5.44	37.12
Facility RVU	**Work**	**PE**	**MP**	**Total**
35523	24.13	7.55	5.44	37.12

	FUD	Status	MUE	Modifiers				IOM Reference
35523	90	A	1(3)	51	50	62*	80	None

* with documentation

Terms To Know

anastomosis. Surgically created connection between ducts, blood vessels, or bowel segments to allow flow from one to the other.

bypass graft. Surgically created alternative blood vessel used to reroute blood flow around an area of obstruction or disease.

35525

35525 Bypass graft, with vein; brachial-brachial

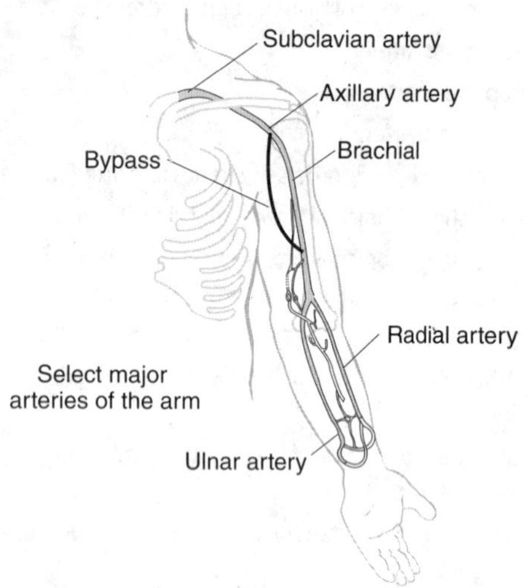

A bypass from the brachial artery to another site along the brachial artery is performed

Explanation

Through an incision in the skin of the upper arm, the physician dissects down to the brachial artery at a site above the diseased or damaged portion of the artery, usually in the mid to distal part, and separates soft tissue and adjacent critical structures. Soft tissue must be cleared for several centimeters. Dissection through the skin and soft tissue at the distal anastomosis site for this bypass graft is also done over the distal brachial artery in the arm, most often below the elbow. Next, a tunnel is made from the exposed proximal brachial site, down the arm to the distal brachial artery site. To create a bypass graft around the section of the artery that is damaged or blocked, the physician uses a harvested vein, usually the greater saphenous. After vascular clamps have been affixed above and below the proximal anastomosis area on the brachial artery, arteriotomy is carried out and the harvested vein is sutured to the brachial artery. When this is completed and checked for hemorrhaging, the arterial clamps are removed. The vein graft is tunneled through the prepared space to the distal site on the brachial artery and arteriotomy and anastomosis are carried out again in the same manner. The clamps are removed, additional sutures may be placed for complete hemostasis, and the patency of the graft is checked. The incisions are closed and the appropriate pulses are checked again before dressings are applied.

Coding Tips

Establishing both inflow and outflow by any method is included. That portion of the operative arteriogram performed by the surgeon is also included. Angioscopy performed during therapeutic intervention should be reported in addition to the code for the primary procedure; see 35400. Harvesting of the saphenous vein graft is included in the description of the work for 35525 and should not be reported as a separate procedure. To report harvesting of an upper extremity vein, use 35500 in addition to the bypass procedure. For harvesting of a femoropopliteal vein segment, use 35572 in addition to the bypass procedure.

ICD-10-CM Diagnostic Codes

I70.92	Chronic total occlusion of artery of the extremities
I73.9	Peripheral vascular disease, unspecified
I74.2	Embolism and thrombosis of arteries of the upper extremities
I74.8	Embolism and thrombosis of other arteries
I75.011	Atheroembolism of right upper extremity ☑
I75.012	Atheroembolism of left upper extremity ☑
I75.013	Atheroembolism of bilateral upper extremities ☑
I77.1	Stricture of artery
I77.2	Rupture of artery
I77.5	Necrosis of artery
I77.89	Other specified disorders of arteries and arterioles
S45.111A	Laceration of brachial artery, right side, initial encounter ☑
S45.112A	Laceration of brachial artery, left side, initial encounter ☑
S45.191A	Other specified injury of brachial artery, right side, initial encounter ☑
S45.192A	Other specified injury of brachial artery, left side, initial encounter ☑

AMA: **35525** 2018,Jan,8; 2017,Jan,8; 2016,Jan,13; 2015,Jan,16; 2014,Jan,11

Relative Value Units/Medicare Edits

Non-Facility RVU	Work	PE	MP	Total
35525	21.69	6.46	4.93	33.08
Facility RVU	**Work**	**PE**	**MP**	**Total**
35525	21.69	6.46	4.93	33.08

	FUD	Status	MUE	Modifiers				IOM Reference
35525	90	A	1(3)	51	50	62*	80	None

* with documentation

Terms To Know

bypass graft. Surgically created alternative blood vessel used to reroute blood flow around an area of obstruction or disease.

thrombosis. Condition arising from the presence or formation of blood clots within a blood vessel that may cause vascular obstruction and insufficient oxygenation.

35526

35526 Bypass graft, with vein; aortosubclavian, aortoinnominate, or aortocarotid

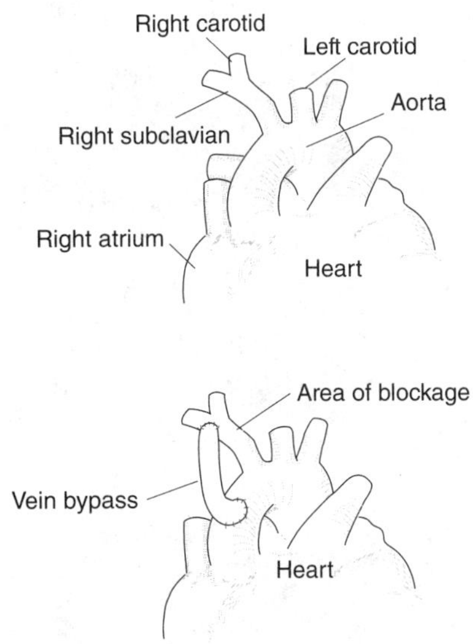

A vein graft is employed to bypass a blockage in the great arteries

Explanation

The physician exposes the aorta by median sternotomy and exposes the aortocarotid, aortoinnominate, or aortosubclavian artery extending this incision in the appropriate direction. The physician clamps the middle part of the right anterolateral aspect of the anterior ascending aorta with a J clamp. The physician makes a 2 cm to 3 cm longitudinal incision in the clamped portion of the aorta and sews the venous graft to the aortic incision. The physician clamps the vein and releases the aortic clamp to assess the anastomosis for leaks. The physician clamps the distal end of the diseased artery. The physician makes a longitudinal incision in the diseased artery, distal to the blockage, and sews the venous graft to the arterial incision. The physician may also use harvested vein to enlarge the arterial lumen (patch graft). The physician removes the clamp from the vein graft. The physician may perform arteriography or use a Doppler probe to establish patency of the graft. The physician closes the sternotomy or thoracotomy, leaving a chest tube in place.

Coding Tips

Establishing both inflow and outflow by any method is included. That portion of the operative arteriogram performed by the surgeon is also included. Angioscopy performed during therapeutic intervention should be reported in addition to the code for the primary procedure; see 35400. If synthetic graft material is used, see 35626. Harvesting of the saphenous vein graft is included in the description of the work for 35526 and should not be reported as a separate procedure. For harvesting of a femoropopliteal vein segment, use 35572 in addition to the bypass procedure. If a composite (combination of vein and synthetic graft) is used, report 35681 in addition to the code for the primary procedure.

ICD-10-CM Diagnostic Codes

G45.1	Carotid artery syndrome (hemispheric)
G45.2	Multiple and bilateral precerebral artery syndromes
G45.3	Amaurosis fugax
G45.8	Other transient cerebral ischemic attacks and related syndromes
G45.9	Transient cerebral ischemic attack, unspecified
I63.031	Cerebral infarction due to thrombosis of right carotid artery ☑
I63.032	Cerebral infarction due to thrombosis of left carotid artery ☑
I63.09	Cerebral infarction due to thrombosis of other precerebral artery
I63.131	Cerebral infarction due to embolism of right carotid artery ☑
I63.132	Cerebral infarction due to embolism of left carotid artery ☑
I63.19	Cerebral infarction due to embolism of other precerebral artery
I63.81	Other cerebral infarction due to occlusion or stenosis of small artery
I63.89	Other cerebral infarction
I65.21	Occlusion and stenosis of right carotid artery ☑
I65.22	Occlusion and stenosis of left carotid artery ☑
I65.23	Occlusion and stenosis of bilateral carotid arteries ☑
I65.8	Occlusion and stenosis of other precerebral arteries
I67.81	Acute cerebrovascular insufficiency
I67.82	Cerebral ischemia
I67.850	Cerebral autosomal dominant arteriopathy with subcortical infarcts and leukoencephalopathy
I67.858	Other hereditary cerebrovascular disease
I67.89	Other cerebrovascular disease
I70.92	Chronic total occlusion of artery of the extremities
I74.2	Embolism and thrombosis of arteries of the upper extremities
I75.011	Atheroembolism of right upper extremity ☑
I75.012	Atheroembolism of left upper extremity ☑
I75.013	Atheroembolism of bilateral upper extremities ☑
I77.1	Stricture of artery
I77.2	Rupture of artery
I77.71	Dissection of carotid artery
I77.79	Dissection of other specified artery
I77.89	Other specified disorders of arteries and arterioles
Q28.1	Other malformations of precerebral vessels
Q28.8	Other specified congenital malformations of circulatory system
S15.011A	Minor laceration of right carotid artery, initial encounter ☑
S15.012A	Minor laceration of left carotid artery, initial encounter ☑
S15.021A	Major laceration of right carotid artery, initial encounter ☑
S15.022A	Major laceration of left carotid artery, initial encounter ☑
S15.091A	Other specified injury of right carotid artery, initial encounter ☑
S15.092A	Other specified injury of left carotid artery, initial encounter ☑
S15.8XXA	Injury of other specified blood vessels at neck level, initial encounter
S25.111A	Minor laceration of right innominate or subclavian artery, initial encounter ☑
S25.112A	Minor laceration of left innominate or subclavian artery, initial encounter ☑
S25.121A	Major laceration of right innominate or subclavian artery, initial encounter ☑
S25.122A	Major laceration of left innominate or subclavian artery, initial encounter ☑
S25.191A	Other specified injury of right innominate or subclavian artery, initial encounter ☑
S25.192A	Other specified injury of left innominate or subclavian artery, initial encounter ☑

AMA: 35526 1999,Mar,6; 1999,Apr,11

Relative Value Units/Medicare Edits

Non-Facility RVU	Work	PE	MP	Total
35526	31.55	11.52	7.43	50.5
Facility RVU	**Work**	**PE**	**MP**	**Total**
35526	31.55	11.52	7.43	50.5

	FUD	Status	MUE	Modifiers				IOM Reference
35526	90	A	1(3)	51	50	62*	80	None

* with documentation

Terms To Know

anastomosis. Surgically created connection between ducts, blood vessels, or bowel segments to allow flow from one to the other.

artery. Vessel through which oxygenated blood passes away from the heart to any part of the body.

sternotomy. Incision into the sternum, the bone that forms the front of the chest cavity and connects with the ribs.

thoracotomy. Surgical procedure for opening the chest wall in order to access the lungs, esophagus, trachea, aorta, heart, and diaphragm.

35531

35531 Bypass graft, with vein; aortoceliac or aortomesenteric

Schematic of an aortomesenteric bypass

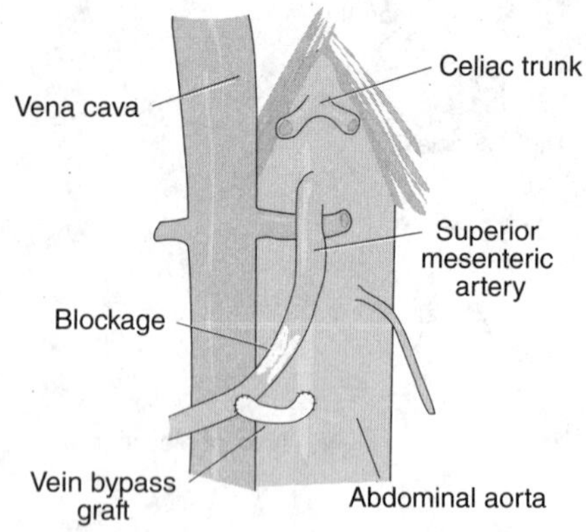

Bypass around blockage of an upper abdominal artery (celiac or mesentary)

Explanation

The physician exposes the involved aortomesenteric or aortoceliac artery using an upper midline abdominal incision, retracting and dissecting past large and small bowel. The physician exposes the distal thoracic aorta, administers heparin for anticoagulation, and clamps the aorta both proximal and distal to the celiac axis origin. The physician cuts out an elliptical disk of aortic wall from the anterior surface of the aorta. The physician exposes the involved vessel (aortomesenteric or aortoceliac artery) and divides it proximal to the occlusion, closing off the proximal stump with suture. The physician sews a venous graft from the clamped aorta to the nondiseased distal artery. The physician may use harvested vein to enlarge the arterial lumen (patch graft). The physician may perform arteriography or use a Doppler probe to establish patency of the graft. The physician closes the abdominal wound, leaving drains in place.

Coding Tips

Establishing both inflow and outflow by any method is included. That portion of the operative arteriogram performed by the surgeon is also included. Angioscopy performed during therapeutic intervention should be reported in addition to the code for the primary procedure; see 35400. Harvesting of the saphenous vein graft is included in the description of the work for 35531 and should not be reported as a separate procedure. For harvesting of a femoropopliteal vein segment, use 35572 in addition to the bypass procedure. If a composite (combination of vein and synthetic graft) is used, report 35681 in addition to the code for the primary procedure. If synthetic graft material is used, see 35631.

ICD-10-CM Diagnostic Codes

I70.8	Atherosclerosis of other arteries
I75.89	Atheroembolism of other site
I77.1	Stricture of artery
I77.4	Celiac artery compression syndrome
I77.5	Necrosis of artery
I77.79	Dissection of other specified artery
I77.89	Other specified disorders of arteries and arterioles
K55.011	Focal (segmental) acute (reversible) ischemia of small intestine
K55.012	Diffuse acute (reversible) ischemia of small intestine

K55.021 Focal (segmental) acute infarction of small intestine
K55.022 Diffuse acute infarction of small intestine
K55.031 Focal (segmental) acute (reversible) ischemia of large intestine
K55.032 Diffuse acute (reversible) ischemia of large intestine
K55.041 Focal (segmental) acute infarction of large intestine
K55.042 Diffuse acute infarction of large intestine
K55.1 Chronic vascular disorders of intestine
K55.8 Other vascular disorders of intestine
S35.211A Minor laceration of celiac artery, initial encounter
S35.212A Major laceration of celiac artery, initial encounter
S35.218A Other injury of celiac artery, initial encounter
S35.221A Minor laceration of superior mesenteric artery, initial encounter
S35.222A Major laceration of superior mesenteric artery, initial encounter
S35.228A Other injury of superior mesenteric artery, initial encounter
S35.231A Minor laceration of inferior mesenteric artery, initial encounter
S35.232A Major laceration of inferior mesenteric artery, initial encounter
S35.238A Other injury of inferior mesenteric artery, initial encounter
S35.291A Minor laceration of branches of celiac and mesenteric artery, initial encounter
S35.292A Major laceration of branches of celiac and mesenteric artery, initial encounter
S35.298A Other injury of branches of celiac and mesenteric artery, initial encounter
S35.8X1A Laceration of other blood vessels at abdomen, lower back and pelvis level, initial encounter
S35.8X8A Other specified injury of other blood vessels at abdomen, lower back and pelvis level, initial encounter
T81.710A Complication of mesenteric artery following a procedure, not elsewhere classified, initial encounter

AMA: 35531 1999,Mar,6; 1999,Apr,11

Relative Value Units/Medicare Edits

Non-Facility RVU	Work	PE	MP	Total
35531	39.11	8.16	9.07	56.34
Facility RVU	**Work**	**PE**	**MP**	**Total**
35531	39.11	8.16	9.07	56.34

	FUD	Status	MUE	Modifiers				IOM Reference
35531	90	A	1(3)	51	50	62*	80	None

* with documentation

35533

35533 Bypass graft, with vein; axillary-femoral-femoral

Axillary-femoral-femoral bypass

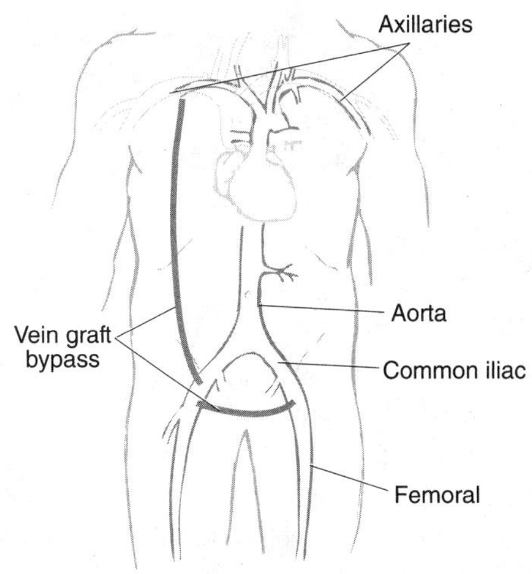

Explanation

Through incisions in the skin of the axilla and both upper thighs, the physician creates a bypass using a harvested vein around the section of diseased or damaged artery. Once vessel clamps have been affixed above and below the area of anastomosis, the harvested vein is sutured to the side of the axillary artery and passed through a subcutaneous tunnel to the upper thigh, where it is sutured end-to-end or end-to-side to the femoral artery. A second harvested vein is sutured end-to-side to the femoral artery or to the vein graft descending from the axilla where it joins the femoral artery, and is passed through another subcutaneous tunnel to the opposite thigh, where it is sutured end-to-end or end-to-side to the femoral artery. When the clamps are removed, the two grafted vein limbs form a new path through which blood can easily bypass the blocked area. The section of the blocked or damaged vessel is not removed. After the graft is complete, the incisions are repaired with layered closures.

Coding Tips

Establishing both inflow and outflow by any method is included. That portion of the operative arteriogram performed by the surgeon is also included. Angioscopy performed during therapeutic intervention should be reported in addition to the code for the primary procedure, see 35400. Harvesting of the saphenous vein graft is included in the description of the work for 35533 and should not be reported as a separate procedure. For harvesting of a femoropopliteal vein segment, use 35572 in addition to the bypass procedure. If a composite (combination of vein and synthetic graft) is used, report 35681 in addition to the code for the primary procedure. If synthetic graft material is used, see 35654.

ICD-10-CM Diagnostic Codes

A52.01 Syphilitic aneurysm of aorta
A52.02 Syphilitic aortitis
I70.0 Atherosclerosis of aorta
I70.92 Chronic total occlusion of artery of the extremities
I71.01 Dissection of thoracic aorta
I71.02 Dissection of abdominal aorta
I71.03 Dissection of thoracoabdominal aorta

I72.2	Aneurysm of renal artery
I72.8	Aneurysm of other specified arteries
I73.89	Other specified peripheral vascular diseases
I74.01	Saddle embolus of abdominal aorta
I74.09	Other arterial embolism and thrombosis of abdominal aorta
I74.19	Embolism and thrombosis of other parts of aorta
I74.5	Embolism and thrombosis of iliac artery
I75.89	Atheroembolism of other site
I76	Septic arterial embolism
I77.1	Stricture of artery
I77.3	Arterial fibromuscular dysplasia
I77.4	Celiac artery compression syndrome
I77.5	Necrosis of artery
I77.72	Dissection of iliac artery
I77.73	Dissection of renal artery
I77.79	Dissection of other specified artery
I77.810	Thoracic aortic ectasia
I77.811	Abdominal aortic ectasia
I77.812	Thoracoabdominal aortic ectasia
I82.0	Budd-Chiari syndrome
K55.011	Focal (segmental) acute (reversible) ischemia of small intestine
K55.012	Diffuse acute (reversible) ischemia of small intestine
K55.021	Focal (segmental) acute infarction of small intestine
K55.022	Diffuse acute infarction of small intestine
K55.031	Focal (segmental) acute (reversible) ischemia of large intestine
K55.032	Diffuse acute (reversible) ischemia of large intestine
K55.041	Focal (segmental) acute infarction of large intestine
K55.042	Diffuse acute infarction of large intestine
K55.1	Chronic vascular disorders of intestine
K55.8	Other vascular disorders of intestine
N28.0	Ischemia and infarction of kidney
Q25.21	Interruption of aortic arch
Q25.41	Absence and aplasia of aorta
Q25.46	Tortuous aortic arch
Q25.47	Right aortic arch
Q25.48	Anomalous origin of subclavian artery
Q25.8	Other congenital malformations of other great arteries
Q27.1	Congenital renal artery stenosis
Q27.2	Other congenital malformations of renal artery
Q79.61	Classical Ehlers-Danlos syndrome
Q79.62	Hypermobile Ehlers-Danlos syndrome
Q79.63	Vascular Ehlers-Danlos syndrome
Q87.418	Marfan's syndrome with other cardiovascular manifestations
S25.01XA	Minor laceration of thoracic aorta, initial encounter
S25.02XA	Major laceration of thoracic aorta, initial encounter
S25.09XA	Other specified injury of thoracic aorta, initial encounter
S25.811A	Laceration of other blood vessels of thorax, right side, initial encounter ☑
S25.812A	Laceration of other blood vessels of thorax, left side, initial encounter ☑
S25.891A	Other specified injury of other blood vessels of thorax, right side, initial encounter ☑
S25.892A	Other specified injury of other blood vessels of thorax, left side, initial encounter ☑
S35.01XA	Minor laceration of abdominal aorta, initial encounter
S35.02XA	Major laceration of abdominal aorta, initial encounter
S35.09XA	Other injury of abdominal aorta, initial encounter
S35.211A	Minor laceration of celiac artery, initial encounter
S35.212A	Major laceration of celiac artery, initial encounter
S35.218A	Other injury of celiac artery, initial encounter
S35.221A	Minor laceration of superior mesenteric artery, initial encounter
S35.222A	Major laceration of superior mesenteric artery, initial encounter
S35.228A	Other injury of superior mesenteric artery, initial encounter
S35.231A	Minor laceration of inferior mesenteric artery, initial encounter
S35.232A	Major laceration of inferior mesenteric artery, initial encounter
S35.238A	Other injury of inferior mesenteric artery, initial encounter
S35.291A	Minor laceration of branches of celiac and mesenteric artery, initial encounter
S35.292A	Major laceration of branches of celiac and mesenteric artery, initial encounter
S35.298A	Other injury of branches of celiac and mesenteric artery, initial encounter
S35.411A	Laceration of right renal artery, initial encounter ☑
S35.412A	Laceration of left renal artery, initial encounter ☑
S35.491A	Other specified injury of right renal artery, initial encounter ☑
S35.492A	Other specified injury of left renal artery, initial encounter ☑
S35.511A	Injury of right iliac artery, initial encounter ☑
S35.512A	Injury of left iliac artery, initial encounter ☑
S35.8X1A	Laceration of other blood vessels at abdomen, lower back and pelvis level, initial encounter
S35.8X8A	Other specified injury of other blood vessels at abdomen, lower back and pelvis level, initial encounter
T81.710A	Complication of mesenteric artery following a procedure, not elsewhere classified, initial encounter

AMA: **35533** 2012,Apr,3-9

Relative Value Units/Medicare Edits

Non-Facility RVU	Work	PE	MP	Total
35533	29.92	6.65	6.92	43.49
Facility RVU	**Work**	**PE**	**MP**	**Total**
35533	29.92	6.65	6.92	43.49

	FUD	Status	MUE	Modifiers				IOM Reference
35533	90	A	1(3)	51	50	62*	80	None

* with documentation

Arteries and Veins

35535

35535 Bypass graft, with vein; hepatorenal

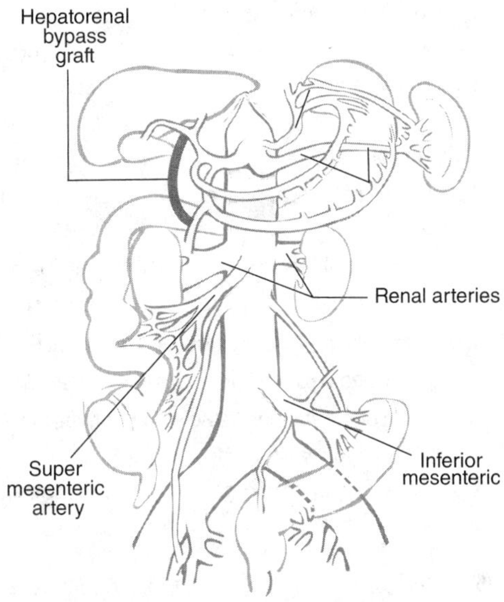

Vein bypass graft from the liver artery to one of the renal arteries

Explanation

The physician performs hepatorenal bypass graft. With the patient placed supine, a right subcostal (beneath the ribs) incision is made and extended through the subcutaneous tissue, fat, and muscle. The abdominal cavity is entered, the stomach is retracted, and the lesser omentum is entered. The physician locates the common hepatic, proper hepatic, and gastroduodenal arteries. These are dissected and encircled with Silastic vessel loops. After the physician mobilizes the right renal vein, the right renal artery is exposed, dissected, and encircled with Silastic vessel loops. The physician harvests a greater saphenous vein segment and forms a proximal end-to-end anastomosis to the common hepatic artery. Distal anastomosis is then performed with the renal artery in either a side-to-side or end-to-end fashion. Bleeding is controlled and Doppler or duplex is performed to verify revascularization. After the graft is complete, the incisions are repaired with layered closure.

Coding Tips

Angioscopy performed during therapeutic intervention should be reported in addition to the code for the primary procedure, see 35400. Harvesting of the saphenous vein graft is included in the description of the work for 35535 and should not be reported as a separate procedure. For harvesting of a femoropopliteal vein segment, use 35572 in addition to the bypass procedure. If a composite (combination of vein and synthetic graft) is used, report 35681 in addition to the code for the primary procedure. Do not report 35535 with 35221, 35251, 35281, 35500, 35536, 35560, 35631, or 35636.

ICD-10-CM Diagnostic Codes

I15.0	Renovascular hypertension
I15.1	Hypertension secondary to other renal disorders
I70.1	Atherosclerosis of renal artery
I72.2	Aneurysm of renal artery
I75.81	Atheroembolism of kidney
I77.1	Stricture of artery
I77.3	Arterial fibromuscular dysplasia
I77.5	Necrosis of artery
I77.73	Dissection of renal artery
I77.89	Other specified disorders of arteries and arterioles
N26.2	Page kidney
N28.0	Ischemia and infarction of kidney
Q27.1	Congenital renal artery stenosis
Q27.2	Other congenital malformations of renal artery
Q27.34	Arteriovenous malformation of renal vessel
S35.411A	Laceration of right renal artery, initial encounter ☑
S35.412A	Laceration of left renal artery, initial encounter ☑
S35.491A	Other specified injury of right renal artery, initial encounter ☑
S35.492A	Other specified injury of left renal artery, initial encounter ☑
T81.711A	Complication of renal artery following a procedure, not elsewhere classified, initial encounter

Relative Value Units/Medicare Edits

Non-Facility RVU	Work	PE	MP	Total
35535	38.13	8.03	8.83	54.99
Facility RVU	**Work**	**PE**	**MP**	**Total**
35535	38.13	8.03	8.83	54.99

	FUD	Status	MUE	Modifiers				IOM Reference
35535	90	A	1(3)	51	50	62*	80	None

* with documentation

Terms To Know

atherosclerosis. Buildup of yellowish plaques composed of cholesterol and lipoid material within the arteries.

occlusion. Constriction, closure, or blockage of a passage.

stenosis. Narrowing or constriction of a passage.

35536

35536 Bypass graft, with vein; splenorenal

Schematic of a splenorenal bypass

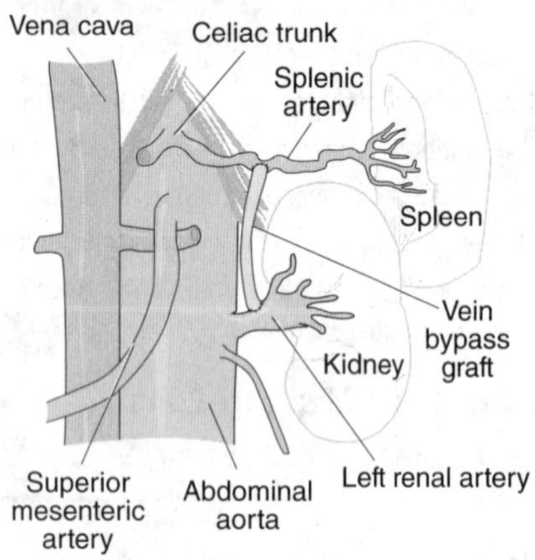

Bypass from the splenic artery to the renal artery

Explanation

The physician performs a bilateral subcostal incision from the right midrectus position extending into the left flank, and dissects past bowel and pancreas to expose the splenic vein. The physician exposes the splenic artery by careful dissection. The physician exposes the left renal artery by dissecting through the posterior parietal peritoneum, partially clamps it, and excises an ellipse of renal artery at its upper border. The physician performs end-to-side anastomosis of vein graft material from the splenic artery to the renal artery. The physician removes the clamps and assesses the anastomotic sites for leaks. The physician may perform Doppler studies or arteriography to establish patency of the graft. The physician closes the abdominal wound, leaving drains in place.

Coding Tips

Establishing both inflow and outflow by any method is included. That portion of the operative arteriogram performed by the surgeon is also included. Angioscopy performed during therapeutic intervention should be reported in addition to the code for the primary procedure; see 35400. Harvesting of the saphenous vein graft is included in the description of the work for 35536 and should not be reported as a separate procedure. For harvesting of a femoropopliteal vein segment, use 35572 in addition to the bypass procedure. If a composite (combination of vein and synthetic graft) is used, report 35681 in addition to the code for the primary procedure. If synthetic graft material is used, see 35636.

ICD-10-CM Diagnostic Codes

D73.5	Infarction of spleen
I70.1	Atherosclerosis of renal artery
I74.8	Embolism and thrombosis of other arteries
I75.81	Atheroembolism of kidney
I76	Septic arterial embolism
I77.1	Stricture of artery
I77.3	Arterial fibromuscular dysplasia
I77.5	Necrosis of artery
I77.73	Dissection of renal artery
I77.89	Other specified disorders of arteries and arterioles
N26.2	Page kidney
N28.0	Ischemia and infarction of kidney
Q27.1	Congenital renal artery stenosis
Q27.2	Other congenital malformations of renal artery
Q27.34	Arteriovenous malformation of renal vessel
S35.291A	Minor laceration of branches of celiac and mesenteric artery, initial encounter
S35.292A	Major laceration of branches of celiac and mesenteric artery, initial encounter
S35.298A	Other injury of branches of celiac and mesenteric artery, initial encounter
S35.411A	Laceration of right renal artery, initial encounter ☑
S35.412A	Laceration of left renal artery, initial encounter ☑
S35.491A	Other specified injury of right renal artery, initial encounter ☑
S35.492A	Other specified injury of left renal artery, initial encounter ☑
S35.8X1A	Laceration of other blood vessels at abdomen, lower back and pelvis level, initial encounter
S35.8X8A	Other specified injury of other blood vessels at abdomen, lower back and pelvis level, initial encounter

AMA: 35536 2018,Jan,8; 2017,Jan,8; 2016,Jan,13; 2015,Jan,16; 2014,Jan,11

Relative Value Units/Medicare Edits

Non-Facility RVU	Work	PE	MP	Total
35536	33.73	7.28	7.82	48.83
Facility RVU	**Work**	**PE**	**MP**	**Total**
35536	33.73	7.28	7.82	48.83

	FUD	Status	MUE	Modifiers				IOM Reference
35536	90	A	1(3)	51	50	62*	80	None

* with documentation

Terms To Know

anastomosis. Surgically created connection between ducts, blood vessels, or bowel segments to allow flow from one to the other.

atherosclerosis. Buildup of yellowish plaques composed of cholesterol and lipoid material within the arteries.

doppler. Ultrasonography used to augment two-dimensional images by registering velocity. When emitted sound waves reflect back off a moving object, the frequency of the reflected sound waves varies in relation to the speed of the moving object and may be used in many different procedures.

hyperplasia. Abnormal proliferation in the number of normal cells in regular tissue arrangement.

patency. State of a tube-like structure or conduit being open and unobstructed.

35537-35538

35537 Bypass graft, with vein; aortoiliac
35538 aortobi-iliac

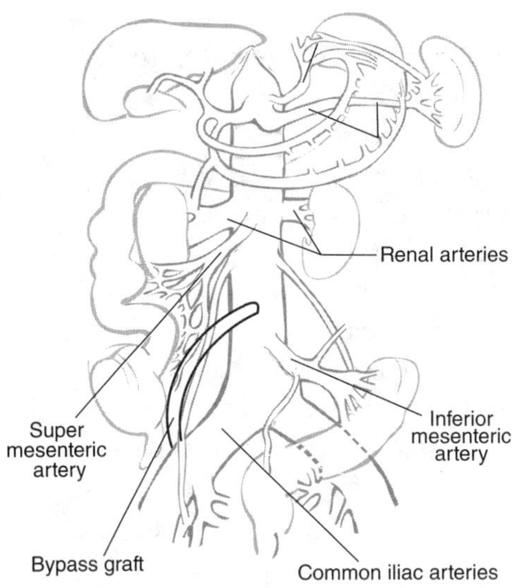

Bypass from the aorta to iliac artery

Explanation

The physician exposes the involved abdominal aorta and iliac arteries using an abdominal incision, retracting and dissecting past large and small bowel. The physician partially clamps the aorta above the diseased area and places a longitudinal incision down the clamped portion of the aorta. The physician sews in a (two) venous graft(s), clamps the graft(s), and removes the aortic clamp to assess the anastomosis(es) for leaks. The physician clamps the iliac artery(ies) distal to the stenosis and incises and attaches the distal venous graft to the iliac artery(ies). The physician may also use harvested vein to enlarge the aortic or arterial lumen (patch graft). The physician may perform arteriography or use a Doppler probe to establish patency of the graft. The physician closes the abdominal wound, leaving drains in place. A bypass graft to a single iliac artery is performed in 35537; both iliac arteries are bypassed in 35538.

Coding Tips

Establishing both inflow and outflow by any method is included. That portion of the operative arteriogram performed by the surgeon is also included. Angioscopy performed during therapeutic intervention should be reported in addition to the code for the primary procedure, see 35400. Harvesting of the saphenous vein graft is included in the description of the work for 35537 and 35538 and should not be reported as a separate procedure. For harvesting of a femoropopliteal vein segment, use 35572 in addition to the bypass procedure. If a composite (combination of vein and synthetic graft) is used, report 35681 in addition to the code for the primary procedure. Do not report 35537 or 35538 with each other. For a bypass graft performed with a synthetic graft, see 35637 or 35638.

ICD-10-CM Diagnostic Codes

A52.01	Syphilitic aneurysm of aorta
A52.02	Syphilitic aortitis
I70.0	Atherosclerosis of aorta
I71.02	Dissection of abdominal aorta
I73.89	Other specified peripheral vascular diseases
I73.9	Peripheral vascular disease, unspecified
I74.01	Saddle embolus of abdominal aorta
I74.09	Other arterial embolism and thrombosis of abdominal aorta
I74.19	Embolism and thrombosis of other parts of aorta
I74.5	Embolism and thrombosis of iliac artery
I75.89	Atheroembolism of other site
I76	Septic arterial embolism
I77.1	Stricture of artery
I77.3	Arterial fibromuscular dysplasia
I77.5	Necrosis of artery
I77.72	Dissection of iliac artery
I77.811	Abdominal aortic ectasia
I77.812	Thoracoabdominal aortic ectasia
I77.89	Other specified disorders of arteries and arterioles
Q25.21	Interruption of aortic arch
Q25.29	Other atresia of aorta
Q25.41	Absence and aplasia of aorta
Q25.42	Hypoplasia of aorta
Q25.43	Congenital aneurysm of aorta
Q25.44	Congenital dilation of aorta
Q25.45	Double aortic arch
Q25.46	Tortuous aortic arch
Q25.47	Right aortic arch
Q25.48	Anomalous origin of subclavian artery
Q25.49	Other congenital malformations of aorta
S35.01XA	Minor laceration of abdominal aorta, initial encounter
S35.02XA	Major laceration of abdominal aorta, initial encounter
S35.09XA	Other injury of abdominal aorta, initial encounter
S35.511A	Injury of right iliac artery, initial encounter ☑
S35.512A	Injury of left iliac artery, initial encounter ☑
S35.59XA	Injury of other iliac blood vessels, initial encounter
S35.8X1A	Laceration of other blood vessels at abdomen, lower back and pelvis level, initial encounter
S35.8X8A	Other specified injury of other blood vessels at abdomen, lower back and pelvis level, initial encounter

AMA: 35537 2018,Jan,8; 2017,Jan,8; 2016,Jan,13; 2015,Jan,16; 2014,Jan,11
35538 2018,Jan,8; 2017,Jan,8; 2016,Jan,13; 2015,Jan,16; 2014,Jan,11

Relative Value Units/Medicare Edits

Non-Facility RVU	Work	PE	MP	Total
35537	41.88	8.67	9.7	60.25
35538	47.03	9.56	10.92	67.51
Facility RVU	**Work**	**PE**	**MP**	**Total**
35537	41.88	8.67	9.7	60.25
35538	47.03	9.56	10.92	67.51

	FUD	Status	MUE	Modifiers				IOM Reference
35537	90	A	1(3)	51	N/A	62*	80	None
35538	90	A	1(3)	51	N/A	62*	80	

* with documentation

35539-35540

35539 Bypass graft, with vein; aortofemoral
35540 aortobifemoral

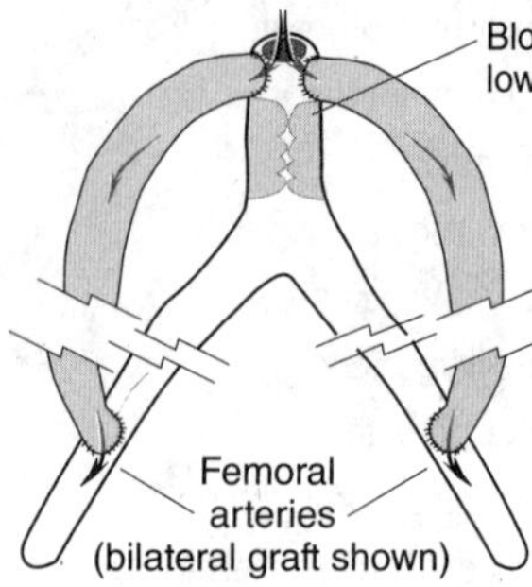

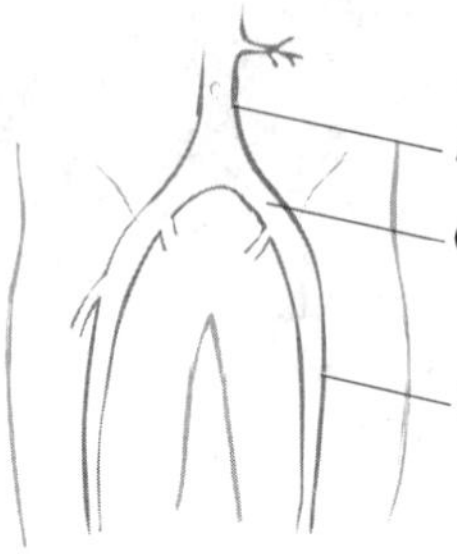

Explanation

The physician makes an incision in the skin of the abdomen over a section of damaged or blocked lower aorta. The artery is isolated and dissected. Through a separate skin incision in the upper thigh, the femoral artery is isolated and dissected from adjacent critical structures. The physician creates a bypass around the damaged or blocked lower aorta using a harvested vein. Once vessel clamps have been affixed above the defect, the lower aorta may be cut through or tied off with sutures above the damaged or blocked area and sutured to one end of the harvested vein in an end-to-end or side-to-side fashion. In 35539, the graft to one femoral artery is passed through a tunnel on the inside of the upper thigh and sutured to the femoral artery. In 35540, a bifemoral bypass is accomplished and a second harvested vein is placed in a similar fashion to the second side. When the clamps are removed, the two grafted vein limbs form a new path through which blood can easily bypass the blocked area. The blocked or damaged portion of artery is not removed. After the graft is complete, the skin incisions are repaired with layered closures.

Coding Tips

Establishing both inflow and outflow by any method is included. That portion of the operative arteriogram performed by the surgeon is also included. Angioscopy performed during therapeutic intervention should be reported in addition to the code for the primary procedure, see 35400. Harvesting of the saphenous vein graft is included in the description of the work for 35539 and 35540 and should not be reported as a separate procedure. For harvesting of a femoropopliteal vein segment, use 35572 in addition to the bypass procedure. If a composite (combination of vein and synthetic graft) is used, report 35681 in addition to the code for the primary procedure. Do not report 35539 or 35540 with each other. For a bypass graft performed with a synthetic graft, see 35646 or 35647.

ICD-10-CM Diagnostic Codes

A52.01	Syphilitic aneurysm of aorta
A52.02	Syphilitic aortitis
I70.0	Atherosclerosis of aorta
I71.02	Dissection of abdominal aorta
I73.89	Other specified peripheral vascular diseases
I73.9	Peripheral vascular disease, unspecified
I74.01	Saddle embolus of abdominal aorta
I74.09	Other arterial embolism and thrombosis of abdominal aorta
I74.19	Embolism and thrombosis of other parts of aorta
I74.5	Embolism and thrombosis of iliac artery
I75.89	Atheroembolism of other site
I76	Septic arterial embolism
I77.1	Stricture of artery
I77.3	Arterial fibromuscular dysplasia
I77.5	Necrosis of artery
I77.72	Dissection of iliac artery
I77.811	Abdominal aortic ectasia
I77.812	Thoracoabdominal aortic ectasia
I77.89	Other specified disorders of arteries and arterioles
I79.0	Aneurysm of aorta in diseases classified elsewhere
Q25.21	Interruption of aortic arch
Q25.29	Other atresia of aorta
Q25.41	Absence and aplasia of aorta
Q25.42	Hypoplasia of aorta
Q25.43	Congenital aneurysm of aorta
Q25.44	Congenital dilation of aorta
Q25.45	Double aortic arch
Q25.46	Tortuous aortic arch
Q25.47	Right aortic arch
Q25.48	Anomalous origin of subclavian artery
Q25.49	Other congenital malformations of aorta
S35.01XA	Minor laceration of abdominal aorta, initial encounter
S35.02XA	Major laceration of abdominal aorta, initial encounter
S35.09XA	Other injury of abdominal aorta, initial encounter
S35.8X1A	Laceration of other blood vessels at abdomen, lower back and pelvis level, initial encounter
S35.8X8A	Other specified injury of other blood vessels at abdomen, lower back and pelvis level, initial encounter

AMA: **35539** 2018,Jan,8; 2017,Jan,8; 2016,Jan,13; 2015,Jan,16; 2014,Jan,11
35540 2018,Jan,8; 2017,Jan,8; 2016,Jan,13; 2015,Jan,16; 2014,Jan,11

Relative Value Units/Medicare Edits

Non-Facility RVU	Work	PE	MP	Total
35539	44.11	9.04	10.24	63.39
35540	49.33	9.89	11.46	70.68
Facility RVU	**Work**	**PE**	**MP**	**Total**
35539	44.11	9.04	10.24	63.39
35540	49.33	9.89	11.46	70.68

	FUD	Status	MUE	Modifiers				IOM Reference
35539	90	A	1(3)	51	50	62*	80	None
35540	90	A	1(3)	51	50	62*	N/A	

* with documentation

35556

35556 Bypass graft, with vein; femoral-popliteal

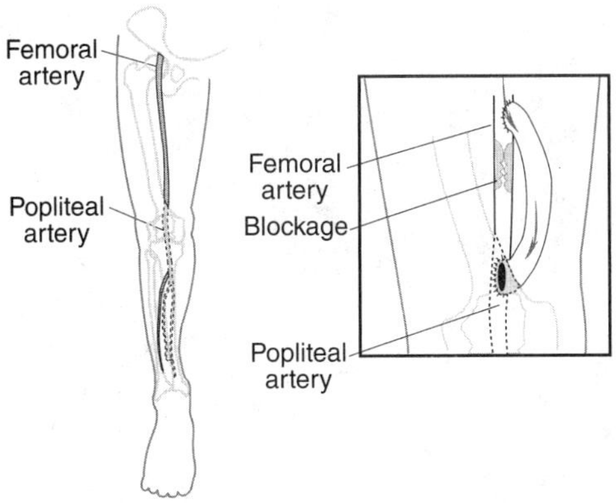

Explanation

Through incisions in the skin of the leg overlying the femoral and popliteal arteries, the physician isolates and dissects a section of artery that is damaged or blocked. The physician creates a bypass around the superficial femoral artery, using a harvested vein and one of two methods of repair. Once vessel clamps have been affixed above and below the defect, the superficial femoral artery may be cut through above the damaged or blocked area and sutured to one end of a harvested vein. The vein is passed through a tunnel down the thigh muscles and behind the knee and sutured to the popliteal artery. In the second method, the ends of the harvested vein are sutured into the side of the femoral and popliteal arterial walls, resulting in a bypass of the damaged area. When the clamps are removed, the section of vein forms a new path through which blood can easily bypass the blocked area. The blocked or damaged portion of artery is not removed. After the graft is complete, the skin incisions are repaired with layered closures.

Coding Tips

Establishing both inflow and outflow by any method is included. That portion of the operative arteriogram performed by the surgeon is also included. Angioscopy performed during therapeutic intervention should be reported in addition to the code for the primary procedure; see 35400. Harvesting of the saphenous vein graft is included in the description of the work for 35556 and should not be reported as a separate procedure. For harvesting of a femoropopliteal vein segment, use 35572 in addition to the bypass procedure. If a composite (combination of vein and synthetic graft) is used, report 35681 in addition to the code for the primary procedure. To report the harvesting and construction of an autogenous composite graft of two segments from two distant locations, report 35682 in addition to the bypass procedure. For autogenous composite of three or more segments from distant sites, see 35683. Report 35700 in addition to 35556 for reoperation more than one month after the original operation. If synthetic graft material is used, see 35656.

ICD-10-CM Diagnostic Codes

I70.211	Atherosclerosis of native arteries of extremities with intermittent claudication, right leg ☑
I70.212	Atherosclerosis of native arteries of extremities with intermittent claudication, left leg ☑
I70.213	Atherosclerosis of native arteries of extremities with intermittent claudication, bilateral legs ☑
I70.221	Atherosclerosis of native arteries of extremities with rest pain, right leg ☑
I70.222	Atherosclerosis of native arteries of extremities with rest pain, left leg ☑
I70.223	Atherosclerosis of native arteries of extremities with rest pain, bilateral legs ☑
I70.231	Atherosclerosis of native arteries of right leg with ulceration of thigh ☑
I70.232	Atherosclerosis of native arteries of right leg with ulceration of calf ☑
I70.233	Atherosclerosis of native arteries of right leg with ulceration of ankle ☑
I70.234	Atherosclerosis of native arteries of right leg with ulceration of heel and midfoot ☑
I70.235	Atherosclerosis of native arteries of right leg with ulceration of other part of foot ☑
I70.238	Atherosclerosis of native arteries of right leg with ulceration of other part of lower leg ☑
I70.241	Atherosclerosis of native arteries of left leg with ulceration of thigh ☑
I70.242	Atherosclerosis of native arteries of left leg with ulceration of calf ☑
I70.243	Atherosclerosis of native arteries of left leg with ulceration of ankle ☑
I70.244	Atherosclerosis of native arteries of left leg with ulceration of heel and midfoot ☑
I70.245	Atherosclerosis of native arteries of left leg with ulceration of other part of foot ☑
I70.248	Atherosclerosis of native arteries of left leg with ulceration of other part of lower leg ☑
I70.261	Atherosclerosis of native arteries of extremities with gangrene, right leg ☑
I70.262	Atherosclerosis of native arteries of extremities with gangrene, left leg ☑
I70.263	Atherosclerosis of native arteries of extremities with gangrene, bilateral legs ☑
I70.291	Other atherosclerosis of native arteries of extremities, right leg ☑
I70.292	Other atherosclerosis of native arteries of extremities, left leg ☑
I70.293	Other atherosclerosis of native arteries of extremities, bilateral legs ☑
I70.461	Atherosclerosis of autologous vein bypass graft(s) of the extremities with gangrene, right leg ☑
I70.462	Atherosclerosis of autologous vein bypass graft(s) of the extremities with gangrene, left leg ☑
I70.511	Atherosclerosis of nonautologous biological bypass graft(s) of the extremities with intermittent claudication, right leg ☑
I70.512	Atherosclerosis of nonautologous biological bypass graft(s) of the extremities with intermittent claudication, left leg ☑
I70.521	Atherosclerosis of nonautologous biological bypass graft(s) of the extremities with rest pain, right leg ☑
I70.522	Atherosclerosis of nonautologous biological bypass graft(s) of the extremities with rest pain, left leg ☑
I70.531	Atherosclerosis of nonautologous biological bypass graft(s) of the right leg with ulceration of thigh ☑
I70.541	Atherosclerosis of nonautologous biological bypass graft(s) of the left leg with ulceration of thigh ☑
I70.561	Atherosclerosis of nonautologous biological bypass graft(s) of the extremities with gangrene, right leg ☑

I70.562	Atherosclerosis of nonautologous biological bypass graft(s) of the extremities with gangrene, left leg ☑
I70.611	Atherosclerosis of nonbiological bypass graft(s) of the extremities with intermittent claudication, right leg ☑
I70.612	Atherosclerosis of nonbiological bypass graft(s) of the extremities with intermittent claudication, left leg ☑
I70.621	Atherosclerosis of nonbiological bypass graft(s) of the extremities with rest pain, right leg ☑
I70.622	Atherosclerosis of nonbiological bypass graft(s) of the extremities with rest pain, left leg ☑
I70.631	Atherosclerosis of nonbiological bypass graft(s) of the right leg with ulceration of thigh ☑
I70.641	Atherosclerosis of nonbiological bypass graft(s) of the left leg with ulceration of thigh ☑
I70.661	Atherosclerosis of nonbiological bypass graft(s) of the extremities with gangrene, right leg ☑
I70.662	Atherosclerosis of nonbiological bypass graft(s) of the extremities with gangrene, left leg ☑
I70.92	Chronic total occlusion of artery of the extremities
I72.4	Aneurysm of artery of lower extremity
I73.89	Other specified peripheral vascular diseases
I74.3	Embolism and thrombosis of arteries of the lower extremities
I75.021	Atheroembolism of right lower extremity ☑
I75.022	Atheroembolism of left lower extremity ☑
I75.023	Atheroembolism of bilateral lower extremities ☑
I76	Septic arterial embolism
I77.1	Stricture of artery
I77.2	Rupture of artery
I77.5	Necrosis of artery
I77.89	Other specified disorders of arteries and arterioles
I79.8	Other disorders of arteries, arterioles and capillaries in diseases classified elsewhere
S75.011A	Minor laceration of femoral artery, right leg, initial encounter ☑
S75.012A	Minor laceration of femoral artery, left leg, initial encounter ☑
S75.021A	Major laceration of femoral artery, right leg, initial encounter ☑
S75.022A	Major laceration of femoral artery, left leg, initial encounter ☑
S75.091A	Other specified injury of femoral artery, right leg, initial encounter ☑
S75.092A	Other specified injury of femoral artery, left leg, initial encounter ☑

AMA: 35556 2018,Jan,8; 2017,Jan,8; 2016,Jan,13; 2015,Jan,16; 2014,Jan,11

Relative Value Units/Medicare Edits

Non-Facility RVU	Work	PE	MP	Total
35556	26.75	7.66	6.11	40.52
Facility RVU	**Work**	**PE**	**MP**	**Total**
35556	26.75	7.66	6.11	40.52

	FUD	Status	MUE	Modifiers				IOM Reference
35556	90	A	1(3)	51	50	62*	80	None

* with documentation

35558

35558 Bypass graft, with vein; femoral-femoral

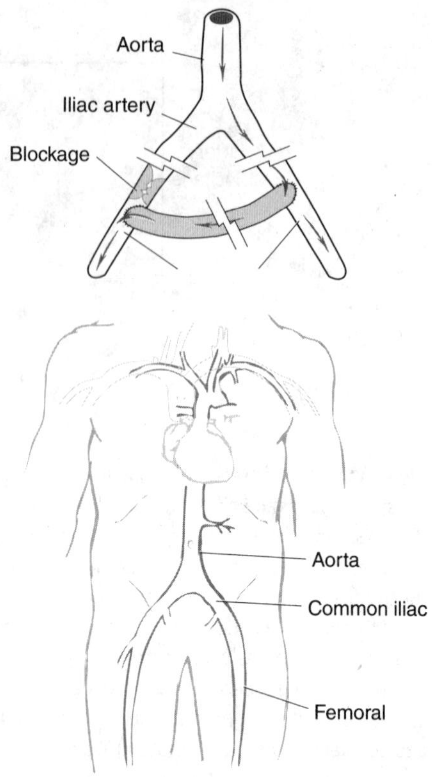

Explanation

Through incisions in the skin of the upper thighs, the physician isolates and dissects a section of the femoral arteries. The physician creates a bypass using a harvested vein. Once vessel clamps have been affixed above and below the area of anastomosis, the femoral artery may be cut through below the damaged area and sutured to one end of a harvested vein, which is sutured to the femoral artery in the opposite leg, resulting in a bypass of the damaged or blocked area. When the clamps are removed, the section of vein forms a new path through which blood can easily bypass the blocked area. The blocked or damaged portion of the artery is not removed. After the graft is complete, the skin incisions are repaired with layered closures.

Coding Tips

Establishing both inflow and outflow by any method is included. That portion of the operative arteriogram performed by the surgeon is also included. Angioscopy performed during therapeutic intervention should be reported in addition to the code for the primary procedure; see 35400. Harvesting of the saphenous vein graft is included in the description of the work for 35558 and should not be reported as a separate procedure. For harvesting of a femoropopliteal vein segment, use 35572 in addition to the bypass procedure. If a composite (combination of vein and synthetic graft) is used, report 35681 in addition to the code for the primary procedure. If synthetic graft material is used, see 35661.

ICD-10-CM Diagnostic Codes

I70.211	Atherosclerosis of native arteries of extremities with intermittent claudication, right leg ☑
I70.212	Atherosclerosis of native arteries of extremities with intermittent claudication, left leg ☑

I70.213 Atherosclerosis of native arteries of extremities with intermittent claudication, bilateral legs ☑
I70.221 Atherosclerosis of native arteries of extremities with rest pain, right leg ☑
I70.222 Atherosclerosis of native arteries of extremities with rest pain, left leg ☑
I70.223 Atherosclerosis of native arteries of extremities with rest pain, bilateral legs ☑
I70.231 Atherosclerosis of native arteries of right leg with ulceration of thigh ☑
I70.232 Atherosclerosis of native arteries of right leg with ulceration of calf ☑
I70.233 Atherosclerosis of native arteries of right leg with ulceration of ankle ☑
I70.234 Atherosclerosis of native arteries of right leg with ulceration of heel and midfoot ☑
I70.235 Atherosclerosis of native arteries of right leg with ulceration of other part of foot ☑
I70.238 Atherosclerosis of native arteries of right leg with ulceration of other part of lower leg ☑
I70.241 Atherosclerosis of native arteries of left leg with ulceration of thigh ☑
I70.242 Atherosclerosis of native arteries of left leg with ulceration of calf ☑
I70.243 Atherosclerosis of native arteries of left leg with ulceration of ankle ☑
I70.244 Atherosclerosis of native arteries of left leg with ulceration of heel and midfoot ☑
I70.245 Atherosclerosis of native arteries of left leg with ulceration of other part of foot ☑
I70.248 Atherosclerosis of native arteries of left leg with ulceration of other part of lower leg ☑
I70.261 Atherosclerosis of native arteries of extremities with gangrene, right leg ☑
I70.262 Atherosclerosis of native arteries of extremities with gangrene, left leg ☑
I70.263 Atherosclerosis of native arteries of extremities with gangrene, bilateral legs ☑
I70.291 Other atherosclerosis of native arteries of extremities, right leg ☑
I70.292 Other atherosclerosis of native arteries of extremities, left leg ☑
I70.293 Other atherosclerosis of native arteries of extremities, bilateral legs ☑
I70.461 Atherosclerosis of autologous vein bypass graft(s) of the extremities with gangrene, right leg ☑
I70.462 Atherosclerosis of autologous vein bypass graft(s) of the extremities with gangrene, left leg ☑
I70.511 Atherosclerosis of nonautologous biological bypass graft(s) of the extremities with intermittent claudication, right leg ☑
I70.512 Atherosclerosis of nonautologous biological bypass graft(s) of the extremities with intermittent claudication, left leg ☑
I70.521 Atherosclerosis of nonautologous biological bypass graft(s) of the extremities with rest pain, right leg ☑
I70.522 Atherosclerosis of nonautologous biological bypass graft(s) of the extremities with rest pain, left leg ☑
I70.531 Atherosclerosis of nonautologous biological bypass graft(s) of the right leg with ulceration of thigh ☑
I70.541 Atherosclerosis of nonautologous biological bypass graft(s) of the left leg with ulceration of thigh ☑
I70.561 Atherosclerosis of nonautologous biological bypass graft(s) of the extremities with gangrene, right leg ☑
I70.562 Atherosclerosis of nonautologous biological bypass graft(s) of the extremities with gangrene, left leg ☑
I70.611 Atherosclerosis of nonbiological bypass graft(s) of the extremities with intermittent claudication, right leg ☑
I70.612 Atherosclerosis of nonbiological bypass graft(s) of the extremities with intermittent claudication, left leg ☑
I70.621 Atherosclerosis of nonbiological bypass graft(s) of the extremities with rest pain, right leg ☑
I70.622 Atherosclerosis of nonbiological bypass graft(s) of the extremities with rest pain, left leg ☑
I70.631 Atherosclerosis of nonbiological bypass graft(s) of the right leg with ulceration of thigh ☑
I70.641 Atherosclerosis of nonbiological bypass graft(s) of the left leg with ulceration of thigh ☑
I70.661 Atherosclerosis of nonbiological bypass graft(s) of the extremities with gangrene, right leg ☑
I70.662 Atherosclerosis of nonbiological bypass graft(s) of the extremities with gangrene, left leg ☑
I70.92 Chronic total occlusion of artery of the extremities
I73.89 Other specified peripheral vascular diseases
I74.3 Embolism and thrombosis of arteries of the lower extremities
I75.021 Atheroembolism of right lower extremity ☑
I75.022 Atheroembolism of left lower extremity ☑
I75.023 Atheroembolism of bilateral lower extremities ☑
I76 Septic arterial embolism
I77.1 Stricture of artery
I77.2 Rupture of artery
I77.5 Necrosis of artery
I77.89 Other specified disorders of arteries and arterioles
I79.8 Other disorders of arteries, arterioles and capillaries in diseases classified elsewhere
S75.011A Minor laceration of femoral artery, right leg, initial encounter ☑
S75.012A Minor laceration of femoral artery, left leg, initial encounter ☑
S75.021A Major laceration of femoral artery, right leg, initial encounter ☑
S75.022A Major laceration of femoral artery, left leg, initial encounter ☑
S75.091A Other specified injury of femoral artery, right leg, initial encounter ☑
S75.092A Other specified injury of femoral artery, left leg, initial encounter ☑

AMA: **35558** 2012,Apr,3-9

Relative Value Units/Medicare Edits

Non-Facility RVU	Work	PE	MP	Total
35558	23.13	7.2	5.3	35.63
Facility RVU	**Work**	**PE**	**MP**	**Total**
35558	23.13	7.2	5.3	35.63

	FUD	Status	MUE	Modifiers				IOM Reference
35558	90	A	1(3)	51	50	62*	80	None

* with documentation

35560

35560 Bypass graft, with vein; aortorenal

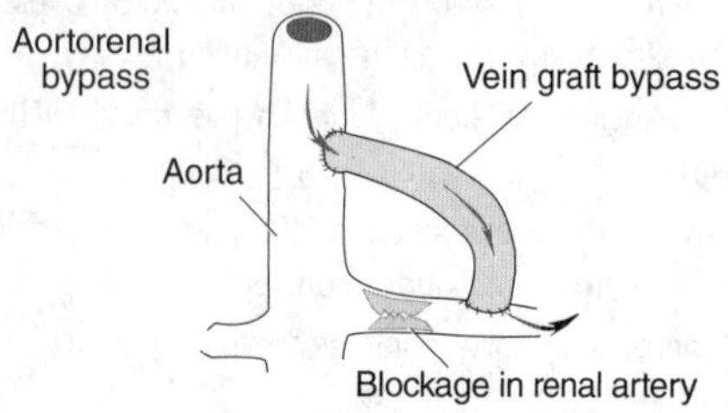

Surgical placement of a vein bypass graft from the aorta to the renal artery

Explanation

The physician exposes the involved abdominal aorta and renal artery using an abdominal incision, retracting and dissecting past large and small bowel. The aorta is partially clamped below the renal takeoff and a small longitudinal incision is performed down the clamped portion of the aorta. The venous graft is sutured and clamped and the aortic clamp is removed to assess the anastomosis for leaks. The renal artery is clamped distal to the stenosis and incised. The distal venous graft is attached to the distal renal artery. A harvested vein may be utilized to enlarge the renal arterial lumen (patch graft). The physician may perform arteriography or use a Doppler probe to establish patency of the graft. The abdominal wound is closed, leaving drains in place.

Coding Tips

Establishing both inflow and outflow by any method is included. That portion of the operative arteriogram performed by the surgeon is also included. Angioscopy performed during therapeutic intervention should be reported in addition to the code for the primary procedure; see 35400. Harvesting of the saphenous vein graft is included in the description of the work for 35560 and should not be reported as a separate procedure. For harvesting of a femoropopliteal vein segment, use 35572 in addition to the bypass procedure. If a composite (combination of vein and synthetic graft) is used, report 35681 in addition to the code for the primary procedure. If synthetic graft material is used, see 35631.

ICD-10-CM Diagnostic Codes

I15.0 Renovascular hypertension
I15.1 Hypertension secondary to other renal disorders
I70.1 Atherosclerosis of renal artery
I72.2 Aneurysm of renal artery
I73.9 Peripheral vascular disease, unspecified
I75.81 Atheroembolism of kidney
I77.1 Stricture of artery
I77.3 Arterial fibromuscular dysplasia
I77.5 Necrosis of artery
I77.73 Dissection of renal artery
I77.89 Other specified disorders of arteries and arterioles
N26.2 Page kidney
N28.0 Ischemia and infarction of kidney
Q27.1 Congenital renal artery stenosis
Q27.2 Other congenital malformations of renal artery
Q27.34 Arteriovenous malformation of renal vessel
S35.411A Laceration of right renal artery, initial encounter ☑
S35.412A Laceration of left renal artery, initial encounter ☑
S35.491A Other specified injury of right renal artery, initial encounter ☑
S35.492A Other specified injury of left renal artery, initial encounter ☑
T81.711A Complication of renal artery following a procedure, not elsewhere classified, initial encounter

AMA: 35560 2018,Jan,8; 2017,Jan,8; 2016,Jan,13; 2015,Jan,16; 2014,Jan,11

Relative Value Units/Medicare Edits

Non-Facility RVU	Work	PE	MP	Total
35560	34.03	7.33	7.89	49.25
Facility RVU	**Work**	**PE**	**MP**	**Total**
35560	34.03	7.33	7.89	49.25

	FUD	Status	MUE	Modifiers				IOM Reference
35560	90	A	1(3)	51	50	62*	80	None

* with documentation

Terms To Know

angioscopy. Visualization of capillary blood vessels with a microscope, or the inside of a blood vessel with a fiberoptic-equipped catheter.

arteriogram. Radiograph of arteries.

atherosclerosis. Buildup of yellowish plaques composed of cholesterol and lipoid material within the arteries.

graft. Tissue implant from another part of the body or another person.

hyperplasia. Abnormal proliferation in the number of normal cells in regular tissue arrangement.

secondary. Second in order of occurrence or importance, or appearing during the course of another disease or condition.

● New ▲ Revised + Add On AMA: CPT Assist [Resequenced] ☑ Laterality

35563

35563 Bypass graft, with vein; ilioiliac

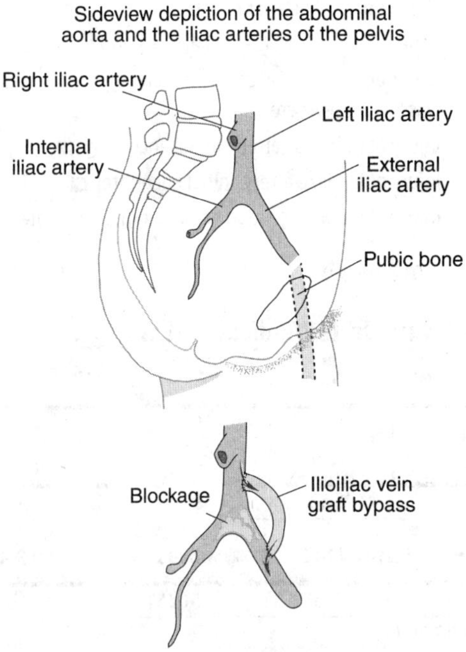

The end-to-side installment of a vein bypass graft from an iliac artery to another point on the iliac artery bypasses a blockage

Explanation

The physician exposes the iliac arteries using an abdominal incision, retracting and dissecting past large and small bowel. The patent (nondiseased) iliac artery is partially clamped and a longitudinal incision is performed down the clamped portion of the aorta. A venous graft is attached and clamped. The iliac clamp is removed to assess the anastomosis for leaks. The diseased iliac artery is clamped distal to the stenosis and a distal incision is performed. The distal venous graft is attached to the diseased iliac artery. A harvested vein may be used to enlarge the aortic or arterial lumen (patch graft). The physician may perform arteriography or use a Doppler probe to establish patency of the graft. The abdominal wound is closed, leaving drains in place.

Coding Tips

Establishing both inflow and outflow by any method is included. That portion of the operative arteriogram performed by the surgeon is also included. Angioscopy performed during therapeutic intervention should be reported in addition to the code for the primary procedure; see 35400. Harvesting of the saphenous vein graft is included in the description of the work for 35563 and should not be reported as a separate procedure. For harvesting of a femoropopliteal vein segment, use 35572 in addition to the bypass procedure. If a composite (combination of vein and synthetic graft) is used, report 35681 in addition to the code for the primary procedure. If synthetic graft material is used, see 35663.

ICD-10-CM Diagnostic Codes

I72.3	Aneurysm of iliac artery
I73.89	Other specified peripheral vascular diseases
I73.9	Peripheral vascular disease, unspecified
I74.5	Embolism and thrombosis of iliac artery
I76	Septic arterial embolism
I77.1	Stricture of artery
I77.5	Necrosis of artery
I77.72	Dissection of iliac artery
S35.511A	Injury of right iliac artery, initial encounter ☑
S35.512A	Injury of left iliac artery, initial encounter ☑
S35.59XA	Injury of other iliac blood vessels, initial encounter

AMA: 35563 1999,Mar,6; 1999,Apr,11

Relative Value Units/Medicare Edits

Non-Facility RVU	Work	PE	MP	Total
35563	26.12	6.04	6.04	38.2
Facility RVU	**Work**	**PE**	**MP**	**Total**
35563	26.12	6.04	6.04	38.2

	FUD	Status	MUE	Modifiers				IOM Reference
35563	90	A	1(3)	51	50	62*	80	None

* with documentation

Terms To Know

anastomosis. Surgically created connection between ducts, blood vessels, or bowel segments to allow flow from one to the other.

aneurysm. Circumscribed dilation or outpouching of an artery wall, often containing blood clots and connecting directly with the lumen of the artery.

angioscopy. Visualization of capillary blood vessels with a microscope, or the inside of a blood vessel with a fiberoptic-equipped catheter.

arteriogram. Radiograph of arteries.

artery. Vessel through which oxygenated blood passes away from the heart to any part of the body.

atherosclerosis. Buildup of yellowish plaques composed of cholesterol and lipoid material within the arteries.

complication. Condition arising after the beginning of observation and treatment that modifies the course of the patient's illness or the medical care required, or an undesired result or misadventure in medical care.

embolism. Obstruction of a blood vessel resulting from a clot or foreign substance.

graft. Tissue implant from another part of the body or another person.

harvest. Removal of cells or tissue from their native site to be used as a graft or transplant to another part of the donor's body or placed into another person.

necrosis. Death of cells or tissue within a living organ or structure.

stricture. Narrowing of an anatomical structure.

thrombosis. Condition arising from the presence or formation of blood clots within a blood vessel that may cause vascular obstruction and insufficient oxygenation.

35565

35565 Bypass graft, with vein; iliofemoral

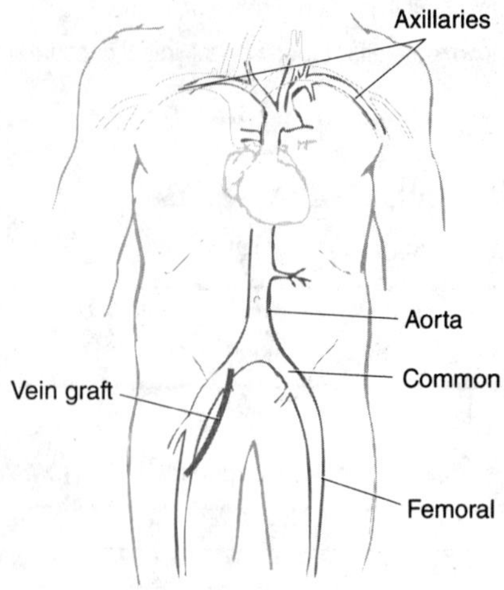

An iliofemoral bypass graft is performed

Explanation

Through incisions in the skin of the lower abdomen overlying the iliac artery and in the skin of the upper thigh overlying the femoral artery, the physician isolates and dissects a section of common iliac artery. The physician creates a bypass around the iliac artery, using a harvested vein and one of two methods of repair. Once vessel clamps have been affixed above and below the defect, the iliac artery may be cut or tied off with sutures above the damaged area and sutured to one end of a harvested vein. The graft is passed through a tunnel on the inside of the upper thigh and is sutured to the side of the femoral artery. In the second method, the end of the harvested vein is sutured to the side of the iliac artery. Either method results in a bypass of the damaged area. When the clamps are removed, the section of vein forms a new path through which blood can easily bypass the blocked area. After the graft is complete, the skin incisions are repaired with layered closures.

Coding Tips

Establishing both inflow and outflow by any method is included. That portion of the operative arteriogram performed by the surgeon is also included. Angioscopy performed during therapeutic intervention should be reported in addition to the code for the primary procedure; see 35400. Harvesting of the saphenous vein graft is included in the description of the work for 35565 and should not be reported as a separate procedure. To report harvesting of an upper extremity vein, use 35500 in addition to the bypass procedure. For harvesting of a femoropopliteal vein segment, use 35572 in addition to the bypass procedure. If a composite (combination of vein and synthetic graft) is used, report 35681 in addition to the code for the primary procedure. If synthetic graft material is used, see 35665.

ICD-10-CM Diagnostic Codes

I70.92 Chronic total occlusion of artery of the extremities
I73.89 Other specified peripheral vascular diseases
I74.3 Embolism and thrombosis of arteries of the lower extremities
I74.5 Embolism and thrombosis of iliac artery
I75.021 Atheroembolism of right lower extremity ☑
I75.022 Atheroembolism of left lower extremity ☑
I75.023 Atheroembolism of bilateral lower extremities ☑
I76 Septic arterial embolism
I77.1 Stricture of artery
I77.2 Rupture of artery
I77.5 Necrosis of artery
I77.72 Dissection of iliac artery
I77.89 Other specified disorders of arteries and arterioles
I79.8 Other disorders of arteries, arterioles and capillaries in diseases classified elsewhere
S35.511A Injury of right iliac artery, initial encounter ☑
S35.512A Injury of left iliac artery, initial encounter ☑
S35.59XA Injury of other iliac blood vessels, initial encounter

AMA: 35565 2012,Apr,3-9

Relative Value Units/Medicare Edits

Non-Facility RVU	Work	PE	MP	Total
35565	25.13	7.19	5.79	38.11
Facility RVU	**Work**	**PE**	**MP**	**Total**
35565	25.13	7.19	5.79	38.11

	FUD	Status	MUE	Modifiers				IOM Reference
35565	90	A	1(3)	51	50	62*	80	None

* with documentation

35566

35566 Bypass graft, with vein; femoral-anterior tibial, posterior tibial, peroneal artery or other distal vessels

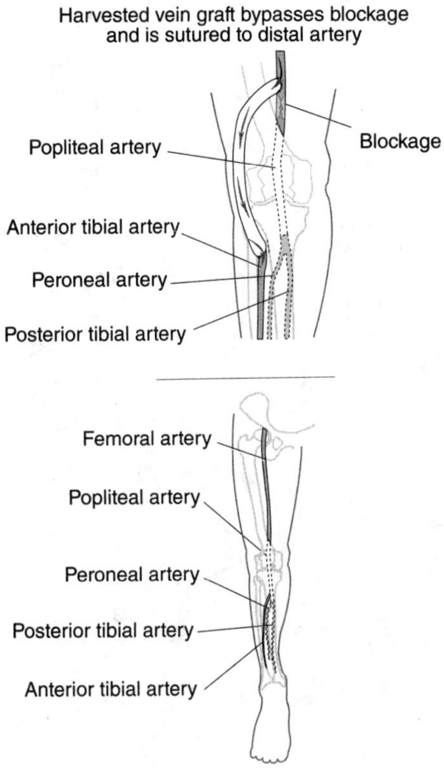

Explanation

Through incisions in the skin of the leg overlying the superficial femoral artery, the physician isolates and dissects sections of the femoral and anterior tibial, posterior tibial, or peroneal arteries. The physician creates a bypass around the affected artery using a harvested vein. Once vessel clamps have been affixed above and below the defect, the superficial femoral artery may be cut through above the damaged area and sutured to one end of a harvested vein, which is passed through an intramuscular tunnel and sutured to the anterior tibial, posterior tibial, peroneal, or other distal vessel. In the second method, the ends of the harvested vein are sutured to the side of the femoral artery and anterior tibial, posterior tibial, peroneal, or other distal vessel wall, resulting in a bypass of the damaged area. When the clamps are removed, the section of vein forms a new path through which blood can easily bypass the blocked area. The blocked or damaged portion of artery is left in place and not removed. After the graft is complete, the skin incisions are repaired with layered closures.

Coding Tips

Establishing both inflow and outflow by any method is included. That portion of the operative arteriogram performed by the surgeon is also included. Angioscopy performed during therapeutic intervention should be reported in addition to the code for the primary procedure; see 35400. Harvesting of the saphenous vein graft is included in the description of the work for 35566 and should not be reported as a separate procedure. For harvesting of a femoropopliteal vein segment, use 35572 in addition to the bypass procedure. To report harvesting of an upper extremity vein, use 35500 in addition to the bypass procedure. If a composite (combination of vein and synthetic graft) is used, report 35681 in addition to the code for the primary procedure. To report the harvesting and construction of an autogenous composite graft of two segments from two distant locations, report 35682 in addition to the bypass procedure. For autogenous composite of three or more segments from distant sites, see 35683. Report 35700 in addition to 35566 for reoperation more than one month after the original operation. If synthetic graft material is used, see 35666.

ICD-10-CM Diagnostic Codes

I70.211	Atherosclerosis of native arteries of extremities with intermittent claudication, right leg ☑
I70.212	Atherosclerosis of native arteries of extremities with intermittent claudication, left leg ☑
I70.221	Atherosclerosis of native arteries of extremities with rest pain, right leg ☑
I70.222	Atherosclerosis of native arteries of extremities with rest pain, left leg ☑
I70.231	Atherosclerosis of native arteries of right leg with ulceration of thigh ☑
I70.232	Atherosclerosis of native arteries of right leg with ulceration of calf ☑
I70.233	Atherosclerosis of native arteries of right leg with ulceration of ankle ☑
I70.234	Atherosclerosis of native arteries of right leg with ulceration of heel and midfoot ☑
I70.241	Atherosclerosis of native arteries of left leg with ulceration of thigh ☑
I70.242	Atherosclerosis of native arteries of left leg with ulceration of calf ☑
I70.243	Atherosclerosis of native arteries of left leg with ulceration of ankle ☑
I70.244	Atherosclerosis of native arteries of left leg with ulceration of heel and midfoot ☑
I70.261	Atherosclerosis of native arteries of extremities with gangrene, right leg ☑
I70.262	Atherosclerosis of native arteries of extremities with gangrene, left leg ☑
I70.461	Atherosclerosis of autologous vein bypass graft(s) of the extremities with gangrene, right leg ☑
I70.462	Atherosclerosis of autologous vein bypass graft(s) of the extremities with gangrene, left leg ☑
I70.511	Atherosclerosis of nonautologous biological bypass graft(s) of the extremities with intermittent claudication, right leg ☑
I70.512	Atherosclerosis of nonautologous biological bypass graft(s) of the extremities with intermittent claudication, left leg ☑
I70.521	Atherosclerosis of nonautologous biological bypass graft(s) of the extremities with rest pain, right leg ☑
I70.522	Atherosclerosis of nonautologous biological bypass graft(s) of the extremities with rest pain, left leg ☑
I70.531	Atherosclerosis of nonautologous biological bypass graft(s) of the right leg with ulceration of thigh ☑
I70.541	Atherosclerosis of nonautologous biological bypass graft(s) of the left leg with ulceration of thigh ☑
I70.561	Atherosclerosis of nonautologous biological bypass graft(s) of the extremities with gangrene, right leg ☑
I70.562	Atherosclerosis of nonautologous biological bypass graft(s) of the extremities with gangrene, left leg ☑
I70.611	Atherosclerosis of nonbiological bypass graft(s) of the extremities with intermittent claudication, right leg ☑

I70.612	Atherosclerosis of nonbiological bypass graft(s) of the extremities with intermittent claudication, left leg ☑
I70.621	Atherosclerosis of nonbiological bypass graft(s) of the extremities with rest pain, right leg ☑
I70.622	Atherosclerosis of nonbiological bypass graft(s) of the extremities with rest pain, left leg ☑
I70.631	Atherosclerosis of nonbiological bypass graft(s) of the right leg with ulceration of thigh ☑
I70.641	Atherosclerosis of nonbiological bypass graft(s) of the left leg with ulceration of thigh ☑
I70.661	Atherosclerosis of nonbiological bypass graft(s) of the extremities with gangrene, right leg ☑
I70.662	Atherosclerosis of nonbiological bypass graft(s) of the extremities with gangrene, left leg ☑
I70.92	Chronic total occlusion of artery of the extremities
I74.3	Embolism and thrombosis of arteries of the lower extremities
I75.021	Atheroembolism of right lower extremity ☑
I75.022	Atheroembolism of left lower extremity ☑
I76	Septic arterial embolism
I77.1	Stricture of artery
I77.2	Rupture of artery
I77.5	Necrosis of artery
S75.021A	Major laceration of femoral artery, right leg, initial encounter ☑
S75.022A	Major laceration of femoral artery, left leg, initial encounter ☑

AMA: 35566 2018,Jan,8; 2017,Jan,8; 2016,Jan,13; 2015,Jan,16; 2014,Jan,11

Relative Value Units/Medicare Edits

Non-Facility RVU	Work	PE	MP	Total
35566	32.35	8.6	7.41	48.36
Facility RVU	**Work**	**PE**	**MP**	**Total**
35566	32.35	8.6	7.41	48.36

	FUD	Status	MUE	Modifiers				IOM Reference
35566	90	A	1(3)	51	50	62*	80	None

* with documentation

Terms To Know

autogenous transplant. Tissue, such as bone, that is harvested from the patient and used for transplantation back into the same patient.

claudication. Lameness, pain, and weakness occurring in the arms or legs during exercise due to muscles not receiving the needed oxygen and nutrients.

embolism. Obstruction of a blood vessel resulting from a clot or foreign substance.

gangrene. Death of tissue, usually resulting from a loss of vascular supply, followed by a bacterial attack or onset of disease.

harvest. Removal of cells or tissue from their native site to be used as a graft or transplant to another part of the donor's body or placed into another person.

thrombosis. Condition arising from the presence or formation of blood clots within a blood vessel that may cause vascular obstruction and insufficient oxygenation.

35570

35570 Bypass graft, with vein; tibial-tibial, peroneal-tibial, or tibial/peroneal trunk-tibial

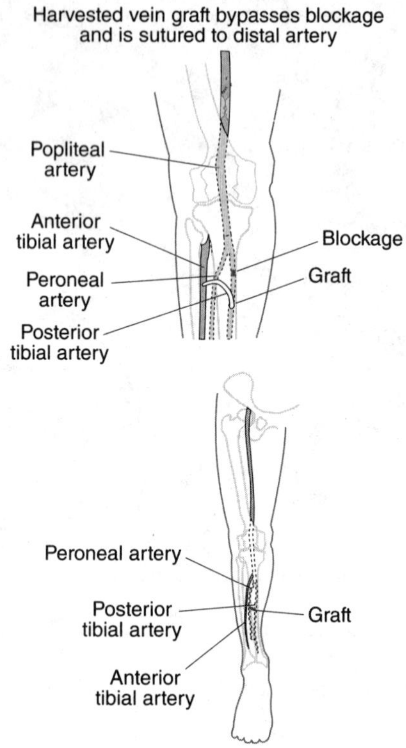

Explanation

The physician performs tibial-tibial, peroneal-tibial, or tibioperoneal trunk-tibial bypass graft. Through incisions in the skin of the leg overlying the affected tibial, peroneal, or tibioperoneal trunk artery, the physician isolates and dissects a section of arteries from adjacent critical structures. The physician creates a bypass around the affected artery using a harvested vein and one of two methods of repair. Once vessel clamps have been affixed above and below the defect, the artery may be cut through above the damaged area and sutured to one end of a harvested vein, which is sutured to the targeted tibial artery. In the second method, the ends of the harvested vein are sutured to the side of the bypassed artery and tibial vessel wall, resulting in a bypass of the damaged area. When the clamps are removed, the section of vein forms a new path through which blood can bypass the blocked area. The blocked or damaged portion of artery is left in place and not removed. After the graft is complete, the skin incisions are repaired with layered closures.

Coding Tips

Establishing both inflow and outflow by any method is included. That portion of the operative arteriogram performed by the surgeon is also included. Angioscopy performed during therapeutic intervention should be reported in addition to the code for the primary procedure, see 35400. Harvesting of the saphenous vein graft is included in the description of the work for 35570 and should not be reported as a separate procedure. For harvesting of a femoropopliteal vein segment, use 35572 in addition to the bypass procedure. If a composite (combination of vein and synthetic graft) is used, report 35681 in addition to the code for the primary procedure. Report 35700 in addition to 35570 for reoperation more than one month after the original operation. Do not report 35570 with 35256 or 35286.

ICD-10-CM Diagnostic Codes

I70.92	Chronic total occlusion of artery of the extremities
I73.89	Other specified peripheral vascular diseases
I74.3	Embolism and thrombosis of arteries of the lower extremities
I75.021	Atheroembolism of right lower extremity ☑
I75.022	Atheroembolism of left lower extremity ☑
I75.023	Atheroembolism of bilateral lower extremities ☑
I76	Septic arterial embolism
I77.1	Stricture of artery
I77.2	Rupture of artery
I77.5	Necrosis of artery
I77.89	Other specified disorders of arteries and arterioles
I79.8	Other disorders of arteries, arterioles and capillaries in diseases classified elsewhere
S85.141A	Laceration of anterior tibial artery, right leg, initial encounter ☑
S85.142A	Laceration of anterior tibial artery, left leg, initial encounter ☑
S85.151A	Other specified injury of anterior tibial artery, right leg, initial encounter ☑
S85.152A	Other specified injury of anterior tibial artery, left leg, initial encounter ☑
S85.171A	Laceration of posterior tibial artery, right leg, initial encounter ☑
S85.172A	Laceration of posterior tibial artery, left leg, initial encounter ☑
S85.181A	Other specified injury of posterior tibial artery, right leg, initial encounter ☑
S85.182A	Other specified injury of posterior tibial artery, left leg, initial encounter ☑
S85.211A	Laceration of peroneal artery, right leg, initial encounter ☑
S85.212A	Laceration of peroneal artery, left leg, initial encounter ☑
S85.291A	Other specified injury of peroneal artery, right leg, initial encounter ☑
S85.292A	Other specified injury of peroneal artery, left leg, initial encounter ☑
S85.811A	Laceration of other blood vessels at lower leg level, right leg, initial encounter ☑
S85.812A	Laceration of other blood vessels at lower leg level, left leg, initial encounter ☑
S85.891A	Other specified injury of other blood vessels at lower leg level, right leg, initial encounter ☑
S85.892A	Other specified injury of other blood vessels at lower leg level, left leg, initial encounter ☑

AMA: 35570 2018,Jan,8; 2017,Jan,8; 2016,Jan,13; 2015,Jan,16; 2014,Jan,11

Relative Value Units/Medicare Edits

Non-Facility RVU	Work	PE	MP	Total
35570	29.15	7.93	6.65	43.73
Facility RVU	**Work**	**PE**	**MP**	**Total**
35570	29.15	7.93	6.65	43.73

	FUD	Status	MUE	Modifiers				IOM Reference
35570	90	A	1(3)	51	50	62*	80	None

* with documentation

35571

35571 Bypass graft, with vein; popliteal-tibial, -peroneal artery or other distal vessels

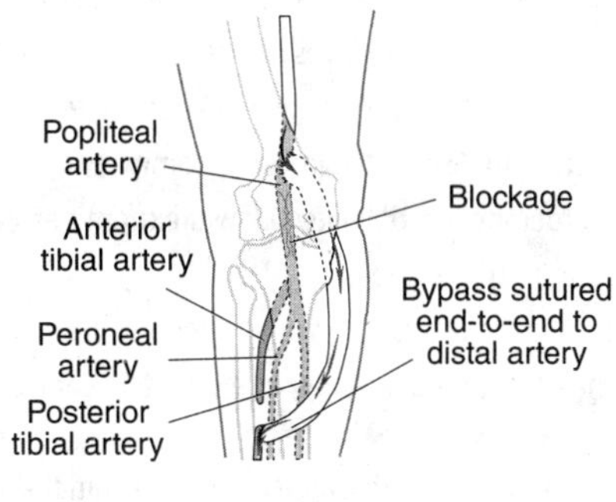

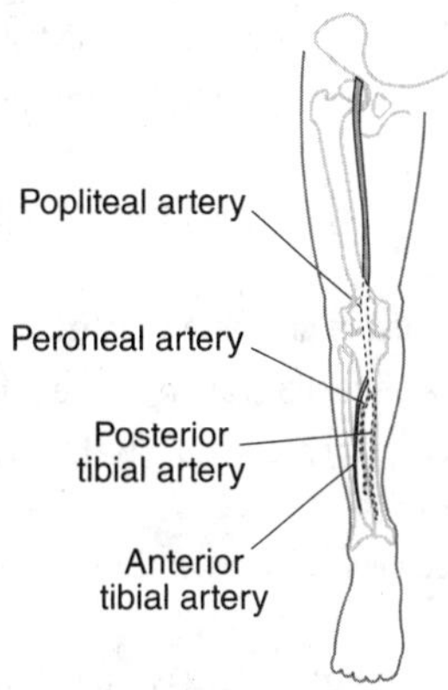

Explanation

Through incisions in the skin of the leg overlying the popliteal arteries, the physician isolates and dissects a section of arteries from adjacent critical structures. The physician creates a bypass around the artery, using a harvested vein and one of two methods of repair. Once vessel clamps have been affixed above and below the defect, the popliteal artery may be cut through above the damaged area and sutured to one end of a harvested vein, which is sutured to the tibial, peroneal, or other distal artery. In the second method, the ends of the harvested vein are sutured into the side of the popliteal and the tibial or peroneal arterial wall resulting in a bypass of the damaged area. When the clamps are removed, the section of vein forms a new path through which blood can easily bypass the blocked area. After the graft is complete, the incisions are repaired with layered closures.

Coding Tips

Establishing both inflow and outflow by any method is included. That portion of the operative arteriogram performed by the surgeon is also included. Angioscopy performed during therapeutic intervention should be reported in addition to the code for the primary procedure; see 35400. Harvesting of the saphenous vein graft is included in the description of the work for 35571 and should not be reported as a separate procedure. To report harvesting of an upper extremity vein, use 35500 in addition to the bypass procedure. For harvesting of a femoropopliteal vein segment, use 35572 in addition to the bypass procedure. If a composite (combination of vein and synthetic graft) is used, report 35681 in addition to the code for the primary procedure. To report the harvesting and construction of an autogenous composite graft of two segments from two distant locations, report 35682 in addition to the bypass procedure. For autogenous composite of three or more segments from distant sites, see 35683. Report 35700 in addition to 35571 for reoperation more than one month after the original operation. If synthetic graft material is used, see 35671.

ICD-10-CM Diagnostic Codes

I70.92	Chronic total occlusion of artery of the extremities
I73.89	Other specified peripheral vascular diseases
I74.3	Embolism and thrombosis of arteries of the lower extremities
I75.021	Atheroembolism of right lower extremity ☑
I75.022	Atheroembolism of left lower extremity ☑
I75.023	Atheroembolism of bilateral lower extremities ☑
I76	Septic arterial embolism
I77.89	Other specified disorders of arteries and arterioles
I79.8	Other disorders of arteries, arterioles and capillaries in diseases classified elsewhere
S85.011A	Laceration of popliteal artery, right leg, initial encounter ☑
S85.012A	Laceration of popliteal artery, left leg, initial encounter ☑
S85.091A	Other specified injury of popliteal artery, right leg, initial encounter ☑
S85.092A	Other specified injury of popliteal artery, left leg, initial encounter ☑
S85.141A	Laceration of anterior tibial artery, right leg, initial encounter ☑
S85.142A	Laceration of anterior tibial artery, left leg, initial encounter ☑
S85.151A	Other specified injury of anterior tibial artery, right leg, initial encounter ☑
S85.152A	Other specified injury of anterior tibial artery, left leg, initial encounter ☑
S85.171A	Laceration of posterior tibial artery, right leg, initial encounter ☑
S85.172A	Laceration of posterior tibial artery, left leg, initial encounter ☑
S85.181A	Other specified injury of posterior tibial artery, right leg, initial encounter ☑
S85.182A	Other specified injury of posterior tibial artery, left leg, initial encounter ☑
S85.211A	Laceration of peroneal artery, right leg, initial encounter ☑
S85.212A	Laceration of peroneal artery, left leg, initial encounter ☑
S85.291A	Other specified injury of peroneal artery, right leg, initial encounter ☑
S85.292A	Other specified injury of peroneal artery, left leg, initial encounter ☑
S85.811A	Laceration of other blood vessels at lower leg level, right leg, initial encounter ☑
S85.812A	Laceration of other blood vessels at lower leg level, left leg, initial encounter ☑
S85.891A	Other specified injury of other blood vessels at lower leg level, right leg, initial encounter ☑
S85.892A	Other specified injury of other blood vessels at lower leg level, left leg, initial encounter ☑

AMA: 35571 2018,Jan,8; 2017,Jan,8; 2016,Jan,13; 2015,Jan,16; 2014,Jan,11

Relative Value Units/Medicare Edits

Non-Facility RVU	Work	PE	MP	Total
35571	25.52	6.99	5.84	38.35
Facility RVU	**Work**	**PE**	**MP**	**Total**
35571	25.52	6.99	5.84	38.35

	FUD	Status	MUE	Modifiers				IOM Reference
35571	90	A	1(3)	51	50	62*	80	None

* with documentation

Terms To Know

artery. Vessel through which oxygenated blood passes away from the heart to any part of the body.

autogenous transplant. Tissue, such as bone, that is harvested from the patient and used for transplantation back into the same patient.

bypass graft. Surgically created alternative blood vessel used to reroute blood flow around an area of obstruction or disease.

embolism. Obstruction of a blood vessel resulting from a clot or foreign substance.

harvest. Removal of cells or tissue from their native site to be used as a graft or transplant to another part of the donor's body or placed into another person.

laceration. Tearing injury; a torn, ragged-edged wound.

thrombosis. Condition arising from the presence or formation of blood clots within a blood vessel that may cause vascular obstruction and insufficient oxygenation.

vein. Vessel through which oxygen-depleted blood passes back to the heart.

35572

+ 35572 Harvest of femoropopliteal vein, 1 segment, for vascular reconstruction procedure (eg, aortic, vena caval, coronary, peripheral artery) (List separately in addition to code for primary procedure)

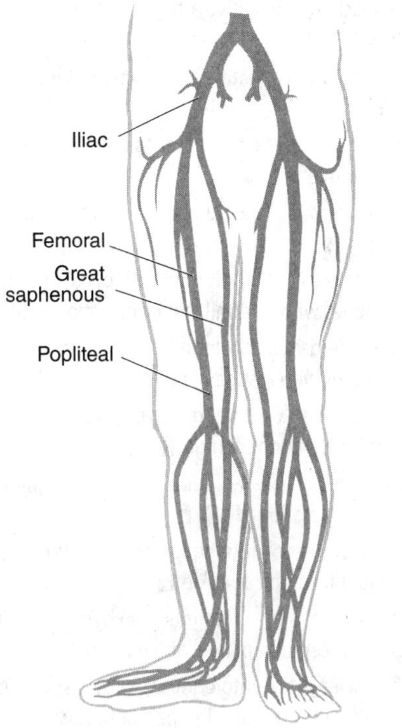

A single segment of femoropopliteal vein is harvested for a vascular reconstruction

Explanation

The physician harvests one segment of the femoropopliteal vein for a vascular reconstructive procedure. The leg is prepared circumferentially to make the leg accessible and provide optimal access. A single incision or multiple incisions can be made to harvest the vein. The vein is first located through an approximately 10 cm incision and dissected. The skin is cut over the course of the vein. If multiple incisions are made, the index finger is used to continue dissection along the anterior surface of the vein, with the incisions made about 2 to 4 cm from the last incision and the physician's finger underneath, or an external vein stripper is used with incisions made where the stripper meets resistance again. Branches of the vein are ligated. Dissection can begin at the proximal or distal end. The length of vein needed is estimated based on its intended purpose and the desired length is mobilized and divided at both ends. The vein is placed in a prepared solution of blood and saline at room temperature and prepared with diluted blood placed to flush the vein. A vascular device is applied, the vein is gently distended, and uncontrolled branches are closed. The vein is returned to the solution until used.

Coding Tips

Code 35572 should be reported twice when performed bilaterally. Do not report with modifier 50. Report 35572 in addition to 33510–33516, 33517–33523, 33533–33536, 34502, 34520, 35001, 35002, 35011–35022, 35102, 35103, 35121–35152, 35231–35256, 35501–35587, and 35879–35907. For endoscopic vein harvest, see 33508.

ICD-10-CM Diagnostic Codes

This/these CPT code(s) are add on code(s). See the primary procedure code that this code is performed with for your ICD-10-CM code selections. Diagnostic code(s) would be the same as the actual procedure performed.

AMA: **35572** 2018,Jan,8; 2017,Jan,8; 2016,Jan,13; 2015,Jan,16; 2014,Jan,11

Relative Value Units/Medicare Edits

Non-Facility RVU	Work	PE	MP	Total
35572	6.81	1.68	1.56	10.05
Facility RVU	**Work**	**PE**	**MP**	**Total**
35572	6.81	1.68	1.56	10.05

	FUD	Status	MUE	Modifiers				IOM Reference
35572	N/A	A	2(3)	N/A	N/A	N/A	80	None

* with documentation

Terms To Know

anterior. Situated in the front area or toward the belly surface of the body; an anatomical reference point used to show the position and relationship of one body structure to another.

dissection. Separating by cutting tissue or body structures apart.

distal. Located farther away from a specified reference point or the trunk.

harvest. Removal of cells or tissue from their native site to be used as a graft or transplant to another part of the donor's body or placed into another person.

incision. Act of cutting into tissue or an organ.

ligate. To tie off a blood vessel or duct with a suture or a soft, thin wire (ligature wire).

proximal. Located closest to a specified reference point, usually the midline or trunk.

reconstruction. Recreating, restoring, or rebuilding a body part or organ.

vein. Vessel through which oxygen-depleted blood passes back to the heart.

35583

35583 In-situ vein bypass; femoral-popliteal

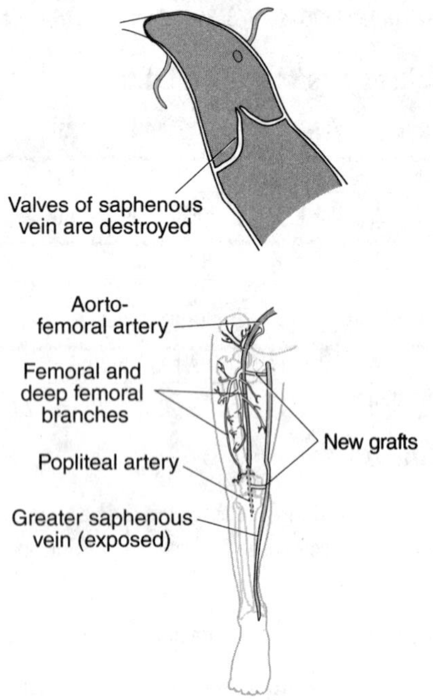

Saphenous vein is attached to femoral (at top) and popliteal arteries, converting it into a defacto artery

Explanation

Through an incision in the skin of the leg overlying the greater saphenous vein, the physician isolates and dissects the greater saphenous vein from adjacent critical structures from the upper thigh to the level of the knee. Vessel clamps are affixed above and below the site of the anastomosis to the femoral and popliteal arteries. All side branches of the saphenous vein are tied off. The vessel's valves are destroyed. The upper end of the saphenous vein is divided and sutured into the femoral artery either end-to-end or end-to-side. The lower end is divided and sutured into the popliteal artery either end-to-end or end-to-side. The clamps are removed, and blood flows backward toward the feet, as if the vein were an artery. When the procedure is complete, the skin incision is repaired with a layered closure.

Coding Tips

Establishing both inflow and outflow by any method is included. That portion of the operative arteriogram performed by the surgeon is also included. Angioscopy performed during therapeutic intervention should be reported in addition to the code for the primary procedure; see 35400. Harvesting of the saphenous vein graft is included in the description of the work for 35583 and should not be reported as a separate procedure. For harvesting of a femoropopliteal vein segment, use 35572 in addition to the bypass procedure. To report harvesting of an upper extremity vein, use 35500 in addition to the bypass procedure. Report 35700 in addition to 35583 for reoperation more than one month after the original operation. Aortobifemoral bypass using synthetic conduit and femoral-popliteal bypass with vein conduit in-situ should be reported with 35646 and 35583. Aorto(uni)femoral bypass with synthetic conduit and femoral popliteal bypass with vein conduit in-situ should be reported with 35647 and 35583. Aortofemoral bypass using vein conduit and femoral-popliteal bypass with vein conduit in-situ should be reported with 35539 and 35583.

ICD-10-CM Diagnostic Codes

I70.211	Atherosclerosis of native arteries of extremities with intermittent claudication, right leg ☑
I70.221	Atherosclerosis of native arteries of extremities with rest pain, right leg ☑
I70.231	Atherosclerosis of native arteries of right leg with ulceration of thigh ☑
I70.232	Atherosclerosis of native arteries of right leg with ulceration of calf ☑
I70.233	Atherosclerosis of native arteries of right leg with ulceration of ankle ☑
I70.234	Atherosclerosis of native arteries of right leg with ulceration of heel and midfoot ☑
I70.261	Atherosclerosis of native arteries of extremities with gangrene, right leg ☑
I70.411	Atherosclerosis of autologous vein bypass graft(s) of the extremities with intermittent claudication, right leg ☑
I70.421	Atherosclerosis of autologous vein bypass graft(s) of the extremities with rest pain, right leg ☑
I70.431	Atherosclerosis of autologous vein bypass graft(s) of the right leg with ulceration of thigh ☑
I70.432	Atherosclerosis of autologous vein bypass graft(s) of the right leg with ulceration of calf ☑
I70.433	Atherosclerosis of autologous vein bypass graft(s) of the right leg with ulceration of ankle ☑
I70.434	Atherosclerosis of autologous vein bypass graft(s) of the right leg with ulceration of heel and midfoot ☑
I70.435	Atherosclerosis of autologous vein bypass graft(s) of the right leg with ulceration of other part of foot ☑
I70.438	Atherosclerosis of autologous vein bypass graft(s) of the right leg with ulceration of other part of lower leg ☑
I70.461	Atherosclerosis of autologous vein bypass graft(s) of the extremities with gangrene, right leg ☑
I70.511	Atherosclerosis of nonautologous biological bypass graft(s) of the extremities with intermittent claudication, right leg ☑
I70.521	Atherosclerosis of nonautologous biological bypass graft(s) of the extremities with rest pain, right leg ☑
I70.531	Atherosclerosis of nonautologous biological bypass graft(s) of the right leg with ulceration of thigh ☑
I70.532	Atherosclerosis of nonautologous biological bypass graft(s) of the right leg with ulceration of calf ☑
I70.533	Atherosclerosis of nonautologous biological bypass graft(s) of the right leg with ulceration of ankle ☑
I70.534	Atherosclerosis of nonautologous biological bypass graft(s) of the right leg with ulceration of heel and midfoot ☑
I70.561	Atherosclerosis of nonautologous biological bypass graft(s) of the extremities with gangrene, right leg ☑
I70.611	Atherosclerosis of nonbiological bypass graft(s) of the extremities with intermittent claudication, right leg ☑
I70.621	Atherosclerosis of nonbiological bypass graft(s) of the extremities with rest pain, right leg ☑
I70.631	Atherosclerosis of nonbiological bypass graft(s) of the right leg with ulceration of thigh ☑
I70.632	Atherosclerosis of nonbiological bypass graft(s) of the right leg with ulceration of calf ☑
I70.633	Atherosclerosis of nonbiological bypass graft(s) of the right leg with ulceration of ankle ☑

I70.634 Atherosclerosis of nonbiological bypass graft(s) of the right leg with ulceration of heel and midfoot ☑
I70.635 Atherosclerosis of nonbiological bypass graft(s) of the right leg with ulceration of other part of foot ☑
I70.638 Atherosclerosis of nonbiological bypass graft(s) of the right leg with ulceration of other part of lower leg ☑
I70.661 Atherosclerosis of nonbiological bypass graft(s) of the extremities with gangrene, right leg ☑
I70.691 Other atherosclerosis of nonbiological bypass graft(s) of the extremities, right leg ☑
I70.711 Atherosclerosis of other type of bypass graft(s) of the extremities with intermittent claudication, right leg ☑
I70.721 Atherosclerosis of other type of bypass graft(s) of the extremities with rest pain, right leg ☑
I70.731 Atherosclerosis of other type of bypass graft(s) of the right leg with ulceration of thigh ☑
I70.732 Atherosclerosis of other type of bypass graft(s) of the right leg with ulceration of calf ☑
I70.733 Atherosclerosis of other type of bypass graft(s) of the right leg with ulceration of ankle ☑
I70.734 Atherosclerosis of other type of bypass graft(s) of the right leg with ulceration of heel and midfoot ☑
I70.761 Atherosclerosis of other type of bypass graft(s) of the extremities with gangrene, right leg ☑
I70.92 Chronic total occlusion of artery of the extremities
I72.4 Aneurysm of artery of lower extremity
I74.3 Embolism and thrombosis of arteries of the lower extremities
I75.021 Atheroembolism of right lower extremity ☑
I76 Septic arterial embolism
I77.1 Stricture of artery
I77.2 Rupture of artery
I77.5 Necrosis of artery
I80.01 Phlebitis and thrombophlebitis of superficial vessels of right lower extremity ☑
I80.11 Phlebitis and thrombophlebitis of right femoral vein ☑
I80.221 Phlebitis and thrombophlebitis of right popliteal vein ☑
I80.231 Phlebitis and thrombophlebitis of right tibial vein ☑
I82.411 Acute embolism and thrombosis of right femoral vein ☑
I82.431 Acute embolism and thrombosis of right popliteal vein ☑
I82.441 Acute embolism and thrombosis of right tibial vein ☑
I82.491 Acute embolism and thrombosis of other specified deep vein of right lower extremity ☑
I82.511 Chronic embolism and thrombosis of right femoral vein ☑
I82.531 Chronic embolism and thrombosis of right popliteal vein ☑
I82.541 Chronic embolism and thrombosis of right tibial vein ☑

AMA: 35583 2018,Jan,8; 2017,Jan,8; 2016,Jan,13; 2015,Jan,16; 2014,Jan,11

Relative Value Units/Medicare Edits

Non-Facility RVU	Work	PE	MP	Total
35583	27.75	7.75	6.34	41.84
Facility RVU	**Work**	**PE**	**MP**	**Total**
35583	27.75	7.75	6.34	41.84

	FUD	Status	MUE	Modifiers				IOM Reference
35583	90	A	1(2)	51	50	62*	80	None

* with documentation

Terms To Know

anastomosis. Surgically created connection between ducts, blood vessels, or bowel segments to allow flow from one to the other.

artery. Vessel through which oxygenated blood passes away from the heart to any part of the body.

bypass graft. Surgically created alternative blood vessel used to reroute blood flow around an area of obstruction or disease.

in situ. Located in the natural position or contained within the origin site, not spread into neighboring tissue.

laceration. Tearing injury; a torn, ragged-edged wound.

thrombosis. Condition arising from the presence or formation of blood clots within a blood vessel that may cause vascular obstruction and insufficient oxygenation.

varicose vein. Abnormal, permanently distended or stretched vein.

vein. Vessel through which oxygen-depleted blood passes back to the heart.

venous. Relating to the veins.

35585

35585 In-situ vein bypass; femoral-anterior tibial, posterior tibial, or peroneal artery

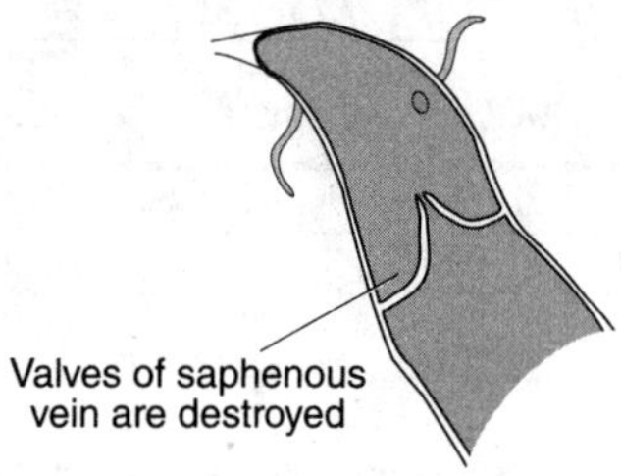

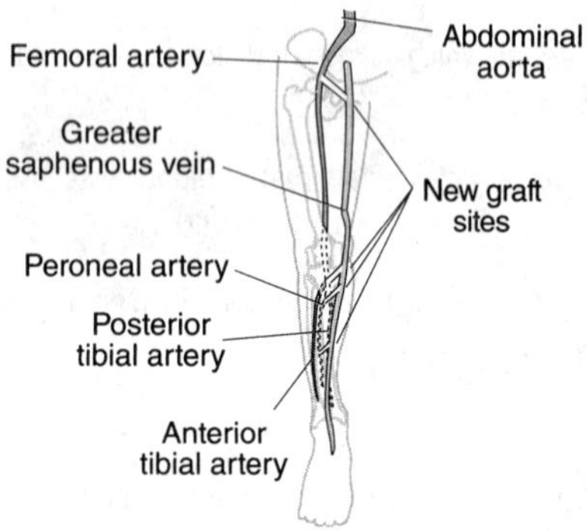

Saphenous vein is attached to femoral (at top) and one of the distal arteries at bottom, thus converting it into a defacto artery

Explanation

Through an incision in the skin of the leg overlying the greater saphenous vein, the physician isolates and dissects the greater saphenous vein from adjacent critical structures. Vessel clamps are affixed above and below the site of anastomosis in the femoral artery and the distal artery. All side branches of the Saphenous are tied off. The vessel's valves are destroyed. The upper end of the saphenous vein is divided and sutured end-to-end or end-to-side in the femoral artery above the blockage. The lower end is divided and sutured end-to-end or end-to-side to the anterior tibial, posterior tibial, or peroneal artery below the blockage. The clamps are removed, and blood flows backward toward the feet, as if the vein were an artery. When the procedure is complete, the skin incision is repaired with a layered closure.

Coding Tips

Establishing both inflow and outflow by any method is included. That portion of the operative arteriogram performed by the surgeon is also included. Angioscopy performed during therapeutic intervention should be reported in addition to the code for the primary procedure; see 35400. Harvesting of the saphenous vein graft is included in the description of the work for 35585 and should not be reported as a separate procedure. To report harvesting of an upper extremity vein, use 35500 in addition to the bypass procedure. For harvesting of a femoropopliteal vein segment, use 35572 in addition to the bypass procedure. If a composite (combination of vein and synthetic graft) is used, report 35681 in addition to the code for the primary procedure. To report the harvesting and construction of an autogenous composite graft of two segments from two distant locations, report 35682 in addition to the bypass procedure. For autogenous composite of three or more segments from distant sites, see 35683. Report 35700 in addition to 35585 for reoperation more than one month after the original operation.

ICD-10-CM Diagnostic Codes

I70.211	Atherosclerosis of native arteries of extremities with intermittent claudication, right leg ☑
I70.221	Atherosclerosis of native arteries of extremities with rest pain, right leg ☑
I70.231	Atherosclerosis of native arteries of right leg with ulceration of thigh ☑
I70.232	Atherosclerosis of native arteries of right leg with ulceration of calf ☑
I70.233	Atherosclerosis of native arteries of right leg with ulceration of ankle ☑
I70.234	Atherosclerosis of native arteries of right leg with ulceration of heel and midfoot ☑
I70.261	Atherosclerosis of native arteries of extremities with gangrene, right leg ☑
I70.411	Atherosclerosis of autologous vein bypass graft(s) of the extremities with intermittent claudication, right leg ☑
I70.421	Atherosclerosis of autologous vein bypass graft(s) of the extremities with rest pain, right leg ☑
I70.431	Atherosclerosis of autologous vein bypass graft(s) of the right leg with ulceration of thigh ☑
I70.432	Atherosclerosis of autologous vein bypass graft(s) of the right leg with ulceration of calf ☑
I70.433	Atherosclerosis of autologous vein bypass graft(s) of the right leg with ulceration of ankle ☑
I70.434	Atherosclerosis of autologous vein bypass graft(s) of the right leg with ulceration of heel and midfoot ☑
I70.435	Atherosclerosis of autologous vein bypass graft(s) of the right leg with ulceration of other part of foot ☑
I70.438	Atherosclerosis of autologous vein bypass graft(s) of the right leg with ulceration of other part of lower leg ☑
I70.461	Atherosclerosis of autologous vein bypass graft(s) of the extremities with gangrene, right leg ☑
I70.511	Atherosclerosis of nonautologous biological bypass graft(s) of the extremities with intermittent claudication, right leg ☑
I70.521	Atherosclerosis of nonautologous biological bypass graft(s) of the extremities with rest pain, right leg ☑
I70.531	Atherosclerosis of nonautologous biological bypass graft(s) of the right leg with ulceration of thigh ☑
I70.532	Atherosclerosis of nonautologous biological bypass graft(s) of the right leg with ulceration of calf ☑
I70.533	Atherosclerosis of nonautologous biological bypass graft(s) of the right leg with ulceration of ankle ☑
I70.534	Atherosclerosis of nonautologous biological bypass graft(s) of the right leg with ulceration of heel and midfoot ☑
I70.561	Atherosclerosis of nonautologous biological bypass graft(s) of the extremities with gangrene, right leg ☑
I70.611	Atherosclerosis of nonbiological bypass graft(s) of the extremities with intermittent claudication, right leg ☑
I70.621	Atherosclerosis of nonbiological bypass graft(s) of the extremities with rest pain, right leg ☑
I70.631	Atherosclerosis of nonbiological bypass graft(s) of the right leg with ulceration of thigh ☑
I70.632	Atherosclerosis of nonbiological bypass graft(s) of the right leg with ulceration of calf ☑
I70.633	Atherosclerosis of nonbiological bypass graft(s) of the right leg with ulceration of ankle ☑

I70.634	Atherosclerosis of nonbiological bypass graft(s) of the right leg with ulceration of heel and midfoot ☑
I70.635	Atherosclerosis of nonbiological bypass graft(s) of the right leg with ulceration of other part of foot ☑
I70.638	Atherosclerosis of nonbiological bypass graft(s) of the right leg with ulceration of other part of lower leg ☑
I70.661	Atherosclerosis of nonbiological bypass graft(s) of the extremities with gangrene, right leg ☑
I70.691	Other atherosclerosis of nonbiological bypass graft(s) of the extremities, right leg ☑
I70.711	Atherosclerosis of other type of bypass graft(s) of the extremities with intermittent claudication, right leg ☑
I70.721	Atherosclerosis of other type of bypass graft(s) of the extremities with rest pain, right leg ☑
I70.731	Atherosclerosis of other type of bypass graft(s) of the right leg with ulceration of thigh ☑
I70.732	Atherosclerosis of other type of bypass graft(s) of the right leg with ulceration of calf ☑
I70.733	Atherosclerosis of other type of bypass graft(s) of the right leg with ulceration of ankle ☑
I70.734	Atherosclerosis of other type of bypass graft(s) of the right leg with ulceration of heel and midfoot ☑
I70.761	Atherosclerosis of other type of bypass graft(s) of the extremities with gangrene, right leg ☑
I70.92	Chronic total occlusion of artery of the extremities
I72.4	Aneurysm of artery of lower extremity
I74.3	Embolism and thrombosis of arteries of the lower extremities
I75.021	Atheroembolism of right lower extremity ☑
I76	Septic arterial embolism
I77.1	Stricture of artery
I77.2	Rupture of artery
I77.5	Necrosis of artery
I80.01	Phlebitis and thrombophlebitis of superficial vessels of right lower extremity ☑
I80.231	Phlebitis and thrombophlebitis of right tibial vein ☑
I82.411	Acute embolism and thrombosis of right femoral vein ☑
I82.441	Acute embolism and thrombosis of right tibial vein ☑
I82.491	Acute embolism and thrombosis of other specified deep vein of right lower extremity ☑
I82.511	Chronic embolism and thrombosis of right femoral vein ☑
I82.541	Chronic embolism and thrombosis of right tibial vein ☑

AMA: 35585 2018,Jan,8; 2017,Jan,8; 2016,Jan,13; 2015,Jan,16; 2014,Jan,11

Relative Value Units/Medicare Edits

Non-Facility RVU	Work	PE	MP	Total
35585	32.35	8.72	7.4	48.47
Facility RVU	**Work**	**PE**	**MP**	**Total**
35585	32.35	8.72	7.4	48.47

	FUD	Status	MUE	Modifiers				IOM Reference
35585	90	A	2(3)	51	50	62*	80	None

* with documentation

35587

35587 In-situ vein bypass; popliteal-tibial, peroneal

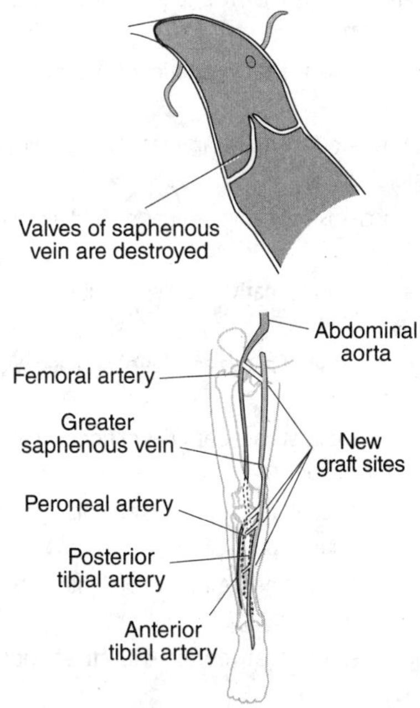

Saphenous vein is attached to the popliteal-tibial (at top) and the peroneal artery at bottom, thus converting the vein into a defacto artery

Explanation

Through an incision in the skin of the leg overlying the greater saphenous vein from the knee to the ankle, the physician isolates and dissects the greater saphenous vein from adjacent critical structures along its length. Vessel clamps are affixed above and below the site of anastomosis on the popliteal and peroneal arteries. All side branches of the saphenous vein are tied off. The vessel's valves are destroyed. The upper end of the saphenous vein is divided and sutured into the popliteal-tibial artery. The lower end is divided and sutured into the peroneal artery. The clamps are removed and blood flows backward through the vein toward the feet, as if it were an artery. When the procedure is complete, the incision is repaired with layered closure.

Coding Tips

Establishing both inflow and outflow by any method is included. That portion of the operative arteriogram performed by the surgeon is also included. Angioscopy performed during therapeutic intervention should be reported in addition to the code for the primary procedure; see 35400. Harvesting of the saphenous vein graft is included in the description of the work for 35587 and should not be reported as a separate procedure. To report harvesting of an upper extremity vein, use 35500 in addition to the bypass procedure. For harvesting of a femoropopliteal vein segment, use 35572 in addition to the bypass procedure. If a composite (combination of vein and synthetic graft) is used, report 35681 in addition to the code for the primary procedure. To report the harvesting and construction of an autogenous composite graft of two segments from two distant locations, report 35682 in addition to the bypass procedure. For autogenous composite of three or more segments from distant sites, see 35683. Report 35700 in addition to 35587 for reoperation more than one month after the original operation.

ICD-10-CM Diagnostic Codes

I70.211	Atherosclerosis of native arteries of extremities with intermittent claudication, right leg ☑

Arteries and Veins

I70.212 Atherosclerosis of native arteries of extremities with intermittent claudication, left leg ☑
I70.213 Atherosclerosis of native arteries of extremities with intermittent claudication, bilateral legs ☑
I70.221 Atherosclerosis of native arteries of extremities with rest pain, right leg ☑
I70.222 Atherosclerosis of native arteries of extremities with rest pain, left leg ☑
I70.223 Atherosclerosis of native arteries of extremities with rest pain, bilateral legs ☑
I70.231 Atherosclerosis of native arteries of right leg with ulceration of thigh ☑
I70.232 Atherosclerosis of native arteries of right leg with ulceration of calf ☑
I70.233 Atherosclerosis of native arteries of right leg with ulceration of ankle ☑
I70.234 Atherosclerosis of native arteries of right leg with ulceration of heel and midfoot ☑
I70.235 Atherosclerosis of native arteries of right leg with ulceration of other part of foot ☑
I70.238 Atherosclerosis of native arteries of right leg with ulceration of other part of lower leg ☑
I70.241 Atherosclerosis of native arteries of left leg with ulceration of thigh ☑
I70.242 Atherosclerosis of native arteries of left leg with ulceration of calf ☑
I70.243 Atherosclerosis of native arteries of left leg with ulceration of ankle ☑
I70.244 Atherosclerosis of native arteries of left leg with ulceration of heel and midfoot ☑
I70.245 Atherosclerosis of native arteries of left leg with ulceration of other part of foot ☑
I70.248 Atherosclerosis of native arteries of left leg with ulceration of other part of lower leg ☑
I70.261 Atherosclerosis of native arteries of extremities with gangrene, right leg ☑
I70.262 Atherosclerosis of native arteries of extremities with gangrene, left leg ☑
I70.263 Atherosclerosis of native arteries of extremities with gangrene, bilateral legs ☑
I70.92 Chronic total occlusion of artery of the extremities
I74.3 Embolism and thrombosis of arteries of the lower extremities
I75.021 Atheroembolism of right lower extremity ☑
I75.022 Atheroembolism of left lower extremity ☑
I75.023 Atheroembolism of bilateral lower extremities ☑
I76 Septic arterial embolism
I77.1 Stricture of artery
I77.2 Rupture of artery
I77.5 Necrosis of artery
I77.89 Other specified disorders of arteries and arterioles
I79.8 Other disorders of arteries, arterioles and capillaries in diseases classified elsewhere
I80.221 Phlebitis and thrombophlebitis of right popliteal vein ☑
I80.222 Phlebitis and thrombophlebitis of left popliteal vein ☑
I80.223 Phlebitis and thrombophlebitis of popliteal vein, bilateral ☑
I80.231 Phlebitis and thrombophlebitis of right tibial vein ☑
I80.232 Phlebitis and thrombophlebitis of left tibial vein ☑
I80.233 Phlebitis and thrombophlebitis of tibial vein, bilateral ☑
I80.291 Phlebitis and thrombophlebitis of other deep vessels of right lower extremity ☑
I80.292 Phlebitis and thrombophlebitis of other deep vessels of left lower extremity ☑
I80.293 Phlebitis and thrombophlebitis of other deep vessels of lower extremity, bilateral ☑
I82.531 Chronic embolism and thrombosis of right popliteal vein ☑
I82.532 Chronic embolism and thrombosis of left popliteal vein ☑
I82.533 Chronic embolism and thrombosis of popliteal vein, bilateral ☑
I82.541 Chronic embolism and thrombosis of right tibial vein ☑
I82.542 Chronic embolism and thrombosis of left tibial vein ☑
I82.543 Chronic embolism and thrombosis of tibial vein, bilateral ☑
I82.591 Chronic embolism and thrombosis of other specified deep vein of right lower extremity ☑
I82.592 Chronic embolism and thrombosis of other specified deep vein of left lower extremity ☑
I82.593 Chronic embolism and thrombosis of other specified deep vein of lower extremity, bilateral ☑

AMA: **35587** 2018,Jan,8; 2017,Jan,8; 2016,Jan,13; 2015,Jan,16; 2014,Jan,11

Relative Value Units/Medicare Edits

Non-Facility RVU	Work	PE	MP	Total
35587	26.21	7.35	5.95	39.51
Facility RVU	**Work**	**PE**	**MP**	**Total**
35587	26.21	7.35	5.95	39.51

	FUD	Status	MUE	Modifiers				IOM Reference
35587	90	A	1(3)	51	50	62*	80	None

* with documentation

Terms To Know

anastomosis. Surgically created connection between ducts, blood vessels, or bowel segments to allow flow from one to the other.

artery. Vessel through which oxygenated blood passes away from the heart to any part of the body.

bypass graft. Surgically created alternative blood vessel used to reroute blood flow around an area of obstruction or disease.

in situ. Located in the natural position or contained within the origin site, not spread into neighboring tissue.

thrombosis. Condition arising from the presence or formation of blood clots within a blood vessel that may cause vascular obstruction and insufficient oxygenation.

varicose vein. Abnormal, permanently distended or stretched vein.

vein. Vessel through which oxygen-depleted blood passes back to the heart.

35600

+ **35600** Harvest of upper extremity artery, 1 segment, for coronary artery bypass procedure (List separately in addition to code for primary procedure)

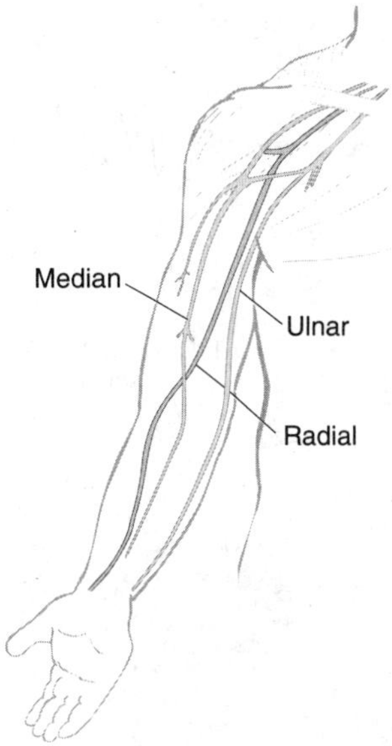

An upper extremity artery or segment is harvested for a coronary artery bypass procedure

Explanation

The physician harvests an artery from an upper extremity (arm) to use for a planned bypass procedure on a coronary artery. An incision is made over the site on the arm. Tissue is dissected to the artery. The portion of the artery to be removed is released from the surrounding structures and is tied off above and below the portion of artery to be removed. The artery is removed. The wound is closed with layered sutures. The portion of artery removed is prepared for use in a bypass graft procedure of a coronary artery (reported separately).

Coding Tips

Report 35600 in addition to 33533–33536.

ICD-10-CM Diagnostic Codes

This/these CPT code(s) are add on code(s). See the primary procedure code that this code is performed with for your ICD-10-CM code selections. Diagnostic code(s) would be the same as the actual procedure performed.

AMA: 35600 2018,Jan,8; 2017,Jan,8; 2016,Jan,13; 2015,Jan,16; 2014,Jan,11

Relative Value Units/Medicare Edits

Non-Facility RVU	Work	PE	MP	Total
35600	4.94	1.37	1.12	7.43
Facility RVU	**Work**	**PE**	**MP**	**Total**
35600	4.94	1.37	1.12	7.43

	FUD	Status	MUE	Modifiers				IOM Reference
35600	N/A	A	2(3)	N/A	N/A	62*	80	None

* with documentation

35601

35601 Bypass graft, with other than vein; common carotid-ipsilateral internal carotid

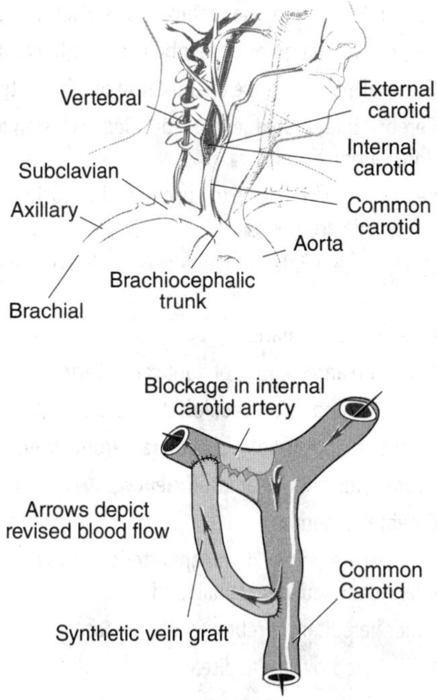

A portion of blocked internal carotid artery is bypassed

Explanation

Through an incision in the skin of the neck in front of the sternocleidomastoid muscle, the physician isolates and dissects the common carotid and internal carotid arteries, separating them from adjacent critical structures. The physician creates a bypass around the section of common carotid artery that is damaged or blocked, using a synthetic vein graft and one of two methods of repair involving the internal carotid artery on the same side of the neck. After vessel clamps have been affixed above and below the damaged area, the common carotid artery may be cut through below the damaged area and sutured to one end of the synthetic vein (end-to-end), which is sutured to the internal carotid artery beyond the affected area. In the second method, the ends of the synthetic vein are sutured into the side of the common carotid arterial wall and the internal carotid arterial wall (end-to-side). Either method results in a bypass of the damaged area. When the clamps are removed, the section of synthetic graft forms a new path through which blood can easily bypass the blocked area. The damaged or blocked carotid artery is not removed. After the graft is complete, the skin incision is repaired with layered closure.

Coding Tips

Establishing both inflow and outflow by any method is included. That portion of the operative arteriogram performed by the surgeon is also included. Angioscopy performed during therapeutic intervention should be reported in addition to the code for the primary procedure, see 35400. If a composite (combination of vein and synthetic graft) is used, report 35681 in addition to the code for the primary procedure. For open transcervical common carotid-common carotid bypass performed in addition to endovascular repair of the descending thoracic aorta, see 33891. For transposition and/or reimplantation of arteries, see 35691–35695.

ICD-10-CM Diagnostic Codes

G45.1	Carotid artery syndrome (hemispheric)
G45.8	Other transient cerebral ischemic attacks and related syndromes
G45.9	Transient cerebral ischemic attack, unspecified
I63.031	Cerebral infarction due to thrombosis of right carotid artery ☑
I63.032	Cerebral infarction due to thrombosis of left carotid artery ☑
I63.131	Cerebral infarction due to embolism of right carotid artery ☑
I63.132	Cerebral infarction due to embolism of left carotid artery ☑
I63.231	Cerebral infarction due to unspecified occlusion or stenosis of right carotid arteries ☑
I63.232	Cerebral infarction due to unspecified occlusion or stenosis of left carotid arteries ☑
I63.81	Other cerebral infarction due to occlusion or stenosis of small artery
I63.89	Other cerebral infarction
I65.21	Occlusion and stenosis of right carotid artery ☑
I65.22	Occlusion and stenosis of left carotid artery ☑
I65.23	Occlusion and stenosis of bilateral carotid arteries ☑
I67.81	Acute cerebrovascular insufficiency
I67.82	Cerebral ischemia
I67.850	Cerebral autosomal dominant arteriopathy with subcortical infarcts and leukoencephalopathy
I67.858	Other hereditary cerebrovascular disease
I67.89	Other cerebrovascular disease
I77.1	Stricture of artery
I77.2	Rupture of artery
I77.89	Other specified disorders of arteries and arterioles
S15.011A	Minor laceration of right carotid artery, initial encounter ☑
S15.012A	Minor laceration of left carotid artery, initial encounter ☑
S15.021A	Major laceration of right carotid artery, initial encounter ☑
S15.022A	Major laceration of left carotid artery, initial encounter ☑
S15.091A	Other specified injury of right carotid artery, initial encounter ☑
S15.092A	Other specified injury of left carotid artery, initial encounter ☑

AMA: 35601 2018,Jan,8; 2017,Jan,8; 2016,Jan,13; 2015,Jan,16; 2014,Jan,11

Relative Value Units/Medicare Edits

Non-Facility RVU	Work	PE	MP	Total
35601	27.09	7.23	6.16	40.48
Facility RVU	**Work**	**PE**	**MP**	**Total**
35601	27.09	7.23	6.16	40.48

	FUD	Status	MUE	Modifiers				IOM Reference
35601	90	A	1(3)	51	50	62*	80	None

* with documentation

35606

35606 Bypass graft, with other than vein; carotid-subclavian

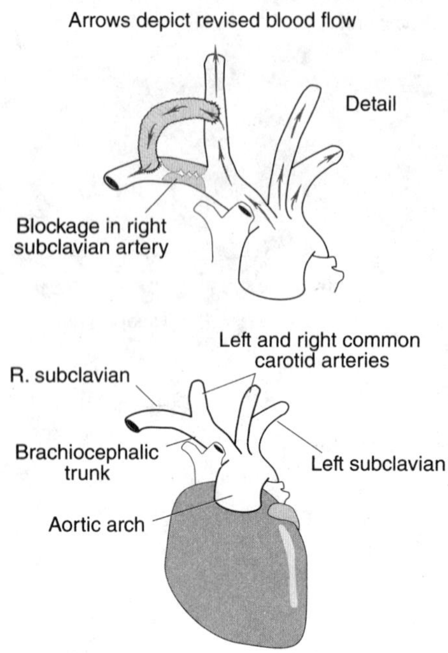

Synthetic material grafted from healthy left subclavian artery to right subclavian artery distal (beyond) to area of blockage or damage

Explanation

Through an incision in the skin at the side of the neck, the physician isolates and dissects the subclavian and carotid arteries, separating them from adjacent critical structures. To create a bypass around a section of subclavian artery that is damaged or blocked, the physician uses a synthetic vein and one of two methods of repair. After vessel clamps have been affixed above and below the damaged area, the graft is sewn to the side of the carotid artery and sewn to the side of the subclavian artery beyond the affected area (end-to-side) or sewn to the cut end of the subclavian artery after dividing it beyond the affected area (end-to-end). The damaged or blocked portion of the subclavian artery is not removed. When the clamps are removed in either case, the section of synthetic graft vein forms a new path through which blood can easily bypass the blocked area. After the graft is complete, the skin incision is repaired with a layered closure.

Coding Tips

Establishing both inflow and outflow by any method is included. That portion of the operative arteriogram performed by the surgeon is also included. Angioscopy performed during therapeutic intervention should be reported in addition to the code for the primary procedure; see 35400. If a composite (combination of vein and synthetic graft) is used, report 35681 in addition to the code for the primary procedure. For transposition and/or reimplantation of arteries, see 35691–35695. Do not report 35606 for open subclavian to carotid artery transposition performed with endovascular thoracic aneurysm repair; use 33889.

ICD-10-CM Diagnostic Codes

G45.2	Multiple and bilateral precerebral artery syndromes
G45.8	Other transient cerebral ischemic attacks and related syndromes
G45.9	Transient cerebral ischemic attack, unspecified
I63.09	Cerebral infarction due to thrombosis of other precerebral artery

I63.19	Cerebral infarction due to embolism of other precerebral artery
I63.29	Cerebral infarction due to unspecified occlusion or stenosis of other precerebral arteries
I63.81	Other cerebral infarction due to occlusion or stenosis of small artery
I63.89	Other cerebral infarction
I65.8	Occlusion and stenosis of other precerebral arteries
I67.81	Acute cerebrovascular insufficiency
I67.850	Cerebral autosomal dominant arteriopathy with subcortical infarcts and leukoencephalopathy
I67.858	Other hereditary cerebrovascular disease
I70.92	Chronic total occlusion of artery of the extremities
I74.2	Embolism and thrombosis of arteries of the upper extremities
I74.8	Embolism and thrombosis of other arteries
I75.011	Atheroembolism of right upper extremity ☑
I75.012	Atheroembolism of left upper extremity ☑
I75.013	Atheroembolism of bilateral upper extremities ☑
I77.1	Stricture of artery
I77.2	Rupture of artery
I77.5	Necrosis of artery
I77.89	Other specified disorders of arteries and arterioles
S15.8XXA	Injury of other specified blood vessels at neck level, initial encounter
S25.111A	Minor laceration of right innominate or subclavian artery, initial encounter ☑
S25.112A	Minor laceration of left innominate or subclavian artery, initial encounter ☑
S25.121A	Major laceration of right innominate or subclavian artery, initial encounter ☑
S25.122A	Major laceration of left innominate or subclavian artery, initial encounter ☑
S25.191A	Other specified injury of right innominate or subclavian artery, initial encounter ☑
S25.192A	Other specified injury of left innominate or subclavian artery, initial encounter ☑

AMA: **35606** 1997,Nov,1

Relative Value Units/Medicare Edits

Non-Facility RVU	Work	PE	MP	Total
35606	22.46	6.41	5.14	34.01
Facility RVU	**Work**	**PE**	**MP**	**Total**
35606	22.46	6.41	5.14	34.01

	FUD	Status	MUE	Modifiers				IOM Reference
35606	90	A	1(3)	51	50	62*	80	None

* with documentation

35612

35612 Bypass graft, with other than vein; subclavian-subclavian

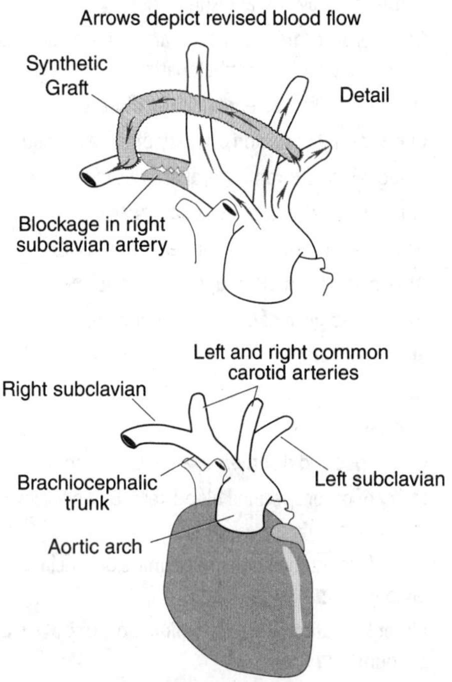

Synthetic material grafted from healthy left subclavian artery to right subclavian artery distal (beyond) to area of blockage or damage

Explanation

Through incisions in the skin at the base of the neck, the physician isolates and dissects the subclavian arteries, separating them from adjacent critical structures. The physician creates a bypass around a section of subclavian artery that is damaged or blocked, using a synthetic vein and one of two methods of repair. Once vessel clamps have been affixed above and below the defect, the ends of the synthetic vein graft are sutured into the sides of the walls of the two subclavian arteries, resulting in a bypass of the damaged area. In the second method, the subclavian artery may be cut through beyond the damaged area and sutured to one end of a synthetic vein, which is sutured to the subclavian artery on the opposite side of the neck. In either case, the blocked or damaged portion of the artery is not removed. When the clamps are removed, the section of synthetic vein graft forms a new path through which blood can easily bypass the blocked area. After the graft is complete, the skin incisions are repaired with a layered closure.

Coding Tips

Establishing both inflow and outflow by any method is included. That portion of the operative arteriogram performed by the surgeon is also included. Angioscopy performed during therapeutic intervention should be reported in addition to the code for the primary procedure, see 35400. For transposition and/or reimplantation of arteries, see 35691–35695.

ICD-10-CM Diagnostic Codes

G45.9	Transient cerebral ischemic attack, unspecified
I63.09	Cerebral infarction due to thrombosis of other precerebral artery
I63.19	Cerebral infarction due to embolism of other precerebral artery
I63.29	Cerebral infarction due to unspecified occlusion or stenosis of other precerebral arteries

I63.81	Other cerebral infarction due to occlusion or stenosis of small artery
I63.89	Other cerebral infarction
I65.8	Occlusion and stenosis of other precerebral arteries
I67.81	Acute cerebrovascular insufficiency
I67.850	Cerebral autosomal dominant arteriopathy with subcortical infarcts and leukoencephalopathy
I67.858	Other hereditary cerebrovascular disease
I70.92	Chronic total occlusion of artery of the extremities
I74.2	Embolism and thrombosis of arteries of the upper extremities
I74.8	Embolism and thrombosis of other arteries
I75.011	Atheroembolism of right upper extremity ☑
I75.012	Atheroembolism of left upper extremity ☑
I75.013	Atheroembolism of bilateral upper extremities ☑
I77.1	Stricture of artery
I77.2	Rupture of artery
I77.5	Necrosis of artery
I77.89	Other specified disorders of arteries and arterioles
S15.8XXA	Injury of other specified blood vessels at neck level, initial encounter
S25.111A	Minor laceration of right innominate or subclavian artery, initial encounter ☑
S25.112A	Minor laceration of left innominate or subclavian artery, initial encounter ☑
S25.121A	Major laceration of right innominate or subclavian artery, initial encounter ☑
S25.122A	Major laceration of left innominate or subclavian artery, initial encounter ☑
S25.191A	Other specified injury of right innominate or subclavian artery, initial encounter ☑
S25.192A	Other specified injury of left innominate or subclavian artery, initial encounter ☑

AMA: 35612 1997,Nov,1

Relative Value Units/Medicare Edits

Non-Facility RVU	Work	PE	MP	Total
35612	20.35	5.08	4.69	30.12
Facility RVU	**Work**	**PE**	**MP**	**Total**
35612	20.35	5.08	4.69	30.12

	FUD	Status	MUE	Modifiers				IOM Reference
35612	90	A	1(3)	51	50	62*	80	None

* with documentation

Terms To Know

angioscopy. Visualization of capillary blood vessels with a microscope, or the inside of a blood vessel with a fiberoptic-equipped catheter.

atherosclerosis. Buildup of yellowish plaques composed of cholesterol and lipoid material within the arteries.

infarction. Area of necrosis in tissue, due to ischemia from lack of circulation, usually from a thrombus or an embolus.

35616

35616 Bypass graft, with other than vein; subclavian-axillary

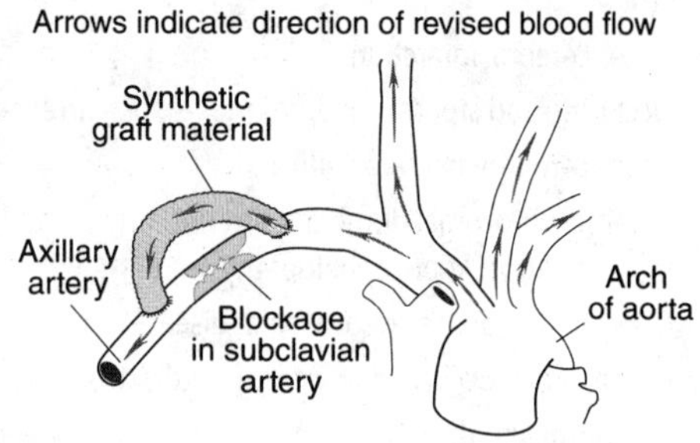

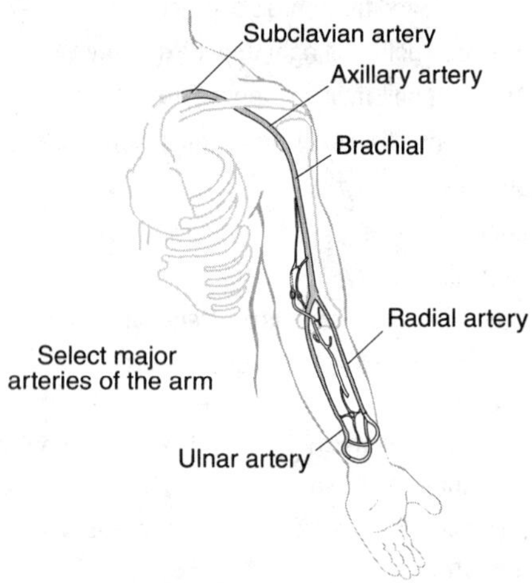

Explanation

Through an incision in the skin at the base of the neck and axilla, the physician isolates and dissects the subclavian and axillary arteries, separating them from adjacent critical structures. The physician creates a bypass around a section of subclavian artery that is damaged or blocked, using a synthetic vein and one of two methods of repair. Once vessel clamps have been affixed above and below the defect, the ends of the synthetic vein are sutured into the sides of the subclavian and axillary arterial walls resulting in a bypass of the damaged area (end-to-side). In the second method, the subclavian artery may be cut through before the damaged area and sutured to one end of a synthetic vein, which is then sutured to the axillary artery (end-to-end). The blocked or damaged portion of the subclavian artery is not removed. When the clamps are removed, the section of synthetic vein graft forms a new path through which blood can easily bypass the blocked area. After the graft is complete, the skin incisions are repaired with a layered closure.

Coding Tips

Establishing both inflow and outflow by any method is included. That portion of the operative arteriogram performed by the surgeon is also included. Angioscopy performed during therapeutic intervention should be reported in addition to the code for the primary procedure; see 35400. For transposition and/or reimplantation of arteries, see 35691–35695.

ICD-10-CM Diagnostic Codes

G45.8	Other transient cerebral ischemic attacks and related syndromes
G45.9	Transient cerebral ischemic attack, unspecified
I63.09	Cerebral infarction due to thrombosis of other precerebral artery
I63.19	Cerebral infarction due to embolism of other precerebral artery

I63.29 Cerebral infarction due to unspecified occlusion or stenosis of other precerebral arteries
I63.81 Other cerebral infarction due to occlusion or stenosis of small artery
I63.89 Other cerebral infarction
I65.8 Occlusion and stenosis of other precerebral arteries
I67.850 Cerebral autosomal dominant arteriopathy with subcortical infarcts and leukoencephalopathy
I67.858 Other hereditary cerebrovascular disease
I70.92 Chronic total occlusion of artery of the extremities
I72.1 Aneurysm of artery of upper extremity
I74.2 Embolism and thrombosis of arteries of the upper extremities
I74.8 Embolism and thrombosis of other arteries
I75.011 Atheroembolism of right upper extremity ☑
I75.012 Atheroembolism of left upper extremity ☑
I75.013 Atheroembolism of bilateral upper extremities ☑
I77.1 Stricture of artery
I77.2 Rupture of artery
I77.5 Necrosis of artery
I77.89 Other specified disorders of arteries and arterioles
S15.8XXA Injury of other specified blood vessels at neck level, initial encounter
S25.111A Minor laceration of right innominate or subclavian artery, initial encounter ☑
S25.112A Minor laceration of left innominate or subclavian artery, initial encounter ☑
S25.121A Major laceration of right innominate or subclavian artery, initial encounter ☑
S25.122A Major laceration of left innominate or subclavian artery, initial encounter ☑
S25.191A Other specified injury of right innominate or subclavian artery, initial encounter ☑
S25.192A Other specified injury of left innominate or subclavian artery, initial encounter ☑

AMA: **35616** 1997,Nov,1

Relative Value Units/Medicare Edits

Non-Facility RVU	Work	PE	MP	Total
35616	21.82	4.96	5.05	31.83
Facility RVU	**Work**	**PE**	**MP**	**Total**
35616	21.82	4.96	5.05	31.83

	FUD	Status	MUE	Modifiers				IOM Reference
35616	90	A	1(3)	51	50	62*	80	None

* with documentation

Terms To Know

angioscopy. Visualization of capillary blood vessels with a microscope, or the inside of a blood vessel with a fiberoptic-equipped catheter.

arteriogram. Radiograph of arteries.

atherosclerosis. Buildup of yellowish plaques composed of cholesterol and lipoid material within the arteries.

35621

35621 Bypass graft, with other than vein; axillary-femoral

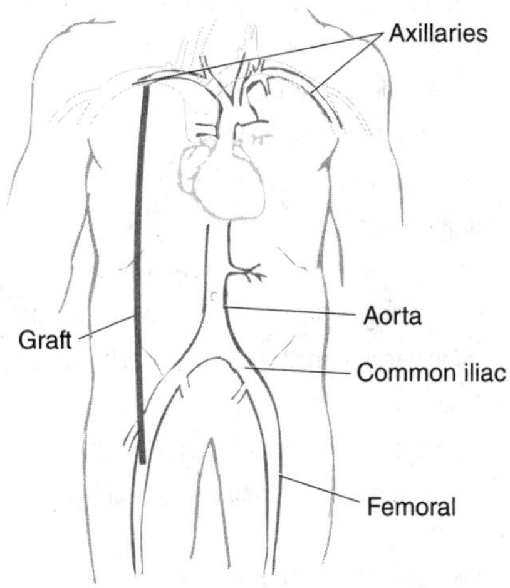

A graft other than vein is used in a bypass procedure from the axillary artery to the femoral artery

Explanation

The physician makes incisions in the skin of the axilla and upper thigh. The artery is isolated and dissected from adjacent critical structures. The physician creates a bypass around a section of artery that is damaged or blocked using a synthetic vein and one of two repair methods. Once vessel clamps have been affixed above and below the areas of anastomosis, the synthetic vein is sutured to an incision in the side of the axillary artery and passed through a subcutaneous tunnel on the side of the body and to the upper thigh. The synthetic vein is sutured to the femoral artery (common, deep, or superficial) in an end-to-side or end-to-end fashion. The blocked or damaged portion of the artery is not removed. When the clamps are removed, the section of synthetic vein graft forms a new path through which blood can easily bypass the blocked area. After the graft is complete, the skin incisions are repaired with layered closures.

Coding Tips

Establishing both inflow and outflow by any method is included. That portion of the operative arteriogram performed by the surgeon is also included. Angioscopy performed during therapeutic intervention should be reported in addition to the code for the primary procedure; see 35400.

ICD-10-CM Diagnostic Codes

A52.02 Syphilitic aortitis
I70.0 Atherosclerosis of aorta
I70.8 Atherosclerosis of other arteries
I70.92 Chronic total occlusion of artery of the extremities
I71.01 Dissection of thoracic aorta
I71.02 Dissection of abdominal aorta
I71.03 Dissection of thoracoabdominal aorta
I74.01 Saddle embolus of abdominal aorta
I74.09 Other arterial embolism and thrombosis of abdominal aorta
I74.19 Embolism and thrombosis of other parts of aorta
I74.5 Embolism and thrombosis of iliac artery
I76 Septic arterial embolism
I77.1 Stricture of artery

I77.3	Arterial fibromuscular dysplasia
I77.5	Necrosis of artery
I77.72	Dissection of iliac artery
I77.89	Other specified disorders of arteries and arterioles
K55.1	Chronic vascular disorders of intestine
K55.8	Other vascular disorders of intestine
Q25.21	Interruption of aortic arch
Q25.41	Absence and aplasia of aorta
Q25.46	Tortuous aortic arch
Q25.47	Right aortic arch
Q25.48	Anomalous origin of subclavian artery
Q25.8	Other congenital malformations of other great arteries
S25.01XA	Minor laceration of thoracic aorta, initial encounter
S25.02XA	Major laceration of thoracic aorta, initial encounter
S25.09XA	Other specified injury of thoracic aorta, initial encounter
S25.811A	Laceration of other blood vessels of thorax, right side, initial encounter ☑
S25.812A	Laceration of other blood vessels of thorax, left side, initial encounter ☑
S25.891A	Other specified injury of other blood vessels of thorax, right side, initial encounter ☑
S25.892A	Other specified injury of other blood vessels of thorax, left side, initial encounter ☑
S35.01XA	Minor laceration of abdominal aorta, initial encounter
S35.02XA	Major laceration of abdominal aorta, initial encounter
S35.09XA	Other injury of abdominal aorta, initial encounter
S35.511A	Injury of right iliac artery, initial encounter ☑
S35.512A	Injury of left iliac artery, initial encounter ☑
S35.59XA	Injury of other iliac blood vessels, initial encounter
S35.8X1A	Laceration of other blood vessels at abdomen, lower back and pelvis level, initial encounter
S35.8X8A	Other specified injury of other blood vessels at abdomen, lower back and pelvis level, initial encounter

AMA: 35621 2018,Jan,8; 2017,Jan,8; 2016,Jan,13; 2015,Jan,16; 2014,Jan,11

Relative Value Units/Medicare Edits

Non-Facility RVU	Work	PE	MP	Total
35621	21.03	5.91	4.81	31.75
Facility RVU	**Work**	**PE**	**MP**	**Total**
35621	21.03	5.91	4.81	31.75

	FUD	Status	MUE	Modifiers				IOM Reference
35621	90	A	1(3)	51	50	62*	80	None

* with documentation

Terms To Know

embolism. Obstruction of a blood vessel resulting from a clot or foreign substance.

thrombosis. Condition arising from the presence or formation of blood clots within a blood vessel that may cause vascular obstruction and insufficient oxygenation.

35623

35623 Bypass graft, with other than vein; axillary-popliteal or -tibial

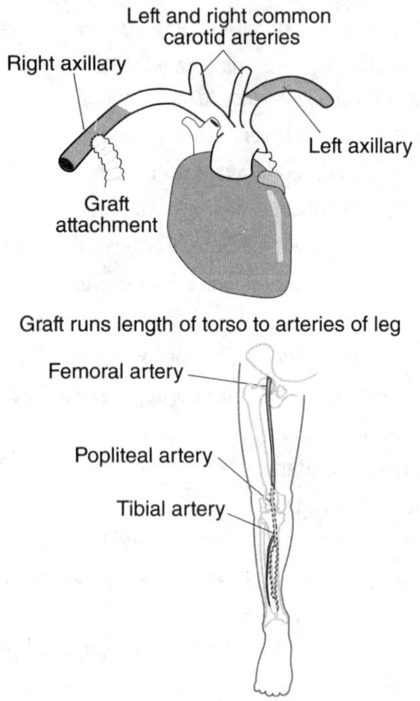

A bypass graft other than vein (synthetic) is surgically attached from the axillary artery to the popliteal or tibial artery of the leg

Explanation

The physician makes incisions in the skin of the axilla and behind the knee or in the lower leg. The artery is isolated and dissected from adjacent critical structures. The physician creates a bypass around a section of artery that is damaged or blocked using a synthetic vein and one of two repair methods. Once vessel clamps have been affixed above and below the areas of anastomosis, the synthetic vein is sutured to an incision in the side of the axillary artery and passed through a subcutaneous tunnel on the side of the body and behind the knee or upper thigh. The synthetic vein is sutured to the popliteal or tibial artery in an end-to-side or end-to-end fashion. The blocked or damaged portion of the artery is not removed. When the clamps are removed, the section of synthetic vein graft forms a new path through which blood can easily bypass the blocked area. After the graft is complete, the skin incisions are repaired with layered closures.

Coding Tips

Establishing both inflow and outflow by any method is included. That portion of the operative arteriogram performed by the surgeon is also included. Angioscopy performed during therapeutic intervention should be reported in addition to the code for the primary procedure; see 35400.

ICD-10-CM Diagnostic Codes

A52.02	Syphilitic aortitis
I70.0	Atherosclerosis of aorta
I70.8	Atherosclerosis of other arteries
I70.92	Chronic total occlusion of artery of the extremities
I71.01	Dissection of thoracic aorta
I71.02	Dissection of abdominal aorta
I71.03	Dissection of thoracoabdominal aorta

I74.01 Saddle embolus of abdominal aorta
I74.09 Other arterial embolism and thrombosis of abdominal aorta
I74.19 Embolism and thrombosis of other parts of aorta
I74.5 Embolism and thrombosis of iliac artery
I76 Septic arterial embolism
I77.1 Stricture of artery
I77.3 Arterial fibromuscular dysplasia
I77.5 Necrosis of artery
I77.72 Dissection of iliac artery
I77.89 Other specified disorders of arteries and arterioles
K55.8 Other vascular disorders of intestine
Q25.41 Absence and aplasia of aorta
Q25.46 Tortuous aortic arch
Q25.47 Right aortic arch
Q25.48 Anomalous origin of subclavian artery
Q25.8 Other congenital malformations of other great arteries
S25.01XA Minor laceration of thoracic aorta, initial encounter
S25.02XA Major laceration of thoracic aorta, initial encounter
S25.09XA Other specified injury of thoracic aorta, initial encounter
S25.811A Laceration of other blood vessels of thorax, right side, initial encounter ☑
S25.812A Laceration of other blood vessels of thorax, left side, initial encounter ☑
S25.891A Other specified injury of other blood vessels of thorax, right side, initial encounter ☑
S25.892A Other specified injury of other blood vessels of thorax, left side, initial encounter ☑
S35.01XA Minor laceration of abdominal aorta, initial encounter
S35.02XA Major laceration of abdominal aorta, initial encounter
S35.09XA Other injury of abdominal aorta, initial encounter
S35.511A Injury of right iliac artery, initial encounter ☑
S35.512A Injury of left iliac artery, initial encounter ☑
S35.59XA Injury of other iliac blood vessels, initial encounter
S35.8X1A Laceration of other blood vessels at abdomen, lower back and pelvis level, initial encounter
S35.8X8A Other specified injury of other blood vessels at abdomen, lower back and pelvis level, initial encounter

AMA: 35623 2012,Apr,3-9

Relative Value Units/Medicare Edits

Non-Facility RVU	Work	PE	MP	Total
35623	25.92	6.01	5.99	37.92
Facility RVU	**Work**	**PE**	**MP**	**Total**
35623	25.92	6.01	5.99	37.92

	FUD	Status	MUE	Modifiers				IOM Reference
35623	90	A	1(3)	51	50	62*	80	None

* with documentation

35626

35626 Bypass graft, with other than vein; aortosubclavian, aortoinnominate, or aortocarotid

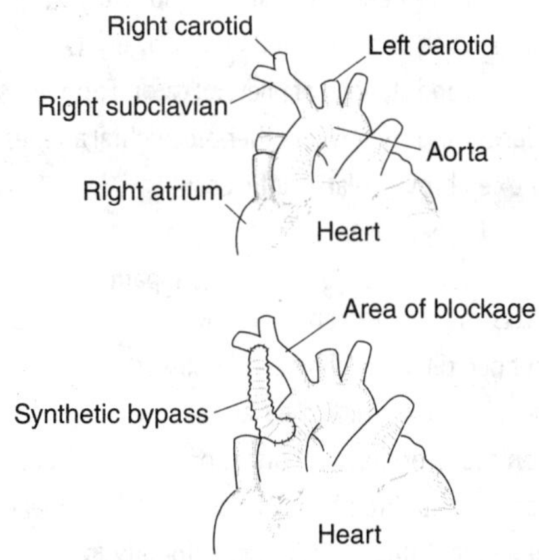

A graft other than vein (e.g., synthetic) is employed to bypass a blockage in the great arteries

Explanation

The physician exposes the aorta by median sternotomy and exposes the aortocarotid, aortoinnominate, or aortosubclavian artery, extending this incision in the appropriate direction. The physician clamps the middle part of the right anterolateral aspect of the anterior ascending aorta with a J clamp. The physician makes a 2 cm to 3 cm longitudinal incision in the clamped portion of the aorta and sews the arterial or synthetic graft to the aortic incision. The physician clamps the graft and releases the aortic clamp to assess the anastomosis for leaks. The physician clamps the distal end of the diseased artery. The physician makes a longitudinal incision in the diseased artery, distal to the blockage, and sews the graft to the arterial incision. The physician may also use graft material to enlarge the arterial lumen (patch graft). The physician removes the clamp from the graft. The physician may perform arteriography or use a Doppler probe to establish patency of the graft. The physician closes the sternotomy or thoracotomy, leaving a chest tube in place.

Coding Tips

Establishing both inflow and outflow by any method is included. That portion of the operative arteriogram performed by the surgeon is also included. Angioscopy performed during therapeutic intervention should be reported in addition to the code for the primary procedure; see 35400. For transposition and/or reimplantation of arteries, see 35691-35695.

ICD-10-CM Diagnostic Codes

G45.1 Carotid artery syndrome (hemispheric)
G45.2 Multiple and bilateral precerebral artery syndromes
G45.8 Other transient cerebral ischemic attacks and related syndromes
I63.031 Cerebral infarction due to thrombosis of right carotid artery ☑
I63.032 Cerebral infarction due to thrombosis of left carotid artery ☑
I63.09 Cerebral infarction due to thrombosis of other precerebral artery
I63.131 Cerebral infarction due to embolism of right carotid artery ☑
I63.132 Cerebral infarction due to embolism of left carotid artery ☑
I63.19 Cerebral infarction due to embolism of other precerebral artery
I63.231 Cerebral infarction due to unspecified occlusion or stenosis of right carotid arteries ☑
I63.232 Cerebral infarction due to unspecified occlusion or stenosis of left carotid arteries ☑

 ● New ▲ Revised + Add On AMA: CPT Assist [Resequenced] ☑ Laterality

I63.29	Cerebral infarction due to unspecified occlusion or stenosis of other precerebral arteries
I63.81	Other cerebral infarction due to occlusion or stenosis of small artery
I63.89	Other cerebral infarction
I65.21	Occlusion and stenosis of right carotid artery ☑
I65.22	Occlusion and stenosis of left carotid artery ☑
I65.23	Occlusion and stenosis of bilateral carotid arteries ☑
I65.8	Occlusion and stenosis of other precerebral arteries
I67.81	Acute cerebrovascular insufficiency
I67.82	Cerebral ischemia
I67.850	Cerebral autosomal dominant arteriopathy with subcortical infarcts and leukoencephalopathy
I67.858	Other hereditary cerebrovascular disease
I67.89	Other cerebrovascular disease
I70.92	Chronic total occlusion of artery of the extremities
I74.2	Embolism and thrombosis of arteries of the upper extremities
I75.011	Atheroembolism of right upper extremity ☑
I75.012	Atheroembolism of left upper extremity ☑
I75.013	Atheroembolism of bilateral upper extremities ☑
I77.1	Stricture of artery
I77.2	Rupture of artery
I77.71	Dissection of carotid artery
I77.76	Dissection of artery of upper extremity
I77.77	Dissection of artery of lower extremity
I77.79	Dissection of other specified artery
I77.89	Other specified disorders of arteries and arterioles
Q28.1	Other malformations of precerebral vessels
Q28.8	Other specified congenital malformations of circulatory system
S15.011A	Minor laceration of right carotid artery, initial encounter ☑
S15.012A	Minor laceration of left carotid artery, initial encounter ☑
S15.021A	Major laceration of right carotid artery, initial encounter ☑
S15.022A	Major laceration of left carotid artery, initial encounter ☑
S15.091A	Other specified injury of right carotid artery, initial encounter ☑
S15.092A	Other specified injury of left carotid artery, initial encounter ☑
S15.8XXA	Injury of other specified blood vessels at neck level, initial encounter
S25.111A	Minor laceration of right innominate or subclavian artery, initial encounter ☑
S25.112A	Minor laceration of left innominate or subclavian artery, initial encounter ☑
S25.121A	Major laceration of right innominate or subclavian artery, initial encounter ☑
S25.122A	Major laceration of left innominate or subclavian artery, initial encounter ☑
S25.191A	Other specified injury of right innominate or subclavian artery, initial encounter ☑
S25.192A	Other specified injury of left innominate or subclavian artery, initial encounter ☑

AMA: **35626** 1997,Nov,1

Relative Value Units/Medicare Edits

Non-Facility RVU	Work	PE	MP	Total
35626	29.14	10.1	6.77	46.01
Facility RVU	**Work**	**PE**	**MP**	**Total**
35626	29.14	10.1	6.77	46.01

	FUD	Status	MUE	Modifiers				IOM Reference
35626	90	A	3(3)	51	50	62*	80	None

* with documentation

Terms To Know

anastomosis. Surgically created connection between ducts, blood vessels, or bowel segments to allow flow from one to the other.

aneurysm. Circumscribed dilation or outpouching of an artery wall, often containing blood clots and connecting directly with the lumen of the artery.

atherosclerosis. Buildup of yellowish plaques composed of cholesterol and lipoid material within the arteries.

stenosis. Narrowing or constriction of a passage.

thoracotomy. Surgical procedure for opening the chest wall in order to access the lungs, esophagus, trachea, aorta, heart, and diaphragm.

35631

35631 Bypass graft, with other than vein; aortoceliac, aortomesenteric, aortorenal

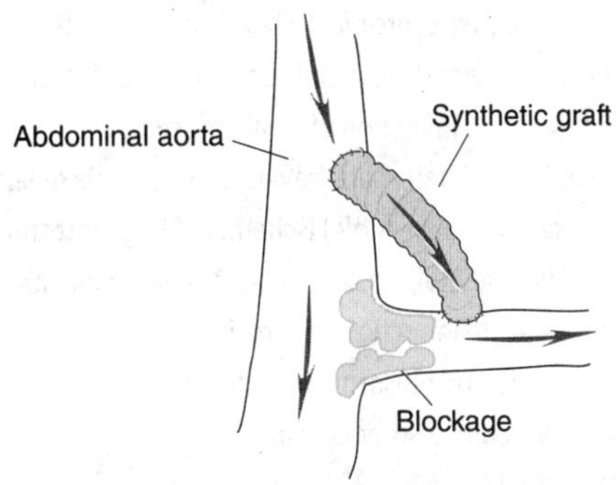

A bypass graft of material other than vein is surgically installed from the aorta to the celiac, mesenteric, or renal arteries. The graft is typically placed in an end-to-side fashion on both the aorta and the recipient vessel downstream from the blockage

Explanation

The physician exposes the involved aortomesenteric, aortoceliac, or aortorenal artery using an upper midline abdominal incision, retracting and dissecting past large and small bowel. The distal thoracic aorta is exposed, heparin is administered for anticoagulation, and the aorta is clamped both proximal and distal to the celiac axis origin. An elliptical disk of aortic wall is cut out from the anterior surface of the aorta. The involved vessel (aortomesenteric, aortoceliac, or aortorenal artery) is exposed and divided proximal to the occlusion, closing off the proximal stump with suture. A synthetic or arterial graft is sewn from the clamped aorta to the undiseased distal artery. Graft material may be utilized to enlarge the arterial lumen (patch graft). The physician may perform arteriography or use a Doppler probe to establish patency of the graft. The abdominal wound is closed, leaving drains in place.

Coding Tips

Establishing both inflow and outflow by any method is included. That portion of the operative arteriogram performed by the surgeon is also included. Angioscopy performed during therapeutic intervention should be reported in addition to the code for the primary procedure, see 35400.

ICD-10-CM Diagnostic Codes

I15.0 Renovascular hypertension
I16.0 Hypertensive urgency
I16.1 Hypertensive emergency
I70.1 Atherosclerosis of renal artery
I75.81 Atheroembolism of kidney
I75.89 Atheroembolism of other site
I77.1 Stricture of artery
I77.3 Arterial fibromuscular dysplasia
I77.4 Celiac artery compression syndrome
I77.5 Necrosis of artery
I77.73 Dissection of renal artery
I77.79 Dissection of other specified artery
K55.011 Focal (segmental) acute (reversible) ischemia of small intestine
K55.012 Diffuse acute (reversible) ischemia of small intestine
K55.021 Focal (segmental) acute infarction of small intestine
K55.022 Diffuse acute infarction of small intestine
K55.031 Focal (segmental) acute (reversible) ischemia of large intestine
K55.032 Diffuse acute (reversible) ischemia of large intestine
K55.041 Focal (segmental) acute infarction of large intestine
K55.042 Diffuse acute infarction of large intestine
K55.1 Chronic vascular disorders of intestine
K55.8 Other vascular disorders of intestine
N26.2 Page kidney
N28.0 Ischemia and infarction of kidney
Q27.1 Congenital renal artery stenosis
Q27.2 Other congenital malformations of renal artery
Q27.34 Arteriovenous malformation of renal vessel
S35.212A Major laceration of celiac artery, initial encounter
S35.218A Other injury of celiac artery, initial encounter
S35.222A Major laceration of superior mesenteric artery, initial encounter
S35.228A Other injury of superior mesenteric artery, initial encounter
S35.232A Major laceration of inferior mesenteric artery, initial encounter
S35.238A Other injury of inferior mesenteric artery, initial encounter
S35.292A Major laceration of branches of celiac and mesenteric artery, initial encounter
S35.298A Other injury of branches of celiac and mesenteric artery, initial encounter
S35.411A Laceration of right renal artery, initial encounter ☑
S35.412A Laceration of left renal artery, initial encounter ☑
S35.491A Other specified injury of right renal artery, initial encounter ☑
S35.492A Other specified injury of left renal artery, initial encounter ☑
S35.8X1A Laceration of other blood vessels at abdomen, lower back and pelvis level, initial encounter
T81.710A Complication of mesenteric artery following a procedure, not elsewhere classified, initial encounter
T81.711A Complication of renal artery following a procedure, not elsewhere classified, initial encounter

AMA: 35631 1997,Nov,1

Relative Value Units/Medicare Edits

Non-Facility RVU	Work	PE	MP	Total
35631	36.03	9.36	8.33	53.72
Facility RVU	**Work**	**PE**	**MP**	**Total**
35631	36.03	9.36	8.33	53.72

	FUD	Status	MUE	Modifiers				IOM Reference
35631	90	A	4(3)	51	50	62*	80	None

* with documentation

 ● New ▲ Revised + Add On AMA: CPT Assist [Resequenced] ☑ Laterality

35632-35634

35632 Bypass graft, with other than vein; ilio-celiac
35633 ilio-mesenteric
35634 iliorenal

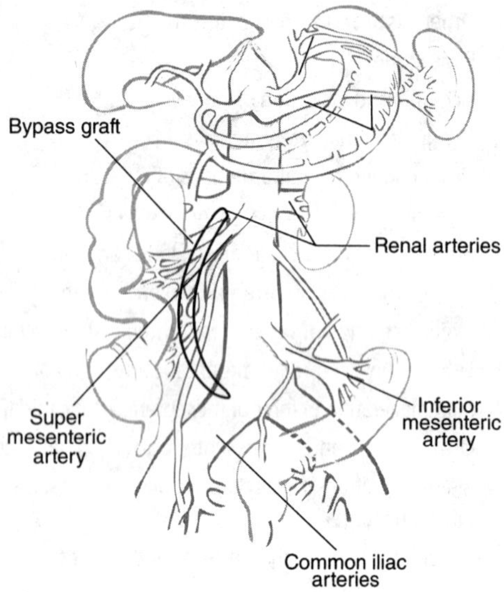

Bypass graft of a material other than vein is placed from the iliac artery to the celiac, mesenteric, or renal arteries

Explanation

The physician performs ilio-celiac (35632), ilio-mesenteric (35633), or iliorenal (35634) bypass using a synthetic graft. Through a midline abdominal incision, the physician retracts the intestines and exposes the common iliac artery and the involved vessel (celiac, mesenteric, or renal artery). The common iliac artery is clamped proximally and distally. The physician makes an oval incision on the anterolateral aspect of the common iliac artery, temporarily releases the distal clamp, and administers heparin for anticoagulation. A synthetic graft is attached to the common iliac artery at the site of the arteriotomy and sutured in place. An end-to-end anastomosis of the synthetic graft to the disease-free portion of the celiac, mesenteric, or renal artery is created. The physician may perform arteriography or Doppler to establish patency of the graft. The physician closes the abdominal wound, leaving drains in place.

Coding Tips

Do not report 35632 or 35633 with 35221, 35251, 35281, 35531, or 35631. Do not report 35634 with 35221, 35251, 35281, 35560, 35536, or 35631. Angioscopy performed during therapeutic intervention should be reported in addition to the code for the primary procedure, see 35400.

ICD-10-CM Diagnostic Codes

I15.0	Renovascular hypertension
I15.1	Hypertension secondary to other renal disorders
I70.1	Atherosclerosis of renal artery
I70.8	Atherosclerosis of other arteries
I74.5	Embolism and thrombosis of iliac artery
I75.81	Atheroembolism of kidney
I75.89	Atheroembolism of other site
I77.1	Stricture of artery
I77.3	Arterial fibromuscular dysplasia
I77.4	Celiac artery compression syndrome
I77.5	Necrosis of artery
I77.72	Dissection of iliac artery
I77.73	Dissection of renal artery
I77.79	Dissection of other specified artery
I77.89	Other specified disorders of arteries and arterioles
K55.011	Focal (segmental) acute (reversible) ischemia of small intestine
K55.012	Diffuse acute (reversible) ischemia of small intestine
K55.021	Focal (segmental) acute infarction of small intestine
K55.022	Diffuse acute infarction of small intestine
K55.031	Focal (segmental) acute (reversible) ischemia of large intestine
K55.032	Diffuse acute (reversible) ischemia of large intestine
K55.041	Focal (segmental) acute infarction of large intestine
K55.042	Diffuse acute infarction of large intestine
K55.1	Chronic vascular disorders of intestine
K55.8	Other vascular disorders of intestine
N26.2	Page kidney
N28.0	Ischemia and infarction of kidney
Q27.1	Congenital renal artery stenosis
S35.211A	Minor laceration of celiac artery, initial encounter
S35.212A	Major laceration of celiac artery, initial encounter
S35.218A	Other injury of celiac artery, initial encounter
S35.221A	Minor laceration of superior mesenteric artery, initial encounter
S35.222A	Major laceration of superior mesenteric artery, initial encounter
S35.228A	Other injury of superior mesenteric artery, initial encounter
S35.231A	Minor laceration of inferior mesenteric artery, initial encounter
S35.232A	Major laceration of inferior mesenteric artery, initial encounter
S35.238A	Other injury of inferior mesenteric artery, initial encounter
S35.291A	Minor laceration of branches of celiac and mesenteric artery, initial encounter
S35.292A	Major laceration of branches of celiac and mesenteric artery, initial encounter
S35.298A	Other injury of branches of celiac and mesenteric artery, initial encounter
S35.411A	Laceration of right renal artery, initial encounter ☑
S35.412A	Laceration of left renal artery, initial encounter ☑
S35.491A	Other specified injury of right renal artery, initial encounter ☑
S35.492A	Other specified injury of left renal artery, initial encounter ☑
S35.8X1A	Laceration of other blood vessels at abdomen, lower back and pelvis level, initial encounter
S35.8X8A	Other specified injury of other blood vessels at abdomen, lower back and pelvis level, initial encounter
T81.710A	Complication of mesenteric artery following a procedure, not elsewhere classified, initial encounter

Relative Value Units/Medicare Edits

Non-Facility RVU	Work	PE	MP	Total
35632	36.13	7.7	8.38	52.21
35633	39.11	9.64	9.06	57.81
35634	35.33	7.58	8.18	51.09
Facility RVU	**Work**	**PE**	**MP**	**Total**
35632	36.13	7.7	8.38	52.21
35633	39.11	9.64	9.06	57.81
35634	35.33	7.58	8.18	51.09

	FUD	Status	MUE	Modifiers				IOM Reference
35632	90	A	1(3)	51	50	62*	80	None
35633	90	A	1(3)	51	50	62*	80	
35634	90	A	1(3)	51	50	62*	80	

* with documentation

Terms To Know

bypass graft. Surgically created alternative blood vessel used to reroute blood flow around an area of obstruction or disease.

doppler. Ultrasonography used to augment two-dimensional images by registering velocity. When emitted sound waves reflect back off a moving object, the frequency of the reflected sound waves varies in relation to the speed of the moving object and may be used in many different procedures.

infarction. Area of necrosis in tissue, due to ischemia from lack of circulation, usually from a thrombus or an embolus.

ischemia. Deficiency in blood supply causing tissues to be deprived of oxygen, resulting from trauma, mechanical or functional constriction of blood vessels, or a physical obstruction.

necrosis. Death of cells or tissue within a living organ or structure.

35636

35636 Bypass graft, with other than vein; splenorenal (splenic to renal arterial anastomosis)

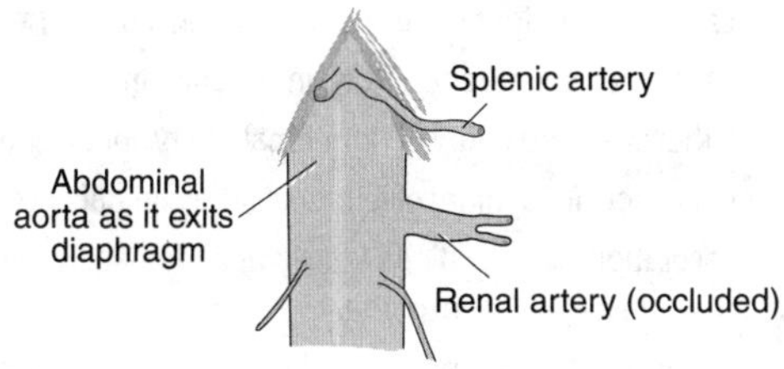

This procedure serves to bypass a diseased or occluded renal artery. The spleen remains perfused by a more distal splenic artery

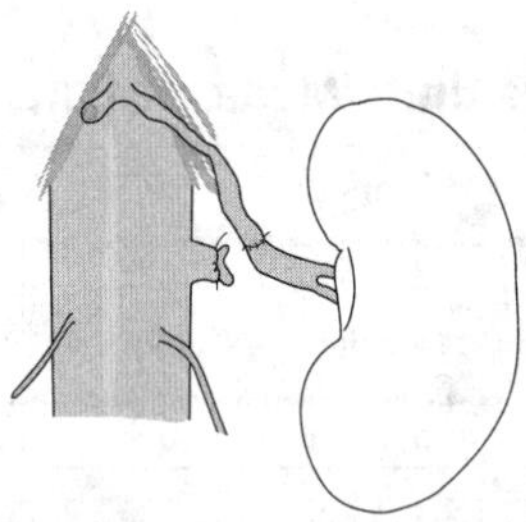

Renal artery is ligated and the splenic artery is anastomosed to remnant renal artery. This procedure is performed on the left kidney

Explanation

The physician performs a bilateral subcostal incision from the right midrectus position extending into the left flank, and dissects past bowel and pancreas to expose the splenic artery. The splenic artery is exposed by careful dissection. The left renal artery is exposed by dissecting through the posterior parietal peritoneum and partially clamped. An ellipse of renal artery is excised at its upper border. An end-to-side anastomosis of synthetic or arterial graft material from the splenic artery to the renal artery is performed. The clamps are removed and the anastomotic sites are assessed for leaks. The physician may perform Doppler studies or arteriography to establish patency of the graft. The abdominal wound is closed, leaving drains in place.

Coding Tips

Establishing both inflow and outflow by any method is included. That portion of the operative arteriogram performed by the surgeon is also included. Angioscopy performed during therapeutic intervention should be reported in addition to the code for the primary procedure; see 35400.

ICD-10-CM Diagnostic Codes

I15.0	Renovascular hypertension
I70.1	Atherosclerosis of renal artery
I73.9	Peripheral vascular disease, unspecified
I74.8	Embolism and thrombosis of other arteries
I75.81	Atheroembolism of kidney
I76	Septic arterial embolism
I77.1	Stricture of artery
I77.3	Arterial fibromuscular dysplasia
I77.5	Necrosis of artery
I77.73	Dissection of renal artery
I77.89	Other specified disorders of arteries and arterioles

N26.2	Page kidney
N28.0	Ischemia and infarction of kidney
Q27.1	Congenital renal artery stenosis
Q27.2	Other congenital malformations of renal artery
Q27.34	Arteriovenous malformation of renal vessel
S35.411A	Laceration of right renal artery, initial encounter ☑
S35.412A	Laceration of left renal artery, initial encounter ☑
S35.491A	Other specified injury of right renal artery, initial encounter ☑
S35.492A	Other specified injury of left renal artery, initial encounter ☑
S35.8X1A	Laceration of other blood vessels at abdomen, lower back and pelvis level, initial encounter
S35.8X8A	Other specified injury of other blood vessels at abdomen, lower back and pelvis level, initial encounter

AMA: **35636** 1997,Nov,1

Relative Value Units/Medicare Edits

Non-Facility RVU	Work	PE	MP	Total
35636	31.75	6.96	7.34	46.05
Facility RVU	**Work**	**PE**	**MP**	**Total**
35636	31.75	6.96	7.34	46.05

	FUD	Status	MUE	Modifiers				IOM Reference
35636	90	A	1(3)	51	50	62*	80	None

* with documentation

Terms To Know

aneurysm. Circumscribed dilation or outpouching of an artery wall, often containing blood clots and connecting directly with the lumen of the artery.

angioscopy. Visualization of capillary blood vessels with a microscope, or the inside of a blood vessel with a fiberoptic-equipped catheter.

arteriogram. Radiograph of arteries.

hyperplasia. Abnormal proliferation in the number of normal cells in regular tissue arrangement.

35637-35638

35637 Bypass graft, with other than vein; aortoiliac
35638 aortobi-iliac

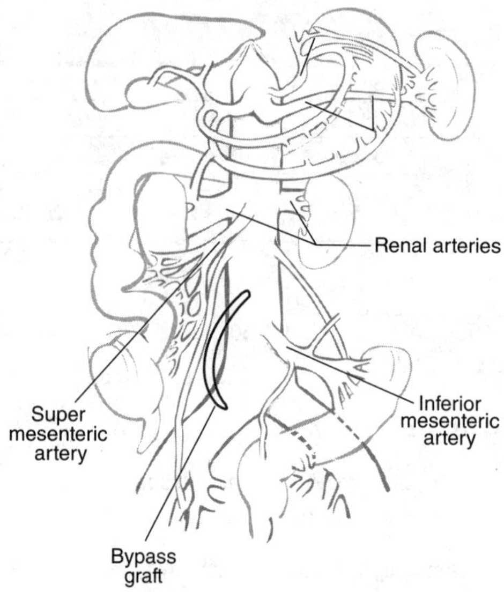

Bypass graft of a material other than vein extending from the aorta to iliac artery

Explanation

The physician makes an incision in the abdominal wall and separates the muscles to expose the internal organs, which are checked for any undetected disease. The aorta and iliac arteries are located and the obstruction is isolated by clamping the vessels. An artificial graft, commonly of polyester or polytetrafluoroethylene, is made ready. Synthetic grafts are preferred in aortoiliac bypass since they more closely match the luminal dimensions of the replaced arteries. The graft is sewn into place, with one end anastomosed to the aorta and the other end to the iliac artery. The clamps are removed, blood flows freely, and the anastomotic sites are assessed for leaks. The physician may perform Doppler studies or arteriography to establish patency of the graft. The abdominal wound is closed in layers. Report 35637 for an artificial bypass graft to a single iliac artery and 35638 when both iliac arteries are bypassed.

Coding Tips

Establishing both inflow and outflow by any method is included. That portion of the operative arteriogram performed by the surgeon is also included. Angioscopy performed during therapeutic intervention should be reported in addition to the code for the primary procedure, see 35400. Do not report 35637 with 35638 or 35646. Do not report 35638 with 35637 or 35646. For open placement of aorto-bi-iliac prosthesis following unsuccessful endovascular repair, see 34831.

ICD-10-CM Diagnostic Codes

A52.01	Syphilitic aneurysm of aorta
A52.02	Syphilitic aortitis
I70.0	Atherosclerosis of aorta
I71.02	Dissection of abdominal aorta
I71.3	Abdominal aortic aneurysm, ruptured
I71.4	Abdominal aortic aneurysm, without rupture
I71.5	Thoracoabdominal aortic aneurysm, ruptured
I71.6	Thoracoabdominal aortic aneurysm, without rupture

I72.3	Aneurysm of iliac artery
I73.89	Other specified peripheral vascular diseases
I73.9	Peripheral vascular disease, unspecified
I74.01	Saddle embolus of abdominal aorta
I74.09	Other arterial embolism and thrombosis of abdominal aorta
I74.19	Embolism and thrombosis of other parts of aorta
I74.5	Embolism and thrombosis of iliac artery
I75.89	Atheroembolism of other site
I76	Septic arterial embolism
I77.1	Stricture of artery
I77.3	Arterial fibromuscular dysplasia
I77.5	Necrosis of artery
I77.72	Dissection of iliac artery
I77.811	Abdominal aortic ectasia
I77.812	Thoracoabdominal aortic ectasia
I77.89	Other specified disorders of arteries and arterioles
I79.0	Aneurysm of aorta in diseases classified elsewhere
Q25.21	Interruption of aortic arch
Q25.29	Other atresia of aorta
Q25.41	Absence and aplasia of aorta
Q25.42	Hypoplasia of aorta
Q25.43	Congenital aneurysm of aorta
Q25.44	Congenital dilation of aorta
Q25.45	Double aortic arch
Q25.46	Tortuous aortic arch
Q25.47	Right aortic arch
Q25.48	Anomalous origin of subclavian artery
Q25.49	Other congenital malformations of aorta
S35.01XA	Minor laceration of abdominal aorta, initial encounter
S35.02XA	Major laceration of abdominal aorta, initial encounter
S35.09XA	Other injury of abdominal aorta, initial encounter
S35.511A	Injury of right iliac artery, initial encounter ☑
S35.512A	Injury of left iliac artery, initial encounter ☑
S35.59XA	Injury of other iliac blood vessels, initial encounter
S35.8X1A	Laceration of other blood vessels at abdomen, lower back and pelvis level, initial encounter
S35.8X8A	Other specified injury of other blood vessels at abdomen, lower back and pelvis level, initial encounter

AMA: 35637 2018,Jan,8; 2017,Jan,8; 2016,Jan,13; 2015,Jan,16; 2014,Jan,11 **35638** 2018,Jan,8; 2017,Jan,8; 2016,Jan,13; 2015,Jan,16; 2014,Jan,11

Relative Value Units/Medicare Edits

Non-Facility RVU	Work	PE	MP	Total
35637	33.05	7.23	7.65	47.93
35638	33.6	9.57	7.75	50.92
Facility RVU	**Work**	**PE**	**MP**	**Total**
35637	33.05	7.23	7.65	47.93
35638	33.6	9.57	7.75	50.92

	FUD	Status	MUE	Modifiers				IOM Reference
35637	90	A	1(3)	51	N/A	62*	80	None
35638	90	A	1(3)	51	N/A	62*	80	

* with documentation

35642-35645

35642 Bypass graft, with other than vein; carotid-vertebral
35645 subclavian-vertebral

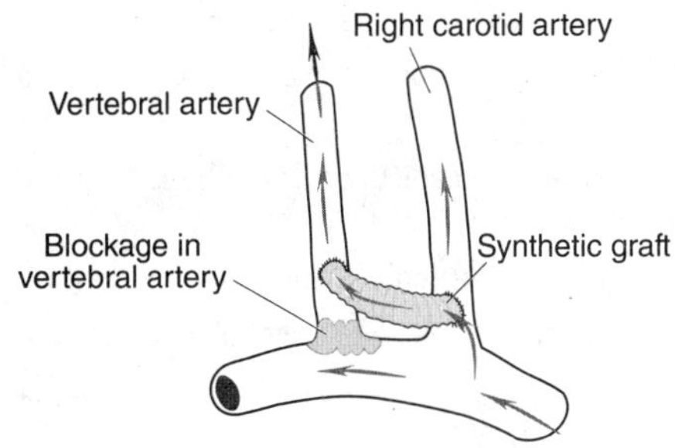

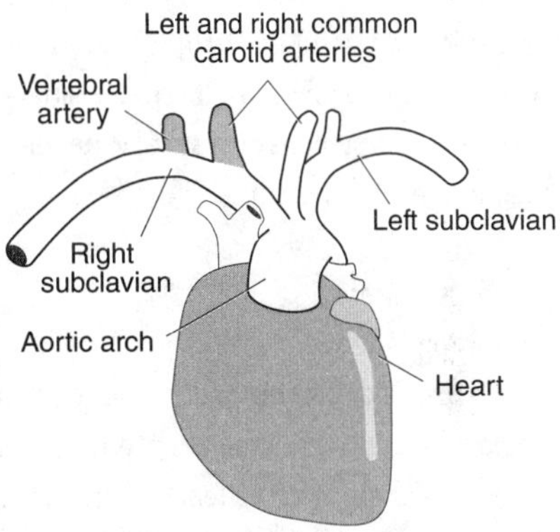

Explanation

Through an incision in the skin of the neck, the physician isolates and dissects the vertebral and carotid arteries, separating them from adjacent critical structures. The physician creates a bypass around a section of vertebral artery that is damaged or blocked, using a synthetic vein and one of two methods of repair. In 35642, after vessel clamps have been affixed above and below the damaged area, the synthetic graft is sewn to the side of the carotid artery and sewn to the side of the vertebral artery beyond the affected area (end-to-side) or sewn to the cut end of the vertebral artery after dividing it beyond the affected area (end-to-end). The damaged or blocked section of the vertebral artery is not removed. In 35645, the physician isolates and dissects the vertebral and subclavian arteries, separating them from adjacent critical structures. Once vessel clamps are affixed above and below the defect, the ends of the synthetic vein are sutured into the sides of the subclavian and vertebral arterial walls resulting in a bypass of the damaged area (end-to-side). In the second method, the vertebral artery can be cut through above the damaged area and sutured to one end of a synthetic vein (end-to-end). The remaining end is sutured to the subclavian artery. In either case, the blocked or damaged vertebral artery is not removed. For both procedures, when the clamps are removed, the section of synthetic vein graft forms a new path through which blood can easily bypass the blocked area. After the graft is complete, the skin incision is repaired with a layered closure.

Coding Tips

Establishing both inflow and outflow by any method is included. That portion of the operative arteriogram performed by the surgeon is also included. Angioscopy performed during therapeutic intervention should be reported in addition to the code for the primary procedure; see 35400. If a subclavian-vertebral bypass graft is performed with harvested vein, see 35515.

If a carotid-vertebral bypass graft is performed with a harvested vein, see 35508.

ICD-10-CM Diagnostic Codes

G45.0	Vertebro-basilar artery syndrome
I63.011	Cerebral infarction due to thrombosis of right vertebral artery ☑
I63.012	Cerebral infarction due to thrombosis of left vertebral artery ☑
I63.013	Cerebral infarction due to thrombosis of bilateral vertebral arteries ☑
I63.033	Cerebral infarction due to thrombosis of bilateral carotid arteries ☑
I63.111	Cerebral infarction due to embolism of right vertebral artery ☑
I63.112	Cerebral infarction due to embolism of left vertebral artery ☑
I63.113	Cerebral infarction due to embolism of bilateral vertebral arteries ☑
I63.133	Cerebral infarction due to embolism of bilateral carotid arteries ☑
I65.01	Occlusion and stenosis of right vertebral artery ☑
I65.02	Occlusion and stenosis of left vertebral artery ☑
I65.03	Occlusion and stenosis of bilateral vertebral arteries ☑
I76	Septic arterial embolism
I77.1	Stricture of artery
I77.2	Rupture of artery
I77.74	Dissection of vertebral artery
I77.89	Other specified disorders of arteries and arterioles
S15.111A	Minor laceration of right vertebral artery, initial encounter ☑
S15.112A	Minor laceration of left vertebral artery, initial encounter ☑
S15.121A	Major laceration of right vertebral artery, initial encounter ☑
S15.122A	Major laceration of left vertebral artery, initial encounter ☑
S15.191A	Other specified injury of right vertebral artery, initial encounter ☑
S15.192A	Other specified injury of left vertebral artery, initial encounter ☑

AMA: **35642** 1997,Nov,1 **35645** 1997,Nov,1

Relative Value Units/Medicare Edits

Non-Facility RVU	Work	PE	MP	Total
35642	18.94	5.13	4.39	28.46
35645	18.43	4.62	4.26	27.31
Facility RVU	**Work**	**PE**	**MP**	**Total**
35642	18.94	5.13	4.39	28.46
35645	18.43	4.62	4.26	27.31

	FUD	Status	MUE	Modifiers				IOM Reference
35642	90	A	1(3)	51	50	62*	80	None
35645	90	A	1(3)	51	50	62*	80	

* with documentation

35646-35647

35646 Bypass graft, with other than vein; aortobifemoral
35647 aortofemoral

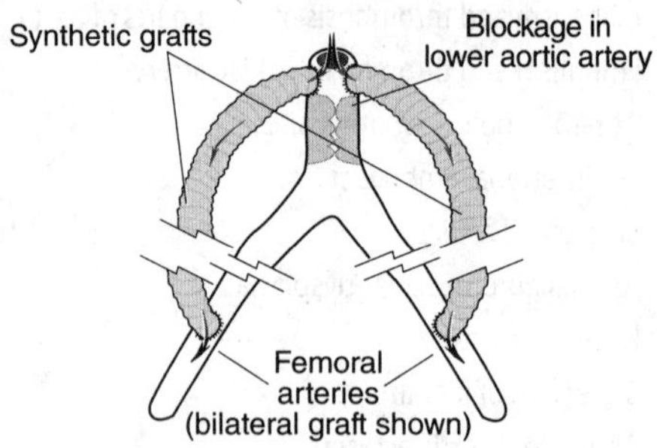

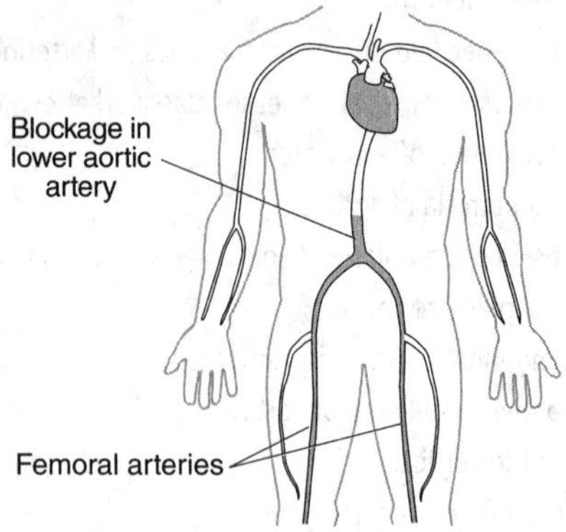

Explanation

The physician makes an incision in the skin of the abdomen over a section of damaged or blocked lower aorta. The artery is isolated and dissected. Through a separate skin incision in the upper thigh, the femoral artery is isolated and dissected from adjacent critical structures. The physician creates a bypass around the damage or blocked lower aorta using a synthetic vein. Once vessel clamps have been affixed above the defect, the lower aorta may be cut through or tied off with sutures above the damaged or blocked area and sutured to one end of the synthetic vein in an end-to-end or side-to-side fashion. The graft to one femoral artery is passed through a tunnel on the inside of the upper thigh and sutured to the femoral artery. A second synthetic vein is placed in a similar fashion to the second side. When the clamps are removed, the two grafted synthetic vein limbs form a new path through which blood can easily bypass the blocked area. The blocked or damaged portion of artery is not removed. After the graft is complete, the skin incisions are repaired with layered closure. Report 35646 when both femoral arteries are bypassed and 35647 when a single femoral artery is bypassed.

Coding Tips

Establishing inflow and outflow by any method is included. That portion of the operative arteriogram performed by the surgeon is also included. Angioscopy performed during therapeutic intervention should be reported in addition to the code for the primary procedure, see 35400. For bypass graft performed with vein graft, see 35540. When 35647 is performed with another separately identifiable procedure, the highest dollar value code is listed as the primary procedure and subsequent procedures are appended with modifier 51. For a bypass graft performed with a vein, see 35539. Do not report 35646 for open placement of aortobifemoral prosthesis following unsuccessful endovascular repair; use 34832.

ICD-10-CM Diagnostic Codes

A52.01	Syphilitic aneurysm of aorta
A52.02	Syphilitic aortitis
I70.0	Atherosclerosis of aorta
I71.02	Dissection of abdominal aorta
I71.3	Abdominal aortic aneurysm, ruptured
I71.4	Abdominal aortic aneurysm, without rupture
I73.89	Other specified peripheral vascular diseases
I73.9	Peripheral vascular disease, unspecified
I74.01	Saddle embolus of abdominal aorta
I74.09	Other arterial embolism and thrombosis of abdominal aorta
I74.19	Embolism and thrombosis of other parts of aorta
I74.5	Embolism and thrombosis of iliac artery
I75.89	Atheroembolism of other site
I76	Septic arterial embolism
I77.1	Stricture of artery
I77.3	Arterial fibromuscular dysplasia
I77.5	Necrosis of artery
I77.72	Dissection of iliac artery
I77.811	Abdominal aortic ectasia
I77.812	Thoracoabdominal aortic ectasia
I77.89	Other specified disorders of arteries and arterioles
I79.0	Aneurysm of aorta in diseases classified elsewhere
Q25.21	Interruption of aortic arch
Q25.29	Other atresia of aorta
Q25.41	Absence and aplasia of aorta
Q25.42	Hypoplasia of aorta
Q25.43	Congenital aneurysm of aorta
Q25.44	Congenital dilation of aorta
Q25.45	Double aortic arch
Q25.46	Tortuous aortic arch
Q25.47	Right aortic arch
Q25.48	Anomalous origin of subclavian artery
Q25.49	Other congenital malformations of aorta
S35.01XA	Minor laceration of abdominal aorta, initial encounter
S35.02XA	Major laceration of abdominal aorta, initial encounter
S35.09XA	Other injury of abdominal aorta, initial encounter
S35.8X1A	Laceration of other blood vessels at abdomen, lower back and pelvis level, initial encounter
S35.8X8A	Other specified injury of other blood vessels at abdomen, lower back and pelvis level, initial encounter

AMA: 35646 2018,Jan,8; 2017,Jan,8; 2016,Jan,13; 2015,Jan,16; 2014,Jan,11
35647 2018,Jan,8; 2017,Jan,8; 2016,Jan,13; 2015,Jan,16; 2014,Jan,11

Relative Value Units/Medicare Edits

Non-Facility RVU	Work	PE	MP	Total
35646	32.98	9.19	7.57	49.74
35647	29.73	8.45	6.85	45.03
Facility RVU	**Work**	**PE**	**MP**	**Total**
35646	32.98	9.19	7.57	49.74
35647	29.73	8.45	6.85	45.03

	FUD	Status	MUE	Modifiers				IOM Reference
35646	90	A	1(3)	51	N/A	62*	80	None
35647	90	A	1(3)	51	50	62*	80	

* with documentation

Terms To Know

bypass graft. Surgically created alternative blood vessel used to reroute blood flow around an area of obstruction or disease.

embolism. Obstruction of a blood vessel resulting from a clot or foreign substance.

graft. Tissue implant from another part of the body or another person.

thrombosis. Condition arising from the presence or formation of blood clots within a blood vessel that may cause vascular obstruction and insufficient oxygenation.

35650

35650 Bypass graft, with other than vein; axillary-axillary

Arrows indicate direction of revised blood flow

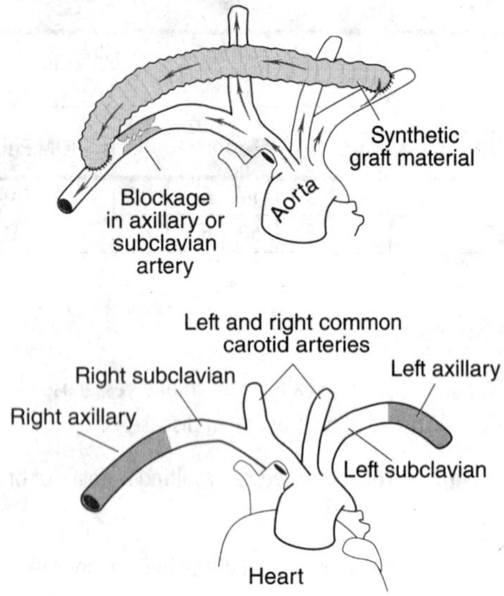

Explanation

The physician makes an incision in the skin of both axillae. The physician creates a bypass around a section of artery that is damaged or blocked, using a synthetic graft and one of two repair methods. Once vessel clamps have been affixed above and below the defect, the ends of the synthetic graft are sutured into the sides of the two axillary arterial walls, resulting in a bypass of the damaged area. In the second method, the axillary artery may be cut through beyond the damaged area and sutured to one end of a synthetic graft, which is passed across the front of the chest under the skin and sutured to the side of the contralateral axillary artery. The blocked or damaged portion of the axillary artery is not removed. When the clamps are removed, the section of synthetic vein graft forms a new path through which blood can easily bypass the blocked area. After the graft is complete, the skin incisions are repaired with layered closures.

Coding Tips

Establishing both inflow and outflow by any method is included. That portion of the operative arteriogram performed by the surgeon is also included. Angioscopy performed during therapeutic intervention should be reported in addition to the code for the primary procedure; see 35400. If a bypass graft is performed with harvested vein, see 35518.

ICD-10-CM Diagnostic Codes

G45.8	Other transient cerebral ischemic attacks and related syndromes
G45.9	Transient cerebral ischemic attack, unspecified
I63.19	Cerebral infarction due to embolism of other precerebral artery
I63.81	Other cerebral infarction due to occlusion or stenosis of small artery
I63.89	Other cerebral infarction
I67.81	Acute cerebrovascular insufficiency
I67.850	Cerebral autosomal dominant arteriopathy with subcortical infarcts and leukoencephalopathy
I67.858	Other hereditary cerebrovascular disease
I70.8	Atherosclerosis of other arteries
I70.92	Chronic total occlusion of artery of the extremities
I73.89	Other specified peripheral vascular diseases
I73.9	Peripheral vascular disease, unspecified
I74.2	Embolism and thrombosis of arteries of the upper extremities
I74.8	Embolism and thrombosis of other arteries
I75.011	Atheroembolism of right upper extremity ☑
I75.012	Atheroembolism of left upper extremity ☑
I75.013	Atheroembolism of bilateral upper extremities ☑
I76	Septic arterial embolism
I77.1	Stricture of artery
I77.2	Rupture of artery
I77.5	Necrosis of artery
I77.79	Dissection of other specified artery
I77.89	Other specified disorders of arteries and arterioles
S15.8XXA	Injury of other specified blood vessels at neck level, initial encounter
S25.111A	Minor laceration of right innominate or subclavian artery, initial encounter ☑
S25.112A	Minor laceration of left innominate or subclavian artery, initial encounter ☑
S25.121A	Major laceration of right innominate or subclavian artery, initial encounter ☑
S25.122A	Major laceration of left innominate or subclavian artery, initial encounter ☑
S25.191A	Other specified injury of right innominate or subclavian artery, initial encounter ☑
S25.192A	Other specified injury of left innominate or subclavian artery, initial encounter ☑
S45.011A	Laceration of axillary artery, right side, initial encounter ☑
S45.012A	Laceration of axillary artery, left side, initial encounter ☑
S45.091A	Other specified injury of axillary artery, right side, initial encounter ☑
S45.092A	Other specified injury of axillary artery, left side, initial encounter ☑

AMA: **35650** 1997,Nov,1

Relative Value Units/Medicare Edits

Non-Facility RVU	Work	PE	MP	Total
35650	20.16	6.62	4.6	31.38
Facility RVU	**Work**	**PE**	**MP**	**Total**
35650	20.16	6.62	4.6	31.38

	FUD	Status	MUE	Modifiers				IOM Reference
35650	90	A	1(3)	51	50	62*	80	None

* with documentation

Terms To Know

angioscopy. Visualization of capillary blood vessels with a microscope, or the inside of a blood vessel with a fiberoptic-equipped catheter.

arteriogram. Radiograph of arteries.

bypass. Auxiliary or diverted route to maintain continuous flow.

claudication. Lameness, pain, and weakness occurring in the arms or legs during exercise due to muscles not receiving the needed oxygen and nutrients.

35654

35654 Bypass graft, with other than vein; axillary-femoral-femoral

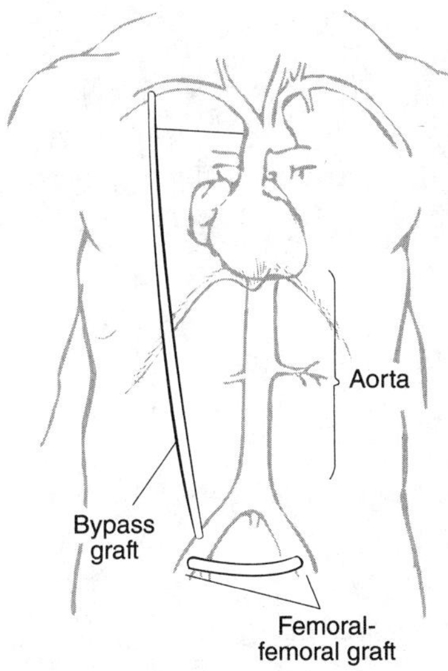

An axillary-femoral-femoral bypass graft is performed

Explanation

Through an incision in the skin of the axilla and both upper thighs, the physician creates a bypass around a section of lower aorta that is damaged or blocked, using a synthetic graft. Once vessel clamps have been affixed above and below the defect, the synthetic graft is sutured to the side of the axillary artery and passed through a subcutaneous tunnel to the upper thigh where it is sutured end-to-end or end-to-side to the femoral artery. A second synthetic graft is sutured end-to-side to the femoral artery and passed through another subcutaneous tunnel to the opposite thigh where it is sutured end-to-end or end-to-side to the femoral artery. The section of blocked artery is not removed. When the clamps are removed, the two synthetic grafted limbs form a new path through which blood can easily bypass the blocked area. After the graft is complete, the skin incisions are repaired with layered closures.

Coding Tips

Establishing both inflow and outflow by any method is included. That portion of the operative arteriogram performed by the surgeon is also included. Angioscopy performed during therapeutic intervention should be reported in addition to the code for the primary procedure; see 35400. If a bypass graft is performed with harvested vein, see 35533.

ICD-10-CM Diagnostic Codes

A52.02	Syphilitic aortitis
I70.0	Atherosclerosis of aorta
I70.92	Chronic total occlusion of artery of the extremities
I71.01	Dissection of thoracic aorta
I71.02	Dissection of abdominal aorta
I71.03	Dissection of thoracoabdominal aorta
I74.01	Saddle embolus of abdominal aorta
I74.09	Other arterial embolism and thrombosis of abdominal aorta
I74.19	Embolism and thrombosis of other parts of aorta
I74.5	Embolism and thrombosis of iliac artery
I75.89	Atheroembolism of other site
I76	Septic arterial embolism
I77.1	Stricture of artery
I77.3	Arterial fibromuscular dysplasia
I77.5	Necrosis of artery
I77.72	Dissection of iliac artery
I77.73	Dissection of renal artery
I77.79	Dissection of other specified artery
I77.810	Thoracic aortic ectasia
I77.811	Abdominal aortic ectasia
I77.812	Thoracoabdominal aortic ectasia
I77.89	Other specified disorders of arteries and arterioles
I79.0	Aneurysm of aorta in diseases classified elsewhere
I82.0	Budd-Chiari syndrome
Q25.41	Absence and aplasia of aorta
Q25.46	Tortuous aortic arch
Q25.47	Right aortic arch
Q25.48	Anomalous origin of subclavian artery
Q25.8	Other congenital malformations of other great arteries
Q27.1	Congenital renal artery stenosis
Q27.2	Other congenital malformations of renal artery
Q28.8	Other specified congenital malformations of circulatory system
Q79.61	Classical Ehlers-Danlos syndrome
Q79.62	Hypermobile Ehlers-Danlos syndrome
Q79.63	Vascular Ehlers-Danlos syndrome
Q87.418	Marfan's syndrome with other cardiovascular manifestations
S25.01XA	Minor laceration of thoracic aorta, initial encounter
S25.02XA	Major laceration of thoracic aorta, initial encounter
S25.09XA	Other specified injury of thoracic aorta, initial encounter
S25.811A	Laceration of other blood vessels of thorax, right side, initial encounter ☑
S25.812A	Laceration of other blood vessels of thorax, left side, initial encounter ☑
S25.891A	Other specified injury of other blood vessels of thorax, right side, initial encounter ☑
S25.892A	Other specified injury of other blood vessels of thorax, left side, initial encounter ☑
S35.01XA	Minor laceration of abdominal aorta, initial encounter
S35.02XA	Major laceration of abdominal aorta, initial encounter
S35.09XA	Other injury of abdominal aorta, initial encounter
S35.8X1A	Laceration of other blood vessels at abdomen, lower back and pelvis level, initial encounter
S35.8X8A	Other specified injury of other blood vessels at abdomen, lower back and pelvis level, initial encounter
T81.710A	Complication of mesenteric artery following a procedure, not elsewhere classified, initial encounter

AMA: 35654 2018,Jan,8; 2017,Jan,8; 2016,Jan,13; 2015,Jan,16; 2014,Jan,11

Relative Value Units/Medicare Edits

Non-Facility RVU	Work	PE	MP	Total
35654	26.28	7.37	6.02	39.67
Facility RVU	**Work**	**PE**	**MP**	**Total**
35654	26.28	7.37	6.02	39.67

	FUD	Status	MUE	Modifiers				IOM Reference
35654	90	A	1(3)	51	N/A	62*	80	None

* with documentation

Terms To Know

Budd-Chiari syndrome. Thrombus or other obstruction of the hepatic vein, with an enlarged liver, intractable ascites, portal hypertension, and the growth of extensive collateral vessels.

dissection. Separating by cutting tissue or body structures apart.

embolus. Any substance, such as air bubbles, cellular masses, calcium fragments, or blood clots, carried through the bloodstream that has become lodged in a vessel, resulting in an obstruction of circulation.

subcutaneous. Below the skin.

35656

35656 Bypass graft, with other than vein; femoral-popliteal

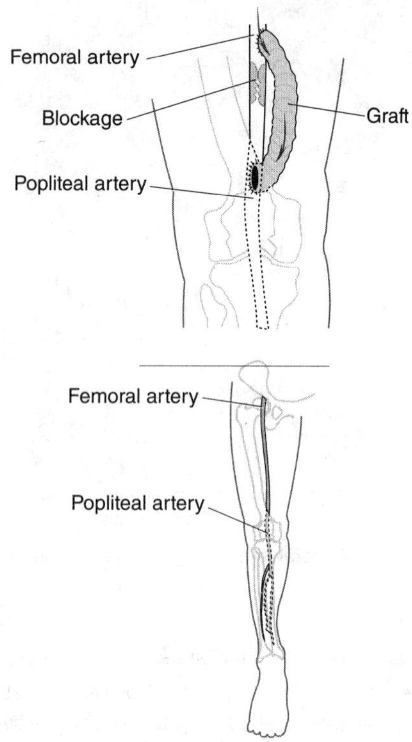

Explanation

Through incisions in the skin of the leg overlying the femoral and popliteal arteries, the physician isolates and dissects a section of artery that is damaged or blocked. The physician creates a bypass around the superficial femoral artery, using a synthetic vein and one of two methods of repair. Once vessel clamps have been affixed above and below the defect, the superficial femoral artery may be cut through above the damaged or blocked area and sutured to one end of a synthetic vein, which is passed through a tunnel down the thigh muscles to behind the knee and sutured to the popliteal artery. In the second method, the ends of the synthetic vein are sutured into the side of the femoral and popliteal arterial walls, resulting in a bypass of the damaged area. When the clamps are removed, the section of synthetic vein forms a new path through which blood can easily bypass the blocked area. The blocked or damaged portion of artery is not removed. After the graft is complete, the skin incisions are repaired with layered closures.

Coding Tips

Establishing both inflow and outflow by any method is included. That portion of the operative arteriogram performed by the surgeon is also included. Angioscopy performed during therapeutic intervention should be reported in addition to the code for the primary procedure, see 35400. Report 35700 in addition to 35656 for reoperation more than one month after the original operation. If in-situ vein bypass is performed, see 35583.

ICD-10-CM Diagnostic Codes

I70.211 Atherosclerosis of native arteries of extremities with intermittent claudication, right leg ☑

I70.212 Atherosclerosis of native arteries of extremities with intermittent claudication, left leg ☑

I70.213 Atherosclerosis of native arteries of extremities with intermittent claudication, bilateral legs ☑

I70.221 Atherosclerosis of native arteries of extremities with rest pain, right leg ☑

I70.222 Atherosclerosis of native arteries of extremities with rest pain, left leg ☑

I70.223 Atherosclerosis of native arteries of extremities with rest pain, bilateral legs ☑

I70.231 Atherosclerosis of native arteries of right leg with ulceration of thigh ☑

I70.232 Atherosclerosis of native arteries of right leg with ulceration of calf ☑

I70.233 Atherosclerosis of native arteries of right leg with ulceration of ankle ☑

I70.234 Atherosclerosis of native arteries of right leg with ulceration of heel and midfoot ☑

I70.235 Atherosclerosis of native arteries of right leg with ulceration of other part of foot ☑

I70.238 Atherosclerosis of native arteries of right leg with ulceration of other part of lower leg ☑

I70.241 Atherosclerosis of native arteries of left leg with ulceration of thigh ☑

I70.242 Atherosclerosis of native arteries of left leg with ulceration of calf ☑

I70.243 Atherosclerosis of native arteries of left leg with ulceration of ankle ☑

I70.244 Atherosclerosis of native arteries of left leg with ulceration of heel and midfoot ☑

I70.245 Atherosclerosis of native arteries of left leg with ulceration of other part of foot ☑

I70.248 Atherosclerosis of native arteries of left leg with ulceration of other part of lower leg ☑

I70.261 Atherosclerosis of native arteries of extremities with gangrene, right leg ☑

I70.262 Atherosclerosis of native arteries of extremities with gangrene, left leg ☑

I70.263 Atherosclerosis of native arteries of extremities with gangrene, bilateral legs ☑

I70.291 Other atherosclerosis of native arteries of extremities, right leg ☑

I70.292 Other atherosclerosis of native arteries of extremities, left leg ☑

I70.293 Other atherosclerosis of native arteries of extremities, bilateral legs ☑

I70.461 Atherosclerosis of autologous vein bypass graft(s) of the extremities with gangrene, right leg ☑

I70.462 Atherosclerosis of autologous vein bypass graft(s) of the extremities with gangrene, left leg ☑

I70.511 Atherosclerosis of nonautologous biological bypass graft(s) of the extremities with intermittent claudication, right leg ☑

I70.512 Atherosclerosis of nonautologous biological bypass graft(s) of the extremities with intermittent claudication, left leg ☑

I70.521 Atherosclerosis of nonautologous biological bypass graft(s) of the extremities with rest pain, right leg ☑

I70.522 Atherosclerosis of nonautologous biological bypass graft(s) of the extremities with rest pain, left leg ☑

I70.531 Atherosclerosis of nonautologous biological bypass graft(s) of the right leg with ulceration of thigh ☑

I70.541 Atherosclerosis of nonautologous biological bypass graft(s) of the left leg with ulceration of thigh ☑

I70.561 Atherosclerosis of nonautologous biological bypass graft(s) of the extremities with gangrene, right leg ☑

I70.562 Atherosclerosis of nonautologous biological bypass graft(s) of the extremities with gangrene, left leg ☑

I70.611 Atherosclerosis of nonbiological bypass graft(s) of the extremities with intermittent claudication, right leg ☑

I70.612 Atherosclerosis of nonbiological bypass graft(s) of the extremities with intermittent claudication, left leg ☑

I70.621 Atherosclerosis of nonbiological bypass graft(s) of the extremities with rest pain, right leg ☑

I70.622 Atherosclerosis of nonbiological bypass graft(s) of the extremities with rest pain, left leg ☑

I70.631 Atherosclerosis of nonbiological bypass graft(s) of the right leg with ulceration of thigh ☑

I70.641 Atherosclerosis of nonbiological bypass graft(s) of the left leg with ulceration of thigh ☑

I70.661 Atherosclerosis of nonbiological bypass graft(s) of the extremities with gangrene, right leg ☑

I70.662 Atherosclerosis of nonbiological bypass graft(s) of the extremities with gangrene, left leg ☑

I70.92 Chronic total occlusion of artery of the extremities

I73.89 Other specified peripheral vascular diseases

I74.3 Embolism and thrombosis of arteries of the lower extremities

I75.021 Atheroembolism of right lower extremity ☑

I75.022 Atheroembolism of left lower extremity ☑

I75.023 Atheroembolism of bilateral lower extremities ☑

I76 Septic arterial embolism

I77.1 Stricture of artery

I77.2 Rupture of artery

I77.5 Necrosis of artery

I77.89 Other specified disorders of arteries and arterioles

I79.8 Other disorders of arteries, arterioles and capillaries in diseases classified elsewhere

S75.011A Minor laceration of femoral artery, right leg, initial encounter ☑

S75.012A Minor laceration of femoral artery, left leg, initial encounter ☑

S75.021A Major laceration of femoral artery, right leg, initial encounter ☑

S75.022A Major laceration of femoral artery, left leg, initial encounter ☑

S75.091A Other specified injury of femoral artery, right leg, initial encounter ☑

S75.092A Other specified injury of femoral artery, left leg, initial encounter ☑

AMA: 35656 2018,Jan,8; 2017,Jan,8; 2016,Jan,13; 2015,Jan,16; 2014,Jan,11

Relative Value Units/Medicare Edits

Non-Facility RVU	Work	PE	MP	Total
35656	20.47	6.19	4.68	31.34
Facility RVU	**Work**	**PE**	**MP**	**Total**
35656	20.47	6.19	4.68	31.34

	FUD	Status	MUE	Modifiers				IOM Reference
35656	90	A	1(3)	51	50	62*	80	None

* with documentation

35661

35661 Bypass graft, with other than vein; femoral-femoral

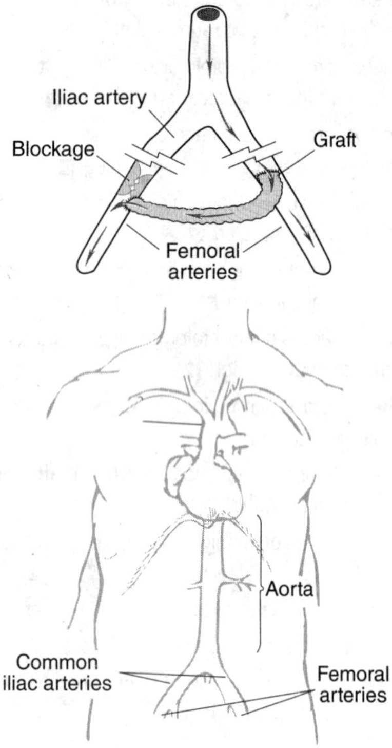

Explanation

Through incisions in the skin of the upper thighs, the physician isolates and dissects a section of the femoral arteries. The physician creates a bypass using a synthetic vein. Once vessel clamps have been affixed above and below the area of anastomosis, the femoral artery may be cut through below the damaged area and sutured to one end of a synthetic vein, which is sutured to the femoral artery in the opposite leg, resulting in a bypass of the damaged or blocked area. When the clamps are removed, the section of synthetic vein forms a new path through which blood can easily bypass the blocked area. The blocked or damaged portion of the artery is not removed. After the graft is complete, the skin incisions are repaired with layered closures.

Coding Tips

Establishing both inflow and outflow by any method is included. That portion of the operative arteriogram performed by the surgeon is also included. Angioscopy performed during therapeutic intervention should be reported in addition to the code for the primary procedure; see 35400. If a bypass graft is performed with harvested vein, see 35558.

ICD-10-CM Diagnostic Codes

I70.211 Atherosclerosis of native arteries of extremities with intermittent claudication, right leg ☑
I70.212 Atherosclerosis of native arteries of extremities with intermittent claudication, left leg ☑
I70.213 Atherosclerosis of native arteries of extremities with intermittent claudication, bilateral legs ☑
I70.221 Atherosclerosis of native arteries of extremities with rest pain, right leg ☑
I70.222 Atherosclerosis of native arteries of extremities with rest pain, left leg ☑
I70.223 Atherosclerosis of native arteries of extremities with rest pain, bilateral legs ☑
I70.231 Atherosclerosis of native arteries of right leg with ulceration of thigh ☑
I70.232 Atherosclerosis of native arteries of right leg with ulceration of calf ☑
I70.233 Atherosclerosis of native arteries of right leg with ulceration of ankle ☑
I70.234 Atherosclerosis of native arteries of right leg with ulceration of heel and midfoot ☑
I70.241 Atherosclerosis of native arteries of left leg with ulceration of thigh ☑
I70.242 Atherosclerosis of native arteries of left leg with ulceration of calf ☑
I70.243 Atherosclerosis of native arteries of left leg with ulceration of ankle ☑
I70.244 Atherosclerosis of native arteries of left leg with ulceration of heel and midfoot ☑
I70.261 Atherosclerosis of native arteries of extremities with gangrene, right leg ☑
I70.262 Atherosclerosis of native arteries of extremities with gangrene, left leg ☑
I70.263 Atherosclerosis of native arteries of extremities with gangrene, bilateral legs ☑
I70.291 Other atherosclerosis of native arteries of extremities, right leg ☑
I70.292 Other atherosclerosis of native arteries of extremities, left leg ☑
I70.293 Other atherosclerosis of native arteries of extremities, bilateral legs ☑
I70.461 Atherosclerosis of autologous vein bypass graft(s) of the extremities with gangrene, right leg ☑
I70.462 Atherosclerosis of autologous vein bypass graft(s) of the extremities with gangrene, left leg ☑
I70.511 Atherosclerosis of nonautologous biological bypass graft(s) of the extremities with intermittent claudication, right leg ☑
I70.512 Atherosclerosis of nonautologous biological bypass graft(s) of the extremities with intermittent claudication, left leg ☑
I70.521 Atherosclerosis of nonautologous biological bypass graft(s) of the extremities with rest pain, right leg ☑
I70.522 Atherosclerosis of nonautologous biological bypass graft(s) of the extremities with rest pain, left leg ☑
I70.531 Atherosclerosis of nonautologous biological bypass graft(s) of the right leg with ulceration of thigh ☑
I70.541 Atherosclerosis of nonautologous biological bypass graft(s) of the left leg with ulceration of thigh ☑
I70.561 Atherosclerosis of nonautologous biological bypass graft(s) of the extremities with gangrene, right leg ☑
I70.562 Atherosclerosis of nonautologous biological bypass graft(s) of the extremities with gangrene, left leg ☑
I70.611 Atherosclerosis of nonbiological bypass graft(s) of the extremities with intermittent claudication, right leg ☑
I70.612 Atherosclerosis of nonbiological bypass graft(s) of the extremities with intermittent claudication, left leg ☑
I70.621 Atherosclerosis of nonbiological bypass graft(s) of the extremities with rest pain, right leg ☑
I70.622 Atherosclerosis of nonbiological bypass graft(s) of the extremities with rest pain, left leg ☑

I70.631 Atherosclerosis of nonbiological bypass graft(s) of the right leg with ulceration of thigh ☑
I70.641 Atherosclerosis of nonbiological bypass graft(s) of the left leg with ulceration of thigh ☑
I70.661 Atherosclerosis of nonbiological bypass graft(s) of the extremities with gangrene, right leg ☑
I70.662 Atherosclerosis of nonbiological bypass graft(s) of the extremities with gangrene, left leg ☑
I70.92 Chronic total occlusion of artery of the extremities
I73.89 Other specified peripheral vascular diseases
I74.3 Embolism and thrombosis of arteries of the lower extremities
I75.021 Atheroembolism of right lower extremity ☑
I75.022 Atheroembolism of left lower extremity ☑
I75.023 Atheroembolism of bilateral lower extremities ☑
I76 Septic arterial embolism
I77.1 Stricture of artery
I77.2 Rupture of artery
I77.5 Necrosis of artery
I77.89 Other specified disorders of arteries and arterioles
I79.8 Other disorders of arteries, arterioles and capillaries in diseases classified elsewhere
S75.011A Minor laceration of femoral artery, right leg, initial encounter ☑
S75.012A Minor laceration of femoral artery, left leg, initial encounter ☑
S75.021A Major laceration of femoral artery, right leg, initial encounter ☑
S75.022A Major laceration of femoral artery, left leg, initial encounter ☑
S75.091A Other specified injury of femoral artery, right leg, initial encounter ☑
S75.092A Other specified injury of femoral artery, left leg, initial encounter ☑

AMA: 35661 2018,Jan,8; 2017,Jan,8; 2016,Jan,13; 2015,Jan,16; 2014,Jan,11

Relative Value Units/Medicare Edits

Non-Facility RVU	Work	PE	MP	Total
35661	20.35	6.44	4.64	31.43
Facility RVU	**Work**	**PE**	**MP**	**Total**
35661	20.35	6.44	4.64	31.43

	FUD	Status	MUE	Modifiers				IOM Reference
35661	90	A	1(3)	51	50	62*	80	None

* with documentation

35663

35663 Bypass graft, with other than vein; ilioiliac

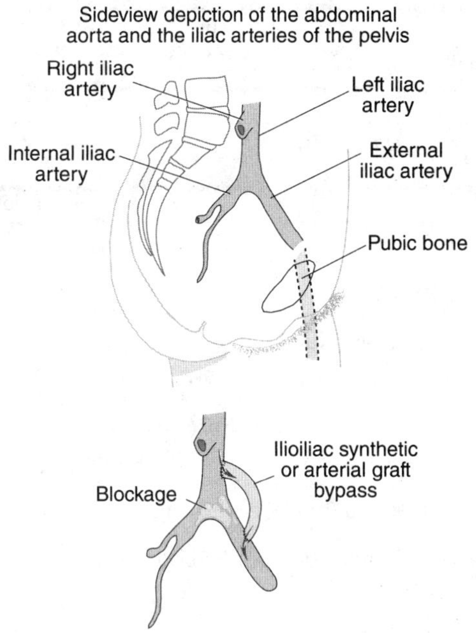

Explanation

The physician exposes the iliac arteries using an abdominal incision, retracting and dissecting past large and small bowel. The patent (nondiseased) iliac artery is partially clamped and a longitudinal incision is performed down the clamped portion of the aorta. A synthetic or arterial graft is sewn in, the graft is clamped, and the iliac clamp is removed to assess patency of the anastomosis. The diseased iliac artery is clamped distal to the stenosis, a distal incision is performed, and the distal graft is attached to the diseased iliac artery. Graft material may be utilized to enlarge the aortic or arterial lumen (patch graft). The physician may perform arteriography or use a Doppler probe to establish patency of the graft. The abdominal wound is closed, leaving drains in place.

Coding Tips

Establishing both inflow and outflow by any method is included. That portion of the operative arteriogram performed by the surgeon is also included. Angioscopy performed during therapeutic intervention should be reported in addition to the code for the primary procedure; see 35400. If a bypass graft is performed with harvested vein, see 35563.

ICD-10-CM Diagnostic Codes

I73.89 Other specified peripheral vascular diseases
I73.9 Peripheral vascular disease, unspecified
I74.5 Embolism and thrombosis of iliac artery
I76 Septic arterial embolism
I77.1 Stricture of artery
I77.5 Necrosis of artery
I77.72 Dissection of iliac artery
S35.50XA Injury of unspecified iliac blood vessel(s), initial encounter
S35.511A Injury of right iliac artery, initial encounter ☑
S35.512A Injury of left iliac artery, initial encounter ☑
S35.513A Injury of unspecified iliac artery, initial encounter
S35.59XA Injury of other iliac blood vessels, initial encounter

AMA: 35663 1997,Nov,1

Relative Value Units/Medicare Edits

Non-Facility RVU	Work	PE	MP	Total
35663	23.93	5.68	5.53	35.14
Facility RVU	**Work**	**PE**	**MP**	**Total**
35663	23.93	5.68	5.53	35.14

	FUD	Status	MUE	Modifiers				IOM Reference
35663	90	A	1(3)	51	50	62*	80	None

* with documentation

Terms To Know

anastomosis. Surgically created connection between ducts, blood vessels, or bowel segments to allow flow from one to the other.

angioscopy. Visualization of capillary blood vessels with a microscope, or the inside of a blood vessel with a fiberoptic-equipped catheter.

arteriogram. Radiograph of arteries.

artery. Vessel through which oxygenated blood passes away from the heart to any part of the body.

atherosclerosis. Buildup of yellowish plaques composed of cholesterol and lipoid material within the arteries.

bypass. Auxiliary or diverted route to maintain continuous flow.

complication. Condition arising after the beginning of observation and treatment that modifies the course of the patient's illness or the medical care required, or an undesired result or misadventure in medical care.

distal. Located farther away from a specified reference point or the trunk.

graft. Tissue implant from another part of the body or another person.

harvest. Removal of cells or tissue from their native site to be used as a graft or transplant to another part of the donor's body or placed into another person.

shunt. Surgically created passage between blood vessels or other natural passages, such as an arteriovenous anastomosis, to divert or bypass blood flow from the normal channel.

stenosis. Narrowing or constriction of a passage.

stricture. Narrowing of an anatomical structure.

35665

35665 Bypass graft, with other than vein; iliofemoral

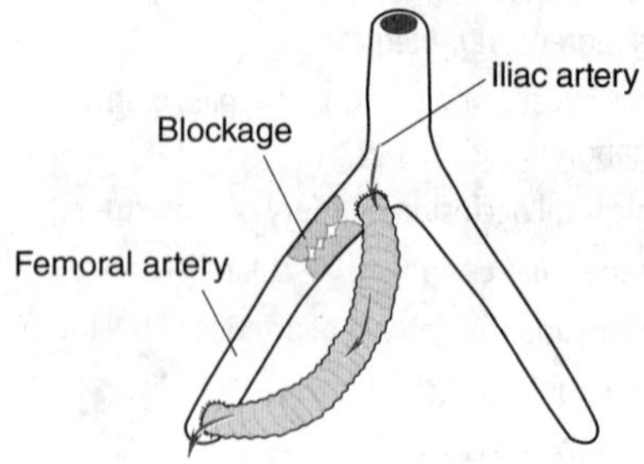

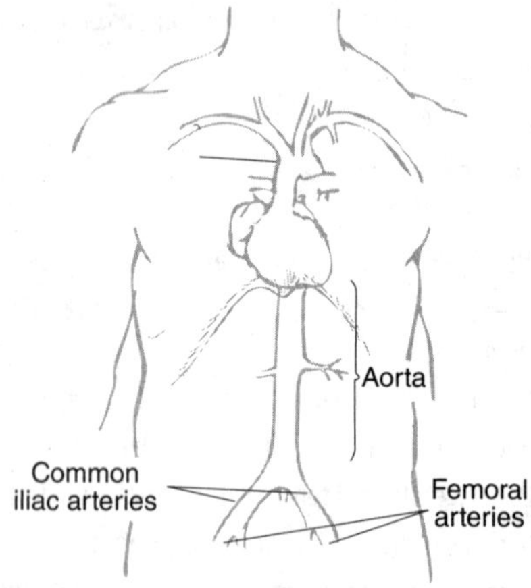

Explanation

Through incisions in the skin of the lower abdomen overlying the iliac artery, and in the skin of the upper thigh overlying the femoral artery, the physician isolates and dissects a section of common iliac artery. The physician creates a bypass around the iliac artery, using a synthetic vein and one of two methods of repair. Once vessel clamps have been affixed above and below the defect, the iliac artery may be cut or tied off with sutures above the damaged area and sutured to one end of a synthetic vein. The graft is passed through a tunnel on the inside of the upper thigh and is sutured to the side of the femoral artery. In the second method, the end of the synthetic vein is sutured to the side of the iliac artery. Either method results in a bypass of the damaged area. When the clamps are removed, the section of synthetic vein forms a new path through which blood can easily bypass the blocked area. After the graft is complete, the skin incisions are repaired with layered closures.

Coding Tips

Establishing both inflow and outflow by any method is included. That portion of the operative arteriogram performed by the surgeon is also included. Angioscopy performed during therapeutic intervention should be reported in addition to the code for the primary procedure; see 35400. If a bypass graft is performed with harvested vein, see 35565.

ICD-10-CM Diagnostic Codes

I70.92	Chronic total occlusion of artery of the extremities
I72.3	Aneurysm of iliac artery
I72.4	Aneurysm of artery of lower extremity
I73.89	Other specified peripheral vascular diseases
I74.3	Embolism and thrombosis of arteries of the lower extremities
I74.5	Embolism and thrombosis of iliac artery
I75.021	Atheroembolism of right lower extremity ☑

I75.022 Atheroembolism of left lower extremity ☑
I75.023 Atheroembolism of bilateral lower extremities ☑
I76 Septic arterial embolism
I77.1 Stricture of artery
I77.2 Rupture of artery
I77.5 Necrosis of artery
I77.72 Dissection of iliac artery
I77.89 Other specified disorders of arteries and arterioles
I79.8 Other disorders of arteries, arterioles and capillaries in diseases classified elsewhere
M79.604 Pain in right leg ☑
M79.605 Pain in left leg ☑
M79.651 Pain in right thigh ☑
M79.652 Pain in left thigh ☑
S35.511A Injury of right iliac artery, initial encounter ☑
S35.512A Injury of left iliac artery, initial encounter ☑
S35.59XA Injury of other iliac blood vessels, initial encounter
S35.8X1A Laceration of other blood vessels at abdomen, lower back and pelvis level, initial encounter
S35.8X8A Other specified injury of other blood vessels at abdomen, lower back and pelvis level, initial encounter

AMA: 35665 2018,Jan,8; 2017,Jan,8; 2016,Jan,13; 2015,Jan,16; 2014,Jan,11

Relative Value Units/Medicare Edits

Non-Facility RVU	Work	PE	MP	Total
35665	22.35	6.58	5.07	34.0
Facility RVU	**Work**	**PE**	**MP**	**Total**
35665	22.35	6.58	5.07	34.0

	FUD	Status	MUE	Modifiers				IOM Reference
35665	90	A	1(3)	51	50	62*	80	None

* with documentation

35666

35666 Bypass graft, with other than vein; femoral-anterior tibial, posterior tibial, or peroneal artery

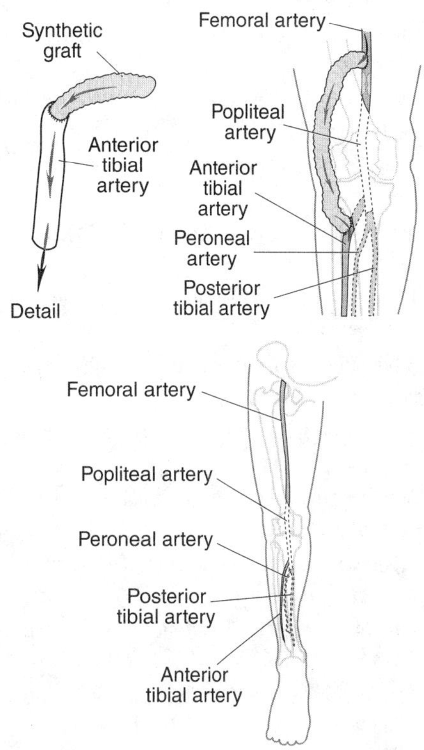

Explanation

Through incisions in the skin of the leg overlying the superficial femoral artery, the physician isolates and dissects sections of the femoral and anterior tibial, posterior tibial or peroneal arteries. The physician creates a bypass around the affected artery using a synthetic vein. Once vessel clamps have been affixed above and below the defect, the superficial femoral artery may be cut through above the damaged area and sutured to one end of a synthetic vein, which is passed through an intramuscular tunnel and sutured to the anterior tibial, posterior tibial, peroneal, or other distal vessel. In the second method, the ends of the synthetic vein are sutured to the side of the femoral artery and anterior tibial, posterior tibial, peroneal, or other distal vessel wall, resulting in a bypass of the damaged area. When the clamps are removed, the section of synthetic vein forms a new path through which blood can easily bypass the blocked area. The blocked or damaged portion of artery is left in place and not removed. After the graft is complete, the skin incisions are repaired with layered closures.

Coding Tips

Establishing both inflow and outflow by any method is included. That portion of the operative arteriogram performed by the surgeon is also included. Angioscopy performed during therapeutic intervention should be reported in addition to the code for the primary procedure; see 35400. Report 35700 in addition to 35666 for reoperation more than one month after the original operation. If a bypass graft is performed with a harvested vein, see 35566. If an in-situ vein bypass is performed, see 35585.

ICD-10-CM Diagnostic Codes

I70.211 Atherosclerosis of native arteries of extremities with intermittent claudication, right leg ☑

I70.212 Atherosclerosis of native arteries of extremities with intermittent claudication, left leg ☑
I70.213 Atherosclerosis of native arteries of extremities with intermittent claudication, bilateral legs ☑
I70.221 Atherosclerosis of native arteries of extremities with rest pain, right leg ☑
I70.222 Atherosclerosis of native arteries of extremities with rest pain, left leg ☑
I70.223 Atherosclerosis of native arteries of extremities with rest pain, bilateral legs ☑
I70.231 Atherosclerosis of native arteries of right leg with ulceration of thigh ☑
I70.232 Atherosclerosis of native arteries of right leg with ulceration of calf ☑
I70.233 Atherosclerosis of native arteries of right leg with ulceration of ankle ☑
I70.234 Atherosclerosis of native arteries of right leg with ulceration of heel and midfoot ☑
I70.235 Atherosclerosis of native arteries of right leg with ulceration of other part of foot ☑
I70.238 Atherosclerosis of native arteries of right leg with ulceration of other part of lower leg ☑
I70.241 Atherosclerosis of native arteries of left leg with ulceration of thigh ☑
I70.242 Atherosclerosis of native arteries of left leg with ulceration of calf ☑
I70.243 Atherosclerosis of native arteries of left leg with ulceration of ankle ☑
I70.244 Atherosclerosis of native arteries of left leg with ulceration of heel and midfoot ☑
I70.245 Atherosclerosis of native arteries of left leg with ulceration of other part of foot ☑
I70.248 Atherosclerosis of native arteries of left leg with ulceration of other part of lower leg ☑
I70.261 Atherosclerosis of native arteries of extremities with gangrene, right leg ☑
I70.262 Atherosclerosis of native arteries of extremities with gangrene, left leg ☑
I70.263 Atherosclerosis of native arteries of extremities with gangrene, bilateral legs ☑
I70.461 Atherosclerosis of autologous vein bypass graft(s) of the extremities with gangrene, right leg ☑
I70.462 Atherosclerosis of autologous vein bypass graft(s) of the extremities with gangrene, left leg ☑
I70.511 Atherosclerosis of nonautologous biological bypass graft(s) of the extremities with intermittent claudication, right leg ☑
I70.512 Atherosclerosis of nonautologous biological bypass graft(s) of the extremities with intermittent claudication, left leg ☑
I70.521 Atherosclerosis of nonautologous biological bypass graft(s) of the extremities with rest pain, right leg ☑
I70.522 Atherosclerosis of nonautologous biological bypass graft(s) of the extremities with rest pain, left leg ☑
I70.531 Atherosclerosis of nonautologous biological bypass graft(s) of the right leg with ulceration of thigh ☑
I70.541 Atherosclerosis of nonautologous biological bypass graft(s) of the left leg with ulceration of thigh ☑
I70.561 Atherosclerosis of nonautologous biological bypass graft(s) of the extremities with gangrene, right leg ☑
I70.562 Atherosclerosis of nonautologous biological bypass graft(s) of the extremities with gangrene, left leg ☑
I70.611 Atherosclerosis of nonbiological bypass graft(s) of the extremities with intermittent claudication, right leg ☑
I70.612 Atherosclerosis of nonbiological bypass graft(s) of the extremities with intermittent claudication, left leg ☑
I70.621 Atherosclerosis of nonbiological bypass graft(s) of the extremities with rest pain, right leg ☑
I70.622 Atherosclerosis of nonbiological bypass graft(s) of the extremities with rest pain, left leg ☑
I70.631 Atherosclerosis of nonbiological bypass graft(s) of the right leg with ulceration of thigh ☑
I70.641 Atherosclerosis of nonbiological bypass graft(s) of the left leg with ulceration of thigh ☑
I70.661 Atherosclerosis of nonbiological bypass graft(s) of the extremities with gangrene, right leg ☑
I70.662 Atherosclerosis of nonbiological bypass graft(s) of the extremities with gangrene, left leg ☑
I70.92 Chronic total occlusion of artery of the extremities
I72.4 Aneurysm of artery of lower extremity
I74.3 Embolism and thrombosis of arteries of the lower extremities
I75.021 Atheroembolism of right lower extremity ☑
I75.022 Atheroembolism of left lower extremity ☑
I75.023 Atheroembolism of bilateral lower extremities ☑
I76 Septic arterial embolism
I77.1 Stricture of artery
I77.2 Rupture of artery
I77.5 Necrosis of artery
S75.021A Major laceration of femoral artery, right leg, initial encounter ☑
S75.022A Major laceration of femoral artery, left leg, initial encounter ☑

AMA: **35666** 2018,Jan,8; 2017,Jan,8; 2016,Jan,13; 2015,Jan,16; 2014,Jan,11

Relative Value Units/Medicare Edits

Non-Facility RVU	Work	PE	MP	Total
35666	23.66	7.57	5.41	36.64
Facility RVU	**Work**	**PE**	**MP**	**Total**
35666	23.66	7.57	5.41	36.64

	FUD	Status	MUE	Modifiers				IOM Reference
35666	90	A	2(3)	51	50	62*	80	None

* with documentation

Arteries and Veins

35671

35671 Bypass graft, with other than vein; popliteal-tibial or -peroneal artery

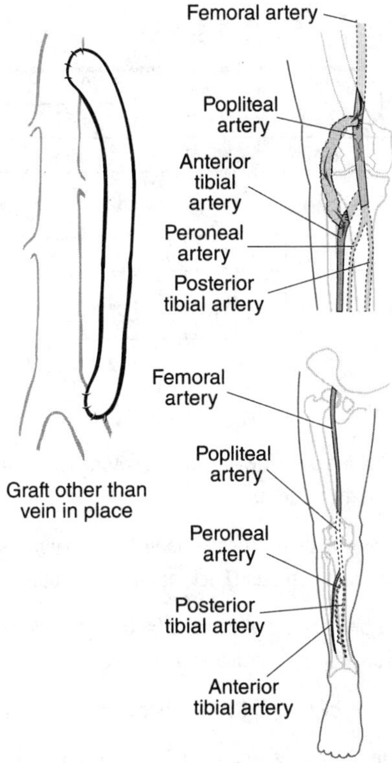

Explanation

Through incisions in the skin of the leg overlying the popliteal arteries, the physician isolates and dissects a section of artery from adjacent critical structures. The physician creates a bypass around the artery, using a synthetic vein and one of two methods of repair. Once vessel clamps have been affixed above and below the defect, the popliteal artery may be cut through above the damaged area and sutured to one end of a synthetic vein, which is sutured to the tibial, peroneal, or other distal artery. In the second method, the ends of the synthetic vein are sutured into the side of the popliteal and the tibial or peroneal arterial wall resulting in a bypass of the damaged area. When the clamps are removed, the section of synthetic vein forms a new path through which blood can easily bypass the blocked area. After the graft is complete, the incision is repaired with layered closures.

Coding Tips

Establishing both inflow and outflow by any method is included. That portion of the operative arteriogram performed by the surgeon is also included. Angioscopy performed during therapeutic intervention should be reported in addition to the code for the primary procedure; see 35400. Report 35700 in addition to 35671 for reoperation more than one month after the original operation. If a bypass graft is performed with a harvested vein, see 35571. If an in-situ vein bypass is performed, see 35587.

ICD-10-CM Diagnostic Codes

I70.92	Chronic total occlusion of artery of the extremities
I73.89	Other specified peripheral vascular diseases
I73.9	Peripheral vascular disease, unspecified
I74.3	Embolism and thrombosis of arteries of the lower extremities
I75.021	Atheroembolism of right lower extremity ☑
I75.022	Atheroembolism of left lower extremity ☑
I75.023	Atheroembolism of bilateral lower extremities ☑
I76	Septic arterial embolism
I77.89	Other specified disorders of arteries and arterioles
I79.8	Other disorders of arteries, arterioles and capillaries in diseases classified elsewhere
S85.011A	Laceration of popliteal artery, right leg, initial encounter ☑
S85.012A	Laceration of popliteal artery, left leg, initial encounter ☑
S85.091A	Other specified injury of popliteal artery, right leg, initial encounter ☑
S85.092A	Other specified injury of popliteal artery, left leg, initial encounter ☑
S85.141A	Laceration of anterior tibial artery, right leg, initial encounter ☑
S85.142A	Laceration of anterior tibial artery, left leg, initial encounter ☑
S85.151A	Other specified injury of anterior tibial artery, right leg, initial encounter ☑
S85.152A	Other specified injury of anterior tibial artery, left leg, initial encounter ☑
S85.171A	Laceration of posterior tibial artery, right leg, initial encounter ☑
S85.172A	Laceration of posterior tibial artery, left leg, initial encounter ☑
S85.181A	Other specified injury of posterior tibial artery, right leg, initial encounter ☑
S85.182A	Other specified injury of posterior tibial artery, left leg, initial encounter ☑
S85.211A	Laceration of peroneal artery, right leg, initial encounter ☑
S85.212A	Laceration of peroneal artery, left leg, initial encounter ☑
S85.291A	Other specified injury of peroneal artery, right leg, initial encounter ☑
S85.292A	Other specified injury of peroneal artery, left leg, initial encounter ☑
S85.811A	Laceration of other blood vessels at lower leg level, right leg, initial encounter ☑
S85.812A	Laceration of other blood vessels at lower leg level, left leg, initial encounter ☑
S85.891A	Other specified injury of other blood vessels at lower leg level, right leg, initial encounter ☑
S85.892A	Other specified injury of other blood vessels at lower leg level, left leg, initial encounter ☑

AMA: 35671 2012,Apr,3-9

Relative Value Units/Medicare Edits

Non-Facility RVU	Work	PE	MP	Total
35671	20.77	6.79	4.73	32.29
Facility RVU	**Work**	**PE**	**MP**	**Total**
35671	20.77	6.79	4.73	32.29

	FUD	Status	MUE	Modifiers				IOM Reference
35671	90	A	2(3)	51	50	62*	80	None

* with documentation

35681-35683

\+ **35681** Bypass graft; composite, prosthetic and vein (List separately in addition to code for primary procedure)

\+ **35682** autogenous composite, 2 segments of veins from 2 locations (List separately in addition to code for primary procedure)

\+ **35683** autogenous composite, 3 or more segments of vein from 2 or more locations (List separately in addition to code for primary procedure)

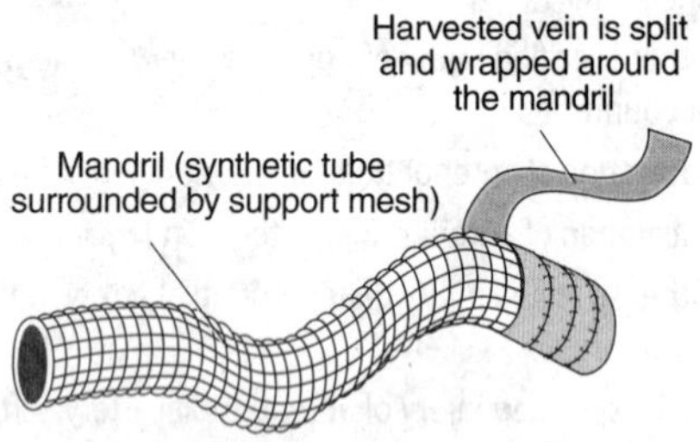

The vein material is harvested from a site distant from the site of the primary procedure

Explanation

In 35681 the physician constructs a composite graft from donor and synthetic materials. One common composite would involve the reconfiguring of a harvested vein into a length of larger diameter graft material. The harvested vein would be split lengthwise and wrapped in a spiral and sutured around a larger diameter mandrill. This length of composite graft would be used to complete the primary procedure. In 35682 a graft is constructed using tissue acquired from two veins at separate locations in the patient's body for the transplantation. In 35683 a graft is constructed using three or more segments of vein from two or more locations in the patient's body. In all three procedures veins are harvested by making an incision over the site where the vein will be removed. Tissues are dissected down to the vein and the vein is released from surrounding tissues. The vein is tied off above and below the area of vein that is to be removed. The vein is removed. The wound is closed with layered sutures. The portion of vein(s) removed is prepared for use in a separately reportable bypass graft procedure.

Coding Tips

Report 35682 and 35683 in addition to 35556, 35566, 35570, 35571, and 35583–35587. Codes 35682–35683 should be reported only when two or more vein segments are harvested from a site distant to the site of the arterial bypass graft. Do not report 35681 with 35682 or 35683; do not report 35682 with 35681 or 35683; do not report 35683 with 35681 or 35682. For harvest of a single upper extremity vein segment for lower extremity bypass, see 35500.

ICD-10-CM Diagnostic Codes

This/these CPT code(s) are add on code(s). See the primary procedure code that this code is performed with for your ICD-10-CM code selections.

AMA: 35681 2018,Jan,8; 2017,Jan,8; 2016,Jan,13; 2015,Jan,16; 2014,Jan,11 **35682** 2018,Jan,8; 2017,Jan,8; 2016,Jan,13; 2015,Jan,16; 2014,Jan,11 **35683** 2018,Jan,8; 2017,Jan,8; 2016,Jan,13; 2015,Jan,16; 2014,Jan,11

Relative Value Units/Medicare Edits

Non-Facility RVU	Work	PE	MP	Total
35681	1.6	0.38	0.36	2.34
35682	7.19	1.41	1.62	10.22
35683	8.49	1.39	1.95	11.83
Facility RVU	**Work**	**PE**	**MP**	**Total**
35681	1.6	0.38	0.36	2.34
35682	7.19	1.41	1.62	10.22
35683	8.49	1.39	1.95	11.83

	FUD	Status	MUE	Modifiers				IOM Reference
35681	N/A	A	1(3)	N/A	N/A	62*	80	None
35682	N/A	A	1(2)	N/A	N/A	62*	80*	
35683	N/A	A	1(2)	N/A	N/A	62*	80*	

* with documentation

Terms To Know

atherosclerosis. Buildup of yellowish plaques composed of cholesterol and lipoid material within the arteries.

autogenous transplant. Tissue, such as bone, that is harvested from the patient and used for transplantation back into the same patient.

bypass graft. Surgically created alternative blood vessel used to reroute blood flow around an area of obstruction or disease.

dissection. Separating by cutting tissue or body structures apart.

graft. Tissue implant from another part of the body or another person.

harvest. Removal of cells or tissue from their native site to be used as a graft or transplant to another part of the donor's body or placed into another person.

incision. Act of cutting into tissue or an organ.

prosthesis. Man-made substitute for a missing body part.

transplantation. Grafting or movement of an organ or tissue from one site or person to another.

venous. Relating to the veins.

35685

+ **35685** Placement of vein patch or cuff at distal anastomosis of bypass graft, synthetic conduit (List separately in addition to code for primary procedure)

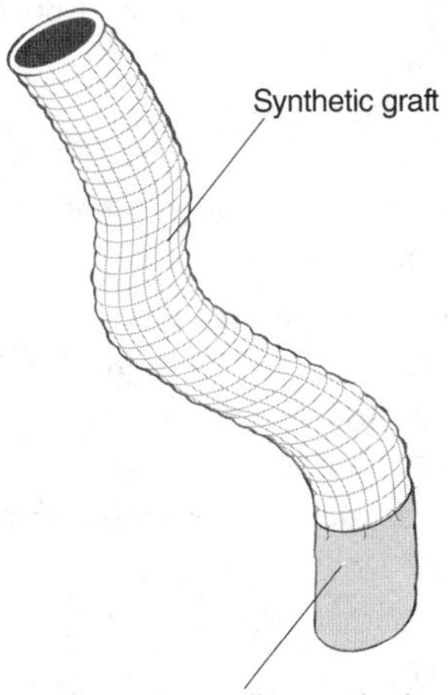

A vein patch or cuff is attached to the distal end of a synthetic graft

Explanation

The physician places a vein patch or cuff at a distal arterial anastomosis site during a bypass graft, synthetic conduit procedure of the lower extremity. The physician harvests the vein to be used for the vein patch from a previously chosen site. The vein patch is positioned and anastomosed between the distal portion of the synthetic vein graft and the native artery, end-to-end or side-to-end. The physician returns to the bypass graft surgery having performed this additional procedure.

Coding Tips

Report 35685 in addition to 35656, 35666, or 35671.

ICD-10-CM Diagnostic Codes

This/these CPT code(s) are add on code(s). See the primary procedure code that this code is performed with for your ICD-10-CM code selections. Diagnostic code(s) would be the same as the actual procedure performed.

AMA: **35685** 2018,Jan,8; 2017,Jan,8; 2016,Jan,13; 2015,Jan,16; 2014,Jan,11

Relative Value Units/Medicare Edits

Non-Facility RVU	Work	PE	MP	Total
35685	4.04	0.79	0.93	5.76
Facility RVU	**Work**	**PE**	**MP**	**Total**
35685	4.04	0.79	0.93	5.76

	FUD	Status	MUE	Modifiers				IOM Reference
35685	N/A	A	2(3)	N/A	N/A	62*	80	None

* with documentation

35686

+ **35686** Creation of distal arteriovenous fistula during lower extremity bypass surgery (non-hemodialysis) (List separately in addition to code for primary procedure)

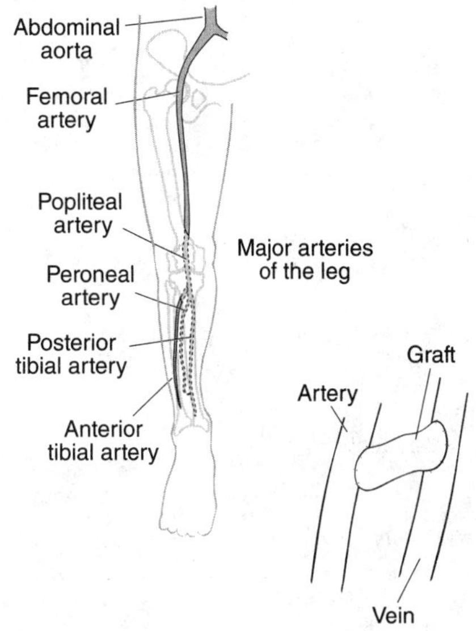

Explanation

The physician creates a fistula between an artery and vein during a lower extremity bypass procedure. The physician harvests the vein to be used for creation of the fistula from a previously chosen site. The vein is anastomosed between the tibial or peroneal artery and a vein at or beyond the distal bypass anastomosis site. The physician returns to the bypass graft surgery having performed this adjuvant (additional) procedure.

Coding Tips

Report 35686 in addition to 35556, 35566, 35570, 35571, 35583–35587, 35623, 35656, 35666, or 35671.

ICD-10-CM Diagnostic Codes

This/these CPT code(s) are add on code(s). See the primary procedure code that this code is performed with for your ICD-10-CM code selections. Diagnostic code(s) would be the same as the actual procedure performed.

AMA: **35686** 2018,Jan,8; 2017,Jan,8; 2016,Jan,13; 2015,Jan,16; 2014,Jan,11

Relative Value Units/Medicare Edits

Non-Facility RVU	Work	PE	MP	Total
35686	3.34	0.55	0.77	4.66
Facility RVU	**Work**	**PE**	**MP**	**Total**
35686	3.34	0.55	0.77	4.66

	FUD	Status	MUE	Modifiers				IOM Reference
35686	N/A	A	1(3)	N/A	N/A	62*	80	None

* with documentation

35691

35691 Transposition and/or reimplantation; vertebral to carotid artery

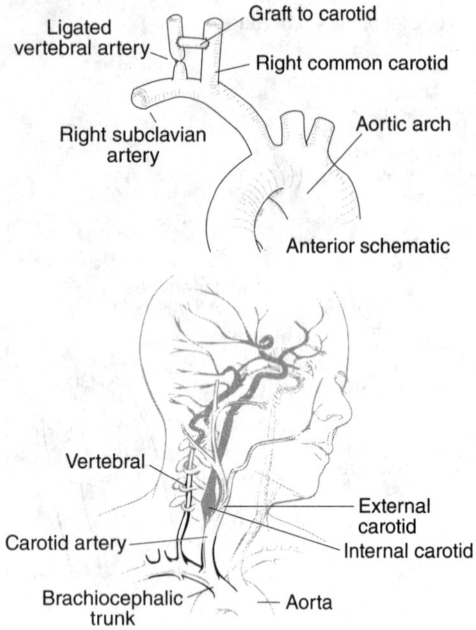

Explanation

The physician performs a supraclavicular incision and exposes the vertebral and carotid arteries by careful dissection. The adventitia of the chosen translocation site in the posterolateral wall of the common carotid artery is cleared. The physician anticoagulates the patient with heparin and divides the vertebral artery above the stenotic area. The proximal vertebral stump is ligated with sutures and a small arteriotomy in the common carotid arterial wall with an aortic punch is performed. The vertebral artery is attached using an end-to-side anastomosis to the carotid artery. The physician may perform arteriography or use a Doppler probe to establish patency of the graft. The supraclavicular wound is closed, leaving a drain in place.

Coding Tips

Establishing both inflow and outflow by any method is included. That portion of the operative arteriogram performed by the surgeon is also included. Angioscopy performed during therapeutic intervention should be reported in addition to the code for the primary procedure, see 35400.

ICD-10-CM Diagnostic Codes

G45.0	Vertebro-basilar artery syndrome
I63.011	Cerebral infarction due to thrombosis of right vertebral artery ☑
I63.012	Cerebral infarction due to thrombosis of left vertebral artery ☑
I63.013	Cerebral infarction due to thrombosis of bilateral vertebral arteries ☑
I63.033	Cerebral infarction due to thrombosis of bilateral carotid arteries ☑
I63.111	Cerebral infarction due to embolism of right vertebral artery ☑
I63.112	Cerebral infarction due to embolism of left vertebral artery ☑
I63.113	Cerebral infarction due to embolism of bilateral vertebral arteries ☑
I63.133	Cerebral infarction due to embolism of bilateral carotid arteries ☑
I63.211	Cerebral infarction due to unspecified occlusion or stenosis of right vertebral artery ☑
I63.212	Cerebral infarction due to unspecified occlusion or stenosis of left vertebral artery ☑
I63.213	Cerebral infarction due to unspecified occlusion or stenosis of bilateral vertebral arteries ☑
I63.233	Cerebral infarction due to unspecified occlusion or stenosis of bilateral carotid arteries ☑
I63.313	Cerebral infarction due to thrombosis of bilateral middle cerebral arteries ☑
I63.323	Cerebral infarction due to thrombosis of bilateral anterior cerebral arteries ☑
I63.333	Cerebral infarction due to thrombosis of bilateral posterior cerebral arteries ☑
I63.343	Cerebral infarction due to thrombosis of bilateral cerebellar arteries ☑
I63.413	Cerebral infarction due to embolism of bilateral middle cerebral arteries ☑
I63.423	Cerebral infarction due to embolism of bilateral anterior cerebral arteries ☑
I63.433	Cerebral infarction due to embolism of bilateral posterior cerebral arteries ☑
I63.443	Cerebral infarction due to embolism of bilateral cerebellar arteries ☑
I65.01	Occlusion and stenosis of right vertebral artery ☑
I65.02	Occlusion and stenosis of left vertebral artery ☑
I65.03	Occlusion and stenosis of bilateral vertebral arteries ☑
I76	Septic arterial embolism
I77.1	Stricture of artery
I77.2	Rupture of artery
I77.74	Dissection of vertebral artery
I77.89	Other specified disorders of arteries and arterioles
S15.111A	Minor laceration of right vertebral artery, initial encounter ☑
S15.112A	Minor laceration of left vertebral artery, initial encounter ☑
S15.121A	Major laceration of right vertebral artery, initial encounter ☑
S15.122A	Major laceration of left vertebral artery, initial encounter ☑
S15.191A	Other specified injury of right vertebral artery, initial encounter ☑
S15.192A	Other specified injury of left vertebral artery, initial encounter ☑

AMA: 35691 1997,Nov,1

Relative Value Units/Medicare Edits

Non-Facility RVU	Work	PE	MP	Total
35691	18.41	4.61	4.25	27.27
Facility RVU	**Work**	**PE**	**MP**	**Total**
35691	18.41	4.61	4.25	27.27

	FUD	Status	MUE	Modifiers				IOM Reference
35691	90	A	1(3)	51	50	62*	80	None

* with documentation

Terms To Know

adventitia. Outermost layer of connective tissue covering an organ or other tissue.

35693

35693 Transposition and/or reimplantation; vertebral to subclavian artery

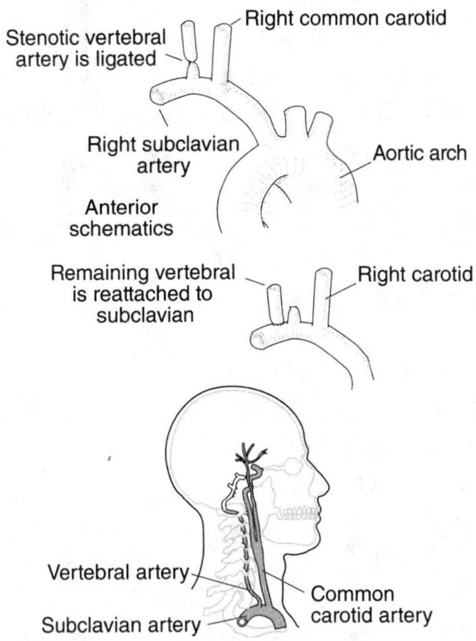

Explanation

The physician performs a supraclavicular incision and exposes the vertebral and subclavian arteries by careful dissection. The adventitia of the chosen translocation site in the subclavian artery lateral to the thyrocervical trunk is cleared. The physician anticoagulates the patient with heparin and divides the vertebral artery above the stenotic area. The proximal vertebral stump is ligated with sutures and a small arteriotomy is made in the subclavian artery wall with an aortic punch. The vertebral artery is attached using an end-to-side anastomosis to the subclavian artery. The physician may perform arteriography or use a Doppler probe to establish patency of the graft. The supraclavicular wound is closed, leaving a drain in place.

Coding Tips

Establishing both inflow and outflow by any method is included. That portion of the operative arteriogram performed by the surgeon is also included. Angioscopy performed during therapeutic intervention should be reported in addition to the code for the primary procedure, see 35400.

ICD-10-CM Diagnostic Codes

G45.0	Vertebro-basilar artery syndrome
I63.011	Cerebral infarction due to thrombosis of right vertebral artery ☑
I63.012	Cerebral infarction due to thrombosis of left vertebral artery ☑
I63.013	Cerebral infarction due to thrombosis of bilateral vertebral arteries ☑
I63.033	Cerebral infarction due to thrombosis of bilateral carotid arteries ☑
I63.111	Cerebral infarction due to embolism of right vertebral artery ☑
I63.112	Cerebral infarction due to embolism of left vertebral artery ☑
I63.113	Cerebral infarction due to embolism of bilateral vertebral arteries ☑
I63.133	Cerebral infarction due to embolism of bilateral carotid arteries ☑
I63.211	Cerebral infarction due to unspecified occlusion or stenosis of right vertebral artery ☑
I63.212	Cerebral infarction due to unspecified occlusion or stenosis of left vertebral artery ☑
I63.213	Cerebral infarction due to unspecified occlusion or stenosis of bilateral vertebral arteries ☑
I63.233	Cerebral infarction due to unspecified occlusion or stenosis of bilateral carotid arteries ☑
I63.313	Cerebral infarction due to thrombosis of bilateral middle cerebral arteries ☑
I63.323	Cerebral infarction due to thrombosis of bilateral anterior cerebral arteries ☑
I63.333	Cerebral infarction due to thrombosis of bilateral posterior cerebral arteries ☑
I63.343	Cerebral infarction due to thrombosis of bilateral cerebellar arteries ☑
I63.413	Cerebral infarction due to embolism of bilateral middle cerebral arteries ☑
I63.423	Cerebral infarction due to embolism of bilateral anterior cerebral arteries ☑
I63.433	Cerebral infarction due to embolism of bilateral posterior cerebral arteries ☑
I63.443	Cerebral infarction due to embolism of bilateral cerebellar arteries ☑
I63.81	Other cerebral infarction due to occlusion or stenosis of small artery
I63.89	Other cerebral infarction
I65.01	Occlusion and stenosis of right vertebral artery ☑
I65.02	Occlusion and stenosis of left vertebral artery ☑
I65.03	Occlusion and stenosis of bilateral vertebral arteries ☑
I76	Septic arterial embolism
I77.1	Stricture of artery
I77.2	Rupture of artery
I77.74	Dissection of vertebral artery
I77.89	Other specified disorders of arteries and arterioles
S15.111A	Minor laceration of right vertebral artery, initial encounter ☑
S15.112A	Minor laceration of left vertebral artery, initial encounter ☑
S15.121A	Major laceration of right vertebral artery, initial encounter ☑
S15.122A	Major laceration of left vertebral artery, initial encounter ☑
S15.191A	Other specified injury of right vertebral artery, initial encounter ☑
S15.192A	Other specified injury of left vertebral artery, initial encounter ☑

AMA: **35693** 1997,Nov,1

Relative Value Units/Medicare Edits

Non-Facility RVU	Work	PE	MP	Total
35693	15.73	4.68	3.64	24.05
Facility RVU	**Work**	**PE**	**MP**	**Total**
35693	15.73	4.68	3.64	24.05

	FUD	Status	MUE	Modifiers				IOM Reference
35693	90	A	1(3)	51	50	62*	80	None

* with documentation

Terms To Know

transposition. Removal or exchange from one side to another; change of position from one place to another.

35694

35694 Transposition and/or reimplantation; subclavian to carotid artery

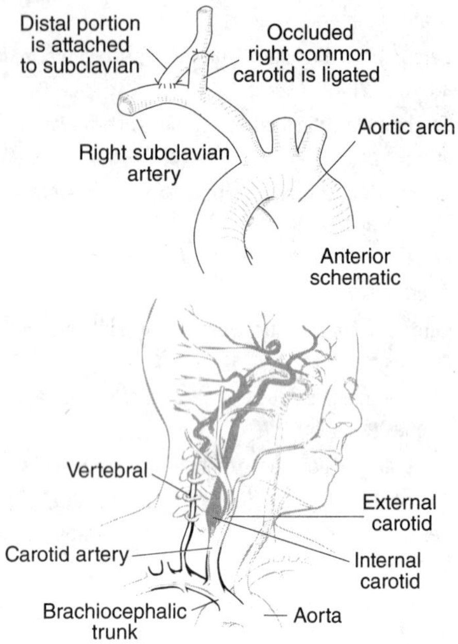

Explanation

The physician performs a supraclavicular incision and exposes the carotid and subclavian arteries by careful dissection. The adventitia of the chosen translocation site in the posterolateral wall of the common carotid artery is cleared. The physician anticoagulates the patient's blood with heparin and divides the subclavian artery distal to the stenotic area. The proximal subclavian stump is ligated with sutures and a small arteriotomy in the common carotid artery wall is performed with an aortic punch. The subclavian artery is attached using an end-to-side anastomosis to the carotid artery. The physician may perform arteriography or use a Doppler probe to establish patency of the graft. The supraclavicular wound is closed, leaving a drain in place.

Coding Tips

Establishing both inflow and outflow by any method is included. That portion of the operative arteriogram performed by the surgeon is also included. Angioscopy performed during therapeutic intervention should be reported in addition to the code for the primary procedure; see 35400. For an open subclavian to carotid artery transposition performed in conjuntion with an endovascular repair of the descending aorta, see 33889. For a bypass graft completed with a harvested vein, subclavian to carotid, see 35506.

ICD-10-CM Diagnostic Codes

G45.1	Carotid artery syndrome (hemispheric)
G45.2	Multiple and bilateral precerebral artery syndromes
G45.3	Amaurosis fugax
G45.8	Other transient cerebral ischemic attacks and related syndromes
G45.9	Transient cerebral ischemic attack, unspecified
I63.031	Cerebral infarction due to thrombosis of right carotid artery ☑
I63.032	Cerebral infarction due to thrombosis of left carotid artery ☑
I63.131	Cerebral infarction due to embolism of right carotid artery ☑
I63.132	Cerebral infarction due to embolism of left carotid artery ☑
I63.231	Cerebral infarction due to unspecified occlusion or stenosis of right carotid arteries ☑
I63.232	Cerebral infarction due to unspecified occlusion or stenosis of left carotid arteries ☑
I63.81	Other cerebral infarction due to occlusion or stenosis of small artery
I63.89	Other cerebral infarction
I65.21	Occlusion and stenosis of right carotid artery ☑
I65.22	Occlusion and stenosis of left carotid artery ☑
I65.23	Occlusion and stenosis of bilateral carotid arteries ☑
I67.81	Acute cerebrovascular insufficiency
I67.82	Cerebral ischemia
I67.850	Cerebral autosomal dominant arteriopathy with subcortical infarcts and leukoencephalopathy
I67.858	Other hereditary cerebrovascular disease
I67.89	Other cerebrovascular disease
I72.0	Aneurysm of carotid artery
I72.6	Aneurysm of vertebral artery
I72.8	Aneurysm of other specified arteries
I77.1	Stricture of artery
I77.2	Rupture of artery
I77.71	Dissection of carotid artery
I77.76	Dissection of artery of upper extremity
I77.89	Other specified disorders of arteries and arterioles
S15.011A	Minor laceration of right carotid artery, initial encounter ☑
S15.012A	Minor laceration of left carotid artery, initial encounter ☑
S15.021A	Major laceration of right carotid artery, initial encounter ☑
S15.022A	Major laceration of left carotid artery, initial encounter ☑
S15.091A	Other specified injury of right carotid artery, initial encounter ☑
S15.092A	Other specified injury of left carotid artery, initial encounter ☑
S15.8XXA	Injury of other specified blood vessels at neck level, initial encounter

AMA: **35694** 1997,Nov,1

Relative Value Units/Medicare Edits

Non-Facility RVU	Work	PE	MP	Total
35694	19.28	4.76	4.46	28.5
Facility RVU	**Work**	**PE**	**MP**	**Total**
35694	19.28	4.76	4.46	28.5

	FUD	Status	MUE	Modifiers				IOM Reference
35694	90	A	1(3)	51	50	62*	80	None

* with documentation

Terms To Know

adventitia. Outermost layer of connective tissue covering an organ or other tissue.

amaurosis fugax. Carotid artery plaque that breaks free and moves to the retinal artery causing decreased blood to the retina and temporary loss of vision. Frequently occurs prior to a stroke.

anastomosis. Surgically created connection between ducts, blood vessels, or bowel segments to allow flow from one to the other.

infarction. Area of necrosis in tissue, due to ischemia from lack of circulation, usually from a thrombus or an embolus.

35695

35695 Transposition and/or reimplantation; carotid to subclavian artery

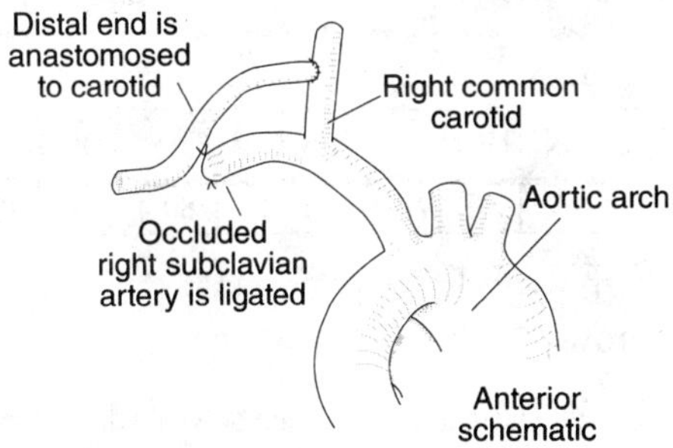

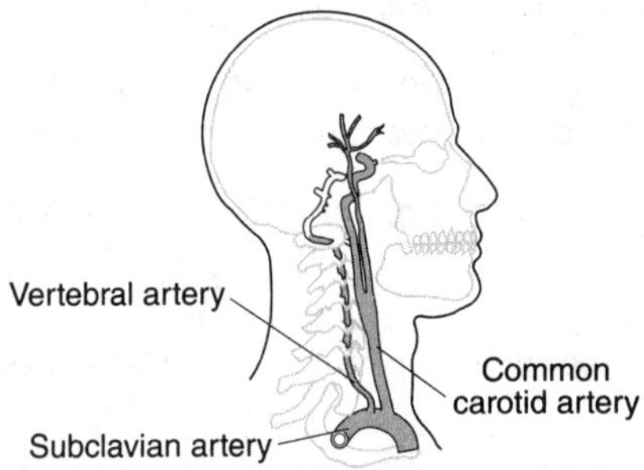

Explanation

The physician performs a supraclavicular incision and exposes the carotid and subclavian arteries by careful dissection. The adventitia of the chosen translocation site in the subclavian artery lateral to the thyrocervical trunk is cleared. The physician anticoagulates the patient's blood with heparin and divides the carotid artery above the stenotic area. The proximal carotid stump is ligated with sutures and a small arteriotomy in the subclavian artery wall is made with an aortic punch. The carotid artery is attached using an end-to-side anastomosis to the subclavian artery. The physician may perform arteriography or use a Doppler probe to establish patency of the graft. The supraclavicular wound is closed, leaving a drain in place.

Coding Tips

Establishing both inflow and outflow by any method is included. That portion of the operative arteriogram performed by the surgeon is also included. Angioscopy performed during therapeutic intervention should be reported in addition to the code for the primary procedure; see 35400. For a bypass graft completed with a harvested vein, carotid to subclavian, see 35506. For a synthetic bypass graft, carotid to subclavian, see 35606.

ICD-10-CM Diagnostic Codes

G45.2 Multiple and bilateral precerebral artery syndromes
G45.3 Amaurosis fugax
G45.8 Other transient cerebral ischemic attacks and related syndromes
I63.09 Cerebral infarction due to thrombosis of other precerebral artery
I63.19 Cerebral infarction due to embolism of other precerebral artery
I63.81 Other cerebral infarction due to occlusion or stenosis of small artery
I63.89 Other cerebral infarction
I65.8 Occlusion and stenosis of other precerebral arteries
I67.81 Acute cerebrovascular insufficiency
I67.850 Cerebral autosomal dominant arteriopathy with subcortical infarcts and leukoencephalopathy
I67.858 Other hereditary cerebrovascular disease
I70.92 Chronic total occlusion of artery of the extremities
I72.1 Aneurysm of artery of upper extremity
I72.6 Aneurysm of vertebral artery
I72.8 Aneurysm of other specified arteries
I74.2 Embolism and thrombosis of arteries of the upper extremities
I74.8 Embolism and thrombosis of other arteries
I75.011 Atheroembolism of right upper extremity ☑
I75.012 Atheroembolism of left upper extremity ☑
I75.013 Atheroembolism of bilateral upper extremities ☑
I77.1 Stricture of artery
I77.2 Rupture of artery
I77.5 Necrosis of artery
I77.79 Dissection of other specified artery
I77.89 Other specified disorders of arteries and arterioles
S15.8XXA Injury of other specified blood vessels at neck level, initial encounter
S25.111A Minor laceration of right innominate or subclavian artery, initial encounter ☑
S25.112A Minor laceration of left innominate or subclavian artery, initial encounter ☑
S25.121A Major laceration of right innominate or subclavian artery, initial encounter ☑
S25.122A Major laceration of left innominate or subclavian artery, initial encounter ☑
S25.191A Other specified injury of right innominate or subclavian artery, initial encounter ☑
S25.192A Other specified injury of left innominate or subclavian artery, initial encounter ☑

AMA: **35695** 1997,Nov,1

Relative Value Units/Medicare Edits

Non-Facility RVU	Work	PE	MP	Total
35695	20.06	4.88	4.63	29.57
Facility RVU	**Work**	**PE**	**MP**	**Total**
35695	20.06	4.88	4.63	29.57

	FUD	Status	MUE	Modifiers				IOM Reference
35695	90	A	1(3)	51	50	62*	80	None

* with documentation

Terms To Know

adventitia. Outermost layer of connective tissue covering an organ or other tissue.

anastomosis. Surgically created connection between ducts, blood vessels, or bowel segments to allow flow from one to the other.

angioscopy. Visualization of capillary blood vessels with a microscope, or the inside of a blood vessel with a fiberoptic-equipped catheter.

ligate. To tie off a blood vessel or duct with a suture or a soft, thin wire (ligature wire).

35697

+ 35697 Reimplantation, visceral artery to infrarenal aortic prosthesis, each artery (List separately in addition to code for primary procedure)

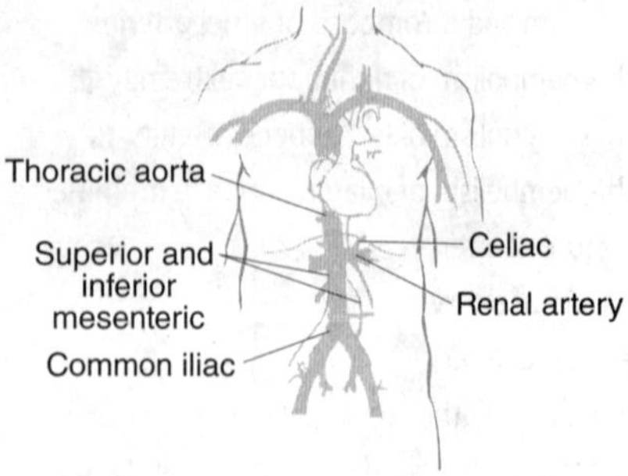

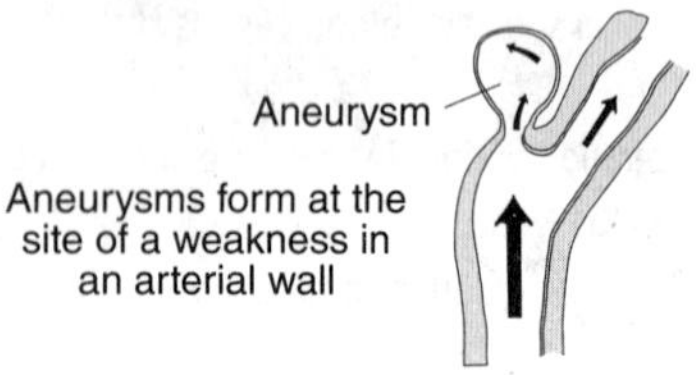

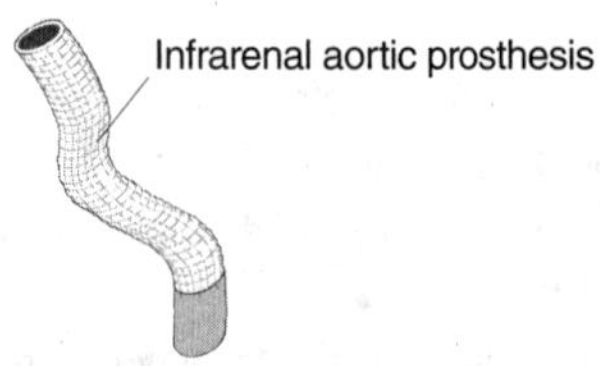

Explanation

A reimplantation of a visceral artery to an infrarenal aortic prosthesis, each artery, is done in addition to the primary procedure of an open aortic aneurysm repair (35081). This surgery is performed when a visceral artery, such as the inferior mesenteric, has been determined not to supply sufficient blood flow to vital organs, after repair of the aortic aneurysm. After the aortic prosthesis has been placed and blood flow is re-established through the aorta, the physician dissects soft tissue from around the origin of the visceral artery in the aorta where it exits. A small button-shaped patch of aortic tissue is removed from this site. Next, a clamp is placed on the aortic prosthesis at the intended site for reimplantation and a hole is cut the size of the button patch, which is anastomosed to the recipient hole in the prosthesis. The suturing is tested by removing the clamps and placing any additional sutures for complete hemostasis.

Coding Tips

Report 35697 in addition to the code for the aortic aneurysm repair (35081–35092). Do not report 35697 with 33877.

ICD-10-CM Diagnostic Codes

This/these CPT code(s) are add on code(s). See the primary procedure code that this code is performed with for your ICD-10-CM code selections.

AMA: 35697 1997,Nov,1

Relative Value Units/Medicare Edits

Non-Facility RVU	Work	PE	MP	Total
35697	3.0	0.61	0.69	4.3
Facility RVU	**Work**	**PE**	**MP**	**Total**
35697	3.0	0.61	0.69	4.3

	FUD	Status	MUE	Modifiers				IOM Reference
35697	N/A	A	2(3)	N/A	N/A	62	80	None

* with documentation

Terms To Know

anastomosis. Surgically created connection between ducts, blood vessels, or bowel segments to allow flow from one to the other.

aneurysm. Circumscribed dilation or outpouching of an artery wall, often containing blood clots and connecting directly with the lumen of the artery.

clamp. Tool used to grip, compress, join, or fasten body parts.

dissection. Separating by cutting tissue or body structures apart.

hemostasis. Interruption of blood flow or the cessation or arrest of bleeding.

prosthesis. Man-made substitute for a missing body part.

reimplant. Reinsert or reattach tissue.

suture. Numerous stitching techniques employed in wound closure.

35700

+ **35700** Reoperation, femoral-popliteal or femoral (popliteal)-anterior tibial, posterior tibial, peroneal artery, or other distal vessels, more than 1 month after original operation (List separately in addition to code for primary procedure)

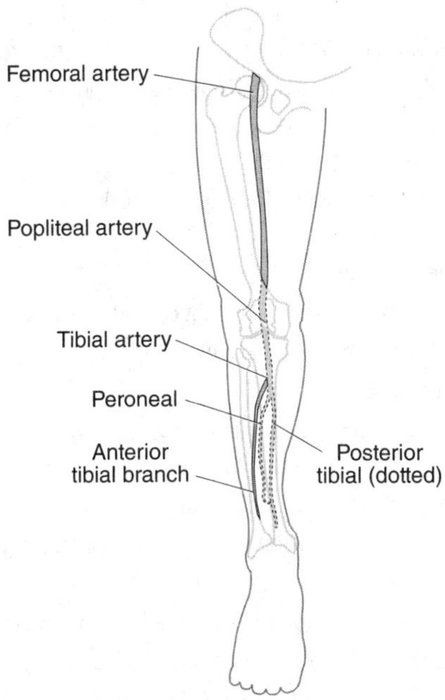

Original grafts may require replacement or patency testing with balloon catheter

Explanation

This code is only used with other codes to identify the reoperation aspect of this procedure, which usually requires more effort when performed again. Through incisions in the skin of the leg, overlying the affected artery, the physician isolates the graft. The physician makes an incision in the proximal portion of the graft and passes a Fogarty balloon catheter through the graft to clear and straighten it. If an arteriograph indicates the graft must be replaced, the physician makes a second incision distal to the inguinal incision, releases the graft, and places vein clamps above and below the stricture. The physician replaces the graft by suturing the ends of a new graft to the side of the arteries to form a bypass of the damaged area. The clamps are removed. After the stricture is controlled or the graft is otherwise complete, the incisions are repaired with layered closures.

Coding Tips

Report 35700 in addition to 35556, 35566, 35570, 35571, 35583, 35585, 35587, 35656, 35666, and 35671. This code is used instead of modifier 22.

ICD-10-CM Diagnostic Codes

This/these CPT code(s) are add on code(s). See the primary procedure code that this code is performed with for your ICD-10-CM code selections. Diagnostic code(s) would be the same as the actual procedure performed.

AMA: 35700 2018,Jan,8; 2017,Jan,8; 2016,Jan,13; 2015,Jan,16; 2014,Jan,11

Relative Value Units/Medicare Edits

Non-Facility RVU	Work	PE	MP	Total
35700	3.08	0.64	0.7	4.42
Facility RVU	**Work**	**PE**	**MP**	**Total**
35700	3.08	0.64	0.7	4.42

	FUD	Status	MUE	Modifiers				IOM Reference
35700	N/A	A	2(3)	N/A	N/A	62*	80	None

* with documentation

Terms To Know

anterior. Situated in the front area or toward the belly surface of the body; an anatomical reference point used to show the position and relationship of one body structure to another.

artery. Vessel through which oxygenated blood passes away from the heart to any part of the body.

bypass. Auxiliary or diverted route to maintain continuous flow.

catheter. Flexible tube inserted into an area of the body for introducing or withdrawing fluid.

distal. Located farther away from a specified reference point or the trunk.

graft. Tissue implant from another part of the body or another person.

incision. Act of cutting into tissue or an organ.

proximal. Located closest to a specified reference point, usually the midline or trunk.

suture. Numerous stitching techniques employed in wound closure.

35701-35703

▲ **35701** Exploration not followed by surgical repair, artery; neck (eg, carotid, subclavian)

● **35702** upper extremity (eg, axillary, brachial, radial, ulnar)

● **35703** lower extremity (eg, common femoral, deep femoral, superficial femoral, popliteal, tibial, peroneal)

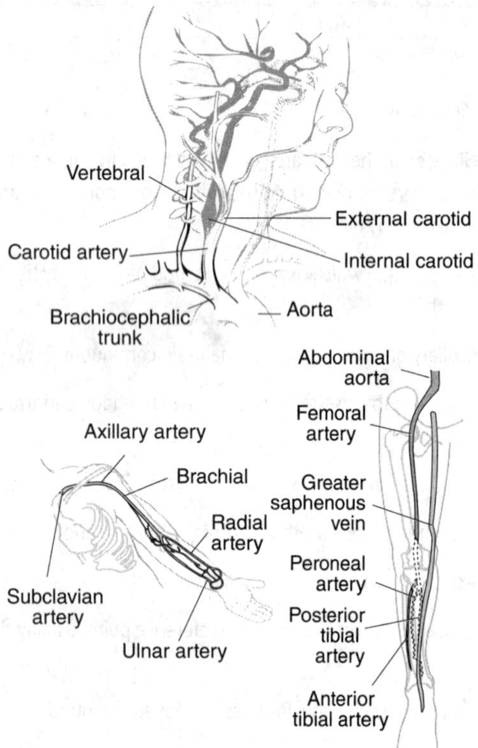

Select vascularity of the right leg

Explanation

Through an incision in the skin overlying the targeted artery, the physician dissects around surrounding structures as necessary to access the artery, freeing it so it can be examined. The artery is released from any surrounding scar tissue that may be compressing it. Finding no perforations or other signs of injury, the physician repairs the skin incision with a layered closure. Report 35701 for exploration of arteries of the neck (e.g., carotid or subclavian); 35702 for those of the upper extremity (e.g., axillary, brachial, radial, or ulnar); and 35703 for those of the lower extremity (e.g., common, deep, or superficial femoral, peroneal, popliteal, or tibial).

Coding Tips

Additional surgical procedures may only be reported if the artery exploration is performed through a separate incision. If the carotid artery is examined through the same incision used for a procedure performed during the same operative session, the exploration is not reported. If the carotid artery is examined and a defect is discovered and repaired, report the repair, not the exploration. Do not report 35702-35703 with 35206, 35207, 35236, 35256, 35266, 35286, or 35860 in the same extremity. For vascular exploration of the chest not followed by surgical repair, see 32100; of the abdomen, see 49000. For an exploration for postoperative hemorrhage, thrombosis, or infection of the neck, see 35800. For excision of an infected graft of the neck, see 35901. For exploration for postoperative hemorrhage, thrombosis, or infection, see 35860. If the procedure is completed through an operating microscope, report 69990 in addition to the primary procedure. However, head gear (e.g., loupes or binoculars) is considered an integral part of this procedure.

ICD-10-CM Diagnostic Codes

G45.1	Carotid artery syndrome (hemispheric)
G45.3	Amaurosis fugax
G45.8	Other transient cerebral ischemic attacks and related syndromes
G45.9	Transient cerebral ischemic attack, unspecified
I63.031	Cerebral infarction due to thrombosis of right carotid artery ☑
I63.131	Cerebral infarction due to embolism of right carotid artery ☑
I63.231	Cerebral infarction due to unspecified occlusion or stenosis of right carotid arteries ☑
I63.81	Other cerebral infarction due to occlusion or stenosis of small artery
I63.89	Other cerebral infarction
I65.21	Occlusion and stenosis of right carotid artery ☑
I67.81	Acute cerebrovascular insufficiency
I67.82	Cerebral ischemia
I67.850	Cerebral autosomal dominant arteriopathy with subcortical infarcts and leukoencephalopathy
I67.858	Other hereditary cerebrovascular disease
I70.92	Chronic total occlusion of artery of the extremities
I73.89	Other specified peripheral vascular diseases
I74.2	Embolism and thrombosis of arteries of the upper extremities
I74.3	Embolism and thrombosis of arteries of the lower extremities
I75.011	Atheroembolism of right upper extremity ☑
I76	Septic arterial embolism
I77.1	Stricture of artery
I77.2	Rupture of artery
I77.71	Dissection of carotid artery
I77.76	Dissection of artery of upper extremity
I77.77	Dissection of artery of lower extremity
I77.89	Other specified disorders of arteries and arterioles
I79.8	Other disorders of arteries, arterioles and capillaries in diseases classified elsewhere
S15.011A	Minor laceration of right carotid artery, initial encounter ☑
S15.021A	Major laceration of right carotid artery, initial encounter ☑
S15.091A	Other specified injury of right carotid artery, initial encounter ☑
S15.8XXA	Injury of other specified blood vessels at neck level, initial encounter
S17.8XXA	Crushing injury of other specified parts of neck, initial encounter
S45.011A	Laceration of axillary artery, right side, initial encounter ☑
S45.091A	Other specified injury of axillary artery, right side, initial encounter ☑
S45.111A	Laceration of brachial artery, right side, initial encounter ☑
S45.191A	Other specified injury of brachial artery, right side, initial encounter ☑
S55.011A	Laceration of ulnar artery at forearm level, right arm, initial encounter ☑
S55.091A	Other specified injury of ulnar artery at forearm level, right arm, initial encounter ☑
S55.111A	Laceration of radial artery at forearm level, right arm, initial encounter ☑
S55.191A	Other specified injury of radial artery at forearm level, right arm, initial encounter ☑

S65.011A Laceration of ulnar artery at wrist and hand level of right arm, initial encounter ☑

S65.091A Other specified injury of ulnar artery at wrist and hand level of right arm, initial encounter ☑

S65.111A Laceration of radial artery at wrist and hand level of right arm, initial encounter ☑

S65.191A Other specified injury of radial artery at wrist and hand level of right arm, initial encounter ☑

S75.001A Unspecified injury of femoral artery, right leg, initial encounter ☑

S75.011A Minor laceration of femoral artery, right leg, initial encounter ☑

S75.021A Major laceration of femoral artery, right leg, initial encounter ☑

S75.091A Other specified injury of femoral artery, right leg, initial encounter ☑

S85.011A Laceration of popliteal artery, right leg, initial encounter ☑

S85.091A Other specified injury of popliteal artery, right leg, initial encounter ☑

S85.111A Laceration of unspecified tibial artery, right leg, initial encounter ☑

S85.121A Other specified injury of unspecified tibial artery, right leg, initial encounter ☑

S85.141A Laceration of anterior tibial artery, right leg, initial encounter ☑

S85.151A Other specified injury of anterior tibial artery, right leg, initial encounter ☑

S85.171A Laceration of posterior tibial artery, right leg, initial encounter ☑

S85.181A Other specified injury of posterior tibial artery, right leg, initial encounter ☑

S85.211A Laceration of peroneal artery, right leg, initial encounter ☑

S85.291A Other specified injury of peroneal artery, right leg, initial encounter ☑

AMA: 35701 1997,Nov,1

Relative Value Units/Medicare Edits

Non-Facility RVU	Work	PE	MP	Total
35701	9.19	5.61	1.6	16.4
35702				
35703				

Facility RVU	Work	PE	MP	Total
35701	9.19	5.61	1.6	16.4
35702				
35703				

	FUD	Status	MUE	Modifiers				IOM Reference
35701	90	A	1(2)	51	50	62*	80	None
35702	N/A		-	N/A	N/A	N/A	N/A	
35703	N/A		-	N/A	N/A	N/A	N/A	

* with documentation

Terms To Know

dissect. Cut apart or separate tissue for surgical purposes or for visual or microscopic study.

stenosis. Narrowing or constriction of a passage.

35800

35800 Exploration for postoperative hemorrhage, thrombosis or infection; neck

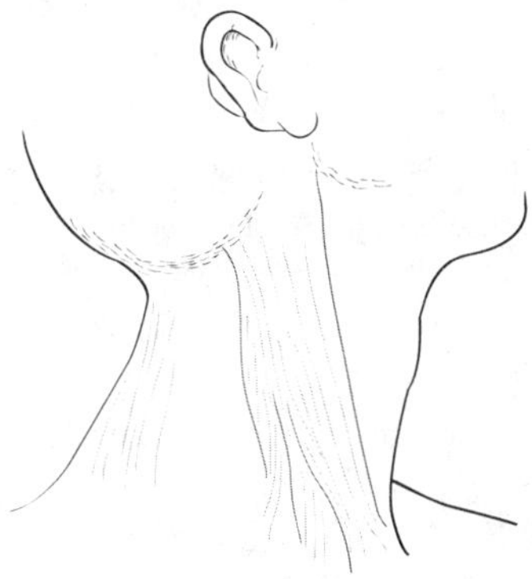

The physician makes an incision in the neck to explore a suspect vessel or to determine where blood loss, clot, or infection is coming from in an attempt to resolve postsurgical complication

Explanation

Through an incision in the neck over the affected area, the physician isolates the vessel and explores it for postoperative complications such as hemorrhage, thrombosis, or infection. The physician dissects any adjacent critical structures as necessary to access the vessel. The complication is identified and corrected. A hemorrhage is controlled by ligation or suture repair of the artery. Thrombosis requires opening of the artery and the removal of the clot. Any infection is drained, and sometimes a temporary tube is placed so the infection can continue to drain. The physician sutures the skin incision with a layered closure once the postsurgical complication has been treated.

Coding Tips

This code is used to report exploration for postoperative hemorrhage, thrombosis, or infection complications of veins and arteries of the neck only, including correction of the problem. For exploration of a vessel (not followed by surgical repair), of the carotid, or for exploration of other vessels of the neck when no other procedure is performed, see 35701. For thrombectomy of an arterial or a venous graft, see 35875–35876. For excision of an infected graft of the neck, see 35901.

ICD-10-CM Diagnostic Codes

G97.51 Postprocedural hemorrhage of a nervous system organ or structure following a nervous system procedure

G97.52 Postprocedural hemorrhage of a nervous system organ or structure following other procedure

G97.61 Postprocedural hematoma of a nervous system organ or structure following a nervous system procedure

G97.62 Postprocedural hematoma of a nervous system organ or structure following other procedure

G97.63 Postprocedural seroma of a nervous system organ or structure following a nervous system procedure

G97.64 Postprocedural seroma of a nervous system organ or structure following other procedure

G97.82 Other postprocedural complications and disorders of nervous system

I77.2 Rupture of artery

I77.71 Dissection of carotid artery

I97.89	Other postprocedural complications and disorders of the circulatory system, not elsewhere classified
T79.2XXA	Traumatic secondary and recurrent hemorrhage and seroma, initial encounter
T79.8XXA	Other early complications of trauma, initial encounter
T80.211A	Bloodstream infection due to central venous catheter, initial encounter
T80.212A	Local infection due to central venous catheter, initial encounter
T80.218A	Other infection due to central venous catheter, initial encounter
T80.29XA	Infection following other infusion, transfusion and therapeutic injection, initial encounter
T81.31XA	Disruption of external operation (surgical) wound, not elsewhere classified, initial encounter
T81.32XA	Disruption of internal operation (surgical) wound, not elsewhere classified, initial encounter
T81.41XA	Infection following a procedure, superficial incisional surgical site, initial encounter
T81.42XA	Infection following a procedure, deep incisional surgical site, initial encounter
T81.43XA	Infection following a procedure, organ and space surgical site, initial encounter
T81.44XA	Sepsis following a procedure, initial encounter
T81.49XA	Infection following a procedure, other surgical site, initial encounter
T81.718A	Complication of other artery following a procedure, not elsewhere classified, initial encounter
T81.72XA	Complication of vein following a procedure, not elsewhere classified, initial encounter
T82.311A	Breakdown (mechanical) of carotid arterial graft (bypass), initial encounter
T82.318A	Breakdown (mechanical) of other vascular grafts, initial encounter
T82.321A	Displacement of carotid arterial graft (bypass), initial encounter
T82.328A	Displacement of other vascular grafts, initial encounter
T82.331A	Leakage of carotid arterial graft (bypass), initial encounter
T82.338A	Leakage of other vascular grafts, initial encounter
T82.391A	Other mechanical complication of carotid arterial graft (bypass), initial encounter
T82.398A	Other mechanical complication of other vascular grafts, initial encounter
T82.518A	Breakdown (mechanical) of other cardiac and vascular devices and implants, initial encounter
T82.528A	Displacement of other cardiac and vascular devices and implants, initial encounter
T82.538A	Leakage of other cardiac and vascular devices and implants, initial encounter
T82.598A	Other mechanical complication of other cardiac and vascular devices and implants, initial encounter
T82.7XXA	Infection and inflammatory reaction due to other cardiac and vascular devices, implants and grafts, initial encounter
T82.818A	Embolism due to vascular prosthetic devices, implants and grafts, initial encounter
T82.828A	Fibrosis due to vascular prosthetic devices, implants and grafts, initial encounter
T82.838A	Hemorrhage due to vascular prosthetic devices, implants and grafts, initial encounter
T82.848A	Pain due to vascular prosthetic devices, implants and grafts, initial encounter
T82.858A	Stenosis of other vascular prosthetic devices, implants and grafts, initial encounter
T82.868A	Thrombosis due to vascular prosthetic devices, implants and grafts, initial encounter
T82.898A	Other specified complication of vascular prosthetic devices, implants and grafts, initial encounter
T88.8XXA	Other specified complications of surgical and medical care, not elsewhere classified, initial encounter

AMA: **35800** 1997,Nov,1

Relative Value Units/Medicare Edits

Non-Facility RVU	Work	PE	MP	Total
35800	12.0	6.43	2.41	20.84
Facility RVU	**Work**	**PE**	**MP**	**Total**
35800	12.0	6.43	2.41	20.84

	FUD	Status	MUE	Modifiers				IOM Reference
35800	90	A	2(3)	51	N/A	62*	80	None

* with documentation

Terms To Know

cautery. Destruction or burning of tissue by means of a hot instrument, an electric current, or a caustic chemical, such as silver nitrate.

complication. Condition arising after the beginning of observation and treatment that modifies the course of the patient's illness or the medical care required, or an undesired result or misadventure in medical care.

exploration. Examination for diagnostic purposes.

hemorrhage. Internal or external bleeding with loss of significant amounts of blood.

infection. Presence of microorganisms in body tissues that may result in cellular damage.

thrombosis. Condition arising from the presence or formation of blood clots within a blood vessel that may cause vascular obstruction and insufficient oxygenation.

35820

35820 Exploration for postoperative hemorrhage, thrombosis or infection; chest

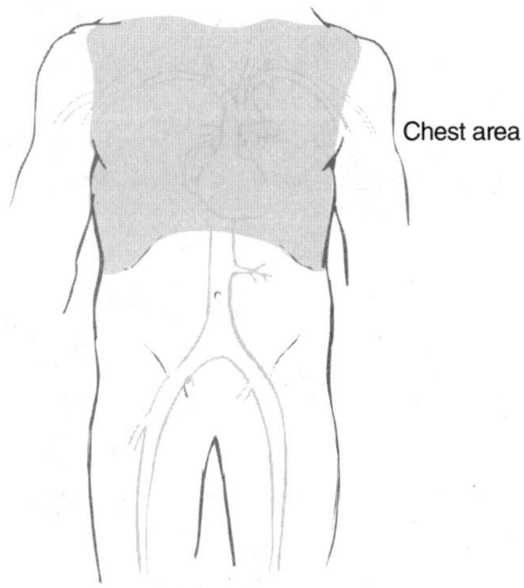

A surgical exploration is performed in the chest cavity to find and identify postoperative hemorrhage, thrombosis (clotting), or infection

Explanation

The physician reopens the original incision site and inspects the operative area for active bleeding, hematoma, thrombus, and exudate. The physician removes or debrides any observed hematoma, thrombus, and infected tissues. The physician looks for and corrects any active bleeding sites using electrocautery or ligation of bleeding vessels. The physician may leave an infected wound open, but generally closes the incision, leaving drains and chest tubes in place.

Coding Tips

This code is used to report exploration for postoperative hemorrhage, thrombosis, or infection complications of veins and arteries of the chest only, including correction of the problem. For thrombectomy of an arterial or a venous graft, see 35875–35876. For excision of an infected graft of the thorax, see 35905.

ICD-10-CM Diagnostic Codes

I26.90	Septic pulmonary embolism without acute cor pulmonale
I26.99	Other pulmonary embolism without acute cor pulmonale
I97.610	Postprocedural hemorrhage of a circulatory system organ or structure following a cardiac catheterization
I97.611	Postprocedural hemorrhage of a circulatory system organ or structure following cardiac bypass
I97.618	Postprocedural hemorrhage of a circulatory system organ or structure following other circulatory system procedure
I97.620	Postprocedural hemorrhage of a circulatory system organ or structure following other procedure
I97.621	Postprocedural hematoma of a circulatory system organ or structure following other procedure
I97.622	Postprocedural seroma of a circulatory system organ or structure following other procedure
I97.630	Postprocedural hematoma of a circulatory system organ or structure following a cardiac catheterization
I97.631	Postprocedural hematoma of a circulatory system organ or structure following cardiac bypass
I97.638	Postprocedural hematoma of a circulatory system organ or structure following other circulatory system procedure
I97.648	Postprocedural seroma of a circulatory system organ or structure following other circulatory system procedure
I97.89	Other postprocedural complications and disorders of the circulatory system, not elsewhere classified
J94.2	Hemothorax
J94.8	Other specified pleural conditions
J95.830	Postprocedural hemorrhage of a respiratory system organ or structure following a respiratory system procedure
J95.831	Postprocedural hemorrhage of a respiratory system organ or structure following other procedure
J95.860	Postprocedural hematoma of a respiratory system organ or structure following a respiratory system procedure
J95.861	Postprocedural hematoma of a respiratory system organ or structure following other procedure
J95.862	Postprocedural seroma of a respiratory system organ or structure following a respiratory system procedure
J95.863	Postprocedural seroma of a respiratory system organ or structure following other procedure
K68.11	Postprocedural retroperitoneal abscess
T80.0XXA	Air embolism following infusion, transfusion and therapeutic injection, initial encounter
T80.211A	Bloodstream infection due to central venous catheter, initial encounter
T80.212A	Local infection due to central venous catheter, initial encounter
T80.218A	Other infection due to central venous catheter, initial encounter
T80.29XA	Infection following other infusion, transfusion and therapeutic injection, initial encounter
T81.11XA	Postprocedural cardiogenic shock, initial encounter
T81.41XA	Infection following a procedure, superficial incisional surgical site, initial encounter
T81.42XA	Infection following a procedure, deep incisional surgical site, initial encounter
T81.43XA	Infection following a procedure, organ and space surgical site, initial encounter
T81.44XA	Sepsis following a procedure, initial encounter
T81.49XA	Infection following a procedure, other surgical site, initial encounter
T81.718A	Complication of other artery following a procedure, not elsewhere classified, initial encounter
T81.72XA	Complication of vein following a procedure, not elsewhere classified, initial encounter
T82.310A	Breakdown (mechanical) of aortic (bifurcation) graft (replacement), initial encounter
T82.318A	Breakdown (mechanical) of other vascular grafts, initial encounter
T82.320A	Displacement of aortic (bifurcation) graft (replacement), initial encounter
T82.328A	Displacement of other vascular grafts, initial encounter
T82.330A	Leakage of aortic (bifurcation) graft (replacement), initial encounter
T82.338A	Leakage of other vascular grafts, initial encounter
T82.390A	Other mechanical complication of aortic (bifurcation) graft (replacement), initial encounter

T82.398A Other mechanical complication of other vascular grafts, initial encounter

T82.518A Breakdown (mechanical) of other cardiac and vascular devices and implants, initial encounter

T82.528A Displacement of other cardiac and vascular devices and implants, initial encounter

T82.538A Leakage of other cardiac and vascular devices and implants, initial encounter

T82.598A Other mechanical complication of other cardiac and vascular devices and implants, initial encounter

T82.7XXA Infection and inflammatory reaction due to other cardiac and vascular devices, implants and grafts, initial encounter

T82.817A Embolism due to cardiac prosthetic devices, implants and grafts, initial encounter

T82.818A Embolism due to vascular prosthetic devices, implants and grafts, initial encounter

T82.828A Fibrosis due to vascular prosthetic devices, implants and grafts, initial encounter

T82.838A Hemorrhage due to vascular prosthetic devices, implants and grafts, initial encounter

T82.848A Pain due to vascular prosthetic devices, implants and grafts, initial encounter

T82.858A Stenosis of other vascular prosthetic devices, implants and grafts, initial encounter

T82.868A Thrombosis due to vascular prosthetic devices, implants and grafts, initial encounter

T82.898A Other specified complication of vascular prosthetic devices, implants and grafts, initial encounter

T88.8XXA Other specified complications of surgical and medical care, not elsewhere classified, initial encounter

AMA: **35820** 1997,Nov,1

Relative Value Units/Medicare Edits

Non-Facility RVU	Work	PE	MP	Total
35820	36.89	13.03	8.4	58.32
Facility RVU	**Work**	**PE**	**MP**	**Total**
35820	36.89	13.03	8.4	58.32

	FUD	Status	MUE	Modifiers				IOM Reference
35820	90	A	2(3)	51	N/A	62*	80	None

* with documentation

Terms To Know

complication. Condition arising after the beginning of observation and treatment that modifies the course of the patient's illness or the medical care required, or an undesired result or misadventure in medical care.

debridement. Removal of dead or contaminated tissue and foreign matter from a wound.

electrocautery. Division or cutting of tissue using high-frequency electrical current to produce heat, which destroys cells.

hematoma. Tumor-like collection of blood in some part of the body caused by a break in a blood vessel wall, usually as a result of trauma.

35840

35840 Exploration for postoperative hemorrhage, thrombosis or infection; abdomen

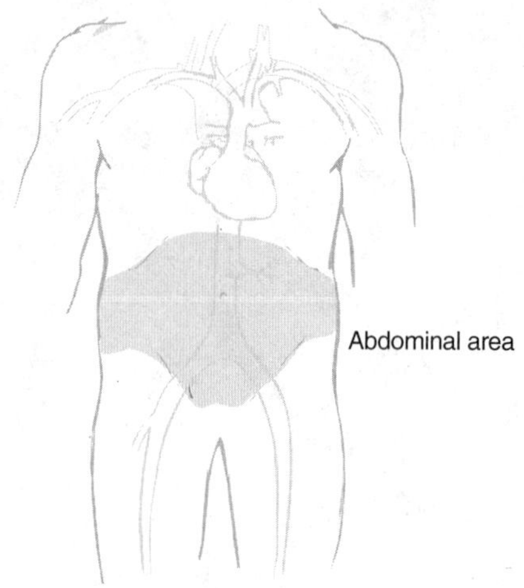

A surgical exploration is performed in the abdominal cavity to find and identify postoperative hemorrhage, thrombosis (clotting), or infection

Explanation

The physician reopens the original incision site and inspects the operative area for active bleeding, hematoma, thrombus, and exudate. The physician removes or debrides any observed hematoma, thrombus, and infected tissues. The physician looks for and corrects any active bleeding sites using electrocautery or ligation of bleeding vessels. The physician may leave an infected wound open, but generally closes the incision, leaving drains in place.

Coding Tips

This code is used to report exploration for postoperative hemorrhage, thrombosis, or infection complications of veins and arteries of the abdomen only, including correction of the problem. For thrombectomy of arterial or venous graft, see 35875–35876. For an excision of an infected graft of the abdomen, see 35907.

ICD-10-CM Diagnostic Codes

D78.21 Postprocedural hemorrhage of the spleen following a procedure on the spleen

D78.22 Postprocedural hemorrhage of the spleen following other procedure

D78.31 Postprocedural hematoma of the spleen following a procedure on the spleen

D78.32 Postprocedural hematoma of the spleen following other procedure

D78.33 Postprocedural seroma of the spleen following a procedure on the spleen

D78.34 Postprocedural seroma of the spleen following other procedure

I77.2 Rupture of artery

K68.11 Postprocedural retroperitoneal abscess

K91.840 Postprocedural hemorrhage of a digestive system organ or structure following a digestive system procedure

K91.841 Postprocedural hemorrhage of a digestive system organ or structure following other procedure

K91.870	Postprocedural hematoma of a digestive system organ or structure following a digestive system procedure
K91.871	Postprocedural hematoma of a digestive system organ or structure following other procedure
K91.872	Postprocedural seroma of a digestive system organ or structure following a digestive system procedure
K91.873	Postprocedural seroma of a digestive system organ or structure following other procedure
K91.89	Other postprocedural complications and disorders of digestive system
N99.0	Postprocedural (acute) (chronic) kidney failure
N99.520	Hemorrhage of incontinent external stoma of urinary tract
N99.521	Infection of incontinent external stoma of urinary tract
N99.522	Malfunction of incontinent external stoma of urinary tract
N99.523	Herniation of incontinent stoma of urinary tract
N99.524	Stenosis of incontinent stoma of urinary tract
N99.528	Other complication of incontinent external stoma of urinary tract
N99.530	Hemorrhage of continent stoma of urinary tract
N99.531	Infection of continent stoma of urinary tract
N99.532	Malfunction of continent stoma of urinary tract
N99.533	Herniation of continent stoma of urinary tract
N99.534	Stenosis of continent stoma of urinary tract
N99.538	Other complication of continent stoma of urinary tract
N99.820	Postprocedural hemorrhage of a genitourinary system organ or structure following a genitourinary system procedure
N99.821	Postprocedural hemorrhage of a genitourinary system organ or structure following other procedure
N99.840	Postprocedural hematoma of a genitourinary system organ or structure following a genitourinary system procedure
N99.841	Postprocedural hematoma of a genitourinary system organ or structure following other procedure
N99.842	Postprocedural seroma of a genitourinary system organ or structure following a genitourinary system procedure
N99.843	Postprocedural seroma of a genitourinary system organ or structure following other procedure
N99.89	Other postprocedural complications and disorders of genitourinary system
T81.31XA	Disruption of external operation (surgical) wound, not elsewhere classified, initial encounter
T81.32XA	Disruption of internal operation (surgical) wound, not elsewhere classified, initial encounter
T81.41XA	Infection following a procedure, superficial incisional surgical site, initial encounter
T81.42XA	Infection following a procedure, deep incisional surgical site, initial encounter
T81.43XA	Infection following a procedure, organ and space surgical site, initial encounter
T81.44XA	Sepsis following a procedure, initial encounter
T81.49XA	Infection following a procedure, other surgical site, initial encounter
T81.710A	Complication of mesenteric artery following a procedure, not elsewhere classified, initial encounter
T81.711A	Complication of renal artery following a procedure, not elsewhere classified, initial encounter
T81.718A	Complication of other artery following a procedure, not elsewhere classified, initial encounter
T81.72XA	Complication of vein following a procedure, not elsewhere classified, initial encounter
T82.7XXA	Infection and inflammatory reaction due to other cardiac and vascular devices, implants and grafts, initial encounter
T82.818A	Embolism due to vascular prosthetic devices, implants and grafts, initial encounter
T82.828A	Fibrosis due to vascular prosthetic devices, implants and grafts, initial encounter
T82.838A	Hemorrhage due to vascular prosthetic devices, implants and grafts, initial encounter
T82.848A	Pain due to vascular prosthetic devices, implants and grafts, initial encounter
T82.856A	Stenosis of peripheral vascular stent, initial encounter
T82.858A	Stenosis of other vascular prosthetic devices, implants and grafts, initial encounter
T82.868A	Thrombosis due to vascular prosthetic devices, implants and grafts, initial encounter
T82.898A	Other specified complication of vascular prosthetic devices, implants and grafts, initial encounter
T88.8XXA	Other specified complications of surgical and medical care, not elsewhere classified, initial encounter

AMA: **35840** 1997,Nov,1; 1997,May,4

Relative Value Units/Medicare Edits

Non-Facility RVU	Work	PE	MP	Total
35840	20.75	9.19	4.7	34.64
Facility RVU	**Work**	**PE**	**MP**	**Total**
35840	20.75	9.19	4.7	34.64

	FUD	Status	MUE	Modifiers				IOM Reference
35840	90	A	2(3)	51	N/A	62*	80	None

* with documentation

Terms To Know

cautery. Destruction or burning of tissue by means of a hot instrument, an electric current, or a caustic chemical, such as silver nitrate.

exudate. Fluid or other material, such as debris from cells, that has escaped blood vessel circulation and is deposited in or on tissues and usually occurs due to inflammation.

hematoma. Tumor-like collection of blood in some part of the body caused by a break in a blood vessel wall, usually as a result of trauma.

seroma. Swelling caused by the collection of serum, or clear fluid, in the tissues.

35860

35860 Exploration for postoperative hemorrhage, thrombosis or infection; extremity

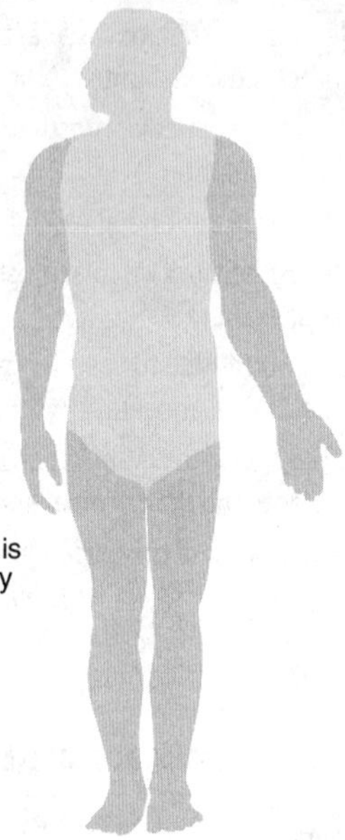

Explanation

Through an incision in the extremity over the affected area, the physician isolates the vessel and explores it for postoperative complications such as hemorrhage, thrombosis, or infection. The physician dissects any adjacent critical structures as necessary to access the vessel. The complication is identified and corrected. A hemorrhage is controlled by ligation or suture repair of the artery. Thrombosis requires opening of the artery and the removal of the clot. Any infection is drained, and sometimes a temporary tube is placed so the infection can continue to drain. The physician sutures the skin incision with a layered closure once the postsurgical complication has been treated.

Coding Tips

This code is used to report exploration for postoperative hemorrhage, thrombosis, and infection complications of veins and arteries of an extremity only, including correction of the problem. For exploration of a vessel of the extremity (not followed by surgical repair) when no other procedure is performed, see 35702 and 35703. For thrombectomy of an arterial or a venous graft, see 35875–35876. For an excision of an infected graft of the extremity, see 35903.

ICD-10-CM Diagnostic Codes

I77.2	Rupture of artery
L76.21	Postprocedural hemorrhage of skin and subcutaneous tissue following a dermatologic procedure
L76.22	Postprocedural hemorrhage of skin and subcutaneous tissue following other procedure
L76.31	Postprocedural hematoma of skin and subcutaneous tissue following a dermatologic procedure
L76.32	Postprocedural hematoma of skin and subcutaneous tissue following other procedure
L76.33	Postprocedural seroma of skin and subcutaneous tissue following a dermatologic procedure
L76.34	Postprocedural seroma of skin and subcutaneous tissue following other procedure
M96.830	Postprocedural hemorrhage of a musculoskeletal structure following a musculoskeletal system procedure
M96.831	Postprocedural hemorrhage of a musculoskeletal structure following other procedure
M96.841	Postprocedural hematoma of a musculoskeletal structure following other procedure
M96.842	Postprocedural seroma of a musculoskeletal structure following a musculoskeletal system procedure
M96.843	Postprocedural seroma of a musculoskeletal structure following other procedure
T81.31XA	Disruption of external operation (surgical) wound, not elsewhere classified, initial encounter
T81.32XA	Disruption of internal operation (surgical) wound, not elsewhere classified, initial encounter
T81.33XA	Disruption of traumatic injury wound repair, initial encounter
T81.41XA	Infection following a procedure, superficial incisional surgical site, initial encounter
T81.42XA	Infection following a procedure, deep incisional surgical site, initial encounter
T81.43XA	Infection following a procedure, organ and space surgical site, initial encounter
T81.44XA	Sepsis following a procedure, initial encounter
T81.49XA	Infection following a procedure, other surgical site, initial encounter
T81.718A	Complication of other artery following a procedure, not elsewhere classified, initial encounter
T81.72XA	Complication of vein following a procedure, not elsewhere classified, initial encounter
T82.312A	Breakdown (mechanical) of femoral arterial graft (bypass), initial encounter
T82.318A	Breakdown (mechanical) of other vascular grafts, initial encounter
T82.322A	Displacement of femoral arterial graft (bypass), initial encounter
T82.328A	Displacement of other vascular grafts, initial encounter
T82.332A	Leakage of femoral arterial graft (bypass), initial encounter
T82.338A	Leakage of other vascular grafts, initial encounter
T82.392A	Other mechanical complication of femoral arterial graft (bypass), initial encounter
T82.398A	Other mechanical complication of other vascular grafts, initial encounter
T82.7XXA	Infection and inflammatory reaction due to other cardiac and vascular devices, implants and grafts, initial encounter
T82.818A	Embolism due to vascular prosthetic devices, implants and grafts, initial encounter
T82.828A	Fibrosis due to vascular prosthetic devices, implants and grafts, initial encounter
T82.838A	Hemorrhage due to vascular prosthetic devices, implants and grafts, initial encounter
T82.848A	Pain due to vascular prosthetic devices, implants and grafts, initial encounter
T82.856A	Stenosis of peripheral vascular stent, initial encounter
T82.858A	Stenosis of other vascular prosthetic devices, implants and grafts, initial encounter

T82.868A Thrombosis due to vascular prosthetic devices, implants and grafts, initial encounter

T82.898A Other specified complication of vascular prosthetic devices, implants and grafts, initial encounter

T88.8XXA Other specified complications of surgical and medical care, not elsewhere classified, initial encounter

AMA: 35860 2018,Jan,8; 2017,Jan,8; 2016,Jan,13; 2015,Jan,16; 2014,Apr,10

Relative Value Units/Medicare Edits

Non-Facility RVU	Work	PE	MP	Total
35860	15.25	5.5	3.5	24.25
Facility RVU	**Work**	**PE**	**MP**	**Total**
35860	15.25	5.5	3.5	24.25

	FUD	Status	MUE	Modifiers				IOM Reference
35860	90	A	2(3)	51	N/A	62*	80	None

* with documentation

Terms To Know

complication. Condition arising after the beginning of observation and treatment that modifies the course of the patient's illness or the medical care required, or an undesired result or misadventure in medical care.

embolism. Obstruction of a blood vessel resulting from a clot or foreign substance.

excision. Surgical removal of an organ or tissue.

hemorrhage. Internal or external bleeding with loss of significant amounts of blood.

infection. Presence of microorganisms in body tissues that may result in cellular damage.

seroma. Swelling caused by the collection of serum, or clear fluid, in the tissues.

thrombosis. Condition arising from the presence or formation of blood clots within a blood vessel that may cause vascular obstruction and insufficient oxygenation.

35870

35870 Repair of graft-enteric fistula

Fistulas sometimes develop at the site of an anastomosis or graft with the communication allowing blood to enter the bowel and digestive juices to further erode the graft site

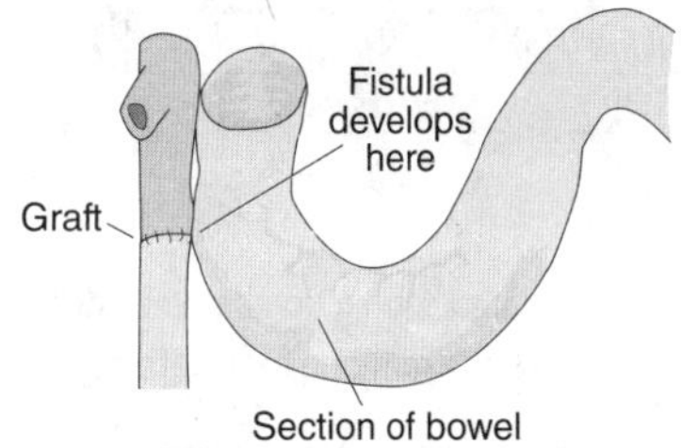

Explanation

The physician opens the abdomen under antibiotic cover and exposes the graft-enteric fistula site by careful dissection (most often aortic/Dacron anastomosis with a fistulous connection to the duodenum). The fistula is disconnected and the enteric defect is repaired using two layers of suture. The vascular prosthesis is examined and removed with an appropriate new bypass graft sewn in if there is obvious graft infection. If there is no obvious infection, the graft is repaired with local sutures. The wound is closed, leaving drains in place.

Coding Tips

When 35870 is performed with another separately identifiable procedure, the highest dollar value code is listed as the primary procedure, and subsequent procedures are appended with modifier 51. For arteriovenous fistula repairs, see 35180–35190.

ICD-10-CM Diagnostic Codes

I77.2 Rupture of artery

T82.818A Embolism due to vascular prosthetic devices, implants and grafts, initial encounter

T82.828A Fibrosis due to vascular prosthetic devices, implants and grafts, initial encounter

T82.838A Hemorrhage due to vascular prosthetic devices, implants and grafts, initial encounter

T82.848A Pain due to vascular prosthetic devices, implants and grafts, initial encounter

T82.858A Stenosis of other vascular prosthetic devices, implants and grafts, initial encounter

T82.868A Thrombosis due to vascular prosthetic devices, implants and grafts, initial encounter

T82.898A Other specified complication of vascular prosthetic devices, implants and grafts, initial encounter

T82.9XXA Unspecified complication of cardiac and vascular prosthetic device, implant and graft, initial encounter

AMA: 35870 1997,Nov,1

Relative Value Units/Medicare Edits

Non-Facility RVU	Work	PE	MP	Total
35870	24.5	5.79	5.66	35.95
Facility RVU	**Work**	**PE**	**MP**	**Total**
35870	24.5	5.79	5.66	35.95

	FUD	Status	MUE	Modifiers				IOM Reference
35870	90	A	1(3)	51	N/A	62*	80	None

* with documentation

Terms To Know

anastomosis. Surgically created connection between ducts, blood vessels, or bowel segments to allow flow from one to the other.

bypass. Auxiliary or diverted route to maintain continuous flow.

complication. Condition arising after the beginning of observation and treatment that modifies the course of the patient's illness or the medical care required, or an undesired result or misadventure in medical care.

fistula. Abnormal tube-like passage between two body cavities or organs or from an organ to the outside surface.

graft. Tissue implant from another part of the body or another person.

infection. Presence of microorganisms in body tissues that may result in cellular damage.

prosthesis. Man-made substitute for a missing body part.

rupture. Tearing or breaking open of tissue.

suture. Numerous stitching techniques employed in wound closure.

buried suture. Continuous or interrupted suture placed under the skin for a layered closure.

continuous suture. Running stitch with tension evenly distributed across a single strand to provide a leakproof closure line.

interrupted suture. Series of single stitches with tension isolated at each stitch, in which all stitches are not affected if one becomes loose, and the isolated sutures cannot act as a wick to transport an infection.

purse-string suture. Continuous suture placed around a tubular structure and tightened, to reduce or close the lumen.

retention suture. Secondary stitching that bridges the primary suture, providing support for the primary repair; a plastic or rubber bolster may be placed over the primary repair and under the retention sutures.

35875-35876

35875 Thrombectomy of arterial or venous graft (other than hemodialysis graft or fistula);

35876 with revision of arterial or venous graft

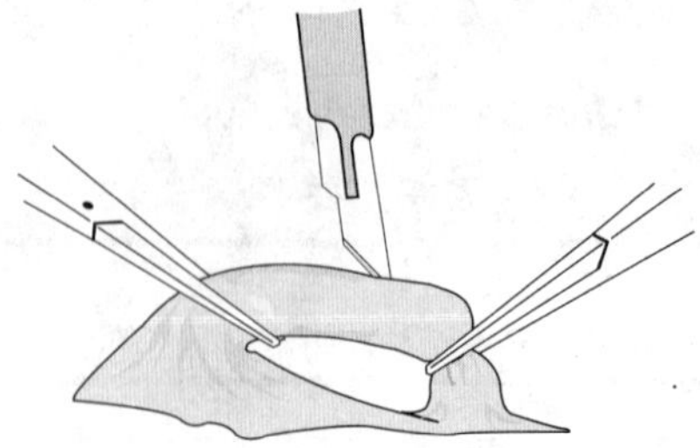

An arterial or venous thrombus is isolated and dissected from graft

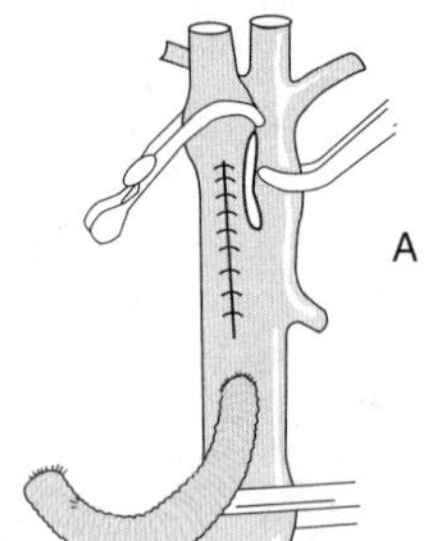

A new graft is placed

Explanation

Through an incision in the skin overlying the arterial or venous graft, the physician isolates the site of the thrombus. The physician dissects any muscle, overlying vessel, and/or adjacent critical structures to access the graft. To excise the thrombus from the graft, the blood vessel is clamped above and below the thrombus, an incision is made into the vessel or graft and the thrombus is removed. The graft or vessel is sutured at the site of the thrombectomy and the clamps are removed. To remove the thrombus with a catheter, the physician makes an incision in the vessel above or below the graft and threads the catheter past the thrombus. A balloon or tool at the tip of the catheter is inflated or extended. The physician withdraws the catheter, repeating as necessary, to capture and retrieve all of the thrombus. The blood vessel is repaired with sutures. After either procedure, the skin incision is repaired with a layered closure. In 35876, the thrombotic graft is removed, the graft site is repaired with sutures, and, avoiding the repair site, a new graft is sutured into place on the vessel. The skin incision is repaired with a layered closure.

Coding Tips

Establishing both inflow and outflow by any method is included. That portion of the operative arteriogram performed by the surgeon is also included. Angioscopy performed during therapeutic intervention should be reported in addition to the code for the primary procedure, see 35400. For thrombectomy of a hemodialysis graft or fistula, see 36831 and 36833. For initial placement of a bypass graft using a vein, see 35501–35571. For an initial in-situ vein graft placement, see 35583–35587. For an initial placement of a bypass graft other than vein, see 35601–35681. For excision of an infected graft, see 35901–35907.

ICD-10-CM Diagnostic Codes

T82.818A	Embolism due to vascular prosthetic devices, implants and grafts, initial encounter
T82.828A	Fibrosis due to vascular prosthetic devices, implants and grafts, initial encounter
T82.848A	Pain due to vascular prosthetic devices, implants and grafts, initial encounter
T82.856A	Stenosis of peripheral vascular stent, initial encounter
T82.858A	Stenosis of other vascular prosthetic devices, implants and grafts, initial encounter
T82.868A	Thrombosis due to vascular prosthetic devices, implants and grafts, initial encounter
T82.898A	Other specified complication of vascular prosthetic devices, implants and grafts, initial encounter
T82.9XXA	Unspecified complication of cardiac and vascular prosthetic device, implant and graft, initial encounter

AMA: **35875** 2018,Jan,8; 2017,Jan,8; 2016,Jan,13; 2015,Jan,16; 2014,Jan,11

Relative Value Units/Medicare Edits

Non-Facility RVU	Work	PE	MP	Total
35875	10.72	4.04	2.49	17.25
35876	17.82	5.56	4.04	27.42
Facility RVU	**Work**	**PE**	**MP**	**Total**
35875	10.72	4.04	2.49	17.25
35876	17.82	5.56	4.04	27.42

	FUD	Status	MUE	Modifiers				IOM Reference
35875	90	A	2(3)	51	N/A	62*	N/A	None
35876	90	A	2(3)	51	N/A	62*	80	

* with documentation

Terms To Know

catheter. Flexible tube inserted into an area of the body for introducing or withdrawing fluid.

complication. Condition arising after the beginning of observation and treatment that modifies the course of the patient's illness or the medical care required, or an undesired result or misadventure in medical care.

dissect. Cut apart or separate tissue for surgical purposes or for visual or microscopic study.

fistula. Abnormal tube-like passage between two body cavities or organs or from an organ to the outside surface.

graft. Tissue implant from another part of the body or another person.

in situ. Located in the natural position or contained within the origin site, not spread into neighboring tissue.

incision. Act of cutting into tissue or an organ.

thrombectomy. Removal of a clot (thrombus) from a blood vessel utilizing various methods.

thrombus. Stationary blood clot inside a blood vessel.

35879-35881

35879 Revision, lower extremity arterial bypass, without thrombectomy, open; with vein patch angioplasty

35881 with segmental vein interposition

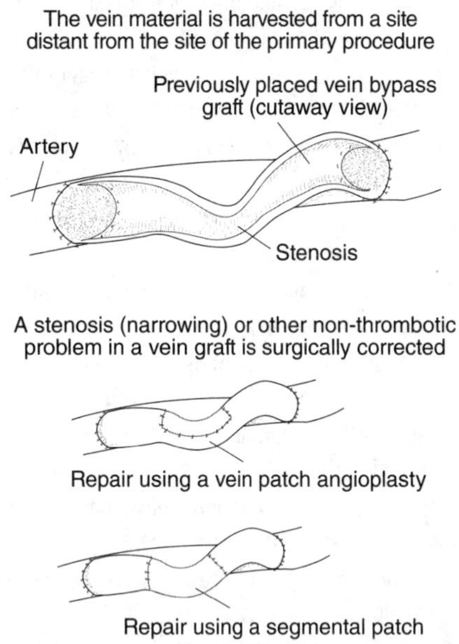

Explanation

The physician revises a lower extremity arterial bypass with vein-patch angioplasty or segmental vein interposition. A previous lower-extremity arterial bypass graft requires open revision due to graft-threatening stenosis. The physician makes an incision in a lower extremity over the site of a previous arterial bypass graft. Dissection is carried down to the graft. In 35879, angioplasty of the stenosed area is performed by excising the area of stenosis and using a patch of vein to close the created wound. In 35881, a segment of vein is excised from another area. The area of stenosis is excised and the vein segment is positioned between the two ends of the graft and anastomosed in an end to end fashion. A thrombectomy is not performed. The wound is closed with layered sutures.

Coding Tips

Codes 35879 and 35881 should be used to report open revision of stenotic arterial bypass grafts when the stenosis is such that it threatens the viability of the previously constructed arterial graft. For thrombectomy with revision of any non-coronary arterial or venous graft (except hemodialysis graft or fistula), including those of the lower extremity, report 35876. For direct repair (other than for fistula) of a lower extremity blood vessel (with or without patch angioplasty), see 35226. For repair of a lower extremity blood vessel using a vein graft, see 35256. For fistula repair of a lower extremity, see 35184 or 35190. For the revision of a femoral anastomosis of a synthetic arterial bypass graft, see 35883 and 35884. For excision of an infected graft, see 35901–35907 and the appropriate revascularization code.

ICD-10-CM Diagnostic Codes

I70.411	Atherosclerosis of autologous vein bypass graft(s) of the extremities with intermittent claudication, right leg ☑
I70.412	Atherosclerosis of autologous vein bypass graft(s) of the extremities with intermittent claudication, left leg ☑
I70.421	Atherosclerosis of autologous vein bypass graft(s) of the extremities with rest pain, right leg ☑

I70.422 Atherosclerosis of autologous vein bypass graft(s) of the extremities with rest pain, left leg ☑

I70.431 Atherosclerosis of autologous vein bypass graft(s) of the right leg with ulceration of thigh ☑

I70.432 Atherosclerosis of autologous vein bypass graft(s) of the right leg with ulceration of calf ☑

I70.433 Atherosclerosis of autologous vein bypass graft(s) of the right leg with ulceration of ankle ☑

I70.434 Atherosclerosis of autologous vein bypass graft(s) of the right leg with ulceration of heel and midfoot ☑

I70.441 Atherosclerosis of autologous vein bypass graft(s) of the left leg with ulceration of thigh ☑

I70.442 Atherosclerosis of autologous vein bypass graft(s) of the left leg with ulceration of calf ☑

I70.443 Atherosclerosis of autologous vein bypass graft(s) of the left leg with ulceration of ankle ☑

I70.444 Atherosclerosis of autologous vein bypass graft(s) of the left leg with ulceration of heel and midfoot ☑

I70.461 Atherosclerosis of autologous vein bypass graft(s) of the extremities with gangrene, right leg ☑

I70.462 Atherosclerosis of autologous vein bypass graft(s) of the extremities with gangrene, left leg ☑

I70.491 Other atherosclerosis of autologous vein bypass graft(s) of the extremities, right leg ☑

I70.492 Other atherosclerosis of autologous vein bypass graft(s) of the extremities, left leg ☑

I70.511 Atherosclerosis of nonautologous biological bypass graft(s) of the extremities with intermittent claudication, right leg ☑

I70.512 Atherosclerosis of nonautologous biological bypass graft(s) of the extremities with intermittent claudication, left leg ☑

I70.521 Atherosclerosis of nonautologous biological bypass graft(s) of the extremities with rest pain, right leg ☑

I70.522 Atherosclerosis of nonautologous biological bypass graft(s) of the extremities with rest pain, left leg ☑

I70.531 Atherosclerosis of nonautologous biological bypass graft(s) of the right leg with ulceration of thigh ☑

I70.532 Atherosclerosis of nonautologous biological bypass graft(s) of the right leg with ulceration of calf ☑

I70.533 Atherosclerosis of nonautologous biological bypass graft(s) of the right leg with ulceration of ankle ☑

I70.534 Atherosclerosis of nonautologous biological bypass graft(s) of the right leg with ulceration of heel and midfoot ☑

I70.541 Atherosclerosis of nonautologous biological bypass graft(s) of the left leg with ulceration of thigh ☑

I70.542 Atherosclerosis of nonautologous biological bypass graft(s) of the left leg with ulceration of calf ☑

I70.543 Atherosclerosis of nonautologous biological bypass graft(s) of the left leg with ulceration of ankle ☑

I70.544 Atherosclerosis of nonautologous biological bypass graft(s) of the left leg with ulceration of heel and midfoot ☑

I70.561 Atherosclerosis of nonautologous biological bypass graft(s) of the extremities with gangrene, right leg ☑

I70.562 Atherosclerosis of nonautologous biological bypass graft(s) of the extremities with gangrene, left leg ☑

I70.611 Atherosclerosis of nonbiological bypass graft(s) of the extremities with intermittent claudication, right leg ☑

I70.612 Atherosclerosis of nonbiological bypass graft(s) of the extremities with intermittent claudication, left leg ☑

I70.621 Atherosclerosis of nonbiological bypass graft(s) of the extremities with rest pain, right leg ☑

I70.622 Atherosclerosis of nonbiological bypass graft(s) of the extremities with rest pain, left leg ☑

I70.631 Atherosclerosis of nonbiological bypass graft(s) of the right leg with ulceration of thigh ☑

I70.632 Atherosclerosis of nonbiological bypass graft(s) of the right leg with ulceration of calf ☑

I70.633 Atherosclerosis of nonbiological bypass graft(s) of the right leg with ulceration of ankle ☑

I70.634 Atherosclerosis of nonbiological bypass graft(s) of the right leg with ulceration of heel and midfoot ☑

I70.641 Atherosclerosis of nonbiological bypass graft(s) of the left leg with ulceration of thigh ☑

I70.642 Atherosclerosis of nonbiological bypass graft(s) of the left leg with ulceration of calf ☑

I70.643 Atherosclerosis of nonbiological bypass graft(s) of the left leg with ulceration of ankle ☑

I70.644 Atherosclerosis of nonbiological bypass graft(s) of the left leg with ulceration of heel and midfoot ☑

I70.661 Atherosclerosis of nonbiological bypass graft(s) of the extremities with gangrene, right leg ☑

I70.662 Atherosclerosis of nonbiological bypass graft(s) of the extremities with gangrene, left leg ☑

AMA: **35879** 2018,Jan,8; 2017,Jan,8; 2016,Jan,13; 2015,Jan,16; 2014,Jan,11 **35881** 2018,Jan,8; 2017,Jan,8; 2016,Jan,13; 2015,Jan,16; 2014,Jan,11

Relative Value Units/Medicare Edits

Non-Facility RVU	Work	PE	MP	Total
35879	17.41	5.44	3.98	26.83
35881	19.35	5.73	4.4	29.48
Facility RVU	**Work**	**PE**	**MP**	**Total**
35879	17.41	5.44	3.98	26.83
35881	19.35	5.73	4.4	29.48

	FUD	Status	MUE	Modifiers				IOM Reference
35879	90	A	2(3)	51	50	62*	80	None
35881	90	A	1(3)	51	50	62*	80	

* with documentation

Terms To Know

anastomosis. Surgically created connection between ducts, blood vessels, or bowel segments to allow flow from one to the other.

angioplasty. Reconstruction or repair of a diseased or damaged blood vessel.

bypass graft. Surgically created alternative blood vessel used to reroute blood flow around an area of obstruction or disease.

35883-35884

35883 Revision, femoral anastomosis of synthetic arterial bypass graft in groin, open; with nonautogenous patch graft (eg, Dacron, ePTFE, bovine pericardium)

35884 with autogenous vein patch graft

A revision of a femoral bypass in the groin is performed due to formation of an anastomotic aneurysm

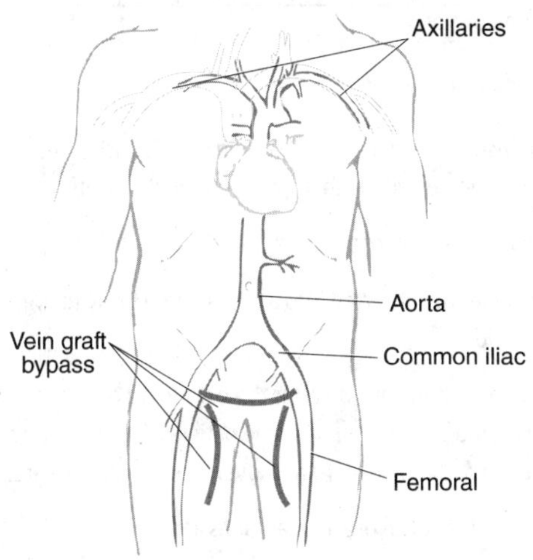

The aneurysm is excised and a patch graft applied

Explanation

An open revision of the femoral anastomosis of a synthetic arterial bypass graft in the groin is performed using a nonautogenous (Dacron, ePTFE, bovine pericardium) patch graft (35883) or an autogenous vein patch graft (35884). This procedure is performed due to formation of an anastomotic aneurysm in the femoral artery. This occurs due to a defect in the anastomosis. Through an incision in the skin of the upper thigh, the physician isolates and dissects the anastomotic aneurysm. An arteriotomy is performed and the aneurysm excised. A patch graft is placed.

Coding Tips

These are unilateral procedures. If performed bilaterally, some payers require that the service be reported twice with modifier 50 appended to the second code, while others require identification of the service only once with modifier 50 appended. Check with individual payers. Modifier 50 identifies a procedure performed identically on the opposite side of the body (mirror image). Do not report 35883 or 35884 with 35700, 35875, or 35876. Do not report these codes with each other.

ICD-10-CM Diagnostic Codes

T81.41XA	Infection following a procedure, superficial incisional surgical site, initial encounter
T81.42XA	Infection following a procedure, deep incisional surgical site, initial encounter
T81.43XA	Infection following a procedure, organ and space surgical site, initial encounter
T81.44XA	Sepsis following a procedure, initial encounter
T81.49XA	Infection following a procedure, other surgical site, initial encounter
T81.718A	Complication of other artery following a procedure, not elsewhere classified, initial encounter
T82.7XXA	Infection and inflammatory reaction due to other cardiac and vascular devices, implants and grafts, initial encounter
T82.818A	Embolism due to vascular prosthetic devices, implants and grafts, initial encounter
T82.828A	Fibrosis due to vascular prosthetic devices, implants and grafts, initial encounter
T82.838A	Hemorrhage due to vascular prosthetic devices, implants and grafts, initial encounter
T82.848A	Pain due to vascular prosthetic devices, implants and grafts, initial encounter
T82.856A	Stenosis of peripheral vascular stent, initial encounter
T82.858A	Stenosis of other vascular prosthetic devices, implants and grafts, initial encounter
T82.868A	Thrombosis due to vascular prosthetic devices, implants and grafts, initial encounter
T82.898A	Other specified complication of vascular prosthetic devices, implants and grafts, initial encounter

AMA: **35883** 2018,Jan,8; 2017,Jan,8; 2016,Jan,13; 2015,Jan,16; 2014,Jan,11 **35884** 2018,Jan,8; 2017,Jan,8; 2016,Jan,13; 2015,Jan,16; 2014,Jan,11

Relative Value Units/Medicare Edits

Non-Facility RVU	Work	PE	MP	Total
35883	23.15	6.38	5.28	34.81
35884	24.65	5.47	5.7	35.82
Facility RVU	**Work**	**PE**	**MP**	**Total**
35883	23.15	6.38	5.28	34.81
35884	24.65	5.47	5.7	35.82

	FUD	Status	MUE	Modifiers				IOM Reference
35883	90	A	1(3)	51	50	62*	80	None
35884	90	A	1(3)	51	50	62*	80	

* with documentation

Terms To Know

anastomosis. Surgically created connection between ducts, blood vessels, or bowel segments to allow flow from one to the other.

aneurysm. Circumscribed dilation or outpouching of an artery wall, often containing blood clots and connecting directly with the lumen of the artery.

arteriotomy. Incision into an artery.

autograft. Any tissue harvested from one anatomical site of a person and grafted to another anatomical site of the same person. Most commonly, blood vessels, skin, tendons, fascia, and bone are used as autografts.

graft. Tissue implant from another part of the body or another person.

pericardium. Thin and slippery case in which the heart lies that is lined with fluid so that the heart is free to pulse and move as it beats.

35901

35901 Excision of infected graft; neck

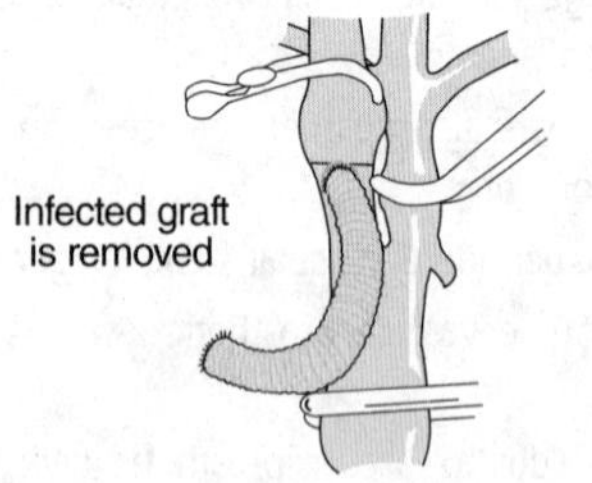

The physician removes an infected graft from the neck and repairs the blood vessel

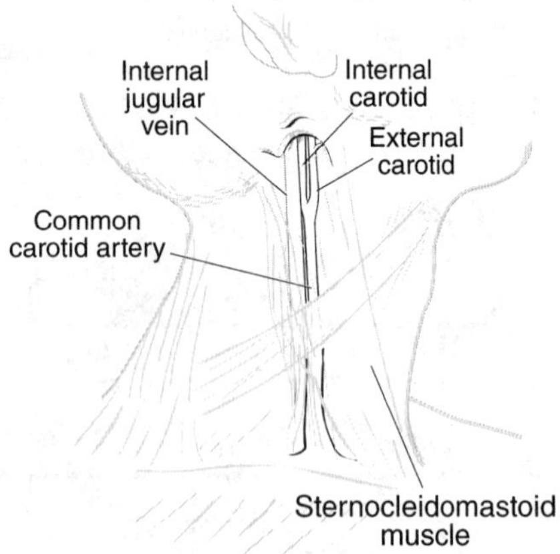

Explanation

Through an incision in the skin of the neck overlying the graft, the physician dissects around any muscle, vessels, or other structures to access the graft site. The physician dissects around the vessel, and applies vessel clamps above and below the graft. The physician excises above and below the existing infected graft. The blood vessel is repaired with sutures. A catheter may be left in place to help drain infection. The skin is loosely closed. If the excised graft is replaced with a new graft, report the appropriate revascularization code.

Coding Tips

Establishing both inflow and outflow by any method is included. That portion of the operative arteriogram performed by the surgeon is also included. Angioscopy performed during therapeutic intervention should be reported in addition to the code for the primary procedure; see 35400. For a thrombectomy of an arterial or venous graft, see 35875–35876. For an initial placement of a bypass graft using a vein, see 35501–35571. For an initial placement of a bypass graft other than vein, see 35601–35681.

ICD-10-CM Diagnostic Codes

T82.7XXA Infection and inflammatory reaction due to other cardiac and vascular devices, implants and grafts, initial encounter

AMA: 35901 1997,Nov,1

Relative Value Units/Medicare Edits

Non-Facility RVU	Work	PE	MP	Total
35901	8.38	3.27	1.92	13.57
Facility RVU	**Work**	**PE**	**MP**	**Total**
35901	8.38	3.27	1.92	13.57

	FUD	Status	MUE	Modifiers				IOM Reference
35901	90	A	1(3)	51	N/A	62*	80	None

* with documentation

Terms To Know

angioscopy. Visualization of capillary blood vessels with a microscope, or the inside of a blood vessel with a fiberoptic-equipped catheter.

arteriogram. Radiograph of arteries.

catheter. Flexible tube inserted into an area of the body for introducing or withdrawing fluid.

complication. Condition arising after the beginning of observation and treatment that modifies the course of the patient's illness or the medical care required, or an undesired result or misadventure in medical care.

excision. Surgical removal of an organ or tissue.

graft. Tissue implant from another part of the body or another person.

incision. Act of cutting into tissue or an organ.

infection. Presence of microorganisms in body tissues that may result in cellular damage.

revascularization. Restoration of blood flow and oxygen supply to a body part. This may apply to an extremity, the heart, or penis.

suture. Numerous stitching techniques employed in wound closure.

35903

35903 Excision of infected graft; extremity

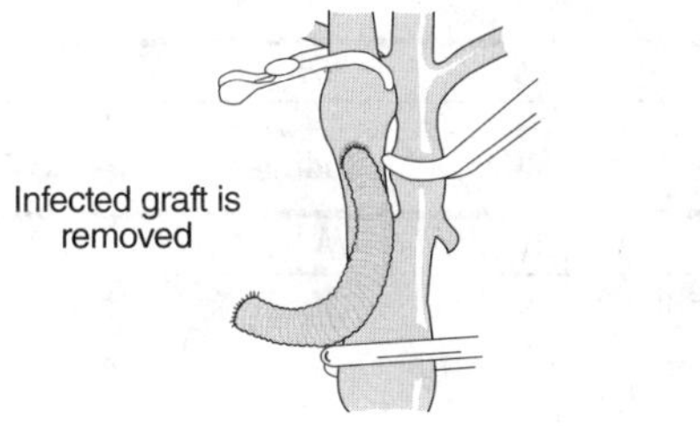

The physician removes an infected graft from an extremity and repairs the blood vessel

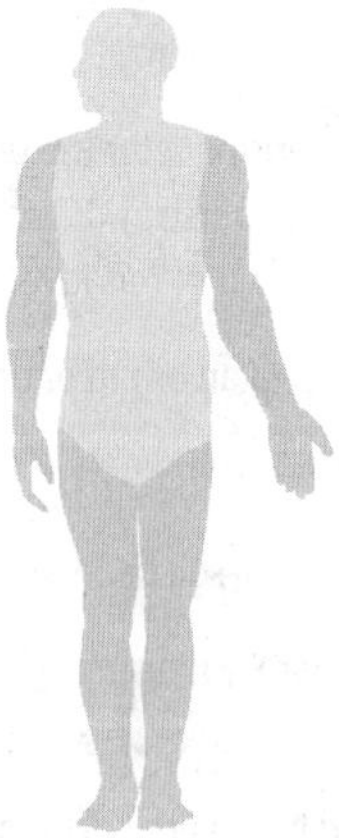

Explanation

Through an incision in the skin of the extremity overlying the graft, the physician dissects around any muscle, vessels or other structures to access the graft site. The physician dissects around the vessel, and applies vessel clamps above and below the graft. The physician excises above and below the existing infected graft. The blood vessel is repaired with sutures. A catheter may be left in place to help drain infection. The skin is loosely closed. If the excised graft is replaced with a new graft, report the appropriate revascularization code.

Coding Tips

Establishing both inflow and outflow by any method is included. That portion of the operative arteriogram performed by the surgeon is also included. Angioscopy performed during therapeutic intervention should be reported in addition to the code for the primary procedure, see 35400. For a thrombectomy of an arterial or venous graft, see 35875–35876. For an initial placement of a bypass graft using a vein, see 35501–35571. For an initial in-situ vein graft placement, see 35583–35587. For an initial placement of a bypass graft other than vein, see 35601–35681.

ICD-10-CM Diagnostic Codes

T81.41XA Infection following a procedure, superficial incisional surgical site, initial encounter

T81.42XA Infection following a procedure, deep incisional surgical site, initial encounter

T81.43XA Infection following a procedure, organ and space surgical site, initial encounter

T81.44XA Sepsis following a procedure, initial encounter

T81.49XA Infection following a procedure, other surgical site, initial encounter

T82.7XXA Infection and inflammatory reaction due to other cardiac and vascular devices, implants and grafts, initial encounter

T88.8XXA Other specified complications of surgical and medical care, not elsewhere classified, initial encounter

AMA: **35903** 2018,Aug,10

Relative Value Units/Medicare Edits

Non-Facility RVU	Work	PE	MP	Total
35903	9.53	4.6	2.2	16.33
Facility RVU	**Work**	**PE**	**MP**	**Total**
35903	9.53	4.6	2.2	16.33

	FUD	Status	MUE	Modifiers				IOM Reference
35903	90	A	2(3)	51	N/A	62*	80	None

* with documentation

Terms To Know

catheter. Flexible tube inserted into an area of the body for introducing or withdrawing fluid.

complication. Condition arising after the beginning of observation and treatment that modifies the course of the patient's illness or the medical care required, or an undesired result or misadventure in medical care.

excision. Surgical removal of an organ or tissue.

graft. Tissue implant from another part of the body or another person.

incision. Act of cutting into tissue or an organ.

infection. Presence of microorganisms in body tissues that may result in cellular damage.

suture. Numerous stitching techniques employed in wound closure.

buried suture. Continuous or interrupted suture placed under the skin for a layered closure.

continuous suture. Running stitch with tension evenly distributed across a single strand to provide a leakproof closure line.

interrupted suture. Series of single stitches with tension isolated at each stitch, in which all stitches are not affected if one becomes loose, and the isolated sutures cannot act as a wick to transport an infection.

purse-string suture. Continuous suture placed around a tubular structure and tightened, to reduce or close the lumen.

retention suture. Secondary stitching that bridges the primary suture, providing support for the primary repair; a plastic or rubber bolster may be placed over the primary repair and under the retention sutures.

35905

35905 Excision of infected graft; thorax

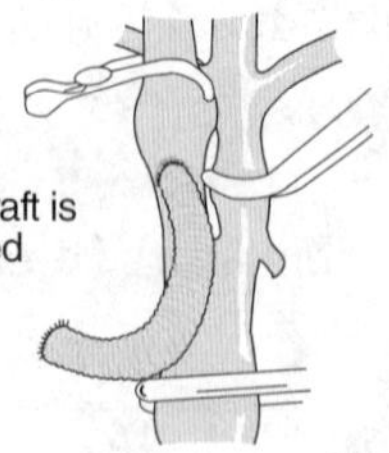

The physician removes an infected graft from the thorax and repairs the blood vessel

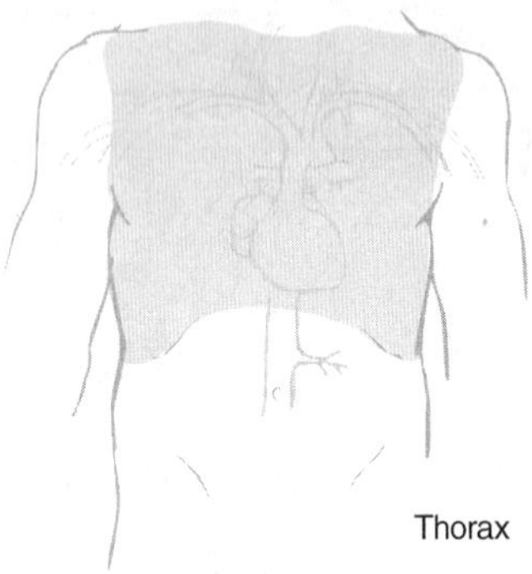

Explanation

Through an incision in the skin of the thorax overlying the graft, the physician dissects around any muscle, vessels or other structures to access the graft site. The physician dissects around the vessel, and applies vessel clamps above and below the graft. The physician excises above and below the existing infected graft. The blood vessel is repaired with sutures. A catheter may be left in place to help drain infection. The skin is loosely closed. If the excised graft is replaced with a new graft, report the appropriate revascularization code.

Coding Tips

Establishing both inflow and outflow by any method is included. That portion of the operative arteriogram performed by the surgeon is also included. Angioscopy performed during therapeutic intervention should be reported in addition to the code for the primary procedure; see 35400. For a thrombectomy of an arterial or a venous graft, see 35875–35876. For an initial placement of a bypass graft using a vein, see 35501–35571. For an initial placement of a bypass graft other than vein, see 35601–35681.

ICD-10-CM Diagnostic Codes

T82.7XXA Infection and inflammatory reaction due to other cardiac and vascular devices, implants and grafts, initial encounter

AMA: **35905** 1997,Nov,1

Relative Value Units/Medicare Edits

Non-Facility RVU	Work	PE	MP	Total
35905	33.52	7.25	7.76	48.53
Facility RVU	**Work**	**PE**	**MP**	**Total**
35905	33.52	7.25	7.76	48.53

	FUD	Status	MUE	Modifiers				IOM Reference
35905	90	A	1(3)	51	N/A	62*	80	None

* with documentation

Terms To Know

angiography. Radiographic imaging of the arteries.

angioscopy. Visualization of capillary blood vessels with a microscope, or the inside of a blood vessel with a fiberoptic-equipped catheter.

complication. Condition arising after the beginning of observation and treatment that modifies the course of the patient's illness or the medical care required, or an undesired result or misadventure in medical care.

excision. Surgical removal of an organ or tissue.

graft. Tissue implant from another part of the body or another person.

incision. Act of cutting into tissue or an organ.

infection. Presence of microorganisms in body tissues that may result in cellular damage.

revascularize. Restoring blood flow or blood supply to a body part.

suture. Numerous stitching techniques employed in wound closure.

buried suture. Continuous or interrupted suture placed under the skin for a layered closure.

continuous suture. Running stitch with tension evenly distributed across a single strand to provide a leakproof closure line.

interrupted suture. Series of single stitches with tension isolated at each stitch, in which all stitches are not affected if one becomes loose, and the isolated sutures cannot act as a wick to transport an infection.

purse-string suture. Continuous suture placed around a tubular structure and tightened, to reduce or close the lumen.

retention suture. Secondary stitching that bridges the primary suture, providing support for the primary repair; a plastic or rubber bolster may be placed over the primary repair and under the retention sutures.

35907

35907 Excision of infected graft; abdomen

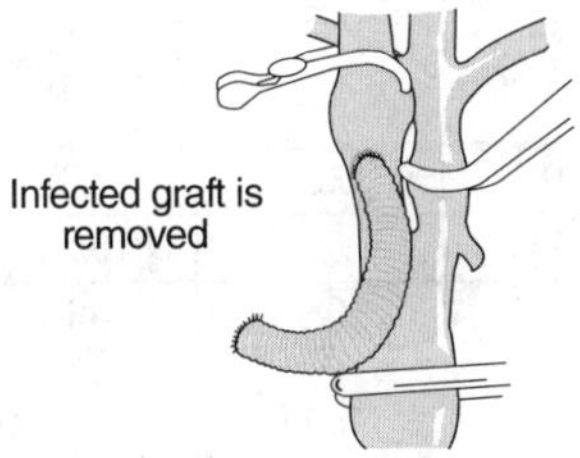

The physician removes an infected graft from the abdomen and repairs the blood vessel

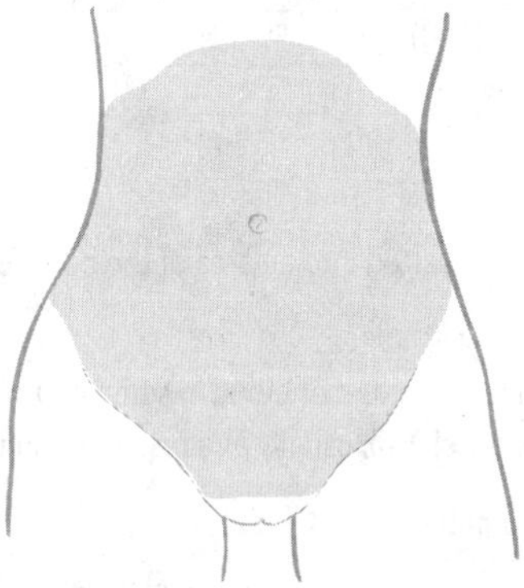

Explanation

Through an incision in the skin of the abdomen overlying the graft, the physician dissects around any muscle, vessels or other structures to access the graft site. The physician dissects around the vessel, and applies vessel clamps above and below the graft. The physician excises above and below the existing infected graft. The blood vessel is repaired with sutures. A catheter may be left in place to help drain infection. The skin is loosely closed. If the excised graft is replaced with a new graft, report the appropriate revascularization code.

Coding Tips

Establishing both inflow and outflow by any method is included. That portion of the operative arteriogram performed by the surgeon is also included. Angioscopy performed during therapeutic intervention should be reported in addition to the code for the primary procedure, see 35400. For a thrombectomy of an arterial or a venous graft, see 35875–35876. For an initial placement of a bypass graft using a vein, see 35501–35571. For an initial in-situ vein graft placement, see 35583–35587. For an initial placement of a bypass graft other than vein, see 35601–35681.

ICD-10-CM Diagnostic Codes

T81.44XA Sepsis following a procedure, initial encounter

T82.7XXA Infection and inflammatory reaction due to other cardiac and vascular devices, implants and grafts, initial encounter

T82.898A Other specified complication of vascular prosthetic devices, implants and grafts, initial encounter

AMA: 35907 1997,Nov,1

Relative Value Units/Medicare Edits

Non-Facility RVU	Work	PE	MP	Total
35907	37.27	9.39	8.59	55.25
Facility RVU	**Work**	**PE**	**MP**	**Total**
35907	37.27	9.39	8.59	55.25

	FUD	Status	MUE	Modifiers				IOM Reference
35907	90	A	1(3)	51	N/A	62*	80	None

* with documentation

Terms To Know

catheter. Flexible tube inserted into an area of the body for introducing or withdrawing fluid.

complication. Condition arising after the beginning of observation and treatment that modifies the course of the patient's illness or the medical care required, or an undesired result or misadventure in medical care.

excision. Surgical removal of an organ or tissue.

graft. Tissue implant from another part of the body or another person.

incision. Act of cutting into tissue or an organ.

infection. Presence of microorganisms in body tissues that may result in cellular damage.

suture. Numerous stitching techniques employed in wound closure.

buried suture. Continuous or interrupted suture placed under the skin for a layered closure.

continuous suture. Running stitch with tension evenly distributed across a single strand to provide a leakproof closure line.

interrupted suture. Series of single stitches with tension isolated at each stitch, in which all stitches are not affected if one becomes loose, and the isolated sutures cannot act as a wick to transport an infection.

purse-string suture. Continuous suture placed around a tubular structure and tightened, to reduce or close the lumen.

retention suture. Secondary stitching that bridges the primary suture, providing support for the primary repair; a plastic or rubber bolster may be placed over the primary repair and under the retention sutures.

36000-36005

36000 Introduction of needle or intracatheter, vein
36002 Injection procedures (eg, thrombin) for percutaneous treatment of extremity pseudoaneurysm
36005 Injection procedure for extremity venography (including introduction of needle or intracatheter)

Explanation

In 36000, the physician places a needle or a catheter through a puncture in the skin and into a peripheral vein. In 36002, the physician injects a pseudoaneurysm, which is a pulsatile hematoma with a fibrous capsule that maintains persistent communication with the adjacent vessel. The vessel wall does not heal and blood flows back and forth between the vessel and hematoma during the cardiac cycle. Under ultrasound control, the physician advances a 22-gauge needle into the lumen of the pseudoaneurysm and injects thrombin to cause thrombosis of the pseudoaneurysm. In 36005, an opaque substance is injected through the catheter for venography. Once the procedure is complete, the catheter is removed and pressure is applied to stop bleeding at the injection site.

Coding Tips

Report 36005 if the catheter is inserted for a venography and 36000 if the catheter is inserted for another purpose. These codes are often incorrectly used to report placement of a routine IV. These codes include local anesthesia, introduction of needles or catheter, injection of contrast material with or without automatic power injection, and/or necessary pre- and postinjection care. See CPT notes for additional guidelines. Supplies (catheters, drugs, and contrast media) are not included in the listed service for the injection procedures. For imaging guidance performed in addition to 36002, see 76942, 77002, 77012, or 77021. For ultrasound guided compression repair of pseudoaneurysms, see 76936. Do not report 36002 for vascular sealant of an arteriotomy site. For radiological supervision and interpretation performed in addition to 36005, see 75820 and 75822. For cardiac catheterizations and injection procedures performed in addition to cardiac catheterization, see 93452–93461 and 93563–93568.

ICD-10-CM Diagnostic Codes

The application of this code is too broad to adequately present ICD-10-CM diagnostic code links here. Refer to your ICD-10-CM book.

AMA: 36000 2019,Aug,8; 2018,Mar,3; 2018,Jan,8; 2017,Jan,8; 2016,Nov,3; 2016,Jan,13; 2015,Jan,16; 2014,Sep,13; 2014,Oct,6; 2014,May,4; 2014,Jan,11 **36002** 2018,Mar,3; 2018,Jan,8; 2017,Jan,8; 2016,Nov,3; 2016,Jan,13; 2015,Jan,16; 2014,Oct,6; 2014,Jan,11; 2013,Nov,6 **36005** 2018,Mar,3; 2018,Jan,8; 2017,Jan,8; 2016,Nov,3; 2016,Jul,6; 2016,Jan,13; 2015,Jan,16; 2014,Oct,6

Relative Value Units/Medicare Edits

Non-Facility RVU	Work	PE	MP	Total
36000	0.18	0.57	0.02	0.77
36002	1.96	2.25	0.28	4.49
36005	0.95	7.66	0.15	8.76
Facility RVU	**Work**	**PE**	**MP**	**Total**
36000	0.18	0.07	0.02	0.27
36002	1.96	0.8	0.28	3.04
36005	0.95	0.3	0.15	1.4

	FUD	Status	MUE	Modifiers				IOM Reference
36000	N/A	B	4(3)	N/A	N/A	N/A	N/A	None
36002	0	A	2(3)	51	50	N/A	N/A	
36005	0	A	2(3)	51	50	N/A	80*	

* with documentation

Terms To Know

catheter. Flexible tube inserted into an area of the body for introducing or withdrawing fluid.

hematoma. Tumor-like collection of blood in some part of the body caused by a break in a blood vessel wall, usually as a result of trauma.

percutaneous. Through the skin.

pseudoaneurysm. False aneurysm produced by a dilated vessel wall, or a ruptured blood vessel that has formed a clot that pulsates, mimicking a true aneurysm.

supervision and interpretation. Radiology services that usually contain an invasive component and are reported by the radiologist for supervision of the procedure and the personnel involved with performing the examination, reading the film, and preparing the written report.

thrombosis. Condition arising from the presence or formation of blood clots within a blood vessel that may cause vascular obstruction and insufficient oxygenation.

ultrasound. Imaging using ultra-high sound frequency bounced off body structures.

vein. Vessel through which oxygen-depleted blood passes back to the heart.

venography. Radiographic study of the veins.

36010

36010 Introduction of catheter, superior or inferior vena cava

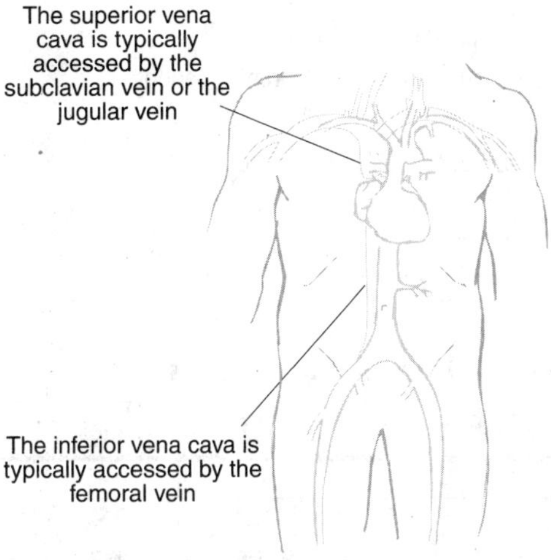

Explanation

The physician punctures a distal vein (typically antecubital, internal jugular, subclavian, or femoral) with a large needle and passes a guidewire via the needle into the punctured vein. The physician removes the needle while leaving the guidewire in place, and enlarges the skin opening slightly with a blade. The physician may slide an introducer sheath over the guidewire into the venous lumen, or may slide the catheter directly into the venous lumen without using an introducer sheath. If using an introducer sheath, the physician inserts the catheter into the vein through an O-ring in the introducer sheath (this prevents blood from leaking around the catheter) into the superior or inferior vena cava. The physician may check the catheter position with fluoroscope or with an x-ray.

Coding Tips

When medically necessary, report moderate (conscious) sedation provided by the performing physician with 99151-99153. When provided by another physician, report 99155-99157. Listed services for injection procedures include necessary local anesthesia, introduction of needles or catheter, injection of contrast material with or without automatic power injection, and/or necessary pre- and postinjection care specifically related to the injection procedure. Supplies (catheters, drugs, and contrast media) are not included in the listed service for the injection procedures. For radiology supervision and interpretation, see 75825–75827. For introduction of catheter, right heart or main pulmonary artery, see 36013; aorta, see 36200. For other cardiac catheterizations and injection procedures performed in addition to cardiac catheterization, see 93452–93461 and 93563–93568.

ICD-10-CM Diagnostic Codes

I26.01	Septic pulmonary embolism with acute cor pulmonale
I26.09	Other pulmonary embolism with acute cor pulmonale
I26.90	Septic pulmonary embolism without acute cor pulmonale
I26.99	Other pulmonary embolism without acute cor pulmonale
I27.0	Primary pulmonary hypertension
I27.20	Pulmonary hypertension, unspecified
I27.21	Secondary pulmonary arterial hypertension
I27.22	Pulmonary hypertension due to left heart disease
I27.23	Pulmonary hypertension due to lung diseases and hypoxia
I27.24	Chronic thromboembolic pulmonary hypertension
I27.29	Other secondary pulmonary hypertension
I27.82	Chronic pulmonary embolism
I27.83	Eisenmenger's syndrome
I27.89	Other specified pulmonary heart diseases
I80.11	Phlebitis and thrombophlebitis of right femoral vein ☑
I80.12	Phlebitis and thrombophlebitis of left femoral vein ☑
I80.13	Phlebitis and thrombophlebitis of femoral vein, bilateral ☑
I82.210	Acute embolism and thrombosis of superior vena cava
I82.211	Chronic embolism and thrombosis of superior vena cava
I82.220	Acute embolism and thrombosis of inferior vena cava
I82.221	Chronic embolism and thrombosis of inferior vena cava
I82.3	Embolism and thrombosis of renal vein
I82.411	Acute embolism and thrombosis of right femoral vein ☑
I82.412	Acute embolism and thrombosis of left femoral vein ☑
I82.413	Acute embolism and thrombosis of femoral vein, bilateral ☑
I82.511	Chronic embolism and thrombosis of right femoral vein ☑
I82.512	Chronic embolism and thrombosis of left femoral vein ☑
I82.513	Chronic embolism and thrombosis of femoral vein, bilateral ☑
I87.1	Compression of vein
I87.8	Other specified disorders of veins
N18.4	Chronic kidney disease, stage 4 (severe)
N18.5	Chronic kidney disease, stage 5
N18.6	End stage renal disease

AMA: 36010 2018,Jan,8; 2017,Jan,8; 2017,Feb,14; 2016,Jul,6; 2016,Jan,13; 2015,Jan,16; 2014,Jan,11

Relative Value Units/Medicare Edits

Non-Facility RVU	Work	PE	MP	Total
36010	2.18	11.73	0.37	14.28
Facility RVU	**Work**	**PE**	**MP**	**Total**
36010	2.18	0.64	0.37	3.19

	FUD	Status	MUE	Modifiers				IOM Reference
36010	N/A	A	2(3)	51	50	N/A	N/A	None

* with documentation

Terms To Know

catheter. Flexible tube inserted into an area of the body for introducing or withdrawing fluid.

fluoroscopy. Radiology technique that allows visual examination of part of the body or a function of an organ using a device that projects an x-ray image on a fluorescent screen.

guidewire. Flexible metal instrument designed to lead another instrument in its proper course.

36011-36012

36011 Selective catheter placement, venous system; first order branch (eg, renal vein, jugular vein)

36012 second order, or more selective, branch (eg, left adrenal vein, petrosal sinus)

A catheter is placed to inject contrast material for venography upstream of the site under investigation

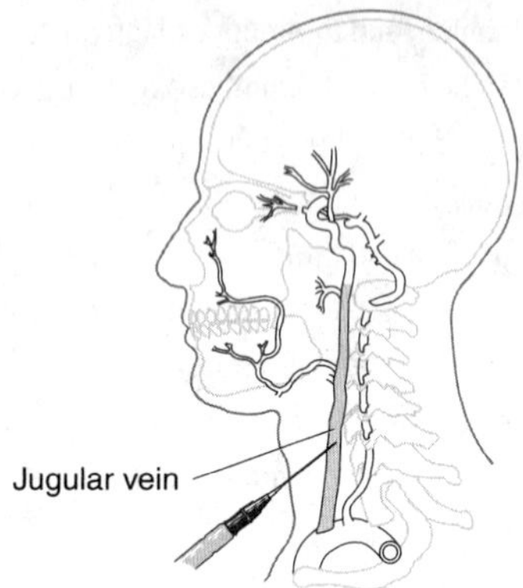

Explanation

Through a puncture through the skin, the physician passes a needle into the vein and threads a guidewire through the needle into the vein. The needle is removed and the wire is passed to the desired location in the venous system. A catheter follows the wire into the selected point in the vein and the wire is removed. A first order branch from the vena cava (36011) is any initial vessel draining directly into the vena cava (e.g., renal vein or jugular vein). A second order branch of the vena cava (36012) is any vein draining into a first order branch (e.g., left adrenal, petrosal sinus). Contrast material for venography is injected into the catheter that has traveled to an area upstream of the site under investigation. Once the procedure is complete, the catheter is removed, and pressure applied to stop bleeding at the injection site.

Coding Tips

These codes include local anesthesia, introduction of needles or catheter, injection of contrast material with or without automatic power injection, and/or necessary pre- and postinjection care specifically related to the injection performed by the physician. Supplies (catheters, drugs, and contrast media) are not included in the listed service for the injection procedures. For chemotherapy of malignant disease, see 96401–96549. For an injection procedure in addition to cardiac catheterization, see 93452–93461 and 93563–93568. For radiological supervision and interpretation of the venography, see 75820–75891. Named or unnamed venous branches beyond a second-order branch should be reported with 36012.

ICD-10-CM Diagnostic Codes

I15.0	Renovascular hypertension
I15.1	Hypertension secondary to other renal disorders
I16.0	Hypertensive urgency
I16.1	Hypertensive emergency
I82.3	Embolism and thrombosis of renal vein
I82.C11	Acute embolism and thrombosis of right internal jugular vein ☑
I82.C12	Acute embolism and thrombosis of left internal jugular vein ☑
I82.C13	Acute embolism and thrombosis of internal jugular vein, bilateral ☑
I82.C21	Chronic embolism and thrombosis of right internal jugular vein ☑
I82.C22	Chronic embolism and thrombosis of left internal jugular vein ☑
I82.C23	Chronic embolism and thrombosis of internal jugular vein, bilateral ☑
I87.1	Compression of vein
I87.2	Venous insufficiency (chronic) (peripheral)
I87.8	Other specified disorders of veins
I87.9	Disorder of vein, unspecified

AMA: 36011 2018,Jan,8; 2017,Jan,8; 2016,Jul,6; 2016,Jan,13; 2015,Jan,16; 2014,Jan,11 **36012** 2018,Oct,3; 2018,Jan,8; 2017,Jan,8; 2016,Jul,6; 2016,Jan,13; 2015,Jan,16; 2014,Jan,11

Relative Value Units/Medicare Edits

Non-Facility RVU	Work	PE	MP	Total
36011	3.14	20.42	0.46	24.02
36012	3.51	20.46	0.53	24.5
Facility RVU	**Work**	**PE**	**MP**	**Total**
36011	3.14	0.94	0.46	4.54
36012	3.51	0.99	0.53	5.03

	FUD	Status	MUE	Modifiers				IOM Reference
36011	N/A	A	4(3)	51	50	N/A	N/A	None
36012	N/A	A	4(3)	51	50	N/A	N/A	

* with documentation

Terms To Know

catheter. Flexible tube inserted into an area of the body for introducing or withdrawing fluid.

contrast material. Radiopaque substance placed into the body to enable a system or body structure to be visualized, such as nonionic and low osmolar contrast media (LOCM), ionic and high osmolar contrast media (HOCM), barium, and gadolinium.

guidewire. Flexible metal instrument designed to lead another instrument in its proper course.

implantable venous access device. Catheter implanted for continuous access to the venous system for long-term parenteral feeding or for the administration of fluids or medications.

vein. Vessel through which oxygen-depleted blood passes back to the heart.

vena cava. Main venous trunk that empties into the right atrium from both the lower and upper regions, beginning at the junction of the common iliac veins inferiorly and the two brachiocephalic veins superiorly.

venography. Radiographic study of the veins.

36013

36013 Introduction of catheter, right heart or main pulmonary artery

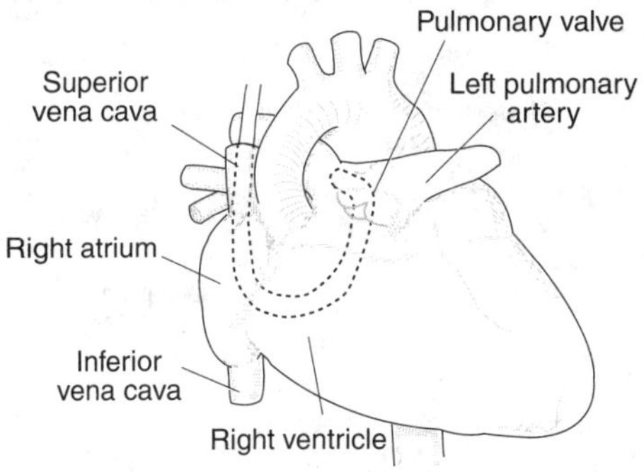

Introduction of a catheter into the right side of the heart or into the main pulmonary artery

Explanation

The physician punctures a distal vein (typically antecubital, internal jugular, subclavian, or femoral) with a large needle and passes a guidewire via the needle into the punctured vein. The physician removes the needle while leaving the guidewire in place, and enlarges the skin opening slightly with a blade. The physician slides an introducer sheath over the guidewire into the venous lumen. The physician inserts the catheter into the vein through an O-ring in the introducer sheath (this prevents blood from leaking around the catheter) and advances the catheter into the right heart or main pulmonary artery, using fluoroscopic guidance or while measuring pressures through the catheter lumen to ensure that the catheter tip is in the desired place. The physician may use the catheter to inject contrast material to perform venography or pulmonary arteriography.

Coding Tips

Listed services for injection procedures include necessary local anesthesia, introduction of needles or catheter, injection of contrast material with or without automatic power injection, and/or necessary pre- and postinjection care specifically related to the injection procedure. Catheters, drugs, and contrast media are not included in the listed service for the injection procedures. For radiology supervision and interpretation, see 75741–75746. For introduction of catheter, superior or inferior vena cava, see 36010; aorta, see 36200. For other cardiac catheterizations and injection procedures in addition to cardiac catheterization, see 93452–93461 and 93563–93568.

ICD-10-CM Diagnostic Codes

I05.0	Rheumatic mitral stenosis
I05.1	Rheumatic mitral insufficiency
I05.2	Rheumatic mitral stenosis with insufficiency
I05.8	Other rheumatic mitral valve diseases
I08.0	Rheumatic disorders of both mitral and aortic valves
I08.1	Rheumatic disorders of both mitral and tricuspid valves
I08.2	Rheumatic disorders of both aortic and tricuspid valves
I08.3	Combined rheumatic disorders of mitral, aortic and tricuspid valves
I08.8	Other rheumatic multiple valve diseases
I25.3	Aneurysm of heart
I25.89	Other forms of chronic ischemic heart disease
I27.0	Primary pulmonary hypertension
I27.21	Secondary pulmonary arterial hypertension
I27.22	Pulmonary hypertension due to left heart disease
I27.23	Pulmonary hypertension due to lung diseases and hypoxia
I27.24	Chronic thromboembolic pulmonary hypertension
I27.29	Other secondary pulmonary hypertension
I27.82	Chronic pulmonary embolism
I27.83	Eisenmenger's syndrome
I27.89	Other specified pulmonary heart diseases
I28.0	Arteriovenous fistula of pulmonary vessels
I28.1	Aneurysm of pulmonary artery
I28.8	Other diseases of pulmonary vessels
I34.0	Nonrheumatic mitral (valve) insufficiency
I34.1	Nonrheumatic mitral (valve) prolapse
I34.2	Nonrheumatic mitral (valve) stenosis
I34.8	Other nonrheumatic mitral valve disorders
I37.0	Nonrheumatic pulmonary valve stenosis
I37.1	Nonrheumatic pulmonary valve insufficiency
I37.2	Nonrheumatic pulmonary valve stenosis with insufficiency
I37.8	Other nonrheumatic pulmonary valve disorders
I42.0	Dilated cardiomyopathy
I42.1	Obstructive hypertrophic cardiomyopathy
I42.2	Other hypertrophic cardiomyopathy
I42.5	Other restrictive cardiomyopathy
I42.6	Alcoholic cardiomyopathy
I42.7	Cardiomyopathy due to drug and external agent
I42.8	Other cardiomyopathies
I50.1	Left ventricular failure, unspecified
I50.21	Acute systolic (congestive) heart failure
I50.22	Chronic systolic (congestive) heart failure
I50.23	Acute on chronic systolic (congestive) heart failure
I50.31	Acute diastolic (congestive) heart failure
I50.32	Chronic diastolic (congestive) heart failure
I50.33	Acute on chronic diastolic (congestive) heart failure
I50.41	Acute combined systolic (congestive) and diastolic (congestive) heart failure
I50.42	Chronic combined systolic (congestive) and diastolic (congestive) heart failure
I50.43	Acute on chronic combined systolic (congestive) and diastolic (congestive) heart failure
I50.811	Acute right heart failure
I50.812	Chronic right heart failure
I50.813	Acute on chronic right heart failure
I50.814	Right heart failure due to left heart failure
I50.82	Biventricular heart failure
I50.83	High output heart failure
I50.84	End stage heart failure
J81.0	Acute pulmonary edema
J81.1	Chronic pulmonary edema
Q21.0	Ventricular septal defect
Q21.1	Atrial septal defect
Q21.3	Tetralogy of Fallot
Q21.4	Aortopulmonary septal defect
Q21.8	Other congenital malformations of cardiac septa

Q22.0	Pulmonary valve atresia
Q22.1	Congenital pulmonary valve stenosis
Q22.2	Congenital pulmonary valve insufficiency
Q22.3	Other congenital malformations of pulmonary valve
Q22.4	Congenital tricuspid stenosis
Q22.5	Ebstein's anomaly
Q22.6	Hypoplastic right heart syndrome
Q22.8	Other congenital malformations of tricuspid valve
Q23.0	Congenital stenosis of aortic valve
Q23.1	Congenital insufficiency of aortic valve
Q23.2	Congenital mitral stenosis
Q23.3	Congenital mitral insufficiency
Q23.4	Hypoplastic left heart syndrome
Q23.8	Other congenital malformations of aortic and mitral valves
Q24.3	Pulmonary infundibular stenosis
Q24.8	Other specified congenital malformations of heart
R57.0	Cardiogenic shock

AMA: **36013** 2019,Jun,3; 2018,Jan,8; 2017,Jan,8; 2016,Jul,6; 2016,Jan,13; 2015,Jan,16; 2014,Jan,11

Relative Value Units/Medicare Edits

Non-Facility RVU	Work	PE	MP	Total
36013	2.52	19.02	0.3	21.84
Facility RVU	**Work**	**PE**	**MP**	**Total**
36013	2.52	0.7	0.3	3.52

	FUD	Status	MUE	Modifiers				IOM Reference
36013	N/A	A	2(3)	51	N/A	N/A	N/A	None

* with documentation

Terms To Know

implantable venous access device. Catheter implanted for continuous access to the venous system for long-term parenteral feeding or for the administration of fluids or medications.

tetralogy of Fallot. Specific combination of congenital cardiac defects: obstruction of the right ventricular outflow tract with pulmonary stenosis, interventricular septal defect, malposition of the aorta, overriding the interventricular septum and receiving blood from both the venous and arterial systems, and enlargement of the right ventricle.

ventricular septal defect. Congenital cardiac anomaly resulting in a continual opening in the septum between the ventricles that, in severe cases, causes oxygenated blood to flow back into the lungs, resulting in pulmonary hypertension.

36014-36015

36014 Selective catheter placement, left or right pulmonary artery

36015 Selective catheter placement, segmental or subsegmental pulmonary artery

Introduction through to the right pulmonary artery shown

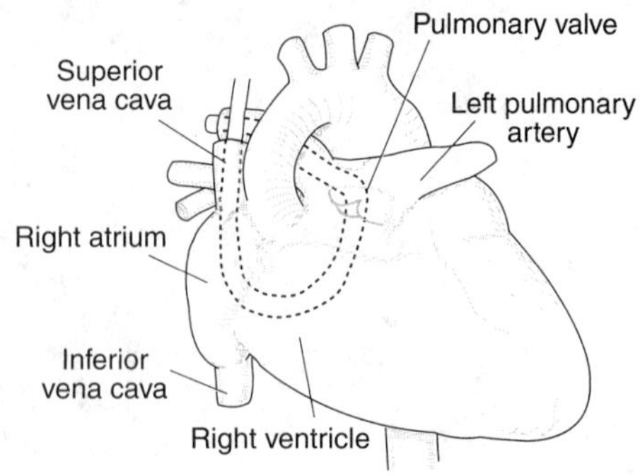

Explanation

The physician punctures a distal vein (typically antecubital, internal jugular, subclavian, or femoral) with a large needle and passes a guidewire via the needle into the punctured vein. The physician removes the needle while leaving the guidewire in place, and enlarges the skin opening slightly with a blade. The physician slides an introducer sheath over the guidewire into the venous lumen. The physician inserts the catheter into the vein through an O-ring in the introducer sheath (this prevents blood from leaking around the catheter) and advances the catheter into one of the main pulmonary arteries (right or left) in 36014 or into one of the segmental or subsegmental pulmonary arteries in 36015, using fluoroscopic guidance and possibly measuring pressures through the catheter lumen to ensure that the catheter tip is in the desired place. The physician may use the catheter to inject contrast material to perform venography or pulmonary arteriography.

Coding Tips

Placement of a CVP line and/or a Swan-Ganz catheter may be reported separately when placed at a different site than the intra-pulmonary catheter for 36014. For an insertion of a flow directed catheter (e.g., Swan-Ganz), see 93503. Listed services for injection procedures include necessary local anesthesia, introduction of needles or catheter, injection of contrast material with or without automatic power injection, and/or necessary pre- and post-injection care specifically related to the injection procedure. Supplies (catheters, drugs, and contrast media) are not included in the listed service for the injection procedures. For venous catheterization for selective organ blood sampling, see 36500. For cardiac catheterizations, injection procedures in addition to cardiac catheterization, see 93452–93461 and 93563–93568.

ICD-10-CM Diagnostic Codes

C34.01	Malignant neoplasm of right main bronchus ☑
C34.02	Malignant neoplasm of left main bronchus ☑
C34.11	Malignant neoplasm of upper lobe, right bronchus or lung ☑
C34.12	Malignant neoplasm of upper lobe, left bronchus or lung ☑
C34.2	Malignant neoplasm of middle lobe, bronchus or lung
C34.31	Malignant neoplasm of lower lobe, right bronchus or lung ☑
C34.32	Malignant neoplasm of lower lobe, left bronchus or lung ☑
C34.81	Malignant neoplasm of overlapping sites of right bronchus and lung ☑

C34.82 Malignant neoplasm of overlapping sites of left bronchus and lung ☑
I26.01 Septic pulmonary embolism with acute cor pulmonale
I26.02 Saddle embolus of pulmonary artery with acute cor pulmonale
I26.09 Other pulmonary embolism with acute cor pulmonale
I26.90 Septic pulmonary embolism without acute cor pulmonale
I26.92 Saddle embolus of pulmonary artery without acute cor pulmonale
I26.93 Single subsegmental pulmonary embolism without acute cor pulmonale
I26.94 Multiple subsegmental pulmonary emboli without acute cor pulmonale
I26.99 Other pulmonary embolism without acute cor pulmonale
I27.0 Primary pulmonary hypertension
I27.21 Secondary pulmonary arterial hypertension
I27.22 Pulmonary hypertension due to left heart disease
I27.23 Pulmonary hypertension due to lung diseases and hypoxia
I27.24 Chronic thromboembolic pulmonary hypertension
I27.29 Other secondary pulmonary hypertension
I27.82 Chronic pulmonary embolism
I27.83 Eisenmenger's syndrome
I27.89 Other specified pulmonary heart diseases
I28.0 Arteriovenous fistula of pulmonary vessels
I28.1 Aneurysm of pulmonary artery
I28.8 Other diseases of pulmonary vessels
I31.4 Cardiac tamponade
I42.0 Dilated cardiomyopathy
I50.1 Left ventricular failure, unspecified
I50.21 Acute systolic (congestive) heart failure
I50.22 Chronic systolic (congestive) heart failure
I50.23 Acute on chronic systolic (congestive) heart failure
I50.31 Acute diastolic (congestive) heart failure
I50.32 Chronic diastolic (congestive) heart failure
I50.33 Acute on chronic diastolic (congestive) heart failure
I50.41 Acute combined systolic (congestive) and diastolic (congestive) heart failure
I50.42 Chronic combined systolic (congestive) and diastolic (congestive) heart failure
I50.43 Acute on chronic combined systolic (congestive) and diastolic (congestive) heart failure
I50.811 Acute right heart failure
I50.812 Chronic right heart failure
I50.813 Acute on chronic right heart failure
I50.814 Right heart failure due to left heart failure
I50.82 Biventricular heart failure
I50.83 High output heart failure
I50.84 End stage heart failure
J44.0 Chronic obstructive pulmonary disease with (acute) lower respiratory infection
J44.1 Chronic obstructive pulmonary disease with (acute) exacerbation
J81.0 Acute pulmonary edema
J81.1 Chronic pulmonary edema
J90 Pleural effusion, not elsewhere classified
J91.0 Malignant pleural effusion
J91.8 Pleural effusion in other conditions classified elsewhere
J98.11 Atelectasis
J98.19 Other pulmonary collapse

AMA: **36014** 2019,Jun,3; 2018,Jan,8; 2017,Jan,8; 2016,Jul,6; 2016,Jan,13; 2015,Jan,16; 2014,Jan,11 **36015** 2019,Jun,3; 2018,Jan,8; 2017,Jan,8; 2016,Jul,6; 2016,Jan,13; 2015,Jan,16; 2014,Jan,11

Relative Value Units/Medicare Edits

Non-Facility RVU	Work	PE	MP	Total
36014	3.02	19.62	0.42	23.06
36015	3.51	21.07	0.4	24.98
Facility RVU	**Work**	**PE**	**MP**	**Total**
36014	3.02	0.94	0.42	4.38
36015	3.51	1.07	0.4	4.98

	FUD	Status	MUE	Modifiers				IOM Reference
36014	N/A	A	2(3)	51	50	N/A	N/A	None
36015	N/A	A	4(3)	51	50	N/A	N/A	

* with documentation

Terms To Know

catheter. Flexible tube inserted into an area of the body for introducing or withdrawing fluid.

contrast material. Radiopaque substance placed into the body to enable a system or body structure to be visualized, such as nonionic and low osmolar contrast media (LOCM), ionic and high osmolar contrast media (HOCM), barium, and gadolinium.

distal. Located farther away from a specified reference point or the trunk.

guidewire. Flexible metal instrument designed to lead another instrument in its proper course.

introducer. Instrument, such as a catheter, needle, or tube, through which another instrument or device is introduced into the body.

36100

36100 Introduction of needle or intracatheter, carotid or vertebral artery

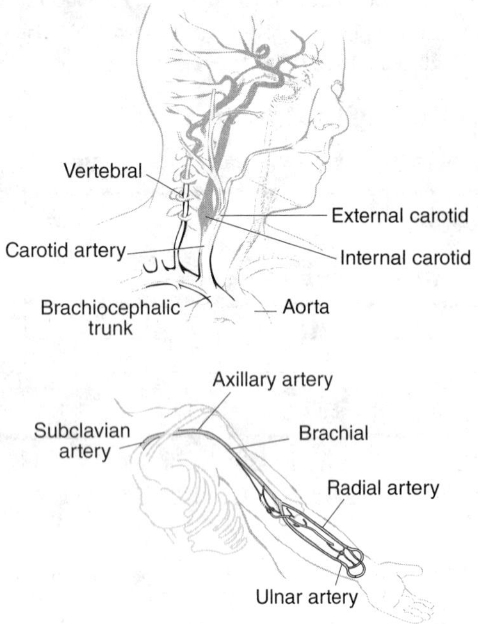

Explanation

Through the skin of the neck, the physician inserts a needle into the carotid or vertebral artery. A guidewire is threaded through the needle into the artery and the needle is removed. A catheter follows the wire into the artery. The wire is removed. Contrast material is injected through the catheter into the artery for arteriography. Once the procedure is complete, the catheter is removed and pressure is applied to the puncture site to stop bleeding.

Coding Tips

Note that 36100 is a unilateral procedure. If performed bilaterally, some payers require that the service be reported twice with modifier 50 appended to the second code, while others require identification of the service only once with modifier 50 appended. Check with individual payers. Modifier 50 identifies a procedure performed identically on the opposite side of the body (mirror image). These codes include local anesthesia, introduction of needles or catheter, injection of contrast material with or without automatic power injection, and/or necessary pre- and postinjection care specifically related to the injection. Supplies (catheters, drugs, and contrast media) are not included in the listed service. For introduction of a needle or intracatheter, vein, see 36000; extremity artery, see 36140; and aortic translumbar, see 36160.

ICD-10-CM Diagnostic Codes

G45.0	Vertebro-basilar artery syndrome
G45.1	Carotid artery syndrome (hemispheric)
G45.8	Other transient cerebral ischemic attacks and related syndromes
G45.9	Transient cerebral ischemic attack, unspecified
I63.011	Cerebral infarction due to thrombosis of right vertebral artery ☑
I63.012	Cerebral infarction due to thrombosis of left vertebral artery ☑
I63.013	Cerebral infarction due to thrombosis of bilateral vertebral arteries ☑
I63.031	Cerebral infarction due to thrombosis of right carotid artery ☑
I63.032	Cerebral infarction due to thrombosis of left carotid artery ☑
I63.033	Cerebral infarction due to thrombosis of bilateral carotid arteries ☑
I63.111	Cerebral infarction due to embolism of right vertebral artery ☑
I63.112	Cerebral infarction due to embolism of left vertebral artery ☑
I63.113	Cerebral infarction due to embolism of bilateral vertebral arteries ☑
I63.131	Cerebral infarction due to embolism of right carotid artery ☑
I63.132	Cerebral infarction due to embolism of left carotid artery ☑
I63.133	Cerebral infarction due to embolism of bilateral carotid arteries ☑
I63.313	Cerebral infarction due to thrombosis of bilateral middle cerebral arteries ☑
I63.323	Cerebral infarction due to thrombosis of bilateral anterior cerebral arteries ☑
I63.333	Cerebral infarction due to thrombosis of bilateral posterior cerebral arteries ☑
I63.343	Cerebral infarction due to thrombosis of bilateral cerebellar arteries ☑
I63.413	Cerebral infarction due to embolism of bilateral middle cerebral arteries ☑
I63.423	Cerebral infarction due to embolism of bilateral anterior cerebral arteries ☑
I63.433	Cerebral infarction due to embolism of bilateral posterior cerebral arteries ☑
I63.443	Cerebral infarction due to embolism of bilateral cerebellar arteries ☑
I63.81	Other cerebral infarction due to occlusion or stenosis of small artery
I63.89	Other cerebral infarction
I65.01	Occlusion and stenosis of right vertebral artery ☑
I65.02	Occlusion and stenosis of left vertebral artery ☑
I65.03	Occlusion and stenosis of bilateral vertebral arteries ☑
I65.21	Occlusion and stenosis of right carotid artery ☑
I65.22	Occlusion and stenosis of left carotid artery ☑
I65.23	Occlusion and stenosis of bilateral carotid arteries ☑
I67.81	Acute cerebrovascular insufficiency
I67.82	Cerebral ischemia
I67.850	Cerebral autosomal dominant arteriopathy with subcortical infarcts and leukoencephalopathy
I67.858	Other hereditary cerebrovascular disease
I72.0	Aneurysm of carotid artery
I76	Septic arterial embolism
I77.1	Stricture of artery
I77.2	Rupture of artery
I77.71	Dissection of carotid artery
I77.74	Dissection of vertebral artery
I77.89	Other specified disorders of arteries and arterioles

AMA: 36100 2000,Oct,4

Relative Value Units/Medicare Edits

Non-Facility RVU	Work	PE	MP	Total
36100	3.02	11.09	0.7	14.81
Facility RVU	**Work**	**PE**	**MP**	**Total**
36100	3.02	0.82	0.7	4.54

	FUD	Status	MUE	Modifiers				IOM Reference
36100	N/A	A	2(3)	51	50	N/A	N/A	None

* with documentation

Terms To Know

aortic arch. Thoracic aorta, ascending/arch.

arteriogram. Radiograph of arteries.

catheter. Flexible tube inserted into an area of the body for introducing or withdrawing fluid.

contrast material. Radiopaque substance placed into the body to enable a system or body structure to be visualized, such as nonionic and low osmolar contrast media (LOCM), ionic and high osmolar contrast media (HOCM), barium, and gadolinium.

guidewire. Flexible metal instrument designed to lead another instrument in its proper course.

36140

36140 Introduction of needle or intracatheter, upper or lower extremity artery

The provider places a needle or catheter into an upper extremity artery to inject contrast material for arteriography

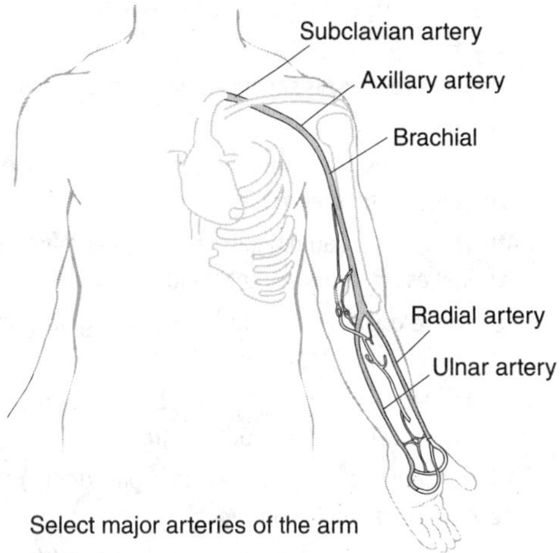

Select major arteries of the arm

Explanation

Through a puncture in the skin over an upper or lower extremity artery, the physician injects a needle into the artery and threads a guidewire through it. The needle is removed. A catheter follows the wire into the artery and the wire is removed. Contrast material for arteriography is injected into the catheter placed upstream of the site under investigation. Once the procedure is complete, the catheter is removed and pressure is applied to stop bleeding at the injection site.

Coding Tips

When medically necessary, report moderate (conscious) sedation provided by the performing physician with 99151-99153. When provided by another physician, report 99155-99157. Note that 36140 includes local anesthesia, introduction of needles or catheter, injection of contrast material with or without automatic power injection, and/or necessary pre- and postinjection care specifically related to the injection. Supplies (catheters, drugs, and contrast media) are not included in this procedure. For introduction of a needle or an intracatheter, vein, see 36000. Chemotherapy codes are reported in addition to intracatheter placements. For an injection procedure in addition to cardiac catheterization, see 93452–93461 and 93563–93568. For radiological supervision and interpretation, see 75710 or 75716. For insertion of an arteriovenous cannula, see 36810–36821.

ICD-10-CM Diagnostic Codes

I70.211	Atherosclerosis of native arteries of extremities with intermittent claudication, right leg ☑
I70.218	Atherosclerosis of native arteries of extremities with intermittent claudication, other extremity
I70.221	Atherosclerosis of native arteries of extremities with rest pain, right leg ☑
I70.228	Atherosclerosis of native arteries of extremities with rest pain, other extremity
I70.231	Atherosclerosis of native arteries of right leg with ulceration of thigh ☑

I70.232 Atherosclerosis of native arteries of right leg with ulceration of calf ☑

I70.233 Atherosclerosis of native arteries of right leg with ulceration of ankle ☑

I70.234 Atherosclerosis of native arteries of right leg with ulceration of heel and midfoot ☑

I70.261 Atherosclerosis of native arteries of extremities with gangrene, right leg ☑

I70.268 Atherosclerosis of native arteries of extremities with gangrene, other extremity

I70.298 Other atherosclerosis of native arteries of extremities, other extremity

I70.411 Atherosclerosis of autologous vein bypass graft(s) of the extremities with intermittent claudication, right leg ☑

I70.418 Atherosclerosis of autologous vein bypass graft(s) of the extremities with intermittent claudication, other extremity

I70.421 Atherosclerosis of autologous vein bypass graft(s) of the extremities with rest pain, right leg ☑

I70.428 Atherosclerosis of autologous vein bypass graft(s) of the extremities with rest pain, other extremity

I70.431 Atherosclerosis of autologous vein bypass graft(s) of the right leg with ulceration of thigh ☑

I70.432 Atherosclerosis of autologous vein bypass graft(s) of the right leg with ulceration of calf ☑

I70.433 Atherosclerosis of autologous vein bypass graft(s) of the right leg with ulceration of ankle ☑

I70.434 Atherosclerosis of autologous vein bypass graft(s) of the right leg with ulceration of heel and midfoot ☑

I70.435 Atherosclerosis of autologous vein bypass graft(s) of the right leg with ulceration of other part of foot ☑

I70.438 Atherosclerosis of autologous vein bypass graft(s) of the right leg with ulceration of other part of lower leg ☑

I70.461 Atherosclerosis of autologous vein bypass graft(s) of the extremities with gangrene, right leg ☑

I70.468 Atherosclerosis of autologous vein bypass graft(s) of the extremities with gangrene, other extremity

I70.491 Other atherosclerosis of autologous vein bypass graft(s) of the extremities, right leg ☑

I70.498 Other atherosclerosis of autologous vein bypass graft(s) of the extremities, other extremity

I70.511 Atherosclerosis of nonautologous biological bypass graft(s) of the extremities with intermittent claudication, right leg ☑

I70.521 Atherosclerosis of nonautologous biological bypass graft(s) of the extremities with rest pain, right leg ☑

I70.528 Atherosclerosis of nonautologous biological bypass graft(s) of the extremities with rest pain, other extremity

I70.531 Atherosclerosis of nonautologous biological bypass graft(s) of the right leg with ulceration of thigh ☑

I70.532 Atherosclerosis of nonautologous biological bypass graft(s) of the right leg with ulceration of calf ☑

I70.533 Atherosclerosis of nonautologous biological bypass graft(s) of the right leg with ulceration of ankle ☑

I70.534 Atherosclerosis of nonautologous biological bypass graft(s) of the right leg with ulceration of heel and midfoot ☑

I70.535 Atherosclerosis of nonautologous biological bypass graft(s) of the right leg with ulceration of other part of foot ☑

I70.538 Atherosclerosis of nonautologous biological bypass graft(s) of the right leg with ulceration of other part of lower leg ☑

I70.561 Atherosclerosis of nonautologous biological bypass graft(s) of the extremities with gangrene, right leg ☑

I70.568 Atherosclerosis of nonautologous biological bypass graft(s) of the extremities with gangrene, other extremity

I70.591 Other atherosclerosis of nonautologous biological bypass graft(s) of the extremities, right leg ☑

I70.598 Other atherosclerosis of nonautologous biological bypass graft(s) of the extremities, other extremity

I70.611 Atherosclerosis of nonbiological bypass graft(s) of the extremities with intermittent claudication, right leg ☑

I70.618 Atherosclerosis of nonbiological bypass graft(s) of the extremities with intermittent claudication, other extremity

I70.621 Atherosclerosis of nonbiological bypass graft(s) of the extremities with rest pain, right leg ☑

I70.628 Atherosclerosis of nonbiological bypass graft(s) of the extremities with rest pain, other extremity

I70.631 Atherosclerosis of nonbiological bypass graft(s) of the right leg with ulceration of thigh ☑

I70.632 Atherosclerosis of nonbiological bypass graft(s) of the right leg with ulceration of calf ☑

I70.633 Atherosclerosis of nonbiological bypass graft(s) of the right leg with ulceration of ankle ☑

I70.634 Atherosclerosis of nonbiological bypass graft(s) of the right leg with ulceration of heel and midfoot ☑

I70.635 Atherosclerosis of nonbiological bypass graft(s) of the right leg with ulceration of other part of foot ☑

I70.638 Atherosclerosis of nonbiological bypass graft(s) of the right leg with ulceration of other part of lower leg ☑

I70.661 Atherosclerosis of nonbiological bypass graft(s) of the extremities with gangrene, right leg ☑

I70.668 Atherosclerosis of nonbiological bypass graft(s) of the extremities with gangrene, other extremity

I70.691 Other atherosclerosis of nonbiological bypass graft(s) of the extremities, right leg ☑

I70.698 Other atherosclerosis of nonbiological bypass graft(s) of the extremities, other extremity

I70.711 Atherosclerosis of other type of bypass graft(s) of the extremities with intermittent claudication, right leg ☑

I70.718 Atherosclerosis of other type of bypass graft(s) of the extremities with intermittent claudication, other extremity

I70.721 Atherosclerosis of other type of bypass graft(s) of the extremities with rest pain, right leg ☑

I70.728 Atherosclerosis of other type of bypass graft(s) of the extremities with rest pain, other extremity

I70.731 Atherosclerosis of other type of bypass graft(s) of the right leg with ulceration of thigh ☑

I70.732 Atherosclerosis of other type of bypass graft(s) of the right leg with ulceration of calf ☑

I70.733 Atherosclerosis of other type of bypass graft(s) of the right leg with ulceration of ankle ☑

I70.734 Atherosclerosis of other type of bypass graft(s) of the right leg with ulceration of heel and midfoot ☑

I70.741 Atherosclerosis of other type of bypass graft(s) of the left leg with ulceration of thigh ☑

I70.742 Atherosclerosis of other type of bypass graft(s) of the left leg with ulceration of calf ☑

I70.743 Atherosclerosis of other type of bypass graft(s) of the left leg with ulceration of ankle ☑

I70.744 Atherosclerosis of other type of bypass graft(s) of the left leg with ulceration of heel and midfoot ☑

I70.745 Atherosclerosis of other type of bypass graft(s) of the left leg with ulceration of other part of foot ☑

I70.761 Atherosclerosis of other type of bypass graft(s) of the extremities with gangrene, right leg ☑

I70.768 Atherosclerosis of other type of bypass graft(s) of the extremities with gangrene, other extremity

I70.791 Other atherosclerosis of other type of bypass graft(s) of the extremities, right leg ☑

I70.798 Other atherosclerosis of other type of bypass graft(s) of the extremities, other extremity

I70.92 Chronic total occlusion of artery of the extremities

I74.2 Embolism and thrombosis of arteries of the upper extremities

I74.3 Embolism and thrombosis of arteries of the lower extremities

I74.4 Embolism and thrombosis of arteries of extremities, unspecified

I75.011 Atheroembolism of right upper extremity ☑

I75.021 Atheroembolism of right lower extremity ☑

I77.1 Stricture of artery

I77.2 Rupture of artery

AMA: 36140 2018,Jan,8; 2017,Jan,8; 2016,Jan,13; 2015,Jan,16; 2014,Jan,11

Relative Value Units/Medicare Edits

Non-Facility RVU	Work	PE	MP	Total
36140	1.76	10.61	0.36	12.73
Facility RVU	**Work**	**PE**	**MP**	**Total**
36140	1.76	0.5	0.36	2.62

	FUD	Status	MUE	Modifiers				IOM Reference
36140	N/A	A	3(3)	51	N/A	N/A	N/A	None

* with documentation

Terms To Know

arteriography. Radiologic study of an artery upon injection of dye.

catheter. Flexible tube inserted into an area of the body for introducing or withdrawing fluid.

36160

36160 Introduction of needle or intracatheter, aortic, translumbar

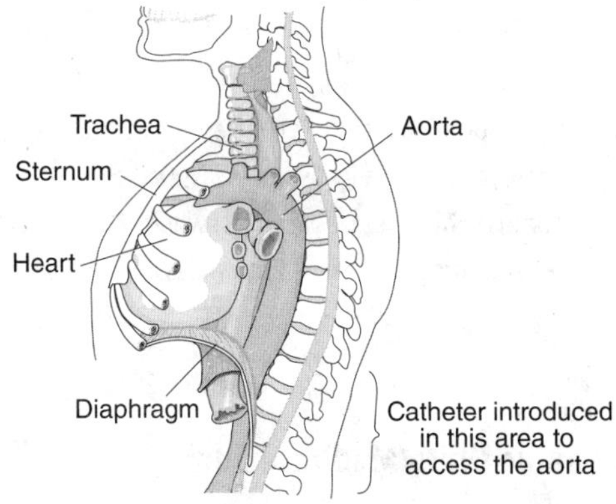

Explanation

The physician punctures the left lumbar area, typically just above a rib, to direct a large needle into the aorta. When pulsatile red blood is obtained through the needle, indicating successful aortic puncture, the physician passes a guidewire via the needle into the punctured aorta. The physician removes the needle while leaving the guidewire in place, and enlarges the skin opening slightly with a blade. The physician slides a catheter over the guidewire into the aortic lumen and secures the catheter in place with suture.

Coding Tips

This code includes local anesthesia, introduction of needles or catheter, injection of contrast material with or without automatic power injection, and/or necessary pre- and postinjection care specifically related to the injection. Other catheters, drugs, and contrast media are not included in the listed service. For introduction of needle or intracatheter, vein, see 36000; carotid or vertebral artery, see 36100; extremity artery, see 36140; chemotherapy of a malignant disease, see 96401–96549; an injection procedure in addition to cardiac catheterization, see 93452–93461 and 93563–93568.

ICD-10-CM Diagnostic Codes

A52.01 Syphilitic aneurysm of aorta

A52.02 Syphilitic aortitis

I70.0 Atherosclerosis of aorta

I71.01 Dissection of thoracic aorta

I71.02 Dissection of abdominal aorta

I71.03 Dissection of thoracoabdominal aorta

I71.1 Thoracic aortic aneurysm, ruptured

I71.2 Thoracic aortic aneurysm, without rupture

I71.3 Abdominal aortic aneurysm, ruptured

I71.4 Abdominal aortic aneurysm, without rupture

I71.5 Thoracoabdominal aortic aneurysm, ruptured

I71.6 Thoracoabdominal aortic aneurysm, without rupture

I74.01 Saddle embolus of abdominal aorta

I74.09 Other arterial embolism and thrombosis of abdominal aorta

I74.11 Embolism and thrombosis of thoracic aorta

I74.19 Embolism and thrombosis of other parts of aorta

I76 Septic arterial embolism

I77.1	Stricture of artery
I77.2	Rupture of artery
I77.3	Arterial fibromuscular dysplasia
I77.5	Necrosis of artery
I77.810	Thoracic aortic ectasia
I77.811	Abdominal aortic ectasia
I77.812	Thoracoabdominal aortic ectasia
I77.89	Other specified disorders of arteries and arterioles
I79.0	Aneurysm of aorta in diseases classified elsewhere
I79.1	Aortitis in diseases classified elsewhere
I79.8	Other disorders of arteries, arterioles and capillaries in diseases classified elsewhere

AMA: **36160** 2018,Jan,8; 2017,Jan,8; 2016,Jan,13; 2015,Jan,16; 2014,Jan,11

Relative Value Units/Medicare Edits

Non-Facility RVU	Work	PE	MP	Total
36160	2.52	11.78	0.31	14.61
Facility RVU	**Work**	**PE**	**MP**	**Total**
36160	2.52	0.76	0.31	3.59

	FUD	Status	MUE	Modifiers				IOM Reference
36160	N/A	A	2(3)	51	N/A	N/A	N/A	None

* with documentation

Terms To Know

aneurysm. Circumscribed dilation or outpouching of an artery wall, often containing blood clots and connecting directly with the lumen of the artery.

atherosclerosis. Buildup of yellowish plaques composed of cholesterol and lipoid material within the arteries.

catheter. Flexible tube inserted into an area of the body for introducing or withdrawing fluid.

guidewire. Flexible metal instrument designed to lead another instrument in its proper course.

lumen. Space inside an intestine, artery, vein, duct, or tube.

retrograde. Moving against the usual direction of flow.

rupture. Tearing or breaking open of tissue.

stricture. Narrowing of an anatomical structure.

36200

36200 Introduction of catheter, aorta

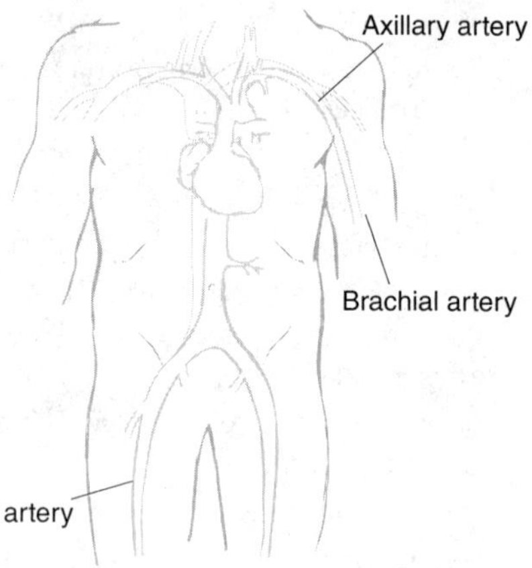

Explanation

The physician punctures a distal artery (typically femoral, brachial, radial, or axillary) with a large needle and passes a guidewire via the needle into the punctured artery. The physician removes the needle while leaving the guidewire in place, and enlarges the skin opening slightly with a blade. The physician slides an introducer sheath over the guidewire into the arterial lumen. The physician inserts a catheter into the artery through an O-ring in the introducer sheath (this prevents blood from leaking around the catheter) and advances the catheter into the aorta. The physician may use the catheter to inject contrast material to perform aortography, measure aortic pressures, or to administer medication.

Coding Tips

When medically necessary, report moderate (conscious) sedation provided by the performing physician with 99151-99153. When provided by another physician, report 99155-99157. Listed services for injection procedures include necessary local anesthesia, introduction of needles or catheter, injection of contrast material with or without automatic power injection, and/or necessary pre- and postinjection care specifically related to the injection procedure. Catheters, drugs, and contrast media are not included in the listed service for the injection procedures. For introduction of a catheter, superior or inferior vena cava, see 36010; for right heart or main artery, see 36013. For other cardiac catheterizations, injection procedures in addition to cardiac catheterization, see 93452–93461 and 93563–93568. For nonselective angiography of the extracranial carotid, cerebral vessels, and cervicocerebral arch, see 36221.

ICD-10-CM Diagnostic Codes

A52.01	Syphilitic aneurysm of aorta
A52.02	Syphilitic aortitis
I70.0	Atherosclerosis of aorta
I70.211	Atherosclerosis of native arteries of extremities with intermittent claudication, right leg ☑
I70.212	Atherosclerosis of native arteries of extremities with intermittent claudication, left leg ☑
I70.221	Atherosclerosis of native arteries of extremities with rest pain, right leg ☑
I70.222	Atherosclerosis of native arteries of extremities with rest pain, left leg ☑
I71.1	Thoracic aortic aneurysm, ruptured

I71.2	Thoracic aortic aneurysm, without rupture
I71.3	Abdominal aortic aneurysm, ruptured
I71.4	Abdominal aortic aneurysm, without rupture
I71.5	Thoracoabdominal aortic aneurysm, ruptured
I71.6	Thoracoabdominal aortic aneurysm, without rupture
I74.01	Saddle embolus of abdominal aorta
I74.09	Other arterial embolism and thrombosis of abdominal aorta
I74.11	Embolism and thrombosis of thoracic aorta
I74.19	Embolism and thrombosis of other parts of aorta
I76	Septic arterial embolism
I77.1	Stricture of artery
I77.2	Rupture of artery
I77.3	Arterial fibromuscular dysplasia
I77.5	Necrosis of artery
I77.810	Thoracic aortic ectasia
I77.811	Abdominal aortic ectasia
I77.812	Thoracoabdominal aortic ectasia
I77.89	Other specified disorders of arteries and arterioles
I79.0	Aneurysm of aorta in diseases classified elsewhere
I79.1	Aortitis in diseases classified elsewhere
I79.8	Other disorders of arteries, arterioles and capillaries in diseases classified elsewhere

AMA: 36200 2018,Jan,8; 2017,Mar,3; 2017,Jan,8; 2016,Jul,6; 2016,Jan,13; 2015,Jan,16; 2014,Jan,11; 2013,Feb,16-17

Relative Value Units/Medicare Edits

Non-Facility RVU	Work	PE	MP	Total
36200	2.77	12.87	0.59	16.23
Facility RVU	**Work**	**PE**	**MP**	**Total**
36200	2.77	0.69	0.59	4.05

	FUD	Status	MUE	Modifiers				IOM Reference
36200	0	A	2(3)	51	50	N/A	N/A	None

* with documentation

Terms To Know

contrast material. Radiopaque substance placed into the body to enable a system or body structure to be visualized, such as nonionic and low osmolar contrast media (LOCM), ionic and high osmolar contrast media (HOCM), barium, and gadolinium.

embolism. Obstruction of a blood vessel resulting from a clot or foreign substance.

guidewire. Flexible metal instrument designed to lead another instrument in its proper course.

sheath. Covering enclosing an organ or part.

thrombus. Stationary blood clot inside a blood vessel.

36215-36216

36215 Selective catheter placement, arterial system; each first order thoracic or brachiocephalic branch, within a vascular family

36216 initial second order thoracic or brachiocephalic branch, within a vascular family

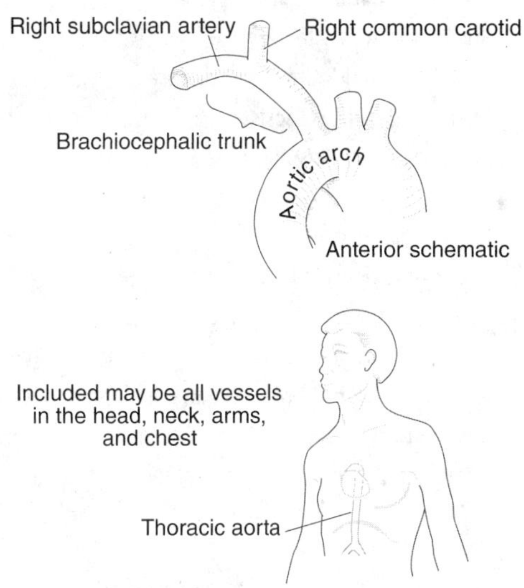

Explanation

The physician passes a needle into the skin into an extremity artery, usually in the upper thigh. A guidewire is threaded through the needle into the vessel. The needle is removed. The wire is threaded into the aorta and up to the thoracic aorta where it is manipulated into a branch off the aortic arch. A catheter follows the wire into a first order thoracic or brachiocephalic artery. The wire is removed. The catheter may pass through the first order vessel into a second order thoracic or brachiocephalic artery. Contrast material for arteriography is injected into the catheter that has been guided to an area upstream of the site under investigation. In 36215, the catheter remains in a first order artery. In 36216, the catheter travels further to a second order artery. Upon completion, the catheter is removed, and pressure applied to stop bleeding at the puncture site.

Coding Tips

These codes include introduction of needles or catheters, injection of contrast material with or without automatic power injection, and/or necessary pre- and postinjection care specifically related to the injection. Supplies (catheters, drugs, and contrast media) are not included in the listed service. Code the highest order vessel cannulated, but not any lesser order vessels cannulated in the approach. Report 36218 for each additional second order, third order, and more selective order vessel cannulated in the same vascular family. Right and left vessels belong to different vascular families; code separate catheterizations when performed. For radiological supervision and interpretation, see 75710. For catheter placement for coronary angiography, see 93454–93461.

ICD-10-CM Diagnostic Codes

C34.01	Malignant neoplasm of right main bronchus ☑
C34.11	Malignant neoplasm of upper lobe, right bronchus or lung ☑
C34.2	Malignant neoplasm of middle lobe, bronchus or lung
C34.31	Malignant neoplasm of lower lobe, right bronchus or lung ☑
C34.81	Malignant neoplasm of overlapping sites of right bronchus and lung ☑

G45.0	Vertebro-basilar artery syndrome
G45.1	Carotid artery syndrome (hemispheric)
G45.2	Multiple and bilateral precerebral artery syndromes
G45.3	Amaurosis fugax
G90.01	Carotid sinus syncope
I05.0	Rheumatic mitral stenosis
I05.1	Rheumatic mitral insufficiency
I05.2	Rheumatic mitral stenosis with insufficiency
I05.8	Other rheumatic mitral valve diseases
I06.0	Rheumatic aortic stenosis
I06.1	Rheumatic aortic insufficiency
I06.2	Rheumatic aortic stenosis with insufficiency
I07.0	Rheumatic tricuspid stenosis
I07.1	Rheumatic tricuspid insufficiency
I07.2	Rheumatic tricuspid stenosis and insufficiency
I08.0	Rheumatic disorders of both mitral and aortic valves
I08.1	Rheumatic disorders of both mitral and tricuspid valves
I08.2	Rheumatic disorders of both aortic and tricuspid valves
I08.3	Combined rheumatic disorders of mitral, aortic and tricuspid valves
I25.3	Aneurysm of heart
I26.01	Septic pulmonary embolism with acute cor pulmonale
I26.02	Saddle embolus of pulmonary artery with acute cor pulmonale
I26.09	Other pulmonary embolism with acute cor pulmonale
I26.90	Septic pulmonary embolism without acute cor pulmonale
I26.92	Saddle embolus of pulmonary artery without acute cor pulmonale
I27.0	Primary pulmonary hypertension
I27.21	Secondary pulmonary arterial hypertension
I27.22	Pulmonary hypertension due to left heart disease
I27.23	Pulmonary hypertension due to lung diseases and hypoxia
I27.24	Chronic thromboembolic pulmonary hypertension
I27.29	Other secondary pulmonary hypertension
I27.82	Chronic pulmonary embolism
I27.83	Eisenmenger's syndrome
I28.0	Arteriovenous fistula of pulmonary vessels
I28.1	Aneurysm of pulmonary artery
I31.4	Cardiac tamponade
I34.0	Nonrheumatic mitral (valve) insufficiency
I34.1	Nonrheumatic mitral (valve) prolapse
I34.2	Nonrheumatic mitral (valve) stenosis
I34.8	Other nonrheumatic mitral valve disorders
I35.0	Nonrheumatic aortic (valve) stenosis
I35.1	Nonrheumatic aortic (valve) insufficiency
I35.2	Nonrheumatic aortic (valve) stenosis with insufficiency
I37.0	Nonrheumatic pulmonary valve stenosis
I37.1	Nonrheumatic pulmonary valve insufficiency
I37.2	Nonrheumatic pulmonary valve stenosis with insufficiency
I42.0	Dilated cardiomyopathy
I42.1	Obstructive hypertrophic cardiomyopathy
I42.6	Alcoholic cardiomyopathy
I42.7	Cardiomyopathy due to drug and external agent
I50.21	Acute systolic (congestive) heart failure
I50.22	Chronic systolic (congestive) heart failure
I50.23	Acute on chronic systolic (congestive) heart failure
I50.31	Acute diastolic (congestive) heart failure
I50.32	Chronic diastolic (congestive) heart failure
I50.33	Acute on chronic diastolic (congestive) heart failure
I50.41	Acute combined systolic (congestive) and diastolic (congestive) heart failure
I50.42	Chronic combined systolic (congestive) and diastolic (congestive) heart failure
I50.43	Acute on chronic combined systolic (congestive) and diastolic (congestive) heart failure
I50.811	Acute right heart failure
I50.812	Chronic right heart failure
I50.813	Acute on chronic right heart failure
I50.814	Right heart failure due to left heart failure
I50.82	Biventricular heart failure
I50.83	High output heart failure
I50.84	End stage heart failure
I63.011	Cerebral infarction due to thrombosis of right vertebral artery ☑
I63.02	Cerebral infarction due to thrombosis of basilar artery
I63.031	Cerebral infarction due to thrombosis of right carotid artery ☑
I63.111	Cerebral infarction due to embolism of right vertebral artery ☑
I63.12	Cerebral infarction due to embolism of basilar artery
I63.131	Cerebral infarction due to embolism of right carotid artery ☑
I65.01	Occlusion and stenosis of right vertebral artery ☑
I65.1	Occlusion and stenosis of basilar artery
I65.21	Occlusion and stenosis of right carotid artery ☑
I67.81	Acute cerebrovascular insufficiency
I67.82	Cerebral ischemia
I67.841	Reversible cerebrovascular vasoconstriction syndrome
I67.850	Cerebral autosomal dominant arteriopathy with subcortical infarcts and leukoencephalopathy
I70.0	Atherosclerosis of aorta
I70.8	Atherosclerosis of other arteries
I70.92	Chronic total occlusion of artery of the extremities
I71.01	Dissection of thoracic aorta
I71.03	Dissection of thoracoabdominal aorta
I71.1	Thoracic aortic aneurysm, ruptured
I71.2	Thoracic aortic aneurysm, without rupture
I71.5	Thoracoabdominal aortic aneurysm, ruptured
I71.6	Thoracoabdominal aortic aneurysm, without rupture
I72.0	Aneurysm of carotid artery
I72.1	Aneurysm of artery of upper extremity
I72.5	Aneurysm of other precerebral arteries
I72.6	Aneurysm of vertebral artery
I74.19	Embolism and thrombosis of other parts of aorta
I74.2	Embolism and thrombosis of arteries of the upper extremities
I75.011	Atheroembolism of right upper extremity ☑
I76	Septic arterial embolism
I77.1	Stricture of artery
I77.2	Rupture of artery
I77.3	Arterial fibromuscular dysplasia
I77.5	Necrosis of artery

I77.71	Dissection of carotid artery
I77.74	Dissection of vertebral artery
I77.75	Dissection of other precerebral arteries
I77.76	Dissection of artery of upper extremity
I77.77	Dissection of artery of lower extremity
I77.810	Thoracic aortic ectasia
I77.812	Thoracoabdominal aortic ectasia
J44.0	Chronic obstructive pulmonary disease with (acute) lower respiratory infection
J44.1	Chronic obstructive pulmonary disease with (acute) exacerbation
J81.0	Acute pulmonary edema
J81.1	Chronic pulmonary edema
J98.11	Atelectasis
Q21.0	Ventricular septal defect
Q21.1	Atrial septal defect
Q21.3	Tetralogy of Fallot
Q21.4	Aortopulmonary septal defect
Q22.5	Ebstein's anomaly
Q22.6	Hypoplastic right heart syndrome
Q23.0	Congenital stenosis of aortic valve
Q23.1	Congenital insufficiency of aortic valve
Q23.2	Congenital mitral stenosis
Q23.3	Congenital mitral insufficiency
R57.0	Cardiogenic shock

AMA: 36215 2018,Jan,8; 2017,Mar,3; 2017,Jan,8; 2016,Jul,6; 2016,Jan,13; 2015,Jan,16; 2014,Jan,11 **36216** 2018,Jan,8; 2017,Jan,8; 2016,Jul,6; 2016,Jan,13; 2015,Jan,16; 2014,Jan,11; 2013,Nov,14

Relative Value Units/Medicare Edits

Non-Facility RVU	Work	PE	MP	Total
36215	4.17	24.64	0.59	29.4
36216	5.27	25.43	0.98	31.68
Facility RVU	**Work**	**PE**	**MP**	**Total**
36215	4.17	1.4	0.59	6.16
36216	5.27	1.68	0.98	7.93

	FUD	Status	MUE	Modifiers				IOM Reference
36215	0	A	6(3)	51	N/A	N/A	N/A	None
36216	0	A	4(3)	51	N/A	N/A	N/A	

* with documentation

Terms To Know

aortic arch. Thoracic aorta, ascending/arch.

first order. First vessel in the arterial or venous system that branches off the main vessel and supplies additional branches within the same vascular family.

second order catheter placement. Catheter manipulation into a vessel that branches off the aorta. May be noted in the record as a second branch or second family placement.

36217-36218

36217 Selective catheter placement, arterial system; initial third order or more selective thoracic or brachiocephalic branch, within a vascular family

\+ **36218** additional second order, third order, and beyond, thoracic or brachiocephalic branch, within a vascular family (List in addition to code for initial second or third order vessel as appropriate)

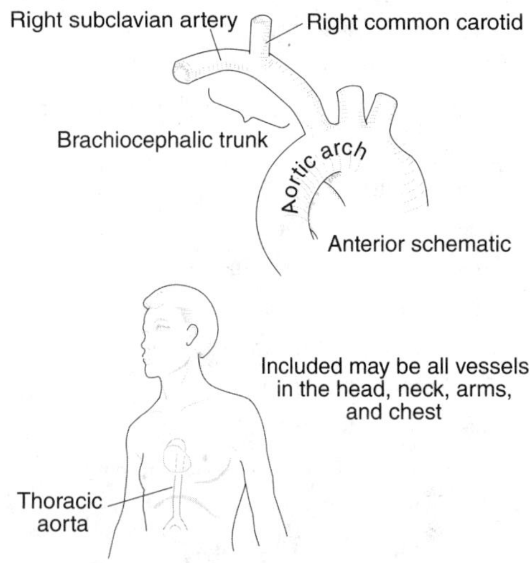

Explanation

The physician punctures the skin and underlying artery with a needle and threads a guidance wire through the needle into the artery. The needle is removed. The guidewire is manipulated into the specific artery. A catheter follows the wire into a first order thoracic or brachiocephalic artery. The catheter passes through the first order vessel into the second order thoracic or brachiocephalic artery. The catheter continues to a third order vessel. Contrast material for arteriography is injected into the catheter that has been guided to the site under investigation. Once the procedure is complete, the catheter is removed, and pressure applied to stop bleeding at the injection site. Use 36218 for an additional second order, third order, and beyond, thoracic or brachiocephalic branch, within a vascular family. Use 36218 in addition to 36216 or 36217.

Coding Tips

These codes include introduction of needles or catheter, injection of contrast material with or without automatic power injection, and/or necessary pre- and postinjection care specifically related to the injection. Supplies (catheters, drugs, and contrast media) are not included in the listed service. Code the highest order vessel cannulated, but not any lesser order vessels cannulated in the approach. Report 36218 for each additional second order, third order, and more selective order vessel cannulated in the same vascular family. Right and left vessels belong to different vascular families; therefore, code separate catheterizations when performed. Report 36218 in addition to 36216, 36217, 36225, and 36226. Do not report 36218 when performing diagnostic angiography of extracranial and intracranial cervicocerebral vessels. Named or unnamed arterial branches beyond a third-order arterial branch should be reported with 36218 or 36248, as appropriate. For angiography, see 36222–36228 and 75600–75774. Transcatheter therapy is reported using 37200, 37211, 37213, 37214, 37236–37239, 37241–37244, 61624, and 61626. For angiography of the coronary artery, arterial conduit, or venous bypass graft performed at the same time as cardiac catheterizations, see 93455, 93457, 93459, 93461, 93530–93533, and 93564. For angiography of the internal mammary artery without concomitant left heart catheterization, see 36216 or 36217.

ICD-10-CM Diagnostic Codes

C34.01	Malignant neoplasm of right main bronchus ☑
C34.11	Malignant neoplasm of upper lobe, right bronchus or lung ☑
C34.2	Malignant neoplasm of middle lobe, bronchus or lung
C34.31	Malignant neoplasm of lower lobe, right bronchus or lung ☑
C34.81	Malignant neoplasm of overlapping sites of right bronchus and lung ☑
G45.0	Vertebro-basilar artery syndrome
G45.1	Carotid artery syndrome (hemispheric)
G45.2	Multiple and bilateral precerebral artery syndromes
G45.3	Amaurosis fugax
G90.01	Carotid sinus syncope
I05.0	Rheumatic mitral stenosis
I05.1	Rheumatic mitral insufficiency
I05.2	Rheumatic mitral stenosis with insufficiency
I05.8	Other rheumatic mitral valve diseases
I06.0	Rheumatic aortic stenosis
I06.1	Rheumatic aortic insufficiency
I06.2	Rheumatic aortic stenosis with insufficiency
I07.0	Rheumatic tricuspid stenosis
I07.1	Rheumatic tricuspid insufficiency
I07.2	Rheumatic tricuspid stenosis and insufficiency
I08.0	Rheumatic disorders of both mitral and aortic valves
I08.1	Rheumatic disorders of both mitral and tricuspid valves
I08.2	Rheumatic disorders of both aortic and tricuspid valves
I08.3	Combined rheumatic disorders of mitral, aortic and tricuspid valves
I25.3	Aneurysm of heart
I26.01	Septic pulmonary embolism with acute cor pulmonale
I26.02	Saddle embolus of pulmonary artery with acute cor pulmonale
I26.09	Other pulmonary embolism with acute cor pulmonale
I26.90	Septic pulmonary embolism without acute cor pulmonale
I26.92	Saddle embolus of pulmonary artery without acute cor pulmonale
I27.0	Primary pulmonary hypertension
I27.21	Secondary pulmonary arterial hypertension
I27.22	Pulmonary hypertension due to left heart disease
I27.23	Pulmonary hypertension due to lung diseases and hypoxia
I27.24	Chronic thromboembolic pulmonary hypertension
I27.29	Other secondary pulmonary hypertension
I27.82	Chronic pulmonary embolism
I27.83	Eisenmenger's syndrome
I28.0	Arteriovenous fistula of pulmonary vessels
I28.1	Aneurysm of pulmonary artery
I31.4	Cardiac tamponade
I34.0	Nonrheumatic mitral (valve) insufficiency
I34.1	Nonrheumatic mitral (valve) prolapse
I34.2	Nonrheumatic mitral (valve) stenosis
I34.8	Other nonrheumatic mitral valve disorders
I35.0	Nonrheumatic aortic (valve) stenosis
I35.1	Nonrheumatic aortic (valve) insufficiency
I35.2	Nonrheumatic aortic (valve) stenosis with insufficiency
I37.0	Nonrheumatic pulmonary valve stenosis
I37.1	Nonrheumatic pulmonary valve insufficiency
I37.2	Nonrheumatic pulmonary valve stenosis with insufficiency
I42.0	Dilated cardiomyopathy
I42.1	Obstructive hypertrophic cardiomyopathy
I42.6	Alcoholic cardiomyopathy
I42.7	Cardiomyopathy due to drug and external agent
I50.21	Acute systolic (congestive) heart failure
I50.22	Chronic systolic (congestive) heart failure
I50.23	Acute on chronic systolic (congestive) heart failure
I50.31	Acute diastolic (congestive) heart failure
I50.32	Chronic diastolic (congestive) heart failure
I50.33	Acute on chronic diastolic (congestive) heart failure
I50.41	Acute combined systolic (congestive) and diastolic (congestive) heart failure
I50.42	Chronic combined systolic (congestive) and diastolic (congestive) heart failure
I50.43	Acute on chronic combined systolic (congestive) and diastolic (congestive) heart failure
I50.811	Acute right heart failure
I50.812	Chronic right heart failure
I50.813	Acute on chronic right heart failure
I50.814	Right heart failure due to left heart failure
I50.82	Biventricular heart failure
I50.83	High output heart failure
I50.84	End stage heart failure
I63.011	Cerebral infarction due to thrombosis of right vertebral artery ☑
I63.02	Cerebral infarction due to thrombosis of basilar artery
I63.031	Cerebral infarction due to thrombosis of right carotid artery ☑
I63.111	Cerebral infarction due to embolism of right vertebral artery ☑
I63.12	Cerebral infarction due to embolism of basilar artery
I63.131	Cerebral infarction due to embolism of right carotid artery ☑
I65.01	Occlusion and stenosis of right vertebral artery ☑
I65.1	Occlusion and stenosis of basilar artery
I65.21	Occlusion and stenosis of right carotid artery ☑
I67.81	Acute cerebrovascular insufficiency
I67.82	Cerebral ischemia
I67.841	Reversible cerebrovascular vasoconstriction syndrome
I67.850	Cerebral autosomal dominant arteriopathy with subcortical infarcts and leukoencephalopathy
I70.0	Atherosclerosis of aorta
I70.8	Atherosclerosis of other arteries
I70.92	Chronic total occlusion of artery of the extremities
I71.01	Dissection of thoracic aorta
I71.03	Dissection of thoracoabdominal aorta
I71.1	Thoracic aortic aneurysm, ruptured
I71.2	Thoracic aortic aneurysm, without rupture
I71.5	Thoracoabdominal aortic aneurysm, ruptured
I71.6	Thoracoabdominal aortic aneurysm, without rupture
I72.0	Aneurysm of carotid artery
I72.1	Aneurysm of artery of upper extremity
I72.5	Aneurysm of other precerebral arteries

I72.6	Aneurysm of vertebral artery
I74.19	Embolism and thrombosis of other parts of aorta
I74.2	Embolism and thrombosis of arteries of the upper extremities
I75.011	Atheroembolism of right upper extremity ☑
I76	Septic arterial embolism
I77.1	Stricture of artery
I77.2	Rupture of artery
I77.3	Arterial fibromuscular dysplasia
I77.5	Necrosis of artery
I77.71	Dissection of carotid artery
I77.74	Dissection of vertebral artery
I77.75	Dissection of other precerebral arteries
I77.76	Dissection of artery of upper extremity
I77.77	Dissection of artery of lower extremity
I77.810	Thoracic aortic ectasia
I77.812	Thoracoabdominal aortic ectasia
J44.0	Chronic obstructive pulmonary disease with (acute) lower respiratory infection
J44.1	Chronic obstructive pulmonary disease with (acute) exacerbation
J81.0	Acute pulmonary edema
J81.1	Chronic pulmonary edema
J98.11	Atelectasis
Q21.0	Ventricular septal defect
Q21.1	Atrial septal defect
Q21.3	Tetralogy of Fallot
Q21.4	Aortopulmonary septal defect
Q22.5	Ebstein's anomaly
Q22.6	Hypoplastic right heart syndrome
Q23.0	Congenital stenosis of aortic valve
Q23.1	Congenital insufficiency of aortic valve
Q23.2	Congenital mitral stenosis
Q23.3	Congenital mitral insufficiency
R57.0	Cardiogenic shock

AMA: **36217** 2018,Jan,8; 2017,Jan,8; 2016,Jul,6; 2016,Jan,13; 2015,Jan,16; 2014,Jan,11 **36218** 2018,Oct,3; 2018,Jan,8; 2017,Jan,8; 2016,Jul,6; 2016,Jan,13; 2015,Jan,16; 2014,Jan,11; 2013,May,3-5

Relative Value Units/Medicare Edits

Non-Facility RVU	Work	PE	MP	Total
36217	6.29	45.62	1.21	53.12
36218	1.01	5.7	0.18	6.89
Facility RVU	**Work**	**PE**	**MP**	**Total**
36217	6.29	2.01	1.21	9.51
36218	1.01	0.32	0.18	1.51

	FUD	Status	MUE	Modifiers				IOM Reference
36217	0	A	2(3)	51	N/A	N/A	N/A	None
36218	N/A	A	6(3)	N/A	N/A	N/A	N/A	

* with documentation

36221

36221 Non-selective catheter placement, thoracic aorta, with angiography of the extracranial carotid, vertebral, and/or intracranial vessels, unilateral or bilateral, and all associated radiological supervision and interpretation, includes angiography of the cervicocerebral arch, when performed

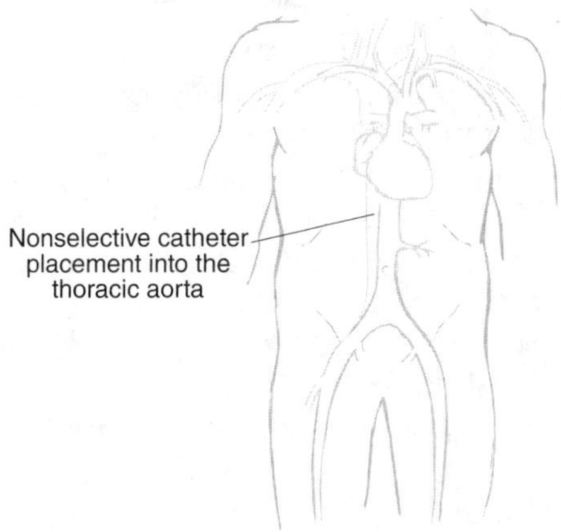

Explanation

The physician punctures a distal artery (typically femoral, brachial, radial, or axillary) with a large needle and passes a guidewire via the needle into the punctured artery. The needle is removed while leaving the guidewire in place, and the skin opening is enlarged slightly with a blade. An introducer sheath is inserted over the guidewire and into the arterial lumen. A catheter is introduced into the artery through an O-ring in the introducer sheath, which prevents blood from leaking around the catheter, and advanced into the thoracic aorta. The physician injects contrast material to perform angiography of the cervicocerebral arch, the extracranial carotid, and the vertebral and/or other intracranial vessels, unilaterally or bilaterally. Upon completion, the catheter is removed and pressure is applied to stop bleeding at the access site.

Coding Tips

When medically necessary, report moderate (conscious) sedation provided by the performing physician with 99151-99153. When provided by another physician, report 99155-99157. This code includes access of the vessel, placement of the catheter(s), injection(s) of the contrast, fluoroscopy, radiologic supervision and interpretation, and closure of the arteriotomy by pressure or by application of an arterial closure device. Diagnostic angiography may be followed by interventional procedures at the same operative session, and may be reported separately using appropriate coding guidelines. Do not report 36221 with 36222–36226. Do not report with the transcatheter placement of an intravascular stent of the common carotid or innominate artery on the same side (37217). For 3D rendering, see 76376–76377. For ultrasound guidance for vascular access, see 76937.

ICD-10-CM Diagnostic Codes

C70.0	Malignant neoplasm of cerebral meninges
C71.0	Malignant neoplasm of cerebrum, except lobes and ventricles
C71.1	Malignant neoplasm of frontal lobe
C71.2	Malignant neoplasm of temporal lobe
C71.3	Malignant neoplasm of parietal lobe
C71.4	Malignant neoplasm of occipital lobe
C71.5	Malignant neoplasm of cerebral ventricle

C71.6 Malignant neoplasm of cerebellum

C71.7 Malignant neoplasm of brain stem

C75.1 Malignant neoplasm of pituitary gland

C75.2 Malignant neoplasm of craniopharyngeal duct

C75.4 Malignant neoplasm of carotid body

C76.0 Malignant neoplasm of head, face and neck

C79.31 Secondary malignant neoplasm of brain

C79.32 Secondary malignant neoplasm of cerebral meninges

D18.02 Hemangioma of intracranial structures

I60.01 Nontraumatic subarachnoid hemorrhage from right carotid siphon and bifurcation ☑

I60.02 Nontraumatic subarachnoid hemorrhage from left carotid siphon and bifurcation ☑

I60.11 Nontraumatic subarachnoid hemorrhage from right middle cerebral artery ☑

I60.12 Nontraumatic subarachnoid hemorrhage from left middle cerebral artery ☑

I60.4 Nontraumatic subarachnoid hemorrhage from basilar artery

I60.51 Nontraumatic subarachnoid hemorrhage from right vertebral artery ☑

I60.52 Nontraumatic subarachnoid hemorrhage from left vertebral artery ☑

I63.311 Cerebral infarction due to thrombosis of right middle cerebral artery ☑

I63.312 Cerebral infarction due to thrombosis of left middle cerebral artery ☑

I63.321 Cerebral infarction due to thrombosis of right anterior cerebral artery ☑

I63.322 Cerebral infarction due to thrombosis of left anterior cerebral artery ☑

I63.331 Cerebral infarction due to thrombosis of right posterior cerebral artery ☑

I63.332 Cerebral infarction due to thrombosis of left posterior cerebral artery ☑

I63.341 Cerebral infarction due to thrombosis of right cerebellar artery ☑

I63.342 Cerebral infarction due to thrombosis of left cerebellar artery ☑

I63.411 Cerebral infarction due to embolism of right middle cerebral artery ☑

I63.412 Cerebral infarction due to embolism of left middle cerebral artery ☑

I63.421 Cerebral infarction due to embolism of right anterior cerebral artery ☑

I63.422 Cerebral infarction due to embolism of left anterior cerebral artery ☑

I63.431 Cerebral infarction due to embolism of right posterior cerebral artery ☑

I63.432 Cerebral infarction due to embolism of left posterior cerebral artery ☑

I63.441 Cerebral infarction due to embolism of right cerebellar artery ☑

I63.442 Cerebral infarction due to embolism of left cerebellar artery ☑

I65.01 Occlusion and stenosis of right vertebral artery ☑

I65.02 Occlusion and stenosis of left vertebral artery ☑

I65.1 Occlusion and stenosis of basilar artery

I65.21 Occlusion and stenosis of right carotid artery ☑

I65.22 Occlusion and stenosis of left carotid artery ☑

I66.01 Occlusion and stenosis of right middle cerebral artery ☑

I66.02 Occlusion and stenosis of left middle cerebral artery ☑

I66.11 Occlusion and stenosis of right anterior cerebral artery ☑

I66.12 Occlusion and stenosis of left anterior cerebral artery ☑

I66.21 Occlusion and stenosis of right posterior cerebral artery ☑

I66.22 Occlusion and stenosis of left posterior cerebral artery ☑

I66.3 Occlusion and stenosis of cerebellar arteries

I67.0 Dissection of cerebral arteries, nonruptured

I67.1 Cerebral aneurysm, nonruptured

I67.2 Cerebral atherosclerosis

I67.81 Acute cerebrovascular insufficiency

I67.82 Cerebral ischemia

I67.841 Reversible cerebrovascular vasoconstriction syndrome

I72.0 Aneurysm of carotid artery

I72.6 Aneurysm of vertebral artery

I76 Septic arterial embolism

I77.1 Stricture of artery

I77.2 Rupture of artery

I77.71 Dissection of carotid artery

I77.74 Dissection of vertebral artery

I97.820 Postprocedural cerebrovascular infarction following cardiac surgery

I97.821 Postprocedural cerebrovascular infarction following other surgery

Q28.2 Arteriovenous malformation of cerebral vessels

S15.011A Minor laceration of right carotid artery, initial encounter ☑

S15.012A Minor laceration of left carotid artery, initial encounter ☑

S15.021A Major laceration of right carotid artery, initial encounter ☑

S15.022A Major laceration of left carotid artery, initial encounter ☑

S15.111A Minor laceration of right vertebral artery, initial encounter ☑

S15.112A Minor laceration of left vertebral artery, initial encounter ☑

S15.121A Major laceration of right vertebral artery, initial encounter ☑

S15.122A Major laceration of left vertebral artery, initial encounter ☑

AMA: 36221 2018,Jan,8; 2017,Jan,8; 2016,Mar,3; 2016,Jan,13; 2015,Nov,3; 2015,May,7; 2015,Jan,16; 2014,Mar,8; 2014,Jan,11; 2013,Oct,18; 2013,May,3-5; 2013,Jun,12; 2013,Feb,16-17

Relative Value Units/Medicare Edits

Non-Facility RVU	Work	PE	MP	Total
36221	3.92	24.59	0.8	29.31
Facility RVU	**Work**	**PE**	**MP**	**Total**
36221	3.92	1.08	0.8	5.8

	FUD	Status	MUE	Modifiers				IOM Reference
36221	0	A	1(3)	51	N/A	N/A	N/A	None

* with documentation

36222-36223

36222 Selective catheter placement, common carotid or innominate artery, unilateral, any approach, with angiography of the ipsilateral extracranial carotid circulation and all associated radiological supervision and interpretation, includes angiography of the cervicocerebral arch, when performed

36223 Selective catheter placement, common carotid or innominate artery, unilateral, any approach, with angiography of the ipsilateral intracranial carotid circulation and all associated radiological supervision and interpretation, includes angiography of the extracranial carotid and cervicocerebral arch, when performed

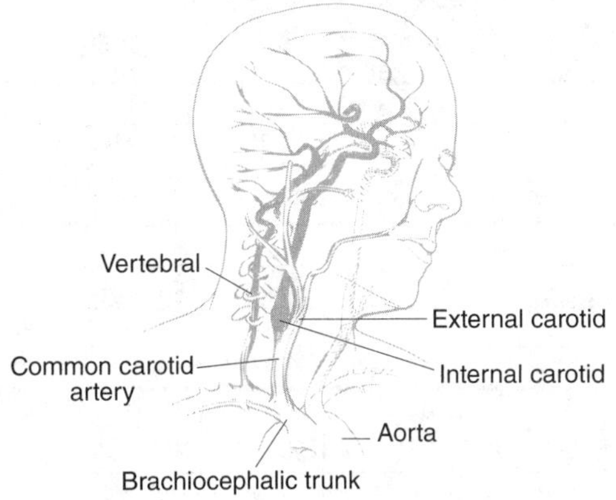

Selective catheter is placed in the common carotid artery

Explanation

The physician passes a needle through the skin and into an extremity artery, usually in the upper thigh. A guidewire is threaded through the needle into the vessel. The needle is removed. The wire is threaded into the aorta and up to the thoracic aorta where it is manipulated into a branch off the aortic arch. A catheter follows the wire into the common carotid or innominate artery on one side. The wire is removed. Contrast material is injected into the catheter for arteriography. Report 36222 when angiography of the ipsilateral extracranial carotid circulation is also included. In 36223, angiography of the ipsilateral extracranial and intracranial carotid circulation is performed. Angiography of the cervicocerebral arch may also be performed. Upon completion, the catheter is removed and pressure is applied to stop bleeding at the access site.

Coding Tips

When medically necessary, report moderate (conscious) sedation provided by the performing physician with 99151-99153. When provided by another physician, report 99155-99157. These procedures include access of the vessel, placement of the catheter(s), injection(s) of the contrast, fluoroscopy, radiologic supervision and interpretation, and closure of the arteriotomy by pressure or by application of an arterial closure device. Diagnostic angiography may be followed by interventional procedures at the same operative session, and may be reported separately using appropriate coding guidelines. These are unilateral procedures. If performed bilaterally, some payers require that the service be reported twice with modifier 50 appended to the second code while others require identification of the service only once with modifier 50 appended. Check with individual payers. Modifier 50 identifies a procedure performed identically on the opposite side of the body (mirror image). Do not report 36222–36224 together to report ipsilateral angiography. Report the single code that represents the most complex service, with 36224 being the most complex and 36222 being the least complex. For 3D rendering, see 76376–76377. For ultrasound guidance for vascular access, see 76937. Do not report 36222 or 36223 with 37215, 37216, 37218 for the treated carotid artery. Do not report 36222 or 36223 with the transcatheter placement of an intravascular stent of the common carotid or innominate artery on the same side (37217).

ICD-10-CM Diagnostic Codes

G45.0	Vertebro-basilar artery syndrome
G45.1	Carotid artery syndrome (hemispheric)
G45.2	Multiple and bilateral precerebral artery syndromes
G45.3	Amaurosis fugax
I60.01	Nontraumatic subarachnoid hemorrhage from right carotid siphon and bifurcation ☑
I60.02	Nontraumatic subarachnoid hemorrhage from left carotid siphon and bifurcation ☑
I60.4	Nontraumatic subarachnoid hemorrhage from basilar artery
I60.51	Nontraumatic subarachnoid hemorrhage from right vertebral artery ☑
I60.52	Nontraumatic subarachnoid hemorrhage from left vertebral artery ☑
I60.6	Nontraumatic subarachnoid hemorrhage from other intracranial arteries
I60.8	Other nontraumatic subarachnoid hemorrhage
I61.8	Other nontraumatic intracerebral hemorrhage
I63.011	Cerebral infarction due to thrombosis of right vertebral artery ☑
I63.012	Cerebral infarction due to thrombosis of left vertebral artery ☑
I63.013	Cerebral infarction due to thrombosis of bilateral vertebral arteries ☑
I63.031	Cerebral infarction due to thrombosis of right carotid artery ☑
I63.032	Cerebral infarction due to thrombosis of left carotid artery ☑
I63.033	Cerebral infarction due to thrombosis of bilateral carotid arteries ☑
I63.09	Cerebral infarction due to thrombosis of other precerebral artery
I63.111	Cerebral infarction due to embolism of right vertebral artery ☑
I63.112	Cerebral infarction due to embolism of left vertebral artery ☑
I63.113	Cerebral infarction due to embolism of bilateral vertebral arteries ☑
I63.131	Cerebral infarction due to embolism of right carotid artery ☑
I63.132	Cerebral infarction due to embolism of left carotid artery ☑
I63.133	Cerebral infarction due to embolism of bilateral carotid arteries ☑
I63.19	Cerebral infarction due to embolism of other precerebral artery
I63.313	Cerebral infarction due to thrombosis of bilateral middle cerebral arteries ☑
I63.323	Cerebral infarction due to thrombosis of bilateral anterior cerebral arteries ☑
I63.333	Cerebral infarction due to thrombosis of bilateral posterior cerebral arteries ☑
I63.343	Cerebral infarction due to thrombosis of bilateral cerebellar arteries ☑
I63.413	Cerebral infarction due to embolism of bilateral middle cerebral arteries ☑
I63.423	Cerebral infarction due to embolism of bilateral anterior cerebral arteries ☑
I63.433	Cerebral infarction due to embolism of bilateral posterior cerebral arteries ☑

I63.443	Cerebral infarction due to embolism of bilateral cerebellar arteries ☑
I65.01	Occlusion and stenosis of right vertebral artery ☑
I65.02	Occlusion and stenosis of left vertebral artery ☑
I65.03	Occlusion and stenosis of bilateral vertebral arteries ☑
I65.1	Occlusion and stenosis of basilar artery
I65.21	Occlusion and stenosis of right carotid artery ☑
I65.22	Occlusion and stenosis of left carotid artery ☑
I65.23	Occlusion and stenosis of bilateral carotid arteries ☑
I65.8	Occlusion and stenosis of other precerebral arteries
I67.1	Cerebral aneurysm, nonruptured
I67.2	Cerebral atherosclerosis
I67.81	Acute cerebrovascular insufficiency
I67.82	Cerebral ischemia
I67.841	Reversible cerebrovascular vasoconstriction syndrome
I67.848	Other cerebrovascular vasospasm and vasoconstriction
I67.89	Other cerebrovascular disease
I72.0	Aneurysm of carotid artery
I72.8	Aneurysm of other specified arteries
I76	Septic arterial embolism
I77.1	Stricture of artery
I77.2	Rupture of artery
I77.71	Dissection of carotid artery
I77.74	Dissection of vertebral artery
I77.79	Dissection of other specified artery
I77.89	Other specified disorders of arteries and arterioles
I97.820	Postprocedural cerebrovascular infarction following cardiac surgery
I97.821	Postprocedural cerebrovascular infarction following other surgery
Q28.1	Other malformations of precerebral vessels
Q28.8	Other specified congenital malformations of circulatory system
S09.0XXA	Injury of blood vessels of head, not elsewhere classified, initial encounter
S15.011A	Minor laceration of right carotid artery, initial encounter ☑
S15.012A	Minor laceration of left carotid artery, initial encounter ☑
S15.021A	Major laceration of right carotid artery, initial encounter ☑
S15.022A	Major laceration of left carotid artery, initial encounter ☑
S15.091A	Other specified injury of right carotid artery, initial encounter ☑
S15.092A	Other specified injury of left carotid artery, initial encounter ☑
S15.111A	Minor laceration of right vertebral artery, initial encounter ☑
S15.112A	Minor laceration of left vertebral artery, initial encounter ☑
S15.121A	Major laceration of right vertebral artery, initial encounter ☑
S15.122A	Major laceration of left vertebral artery, initial encounter ☑
S15.191A	Other specified injury of right vertebral artery, initial encounter ☑
S15.192A	Other specified injury of left vertebral artery, initial encounter ☑
S15.8XXA	Injury of other specified blood vessels at neck level, initial encounter
S25.111A	Minor laceration of right innominate or subclavian artery, initial encounter ☑
S25.112A	Minor laceration of left innominate or subclavian artery, initial encounter ☑
S25.121A	Major laceration of right innominate or subclavian artery, initial encounter ☑
S25.122A	Major laceration of left innominate or subclavian artery, initial encounter ☑
S25.191A	Other specified injury of right innominate or subclavian artery, initial encounter ☑
S25.192A	Other specified injury of left innominate or subclavian artery, initial encounter ☑

AMA: 36222 2018,Jan,8; 2017,Jan,8; 2016,Mar,3; 2016,Jan,13; 2015,Nov,3; 2015,Nov,10; 2015,May,7; 2015,Jan,16; 2014,Mar,8; 2014,Jan,11; 2013,Oct,18; 2013,Nov,14; 2013,May,3-5; 2013,Jun,12; 2013,Feb,16-17 **36223** 2018,Jan,8; 2017,Jan,8; 2016,Mar,3; 2016,Jan,13; 2015,Nov,3; 2015,Jan,16; 2014,Mar,8; 2014,Jan,11; 2013,Oct,18; 2013,May,3-5; 2013,Jun,12; 2013,Feb,16-17

Relative Value Units/Medicare Edits

Non-Facility RVU	Work	PE	MP	Total
36222	5.28	28.25	1.2	34.73
36223	5.75	36.86	1.34	43.95
Facility RVU	**Work**	**PE**	**MP**	**Total**
36222	5.28	1.74	1.2	8.22
36223	5.75	2.09	1.34	9.18

	FUD	Status	MUE	Modifiers				IOM Reference
36222	0	A	1(3)	51	50	N/A	N/A	None
36223	0	A	1(3)	51	50	N/A	N/A	

* with documentation

Terms To Know

angiography. Radiographic imaging of the arteries.

guidewire. Flexible metal instrument designed to lead another instrument in its proper course.

ipsilateral. Located on, or affecting, the same side of the body, usually as it relates to a bilateral body part.

selective placement. Introduction and manipulation of a catheter or guidewire within a vascular tree or family into a specified target area that is identified and monitored by radiographic imaging in order to carry out a diagnostic or therapeutic procedure.

36224

36224 Selective catheter placement, internal carotid artery, unilateral, with angiography of the ipsilateral intracranial carotid circulation and all associated radiological supervision and interpretation, includes angiography of the extracranial carotid and cervicocerebral arch, when performed

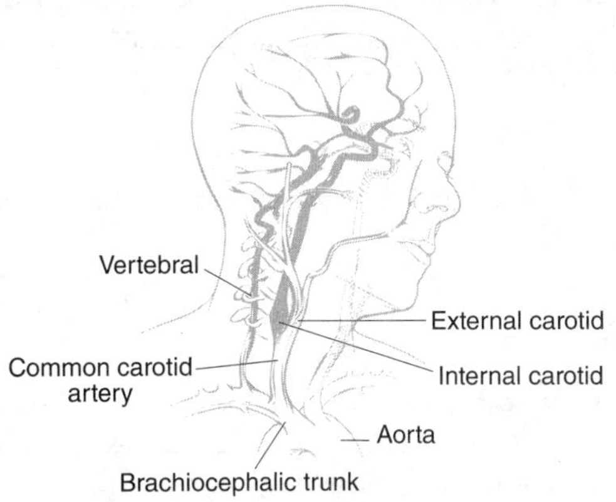

Selective catheter is placed in the internal carotid artery

Explanation

The physician passes a needle through the skin and into an extremity artery, usually in the upper thigh. A guidewire is threaded through the needle into the vessel. The needle is removed. The wire is threaded into the aorta and up to the thoracic aorta where it is manipulated into a branch off the aortic arch. A catheter follows the wire into the internal carotid artery on one side. The wire is removed. Contrast material is injected into the catheter for arteriography, including the intracranial carotid circulation. Angiography of the ipsilateral extracranial carotid circulation and the cervicocerebral arch may also be performed. Upon completion, the catheter is removed and pressure is applied to stop bleeding at the access site.

Coding Tips

When medically necessary, report moderate (conscious) sedation provided by the performing physician with 99151-99153. When provided by another physician, report 99155-99157. This code includes access of the vessel, placement of the catheter(s), injection(s) of the contrast, fluoroscopy, radiologic supervision and interpretation, and closure of the arteriotomy by pressure or by application of an arterial closure device. Diagnostic angiography may be followed by interventional procedures at the same operative session, and may be reported separately using appropriate coding guidelines. Do not report 36222–36224 together to report ipsilateral angiography. Do not report 36224 with 37215, 37216, or 37218 for the treated carotid artery. Do not report these codes with transcatheter placement of an intravascular stent of the common carotid or innominate artery on the same side (37217). Report the single code that represents the most complex service, with 36224 being the most complex and 36222 being the least complex. For 3D rendering, see 76376–76377. For ultrasound guidance for vascular access, see 76937.

ICD-10-CM Diagnostic Codes

G45.0	Vertebro-basilar artery syndrome
G45.1	Carotid artery syndrome (hemispheric)
G45.2	Multiple and bilateral precerebral artery syndromes
G45.3	Amaurosis fugax
I60.01	Nontraumatic subarachnoid hemorrhage from right carotid siphon and bifurcation ☑
I60.02	Nontraumatic subarachnoid hemorrhage from left carotid siphon and bifurcation ☑
I60.4	Nontraumatic subarachnoid hemorrhage from basilar artery
I60.51	Nontraumatic subarachnoid hemorrhage from right vertebral artery ☑
I60.52	Nontraumatic subarachnoid hemorrhage from left vertebral artery ☑
I60.6	Nontraumatic subarachnoid hemorrhage from other intracranial arteries
I60.8	Other nontraumatic subarachnoid hemorrhage
I63.011	Cerebral infarction due to thrombosis of right vertebral artery ☑
I63.012	Cerebral infarction due to thrombosis of left vertebral artery ☑
I63.013	Cerebral infarction due to thrombosis of bilateral vertebral arteries ☑
I63.031	Cerebral infarction due to thrombosis of right carotid artery ☑
I63.032	Cerebral infarction due to thrombosis of left carotid artery ☑
I63.033	Cerebral infarction due to thrombosis of bilateral carotid arteries ☑
I63.09	Cerebral infarction due to thrombosis of other precerebral artery
I63.111	Cerebral infarction due to embolism of right vertebral artery ☑
I63.112	Cerebral infarction due to embolism of left vertebral artery ☑
I63.113	Cerebral infarction due to embolism of bilateral vertebral arteries ☑
I63.131	Cerebral infarction due to embolism of right carotid artery ☑
I63.132	Cerebral infarction due to embolism of left carotid artery ☑
I63.133	Cerebral infarction due to embolism of bilateral carotid arteries ☑
I63.19	Cerebral infarction due to embolism of other precerebral artery
I63.211	Cerebral infarction due to unspecified occlusion or stenosis of right vertebral artery ☑
I63.313	Cerebral infarction due to thrombosis of bilateral middle cerebral arteries ☑
I63.323	Cerebral infarction due to thrombosis of bilateral anterior cerebral arteries ☑
I63.333	Cerebral infarction due to thrombosis of bilateral posterior cerebral arteries ☑
I63.343	Cerebral infarction due to thrombosis of bilateral cerebellar arteries ☑
I63.413	Cerebral infarction due to embolism of bilateral middle cerebral arteries ☑
I63.423	Cerebral infarction due to embolism of bilateral anterior cerebral arteries ☑
I63.433	Cerebral infarction due to embolism of bilateral posterior cerebral arteries ☑
I63.443	Cerebral infarction due to embolism of bilateral cerebellar arteries ☑
I65.01	Occlusion and stenosis of right vertebral artery ☑
I65.02	Occlusion and stenosis of left vertebral artery ☑
I65.03	Occlusion and stenosis of bilateral vertebral arteries ☑
I65.1	Occlusion and stenosis of basilar artery
I65.21	Occlusion and stenosis of right carotid artery ☑
I65.22	Occlusion and stenosis of left carotid artery ☑
I65.23	Occlusion and stenosis of bilateral carotid arteries ☑
I65.8	Occlusion and stenosis of other precerebral arteries

 ● New ▲ Revised + Add On AMA: CPT Assist [Resequenced] ☑ Laterality

I67.1	Cerebral aneurysm, nonruptured
I67.2	Cerebral atherosclerosis
I67.81	Acute cerebrovascular insufficiency
I67.82	Cerebral ischemia
I67.841	Reversible cerebrovascular vasoconstriction syndrome
I67.848	Other cerebrovascular vasospasm and vasoconstriction
I67.89	Other cerebrovascular disease
I72.0	Aneurysm of carotid artery
I72.6	Aneurysm of vertebral artery
I76	Septic arterial embolism
I77.1	Stricture of artery
I77.2	Rupture of artery
I77.71	Dissection of carotid artery
I77.74	Dissection of vertebral artery
I77.79	Dissection of other specified artery
I77.89	Other specified disorders of arteries and arterioles
I97.820	Postprocedural cerebrovascular infarction following cardiac surgery
I97.821	Postprocedural cerebrovascular infarction following other surgery
Q28.1	Other malformations of precerebral vessels
Q28.8	Other specified congenital malformations of circulatory system
S09.0XXA	Injury of blood vessels of head, not elsewhere classified, initial encounter
S15.011A	Minor laceration of right carotid artery, initial encounter ☑
S15.012A	Minor laceration of left carotid artery, initial encounter ☑
S15.021A	Major laceration of right carotid artery, initial encounter ☑
S15.022A	Major laceration of left carotid artery, initial encounter ☑
S15.091A	Other specified injury of right carotid artery, initial encounter ☑
S15.092A	Other specified injury of left carotid artery, initial encounter ☑
S15.111A	Minor laceration of right vertebral artery, initial encounter ☑
S15.112A	Minor laceration of left vertebral artery, initial encounter ☑
S15.121A	Major laceration of right vertebral artery, initial encounter ☑
S15.122A	Major laceration of left vertebral artery, initial encounter ☑
S15.191A	Other specified injury of right vertebral artery, initial encounter ☑
S15.192A	Other specified injury of left vertebral artery, initial encounter ☑
S15.8XXA	Injury of other specified blood vessels at neck level, initial encounter
S25.111A	Minor laceration of right innominate or subclavian artery, initial encounter ☑
S25.112A	Minor laceration of left innominate or subclavian artery, initial encounter ☑
S25.121A	Major laceration of right innominate or subclavian artery, initial encounter ☑
S25.122A	Major laceration of left innominate or subclavian artery, initial encounter ☑
S25.191A	Other specified injury of right innominate or subclavian artery, initial encounter ☑
S25.192A	Other specified injury of left innominate or subclavian artery, initial encounter ☑

AMA: 36224 2018,Jan,8; 2017,Jan,8; 2016,Mar,3; 2016,Jan,13; 2015,Nov,3; 2015,Jan,16; 2014,Mar,8; 2014,Jan,11; 2013,Oct,18; 2013,May,3-5; 2013,Jun,12; 2013,Feb,16-17

Relative Value Units/Medicare Edits

Non-Facility RVU	Work	PE	MP	Total
36224	6.25	48.95	1.67	56.87
Facility RVU	**Work**	**PE**	**MP**	**Total**
36224	6.25	2.56	1.67	10.48

	FUD	Status	MUE	Modifiers				IOM Reference
36224	0	A	1(3)	51	50	N/A	N/A	None

* with documentation

Terms To Know

guidewire. Flexible metal instrument designed to lead another instrument in its proper course.

ipsilateral. Located on, or affecting, the same side of the body, usually as it relates to a bilateral body part.

selective placement. Introduction and manipulation of a catheter or guidewire within a vascular tree or family into a specified target area that is identified and monitored by radiographic imaging in order to carry out a diagnostic or therapeutic procedure.

36225

36225 Selective catheter placement, subclavian or innominate artery, unilateral, with angiography of the ipsilateral vertebral circulation and all associated radiological supervision and interpretation, includes angiography of the cervicocerebral arch, when performed

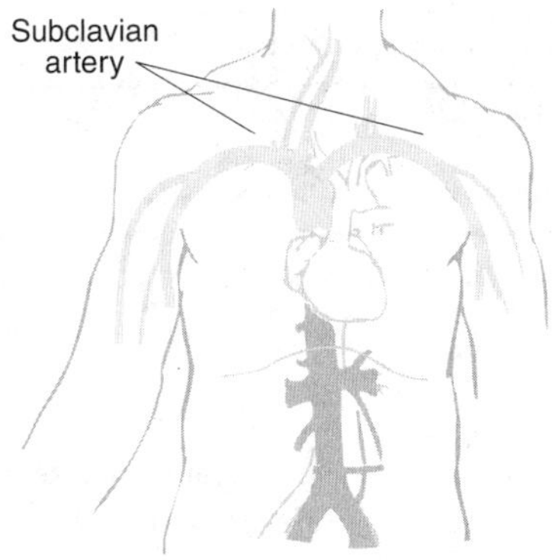

Selective cather is placed in the subclavian artery

Explanation

The physician passes a needle through the skin and into an extremity artery. A guidewire is threaded through the needle into the vessel. The needle is removed. The wire is threaded into the thoracic aorta where it is manipulated into a branch off the aortic arch. A catheter follows the wire into the subclavian or innominate artery on one side. The wire is removed. Contrast material is injected into the catheter for arteriography, including the ipsilateral vertebral circulation. Angiography of the cervicocerebral arch may also be performed. Upon completion, the catheter is removed and pressure is applied to stop bleeding at the access site.

Coding Tips

When medically necessary, report moderate (conscious) sedation provided by the performing physician with 99151-99153. When provided by another physician, report 99155-99157. This code includes access of the vessel, placement of the catheter(s), injection(s) of the contrast, fluoroscopy, radiologic supervision and interpretation, and closure of the arteriotomy by pressure or by application of an arterial closure device. Diagnostic angiography may be followed by interventional procedures at the same operative session, and may be reported separately using appropriate coding guidelines. Do not report 36225 and 36226 together to report ipsilateral angiography. Report the single code that represents the most complex service, with 36226 being the most complex. Do not report with the transcatheter placement of an intravascular stent of the common carotid or innominate artery on the same side (37217). For 3D rendering, see 76376–76377. For ultrasound guidance for vascular access, see 76937.

ICD-10-CM Diagnostic Codes

G45.0	Vertebro-basilar artery syndrome
G45.1	Carotid artery syndrome (hemispheric)
G45.2	Multiple and bilateral precerebral artery syndromes
G45.3	Amaurosis fugax
G45.8	Other transient cerebral ischemic attacks and related syndromes
G45.9	Transient cerebral ischemic attack, unspecified
I60.01	Nontraumatic subarachnoid hemorrhage from right carotid siphon and bifurcation ☑
I60.02	Nontraumatic subarachnoid hemorrhage from left carotid siphon and bifurcation ☑
I60.4	Nontraumatic subarachnoid hemorrhage from basilar artery
I60.51	Nontraumatic subarachnoid hemorrhage from right vertebral artery ☑
I60.52	Nontraumatic subarachnoid hemorrhage from left vertebral artery ☑
I60.6	Nontraumatic subarachnoid hemorrhage from other intracranial arteries
I60.8	Other nontraumatic subarachnoid hemorrhage
I61.8	Other nontraumatic intracerebral hemorrhage
I63.011	Cerebral infarction due to thrombosis of right vertebral artery ☑
I63.012	Cerebral infarction due to thrombosis of left vertebral artery ☑
I63.013	Cerebral infarction due to thrombosis of bilateral vertebral arteries ☑
I63.031	Cerebral infarction due to thrombosis of right carotid artery ☑
I63.032	Cerebral infarction due to thrombosis of left carotid artery ☑
I63.033	Cerebral infarction due to thrombosis of bilateral carotid arteries ☑
I63.09	Cerebral infarction due to thrombosis of other precerebral artery
I63.111	Cerebral infarction due to embolism of right vertebral artery ☑
I63.112	Cerebral infarction due to embolism of left vertebral artery ☑
I63.113	Cerebral infarction due to embolism of bilateral vertebral arteries ☑
I63.131	Cerebral infarction due to embolism of right carotid artery ☑
I63.132	Cerebral infarction due to embolism of left carotid artery ☑
I63.133	Cerebral infarction due to embolism of bilateral carotid arteries ☑
I63.19	Cerebral infarction due to embolism of other precerebral artery
I63.313	Cerebral infarction due to thrombosis of bilateral middle cerebral arteries ☑
I63.323	Cerebral infarction due to thrombosis of bilateral anterior cerebral arteries ☑
I63.333	Cerebral infarction due to thrombosis of bilateral posterior cerebral arteries ☑
I63.343	Cerebral infarction due to thrombosis of bilateral cerebellar arteries ☑
I63.413	Cerebral infarction due to embolism of bilateral middle cerebral arteries ☑
I63.423	Cerebral infarction due to embolism of bilateral anterior cerebral arteries ☑
I63.433	Cerebral infarction due to embolism of bilateral posterior cerebral arteries ☑
I63.443	Cerebral infarction due to embolism of bilateral cerebellar arteries ☑
I63.81	Other cerebral infarction due to occlusion or stenosis of small artery
I63.89	Other cerebral infarction
I65.01	Occlusion and stenosis of right vertebral artery ☑
I65.02	Occlusion and stenosis of left vertebral artery ☑
I65.03	Occlusion and stenosis of bilateral vertebral arteries ☑
I65.1	Occlusion and stenosis of basilar artery
I65.21	Occlusion and stenosis of right carotid artery ☑
I65.22	Occlusion and stenosis of left carotid artery ☑
I65.23	Occlusion and stenosis of bilateral carotid arteries ☑
I65.8	Occlusion and stenosis of other precerebral arteries

I67.1 Cerebral aneurysm, nonruptured
I67.2 Cerebral atherosclerosis
I67.81 Acute cerebrovascular insufficiency
I67.82 Cerebral ischemia
I67.841 Reversible cerebrovascular vasoconstriction syndrome
I67.848 Other cerebrovascular vasospasm and vasoconstriction
I67.850 Cerebral autosomal dominant arteriopathy with subcortical infarcts and leukoencephalopathy
I67.858 Other hereditary cerebrovascular disease
I67.89 Other cerebrovascular disease
I72.0 Aneurysm of carotid artery
I72.6 Aneurysm of vertebral artery
I72.8 Aneurysm of other specified arteries
I76 Septic arterial embolism
I77.1 Stricture of artery
I77.2 Rupture of artery
I77.71 Dissection of carotid artery
I77.74 Dissection of vertebral artery
I77.79 Dissection of other specified artery
I77.89 Other specified disorders of arteries and arterioles
I97.820 Postprocedural cerebrovascular infarction following cardiac surgery
I97.821 Postprocedural cerebrovascular infarction following other surgery
Q28.1 Other malformations of precerebral vessels
Q28.8 Other specified congenital malformations of circulatory system
S09.0XXA Injury of blood vessels of head, not elsewhere classified, initial encounter
S15.011A Minor laceration of right carotid artery, initial encounter ☑
S15.012A Minor laceration of left carotid artery, initial encounter ☑
S15.021A Major laceration of right carotid artery, initial encounter ☑
S15.022A Major laceration of left carotid artery, initial encounter ☑
S15.091A Other specified injury of right carotid artery, initial encounter ☑
S15.092A Other specified injury of left carotid artery, initial encounter ☑
S15.111A Minor laceration of right vertebral artery, initial encounter ☑
S15.112A Minor laceration of left vertebral artery, initial encounter ☑
S15.121A Major laceration of right vertebral artery, initial encounter ☑
S15.122A Major laceration of left vertebral artery, initial encounter ☑
S15.191A Other specified injury of right vertebral artery, initial encounter ☑
S15.192A Other specified injury of left vertebral artery, initial encounter ☑
S15.8XXA Injury of other specified blood vessels at neck level, initial encounter
S25.111A Minor laceration of right innominate or subclavian artery, initial encounter ☑
S25.112A Minor laceration of left innominate or subclavian artery, initial encounter ☑
S25.121A Major laceration of right innominate or subclavian artery, initial encounter ☑
S25.122A Major laceration of left innominate or subclavian artery, initial encounter ☑
S25.191A Other specified injury of right innominate or subclavian artery, initial encounter ☑
S25.192A Other specified injury of left innominate or subclavian artery, initial encounter ☑

AMA: 36225 2018,Jan,8; 2017,Jan,8; 2016,Mar,3; 2016,Jan,13; 2015,Nov,3; 2015,Jan,16; 2014,Mar,8; 2014,Jan,11; 2013,Oct,18; 2013,Nov,14; 2013,May,3-5; 2013,Jun,12

Relative Value Units/Medicare Edits

Non-Facility RVU	Work	PE	MP	Total
36225	5.75	35.22	1.37	42.34
Facility RVU	**Work**	**PE**	**MP**	**Total**
36225	5.75	2.04	1.37	9.16

	FUD	Status	MUE	Modifiers				IOM Reference
36225	0	A	1(3)	51	50	N/A	N/A	None

* with documentation

Terms To Know

angiography. Radiographic imaging of the arteries. Imaging may be performed to study the vasculature of any given organ, body system, or area of circulation such as the brain, heart, chest, kidneys, limbs, gastrointestinal tract, aorta, and pulmonary circulation to visualize the formation and the function of the blood vessels to detect problems such as a blockage or stricture. A catheter is inserted through an accessible blood vessel and the artery is injected with a radiopaque contrast material after which x-rays are taken.

catheter. Flexible tube inserted into an area of the body for introducing or withdrawing fluid.

guidewire. Flexible metal instrument designed to lead another instrument in its proper course.

36226

36226 Selective catheter placement, vertebral artery, unilateral, with angiography of the ipsilateral vertebral circulation and all associated radiological supervision and interpretation, includes angiography of the cervicocerebral arch, when performed

A catheter is placed in the vertebral artery to inject contrast material

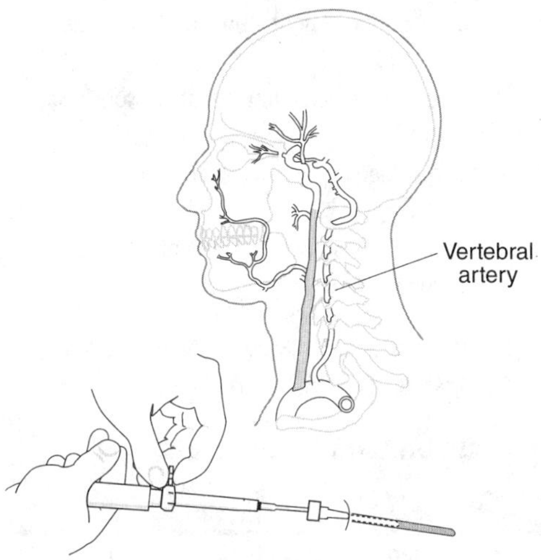

Explanation

The physician passes a needle through the skin and into an extremity artery. A guidewire is threaded through the needle into the vessel. The needle is removed. The wire is threaded into the thoracic aorta where it is manipulated into a branch off the aortic arch. A catheter follows the wire into the vertebral artery on one side. The wire is removed. Contrast material is injected into the catheter for arteriography, including the ipsilateral vertebral circulation. Angiography of the cervicocerebral arch may also be performed. Upon completion, the catheter is removed and pressure is applied to stop bleeding at the access site.

Coding Tips

When medically necessary, report moderate (conscious) sedation provided by the performing physician with 99151-99153. When provided by another physician, report 99155-99157. This code includes access of the vessel, placement of the catheter(s), injection(s) of the contrast, fluoroscopy, radiologic supervision and interpretation, and closure of the arteriotomy by pressure or by application of an arterial closure device. Diagnostic angiography may be followed by interventional procedures at the same operative session, and may be reported separately using appropriate coding guidelines. Do not report 36226 with transcatheter placement of an intravascular stent of the common carotid or innominate artery on the same side (37217). Do not report 36225 and 36226 together to report ipsilateral angiography. Report the single code that represents the most complex service, with 36226 being the most complex. For 3D rendering, see 76376–76377. For ultrasound guidance for vascular access, see 76937.

ICD-10-CM Diagnostic Codes

G45.0	Vertebro-basilar artery syndrome
G45.1	Carotid artery syndrome (hemispheric)
G45.2	Multiple and bilateral precerebral artery syndromes
G45.3	Amaurosis fugax
G45.8	Other transient cerebral ischemic attacks and related syndromes
G45.9	Transient cerebral ischemic attack, unspecified
I60.01	Nontraumatic subarachnoid hemorrhage from right carotid siphon and bifurcation ☑
I60.02	Nontraumatic subarachnoid hemorrhage from left carotid siphon and bifurcation ☑
I60.4	Nontraumatic subarachnoid hemorrhage from basilar artery
I60.51	Nontraumatic subarachnoid hemorrhage from right vertebral artery ☑
I60.52	Nontraumatic subarachnoid hemorrhage from left vertebral artery ☑
I60.6	Nontraumatic subarachnoid hemorrhage from other intracranial arteries
I60.8	Other nontraumatic subarachnoid hemorrhage
I61.8	Other nontraumatic intracerebral hemorrhage
I63.011	Cerebral infarction due to thrombosis of right vertebral artery ☑
I63.012	Cerebral infarction due to thrombosis of left vertebral artery ☑
I63.013	Cerebral infarction due to thrombosis of bilateral vertebral arteries ☑
I63.031	Cerebral infarction due to thrombosis of right carotid artery ☑
I63.032	Cerebral infarction due to thrombosis of left carotid artery ☑
I63.033	Cerebral infarction due to thrombosis of bilateral carotid arteries ☑
I63.09	Cerebral infarction due to thrombosis of other precerebral artery
I63.111	Cerebral infarction due to embolism of right vertebral artery ☑
I63.112	Cerebral infarction due to embolism of left vertebral artery ☑
I63.113	Cerebral infarction due to embolism of bilateral vertebral arteries ☑
I63.131	Cerebral infarction due to embolism of right carotid artery ☑
I63.132	Cerebral infarction due to embolism of left carotid artery ☑
I63.133	Cerebral infarction due to embolism of bilateral carotid arteries ☑
I63.19	Cerebral infarction due to embolism of other precerebral artery
I63.211	Cerebral infarction due to unspecified occlusion or stenosis of right vertebral artery ☑
I63.212	Cerebral infarction due to unspecified occlusion or stenosis of left vertebral artery ☑
I63.213	Cerebral infarction due to unspecified occlusion or stenosis of bilateral vertebral arteries ☑
I63.231	Cerebral infarction due to unspecified occlusion or stenosis of right carotid arteries ☑
I63.232	Cerebral infarction due to unspecified occlusion or stenosis of left carotid arteries ☑
I63.233	Cerebral infarction due to unspecified occlusion or stenosis of bilateral carotid arteries ☑
I63.29	Cerebral infarction due to unspecified occlusion or stenosis of other precerebral arteries
I63.313	Cerebral infarction due to thrombosis of bilateral middle cerebral arteries ☑
I63.323	Cerebral infarction due to thrombosis of bilateral anterior cerebral arteries ☑
I63.333	Cerebral infarction due to thrombosis of bilateral posterior cerebral arteries ☑
I63.343	Cerebral infarction due to thrombosis of bilateral cerebellar arteries ☑

I63.413	Cerebral infarction due to embolism of bilateral middle cerebral arteries ☑
I63.423	Cerebral infarction due to embolism of bilateral anterior cerebral arteries ☑
I63.433	Cerebral infarction due to embolism of bilateral posterior cerebral arteries ☑
I63.443	Cerebral infarction due to embolism of bilateral cerebellar arteries ☑
I63.81	Other cerebral infarction due to occlusion or stenosis of small artery
I63.89	Other cerebral infarction
I65.01	Occlusion and stenosis of right vertebral artery ☑
I65.02	Occlusion and stenosis of left vertebral artery ☑
I65.03	Occlusion and stenosis of bilateral vertebral arteries ☑
I65.1	Occlusion and stenosis of basilar artery
I65.21	Occlusion and stenosis of right carotid artery ☑
I65.22	Occlusion and stenosis of left carotid artery ☑
I65.23	Occlusion and stenosis of bilateral carotid arteries ☑
I65.8	Occlusion and stenosis of other precerebral arteries
I67.1	Cerebral aneurysm, nonruptured
I67.2	Cerebral atherosclerosis
I67.81	Acute cerebrovascular insufficiency
I67.82	Cerebral ischemia
I67.841	Reversible cerebrovascular vasoconstriction syndrome
I67.848	Other cerebrovascular vasospasm and vasoconstriction
I67.850	Cerebral autosomal dominant arteriopathy with subcortical infarcts and leukoencephalopathy
I67.858	Other hereditary cerebrovascular disease
I67.89	Other cerebrovascular disease
I72.0	Aneurysm of carotid artery
I72.6	Aneurysm of vertebral artery
I72.8	Aneurysm of other specified arteries
I76	Septic arterial embolism
I77.1	Stricture of artery
I77.2	Rupture of artery
I77.71	Dissection of carotid artery
I77.74	Dissection of vertebral artery
I77.79	Dissection of other specified artery
I77.89	Other specified disorders of arteries and arterioles
I97.820	Postprocedural cerebrovascular infarction following cardiac surgery
I97.821	Postprocedural cerebrovascular infarction following other surgery
Q28.1	Other malformations of precerebral vessels
Q28.8	Other specified congenital malformations of circulatory system
S09.0XXA	Injury of blood vessels of head, not elsewhere classified, initial encounter
S15.011A	Minor laceration of right carotid artery, initial encounter ☑
S15.012A	Minor laceration of left carotid artery, initial encounter ☑
S15.021A	Major laceration of right carotid artery, initial encounter ☑
S15.022A	Major laceration of left carotid artery, initial encounter ☑
S15.091A	Other specified injury of right carotid artery, initial encounter ☑
S15.092A	Other specified injury of left carotid artery, initial encounter ☑
S15.111A	Minor laceration of right vertebral artery, initial encounter ☑
S15.112A	Minor laceration of left vertebral artery, initial encounter ☑
S15.121A	Major laceration of right vertebral artery, initial encounter ☑
S15.122A	Major laceration of left vertebral artery, initial encounter ☑
S15.191A	Other specified injury of right vertebral artery, initial encounter ☑
S15.192A	Other specified injury of left vertebral artery, initial encounter ☑
S15.8XXA	Injury of other specified blood vessels at neck level, initial encounter
S25.111A	Minor laceration of right innominate or subclavian artery, initial encounter ☑
S25.112A	Minor laceration of left innominate or subclavian artery, initial encounter ☑
S25.121A	Major laceration of right innominate or subclavian artery, initial encounter ☑
S25.122A	Major laceration of left innominate or subclavian artery, initial encounter ☑
S25.191A	Other specified injury of right innominate or subclavian artery, initial encounter ☑
S25.192A	Other specified injury of left innominate or subclavian artery, initial encounter ☑

AMA: 36226 2018,Jan,8; 2017,Jan,8; 2016,Mar,3; 2016,Jan,13; 2015,Nov,3; 2015,Jan,16; 2014,Mar,8; 2013,Oct,18; 2013,May,3-5; 2013,Jun,12

Relative Value Units/Medicare Edits

Non-Facility RVU	Work	PE	MP	Total
36226	6.25	45.93	1.6	53.78
Facility RVU	**Work**	**PE**	**MP**	**Total**
36226	6.25	2.48	1.6	10.33

	FUD	Status	MUE	Modifiers				IOM Reference
36226	0	A	1(3)	51	50	N/A	N/A	None

* with documentation

36227-36228

+ 36227 Selective catheter placement, external carotid artery, unilateral, with angiography of the ipsilateral external carotid circulation and all associated radiological supervision and interpretation (List separately in addition to code for primary procedure)

+ 36228 Selective catheter placement, each intracranial branch of the internal carotid or vertebral arteries, unilateral, with angiography of the selected vessel circulation and all associated radiological supervision and interpretation (eg, middle cerebral artery, posterior inferior cerebellar artery) (List separately in addition to code for primary procedure)

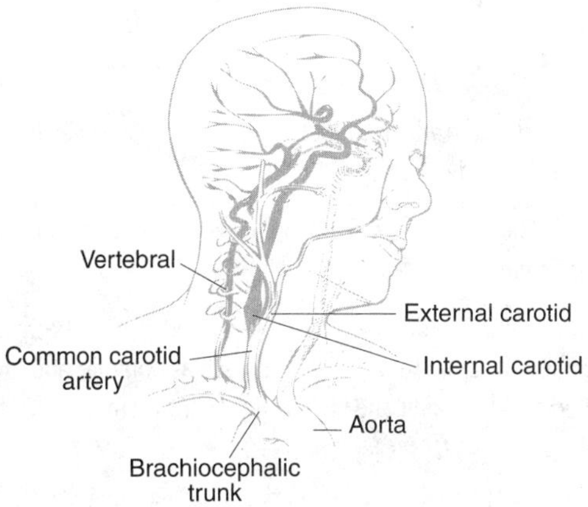

Explanation

In 36227, during selective angiography of the common carotid, internal carotid, or innominate artery, the physician also manipulates the catheter to the external carotid artery. Contrast material is injected into the catheter for arteriography, including the ipsilateral external carotid circulation. In 36228, during selective angiography of the internal carotid or vertebral artery, the physician further manipulates the catheter into additional intracranial branches of the artery, such as the middle cerebral or posterior inferior cerebellar arteries. Contrast material is injected into the catheter for arteriography, including the selected vessels circulation.

Coding Tips

When medically necessary, report moderate (conscious) sedation provided by the performing physician with 99151-99153. When provided by another physician, report 99155-99157. These codes include accessing the vessel, catheter placement(s), injection(s) of contrast, fluoroscopy, and radiological supervision and interpretation. Although it includes any additional second or third order selective catheter placements in the affected vessels, 36228 cannot be reported more than twice per side at the same operative session. Report 36227 in addition to 36222-36224. Report 36228 in addition to 36223-36226. Do not report these codes with transcatheter placement of an intravascular stent of the common carotid or innominate artery on the same side (37217).

ICD-10-CM Diagnostic Codes

This/these CPT code(s) are add on code(s). See the primary procedure code that this code is performed with for your ICD-10-CM code selections. Diagnostic code(s) would be the same as the actual procedure performed.

AMA: 36227 2018,Jan,8; 2017,Jan,8; 2016,Jan,13; 2015,Nov,10; 2015,Jan,16; 2014,Mar,8; 2014,Jan,11; 2013,Oct,18; 2013,May,3-5; 2013,Jun,12; 2013,Feb,16-17 **36228** 2018,Jan,8; 2017,Jan,8; 2016,Jan,13; 2015,Nov,3; 2015,Jan,16; 2014,Jan,11; 2013,Oct,18; 2013,May,3-5; 2013,Jun,12; 2013,Feb,16-17

Relative Value Units/Medicare Edits

Non-Facility RVU	Work	PE	MP	Total
36227	2.09	4.61	0.53	7.23
36228	4.25	32.25	1.14	37.64
Facility RVU	**Work**	**PE**	**MP**	**Total**
36227	2.09	0.79	0.53	3.41
36228	4.25	1.64	1.14	7.03

	FUD	Status	MUE	Modifiers				IOM Reference
36227	N/A	A	1(3)	N/A	50	N/A	N/A	None
36228	N/A	A	4(3)	N/A	50	N/A	N/A	

* with documentation

Terms To Know

angiography. Radiographic imaging of the arteries. Imaging may be performed to study the vasculature of any given organ, body system, or area of circulation such as the brain, heart, chest, kidneys, limbs, gastrointestinal tract, aorta, and pulmonary circulation to visualize the formation and the function of the blood vessels to detect problems such as a blockage or stricture. A catheter is inserted through an accessible blood vessel and the artery is injected with a radiopaque contrast material after which x-rays are taken.

catheter. Flexible tube inserted into an area of the body for introducing or withdrawing fluid.

cerebellum. Portion of the brain in the rear cranial fossa behind the brain stem responsible for movement coordination.

contrast material. Any internally administered substance that has a different opacity from soft tissue on radiography or computed tomograph; includes barium, used to opacify parts of the gastrointestinal tract; water-soluble iodinated compounds, used to opacify blood vessels or the genitourinary tract; may refer to air occurring naturally or introduced into the body; also, paramagnetic substances used in magnetic resonance imaging. Substances may also be documented as contrast agent or contrast medium.

selective placement. Introduction and manipulation of a catheter or guidewire within a vascular tree or family into a specified target area that is identified and monitored by radiographic imaging in order to carry out a diagnostic or therapeutic procedure.

36245-36246

36245 Selective catheter placement, arterial system; each first order abdominal, pelvic, or lower extremity artery branch, within a vascular family

36246 initial second order abdominal, pelvic, or lower extremity artery branch, within a vascular family

Selective catheter placement, arterial system

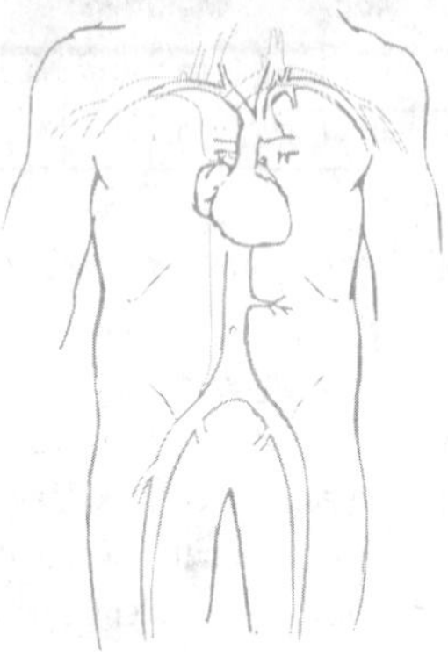

Explanation

The physician inserts a needle through the skin and into an underlying artery, usually a lower extremity artery, and threads a guidewire through the needle and into the artery. The needle is removed. The wire is threaded into the specific vessel. A catheter follows the wire into the artery branch. The wire is removed. Contrast material for arteriography is injected into the catheter that has been guided to the site under investigation. In 36245, the catheter remains in a first order artery. In 36246, the catheter travels to a second order artery. Once the procedure is complete, the catheter is removed and pressure applied to stop bleeding at the injection site.

Coding Tips

When medically necessary, report moderate (conscious) sedation provided by the performing physician with 99151-99153. When provided by another physician, report 99155-99157. These codes include introduction of needles or a catheter, injection of contrast material with or without automatic power injection, and/or necessary pre- and postinjection care specifically related to the injection. Supplies (catheters, drugs, and contrast media) are not included in the listed service. Report only the highest order vessel cannulated in each vascular family, but not any lesser order vessels cannulated in the approach. Report 36248 for each additional second order, third order, and more selective order vessel cannulated in the same vascular family. Right and left vessels belong to different vascular families; therefore, code separate catheterizations when performed.

ICD-10-CM Diagnostic Codes

The application of this code is too broad to adequately present ICD-10-CM diagnostic code links here. Refer to your ICD-10-CM book.

AMA: 36245 2018,Jan,8; 2017,Jan,8; 2016,Jul,6; 2016,Jan,13; 2015,Jan,16; 2014,Jan,11; 2013,Nov,14 **36246** 2018,Jan,8; 2017,Jan,8; 2016,Jul,6; 2016,Jan,13; 2015,Jan,16; 2014,Jan,11; 2013,Nov,14

Relative Value Units/Medicare Edits

Non-Facility RVU	Work	PE	MP	Total
36245	4.65	32.01	0.77	37.43
36246	5.02	17.81	0.97	23.8
Facility RVU	**Work**	**PE**	**MP**	**Total**
36245	4.65	1.47	0.77	6.89
36246	5.02	1.4	0.97	7.39

	FUD	Status	MUE	Modifiers				IOM Reference
36245	N/A	A	6(3)	51	50	N/A	N/A	None
36246	0	A	4(3)	51	50	N/A	N/A	

* with documentation

Terms To Know

artery. Vessel through which oxygenated blood passes away from the heart to any part of the body.

catheter. Flexible tube inserted into an area of the body for introducing or withdrawing fluid.

contrast material. Radiopaque substance placed into the body to enable a system or body structure to be visualized, such as nonionic and low osmolar contrast media (LOCM), ionic and high osmolar contrast media (HOCM), barium, and gadolinium.

first order. First vessel in the arterial or venous system that branches off the main vessel and supplies additional branches within the same vascular family.

guidewire. Flexible metal instrument designed to lead another instrument in its proper course.

second order catheter placement. Catheter manipulation into a vessel that branches off the aorta. May be noted in the record as a second branch or second family placement.

36247-36248

36247 Selective catheter placement, arterial system; initial third order or more selective abdominal, pelvic, or lower extremity artery branch, within a vascular family

+ **36248** additional second order, third order, and beyond, abdominal, pelvic, or lower extremity artery branch, within a vascular family (List in addition to code for initial second or third order vessel as appropriate)

Selective catheter placement, arterial system

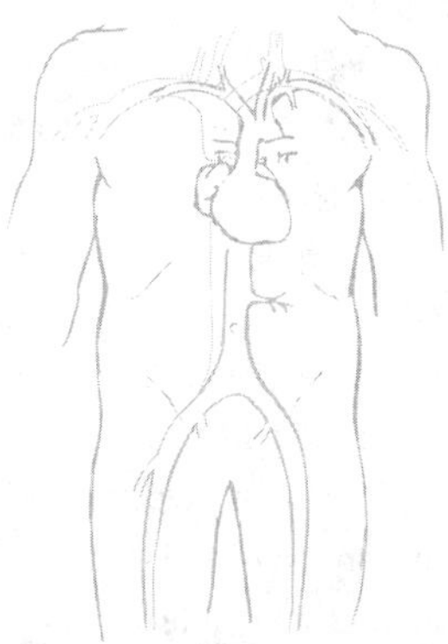

Explanation

The physician inserts a needle through the skin and into an underlying artery. A guidewire is threaded through the needle into the artery and the needle is removed. The guidewire is manipulated into the specific artery. A catheter follows the wire into the third order abdominal, pelvic, or lower extremity artery branch. Contrast material for arteriography is injected into the catheter that has been guided to the site under investigation. Once the procedure is complete, the catheter is removed and pressure applied at the injection site. Report 36247 for a placement in the initial third order or more selective abdominal, pelvic, or lower extremity artery branch, within a vascular family. Report 36248 for any additional second order, third order, and beyond, abdominal, pelvic, or lower extremity artery branch, within a vascular family.

Coding Tips

When medically necessary, report moderate (conscious) sedation provided by the performing physician with 99151-99153. When provided by another physician, report 99155-99157. These codes include introduction of needles or a catheter, injection of contrast material with or without automatic power injection, and/or necessary pre- and postinjection care specifically related to the injection. Supplies (catheters, drugs, and contrast media) are not included in the listed service. Report only the highest order vessel cannulated in each vascular family, but not any lesser order vessels cannulated in the approach. Report 36248 for each additional second order, third order, and more selective order vessel cannulated in the same vascular family. Right and left vessels belong to different vascular families; therefore, code separate catheterizations when performed. Report 36248 with 36246 and 36247. Named or unnamed arterial branches beyond a third-order arterial branch should be reported with 36218 or 36248, as appropriate.

ICD-10-CM Diagnostic Codes

The application of this code is too broad to adequately present ICD-10-CM diagnostic code links here. Refer to your ICD-10-CM book.

AMA: 36247 2018,Jan,8; 2017,Jan,8; 2016,Jul,6; 2016,Jan,13; 2015,Jan,16; 2014,Jan,11; 2013,Nov,14 **36248** 2018,Oct,3; 2018,Jan,8; 2017,Jan,8; 2016,Jul,6; 2016,Jan,13; 2015,Jan,16; 2014,Jan,11

Relative Value Units/Medicare Edits

Non-Facility RVU	Work	PE	MP	Total
36247	6.04	35.53	1.03	42.6
36248	1.01	2.99	0.11	4.11
Facility RVU	**Work**	**PE**	**MP**	**Total**
36247	6.04	1.71	1.03	8.78
36248	1.01	0.3	0.11	1.42

	FUD	Status	MUE	Modifiers				IOM Reference
36247	0	A	3(3)	51	50	N/A	N/A	None
36248	N/A	A	6(3)	N/A	N/A	N/A	N/A	

* with documentation

Terms To Know

artery. Vessel through which oxygenated blood passes away from the heart to any part of the body.

catheter. Flexible tube inserted into an area of the body for introducing or withdrawing fluid.

contrast material. Radiopaque substance placed into the body to enable a system or body structure to be visualized, such as nonionic and low osmolar contrast media (LOCM), ionic and high osmolar contrast media (HOCM), barium, and gadolinium.

guidewire. Flexible metal instrument designed to lead another instrument in its proper course.

36251-36252

36251 Selective catheter placement (first-order), main renal artery and any accessory renal artery(s) for renal angiography, including arterial puncture and catheter placement(s), fluoroscopy, contrast injection(s), image postprocessing, permanent recording of images, and radiological supervision and interpretation, including pressure gradient measurements when performed, and flush aortogram when performed; unilateral

36252 bilateral

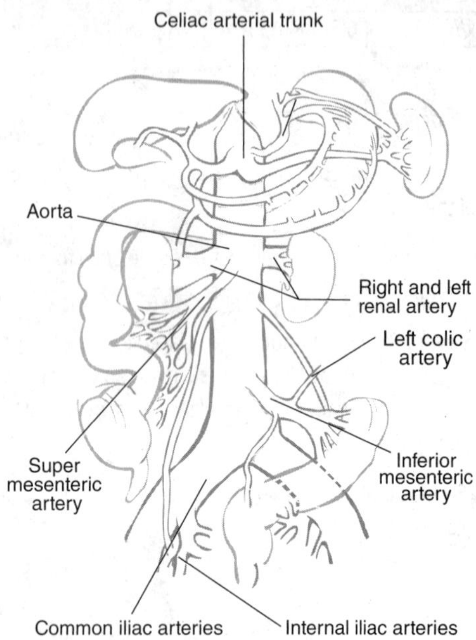

Explanation

The physician inserts a needle through the skin and into an underlying artery, usually a lower extremity artery, and threads a guidewire through the needle and into the artery. The needle is removed. The wire is threaded into the main renal artery and any accessory renal arteries, first order (branch) only. A catheter follows the wire into the arteries. The wire is removed. Contrast material for arteriography is injected into the catheter. Images are taken, the catheter is removed, and pressure applied to stop bleeding at the injection site. These codes include image postprocessing, permanent recording of images, and radiological supervision and interpretation (e.g., pressure gradient measurements and flush aortogram). Report 36251 for a unilateral procedure and 36252 for a bilateral procedure.

Coding Tips

When medically necessary, report moderate (conscious) sedation provided by the performing physician with 99151-99153. When provided by another physician, report 99155-99157. These codes include introduction of needles or a catheter, injection of contrast material, fluoroscopic guidance, image postprocessing and permanent recording, radiological supervision and interpretation with or without pressure gradient measurement, and flush aortogram. Do not report closure device placement at the vascular access site separately. Do not report 36253 with 36251 when the procedure is performed on the same kidney. Do not report these codes with 0338T or 0339T.

ICD-10-CM Diagnostic Codes

C64.1	Malignant neoplasm of right kidney, except renal pelvis ☑
C64.2	Malignant neoplasm of left kidney, except renal pelvis ☑
C65.1	Malignant neoplasm of right renal pelvis ☑
C65.2	Malignant neoplasm of left renal pelvis ☑
C79.01	Secondary malignant neoplasm of right kidney and renal pelvis ☑
C79.02	Secondary malignant neoplasm of left kidney and renal pelvis ☑
D09.19	Carcinoma in situ of other urinary organs
D30.01	Benign neoplasm of right kidney ☑
D30.02	Benign neoplasm of left kidney ☑
D30.11	Benign neoplasm of right renal pelvis ☑
D30.12	Benign neoplasm of left renal pelvis ☑
D41.01	Neoplasm of uncertain behavior of right kidney ☑
D41.02	Neoplasm of uncertain behavior of left kidney ☑
D41.11	Neoplasm of uncertain behavior of right renal pelvis ☑
D41.12	Neoplasm of uncertain behavior of left renal pelvis ☑
D41.21	Neoplasm of uncertain behavior of right ureter ☑
D41.22	Neoplasm of uncertain behavior of left ureter ☑
D49.511	Neoplasm of unspecified behavior of right kidney ☑
D49.512	Neoplasm of unspecified behavior of left kidney ☑
I15.0	Renovascular hypertension
I15.1	Hypertension secondary to other renal disorders
I15.8	Other secondary hypertension
I70.1	Atherosclerosis of renal artery
I72.2	Aneurysm of renal artery
I75.81	Atheroembolism of kidney
I77.73	Dissection of renal artery
N17.0	Acute kidney failure with tubular necrosis
N17.1	Acute kidney failure with acute cortical necrosis
N17.2	Acute kidney failure with medullary necrosis
N17.8	Other acute kidney failure
N17.9	Acute kidney failure, unspecified
N26.1	Atrophy of kidney (terminal)
N26.2	Page kidney
N27.0	Small kidney, unilateral
N27.1	Small kidney, bilateral
N28.0	Ischemia and infarction of kidney
N28.82	Megaloureter
N28.89	Other specified disorders of kidney and ureter
Q27.1	Congenital renal artery stenosis
Q27.2	Other congenital malformations of renal artery
S35.411A	Laceration of right renal artery, initial encounter ☑
S35.412A	Laceration of left renal artery, initial encounter ☑
S35.491A	Other specified injury of right renal artery, initial encounter ☑
S35.492A	Other specified injury of left renal artery, initial encounter ☑
S37.011A	Minor contusion of right kidney, initial encounter ☑
S37.012A	Minor contusion of left kidney, initial encounter ☑
S37.021A	Major contusion of right kidney, initial encounter ☑
S37.022A	Major contusion of left kidney, initial encounter ☑
S37.061A	Major laceration of right kidney, initial encounter ☑
S37.062A	Major laceration of left kidney, initial encounter ☑
S37.091A	Other injury of right kidney, initial encounter ☑
S37.092A	Other injury of left kidney, initial encounter ☑

AMA: **36251** 2018,Jan,8; 2017,Jan,8; 2016,Jan,13; 2015,Jan,16; 2014,Jan,11; 2013,Nov,14 **36252** 2018,Jan,8; 2017,Jan,8; 2016,Jan,13; 2015,Jan,16; 2014,Jan,11

Relative Value Units/Medicare Edits

Non-Facility RVU	Work	PE	MP	Total
36251	5.1	33.23	0.89	39.22
36252	6.74	34.22	1.47	42.43
Facility RVU	**Work**	**PE**	**MP**	**Total**
36251	5.1	1.56	0.89	7.55
36252	6.74	2.28	1.47	10.49

	FUD	Status	MUE	Modifiers				IOM Reference
36251	0	A	1(3)	51	N/A	N/A	N/A	None
36252	0	A	1(3)	51	N/A	N/A	N/A	

* with documentation

Terms To Know

angiography. Radiographic imaging of the arteries. Imaging may be performed to study the vasculature of any given organ, body system, or area of circulation such as the brain, heart, chest, kidneys, limbs, gastrointestinal tract, aorta, and pulmonary circulation to visualize the formation and the function of the blood vessels to detect problems such as a blockage or stricture. A catheter is inserted through an accessible blood vessel and the artery is injected with a radiopaque contrast material after which x-rays are taken.

aortography. Radiographic visualization of the aorta and its branches by injecting contrast medium through percutaneous puncture or catheterization technique.

first order selective. Catheter placement into the first vessel that branches off the aorta; catheter placement into the first vessel that branches off the vessel into which percutaneous insertion was made.

36253-36254

36253 Superselective catheter placement (one or more second order or higher renal artery branches) renal artery and any accessory renal artery(s) for renal angiography, including arterial puncture, catheterization, fluoroscopy, contrast injection(s), image postprocessing, permanent recording of images, and radiological supervision and interpretation, including pressure gradient measurements when performed, and flush aortogram when performed; unilateral

36254 bilateral

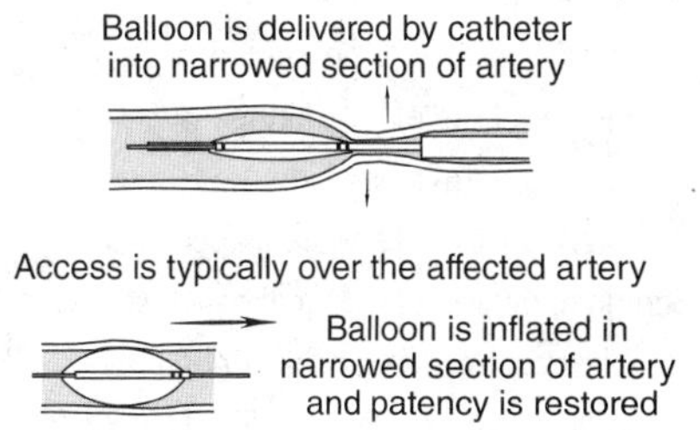

An open transluminal angioplasty is performed

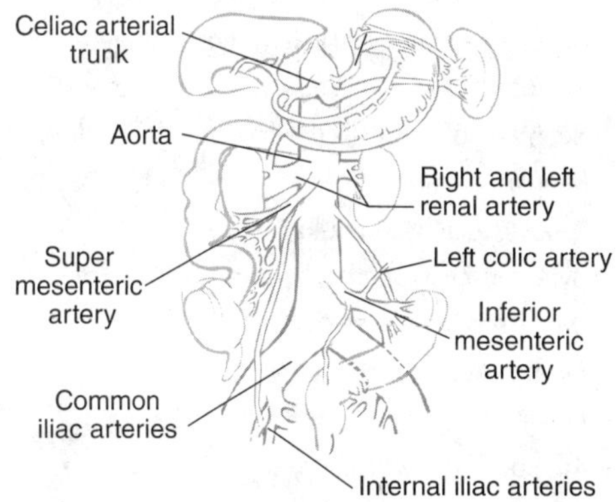

Explanation

A superselective catheterization is performed on one or more of the second order (branch) or higher of the renal artery branches. Superselective catheterization is needed for extremely small vessels or vessels that have sharp angles when branching to another order. The physician inserts a needle through the skin and into an underlying artery, usually a lower extremity artery, and threads a guidewire through the needle and into the artery. The needle is removed. The wire is threaded into the targeted artery and any accessory renal arteries of the second order or higher. A super fine and small catheter follows the wire into the arteries. The wire is removed. Contrast material for arteriography is injected into the catheter. Images are taken, the catheter is removed, and pressure is applied to stop bleeding at the injection site. These codes include image postprocessing, permanent recording of images, and radiological supervision and interpretation (e.g., pressure gradient measurements and flush aortogram). Report 36253 for a unilateral procedure and 36254 for a bilateral procedure.

Coding Tips

When medically necessary, report moderate (conscious) sedation provided by the performing physician with 99151-99153. When provided by another physician, report 99155-99157. These codes include needle or catheter placement, injection of contrast material, fluoroscopic guidance, image postprocessing and permanent storage of images, radiologic supervision and interpretation with or without pressure gradient measurements, and flush aortogram. Do not report closure device placement at the vascular access site separately. Do not report 36253 with 36251 when the procedure is performed on the same kidney. Do not report 36254 with 36252. Do not report these codes with 0338T or 0339T.

ICD-10-CM Diagnostic Codes

C64.1 Malignant neoplasm of right kidney, except renal pelvis ☑
C64.2 Malignant neoplasm of left kidney, except renal pelvis ☑
C65.1 Malignant neoplasm of right renal pelvis ☑
C65.2 Malignant neoplasm of left renal pelvis ☑
C79.01 Secondary malignant neoplasm of right kidney and renal pelvis ☑
C79.02 Secondary malignant neoplasm of left kidney and renal pelvis ☑
D09.19 Carcinoma in situ of other urinary organs
D30.01 Benign neoplasm of right kidney ☑
D30.02 Benign neoplasm of left kidney ☑
D30.11 Benign neoplasm of right renal pelvis ☑
D30.12 Benign neoplasm of left renal pelvis ☑
D41.01 Neoplasm of uncertain behavior of right kidney ☑
D41.02 Neoplasm of uncertain behavior of left kidney ☑
D41.11 Neoplasm of uncertain behavior of right renal pelvis ☑
D41.12 Neoplasm of uncertain behavior of left renal pelvis ☑
D41.21 Neoplasm of uncertain behavior of right ureter ☑
D41.22 Neoplasm of uncertain behavior of left ureter ☑
D49.511 Neoplasm of unspecified behavior of right kidney ☑
D49.512 Neoplasm of unspecified behavior of left kidney ☑
I15.0 Renovascular hypertension
I15.1 Hypertension secondary to other renal disorders
I15.8 Other secondary hypertension
I70.1 Atherosclerosis of renal artery
I72.2 Aneurysm of renal artery
I75.81 Atheroembolism of kidney
I77.73 Dissection of renal artery
N17.0 Acute kidney failure with tubular necrosis
N17.1 Acute kidney failure with acute cortical necrosis
N17.2 Acute kidney failure with medullary necrosis
N17.8 Other acute kidney failure
N26.1 Atrophy of kidney (terminal)
N26.2 Page kidney
N27.0 Small kidney, unilateral
N27.1 Small kidney, bilateral
N28.0 Ischemia and infarction of kidney
N28.82 Megaloureter
N28.89 Other specified disorders of kidney and ureter
Q27.1 Congenital renal artery stenosis
Q27.2 Other congenital malformations of renal artery
S35.411A Laceration of right renal artery, initial encounter ☑
S35.412A Laceration of left renal artery, initial encounter ☑
S35.491A Other specified injury of right renal artery, initial encounter ☑
S35.492A Other specified injury of left renal artery, initial encounter ☑
S37.011A Minor contusion of right kidney, initial encounter ☑
S37.012A Minor contusion of left kidney, initial encounter ☑
S37.021A Major contusion of right kidney, initial encounter ☑
S37.022A Major contusion of left kidney, initial encounter ☑
S37.061A Major laceration of right kidney, initial encounter ☑
S37.062A Major laceration of left kidney, initial encounter ☑
S37.091A Other injury of right kidney, initial encounter ☑
S37.092A Other injury of left kidney, initial encounter ☑

AMA: 36253 2018,Jan,8; 2017,Jan,8; 2016,Jan,13; 2015,Jan,16; 2014,Jan,11; 2013,Nov,14 **36254** 2018,Jan,8; 2017,Jan,8; 2016,Jan,13; 2015,Jan,16; 2014,Jan,11

Relative Value Units/Medicare Edits

Non-Facility RVU	Work	PE	MP	Total
36253	7.3	54.51	0.79	62.6
36254	7.9	51.25	1.67	60.82
Facility RVU	**Work**	**PE**	**MP**	**Total**
36253	7.3	2.28	0.79	10.37
36254	7.9	2.56	1.67	12.13

	FUD	Status	MUE	Modifiers				IOM Reference
36253	0	A	1(3)	51	N/A	N/A	N/A	None
36254	0	A	1(3)	51	N/A	N/A	N/A	

* with documentation

Terms To Know

aneurysm. Circumscribed dilation or outpouching of an artery wall, often containing blood clots and connecting directly with the lumen of the artery.

36260

36260 Insertion of implantable intra-arterial infusion pump (eg, for chemotherapy of liver)

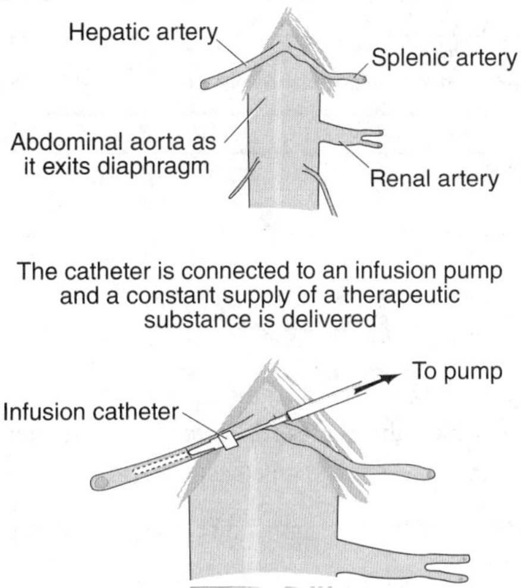

Explanation

The physician performs an upper abdominal incision and exposes the hepatic artery. The physician punctures the hepatic artery with a large needle and passes a guidewire via the needle into the punctured artery. The physician removes the needle while leaving the guidewire in place. The physician slides the infusion catheter over the guidewire into the arterial lumen. The physician secures the catheter with suture and closes the abdominal wound around the proximal end of the infusion catheter. The physician may use the catheter to administer chemotherapeutic medication.

Coding Tips

For removal of an intra-arterial infusion pump, see 36262. Supplies used when providing this procedure may be reported with C1772. Check with the specific payer to determine coverage. For revision of an implanted intra-arterial infusion pump, see 36261.

ICD-10-CM Diagnostic Codes

C22.0	Liver cell carcinoma
C22.1	Intrahepatic bile duct carcinoma
C22.2	Hepatoblastoma
C22.3	Angiosarcoma of liver
C22.4	Other sarcomas of liver
C22.7	Other specified carcinomas of liver
C78.7	Secondary malignant neoplasm of liver and intrahepatic bile duct
C7B.02	Secondary carcinoid tumors of liver
D01.5	Carcinoma in situ of liver, gallbladder and bile ducts
D01.7	Carcinoma in situ of other specified digestive organs
D37.6	Neoplasm of uncertain behavior of liver, gallbladder and bile ducts

Associated HCPCS Codes

C1772	Infusion pump, programmable (implantable)

AMA: **36260** 2018,Jan,8; 2017,Jan,8; 2016,Jan,13; 2015,Jan,16; 2014,Jan,11

Relative Value Units/Medicare Edits

Non-Facility RVU	Work	PE	MP	Total
36260	9.91	6.49	2.4	18.8
Facility RVU	**Work**	**PE**	**MP**	**Total**
36260	9.91	6.49	2.4	18.8

	FUD	Status	MUE	Modifiers				IOM Reference
36260	90	A	1(2)	51	N/A	N/A	N/A	None

* with documentation

Terms To Know

artery. Vessel through which oxygenated blood passes away from the heart to any part of the body.

carcinoma in situ. Malignancy that arises from the cells of the vessel, gland, or organ of origin that remains confined to that site or has not invaded neighboring tissue.

catheter. Flexible tube inserted into an area of the body for introducing or withdrawing fluid.

in situ. Located in the natural position or contained within the origin site, not spread into neighboring tissue.

malignant. Any condition tending to progress toward death, specifically an invasive tumor with a loss of cellular differentiation that has the ability to spread or metastasize to other body areas.

proximal. Located closest to a specified reference point, usually the midline or trunk.

36261

36261 Revision of implanted intra-arterial infusion pump

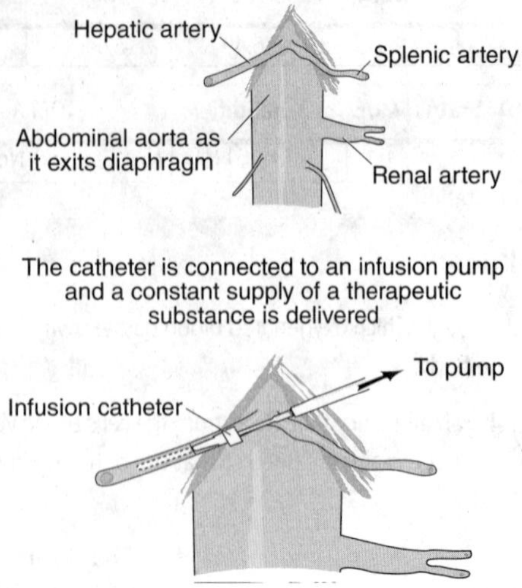

Explanation

The physician performs an upper abdominal incision and exposes the hepatic artery, locating the previously implanted infusion catheter. The physician may unkink the catheter or replace it over a wire. The physician secures the catheter with suture and closes the abdominal wound around the proximal end of the infusion catheter. The physician may use the catheter to administer chemotherapeutic medication.

Coding Tips

Supplies used when providing this procedure may be reported with the appropriate HCPCS Level II code. Check with the specific payer to determine coverage. For insertion of an implantable intra-arterial infusion pump, see 36260. For removal of an implanted intra-arterial infusion pump, see 36262.

ICD-10-CM Diagnostic Codes

C22.0	Liver cell carcinoma
C22.1	Intrahepatic bile duct carcinoma
C22.2	Hepatoblastoma
C22.3	Angiosarcoma of liver
C22.4	Other sarcomas of liver
C22.7	Other specified carcinomas of liver
C78.7	Secondary malignant neoplasm of liver and intrahepatic bile duct
C7B.02	Secondary carcinoid tumors of liver
D01.5	Carcinoma in situ of liver, gallbladder and bile ducts
D01.7	Carcinoma in situ of other specified digestive organs
D37.6	Neoplasm of uncertain behavior of liver, gallbladder and bile ducts
Z45.2	Encounter for adjustment and management of vascular access device
Z95.828	Presence of other vascular implants and grafts

AMA: **36261** 2000,Oct,4

Relative Value Units/Medicare Edits

Non-Facility RVU	Work	PE	MP	Total
36261	5.63	4.66	1.35	11.64
Facility RVU	**Work**	**PE**	**MP**	**Total**
36261	5.63	4.66	1.35	11.64

	FUD	Status	MUE	Modifiers				IOM Reference
36261	90	A	1(2)	51	N/A	N/A	80	None

* with documentation

Terms To Know

catheter. Flexible tube inserted into an area of the body for introducing or withdrawing fluid.

complication. Condition arising after the beginning of observation and treatment that modifies the course of the patient's illness or the medical care required, or an undesired result or misadventure in medical care.

infection. Presence of microorganisms in body tissues that may result in cellular damage.

proximal. Located closest to a specified reference point, usually the midline or trunk.

suture. Numerous stitching techniques employed in wound closure.

buried suture. Continuous or interrupted suture placed under the skin for a layered closure.

continuous suture. Running stitch with tension evenly distributed across a single strand to provide a leakproof closure line.

interrupted suture. Series of single stitches with tension isolated at each stitch, in which all stitches are not affected if one becomes loose, and the isolated sutures cannot act as a wick to transport an infection.

purse-string suture. Continuous suture placed around a tubular structure and tightened, to reduce or close the lumen.

retention suture. Secondary stitching that bridges the primary suture, providing support for the primary repair; a plastic or rubber bolster may be placed over the primary repair and under the retention sutures.

36262

36262 Removal of implanted intra-arterial infusion pump

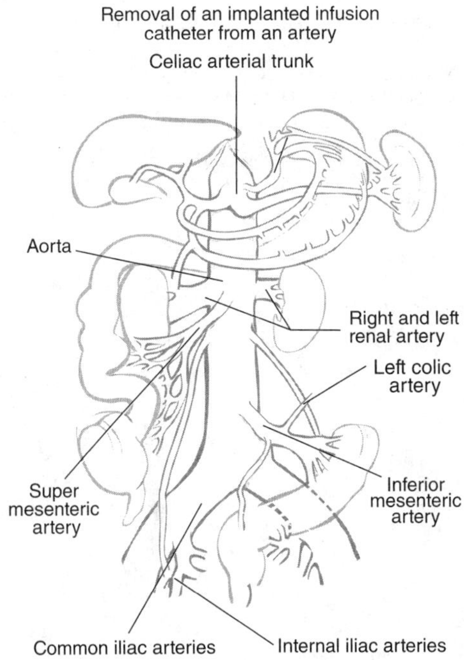

Explanation

The physician performs an upper abdominal incision and exposes the hepatic artery while dissecting free the previously implanted infusion catheter. The physician removes the catheter, and may repair the arteriotomy with suture. The physician closes the abdominal wound, and may leave a drain in place.

Coding Tips

For insertion of an implantable intra-arterial infusion pump, see 36260. For revision of an implanted intra-arterial infusion pump, see 36261.

ICD-10-CM Diagnostic Codes

T82.514A	Breakdown (mechanical) of infusion catheter, initial encounter
T82.518A	Breakdown (mechanical) of other cardiac and vascular devices and implants, initial encounter
T82.524A	Displacement of infusion catheter, initial encounter
T82.528A	Displacement of other cardiac and vascular devices and implants, initial encounter
T82.534A	Leakage of infusion catheter, initial encounter
T82.538A	Leakage of other cardiac and vascular devices and implants, initial encounter
T82.594A	Other mechanical complication of infusion catheter, initial encounter
T82.598A	Other mechanical complication of other cardiac and vascular devices and implants, initial encounter
T82.7XXA	Infection and inflammatory reaction due to other cardiac and vascular devices, implants and grafts, initial encounter
T82.818A	Embolism due to vascular prosthetic devices, implants and grafts, initial encounter
T82.828A	Fibrosis due to vascular prosthetic devices, implants and grafts, initial encounter
T82.838A	Hemorrhage due to vascular prosthetic devices, implants and grafts, initial encounter
T82.848A	Pain due to vascular prosthetic devices, implants and grafts, initial encounter
T82.858A	Stenosis of other vascular prosthetic devices, implants and grafts, initial encounter
T82.868A	Thrombosis due to vascular prosthetic devices, implants and grafts, initial encounter
T82.898A	Other specified complication of vascular prosthetic devices, implants and grafts, initial encounter
Z45.2	Encounter for adjustment and management of vascular access device
Z95.828	Presence of other vascular implants and grafts

AMA: **36262** 2000,Oct,4

Relative Value Units/Medicare Edits

Non-Facility RVU	Work	PE	MP	Total
36262	4.11	3.79	1.0	8.9
Facility RVU	**Work**	**PE**	**MP**	**Total**
36262	4.11	3.79	1.0	8.9

	FUD	Status	MUE	Modifiers				IOM Reference
36262	90	A	1(2)	51	N/A	N/A	N/A	None

* with documentation

Terms To Know

arteriotomy. Incision into an artery.

catheter. Flexible tube inserted into an area of the body for introducing or withdrawing fluid.

complication. Condition arising after the beginning of observation and treatment that modifies the course of the patient's illness or the medical care required, or an undesired result or misadventure in medical care.

incision. Act of cutting into tissue or an organ.

infection. Presence of microorganisms in body tissues that may result in cellular damage.

malignant. Any condition tending to progress toward death, specifically an invasive tumor with a loss of cellular differentiation that has the ability to spread or metastasize to other body areas.

36468

36468 Injection(s) of sclerosant for spider veins (telangiectasia), limb or trunk

A solution is injected directly into the tiny distended veins in the arms, legs, or body trunk causing the walls of the vein to close

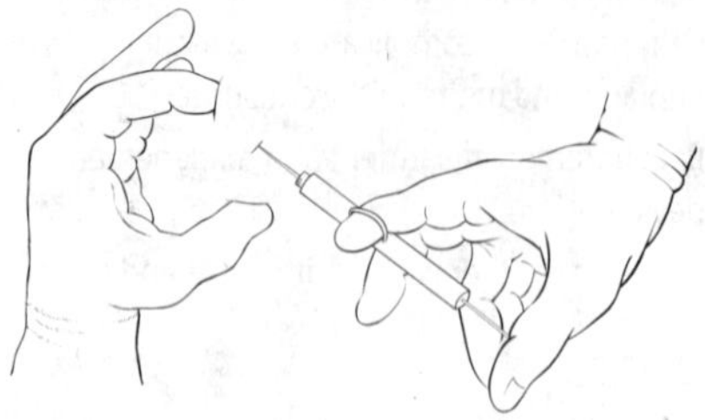

Explanation

The physician inserts a tiny needle through the skin and directly into the tiny, distended veins in the arm, leg, or trunk. A sclerosant for telangiectasias (spider veins) is injected into these veins. The solution causes the walls of the veins to become inflamed, collapse, and stick together so the veins close.

Coding Tips

This code should only be reported once per extremity. Do not report 36468 with 37241 for the same surgical field. Because this procedure usually is not done out of medical necessity, the patient may be responsible for charges. Verify with the insurance carrier for coverage. For ultrasound guidance performed with 36468, see 76942. Do not report 36468 with 29520, 29530, 29540, 29550, 29580, 29581, or 29584 for the same extremity. For treatment of larger varicose veins in the leg, with sclerosing solutions, see 36470–36471. For removal of a varicose vein/vein cluster, see 37785.

ICD-10-CM Diagnostic Codes

I78.0	Hereditary hemorrhagic telangiectasia
I78.8	Other diseases of capillaries
I78.9	Disease of capillaries, unspecified
I79.8	Other disorders of arteries, arterioles and capillaries in diseases classified elsewhere
Z41.1	Encounter for cosmetic surgery

AMA: **36468** 2018,Mar,3; 2018,Jan,8; 2017,Jan,8; 2016,Nov,3; 2016,Jan,13; 2015,Jan,16; 2015,Apr,10; 2014,Oct,6; 2014,Aug,14; 2013,Nov,6

Relative Value Units/Medicare Edits

Non-Facility RVU	Work	PE	MP	Total
36468	0.0	0.0	0.0	0.0
Facility RVU	**Work**	**PE**	**MP**	**Total**
36468	0.0	0.0	0.0	0.0

	FUD	Status	MUE	Modifiers				IOM Reference
36468	0	R	2(3)	51	N/A	N/A	80*	100-02,16,10; 100-02,16,120; 100-02,16,180

* with documentation

36470-36471

36470 Injection of sclerosant; single incompetent vein (other than telangiectasia)

36471 multiple incompetent veins (other than telangiectasia), same leg

A solution is injected directly into the tiny distended veins in the leg causing the walls of the vein to close

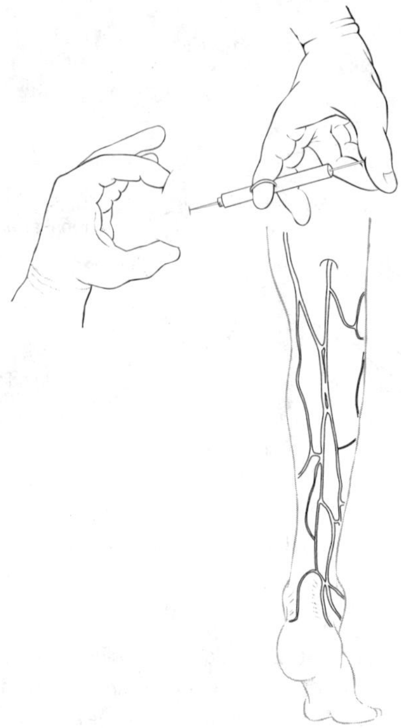

Explanation

The physician inserts a tiny needle through the skin and injects sclerosant into a single, incompetent vein, other than telangiectasias (spider veins), of the leg. The patient stands while the sclerosant injection is given. The leg is elevated and wrapped in an elastic dressing. The solution causes the walls of the veins to become inflamed, collapse, and stick together so the veins close. Report 36471 for injection of sclerosant into multiple incompetent veins, other than telangiectasias, of the same leg.

Coding Tips

Note that 36471 is a unilateral procedure. If performed bilaterally, some payers require that the service be reported twice with modifier 50 appended to the second code, while others require identification of the service only once with modifier 50 appended. Check with individual payers. Modifier 50 identifies a procedure performed identically on the opposite side of the body (mirror image). For ultrasound guidance performed with 36470-36471, see 76942. Do not report these codes with 29520, 29530, 29540, 29550, 29580, 29581, or 29584 for the same extremity. Do not report these codes with 37241 for the same surgical field. Do not report 36471 more than once per extremity. If extremity truncal vein injection of noncompounded foam sclerosant with ultrasound guided compression maneuvers to guide dispersion of the injectate is performed, see 36465-36466. For injections of spider veins (telangiectasia) of the arm, limb, or trunk, see 36468. Because this procedure usually is not done out of medical necessity, the patient may be responsible for charges. Verify with the insurance carrier for coverage.

ICD-10-CM Diagnostic Codes

I83.011 Varicose veins of right lower extremity with ulcer of thigh ☑

I83.012 Varicose veins of right lower extremity with ulcer of calf ☑
I83.013 Varicose veins of right lower extremity with ulcer of ankle ☑
I83.014 Varicose veins of right lower extremity with ulcer of heel and midfoot ☑
I83.015 Varicose veins of right lower extremity with ulcer other part of foot ☑
I83.018 Varicose veins of right lower extremity with ulcer other part of lower leg ☑
I83.021 Varicose veins of left lower extremity with ulcer of thigh ☑
I83.022 Varicose veins of left lower extremity with ulcer of calf ☑
I83.023 Varicose veins of left lower extremity with ulcer of ankle ☑
I83.024 Varicose veins of left lower extremity with ulcer of heel and midfoot ☑
I83.025 Varicose veins of left lower extremity with ulcer other part of foot ☑
I83.028 Varicose veins of left lower extremity with ulcer other part of lower leg ☑
I83.11 Varicose veins of right lower extremity with inflammation ☑
I83.12 Varicose veins of left lower extremity with inflammation ☑
I83.211 Varicose veins of right lower extremity with both ulcer of thigh and inflammation ☑
I83.212 Varicose veins of right lower extremity with both ulcer of calf and inflammation ☑
I83.213 Varicose veins of right lower extremity with both ulcer of ankle and inflammation ☑
I83.214 Varicose veins of right lower extremity with both ulcer of heel and midfoot and inflammation ☑
I83.215 Varicose veins of right lower extremity with both ulcer other part of foot and inflammation ☑
I83.218 Varicose veins of right lower extremity with both ulcer of other part of lower extremity and inflammation ☑
I83.221 Varicose veins of left lower extremity with both ulcer of thigh and inflammation ☑
I83.222 Varicose veins of left lower extremity with both ulcer of calf and inflammation ☑
I83.223 Varicose veins of left lower extremity with both ulcer of ankle and inflammation ☑
I83.224 Varicose veins of left lower extremity with both ulcer of heel and midfoot and inflammation ☑
I83.225 Varicose veins of left lower extremity with both ulcer other part of foot and inflammation ☑
I83.228 Varicose veins of left lower extremity with both ulcer of other part of lower extremity and inflammation ☑
I83.811 Varicose veins of right lower extremity with pain ☑
I83.812 Varicose veins of left lower extremity with pain ☑
I83.813 Varicose veins of bilateral lower extremities with pain ☑
I83.891 Varicose veins of right lower extremity with other complications ☑
I83.892 Varicose veins of left lower extremity with other complications ☑
I83.893 Varicose veins of bilateral lower extremities with other complications ☑
I83.91 Asymptomatic varicose veins of right lower extremity ☑
I83.92 Asymptomatic varicose veins of left lower extremity ☑
I83.93 Asymptomatic varicose veins of bilateral lower extremities ☑

AMA: **36470** 2018,Mar,3; 2018,Jan,8; 2018,Dec,10; 2018,Dec,10; 2017,Jan,8; 2016,Nov,3; 2016,Jan,13; 2015,Nov,10; 2015,Jan,16; 2015,Apr,10; 2014,Oct,6; 2014,Aug,14; 2013,Nov,6 **36471** 2018,Mar,3; 2018,Jan,8; 2018,Dec,10; 2018,Dec,10; 2017,Jan,8; 2016,Nov,3; 2016,Jan,13; 2015,Nov,10; 2015,Jan,16; 2015,Aug,8; 2015,Apr,10; 2014,Oct,6; 2014,Aug,14; 2013,Nov,6

Relative Value Units/Medicare Edits

Non-Facility RVU	Work	PE	MP	Total
36470	0.75	2.13	0.14	3.02
36471	1.5	3.71	0.26	5.47
Facility RVU	**Work**	**PE**	**MP**	**Total**
36470	0.75	0.22	0.14	1.11
36471	1.5	0.45	0.26	2.21

	FUD	Status	MUE	Modifiers				IOM Reference
36470	0	A	1(2)	51	50	N/A	N/A	100-02,16,10; 100-02,16,120; 100-03,150.7
36471	0	A	1(2)	51	50	N/A	N/A	

* with documentation

Terms To Know

cosmetic. Superficial or external, having no medical necessity.

distention. Enlarged or expanded due to pressure from inside.

edema. Swelling due to fluid accumulation in the intercellular spaces.

inflammation. Cytologic and chemical reactions that occur in affected blood vessels and adjacent tissues in response to injury or abnormal stimulation from a physical, chemical, or biologic agent.

sclerose. To become hard or firm and indurated from increased formation of connective tissue or disease.

ulcer. Open sore or excavating lesion of skin or the tissue on the surface of an organ from the sloughing of chronically inflamed and necrosing tissue.

varicose vein. Abnormal, permanently distended or stretched vein.

[36465, 36466]

36465 Injection of non-compounded foam sclerosant with ultrasound compression maneuvers to guide dispersion of the injectate, inclusive of all imaging guidance and monitoring; single incompetent extremity truncal vein (eg, great saphenous vein, accessory saphenous vein)

36466 Injection of non-compounded foam sclerosant with ultrasound compression maneuvers to guide dispersion of the injectate, inclusive of all imaging guidance and monitoring; multiple incompetent truncal veins (eg, great saphenous vein, accessory saphenous vein), same leg

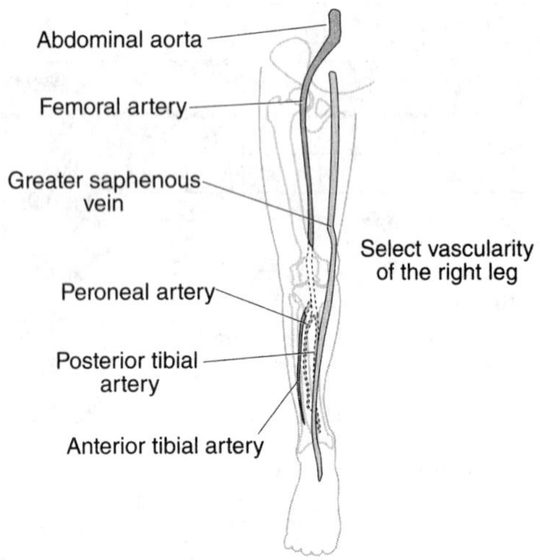

Explanation

The physician performs ultrasound guided foam sclerotherapy (UGFS) of varicose veins. UGFS is a minimally invasive and relatively safe treatment of restricted amounts of small varicose veins. In UGFS, a non-compounded foam sclerosant is injected into an extremity truncal vein (e.g., great saphenous vein, accessory saphenous vein) using ultrasound-guided compression of the junction of the central vein (saphenofemoral junction or saphenopopliteal junction) to limit the dispersion of the injectate. The physician creates a detailed outline or mapping of the veins in the lower legs to identify all vein abnormalities along with additional nearby structures to include deep veins and arteries via duplex ultrasound examination. Once completed, the patient is placed in the supine position and the leg being treated is exposed. The physician guides the needle into the vein using ultrasonic guidance and injects a non-compounded foam. Foam volumes vary from 1 mL to 16 mL per treatment. The injected vein collapses and is eventually absorbed by the body. The physician may need to repeat the injection process a number of times along the vein in order to completely target the incompetent truncal vein. Report 36465 for injection of a non-compounded foam sclerosant into a single incompetent extremity truncal vein and 36466 for multiple incompetent truncal veins of the same leg.

Coding Tips

When these procedures are performed in the office, all supplies and equipment are included. Codes may be reported only once per extremity per day. Application of compression bandages and/or stockings is included and may not be reported separately. Do not report 36465 or 36466 with 29520, 29530, 29540, 29550, 29580, 29581, or 29584 for the same extremity. Do not report 36465 or 36466 with 37241 when performed in the same surgical field. For a truncal vein injection in an extremity using compounded foam sclerosants or injection of a sclerosant into an incompetent vein without compression maneuvers to guide dispersion of the injectate, see 36470 and 36471. For endovenous ablation therapy of incompetent veins by transcatheter delivery of a chemical adhesive, see 36482 or 36483. For vascular embolization and occlusion procedures, see 37241-37244.

ICD-10-CM Diagnostic Codes

I78.0	Hereditary hemorrhagic telangiectasia
I82.491	Acute embolism and thrombosis of other specified deep vein of right lower extremity ☑
I82.492	Acute embolism and thrombosis of other specified deep vein of left lower extremity ☑
I82.499	Acute embolism and thrombosis of other specified deep vein of unspecified lower extremity
I82.591	Chronic embolism and thrombosis of other specified deep vein of right lower extremity ☑
I82.592	Chronic embolism and thrombosis of other specified deep vein of left lower extremity ☑
I82.811	Embolism and thrombosis of superficial veins of right lower extremity ☑
I82.812	Embolism and thrombosis of superficial veins of left lower extremity ☑
I83.011	Varicose veins of right lower extremity with ulcer of thigh ☑
I83.012	Varicose veins of right lower extremity with ulcer of calf ☑
I83.013	Varicose veins of right lower extremity with ulcer of ankle ☑
I83.014	Varicose veins of right lower extremity with ulcer of heel and midfoot ☑
I83.015	Varicose veins of right lower extremity with ulcer other part of foot ☑
I83.018	Varicose veins of right lower extremity with ulcer other part of lower leg ☑
I83.021	Varicose veins of left lower extremity with ulcer of thigh ☑
I83.022	Varicose veins of left lower extremity with ulcer of calf ☑
I83.023	Varicose veins of left lower extremity with ulcer of ankle ☑
I83.024	Varicose veins of left lower extremity with ulcer of heel and midfoot ☑
I83.025	Varicose veins of left lower extremity with ulcer other part of foot ☑
I83.028	Varicose veins of left lower extremity with ulcer other part of lower leg ☑
I83.11	Varicose veins of right lower extremity with inflammation ☑
I83.12	Varicose veins of left lower extremity with inflammation ☑
I83.211	Varicose veins of right lower extremity with both ulcer of thigh and inflammation ☑
I83.212	Varicose veins of right lower extremity with both ulcer of calf and inflammation ☑
I83.213	Varicose veins of right lower extremity with both ulcer of ankle and inflammation ☑
I83.214	Varicose veins of right lower extremity with both ulcer of heel and midfoot and inflammation ☑
I83.215	Varicose veins of right lower extremity with both ulcer other part of foot and inflammation ☑
I83.218	Varicose veins of right lower extremity with both ulcer of other part of lower extremity and inflammation ☑
I83.219	Varicose veins of right lower extremity with both ulcer of unspecified site and inflammation ☑
I83.221	Varicose veins of left lower extremity with both ulcer of thigh and inflammation ☑

I83.222 Varicose veins of left lower extremity with both ulcer of calf and inflammation ☑
I83.223 Varicose veins of left lower extremity with both ulcer of ankle and inflammation ☑
I83.224 Varicose veins of left lower extremity with both ulcer of heel and midfoot and inflammation ☑
I83.225 Varicose veins of left lower extremity with both ulcer other part of foot and inflammation ☑
I83.228 Varicose veins of left lower extremity with both ulcer of other part of lower extremity and inflammation ☑
I83.811 Varicose veins of right lower extremity with pain ☑
I83.812 Varicose veins of left lower extremity with pain ☑
I83.891 Varicose veins of right lower extremity with other complications ☑
I83.892 Varicose veins of left lower extremity with other complications ☑
I83.91 Asymptomatic varicose veins of right lower extremity ☑
I83.92 Asymptomatic varicose veins of left lower extremity ☑
I86.8 Varicose veins of other specified sites
I87.2 Venous insufficiency (chronic) (peripheral)

AMA: **36465** 2019,Feb,9; 2018,Mar,3; 2018,Dec,10; 2018,Dec,10 **36466** 2019,Feb,9; 2018,Mar,3; 2018,Dec,10; 2018,Dec,10

Relative Value Units/Medicare Edits

Non-Facility RVU	Work	PE	MP	Total
36465	2.35	40.82	0.47	43.64
36466	3.0	42.27	0.6	45.87
Facility RVU	**Work**	**PE**	**MP**	**Total**
36465	2.35	0.63	0.47	3.45
36466	3.0	0.79	0.6	4.39

	FUD	Status	MUE	Modifiers				IOM Reference
36465	0	A	1(2)	51	50	N/A	N/A	None
36466	0	A	1(2)	51	50	N/A	N/A	

* with documentation

Terms To Know

sclerotherapy. Injection of a chemical agent that will irritate, inflame, and cause fibrosis in a vein, eventually obliterating hemorrhoids or varicose veins.

varicose vein. Abnormal, permanently distended or stretched vein.

36473-36474

36473 Endovenous ablation therapy of incompetent vein, extremity, inclusive of all imaging guidance and monitoring, percutaneous, mechanochemical; first vein treated

+ **36474** subsequent vein(s) treated in a single extremity, each through separate access sites (List separately in addition to code for primary procedure)

Incompetent veins are treated with endovenous ablation including imaging guidance and monitoring

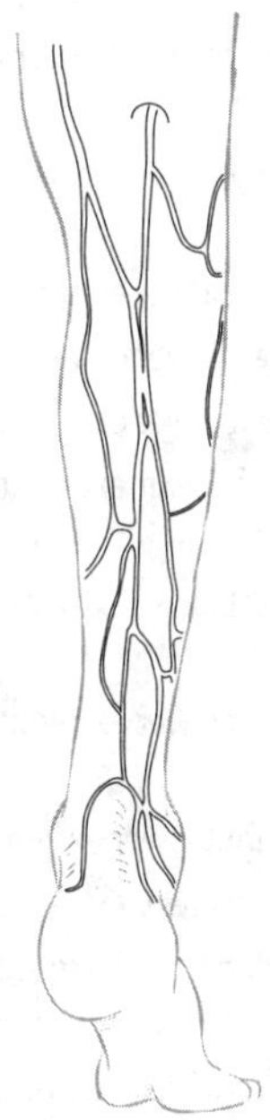

Explanation

The physician uses endovenous ablation therapy to treat venous incompetence in an extremity vein. Mechanochemical endovenous ablation (MOCA) uses a rotating wire in conjunction with an infused sclerosing agent to damage the wall of the vein. The most common site of treatment is the greater saphenous vein. The procedure includes any imaging guidance and monitoring. The leg is prepared and draped and a local anesthetic is applied to the puncture site. A needle is inserted into the access site. A guidewire is placed into the vessel using ultrasound guidance. An introducer sheath is placed over the guidewire and the guidewire is removed. A wire catheter system is introduced and the tip is advanced to the site of the venous incompetence under ultrasound guidance. The wire catheter system is connected to a handle with a motor that provides the rotation to the wire. The system is started for about 10 seconds to create vasospasm and slowly withdrawn with continuous infusion of sclerosing agent. The ablation catheter and introducer sheath are removed and pressure is applied to the puncture site. A compression stocking is applied for the immediate 24 hours and replaced daily for the following two weeks. Report 36473 for the initial vein treated and 36474 for subsequent veins treated in the same extremity via different access sites.

Coding Tips

When these procedures are performed in an office setting, required supplies and equipment are included and may not be reported separately. Codes may be reported only once per extremity per day. Application of compression bandages and/or stockings are included, when performed, and may not be reported separately. Report 36474 in addition to 36473. Report 36474 for subsequent veins treated in the same extremity; it may only be reported once per extremity. Do not report 36473 or 36474 with 36000-36005, 36410, 36425, 36475-36479, 37241, 75894, 76000, 76937, 76942, 76998, 77022, 93970, or 93971 for the same surgical field. Do not report these codes with 29520, 29530, 29540, 29550, 29580, 29581, or 29584 for the same extremity. For injection of an adhesive via catheter, see 37799.

ICD-10-CM Diagnostic Codes

I83.011 Varicose veins of right lower extremity with ulcer of thigh ☑
I83.012 Varicose veins of right lower extremity with ulcer of calf ☑
I83.013 Varicose veins of right lower extremity with ulcer of ankle ☑
I83.014 Varicose veins of right lower extremity with ulcer of heel and midfoot ☑
I83.015 Varicose veins of right lower extremity with ulcer other part of foot ☑
I83.018 Varicose veins of right lower extremity with ulcer other part of lower leg ☑
I83.021 Varicose veins of left lower extremity with ulcer of thigh ☑
I83.022 Varicose veins of left lower extremity with ulcer of calf ☑
I83.023 Varicose veins of left lower extremity with ulcer of ankle ☑
I83.024 Varicose veins of left lower extremity with ulcer of heel and midfoot ☑
I83.025 Varicose veins of left lower extremity with ulcer other part of foot ☑
I83.028 Varicose veins of left lower extremity with ulcer other part of lower leg ☑
I83.11 Varicose veins of right lower extremity with inflammation ☑
I83.12 Varicose veins of left lower extremity with inflammation ☑
I83.211 Varicose veins of right lower extremity with both ulcer of thigh and inflammation ☑
I83.212 Varicose veins of right lower extremity with both ulcer of calf and inflammation ☑
I83.213 Varicose veins of right lower extremity with both ulcer of ankle and inflammation ☑
I83.214 Varicose veins of right lower extremity with both ulcer of heel and midfoot and inflammation ☑
I83.215 Varicose veins of right lower extremity with both ulcer other part of foot and inflammation ☑
I83.218 Varicose veins of right lower extremity with both ulcer of other part of lower extremity and inflammation ☑
I83.221 Varicose veins of left lower extremity with both ulcer of thigh and inflammation ☑
I83.222 Varicose veins of left lower extremity with both ulcer of calf and inflammation ☑
I83.223 Varicose veins of left lower extremity with both ulcer of ankle and inflammation ☑
I83.224 Varicose veins of left lower extremity with both ulcer of heel and midfoot and inflammation ☑
I83.225 Varicose veins of left lower extremity with both ulcer other part of foot and inflammation ☑
I83.228 Varicose veins of left lower extremity with both ulcer of other part of lower extremity and inflammation ☑
I83.811 Varicose veins of right lower extremity with pain ☑
I83.812 Varicose veins of left lower extremity with pain ☑
I83.813 Varicose veins of bilateral lower extremities with pain ☑
I83.891 Varicose veins of right lower extremity with other complications ☑
I83.892 Varicose veins of left lower extremity with other complications ☑
I83.893 Varicose veins of bilateral lower extremities with other complications ☑
I83.91 Asymptomatic varicose veins of right lower extremity ☑
I83.92 Asymptomatic varicose veins of left lower extremity ☑
I83.93 Asymptomatic varicose veins of bilateral lower extremities ☑
I86.8 Varicose veins of other specified sites

AMA: 36473 2019,Feb,9; 2018,Mar,3; 2018,Jan,8; 2017,Jan,8; 2016,Nov,3
36474 2019,Feb,9; 2018,Mar,3; 2018,Jan,8; 2017,Jan,8; 2016,Nov,3

Relative Value Units/Medicare Edits

Non-Facility RVU	Work	PE	MP	Total
36473	3.5	37.21	0.69	41.4
36474	1.75	5.76	0.36	7.87
Facility RVU	**Work**	**PE**	**MP**	**Total**
36473	3.5	0.96	0.69	5.15
36474	1.75	0.46	0.36	2.57

	FUD	Status	MUE	Modifiers				IOM Reference
36473	0	A	1(3)	51	50	N/A	N/A	None
36474	N/A	A	1(3)	N/A	50	N/A	N/A	

* with documentation

Terms To Know

ablation. Removal or destruction of a body part or tissue or its function. Ablation may be performed by surgical means, hormones, drugs, radiofrequency, heat, chemical application, or other methods.

incompetent. Inability of a valve or structure to perform its normal function.

percutaneous approach. Method used to gain access to a body organ or specific area by puncture or minor incision through the skin or mucous membrane and/or any other body layers necessary to reach the procedure site.

36475-36476

36475 Endovenous ablation therapy of incompetent vein, extremity, inclusive of all imaging guidance and monitoring, percutaneous, radiofrequency; first vein treated

\+ **36476** subsequent vein(s) treated in a single extremity, each through separate access sites (List separately in addition to code for primary procedure)

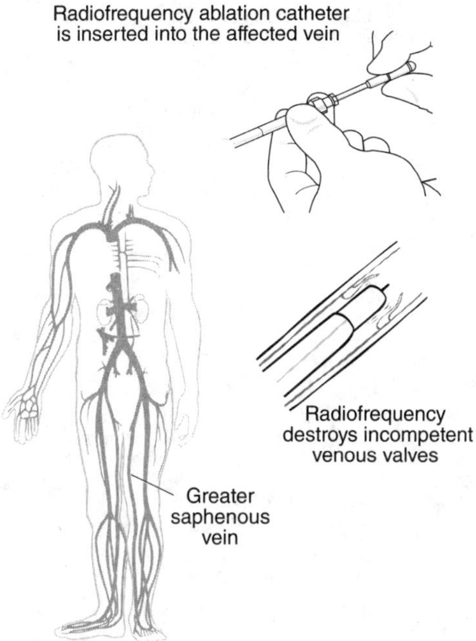

Radiofrequency endovenous ablation therapy is performed on a site in an extremity

Explanation

The physician uses percutaneous, radiofrequency, endovenous ablation therapy to treat venous incompetence in an extremity vein. Radiofrequency energy is used to heat and seal the vein closed. The most common site of treatment is the greater saphenous vein. The procedure includes any imaging guidance and monitoring. The leg is prepared and draped and a local anesthetic is applied to the puncture site. A needle is inserted into the access site. A guidewire is placed into the vessel using ultrasound guidance. An introducer sheath is placed over the guidewire and the guidewire is removed. The radiofrequency ablation catheter system is introduced and the tip is advanced to the site of the venous incompetence under ultrasound guidance. A local anesthetic agent is injected into the tissues surrounding the vein within its fascial sheath along the course of the vein. Ultrasonography is used to position the catheter tip at the level of the terminal valve and the catheter electrodes are deployed. The electrodes should be just distal to the valve cusps of the terminal valve. Radiofrequency energy is applied until the thermocouple temperature rises to 80° to 85°C and remains at this temperature for 10 to 15 seconds. Once this temperature is reached, the catheter tip is slowly withdrawn until it reaches the introducer sheath in the distal vein. The ablation catheter and introducer sheath are removed and pressure is applied to the puncture site. Report 36475 for the first vein treated in a single extremity and 36476 for each additional vein treated through a separate access site in the same extremity.

Coding Tips

When these procedures are performed in an office setting, required supplies and equipment are included and may not be reported separately. Application of compression bandages and/or stockings are included, when performed, and may not be reported separately. Report 36476 for subsequent veins treated in the same extremity; it may only be reported once per extremity. Report 36476 in addition to 36475. Do not report 36475 or 36476 with 36000–36005, 36410, 36425, 36478, 36479, 36482, 36483, 37241–37244, 75894, 76000, 76937, 76942, 76998, 77022, 93970, or 93971 in the same surgical field. Do not report 36468 with 29520, 29530, 29540, 29550, 29580, 29581, or 29584 for the same extremity.

ICD-10-CM Diagnostic Codes

I83.011	Varicose veins of right lower extremity with ulcer of thigh ☑
I83.012	Varicose veins of right lower extremity with ulcer of calf ☑
I83.013	Varicose veins of right lower extremity with ulcer of ankle ☑
I83.014	Varicose veins of right lower extremity with ulcer of heel and midfoot ☑
I83.015	Varicose veins of right lower extremity with ulcer other part of foot ☑
I83.018	Varicose veins of right lower extremity with ulcer other part of lower leg ☑
I83.021	Varicose veins of left lower extremity with ulcer of thigh ☑
I83.022	Varicose veins of left lower extremity with ulcer of calf ☑
I83.023	Varicose veins of left lower extremity with ulcer of ankle ☑
I83.024	Varicose veins of left lower extremity with ulcer of heel and midfoot ☑
I83.025	Varicose veins of left lower extremity with ulcer other part of foot ☑
I83.028	Varicose veins of left lower extremity with ulcer other part of lower leg ☑
I83.11	Varicose veins of right lower extremity with inflammation ☑
I83.12	Varicose veins of left lower extremity with inflammation ☑
I83.211	Varicose veins of right lower extremity with both ulcer of thigh and inflammation ☑
I83.212	Varicose veins of right lower extremity with both ulcer of calf and inflammation ☑
I83.213	Varicose veins of right lower extremity with both ulcer of ankle and inflammation ☑
I83.214	Varicose veins of right lower extremity with both ulcer of heel and midfoot and inflammation ☑
I83.215	Varicose veins of right lower extremity with both ulcer other part of foot and inflammation ☑
I83.218	Varicose veins of right lower extremity with both ulcer of other part of lower extremity and inflammation ☑
I83.221	Varicose veins of left lower extremity with both ulcer of thigh and inflammation ☑
I83.222	Varicose veins of left lower extremity with both ulcer of calf and inflammation ☑
I83.223	Varicose veins of left lower extremity with both ulcer of ankle and inflammation ☑
I83.224	Varicose veins of left lower extremity with both ulcer of heel and midfoot and inflammation ☑
I83.225	Varicose veins of left lower extremity with both ulcer other part of foot and inflammation ☑
I83.228	Varicose veins of left lower extremity with both ulcer of other part of lower extremity and inflammation ☑
I83.811	Varicose veins of right lower extremity with pain ☑
I83.812	Varicose veins of left lower extremity with pain ☑
I83.813	Varicose veins of bilateral lower extremities with pain ☑

I83.891	Varicose veins of right lower extremity with other complications ☑
I83.892	Varicose veins of left lower extremity with other complications ☑
I83.893	Varicose veins of bilateral lower extremities with other complications ☑
I83.91	Asymptomatic varicose veins of right lower extremity ☑
I83.92	Asymptomatic varicose veins of left lower extremity ☑
I83.93	Asymptomatic varicose veins of bilateral lower extremities ☑
I86.8	Varicose veins of other specified sites

AMA: **36475** 2018,Mar,3; 2018,Jan,8; 2017,Jan,8; 2016,Nov,3; 2016,Jan,13; 2016,Aug,3; 2015,Jan,16; 2015,Apr,10; 2014,Oct,6; 2014,Mar,4; 2014,Jan,11; 2014,Aug,14; 2013,Nov,6 **36476** 2018,Mar,3; 2018,Jan,8; 2017,Jan,8; 2016,Nov,3; 2016,Jan,13; 2016,Aug,3; 2015,Jan,16; 2015,Apr,10; 2014,Oct,6; 2014,Mar,4; 2014,Jan,11; 2014,Aug,14; 2013,Nov,6

Relative Value Units/Medicare Edits

Non-Facility RVU	Work	PE	MP	Total
36475	5.3	34.22	1.08	40.6
36476	2.65	5.35	0.55	8.55
Facility RVU	**Work**	**PE**	**MP**	**Total**
36475	5.3	1.73	1.08	8.11
36476	2.65	0.73	0.55	3.93

	FUD	Status	MUE	Modifiers				IOM Reference
36475	0	A	1(3)	51	50	N/A	N/A	None
36476	N/A	A	2(3)	N/A	50	N/A	N/A	

* with documentation

Terms To Know

ablation. Removal or destruction of tissue by cutting, electrical energy, chemical substances, or excessive heat application.

guidewire. Flexible metal instrument designed to lead another instrument in its proper course.

incompetent. Inability of a valve or structure to perform its normal function.

percutaneous. Through the skin.

radiofrequency ablation. To destroy by electromagnetic wave frequencies.

ulcer. Open sore or excavating lesion of skin or the tissue on the surface of an organ from the sloughing of chronically inflamed and necrosing tissue.

ultrasound. Imaging using ultra-high sound frequency bounced off body structures.

varicose vein. Abnormal, permanently distended or stretched vein.

36478-36479

36478 Endovenous ablation therapy of incompetent vein, extremity, inclusive of all imaging guidance and monitoring, percutaneous, laser; first vein treated

\+ **36479** subsequent vein(s) treated in a single extremity, each through separate access sites (List separately in addition to code for primary procedure)

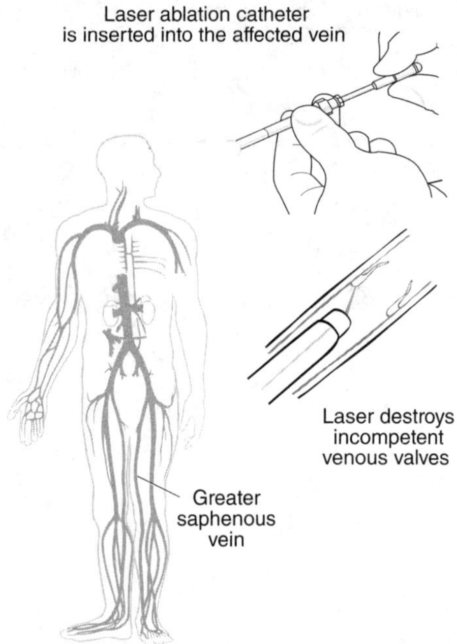

Laser endovenous ablation therapy is performed on a site in an extremity

Explanation

The physician uses percutaneous, laser, endovenous ablation therapy to treat venous incompetence in an extremity vein. Laser energy is used to heat the vein and seal the vein closed. The most common site of treatment is the greater saphenous vein. The procedure includes any imaging guidance and monitoring. The leg is prepared and draped and a local anesthetic is applied to the puncture site. A needle is inserted into the access site. A guidewire is placed into the vessel using ultrasound guidance. An introducer sheath is placed over the guidewire and the guidewire is removed. The laser ablation catheter system is introduced and the tip is advanced to the site of the venous incompetence under ultrasound guidance. A local anesthetic agent is injected into the tissues surrounding the vein within its fascial sheath. The anesthetic is injected along the course of the vein. Ultrasonography is used to position the catheter tip at the level of the terminal valve and laser energy is applied via a laser fiber along the length of the vein as the catheter is slowly withdrawn. When the laser catheter tip reaches the introducer sheath in the distal vein, the laser energy is terminated. The ablation catheter and introducer sheath are removed and pressure is applied at the puncture site. Report 36478 for the first vein treated in a single extremity and 36479 for each additional vein treated through a separate access site in the same extremity.

Coding Tips

When these procedures are performed in an office setting, required supplies and equipment are included and may not be reported separately. Application of compression bandages and/or stockings are included, when performed, and may not be reported separately. Report 36479 for subsequent veins treated in the same extremity; it may only be reported once per extremity. Report 36479 in addition to 36478. Do not report 36478 or 36479 with 36000–36005,

36410, 36425, 36475, 36476, 36482, 36483, 37241, 75894, 76000, 76937, 76942, 76998, 77022, 93970, or 93971 in the same surgical field. Do not report 36468 with 29520, 29530, 29540, 29550, 29580, 29581, or 29584 for the same extremity.

ICD-10-CM Diagnostic Codes

I83.011	Varicose veins of right lower extremity with ulcer of thigh ☑
I83.012	Varicose veins of right lower extremity with ulcer of calf ☑
I83.013	Varicose veins of right lower extremity with ulcer of ankle ☑
I83.014	Varicose veins of right lower extremity with ulcer of heel and midfoot ☑
I83.015	Varicose veins of right lower extremity with ulcer other part of foot ☑
I83.018	Varicose veins of right lower extremity with ulcer other part of lower leg ☑
I83.021	Varicose veins of left lower extremity with ulcer of thigh ☑
I83.022	Varicose veins of left lower extremity with ulcer of calf ☑
I83.023	Varicose veins of left lower extremity with ulcer of ankle ☑
I83.024	Varicose veins of left lower extremity with ulcer of heel and midfoot ☑
I83.025	Varicose veins of left lower extremity with ulcer other part of foot ☑
I83.028	Varicose veins of left lower extremity with ulcer other part of lower leg ☑
I83.11	Varicose veins of right lower extremity with inflammation ☑
I83.12	Varicose veins of left lower extremity with inflammation ☑
I83.211	Varicose veins of right lower extremity with both ulcer of thigh and inflammation ☑
I83.212	Varicose veins of right lower extremity with both ulcer of calf and inflammation ☑
I83.213	Varicose veins of right lower extremity with both ulcer of ankle and inflammation ☑
I83.214	Varicose veins of right lower extremity with both ulcer of heel and midfoot and inflammation ☑
I83.215	Varicose veins of right lower extremity with both ulcer other part of foot and inflammation ☑
I83.218	Varicose veins of right lower extremity with both ulcer of other part of lower extremity and inflammation ☑
I83.221	Varicose veins of left lower extremity with both ulcer of thigh and inflammation ☑
I83.222	Varicose veins of left lower extremity with both ulcer of calf and inflammation ☑
I83.223	Varicose veins of left lower extremity with both ulcer of ankle and inflammation ☑
I83.224	Varicose veins of left lower extremity with both ulcer of heel and midfoot and inflammation ☑
I83.225	Varicose veins of left lower extremity with both ulcer other part of foot and inflammation ☑
I83.228	Varicose veins of left lower extremity with both ulcer of other part of lower extremity and inflammation ☑
I83.811	Varicose veins of right lower extremity with pain ☑
I83.812	Varicose veins of left lower extremity with pain ☑
I83.813	Varicose veins of bilateral lower extremities with pain ☑
I83.891	Varicose veins of right lower extremity with other complications ☑
I83.892	Varicose veins of left lower extremity with other complications ☑
I83.893	Varicose veins of bilateral lower extremities with other complications ☑
I83.91	Asymptomatic varicose veins of right lower extremity ☑
I83.92	Asymptomatic varicose veins of left lower extremity ☑
I83.93	Asymptomatic varicose veins of bilateral lower extremities ☑
I86.8	Varicose veins of other specified sites

AMA: 36478 2018,Mar,3; 2018,Jan,8; 2017,Jan,8; 2016,Nov,3; 2016,Jan,13; 2016,Aug,3; 2015,Jan,16; 2015,Apr,10; 2014,Oct,6; 2014,Mar,4; 2014,Jan,11; 2014,Aug,14; 2013,Nov,6 **36479** 2018,Mar,3; 2018,Jan,8; 2017,Jan,8; 2016,Nov,3; 2016,Jan,13; 2016,Aug,3; 2015,Jan,16; 2015,Apr,10; 2014,Oct,6; 2014,Mar,4; 2014,Jan,11; 2014,Aug,14; 2013,Nov,6

Relative Value Units/Medicare Edits

Non-Facility RVU	Work	PE	MP	Total
36478	5.3	25.8	1.0	32.1
36479	2.65	5.87	0.51	9.03
Facility RVU	**Work**	**PE**	**MP**	**Total**
36478	5.3	1.76	1.0	8.06
36479	2.65	0.79	0.51	3.95

	FUD	Status	MUE	Modifiers				IOM Reference
36478	0	A	1(3)	51	50	N/A	N/A	None
36479	N/A	A	2(3)	N/A	50	N/A	N/A	

* with documentation

Terms To Know

ablation. Removal or destruction of a body part or tissue or its function. Ablation may be performed by surgical means, hormones, drugs, radiofrequency, heat, chemical application, or other methods.

guidewire. Flexible metal instrument designed to lead another instrument in its proper course.

varicose vein. Abnormal, permanently distended or stretched vein.

[36482, 36483]

36482 Endovenous ablation therapy of incompetent vein, extremity, by transcatheter delivery of a chemical adhesive (eg, cyanoacrylate) remote from the access site, inclusive of all imaging guidance and monitoring, percutaneous; first vein treated

+ **36483** Endovenous ablation therapy of incompetent vein, extremity, by transcatheter delivery of a chemical adhesive (eg, cyanoacrylate) remote from the access site, inclusive of all imaging guidance and monitoring, percutaneous; subsequent vein(s) treated in a single extremity, each through separate access sites (List separately in addition to code for primary procedure)

Incompetent veins treated with chemical adhesive

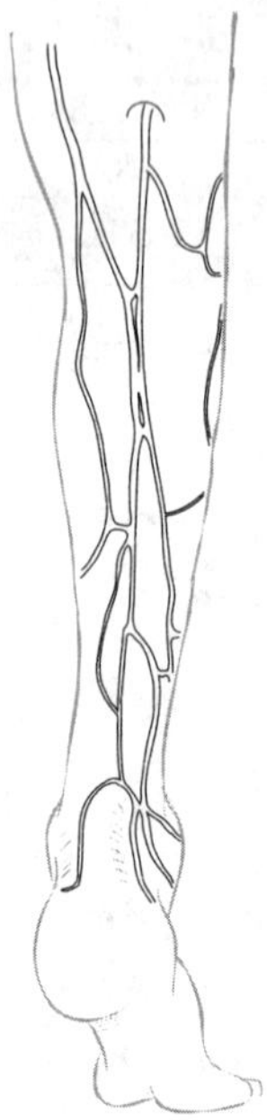

Explanation

The physician creates a detailed outline or mapping of the veins in the lower legs to identify all vein abnormalities, along with additional nearby structures to include deep veins and arteries, via duplex ultrasound examination. The patient is placed in the supine position and the leg being treated is exposed. A local anesthetic is administered. Through a small incision, the physician uses a needle to position an intravenous catheter the length of the incompetent vein. A chemical adhesive, such as cyanoacrylate, is injected through the catheter via a special type of applicator and into the vein under imaging guidance. A small amount of the chemical adhesive is injected approximately every 3 cm along the vein causing sclerosis or a hardening of the vein. To minimize dispersing of the chemical adhesive, ultrasound compression of the outflow vein is often included in these procedures. Imaging guidance and monitoring are included in these procedures. Report 36482 for the first vein treated and 36483 for subsequent veins treated in a single extremity, each through separate access sites.

Coding Tips

When these procedures are performed in the office, all supplies and equipment are included. Codes may be reported only once per extremity per day. Application of compression bandages and/or stockings is included and may not be reported separately. Report 36483 in addition to 36482. Report 36483 only once per extremity. Do not report 36482 or 36483 with 36000, 36002, 36005, 36410, 36425, 36475, 36476, 36478, 36479, 37241, 75894, 76000, 76937, 76942, 76998, 77022, 93970, or 93971 when performed in the same surgical field. Do not report 36468 with 29520, 29530, 29540, 29550, 29580, 29581, or 29584 for the same extremity.

ICD-10-CM Diagnostic Codes

I82.491	Acute embolism and thrombosis of other specified deep vein of right lower extremity ☑
I82.492	Acute embolism and thrombosis of other specified deep vein of left lower extremity ☑
I82.591	Chronic embolism and thrombosis of other specified deep vein of right lower extremity ☑
I82.592	Chronic embolism and thrombosis of other specified deep vein of left lower extremity ☑
I82.811	Embolism and thrombosis of superficial veins of right lower extremity ☑
I82.812	Embolism and thrombosis of superficial veins of left lower extremity ☑
I83.011	Varicose veins of right lower extremity with ulcer of thigh ☑
I83.012	Varicose veins of right lower extremity with ulcer of calf ☑
I83.013	Varicose veins of right lower extremity with ulcer of ankle ☑
I83.014	Varicose veins of right lower extremity with ulcer of heel and midfoot ☑
I83.015	Varicose veins of right lower extremity with ulcer other part of foot ☑
I83.018	Varicose veins of right lower extremity with ulcer other part of lower leg ☑
I83.021	Varicose veins of left lower extremity with ulcer of thigh ☑
I83.022	Varicose veins of left lower extremity with ulcer of calf ☑
I83.023	Varicose veins of left lower extremity with ulcer of ankle ☑
I83.024	Varicose veins of left lower extremity with ulcer of heel and midfoot ☑
I83.025	Varicose veins of left lower extremity with ulcer other part of foot ☑
I83.028	Varicose veins of left lower extremity with ulcer other part of lower leg ☑
I83.11	Varicose veins of right lower extremity with inflammation ☑
I83.12	Varicose veins of left lower extremity with inflammation ☑
I83.211	Varicose veins of right lower extremity with both ulcer of thigh and inflammation ☑
I83.212	Varicose veins of right lower extremity with both ulcer of calf and inflammation ☑
I83.213	Varicose veins of right lower extremity with both ulcer of ankle and inflammation ☑
I83.214	Varicose veins of right lower extremity with both ulcer of heel and midfoot and inflammation ☑
I83.215	Varicose veins of right lower extremity with both ulcer other part of foot and inflammation ☑
I83.218	Varicose veins of right lower extremity with both ulcer of other part of lower extremity and inflammation ☑
I83.221	Varicose veins of left lower extremity with both ulcer of thigh and inflammation ☑
I83.222	Varicose veins of left lower extremity with both ulcer of calf and inflammation ☑
I83.223	Varicose veins of left lower extremity with both ulcer of ankle and inflammation ☑
I83.224	Varicose veins of left lower extremity with both ulcer of heel and midfoot and inflammation ☑

I83.225	Varicose veins of left lower extremity with both ulcer other part of foot and inflammation ☑
I83.228	Varicose veins of left lower extremity with both ulcer of other part of lower extremity and inflammation ☑
I83.811	Varicose veins of right lower extremity with pain ☑
I83.812	Varicose veins of left lower extremity with pain ☑
I83.891	Varicose veins of right lower extremity with other complications ☑
I83.892	Varicose veins of left lower extremity with other complications ☑
I83.91	Asymptomatic varicose veins of right lower extremity ☑
I83.92	Asymptomatic varicose veins of left lower extremity ☑
I86.8	Varicose veins of other specified sites
I87.2	Venous insufficiency (chronic) (peripheral)

AMA: **36482** 2019,Feb,9; 2018,Mar,3 **36483** 2019,Feb,9; 2018,Mar,3

Relative Value Units/Medicare Edits

Non-Facility RVU	Work	PE	MP	Total
36482	3.5	53.79	0.7	57.99
36483	1.75	2.16	0.35	4.26
Facility RVU	**Work**	**PE**	**MP**	**Total**
36482	3.5	0.92	0.7	5.12
36483	1.75	0.47	0.35	2.57

	FUD	Status	MUE	Modifiers				IOM Reference
36482	0	A	1(3)	51	50	N/A	N/A	None
36483	N/A	A	2(3)	N/A	50	N/A	N/A	

* with documentation

36481

36481 Percutaneous portal vein catheterization by any method

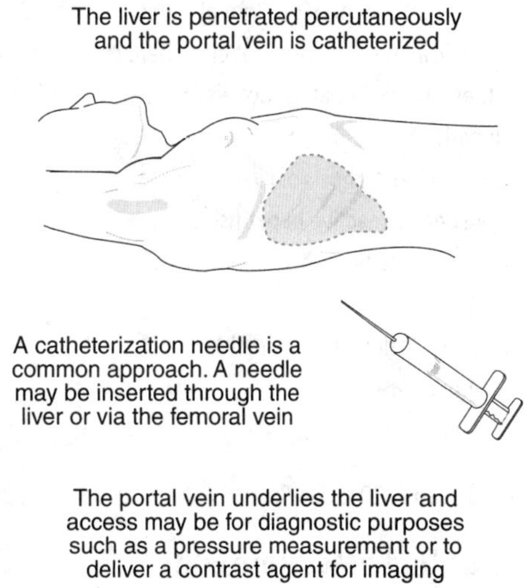

Explanation

The physician numbs the right lateral abdominal wall with local anesthetic. The physician places a large needle through the skin into the liver, maneuvering the needle through the liver into the intrahepatic portal vein, injecting contrast under fluoroscope for localization. The physician places a wire through the needle, retrograde into the portal vein. The physician removes the wire over the needle, and advances a catheter over the wire, through the skin and liver into the portal vein. The physician secures the catheter with suture. Alternative methods include placing a catheter via the internal jugular vein or using a transsplenic approach.

Coding Tips

When medically necessary, report moderate (conscious) sedation provided by the performing physician with 99151-99153. When provided by another physician, report 99155-99157. Listed services for injection procedures include necessary local anesthesia, introduction of needles or catheter, injection of contrast material with or without automatic power injection, and/or necessary pre- and postinjection care specifically related to the injection procedure. Supplies (catheters, drugs, and contrast media) are not included in the listed service for the injection procedures. For selective catheter placement, venous system, see 36011–36012. For radiological supervision and interpretation, see 75885 and 75887.

ICD-10-CM Diagnostic Codes

B15.0	Hepatitis A with hepatic coma
B15.9	Hepatitis A without hepatic coma
B17.10	Acute hepatitis C without hepatic coma
B17.11	Acute hepatitis C with hepatic coma
B17.2	Acute hepatitis E
B17.8	Other specified acute viral hepatitis
B18.1	Chronic viral hepatitis B without delta-agent
B18.2	Chronic viral hepatitis C
B18.8	Other chronic viral hepatitis
B25.1	Cytomegaloviral hepatitis
B58.1	Toxoplasma hepatitis
I81	Portal vein thrombosis
I85.01	Esophageal varices with bleeding

I85.11	Secondary esophageal varices with bleeding
K70.10	Alcoholic hepatitis without ascites
K70.11	Alcoholic hepatitis with ascites
K73.0	Chronic persistent hepatitis, not elsewhere classified
K73.1	Chronic lobular hepatitis, not elsewhere classified
K73.2	Chronic active hepatitis, not elsewhere classified
K73.8	Other chronic hepatitis, not elsewhere classified
K74.0	Hepatic fibrosis
K74.60	Unspecified cirrhosis of liver
K75.2	Nonspecific reactive hepatitis
K75.4	Autoimmune hepatitis
K76.6	Portal hypertension
K76.89	Other specified diseases of liver
R18.0	Malignant ascites
R18.8	Other ascites

AMA: **36481** 2018,Jan,8; 2017,Jan,8; 2016,Jan,13; 2015,Jan,16; 2014,Jan,11

Relative Value Units/Medicare Edits

Non-Facility RVU	Work	PE	MP	Total
36481	6.73	48.04	0.67	55.44
Facility RVU	**Work**	**PE**	**MP**	**Total**
36481	6.73	2.27	0.67	9.67

	FUD	Status	MUE	Modifiers				IOM Reference
36481	0	A	1(3)	51	N/A	N/A	N/A	None

* with documentation

Terms To Know

catheter. Flexible tube inserted into an area of the body for introducing or withdrawing fluid.

fluoroscopy. Radiology technique that allows visual examination of part of the body or a function of an organ using a device that projects an x-ray image on a fluorescent screen.

guidewire. Flexible metal instrument designed to lead another instrument in its proper course.

local anesthesia. Induced loss of feeling or sensation restricted to a certain area of the body, including topical, local tissue infiltration, field block, or nerve block methods.

moderate sedation. Medically controlled state of depressed consciousness, with or without analgesia, while maintaining the patient's airway, protective reflexes, and ability to respond to stimulation or verbal commands.

36500

36500 Venous catheterization for selective organ blood sampling

Explanation

The physician inserts a needle through the skin and into a peripheral vein. A guidewire is threaded through the needle into the vessel. The needle is removed. The wire is manipulated into the vein draining from the organ to be sampled. The catheter follows the guidewire into the vein. Once the catheter has been placed, the guidewire is removed and the blood sample obtained. The catheter is removed and pressure is applied to the puncture site to stop the flow of blood.

Coding Tips

This procedure does not include laboratory analysis. If a specimen is transported to an outside laboratory, report 99000 for handling or conveyance. For catheterization in the superior or inferior vena cava, see 36010. For radiological supervision and interpretation, see 75893.

ICD-10-CM Diagnostic Codes

C25.0	Malignant neoplasm of head of pancreas
C25.1	Malignant neoplasm of body of pancreas
C25.2	Malignant neoplasm of tail of pancreas
C25.3	Malignant neoplasm of pancreatic duct
C25.4	Malignant neoplasm of endocrine pancreas
C25.7	Malignant neoplasm of other parts of pancreas
C25.8	Malignant neoplasm of overlapping sites of pancreas
C56.1	Malignant neoplasm of right ovary ☑
C56.2	Malignant neoplasm of left ovary ☑
C74.01	Malignant neoplasm of cortex of right adrenal gland ☑
C74.02	Malignant neoplasm of cortex of left adrenal gland ☑
C75.0	Malignant neoplasm of parathyroid gland
C79.61	Secondary malignant neoplasm of right ovary ☑
C79.62	Secondary malignant neoplasm of left ovary ☑
D13.6	Benign neoplasm of pancreas
D13.7	Benign neoplasm of endocrine pancreas
D27.0	Benign neoplasm of right ovary ☑
D27.1	Benign neoplasm of left ovary ☑
D35.01	Benign neoplasm of right adrenal gland ☑
D35.02	Benign neoplasm of left adrenal gland ☑
D35.1	Benign neoplasm of parathyroid gland
D35.2	Benign neoplasm of pituitary gland
D37.8	Neoplasm of uncertain behavior of other specified digestive organs
D44.2	Neoplasm of uncertain behavior of parathyroid gland
D44.3	Neoplasm of uncertain behavior of pituitary gland
D44.4	Neoplasm of uncertain behavior of craniopharyngeal duct
E21.0	Primary hyperparathyroidism
E21.1	Secondary hyperparathyroidism, not elsewhere classified
E21.2	Other hyperparathyroidism
E22.0	Acromegaly and pituitary gigantism
E22.8	Other hyperfunction of pituitary gland
E24.0	Pituitary-dependent Cushing's disease
E24.2	Drug-induced Cushing's syndrome

E24.3	Ectopic ACTH syndrome
E24.4	Alcohol-induced pseudo-Cushing's syndrome
E24.8	Other Cushing's syndrome
E26.01	Conn's syndrome
E26.02	Glucocorticoid-remediable aldosteronism
E26.09	Other primary hyperaldosteronism
E26.1	Secondary hyperaldosteronism
E26.89	Other hyperaldosteronism
E28.1	Androgen excess
E28.2	Polycystic ovarian syndrome

AMA: 36500 2014,Jan,11

Relative Value Units/Medicare Edits

Non-Facility RVU	Work	PE	MP	Total
36500	3.51	1.19	0.6	5.3
Facility RVU	**Work**	**PE**	**MP**	**Total**
36500	3.51	1.19	0.6	5.3

	FUD	Status	MUE	Modifiers				IOM Reference
36500	0	A	4(3)	51	N/A	N/A	N/A	None

* with documentation

Terms To Know

cannula. Tube inserted into a blood vessel, duct, or body cavity to facilitate passage.

catheter. Flexible tube inserted into an area of the body for introducing or withdrawing fluid.

guidewire. Flexible metal instrument designed to lead another instrument in its proper course.

peripheral. Outside of a structure or organ.

puncture. Creating a hole.

specimen. Tissue cells or sample of fluid taken for analysis, pathologic examination, and diagnosis.

supervision and interpretation. Radiology services that usually contain an invasive component and are reported by the radiologist for supervision of the procedure and the personnel involved with performing the examination, reading the film, and preparing the written report.

vena cava. Main venous trunk that empties into the right atrium from both the lower and upper regions, beginning at the junction of the common iliac veins inferiorly and the two brachiocephalic veins superiorly.

venous. Relating to the veins.

36511-36513

36511 Therapeutic apheresis; for white blood cells
36512 for red blood cells
36513 for platelets

Explanation

Therapeutic apheresis is the removal of some specific circulating blood component, cells or plasma solute, that is directly responsible for a disease process. Cells and plasma components may also be mobilized from other tissue storage during apheresis, such as from the spleen and lymph nodes, for enhanced clearance of the undesired element. The patient is prepared much the same as giving a regular blood donation. Whole blood is drawn out of one arm and into an instrument called a separator, which uses a microprocessing technique to draw the blood, anticoagulate it, and separate the component to be removed by centrifugal spinning, filtration, or column adsorption with the help of computerized calibration. The cells to be removed are collected while the remainder of the blood is recombined and returned to the patient through a tube and needle in the other arm. Report 36511 for white blood cell isolation and removal (leukapheresis or lymphocytapheresis), 36512 for red blood cell removal, and 36513 for removal of platelets.

Coding Tips

For therapeutic plasma pheresis, see 36514. For therapeutic apheresis with extracorporeal immunoadsorption or selective adsorption or filtration with plasma reinfusion, see 36516. Do not report 36513 for donor platelet collections, only report for treatment of the patient when platelets are removed using apheresis.

ICD-10-CM Diagnostic Codes

The application of this code is too broad to adequately present ICD-10-CM diagnostic code links here. Refer to your ICD-10-CM book.

AMA: 36511 2018,Jan,8; 2017,Jan,8; 2016,Jan,13; 2015,Jan,16; 2014,Jan,11; 2013,Oct,3 **36512** 2018,Jan,8; 2017,Jan,8; 2016,Jan,13; 2015,Jan,16; 2014,Jan,11; 2013,Oct,3 **36513** 2018,Jan,8; 2017,Jan,8; 2016,Jan,13; 2015,Jan,16; 2014,Jan,11; 2013,Oct,3

Relative Value Units/Medicare Edits

Non-Facility RVU	Work	PE	MP	Total
36511	2.0	0.96	0.14	3.1
36512	2.0	0.97	0.14	3.11
36513	2.0	0.91	0.25	3.16
Facility RVU	**Work**	**PE**	**MP**	**Total**
36511	2.0	0.96	0.14	3.1
36512	2.0	0.97	0.14	3.11
36513	2.0	0.91	0.25	3.16

	FUD	Status	MUE	Modifiers				IOM Reference
36511	0	A	1(3)	51	N/A	N/A	N/A	100-03,110.14; 100-04,4,231.9
36512	0	A	1(3)	51	N/A	N/A	N/A	
36513	0	A	1(3)	51	N/A	N/A	N/A	

* with documentation

Terms To Know

centrifuge. Machine used to simulate gravitational effects or centrifugal force to separate substances of different densities.

36514-36516

36514 Therapeutic apheresis; for plasma pheresis
36516 with extracorporeal immunoadsorption, selective adsorption or selective filtration and plasma reinfusion

Explanation

Therapeutic apheresis is the removal of specific circulating blood components, cells, or plasma solute that is directly responsible for a disease process. Cells and plasma components may also be mobilized from other tissue storage during apheresis, such as from the spleen and lymph nodes, for enhanced clearance of the undesired element. The patient is prepared much the same as giving a regular blood donation. Whole blood is drawn out of one arm and into an instrument called a separator, which uses a microprocessing technique to draw the blood, anticoagulate it, and separate the component to be removed by centrifugal spinning, filtration, or column adsorption with the help of computerized calibration. Plasmapheresis, reported with 36514, is the isolation of the plasma from the blood. Plasma exchange isolates, discards, and replaces the plasma with a substitute fluid, like albumin. Plasma exchange is nonspecific since the plasma is discarded on the basis that toxins and antibodies accumulate in the plasma. The best method requires treating a disorder by removing the offending abnormal plasma component selectively. Report 36516 for extracorporeal immunoadsorption, selective adsorption, or selective filtration, such as dextran sulfate cellulose columns, to selectively remove low-density lipoproteins with plasma reinfusion.

Coding Tips

For therapeutic apheresis for white blood cells, see 36511; red blood cells, see 36512; and platelets, see 36513. For professional supervision only for 36516, append modifier 26.

ICD-10-CM Diagnostic Codes

C90.00	Multiple myeloma not having achieved remission
C90.02	Multiple myeloma in relapse
C90.10	Plasma cell leukemia not having achieved remission
C90.12	Plasma cell leukemia in relapse
C90.20	Extramedullary plasmacytoma not having achieved remission
C90.22	Extramedullary plasmacytoma in relapse
C90.30	Solitary plasmacytoma not having achieved remission
C90.32	Solitary plasmacytoma in relapse
C91.00	Acute lymphoblastic leukemia not having achieved remission
C91.01	Acute lymphoblastic leukemia, in remission
C91.02	Acute lymphoblastic leukemia, in relapse
C91.10	Chronic lymphocytic leukemia of B-cell type not having achieved remission
C91.11	Chronic lymphocytic leukemia of B-cell type in remission
C91.12	Chronic lymphocytic leukemia of B-cell type in relapse
C91.30	Prolymphocytic leukemia of B-cell type not having achieved remission
C91.31	Prolymphocytic leukemia of B-cell type, in remission
C91.32	Prolymphocytic leukemia of B-cell type, in relapse
C91.40	Hairy cell leukemia not having achieved remission
C91.41	Hairy cell leukemia, in remission
C91.42	Hairy cell leukemia, in relapse
C91.50	Adult T-cell lymphoma/leukemia (HTLV-1-associated) not having achieved remission
C91.51	Adult T-cell lymphoma/leukemia (HTLV-1-associated), in remission
C91.52	Adult T-cell lymphoma/leukemia (HTLV-1-associated), in relapse
C91.60	Prolymphocytic leukemia of T-cell type not having achieved remission
C91.61	Prolymphocytic leukemia of T-cell type, in remission
C91.62	Prolymphocytic leukemia of T-cell type, in relapse
C91.A0	Mature B-cell leukemia Burkitt-type not having achieved remission
C91.A1	Mature B-cell leukemia Burkitt-type, in remission
C91.A2	Mature B-cell leukemia Burkitt-type, in relapse
C92.00	Acute myeloblastic leukemia, not having achieved remission
C92.01	Acute myeloblastic leukemia, in remission
C92.02	Acute myeloblastic leukemia, in relapse
C92.10	Chronic myeloid leukemia, BCR/ABL-positive, not having achieved remission
C92.11	Chronic myeloid leukemia, BCR/ABL-positive, in remission
C92.12	Chronic myeloid leukemia, BCR/ABL-positive, in relapse
C92.20	Atypical chronic myeloid leukemia, BCR/ABL-negative, not having achieved remission
C92.21	Atypical chronic myeloid leukemia, BCR/ABL-negative, in remission
C92.22	Atypical chronic myeloid leukemia, BCR/ABL-negative, in relapse
C92.40	Acute promyelocytic leukemia, not having achieved remission
C92.41	Acute promyelocytic leukemia, in remission
C92.42	Acute promyelocytic leukemia, in relapse
C92.50	Acute myelomonocytic leukemia, not having achieved remission
C92.51	Acute myelomonocytic leukemia, in remission
C92.52	Acute myelomonocytic leukemia, in relapse
C92.60	Acute myeloid leukemia with 11q23-abnormality not having achieved remission
C92.61	Acute myeloid leukemia with 11q23-abnormality in remission
C92.62	Acute myeloid leukemia with 11q23-abnormality in relapse
C92.A0	Acute myeloid leukemia with multilineage dysplasia, not having achieved remission
C92.A1	Acute myeloid leukemia with multilineage dysplasia, in remission
C92.A2	Acute myeloid leukemia with multilineage dysplasia, in relapse
C93.00	Acute monoblastic/monocytic leukemia, not having achieved remission
C93.01	Acute monoblastic/monocytic leukemia, in remission
C93.02	Acute monoblastic/monocytic leukemia, in relapse
C93.10	Chronic myelomonocytic leukemia not having achieved remission
C93.11	Chronic myelomonocytic leukemia, in remission
C93.12	Chronic myelomonocytic leukemia, in relapse
C93.30	Juvenile myelomonocytic leukemia, not having achieved remission
C93.31	Juvenile myelomonocytic leukemia, in remission
C93.32	Juvenile myelomonocytic leukemia, in relapse
C94.00	Acute erythroid leukemia, not having achieved remission
C94.01	Acute erythroid leukemia, in remission
C94.02	Acute erythroid leukemia, in relapse
C94.20	Acute megakaryoblastic leukemia not having achieved remission
C94.21	Acute megakaryoblastic leukemia, in remission
C94.22	Acute megakaryoblastic leukemia, in relapse

C94.30	Mast cell leukemia not having achieved remission
C94.31	Mast cell leukemia, in remission
C94.32	Mast cell leukemia, in relapse
D47.1	Chronic myeloproliferative disease
D47.2	Monoclonal gammopathy
D47.3	Essential (hemorrhagic) thrombocythemia
D57.211	Sickle-cell/Hb-C disease with acute chest syndrome
D57.212	Sickle-cell/Hb-C disease with splenic sequestration
D59.0	Drug-induced autoimmune hemolytic anemia
D59.3	Hemolytic-uremic syndrome
D61.01	Constitutional (pure) red blood cell aplasia
D61.3	Idiopathic aplastic anemia
D69.1	Qualitative platelet defects
D69.3	Immune thrombocytopenic purpura
D69.42	Congenital and hereditary thrombocytopenia purpura
D69.51	Posttransfusion purpura
D72.823	Leukemoid reaction
D75.1	Secondary polycythemia
D89.1	Cryoglobulinemia
D89.41	Monoclonal mast cell activation syndrome
D89.42	Idiopathic mast cell activation syndrome
T80.310A	ABO incompatibility with acute hemolytic transfusion reaction, initial encounter
T80.311A	ABO incompatibility with delayed hemolytic transfusion reaction, initial encounter
T86.01	Bone marrow transplant rejection
T86.02	Bone marrow transplant failure
T86.03	Bone marrow transplant infection

AMA: 36514 2018,May,10; 2018,Jan,8; 2017,Jan,8; 2016,Jan,13; 2015,Jan,16; 2014,Jan,11; 2013,Oct,3 **36516** 2018,Jan,8; 2017,Jan,8; 2016,Jan,13; 2015,Jan,16; 2014,Jan,11; 2013,Oct,3

Relative Value Units/Medicare Edits

Non-Facility RVU	Work	PE	MP	Total
36514	1.81	18.52	0.17	20.5
36516	1.56	54.44	0.27	56.27
Facility RVU	**Work**	**PE**	**MP**	**Total**
36514	1.81	0.78	0.17	2.76
36516	1.56	0.63	0.27	2.46

	FUD	Status	MUE	Modifiers				IOM Reference
36514	0	A	1(3)	51	N/A	N/A	N/A	None
36516	0	A	1(3)	51	N/A	N/A	N/A	

* with documentation

Terms To Know

apheresis. Process of extracting blood from a donor, centrifuging or separating the desired part of the blood, and transfusing the remainder back into the donor.

centrifuge. Machine used to simulate gravitational effects or centrifugal force to separate substances of different densities.

extracorporeal. Located or taking place outside the body.

36555-36556

36555 Insertion of non-tunneled centrally inserted central venous catheter; younger than 5 years of age

36556 age 5 years or older

A non-tunneled centrally inserted CVC is inserted

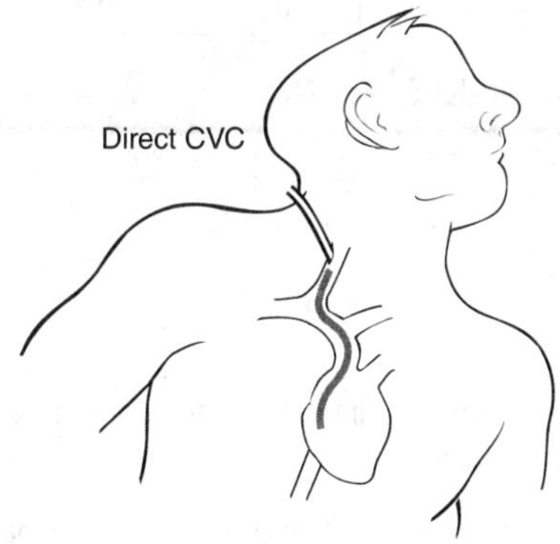

Explanation

A central venous access device (CVAD) or catheter is one in which the tip terminates in the subclavian, brachiocephalic, or iliac vein; the superior or inferior vena cava; or the right atrium. A centrally inserted CVAD has an entry site in the inferior vena cava or the jugular, subclavian, or femoral vein. For insertion of a non-tunneled, centrally inserted CVAD, the site over the access vein (e.g., subclavian, jugular) is injected with local anesthesia and punctured with a needle. A guidewire is inserted. The central venous catheter is placed over the guidewire. Ultrasound guidance may be used to gain venous access and/or fluoroscopy to check the positioning of the catheter tip. The catheter is secured into position and dressed. Non-tunneled catheters are percutaneously inserted for short term (five to seven days) use; to infuse medications, fluids, blood products, and parenteral nutrition; and to take blood draws. Report 36555 for insertion for children younger than 5 years of age and 36556 for a patient 5 years of age or older.

Coding Tips

When medically necessary, report moderate (conscious) sedation provided by the performing physician with 99151-99153. When provided by another physician, report 99155-99157. If imaging guidance is used, either for obtaining access to the venous access site or for manipulating the catheter into its final end position, see 76937 or 77001. For central venous catheter without a subcutaneous port or pump inserted peripherally in patients younger than 5 years old, see 36568. For central venous catheter without a subcutaneous port or pump inserted peripherally in patients older than age 5, see 36569.

ICD-10-CM Diagnostic Codes

The application of this code is too broad to adequately present ICD-10-CM diagnostic code links here. Refer to your ICD-10-CM book.

AMA: 36555 2019,May,3; 2018,Jan,8; 2017,Jan,8; 2016,Jan,13; 2015,Jan,16; 2014,Jan,11 **36556** 2019,May,3; 2018,Nov,11; 2018,Jan,8; 2017,Jan,8; 2016,Jan,13; 2015,Jan,16; 2014,Jan,11

Relative Value Units/Medicare Edits

Non-Facility RVU	Work	PE	MP	Total
36555	1.93	3.25	0.15	5.33
36556	1.75	4.04	0.2	5.99
Facility RVU	**Work**	**PE**	**MP**	**Total**
36555	1.93	0.38	0.15	2.46
36556	1.75	0.5	0.2	2.45

	FUD	Status	MUE	Modifiers				IOM Reference
36555	0	A	2(3)	N/A	N/A	N/A	N/A	None
36556	0	A	2(3)	N/A	N/A	N/A	N/A	

* with documentation

Terms To Know

catheter. Flexible tube inserted into an area of the body for introducing or withdrawing fluid.

fluoroscopy. Radiology technique that allows visual examination of part of the body or a function of an organ using a device that projects an x-ray image on a fluorescent screen.

guidewire. Flexible metal instrument designed to lead another instrument in its proper course.

infusion. Introduction of a therapeutic fluid, other than blood, into the bloodstream.

insertion. Placement or implantation into a body part.

jugular vein. Two pairs of veins on either side of the neck that open into the subclavian, sending blood from the head and neck to the heart.

parenteral nutrition. Nutrients provided subcutaneously, intravenously, intramuscularly, or intradermally for patients during the postoperative period and in other conditions, such as shock, coma, and renal failure.

vena cava. Main venous trunk that empties into the right atrium from both the lower and upper regions, beginning at the junction of the common iliac veins inferiorly and the two brachiocephalic veins superiorly.

36557-36558

36557 Insertion of tunneled centrally inserted central venous catheter, without subcutaneous port or pump; younger than 5 years of age

36558 age 5 years or older

A tunneled centrally inserted CVC is inserted

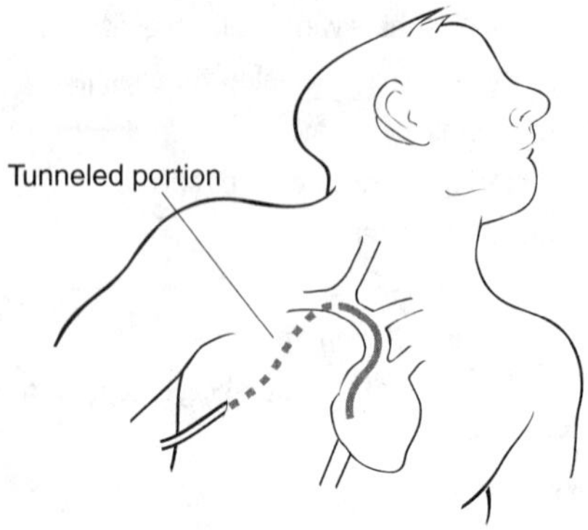

Explanation

A central venous access device (CVAD) or catheter is one in which the tip terminates in the subclavian, brachiocephalic, or iliac vein; the superior or inferior vena cava; or the right atrium. A centrally inserted CVAD has an entry site in the inferior vena cava or the jugular, subclavian, or femoral vein. A tunneled catheter has an entrance site at a distance from its entrance into the vascular system; they are "tunneled" through the skin and subcutaneous tissue to a great vein. For insertion of a tunneled, centrally inserted CVAD, without subcutaneous port or pump, standard preparations are made and the site over the access vein (e.g., subclavian, jugular) is injected with local anesthesia and punctured with a needle or accessed by cutdown approach. A guidewire is inserted. A subcutaneous tunnel is created using a blunt pair of forceps or sharp tunneling tools, over the clavicle from the anterior chest wall to the venotomy site, which is dilated to the right size. The catheter is passed through this tunnel over the guidewire and into the target vein. Ultrasound guidance may be used to gain venous access and/or fluoroscopy to check the positioning of the catheter tip. The catheter is secured into position and any incisions are sutured. Report 36557 for insertion for children younger than 5 years of age and 36558 for a patient 5 years of age or older.

Coding Tips

When medically necessary, report moderate (conscious) sedation provided by the performing physician with 99151-99153. When provided by another physician, report 99155-99157. If imaging guidance is used, either for obtaining access to the venous access site or for manipulating the catheter into its final end position, see 76937 or 77001. For central venous catheter with a port inserted peripherally on patients age 5 years or older, see 36571.

ICD-10-CM Diagnostic Codes

The application of this code is too broad to adequately present ICD-10-CM diagnostic code links here. Refer to your ICD-10-CM book.

AMA: 36557 2018,Jan,8; 2017,Jan,8; 2016,Jan,13; 2015,Jan,16; 2014,Jan,11
36558 2018,Jan,8; 2017,Jan,8; 2016,Jan,13; 2015,Jan,13; 2015,Jan,16; 2014,Jan,11

Arteries and Veins

Relative Value Units/Medicare Edits

Non-Facility RVU	Work	PE	MP	Total
36557	4.89	23.01	1.19	29.09
36558	4.59	16.52	0.59	21.7
Facility RVU	**Work**	**PE**	**MP**	**Total**
36557	4.89	3.13	1.19	9.21
36558	4.59	2.36	0.59	7.54

	FUD	Status	MUE	Modifiers				IOM Reference
36557	10	A	2(3)	51	50	N/A	80*	None
36558	10	A	2(3)	51	50	N/A	80*	

* with documentation

Terms To Know

anterior. Situated in the front area or toward the belly surface of the body.

catheter. Flexible tube inserted into an area of the body for introducing or withdrawing fluid.

cutdown. Small, incised opening in the skin to expose a blood vessel, especially over a vein (venous cutdown) to allow venipuncture and permit a needle or cannula to be inserted for the withdrawal of blood or administration of fluids.

forceps. Tool used for grasping or compressing tissue.

guidewire. Flexible metal instrument designed to lead another instrument in its proper course.

jugular vein. Two pairs of veins on either side of the neck that open into the subclavian, sending blood from the head and neck to the heart.

vascular. Pertaining to blood vessels.

venotomy. Incision or puncture of a vein.

36560-36563

36560 Insertion of tunneled centrally inserted central venous access device, with subcutaneous port; younger than 5 years of age

36561 age 5 years or older

36563 Insertion of tunneled centrally inserted central venous access device with subcutaneous pump

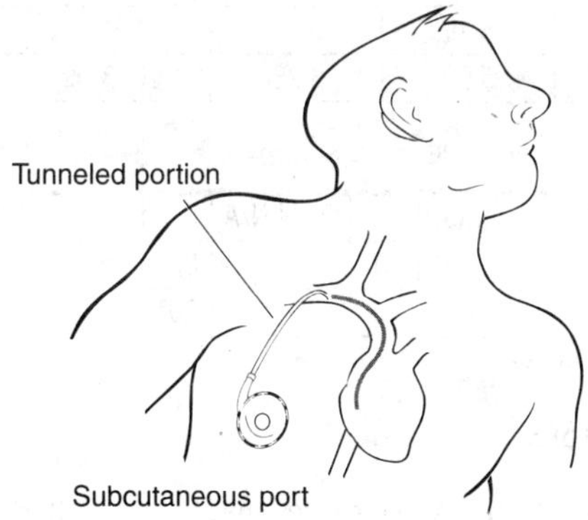

Explanation

For insertion of a tunneled, centrally inserted CVAD, with subcutaneous port/pump, the site over the access vein (e.g., subclavian, jugular) is injected with local anesthesia and punctured with a needle or accessed by cutdown approach. A guidewire is inserted. A subcutaneous tunnel is created using a blunt pair of forceps or sharp tunneling tools, over the clavicle, from the anterior chest wall to the venotomy site, which is dilated to the right size. The catheter is passed through this tunnel over the guidewire and into the target vein. The subcutaneous pocket for the port/pump is created with an incision through the skin overlying the second rib, a few centimeters from the midline. Blunt dissection and cautery are used to create the pocket in the chest wall and the port/pump is placed. The catheter is connected to the port/pump and checked by injection. Ultrasound guidance may be used to gain venous access and/or fluoroscopy to check the positioning of the catheter tip. The catheter and port/pump are secured into position and any incisions are sutured. Report 36560 for insertion with a port for children younger than 5 years of age and 36561 for a patient 5 years of age or older. Report 36563 for insertion with a pump.

Coding Tips

When medically necessary, report moderate (conscious) sedation provided by the performing physician with 99151-99153. When provided by another physician, report 99155-99157. If imaging guidance is used, either for obtaining access to the venous access site or for manipulating the catheter into its final end position, see 76937 or 77001. For a peripherally inserted central venous access device with subcutaneous port, younger than 5 years of age, see 36570; 5 years or older, see 36571.

ICD-10-CM Diagnostic Codes

The application of this code is too broad to adequately present ICD-10-CM diagnostic code links here. Refer to your ICD-10-CM book.

AMA: 36560 2018,Jan,8; 2017,Jan,8; 2016,Jan,13; 2015,Jan,16; 2014,Jan,11 **36561** 2018,Jan,8; 2017,Jan,8; 2016,Jan,13; 2015,Jan,16; 2014,Jan,11 **36563** 2018,Jan,8; 2017,Jan,8; 2016,Jan,13; 2015,Jan,16; 2014,Jan,11

Relative Value Units/Medicare Edits

Non-Facility RVU	Work	PE	MP	Total
36560	6.04	29.65	1.46	37.15
36561	5.79	23.88	0.94	30.61
36563	5.99	27.15	1.33	34.47
Facility RVU	**Work**	**PE**	**MP**	**Total**
36560	6.04	3.54	1.46	11.04
36561	5.79	3.01	0.94	9.74
36563	5.99	3.28	1.33	10.6

	FUD	Status	MUE	Modifiers				IOM Reference
36560	10	A	2(3)	51	50	N/A	80*	None
36561	10	A	2(3)	51	50	N/A	80*	
36563	10	A	1(3)	51	N/A	N/A	80*	

* with documentation

Terms To Know

guidewire. Flexible metal instrument designed to lead another instrument in its proper course.

injection. Forcing a liquid substance into a body part such as a joint or muscle.

puncture. Creating a hole.

subcutaneous. Below the skin.

36565-36566

36565 Insertion of tunneled centrally inserted central venous access device, requiring 2 catheters via 2 separate venous access sites; without subcutaneous port or pump (eg, Tesio type catheter)

36566 with subcutaneous port(s)

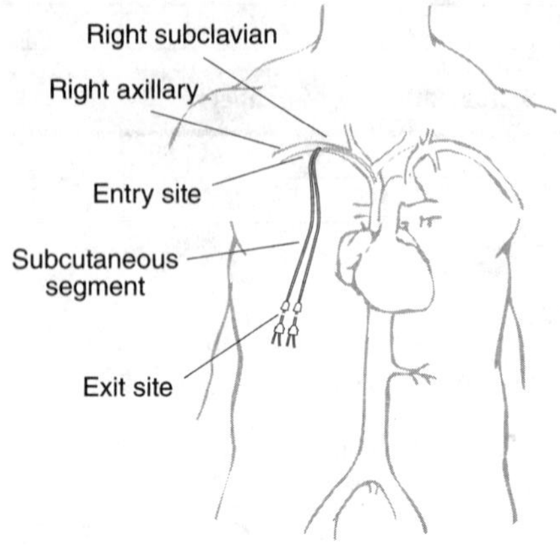

Tesio type catheters are double lumen devices. They are typically inserted into the superior vena cava and positioned before tunneling to an exit site or connecting to a subcutaneous port

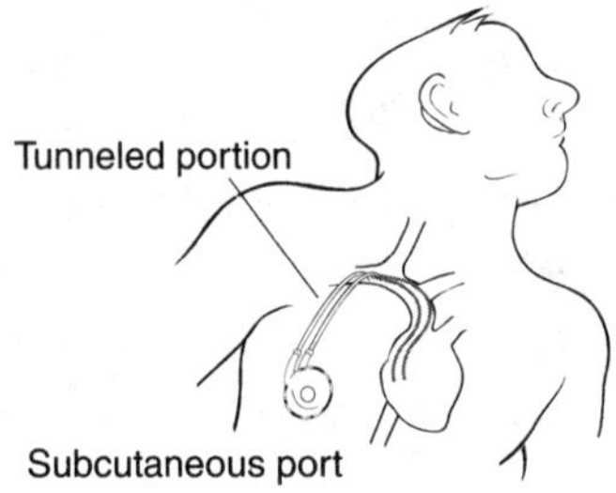

Explanation

For insertion of a tunneled, centrally inserted CVAD, requiring two catheters via two separate venous access sites, the sites of access (e.g., subclavian, jugular vein) for each catheter are injected with local anesthesia and two punctures are made with a needle or cutdown approach. Guidewires are inserted. Two subcutaneous tunnels are created using a blunt pair of forceps or sharp tunneling tools, over the clavicle, from the anterior chest wall to the venotomy sites, which are dilated to the right size. The catheters are each passed through their tunnel, over the guidewires, and into their venotomy sites. Ultrasound guidance may be used to gain venous access and/or fluoroscopy to check the positioning of the catheter tip. In 36565, the catheters are secured into position and any incisions are sutured. In 36566, two subcutaneous pockets for the ports are created with incisions through the skin in the chest wall, a few centimeters from the midline. Blunt dissection and cautery are used to create the pockets in the chest wall and the ports are placed. The catheters are connected to their respective ports and checked by injection. The catheters and ports are secured into position and any incisions are sutured.

Coding Tips

When medically necessary, report moderate (conscious) sedation provided by the performing physician with 99151-99153. When provided by another physician, report 99155-99157. If imaging guidance is used, either for obtaining access to the venous access site or for manipulating the catheter into its final end position, see 76937 or 77001.

ICD-10-CM Diagnostic Codes

The application of this code is too broad to adequately present ICD-10-CM diagnostic code links here. Refer to your ICD-10-CM book.

AMA: **36565** 2018,Jan,8; 2017,Jan,8; 2016,Jan,13; 2015,Jan,16; 2014,Jan,11
36566 2018,Jan,8; 2017,Jan,8; 2016,Jan,13; 2015,Jan,16; 2014,Jan,11

Relative Value Units/Medicare Edits

Non-Facility RVU	Work	PE	MP	Total
36565	5.79	17.82	1.24	24.85
36566	6.29	128.25	1.23	135.77
Facility RVU	**Work**	**PE**	**MP**	**Total**
36565	5.79	2.6	1.24	9.63
36566	6.29	2.94	1.23	10.46

	FUD	Status	MUE	Modifiers				IOM Reference
36565	10	A	1(3)	51	50	N/A	80*	None
36566	10	A	1(3)	51	50	N/A	80*	

* with documentation

Terms To Know

fluoroscopy. Radiology technique that allows visual examination of part of the body or a function of an organ using a device that projects an x-ray image on a fluorescent screen.

guidewire. Flexible metal instrument designed to lead another instrument in its proper course.

injection. Forcing a liquid substance into a body part such as a joint or muscle.

moderate sedation. Medically controlled state of depressed consciousness, with or without analgesia, while maintaining the patient's airway, protective reflexes, and ability to respond to stimulation or verbal commands.

puncture. Creating a hole.

subcutaneous. Below the skin.

vena cava. Main venous trunk that empties into the right atrium from both the lower and upper regions, beginning at the junction of the common iliac veins inferiorly and the two brachiocephalic veins superiorly.

venotomy. Incision or puncture of a vein.

36568-36569 [36572, 36573]

36568 Insertion of peripherally inserted central venous catheter (PICC), without subcutaneous port or pump, without imaging guidance; younger than 5 years of age

36569 age 5 years or older

36572 Insertion of peripherally inserted central venous catheter (PICC), without subcutaneous port or pump, including all imaging guidance, image documentation, and all associated radiological supervision and interpretation required to perform the insertion; younger than 5 years of age

36573 Insertion of peripherally inserted central venous catheter (PICC), without subcutaneous port or pump, including all imaging guidance, image documentation, and all associated radiological supervision and interpretation required to perform the insertion; age 5 years or older

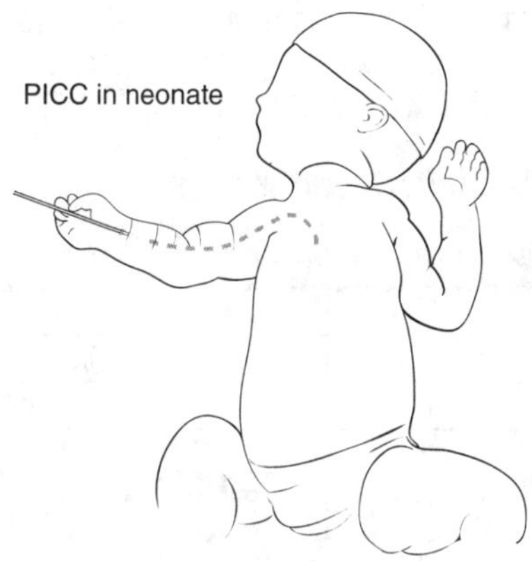

A central venous catheter is inserted from a periphery

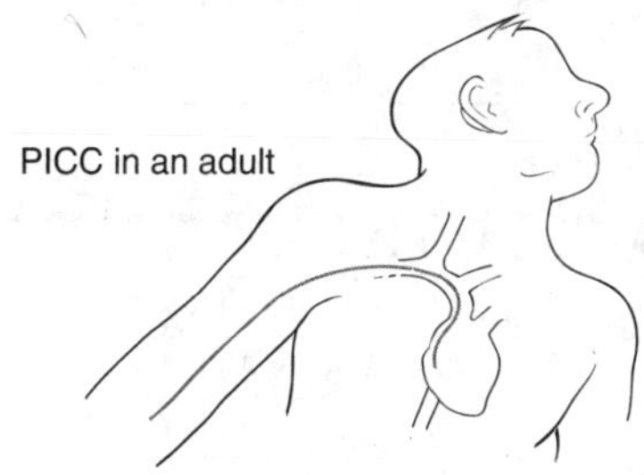

Explanation

A central venous access device or catheter is one in which the tip terminates in the subclavian, brachiocephalic, or iliac vein; the superior or inferior vena cava; or the right atrium. A peripherally inserted central venous catheter (PICC) has an entry site in the basilic or cephalic vein in the arm and is threaded into the superior vena cava above the right atrium. PICC lines are used for antibiotic therapy, chemotherapy, total parenteral nutrition, lab work, pain medications, blood transfusions, and hydration the same as a central line. For insertion of a (non-tunneled) peripherally inserted central venous catheter, without subcutaneous port or pump, the access vein (basilic or cephalic) is injected with local anesthesia and punctured with a needle. A guidewire is inserted. The central venous catheter is placed over the guidewire. The catheter is secured into position and dressed. Report 36568 for insertion of a PICC, without imaging, for children younger than 5 years of age; for a patient 5 years of age or older, report 36569. Report 36572 for insertion of a PICC, with imaging, for children younger than 5 years age; for a patient 5 years of age or older, report 36573.

Coding Tips

When medically necessary, report moderate (conscious) sedation provided by the performing physician with 99151-99153. When provided by another physician, report 99155-99157. Do not report 36568, 36569, 36572, or 36573 with 76937 or 77001. Do not report 36572 or 36573 with 71045-71048 as these services include confirming the catheter tip location. Report 36572 or 36573 for non-tunneled central venous catheter placement. If confirmation of catheter tip placement is not performed by the provider inserting the PICC line, append modifier 52 to 36572 or 36573. For midline catheter placement, see 36400, 36405, 36406, and 36410.

ICD-10-CM Diagnostic Codes

The application of this code is too broad to adequately present ICD-10-CM diagnostic code links here. Refer to your ICD-10-CM book.

AMA: **36568** 2019,May,3; 2018,Jan,8; 2017,Jan,8; 2016,Jan,13; 2015,Jan,16; 2014,Jan,11 **36569** 2019,May,3; 2018,Jan,8; 2017,Jan,8; 2016,Jan,13; 2015,Jan,16; 2014,Sep,13; 2014,Jan,11; 2013,Sep,17 **36572** 2019,May,3; 2019,Mar,10 **36573** 2019,May,3; 2019,Mar,10

Relative Value Units/Medicare Edits

Non-Facility RVU	Work	PE	MP	Total
36568	2.11	0.36	0.18	2.65
36569	1.9	0.65	0.17	2.72
36572	1.82	9.92	0.16	11.9
36573	1.7	9.32	0.18	11.2
Facility RVU	**Work**	**PE**	**MP**	**Total**
36568	2.11	0.36	0.18	2.65
36569	1.9	0.65	0.17	2.72
36572	1.82	0.67	0.16	2.65
36573	1.7	0.57	0.18	2.45

	FUD	Status	MUE	Modifiers				IOM Reference
36568	0	A	2(3)	N/A	N/A	N/A	N/A	None
36569	0	A	2(3)	N/A	N/A	N/A	N/A	
36572	0	A	1(3)	N/A	N/A	N/A	N/A	
36573	0	A	1(3)	N/A	N/A	N/A	N/A	

* with documentation

Terms To Know

guidewire. Flexible metal instrument designed to lead another instrument in its proper course.

injection. Forcing a liquid substance into a body part such as a joint or muscle.

subcutaneous. Below the skin.

ultrasound. Imaging using ultra-high sound frequency bounced off body structures.

vena cava. Main venous trunk that empties into the right atrium from both the lower and upper regions, beginning at the junction of the common iliac veins inferiorly and the two brachiocephalic veins superiorly.

36570-36571

36570 Insertion of peripherally inserted central venous access device, with subcutaneous port; younger than 5 years of age

36571 age 5 years or older

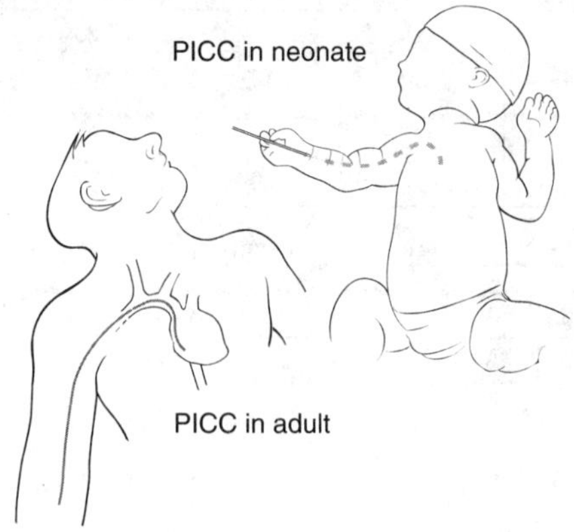

A central venous catheter is inserted from a periphery, with use of a subcutaneous port

Explanation

A central venous access device or catheter is one in which the tip terminates in the subclavian, brachiocephalic, or iliac vein; the superior or inferior vena cava; or the right atrium. A peripherally inserted central venous catheter (PICC) has an entry site in the basilic or cephalic vein in the arm and is threaded into the superior vena cava above the right atrium. PICC lines are used for antibiotic therapy, chemotherapy, total parenteral nutrition, lab work, pain medications, blood transfusions, and hydration the same as a central line. For insertion of a peripherally inserted central venous catheter with a subcutaneous port, the site over the access vein (basilic or cephalic) is injected with local anesthesia and punctured with a needle. A guidewire is inserted. The central venous catheter is placed over the guidewire and fed through the vein in the arm into the superior vena cava. The port may be placed in the chest in a subcutaneous pocket created through an incision in the chest wall, or placed in the arm through a small incision just above or halfway between the elbow crease and the shoulder on the inside of the arm. The port is attached to the catheter and checked. Ultrasound guidance may be used to gain venous access and/or fluoroscopy to check the positioning of the catheter tip. The catheter and port are secured into position and incisions are closed and dressed. Report 36570 for insertion for children younger than 5 years of age and 36571 for a patient 5 years of age or older.

Coding Tips

When medically necessary, report moderate (conscious) sedation provided by the performing physician with 99151-99153. When provided by another physician, report 99155-99157. If imaging guidance is used, either for obtaining access to the venous access site or for manipulating the catheter into its final end position, see 76937 or 77001. For insertion of a tunneled, centrally inserted central venous access device with subcutaneous port for patients younger than 5 years of age, see 36560; 5 years of age or older, see 36561.

ICD-10-CM Diagnostic Codes

The application of this code is too broad to adequately present ICD-10-CM diagnostic code links here. Refer to your ICD-10-CM book.

AMA: **36570** 2018,Jan,8; 2017,Jan,8; 2016,Jan,13; 2015,Jan,16; 2014,Jan,11 **36571** 2018,Jan,8; 2017,Jan,8; 2016,Jan,13; 2015,Jan,16; 2014,Jan,11

Relative Value Units/Medicare Edits

Non-Facility RVU	Work	PE	MP	Total
36570	5.11	34.53	1.24	40.88
36571	5.09	29.83	0.96	35.88
Facility RVU	**Work**	**PE**	**MP**	**Total**
36570	5.11	3.21	1.24	9.56
36571	5.09	2.95	0.96	9.0

	FUD	Status	MUE	Modifiers				IOM Reference
36570	10	A	2(3)	51	50	N/A	80*	None
36571	10	A	2(3)	51	50	N/A	80*	

* with documentation

Terms To Know

chemotherapy. Treatment of disease, especially cancerous conditions, using chemical agents.

fluoroscopy. Radiology technique that allows visual examination of part of the body or a function of an organ using a device that projects an x-ray image on a fluorescent screen.

guidewire. Flexible metal instrument designed to lead another instrument in its proper course.

incision. Act of cutting into tissue or an organ.

injection. Forcing a liquid substance into a body part such as a joint or muscle.

insertion. Placement or implantation into a body part.

parenteral nutrition. Nutrients provided subcutaneously, intravenously, intramuscularly, or intradermally for patients during the postoperative period and in other conditions, such as shock, coma, and renal failure.

36575-36576

36575 Repair of tunneled or non-tunneled central venous access catheter, without subcutaneous port or pump, central or peripheral insertion site

36576 Repair of central venous access device, with subcutaneous port or pump, central or peripheral insertion site

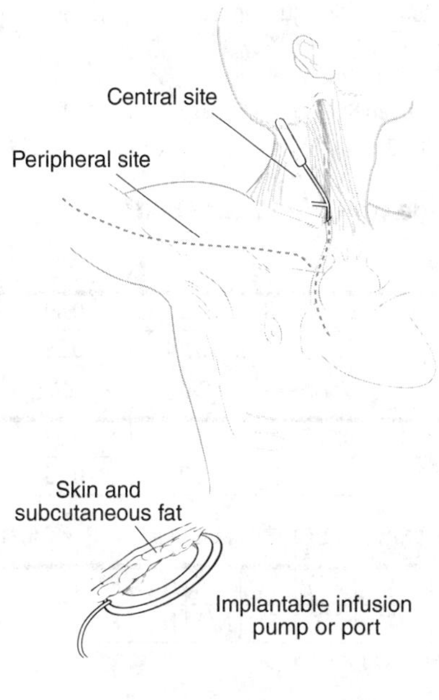

A CVA catheter or device, central or peripheral access, is repaired

Explanation

Code 36575 reports repair of a central venous access device (CVAD) that has external catheters with the access ports outside the body, and no subcutaneous ports or pumps, whether centrally or peripherally inserted, tunneled or non-tunneled. The repair is done on the catheter that is placed without any replacement of components. A Hickman catheter is an example of a tunneled CVAD with an external port. Code 36576 reports repair of a central venous access device (CVAD) that has an internal access port/pump in a subcutaneous pocket that is connected to the catheter, whether centrally or peripherally inserted. The repair is done on the device as it is placed within the patient, without any replacement of components, catheter or subcutaneous port/pump.

Coding Tips

When medically necessary, report moderate (conscious) sedation provided by the performing physician with 99151-99153. When provided by another physician, report 99155-99157. If imaging guidance is used, either for obtaining access to the venous access site or for manipulating the catheter into its final end position, see 76937 or 77001. For mechanical removal of pericatheter obstructive material, see 36595. For mechanical removal of intracatheter obstructive material, see 36596.

ICD-10-CM Diagnostic Codes

T82.41XA	Breakdown (mechanical) of vascular dialysis catheter, initial encounter
T82.42XA	Displacement of vascular dialysis catheter, initial encounter
T82.43XA	Leakage of vascular dialysis catheter, initial encounter
T82.49XA	Other complication of vascular dialysis catheter, initial encounter
T82.514A	Breakdown (mechanical) of infusion catheter, initial encounter

T82.524A Displacement of infusion catheter, initial encounter
T82.534A Leakage of infusion catheter, initial encounter
T82.594A Other mechanical complication of infusion catheter, initial encounter
T82.598A Other mechanical complication of other cardiac and vascular devices and implants, initial encounter
T82.898A Other specified complication of vascular prosthetic devices, implants and grafts, initial encounter
Z45.2 Encounter for adjustment and management of vascular access device

AMA: 36575 2018,Jan,8; 2017,Jan,8; 2016,Jan,13; 2015,Jan,16; 2014,Jan,11
36576 2018,Jan,8; 2017,Jan,8; 2016,Jan,13; 2015,Jan,16; 2014,Jan,11

Relative Value Units/Medicare Edits

Non-Facility RVU	Work	PE	MP	Total
36575	0.67	3.83	0.09	4.59
36576	2.99	5.77	0.55	9.31
Facility RVU	**Work**	**PE**	**MP**	**Total**
36575	0.67	0.25	0.09	1.01
36576	2.99	1.79	0.55	5.33

	FUD	Status	MUE	Modifiers				IOM Reference
36575	0	A	2(3)	51	N/A	N/A	80*	None
36576	10	A	2(3)	51	N/A	N/A	80*	

* with documentation

Terms To Know

anesthesia. Loss of feeling or sensation, usually induced to permit the performance of surgery or other painful procedures.

Hickman catheter. Central venous catheter used for long-term delivery of medications, such as antibiotics, nutritional substances, or chemotherapeutic agents.

moderate sedation. Medically controlled state of depressed consciousness, with or without analgesia, while maintaining the patient's airway, protective reflexes, and ability to respond to stimulation or verbal commands.

peripheral. Outside of a structure or organ.

subcutaneous. Below the skin.

36578

36578 Replacement, catheter only, of central venous access device, with subcutaneous port or pump, central or peripheral insertion site

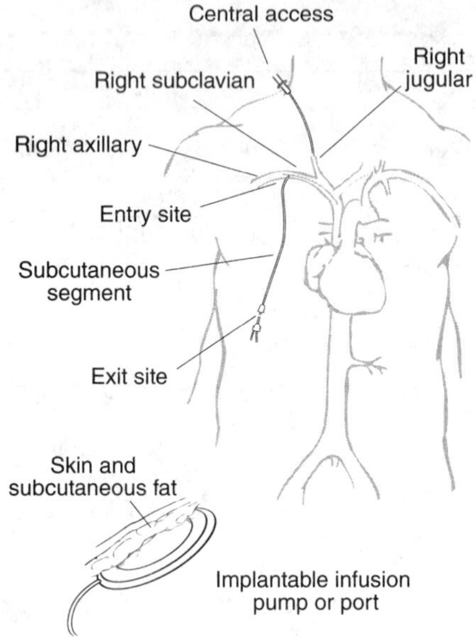

The catheter alone is replaced in a CVA device, with subcutaneous port or pump, central or peripheral access site

Explanation

The catheter only of a central venous access device with a subcutaneous port or pump is replaced, whether centrally or peripherally inserted. Local anesthesia is given and the subcutaneous pocket over the port is incised. The catheter is disconnected. A guidewire is placed through the existing catheter, which is removed over the guidewire. A new central venous catheter of correct length is placed into position and connected to the port/pump device that has not been removed or replaced. The connection with the new catheter is checked, as well as the catheter and port secured, and the wound is dressed.

Coding Tips

When medically necessary, report moderate (conscious) sedation provided by the performing physician with 99151-99153. When provided by another physician, report 99155-99157. For complete replacement of an entire device through the same venous access, see 36582 or 36583. If imaging guidance is used, either for obtaining access to the venous access site or for manipulating the catheter into its final end position, see 76937 or 77001.

ICD-10-CM Diagnostic Codes

T80.211A Bloodstream infection due to central venous catheter, initial encounter
T80.212A Local infection due to central venous catheter, initial encounter
T80.218A Other infection due to central venous catheter, initial encounter
T82.41XA Breakdown (mechanical) of vascular dialysis catheter, initial encounter
T82.42XA Displacement of vascular dialysis catheter, initial encounter
T82.43XA Leakage of vascular dialysis catheter, initial encounter
T82.49XA Other complication of vascular dialysis catheter, initial encounter
T82.514A Breakdown (mechanical) of infusion catheter, initial encounter
T82.524A Displacement of infusion catheter, initial encounter
T82.534A Leakage of infusion catheter, initial encounter

T82.594A	Other mechanical complication of infusion catheter, initial encounter
T82.598A	Other mechanical complication of other cardiac and vascular devices and implants, initial encounter
T82.7XXA	Infection and inflammatory reaction due to other cardiac and vascular devices, implants and grafts, initial encounter
T82.818A	Embolism due to vascular prosthetic devices, implants and grafts, initial encounter
T82.828A	Fibrosis due to vascular prosthetic devices, implants and grafts, initial encounter
T82.838A	Hemorrhage due to vascular prosthetic devices, implants and grafts, initial encounter
T82.848A	Pain due to vascular prosthetic devices, implants and grafts, initial encounter
T82.858A	Stenosis of other vascular prosthetic devices, implants and grafts, initial encounter
T82.868A	Thrombosis due to vascular prosthetic devices, implants and grafts, initial encounter
T82.898A	Other specified complication of vascular prosthetic devices, implants and grafts, initial encounter
Z45.2	Encounter for adjustment and management of vascular access device

AMA: 36578 2018,Jan,8; 2017,Jan,8; 2016,Jan,13; 2015,Jan,16; 2014,Jan,11

Relative Value Units/Medicare Edits

Non-Facility RVU	Work	PE	MP	Total
36578	3.29	9.23	0.54	13.06
Facility RVU	**Work**	**PE**	**MP**	**Total**
36578	3.29	2.03	0.54	5.86

	FUD	Status	MUE	Modifiers				IOM Reference
36578	10	A	2(3)	51	N/A	N/A	80*	None

* with documentation

Terms To Know

anesthesia. Loss of feeling or sensation, usually induced to permit the performance of surgery or other painful procedures.

catheter. Flexible tube inserted into an area of the body for introducing or withdrawing fluid.

complication. Condition arising after the beginning of observation and treatment that modifies the course of the patient's illness or the medical care required, or an undesired result or misadventure in medical care.

guidewire. Flexible metal instrument designed to lead another instrument in its proper course.

36580-36581

36580 Replacement, complete, of a non-tunneled centrally inserted central venous catheter, without subcutaneous port or pump, through same venous access

36581 Replacement, complete, of a tunneled centrally inserted central venous catheter, without subcutaneous port or pump, through same venous access

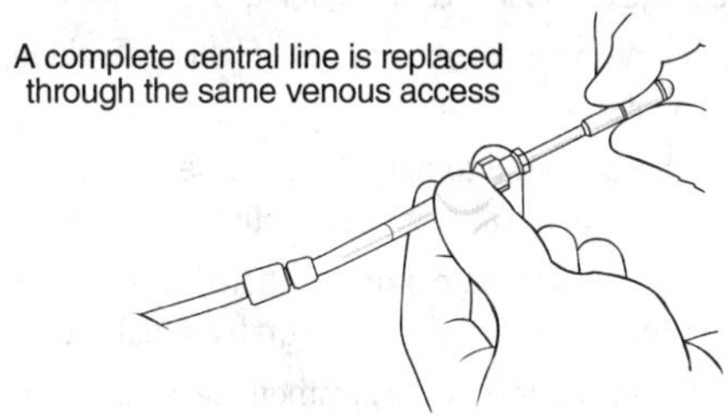

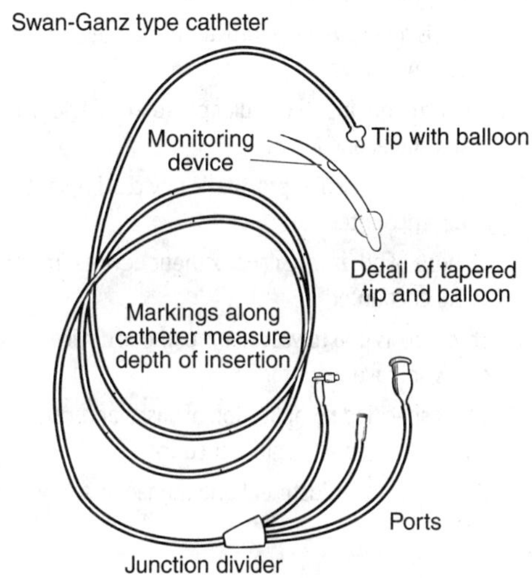

Explanation

In 36580, a non-tunneled, centrally inserted central venous catheter, without subcutaneous port or pump, is replaced through the same venous access site. Local anesthesia is given. In 36581, sutures securing the cuff of the indwelling catheter are freed from the skin. A guidewire is first passed through the existing central line catheter and the catheter is removed. A new central venous catheter is placed back into position over the guidewire, secured into position, and the wound dressed.

Coding Tips

When medically necessary, report moderate (conscious) sedation provided by the performing physician with 99151-99153. When provided by another physician, report 99155-99157. If imaging guidance is used for obtaining access to the venous access site or for manipulating the replacement catheter into its final end position, see 76937 or 77001. For replacement of a multicatheter device placed at separate venous access sites, use the appropriate code and indicate a frequency of two in the units column. If a venous access device is removed and a new one placed at a different access site, do not report 36580 or 36581; use the appropriate codes for the removal of the old device (if a removal code exists) and the insertion of the new device.

ICD-10-CM Diagnostic Codes

T80.211A	Bloodstream infection due to central venous catheter, initial encounter
T80.212A	Local infection due to central venous catheter, initial encounter

T80.218A	Other infection due to central venous catheter, initial encounter
T82.41XA	Breakdown (mechanical) of vascular dialysis catheter, initial encounter
T82.42XA	Displacement of vascular dialysis catheter, initial encounter
T82.43XA	Leakage of vascular dialysis catheter, initial encounter
T82.49XA	Other complication of vascular dialysis catheter, initial encounter
T82.514A	Breakdown (mechanical) of infusion catheter, initial encounter
T82.524A	Displacement of infusion catheter, initial encounter
T82.534A	Leakage of infusion catheter, initial encounter
T82.594A	Other mechanical complication of infusion catheter, initial encounter
T82.598A	Other mechanical complication of other cardiac and vascular devices and implants, initial encounter
T82.7XXA	Infection and inflammatory reaction due to other cardiac and vascular devices, implants and grafts, initial encounter
T82.818A	Embolism due to vascular prosthetic devices, implants and grafts, initial encounter
T82.828A	Fibrosis due to vascular prosthetic devices, implants and grafts, initial encounter
T82.838A	Hemorrhage due to vascular prosthetic devices, implants and grafts, initial encounter
T82.848A	Pain due to vascular prosthetic devices, implants and grafts, initial encounter
T82.858A	Stenosis of other vascular prosthetic devices, implants and grafts, initial encounter
T82.868A	Thrombosis due to vascular prosthetic devices, implants and grafts, initial encounter
T82.898A	Other specified complication of vascular prosthetic devices, implants and grafts, initial encounter
Z45.2	Encounter for adjustment and management of vascular access device

AMA: **36580** 2018,Jan,8; 2017,Jan,8; 2016,Jan,13; 2015,Jan,16; 2014,Jan,11 **36581** 2018,Jan,8; 2017,Jan,8; 2016,Jan,13; 2015,Jan,16; 2014,Jan,11

Relative Value Units/Medicare Edits

Non-Facility RVU	Work	PE	MP	Total
36580	1.31	4.67	0.15	6.13
36581	3.23	17.85	0.4	21.48
Facility RVU	**Work**	**PE**	**MP**	**Total**
36580	1.31	0.46	0.15	1.92
36581	3.23	1.68	0.4	5.31

	FUD	Status	MUE	Modifiers				IOM Reference
36580	0	A	2(3)	N/A	N/A	N/A	N/A	None
36581	10	A	2(3)	51	N/A	N/A	80*	

* with documentation

Terms To Know

catheter. Flexible tube inserted into an area of the body for introducing or withdrawing fluid.

guidewire. Flexible metal instrument designed to lead another instrument in its proper course.

36582-36583

36582 Replacement, complete, of a tunneled centrally inserted central venous access device, with subcutaneous port, through same venous access

36583 Replacement, complete, of a tunneled centrally inserted central venous access device, with subcutaneous pump, through same venous access

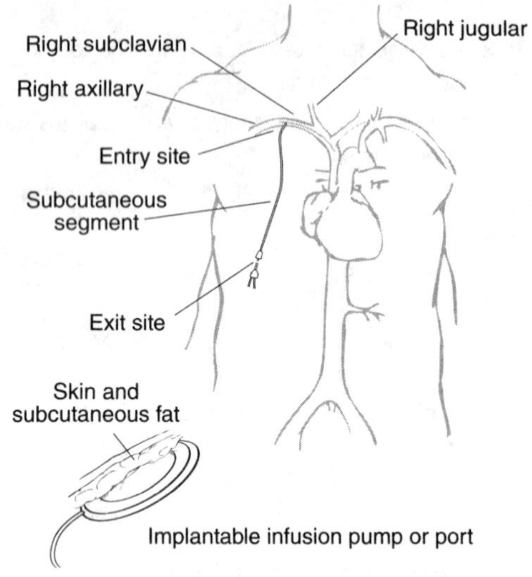

A complete replacement is performed for a tunneled CVA device, with subcutaneous port or pump, through the same venous access

Explanation

A tunneled, centrally inserted central venous catheter, along with a subcutaneous port (36582) or pump (36583) device is replaced. Local anesthesia is given and the subcutaneous pocket over the port/pump device is incised. The pump/port is dissected free and tested. The catheter is disconnected and the pump/port device is removed from its pocket. A guidewire is placed over the existing catheter, which is removed, and a new central venous catheter is threaded into position over the guidewire. A new pump/port device is inserted into the subcutaneous pocket and the catheter is connected. The connection is checked with an injection. The new pump/port is secured into the pocket, incisions are closed, and the wound is dressed.

Coding Tips

When medically necessary, report moderate (conscious) sedation provided by the performing physician with 99151-99153. When provided by another physician, report 99155-99157. If imaging guidance is used, either for obtaining access to the venous access site or for manipulating the catheter into its final end position, see 76937 or 77001. Supplies used when providing this procedure may be reported with HCPCS Level II code C1751. Check with the specific payer to determine coverage.

ICD-10-CM Diagnostic Codes

T80.211A	Bloodstream infection due to central venous catheter, initial encounter
T80.212A	Local infection due to central venous catheter, initial encounter
T80.218A	Other infection due to central venous catheter, initial encounter
T82.41XA	Breakdown (mechanical) of vascular dialysis catheter, initial encounter
T82.42XA	Displacement of vascular dialysis catheter, initial encounter

T82.43XA Leakage of vascular dialysis catheter, initial encounter
T82.49XA Other complication of vascular dialysis catheter, initial encounter
T82.514A Breakdown (mechanical) of infusion catheter, initial encounter
T82.524A Displacement of infusion catheter, initial encounter
T82.534A Leakage of infusion catheter, initial encounter
T82.594A Other mechanical complication of infusion catheter, initial encounter
T82.598A Other mechanical complication of other cardiac and vascular devices and implants, initial encounter
T82.7XXA Infection and inflammatory reaction due to other cardiac and vascular devices, implants and grafts, initial encounter
T82.818A Embolism due to vascular prosthetic devices, implants and grafts, initial encounter
T82.828A Fibrosis due to vascular prosthetic devices, implants and grafts, initial encounter
T82.838A Hemorrhage due to vascular prosthetic devices, implants and grafts, initial encounter
T82.848A Pain due to vascular prosthetic devices, implants and grafts, initial encounter
T82.858A Stenosis of other vascular prosthetic devices, implants and grafts, initial encounter
T82.868A Thrombosis due to vascular prosthetic devices, implants and grafts, initial encounter
T82.898A Other specified complication of vascular prosthetic devices, implants and grafts, initial encounter
Z45.2 Encounter for adjustment and management of vascular access device

AMA: 36582 2018,Jan,8; 2017,Jan,8; 2016,Jan,13; 2015,Jan,16; 2014,Jan,11
36583 2018,Jan,8; 2017,Jan,8; 2016,Jan,13; 2015,Jan,16; 2014,Jan,11

Relative Value Units/Medicare Edits

Non-Facility RVU	Work	PE	MP	Total
36582	4.99	22.55	0.81	28.35
36583	5.04	29.65	1.22	35.91
Facility RVU	**Work**	**PE**	**MP**	**Total**
36582	4.99	2.58	0.81	8.38
36583	5.04	3.19	1.22	9.45

	FUD	Status	MUE	Modifiers				IOM Reference
36582	10	A	2(3)	51	N/A	N/A	80*	None
36583	10	A	2(3)	51	N/A	N/A	80*	

* with documentation

Terms To Know

anesthesia. Loss of feeling or sensation, usually induced to permit the performance of surgery or other painful procedures.

catheter. Flexible tube inserted into an area of the body for introducing or withdrawing fluid.

complication. Condition arising after the beginning of observation and treatment that modifies the course of the patient's illness or the medical care required, or an undesired result or misadventure in medical care.

36584-36585

36584 Replacement, complete, of a peripherally inserted central venous catheter (PICC), without subcutaneous port or pump, through same venous access, including all imaging guidance, image documentation, and all associated radiological supervision and interpretation required to perform the replacement

36585 Replacement, complete, of a peripherally inserted central venous access device, with subcutaneous port, through same venous access

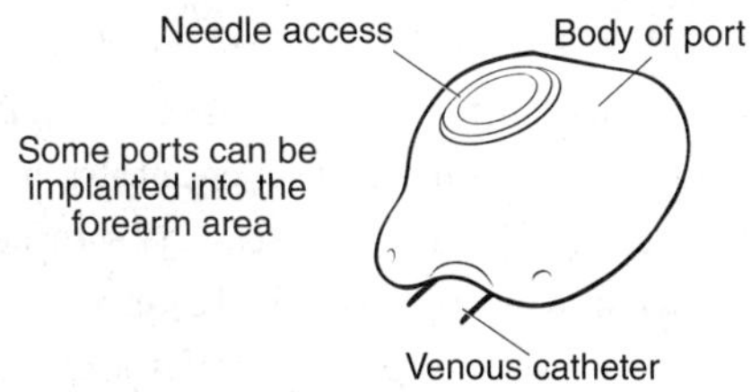

A PICC system is replaced in its entirety. The replacement is accomplished through the same venous access as the previous catheter previous catheter system

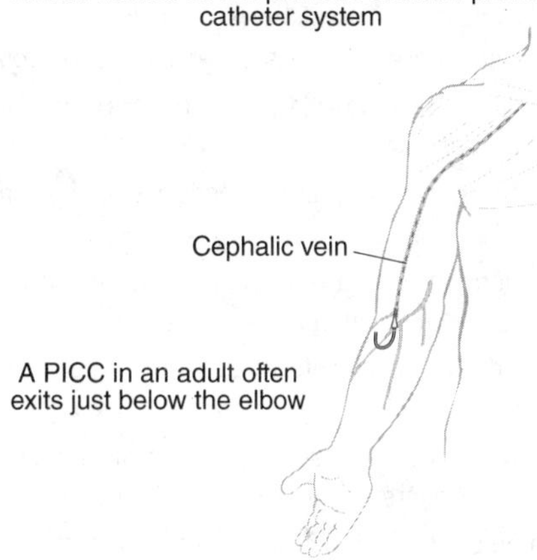

Explanation

In 36584, a peripherally inserted central venous catheter (PICC), without subcutaneous port or pump, is replaced through the same venous access site. Local anesthesia is given and the sutures securing the cuff of the catheter with external port are freed from the skin and it is partially withdrawn. This service includes all imaging guidance and documentation, as well as the supervision and interpretation. In 36585, a peripherally inserted central venous catheter (PICC), along with a subcutaneous port, is replaced through the same venous access site. Local anesthesia is given, the skin over the subcutaneous pocket is incised, and the port is dissected free. In both cases, a sheath is placed over the nonfunctioning catheter and it is completely withdrawn. A guidewire is inserted into the access site through the sheath and advanced. A new catheter of correct length is placed over the guidewire and the sheath and guidewire are removed. The catheter is fastened in position and the wound is dressed.

Coding Tips

Complete replacement, also referred to as complete exchange, involves removal of the entire device via the same access site. When medically necessary, report moderate (conscious) sedation provided by the performing physician with 99151-99153. When provided by another physician, report 99155-99157. Imaging guidance is included in 36584 and is not reported separately. If confirmation of catheter tip placement is not performed by the provider inserting the PICC line, append modifier 52 to 36584. For replacement of a peripherally inserted central venous catheter without subcutaneous port or pump, through the same venous access, without imaging guidance, see 37799. Do not report 36584 with 76937 or 77001.

ICD-10-CM Diagnostic Codes

T80.211A	Bloodstream infection due to central venous catheter, initial encounter
T80.212A	Local infection due to central venous catheter, initial encounter
T80.218A	Other infection due to central venous catheter, initial encounter
T82.41XA	Breakdown (mechanical) of vascular dialysis catheter, initial encounter
T82.42XA	Displacement of vascular dialysis catheter, initial encounter
T82.43XA	Leakage of vascular dialysis catheter, initial encounter
T82.49XA	Other complication of vascular dialysis catheter, initial encounter
T82.514A	Breakdown (mechanical) of infusion catheter, initial encounter
T82.524A	Displacement of infusion catheter, initial encounter
T82.534A	Leakage of infusion catheter, initial encounter
T82.594A	Other mechanical complication of infusion catheter, initial encounter
T82.598A	Other mechanical complication of other cardiac and vascular devices and implants, initial encounter
T82.7XXA	Infection and inflammatory reaction due to other cardiac and vascular devices, implants and grafts, initial encounter
T82.818A	Embolism due to vascular prosthetic devices, implants and grafts, initial encounter
T82.828A	Fibrosis due to vascular prosthetic devices, implants and grafts, initial encounter
T82.838A	Hemorrhage due to vascular prosthetic devices, implants and grafts, initial encounter
T82.848A	Pain due to vascular prosthetic devices, implants and grafts, initial encounter
T82.858A	Stenosis of other vascular prosthetic devices, implants and grafts, initial encounter
T82.868A	Thrombosis due to vascular prosthetic devices, implants and grafts, initial encounter
T82.898A	Other specified complication of vascular prosthetic devices, implants and grafts, initial encounter
Z45.2	Encounter for adjustment and management of vascular access device

AMA: 36584 2019,May,3; 2019,Mar,10; 2018,Jan,8; 2017,Jan,8; 2016,Jan,13; 2015,Jan,16; 2014,Jan,11 **36585** 2018,Jan,8; 2017,Jan,8; 2016,Jan,13; 2015,Jan,16; 2014,Jan,11

Relative Value Units/Medicare Edits

Non-Facility RVU	Work	PE	MP	Total
36584	1.2	8.47	0.11	9.78
36585	4.59	25.12	0.8	30.51
Facility RVU	**Work**	**PE**	**MP**	**Total**
36584	1.2	0.42	0.11	1.73
36585	4.59	2.41	0.8	7.8

	FUD	Status	MUE	Modifiers				IOM Reference
36584	0	A	2(3)	N/A	N/A	N/A	N/A	None
36585	10	A	2(3)	51	N/A	N/A	80*	

* with documentation

36589-36590

36589 Removal of tunneled central venous catheter, without subcutaneous port or pump

36590 Removal of tunneled central venous access device, with subcutaneous port or pump, central or peripheral insertion

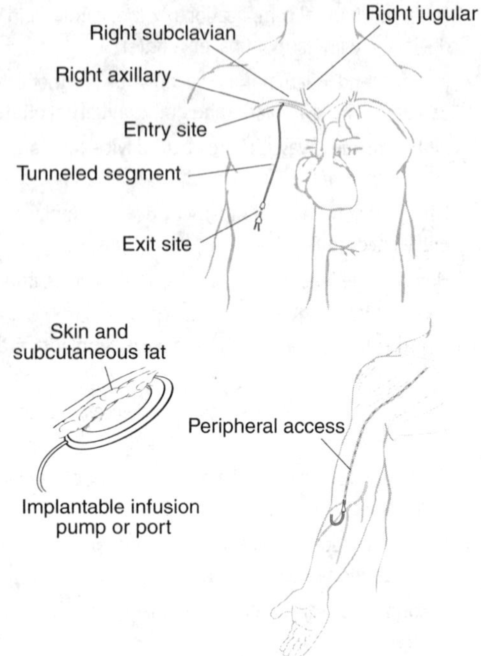

Explanation

In 36589, a tunneled central venous catheter without subcutaneous port or pump is removed. Local anesthesia is given and the sutures securing the cuff of the tunneled catheter's external port are freed from the skin. In 36590, a tunneled central venous access device, both catheter and subcutaneous port or pump, is removed. Local anesthesia is given and the subcutaneous pocket over the port/pump device is incised and the pump/port is dissected free. The catheter is disconnected and the pump/port device is removed from its pocket. In both cases, a guidewire is placed over the existing catheter, which is withdrawn over the guidewire, and the guidewire is removed. The incisions are closed and the wound is dressed.

Coding Tips

When medically necessary, report moderate (conscious) sedation provided by the performing physician with 99151-99153. When provided by another physician, report 99155-99157. Do not report 36589 or 36590 for removal of non-tunneled central venous catheters. If imaging guidance is used, either for obtaining access to the venous access site or for manipulating the catheter into its final end position, see 76937 or 77001.

ICD-10-CM Diagnostic Codes

T80.211A	Bloodstream infection due to central venous catheter, initial encounter
T80.212A	Local infection due to central venous catheter, initial encounter
T80.218A	Other infection due to central venous catheter, initial encounter
T82.41XA	Breakdown (mechanical) of vascular dialysis catheter, initial encounter
T82.42XA	Displacement of vascular dialysis catheter, initial encounter
T82.43XA	Leakage of vascular dialysis catheter, initial encounter

T82.49XA	Other complication of vascular dialysis catheter, initial encounter
T82.514A	Breakdown (mechanical) of infusion catheter, initial encounter
T82.524A	Displacement of infusion catheter, initial encounter
T82.534A	Leakage of infusion catheter, initial encounter
T82.594A	Other mechanical complication of infusion catheter, initial encounter
T82.598A	Other mechanical complication of other cardiac and vascular devices and implants, initial encounter
T82.7XXA	Infection and inflammatory reaction due to other cardiac and vascular devices, implants and grafts, initial encounter
T82.818A	Embolism due to vascular prosthetic devices, implants and grafts, initial encounter
T82.828A	Fibrosis due to vascular prosthetic devices, implants and grafts, initial encounter
T82.838A	Hemorrhage due to vascular prosthetic devices, implants and grafts, initial encounter
T82.848A	Pain due to vascular prosthetic devices, implants and grafts, initial encounter
T82.858A	Stenosis of other vascular prosthetic devices, implants and grafts, initial encounter
T82.868A	Thrombosis due to vascular prosthetic devices, implants and grafts, initial encounter
T82.898A	Other specified complication of vascular prosthetic devices, implants and grafts, initial encounter
Z45.2	Encounter for adjustment and management of vascular access device

AMA: 36589 2018,Jan,8; 2017,Jan,8; 2016,Jan,13; 2015,Nov,10; 2015,Jan,16; 2014,Jan,11 **36590** 2018,Jan,8; 2017,Jan,8; 2016,Jan,13; 2015,Jan,16; 2014,Jan,11

Relative Value Units/Medicare Edits

Non-Facility RVU	Work	PE	MP	Total
36589	2.28	2.11	0.32	4.71
36590	3.1	2.71	0.53	6.34
Facility RVU	**Work**	**PE**	**MP**	**Total**
36589	2.28	1.36	0.32	3.96
36590	3.1	1.86	0.53	5.49

	FUD	Status	MUE	Modifiers				IOM Reference
36589	10	A	2(3)	51	N/A	N/A	80*	None
36590	10	A	2(3)	51	N/A	N/A	80*	

* with documentation

36591

36591 Collection of blood specimen from a completely implantable venous access device

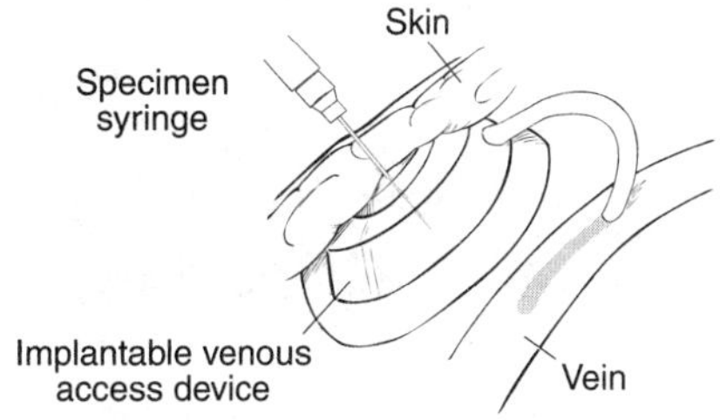

A blood specimen is collected from a partially or completely implantable venous access device

Explanation

The physician obtains a blood specimen from a previously placed, completely implantable venous access device. Completely implanted devices are those that have access through a subcutaneous port (e.g., Port-A-Cath, Infusaport). An implantable access device requires a percutaneous noncoring needle to accomplish the blood draw. The skin is cleansed with alcohol or iodine solution. The needle is placed into the port. Heparin is withdrawn. A second needle is inserted and the blood specimen obtained. The port is flushed with heparin solution.

Coding Tips

This service may only be reported in addition to laboratory services. To report collection of venous blood by venipuncture, see 36415. Medicare and some payers may require HCPCS Level II code G0471 to report this service when provided in a federally qualified health center (FQHC). To report collection of capillary blood, see 36416. Code 36591 is included in the codes for critical care services 99291–99292. Surgical trays, A4550, are not separately reimbursed by Medicare; however, other third-party payers may cover them. Check with the specific payer to determine coverage.

ICD-10-CM Diagnostic Codes

The application of this code is too broad to adequately present ICD-10-CM diagnostic code links here. Refer to your ICD-10-CM book.

AMA: 36591 2019,Aug,8; 2018,Jan,8; 2017,Jan,8; 2016,Jan,13; 2015,Jan,16; 2014,May,4; 2014,Jan,11

Relative Value Units/Medicare Edits

Non-Facility RVU	Work	PE	MP	Total
36591	0.0	0.68	0.01	0.69
Facility RVU	**Work**	**PE**	**MP**	**Total**
36591	0.0	0.68	0.01	0.69

	FUD	Status	MUE	Modifiers				IOM Reference
36591	N/A	T	2(3)	N/A	N/A	N/A	80*	None

* with documentation

36592

36592 Collection of blood specimen using established central or peripheral catheter, venous, not otherwise specified

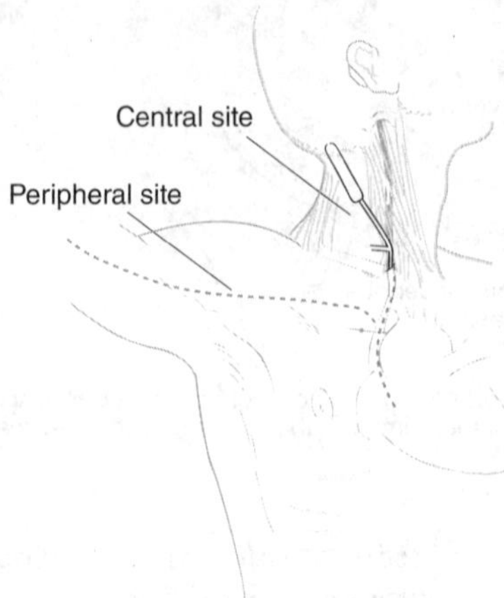

Blood specimen is collected from established catheter

Explanation

The physician obtains a blood specimen from an established central venous or peripheral venous catheter. A central venous catheter (CVC) is one that is inserted through the skin into central veins, such as the femoral, internal jugular, or subclavian veins. Peripheral catheters include those inserted in the arm veins (basilic or cephalic), such as a PICC line, saline lock, or heparin lock. In order to clear the catheter of any material that could contaminate the sample and affect the test results, a specific volume of infusing fluid and blood must be discarded before a blood specimen is obtained; this volume will vary depending on the type of catheter utilized. With a central venous catheter, a three-way stopcock is attached to the catheter's hub and two syringes attached to the stopcock. Using one syringe, the catheter is flushed with normal saline. A specific amount of blood is aspirated into the same syringe used for the saline flush and discarded. The blood sample is then withdrawn using the other syringe and placed into an appropriate tube for laboratory analysis. If using a peripheral venous catheter, a specific amount of blood is also aspirated and discarded before the blood sample is drawn.

Coding Tips

This service may only be reported in addition to laboratory services. To report blood collection from an established arterial catheter, see 37799.

ICD-10-CM Diagnostic Codes

The application of this code is too broad to adequately present ICD-10-CM diagnostic code links here. Refer to your ICD-10-CM book.

AMA: 36592 2018,Jan,8; 2017,Jan,8; 2016,Jan,13; 2015,Jan,16; 2014,Jan,11

Relative Value Units/Medicare Edits

Non-Facility RVU	Work	PE	MP	Total
36592	0.0	0.76	0.01	0.77
Facility RVU	**Work**	**PE**	**MP**	**Total**
36592	0.0	0.76	0.01	0.77

	FUD	Status	MUE	Modifiers				IOM Reference
36592	N/A	T	1(3)	N/A	N/A	N/A	80*	None

* with documentation

36593

36593 Declotting by thrombolytic agent of implanted vascular access device or catheter

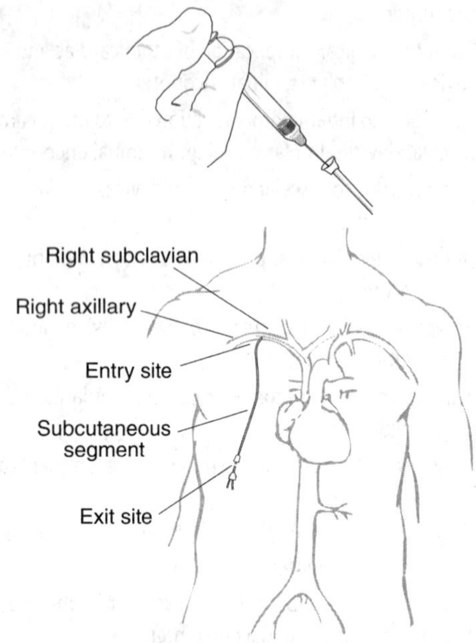

A thrombolytic agent is used to declot a catheter or implanted vascular access device

Explanation

To remove a clot from an implanted vascular access device or catheter, the physician injects a thrombolytic agent (e.g., Streptokinase) into the catheter to dissolve the clot. The patient is observed for any abnormal signs of bleeding.

Coding Tips

When 36593 is performed with another separately identifiable procedure, the highest dollar value code is listed as the primary procedure and subsequent procedures are appended with modifier 51. Supplies used when providing this procedure may be reported with HCPCS Level II code J2995. Check with the specific payer to determine coverage.

ICD-10-CM Diagnostic Codes

T82.818A	Embolism due to vascular prosthetic devices, implants and grafts, initial encounter
T82.848A	Pain due to vascular prosthetic devices, implants and grafts, initial encounter
T82.856A	Stenosis of peripheral vascular stent, initial encounter
T82.858A	Stenosis of other vascular prosthetic devices, implants and grafts, initial encounter
T82.868A	Thrombosis due to vascular prosthetic devices, implants and grafts, initial encounter
T82.898A	Other specified complication of vascular prosthetic devices, implants and grafts, initial encounter

AMA: 36593 2018,Jan,8; 2017,Jan,8; 2016,Jan,13; 2015,Jan,16; 2014,Jan,11; 2013,Feb,3-6

Relative Value Units/Medicare Edits

Non-Facility RVU	Work	PE	MP	Total
36593	0.0	0.87	0.02	0.89
Facility RVU	**Work**	**PE**	**MP**	**Total**
36593	0.0	0.87	0.02	0.89

	FUD	Status	MUE	Modifiers				IOM Reference
36593	N/A	A	2(3)	N/A	N/A	N/A	80*	None

* with documentation

Terms To Know

catheter. Flexible tube inserted into an area of the body for introducing or withdrawing fluid.

complication. Condition arising after the beginning of observation and treatment that modifies the course of the patient's illness or the medical care required, or an undesired result or misadventure in medical care.

embolism. Obstruction of a blood vessel resulting from a clot or foreign substance.

implantable venous access device. Catheter implanted for continuous access to the venous system for long-term parenteral feeding or for the administration of fluids or medications.

stenosis. Narrowing or constriction of a passage.

thrombolytic agent. Drugs or other substances used to dissolve blood clots in blood vessels or in tubes that have been placed into the body.

thrombosis. Condition arising from the presence or formation of blood clots within a blood vessel that may cause vascular obstruction and insufficient oxygenation.

36595

36595 Mechanical removal of pericatheter obstructive material (eg, fibrin sheath) from central venous device via separate venous access

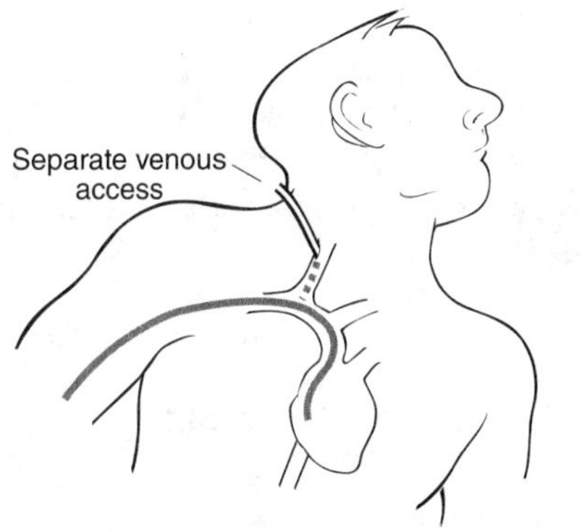

A CVC that has become obstructed is addressed mechanically via a second venous access site. The obstructive matter is on the exterior of the catheter lumen

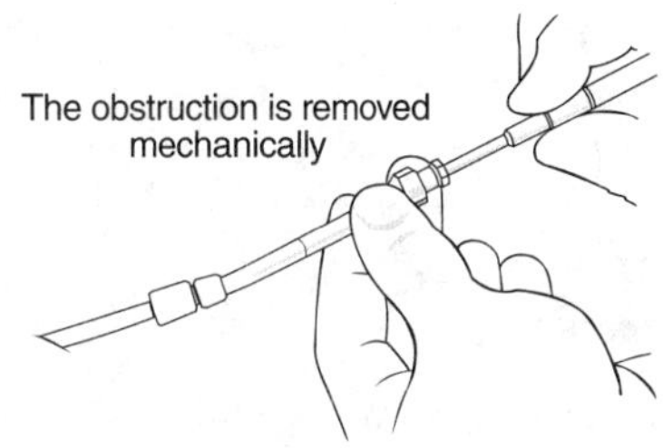

Explanation

Pericatheter obstructive material such as a fibrin sheath is removed from around a central venous device via separate venous access. Central venous catheters often fail because of the accumulation of an obstructing thrombus or fibrin sheath around the tip of the catheter. The catheter is first checked that it can aspirate and flush forward. The pericatheter material is identified by contrast material injection. Generally, a right femoral vein access is used. A guidewire followed by an angiographic catheter are advanced into the superior vena cava and exchanged for a loop snare with its catheter, which are advanced cephalad along the length of the central venous catheter beyond the ports. The loop snare is tightly closed about the central venous catheter to encircle it and slowly pulled down and off the tip of the catheter, stripping off the pericatheter obstructive material. This is repeated a few times and the catheter is rechecked for infusion and injection ability of the ports. A contrast study is done again to identify any fibrin and the process may be repeated until the fibrin sheath is completely removed.

Coding Tips

Do not report 36593 in addition to 36595. For venous catheterization, see 36010–36012. For radiological supervision and interpretation, see 75901.

ICD-10-CM Diagnostic Codes

T82.49XA	Other complication of vascular dialysis catheter, initial encounter
T82.594A	Other mechanical complication of infusion catheter, initial encounter
T82.598A	Other mechanical complication of other cardiac and vascular devices and implants, initial encounter
T82.818A	Embolism due to vascular prosthetic devices, implants and grafts, initial encounter

T82.828A Fibrosis due to vascular prosthetic devices, implants and grafts, initial encounter

T82.856A Stenosis of peripheral vascular stent, initial encounter

T82.858A Stenosis of other vascular prosthetic devices, implants and grafts, initial encounter

T82.868A Thrombosis due to vascular prosthetic devices, implants and grafts, initial encounter

T82.898A Other specified complication of vascular prosthetic devices, implants and grafts, initial encounter

Z45.2 Encounter for adjustment and management of vascular access device

AMA: 36595 2018,Jan,8; 2017,Jan,8; 2016,Jan,13; 2015,Jan,16; 2014,Jan,11

Relative Value Units/Medicare Edits

Non-Facility RVU	Work	PE	MP	Total
36595	3.59	13.32	0.39	17.3
Facility RVU	**Work**	**PE**	**MP**	**Total**
36595	3.59	1.32	0.39	5.3

	FUD	Status	MUE	Modifiers				IOM Reference
36595	0	A	2(3)	51	N/A	N/A	N/A	None

* with documentation

Terms To Know

aspiration. Drawing fluid out by suction.

cephalad. Toward the head.

fibrin. Main fibrous composition of blood clots.

guidewire. Flexible metal instrument designed to lead another instrument in its proper course.

infection. Presence of microorganisms in body tissues that may result in cellular damage.

infusion. Introduction of a therapeutic fluid, other than blood, into the bloodstream.

injection. Forcing a liquid substance into a body part such as a joint or muscle.

snare. Wire used as a loop to excise a polyp or lesion.

thrombus. Stationary blood clot inside a blood vessel.

vena cava. Main venous trunk that empties into the right atrium from both the lower and upper regions, beginning at the junction of the common iliac veins inferiorly and the two brachiocephalic veins superiorly.

36596

36596 Mechanical removal of intraluminal (intracatheter) obstructive material from central venous device through device lumen

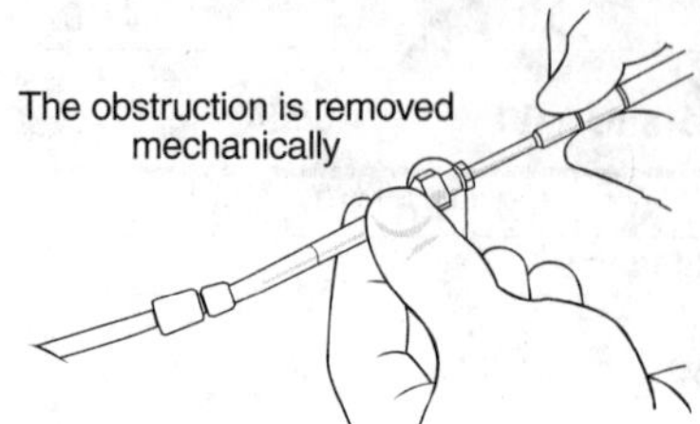

A CVA that has become obstructed is addressed mechanically through the catheter lumen. The obstructive matter is on the interior of the catheter lumen

Explanation

Intraluminal obstructive material, such as a thrombus or fibrin sheath, is removed from inside a central venous device through the lumen of the device. This does not require a separate access incision. The central venous catheter is first checked that it can aspirate and flush forward. The obstructing material is disrupted and removed mechanically by using an angioplasty balloon or other catheter introduced into the central venous catheter through its entry site on the skin. The catheter is checked for unimpeded, restored flow and the process may be repeated until the central venous catheter is cleared.

Coding Tips

Do not report 36593 in addition to 36596. For venous catheterization, see 36010–36012. For radiological supervision and interpretation, see 75902.

ICD-10-CM Diagnostic Codes

T82.49XA Other complication of vascular dialysis catheter, initial encounter

T82.594A Other mechanical complication of infusion catheter, initial encounter

T82.598A Other mechanical complication of other cardiac and vascular devices and implants, initial encounter

T82.818A Embolism due to vascular prosthetic devices, implants and grafts, initial encounter

T82.828A Fibrosis due to vascular prosthetic devices, implants and grafts, initial encounter

T82.856A Stenosis of peripheral vascular stent, initial encounter

T82.858A Stenosis of other vascular prosthetic devices, implants and grafts, initial encounter

T82.868A Thrombosis due to vascular prosthetic devices, implants and grafts, initial encounter

T82.898A Other specified complication of vascular prosthetic devices, implants and grafts, initial encounter

Z45.2 Encounter for adjustment and management of vascular access device

AMA: 36596 2018,Jan,8; 2017,Jan,8; 2016,Jan,13; 2015,Jan,16; 2014,Jan,11

Relative Value Units/Medicare Edits

Non-Facility RVU	Work	PE	MP	Total
36596	0.75	2.72	0.1	3.57
Facility RVU	**Work**	**PE**	**MP**	**Total**
36596	0.75	0.43	0.1	1.28

	FUD	Status	MUE	Modifiers				IOM Reference
36596	0	A	2(3)	51	N/A	N/A	N/A	None

* with documentation

Terms To Know

angioplasty. Reconstruction or repair of a diseased or damaged blood vessel.

aspiration. Drawing fluid out by suction.

complication. Condition arising after the beginning of observation and treatment that modifies the course of the patient's illness or the medical care required, or an undesired result or misadventure in medical care.

incision. Act of cutting into tissue or an organ.

lumen. Space inside an intestine, artery, vein, duct, or tube.

thrombus. Stationary blood clot inside a blood vessel.

36597

36597 Repositioning of previously placed central venous catheter under fluoroscopic guidance

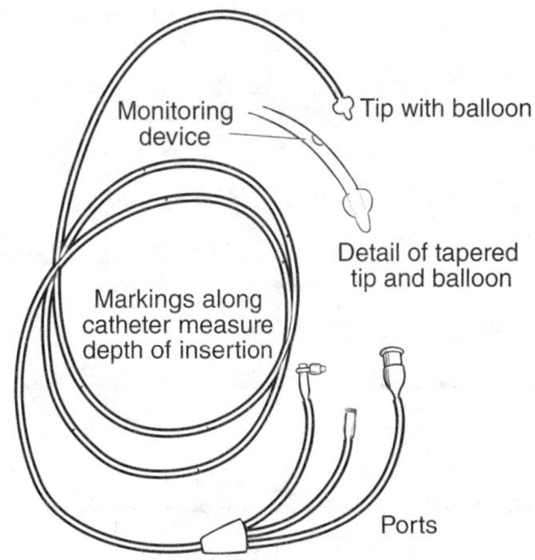

A central venous catheter is repositioned using fluoroscopic guidance, a type of live-image radiology

Explanation

A previously placed central venous catheter needs to be repositioned. It is possible for a catheter position to change significantly after the procedure is completed. Catheter position change and tip migration occur most often with subclavian venous access in women and obese patients, because the soft tissues of the chest wall move inferiorly with standing and often cause the catheter to get pulled back. When a catheter tip is incorrectly placed, it can increase the risks of thrombosis, fibrin sheath formation, perforation of the vein, and even arrhythmias. Fluoroscopy is used to check the positioning of the catheter tip and guide it to its correct position. Local anesthesia is given, and the sutures securing the cuff of the catheter may be freed from the skin. The catheter is partially withdrawn, and a sheath may be placed over the catheter at the existing venous access site. A guidewire is inserted through the catheter and advanced. The central venous catheter is maneuvered back into correct position and monitored with fluoroscopy to view correct placement of the tip.

Coding Tips

For fluoroscopic guidance, see 76000.

ICD-10-CM Diagnostic Codes

T82.41XA	Breakdown (mechanical) of vascular dialysis catheter, initial encounter
T82.42XA	Displacement of vascular dialysis catheter, initial encounter
T82.43XA	Leakage of vascular dialysis catheter, initial encounter
T82.49XA	Other complication of vascular dialysis catheter, initial encounter
T82.514A	Breakdown (mechanical) of infusion catheter, initial encounter
T82.524A	Displacement of infusion catheter, initial encounter
T82.534A	Leakage of infusion catheter, initial encounter
T82.594A	Other mechanical complication of infusion catheter, initial encounter
T82.598A	Other mechanical complication of other cardiac and vascular devices and implants, initial encounter

T82.898A	Other specified complication of vascular prosthetic devices, implants and grafts, initial encounter
Z45.2	Encounter for adjustment and management of vascular access device
Z45.89	Encounter for adjustment and management of other implanted devices
Z46.89	Encounter for fitting and adjustment of other specified devices

AMA: **36597** 2018,Jan,8; 2017,Jan,8; 2016,Jan,13; 2015,Jan,16; 2014,Sep,5; 2014,Jan,11

Relative Value Units/Medicare Edits

Non-Facility RVU	Work	PE	MP	Total
36597	1.21	2.35	0.13	3.69
Facility RVU	**Work**	**PE**	**MP**	**Total**
36597	1.21	0.43	0.13	1.77

	FUD	Status	MUE	Modifiers				IOM Reference
36597	0	A	2(3)	51	N/A	N/A	N/A	None

* with documentation

Terms To Know

arrhythmias. Heart disorder of rhythm or rate, due to an electrical conduction system malfunction.

catheter. Flexible tube inserted into an area of the body for introducing or withdrawing fluid.

fluoroscopy. Radiology technique that allows visual examination of part of the body or a function of an organ using a device that projects an x-ray image on a fluorescent screen.

guidewire. Flexible metal instrument designed to lead another instrument in its proper course.

introducer. Instrument, such as a catheter, needle, or tube, through which another instrument or device is introduced into the body.

soft tissue. Nonepithelial tissues outside of the skeleton that includes subcutaneous adipose tissue, fibrous tissue, fascia, muscles, blood and lymph vessels, and peripheral nervous system tissue.

thrombosis. Condition arising from the presence or formation of blood clots within a blood vessel that may cause vascular obstruction and insufficient oxygenation.

36598

36598 Contrast injection(s) for radiologic evaluation of existing central venous access device, including fluoroscopy, image documentation and report

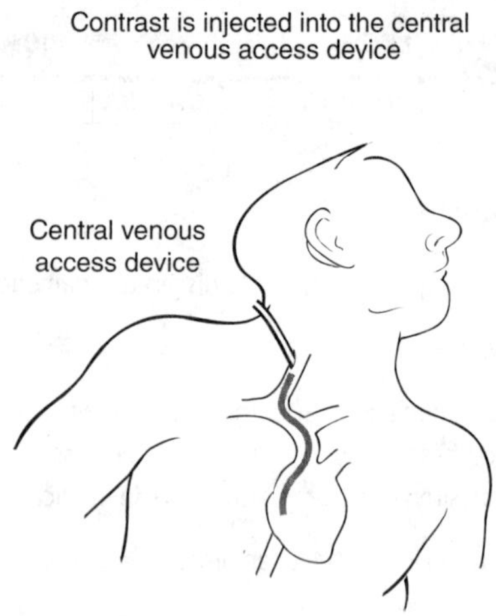

Explanation

A previously placed central venous access device is evaluated for complications that may be interfering with its proper functioning or the ability to draw blood from the catheter. Complications may include the presence of a fibrin sheath around the end of the catheter, migration of the catheter tip, patency of the tubing, kinking, fracture, or leaks. A small amount of contrast agent is injected into the catheter and the central venous access device is examined under fluoroscopy as the flow is evaluated. Images are documented and a radiological report is prepared.

Coding Tips

Fluoroscopic guidance is included in 36598. Do not report 36598 with 76000. Do not report mechanical removal of pericatheter obstructive material separately (36595). Do not report mechanical removal of intraluminal (intracatheter) obstructive material separately (36596). For complete diagnostic studies (venography), see 75820, 75825, and 75827.

ICD-10-CM Diagnostic Codes

T80.211A	Bloodstream infection due to central venous catheter, initial encounter
T80.212A	Local infection due to central venous catheter, initial encounter
T82.41XA	Breakdown (mechanical) of vascular dialysis catheter, initial encounter
T82.42XA	Displacement of vascular dialysis catheter, initial encounter
T82.43XA	Leakage of vascular dialysis catheter, initial encounter
T82.514A	Breakdown (mechanical) of infusion catheter, initial encounter
T82.524A	Displacement of infusion catheter, initial encounter
T82.534A	Leakage of infusion catheter, initial encounter
T82.594A	Other mechanical complication of infusion catheter, initial encounter
T82.598A	Other mechanical complication of other cardiac and vascular devices and implants, initial encounter
T82.7XXA	Infection and inflammatory reaction due to other cardiac and vascular devices, implants and grafts, initial encounter
T82.818A	Embolism due to vascular prosthetic devices, implants and grafts, initial encounter

T82.828A	Fibrosis due to vascular prosthetic devices, implants and grafts, initial encounter
T82.838A	Hemorrhage due to vascular prosthetic devices, implants and grafts, initial encounter
T82.848A	Pain due to vascular prosthetic devices, implants and grafts, initial encounter
T82.858A	Stenosis of other vascular prosthetic devices, implants and grafts, initial encounter
T82.868A	Thrombosis due to vascular prosthetic devices, implants and grafts, initial encounter
T82.898A	Other specified complication of vascular prosthetic devices, implants and grafts, initial encounter
Z45.2	Encounter for adjustment and management of vascular access device

AMA: 36598 2014,Jan,11

Relative Value Units/Medicare Edits

Non-Facility RVU	Work	PE	MP	Total
36598	0.74	2.49	0.07	3.3
Facility RVU	**Work**	**PE**	**MP**	**Total**
36598	0.74	0.25	0.07	1.06

	FUD	Status	MUE	Modifiers				IOM Reference
36598	0	T	2(3)	51	50	N/A	80*	None

* with documentation

Terms To Know

central venous access device. Catheter or other device introduced through a large vein, such as the subclavian or femoral vein, terminating in the superior or inferior vena cava or the right atrium and used to measure venous pressure or administer medication or fluids.

contrast material. Radiopaque substance placed into the body to enable a system or body structure to be visualized, such as nonionic and low osmolar contrast media (LOCM), ionic and high osmolar contrast media (HOCM), barium, and gadolinium.

embolism. Obstruction of a blood vessel resulting from a clot or foreign substance.

fluoroscopy. Radiology technique that allows visual examination of part of the body or a function of an organ using a device that projects an x-ray image on a fluorescent screen.

injection. Forcing a liquid substance into a body part such as a joint or muscle.

stenosis. Narrowing or constriction of a passage.

36600

36600 Arterial puncture, withdrawal of blood for diagnosis

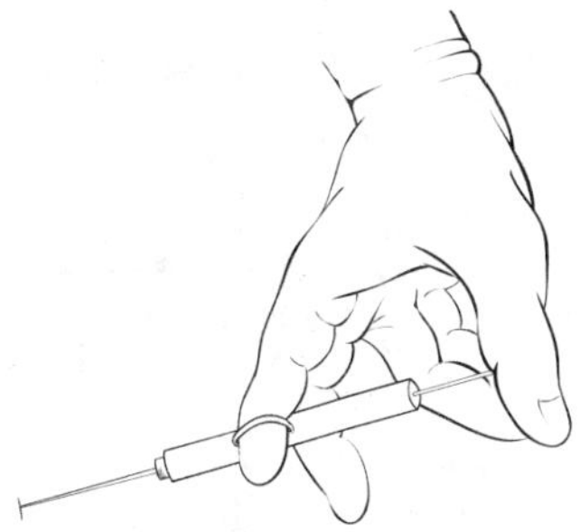

Any artery is punctured by a needle to withdraw blood for testing

Explanation

The physician inserts a needle through the skin and punctures the artery to withdraw blood for testing. No catheter is left in the artery. Pressure is applied to the puncture site to stop the flow of blood.

Coding Tips

Report 36600 only once when multiple tests are performed on the same arterial blood draw. This procedure does not include laboratory analysis. If specimen is transported to an outside laboratory, report 99000 for handling or conveyance. This service is included in the codes for critical care services including 99291-99292 and 99468-99476.

ICD-10-CM Diagnostic Codes

The application of this code is too broad to adequately present ICD-10-CM diagnostic code links here. Refer to your ICD-10-CM book.

AMA: 36600 2019,Aug,8; 2018,Jan,8; 2017,Jan,8; 2016,Jan,13; 2015,Jan,16; 2014,May,4; 2014,Jan,11

Relative Value Units/Medicare Edits

Non-Facility RVU	Work	PE	MP	Total
36600	0.32	0.52	0.03	0.87
Facility RVU	**Work**	**PE**	**MP**	**Total**
36600	0.32	0.1	0.03	0.45

	FUD	Status	MUE	Modifiers				IOM Reference
36600	N/A	A	4(3)	51	N/A	N/A	N/A	None

* with documentation

36620-36640

36620 Arterial catheterization or cannulation for sampling, monitoring or transfusion (separate procedure); percutaneous

36625 cutdown

36640 Arterial catheterization for prolonged infusion therapy (chemotherapy), cutdown

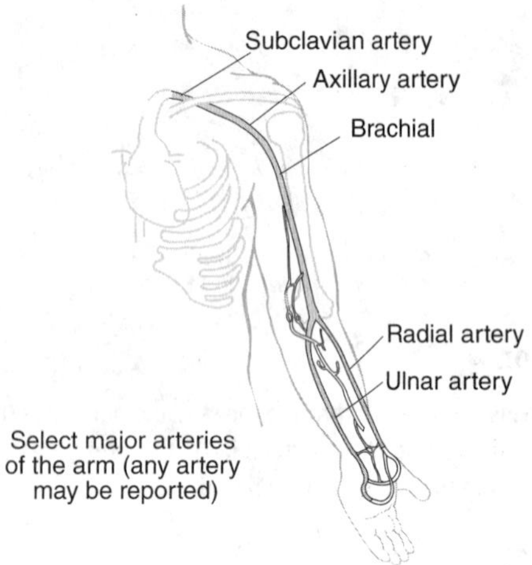

An artery is percutaneously catheterized or cannulized for sampling, monitoring, or for transfusion

Explanation

The physician accesses, in most cases, the ulnar or radial artery to insert a cannula, or tube-shaped portal. In 36620, the physician inserts a needle through the skin to puncture the artery, and then inserts a cannula. In 36625, the physician makes an incision in the skin overlying the artery and dissects the surrounding tissue to access it. The artery is sometimes nicked with a thin-bladed scalpel before the physician inserts the cannula. This cannula acts as a portal for sampling, monitoring or transfusion. Once the procedure is complete, the cannula is removed. In an open procedure, the opening in the artery may be sutured and the incision repaired with a layered closure. Pressure is applied to the puncture if a percutaneous approach is used. In 36640, the physician accesses the artery supplying the area to be treated. To insert a cannula, or tube-shaped portal for prolonged infusion therapy, the physician makes an incision above the artery and dissects the surrounding tissue to access it. The artery is sometimes nicked with a thin-bladed scalpel before the physician inserts the catheter. The catheter may be advanced to a site immediately upstream of the site to be treated. This catheter acts as a portal for the infusion of chemotherapy drugs and will remain in place until chemotherapy is completed. The catheter is removed, the hole in the artery is repaired, and the incision is repaired with a layered closure.

Coding Tips

Codes 36620 and 36625, separate procedures by definition, are usually a component of a more complex service and are not identified separately. When performed alone or with other unrelated procedures/services, they may be reported. If performed alone, list the code; if performed with other procedures/services, list the code and append modifier 59 or an X{EPSU} modifier. As exempt from modifier 51, 36620 has not been designated in CPT as an add-on service/procedure. However, codes identified as exempt from modifier 51 are not subject to multiple procedure rules. No reimbursement reduction or modifier 51 is applied. Code 36620 is included in critical care codes 99468–99476. These codes include only the insertion of the catheter. For transfusion via venous access, see 36430–36460. For occlusion therapy via arterial catheterization, see 75894. For chemotherapy administration, see 96420–96425.

ICD-10-CM Diagnostic Codes

The application of this code is too broad to adequately present ICD-10-CM diagnostic code links here. Refer to your ICD-10-CM book.

AMA: **36620** 2018,Jan,8; 2017,Jan,8; 2016,Jan,13; 2015,Jan,16; 2014,Jan,11 **36625** 2018,Jan,8; 2017,Jan,8; 2016,Jan,13; 2015,Jan,16; 2014,Jan,11 **36640** 2018,Jan,8; 2017,Jan,8; 2016,Jan,13; 2015,Jan,16; 2014,Jan,11

Relative Value Units/Medicare Edits

Non-Facility RVU	Work	PE	MP	Total
36620	1.0	0.2	0.08	1.28
36625	2.11	0.61	0.33	3.05
36640	2.1	1.05	0.15	3.3
Facility RVU	**Work**	**PE**	**MP**	**Total**
36620	1.0	0.2	0.08	1.28
36625	2.11	0.61	0.33	3.05
36640	2.1	1.05	0.15	3.3

	FUD	Status	MUE	Modifiers				IOM Reference
36620	0	A	3(3)	N/A	N/A	N/A	N/A	100-03,110.7; 100-03,110.8
36625	0	A	2(3)	N/A	N/A	N/A	N/A	
36640	0	A	1(3)	51	N/A	N/A	N/A	

* with documentation

Terms To Know

artery. Vessel through which oxygenated blood passes away from the heart to any part of the body.

cannula. Tube inserted into a blood vessel, duct, or body cavity to facilitate passage.

chemotherapy. Treatment of disease, especially cancerous conditions, using chemical agents.

incision. Act of cutting into tissue or an organ.

infusion. Introduction of a therapeutic fluid, other than blood, into the bloodstream.

percutaneous. Through the skin.

suture. Numerous stitching techniques employed in wound closure.

transfusion. Process of transferring whole blood or blood components from one person, the donor, to another person, the recipient, or the process of taking liquid from one vessel and putting it into another.

36680

36680 Placement of needle for intraosseous infusion

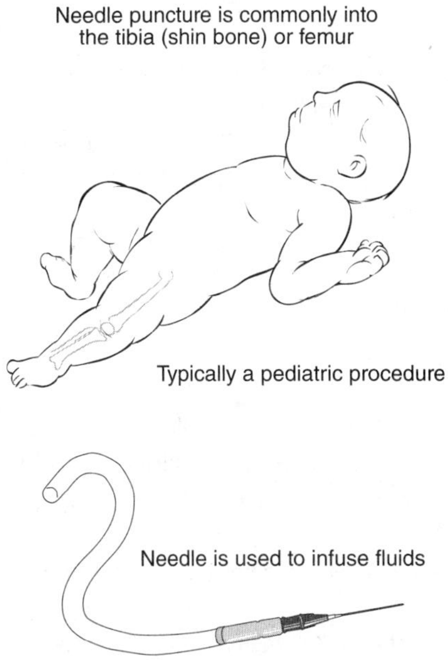

Explanation

The physician inserts a hollow needle through the skin and through the muscle tissue to puncture the bone marrow cavity, usually in the tibia or femur, of a patient whose vessels otherwise seem inaccessible. This needle is used as a method of infusing fluids into the blood vessels in the bone marrow.

Coding Tips

This is typically a pediatric procedure for severe dehydration. When 36680 is performed with another distinct or independent procedure, in which the procedures are not normally performed on the same day, and another modifier does not apply (e.g., modifier 51), the highest dollar value code is listed as the primary procedure and subsequent procedures are appended with modifier 59 or an X{EPSU} modifier. For IV infusion for hydration, see 96360–96361. For IV infusion for therapy/diagnosis, administered by physician or under direct supervision of a physician, see 96365–96368.

ICD-10-CM Diagnostic Codes

E66.01	Morbid (severe) obesity due to excess calories
E66.09	Other obesity due to excess calories
E66.1	Drug-induced obesity
E66.2	Morbid (severe) obesity with alveolar hypoventilation
E66.8	Other obesity
E86.0	Dehydration
E86.1	Hypovolemia
G40.001	Localization-related (focal) (partial) idiopathic epilepsy and epileptic syndromes with seizures of localized onset, not intractable, with status epilepticus
G40.011	Localization-related (focal) (partial) idiopathic epilepsy and epileptic syndromes with seizures of localized onset, intractable, with status epilepticus
G40.101	Localization-related (focal) (partial) symptomatic epilepsy and epileptic syndromes with simple partial seizures, not intractable, with status epilepticus
G40.111	Localization-related (focal) (partial) symptomatic epilepsy and epileptic syndromes with simple partial seizures, intractable, with status epilepticus
G40.201	Localization-related (focal) (partial) symptomatic epilepsy and epileptic syndromes with complex partial seizures, not intractable, with status epilepticus
G40.211	Localization-related (focal) (partial) symptomatic epilepsy and epileptic syndromes with complex partial seizures, intractable, with status epilepticus
G40.301	Generalized idiopathic epilepsy and epileptic syndromes, not intractable, with status epilepticus
G40.311	Generalized idiopathic epilepsy and epileptic syndromes, intractable, with status epilepticus
G40.401	Other generalized epilepsy and epileptic syndromes, not intractable, with status epilepticus
G40.411	Other generalized epilepsy and epileptic syndromes, intractable, with status epilepticus
G40.501	Epileptic seizures related to external causes, not intractable, with status epilepticus
G40.801	Other epilepsy, not intractable, with status epilepticus
G40.803	Other epilepsy, intractable, with status epilepticus
G40.811	Lennox-Gastaut syndrome, not intractable, with status epilepticus
G40.813	Lennox-Gastaut syndrome, intractable, with status epilepticus
G40.821	Epileptic spasms, not intractable, with status epilepticus
G40.823	Epileptic spasms, intractable, with status epilepticus
G40.89	Other seizures
G40.A01	Absence epileptic syndrome, not intractable, with status epilepticus
G40.A11	Absence epileptic syndrome, intractable, with status epilepticus
G40.B01	Juvenile myoclonic epilepsy, not intractable, with status epilepticus
G40.B11	Juvenile myoclonic epilepsy, intractable, with status epilepticus
P28.5	Respiratory failure of newborn
P28.81	Respiratory arrest of newborn
P29.81	Cardiac arrest of newborn
P29.89	Other cardiovascular disorders originating in the perinatal period
R09.2	Respiratory arrest
R57.1	Hypovolemic shock

AMA: **36680** 2018,Jan,8; 2017,Jan,8; 2016,Jan,13; 2015,Jan,16; 2014,Jan,11

Relative Value Units/Medicare Edits

Non-Facility RVU	Work	PE	MP	Total
36680	1.2	0.31	0.18	1.69
Facility RVU	**Work**	**PE**	**MP**	**Total**
36680	1.2	0.31	0.18	1.69

	FUD	Status	MUE	Modifiers				IOM Reference
36680	0	A	1(3)	51	N/A	N/A	80*	None

* with documentation

36800

36800 Insertion of cannula for hemodialysis, other purpose (separate procedure); vein to vein

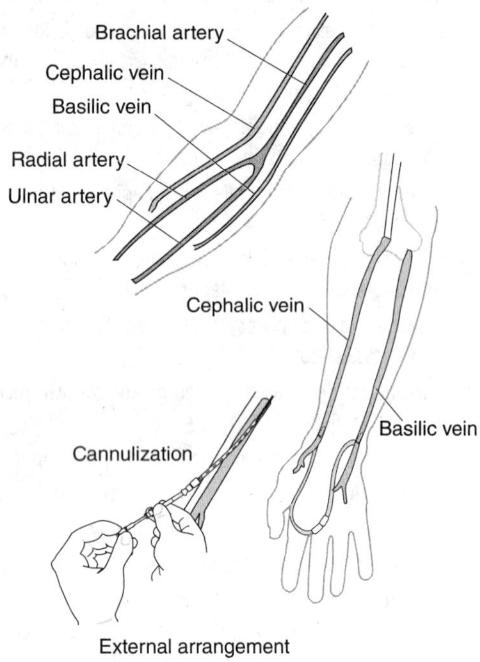

Vein-to-vein cannulization is established, usually for dialysis

Explanation

The physician isolates two veins, usually in the nondominant forearm, and inserts a needle through the skin and into each vessel. A guidance wire may be threaded through the needle into each vessel. The needle is removed. An end of a single cannula is inserted into each puncture, and any guidance wire removed. The cannula remains external, and may be left in place for several days. (This hemodialysis cannula is used to remove blood from the vein, route it through the dialysis machine, then reinfuse it.)

Coding Tips

This separate procedure by definition is usually a component of a more complex service and is not identified separately. When performed alone or with other unrelated procedures/services, it may be reported. If performed alone, list the code; if performed with other procedures/services, list the code and append modifier 59 or X{EPSU}. This type of hemodialysis cannula is infrequently used; verify this is the correct code by obtaining a copy of the cannula label from the medical record. This code includes venipuncture when performed by the physician. If the hemodialysis procedure is done intraoperatively and is a standard and necessary part of the main procedure during the same surgical session, the cannula insertion should not be reported separately.

ICD-10-CM Diagnostic Codes

D59.3	Hemolytic-uremic syndrome
E87.2	Acidosis
E87.5	Hyperkalemia
I12.0	Hypertensive chronic kidney disease with stage 5 chronic kidney disease or end stage renal disease
I12.9	Hypertensive chronic kidney disease with stage 1 through stage 4 chronic kidney disease, or unspecified chronic kidney disease
I13.0	Hypertensive heart and chronic kidney disease with heart failure and stage 1 through stage 4 chronic kidney disease, or unspecified chronic kidney disease
I13.10	Hypertensive heart and chronic kidney disease without heart failure, with stage 1 through stage 4 chronic kidney disease, or unspecified chronic kidney disease
I13.11	Hypertensive heart and chronic kidney disease without heart failure, with stage 5 chronic kidney disease, or end stage renal disease
I13.2	Hypertensive heart and chronic kidney disease with heart failure and with stage 5 chronic kidney disease, or end stage renal disease
I16.0	Hypertensive urgency
I16.1	Hypertensive emergency
I82.3	Embolism and thrombosis of renal vein
N00.0	Acute nephritic syndrome with minor glomerular abnormality
N00.1	Acute nephritic syndrome with focal and segmental glomerular lesions
N00.2	Acute nephritic syndrome with diffuse membranous glomerulonephritis
N00.3	Acute nephritic syndrome with diffuse mesangial proliferative glomerulonephritis
N00.4	Acute nephritic syndrome with diffuse endocapillary proliferative glomerulonephritis
N00.5	Acute nephritic syndrome with diffuse mesangiocapillary glomerulonephritis
N00.6	Acute nephritic syndrome with dense deposit disease
N00.7	Acute nephritic syndrome with diffuse crescentic glomerulonephritis
N01.0	Rapidly progressive nephritic syndrome with minor glomerular abnormality
N01.1	Rapidly progressive nephritic syndrome with focal and segmental glomerular lesions
N01.2	Rapidly progressive nephritic syndrome with diffuse membranous glomerulonephritis
N01.3	Rapidly progressive nephritic syndrome with diffuse mesangial proliferative glomerulonephritis
N01.4	Rapidly progressive nephritic syndrome with diffuse endocapillary proliferative glomerulonephritis
N01.5	Rapidly progressive nephritic syndrome with diffuse mesangiocapillary glomerulonephritis
N01.6	Rapidly progressive nephritic syndrome with dense deposit disease
N01.7	Rapidly progressive nephritic syndrome with diffuse crescentic glomerulonephritis
N03.0	Chronic nephritic syndrome with minor glomerular abnormality
N03.1	Chronic nephritic syndrome with focal and segmental glomerular lesions
N03.2	Chronic nephritic syndrome with diffuse membranous glomerulonephritis
N03.3	Chronic nephritic syndrome with diffuse mesangial proliferative glomerulonephritis
N03.4	Chronic nephritic syndrome with diffuse endocapillary proliferative glomerulonephritis

N03.5	Chronic nephritic syndrome with diffuse mesangiocapillary glomerulonephritis
N03.6	Chronic nephritic syndrome with dense deposit disease
N03.7	Chronic nephritic syndrome with diffuse crescentic glomerulonephritis
N04.0	Nephrotic syndrome with minor glomerular abnormality
N04.1	Nephrotic syndrome with focal and segmental glomerular lesions
N04.2	Nephrotic syndrome with diffuse membranous glomerulonephritis
N04.3	Nephrotic syndrome with diffuse mesangial proliferative glomerulonephritis
N04.4	Nephrotic syndrome with diffuse endocapillary proliferative glomerulonephritis
N04.5	Nephrotic syndrome with diffuse mesangiocapillary glomerulonephritis
N04.6	Nephrotic syndrome with dense deposit disease
N04.7	Nephrotic syndrome with diffuse crescentic glomerulonephritis
N08	Glomerular disorders in diseases classified elsewhere
N10	Acute pyelonephritis
N11.0	Nonobstructive reflux-associated chronic pyelonephritis
N11.1	Chronic obstructive pyelonephritis
N12	Tubulo-interstitial nephritis, not specified as acute or chronic
N15.8	Other specified renal tubulo-interstitial diseases
N16	Renal tubulo-interstitial disorders in diseases classified elsewhere
N17.0	Acute kidney failure with tubular necrosis
N17.1	Acute kidney failure with acute cortical necrosis
N17.2	Acute kidney failure with medullary necrosis
N17.8	Other acute kidney failure
N18.4	Chronic kidney disease, stage 4 (severe)
N18.5	Chronic kidney disease, stage 5
N18.6	End stage renal disease

AMA: 36800 2018,Jan,8; 2017,Jan,8; 2016,Jan,13; 2015,Jan,16; 2014,Jan,11

Relative Value Units/Medicare Edits

Non-Facility RVU	Work	PE	MP	Total
36800	2.43	0.78	0.32	3.53
Facility RVU	**Work**	**PE**	**MP**	**Total**
36800	2.43	0.78	0.32	3.53

	FUD	Status	MUE	Modifiers				IOM Reference
36800	0	A	1(3)	51	N/A	N/A	N/A	None

* with documentation

Terms To Know

cannula. Tube inserted into a blood vessel, duct, or body cavity to facilitate passage.

nephrotic syndrome. Condition where levels of albumin in the blood and urine are far below the norm.

36810

36810 Insertion of cannula for hemodialysis, other purpose (separate procedure); arteriovenous, external (Scribner type)

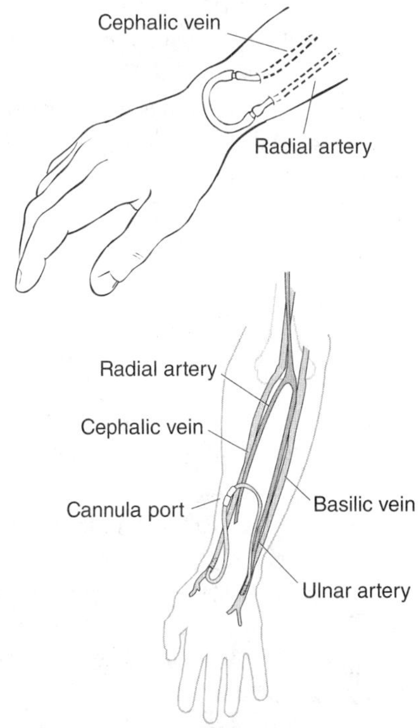

One end of the cannula is inserted into the artery and the other end is inserted into the vein to create a portal for hemodialysis

Explanation

The physician isolates an artery and a vein, usually in the nondominant forearm, and inserts a needle through the skin and into each vessel. A guidewire may be threaded through the needle into each vessel. The needle is removed. An end of a single cannula is inserted into each puncture, and any guidance wire removed. The Scribner cannula remains external, and may be left in place for several days. (This hemodialysis cannula is used to remove blood from the vessel, route it through the dialysis machine, then reinfuse it.)

Coding Tips

This separate procedure by definition is usually a component of a more complex service and is not identified separately. When performed alone or with other unrelated procedures/services, it may be reported. If performed alone, list the code; if performed with other procedures/services, list the code and append modifier 59 or an X{EPSU} modifier. This type of hemodialysis cannula is infrequently used; verify this is the correct code by obtaining a copy of the cannula label from the medical record. This code includes venipuncture when performed by the physician. If the hemodialysis procedure is done intraoperatively and is a standard and necessary part of the main procedure during the same surgical session, the cannula insertion should not be reported separately.

ICD-10-CM Diagnostic Codes

D59.3	Hemolytic-uremic syndrome
E87.2	Acidosis
E87.5	Hyperkalemia
I12.0	Hypertensive chronic kidney disease with stage 5 chronic kidney disease or end stage renal disease

I12.9 Hypertensive chronic kidney disease with stage 1 through stage 4 chronic kidney disease, or unspecified chronic kidney disease

I13.0 Hypertensive heart and chronic kidney disease with heart failure and stage 1 through stage 4 chronic kidney disease, or unspecified chronic kidney disease

I13.10 Hypertensive heart and chronic kidney disease without heart failure, with stage 1 through stage 4 chronic kidney disease, or unspecified chronic kidney disease

I13.11 Hypertensive heart and chronic kidney disease without heart failure, with stage 5 chronic kidney disease, or end stage renal disease

I13.2 Hypertensive heart and chronic kidney disease with heart failure and with stage 5 chronic kidney disease, or end stage renal disease

I16.0 Hypertensive urgency

I16.1 Hypertensive emergency

I82.3 Embolism and thrombosis of renal vein

N00.0 Acute nephritic syndrome with minor glomerular abnormality

N00.1 Acute nephritic syndrome with focal and segmental glomerular lesions

N00.2 Acute nephritic syndrome with diffuse membranous glomerulonephritis

N00.3 Acute nephritic syndrome with diffuse mesangial proliferative glomerulonephritis

N00.4 Acute nephritic syndrome with diffuse endocapillary proliferative glomerulonephritis

N00.5 Acute nephritic syndrome with diffuse mesangiocapillary glomerulonephritis

N00.6 Acute nephritic syndrome with dense deposit disease

N00.7 Acute nephritic syndrome with diffuse crescentic glomerulonephritis

N01.0 Rapidly progressive nephritic syndrome with minor glomerular abnormality

N01.1 Rapidly progressive nephritic syndrome with focal and segmental glomerular lesions

N01.2 Rapidly progressive nephritic syndrome with diffuse membranous glomerulonephritis

N01.3 Rapidly progressive nephritic syndrome with diffuse mesangial proliferative glomerulonephritis

N01.4 Rapidly progressive nephritic syndrome with diffuse endocapillary proliferative glomerulonephritis

N01.5 Rapidly progressive nephritic syndrome with diffuse mesangiocapillary glomerulonephritis

N01.6 Rapidly progressive nephritic syndrome with dense deposit disease

N01.7 Rapidly progressive nephritic syndrome with diffuse crescentic glomerulonephritis

N03.0 Chronic nephritic syndrome with minor glomerular abnormality

N03.1 Chronic nephritic syndrome with focal and segmental glomerular lesions

N03.2 Chronic nephritic syndrome with diffuse membranous glomerulonephritis

N03.3 Chronic nephritic syndrome with diffuse mesangial proliferative glomerulonephritis

N03.4 Chronic nephritic syndrome with diffuse endocapillary proliferative glomerulonephritis

N03.5 Chronic nephritic syndrome with diffuse mesangiocapillary glomerulonephritis

N03.6 Chronic nephritic syndrome with dense deposit disease

N03.7 Chronic nephritic syndrome with diffuse crescentic glomerulonephritis

N04.0 Nephrotic syndrome with minor glomerular abnormality

N04.1 Nephrotic syndrome with focal and segmental glomerular lesions

N04.2 Nephrotic syndrome with diffuse membranous glomerulonephritis

N04.3 Nephrotic syndrome with diffuse mesangial proliferative glomerulonephritis

N04.4 Nephrotic syndrome with diffuse endocapillary proliferative glomerulonephritis

N04.5 Nephrotic syndrome with diffuse mesangiocapillary glomerulonephritis

N04.6 Nephrotic syndrome with dense deposit disease

N04.7 Nephrotic syndrome with diffuse crescentic glomerulonephritis

N08 Glomerular disorders in diseases classified elsewhere

N10 Acute pyelonephritis

N11.0 Nonobstructive reflux-associated chronic pyelonephritis

N11.1 Chronic obstructive pyelonephritis

N12 Tubulo-interstitial nephritis, not specified as acute or chronic

N15.8 Other specified renal tubulo-interstitial diseases

N16 Renal tubulo-interstitial disorders in diseases classified elsewhere

N17.0 Acute kidney failure with tubular necrosis

N17.1 Acute kidney failure with acute cortical necrosis

N17.2 Acute kidney failure with medullary necrosis

N17.8 Other acute kidney failure

N18.4 Chronic kidney disease, stage 4 (severe)

N18.5 Chronic kidney disease, stage 5

N18.6 End stage renal disease

AMA: **36810** 2018,Jan,8; 2017,Jan,8; 2016,Jan,13; 2015,Jan,16; 2014,Jan,11

Relative Value Units/Medicare Edits

Non-Facility RVU	Work	PE	MP	Total
36810	3.96	1.54	0.55	6.05
Facility RVU	**Work**	**PE**	**MP**	**Total**
36810	3.96	1.54	0.55	6.05

	FUD	Status	MUE	Modifiers				IOM Reference
36810	0	A	1(3)	51	N/A	N/A	N/A	None

* with documentation

Terms To Know

cannula. Tube inserted into a blood vessel, duct, or body cavity to facilitate passage.

guidewire. Flexible metal instrument designed to lead another instrument in its proper course.

36815

36815 Insertion of cannula for hemodialysis, other purpose (separate procedure); arteriovenous, external revision, or closure

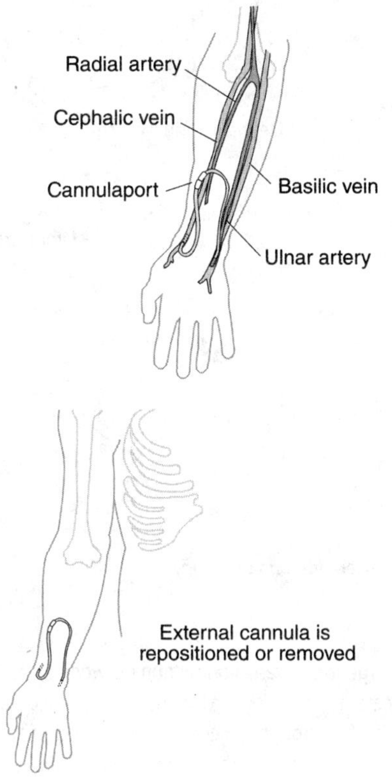

Explanation

The physician repositions an external cannula or removes it. The cannula forms a ready connection between the artery and vein or vein and vein for hemodialysis or another purpose. Closure of the insertion site is performed using sutures on the vessels or skin as necessary.

Coding Tips

This separate procedure by definition is usually a component of a more complex service and is not identified separately. When performed alone or with other unrelated procedures/services, it may be reported. If performed alone, list the code; if performed with other procedures/services, list the code and append modifier 59 or an X{EPSU} modifier. This type of hemodialysis cannula is infrequently used; verify this is the correct code by obtaining a copy of the cannula label from the medical record. This code includes venipuncture when performed by the physician. If the hemodialysis procedure is done intraoperatively and is a standard and necessary part of the main procedure during the same surgical session, the cannula insertion should not be reported separately.

ICD-10-CM Diagnostic Codes

D59.3	Hemolytic-uremic syndrome
E87.2	Acidosis
E87.5	Hyperkalemia
I12.0	Hypertensive chronic kidney disease with stage 5 chronic kidney disease or end stage renal disease
I12.9	Hypertensive chronic kidney disease with stage 1 through stage 4 chronic kidney disease, or unspecified chronic kidney disease
I13.0	Hypertensive heart and chronic kidney disease with heart failure and stage 1 through stage 4 chronic kidney disease, or unspecified chronic kidney disease
I13.10	Hypertensive heart and chronic kidney disease without heart failure, with stage 1 through stage 4 chronic kidney disease, or unspecified chronic kidney disease
I13.11	Hypertensive heart and chronic kidney disease without heart failure, with stage 5 chronic kidney disease, or end stage renal disease
I13.2	Hypertensive heart and chronic kidney disease with heart failure and with stage 5 chronic kidney disease, or end stage renal disease
I16.0	Hypertensive urgency
I16.1	Hypertensive emergency
I82.3	Embolism and thrombosis of renal vein
N00.0	Acute nephritic syndrome with minor glomerular abnormality
N00.1	Acute nephritic syndrome with focal and segmental glomerular lesions
N00.2	Acute nephritic syndrome with diffuse membranous glomerulonephritis
N00.3	Acute nephritic syndrome with diffuse mesangial proliferative glomerulonephritis
N00.4	Acute nephritic syndrome with diffuse endocapillary proliferative glomerulonephritis
N00.5	Acute nephritic syndrome with diffuse mesangiocapillary glomerulonephritis
N00.6	Acute nephritic syndrome with dense deposit disease
N00.7	Acute nephritic syndrome with diffuse crescentic glomerulonephritis
N01.0	Rapidly progressive nephritic syndrome with minor glomerular abnormality
N01.1	Rapidly progressive nephritic syndrome with focal and segmental glomerular lesions
N01.2	Rapidly progressive nephritic syndrome with diffuse membranous glomerulonephritis
N01.3	Rapidly progressive nephritic syndrome with diffuse mesangial proliferative glomerulonephritis
N01.4	Rapidly progressive nephritic syndrome with diffuse endocapillary proliferative glomerulonephritis
N01.5	Rapidly progressive nephritic syndrome with diffuse mesangiocapillary glomerulonephritis
N01.6	Rapidly progressive nephritic syndrome with dense deposit disease
N01.7	Rapidly progressive nephritic syndrome with diffuse crescentic glomerulonephritis
N03.0	Chronic nephritic syndrome with minor glomerular abnormality
N03.1	Chronic nephritic syndrome with focal and segmental glomerular lesions
N03.2	Chronic nephritic syndrome with diffuse membranous glomerulonephritis
N03.3	Chronic nephritic syndrome with diffuse mesangial proliferative glomerulonephritis
N03.4	Chronic nephritic syndrome with diffuse endocapillary proliferative glomerulonephritis
N03.5	Chronic nephritic syndrome with diffuse mesangiocapillary glomerulonephritis
N03.6	Chronic nephritic syndrome with dense deposit disease

N03.7	Chronic nephritic syndrome with diffuse crescentic glomerulonephritis
N04.0	Nephrotic syndrome with minor glomerular abnormality
N04.1	Nephrotic syndrome with focal and segmental glomerular lesions
N04.2	Nephrotic syndrome with diffuse membranous glomerulonephritis
N04.3	Nephrotic syndrome with diffuse mesangial proliferative glomerulonephritis
N04.4	Nephrotic syndrome with diffuse endocapillary proliferative glomerulonephritis
N04.5	Nephrotic syndrome with diffuse mesangiocapillary glomerulonephritis
N04.6	Nephrotic syndrome with dense deposit disease
N04.7	Nephrotic syndrome with diffuse crescentic glomerulonephritis
N10	Acute pyelonephritis
N11.0	Nonobstructive reflux-associated chronic pyelonephritis
N11.1	Chronic obstructive pyelonephritis
N17.0	Acute kidney failure with tubular necrosis
N17.1	Acute kidney failure with acute cortical necrosis
N17.2	Acute kidney failure with medullary necrosis
N18.4	Chronic kidney disease, stage 4 (severe)
N18.5	Chronic kidney disease, stage 5
N18.6	End stage renal disease

AMA: **36815** 2018,Jan,8; 2017,Jan,8; 2016,Jan,13; 2015,Jan,16; 2014,Jan,11

Relative Value Units/Medicare Edits

Non-Facility RVU	Work	PE	MP	Total
36815	2.62	0.69	0.6	3.91
Facility RVU	**Work**	**PE**	**MP**	**Total**
36815	2.62	0.69	0.6	3.91

	FUD	Status	MUE	Modifiers				IOM Reference
36815	0	A	1(3)	51	N/A	N/A	N/A	None

* with documentation

Terms To Know

cannulation. Insertion of a flexible length of hollow tubing into a blood vessel, duct, or body cavity, usually for extracorporeal circulation or chemotherapy infusion to a particular region of the body.

complication. Condition arising after the beginning of observation and treatment that modifies the course of the patient's illness or the medical care required, or an undesired result or misadventure in medical care.

glomerulonephritis. Disease of the kidney with diffuse inflammation of the capillary loops of the glomeruli. It may be a complication of bacterial infection or immune disorders and can lead to renal failure and may be associated with hypertension or diabetes.

nephrotic syndrome. Condition where levels of albumin in the blood and urine are far below the norm.

renal glomerulohyalinosis-diabetic syndrome. High blood pressure and kidney failure resulting from a form of diabetes in which carbohydrate utilization is reduced and that of lipid and protein enhanced.

36818

36818 Arteriovenous anastomosis, open; by upper arm cephalic vein transposition

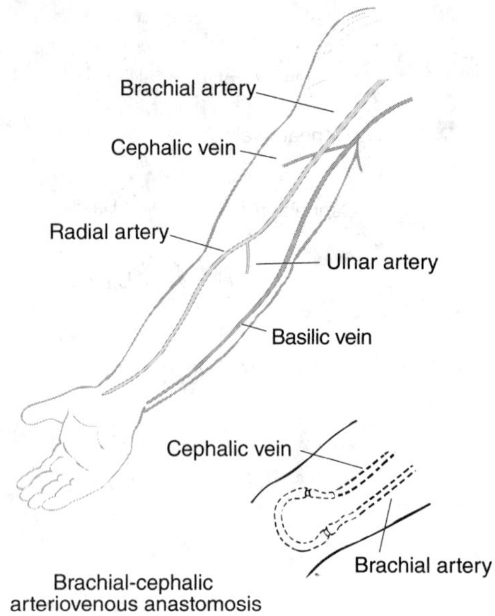

Explanation

A vascular surgeon creates a connection between an artery and a vein for a vascular access site in patients with end stage renal disease that require hemodialysis. The surgeon dissects down to the cephalic vein on the medial side of the upper arm and mobilizes the vein. A subcutaneous tunnel on the anterior side of the arm is created, and the mobilized cephalic vein is transposed to this tunnel and anastomosed to the brachial artery.

Coding Tips

This is a unilateral procedure. If performed bilaterally, some payers require that the service be reported twice with modifier 50 appended to the second code, while others require identification of the service only once with modifier 50 appended. Check with individual payers. Modifier 50 identifies a procedure performed identically on the opposite side of the body (mirror image). Do not report 36818 with 36819, 36820, 36821, or 36830 during a unilateral upper extremity procedure. For bilateral, upper extremity, open arteriovenous anastomosis performed at the same operative session, use modifier 50 or 59 as appropriate. When central dialysis segment angioplasty is performed with 36818–36833, see 36907. When central dialysis segment stent placement is performed with 36818–36833, see 36908.

ICD-10-CM Diagnostic Codes

D59.3	Hemolytic-uremic syndrome
I12.0	Hypertensive chronic kidney disease with stage 5 chronic kidney disease or end stage renal disease
I13.0	Hypertensive heart and chronic kidney disease with heart failure and stage 1 through stage 4 chronic kidney disease, or unspecified chronic kidney disease
I13.11	Hypertensive heart and chronic kidney disease without heart failure, with stage 5 chronic kidney disease, or end stage renal disease
I13.2	Hypertensive heart and chronic kidney disease with heart failure and with stage 5 chronic kidney disease, or end stage renal disease

I16.0 Hypertensive urgency
I16.1 Hypertensive emergency
I82.3 Embolism and thrombosis of renal vein
N00.0 Acute nephritic syndrome with minor glomerular abnormality
N00.1 Acute nephritic syndrome with focal and segmental glomerular lesions
N00.2 Acute nephritic syndrome with diffuse membranous glomerulonephritis
N00.3 Acute nephritic syndrome with diffuse mesangial proliferative glomerulonephritis
N00.4 Acute nephritic syndrome with diffuse endocapillary proliferative glomerulonephritis
N00.5 Acute nephritic syndrome with diffuse mesangiocapillary glomerulonephritis
N00.6 Acute nephritic syndrome with dense deposit disease
N00.7 Acute nephritic syndrome with diffuse crescentic glomerulonephritis
N00.8 Acute nephritic syndrome with other morphologic changes
N01.0 Rapidly progressive nephritic syndrome with minor glomerular abnormality
N01.1 Rapidly progressive nephritic syndrome with focal and segmental glomerular lesions
N01.2 Rapidly progressive nephritic syndrome with diffuse membranous glomerulonephritis
N01.3 Rapidly progressive nephritic syndrome with diffuse mesangial proliferative glomerulonephritis
N01.4 Rapidly progressive nephritic syndrome with diffuse endocapillary proliferative glomerulonephritis
N01.5 Rapidly progressive nephritic syndrome with diffuse mesangiocapillary glomerulonephritis
N01.6 Rapidly progressive nephritic syndrome with dense deposit disease
N01.7 Rapidly progressive nephritic syndrome with diffuse crescentic glomerulonephritis
N01.8 Rapidly progressive nephritic syndrome with other morphologic changes
N03.0 Chronic nephritic syndrome with minor glomerular abnormality
N03.1 Chronic nephritic syndrome with focal and segmental glomerular lesions
N03.2 Chronic nephritic syndrome with diffuse membranous glomerulonephritis
N03.3 Chronic nephritic syndrome with diffuse mesangial proliferative glomerulonephritis
N03.4 Chronic nephritic syndrome with diffuse endocapillary proliferative glomerulonephritis
N03.5 Chronic nephritic syndrome with diffuse mesangiocapillary glomerulonephritis
N03.6 Chronic nephritic syndrome with dense deposit disease
N03.7 Chronic nephritic syndrome with diffuse crescentic glomerulonephritis
N03.8 Chronic nephritic syndrome with other morphologic changes
N04.0 Nephrotic syndrome with minor glomerular abnormality
N04.1 Nephrotic syndrome with focal and segmental glomerular lesions
N04.2 Nephrotic syndrome with diffuse membranous glomerulonephritis
N04.3 Nephrotic syndrome with diffuse mesangial proliferative glomerulonephritis
N04.4 Nephrotic syndrome with diffuse endocapillary proliferative glomerulonephritis
N04.5 Nephrotic syndrome with diffuse mesangiocapillary glomerulonephritis
N04.6 Nephrotic syndrome with dense deposit disease
N04.7 Nephrotic syndrome with diffuse crescentic glomerulonephritis
N04.8 Nephrotic syndrome with other morphologic changes
N07.0 Hereditary nephropathy, not elsewhere classified with minor glomerular abnormality
N07.1 Hereditary nephropathy, not elsewhere classified with focal and segmental glomerular lesions
N07.2 Hereditary nephropathy, not elsewhere classified with diffuse membranous glomerulonephritis
N07.3 Hereditary nephropathy, not elsewhere classified with diffuse mesangial proliferative glomerulonephritis
N07.4 Hereditary nephropathy, not elsewhere classified with diffuse endocapillary proliferative glomerulonephritis
N07.5 Hereditary nephropathy, not elsewhere classified with diffuse mesangiocapillary glomerulonephritis
N07.6 Hereditary nephropathy, not elsewhere classified with dense deposit disease
N07.7 Hereditary nephropathy, not elsewhere classified with diffuse crescentic glomerulonephritis
N07.8 Hereditary nephropathy, not elsewhere classified with other morphologic lesions
N08 Glomerular disorders in diseases classified elsewhere
N10 Acute pyelonephritis
N11.0 Nonobstructive reflux-associated chronic pyelonephritis
N11.1 Chronic obstructive pyelonephritis
N11.8 Other chronic tubulo-interstitial nephritis
N12 Tubulo-interstitial nephritis, not specified as acute or chronic
N15.8 Other specified renal tubulo-interstitial diseases
N16 Renal tubulo-interstitial disorders in diseases classified elsewhere
N17.0 Acute kidney failure with tubular necrosis
N17.1 Acute kidney failure with acute cortical necrosis
N17.2 Acute kidney failure with medullary necrosis
N17.8 Other acute kidney failure
N18.4 Chronic kidney disease, stage 4 (severe)
N18.5 Chronic kidney disease, stage 5
N18.6 End stage renal disease

AMA: 36818 2018,Jan,8; 2017,Mar,3; 2017,Jan,8; 2016,Mar,10; 2016,Jan,13; 2015,Jan,16; 2014,Jan,11

Relative Value Units/Medicare Edits

Non-Facility RVU	Work	PE	MP	Total
36818	12.39	4.84	2.88	20.11
Facility RVU	**Work**	**PE**	**MP**	**Total**
36818	12.39	4.84	2.88	20.11

	FUD	Status	MUE	Modifiers				IOM Reference
36818	90	A	1(3)	51	N/A	62*	80	None

* with documentation

36819

36819 Arteriovenous anastomosis, open; by upper arm basilic vein transposition

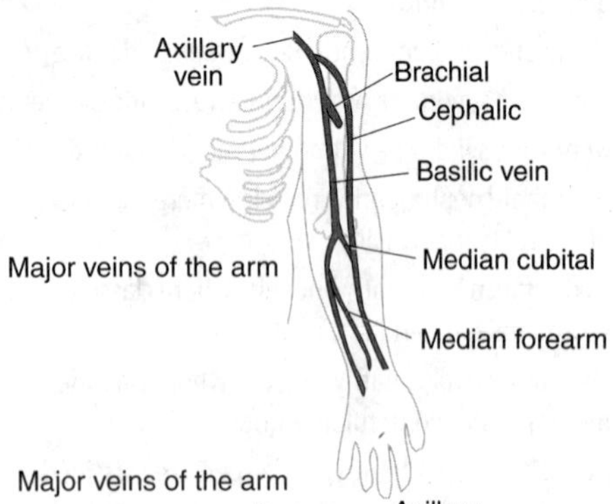

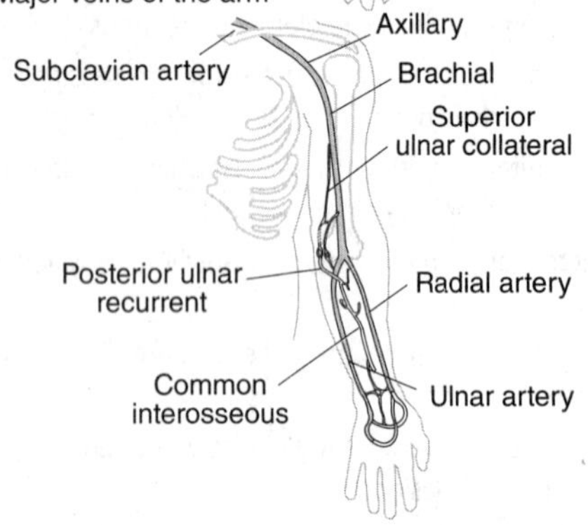

The basilic vein is transposed in an open arteriovenous anastomosis

Explanation

A vascular surgeon creates a connection between an artery and a vein for a vascular access site in patients with end-stage renal disease that require hemodialysis. The surgeon dissects down to the basilic vein on the medial side of the upper arm and mobilizes the vein. A subcutaneous tunnel on the anterior side of the arm is created and the mobilized basilic vein is transposed to this tunnel and anastomosed to the brachial artery.

Coding Tips

This is a unilateral procedure. If performed bilaterally, some payers require that the service be reported twice with modifier 50 appended to the second code, while others require identification of the service only once with modifier 50 appended. Check with individual payers. Modifier 50 identifies a procedure performed identically on the opposite side of the body (mirror image). Do not report 36819 with 36818, 36820, 36821, or 36830 during a unilateral upper extremity procedure. For bilateral, upper extremity, open arteriovenous anastomoses performed at the same operative session, use modifier 50 or 59 as appropriate. When central dialysis segment angioplasty is performed with 36818-36833, use 36907. When central dialysis segment stent placement is performed with 36818-36833, use 36908.

ICD-10-CM Diagnostic Codes

D59.3	Hemolytic-uremic syndrome
I12.0	Hypertensive chronic kidney disease with stage 5 chronic kidney disease or end stage renal disease
I13.0	Hypertensive heart and chronic kidney disease with heart failure and stage 1 through stage 4 chronic kidney disease, or unspecified chronic kidney disease
I13.11	Hypertensive heart and chronic kidney disease without heart failure, with stage 5 chronic kidney disease, or end stage renal disease
I13.2	Hypertensive heart and chronic kidney disease with heart failure and with stage 5 chronic kidney disease, or end stage renal disease
I16.0	Hypertensive urgency
I16.1	Hypertensive emergency
I82.3	Embolism and thrombosis of renal vein
N00.0	Acute nephritic syndrome with minor glomerular abnormality
N00.1	Acute nephritic syndrome with focal and segmental glomerular lesions
N00.2	Acute nephritic syndrome with diffuse membranous glomerulonephritis
N00.3	Acute nephritic syndrome with diffuse mesangial proliferative glomerulonephritis
N00.4	Acute nephritic syndrome with diffuse endocapillary proliferative glomerulonephritis
N00.5	Acute nephritic syndrome with diffuse mesangiocapillary glomerulonephritis
N00.6	Acute nephritic syndrome with dense deposit disease
N00.7	Acute nephritic syndrome with diffuse crescentic glomerulonephritis
N00.8	Acute nephritic syndrome with other morphologic changes
N01.0	Rapidly progressive nephritic syndrome with minor glomerular abnormality
N01.1	Rapidly progressive nephritic syndrome with focal and segmental glomerular lesions
N01.2	Rapidly progressive nephritic syndrome with diffuse membranous glomerulonephritis
N01.3	Rapidly progressive nephritic syndrome with diffuse mesangial proliferative glomerulonephritis
N01.4	Rapidly progressive nephritic syndrome with diffuse endocapillary proliferative glomerulonephritis
N01.5	Rapidly progressive nephritic syndrome with diffuse mesangiocapillary glomerulonephritis
N01.6	Rapidly progressive nephritic syndrome with dense deposit disease
N01.7	Rapidly progressive nephritic syndrome with diffuse crescentic glomerulonephritis
N01.8	Rapidly progressive nephritic syndrome with other morphologic changes
N03.0	Chronic nephritic syndrome with minor glomerular abnormality
N03.1	Chronic nephritic syndrome with focal and segmental glomerular lesions
N03.2	Chronic nephritic syndrome with diffuse membranous glomerulonephritis
N03.3	Chronic nephritic syndrome with diffuse mesangial proliferative glomerulonephritis
N03.4	Chronic nephritic syndrome with diffuse endocapillary proliferative glomerulonephritis
N03.5	Chronic nephritic syndrome with diffuse mesangiocapillary glomerulonephritis
N03.6	Chronic nephritic syndrome with dense deposit disease
N03.7	Chronic nephritic syndrome with diffuse crescentic glomerulonephritis

N03.8	Chronic nephritic syndrome with other morphologic changes
N04.0	Nephrotic syndrome with minor glomerular abnormality
N04.1	Nephrotic syndrome with focal and segmental glomerular lesions
N04.2	Nephrotic syndrome with diffuse membranous glomerulonephritis
N04.3	Nephrotic syndrome with diffuse mesangial proliferative glomerulonephritis
N04.4	Nephrotic syndrome with diffuse endocapillary proliferative glomerulonephritis
N04.5	Nephrotic syndrome with diffuse mesangiocapillary glomerulonephritis
N04.6	Nephrotic syndrome with dense deposit disease
N04.7	Nephrotic syndrome with diffuse crescentic glomerulonephritis
N04.8	Nephrotic syndrome with other morphologic changes
N07.0	Hereditary nephropathy, not elsewhere classified with minor glomerular abnormality
N07.1	Hereditary nephropathy, not elsewhere classified with focal and segmental glomerular lesions
N07.2	Hereditary nephropathy, not elsewhere classified with diffuse membranous glomerulonephritis
N07.3	Hereditary nephropathy, not elsewhere classified with diffuse mesangial proliferative glomerulonephritis
N07.4	Hereditary nephropathy, not elsewhere classified with diffuse endocapillary proliferative glomerulonephritis
N07.5	Hereditary nephropathy, not elsewhere classified with diffuse mesangiocapillary glomerulonephritis
N07.6	Hereditary nephropathy, not elsewhere classified with dense deposit disease
N07.7	Hereditary nephropathy, not elsewhere classified with diffuse crescentic glomerulonephritis
N07.8	Hereditary nephropathy, not elsewhere classified with other morphologic lesions
N08	Glomerular disorders in diseases classified elsewhere
N10	Acute pyelonephritis
N11.0	Nonobstructive reflux-associated chronic pyelonephritis
N11.1	Chronic obstructive pyelonephritis
N11.8	Other chronic tubulo-interstitial nephritis
N12	Tubulo-interstitial nephritis, not specified as acute or chronic
N15.8	Other specified renal tubulo-interstitial diseases
N16	Renal tubulo-interstitial disorders in diseases classified elsewhere
N17.0	Acute kidney failure with tubular necrosis
N17.1	Acute kidney failure with acute cortical necrosis
N17.2	Acute kidney failure with medullary necrosis
N17.8	Other acute kidney failure
N18.4	Chronic kidney disease, stage 4 (severe)
N18.5	Chronic kidney disease, stage 5
N18.6	End stage renal disease

AMA: 36819 2018,Jan,8; 2017,Mar,3; 2017,Jan,8; 2016,Jan,13; 2015,Jan,16; 2014,Jan,11

Relative Value Units/Medicare Edits

Non-Facility RVU	Work	PE	MP	Total
36819	13.29	4.83	3.07	21.19
Facility RVU	**Work**	**PE**	**MP**	**Total**
36819	13.29	4.83	3.07	21.19

	FUD	Status	MUE	Modifiers				IOM Reference
36819	90	A	1(3)	51	N/A	62*	80	None

* with documentation

Terms To Know

anastomosis. Surgically created connection between ducts, blood vessels, or bowel segments to allow flow from one to the other.

arteriovenous fistula. Connecting passage between an artery and a vein.

end-stage renal disease. Chronic, advanced kidney disease requiring renal dialysis or a kidney transplant to prevent imminent death.

hemodialysis. Cleansing of wastes and contaminating elements from the blood by virtue of different diffusion rates through a semipermeable membrane, which separates blood from a filtration solution that diffuses other elements out of the blood.

transposition. Removal or exchange from one side to another; change of position from one place to another.

36820

36820 Arteriovenous anastomosis, open; by forearm vein transposition

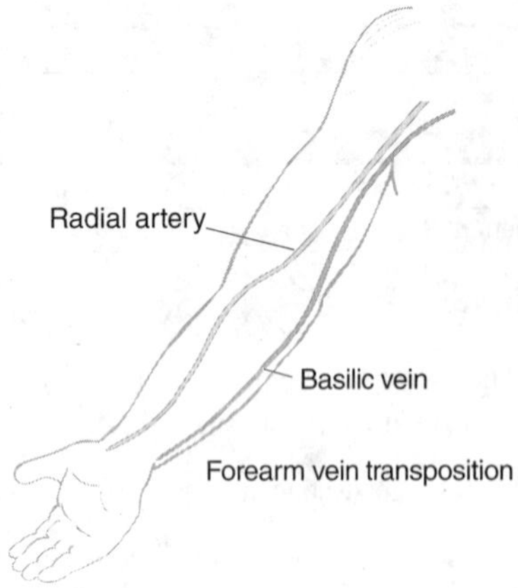

Explanation

The physician creates a connection between an artery or vein, using a forearm vein in the arm-inverted end to end. The physician dissects down to the vein and artery. The subfascial plane is identified and elevated laterally to the flexor carpi radialis (FCR) and medially to the brachioradialis (BR). The plane between the BR and FCR is dissected and the perforating vessels are identified and cauterized. The pedicle is followed to the antecubital fossa. The tourniquet is released, and the vessels are further cleaned of their adventitia under loupe visualization. Using microvascular techniques, a suture for the arterial anastomosis is performed and closure is completed. Suction drains are placed in the neck. If a Doppler is to be used for postoperative assessment, a suture is placed to mark the pedicle site. A splint is fabricated and secured to the arm with an elastic bandage.

Coding Tips

When this procedure is performed on the upper arm, basilic vein, see 36819; on the upper arm cephalic vein, see 36818. For insertion of a cannula for hemodialysis, other purpose (separate procedure), see 36800–36815. When central dialysis segment angioplasty is performed with 36818-36833, use 36907. When central dialysis segment stent placement is performed with 36818-36833, use 36908.

ICD-10-CM Diagnostic Codes

D59.3	Hemolytic-uremic syndrome
I12.0	Hypertensive chronic kidney disease with stage 5 chronic kidney disease or end stage renal disease
I13.0	Hypertensive heart and chronic kidney disease with heart failure and stage 1 through stage 4 chronic kidney disease, or unspecified chronic kidney disease
I13.11	Hypertensive heart and chronic kidney disease without heart failure, with stage 5 chronic kidney disease, or end stage renal disease
I13.2	Hypertensive heart and chronic kidney disease with heart failure and with stage 5 chronic kidney disease, or end stage renal disease
I16.0	Hypertensive urgency
I16.1	Hypertensive emergency
I82.3	Embolism and thrombosis of renal vein
N00.0	Acute nephritic syndrome with minor glomerular abnormality
N00.1	Acute nephritic syndrome with focal and segmental glomerular lesions
N00.2	Acute nephritic syndrome with diffuse membranous glomerulonephritis
N00.3	Acute nephritic syndrome with diffuse mesangial proliferative glomerulonephritis
N00.4	Acute nephritic syndrome with diffuse endocapillary proliferative glomerulonephritis
N00.5	Acute nephritic syndrome with diffuse mesangiocapillary glomerulonephritis
N00.6	Acute nephritic syndrome with dense deposit disease
N00.7	Acute nephritic syndrome with diffuse crescentic glomerulonephritis
N00.8	Acute nephritic syndrome with other morphologic changes
N01.0	Rapidly progressive nephritic syndrome with minor glomerular abnormality
N01.1	Rapidly progressive nephritic syndrome with focal and segmental glomerular lesions
N01.2	Rapidly progressive nephritic syndrome with diffuse membranous glomerulonephritis
N01.3	Rapidly progressive nephritic syndrome with diffuse mesangial proliferative glomerulonephritis
N01.4	Rapidly progressive nephritic syndrome with diffuse endocapillary proliferative glomerulonephritis
N01.5	Rapidly progressive nephritic syndrome with diffuse mesangiocapillary glomerulonephritis
N01.6	Rapidly progressive nephritic syndrome with dense deposit disease
N01.7	Rapidly progressive nephritic syndrome with diffuse crescentic glomerulonephritis
N01.8	Rapidly progressive nephritic syndrome with other morphologic changes
N03.0	Chronic nephritic syndrome with minor glomerular abnormality
N03.1	Chronic nephritic syndrome with focal and segmental glomerular lesions
N03.2	Chronic nephritic syndrome with diffuse membranous glomerulonephritis
N03.3	Chronic nephritic syndrome with diffuse mesangial proliferative glomerulonephritis
N03.4	Chronic nephritic syndrome with diffuse endocapillary proliferative glomerulonephritis
N03.5	Chronic nephritic syndrome with diffuse mesangiocapillary glomerulonephritis
N03.6	Chronic nephritic syndrome with dense deposit disease
N03.7	Chronic nephritic syndrome with diffuse crescentic glomerulonephritis
N03.8	Chronic nephritic syndrome with other morphologic changes
N04.0	Nephrotic syndrome with minor glomerular abnormality
N04.1	Nephrotic syndrome with focal and segmental glomerular lesions
N04.2	Nephrotic syndrome with diffuse membranous glomerulonephritis
N04.3	Nephrotic syndrome with diffuse mesangial proliferative glomerulonephritis
N04.4	Nephrotic syndrome with diffuse endocapillary proliferative glomerulonephritis

N04.5	Nephrotic syndrome with diffuse mesangiocapillary glomerulonephritis
N04.6	Nephrotic syndrome with dense deposit disease
N04.7	Nephrotic syndrome with diffuse crescentic glomerulonephritis
N04.8	Nephrotic syndrome with other morphologic changes
N07.0	Hereditary nephropathy, not elsewhere classified with minor glomerular abnormality
N07.1	Hereditary nephropathy, not elsewhere classified with focal and segmental glomerular lesions
N07.2	Hereditary nephropathy, not elsewhere classified with diffuse membranous glomerulonephritis
N07.3	Hereditary nephropathy, not elsewhere classified with diffuse mesangial proliferative glomerulonephritis
N07.4	Hereditary nephropathy, not elsewhere classified with diffuse endocapillary proliferative glomerulonephritis
N07.5	Hereditary nephropathy, not elsewhere classified with diffuse mesangiocapillary glomerulonephritis
N07.6	Hereditary nephropathy, not elsewhere classified with dense deposit disease
N07.7	Hereditary nephropathy, not elsewhere classified with diffuse crescentic glomerulonephritis
N07.8	Hereditary nephropathy, not elsewhere classified with other morphologic lesions
N08	Glomerular disorders in diseases classified elsewhere
N10	Acute pyelonephritis
N11.0	Nonobstructive reflux-associated chronic pyelonephritis
N11.1	Chronic obstructive pyelonephritis
N11.8	Other chronic tubulo-interstitial nephritis
N12	Tubulo-interstitial nephritis, not specified as acute or chronic
N15.8	Other specified renal tubulo-interstitial diseases
N16	Renal tubulo-interstitial disorders in diseases classified elsewhere
N17.0	Acute kidney failure with tubular necrosis
N17.1	Acute kidney failure with acute cortical necrosis
N17.2	Acute kidney failure with medullary necrosis
N17.8	Other acute kidney failure
N18.4	Chronic kidney disease, stage 4 (severe)
N18.5	Chronic kidney disease, stage 5
N18.6	End stage renal disease

AMA: 36820 2018,Jan,8; 2017,Mar,3; 2017,Jan,8; 2016,Jan,13; 2015,Jan,16; 2014,Jan,11

Relative Value Units/Medicare Edits

Non-Facility RVU	Work	PE	MP	Total
36820	13.07	5.17	3.01	21.25
Facility RVU	**Work**	**PE**	**MP**	**Total**
36820	13.07	5.17	3.01	21.25

	FUD	Status	MUE	Modifiers				IOM Reference
36820	90	A	1(3)	51	50	62*	80	None

* with documentation

36821

36821 Arteriovenous anastomosis, open; direct, any site (eg, Cimino type) (separate procedure)

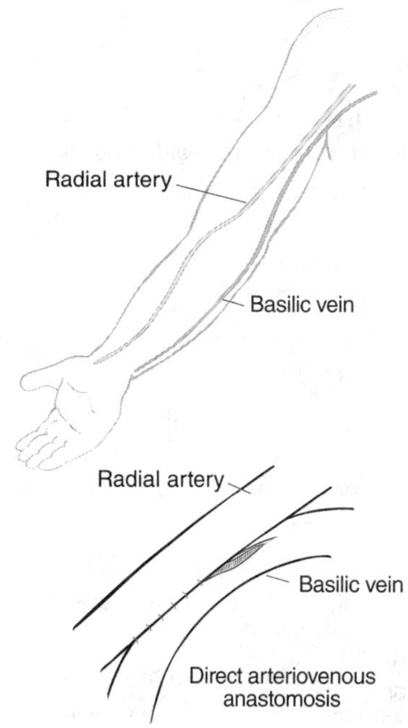

Explanation

Through an incision, usually in the skin over an artery in the nondominant wrist or antecubital fossa, the physician isolates a desired section of artery and neighboring vein. Vessel clamps are placed on the vein and adjacent artery. The vein is dissected free, divided, and the downstream portion of the vein is sutured to an opening created in the adjacent artery, usually in an end-to-side fashion, allowing blood to flow both down the artery and into the vein. Large branches of the vein may be tied off to cause flow down a single vein. The skin incision is repaired with a layered closure. This arteriovenous anastomosis will allow an increased blood flow through the vein, usually for hemodialysis.

Coding Tips

This separate procedure by definition is usually a component of a more complex service and is not identified separately. When performed alone or with other unrelated procedures/services, it may be reported. If performed alone, list the code; if performed with other procedures/services, list the code and append modifier 59 or an X{EPSU} modifier. For insertion of cannula for hemodialysis, other purpose (separate procedure), see 36800–36815. When central dialysis segment angioplasty is performed with 36818-36833, use 36907. When central dialysis segment stent placement is performed with 36818-36833, use 36908.

ICD-10-CM Diagnostic Codes

D59.3	Hemolytic-uremic syndrome
E87.2	Acidosis
E87.5	Hyperkalemia
I12.0	Hypertensive chronic kidney disease with stage 5 chronic kidney disease or end stage renal disease
I13.0	Hypertensive heart and chronic kidney disease with heart failure and stage 1 through stage 4 chronic kidney disease, or unspecified chronic kidney disease

I13.11 Hypertensive heart and chronic kidney disease without heart failure, with stage 5 chronic kidney disease, or end stage renal disease
I13.2 Hypertensive heart and chronic kidney disease with heart failure and with stage 5 chronic kidney disease, or end stage renal disease
I16.0 Hypertensive urgency
I16.1 Hypertensive emergency
I82.3 Embolism and thrombosis of renal vein
N00.0 Acute nephritic syndrome with minor glomerular abnormality
N00.1 Acute nephritic syndrome with focal and segmental glomerular lesions
N00.2 Acute nephritic syndrome with diffuse membranous glomerulonephritis
N00.3 Acute nephritic syndrome with diffuse mesangial proliferative glomerulonephritis
N00.4 Acute nephritic syndrome with diffuse endocapillary proliferative glomerulonephritis
N00.5 Acute nephritic syndrome with diffuse mesangiocapillary glomerulonephritis
N00.6 Acute nephritic syndrome with dense deposit disease
N00.7 Acute nephritic syndrome with diffuse crescentic glomerulonephritis
N00.8 Acute nephritic syndrome with other morphologic changes
N01.0 Rapidly progressive nephritic syndrome with minor glomerular abnormality
N01.1 Rapidly progressive nephritic syndrome with focal and segmental glomerular lesions
N01.2 Rapidly progressive nephritic syndrome with diffuse membranous glomerulonephritis
N01.3 Rapidly progressive nephritic syndrome with diffuse mesangial proliferative glomerulonephritis
N01.4 Rapidly progressive nephritic syndrome with diffuse endocapillary proliferative glomerulonephritis
N01.5 Rapidly progressive nephritic syndrome with diffuse mesangiocapillary glomerulonephritis
N01.6 Rapidly progressive nephritic syndrome with dense deposit disease
N01.7 Rapidly progressive nephritic syndrome with diffuse crescentic glomerulonephritis
N01.8 Rapidly progressive nephritic syndrome with other morphologic changes
N03.0 Chronic nephritic syndrome with minor glomerular abnormality
N03.1 Chronic nephritic syndrome with focal and segmental glomerular lesions
N03.2 Chronic nephritic syndrome with diffuse membranous glomerulonephritis
N03.3 Chronic nephritic syndrome with diffuse mesangial proliferative glomerulonephritis
N03.4 Chronic nephritic syndrome with diffuse endocapillary proliferative glomerulonephritis
N03.5 Chronic nephritic syndrome with diffuse mesangiocapillary glomerulonephritis
N03.6 Chronic nephritic syndrome with dense deposit disease
N03.7 Chronic nephritic syndrome with diffuse crescentic glomerulonephritis
N03.8 Chronic nephritic syndrome with other morphologic changes
N04.0 Nephrotic syndrome with minor glomerular abnormality
N04.1 Nephrotic syndrome with focal and segmental glomerular lesions
N04.2 Nephrotic syndrome with diffuse membranous glomerulonephritis
N04.3 Nephrotic syndrome with diffuse mesangial proliferative glomerulonephritis
N04.4 Nephrotic syndrome with diffuse endocapillary proliferative glomerulonephritis
N04.5 Nephrotic syndrome with diffuse mesangiocapillary glomerulonephritis
N04.6 Nephrotic syndrome with dense deposit disease
N04.7 Nephrotic syndrome with diffuse crescentic glomerulonephritis
N04.8 Nephrotic syndrome with other morphologic changes
N07.0 Hereditary nephropathy, not elsewhere classified with minor glomerular abnormality
N07.1 Hereditary nephropathy, not elsewhere classified with focal and segmental glomerular lesions
N07.2 Hereditary nephropathy, not elsewhere classified with diffuse membranous glomerulonephritis
N07.3 Hereditary nephropathy, not elsewhere classified with diffuse mesangial proliferative glomerulonephritis
N07.4 Hereditary nephropathy, not elsewhere classified with diffuse endocapillary proliferative glomerulonephritis
N07.5 Hereditary nephropathy, not elsewhere classified with diffuse mesangiocapillary glomerulonephritis
N07.6 Hereditary nephropathy, not elsewhere classified with dense deposit disease
N07.7 Hereditary nephropathy, not elsewhere classified with diffuse crescentic glomerulonephritis
N07.8 Hereditary nephropathy, not elsewhere classified with other morphologic lesions
N08 Glomerular disorders in diseases classified elsewhere
N10 Acute pyelonephritis
N11.0 Nonobstructive reflux-associated chronic pyelonephritis
N11.1 Chronic obstructive pyelonephritis
N11.8 Other chronic tubulo-interstitial nephritis
N12 Tubulo-interstitial nephritis, not specified as acute or chronic
N15.8 Other specified renal tubulo-interstitial diseases
N16 Renal tubulo-interstitial disorders in diseases classified elsewhere
N17.0 Acute kidney failure with tubular necrosis
N17.1 Acute kidney failure with acute cortical necrosis
N17.2 Acute kidney failure with medullary necrosis
N17.8 Other acute kidney failure
N18.4 Chronic kidney disease, stage 4 (severe)
N18.5 Chronic kidney disease, stage 5
N18.6 End stage renal disease

AMA: 36821 2018,Jan,8; 2017,Mar,3; 2017,Jan,8; 2016,Jan,13; 2015,Jan,16; 2015,Aug,8; 2014,Jan,11

Relative Value Units/Medicare Edits

Non-Facility RVU	Work	PE	MP	Total
36821	11.9	4.59	2.76	19.25
Facility RVU	**Work**	**PE**	**MP**	**Total**
36821	11.9	4.59	2.76	19.25

	FUD	Status	MUE	Modifiers				IOM Reference
36821	90	A	2(3)	51	N/A	62*	80	None

* with documentation

Terms To Know

anastomosis. Surgically created connection between ducts, blood vessels, or bowel segments to allow flow from one to the other.

arteriovenous fistula. Connecting passage between an artery and a vein.

end-stage renal disease. Chronic, advanced kidney disease requiring renal dialysis or a kidney transplant to prevent imminent death.

hemodialysis. Cleansing of wastes and contaminating elements from the blood by virtue of different diffusion rates through a semipermeable membrane, which separates blood from a filtration solution that diffuses other elements out of the blood.

transposition. Removal or exchange from one side to another; change of position from one place to another.

36823

36823 Insertion of arterial and venous cannula(s) for isolated extracorporeal circulation including regional chemotherapy perfusion to an extremity, with or without hyperthermia, with removal of cannula(s) and repair of arteriotomy and venotomy sites

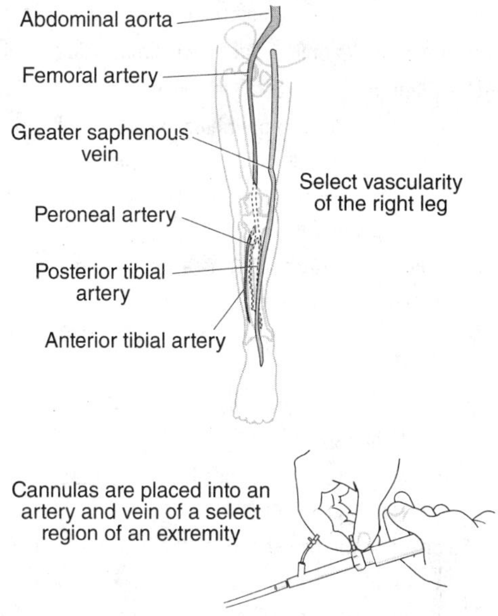

Explanation

The physician inserts arterial and venous cannula(s) for isolated extracorporeal circulation to an extremity to provide regional perfusion chemotherapy (RPC) with or without hyperthermia. The external iliac, common femoral, or subclavian artery and vein are isolated depending on the site of the tumor. A cannula is inserted into the selected artery and vein to isolate blood flow to and from the extremity. The blood flow from the isolated extremity is connected to a perfusion pump where the blood is oxygenated. The blood may be heated to between 40°-40.5° C (104°-105° F). One or more high dose chemotherapy agents are injected and perfused over an hour or more with flow rates monitored and adjusted to minimize leakage into the systemic circulation. The combination of heat and the chemotherapy agent act to destroy the cancer cells. After completion of the perfusion procedure, the cannula(s) are removed and the artery and vein repaired.

Coding Tips

Chemotherapy perfusion supported by a membrane oxygenator/perfusion pump, is included in 36823. Do not report chemotherapy administration codes 96409–96425 with 36823. Report chemotherapy drugs and supplies separately. When central dialysis segment angioplasty is performed with 36818–36833, use 36907. When central dialysis segment stent placement is performed with 36818–36833, use 36908.

ICD-10-CM Diagnostic Codes

C40.01	Malignant neoplasm of scapula and long bones of right upper limb ☑
C40.02	Malignant neoplasm of scapula and long bones of left upper limb ☑
C40.11	Malignant neoplasm of short bones of right upper limb ☑
C40.12	Malignant neoplasm of short bones of left upper limb ☑
C40.21	Malignant neoplasm of long bones of right lower limb ☑
C40.22	Malignant neoplasm of long bones of left lower limb ☑

C40.31 Malignant neoplasm of short bones of right lower limb ☑
C40.32 Malignant neoplasm of short bones of left lower limb ☑
C40.81 Malignant neoplasm of overlapping sites of bone and articular cartilage of right limb ☑
C40.82 Malignant neoplasm of overlapping sites of bone and articular cartilage of left limb ☑
C43.61 Malignant melanoma of right upper limb, including shoulder ☑
C43.62 Malignant melanoma of left upper limb, including shoulder ☑
C43.71 Malignant melanoma of right lower limb, including hip ☑
C43.72 Malignant melanoma of left lower limb, including hip ☑
C47.11 Malignant neoplasm of peripheral nerves of right upper limb, including shoulder ☑
C47.12 Malignant neoplasm of peripheral nerves of left upper limb, including shoulder ☑
C47.21 Malignant neoplasm of peripheral nerves of right lower limb, including hip ☑
C47.22 Malignant neoplasm of peripheral nerves of left lower limb, including hip ☑
C49.11 Malignant neoplasm of connective and soft tissue of right upper limb, including shoulder ☑
C49.12 Malignant neoplasm of connective and soft tissue of left upper limb, including shoulder ☑
C49.21 Malignant neoplasm of connective and soft tissue of right lower limb, including hip ☑
C49.22 Malignant neoplasm of connective and soft tissue of left lower limb, including hip ☑
C76.41 Malignant neoplasm of right upper limb ☑
C76.42 Malignant neoplasm of left upper limb ☑
C76.51 Malignant neoplasm of right lower limb ☑
C76.52 Malignant neoplasm of left lower limb ☑
D04.61 Carcinoma in situ of skin of right upper limb, including shoulder ☑
D04.62 Carcinoma in situ of skin of left upper limb, including shoulder ☑
D04.71 Carcinoma in situ of skin of right lower limb, including hip ☑
D04.72 Carcinoma in situ of skin of left lower limb, including hip ☑
D48.0 Neoplasm of uncertain behavior of bone and articular cartilage

AMA: 36823 2018,Jan,8; 2017,Mar,3; 2014,Jan,11

Relative Value Units/Medicare Edits

Non-Facility RVU	Work	PE	MP	Total
36823	22.98	11.95	5.57	40.5
Facility RVU	**Work**	**PE**	**MP**	**Total**
36823	22.98	11.95	5.57	40.5

	FUD	Status	MUE	Modifiers				IOM Reference
36823	90	A	1(3)	51	N/A	N/A	N/A	None

* with documentation

36825-36830

36825 Creation of arteriovenous fistula by other than direct arteriovenous anastomosis (separate procedure); autogenous graft
36830 nonautogenous graft (eg, biological collagen, thermoplastic graft)

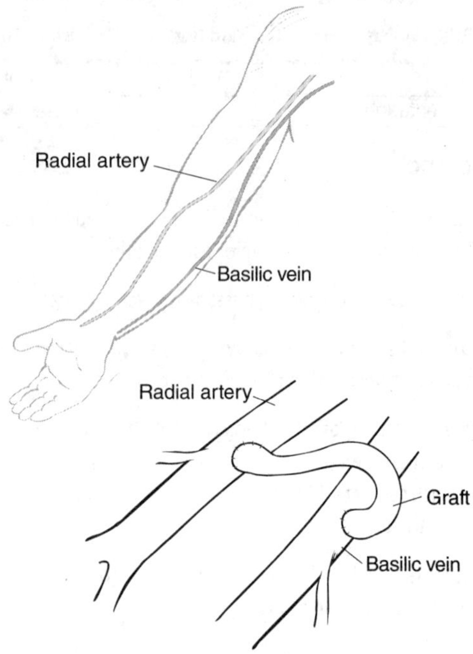

Explanation

The physician creates an arteriovenous fistula by other than direct anastomosis. The physician makes an incision in the skin over an artery and vein, and the vein and artery are dissected free. A vessel clamp is affixed to each. A length of harvested vein from the patient is used for an autogenous graft in 36825 and is sutured to the incised artery and vein, usually in an end-to-side fashion. The graft is passed in a superficial subcutaneous tunnel that is created bluntly and connects the arterial and venous sites. The clamps are removed, allowing the blood to flow through the graft, creating an arteriovenous fistula. The skin incision is repaired with a layered closure. Report 36830 if a nonautogenous graft, such as biological collagen or a thermoplastic graft, is used.

Coding Tips

These separate procedures by definition are usually a component of a more complex service and are not identified separately. When performed alone or with other unrelated procedures/services, they may be reported. If performed alone, list the code; if performed with other procedures/services, list the code and append modifier 59 or an X{EPSU} modifier. For direct arteriovenous anastomosis, see 36821. When central dialysis segment angioplasty is performed with 36818-36833, use 36907. When central dialysis segment stent placement is performed with 36818-36833, use 36908.

ICD-10-CM Diagnostic Codes

D59.3 Hemolytic-uremic syndrome
E87.2 Acidosis
E87.5 Hyperkalemia
I12.0 Hypertensive chronic kidney disease with stage 5 chronic kidney disease or end stage renal disease
I13.0 Hypertensive heart and chronic kidney disease with heart failure and stage 1 through stage 4 chronic kidney disease, or unspecified chronic kidney disease

I13.10	Hypertensive heart and chronic kidney disease without heart failure, with stage 1 through stage 4 chronic kidney disease, or unspecified chronic kidney disease
I13.11	Hypertensive heart and chronic kidney disease without heart failure, with stage 5 chronic kidney disease, or end stage renal disease
I13.2	Hypertensive heart and chronic kidney disease with heart failure and with stage 5 chronic kidney disease, or end stage renal disease
I16.0	Hypertensive urgency
I16.1	Hypertensive emergency
I82.3	Embolism and thrombosis of renal vein
N00.0	Acute nephritic syndrome with minor glomerular abnormality
N00.1	Acute nephritic syndrome with focal and segmental glomerular lesions
N00.2	Acute nephritic syndrome with diffuse membranous glomerulonephritis
N00.3	Acute nephritic syndrome with diffuse mesangial proliferative glomerulonephritis
N00.4	Acute nephritic syndrome with diffuse endocapillary proliferative glomerulonephritis
N00.5	Acute nephritic syndrome with diffuse mesangiocapillary glomerulonephritis
N00.6	Acute nephritic syndrome with dense deposit disease
N00.7	Acute nephritic syndrome with diffuse crescentic glomerulonephritis
N00.8	Acute nephritic syndrome with other morphologic changes
N01.0	Rapidly progressive nephritic syndrome with minor glomerular abnormality
N01.1	Rapidly progressive nephritic syndrome with focal and segmental glomerular lesions
N01.2	Rapidly progressive nephritic syndrome with diffuse membranous glomerulonephritis
N01.3	Rapidly progressive nephritic syndrome with diffuse mesangial proliferative glomerulonephritis
N01.4	Rapidly progressive nephritic syndrome with diffuse endocapillary proliferative glomerulonephritis
N01.5	Rapidly progressive nephritic syndrome with diffuse mesangiocapillary glomerulonephritis
N01.6	Rapidly progressive nephritic syndrome with dense deposit disease
N01.7	Rapidly progressive nephritic syndrome with diffuse crescentic glomerulonephritis
N01.8	Rapidly progressive nephritic syndrome with other morphologic changes
N03.0	Chronic nephritic syndrome with minor glomerular abnormality
N03.1	Chronic nephritic syndrome with focal and segmental glomerular lesions
N03.2	Chronic nephritic syndrome with diffuse membranous glomerulonephritis
N03.3	Chronic nephritic syndrome with diffuse mesangial proliferative glomerulonephritis
N03.4	Chronic nephritic syndrome with diffuse endocapillary proliferative glomerulonephritis
N03.5	Chronic nephritic syndrome with diffuse mesangiocapillary glomerulonephritis
N03.6	Chronic nephritic syndrome with dense deposit disease
N03.7	Chronic nephritic syndrome with diffuse crescentic glomerulonephritis
N03.8	Chronic nephritic syndrome with other morphologic changes
N04.0	Nephrotic syndrome with minor glomerular abnormality
N04.1	Nephrotic syndrome with focal and segmental glomerular lesions
N04.2	Nephrotic syndrome with diffuse membranous glomerulonephritis
N04.3	Nephrotic syndrome with diffuse mesangial proliferative glomerulonephritis
N04.4	Nephrotic syndrome with diffuse endocapillary proliferative glomerulonephritis
N04.5	Nephrotic syndrome with diffuse mesangiocapillary glomerulonephritis
N04.6	Nephrotic syndrome with dense deposit disease
N04.7	Nephrotic syndrome with diffuse crescentic glomerulonephritis
N04.8	Nephrotic syndrome with other morphologic changes
N07.0	Hereditary nephropathy, not elsewhere classified with minor glomerular abnormality
N07.1	Hereditary nephropathy, not elsewhere classified with focal and segmental glomerular lesions
N07.2	Hereditary nephropathy, not elsewhere classified with diffuse membranous glomerulonephritis
N07.3	Hereditary nephropathy, not elsewhere classified with diffuse mesangial proliferative glomerulonephritis
N07.4	Hereditary nephropathy, not elsewhere classified with diffuse endocapillary proliferative glomerulonephritis
N07.5	Hereditary nephropathy, not elsewhere classified with diffuse mesangiocapillary glomerulonephritis
N07.6	Hereditary nephropathy, not elsewhere classified with dense deposit disease
N07.7	Hereditary nephropathy, not elsewhere classified with diffuse crescentic glomerulonephritis
N07.8	Hereditary nephropathy, not elsewhere classified with other morphologic lesions
N08	Glomerular disorders in diseases classified elsewhere
N10	Acute pyelonephritis
N11.0	Nonobstructive reflux-associated chronic pyelonephritis
N11.1	Chronic obstructive pyelonephritis
N11.8	Other chronic tubulo-interstitial nephritis
N12	Tubulo-interstitial nephritis, not specified as acute or chronic
N15.8	Other specified renal tubulo-interstitial diseases
N16	Renal tubulo-interstitial disorders in diseases classified elsewhere
N17.0	Acute kidney failure with tubular necrosis
N17.1	Acute kidney failure with acute cortical necrosis
N17.2	Acute kidney failure with medullary necrosis
N17.8	Other acute kidney failure
N18.4	Chronic kidney disease, stage 4 (severe)
N18.5	Chronic kidney disease, stage 5
N18.6	End stage renal disease

Associated HCPCS Codes

G0365	Vessel mapping of vessels for hemodialysis access (services for preoperative vessel mapping prior to creation of hemodialysis access using an autogenous hemodialysis conduit, including arterial inflow and venous outflow)

AMA: **36825** 2018,Jan,8; 2017,Mar,3; 2017,Jan,8; 2016,Jan,13; 2015,Jan,16; 2014,Jan,11 **36830** 2018,Jan,8; 2017,Mar,3; 2017,Jan,8; 2016,Jan,13; 2015,Jan,13; 2015,Jan,16; 2014,Jan,11

Relative Value Units/Medicare Edits

Non-Facility RVU	Work	PE	MP	Total
36825	14.17	5.58	3.3	23.05
36830	12.03	4.52	2.79	19.34
Facility RVU	**Work**	**PE**	**MP**	**Total**
36825	14.17	5.58	3.3	23.05
36830	12.03	4.52	2.79	19.34

	FUD	Status	MUE	Modifiers				IOM Reference
36825	90	A	1(3)	51	N/A	62*	80	None
36830	90	A	2(3)	51	N/A	62*	80	

* with documentation

Terms To Know

anastomosis. Surgically created connection between ducts, blood vessels, or bowel segments to allow flow from one to the other.

arteriovenous fistula. Connecting passage between an artery and a vein.

nonautogenous. Derived from a source other than the same individual or recipient (e.g., cells, tissue, blood vessels, and other organs donated from another human).

36831

36831 Thrombectomy, open, arteriovenous fistula without revision, autogenous or nonautogenous dialysis graft (separate procedure)

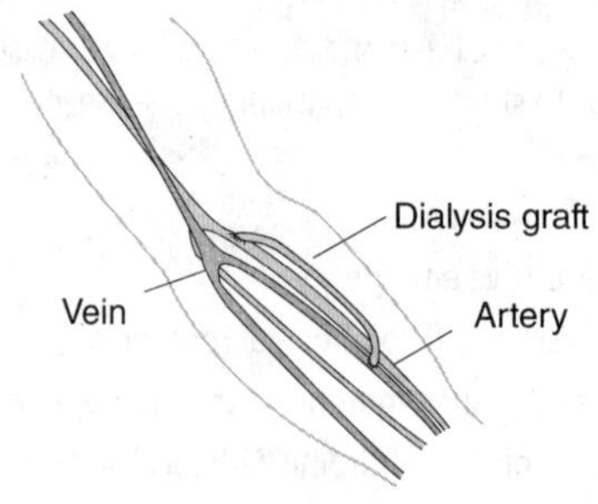

A previously placed dialysis graft, autogenous or nonautogenous, has developed a thrombus

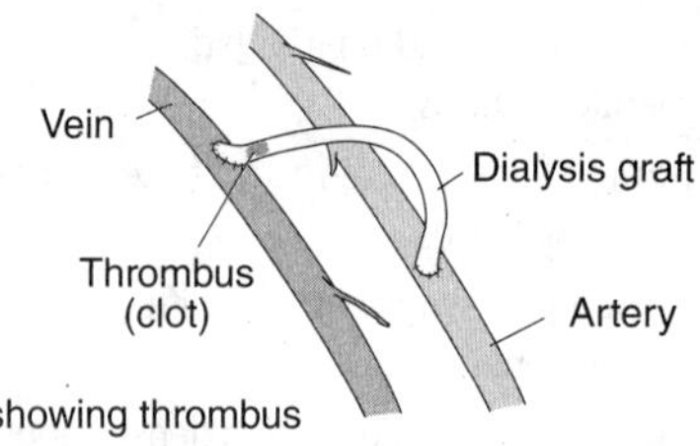

Detail showing thrombus

Explanation

The physician removes a blood clot from a surgically created connection between an artery and a vein (arteriovenous fistula). The procedure involves making an incision over the site of an existing fistula. The fistula is isolated and dissected free. Vessel clamps are affixed above and below the fistula. The blood clot is removed, the clamps are taken off, and the incision is repaired by layered sutures. The procedure may involve a vein acquired from the patient or the construction of a synthetic graft.

Coding Tips

This separate procedure by definition is usually a component of a more complex service and is not identified separately. When performed alone or with other unrelated procedures/services, it may be reported. If performed alone, list the code; if performed with other procedures/services, list the code and append modifier 59 of an X{EPSU} modifier. Use this procedure for thrombectomy associated with reduced flow. If a vein is acquired from the patient or the construction of a synthetic graft is performed, it may be reported with a separate code. For cannula declotting, see 36860–36861. For thrombectomy with revision of an arteriovenous fistula, see 36833. When central dialysis segment angioplasty is performed with 36818-36833, use 36907. When central dialysis segment stent placement is performed with 36818-36833, use 36908.

ICD-10-CM Diagnostic Codes

T82.818A Embolism due to vascular prosthetic devices, implants and grafts, initial encounter

T82.828A Fibrosis due to vascular prosthetic devices, implants and grafts, initial encounter

T82.848A Pain due to vascular prosthetic devices, implants and grafts, initial encounter

T82.856A Stenosis of peripheral vascular stent, initial encounter

T82.858A Stenosis of other vascular prosthetic devices, implants and grafts, initial encounter

T82.868A Thrombosis due to vascular prosthetic devices, implants and grafts, initial encounter

T82.898A Other specified complication of vascular prosthetic devices, implants and grafts, initial encounter

AMA: **36831** 2018,Jan,8; 2017,Mar,3; 2017,Jan,8; 2016,Jan,13; 2015,Jan,16; 2014,Jan,11

Relative Value Units/Medicare Edits

Non-Facility RVU	Work	PE	MP	Total
36831	11.0	4.3	2.55	17.85
Facility RVU	**Work**	**PE**	**MP**	**Total**
36831	11.0	4.3	2.55	17.85

	FUD	Status	MUE	Modifiers				IOM Reference
36831	90	A	1(3)	51	N/A	62*	80	None

* with documentation

Terms To Know

chronic. Persistent, continuing, or recurring.

complication. Condition arising after the beginning of observation and treatment that modifies the course of the patient's illness or the medical care required, or an undesired result or misadventure in medical care.

fistula. Abnormal tube-like passage between two body cavities or organs or from an organ to the outside surface.

graft. Tissue implant from another part of the body or another person.

incision. Act of cutting into tissue or an organ.

renal failure. Inability of a kidney to eliminate metabolites and retain electrolytes at a normal level.

thrombus. Stationary blood clot inside a blood vessel.

36832-36833

36832 Revision, open, arteriovenous fistula; without thrombectomy, autogenous or nonautogenous dialysis graft (separate procedure)

36833 with thrombectomy, autogenous or nonautogenous dialysis graft (separate procedure)

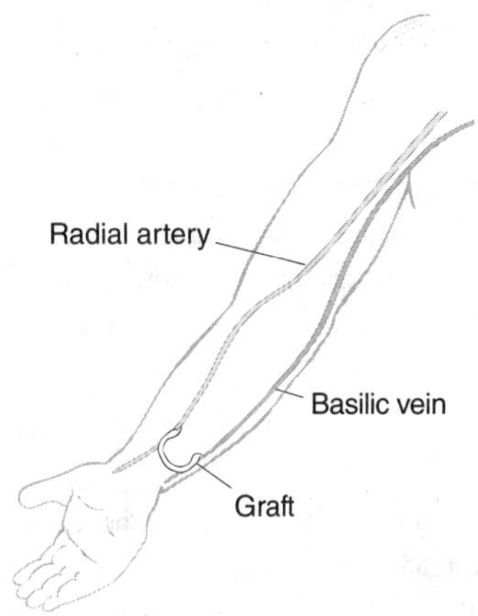

Explanation

In 36832, the physician makes an incision at the site of an already existing artificial fistula between an artery and a vein. The fistula is dissected free. Vessel clamps are affixed above and below the fistula, which is incised. Revisions are made to the fistula at its juncture to the vein and/or artery and may require creating a new anastomosis with a graft obtained from a separate site or created with synthetic material. After the repair has been made, the fistula is sutured, the clamps removed, and the skin incision repaired with a layered closure. Report 36833 when the physician removes a blood clot at the fistula site in addition to revising the existing arteriovenous fistula.

Coding Tips

These codes should be reported only for open revision of an arteriovenous fistula. These separate procedures by definition are usually a component of a more complex service and are not identified separately. When performed alone or with other unrelated procedures/services, they may be reported. If performed alone, list the code; if performed with other procedures/services, list the code and append modifier 59 or an X{EPSU} modifier. For cannula declotting, see 36860–36861. For open thrombectomy without revision of an arteriovenous fistula, see 36831. When central dialysis segment angioplasty is performed with 36818-36833, use 36907. When central dialysis segment stent placement is performed with 36818-36833, use 36908. When percutaneous thrombectomy is performed within the dialysis circuit, see 36904-36906. Do not report 36832 or 36833 with 36901-36906 for revision of the dialysis circuit.

ICD-10-CM Diagnostic Codes

T82.318A Breakdown (mechanical) of other vascular grafts, initial encounter

T82.328A Displacement of other vascular grafts, initial encounter

T82.338A Leakage of other vascular grafts, initial encounter

T82.398A Other mechanical complication of other vascular grafts, initial encounter

T82.510A Breakdown (mechanical) of surgically created arteriovenous fistula, initial encounter

T82.518A	Breakdown (mechanical) of other cardiac and vascular devices and implants, initial encounter
T82.520A	Displacement of surgically created arteriovenous fistula, initial encounter
T82.528A	Displacement of other cardiac and vascular devices and implants, initial encounter
T82.530A	Leakage of surgically created arteriovenous fistula, initial encounter
T82.538A	Leakage of other cardiac and vascular devices and implants, initial encounter
T82.590A	Other mechanical complication of surgically created arteriovenous fistula, initial encounter
T82.598A	Other mechanical complication of other cardiac and vascular devices and implants, initial encounter
T82.7XXA	Infection and inflammatory reaction due to other cardiac and vascular devices, implants and grafts, initial encounter
T82.818A	Embolism due to vascular prosthetic devices, implants and grafts, initial encounter
T82.828A	Fibrosis due to vascular prosthetic devices, implants and grafts, initial encounter
T82.838A	Hemorrhage due to vascular prosthetic devices, implants and grafts, initial encounter
T82.848A	Pain due to vascular prosthetic devices, implants and grafts, initial encounter
T82.856A	Stenosis of peripheral vascular stent, initial encounter
T82.858A	Stenosis of other vascular prosthetic devices, implants and grafts, initial encounter
T82.868A	Thrombosis due to vascular prosthetic devices, implants and grafts, initial encounter
T82.898A	Other specified complication of vascular prosthetic devices, implants and grafts, initial encounter
Z45.89	Encounter for adjustment and management of other implanted devices
Z46.89	Encounter for fitting and adjustment of other specified devices

AMA: 36832 2018,Jan,8; 2017,Mar,3; 2017,Jan,8; 2016,Jan,13; 2015,Jan,16; 2014,Jan,11 **36833** 2018,Jan,8; 2017,Mar,3; 2017,Jan,8; 2016,Jan,13; 2015,Jan,16; 2014,Jan,11

Relative Value Units/Medicare Edits

Non-Facility RVU	Work	PE	MP	Total
36832	13.5	5.3	3.1	21.9
36833	14.5	5.67	3.37	23.54
Facility RVU	**Work**	**PE**	**MP**	**Total**
36832	13.5	5.3	3.1	21.9
36833	14.5	5.67	3.37	23.54

	FUD	Status	MUE	Modifiers				IOM Reference
36832	90	A	2(3)	51	N/A	62*	80	None
36833	90	A	1(3)	51	N/A	62*	80	

* with documentation

36835

36835 Insertion of Thomas shunt (separate procedure)

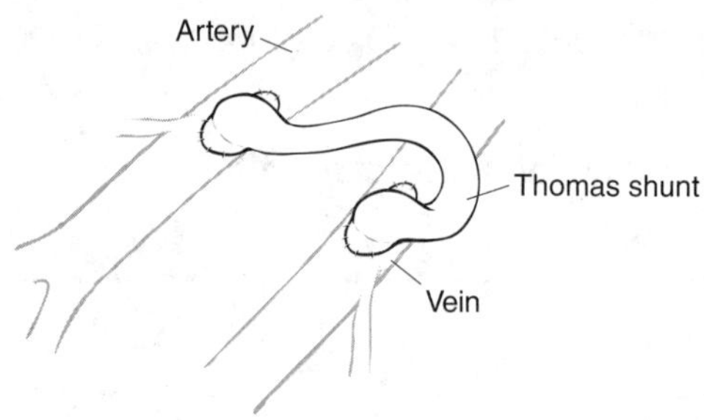

The Thomas shunt is a specialized synthetic graft and is typically used for infant and pediatric patients

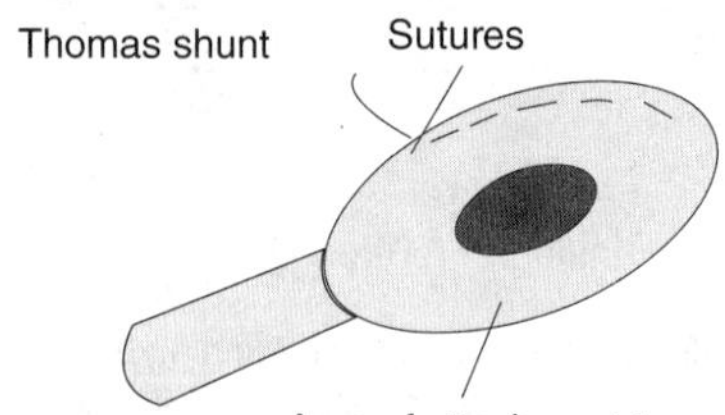

Explanation

Through an incision in the skin overlying a large vein or artery of a child, the physician dissects the vessel that will receive a synthetic shunt. The vessel may be clamped. The vessel is nicked, and a needle threads a guidance wire into the vein or artery. The shunt follows, and the wire is removed. The physician sutures the synthetic shunt either end-to-end, or end-to-side, to the vein or artery. The shunt is most often used for access in hemodialysis.

Coding Tips

This separate procedure by definition is usually a component of a more complex service and is not identified separately. When performed alone or with other unrelated procedures/services, it may be reported. If performed alone, list the code; if performed with other procedures/services, list the code and append modifier 59 or an X{EPSU} modifier. This type of shunt is infrequently used; verify this is the correct code by obtaining a copy of the shunt label from the medical record. This code includes venipuncture performed by the physician. Supplies used when providing this procedure may be reported with C1750. Check with the specific payer to determine coverage.

ICD-10-CM Diagnostic Codes

D59.3	Hemolytic-uremic syndrome
E87.2	Acidosis
E87.5	Hyperkalemia
I12.0	Hypertensive chronic kidney disease with stage 5 chronic kidney disease or end stage renal disease
I13.0	Hypertensive heart and chronic kidney disease with heart failure and stage 1 through stage 4 chronic kidney disease, or unspecified chronic kidney disease
I13.10	Hypertensive heart and chronic kidney disease without heart failure, with stage 1 through stage 4 chronic kidney disease, or unspecified chronic kidney disease

I13.11	Hypertensive heart and chronic kidney disease without heart failure, with stage 5 chronic kidney disease, or end stage renal disease
I13.2	Hypertensive heart and chronic kidney disease with heart failure and with stage 5 chronic kidney disease, or end stage renal disease
I16.0	Hypertensive urgency
I16.1	Hypertensive emergency
I82.3	Embolism and thrombosis of renal vein
N00.0	Acute nephritic syndrome with minor glomerular abnormality
N00.1	Acute nephritic syndrome with focal and segmental glomerular lesions
N00.2	Acute nephritic syndrome with diffuse membranous glomerulonephritis
N00.3	Acute nephritic syndrome with diffuse mesangial proliferative glomerulonephritis
N00.4	Acute nephritic syndrome with diffuse endocapillary proliferative glomerulonephritis
N00.5	Acute nephritic syndrome with diffuse mesangiocapillary glomerulonephritis
N00.6	Acute nephritic syndrome with dense deposit disease
N00.7	Acute nephritic syndrome with diffuse crescentic glomerulonephritis
N01.0	Rapidly progressive nephritic syndrome with minor glomerular abnormality
N01.1	Rapidly progressive nephritic syndrome with focal and segmental glomerular lesions
N01.2	Rapidly progressive nephritic syndrome with diffuse membranous glomerulonephritis
N01.3	Rapidly progressive nephritic syndrome with diffuse mesangial proliferative glomerulonephritis
N01.4	Rapidly progressive nephritic syndrome with diffuse endocapillary proliferative glomerulonephritis
N01.5	Rapidly progressive nephritic syndrome with diffuse mesangiocapillary glomerulonephritis
N01.6	Rapidly progressive nephritic syndrome with dense deposit disease
N01.7	Rapidly progressive nephritic syndrome with diffuse crescentic glomerulonephritis
N03.0	Chronic nephritic syndrome with minor glomerular abnormality
N03.1	Chronic nephritic syndrome with focal and segmental glomerular lesions
N03.2	Chronic nephritic syndrome with diffuse membranous glomerulonephritis
N03.3	Chronic nephritic syndrome with diffuse mesangial proliferative glomerulonephritis
N03.4	Chronic nephritic syndrome with diffuse endocapillary proliferative glomerulonephritis
N03.5	Chronic nephritic syndrome with diffuse mesangiocapillary glomerulonephritis
N03.6	Chronic nephritic syndrome with dense deposit disease
N03.7	Chronic nephritic syndrome with diffuse crescentic glomerulonephritis
N04.0	Nephrotic syndrome with minor glomerular abnormality
N04.1	Nephrotic syndrome with focal and segmental glomerular lesions
N04.2	Nephrotic syndrome with diffuse membranous glomerulonephritis
N04.3	Nephrotic syndrome with diffuse mesangial proliferative glomerulonephritis
N04.4	Nephrotic syndrome with diffuse endocapillary proliferative glomerulonephritis
N04.5	Nephrotic syndrome with diffuse mesangiocapillary glomerulonephritis
N04.6	Nephrotic syndrome with dense deposit disease
N04.7	Nephrotic syndrome with diffuse crescentic glomerulonephritis
N10	Acute pyelonephritis
N11.0	Nonobstructive reflux-associated chronic pyelonephritis
N11.1	Chronic obstructive pyelonephritis
N17.0	Acute kidney failure with tubular necrosis
N17.1	Acute kidney failure with acute cortical necrosis
N17.2	Acute kidney failure with medullary necrosis
N18.1	Chronic kidney disease, stage 1
N18.2	Chronic kidney disease, stage 2 (mild)
N18.3	Chronic kidney disease, stage 3 (moderate)
N18.4	Chronic kidney disease, stage 4 (severe)
N18.5	Chronic kidney disease, stage 5
N18.6	End stage renal disease
T80.211A	Bloodstream infection due to central venous catheter, initial encounter
T80.212A	Local infection due to central venous catheter, initial encounter
T82.318A	Breakdown (mechanical) of other vascular grafts, initial encounter
T82.41XA	Breakdown (mechanical) of vascular dialysis catheter, initial encounter
T82.42XA	Displacement of vascular dialysis catheter, initial encounter
T82.43XA	Leakage of vascular dialysis catheter, initial encounter
T82.510A	Breakdown (mechanical) of surgically created arteriovenous fistula, initial encounter
T82.514A	Breakdown (mechanical) of infusion catheter, initial encounter
T82.518A	Breakdown (mechanical) of other cardiac and vascular devices and implants, initial encounter
T82.520A	Displacement of surgically created arteriovenous fistula, initial encounter
T82.524A	Displacement of infusion catheter, initial encounter
T82.528A	Displacement of other cardiac and vascular devices and implants, initial encounter
T82.530A	Leakage of surgically created arteriovenous fistula, initial encounter
T82.534A	Leakage of infusion catheter, initial encounter
T82.538A	Leakage of other cardiac and vascular devices and implants, initial encounter
T82.7XXA	Infection and inflammatory reaction due to other cardiac and vascular devices, implants and grafts, initial encounter
T82.818A	Embolism due to vascular prosthetic devices, implants and grafts, initial encounter
T82.828A	Fibrosis due to vascular prosthetic devices, implants and grafts, initial encounter
T82.838A	Hemorrhage due to vascular prosthetic devices, implants and grafts, initial encounter
T82.848A	Pain due to vascular prosthetic devices, implants and grafts, initial encounter

T82.856A Stenosis of peripheral vascular stent, initial encounter

T82.858A Stenosis of other vascular prosthetic devices, implants and grafts, initial encounter

T82.868A Thrombosis due to vascular prosthetic devices, implants and grafts, initial encounter

AMA: **36835** 2014,Jan,11

Relative Value Units/Medicare Edits

Non-Facility RVU	Work	PE	MP	Total
36835	7.51	4.56	1.78	13.85
Facility RVU	**Work**	**PE**	**MP**	**Total**
36835	7.51	4.56	1.78	13.85

	FUD	Status	MUE	Modifiers				IOM Reference
36835	90	A	1(3)	51	N/A	N/A	N/A	None

* with documentation

Terms To Know

artery. Vessel through which oxygenated blood passes away from the heart to any part of the body.

guidewire. Flexible metal instrument designed to lead another instrument in its proper course.

hemodialysis. Cleansing of wastes and contaminating elements from the blood by virtue of different diffusion rates through a semipermeable membrane, which separates blood from a filtration solution that diffuses other elements out of the blood.

vein. Vessel through which oxygen-depleted blood passes back to the heart.

36838

36838 Distal revascularization and interval ligation (DRIL), upper extremity hemodialysis access (steal syndrome)

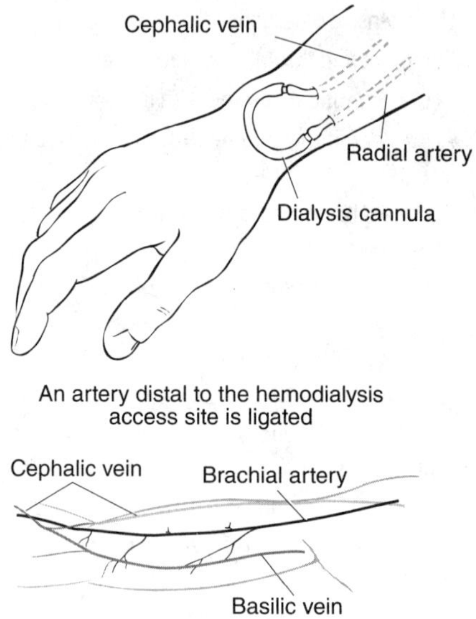

Explanation

A DRIL procedure, distal revascularization and interval ligation, is done to treat Steal syndrome occurring in patients with a permanent indwelling access site in the arm for hemodialysis. In Steal syndrome, the hand becomes cold and painful, due to ischemia because the hemodialysis access is taking the arm's blood supply. The DRIL procedure restores blood flow to the hand and preserves the access site. It is a two-step procedure. The surgeon first creates a bypass graft around the access site, using a harvested vein conduit, usually the greater saphenous. An incision is made in the upper arm for the proximal anastomosis, which is placed above the dialysis access site, nearer to the axilla. Soft tissue is dissected to expose the brachial artery. An incision is also made lower in the arm for the site of the distal anastomosis, which is placed below the dialysis access site, down in the forearm. A tunnel is created from one site to the other and the graft is completed using the harvested vein. This is the revascularization portion of the procedure and allows a good flow of blood around the access site. The second part of the procedure is the ligation. The brachial artery is tied off at a point between the dialysis access and the distal anastomosis site of the bypass graft. Now the arterial blood flow being pumped from the heart runs through the bypass, supplying the hand with oxygen before entering the access site. The incisions are closed and pulses are checked for good perfusion before applying dressings.

Coding Tips

Do not report 36838 with 35512, 35522, 35523, 36832, 37607, or 37618.

ICD-10-CM Diagnostic Codes

T80.211A Bloodstream infection due to central venous catheter, initial encounter

T80.212A Local infection due to central venous catheter, initial encounter

T80.218A Other infection due to central venous catheter, initial encounter

T82.318A Breakdown (mechanical) of other vascular grafts, initial encounter

T82.328A Displacement of other vascular grafts, initial encounter

T82.338A Leakage of other vascular grafts, initial encounter

T82.398A Other mechanical complication of other vascular grafts, initial encounter

T82.41XA Breakdown (mechanical) of vascular dialysis catheter, initial encounter

T82.42XA Displacement of vascular dialysis catheter, initial encounter

T82.43XA Leakage of vascular dialysis catheter, initial encounter

T82.49XA Other complication of vascular dialysis catheter, initial encounter

T82.510A Breakdown (mechanical) of surgically created arteriovenous fistula, initial encounter

T82.514A Breakdown (mechanical) of infusion catheter, initial encounter

T82.518A Breakdown (mechanical) of other cardiac and vascular devices and implants, initial encounter

T82.520A Displacement of surgically created arteriovenous fistula, initial encounter

T82.524A Displacement of infusion catheter, initial encounter

T82.528A Displacement of other cardiac and vascular devices and implants, initial encounter

T82.530A Leakage of surgically created arteriovenous fistula, initial encounter

T82.534A Leakage of infusion catheter, initial encounter

T82.538A Leakage of other cardiac and vascular devices and implants, initial encounter

T82.590A Other mechanical complication of surgically created arteriovenous fistula, initial encounter

T82.594A Other mechanical complication of infusion catheter, initial encounter

T82.598A Other mechanical complication of other cardiac and vascular devices and implants, initial encounter

T82.7XXA Infection and inflammatory reaction due to other cardiac and vascular devices, implants and grafts, initial encounter

T82.818A Embolism due to vascular prosthetic devices, implants and grafts, initial encounter

T82.828A Fibrosis due to vascular prosthetic devices, implants and grafts, initial encounter

T82.838A Hemorrhage due to vascular prosthetic devices, implants and grafts, initial encounter

T82.848A Pain due to vascular prosthetic devices, implants and grafts, initial encounter

T82.856A Stenosis of peripheral vascular stent, initial encounter

T82.858A Stenosis of other vascular prosthetic devices, implants and grafts, initial encounter

T82.868A Thrombosis due to vascular prosthetic devices, implants and grafts, initial encounter

T82.898A Other specified complication of vascular prosthetic devices, implants and grafts, initial encounter

Z45.89 Encounter for adjustment and management of other implanted devices

AMA: **36838** 2014,Jan,11

Relative Value Units/Medicare Edits

Non-Facility RVU	Work	PE	MP	Total
36838	21.69	6.47	4.99	33.15
Facility RVU	**Work**	**PE**	**MP**	**Total**
36838	21.69	6.47	4.99	33.15

	FUD	Status	MUE	Modifiers				IOM Reference
36838	90	A	1(3)	51	50	62*	80	None

* with documentation

Terms To Know

bypass graft. Surgically created alternative blood vessel used to reroute blood flow around an area of obstruction or disease.

conduit. Surgically created channel for the passage of fluids.

harvest. Removal of cells or tissue from their native site to be used as a graft or transplant to another part of the donor's body or placed into another person.

hemodialysis. Cleansing of wastes and contaminating elements from the blood by virtue of different diffusion rates through a semipermeable membrane, which separates blood from a filtration solution that diffuses other elements out of the blood.

hypertension. Abnormally increased pressure, usually referring to arterial pressure, exceeding an acceptable range.

ligation. Tying off a blood vessel or duct with a suture or a soft, thin wire.

perfusion. Act of pouring over or through, especially the passage of a fluid through the vessels of a specific organ.

revascularize. Restoring blood flow or blood supply to a body part.

36860-36861

36860 External cannula declotting (separate procedure); without balloon catheter

36861 with balloon catheter

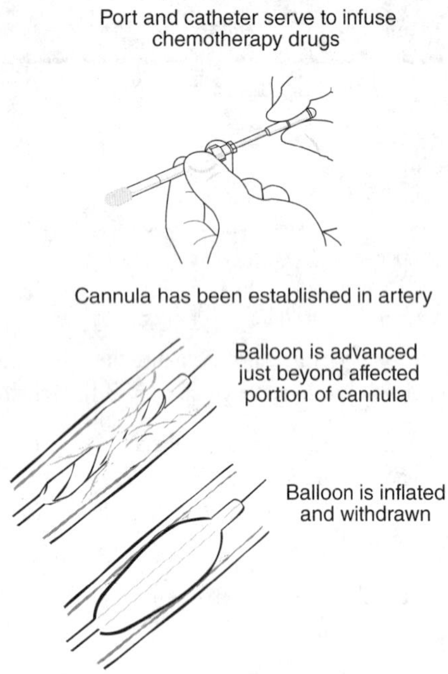

Explanation

To remove a blood clot lodged in a previously placed cannula, the physician may inject a solution containing enzymes into the cannula to dissolve the clot (in 36860) or the physician may, after injecting a solution containing enzymes, insert a balloon catheter (in 36861) into the cannula to retrieve a clot there. The balloon is inserted and inflated beyond the clot. The catheter is slowly pulled out, capturing and retrieving the clot. Once the clot is dissolved or retrieved, the catheter is removed and the cannula is left in place.

Coding Tips

These separate procedures by definition are usually a component of a more complex service and are not identified separately. When performed alone or with other unrelated procedures/services, they may be reported. If performed alone, list the code; if performed with other procedures/services, list the code and append modifier 59 or an X{EPSU} modifier. If imaging guidance is performed with 36861, see 76000.

ICD-10-CM Diagnostic Codes

T82.49XA Other complication of vascular dialysis catheter, initial encounter

T82.594A Other mechanical complication of infusion catheter, initial encounter

T82.818A Embolism due to vascular prosthetic devices, implants and grafts, initial encounter

T82.828A Fibrosis due to vascular prosthetic devices, implants and grafts, initial encounter

T82.848A Pain due to vascular prosthetic devices, implants and grafts, initial encounter

T82.856A Stenosis of peripheral vascular stent, initial encounter

T82.858A Stenosis of other vascular prosthetic devices, implants and grafts, initial encounter

T82.868A Thrombosis due to vascular prosthetic devices, implants and grafts, initial encounter

T82.898A Other specified complication of vascular prosthetic devices, implants and grafts, initial encounter

T82.9XXA Unspecified complication of cardiac and vascular prosthetic device, implant and graft, initial encounter

AMA: 36860 2018,Jan,8; 2017,Jan,8; 2016,Jan,13; 2015,Jan,16; 2014,Jan,11 **36861** 2018,Jan,8; 2017,Jan,8; 2016,Jan,13; 2015,Jan,16; 2014,Jan,11

Relative Value Units/Medicare Edits

Non-Facility RVU	Work	PE	MP	Total
36860	2.01	4.68	0.48	7.17
36861	2.52	0.89	0.61	4.02
Facility RVU	**Work**	**PE**	**MP**	**Total**
36860	2.01	0.71	0.48	3.2
36861	2.52	0.89	0.61	4.02

	FUD	Status	MUE	Modifiers				IOM Reference
36860	0	A	2(3)	51	N/A	N/A	N/A	None
36861	0	A	2(3)	51	N/A	N/A	N/A	

* with documentation

Terms To Know

cannula. Tube inserted into a blood vessel, duct, or body cavity to facilitate passage.

catheter. Flexible tube inserted into an area of the body for introducing or withdrawing fluid.

complication. Condition arising after the beginning of observation and treatment that modifies the course of the patient's illness or the medical care required, or an undesired result or misadventure in medical care.

embolism. Obstruction of a blood vessel resulting from a clot or foreign substance.

thrombosis. Condition arising from the presence or formation of blood clots within a blood vessel that may cause vascular obstruction and insufficient oxygenation.

36901-36903

36901 Introduction of needle(s) and/or catheter(s), dialysis circuit, with diagnostic angiography of the dialysis circuit, including all direct puncture(s) and catheter placement(s), injection(s) of contrast, all necessary imaging from the arterial anastomosis and adjacent artery through entire venous outflow including the inferior or superior vena cava, fluoroscopic guidance, radiological supervision and interpretation and image documentation and report;

36902 with transluminal balloon angioplasty, peripheral dialysis segment, including all imaging and radiological supervision and interpretation necessary to perform the angioplasty

36903 with transcatheter placement of intravascular stent(s), peripheral dialysis segment, including all imaging and radiological supervision and interpretation necessary to perform the stenting, and all angioplasty within the peripheral dialysis segment

Major arteries of the arm

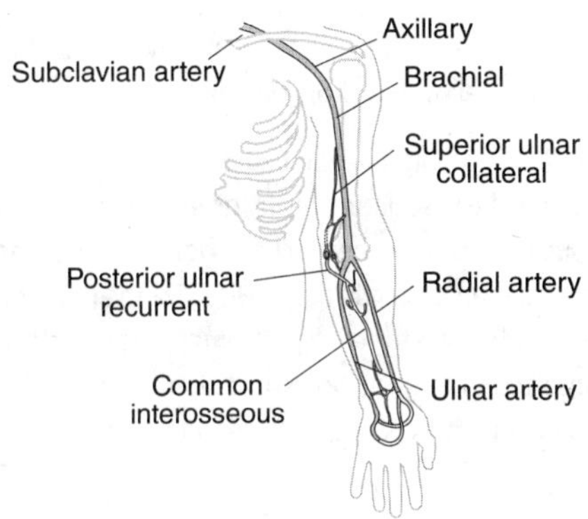

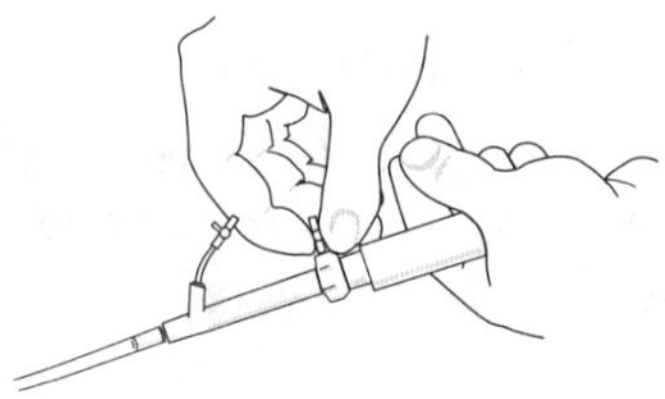

Needles or catheter are inserted into the dialysis circuit for diagnostic angiography

Explanation

The physician inserts a needle or catheter into a dialysis circuit via a puncture in the skin overlying the circuit of a dialysis patient. The catheter is guided into the circuit and vessel to an area upstream of the site under investigation, and contrast material is injected into it. Report 36901 for the initial access, including shunt access, contrast injections, and all fluoroscopic imaging deemed necessary from the arterial anastomosis and adjacent artery through the entire venous outflow (inferior and superior vena cava included). In 36902, a catheter with a balloon attached is inserted into the peripheral dialysis segment and fed into the narrowed portion where its balloon may be inflated several times in order to stretch the diameter, allowing a more normal flow of blood through the area. In 36903, a catheter with a stent-transporting tip is threaded over the guidewire into the peripheral dialysis segment and the wire is extracted. The catheter travels to the point where the vessel needs additional support. The compressed stent is passed from the catheter into the vessel, where it deploys, expanding to support the vessel walls. Once the procedure is complete, the catheter is removed and pressure is applied over the puncture site.

Coding Tips

Direct access, imaging of the dialysis circuit, catheter manipulation, catheter advancement to the vena cava for imaging, all dialysis circuit punctures, and venous side branches communicating with the dialysis circuit that require catheterization are included in 36901. If ultrasound guidance is required to safely puncture the dialysis circuit for evaluation, it may be reported separately, see 76937. Report 36902 once per encounter for all angioplasty services performed in the peripheral segment of the circuit. Report 36903 once per encounter regardless of the number of stents placed in the peripheral segment. Do not report 36901-36903 with 36833, 36904-36906, or with each other.

ICD-10-CM Diagnostic Codes

E08.21	Diabetes mellitus due to underlying condition with diabetic nephropathy
E08.22	Diabetes mellitus due to underlying condition with diabetic chronic kidney disease
E08.29	Diabetes mellitus due to underlying condition with other diabetic kidney complication
E08.65	Diabetes mellitus due to underlying condition with hyperglycemia
E09.21	Drug or chemical induced diabetes mellitus with diabetic nephropathy
E09.22	Drug or chemical induced diabetes mellitus with diabetic chronic kidney disease
E09.29	Drug or chemical induced diabetes mellitus with other diabetic kidney complication
E10.21	Type 1 diabetes mellitus with diabetic nephropathy
E10.22	Type 1 diabetes mellitus with diabetic chronic kidney disease
E10.29	Type 1 diabetes mellitus with other diabetic kidney complication
E10.65	Type 1 diabetes mellitus with hyperglycemia
E11.21	Type 2 diabetes mellitus with diabetic nephropathy
E11.22	Type 2 diabetes mellitus with diabetic chronic kidney disease
E11.29	Type 2 diabetes mellitus with other diabetic kidney complication
E11.65	Type 2 diabetes mellitus with hyperglycemia
E13.21	Other specified diabetes mellitus with diabetic nephropathy
E13.22	Other specified diabetes mellitus with diabetic chronic kidney disease
E13.29	Other specified diabetes mellitus with other diabetic kidney complication
I12.0	Hypertensive chronic kidney disease with stage 5 chronic kidney disease or end stage renal disease
I12.9	Hypertensive chronic kidney disease with stage 1 through stage 4 chronic kidney disease, or unspecified chronic kidney disease
I13.0	Hypertensive heart and chronic kidney disease with heart failure and stage 1 through stage 4 chronic kidney disease, or unspecified chronic kidney disease
I13.10	Hypertensive heart and chronic kidney disease without heart failure, with stage 1 through stage 4 chronic kidney disease, or unspecified chronic kidney disease
I13.11	Hypertensive heart and chronic kidney disease without heart failure, with stage 5 chronic kidney disease, or end stage renal disease
I13.2	Hypertensive heart and chronic kidney disease with heart failure and with stage 5 chronic kidney disease, or end stage renal disease
I16.0	Hypertensive urgency
I16.1	Hypertensive emergency

I16.9 Hypertensive crisis, unspecified
I87.1 Compression of vein
N17.0 Acute kidney failure with tubular necrosis
N17.1 Acute kidney failure with acute cortical necrosis
N17.2 Acute kidney failure with medullary necrosis
N17.8 Other acute kidney failure
N17.9 Acute kidney failure, unspecified
N18.4 Chronic kidney disease, stage 4 (severe)
N18.5 Chronic kidney disease, stage 5
N18.6 End stage renal disease
N18.9 Chronic kidney disease, unspecified
T82.510A Breakdown (mechanical) of surgically created arteriovenous fistula, initial encounter
T82.511A Breakdown (mechanical) of surgically created arteriovenous shunt, initial encounter
T82.530A Leakage of surgically created arteriovenous fistula, initial encounter
T82.531A Leakage of surgically created arteriovenous shunt, initial encounter
T82.590A Other mechanical complication of surgically created arteriovenous fistula, initial encounter
T82.591A Other mechanical complication of surgically created arteriovenous shunt, initial encounter
T82.818A Embolism due to vascular prosthetic devices, implants and grafts, initial encounter
T82.828A Fibrosis due to vascular prosthetic devices, implants and grafts, initial encounter
T82.838A Hemorrhage due to vascular prosthetic devices, implants and grafts, initial encounter
T82.848A Pain due to vascular prosthetic devices, implants and grafts, initial encounter
T82.856A Stenosis of peripheral vascular stent, initial encounter
T82.858A Stenosis of other vascular prosthetic devices, implants and grafts, initial encounter
T82.868A Thrombosis due to vascular prosthetic devices, implants and grafts, initial encounter
T82.898A Other specified complication of vascular prosthetic devices, implants and grafts, initial encounter

AMA: 36901 2018,Jan,8; 2017,Mar,3 **36902** 2018,Jan,8; 2017,Mar,3; 2017,Jul,3 **36903** 2018,Jan,8; 2017,Mar,3; 2017,Jul,3

Relative Value Units/Medicare Edits

Non-Facility RVU	Work	PE	MP	Total
36901	3.36	14.5	0.47	18.33
36902	4.83	30.59	0.67	36.09
36903	6.39	144.87	0.95	152.21
Facility RVU	**Work**	**PE**	**MP**	**Total**
36901	3.36	1.05	0.47	4.88
36902	4.83	1.48	0.67	6.98
36903	6.39	1.89	0.95	9.23

	FUD	Status	MUE	Modifiers				IOM Reference
36901	0	A	1(3)	51	N/A	N/A	N/A	None
36902	0	A	1(3)	51	N/A	N/A	N/A	
36903	0	A	1(3)	51	N/A	N/A	N/A	

* with documentation

Terms To Know

anastomosis. Surgically created connection between ducts, blood vessels, or bowel segments to allow flow from one to the other.

angiography. Radiographic imaging of the arteries. Imaging may be performed to study the vasculature of any given organ, body system, or area of circulation such as the brain, heart, chest, kidneys, limbs, gastrointestinal tract, aorta, and pulmonary circulation to visualize the formation and the function of the blood vessels to detect problems such as a blockage or stricture. A catheter is inserted through an accessible blood vessel and the artery is injected with a radiopaque contrast material after which x-rays are taken.

stent. Tube to provide support in a body cavity or lumen.

transcatheter. Procedure or treatment performed via a catheter.

transluminal balloon angioplasty. Balloon-tipped catheter is placed within a narrowed artery or vein and the balloon is inflated to stretch the vessel to a larger diameter for increased blood flow.

36904-36906

36904 Percutaneous transluminal mechanical thrombectomy and/or infusion for thrombolysis, dialysis circuit, any method, including all imaging and radiological supervision and interpretation, diagnostic angiography, fluoroscopic guidance, catheter placement(s), and intraprocedural pharmacological thrombolytic injection(s);

36905 with transluminal balloon angioplasty, peripheral dialysis segment, including all imaging and radiological supervision and interpretation necessary to perform the angioplasty

36906 with transcatheter placement of intravascular stent(s), peripheral dialysis segment, including all imaging and radiological supervision and interpretation necessary to perform the stenting, and all angioplasty within the peripheral dialysis circuit

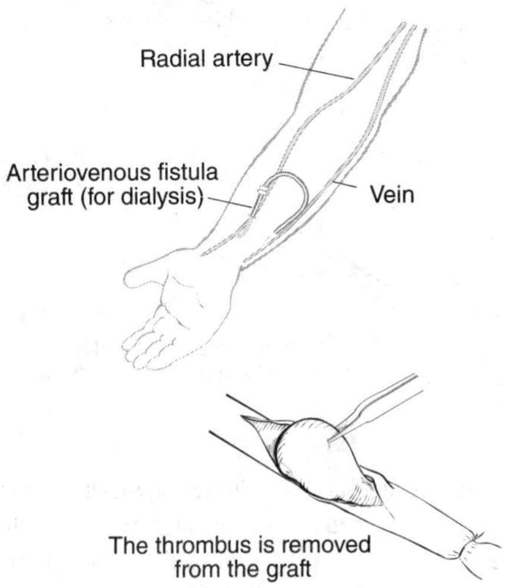

A thrombus (clot) is removed percutaneously from the dialysis circuit

Explanation

The physician treats the dialysis circuit occlusion with mechanical thrombectomy and/or thrombolysis infusion. The devices used for mechanical thrombectomy include those that fragment the thrombus with or without removal of the clot, as well as those that come into contact with the vessel wall. The dialysis circuit is cannulated to gain access and 5,000 units of heparin are administered. Angiography is performed to confirm the occluded segment. A hydrophilic wire is passed across the occlusion, followed by passing of the Trellis device over a stiff exchange length wire. The distal and proximal balloons are inflated in the segment on either side of a treatment zone containing infusion to isolate the treatment zone and to sustain the fluid concentration that is infused. One milligram of tissue plasminogen activator (TPA) is infused into the treatment zone. The Turbo Trellis is run at 4,000 rpm for five minutes. After the proximal balloon is deflated, small clots are removed via the integral aspiration port to prevent embolization. Thrombolysis infusion may be performed with a catheter threaded over the wire for pharmaceutical administration directly within the thrombosis. When the procedure is complete, the instruments are removed and pressure is applied over the puncture site to stop the bleeding. This procedure is reported with 36904 and includes imaging guidance, diagnostic angiography, catheter placement, and intraprocedural pharmacological thrombolytic injections. Report 36905 when the peripheral dialysis segment is treated with balloon angioplasty. A catheter with a balloon attached is inserted into the segment and fed into the narrowed portion, where its balloon may be inflated several times in order to stretch the diameter allowing a more normal flow of blood through the area. Report 36906 when the peripheral dialysis segment is treated with an intravascular stent. A catheter with a stent-transporting tip is threaded over the guidewire into the vessel and the wire is extracted. The catheter travels to the point where the vessel needs additional support. The compressed stent is passed from the catheter into the vessel, where it deploys, expanding to support the vessel walls. Once the procedure is complete, the catheter is removed and pressure is applied over the puncture site.

Coding Tips

Diagnostic angiography, fluoroscopy, all manipulation required to remove a thrombus, and catheter placements are included in 36904. Report 36905 once per encounter for all angioplasty services performed in the peripheral segment of the circuit. Report 36906 once per encounter regardless of the number of stents placed in the peripheral segment. Do not report 36905 with 36904. Do not report 36906 with 36901-36905. For transluminal balloon angioplasty, see 36907. For transcatheter placement of intravascular stents within the central vein of the dialysis circuit, see 36908.

ICD-10-CM Diagnostic Codes

T82.328A	Displacement of other vascular grafts, initial encounter
T82.338A	Leakage of other vascular grafts, initial encounter
T82.398A	Other mechanical complication of other vascular grafts, initial encounter
T82.41XA	Breakdown (mechanical) of vascular dialysis catheter, initial encounter
T82.42XA	Displacement of vascular dialysis catheter, initial encounter
T82.43XA	Leakage of vascular dialysis catheter, initial encounter
T82.49XA	Other complication of vascular dialysis catheter, initial encounter
T82.510A	Breakdown (mechanical) of surgically created arteriovenous fistula, initial encounter
T82.511A	Breakdown (mechanical) of surgically created arteriovenous shunt, initial encounter
T82.520A	Displacement of surgically created arteriovenous fistula, initial encounter
T82.521A	Displacement of surgically created arteriovenous shunt, initial encounter
T82.530A	Leakage of surgically created arteriovenous fistula, initial encounter
T82.531A	Leakage of surgically created arteriovenous shunt, initial encounter
T82.590A	Other mechanical complication of surgically created arteriovenous fistula, initial encounter
T82.591A	Other mechanical complication of surgically created arteriovenous shunt, initial encounter
T82.818A	Embolism due to vascular prosthetic devices, implants and grafts, initial encounter
T82.828A	Fibrosis due to vascular prosthetic devices, implants and grafts, initial encounter
T82.838A	Hemorrhage due to vascular prosthetic devices, implants and grafts, initial encounter
T82.848A	Pain due to vascular prosthetic devices, implants and grafts, initial encounter
T82.856A	Stenosis of peripheral vascular stent, initial encounter
T82.858A	Stenosis of other vascular prosthetic devices, implants and grafts, initial encounter
T82.868A	Thrombosis due to vascular prosthetic devices, implants and grafts, initial encounter
T82.898A	Other specified complication of vascular prosthetic devices, implants and grafts, initial encounter

AMA: 36904 2018,Jan,8; 2017,Mar,3; 2017,Jul,3 **36905** 2018,Jan,8; 2017,Mar,3; 2017,Jul,3 **36906** 2018,Jan,8; 2017,Mar,3; 2017,Jul,3

Relative Value Units/Medicare Edits

Non-Facility RVU	Work	PE	MP	Total
36904	7.5	44.57	1.04	53.11
36905	9.0	56.58	1.22	66.8
36906	10.42	174.72	1.42	186.56
Facility RVU	**Work**	**PE**	**MP**	**Total**
36904	7.5	2.23	1.04	10.77
36905	9.0	2.69	1.22	12.91
36906	10.42	3.06	1.42	14.9

	FUD	Status	MUE	Modifiers				IOM Reference
36904	0	A	1(3)	51	N/A	62*	N/A	None
36905	0	A	1(3)	51	N/A	62*	N/A	
36906	0	A	1(3)	51	N/A	62*	N/A	

* with documentation

Terms To Know

cannulation. Insertion of a flexible length of hollow tubing into a blood vessel, duct, or body cavity, usually for extracorporeal circulation or chemotherapy infusion to a particular region of the body.

thrombectomy. Removal of a clot (thrombus) from a blood vessel utilizing various methods.

thrombolysis. Chemical process of dissolving or breaking down a blood clot by inducing a complex chain of events involving the action of plasminogen to solubilize fibrin clots and degrade fibrinogen.

transluminal balloon angioplasty. Balloon-tipped catheter is placed within a narrowed artery or vein and the balloon is inflated to stretch the vessel to a larger diameter for increased blood flow.

36907-36908

+ 36907 Transluminal balloon angioplasty, central dialysis segment, performed through dialysis circuit, including all imaging and radiological supervision and interpretation required to perform the angioplasty (List separately in addition to code for primary procedure)

+ 36908 Transcatheter placement of intravascular stent(s), central dialysis segment, performed through dialysis circuit, including all imaging and radiological supervision and interpretation required to perform the stenting, and all angioplasty in the central dialysis segment (List separately in addition to code for primary procedure)

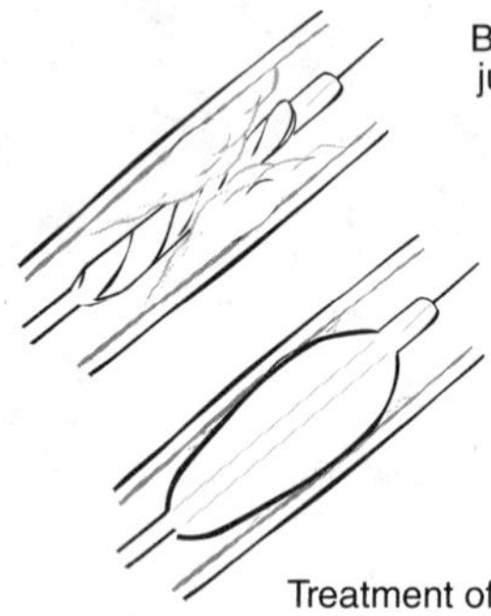

Treatment of the central dialysis segment by balloon angioplasty or stent

Explanation

The physician inserts a needle or catheter into a dialysis circuit via a puncture in the skin. The catheter is guided into the circuit to an area upstream of the investigation site and contrast material is injected. In 36907, a catheter with a balloon attached is inserted into the central dialysis segment and fed into the narrowed portion, where its balloon may be inflated several times in order to stretch the diameter, allowing a more normal blood flow through the area. In 36908, a catheter with a stent-transporting tip is threaded over the guidewire into the central dialysis segment and the wire is extracted. The catheter travels to the point where the vessel needs additional support. The compressed stent is passed from the catheter out into the vessel, where it deploys, expanding to support the vessel walls. Once the procedure is complete, the catheter is removed and pressure is applied over the puncture site. All imaging and radiological supervision and interpretation is included.

Coding Tips

Report 36907 and 36908 in addition to 36818-36833, or 36901-36906. Report 36907 once for all angioplasty performed within the central dialysis segment. Report 36908 once per encounter for all stenting performed within the central dialysis segment. Report 36908 once per encounter regardless of the number of stents placed or lesions treated. Do not report 36908 with 36907.

ICD-10-CM Diagnostic Codes

This/these CPT code(s) are add on code(s). See the primary procedure code that this code is performed with for your ICD-10-CM code selections. Diagnostic code(s) would be the same as the actual procedure performed.

AMA: 36907 2018,Jan,8; 2017,Mar,3; 2017,Jul,3 **36908** 2018,Jan,8; 2017,Mar,3; 2017,Jul,3

Relative Value Units/Medicare Edits

Non-Facility RVU	Work	PE	MP	Total
36907	3.0	17.01	0.42	20.43
36908	4.25	63.14	0.63	68.02
Facility RVU	**Work**	**PE**	**MP**	**Total**
36907	3.0	0.84	0.42	4.26
36908	4.25	1.15	0.63	6.03

	FUD	Status	MUE	Modifiers				IOM Reference
36907	N/A	A	1(3)	N/A	N/A	N/A	N/A	None
36908	N/A	A	1(3)	N/A	N/A	N/A	N/A	

* with documentation

Terms To Know

angioplasty. Reconstruction or repair of a diseased or damaged blood vessel.

dialysis. Artificial filtering of the blood to remove contaminating waste elements and restore normal balance.

guidewire. Flexible metal instrument designed to lead another instrument in its proper course.

stent. Tube to provide support in a body cavity or lumen.

supervision and interpretation. Radiology services that usually contain an invasive component and are reported by the radiologist for supervision of the procedure and the personnel involved with performing the examination, reading the film, and preparing the written report.

36909

\+ **36909** Dialysis circuit permanent vascular embolization or occlusion (including main circuit or any accessory veins), endovascular, including all imaging and radiological supervision and interpretation necessary to complete the intervention (List separately in addition to code for primary procedure)

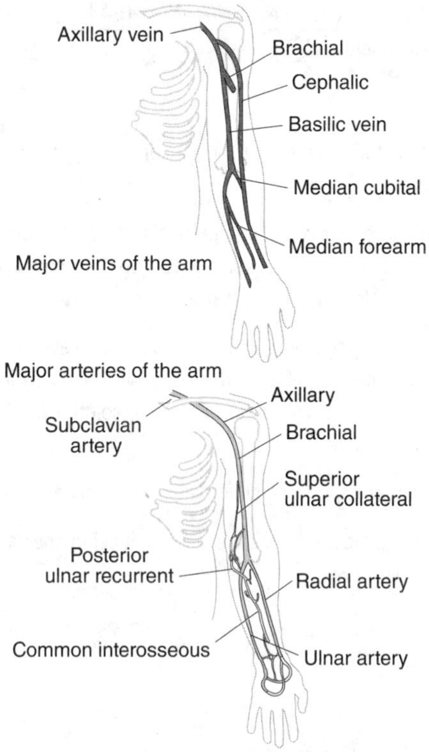

Endovascular embolization or occlusion of dialysis circuit

Explanation

The physician performs embolization or occlusion of a dialysis circuit (main circuit or any accessory vein) due to complications or to assist in circuit maturity and/or patency. A needle is inserted through the skin and into a blood vessel. A guidewire is threaded through the needle into the vessel. The needle is removed. A catheter is threaded into the vessel and the wire is extracted. The catheter travels to the appropriate blood vessel and beads, coils, or another vessel-blocking device are released. The beads or other device block the vessel. The catheter is removed and pressure is applied over the puncture site to stop bleeding.

Coding Tips

Report 36909 in addition to 36901-36906. Report 36909 once per encounter/day for all permanent vascular occlusions within the circuit. For open ligation/occlusion of dialysis access, see 37607.

ICD-10-CM Diagnostic Codes

This/these CPT code(s) are add on code(s). See the primary procedure code that this code is performed with for your ICD-10-CM code selections. Diagnostic code(s) would be the same as the actual procedure performed.

AMA: 36909 2018,Jan,8; 2017,Mar,3

Relative Value Units/Medicare Edits

Non-Facility RVU	Work	PE	MP	Total
36909	4.12	50.25	0.61	54.98
Facility RVU	**Work**	**PE**	**MP**	**Total**
36909	4.12	1.11	0.61	5.84

	FUD	Status	MUE	Modifiers				IOM Reference
36909	N/A	A	1(3)	N/A	N/A	N/A	N/A	None

* with documentation

Terms To Know

catheter. Flexible tube inserted into an area of the body for introducing or withdrawing fluid.

embolization. Placement of a clotting agent, such as a coil, plastic particles, gel, foam, etc., into an area of hemorrhage to stop the bleeding or to block blood flow to a problem area, such as an aneurysm or a tumor.

hemodialysis. Cleansing of wastes and contaminating elements from the blood by virtue of different diffusion rates through a semipermeable membrane, which separates blood from a filtration solution that diffuses other elements out of the blood.

occlusion. Constriction, closure, or blockage of a passage.

patency. State of a tube-like structure or conduit being open and unobstructed.

37140

37140 Venous anastomosis, open; portocaval

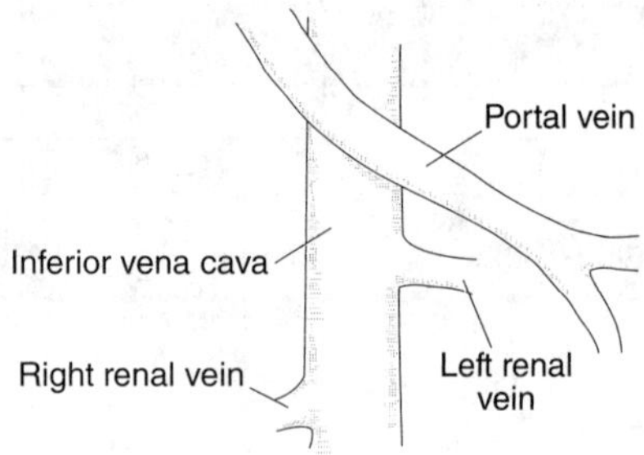

Schematic of portocaval anatomy

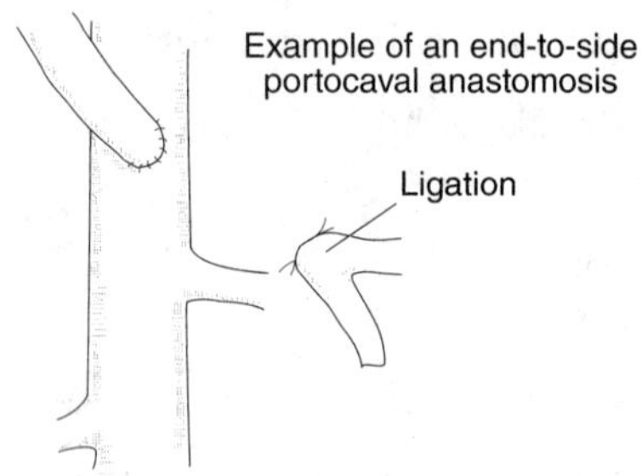

Explanation

The physician performs portacaval venous anastomosis. The physician places a long right thoracoabdominal incision and exposes the liver. The physician exposes the inferior vena cava and portal vein through careful dissection. The physician places a plastic sling around the portal vein and ties it closed, just proximal to its bifurcation. The physician clamps and divides the portal vein. The physician applies a partial exclusion vascular clamp to the front of the vena cava and removes a small oval of tissue from the vena cava to allow end-to-side anastomosis of portal vein to the inferior vena cava. The physician removes the clamps and checks for appropriate flow without anastomotic leakage. The physician closes the incision, leaving a chest tube in place (but no abdominal drains, as this may lead to protein loss from postoperative drainage of ascites).

Coding Tips

When 37140 is performed with another separately identifiable procedure, the highest dollar value code is listed as the primary procedure and subsequent procedures are appended with modifier 51. For a percutaneous procedure, see 37182. For a peritoneal-venous shunt, see 49425. For venous anastomosis, renoportal, see 37145.

ICD-10-CM Diagnostic Codes

I81	Portal vein thrombosis
I82.0	Budd-Chiari syndrome
I85.11	Secondary esophageal varices with bleeding
I87.1	Compression of vein
K70.0	Alcoholic fatty liver
K70.30	Alcoholic cirrhosis of liver without ascites
K70.31	Alcoholic cirrhosis of liver with ascites
K74.69	Other cirrhosis of liver
K75.1	Phlebitis of portal vein
K76.0	Fatty (change of) liver, not elsewhere classified

K76.1	Chronic passive congestion of liver
K76.3	Infarction of liver
K76.5	Hepatic veno-occlusive disease
K76.6	Portal hypertension
K76.89	Other specified diseases of liver

AMA: **37140** 2014,Jan,11

Relative Value Units/Medicare Edits

Non-Facility RVU	Work	PE	MP	Total
37140	40.0	17.67	9.73	67.4
Facility RVU	**Work**	**PE**	**MP**	**Total**
37140	40.0	17.67	9.73	67.4

	FUD	Status	MUE	Modifiers				IOM Reference
37140	90	A	1(2)	51	N/A	62*	N/A	None

* with documentation

Terms To Know

anastomosis. Surgically created connection between ducts, blood vessels, or bowel segments to allow flow from one to the other.

bifurcated. Having two branches or divisions, such as the left pulmonary veins that split off from the left atrium to carry oxygenated blood away from the heart.

Budd-Chiari syndrome. Thrombus or other obstruction of the hepatic vein, with an enlarged liver, intractable ascites, portal hypertension, and the growth of extensive collateral vessels.

dissection. Separating by cutting tissue or body structures apart.

hypertension. Abnormally increased pressure, usually referring to arterial pressure, exceeding an acceptable range.

incision. Act of cutting into tissue or an organ.

portal hypertension. Abnormally high blood pressure in the portal vein.

shunt. Surgically created passage between blood vessels or other natural passages, such as an arteriovenous anastomosis, to divert or bypass blood flow from the normal channel.

thrombosis. Condition arising from the presence or formation of blood clots within a blood vessel that may cause vascular obstruction and insufficient oxygenation.

thrombus. Stationary blood clot inside a blood vessel.

varices. Enlarged, dilated, or twisted turning veins.

37145

37145 Venous anastomosis, open; renoportal

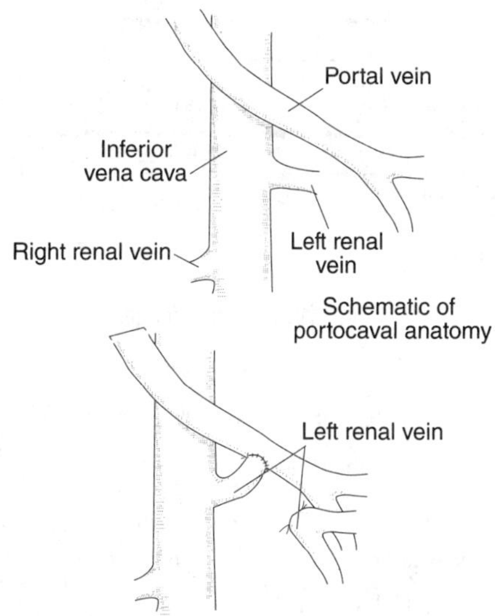

Example of a renoportal anastomosis

Explanation

The physician performs an abdominal incision and exposes the left renal vein and inferior vena cava. The physician transects the left renal vein and attaches it to the portal circulation by sewing the vena caval end to the portal vein, the superior mesenteric vein, or the splenic vein. Alternatively, the physician may divide the portal vein and attach its splanchnic end to the end of the transected renal vein. The physician assesses patency of the anastomosis and may measure venous pressures before closing the abdomen.

Coding Tips

When 37145 is performed with another separately identifiable procedure, the highest dollar value code is listed as the primary procedure, and subsequent procedures are appended with modifier 51. For venous anastomosis, portocaval, see 37140.

ICD-10-CM Diagnostic Codes

I81	Portal vein thrombosis
I82.0	Budd-Chiari syndrome
I82.3	Embolism and thrombosis of renal vein
I85.11	Secondary esophageal varices with bleeding
N26.9	Renal sclerosis, unspecified
N28.0	Ischemia and infarction of kidney
Q27.34	Arteriovenous malformation of renal vessel
Q27.8	Other specified congenital malformations of peripheral vascular system
S35.311A	Laceration of portal vein, initial encounter
S35.318A	Other specified injury of portal vein, initial encounter
S35.319A	Unspecified injury of portal vein, initial encounter

AMA: **37145** 2014,Jan,11

Relative Value Units/Medicare Edits

Non-Facility RVU	Work	PE	MP	Total
37145	37.0	16.51	8.99	62.5
Facility RVU	**Work**	**PE**	**MP**	**Total**
37145	37.0	16.51	8.99	62.5

	FUD	Status	MUE	Modifiers				IOM Reference
37145	90	A	1(3)	51	N/A	N/A	80	None

* with documentation

Terms To Know

anastomosis. Surgically created connection between ducts, blood vessels, or bowel segments to allow flow from one to the other.

anomaly. Irregularity in the structure or position of an organ or tissue.

benign. Mild or nonmalignant in nature.

Budd-Chiari syndrome. Thrombus or other obstruction of the hepatic vein, with an enlarged liver, intractable ascites, portal hypertension, and the growth of extensive collateral vessels.

congenital. Present at birth, occurring through heredity or an influence during gestation up to the moment of birth.

embolism. Obstruction of a blood vessel resulting from a clot or foreign substance.

incision. Act of cutting into tissue or an organ.

malignant. Any condition tending to progress toward death, specifically an invasive tumor with a loss of cellular differentiation that has the ability to spread or metastasize to other body areas.

patency. State of a tube-like structure or conduit being open and unobstructed.

renal failure. Inability of a kidney to eliminate metabolites and retain electrolytes at a normal level.

shunt. Surgically created passage between blood vessels or other natural passages, such as an arteriovenous anastomosis, to divert or bypass blood flow from the normal channel.

thrombosis. Condition arising from the presence or formation of blood clots within a blood vessel that may cause vascular obstruction and insufficient oxygenation.

37160

37160 Venous anastomosis, open; caval-mesenteric

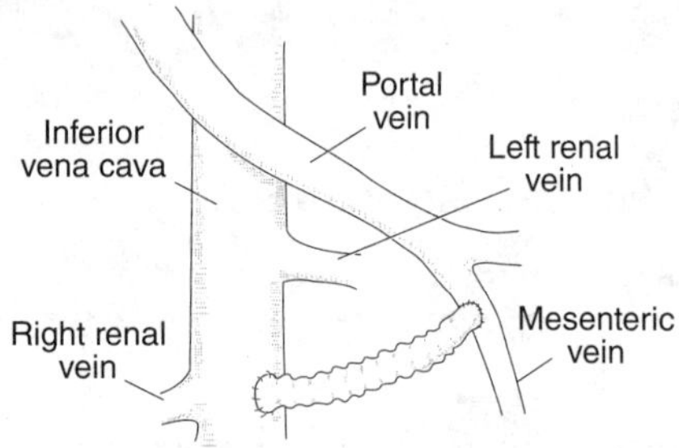

Example of a synthetic side-to-side caval-mesenteric anastomosis

This shunting procedure is designed to reduce pressure in the portal system and as therapy for esophagogastric varices

Explanation

The physician performs an upper midline vertical abdominal incision and retracts the transverse colon in a cephalad direction. The physician exposes the anterior surface of the inferior vena cava and frees the posterior surface of the superior mesenteric vein after careful dissection through the root of the transverse mesocolon. The physician isolates a long segment of the superior mesenteric vein with ties and partially occludes the inferior vena cava. The physician removes an ellipse of tissue from the inferior vena cava and performs and end-to-side anastomosis of Dacron graft to the inferior vena cava. The physician occludes the superior mesenteric vein, cuts an ellipse from its anterior surface, and sews the end of the Dacron graft to the side of the superior mesenteric vein. The physician assesses patency of the anastomosis and may measure venous pressures before closing the abdomen.

Coding Tips

When 37160 is performed with another separately identifiable procedure, the highest dollar value code is listed as the primary procedure, and subsequent procedures are appended with modifier 51. For venous anastomosis, portocaval, see 37140. For venous anastomosis, renoportal, see 37145.

ICD-10-CM Diagnostic Codes

I81	Portal vein thrombosis
I82.890	Acute embolism and thrombosis of other specified veins
I82.891	Chronic embolism and thrombosis of other specified veins
I85.11	Secondary esophageal varices with bleeding
I87.1	Compression of vein
K70.0	Alcoholic fatty liver
K70.30	Alcoholic cirrhosis of liver without ascites
K70.31	Alcoholic cirrhosis of liver with ascites
K74.60	Unspecified cirrhosis of liver
K74.69	Other cirrhosis of liver
K76.0	Fatty (change of) liver, not elsewhere classified
K76.1	Chronic passive congestion of liver
K76.3	Infarction of liver
K76.5	Hepatic veno-occlusive disease
K76.6	Portal hypertension
K76.89	Other specified diseases of liver
K76.9	Liver disease, unspecified

R16.0 Hepatomegaly, not elsewhere classified

R16.2 Hepatomegaly with splenomegaly, not elsewhere classified

AMA: **37160** 2014,Jan,11

Relative Value Units/Medicare Edits

Non-Facility RVU	Work	PE	MP	Total
37160	38.0	16.97	9.25	64.22
Facility RVU	**Work**	**PE**	**MP**	**Total**
37160	38.0	16.97	9.25	64.22

	FUD	Status	MUE	Modifiers				IOM Reference
37160	90	A	1(3)	51	N/A	62*	80	None

* with documentation

Terms To Know

acute. Sudden, severe. Documentation and reporting of an acute condition is important to establishing medical necessity.

anastomosis. Surgically created connection between ducts, blood vessels, or bowel segments to allow flow from one to the other.

cephalad. Toward the head.

chronic. Persistent, continuing, or recurring.

dissection. Separating by cutting tissue or body structures apart.

embolism. Obstruction of a blood vessel resulting from a clot or foreign substance.

graft. Tissue implant from another part of the body or another person.

incision. Act of cutting into tissue or an organ.

patency. State of a tube-like structure or conduit being open and unobstructed.

shunt. Surgically created passage between blood vessels or other natural passages, such as an arteriovenous anastomosis, to divert or bypass blood flow from the normal channel.

vascular insufficiency. Inadequate blood flow and oxygenation.

37180

37180 Venous anastomosis, open; splenorenal, proximal

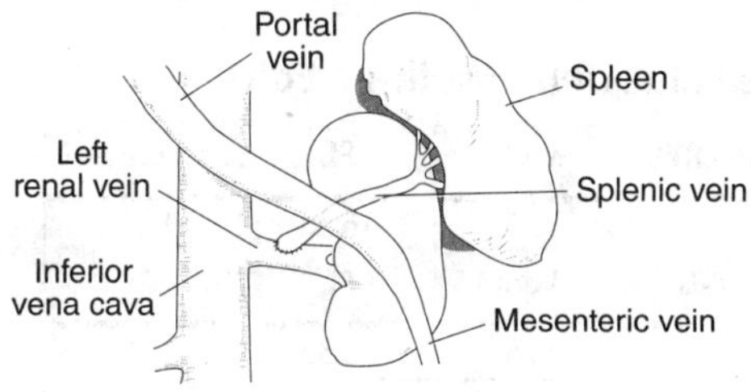

Example of a splenorenal anastomosis

A shunting procedure designed to reduce pressure in the portal system and as therapy for esophagogastric varices

Explanation

The physician performs a bilateral subcostal incision from the right midrectus position extending into the left flank, and dissects past bowel and pancreas to expose the splenic vein. The physician dissects the splenic vein free, ligating the splenic vein toward the left and using the central (right) end of the vein for the anastomosis. The physician exposes the left renal vein by dissecting through the posterior parietal peritoneum. The physician exposes the left renal vein, partially clamps it, and excises an ellipse of renal vein at its upper border. The physician performs and end-to-side anastomosis of the splenic vein to the renal vein, using harvested vein graft material if extension is required. The physician removes the clamps. The physician may measure superior mesenteric (portal), renal, and splenic venous pressures. The physician may perform venography to establish patency of the graft. The physician closes the abdominal wound.

Coding Tips

When 37180 is performed with another separately identifiable procedure, the highest dollar value code is listed as the primary procedure, and subsequent procedures are appended with modifier 51. For venous anastomosis, splenorenal, distal, see 37181. For venous anastomosis, portocaval, see 37140. For venous anastomosis, renoportal, see 37145. For venous anastomosis, caval-mesenteric, see 37160.

ICD-10-CM Diagnostic Codes

D73.1 Hypersplenism

I81 Portal vein thrombosis

I85.11 Secondary esophageal varices with bleeding

I87.1 Compression of vein

K70.0 Alcoholic fatty liver

K70.30 Alcoholic cirrhosis of liver without ascites

K70.31 Alcoholic cirrhosis of liver with ascites

K74.60 Unspecified cirrhosis of liver

K74.69 Other cirrhosis of liver

K76.0 Fatty (change of) liver, not elsewhere classified

K76.1 Chronic passive congestion of liver

K76.3 Infarction of liver

K76.5 Hepatic veno-occlusive disease

K76.6 Portal hypertension

K76.89 Other specified diseases of liver

K76.9 Liver disease, unspecified

R16.0 Hepatomegaly, not elsewhere classified
R16.1 Splenomegaly, not elsewhere classified
R16.2 Hepatomegaly with splenomegaly, not elsewhere classified

AMA: **37180** 2014,Jan,11

Relative Value Units/Medicare Edits

Non-Facility RVU	Work	PE	MP	Total
37180	36.5	16.36	8.87	61.73
Facility RVU	**Work**	**PE**	**MP**	**Total**
37180	36.5	16.36	8.87	61.73

	FUD	Status	MUE	Modifiers				IOM Reference
37180	90	A	1(2)	51	N/A	62*	80	None

* with documentation

Terms To Know

cirrhosis of liver. Chronic disease of the liver that characteristically produces intertwining bands of fibrotic tissue that change the normal structure of the lobes of the liver and destroys normal cells, which then regenerate into nodules and cause the liver to stop functioning over time. This form of cirrhosis is not alcohol related.

embolism. Obstruction of a blood vessel resulting from a clot or foreign substance.

portal hypertension. Abnormally high blood pressure in the portal vein.

thrombosis. Condition arising from the presence or formation of blood clots within a blood vessel that may cause vascular obstruction and insufficient oxygenation.

37181

37181 Venous anastomosis, open; splenorenal, distal (selective decompression of esophagogastric varices, any technique)

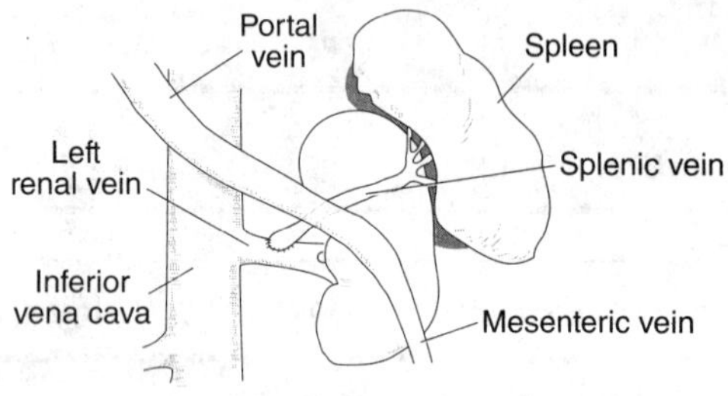

Example of a distal splenorenal anastomosis, also known as a DSR

A shunting procedure designed to reduce pressure in the portal system and as therapy for esophagogastric varices

Explanation

The physician performs a bilateral subcostal incision from the right midrectus position extending into the left flank, and dissects past bowel and pancreas to expose the splenic vein. The physician dissects the splenic vein free, ligating or clipping any vessels in continuity to the vein. The physician exposes the left renal vein by dissecting through the posterior parietal peritoneum. The physician exposes the left renal vein, partially clamps it, and excises an ellipse of renal vein at its upper border. The physician performs and end-to-side anastomosis of the splenic vein to the renal vein, using harvested vein graft material if extension is required. The physician removes the clamps and divides the coronary (right gastric) vein, left gastric vein, and gastroepiploic veins. The physician may measure superior mesenteric (portal), renal, and splenic venous pressures. The physician may perform venography to establish patency of the graft. The physician closes the abdominal wound.

Coding Tips

When 37181 is performed with another separately identifiable procedure, the highest dollar value code is listed as the primary procedure, and subsequent procedures are appended with modifier 51. For venous anastomosis, splenorenal, proximal, see 37180; portocaval, see 37140; and renoportal, see 37145. For venous anastomosis, caval-mesenteric, see 37160. For percutaneous approach, see 37182.

ICD-10-CM Diagnostic Codes

D73.1 Hypersplenism
I81 Portal vein thrombosis
I85.11 Secondary esophageal varices with bleeding
I87.1 Compression of vein
K70.0 Alcoholic fatty liver
K70.30 Alcoholic cirrhosis of liver without ascites
K70.31 Alcoholic cirrhosis of liver with ascites
K74.60 Unspecified cirrhosis of liver
K74.69 Other cirrhosis of liver
K76.0 Fatty (change of) liver, not elsewhere classified
K76.1 Chronic passive congestion of liver
K76.3 Infarction of liver
K76.5 Hepatic veno-occlusive disease
K76.6 Portal hypertension

K76.89	Other specified diseases of liver
K76.9	Liver disease, unspecified
R16.0	Hepatomegaly, not elsewhere classified
R16.1	Splenomegaly, not elsewhere classified
R16.2	Hepatomegaly with splenomegaly, not elsewhere classified
R18.8	Other ascites

AMA: **37181** 2014,Jan,11

Relative Value Units/Medicare Edits

Non-Facility RVU	Work	PE	MP	Total
37181	40.0	17.67	9.73	67.4
Facility RVU	**Work**	**PE**	**MP**	**Total**
37181	40.0	17.67	9.73	67.4

	FUD	Status	MUE	Modifiers				IOM Reference
37181	90	A	1(2)	51	N/A	62*	80	None

* with documentation

Terms To Know

cirrhosis of liver. Chronic disease of the liver that characteristically produces intertwining bands of fibrotic tissue that change the normal structure of the lobes of the liver and destroys normal cells, which then regenerate into nodules and cause the liver to stop functioning over time. This form of cirrhosis is not alcohol related.

esophageal varices. Distended, tortuous varicose veins in the lower esophagus. Esophageal varices are frequently a cause of esophageal hemorrhaging and commonly a symptom of portal hypertension from chronic liver disease, especially alcoholic cirrhosis.

portal hypertension. Abnormally high blood pressure in the portal vein.

37182-37183

37182 Insertion of transvenous intrahepatic portosystemic shunt(s) (TIPS) (includes venous access, hepatic and portal vein catheterization, portography with hemodynamic evaluation, intrahepatic tract formation/dilatation, stent placement and all associated imaging guidance and documentation)

37183 Revision of transvenous intrahepatic portosystemic shunt(s) (TIPS) (includes venous access, hepatic and portal vein catheterization, portography with hemodynamic evaluation, intrahepatic tract recanulization/dilatation, stent placement and all associated imaging guidance and documentation)

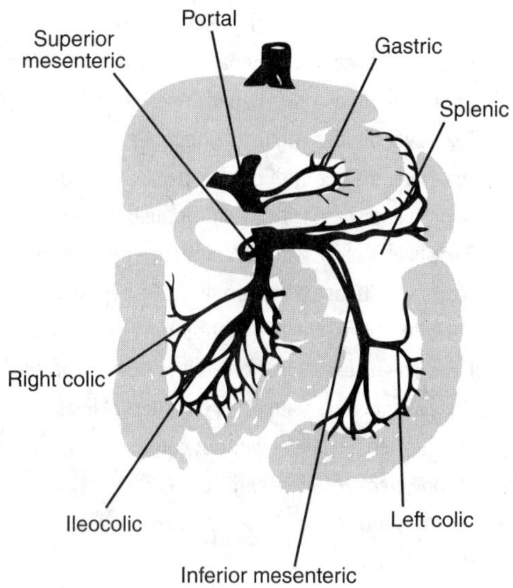

Explanation

A transvenous intrahepatic portosystemic shunt (TIPS) is inserted in 37182 and replaced in 37183. Shunts are placed percutaneously to manage the complications of portal hypertension and control variceal bleeding and ascites. Once the patient is under general anesthesia or conscious sedation, the right internal jugular vein is accessed and a catheter is placed into the right hepatic vein. Catheter placement is verified using venography. A Colapinto needle is advanced through the catheter into the wall of the right hepatic vein to access the right portal vein. A guidewire and catheter are advanced along this route into the portal vein and venography is performed again to verify placement. A self-expanding metallic stent is deployed through the catheter and dilated to the desired diameter where it bridges the portal and hepatic veins, using an angioplastic balloon. Postplacement venography and pressure measurements confirm adequate position and flow through the TIPS. The balloon, catheter, and other endoscopic tools are removed and pressure is applied to the insertion site, which may require suture. In 37183, the existing shunt is collapsed and removed through the catheter before a new one is inserted and dilated.

Coding Tips

When medically necessary, report moderate (conscious) sedation provided by the performing physician with 99151-99153. When provided by another physician, report 99155-99157. Do not report 75885 or 75887 with 37182 or 37183. For open portocaval venous anastomosis, see 37140. For repair of an arteriovenous aneurysm, see 36832.

ICD-10-CM Diagnostic Codes

I81	Portal vein thrombosis

I82.0 Budd-Chiari syndrome
I85.01 Esophageal varices with bleeding
I85.11 Secondary esophageal varices with bleeding
I87.1 Compression of vein
K70.0 Alcoholic fatty liver
K70.10 Alcoholic hepatitis without ascites
K70.11 Alcoholic hepatitis with ascites
K70.2 Alcoholic fibrosis and sclerosis of liver
K70.30 Alcoholic cirrhosis of liver without ascites
K70.31 Alcoholic cirrhosis of liver with ascites
K70.40 Alcoholic hepatic failure without coma
K70.41 Alcoholic hepatic failure with coma
K71.0 Toxic liver disease with cholestasis
K71.10 Toxic liver disease with hepatic necrosis, without coma
K71.11 Toxic liver disease with hepatic necrosis, with coma
K71.2 Toxic liver disease with acute hepatitis
K71.3 Toxic liver disease with chronic persistent hepatitis
K71.4 Toxic liver disease with chronic lobular hepatitis
K71.50 Toxic liver disease with chronic active hepatitis without ascites
K71.51 Toxic liver disease with chronic active hepatitis with ascites
K71.6 Toxic liver disease with hepatitis, not elsewhere classified
K71.7 Toxic liver disease with fibrosis and cirrhosis of liver
K71.8 Toxic liver disease with other disorders of liver
K72.10 Chronic hepatic failure without coma
K72.11 Chronic hepatic failure with coma
K74.0 Hepatic fibrosis
K74.1 Hepatic sclerosis
K74.2 Hepatic fibrosis with hepatic sclerosis
K74.69 Other cirrhosis of liver
K75.1 Phlebitis of portal vein
K75.89 Other specified inflammatory liver diseases
K76.0 Fatty (change of) liver, not elsewhere classified
K76.1 Chronic passive congestion of liver
K76.2 Central hemorrhagic necrosis of liver
K76.3 Infarction of liver
K76.5 Hepatic veno-occlusive disease
K76.6 Portal hypertension
K76.7 Hepatorenal syndrome
K76.89 Other specified diseases of liver
K91.82 Postprocedural hepatic failure
K91.83 Postprocedural hepatorenal syndrome
K91.89 Other postprocedural complications and disorders of digestive system
R18.0 Malignant ascites
R18.8 Other ascites
S35.11XA Minor laceration of inferior vena cava, initial encounter
S35.12XA Major laceration of inferior vena cava, initial encounter
S35.19XA Other injury of inferior vena cava, initial encounter
T82.598A Other mechanical complication of other cardiac and vascular devices and implants, initial encounter
T82.7XXA Infection and inflammatory reaction due to other cardiac and vascular devices, implants and grafts, initial encounter
T82.818A Embolism due to vascular prosthetic devices, implants and grafts, initial encounter
T82.828A Fibrosis due to vascular prosthetic devices, implants and grafts, initial encounter
T82.838A Hemorrhage due to vascular prosthetic devices, implants and grafts, initial encounter
T82.848A Pain due to vascular prosthetic devices, implants and grafts, initial encounter
T82.856A Stenosis of peripheral vascular stent, initial encounter
T82.858A Stenosis of other vascular prosthetic devices, implants and grafts, initial encounter
T82.868A Thrombosis due to vascular prosthetic devices, implants and grafts, initial encounter
T82.898A Other specified complication of vascular prosthetic devices, implants and grafts, initial encounter

AMA: **37182** 2018,Jan,8; 2017,Jan,8; 2016,Jan,13; 2015,Jan,16; 2014,Jan,11; 2013,Sep,17 **37183** 2018,Jan,8; 2017,Jan,8; 2016,Jan,13; 2015,Jan,16; 2014,Jan,11

Relative Value Units/Medicare Edits

Non-Facility RVU	Work	PE	MP	Total
37182	16.97	5.36	1.46	23.79
37183	7.74	161.95	0.67	170.36
Facility RVU	**Work**	**PE**	**MP**	**Total**
37182	16.97	5.36	1.46	23.79
37183	7.74	2.47	0.67	10.88

	FUD	Status	MUE	Modifiers				IOM Reference
37182	0	A	1(2)	51	N/A	N/A	80*	None
37183	0	A	1(2)	51	N/A	N/A	80*	

* with documentation

Terms To Know

ascites. Abnormal accumulation of free fluid in the abdominal cavity, causing distention and tightness in addition to shortness of breath as the fluid accumulates. Ascites is usually an underlying disorder and can be a manifestation of any number of diseases.

Budd-Chiari syndrome. Thrombus or other obstruction of the hepatic vein, with an enlarged liver, intractable ascites, portal hypertension, and the growth of extensive collateral vessels.

portal hypertension. Abnormally high blood pressure in the portal vein.

37184-37185

37184 Primary percutaneous transluminal mechanical thrombectomy, noncoronary, non-intracranial, arterial or arterial bypass graft, including fluoroscopic guidance and intraprocedural pharmacological thrombolytic injection(s); initial vessel

\+ **37185** second and all subsequent vessel(s) within the same vascular family (List separately in addition to code for primary mechanical thrombectomy procedure)

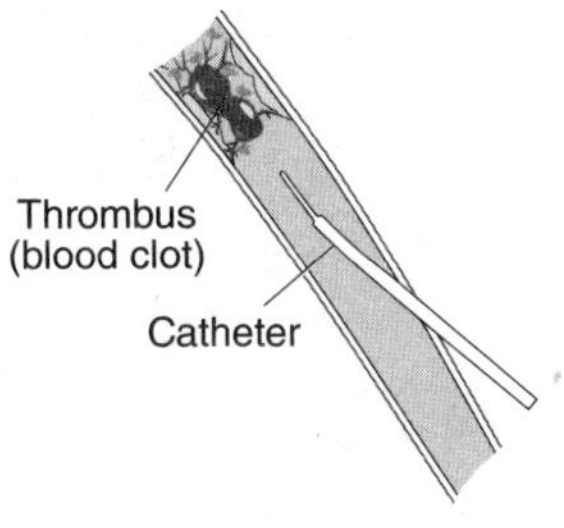

A transluminal device removes a blood clot from an artery or artery graft other than from the heart

Explanation

The physician treats an acute noncoronary, nonintracranial arterial occlusion with a combination of thrombolytic drugs and percutaneous mechanical thrombectomy. The devices used for mechanical thrombectomy include those that fragment the thrombus with or without removal of the clot, as well as those that come into contact with the wall of the vessel. For the procedure using the Trellis device, the artery is cannulated to gain access and 5,000 units of heparin are administered. Angiography is performed to confirm the occluded arteries. A hydrophilic wire is passed across the occlusion, followed by passing of the Trellis device over a stiff exchange length wire. The distal and proximal balloons are inflated in the artery on either side of a treatment zone containing infusion to isolate the treatment zone and to sustain the fluid concentration that is infused. One milligram of tissue plasminogen activator (TPA) is infused into the treatment zone. The Turbo Trellis is run at 4,000 rpm for five minutes. After the proximal balloon is deflated, small clots are removed via the integral aspiration port to prevent embolization. Fluoroscopic guidance services and injections administered during the course of the procedure are included in the service. Separately reportable procedures include other percutaneous interventions such as stent placement and diagnostic studies. Report 37184 for the first vessel and 37185 for the second and subsequent vessels in the same vascular family.

Coding Tips

Do not report 37184 with 61645, 76000 or 96374. Do not report 37185 with 76000 or 96375. Do not report 37185 with 61645 when treating the same vascular territory. Codes 37184 and 37185 should not be used to report mechanical thrombectomy performed to remove short segments of thrombus or embolus discovered during other percutaneous interventional procedures, see 37186.

ICD-10-CM Diagnostic Codes

I26.01	Septic pulmonary embolism with acute cor pulmonale
I26.02	Saddle embolus of pulmonary artery with acute cor pulmonale
I26.90	Septic pulmonary embolism without acute cor pulmonale
I26.92	Saddle embolus of pulmonary artery without acute cor pulmonale
I26.93	Single subsegmental pulmonary embolism without acute cor pulmonale
I26.94	Multiple subsegmental pulmonary emboli without acute cor pulmonale
I72.8	Aneurysm of other specified arteries
I73.89	Other specified peripheral vascular diseases
I74.01	Saddle embolus of abdominal aorta
I74.09	Other arterial embolism and thrombosis of abdominal aorta
I74.11	Embolism and thrombosis of thoracic aorta
I74.19	Embolism and thrombosis of other parts of aorta
I74.2	Embolism and thrombosis of arteries of the upper extremities
I74.3	Embolism and thrombosis of arteries of the lower extremities
I74.5	Embolism and thrombosis of iliac artery
I74.8	Embolism and thrombosis of other arteries
I75.011	Atheroembolism of right upper extremity ☑
I75.012	Atheroembolism of left upper extremity ☑
I75.013	Atheroembolism of bilateral upper extremities ☑
I75.021	Atheroembolism of right lower extremity ☑
I75.022	Atheroembolism of left lower extremity ☑
I75.023	Atheroembolism of bilateral lower extremities ☑
I75.81	Atheroembolism of kidney
I75.89	Atheroembolism of other site
I76	Septic arterial embolism
K55.011	Focal (segmental) acute (reversible) ischemia of small intestine
K55.012	Diffuse acute (reversible) ischemia of small intestine
K55.021	Focal (segmental) acute infarction of small intestine
K55.022	Diffuse acute infarction of small intestine
K55.031	Focal (segmental) acute (reversible) ischemia of large intestine
K55.032	Diffuse acute (reversible) ischemia of large intestine
K55.041	Focal (segmental) acute infarction of large intestine
K55.042	Diffuse acute infarction of large intestine
K55.1	Chronic vascular disorders of intestine
K55.8	Other vascular disorders of intestine
N28.0	Ischemia and infarction of kidney
T82.818A	Embolism due to vascular prosthetic devices, implants and grafts, initial encounter
T82.868A	Thrombosis due to vascular prosthetic devices, implants and grafts, initial encounter

AMA: 37184 2019,Sep,5; 2018,Jan,8; 2017,Jan,8; 2016,Mar,3; 2016,Jul,6; 2016,Jan,13; 2015,Nov,3; 2015,Jan,16; 2015,Apr,10; 2014,Jan,11; 2013,Feb,3-6 **37185** 2019,Sep,5; 2018,Jan,8; 2017,Jan,8; 2016,Jul,6; 2016,Jan,13; 2015,Nov,3; 2015,Jan,16; 2015,Apr,10; 2014,Jan,11; 2013,Feb,3-6

Relative Value Units/Medicare Edits

Non-Facility RVU	Work	PE	MP	Total
37184	8.41	50.1	1.73	60.24
37185	3.28	14.62	0.66	18.56
Facility RVU	**Work**	**PE**	**MP**	**Total**
37184	8.41	2.83	1.73	12.97
37185	3.28	0.91	0.66	4.85

	FUD	Status	MUE	Modifiers				IOM Reference
37184	0	A	1(2)	51	50	62	N/A	None
37185	N/A	A	2(3)	N/A	N/A	62	N/A	

* with documentation

37186

\+ **37186** Secondary percutaneous transluminal thrombectomy (eg, nonprimary mechanical, snare basket, suction technique), noncoronary, non-intracranial, arterial or arterial bypass graft, including fluoroscopic guidance and intraprocedural pharmacological thrombolytic injections, provided in conjunction with another percutaneous intervention other than primary mechanical thrombectomy (List separately in addition to code for primary procedure)

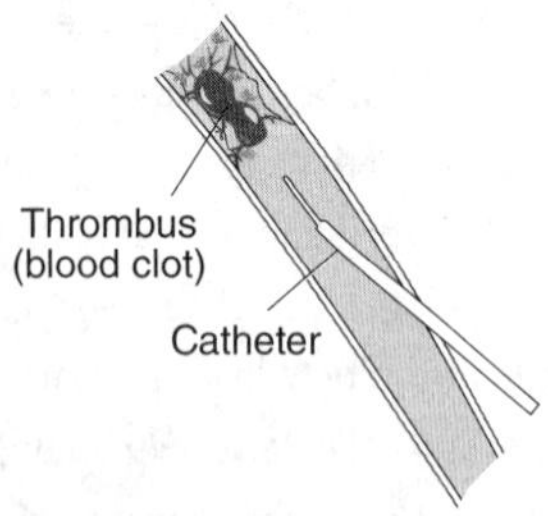

Secondary percutaneous transluminal thombectomy occurs prior to, or after, the primary procedure

Explanation

The physician performs a secondary thrombectomy of a noncoronary, non-intracranial arterial occlusion. Prior to or after a percutaneous intervention is performed, such as balloon angioplasty or placement of a stent, the transcatheter removal of small sections of the thrombus or embolism is performed using suction, a snare basket, or a mechanical thrombectomy device under fluoroscopic guidance. Thrombolytic injections may also be used during the procedure.

Coding Tips

When medically necessary, report moderate (conscious) sedation provided by the performing physician with 99151-99153. When provided by another physician, report 99155-99157. Do not report 37186 with 76000 or 96375. Do not report 37186 with 61645 when treating the same vascular territory.

ICD-10-CM Diagnostic Codes

This/these CPT code(s) are add on code(s). See the primary procedure code that this code is performed with for your ICD-10-CM code selections.

AMA: 37186 2019,Sep,5; 2018,Jan,8; 2017,Jan,8; 2016,Jul,6; 2016,Jan,13; 2015,Nov,3; 2015,Jan,16; 2014,Jan,11; 2013,Feb,3-6

Relative Value Units/Medicare Edits

Non-Facility RVU	Work	PE	MP	Total
37186	4.92	31.59	0.95	37.46
Facility RVU	**Work**	**PE**	**MP**	**Total**
37186	4.92	1.23	0.95	7.1

	FUD	Status	MUE	Modifiers				IOM Reference
37186	N/A	A	2(3)	N/A	N/A	62	N/A	None

* with documentation

37187-37188

37187 Percutaneous transluminal mechanical thrombectomy, vein(s), including intraprocedural pharmacological thrombolytic injections and fluoroscopic guidance

37188 Percutaneous transluminal mechanical thrombectomy, vein(s), including intraprocedural pharmacological thrombolytic injections and fluoroscopic guidance, repeat treatment on subsequent day during course of thrombolytic therapy

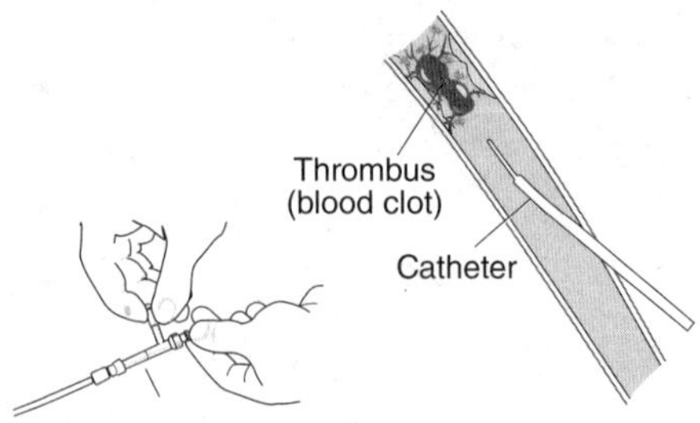

Explanation

The physician performs a percutaneous transluminal mechanical venous thrombectomy. A catheter sheath is inserted through a small incision in the vein, most commonly a groin incision in the femoral vein or an incision below the knee in the popliteal vein. Contrast is injected through the sheath and a separately reportable venography is performed to visualize the area of the vein being treated. Fluoroscopic guidance may be used. A guidewire is inserted through the sheath and advanced past the clot. A catheter is passed over the wire to the blocked area. A device at the tip of the catheter, a mechanical tool or a high-velocity liquid jet, is used to break the clot. A thrombolytic agent may be injected. When the procedure is completed, all instruments are removed and a compression bandage is applied. Report 37187 for the initial treatment. Report 37188 for repeat treatment on a subsequent day during the course of thrombolytic therapy.

Coding Tips

When medically necessary, report moderate (conscious) sedation provided by the performing physician with 99151-99153. When provided by another physician, report 99155-99157. Do not report 37187 or 37188 with 76000 or 96375. Supplies used when providing this procedure may be reported with A4300. Check with the specific payer to determine coverage.

ICD-10-CM Diagnostic Codes

I80.01	Phlebitis and thrombophlebitis of superficial vessels of right lower extremity ☑
I80.02	Phlebitis and thrombophlebitis of superficial vessels of left lower extremity ☑
I80.03	Phlebitis and thrombophlebitis of superficial vessels of lower extremities, bilateral ☑
I80.11	Phlebitis and thrombophlebitis of right femoral vein ☑
I80.12	Phlebitis and thrombophlebitis of left femoral vein ☑
I80.13	Phlebitis and thrombophlebitis of femoral vein, bilateral ☑
I80.211	Phlebitis and thrombophlebitis of right iliac vein ☑
I80.212	Phlebitis and thrombophlebitis of left iliac vein ☑
I80.213	Phlebitis and thrombophlebitis of iliac vein, bilateral ☑
I80.221	Phlebitis and thrombophlebitis of right popliteal vein ☑
I80.222	Phlebitis and thrombophlebitis of left popliteal vein ☑
I80.223	Phlebitis and thrombophlebitis of popliteal vein, bilateral ☑

I80.231 Phlebitis and thrombophlebitis of right tibial vein ☑
I80.232 Phlebitis and thrombophlebitis of left tibial vein ☑
I80.233 Phlebitis and thrombophlebitis of tibial vein, bilateral ☑
I80.291 Phlebitis and thrombophlebitis of other deep vessels of right lower extremity ☑
I80.292 Phlebitis and thrombophlebitis of other deep vessels of left lower extremity ☑
I80.293 Phlebitis and thrombophlebitis of other deep vessels of lower extremity, bilateral ☑
I80.8 Phlebitis and thrombophlebitis of other sites
I82.0 Budd-Chiari syndrome
I82.1 Thrombophlebitis migrans
I82.210 Acute embolism and thrombosis of superior vena cava
I82.211 Chronic embolism and thrombosis of superior vena cava
I82.220 Acute embolism and thrombosis of inferior vena cava
I82.221 Chronic embolism and thrombosis of inferior vena cava
I82.290 Acute embolism and thrombosis of other thoracic veins
I82.291 Chronic embolism and thrombosis of other thoracic veins
I82.3 Embolism and thrombosis of renal vein
I82.411 Acute embolism and thrombosis of right femoral vein ☑
I82.412 Acute embolism and thrombosis of left femoral vein ☑
I82.413 Acute embolism and thrombosis of femoral vein, bilateral ☑
I82.421 Acute embolism and thrombosis of right iliac vein ☑
I82.422 Acute embolism and thrombosis of left iliac vein ☑
I82.423 Acute embolism and thrombosis of iliac vein, bilateral ☑
I82.431 Acute embolism and thrombosis of right popliteal vein ☑
I82.432 Acute embolism and thrombosis of left popliteal vein ☑
I82.433 Acute embolism and thrombosis of popliteal vein, bilateral ☑
I82.441 Acute embolism and thrombosis of right tibial vein ☑
I82.442 Acute embolism and thrombosis of left tibial vein ☑
I82.443 Acute embolism and thrombosis of tibial vein, bilateral ☑
I82.491 Acute embolism and thrombosis of other specified deep vein of right lower extremity ☑
I82.492 Acute embolism and thrombosis of other specified deep vein of left lower extremity ☑
I82.493 Acute embolism and thrombosis of other specified deep vein of lower extremity, bilateral ☑
I82.511 Chronic embolism and thrombosis of right femoral vein ☑
I82.512 Chronic embolism and thrombosis of left femoral vein ☑
I82.513 Chronic embolism and thrombosis of femoral vein, bilateral ☑
I82.521 Chronic embolism and thrombosis of right iliac vein ☑
I82.522 Chronic embolism and thrombosis of left iliac vein ☑
I82.523 Chronic embolism and thrombosis of iliac vein, bilateral ☑
I82.531 Chronic embolism and thrombosis of right popliteal vein ☑
I82.532 Chronic embolism and thrombosis of left popliteal vein ☑
I82.533 Chronic embolism and thrombosis of popliteal vein, bilateral ☑
I82.541 Chronic embolism and thrombosis of right tibial vein ☑
I82.542 Chronic embolism and thrombosis of left tibial vein ☑
I82.543 Chronic embolism and thrombosis of tibial vein, bilateral ☑
I82.591 Chronic embolism and thrombosis of other specified deep vein of right lower extremity ☑
I82.592 Chronic embolism and thrombosis of other specified deep vein of left lower extremity ☑
I82.593 Chronic embolism and thrombosis of other specified deep vein of lower extremity, bilateral ☑
I82.611 Acute embolism and thrombosis of superficial veins of right upper extremity ☑
I82.612 Acute embolism and thrombosis of superficial veins of left upper extremity ☑
I82.613 Acute embolism and thrombosis of superficial veins of upper extremity, bilateral ☑
I82.621 Acute embolism and thrombosis of deep veins of right upper extremity ☑
I82.622 Acute embolism and thrombosis of deep veins of left upper extremity ☑
I82.623 Acute embolism and thrombosis of deep veins of upper extremity, bilateral ☑
I82.711 Chronic embolism and thrombosis of superficial veins of right upper extremity ☑
I82.712 Chronic embolism and thrombosis of superficial veins of left upper extremity ☑
I82.713 Chronic embolism and thrombosis of superficial veins of upper extremity, bilateral ☑
I82.721 Chronic embolism and thrombosis of deep veins of right upper extremity ☑
I82.722 Chronic embolism and thrombosis of deep veins of left upper extremity ☑
I82.723 Chronic embolism and thrombosis of deep veins of upper extremity, bilateral ☑
I82.811 Embolism and thrombosis of superficial veins of right lower extremity ☑
I82.812 Embolism and thrombosis of superficial veins of left lower extremity ☑
I82.813 Embolism and thrombosis of superficial veins of lower extremities, bilateral ☑
I82.890 Acute embolism and thrombosis of other specified veins
I82.891 Chronic embolism and thrombosis of other specified veins
I82.A11 Acute embolism and thrombosis of right axillary vein ☑
I82.A12 Acute embolism and thrombosis of left axillary vein ☑
I82.A13 Acute embolism and thrombosis of axillary vein, bilateral ☑
I82.A21 Chronic embolism and thrombosis of right axillary vein ☑
I82.A22 Chronic embolism and thrombosis of left axillary vein ☑
I82.A23 Chronic embolism and thrombosis of axillary vein, bilateral ☑
I82.B11 Acute embolism and thrombosis of right subclavian vein ☑
I82.B12 Acute embolism and thrombosis of left subclavian vein ☑
I82.B13 Acute embolism and thrombosis of subclavian vein, bilateral ☑
I82.B21 Chronic embolism and thrombosis of right subclavian vein ☑
I82.B22 Chronic embolism and thrombosis of left subclavian vein ☑
I82.B23 Chronic embolism and thrombosis of subclavian vein, bilateral ☑
I82.C11 Acute embolism and thrombosis of right internal jugular vein ☑
I82.C12 Acute embolism and thrombosis of left internal jugular vein ☑
I82.C13 Acute embolism and thrombosis of internal jugular vein, bilateral ☑
I82.C21 Chronic embolism and thrombosis of right internal jugular vein ☑
I82.C22 Chronic embolism and thrombosis of left internal jugular vein ☑
I82.C23 Chronic embolism and thrombosis of internal jugular vein, bilateral ☑

AMA: **37187** 2018,Jan,8; 2017,Jan,8; 2016,Mar,3; 2016,Jul,6; 2016,Jan,13; 2015,Nov,3; 2015,Jan,16; 2014,Jan,11; 2013,Feb,3-6 **37188** 2018,Jan,8; 2017,Jan,8; 2016,Mar,3; 2016,Jul,6; 2016,Jan,13; 2015,Nov,3; 2015,Jan,16; 2014,Jan,11; 2013,Feb,3-6

Relative Value Units/Medicare Edits

Non-Facility RVU	Work	PE	MP	Total
37187	7.78	46.63	1.15	55.56
37188	5.46	40.47	0.8	46.73
Facility RVU	**Work**	**PE**	**MP**	**Total**
37187	7.78	2.47	1.15	11.4
37188	5.46	1.77	0.8	8.03

	FUD	Status	MUE	Modifiers				IOM Reference
37187	0	A	1(3)	51	50	62	N/A	None
37188	0	A	1(3)	N/A	50	62	N/A	

* with documentation

Terms To Know

Budd-Chiari syndrome. Thrombus or other obstruction of the hepatic vein, with an enlarged liver, intractable ascites, portal hypertension, and the growth of extensive collateral vessels.

embolism. Obstruction of a blood vessel resulting from a clot or foreign substance.

fluoroscopy. Radiology technique that allows visual examination of part of the body or a function of an organ using a device that projects an x-ray image on a fluorescent screen.

moderate sedation. Medically controlled state of depressed consciousness, with or without analgesia, while maintaining the patient's airway, protective reflexes, and ability to respond to stimulation or verbal commands.

thrombolysis. Chemical process of dissolving or breaking down a blood clot by inducing a complex chain of events involving the action of plasminogen to solubilize fibrin clots and degrade fibrinogen.

37191-37193

37191 Insertion of intravascular vena cava filter, endovascular approach including vascular access, vessel selection, and radiological supervision and interpretation, intraprocedural roadmapping, and imaging guidance (ultrasound and fluoroscopy), when performed

37192 Repositioning of intravascular vena cava filter, endovascular approach including vascular access, vessel selection, and radiological supervision and interpretation, intraprocedural roadmapping, and imaging guidance (ultrasound and fluoroscopy), when performed

37193 Retrieval (removal) of intravascular vena cava filter, endovascular approach including vascular access, vessel selection, and radiological supervision and interpretation, intraprocedural roadmapping, and imaging guidance (ultrasound and fluoroscopy), when performed

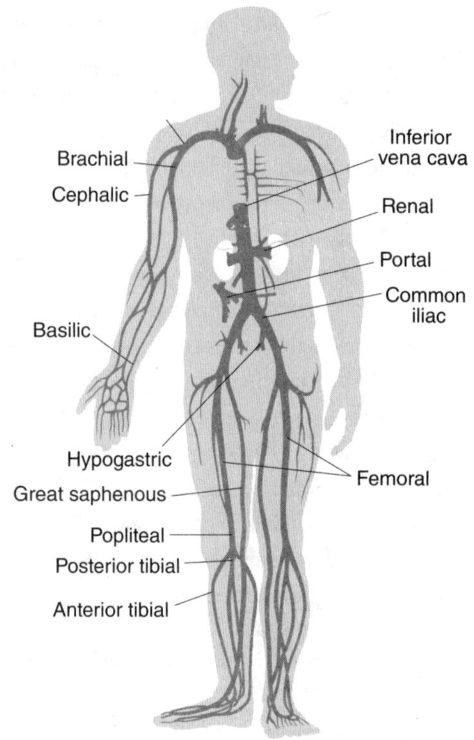

Explanation

An inferior vena cava (IVC) filter is placed most commonly for refractory deep vein thrombosis and pulmonary embolism or when anticoagulation is contraindicated. In 37191, the physician places a needle in the femoral (or internal jugular) vein, advances a guidewire through the needle, removes the needle over the wire, and advances an introducer sheath over the wire into the femoral vein. The physician advances the filter through the introducer sheath into the inferior vena cava under fluoroscopic guidance. The physician removes the introducer sheath and compresses the femoral vein manually until hemostasis is achieved. Report 37192 for the repositioning of an already placed filter utilizing an endovascular approach and associated radiologic guidance when applicable. In 37193, the physician utilizes the same approach to remove the filter.

Coding Tips

When medically necessary, report moderate (conscious) sedation provided by the performing physician with 99151-99153. When provided by another physician, report 99155-99157. These codes include access and vessel selection, radiological supervision and interpretation, roadmapping, and imaging guidance by ultrasound and/or fluoroscopy. For open surgical interruption of the inferior vena cava through laparotomy or retroperitoneal exposure, see 37619. Do not report 37192 with 37191. Do not report 37193 with 37197.

ICD-10-CM Diagnostic Codes

I26.01	Septic pulmonary embolism with acute cor pulmonale
I26.09	Other pulmonary embolism with acute cor pulmonale
I26.90	Septic pulmonary embolism without acute cor pulmonale
I26.99	Other pulmonary embolism without acute cor pulmonale
I27.82	Chronic pulmonary embolism
I82.220	Acute embolism and thrombosis of inferior vena cava
I82.221	Chronic embolism and thrombosis of inferior vena cava
I82.290	Acute embolism and thrombosis of other thoracic veins
I82.291	Chronic embolism and thrombosis of other thoracic veins
I82.3	Embolism and thrombosis of renal vein
I82.411	Acute embolism and thrombosis of right femoral vein ☑
I82.412	Acute embolism and thrombosis of left femoral vein ☑
I82.413	Acute embolism and thrombosis of femoral vein, bilateral ☑
I82.421	Acute embolism and thrombosis of right iliac vein ☑
I82.422	Acute embolism and thrombosis of left iliac vein ☑
I82.423	Acute embolism and thrombosis of iliac vein, bilateral ☑
I82.431	Acute embolism and thrombosis of right popliteal vein ☑
I82.432	Acute embolism and thrombosis of left popliteal vein ☑
I82.433	Acute embolism and thrombosis of popliteal vein, bilateral ☑
I82.441	Acute embolism and thrombosis of right tibial vein ☑
I82.442	Acute embolism and thrombosis of left tibial vein ☑
I82.443	Acute embolism and thrombosis of tibial vein, bilateral ☑
I82.491	Acute embolism and thrombosis of other specified deep vein of right lower extremity ☑
I82.492	Acute embolism and thrombosis of other specified deep vein of left lower extremity ☑
I82.493	Acute embolism and thrombosis of other specified deep vein of lower extremity, bilateral ☑
I82.511	Chronic embolism and thrombosis of right femoral vein ☑
I82.512	Chronic embolism and thrombosis of left femoral vein ☑
I82.513	Chronic embolism and thrombosis of femoral vein, bilateral ☑
I82.521	Chronic embolism and thrombosis of right iliac vein ☑
I82.522	Chronic embolism and thrombosis of left iliac vein ☑
I82.523	Chronic embolism and thrombosis of iliac vein, bilateral ☑
I82.531	Chronic embolism and thrombosis of right popliteal vein ☑
I82.532	Chronic embolism and thrombosis of left popliteal vein ☑
I82.533	Chronic embolism and thrombosis of popliteal vein, bilateral ☑
I82.541	Chronic embolism and thrombosis of right tibial vein ☑
I82.542	Chronic embolism and thrombosis of left tibial vein ☑
I82.543	Chronic embolism and thrombosis of tibial vein, bilateral ☑
I82.591	Chronic embolism and thrombosis of other specified deep vein of right lower extremity ☑
I82.592	Chronic embolism and thrombosis of other specified deep vein of left lower extremity ☑
I82.593	Chronic embolism and thrombosis of other specified deep vein of lower extremity, bilateral ☑
I82.5Y1	Chronic embolism and thrombosis of unspecified deep veins of right proximal lower extremity ☑
I82.5Y2	Chronic embolism and thrombosis of unspecified deep veins of left proximal lower extremity ☑
I82.5Y3	Chronic embolism and thrombosis of unspecified deep veins of proximal lower extremity, bilateral ☑
I82.5Z1	Chronic embolism and thrombosis of unspecified deep veins of right distal lower extremity ☑
I82.5Z2	Chronic embolism and thrombosis of unspecified deep veins of left distal lower extremity ☑
I82.5Z3	Chronic embolism and thrombosis of unspecified deep veins of distal lower extremity, bilateral ☑
I82.811	Embolism and thrombosis of superficial veins of right lower extremity ☑
I82.812	Embolism and thrombosis of superficial veins of left lower extremity ☑
I82.813	Embolism and thrombosis of superficial veins of lower extremities, bilateral ☑
T82.515A	Breakdown (mechanical) of umbrella device, initial encounter
T82.518A	Breakdown (mechanical) of other cardiac and vascular devices and implants, initial encounter
T82.525A	Displacement of umbrella device, initial encounter
T82.528A	Displacement of other cardiac and vascular devices and implants, initial encounter
T82.535A	Leakage of umbrella device, initial encounter
T82.538A	Leakage of other cardiac and vascular devices and implants, initial encounter
T82.595A	Other mechanical complication of umbrella device, initial encounter
T82.598A	Other mechanical complication of other cardiac and vascular devices and implants, initial encounter
T82.7XXA	Infection and inflammatory reaction due to other cardiac and vascular devices, implants and grafts, initial encounter
T82.818A	Embolism due to vascular prosthetic devices, implants and grafts, initial encounter
T82.828A	Fibrosis due to vascular prosthetic devices, implants and grafts, initial encounter
T82.848A	Pain due to vascular prosthetic devices, implants and grafts, initial encounter
T82.858A	Stenosis of other vascular prosthetic devices, implants and grafts, initial encounter
T82.868A	Thrombosis due to vascular prosthetic devices, implants and grafts, initial encounter
T82.898A	Other specified complication of vascular prosthetic devices, implants and grafts, initial encounter

AMA: **37191** 2018,Jan,8; 2017,Jan,8; 2017,Feb,14; 2016,May,11; 2016,Jan,13; 2015,Jan,16; 2014,Jan,11; 2013,Feb,3-6 **37192** 2018,Jan,8; 2017,Jan,8; 2016,May,11; 2016,Jan,13; 2015,Jan,16; 2014,Jan,11; 2013,Feb,3-6 **37193** 2018,Jan,8; 2017,Jan,8; 2016,May,11; 2016,Jan,13; 2015,Jan,16; 2014,Jan,11; 2013,Feb,3-6

Relative Value Units/Medicare Edits

Non-Facility RVU	Work	PE	MP	Total
37191	4.46	64.89	0.6	69.95
37192	7.1	28.75	1.64	37.49
37193	7.1	36.0	0.96	44.06
Facility RVU	**Work**	**PE**	**MP**	**Total**
37191	4.46	1.43	0.6	6.49
37192	7.1	1.24	1.64	9.98
37193	7.1	2.09	0.96	10.15

	FUD	Status	MUE	Modifiers				IOM Reference
37191	0	A	1(3)	51	N/A	N/A	N/A	None
37192	0	A	1(3)	51	N/A	N/A	N/A	
37193	0	A	1(3)	51	N/A	N/A	N/A	

* with documentation

Terms To Know

embolism. Obstruction of a blood vessel resulting from a clot or foreign substance.

fluoroscopy. Radiology technique that allows visual examination of part of the body or a function of an organ using a device that projects an x-ray image on a fluorescent screen.

thrombosis. Condition arising from the presence or formation of blood clots within a blood vessel that may cause vascular obstruction and insufficient oxygenation.

ultrasound. Imaging using ultra-high sound frequency bounced off body structures.

37195

37195 Thrombolysis, cerebral, by intravenous infusion

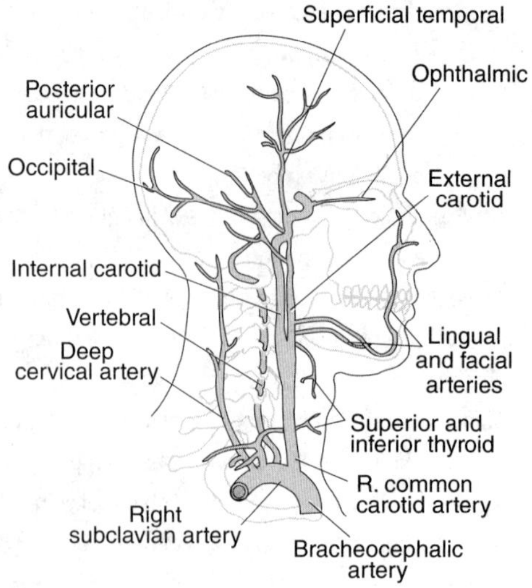

Explanation

The physician remedies a stroke-causing blood clot obstructing blood flow to the brain. The physician infuses a thrombolytic ("clot-busting") drug through an intravenous catheter to help dissolve the clot and restore normal blood flow to the brain.

Coding Tips

For transcatheter therapy, infusion for thrombolysis other than coronary (or cerebral), see 37211-37214. For thrombolysis of the coronary vessels, see 92975 and 92977.

ICD-10-CM Diagnostic Codes

G45.8	Other transient cerebral ischemic attacks and related syndromes
G45.9	Transient cerebral ischemic attack, unspecified
G46.0	Middle cerebral artery syndrome
G46.1	Anterior cerebral artery syndrome
G46.2	Posterior cerebral artery syndrome
I63.311	Cerebral infarction due to thrombosis of right middle cerebral artery ☑
I63.312	Cerebral infarction due to thrombosis of left middle cerebral artery ☑
I63.321	Cerebral infarction due to thrombosis of right anterior cerebral artery ☑
I63.322	Cerebral infarction due to thrombosis of left anterior cerebral artery ☑
I63.331	Cerebral infarction due to thrombosis of right posterior cerebral artery ☑
I63.332	Cerebral infarction due to thrombosis of left posterior cerebral artery ☑
I63.39	Cerebral infarction due to thrombosis of other cerebral artery
I63.411	Cerebral infarction due to embolism of right middle cerebral artery ☑
I63.412	Cerebral infarction due to embolism of left middle cerebral artery ☑

I63.421 Cerebral infarction due to embolism of right anterior cerebral artery ☑
I63.422 Cerebral infarction due to embolism of left anterior cerebral artery ☑
I63.431 Cerebral infarction due to embolism of right posterior cerebral artery ☑
I63.432 Cerebral infarction due to embolism of left posterior cerebral artery ☑
I63.511 Cerebral infarction due to unspecified occlusion or stenosis of right middle cerebral artery ☑
I63.512 Cerebral infarction due to unspecified occlusion or stenosis of left middle cerebral artery ☑
I63.521 Cerebral infarction due to unspecified occlusion or stenosis of right anterior cerebral artery ☑
I63.522 Cerebral infarction due to unspecified occlusion or stenosis of left anterior cerebral artery ☑
I63.531 Cerebral infarction due to unspecified occlusion or stenosis of right posterior cerebral artery ☑
I63.532 Cerebral infarction due to unspecified occlusion or stenosis of left posterior cerebral artery ☑
I63.59 Cerebral infarction due to unspecified occlusion or stenosis of other cerebral artery
I63.6 Cerebral infarction due to cerebral venous thrombosis, nonpyogenic
I63.81 Other cerebral infarction due to occlusion or stenosis of small artery
I63.89 Other cerebral infarction
I66.01 Occlusion and stenosis of right middle cerebral artery ☑
I66.02 Occlusion and stenosis of left middle cerebral artery ☑
I66.03 Occlusion and stenosis of bilateral middle cerebral arteries ☑
I66.11 Occlusion and stenosis of right anterior cerebral artery ☑
I66.12 Occlusion and stenosis of left anterior cerebral artery ☑
I66.13 Occlusion and stenosis of bilateral anterior cerebral arteries ☑
I66.21 Occlusion and stenosis of right posterior cerebral artery ☑
I66.22 Occlusion and stenosis of left posterior cerebral artery ☑
I66.23 Occlusion and stenosis of bilateral posterior cerebral arteries ☑
I66.8 Occlusion and stenosis of other cerebral arteries
I67.848 Other cerebrovascular vasospasm and vasoconstriction
I67.850 Cerebral autosomal dominant arteriopathy with subcortical infarcts and leukoencephalopathy
I67.858 Other hereditary cerebrovascular disease
I97.810 Intraoperative cerebrovascular infarction during cardiac surgery
I97.811 Intraoperative cerebrovascular infarction during other surgery
I97.820 Postprocedural cerebrovascular infarction following cardiac surgery
I97.821 Postprocedural cerebrovascular infarction following other surgery

AMA: **37195** 2014,Jan,11

Relative Value Units/Medicare Edits

Non-Facility RVU	Work	PE	MP	Total
37195	0.0	0.0	0.0	0.0
Facility RVU	**Work**	**PE**	**MP**	**Total**
37195	0.0	0.0	0.0	0.0

	FUD	Status	MUE	Modifiers				IOM Reference
37195	N/A	C	1(3)	N/A	N/A	N/A	80*	None

* with documentation

Terms To Know

embolism. Obstruction of a blood vessel resulting from a clot or foreign substance.

infarction. Area of necrosis in tissue, due to ischemia from lack of circulation, usually from a thrombus or an embolus.

stenosis. Narrowing or constriction of a passage.

thrombolysis. Chemical process of dissolving or breaking down a blood clot by inducing a complex chain of events involving the action of plasminogen to solubilize fibrin clots and degrade fibrinogen.

thrombosis. Condition arising from the presence or formation of blood clots within a blood vessel that may cause vascular obstruction and insufficient oxygenation.

37197

37197 Transcatheter retrieval, percutaneous, of intravascular foreign body (eg, fractured venous or arterial catheter), includes radiological supervision and interpretation, and imaging guidance (ultrasound or fluoroscopy), when performed

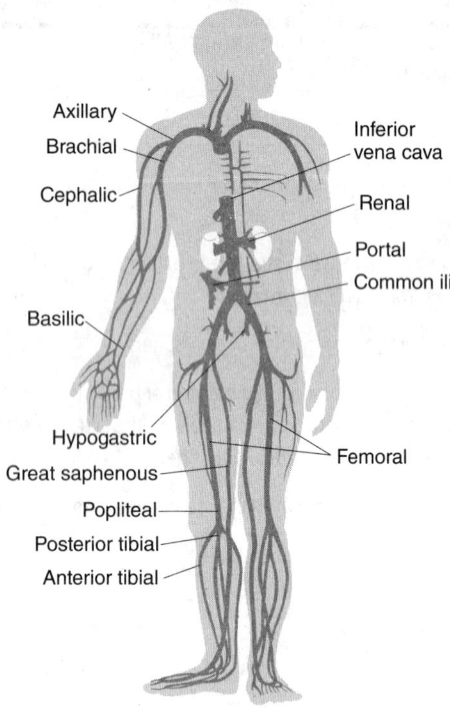

Select major veins

Explanation

The physician places a needle into a blood vessel. A guidewire is threaded through the needle into the vessel and the needle is removed. A catheter is threaded into the vessel and the wire is extracted. The catheter, equipped with a grasping instrument, travels to the site of the foreign body typically using imaging guidance. The instrument grasps the foreign body, typically a fractured catheter, and retrieves it. The catheter is removed and pressure is applied over the puncture site to stop the bleeding.

Coding Tips

When medically necessary, report moderate (conscious) sedation provided by the performing physician with 99151-99153. When provided by another physician, report 99155-99157. For percutaneous retrieval of a vena cava filter, see 37193. For transcatheter removal of a permanent leadless pacemaker, see 33275.

ICD-10-CM Diagnostic Codes

T81.510A	Adhesions due to foreign body accidentally left in body following surgical operation, initial encounter
T81.511A	Adhesions due to foreign body accidentally left in body following infusion or transfusion, initial encounter
T81.512A	Adhesions due to foreign body accidentally left in body following kidney dialysis, initial encounter
T81.513A	Adhesions due to foreign body accidentally left in body following injection or immunization, initial encounter
T81.515A	Adhesions due to foreign body accidentally left in body following heart catheterization, initial encounter
T81.517A	Adhesions due to foreign body accidentally left in body following removal of catheter or packing, initial encounter
T81.518A	Adhesions due to foreign body accidentally left in body following other procedure, initial encounter
T81.520A	Obstruction due to foreign body accidentally left in body following surgical operation, initial encounter
T81.521A	Obstruction due to foreign body accidentally left in body following infusion or transfusion, initial encounter
T81.522A	Obstruction due to foreign body accidentally left in body following kidney dialysis, initial encounter
T81.523A	Obstruction due to foreign body accidentally left in body following injection or immunization, initial encounter
T81.525A	Obstruction due to foreign body accidentally left in body following heart catheterization, initial encounter
T81.527A	Obstruction due to foreign body accidentally left in body following removal of catheter or packing, initial encounter
T81.528A	Obstruction due to foreign body accidentally left in body following other procedure, initial encounter
T81.530A	Perforation due to foreign body accidentally left in body following surgical operation, initial encounter
T81.531A	Perforation due to foreign body accidentally left in body following infusion or transfusion, initial encounter
T81.532A	Perforation due to foreign body accidentally left in body following kidney dialysis, initial encounter
T81.533A	Perforation due to foreign body accidentally left in body following injection or immunization, initial encounter
T81.535A	Perforation due to foreign body accidentally left in body following heart catheterization, initial encounter
T81.537A	Perforation due to foreign body accidentally left in body following removal of catheter or packing, initial encounter
T81.538A	Perforation due to foreign body accidentally left in body following other procedure, initial encounter
T81.590A	Other complications of foreign body accidentally left in body following surgical operation, initial encounter
T81.591A	Other complications of foreign body accidentally left in body following infusion or transfusion, initial encounter
T81.592A	Other complications of foreign body accidentally left in body following kidney dialysis, initial encounter
T81.593A	Other complications of foreign body accidentally left in body following injection or immunization, initial encounter
T81.595A	Other complications of foreign body accidentally left in body following heart catheterization, initial encounter
T81.597A	Other complications of foreign body accidentally left in body following removal of catheter or packing, initial encounter
T81.598A	Other complications of foreign body accidentally left in body following other procedure, initial encounter
T82.310A	Breakdown (mechanical) of aortic (bifurcation) graft (replacement), initial encounter
T82.311A	Breakdown (mechanical) of carotid arterial graft (bypass), initial encounter
T82.312A	Breakdown (mechanical) of femoral arterial graft (bypass), initial encounter
T82.318A	Breakdown (mechanical) of other vascular grafts, initial encounter
T82.390A	Other mechanical complication of aortic (bifurcation) graft (replacement), initial encounter
T82.391A	Other mechanical complication of carotid arterial graft (bypass), initial encounter

T82.392A	Other mechanical complication of femoral arterial graft (bypass), initial encounter
T82.398A	Other mechanical complication of other vascular grafts, initial encounter
T82.41XA	Breakdown (mechanical) of vascular dialysis catheter, initial encounter
T82.49XA	Other complication of vascular dialysis catheter, initial encounter
T82.513A	Breakdown (mechanical) of balloon (counterpulsation) device, initial encounter
T82.514A	Breakdown (mechanical) of infusion catheter, initial encounter
T82.515A	Breakdown (mechanical) of umbrella device, initial encounter
T82.518A	Breakdown (mechanical) of other cardiac and vascular devices and implants, initial encounter
T82.593A	Other mechanical complication of balloon (counterpulsation) device, initial encounter
T82.594A	Other mechanical complication of infusion catheter, initial encounter
T82.595A	Other mechanical complication of umbrella device, initial encounter
T82.598A	Other mechanical complication of other cardiac and vascular devices and implants, initial encounter
T82.898A	Other specified complication of vascular prosthetic devices, implants and grafts, initial encounter

AMA: 37197 2018,Jan,8; 2017,Jan,8; 2017,Feb,14; 2016,May,11; 2016,Jan,13; 2015,Jan,16; 2014,Jan,11; 2013,Feb,3-6

Relative Value Units/Medicare Edits

Non-Facility RVU	Work	PE	MP	Total
37197	6.04	36.43	0.93	43.4
Facility RVU	**Work**	**PE**	**MP**	**Total**
37197	6.04	1.81	0.93	8.78

	FUD	Status	MUE	Modifiers				IOM Reference
37197	0	A	2(3)	51	N/A	N/A	N/A	None

* with documentation

37200

37200 Transcatheter biopsy

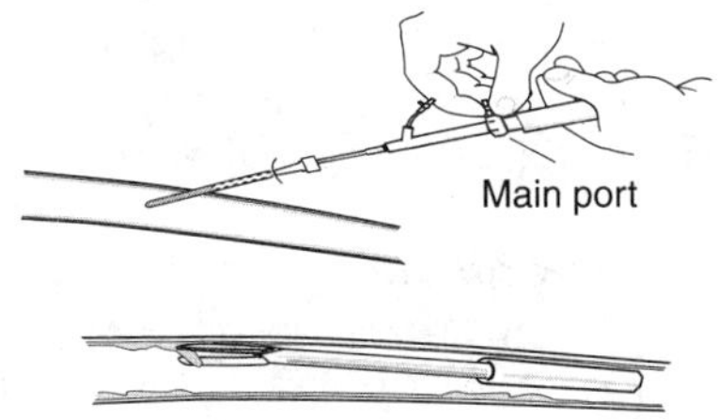

A biopsy instrument extracts tissue from vessel wall for biopsy

Explanation

A needle is inserted through the skin and into a blood vessel, and a guidewire is threaded through the needle into the vessel. The needle is removed. A catheter is threaded into the vessel, and the wire extracted. The catheter equipped with a biopsy instrument travels to the area to be sampled. The instrument extracts for biopsy tissue affixed to the vessel wall. Pressure is applied over the puncture site to stop bleeding after the catheter is removed. This procedure may also be performed through a skin incision with direct exposure of the access vessel.

Coding Tips

When 37200 is performed with another separately identifiable procedure, the highest dollar value code is listed as the primary procedure, and subsequent procedures are appended with modifier 51. For radiological supervision and interpretation, see 75970.

ICD-10-CM Diagnostic Codes

The application of this code is too broad to adequately present ICD-10-CM diagnostic code links here. Refer to your ICD-10-CM book.

AMA: 37200 2014,Jan,11

Relative Value Units/Medicare Edits

Non-Facility RVU	Work	PE	MP	Total
37200	4.55	1.35	0.4	6.3
Facility RVU	**Work**	**PE**	**MP**	**Total**
37200	4.55	1.35	0.4	6.3

	FUD	Status	MUE	Modifiers				IOM Reference
37200	0	A	2(3)	51	N/A	N/A	N/A	None

* with documentation

Terms To Know

biopsy. Tissue or fluid removed for diagnostic purposes through analysis of the cells in the biopsy material.

catheter. Flexible tube inserted into an area of the body for introducing or withdrawing fluid.

guidewire. Flexible metal instrument designed to lead another instrument in its proper course.

incision. Act of cutting into tissue or an organ.

37211-37214

37211 Transcatheter therapy, arterial infusion for thrombolysis other than coronary or intracranial, any method, including radiological supervision and interpretation, initial treatment day

37212 Transcatheter therapy, venous infusion for thrombolysis, any method, including radiological supervision and interpretation, initial treatment day

37213 Transcatheter therapy, arterial or venous infusion for thrombolysis other than coronary, any method, including radiological supervision and interpretation, continued treatment on subsequent day during course of thrombolytic therapy, including follow-up catheter contrast injection, position change, or exchange, when performed;

37214 cessation of thrombolysis including removal of catheter and vessel closure by any method

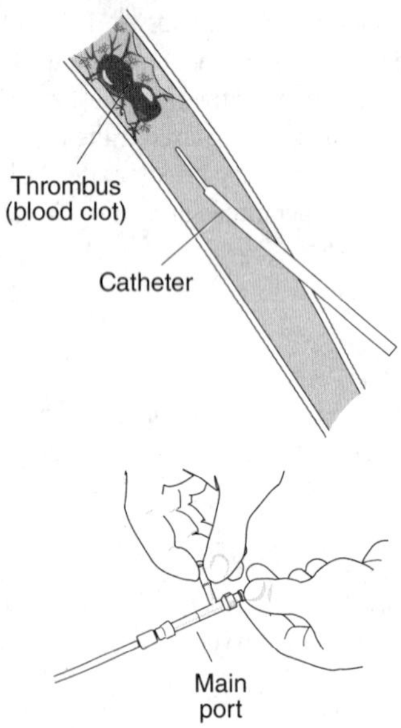

Thrombolysis is performed using intraarterial or intravenous infusion

Explanation

Transcatheter thrombolysis infusion is most commonly used to treat symptomatic inferior vena cava thrombosis that is responding poorly to the routine anticoagulation regimen or symptomatic iliofemoral or femoropopliteal deep vein thrombosis (DVT) in patients with a low risk of bleeding. A diagnostic arteriography or venography is performed to pinpoint the extent of the thrombosis. The physician places a needle into the blood vessel. A guidewire is threaded through the needle to the site of the clot using fluoroscopic guidance and the needle is removed. An infusion catheter is threaded to the site and the wire is extracted. A thrombolytic pharmaceutical is administered directly to the thrombosis. During the infusion, the patient is on bed rest with frequent monitoring. Once the thrombosis has dissipated satisfactorily, the infusion is stopped and the catheter removed. Pressure is applied over the puncture site to stop the bleeding. Report 37211 for the first day of arterial transcatheter therapy; 37212 for the first day of venous transcatheter therapy; 37213 for each subsequent day of arterial or venous therapy, including follow-up catheter contrast injection, position change, or exchange, if applicable; and 37214 for the last day the thrombolysis is administered, including removal of the catheter and closure of the access site. These codes are not for use when thrombolysis is performed on coronary or intracranial arteries.

Coding Tips

When medically necessary, report moderate (conscious) sedation provided by the performing physician with 99151-99153. When provided by another physician, report 99155-99157. Codes 37211–37214 are resequenced codes and will not display in numeric order. These are unilateral procedures. If performed bilaterally, some payers require that the service be reported twice with modifier 50 appended to the second code while others require identification of the service only once with modifier 50 appended. Check with individual payers. Modifier 50 identifies a procedure performed identically on the opposite side of the body (mirror image). Catheter placement, diagnostic studies, and any other percutaneous interventions performed are separately reportable. Fluoroscopic guidance and radiological supervision and interpretation are included in 37211–37214. These codes should only be reported once per treatment day. For ultrasound guidance for vascular access, see 76937. For declotting of an implanted vascular access device or catheter by thrombolytic agent, see 36593. For mechanical thrombectomy and/or thrombolysis infusion performed on an intracranial artery, see 61645.

ICD-10-CM Diagnostic Codes

G45.2	Multiple and bilateral precerebral artery syndromes
I26.01	Septic pulmonary embolism with acute cor pulmonale
I26.02	Saddle embolus of pulmonary artery with acute cor pulmonale
I26.90	Septic pulmonary embolism without acute cor pulmonale
I26.92	Saddle embolus of pulmonary artery without acute cor pulmonale
I26.93	Single subsegmental pulmonary embolism without acute cor pulmonale
I26.94	Multiple subsegmental pulmonary emboli without acute cor pulmonale
I63.012	Cerebral infarction due to thrombosis of left vertebral artery ☑
I63.02	Cerebral infarction due to thrombosis of basilar artery
I63.032	Cerebral infarction due to thrombosis of left carotid artery ☑
I63.112	Cerebral infarction due to embolism of left vertebral artery ☑
I63.12	Cerebral infarction due to embolism of basilar artery
I63.132	Cerebral infarction due to embolism of left carotid artery ☑
I63.6	Cerebral infarction due to cerebral venous thrombosis, nonpyogenic
I65.02	Occlusion and stenosis of left vertebral artery ☑
I65.1	Occlusion and stenosis of basilar artery
I65.22	Occlusion and stenosis of left carotid artery ☑
I72.6	Aneurysm of vertebral artery
I74.01	Saddle embolus of abdominal aorta
I74.11	Embolism and thrombosis of thoracic aorta
I74.2	Embolism and thrombosis of arteries of the upper extremities
I74.3	Embolism and thrombosis of arteries of the lower extremities
I74.5	Embolism and thrombosis of iliac artery
I75.012	Atheroembolism of left upper extremity ☑
I75.022	Atheroembolism of left lower extremity ☑
I75.81	Atheroembolism of kidney
I76	Septic arterial embolism
I80.02	Phlebitis and thrombophlebitis of superficial vessels of left lower extremity ☑
I80.12	Phlebitis and thrombophlebitis of left femoral vein ☑
I80.212	Phlebitis and thrombophlebitis of left iliac vein ☑
I80.222	Phlebitis and thrombophlebitis of left popliteal vein ☑
I80.232	Phlebitis and thrombophlebitis of left tibial vein ☑

I81 Portal vein thrombosis
I82.0 Budd-Chiari syndrome
I82.1 Thrombophlebitis migrans
I82.210 Acute embolism and thrombosis of superior vena cava
I82.211 Chronic embolism and thrombosis of superior vena cava
I82.220 Acute embolism and thrombosis of inferior vena cava
I82.221 Chronic embolism and thrombosis of inferior vena cava
I82.3 Embolism and thrombosis of renal vein
I82.412 Acute embolism and thrombosis of left femoral vein ☑
I82.422 Acute embolism and thrombosis of left iliac vein ☑
I82.432 Acute embolism and thrombosis of left popliteal vein ☑
I82.442 Acute embolism and thrombosis of left tibial vein ☑
I82.512 Chronic embolism and thrombosis of left femoral vein ☑
I82.522 Chronic embolism and thrombosis of left iliac vein ☑
I82.532 Chronic embolism and thrombosis of left popliteal vein ☑
I82.542 Chronic embolism and thrombosis of left tibial vein ☑
I82.612 Acute embolism and thrombosis of superficial veins of left upper extremity ☑
I82.622 Acute embolism and thrombosis of deep veins of left upper extremity ☑
I82.712 Chronic embolism and thrombosis of superficial veins of left upper extremity ☑
I82.722 Chronic embolism and thrombosis of deep veins of left upper extremity ☑
I82.812 Embolism and thrombosis of superficial veins of left lower extremity ☑
I82.A12 Acute embolism and thrombosis of left axillary vein ☑
I82.A22 Chronic embolism and thrombosis of left axillary vein ☑
I82.B12 Acute embolism and thrombosis of left subclavian vein ☑
I82.B22 Chronic embolism and thrombosis of left subclavian vein ☑
I82.C12 Acute embolism and thrombosis of left internal jugular vein ☑
I82.C22 Chronic embolism and thrombosis of left internal jugular vein ☑
K55.011 Focal (segmental) acute (reversible) ischemia of small intestine
K55.012 Diffuse acute (reversible) ischemia of small intestine
K55.021 Focal (segmental) acute infarction of small intestine
K55.022 Diffuse acute infarction of small intestine
K55.031 Focal (segmental) acute (reversible) ischemia of large intestine
K55.032 Diffuse acute (reversible) ischemia of large intestine
K55.041 Focal (segmental) acute infarction of large intestine
K55.042 Diffuse acute infarction of large intestine
K55.1 Chronic vascular disorders of intestine
N28.0 Ischemia and infarction of kidney
T82.818A Embolism due to vascular prosthetic devices, implants and grafts, initial encounter
T82.868A Thrombosis due to vascular prosthetic devices, implants and grafts, initial encounter

AMA: **37211** 2019,Sep,6; 2018,Jan,8; 2017,Jan,8; 2016,Mar,3; 2016,Jul,6; 2016,Jan,13; 2015,Nov,3; 2015,Jan,16; 2014,Jan,11; 2013,Feb,3-6 **37212** 2019,Sep,6; 2018,Jan,8; 2017,Jan,8; 2016,Mar,3; 2016,Jul,6; 2016,Jan,13; 2015,Nov,3; 2015,Jan,16; 2014,Jan,11; 2013,Feb,3-6 **37213** 2019,Sep,6; 2018,Jan,8; 2017,Jan,8; 2016,Mar,3; 2016,Jul,6; 2016,Jan,13; 2015,Nov,3; 2015,Jan,16; 2014,Jan,11; 2013,Feb,3-6 **37214** 2019,Sep,6; 2018,Jan,8; 2017,Jan,8; 2016,Mar,3; 2016,Jul,6; 2016,Jan,13; 2015,Nov,3; 2015,Jan,16; 2014,Jan,11; 2013,Feb,3-6

Relative Value Units/Medicare Edits

Non-Facility RVU	Work	PE	MP	Total
37211	7.75	2.13	1.33	11.21
37212	6.81	1.93	1.07	9.81
37213	4.75	1.32	0.69	6.76
37214	2.49	0.69	0.39	3.57
Facility RVU	**Work**	**PE**	**MP**	**Total**
37211	7.75	2.13	1.33	11.21
37212	6.81	1.93	1.07	9.81
37213	4.75	1.32	0.69	6.76
37214	2.49	0.69	0.39	3.57

	FUD	Status	MUE	Modifiers				IOM Reference
37211	0	A	1(2)	51	50	N/A	N/A	None
37212	0	A	1(2)	51	50	N/A	N/A	
37213	0	A	1(2)	51	N/A	N/A	N/A	
37214	0	A	1(2)	51	N/A	N/A	N/A	

* with documentation

Terms To Know

artery. Vessel through which oxygenated blood passes away from the heart to any part of the body.

infusion. Introduction of a therapeutic fluid, other than blood, into the bloodstream.

thrombolysis. Chemical process of dissolving or breaking down a blood clot by inducing a complex chain of events involving the action of plasminogen to solubilize fibrin clots and degrade fibrinogen.

transcatheter therapy. Therapeutic procedure or treatment performed via a catheter as opposed to open access.

vein. Vessel through which oxygen-depleted blood passes back to the heart.

37215-37216

37215 Transcatheter placement of intravascular stent(s), cervical carotid artery, open or percutaneous, including angioplasty, when performed, and radiological supervision and interpretation; with distal embolic protection

37216 without distal embolic protection

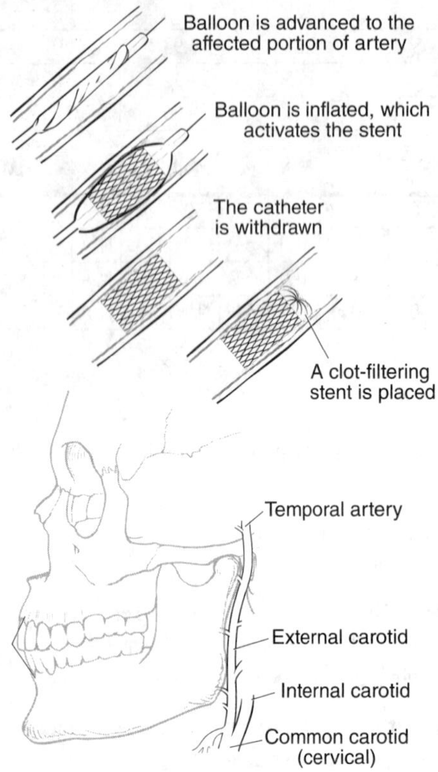

Explanation

The physician places an intravascular stent via open or percutaneous approach through a catheter into the cervical carotid artery. The open procedure is carried out by making an incision exposing the cervical carotid artery and creating an arteriotomy. In the percutaneous approach, a needle is inserted through the skin into the access blood vessel, usually the brachial or femoral artery. A guidewire is threaded through the needle into the cervical carotid artery and the needle is removed. Long sheaths or guiding catheters are advanced into the stenosed cervical carotid artery. A filter protection device may be inserted distal to the stenosis to capture emboli. After filter opening, predilation of the stenosis with angioplasty balloons may be performed. A catheter with a stent-transporting tip is threaded over the guidewire into the vessel and the wire is extracted. The catheter travels to the point where the vessel needs additional support. The compressed stent is passed from the catheter out into the vessel, where it deploys, expanding to support the vessel walls. The catheter is removed and pressure is applied over the puncture site. Report 37215 when stenting is performed with a filter protection device (distal embolic protection) and 37216 when stenting is performed without a filter protection device. The procedures include radiologic supervision and interpretation, as well as angioplasty, when performed.

Coding Tips

When medically necessary, report moderate (conscious) sedation provided by the performing physician with 99151-99153. When provided by another physician, report 99155-99157. These procedures include all ipsilateral selective carotid catheterization; all diagnostic imaging for ipsilateral, cervical, and cerebral carotid arteriography; and all related radiological supervision and interpretation. When ipsilateral carotid arteriogram (including imaging and selective catheterization) confirms the need for carotid stenting, 37215 and 37216 are inclusive of these services. If carotid stenting is not indicated, then the appropriate codes for carotid catheterization and imaging should be reported in lieu of 37215 and 37216. Do not report 37215 or 37216 with 36222–36224 for the carotid artery being treated. For transcatheter placement of an extracranial vertebral artery stent(s), see Category III codes 0075T–0076T. For percutaneous transcatheter placement of intravascular stents other than coronary, carotid, or vertebral, see 37236–37239. Supplies used when providing this procedure may be reported with HCPCS Level II code C1884 or C1886. Check with the specific payer to determine coverage.

ICD-10-CM Diagnostic Codes

G45.1	Carotid artery syndrome (hemispheric)
G45.8	Other transient cerebral ischemic attacks and related syndromes
G45.9	Transient cerebral ischemic attack, unspecified
I63.031	Cerebral infarction due to thrombosis of right carotid artery ☑
I63.032	Cerebral infarction due to thrombosis of left carotid artery ☑
I63.131	Cerebral infarction due to embolism of right carotid artery ☑
I63.132	Cerebral infarction due to embolism of left carotid artery ☑
I63.231	Cerebral infarction due to unspecified occlusion or stenosis of right carotid arteries ☑
I63.232	Cerebral infarction due to unspecified occlusion or stenosis of left carotid arteries ☑
I63.81	Other cerebral infarction due to occlusion or stenosis of small artery
I63.89	Other cerebral infarction
I65.21	Occlusion and stenosis of right carotid artery ☑
I65.22	Occlusion and stenosis of left carotid artery ☑
I65.23	Occlusion and stenosis of bilateral carotid arteries ☑
I67.81	Acute cerebrovascular insufficiency
I67.82	Cerebral ischemia
I67.848	Other cerebrovascular vasospasm and vasoconstriction
I67.850	Cerebral autosomal dominant arteriopathy with subcortical infarcts and leukoencephalopathy
I67.858	Other hereditary cerebrovascular disease
I67.89	Other cerebrovascular disease
I72.0	Aneurysm of carotid artery
I76	Septic arterial embolism
I77.1	Stricture of artery
I77.3	Arterial fibromuscular dysplasia
I77.89	Other specified disorders of arteries and arterioles

AMA: 37215 2018,Jan,8; 2017,Jul,3; 2017,Jan,8; 2016,Jan,13; 2015,Jan,16; 2014,Mar,8; 2014,Jan,11; 2013,Feb,3-6 **37216** 2018,Jan,8; 2017,Jul,3; 2017,Jan,8; 2016,Jan,13; 2015,Jan,16; 2014,Mar,8; 2014,Jan,11; 2013,Feb,3-6

Relative Value Units/Medicare Edits

Non-Facility RVU	Work	PE	MP	Total
37215	17.75	7.2	4.26	29.21
37216	17.98	8.87	2.44	29.29
Facility RVU	**Work**	**PE**	**MP**	**Total**
37215	17.75	7.2	4.26	29.21
37216	17.98	8.87	2.44	29.29

	FUD	Status	MUE	Modifiers				IOM Reference
37215	90	R	1(2)	51	50	N/A	80*	None
37216	90	N	0(3)	N/A	N/A	N/A	N/A	

* with documentation

Terms To Know

angioplasty. Reconstruction or repair of a diseased or damaged blood vessel.

cerebrovascular accident. Disruption in blood flow to the brain caused by an embolism, thrombosis, or other occlusion, resulting in a lack of perfusion and infarction of brain tissue. Sequelae or late effects of CVA can include paralysis, weakness, speech problems, and aphasia.

embolism. Obstruction of a blood vessel resulting from a clot or foreign substance.

guidewire. Flexible metal instrument designed to lead another instrument in its proper course.

infarction. Area of necrosis in tissue, due to ischemia from lack of circulation, usually from a thrombus or an embolus.

intravascular. Within a blood vessel.

ipsilateral. Located on, or affecting, the same side of the body, usually as it relates to a bilateral body part.

sheath. Covering enclosing an organ or part.

stent. Tube to provide support in a body cavity or lumen.

supervision and interpretation. Radiology services that usually contain an invasive component and are reported by the radiologist for supervision of the procedure and the personnel involved with performing the examination, reading the film, and preparing the written report.

transcatheter. Procedure or treatment performed via a catheter.

37217

37217 Transcatheter placement of intravascular stent(s), intrathoracic common carotid artery or innominate artery by retrograde treatment, open ipsilateral cervical carotid artery exposure, including angioplasty, when performed, and radiological supervision and interpretation

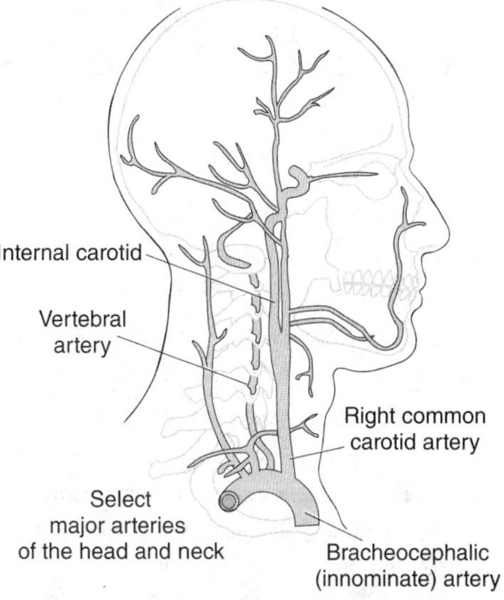

Intravascular stents are placed into the common carotid or innominate artery

Explanation

Placing stents into the intrathoracic common carotid artery or innominate artery via a catheter is a less invasive alternative to open endarterectomy. The procedure is carried out by making an incision exposing the cervical carotid artery and creating an arteriotomy. A catheter is inserted through the artery and threaded to the target. A stent delivery system, which may also include an embolic capturing device, is loaded into a delivery pod and advanced to the blocked or narrowed artery through the catheter. The embolic protection device is deployed first, distal to the lesion so that any emboli are collected as the blood passes through the device. The stent is advanced out of the pod until it expands to open the narrowing. The instruments are removed. The artery and overlying tissues are closed. The procedure includes radiologic supervision and interpretation, as well as angioplasty, when performed.

Coding Tips

This procedure includes all open vessel exposure and vascular access closure, access to and selective catheterization of the vessel being treated, traversing of the lesion, supervision and interpretation of radiology services that are related to the intervention when applicable including imaging performed to document completion of the intervention, and standard closure by suture of the arteriotomy site. None of these services can be reported separately. Carotid artery revascularization services, such as 33891, 35301, 35509–35510, 35601, and 35606, may be reported separately when performed during the same session. Do not report 37217 with 35201, 36221–36227, 37246, or 37247 when ipsilateral services are performed. For percutaneous or open transcatheter placement of an intravascular cervical carotid artery stent, see 37215–37216. For transcatheter placement of an intracranial stent, see 61635. For percutaneous or open transcatheter placement of an extracranial vertebral artery stent(s), see 0075T–0076T. For percutaneous or open antegrade transcatheter placement of innominate and/or intrathoracic carotid artery stent(s), see 37218.

ICD-10-CM Diagnostic Codes

G45.1	Carotid artery syndrome (hemispheric)
G45.9	Transient cerebral ischemic attack, unspecified
I63.031	Cerebral infarction due to thrombosis of right carotid artery ☑
I63.032	Cerebral infarction due to thrombosis of left carotid artery ☑
I63.131	Cerebral infarction due to embolism of right carotid artery ☑
I63.132	Cerebral infarction due to embolism of left carotid artery ☑
I63.231	Cerebral infarction due to unspecified occlusion or stenosis of right carotid arteries ☑
I63.232	Cerebral infarction due to unspecified occlusion or stenosis of left carotid arteries ☑
I63.81	Other cerebral infarction due to occlusion or stenosis of small artery
I63.89	Other cerebral infarction
I65.21	Occlusion and stenosis of right carotid artery ☑
I65.22	Occlusion and stenosis of left carotid artery ☑
I65.23	Occlusion and stenosis of bilateral carotid arteries ☑
I65.8	Occlusion and stenosis of other precerebral arteries
I67.81	Acute cerebrovascular insufficiency
I67.82	Cerebral ischemia
I67.848	Other cerebrovascular vasospasm and vasoconstriction
I67.850	Cerebral autosomal dominant arteriopathy with subcortical infarcts and leukoencephalopathy
I67.858	Other hereditary cerebrovascular disease
I67.89	Other cerebrovascular disease
I72.0	Aneurysm of carotid artery
I76	Septic arterial embolism
I77.1	Stricture of artery
I77.3	Arterial fibromuscular dysplasia
I77.71	Dissection of carotid artery
I77.89	Other specified disorders of arteries and arterioles

AMA: 37217 2018,Jan,8; 2017,Jul,3; 2017,Jan,8; 2016,Jan,13; 2015,May,7; 2015,Jan,16; 2014,Mar,8; 2014,Jan,11

Relative Value Units/Medicare Edits

Non-Facility RVU	Work	PE	MP	Total
37217	20.38	6.41	4.6	31.39
Facility RVU	**Work**	**PE**	**MP**	**Total**
37217	20.38	6.41	4.6	31.39

	FUD	Status	MUE	Modifiers				IOM Reference
37217	90	A	1(2)	51	50	N/A	80*	None

* with documentation

Terms To Know

stent. Tube to provide support in a body cavity or lumen.

transcatheter. Procedure or treatment performed via a catheter.

37218

37218 Transcatheter placement of intravascular stent(s), intrathoracic common carotid artery or innominate artery, open or percutaneous antegrade approach, including angioplasty, when performed, and radiological supervision and interpretation

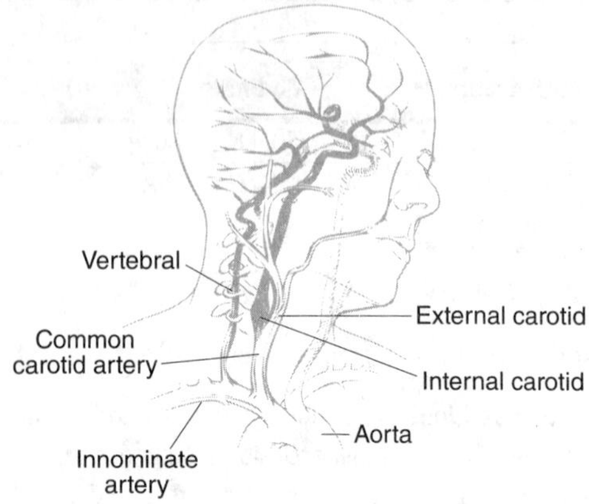

Explanation

The physician places an intravascular stent via open or percutaneous antegrade approach through a catheter into the intrathoracic common carotid artery or innominate artery. A catheter is inserted through the artery and threaded to the target. A stent delivery system, which may also include an embolic capturing device, is loaded into a delivery pod and advanced to the blocked or narrowed artery through the catheter. The embolic protection device is deployed first, distal to the lesion, so that any emboli are collected as the blood passes through the device. The stent is advanced out of the pod until it expands to open the narrowing. The instruments are removed. The artery and overlying tissues are closed. The procedure includes radiologic supervision and interpretation, as well as angioplasty, when performed.

Coding Tips

When medically necessary, report moderate (conscious) sedation provided by the performing physician with 99151-99153. When provided by another physician, report 99155-99157. This code includes all ipsilateral, extracranial, intrathoracic, selective innominate, and carotid catheterization, imaging for stent deployment, and radiological supervision and interpretation. Report this code when arteriogram determines the need for the stent; however, if stenting is not medically necessary, see codes for selective catheterization and imaging. For percutaneous or open transcatheter placement of intravascular cervical carotid artery stent, see 37215 and 37216. For percutaneous or open transcatheter placement of an extracranial vertebral artery stent, see 0075T and 0076T. For transcatheter placement of an intracranial stent, see 61635. Do not report 37218 with 36222-36224.

ICD-10-CM Diagnostic Codes

G45.1	Carotid artery syndrome (hemispheric)
G45.9	Transient cerebral ischemic attack, unspecified
I63.031	Cerebral infarction due to thrombosis of right carotid artery ☑
I63.032	Cerebral infarction due to thrombosis of left carotid artery ☑
I63.131	Cerebral infarction due to embolism of right carotid artery ☑
I63.132	Cerebral infarction due to embolism of left carotid artery ☑
I63.231	Cerebral infarction due to unspecified occlusion or stenosis of right carotid arteries ☑
I63.232	Cerebral infarction due to unspecified occlusion or stenosis of left carotid arteries ☑

I63.81	Other cerebral infarction due to occlusion or stenosis of small artery
I63.89	Other cerebral infarction
I65.21	Occlusion and stenosis of right carotid artery ☑
I65.22	Occlusion and stenosis of left carotid artery ☑
I65.23	Occlusion and stenosis of bilateral carotid arteries ☑
I65.8	Occlusion and stenosis of other precerebral arteries
I67.81	Acute cerebrovascular insufficiency
I67.82	Cerebral ischemia
I67.848	Other cerebrovascular vasospasm and vasoconstriction
I67.850	Cerebral autosomal dominant arteriopathy with subcortical infarcts and leukoencephalopathy
I67.858	Other hereditary cerebrovascular disease
I67.89	Other cerebrovascular disease
I72.0	Aneurysm of carotid artery
I76	Septic arterial embolism
I77.1	Stricture of artery
I77.3	Arterial fibromuscular dysplasia
I77.71	Dissection of carotid artery
I77.89	Other specified disorders of arteries and arterioles

AMA: **37218** 2018,Jan,8; 2017,Jul,3; 2017,Jan,8; 2016,Jan,13; 2015,May,7

Relative Value Units/Medicare Edits

Non-Facility RVU	Work	PE	MP	Total
37218	14.75	5.75	3.24	23.74
Facility RVU	**Work**	**PE**	**MP**	**Total**
37218	14.75	5.75	3.24	23.74

	FUD	Status	MUE	Modifiers				IOM Reference
37218	90	A	1(2)	51	50	N/A	80*	None

* with documentation

Terms To Know

arteriography. Radiologic study of an artery upon injection of dye.

ipsilateral. Located on, or affecting, the same side of the body, usually as it relates to a bilateral body part.

37220-37223

37220 Revascularization, endovascular, open or percutaneous, iliac artery, unilateral, initial vessel; with transluminal angioplasty

37221 with transluminal stent placement(s), includes angioplasty within the same vessel, when performed

+ **37222** Revascularization, endovascular, open or percutaneous, iliac artery, each additional ipsilateral iliac vessel; with transluminal angioplasty (List separately in addition to code for primary procedure)

+ **37223** with transluminal stent placement(s), includes angioplasty within the same vessel, when performed (List separately in addition to code for primary procedure)

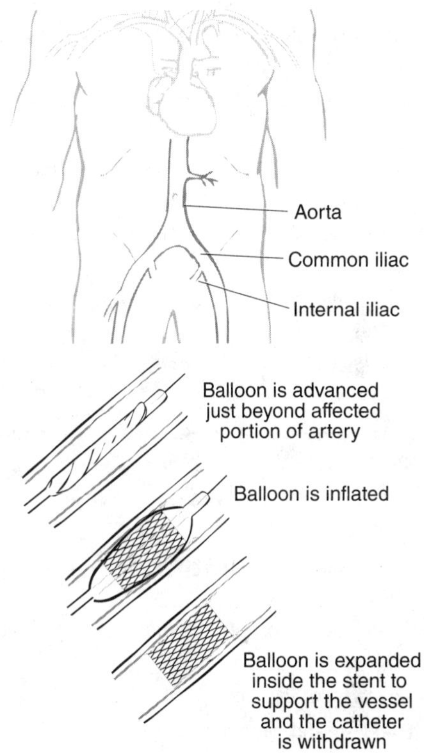

Explanation

The physician treats an iliac artery occlusion or stenosis by endovascular revascularization (restoration of blood supply) in 37220. Access is gained using a small open incision or a percutaneous sheath. Typically, a femoral approach under local anesthesia is used. After sheath placement, intra-arterial heparin is administered. Using a retrograde approach and under angiographic guidance, the occlusion is crossed using a catheter and guidewire. The balloon catheter is inflated in order to dilate the vessel to a larger diameter. Report 37220 for revascularization of the initial vessel and 37222 for each additional vessel on the same side (ipsilateral). Report 37221 if stent placement follows; angioplasty within the same vessel is included in this code. Following dilation and stent deployment, an angiogram is performed to assure appropriate placement and to evaluate the final result. Report 37223 for each additional ipsilateral vessel into which a stent is placed.

Coding Tips

When medically necessary, report moderate (conscious) sedation provided by the performing physician with 99151-99153. When provided by another physician, report 99155-99157. There are up to three vessels within the iliac region that can be treated within the same surgical session; report 37220 or

37221 for the initial vessel treated within one leg and 37222 and 37223 for other vessels when treated. Codes 37222–37223 are specific to additional vessels treated, not separate lesions within the same vessel. These procedures include accessing and selective catheterization of the vessel, traversing the lesion, radiological supervision and interpretation related to the vessel, embolic protection if utilized, closure of the arteriotomy, and imaging related to the completion of the procedure. Report 37220-37223 in addition to 34701-34711, 34718, or 34845-34848 when performed outside the treatment area of the endograft.

ICD-10-CM Diagnostic Codes

I70.211	Atherosclerosis of native arteries of extremities with intermittent claudication, right leg ☑
I70.212	Atherosclerosis of native arteries of extremities with intermittent claudication, left leg ☑
I70.213	Atherosclerosis of native arteries of extremities with intermittent claudication, bilateral legs ☑
I70.221	Atherosclerosis of native arteries of extremities with rest pain, right leg ☑
I70.222	Atherosclerosis of native arteries of extremities with rest pain, left leg ☑
I70.223	Atherosclerosis of native arteries of extremities with rest pain, bilateral legs ☑
I70.231	Atherosclerosis of native arteries of right leg with ulceration of thigh ☑
I70.232	Atherosclerosis of native arteries of right leg with ulceration of calf ☑
I70.233	Atherosclerosis of native arteries of right leg with ulceration of ankle ☑
I70.241	Atherosclerosis of native arteries of left leg with ulceration of thigh ☑
I70.242	Atherosclerosis of native arteries of left leg with ulceration of calf ☑
I70.243	Atherosclerosis of native arteries of left leg with ulceration of ankle ☑
I72.3	Aneurysm of iliac artery
I74.5	Embolism and thrombosis of iliac artery
I76	Septic arterial embolism
I77.1	Stricture of artery
I77.2	Rupture of artery
I77.3	Arterial fibromuscular dysplasia
I77.5	Necrosis of artery
I77.72	Dissection of iliac artery
I77.89	Other specified disorders of arteries and arterioles
S35.511A	Injury of right iliac artery, initial encounter ☑
S35.512A	Injury of left iliac artery, initial encounter ☑
S35.59XA	Injury of other iliac blood vessels, initial encounter
S35.8X1A	Laceration of other blood vessels at abdomen, lower back and pelvis level, initial encounter
S35.8X8A	Other specified injury of other blood vessels at abdomen, lower back and pelvis level, initial encounter

AMA: **37220** 2019,Jun,14; 2018,Jan,8; 2017,Jul,3; 2017,Jan,8; 2016,Jul,8; 2016,Jan,13; 2015,Jan,16; 2014,Jan,11; 2013,Dec,8 **37221** 2019,Jun,14; 2018,Jan,8; 2017,Jul,3; 2017,Jan,8; 2017,Dec,3; 2016,Jul,6; 2016,Jul,8; 2016,Jan,13; 2015,Jan,16; 2015,Jan,13; 2014,Jan,11; 2013,Dec,8 **37222** 2019,Jun,14; 2018,Jan,8; 2017,Jul,3; 2017,Jan,8; 2016,Jul,8; 2016,Jan,13; 2015,Jan,16; 2014,Jan,11; 2013,Dec,8 **37223** 2019,Jun,14; 2018,Jan,8; 2017,Jul,3; 2017,Jan,8; 2017,Dec,3; 2016,Jul,6; 2016,Jul,8; 2016,Jan,13; 2015,Jan,16; 2014,Jan,11; 2013,Dec,8

Relative Value Units/Medicare Edits

Non-Facility RVU	Work	PE	MP	Total
37220	7.9	74.16	1.7	83.76
37221	9.75	107.03	2.09	118.87
37222	3.73	18.11	0.8	22.64
37223	4.25	57.45	0.91	62.61
Facility RVU	**Work**	**PE**	**MP**	**Total**
37220	7.9	2.08	1.7	11.68
37221	9.75	2.59	2.09	14.43
37222	3.73	0.89	0.8	5.42
37223	4.25	1.04	0.91	6.2

	FUD	Status	MUE	Modifiers				IOM Reference
37220	0	A	1(2)	51	50	N/A	N/A	None
37221	0	A	1(2)	51	50	N/A	80*	
37222	N/A	A	2(2)	N/A	50	N/A	80*	
37223	N/A	A	2(2)	N/A	50	N/A	80*	

* with documentation

Terms To Know

revascularization. Restoration of blood flow and oxygen supply to a body part. This may apply to an extremity, the heart, or penis.

stent. Tube to provide support in a body cavity or lumen.

transluminal balloon angioplasty. Balloon-tipped catheter is placed within a narrowed artery or vein and the balloon is inflated to stretch the vessel to a larger diameter for increased blood flow.

37224-37227

37224 Revascularization, endovascular, open or percutaneous, femoral, popliteal artery(s), unilateral; with transluminal angioplasty
37225 with atherectomy, includes angioplasty within the same vessel, when performed
37226 with transluminal stent placement(s), includes angioplasty within the same vessel, when performed
37227 with transluminal stent placement(s) and atherectomy, includes angioplasty within the same vessel, when performed

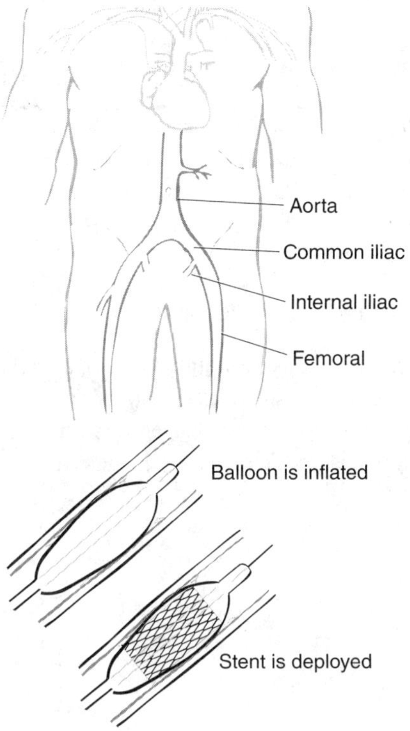

Explanation

The physician treats occlusive disease of a unilateral femoral or popliteal artery by endovascular revascularization (restoration of blood supply) using angioplasty in 37224. Access is gained using a femoral cutdown incision or a percutaneous sheath. Under local anesthesia, the physician accesses the femoral artery. After sheath or needle placement, intra-arterial heparin may be administered. A guidewire is inserted into the artery, followed by a catheter with an attached balloon. The catheter is advanced through the arterial system and into the narrowed portion of the targeted artery. There, the balloon is inflated in order to dilate the vessel to a larger diameter; several inflations may be necessary to achieve maximal results. The physician withdraws the deflated catheter and applies pressure to the puncture site to staunch the bleeding or closes the arteriotomy with suture. In 37225, the physician also performs atherectomy. The physician slides a guidewire through the atherectomy catheter or device, and inserts the guidewire/atherectomy catheter combination through the introducer sheath. The atherectomy device is fluoroscopically positioned at the site of the stenosis. The physician activates the device to remove the stenotic tissue and rechecks the diameter of the lesion by angiography. Several passes with the atherectomy device may be required. The physician removes the atherectomy catheter, guidewire, and introducer sheath. In 37226, the physician places one or more transluminal stents percutaneously using a guidewire or by incision. A catheter with a stent-transporting tip is threaded into the vessel. The catheter travels to the point where the vessel needs additional support, and the compressed stent is passed from the catheter into the vessel, where it deploys and expands to support the vessel walls. The catheter is removed. Pressure is applied over the percutaneous puncture site or, if performed via open approach, the vessel may be repaired and the skin incision closed by sutures. Angioplasty within the same vessel is included in 37226. Report 37227 if the physician performs both stent placement and atherectomy.

Coding Tips

When medically necessary, report moderate (conscious) sedation provided by the performing physician with 99151-99153. When provided by another physician, report 99155-99157. These procedures include accessing and selective catheterization of the vessel, traversing the lesion, radiological supervision and interpretation related to the vessel, embolic protection if utilized, closure of the arteriotomy, and imaging related to the completion of the procedure. These codes pertain to open and/or percutaneous access. There is only one vessel within the femoral/popliteal region that can be treated within the same surgical session. A single code is reported based on the specific procedures performed in this area, including the common, deep, and superficial femoral arteries and the popliteal artery. Do not report these codes in addition to 0505T, when performed in the femoral-popliteal. Supplies used when providing 37224 or 37226 may be reported with HCPCS Level II code C2623. Check with the specific payer to determine coverage.

ICD-10-CM Diagnostic Codes

I70.211	Atherosclerosis of native arteries of extremities with intermittent claudication, right leg ☑
I70.212	Atherosclerosis of native arteries of extremities with intermittent claudication, left leg ☑
I70.213	Atherosclerosis of native arteries of extremities with intermittent claudication, bilateral legs ☑
I70.221	Atherosclerosis of native arteries of extremities with rest pain, right leg ☑
I70.222	Atherosclerosis of native arteries of extremities with rest pain, left leg ☑
I70.223	Atherosclerosis of native arteries of extremities with rest pain, bilateral legs ☑
I70.231	Atherosclerosis of native arteries of right leg with ulceration of thigh ☑
I70.232	Atherosclerosis of native arteries of right leg with ulceration of calf ☑
I70.233	Atherosclerosis of native arteries of right leg with ulceration of ankle ☑
I70.241	Atherosclerosis of native arteries of left leg with ulceration of thigh ☑
I70.242	Atherosclerosis of native arteries of left leg with ulceration of calf ☑
I70.243	Atherosclerosis of native arteries of left leg with ulceration of ankle ☑
I70.244	Atherosclerosis of native arteries of left leg with ulceration of heel and midfoot ☑
I70.261	Atherosclerosis of native arteries of extremities with gangrene, right leg ☑
I70.262	Atherosclerosis of native arteries of extremities with gangrene, left leg ☑
I70.263	Atherosclerosis of native arteries of extremities with gangrene, bilateral legs ☑
I70.512	Atherosclerosis of nonautologous biological bypass graft(s) of the extremities with intermittent claudication, left leg ☑

I70.522	Atherosclerosis of nonautologous biological bypass graft(s) of the extremities with rest pain, left leg ☑
I70.541	Atherosclerosis of nonautologous biological bypass graft(s) of the left leg with ulceration of thigh ☑
I70.542	Atherosclerosis of nonautologous biological bypass graft(s) of the left leg with ulceration of calf ☑
I70.543	Atherosclerosis of nonautologous biological bypass graft(s) of the left leg with ulceration of ankle ☑
I70.544	Atherosclerosis of nonautologous biological bypass graft(s) of the left leg with ulceration of heel and midfoot ☑
I70.562	Atherosclerosis of nonautologous biological bypass graft(s) of the extremities with gangrene, left leg ☑
I70.612	Atherosclerosis of nonbiological bypass graft(s) of the extremities with intermittent claudication, left leg ☑
I70.622	Atherosclerosis of nonbiological bypass graft(s) of the extremities with rest pain, left leg ☑
I70.641	Atherosclerosis of nonbiological bypass graft(s) of the left leg with ulceration of thigh ☑
I70.642	Atherosclerosis of nonbiological bypass graft(s) of the left leg with ulceration of calf ☑
I70.643	Atherosclerosis of nonbiological bypass graft(s) of the left leg with ulceration of ankle ☑
I70.644	Atherosclerosis of nonbiological bypass graft(s) of the left leg with ulceration of heel and midfoot ☑
I70.662	Atherosclerosis of nonbiological bypass graft(s) of the extremities with gangrene, left leg ☑
I70.92	Chronic total occlusion of artery of the extremities
I72.4	Aneurysm of artery of lower extremity
I74.3	Embolism and thrombosis of arteries of the lower extremities
I75.022	Atheroembolism of left lower extremity ☑
I76	Septic arterial embolism
I77.1	Stricture of artery
I77.2	Rupture of artery
I77.3	Arterial fibromuscular dysplasia
I77.5	Necrosis of artery
S75.012A	Minor laceration of femoral artery, left leg, initial encounter ☑
S75.022A	Major laceration of femoral artery, left leg, initial encounter ☑
S85.012A	Laceration of popliteal artery, left leg, initial encounter ☑

AMA: 37224 2019,Jun,14; 2018,Jan,8; 2017,Jul,3; 2017,Jan,8; 2016,Jul,8; 2016,Jan,13; 2015,Jan,16; 2014,Jan,11 **37225** 2019,Jun,14; 2018,Jan,8; 2017,Jul,3; 2017,Jan,8; 2016,Jul,8; 2016,Jan,13; 2015,Jan,16; 2014,Jan,11 **37226** 2019,Jun,14; 2018,Jan,8; 2017,Jul,3; 2017,Jan,8; 2016,Jul,6; 2016,Jul,8; 2016,Jan,13; 2015,Jan,16; 2014,Jan,11 **37227** 2019,Jun,14; 2018,Jan,8; 2017,Jul,3; 2017,Jan,8; 2016,Jul,6; 2016,Jul,8; 2016,Jan,13; 2015,Jan,16; 2014,Jan,11

Relative Value Units/Medicare Edits

Non-Facility RVU	Work	PE	MP	Total
37224	8.75	90.1	1.83	100.68
37225	11.75	331.01	2.53	345.29
37226	10.24	287.05	2.2	299.49
37227	14.25	427.61	3.04	444.9
Facility RVU	**Work**	**PE**	**MP**	**Total**
37224	8.75	2.36	1.83	12.94
37225	11.75	3.33	2.53	17.61
37226	10.24	2.74	2.2	15.18
37227	14.25	3.88	3.04	21.17

	FUD	Status	MUE	Modifiers				IOM Reference
37224	0	A	1(2)	51	50	N/A	80*	None
37225	0	A	1(2)	51	50	N/A	80*	
37226	0	A	1(2)	51	50	N/A	80*	
37227	0	A	1(2)	51	50	N/A	80*	

* with documentation

Terms To Know

atherectomy. Surgical removal of arterial plaque from inside an artery. The procedure may be performed percutaneously, using a special catheter with a high-speed burr at the tip to bore through the sclerotic deposits, or transluminally by open incision.

37228-37231

37228 Revascularization, endovascular, open or percutaneous, tibial, peroneal artery, unilateral, initial vessel; with transluminal angioplasty

37229 with atherectomy, includes angioplasty within the same vessel, when performed

37230 with transluminal stent placement(s), includes angioplasty within the same vessel, when performed

37231 with transluminal stent placement(s) and atherectomy, includes angioplasty within the same vessel, when performed

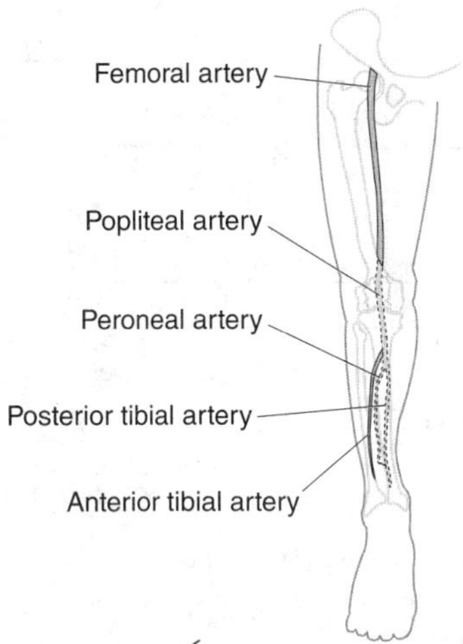

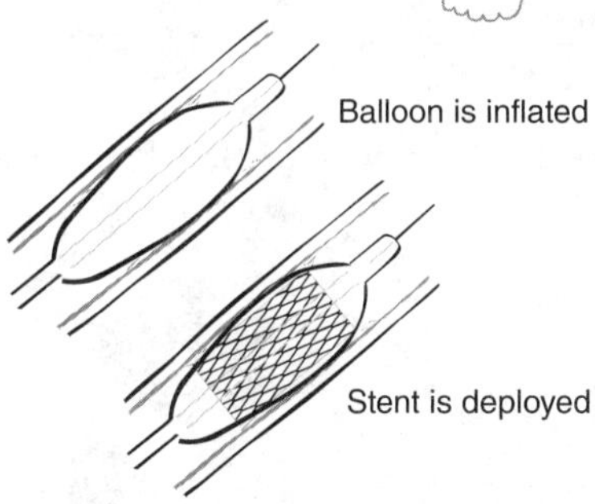

Explanation

The physician treats occlusive disease of a unilateral tibial or peroneal artery by endovascular revascularization (restoration of blood supply) using angioplasty in 37228. Access is gained using a femoral cutdown incision or a percutaneous sheath. Under local anesthesia, the physician accesses the femoral artery. After sheath or needle placement, intra-arterial heparin may be administered. A guidewire is inserted into the artery, followed by a catheter with an attached balloon. The catheter is advanced through the arterial system and into the narrowed portion of the targeted artery. There, the balloon is inflated in order to dilate the vessel to a larger diameter; several inflations may be necessary to achieve maximal results. The physician withdraws the deflated catheter and applies pressure to the puncture site to staunch the bleeding or closes the arteriotomy with suture. In 37229, the physician also performs atherectomy. The physician slides a guidewire through the atherectomy catheter or device, and inserts the guidewire/atherectomy catheter combination through the introducer sheath. The atherectomy device is fluoroscopically positioned at the site of the stenosis. The physician activates the device to remove the stenotic tissue and then rechecks the diameter of the lesion by angiography. Several passes with the atherectomy device may be required. The physician removes the atherectomy catheter, guidewire, and introducer sheath. In 37230, the physician places one or more transluminal stents percutaneously using a guidewire or by incision. A catheter with a stent-transporting tip is threaded into the vessel. The catheter travels to the point where the vessel needs additional support, and the compressed stent is passed from the catheter into the vessel, where it deploys and expands to support the vessel walls. The catheter is removed. Pressure is applied over the percutaneous puncture site or, if performed via open approach, the vessel may be repaired and the skin incision closed by sutures. Angioplasty within the same vessel is included in 37230. Report 37231 if the physician performs both stent placement and atherectomy.

Coding Tips

When medically necessary, report moderate (conscious) sedation provided by the performing physician with 99151-99153. When provided by another physician, report 99155-99157. These procedures include accessing and selective catheterization of the vessel, traversing the lesion, radiological supervision and interpretation related to the vessel, embolic protection if utilized, closure of the arteriotomy, and imaging related to the completion of the procedure. These codes pertain to open and/or percutaneous access. There are up to three vessels within the tibial/peroneal region that can be treated within the same surgical session. Report 37227, 37228, 37229, or 37230 for the initial vessel treated within one leg. Report add-on codes 37232–37235 for other vessels when treated.

ICD-10-CM Diagnostic Codes

I70.211	Atherosclerosis of native arteries of extremities with intermittent claudication, right leg ☑
I70.212	Atherosclerosis of native arteries of extremities with intermittent claudication, left leg ☑
I70.213	Atherosclerosis of native arteries of extremities with intermittent claudication, bilateral legs ☑
I70.221	Atherosclerosis of native arteries of extremities with rest pain, right leg ☑
I70.222	Atherosclerosis of native arteries of extremities with rest pain, left leg ☑
I70.223	Atherosclerosis of native arteries of extremities with rest pain, bilateral legs ☑
I70.231	Atherosclerosis of native arteries of right leg with ulceration of thigh ☑
I70.232	Atherosclerosis of native arteries of right leg with ulceration of calf ☑
I70.233	Atherosclerosis of native arteries of right leg with ulceration of ankle ☑
I70.241	Atherosclerosis of native arteries of left leg with ulceration of thigh ☑
I70.242	Atherosclerosis of native arteries of left leg with ulceration of calf ☑
I70.243	Atherosclerosis of native arteries of left leg with ulceration of ankle ☑
I70.244	Atherosclerosis of native arteries of left leg with ulceration of heel and midfoot ☑
I70.261	Atherosclerosis of native arteries of extremities with gangrene, right leg ☑
I70.262	Atherosclerosis of native arteries of extremities with gangrene, left leg ☑
I70.263	Atherosclerosis of native arteries of extremities with gangrene, bilateral legs ☑
I70.512	Atherosclerosis of nonautologous biological bypass graft(s) of the extremities with intermittent claudication, left leg ☑
I70.522	Atherosclerosis of nonautologous biological bypass graft(s) of the extremities with rest pain, left leg ☑

I70.541	Atherosclerosis of nonautologous biological bypass graft(s) of the left leg with ulceration of thigh ☑
I70.542	Atherosclerosis of nonautologous biological bypass graft(s) of the left leg with ulceration of calf ☑
I70.543	Atherosclerosis of nonautologous biological bypass graft(s) of the left leg with ulceration of ankle ☑
I70.544	Atherosclerosis of nonautologous biological bypass graft(s) of the left leg with ulceration of heel and midfoot ☑
I70.562	Atherosclerosis of nonautologous biological bypass graft(s) of the extremities with gangrene, left leg ☑
I70.612	Atherosclerosis of nonbiological bypass graft(s) of the extremities with intermittent claudication, left leg ☑
I70.622	Atherosclerosis of nonbiological bypass graft(s) of the extremities with rest pain, left leg ☑
I70.641	Atherosclerosis of nonbiological bypass graft(s) of the left leg with ulceration of thigh ☑
I70.642	Atherosclerosis of nonbiological bypass graft(s) of the left leg with ulceration of calf ☑
I70.643	Atherosclerosis of nonbiological bypass graft(s) of the left leg with ulceration of ankle ☑
I70.644	Atherosclerosis of nonbiological bypass graft(s) of the left leg with ulceration of heel and midfoot ☑
I70.662	Atherosclerosis of nonbiological bypass graft(s) of the extremities with gangrene, left leg ☑
I70.92	Chronic total occlusion of artery of the extremities
I72.4	Aneurysm of artery of lower extremity
I74.3	Embolism and thrombosis of arteries of the lower extremities
I75.022	Atheroembolism of left lower extremity ☑
I76	Septic arterial embolism
I77.1	Stricture of artery
I77.2	Rupture of artery
I77.3	Arterial fibromuscular dysplasia
I77.5	Necrosis of artery
S85.142A	Laceration of anterior tibial artery, left leg, initial encounter ☑
S85.172A	Laceration of posterior tibial artery, left leg, initial encounter ☑
S85.212A	Laceration of peroneal artery, left leg, initial encounter ☑

AMA: **37228** 2019,Jun,14; 2018,Jan,8; 2017,Jul,3; 2017,Jan,8; 2016,Jul,8; 2016,Jan,13; 2015,Jan,16; 2014,Jan,11 **37229** 2019,Jun,14; 2018,Jan,8; 2017,Jul,3; 2017,Jan,8; 2016,Jul,8; 2016,Jan,13; 2015,Jan,16; 2014,Jan,11 **37230** 2019,Jun,14; 2018,Jan,8; 2017,Jul,3; 2017,Jan,8; 2016,Jul,6; 2016,Jul,8; 2016,Jan,13; 2015,Jan,16; 2014,Jan,11 **37231** 2019,Jun,14; 2018,Jan,8; 2017,Jul,3; 2017,Jan,8; 2016,Jul,8; 2016,Jul,6; 2016,Jan,13; 2015,Jan,16; 2014,Jan,11

Relative Value Units/Medicare Edits

Non-Facility RVU	Work	PE	MP	Total
37228	10.75	132.93	2.26	145.94
37229	13.8	328.78	2.9	345.48
37230	13.55	277.65	2.93	294.13
37231	14.75	404.75	3.1	422.6
Facility RVU	**Work**	**PE**	**MP**	**Total**
37228	10.75	2.8	2.26	15.81
37229	13.8	3.86	2.9	20.56
37230	13.55	3.91	2.93	20.39
37231	14.75	4.31	3.1	22.16

	FUD	Status	MUE	Modifiers				IOM Reference
37228	0	A	1(2)	51	50	N/A	80*	None
37229	0	A	1(2)	51	50	N/A	80*	
37230	0	A	1(2)	51	50	N/A	80*	
37231	0	A	1(2)	51	50	N/A	80*	

* with documentation

Terms To Know

angioplasty. Reconstruction or repair of a diseased or damaged blood vessel.

atherectomy. Surgical removal of arterial plaque from inside an artery. The procedure may be performed percutaneously, using a special catheter with a high-speed burr at the tip to bore through the sclerotic deposits, or transluminally by open incision.

endovascular therapy. Intravascular catheters, scopes, stents, balloons, and other devices or methods used to treat vascular disease.

37232-37235

- **+ 37232** Revascularization, endovascular, open or percutaneous, tibial/peroneal artery, unilateral, each additional vessel; with transluminal angioplasty (List separately in addition to code for primary procedure)
- **+ 37233** with atherectomy, includes angioplasty within the same vessel, when performed (List separately in addition to code for primary procedure)
- **+ 37234** with transluminal stent placement(s), includes angioplasty within the same vessel, when performed (List separately in addition to code for primary procedure)
- **+ 37235** with transluminal stent placement(s) and atherectomy, includes angioplasty within the same vessel, when performed (List separately in addition to code for primary procedure)

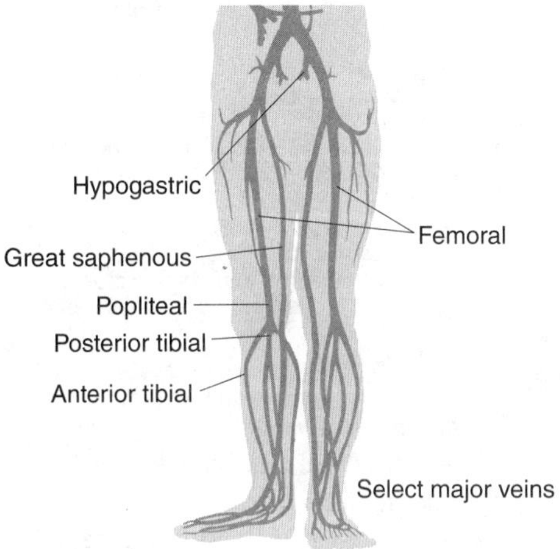

Explanation

The physician treats occlusive disease of unilateral tibial or peroneal arteries by endovascular revascularization (restoration of blood supply) using angioplasty. Access is gained using a femoral cutdown incision or a percutaneous sheath. Under local anesthesia, the physician accesses the femoral artery. After sheath or needle placement, intra-arterial heparin may be administered. A guidewire is inserted into the artery, followed by a catheter with an attached balloon. The catheter is advanced through the arterial system and into the narrowed portion of the targeted artery. The balloon is inflated in order to dilate the vessel to a larger diameter; several inflations may be necessary to achieve maximal results. The physician withdraws the deflated catheter and applies pressure to the puncture site to staunch the bleeding or closes the arteriotomy with suture. In some cases, the physician also performs atherectomy. The physician slides a guidewire through the atherectomy catheter or device and inserts the guidewire/atherectomy catheter combination through the introducer sheath. The atherectomy device is fluoroscopically positioned at the site of the stenosis. The physician activates the device to remove the stenotic tissue and rechecks the diameter of the lesion by angiography. Several passes with the atherectomy device may be required. The physician removes the atherectomy catheter, guidewire, and introducer sheath. In other cases, the physician places one or more transluminal stents percutaneously using a guidewire or by incision. A catheter with a stent-transporting tip is threaded into the vessel. The catheter travels to the point where the vessel needs additional support, and the compressed stent is passed from the catheter into the vessel, where it deploys and expands to support the vessel walls. The catheter is removed. Pressure is applied over the percutaneous puncture site or, if performed via open approach, the vessel may be repaired and the skin incision closed by sutures. Angioplasty within the same vessel is included in the codes for this procedure.

Coding Tips

When medically necessary, report moderate (conscious) sedation provided by the performing physician with 99151-99153. When provided by another physician, report 99155-99157. These procedures include accessing and selective catheterization of the vessel, traversing the lesion, radiological supervision and interpretation related to the vessel, embolic protection if utilized, closure of the arteriotomy, and imaging related to the completion of the procedure. These codes pertain to open and/or percutaneous access. These codes are based on the degree of progression where a code with more intensive procedures includes less intensive procedures (i.e., angioplasty, stent placement, atherectomy). Stent placement includes angioplasty when performed by the physician. Report 37232 with applicable codes in range 37228-37231 for each additional vessel. Report 37233 with 37229 and 37231 for each additional vessel. Report 37234 with 37229, 37230, and 37231 for each additional vessel. Report 37235 with 37231 when the physician performs both stent placement and atherectomy on more than one vessel. There are up to three vessels within the tibial/peroneal region that can be treated within the same surgical session. Report 37227-37230 for the initial vessel treated within one leg. Report add-on codes 37232–37235 for other vessels when treated.

ICD-10-CM Diagnostic Codes

I70.212	Atherosclerosis of native arteries of extremities with intermittent claudication, left leg ☑
I70.222	Atherosclerosis of native arteries of extremities with rest pain, left leg ☑
I70.241	Atherosclerosis of native arteries of left leg with ulceration of thigh ☑
I70.242	Atherosclerosis of native arteries of left leg with ulceration of calf ☑
I70.243	Atherosclerosis of native arteries of left leg with ulceration of ankle ☑
I70.244	Atherosclerosis of native arteries of left leg with ulceration of heel and midfoot ☑
I70.262	Atherosclerosis of native arteries of extremities with gangrene, left leg ☑
I70.512	Atherosclerosis of nonautologous biological bypass graft(s) of the extremities with intermittent claudication, left leg ☑
I70.522	Atherosclerosis of nonautologous biological bypass graft(s) of the extremities with rest pain, left leg ☑
I70.541	Atherosclerosis of nonautologous biological bypass graft(s) of the left leg with ulceration of thigh ☑
I70.542	Atherosclerosis of nonautologous biological bypass graft(s) of the left leg with ulceration of calf ☑
I70.543	Atherosclerosis of nonautologous biological bypass graft(s) of the left leg with ulceration of ankle ☑
I70.544	Atherosclerosis of nonautologous biological bypass graft(s) of the left leg with ulceration of heel and midfoot ☑
I70.562	Atherosclerosis of nonautologous biological bypass graft(s) of the extremities with gangrene, left leg ☑
I70.612	Atherosclerosis of nonbiological bypass graft(s) of the extremities with intermittent claudication, left leg ☑
I70.622	Atherosclerosis of nonbiological bypass graft(s) of the extremities with rest pain, left leg ☑
I70.641	Atherosclerosis of nonbiological bypass graft(s) of the left leg with ulceration of thigh ☑

I70.642	Atherosclerosis of nonbiological bypass graft(s) of the left leg with ulceration of calf ☑
I70.643	Atherosclerosis of nonbiological bypass graft(s) of the left leg with ulceration of ankle ☑
I70.644	Atherosclerosis of nonbiological bypass graft(s) of the left leg with ulceration of heel and midfoot ☑
I70.662	Atherosclerosis of nonbiological bypass graft(s) of the extremities with gangrene, left leg ☑
I70.92	Chronic total occlusion of artery of the extremities
I72.4	Aneurysm of artery of lower extremity
I74.3	Embolism and thrombosis of arteries of the lower extremities
I75.022	Atheroembolism of left lower extremity ☑
I76	Septic arterial embolism
I77.1	Stricture of artery
I77.2	Rupture of artery
I77.3	Arterial fibromuscular dysplasia
I77.5	Necrosis of artery
S85.142A	Laceration of anterior tibial artery, left leg, initial encounter ☑
S85.172A	Laceration of posterior tibial artery, left leg, initial encounter ☑
S85.212A	Laceration of peroneal artery, left leg, initial encounter ☑

AMA: **37232** 2019,Jun,14; 2018,Jan,8; 2017,Jul,3; 2017,Jan,8; 2016,Jul,8; 2016,Jan,13; 2015,Jan,16; 2014,Jan,11 **37233** 2019,Jun,14; 2018,Jan,8; 2017,Jul,3; 2017,Jan,8; 2016,Jul,8; 2016,Jan,13; 2015,Jan,16; 2014,Jan,11 **37234** 2019,Jun,14; 2018,Jan,8; 2017,Jul,3; 2017,Jan,8; 2016,Jul,6; 2016,Jul,8; 2016,Jan,13; 2015,Jan,16; 2014,Jan,11 **37235** 2019,Jun,14; 2018,Jan,8; 2017,Jul,3; 2017,Jan,8; 2016,Jul,6; 2016,Jul,8; 2016,Jan,13; 2015,Jan,16; 2014,Jan,11

Relative Value Units/Medicare Edits

Non-Facility RVU	Work	PE	MP	Total
37232	4.0	26.33	0.8	31.13
37233	6.5	30.1	1.33	37.93
37234	5.5	103.06	1.19	109.75
37235	7.8	109.64	1.63	119.07
Facility RVU	**Work**	**PE**	**MP**	**Total**
37232	4.0	1.05	0.8	5.85
37233	6.5	1.7	1.33	9.53
37234	5.5	1.63	1.19	8.32
37235	7.8	2.25	1.63	11.68

	FUD	Status	MUE	Modifiers				IOM Reference
37232	N/A	A	2(3)	N/A	50	N/A	80*	None
37233	N/A	A	2(3)	N/A	50	N/A	80*	
37234	N/A	A	2(3)	N/A	50	N/A	80*	
37235	N/A	A	2(3)	N/A	50	N/A	80*	

* with documentation

[37246, 37247]

37246 Transluminal balloon angioplasty (except lower extremity artery(ies) for occlusive disease, intracranial, coronary, pulmonary, or dialysis circuit), open or percutaneous, including all imaging and radiological supervision and interpretation necessary to perform the angioplasty within the same artery; initial artery

\+ **37247** Transluminal balloon angioplasty (except lower extremity artery(ies) for occlusive disease, intracranial, coronary, pulmonary, or dialysis circuit), open or percutaneous, including all imaging and radiological supervision and interpretation necessary to perform the angioplasty within the same artery; each additional artery (List separately in addition to code for primary procedure)

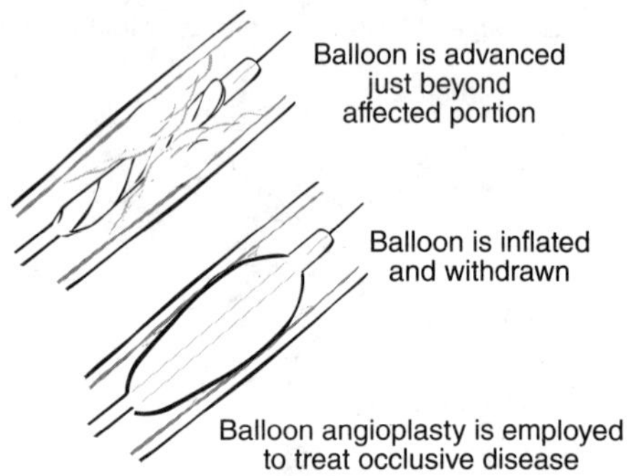

Explanation

Transluminal balloon angioplasty is performed by open or percutaneous approach (except lower limb arterial occlusion, intracranial, coronary, pulmonary, or dialysis circuit). In an open procedure, the physician makes an incision in the skin overlying the vessel. The vessel is dissected from adjacent critical structures, and vessel clamps are applied. The physician may nick the vessel to create an opening into which a catheter with a balloon attached is inserted into the vessel and threaded. The catheter is fed into the narrowed portion of the vessel, where its balloon is inflated in the narrowed area. The blood vessel is stretched to a larger diameter, allowing a more normal outflow of blood through the area. Several inflations may be performed along the narrowed area. The catheter is slowly withdrawn after deflation. Occasionally, the opening in the vessel is repaired with sutures. In a percutaneous approach, the physician isolates the vessel and inserts a large needle through the skin and into the vessel. A guidewire is threaded through the needle into the vessel. The needle is removed. A catheter with a balloon attached follows the wire into the vessel. The wire is removed. The catheter is fed through the vascular system and into the narrowed portion of the affected vessel and the balloon is inflated. The blood vessel is stretched to a larger diameter, allowing a more normal outflow of blood through the area. Several inflations may be performed along the narrowed area. The catheter is slowly withdrawn after deflation. Pressure is applied to the puncture site to stop the bleeding after the catheter is removed. These codes include all radiological imaging within the same artery. Report 37246 for the initial artery treated and 37247 for each additional artery.

Coding Tips

Report 37247 in addition to 37246. Radiological supervision and interpretation and imaging used to record the completion of the intervention are included in these codes. Do not report these codes with 37215-37218 or 37220-37237 during the same operative encounter in the same artery. Do not report these codes with 34841-34848 for angioplasty for insertion of bare metal/covered stent into the visceral branches within the endoprosthesis target zone.

ICD-10-CM Diagnostic Codes

G45.3	Amaurosis fugax
I10	Essential (primary) hypertension
I15.0	Renovascular hypertension
I15.1	Hypertension secondary to other renal disorders
I16.0	Hypertensive urgency
I16.1	Hypertensive emergency
I70.1	Atherosclerosis of renal artery
I77.1	Stricture of artery
I77.2	Rupture of artery
I77.3	Arterial fibromuscular dysplasia
I77.4	Celiac artery compression syndrome
I77.89	Other specified disorders of arteries and arterioles
I81	Portal vein thrombosis
I82.0	Budd-Chiari syndrome
I82.1	Thrombophlebitis migrans
I82.291	Chronic embolism and thrombosis of other thoracic veins
I82.3	Embolism and thrombosis of renal vein
I82.890	Acute embolism and thrombosis of other specified veins
I82.891	Chronic embolism and thrombosis of other specified veins
K55.011	Focal (segmental) acute (reversible) ischemia of small intestine
K55.012	Diffuse acute (reversible) ischemia of small intestine
K55.021	Focal (segmental) acute infarction of small intestine
K55.022	Diffuse acute infarction of small intestine
K55.031	Focal (segmental) acute (reversible) ischemia of large intestine
K55.032	Diffuse acute (reversible) ischemia of large intestine
K55.041	Focal (segmental) acute infarction of large intestine
K55.042	Diffuse acute infarction of large intestine
K55.051	Focal (segmental) acute (reversible) ischemia of intestine, part unspecified
K55.052	Diffuse acute (reversible) ischemia of intestine, part unspecified
K55.1	Chronic vascular disorders of intestine
K55.8	Other vascular disorders of intestine
N17.0	Acute kidney failure with tubular necrosis
N17.1	Acute kidney failure with acute cortical necrosis
N17.2	Acute kidney failure with medullary necrosis
N17.8	Other acute kidney failure
N26.2	Page kidney
N28.0	Ischemia and infarction of kidney
Q27.1	Congenital renal artery stenosis
Q27.2	Other congenital malformations of renal artery

AMA: 37246 2018,Jan,8; 2017,Jul,3; 2017,Aug,10 **37247** 2018,Jan,8; 2017,Jul,3; 2017,Aug,10

Relative Value Units/Medicare Edits

Non-Facility RVU	Work	PE	MP	Total
37246	7.0	51.17	1.11	59.28
37247	3.5	18.57	0.52	22.59
Facility RVU	**Work**	**PE**	**MP**	**Total**
37246	7.0	2.01	1.11	10.12
37247	3.5	0.95	0.52	4.97

	FUD	Status	MUE	Modifiers				IOM Reference
37246	0	A	1(2)	51	50	N/A	N/A	None
37247	N/A	A	2(3)	N/A	50	N/A	N/A	

* with documentation

Terms To Know

hypertension. Abnormally increased pressure, usually referring to arterial pressure, exceeding an acceptable range.

ischemia. Deficiency in blood supply causing tissues to be deprived of oxygen, resulting from trauma, mechanical or functional constriction of blood vessels, or a physical obstruction.

occlusion. Constriction, closure, or blockage of a passage.

transluminal balloon angioplasty. Balloon-tipped catheter is placed within a narrowed artery or vein and the balloon is inflated to stretch the vessel to a larger diameter for increased blood flow.

[37248, 37249]

37248 Transluminal balloon angioplasty (except dialysis circuit), open or percutaneous, including all imaging and radiological supervision and interpretation necessary to perform the angioplasty within the same vein; initial vein

\+ **37249** Transluminal balloon angioplasty (except dialysis circuit), open or percutaneous, including all imaging and radiological supervision and interpretation necessary to perform the angioplasty within the same vein; each additional vein (List separately in addition to code for primary procedure)

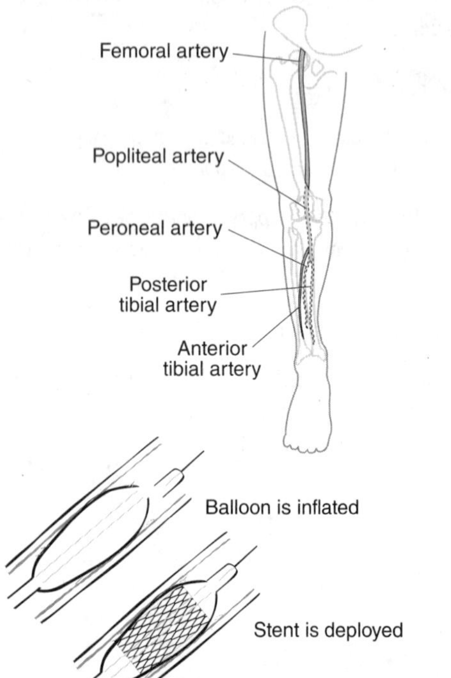

Open or percutaneous balloon angioplasty including imaging

Explanation

Transluminal balloon angioplasty is performed by open or percutaneous approach (except dialysis circuit). In an open procedure, the physician makes an incision in the skin overlying the vessel. The vessel is dissected from adjacent critical structures and vessel clamps are applied. The physician may nick the vessel to create an opening into which a catheter with a balloon attached is inserted into the vessel and threaded. The catheter is fed into the narrowed portion of the vessel, where its balloon is inflated in the narrowed area. The blood vessel is stretched to a larger diameter, allowing a more normal outflow of blood through the area. Several inflations may be performed along the narrowed area. The catheter is slowly withdrawn after deflation. Occasionally, the opening in the vessel is repaired with sutures. In a percutaneous approach, the physician isolates the vessel and inserts a large needle through the skin and into the vessel. A guidewire is threaded through the needle into the vessel. The needle is removed. A catheter with a balloon attached follows the wire into the vessel. The wire is removed. The catheter is fed through the vascular system and into the narrowed portion of the affected vessel and the balloon is inflated. The blood vessel is stretched to a larger diameter, allowing a more normal outflow of blood through the area. Several inflations may be performed along the narrowed area. The catheter is slowly withdrawn after deflation. Pressure is applied to the puncture site to stop the bleeding after the catheter is removed. These codes include all radiological imaging within the same vein. Report 37248 for the initial vein treated and 37249 for each additional vein.

Coding Tips

Report 37249 in addition to 37248. Radiological supervision and interpretation and imaging used to record the completion of the intervention are included in these codes. Do not report these codes with 37238 or 37239 during the same operative encounter in the same vein. Intravascular ultrasound may be reported separately, see 37252 and 37253. Do not report these codes in addition to 0505T, when performed in the femoral-popliteal. For balloon angioplasty performed through the dialysis circuit, see 36902-36908. For transluminal balloon angioplasty in aorta/visceral artery during fenestrated endovascular repair, see 34841-34848; in the iliac, femoral, popliteal, or tibial/peroneal artery due to occlusive disease, see 37220-37235; in an intracranial artery, see 61630 or 61635.

ICD-10-CM Diagnostic Codes

The application of this code is too broad to adequately present ICD-10-CM diagnostic code links here. Refer to your ICD-10-CM book.

AMA: **37248** 2018,Jan,8; 2017,Mar,3; 2017,Jul,3; 2017,Aug,10 **37249** 2018,Jan,8; 2017,Mar,3; 2017,Jul,3; 2017,Aug,10

Relative Value Units/Medicare Edits

Non-Facility RVU	Work	PE	MP	Total
37248	6.0	35.54	0.84	42.38
37249	2.97	13.38	0.42	16.77
Facility RVU	**Work**	**PE**	**MP**	**Total**
37248	6.0	1.82	0.84	8.66
37249	2.97	0.83	0.42	4.22

	FUD	Status	MUE	Modifiers				IOM Reference
37248	0	A	1(2)	51	50	N/A	N/A	None
37249	N/A	A	3(3)	N/A	50	N/A	N/A	

* with documentation

37236-37237

37236 Transcatheter placement of an intravascular stent(s) (except lower extremity artery(s) for occlusive disease, cervical carotid, extracranial vertebral or intrathoracic carotid, intracranial, or coronary), open or percutaneous, including radiological supervision and interpretation and including all angioplasty within the same vessel, when performed; initial artery

\+ **37237** each additional artery (List separately in addition to code for primary procedure)

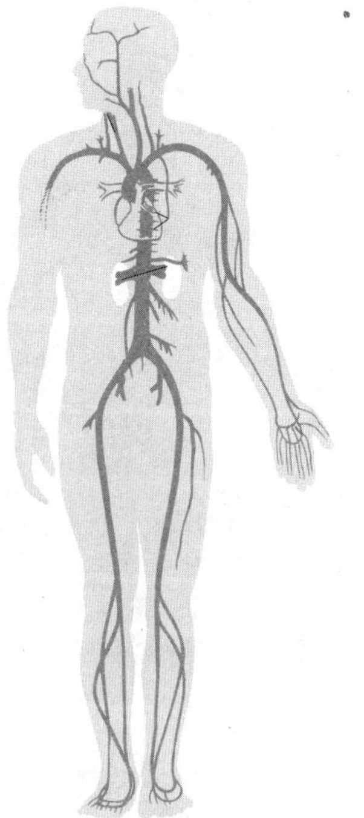

Map of major arteries

Explanation

The physician places one or more intravascular stents through a catheter into an artery other than a coronary, cervical or intrathoracic carotid, extracranial vertebral, iliac, intracranial, or lower extremity artery. The procedure may be performed via a percutaneous or an open approach. In the percutaneous approach, a guidewire is threaded through the needle into the blood vessel and the needle is removed. In the open approach, the physician makes an incision in the skin overlying the vessel to be catheterized. The vessel is dissected and nicked with a small blade. After the approach, a catheter with a stent-transporting tip is threaded over the guidewire into the vessel and the wire is extracted. The catheter travels to the point where the vessel needs additional support. The compressed stent is passed from the catheter out into the vessel, where it deploys, expanding to support the vessel walls. The catheter is removed and pressure is applied over the puncture site or layered closure is performed. Report 37236 for stents placed in the initial artery and 37237 for each additional artery where a stent is placed. These procedures include radiologic supervision and interpretation, as well as angioplasty, when performed.

Coding Tips

When medically necessary, report moderate (conscious) sedation provided by the performing physician with 99151-99153. When provided by another physician, report 99155-99157. Report 37237 in addition to 37236. These codes include all balloon angioplasty procedures performed in the treated vessel including pre- and postdilation, treatment of lesions outside of the stented segment but within the same vessel, and use of a smaller or larger balloon to achieve the same therapeutic result. Angioplasty performed in vessels other than the one being reported with this code can be reported separately. Selective and/or nonselective catheterization is reported separately in addition to 37236–37237. These codes include supervision and interpretation of radiology services related to the intervention, as well as imaging to document completion of the intervention. Also included are closure of the arteriotomy via pressure and application of an arterial closure device or standard closure of the puncture site by suture. Extensive repairs or replacement of the artery may be reported separately, see 35226 or 35286. Ultrasound guidance for vascular access (76937) may be reported separately, as well as intravascular ultrasound (37252–37253). If a stent is being deployed for the purpose of serving as a lattice work for embolization coils, use the embolization code and not the stent deployment code. Do not report 37236–37237 with 34841–34848 for bare metal or covered stents placed into the visceral branches within the endoprosthesis target zone. For transcatheter placement of intravascular stent in the intracranial vessels, see 61635. For stent placement in iliac, femoral, popliteal, or tibial/peroneal artery for occlusive disease, see 37221, 37223, 37226, 37227, 37230, 37231, 37234, and 37235. For open or percutaneous antegrade transcatheter placement of intrathoracic carotid/innominate artery stent, see 37218. For open or percutaneous transcatheter placement of extracranial vertebral artery stent, see 0075T and 0076T. For placement of stent at arterial anastomosis of the dialysis circuit, see 36903 or 36906.

ICD-10-CM Diagnostic Codes

A52.01	Syphilitic aneurysm of aorta
I15.0	Renovascular hypertension
I70.0	Atherosclerosis of aorta
I70.1	Atherosclerosis of renal artery
I70.218	Atherosclerosis of native arteries of extremities with intermittent claudication, other extremity
I70.228	Atherosclerosis of native arteries of extremities with rest pain, other extremity
I70.25	Atherosclerosis of native arteries of other extremities with ulceration
I70.268	Atherosclerosis of native arteries of extremities with gangrene, other extremity
I70.92	Chronic total occlusion of artery of the extremities
I71.02	Dissection of abdominal aorta
I71.03	Dissection of thoracoabdominal aorta
I71.3	Abdominal aortic aneurysm, ruptured
I71.4	Abdominal aortic aneurysm, without rupture
I72.1	Aneurysm of artery of upper extremity
I74.01	Saddle embolus of abdominal aorta
I74.2	Embolism and thrombosis of arteries of the upper extremities
I74.5	Embolism and thrombosis of iliac artery
I75.011	Atheroembolism of right upper extremity ☑
I75.012	Atheroembolism of left upper extremity ☑
I75.81	Atheroembolism of kidney
I77.1	Stricture of artery
I77.3	Arterial fibromuscular dysplasia
I77.72	Dissection of iliac artery
I77.73	Dissection of renal artery
K55.011	Focal (segmental) acute (reversible) ischemia of small intestine
K55.012	Diffuse acute (reversible) ischemia of small intestine
K55.021	Focal (segmental) acute infarction of small intestine
K55.022	Diffuse acute infarction of small intestine

K55.031	Focal (segmental) acute (reversible) ischemia of large intestine
K55.032	Diffuse acute (reversible) ischemia of large intestine
K55.041	Focal (segmental) acute infarction of large intestine
K55.042	Diffuse acute infarction of large intestine
K55.1	Chronic vascular disorders of intestine
Q25.21	Interruption of aortic arch
Q25.29	Other atresia of aorta
Q25.3	Supravalvular aortic stenosis
Q25.41	Absence and aplasia of aorta
Q25.42	Hypoplasia of aorta
Q25.43	Congenital aneurysm of aorta
Q25.44	Congenital dilation of aorta
Q25.45	Double aortic arch
Q25.46	Tortuous aortic arch
Q25.47	Right aortic arch
Q25.48	Anomalous origin of subclavian artery
Q25.5	Atresia of pulmonary artery
Q25.71	Coarctation of pulmonary artery
Q27.1	Congenital renal artery stenosis
Q27.34	Arteriovenous malformation of renal vessel

AMA: 37236 2018,Jan,8; 2017,Jul,3; 2017,Jan,8; 2017,Dec,3; 2016,Mar,5; 2016,Jul,3; 2016,Jul,6; 2016,Jan,13; 2015,May,7; 2015,Jan,16; 2014,Jan,11; 2013,Dec,8 **37237** 2018,Jan,8; 2017,Jul,3; 2017,Jan,8; 2017,Dec,3; 2016,Mar,5; 2016,Jul,6; 2016,Jan,13; 2015,Jan,16; 2014,Jan,11; 2013,Dec,8

Relative Value Units/Medicare Edits

Non-Facility RVU	Work	PE	MP	Total
37236	8.75	91.1	1.77	101.62
37237	4.25	55.2	0.89	60.34
Facility RVU	**Work**	**PE**	**MP**	**Total**
37236	8.75	2.42	1.77	12.94
37237	4.25	1.05	0.89	6.19

	FUD	Status	MUE	Modifiers				IOM Reference
37236	0	A	1(2)	51	50	N/A	80*	None
37237	N/A	A	2(3)	N/A	50	N/A	80*	

* with documentation

37238-37239

37238 Transcatheter placement of an intravascular stent(s), open or percutaneous, including radiological supervision and interpretation and including angioplasty within the same vessel, when performed; initial vein

+ **37239** each additional vein (List separately in addition to code for primary procedure)

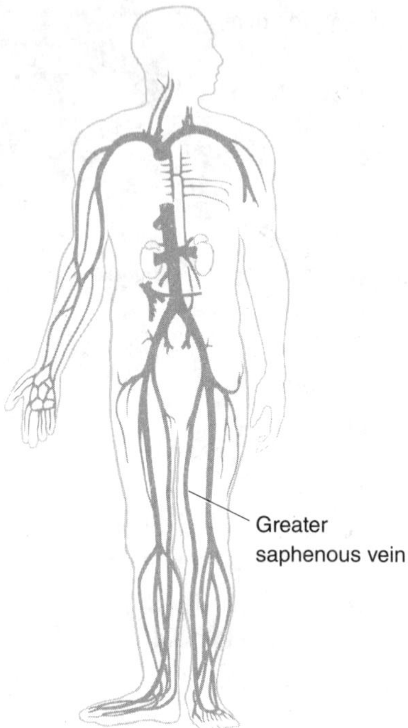

Map of major veins

Explanation

The physician places one or more intravascular stents through a catheter into a vein. The procedure may be performed via a percutaneous or an open approach. In the percutaneous approach, a guidewire is threaded through the needle into the blood vessel and the needle is removed. In the open approach, the physician makes an incision in the skin overlying the vessel to be catheterized. The vessel is dissected and nicked with a small blade. After the approach, a catheter with a stent-transporting tip is threaded over the guidewire into the vessel and the wire is extracted. The catheter travels to the point where the vessel needs additional support. The compressed stent is passed from the catheter out into the vessel, where it deploys, expanding to support the vessel walls. The catheter is removed and pressure is applied over the puncture site or layered closure is performed. Report 37238 for stents placed in the initial vein and 37239 for each additional vein where a stent is placed.

Coding Tips

When medically necessary, report moderate (conscious) sedation provided by the performing physician with 99151-99153. When provided by another physician, report 99155-99157. Report 37239 in addition to 37238. These codes include all balloon angioplasty procedures performed in the treated vessel including pre- and postdilation, treatment of lesions outside of the stented segment but within the same vessel, and use of a smaller or larger balloon to achieve the same therapeutic result. Angioplasty performed in vessels other than the one being reported with this code can be reported separately. Selective and/or nonselective catheterization is reported separately in addition to 37238–37239. These codes include supervision and interpretation of radiology services related to the intervention, as well as imaging to document completion of the intervention. Also included is closure of the arteriotomy via pressure and application of an arterial closure device or standard closure of the puncture site by suture. Extensive repairs or replacement of the artery may be reported separately, see 35226 or 35286. Ultrasound guidance for vascular access (76937) may be reported separately, as well as intravascular ultrasound (37252–37253). If a stent is being deployed for the purpose of serving as a lattice work for embolization coils, use the embolization code and not the stent deployment code. Do not report these codes in addition to 0505T, when performed in the femoral-popliteal. For transcatheter placement of intravascular stent in the intracranial vessels, see 61635. For stent placement in iliac, femoral, popliteal, or tibial/peroneal artery for occlusive disease, see 37221, 37223, 37226, 37227, 37230, 37231, 37234, 37235; for cervical carotid, see 37215, 37216; for intracoronary, see 92928, 92929, 92933, 92934, 92937, 92938, 92941, 92943, 92944; for open retrograde intrathoracic common carotid or innominate vessels, see 37217. For open or percutaneous antegrade transcatheter placement of intrathoracic carotid/innominate artery stent, see 37218. For open or percutaneous transcatheter placement of extracranial vertebral artery stent, see 0075T and 0076T. For placement of stent within the peripheral segment of dialysis segment, see 36903 or 36906. For transcatheter placement of an intravascular stent within the central dialysis segment performed through the dialysis segment, see 36908.

ICD-10-CM Diagnostic Codes

I80.11	Phlebitis and thrombophlebitis of right femoral vein ☑
I80.12	Phlebitis and thrombophlebitis of left femoral vein ☑
I80.211	Phlebitis and thrombophlebitis of right iliac vein ☑
I80.212	Phlebitis and thrombophlebitis of left iliac vein ☑
I80.221	Phlebitis and thrombophlebitis of right popliteal vein ☑
I80.222	Phlebitis and thrombophlebitis of left popliteal vein ☑
I80.231	Phlebitis and thrombophlebitis of right tibial vein ☑
I80.232	Phlebitis and thrombophlebitis of left tibial vein ☑
I80.241	Phlebitis and thrombophlebitis of right peroneal vein ☑
I81	Portal vein thrombosis
I82.210	Acute embolism and thrombosis of superior vena cava
I82.220	Acute embolism and thrombosis of inferior vena cava
I82.221	Chronic embolism and thrombosis of inferior vena cava
I82.411	Acute embolism and thrombosis of right femoral vein ☑
I82.412	Acute embolism and thrombosis of left femoral vein ☑
I82.421	Acute embolism and thrombosis of right iliac vein ☑
I82.422	Acute embolism and thrombosis of left iliac vein ☑
I82.451	Acute embolism and thrombosis of right peroneal vein ☑
I82.511	Chronic embolism and thrombosis of right femoral vein ☑
I82.512	Chronic embolism and thrombosis of left femoral vein ☑
I82.521	Chronic embolism and thrombosis of right iliac vein ☑
I82.522	Chronic embolism and thrombosis of left iliac vein ☑
I82.621	Acute embolism and thrombosis of deep veins of right upper extremity ☑
I82.622	Acute embolism and thrombosis of deep veins of left upper extremity ☑
I82.721	Chronic embolism and thrombosis of deep veins of right upper extremity ☑
I82.722	Chronic embolism and thrombosis of deep veins of left upper extremity ☑
I82.A11	Acute embolism and thrombosis of right axillary vein ☑
I82.A12	Acute embolism and thrombosis of left axillary vein ☑
I82.B11	Acute embolism and thrombosis of right subclavian vein ☑
I82.B12	Acute embolism and thrombosis of left subclavian vein ☑
I87.001	Postthrombotic syndrome without complications of right lower extremity ☑
I87.002	Postthrombotic syndrome without complications of left lower extremity ☑
I87.091	Postthrombotic syndrome with other complications of right lower extremity ☑
I87.092	Postthrombotic syndrome with other complications of left lower extremity ☑
I87.1	Compression of vein
Q26.0	Congenital stenosis of vena cava
Q26.1	Persistent left superior vena cava

AMA: **37238** 2018,Jan,8; 2017,Mar,3; 2017,Jul,3; 2017,Jan,8; 2016,Jun,8; 2016,Jul,6; 2014,Jan,11 **37239** 2018,Jan,8; 2017,Mar,3; 2017,Jul,3; 2017,Jan,8; 2016,Jul,6; 2014,Jan,11

Relative Value Units/Medicare Edits

Non-Facility RVU	Work	PE	MP	Total
37238	6.04	95.6	1.0	102.64
37239	2.97	45.4	0.6	48.97
Facility RVU	**Work**	**PE**	**MP**	**Total**
37238	6.04	1.78	1.0	8.82
37239	2.97	0.85	0.6	4.42

	FUD	Status	MUE	Modifiers				IOM Reference
37238	0	A	1(2)	51	50	N/A	80*	None
37239	N/A	A	2(3)	N/A	50	N/A	80*	

* with documentation

Terms To Know

catheter. Flexible tube inserted into an area of the body for introducing or withdrawing fluid.

guidewire. Flexible metal instrument designed to lead another instrument in its proper course.

stent. Tube to provide support in a body cavity or lumen.

37241-37242

37241 Vascular embolization or occlusion, inclusive of all radiological supervision and interpretation, intraprocedural roadmapping, and imaging guidance necessary to complete the intervention; venous, other than hemorrhage (eg, congenital or acquired venous malformations, venous and capillary hemangiomas, varices, varicoceles)

37242 arterial, other than hemorrhage or tumor (eg, congenital or acquired arterial malformations, arteriovenous malformations, arteriovenous fistulas, aneurysms, pseudoaneurysms)

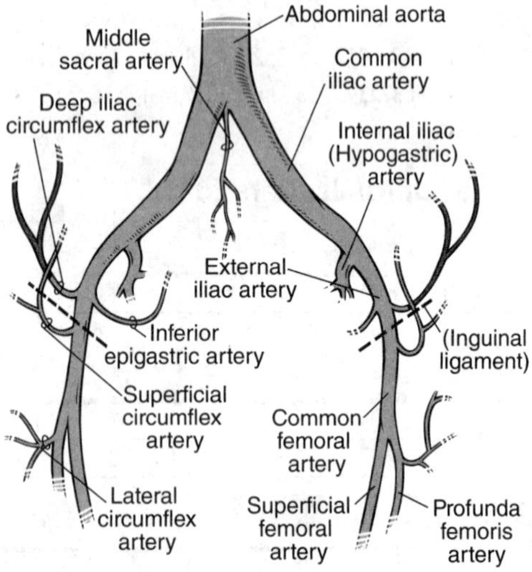

Pelvic arterial anatomy

Explanation

Embolization or occlusion of a blood vessel is performed. A needle is inserted through the skin and into a blood vessel. A guidewire is threaded through the needle into the vessel. The needle is removed. A catheter is threaded into the vessel and the wire is extracted. The catheter travels to the appropriate blood vessel and beads, coils, or another vessel-blocking device are released. The beads or other device block the vessel. The catheter is removed and pressure is applied over the puncture site to stop bleeding. Report 37241 for occlusion of a vein for any condition other than hemorrhage. Report 37242 when the occlusion is of an artery to treat a condition other than hemorrhage or tumor.

Coding Tips

When medically necessary, report moderate (conscious) sedation provided by the performing physician with 99151-99153. When provided by another physician, report 99155-99157. Only one embolization code should be reported for each surgical field, including the entire area directly involved in and immediately surrounding the procedure. If an intravascular stent is deployed for the purpose of providing a lattice work for embolization coils, report the embolization codes. The code representing the immediate cause for the embolization should be used. Diagnostic angiography and catheter placement may be reported separately. Report with an appropriate modifier. Do not report 37241 for treatment of incompetent veins. Do not report 37241 with 36465, 36466, 36468, 36470, 36471, 36473-36479, 75894, or 75898 in the same surgical field. Do not report 37242 with 75894 or 75898 in the same surgical field. For sclerosis of veins or endovenous ablation of incompetent extremity veins, see 36468–36479. For percutaneous treatment of an extremity pseudoaneurysms, see 36002. For permanent endovascular embolization or occlusion within the dialysis circuit, see 36909.

ICD-10-CM Diagnostic Codes

D18.01	Hemangioma of skin and subcutaneous tissue
D18.02	Hemangioma of intracranial structures
D18.03	Hemangioma of intra-abdominal structures
I28.0	Arteriovenous fistula of pulmonary vessels
I28.1	Aneurysm of pulmonary artery
I71.1	Thoracic aortic aneurysm, ruptured
I71.2	Thoracic aortic aneurysm, without rupture
I71.3	Abdominal aortic aneurysm, ruptured
I71.4	Abdominal aortic aneurysm, without rupture
I71.5	Thoracoabdominal aortic aneurysm, ruptured
I71.6	Thoracoabdominal aortic aneurysm, without rupture
I72.0	Aneurysm of carotid artery
I72.1	Aneurysm of artery of upper extremity
I72.2	Aneurysm of renal artery
I72.3	Aneurysm of iliac artery
I72.4	Aneurysm of artery of lower extremity
I72.6	Aneurysm of vertebral artery
I77.0	Arteriovenous fistula, acquired
I83.011	Varicose veins of right lower extremity with ulcer of thigh ☑
I83.012	Varicose veins of right lower extremity with ulcer of calf ☑
I83.013	Varicose veins of right lower extremity with ulcer of ankle ☑
I83.014	Varicose veins of right lower extremity with ulcer of heel and midfoot ☑
I83.018	Varicose veins of right lower extremity with ulcer other part of lower leg ☑
I83.11	Varicose veins of right lower extremity with inflammation ☑
I83.211	Varicose veins of right lower extremity with both ulcer of thigh and inflammation ☑
I83.212	Varicose veins of right lower extremity with both ulcer of calf and inflammation ☑
I83.213	Varicose veins of right lower extremity with both ulcer of ankle and inflammation ☑
I83.214	Varicose veins of right lower extremity with both ulcer of heel and midfoot and inflammation ☑
I83.811	Varicose veins of right lower extremity with pain ☑
I83.813	Varicose veins of bilateral lower extremities with pain ☑
I83.891	Varicose veins of right lower extremity with other complications ☑
I83.92	Asymptomatic varicose veins of left lower extremity ☑
I85.00	Esophageal varices without bleeding
I85.01	Esophageal varices with bleeding
I85.10	Secondary esophageal varices without bleeding
I85.11	Secondary esophageal varices with bleeding
I86.0	Sublingual varices
I86.1	Scrotal varices
I86.2	Pelvic varices
I86.3	Vulval varices
I86.4	Gastric varices
Q24.5	Malformation of coronary vessels
Q25.0	Patent ductus arteriosus
Q25.1	Coarctation of aorta
Q25.21	Interruption of aortic arch

Q25.3 Supravalvular aortic stenosis
Q25.41 Absence and aplasia of aorta
Q25.42 Hypoplasia of aorta
Q25.43 Congenital aneurysm of aorta
Q25.44 Congenital dilation of aorta
Q25.45 Double aortic arch
Q25.46 Tortuous aortic arch
Q25.47 Right aortic arch
Q25.48 Anomalous origin of subclavian artery
Q25.5 Atresia of pulmonary artery
Q25.6 Stenosis of pulmonary artery
Q25.71 Coarctation of pulmonary artery
Q25.72 Congenital pulmonary arteriovenous malformation
Q26.0 Congenital stenosis of vena cava
Q26.1 Persistent left superior vena cava
Q26.2 Total anomalous pulmonary venous connection
Q26.3 Partial anomalous pulmonary venous connection
Q26.5 Anomalous portal venous connection
Q27.31 Arteriovenous malformation of vessel of upper limb
Q27.32 Arteriovenous malformation of vessel of lower limb
Q27.33 Arteriovenous malformation of digestive system vessel
Q27.34 Arteriovenous malformation of renal vessel
Q28.0 Arteriovenous malformation of precerebral vessels
Q28.2 Arteriovenous malformation of cerebral vessels

AMA: **37241** 2019,Sep,6; 2018,Mar,3; 2018,Jan,8; 2017,Mar,3; 2017,Jan,8; 2016,Nov,3; 2016,Jan,13; 2015,Nov,3; 2015,Jan,16; 2015,Aug,8; 2015,Apr,10; 2014,Oct,6; 2014,Jan,11; 2014,Aug,14; 2013,Nov,6; 2013,Nov,14 **37242** 2019,Sep,6; 2018,Mar,3; 2018,Jul,14; 2018,Jan,8; 2017,Jan,8; 2016,Jan,13; 2015,Nov,3; 2015,Jan,16; 2014,Oct,6; 2014,Jan,11; 2013,Nov,6; 2013,Nov,14

Relative Value Units/Medicare Edits

Non-Facility RVU	Work	PE	MP	Total
37241	8.75	127.12	1.47	137.34
37242	9.8	200.36	1.34	211.5
Facility RVU	**Work**	**PE**	**MP**	**Total**
37241	8.75	2.64	1.47	12.86
37242	9.8	2.72	1.34	13.86

	FUD	Status	MUE	Modifiers				IOM Reference
37241	0	A	2(3)	51	N/A	N/A	N/A	None
37242	0	A	2(3)	51	N/A	N/A	N/A	

* with documentation

Terms To Know

catheter. Flexible tube inserted into an area of the body for introducing or withdrawing fluid.

embolization. Placement of a clotting agent, such as a coil, plastic particles, gel, foam, etc., into an area of hemorrhage to stop the bleeding or to block blood flow to a problem area, such as an aneurysm or a tumor.

occlusion. Constriction, closure, or blockage of a passage.

37243

37243 Vascular embolization or occlusion, inclusive of all radiological supervision and interpretation, intraprocedural roadmapping, and imaging guidance necessary to complete the intervention; for tumors, organ ischemia, or infarction

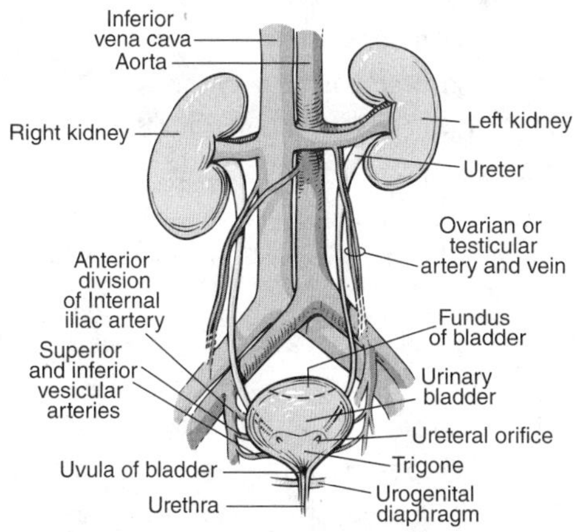

Embolization or occlusion for tumors, organ ischemia, or infarction

Explanation

Embolization or occlusion of an artery is performed to treat tumors or organ infarction/ischemia. A needle is inserted through the skin and into the artery. A guidewire is threaded through the needle and the needle is removed. A catheter is threaded into the vessel over the guidewire and the wire is extracted. The catheter travels to the appropriate site and beads, coils, or another vessel-blocking device are released. The beads or other device block the artery that supplies the tumor or that portion of the organ with blood. The catheter is removed and pressure is applied over the puncture site to stop bleeding.

Coding Tips

When medically necessary, report moderate (conscious) sedation provided by the performing physician with 99151-99153. When provided by another physician, report 99155-99157. Only one embolization code should be reported for each surgical field, including the entire area directly involved in and immediately surrounding the procedure. If chemotherapy or radioisotopes are used with the embolization procedure, additional codes such as 79445 or 96420 may be reported. The code representing the immediate cause for the embolization should be used. Diagnostic angiography and catheter placement may be reported separately. Report with an appropriate modifier. Do not report 37243 with 75894 or 75898 in the same surgical field.

ICD-10-CM Diagnostic Codes

C22.0 Liver cell carcinoma
C23 Malignant neoplasm of gallbladder
C24.0 Malignant neoplasm of extrahepatic bile duct
C24.1 Malignant neoplasm of ampulla of Vater
C41.0 Malignant neoplasm of bones of skull and face
C41.1 Malignant neoplasm of mandible
C41.2 Malignant neoplasm of vertebral column
C41.3 Malignant neoplasm of ribs, sternum and clavicle
C41.4 Malignant neoplasm of pelvic bones, sacrum and coccyx
C64.1 Malignant neoplasm of right kidney, except renal pelvis ☑
C64.2 Malignant neoplasm of left kidney, except renal pelvis ☑

C65.1	Malignant neoplasm of right renal pelvis ☑
C65.2	Malignant neoplasm of left renal pelvis ☑
C71.0	Malignant neoplasm of cerebrum, except lobes and ventricles
C71.1	Malignant neoplasm of frontal lobe
C71.2	Malignant neoplasm of temporal lobe
C71.3	Malignant neoplasm of parietal lobe
C71.4	Malignant neoplasm of occipital lobe
C71.5	Malignant neoplasm of cerebral ventricle
C71.6	Malignant neoplasm of cerebellum
C71.7	Malignant neoplasm of brain stem
C72.0	Malignant neoplasm of spinal cord
C76.0	Malignant neoplasm of head, face and neck
C78.7	Secondary malignant neoplasm of liver and intrahepatic bile duct
D16.01	Benign neoplasm of scapula and long bones of right upper limb ☑
D16.02	Benign neoplasm of scapula and long bones of left upper limb ☑
D16.11	Benign neoplasm of short bones of right upper limb ☑
D16.12	Benign neoplasm of short bones of left upper limb ☑
D18.02	Hemangioma of intracranial structures
D25.0	Submucous leiomyoma of uterus
D25.1	Intramural leiomyoma of uterus
D25.2	Subserosal leiomyoma of uterus
D32.0	Benign neoplasm of cerebral meninges
D32.1	Benign neoplasm of spinal meninges
D36.11	Benign neoplasm of peripheral nerves and autonomic nervous system of face, head, and neck
D36.12	Benign neoplasm of peripheral nerves and autonomic nervous system, upper limb, including shoulder
D36.13	Benign neoplasm of peripheral nerves and autonomic nervous system of lower limb, including hip
D36.14	Benign neoplasm of peripheral nerves and autonomic nervous system of thorax
D36.15	Benign neoplasm of peripheral nerves and autonomic nervous system of abdomen
D36.16	Benign neoplasm of peripheral nerves and autonomic nervous system of pelvis
D44.7	Neoplasm of uncertain behavior of aortic body and other paraganglia
D73.1	Hypersplenism
I15.0	Renovascular hypertension
N18.6	End stage renal disease

AMA: 37243 2019,Sep,6; 2018,Mar,3; 2018,Jan,8; 2017,Jan,8; 2016,Jan,13; 2015,Nov,3; 2015,Jan,16; 2014,Oct,6; 2014,Jan,11; 2013,Nov,6; 2013,Nov,14

Relative Value Units/Medicare Edits

Non-Facility RVU	Work	PE	MP	Total
37243	11.74	260.86	1.02	273.62
Facility RVU	**Work**	**PE**	**MP**	**Total**
37243	11.74	3.57	1.02	16.33

	FUD	Status	MUE	Modifiers				IOM Reference
37243	0	A	1(3)	51	N/A	N/A	N/A	None

* with documentation

37244

37244 Vascular embolization or occlusion, inclusive of all radiological supervision and interpretation, intraprocedural roadmapping, and imaging guidance necessary to complete the intervention; for arterial or venous hemorrhage or lymphatic extravasation

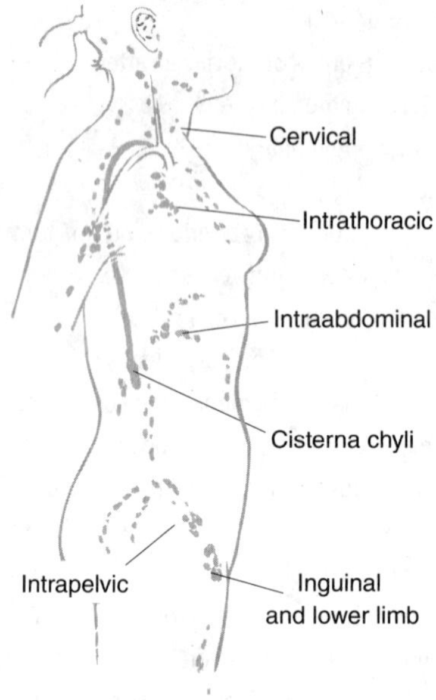

Lymphatic system

Explanation

Embolization or occlusion of a blood vessel is performed to treat hemorrhage. A needle is inserted through the skin and into a blood vessel. A guidewire is threaded through the needle and the needle is removed. A catheter is threaded into the vessel over the guidewire and the wire is extracted. The catheter travels to the appropriate site and beads, coils, or another vessel-blocking device are released. The beads or other device block the vessel. The catheter is removed and pressure is applied over the puncture site to stop the bleeding.

Coding Tips

When medically necessary, report moderate (conscious) sedation provided by the performing physician with 99151-99153. When provided by another physician, report 99155-99157. Only one embolization code should be reported for each surgical field, including the entire area directly involved in and immediately surrounding the procedure. The code representing the immediate cause for the embolization should be used. Diagnostic angiography and catheter placement may be reported separately. Report with an appropriate modifier. Do not report 37244 with 75894 or 75898 in the same surgical field. For embolization procedures of the head and neck, see 61626 or 61710.

ICD-10-CM Diagnostic Codes

I61.0	Nontraumatic intracerebral hemorrhage in hemisphere, subcortical
I61.1	Nontraumatic intracerebral hemorrhage in hemisphere, cortical
I61.3	Nontraumatic intracerebral hemorrhage in brain stem
I61.4	Nontraumatic intracerebral hemorrhage in cerebellum
I61.5	Nontraumatic intracerebral hemorrhage, intraventricular
I62.01	Nontraumatic acute subdural hemorrhage
I62.02	Nontraumatic subacute subdural hemorrhage
I62.03	Nontraumatic chronic subdural hemorrhage

I62.1	Nontraumatic extradural hemorrhage
N99.820	Postprocedural hemorrhage of a genitourinary system organ or structure following a genitourinary system procedure
O72.0	Third-stage hemorrhage
O72.2	Delayed and secondary postpartum hemorrhage
O72.3	Postpartum coagulation defects
R04.0	Epistaxis
R04.2	Hemoptysis
S15.011A	Minor laceration of right carotid artery, initial encounter ☑
S15.012A	Minor laceration of left carotid artery, initial encounter ☑
S15.021A	Major laceration of right carotid artery, initial encounter ☑
S15.022A	Major laceration of left carotid artery, initial encounter ☑
S15.111A	Minor laceration of right vertebral artery, initial encounter ☑
S15.112A	Minor laceration of left vertebral artery, initial encounter ☑
S15.121A	Major laceration of right vertebral artery, initial encounter ☑
S15.122A	Major laceration of left vertebral artery, initial encounter ☑
S25.01XA	Minor laceration of thoracic aorta, initial encounter
S25.02XA	Major laceration of thoracic aorta, initial encounter
S25.411A	Minor laceration of right pulmonary blood vessels, initial encounter ☑
S25.412A	Minor laceration of left pulmonary blood vessels, initial encounter ☑
S25.421A	Major laceration of right pulmonary blood vessels, initial encounter ☑
S25.422A	Major laceration of left pulmonary blood vessels, initial encounter ☑
S25.511A	Laceration of intercostal blood vessels, right side, initial encounter ☑
S25.512A	Laceration of intercostal blood vessels, left side, initial encounter ☑
S35.01XA	Minor laceration of abdominal aorta, initial encounter
S35.02XA	Major laceration of abdominal aorta, initial encounter
S35.11XA	Minor laceration of inferior vena cava, initial encounter
S35.12XA	Major laceration of inferior vena cava, initial encounter
S45.011A	Laceration of axillary artery, right side, initial encounter ☑
S45.012A	Laceration of axillary artery, left side, initial encounter ☑

AMA: **37244** 2019,Sep,6; 2018,Mar,3; 2018,Jul,14; 2018,Jan,8; 2017,Oct,9; 2017,Jan,8; 2016,Jan,13; 2015,Nov,3; 2015,Jan,16; 2014,Oct,6; 2014,Jan,11; 2014,Aug,14; 2013,Nov,6; 2013,Nov,14

Relative Value Units/Medicare Edits

Non-Facility RVU	Work	PE	MP	Total
37244	13.75	180.66	1.26	195.67
Facility RVU	**Work**	**PE**	**MP**	**Total**
37244	13.75	4.3	1.26	19.31

	FUD	Status	MUE	Modifiers				IOM Reference
37244	0	A	2(3)	51	N/A	N/A	N/A	None

* with documentation

Terms To Know

embolization. Placement of a clotting agent, such as a coil, plastic particles, gel, foam, etc., into an area of hemorrhage to stop the bleeding or to block blood flow to a problem area, such as an aneurysm or a tumor.

37252-37253

\+ **37252** Intravascular ultrasound (noncoronary vessel) during diagnostic evaluation and/or therapeutic intervention, including radiological supervision and interpretation; initial noncoronary vessel (List separately in addition to code for primary procedure)

\+ **37253** each additional noncoronary vessel (List separately in addition to code for primary procedure)

Explanation

Intravascular ultrasound may be used during diagnostic evaluation of the noncoronary artery or vein. It may also be used before and after a therapeutic intervention upon a noncoronary artery or vein to assess patency and integrity of the vessel. A needle is inserted through the skin and into a blood vessel. A guidewire is threaded through the needle into a noncoronary blood vessel. The needle is removed. An intravascular ultrasound catheter is placed over the guidewire. The ultrasound catheter is used to obtain images from inside the vessel to assess area and extent of disease prior to interventional therapy, as well as adequacy of therapy after interventional therapy. Report 37252 for the initial noncoronary vessel. In 37253, the physician advances the ultrasound catheter into additional noncoronary vessels to assess patency and structure. The catheter and guidewire are removed and pressure is applied over the puncture site to stop bleeding. These codes include radiological supervision and interpretation.

Coding Tips

When medically necessary, report moderate (conscious) sedation provided by the performing physician with 99151-99153. When provided by another physician, report 99155-99157. Use 37253 in addition to 37252. Intravascular ultrasound services include all transducer manipulations within the specific vessel being examined, before and after therapeutic intervention. Catheterization may be reported separately, see 36005–36248. Do not report 37252–37253 with 37191–37193 or 37197. These codes may be reported with an extensive number of primary procedures ranging from 33361-34848, 36010-37249, 61623, 75600-77001, and 0075T-0338T. Refer to the CPT manual for details.

ICD-10-CM Diagnostic Codes

This/these CPT code(s) are add on code(s). See the primary procedure code that this code is performed with for your ICD-10-CM code selections.

AMA: **37252** 2018,Jan,8; 2017,Mar,3; 2017,Jan,8; 2017,Dec,3; 2017,Aug,10; 2016,May,11; 2016,Jul,6 **37253** 2018,Jan,8; 2017,Mar,3; 2017,Jan,8; 2017,Dec,3; 2017,Aug,10; 2016,May,11; 2016,Jul,6

Relative Value Units/Medicare Edits

Non-Facility RVU	Work	PE	MP	Total
37252	1.8	33.6	0.38	35.78
37253	1.44	3.85	0.31	5.6
Facility RVU	**Work**	**PE**	**MP**	**Total**
37252	1.8	0.47	0.38	2.65
37253	1.44	0.38	0.31	2.13

	FUD	Status	MUE	Modifiers				IOM Reference
37252	N/A	A	1(2)	N/A	N/A	62*	80*	None
37253	N/A	A	5(3)	N/A	N/A	62*	80*	

* with documentation

Arteries and Veins

37500

37500 Vascular endoscopy, surgical, with ligation of perforator veins, subfascial (SEPS)

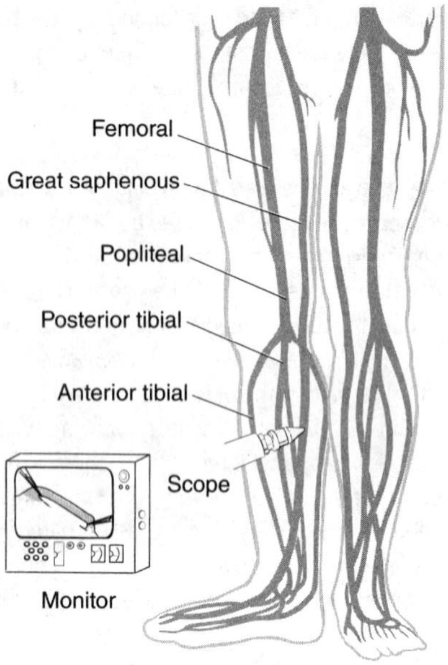

Incompetent perforator veins are treated endoscopically in the subfascial plane of the lower leg. The veins are typically ligated or transected

Explanation

Subfascial endoscopic perforator surgery (SEPS) is performed as a minimally invasive way to treat patients with chronic venous insufficiency (CVI) of the lower extremities. Incompetent calf perforator veins are ligated in this procedure. Perforator veins are an irregular group of veins growing as tributaries of the greater saphenous vein, which connect between it and other veins in the lower leg. They are considered incompetent when the direction of blood flow within the perforator vein changes upon applying distal pressure. SEP is carried out under regional or general anesthesia. A rollover tourniquet technique is used to exsanguinate the leg and a single stab incision is made over the medial aspect of the calf through which the operating telescope is inserted. The subfascial plane is created with blunt dissection and maintained open by insufflating with carbon dioxide gas at low pressure. The perforators are identified and ligated, or transected, with a 5 mm ultrasonic scalpel. Patients may be given elastic stockings to wear for the next two weeks.

Coding Tips

This is a unilateral procedure. If performed bilaterally, some payers require that the service be reported twice with modifier 50 appended to the second code, while others require identification of the service only once with modifier 50 appended. Check with individual payers. Modifier 50 identifies a procedure performed identically on the opposite side of the body (mirror image). For other treatment of long and/or short saphenous veins, see 37700–37735 and 37780. For open radical ligation of perforators (Linton type), with or without a skin graft, see 37760. For injection of a sclerosing solution, spider veins (telangiectasia), see 36468. For injection of a sclerosing solution for larger veins, see 36470–36471.

ICD-10-CM Diagnostic Codes

I83.011	Varicose veins of right lower extremity with ulcer of thigh ☑
I83.012	Varicose veins of right lower extremity with ulcer of calf ☑
I83.013	Varicose veins of right lower extremity with ulcer of ankle ☑
I83.014	Varicose veins of right lower extremity with ulcer of heel and midfoot ☑
I83.015	Varicose veins of right lower extremity with ulcer other part of foot ☑
I83.018	Varicose veins of right lower extremity with ulcer other part of lower leg ☑
I83.021	Varicose veins of left lower extremity with ulcer of thigh ☑
I83.022	Varicose veins of left lower extremity with ulcer of calf ☑
I83.023	Varicose veins of left lower extremity with ulcer of ankle ☑
I83.024	Varicose veins of left lower extremity with ulcer of heel and midfoot ☑
I83.025	Varicose veins of left lower extremity with ulcer other part of foot ☑
I83.028	Varicose veins of left lower extremity with ulcer other part of lower leg ☑
I83.11	Varicose veins of right lower extremity with inflammation ☑
I83.12	Varicose veins of left lower extremity with inflammation ☑
I83.211	Varicose veins of right lower extremity with both ulcer of thigh and inflammation ☑
I83.212	Varicose veins of right lower extremity with both ulcer of calf and inflammation ☑
I83.213	Varicose veins of right lower extremity with both ulcer of ankle and inflammation ☑
I83.214	Varicose veins of right lower extremity with both ulcer of heel and midfoot and inflammation ☑
I83.215	Varicose veins of right lower extremity with both ulcer other part of foot and inflammation ☑
I83.218	Varicose veins of right lower extremity with both ulcer of other part of lower extremity and inflammation ☑
I83.221	Varicose veins of left lower extremity with both ulcer of thigh and inflammation ☑
I83.222	Varicose veins of left lower extremity with both ulcer of calf and inflammation ☑
I83.223	Varicose veins of left lower extremity with both ulcer of ankle and inflammation ☑
I83.224	Varicose veins of left lower extremity with both ulcer of heel and midfoot and inflammation ☑
I83.225	Varicose veins of left lower extremity with both ulcer other part of foot and inflammation ☑
I83.228	Varicose veins of left lower extremity with both ulcer of other part of lower extremity and inflammation ☑
I83.811	Varicose veins of right lower extremity with pain ☑
I83.812	Varicose veins of left lower extremity with pain ☑
I83.813	Varicose veins of bilateral lower extremities with pain ☑
I83.891	Varicose veins of right lower extremity with other complications ☑
I83.892	Varicose veins of left lower extremity with other complications ☑
I83.893	Varicose veins of bilateral lower extremities with other complications ☑
I87.1	Compression of vein
I87.2	Venous insufficiency (chronic) (peripheral)

AMA: 37500 2018,Jan,8; 2017,Jan,8; 2016,Jan,13; 2015,Jan,16; 2014,Jan,11

Relative Value Units/Medicare Edits

Non-Facility RVU	Work	PE	MP	Total
37500	11.67	3.92	2.71	18.3
Facility RVU	**Work**	**PE**	**MP**	**Total**
37500	11.67	3.92	2.71	18.3

	FUD	Status	MUE	Modifiers				IOM Reference
37500	90	A	1(3)	51	50	62*	N/A	None

* with documentation

Terms To Know

incompetent. Inability of a valve or structure to perform its normal function.

inflammation. Cytologic and chemical reactions that occur in affected blood vessels and adjacent tissues in response to injury or abnormal stimulation from a physical, chemical, or biologic agent.

ligate. To tie off a blood vessel or duct with a suture or a soft, thin wire (ligature wire).

subfascial. Beneath the band of fibrous tissue that lies deep to the skin, encloses muscles, and separates their layers.

transection. Transverse dissection; to cut across a long axis; cross section.

ulcer. Open sore or excavating lesion of skin or the tissue on the surface of an organ from the sloughing of chronically inflamed and necrosing tissue.

varicose vein. Abnormal, permanently distended or stretched vein.

vascular. Pertaining to blood vessels.

venous. Relating to the veins.

37565

37565 Ligation, internal jugular vein

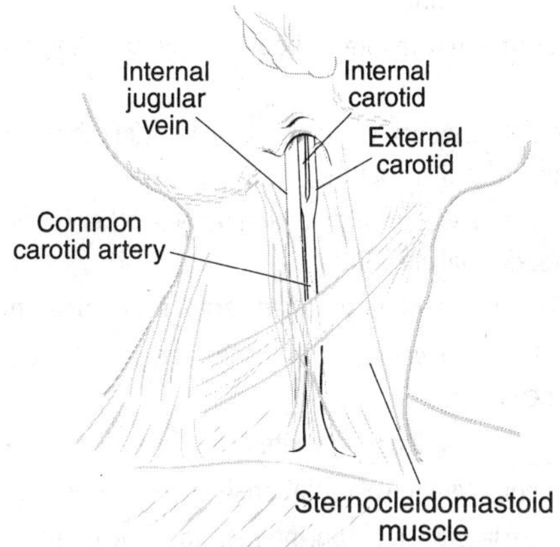

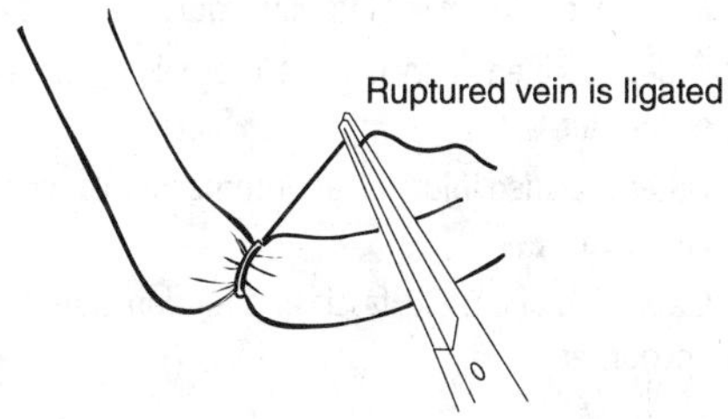

Explanation

Through an incision in the skin at side of neck in front of the sternocleidomastoid muscle, the physician isolates and dissects the internal jugular vein, separating it from critical structures. Using a vascular clip or ligature, the blood flow is reduced and the vein is ligated. Once the vein has been tied off, the skin incision is repaired with a layered closure.

Coding Tips

For ligation of the internal or common carotid artery, see 37605 and 37606.

ICD-10-CM Diagnostic Codes

G97.31	Intraoperative hemorrhage and hematoma of a nervous system organ or structure complicating a nervous system procedure
G97.48	Accidental puncture and laceration of other nervous system organ or structure during a nervous system procedure
G97.51	Postprocedural hemorrhage of a nervous system organ or structure following a nervous system procedure
G97.61	Postprocedural hematoma of a nervous system organ or structure following a nervous system procedure
G97.63	Postprocedural seroma of a nervous system organ or structure following a nervous system procedure
H93.11	Tinnitus, right ear ☑
H93.A1	Pulsatile tinnitus, right ear ☑
I82.C11	Acute embolism and thrombosis of right internal jugular vein ☑
I82.C12	Acute embolism and thrombosis of left internal jugular vein ☑
I82.C13	Acute embolism and thrombosis of internal jugular vein, bilateral ☑
I82.C21	Chronic embolism and thrombosis of right internal jugular vein ☑
I82.C22	Chronic embolism and thrombosis of left internal jugular vein ☑

I82.C23	Chronic embolism and thrombosis of internal jugular vein, bilateral ☑
R58	Hemorrhage, not elsewhere classified
S11.81XA	Laceration without foreign body of other specified part of neck, initial encounter
S11.82XA	Laceration with foreign body of other specified part of neck, initial encounter
S11.83XA	Puncture wound without foreign body of other specified part of neck, initial encounter
S11.84XA	Puncture wound with foreign body of other specified part of neck, initial encounter
S11.85XA	Open bite of other specified part of neck, initial encounter
S11.89XA	Other open wound of other specified part of neck, initial encounter
S15.311A	Minor laceration of right internal jugular vein, initial encounter ☑
S15.312A	Minor laceration of left internal jugular vein, initial encounter ☑
S15.321A	Major laceration of right internal jugular vein, initial encounter ☑
S15.322A	Major laceration of left internal jugular vein, initial encounter ☑
S15.391A	Other specified injury of right internal jugular vein, initial encounter ☑
S15.392A	Other specified injury of left internal jugular vein, initial encounter ☑
S16.2XXA	Laceration of muscle, fascia and tendon at neck level, initial encounter

AMA: **37565** 2014,Jan,11

Relative Value Units/Medicare Edits

Non-Facility RVU	Work	PE	MP	Total
37565	12.05	6.36	2.37	20.78
Facility RVU	**Work**	**PE**	**MP**	**Total**
37565	12.05	6.36	2.37	20.78

	FUD	Status	MUE	Modifiers				IOM Reference
37565	90	A	1(2)	51	50	62*	80*	100-03,160.8

* with documentation

Terms To Know

dissect. Cut apart or separate tissue for surgical purposes or for visual or microscopic study.

embolism. Obstruction of a blood vessel resulting from a clot or foreign substance.

hemorrhage syndrome. Fulminating meningococcal septicemia occurring in children younger than 10 years of age with vomiting, cyanosis, diarrhea, purpura, convulsions, circulatory collapse, meningitis, and hemorrhaging into adrenal glands.

ligation. Tying off a blood vessel or duct with a suture or a soft, thin wire.

seroma. Swelling caused by the collection of serum, or clear fluid, in the tissues.

37600

37600 Ligation; external carotid artery

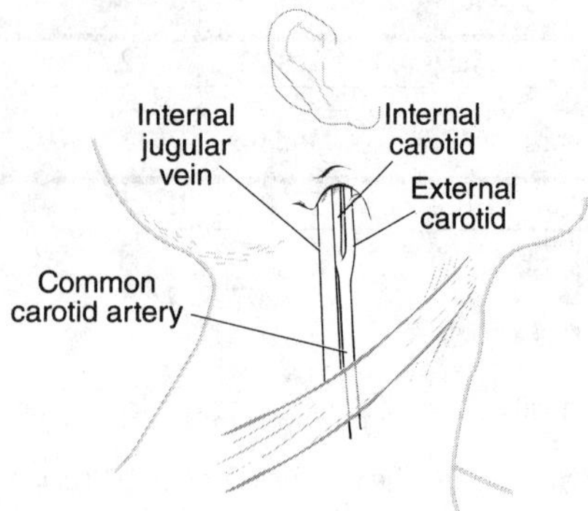

Deep dissection showing bifurcation of carotid arteries

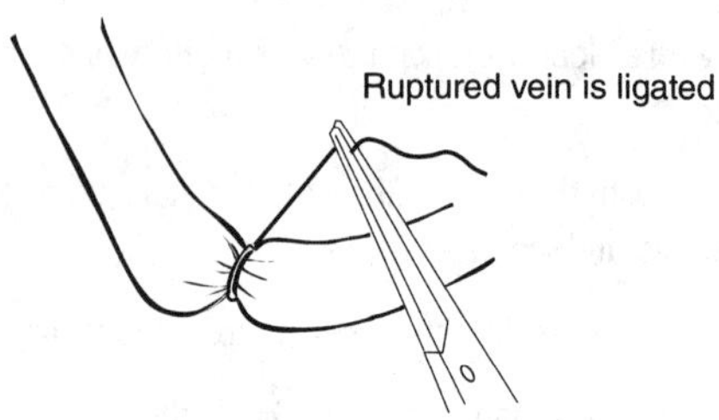

Explanation

Through an incision in the skin at the side of the neck in front of the sternocleidomastoid muscle, the physician isolates and dissects the external carotid artery, separating it from critical structures. Using a vascular clip or ligature, the blood flow is reduced and the artery is ligated. Once the artery has been tied off, the skin incision is repaired with a layered closure.

Coding Tips

Angioscopy during therapeutic intervention is listed separately, see 35400. For ligation of the internal or common carotid artery, see 37605 or 37606.

ICD-10-CM Diagnostic Codes

S15.011A	Minor laceration of right carotid artery, initial encounter ☑
S15.012A	Minor laceration of left carotid artery, initial encounter ☑
S15.021A	Major laceration of right carotid artery, initial encounter ☑
S15.022A	Major laceration of left carotid artery, initial encounter ☑
S15.091A	Other specified injury of right carotid artery, initial encounter ☑
S15.092A	Other specified injury of left carotid artery, initial encounter ☑

AMA: **37600** 2014,Jan,11

Relative Value Units/Medicare Edits

Non-Facility RVU	Work	PE	MP	Total
37600	12.42	6.49	2.16	21.07
Facility RVU	**Work**	**PE**	**MP**	**Total**
37600	12.42	6.49	2.16	21.07

	FUD	Status	MUE	Modifiers				IOM Reference
37600	90	A	1(3)	51	N/A	62*	80	None

* with documentation

37605-37606

37605 Ligation; internal or common carotid artery
37606 internal or common carotid artery, with gradual occlusion, as with Selverstone or Crutchfield clamp

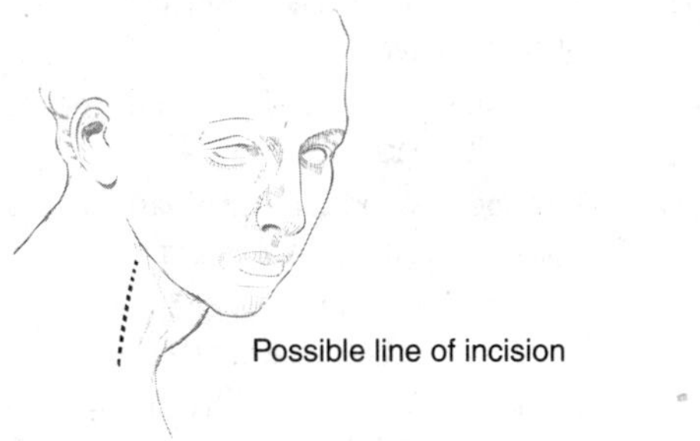

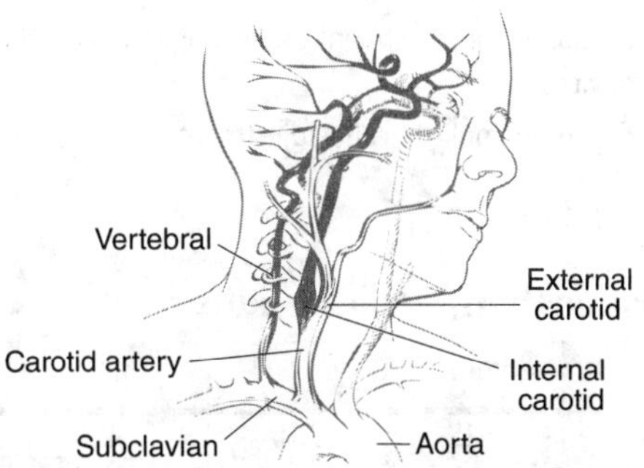

Explanation

Through an incision in the skin at the side of the neck, the physician isolates and dissects the internal or common carotid artery, separating it from critical structures. After vessel clamps have been affixed above and below the injured or affected artery, the physician sutures the artery to permanently stop the flow of blood through it (37605). The physician may apply a gradual occluding clamp (37606) to assess the effect of a ligation prior to complete occlusion (37605). Once the artery has been ligated or the occluding clamp has been placed, the vessel clamp is removed and the skin incision is repaired with a layered closure.

Coding Tips

Angioscopy during therapeutic intervention is listed separately, see 35400. Neurologic monitoring of the patient is normally a function of the anesthesiologist or neurologist. This code includes any neurologic monitoring performed by the physician. For ligation of the external carotid artery, see 37600. For ligation treatment of intracranial aneurysm, see 61703. For transcatheter permanent arterial occlusion or embolization, see 61624 and 61626. For temporary endovascular arterial balloon occlusion, see 61623.

ICD-10-CM Diagnostic Codes

S11.81XA Laceration without foreign body of other specified part of neck, initial encounter
S11.82XA Laceration with foreign body of other specified part of neck, initial encounter
S11.83XA Puncture wound without foreign body of other specified part of neck, initial encounter
S11.84XA Puncture wound with foreign body of other specified part of neck, initial encounter
S11.85XA Open bite of other specified part of neck, initial encounter
S11.89XA Other open wound of other specified part of neck, initial encounter
S15.011A Minor laceration of right carotid artery, initial encounter ☑
S15.012A Minor laceration of left carotid artery, initial encounter ☑
S15.021A Major laceration of right carotid artery, initial encounter ☑
S15.022A Major laceration of left carotid artery, initial encounter ☑
S15.091A Other specified injury of right carotid artery, initial encounter ☑
S15.092A Other specified injury of left carotid artery, initial encounter ☑
S16.2XXA Laceration of muscle, fascia and tendon at neck level, initial encounter

AMA: **37605** 2014,Jan,11 **37606** 2014,Jan,11

Relative Value Units/Medicare Edits

Non-Facility RVU	Work	PE	MP	Total
37605	14.28	3.72	3.31	21.31
37606	8.81	8.5	3.65	20.96
Facility RVU	**Work**	**PE**	**MP**	**Total**
37605	14.28	3.72	3.31	21.31
37606	8.81	8.5	3.65	20.96

	FUD	Status	MUE	Modifiers				IOM Reference
37605	90	A	1(3)	51	N/A	62*	80	None
37606	90	A	1(3)	51	N/A	N/A	80	

* with documentation

Terms To Know

dissect. Cut apart or separate tissue for surgical purposes or for visual or microscopic study.

ligation. Tying off a blood vessel or duct with a suture or a soft, thin wire.

occlusion. Constriction, closure, or blockage of a passage.

37607

37607 Ligation or banding of angioaccess arteriovenous fistula

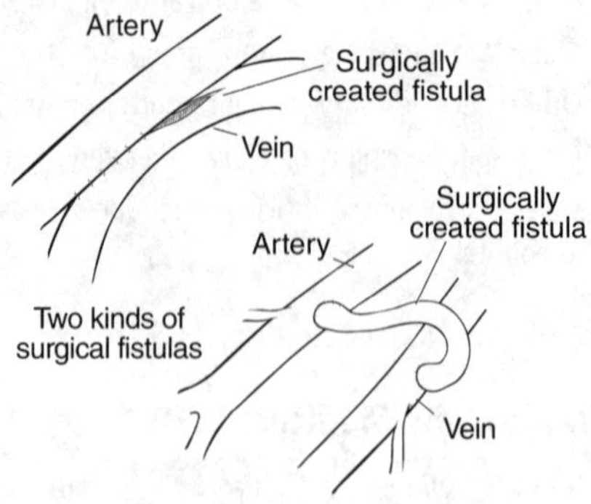

An arteriovenous fistula that occurs at the site of an access is ligated or banded

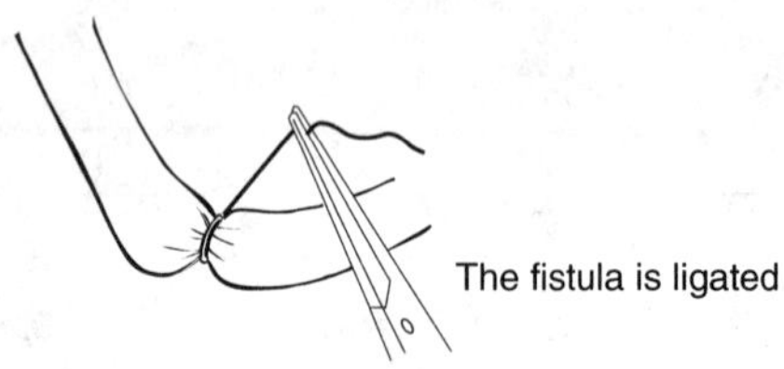

Explanation

The physician exposes a surgically created arteriovenous fistula by careful dissection. The physician isolates the fistula with ties or clamps. The physician may tie the arteriovenous fistula off completely (ligation) with suture, or the physician may partially obstruct (banding) the lumen of the fistula with a broader band in order to reduce flow. The physician closes the skin incision.

Coding Tips

This code is used to report ligation or banding of a surgically created arteriovenous fistula. It should not be used to report repair of traumatic or congenital arteriovenous fistulas. For repair of traumatic or congenital arteriovenous fistulas, see 35180–35190. For creation of an arteriovenous fistula by other than direct arteriovenous anastomosis, see 36825–36830.

ICD-10-CM Diagnostic Codes

T82.318A Breakdown (mechanical) of other vascular grafts, initial encounter
T82.338A Leakage of other vascular grafts, initial encounter
T82.398A Other mechanical complication of other vascular grafts, initial encounter
T82.510A Breakdown (mechanical) of surgically created arteriovenous fistula, initial encounter
T82.518A Breakdown (mechanical) of other cardiac and vascular devices and implants, initial encounter
T82.530A Leakage of surgically created arteriovenous fistula, initial encounter
T82.538A Leakage of other cardiac and vascular devices and implants, initial encounter
T82.590A Other mechanical complication of surgically created arteriovenous fistula, initial encounter
T82.598A Other mechanical complication of other cardiac and vascular devices and implants, initial encounter
T82.7XXA Infection and inflammatory reaction due to other cardiac and vascular devices, implants and grafts, initial encounter
T82.818A Embolism due to vascular prosthetic devices, implants and grafts, initial encounter
T82.828A Fibrosis due to vascular prosthetic devices, implants and grafts, initial encounter
T82.838A Hemorrhage due to vascular prosthetic devices, implants and grafts, initial encounter
T82.858A Stenosis of other vascular prosthetic devices, implants and grafts, initial encounter
T82.868A Thrombosis due to vascular prosthetic devices, implants and grafts, initial encounter
T82.898A Other specified complication of vascular prosthetic devices, implants and grafts, initial encounter
T82.9XXA Unspecified complication of cardiac and vascular prosthetic device, implant and graft, initial encounter
Z45.2 Encounter for adjustment and management of vascular access device
Z45.89 Encounter for adjustment and management of other implanted devices
Z46.89 Encounter for fitting and adjustment of other specified devices

AMA: **37607** 2014,Jan,11

Relative Value Units/Medicare Edits

Non-Facility RVU	Work	PE	MP	Total
37607	6.25	3.16	1.42	10.83
Facility RVU	**Work**	**PE**	**MP**	**Total**
37607	6.25	3.16	1.42	10.83

	FUD	Status	MUE	Modifiers				IOM Reference
37607	90	A	1(3)	51	N/A	62*	N/A	None

* with documentation

Terms To Know

anastomosis. Surgically created connection between ducts, blood vessels, or bowel segments to allow flow from one to the other.

clamp. Tool used to grip, compress, join, or fasten body parts.

complication. Condition arising after the beginning of observation and treatment that modifies the course of the patient's illness or the medical care required, or an undesired result or misadventure in medical care.

dissection. Separating by cutting tissue or body structures apart.

fistula. Abnormal tube-like passage between two body cavities or organs or from an organ to the outside surface.

incision. Act of cutting into tissue or an organ.

revision. Reordering or rearrangement of tissue to suit a particular need or function.

37609

37609 Ligation or biopsy, temporal artery

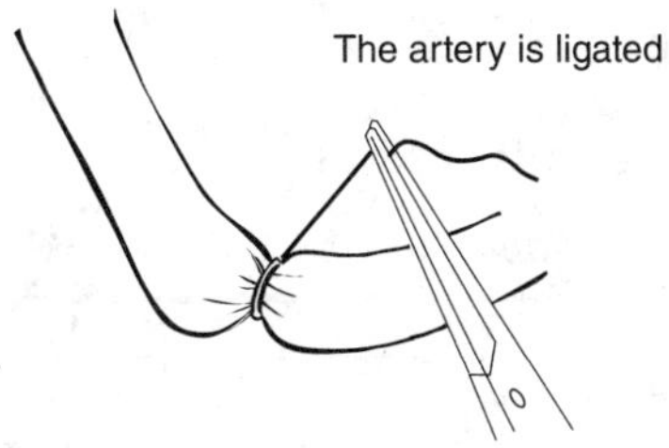

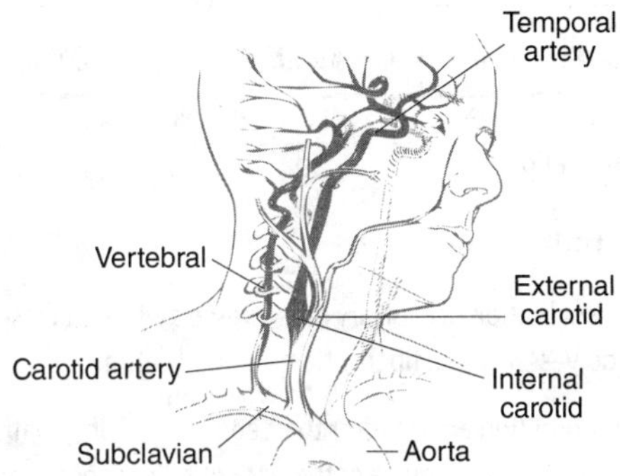

Explanation

Through an incision in the skin in front of the ear, the physician isolates and dissects the temporal artery, separating it from critical structures. Using a vascular clip or ligature, the artery is ligated or tissue samples are taken for biopsy. Once the artery has been tied off, the skin incision is repaired with a layered closure.

Coding Tips

Angioscopy during therapeutic intervention is listed separately, see 35400. For ligation of the external, internal, or common carotid artery, see 37600–37606.

ICD-10-CM Diagnostic Codes

G43.011	Migraine without aura, intractable, with status migrainosus
G43.019	Migraine without aura, intractable, without status migrainosus
G43.111	Migraine with aura, intractable, with status migrainosus
G43.119	Migraine with aura, intractable, without status migrainosus
G43.411	Hemiplegic migraine, intractable, with status migrainosus
G43.419	Hemiplegic migraine, intractable, without status migrainosus
G43.711	Chronic migraine without aura, intractable, with status migrainosus
G43.719	Chronic migraine without aura, intractable, without status migrainosus
G43.811	Other migraine, intractable, with status migrainosus
G43.819	Other migraine, intractable, without status migrainosus
G44.1	Vascular headache, not elsewhere classified
M31.5	Giant cell arteritis with polymyalgia rheumatica
M31.6	Other giant cell arteritis

AMA: 37609 2014,Jan,11

Relative Value Units/Medicare Edits

Non-Facility RVU	Work	PE	MP	Total
37609	3.05	5.21	0.61	8.87
Facility RVU	**Work**	**PE**	**MP**	**Total**
37609	3.05	2.28	0.61	5.94

	FUD	Status	MUE	Modifiers				IOM Reference
37609	10	A	1(2)	51	50	N/A	N/A	None

* with documentation

Terms To Know

angioscopy. Visualization of capillary blood vessels with a microscope, or the inside of a blood vessel with a fiberoptic-equipped catheter.

anomaly. Irregularity in the structure or position of an organ or tissue.

atherosclerosis. Buildup of yellowish plaques composed of cholesterol and lipoid material within the arteries.

biopsy. Tissue or fluid removed for diagnostic purposes through analysis of the cells in the biopsy material.

congenital. Present at birth, occurring through heredity or an influence during gestation up to the moment of birth.

dissect. Cut apart or separate tissue for surgical purposes or for visual or microscopic study.

incision. Act of cutting into tissue or an organ.

ligation. Tying off a blood vessel or duct with a suture or a soft, thin wire.

syncope. Light-headedness or fainting caused by insufficient blood supply to the brain.

37615

37615 Ligation, major artery (eg, post-traumatic, rupture); neck

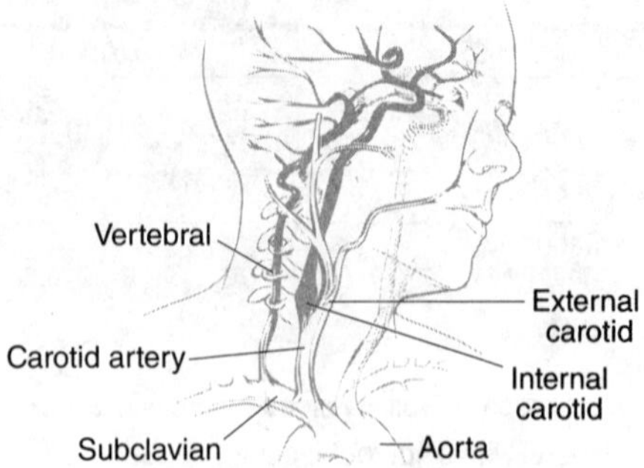

A major artery of the neck is ligated

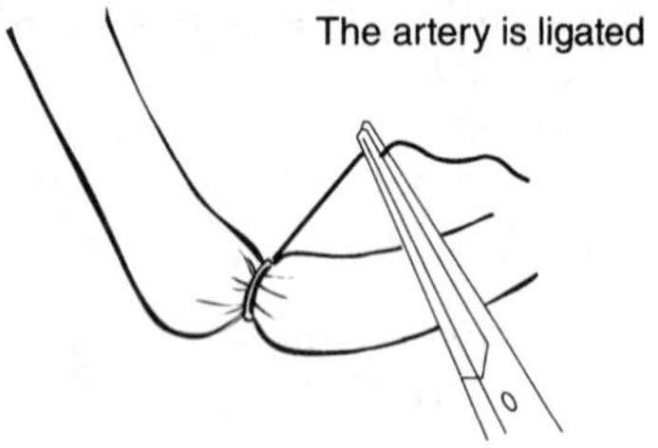

Explanation

Through an incision in the skin in the side of the neck, usually in front of the sternocleidomastoid muscle, the physician isolates and dissects the ruptured or otherwise traumatized vessel, separating it from critical structures. Using a vascular clip or ligature, the vessel is ligated with sutures. Once the vessel has been tied off, the skin incision is repaired with a layered closure.

Coding Tips

Angioscopy during therapeutic intervention is listed separately, see 35400. For ligation, major artery (e.g., post-traumatic, rupture), chest, see 37616; abdomen, see 37617; extremity, see 37618. For ligation of the external, internal, or common carotid artery for reasons other than trauma, see 37600–37606. If an artery is ligated in the course of dissecting another structure, or if a vessel is accidentally injured during dissection, requiring ligation, the procedure is not reported separately.

ICD-10-CM Diagnostic Codes

S11.81XA Laceration without foreign body of other specified part of neck, initial encounter
S11.82XA Laceration with foreign body of other specified part of neck, initial encounter
S11.83XA Puncture wound without foreign body of other specified part of neck, initial encounter
S11.84XA Puncture wound with foreign body of other specified part of neck, initial encounter
S11.85XA Open bite of other specified part of neck, initial encounter
S11.89XA Other open wound of other specified part of neck, initial encounter
S15.111A Minor laceration of right vertebral artery, initial encounter ☑
S15.112A Minor laceration of left vertebral artery, initial encounter ☑
S15.121A Major laceration of right vertebral artery, initial encounter ☑
S15.122A Major laceration of left vertebral artery, initial encounter ☑
S15.191A Other specified injury of right vertebral artery, initial encounter ☑
S15.192A Other specified injury of left vertebral artery, initial encounter ☑
S15.8XXA Injury of other specified blood vessels at neck level, initial encounter

AMA: 37615 2014,Jan,11

Relative Value Units/Medicare Edits

Non-Facility RVU	Work	PE	MP	Total
37615	7.8	5.52	1.89	15.21
Facility RVU	**Work**	**PE**	**MP**	**Total**
37615	7.8	5.52	1.89	15.21

	FUD	Status	MUE	Modifiers				IOM Reference
37615	90	A	2(3)	51	N/A	62*	80	None

* with documentation

Terms To Know

angioscopy. Visualization of capillary blood vessels with a microscope, or the inside of a blood vessel with a fiberoptic-equipped catheter.

complication. Condition arising after the beginning of observation and treatment that modifies the course of the patient's illness or the medical care required, or an undesired result or misadventure in medical care.

hematoma. Tumor-like collection of blood in some part of the body caused by a break in a blood vessel wall, usually as a result of trauma.

ligation. Tying off a blood vessel or duct with a suture or a soft, thin wire.

seroma. Swelling caused by the collection of serum, or clear fluid, in the tissues.

37616

37616 Ligation, major artery (eg, post-traumatic, rupture); chest

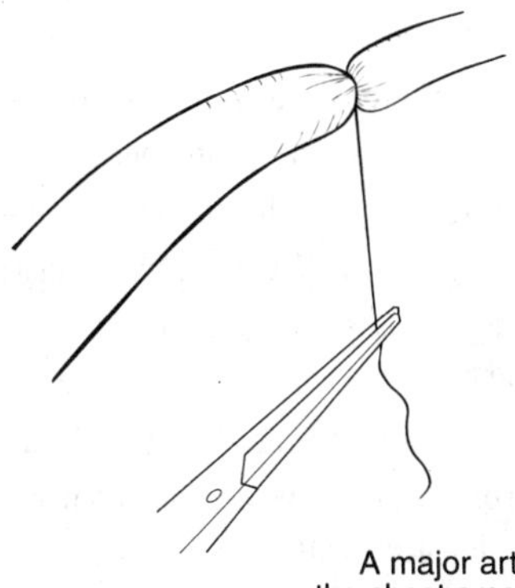

A major artery of the chest area is ligated

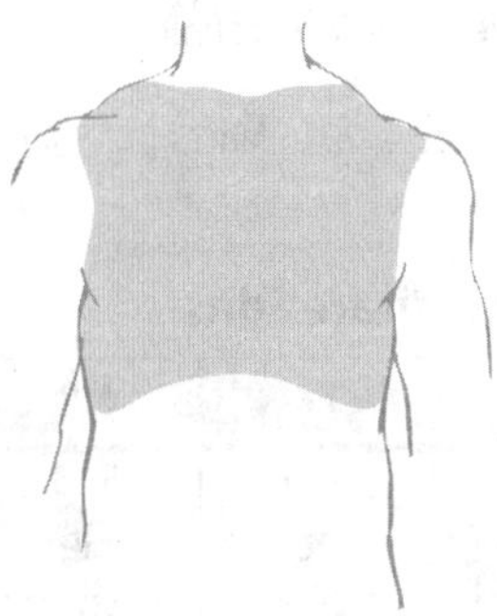

Explanation

The physician performs an incision of the chest wall (thoracotomy or median sternotomy) to best expose the involved artery. The physician identifies the injured artery and quickly clamps it to reduce blood loss. The physician then ties off the artery completely (ligation), proximal and distal to the site of injury. The physician closes the chest, leaving chest tubes in place.

Coding Tips

Angioscopy during therapeutic intervention is listed separately, see 35400. For ligation, major artery (e.g., posttraumatic, rupture) of the neck, see 37615; abdomen, see 37617; extremity, see 37618. If an artery is ligated in the course of dissecting another structure, or if a vessel is accidentally injured during dissection, requiring ligation, it is not reported separately.

ICD-10-CM Diagnostic Codes

S21.121A Laceration with foreign body of right front wall of thorax without penetration into thoracic cavity, initial encounter ☑
S21.122A Laceration with foreign body of left front wall of thorax without penetration into thoracic cavity, initial encounter ☑
S21.141A Puncture wound with foreign body of right front wall of thorax without penetration into thoracic cavity, initial encounter ☑
S21.142A Puncture wound with foreign body of left front wall of thorax without penetration into thoracic cavity, initial encounter ☑
S25.01XA Minor laceration of thoracic aorta, initial encounter
S25.02XA Major laceration of thoracic aorta, initial encounter
S25.09XA Other specified injury of thoracic aorta, initial encounter
S25.411A Minor laceration of right pulmonary blood vessels, initial encounter ☑
S25.412A Minor laceration of left pulmonary blood vessels, initial encounter ☑
S25.421A Major laceration of right pulmonary blood vessels, initial encounter ☑
S25.422A Major laceration of left pulmonary blood vessels, initial encounter ☑
S25.491A Other specified injury of right pulmonary blood vessels, initial encounter ☑
S25.492A Other specified injury of left pulmonary blood vessels, initial encounter ☑
S25.511A Laceration of intercostal blood vessels, right side, initial encounter ☑
S25.512A Laceration of intercostal blood vessels, left side, initial encounter ☑
S25.591A Other specified injury of intercostal blood vessels, right side, initial encounter ☑
S25.592A Other specified injury of intercostal blood vessels, left side, initial encounter ☑
S25.811A Laceration of other blood vessels of thorax, right side, initial encounter ☑
S25.812A Laceration of other blood vessels of thorax, left side, initial encounter ☑
S25.891A Other specified injury of other blood vessels of thorax, right side, initial encounter ☑
S25.892A Other specified injury of other blood vessels of thorax, left side, initial encounter ☑

AMA: **37616** 2014,Jan,11

Relative Value Units/Medicare Edits

Non-Facility RVU	Work	PE	MP	Total
37616	18.97	8.73	4.35	32.05
Facility RVU	**Work**	**PE**	**MP**	**Total**
37616	18.97	8.73	4.35	32.05

	FUD	Status	MUE	Modifiers				IOM Reference
37616	90	A	1(3)	51	N/A	62*	80	None

* with documentation

Terms To Know

angioscopy. Visualization of capillary blood vessels with a microscope, or the inside of a blood vessel with a fiberoptic-equipped catheter.

distal. Located farther away from a specified reference point or the trunk.

hemorrhage syndrome. Fulminating meningococcal septicemia occurring in children younger than 10 years of age with vomiting, cyanosis, diarrhea, purpura, convulsions, circulatory collapse, meningitis, and hemorrhaging into adrenal glands.

ligation. Tying off a blood vessel or duct with a suture or a soft, thin wire.

proximal. Located closest to a specified reference point, usually the midline or trunk.

sternotomy. Incision into the sternum, the bone that forms the front of the chest cavity and connects with the ribs.

thoracotomy. Surgical procedure for opening the chest wall in order to access the lungs, esophagus, trachea, aorta, heart, and diaphragm.

37617

37617 Ligation, major artery (eg, post-traumatic, rupture); abdomen

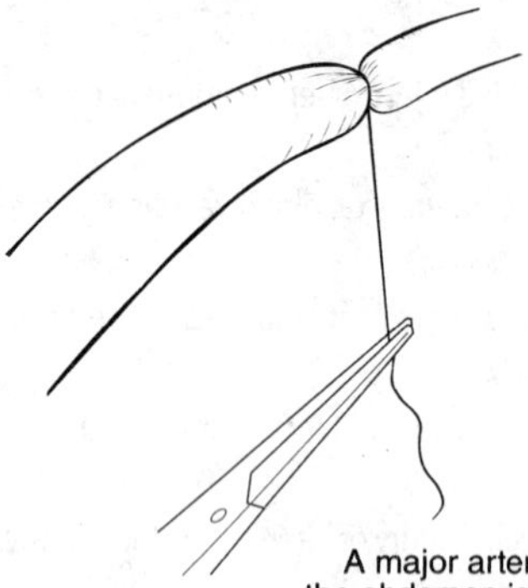

A major artery of the abdomen is ligated

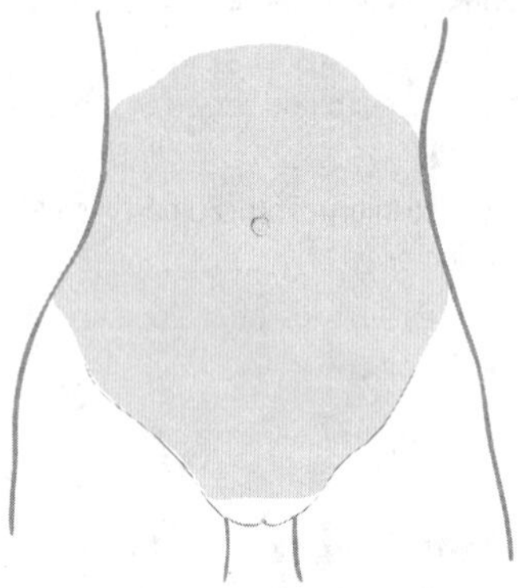

Explanation

The physician performs an abdominal incision to best expose the involved artery. The physician identifies the injured artery and quickly clamps it to reduce blood loss. The physician ties off the artery completely (ligation), proximal and distal to the site of injury. The physician closes the abdomen, leaving drains in place.

Coding Tips

Angioscopy during therapeutic intervention is listed separately, see 35400. For ligation, major artery (e.g., post-traumatic, rupture) of the neck, see 37615; chest, see 37616; extremity, see 37618. If an artery is ligated in the course of dissecting another structure, or if a vessel is accidentally injured during dissection, requiring ligation, it is not reported separately.

ICD-10-CM Diagnostic Codes

S35.01XA Minor laceration of abdominal aorta, initial encounter
S35.02XA Major laceration of abdominal aorta, initial encounter
S35.09XA Other injury of abdominal aorta, initial encounter
S35.211A Minor laceration of celiac artery, initial encounter
S35.212A Major laceration of celiac artery, initial encounter
S35.218A Other injury of celiac artery, initial encounter
S35.221A Minor laceration of superior mesenteric artery, initial encounter
S35.222A Major laceration of superior mesenteric artery, initial encounter
S35.228A Other injury of superior mesenteric artery, initial encounter
S35.231A Minor laceration of inferior mesenteric artery, initial encounter
S35.232A Major laceration of inferior mesenteric artery, initial encounter
S35.238A Other injury of inferior mesenteric artery, initial encounter
S35.291A Minor laceration of branches of celiac and mesenteric artery, initial encounter
S35.292A Major laceration of branches of celiac and mesenteric artery, initial encounter
S35.298A Other injury of branches of celiac and mesenteric artery, initial encounter
S35.411A Laceration of right renal artery, initial encounter ☑
S35.412A Laceration of left renal artery, initial encounter ☑
S35.491A Other specified injury of right renal artery, initial encounter ☑
S35.492A Other specified injury of left renal artery, initial encounter ☑
S35.511A Injury of right iliac artery, initial encounter ☑
S35.512A Injury of left iliac artery, initial encounter ☑
S35.59XA Injury of other iliac blood vessels, initial encounter
S35.8X1A Laceration of other blood vessels at abdomen, lower back and pelvis level, initial encounter
S35.8X8A Other specified injury of other blood vessels at abdomen, lower back and pelvis level, initial encounter

AMA: **37617** 2018,Jan,8; 2017,Jan,8; 2016,Jan,13; 2015,Jan,16; 2014,Jan,11; 2013,Aug,13

Relative Value Units/Medicare Edits

Non-Facility RVU	Work	PE	MP	Total
37617	23.79	9.79	5.26	38.84
Facility RVU	**Work**	**PE**	**MP**	**Total**
37617	23.79	9.79	5.26	38.84

	FUD	Status	MUE	Modifiers				IOM Reference
37617	90	A	3(3)	51	N/A	62*	80	None

* with documentation

Terms To Know

aneurysm. Circumscribed dilation or outpouching of an artery wall, often containing blood clots and connecting directly with the lumen of the artery.

angioscopy. Visualization of capillary blood vessels with a microscope, or the inside of a blood vessel with a fiberoptic-equipped catheter.

dissection. Separating by cutting tissue or body structures apart.

distal. Located farther away from a specified reference point or the trunk.

hematoma. Tumor-like collection of blood in some part of the body caused by a break in a blood vessel wall, usually as a result of trauma.

ligation. Tying off a blood vessel or duct with a suture or a soft, thin wire.

proximal. Located closest to a specified reference point, usually the midline or trunk.

37618

37618 Ligation, major artery (eg, post-traumatic, rupture); extremity

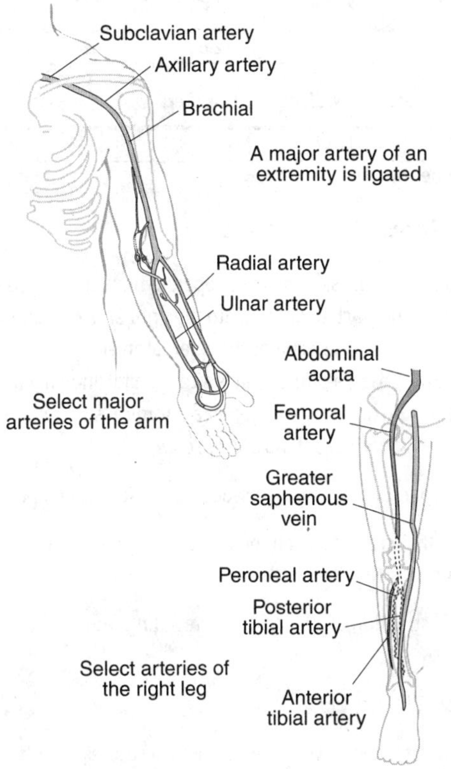

Explanation

Through an incision in the skin of an extremity, usually over the damaged or traumatized vessel, the physician isolates and dissects the vessel, separating it from critical structures. Using a vascular clip or ligature, the vessel is ligated with sutures or vascular clips. Once the vessel has been tied off, the skin incision is repaired with a layered closure.

Coding Tips

Angioscopy during therapeutic intervention is listed separately, see 35400. For ligation, major artery (e.g., post-traumatic, rupture) of the neck, see 37615; chest, see 37616; abdomen, see 37617. If an artery is ligated in the course of dissecting another structure, or if a vessel is accidentally injured during dissection, requiring ligation, it is not reported separately.

ICD-10-CM Diagnostic Codes

S45.011A Laceration of axillary artery, right side, initial encounter ☑
S45.091A Other specified injury of axillary artery, right side, initial encounter ☑
S45.111A Laceration of brachial artery, right side, initial encounter ☑
S45.191A Other specified injury of brachial artery, right side, initial encounter ☑
S45.811A Laceration of other specified blood vessels at shoulder and upper arm level, right arm, initial encounter ☑
S55.011A Laceration of ulnar artery at forearm level, right arm, initial encounter ☑
S55.091A Other specified injury of ulnar artery at forearm level, right arm, initial encounter ☑
S55.111A Laceration of radial artery at forearm level, right arm, initial encounter ☑
S55.191A Other specified injury of radial artery at forearm level, right arm, initial encounter ☑
S55.811A Laceration of other blood vessels at forearm level, right arm, initial encounter ☑
S55.891A Other specified injury of other blood vessels at forearm level, right arm, initial encounter ☑
S65.011A Laceration of ulnar artery at wrist and hand level of right arm, initial encounter ☑
S65.091A Other specified injury of ulnar artery at wrist and hand level of right arm, initial encounter ☑
S65.111A Laceration of radial artery at wrist and hand level of right arm, initial encounter ☑
S65.191A Other specified injury of radial artery at wrist and hand level of right arm, initial encounter ☑
S65.811A Laceration of other blood vessels at wrist and hand level of right arm, initial encounter ☑
S75.011A Minor laceration of femoral artery, right leg, initial encounter ☑
S75.021A Major laceration of femoral artery, right leg, initial encounter ☑
S75.091A Other specified injury of femoral artery, right leg, initial encounter ☑
S75.811A Laceration of other blood vessels at hip and thigh level, right leg, initial encounter ☑
S85.011A Laceration of popliteal artery, right leg, initial encounter ☑
S85.091A Other specified injury of popliteal artery, right leg, initial encounter ☑
S85.141A Laceration of anterior tibial artery, right leg, initial encounter ☑
S85.151A Other specified injury of anterior tibial artery, right leg, initial encounter ☑
S85.171A Laceration of posterior tibial artery, right leg, initial encounter ☑
S85.181A Other specified injury of posterior tibial artery, right leg, initial encounter ☑
S85.211A Laceration of peroneal artery, right leg, initial encounter ☑
S85.291A Other specified injury of peroneal artery, right leg, initial encounter ☑
S85.811A Laceration of other blood vessels at lower leg level, right leg, initial encounter ☑
S95.011A Laceration of dorsal artery of right foot, initial encounter ☑
S95.091A Other specified injury of dorsal artery of right foot, initial encounter ☑
S95.111A Laceration of plantar artery of right foot, initial encounter ☑
S95.191A Other specified injury of plantar artery of right foot, initial encounter ☑

AMA: 37618 2014,Jan,11

Relative Value Units/Medicare Edits

Non-Facility RVU	Work	PE	MP	Total
37618	6.03	3.76	1.32	11.11
Facility RVU	**Work**	**PE**	**MP**	**Total**
37618	6.03	3.76	1.32	11.11

	FUD	Status	MUE	Modifiers				IOM Reference
37618	90	A	2(3)	51	N/A	62*	80	None

* with documentation

37619

37619 Ligation of inferior vena cava

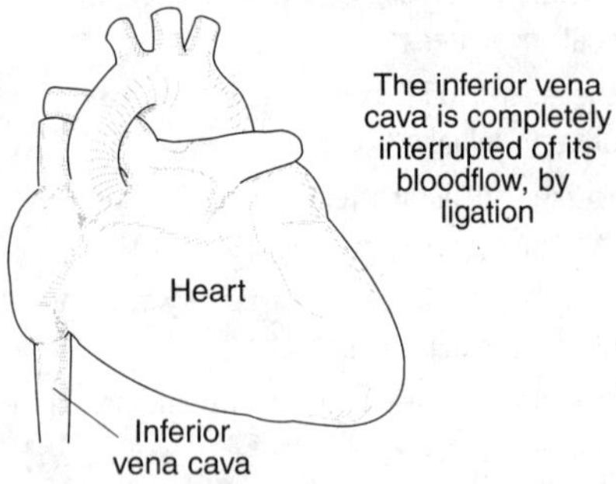

The inferior vena cava (or IVC) is the major return vessel of the lower body. It extends from the right atrium of the heart down to the bifurcation of the iliac veins

Explanation

The physician performs an upper midline abdominal incision and dissects to expose the inferior vena cava. The physician interrupts vena caval flow by tying the cava off with suture or clipping it. The physician closes the abdomen, leaving drains in place.

Coding Tips

For endovascular placement of an intravascular filter, see 37191. For phleborrhaphy and arteriorrhaphy, see 35201–35286.

ICD-10-CM Diagnostic Codes

I26.01	Septic pulmonary embolism with acute cor pulmonale
I26.90	Septic pulmonary embolism without acute cor pulmonale
I27.82	Chronic pulmonary embolism
I82.220	Acute embolism and thrombosis of inferior vena cava
I82.221	Chronic embolism and thrombosis of inferior vena cava
I82.3	Embolism and thrombosis of renal vein
I82.412	Acute embolism and thrombosis of left femoral vein ☑
I82.422	Acute embolism and thrombosis of left iliac vein ☑
I82.432	Acute embolism and thrombosis of left popliteal vein ☑
I82.442	Acute embolism and thrombosis of left tibial vein ☑
I82.512	Chronic embolism and thrombosis of left femoral vein ☑
I82.522	Chronic embolism and thrombosis of left iliac vein ☑
I82.532	Chronic embolism and thrombosis of left popliteal vein ☑
I82.542	Chronic embolism and thrombosis of left tibial vein ☑
I82.812	Embolism and thrombosis of superficial veins of left lower extremity ☑
O86.81	Puerperal septic thrombophlebitis
O87.1	Deep phlebothrombosis in the puerperium
S35.11XA	Minor laceration of inferior vena cava, initial encounter
S35.12XA	Major laceration of inferior vena cava, initial encounter
S35.19XA	Other injury of inferior vena cava, initial encounter

AMA: 37619 2018,Jan,8; 2017,Jan,8; 2016,Jan,13; 2015,Jan,16; 2014,Jan,11

Relative Value Units/Medicare Edits

Non-Facility RVU	Work	PE	MP	Total
37619	30.0	12.86	7.29	50.15
Facility RVU	**Work**	**PE**	**MP**	**Total**
37619	30.0	12.86	7.29	50.15

	FUD	Status	MUE	Modifiers				IOM Reference
37619	90	A	1(2)	51	N/A	N/A	80	None

* with documentation

Terms To Know

bifurcation. Point of division into two separate branches or structures, such as the site where the trachea divides into the right and left main bronchi or the common carotid artery becomes the external and internal carotid arteries. For diagnostic purposes, a bifurcation is a congenital anomaly that results in an imperfect closure of an organ or other anatomical structure, such as the ureter, renal pelvis, hard or soft palate, lip, etc.

dissection. Separating by cutting tissue or body structures apart.

drain. Device that creates a channel to allow fluid from a cavity, wound, or infected area to exit the body.

embolism. Obstruction of a blood vessel resulting from a clot or foreign substance.

intravascular. Within a blood vessel.

ligation. Tying off a blood vessel or duct with a suture or a soft, thin wire.

phlebo-. Relating to the vein.

suture. Numerous stitching techniques employed in wound closure.

thrombosis. Condition arising from the presence or formation of blood clots within a blood vessel that may cause vascular obstruction and insufficient oxygenation.

vena cava. Main venous trunk that empties into the right atrium from both the lower and upper regions, beginning at the junction of the common iliac veins inferiorly and the two brachiocephalic veins superiorly.

37650

37650 Ligation of femoral vein

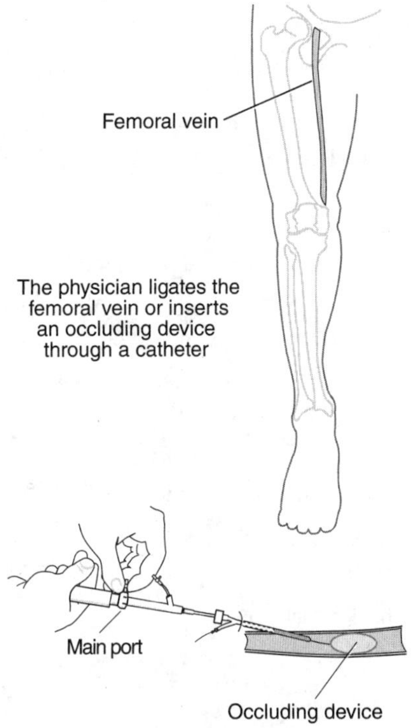

Explanation

Through a small incision in the skin of the upper leg overlying the femoral vein, the physician isolates and dissects the femoral vein from other critical structures. After affixing vessel clamps, the physician either ligates the vein or inserts a catheter into the femoral vein. A guidewire may be inserted prior to the catheter, then removed. Through the catheter, the physician places an occluding device (one that blocks blood flow) in the vein. The catheter is removed and the skin incision is repaired with a layered closure.

Coding Tips

This is a unilateral procedure. If performed bilaterally, some payers require that the service be reported twice with modifier 50 appended to the second code, while others require identification of the service only once with modifier 50 appended. Check with individual payers. Modifier 50 identifies a procedure performed identically on the opposite side of the body (mirror image). For femoral vein repair, see 35226, 36256, or 35286. For ligation of the common iliac vein, see 37660.

ICD-10-CM Diagnostic Codes

I26.01	Septic pulmonary embolism with acute cor pulmonale
I26.09	Other pulmonary embolism with acute cor pulmonale
I26.90	Septic pulmonary embolism without acute cor pulmonale
I26.99	Other pulmonary embolism without acute cor pulmonale
I27.82	Chronic pulmonary embolism
I80.11	Phlebitis and thrombophlebitis of right femoral vein ☑
I80.12	Phlebitis and thrombophlebitis of left femoral vein ☑
I80.13	Phlebitis and thrombophlebitis of femoral vein, bilateral ☑
I82.411	Acute embolism and thrombosis of right femoral vein ☑
I82.412	Acute embolism and thrombosis of left femoral vein ☑
I82.413	Acute embolism and thrombosis of femoral vein, bilateral ☑
I82.511	Chronic embolism and thrombosis of right femoral vein ☑
I82.512	Chronic embolism and thrombosis of left femoral vein ☑
I82.513	Chronic embolism and thrombosis of femoral vein, bilateral ☑
I83.011	Varicose veins of right lower extremity with ulcer of thigh ☑
I83.012	Varicose veins of right lower extremity with ulcer of calf ☑
I83.013	Varicose veins of right lower extremity with ulcer of ankle ☑
I83.014	Varicose veins of right lower extremity with ulcer of heel and midfoot ☑
I83.015	Varicose veins of right lower extremity with ulcer other part of foot ☑
I83.018	Varicose veins of right lower extremity with ulcer other part of lower leg ☑
I83.021	Varicose veins of left lower extremity with ulcer of thigh ☑
I83.022	Varicose veins of left lower extremity with ulcer of calf ☑
I83.023	Varicose veins of left lower extremity with ulcer of ankle ☑
I83.024	Varicose veins of left lower extremity with ulcer of heel and midfoot ☑
I83.025	Varicose veins of left lower extremity with ulcer other part of foot ☑
I83.028	Varicose veins of left lower extremity with ulcer other part of lower leg ☑
I83.11	Varicose veins of right lower extremity with inflammation ☑
I83.12	Varicose veins of left lower extremity with inflammation ☑
I83.211	Varicose veins of right lower extremity with both ulcer of thigh and inflammation ☑
I83.212	Varicose veins of right lower extremity with both ulcer of calf and inflammation ☑
I83.213	Varicose veins of right lower extremity with both ulcer of ankle and inflammation ☑
I83.214	Varicose veins of right lower extremity with both ulcer of heel and midfoot and inflammation ☑
I83.215	Varicose veins of right lower extremity with both ulcer other part of foot and inflammation ☑
I83.218	Varicose veins of right lower extremity with both ulcer of other part of lower extremity and inflammation ☑
I83.221	Varicose veins of left lower extremity with both ulcer of thigh and inflammation ☑
I83.222	Varicose veins of left lower extremity with both ulcer of calf and inflammation ☑
I83.223	Varicose veins of left lower extremity with both ulcer of ankle and inflammation ☑
I83.224	Varicose veins of left lower extremity with both ulcer of heel and midfoot and inflammation ☑
I83.225	Varicose veins of left lower extremity with both ulcer other part of foot and inflammation ☑
I83.228	Varicose veins of left lower extremity with both ulcer of other part of lower extremity and inflammation ☑
I83.811	Varicose veins of right lower extremity with pain ☑
I83.812	Varicose veins of left lower extremity with pain ☑
I83.813	Varicose veins of bilateral lower extremities with pain ☑
I83.891	Varicose veins of right lower extremity with other complications ☑
I83.892	Varicose veins of left lower extremity with other complications ☑
I83.893	Varicose veins of bilateral lower extremities with other complications ☑

I83.91 Asymptomatic varicose veins of right lower extremity ☑
I83.92 Asymptomatic varicose veins of left lower extremity ☑
I83.93 Asymptomatic varicose veins of bilateral lower extremities ☑
I87.001 Postthrombotic syndrome without complications of right lower extremity ☑
I87.002 Postthrombotic syndrome without complications of left lower extremity ☑
I87.003 Postthrombotic syndrome without complications of bilateral lower extremity ☑
I87.011 Postthrombotic syndrome with ulcer of right lower extremity ☑
I87.012 Postthrombotic syndrome with ulcer of left lower extremity ☑
I87.013 Postthrombotic syndrome with ulcer of bilateral lower extremity ☑
I87.021 Postthrombotic syndrome with inflammation of right lower extremity ☑
I87.022 Postthrombotic syndrome with inflammation of left lower extremity ☑
I87.023 Postthrombotic syndrome with inflammation of bilateral lower extremity ☑
I87.031 Postthrombotic syndrome with ulcer and inflammation of right lower extremity ☑
I87.032 Postthrombotic syndrome with ulcer and inflammation of left lower extremity ☑
I87.033 Postthrombotic syndrome with ulcer and inflammation of bilateral lower extremity ☑
I87.091 Postthrombotic syndrome with other complications of right lower extremity ☑
I87.092 Postthrombotic syndrome with other complications of left lower extremity ☑
I87.093 Postthrombotic syndrome with other complications of bilateral lower extremity ☑
I87.2 Venous insufficiency (chronic) (peripheral)
S75.111A Minor laceration of femoral vein at hip and thigh level, right leg, initial encounter ☑
S75.112A Minor laceration of femoral vein at hip and thigh level, left leg, initial encounter ☑
S75.121A Major laceration of femoral vein at hip and thigh level, right leg, initial encounter ☑
S75.122A Major laceration of femoral vein at hip and thigh level, left leg, initial encounter ☑

AMA: 37650 2014,Jan,11

Relative Value Units/Medicare Edits

Non-Facility RVU	Work	PE	MP	Total
37650	8.49	2.78	1.95	13.22
Facility RVU	**Work**	**PE**	**MP**	**Total**
37650	8.49	2.78	1.95	13.22

	FUD	Status	MUE	Modifiers				IOM Reference
37650	90	A	1(2)	51	50	62*	N/A	None

* with documentation

37660

37660 Ligation of common iliac vein

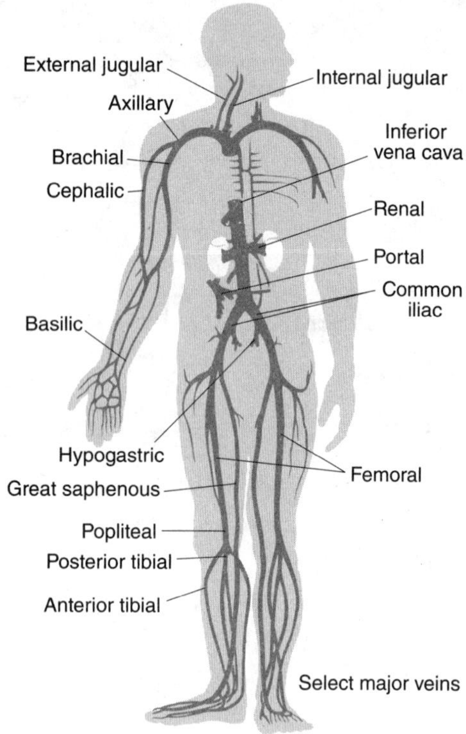

Explanation

The physician performs a lower midline abdominal incision and dissects to expose the common iliac vein. The physician interrupts common iliac venous flow by tying the common iliac vein off with suture. The physician closes the abdomen, leaving drains in place.

Coding Tips

This is a unilateral procedure. If performed bilaterally, some payers require that the service be reported twice with modifier 50 appended to the second code, while others require identification of the service only once with modifier 50 appended. Check with individual payers. Modifier 50 identifies a procedure performed identically on the opposite side of the body (mirror image).

ICD-10-CM Diagnostic Codes

I80.211 Phlebitis and thrombophlebitis of right iliac vein ☑
I80.212 Phlebitis and thrombophlebitis of left iliac vein ☑
I80.213 Phlebitis and thrombophlebitis of iliac vein, bilateral ☑
I82.421 Acute embolism and thrombosis of right iliac vein ☑
I82.422 Acute embolism and thrombosis of left iliac vein ☑
I82.423 Acute embolism and thrombosis of iliac vein, bilateral ☑
I82.521 Chronic embolism and thrombosis of right iliac vein ☑
I82.522 Chronic embolism and thrombosis of left iliac vein ☑
I82.523 Chronic embolism and thrombosis of iliac vein, bilateral ☑
K91.71 Accidental puncture and laceration of a digestive system organ or structure during a digestive system procedure
K91.72 Accidental puncture and laceration of a digestive system organ or structure during other procedure
K91.840 Postprocedural hemorrhage of a digestive system organ or structure following a digestive system procedure

K91.841	Postprocedural hemorrhage of a digestive system organ or structure following other procedure
K91.870	Postprocedural hematoma of a digestive system organ or structure following a digestive system procedure
K91.871	Postprocedural hematoma of a digestive system organ or structure following other procedure
K91.872	Postprocedural seroma of a digestive system organ or structure following a digestive system procedure
K91.873	Postprocedural seroma of a digestive system organ or structure following other procedure
M96.810	Intraoperative hemorrhage and hematoma of a musculoskeletal structure complicating a musculoskeletal system procedure
M96.811	Intraoperative hemorrhage and hematoma of a musculoskeletal structure complicating other procedure
M96.820	Accidental puncture and laceration of a musculoskeletal structure during a musculoskeletal system procedure
M96.821	Accidental puncture and laceration of a musculoskeletal structure during other procedure
S35.514A	Injury of right iliac vein, initial encounter ☑
S35.515A	Injury of left iliac vein, initial encounter ☑

AMA: **37660** 2014,Jan,11

Relative Value Units/Medicare Edits

Non-Facility RVU	Work	PE	MP	Total
37660	22.28	10.5	5.4	38.18
Facility RVU	**Work**	**PE**	**MP**	**Total**
37660	22.28	10.5	5.4	38.18

	FUD	Status	MUE	Modifiers				IOM Reference
37660	90	A	1(2)	51	50	62*	80	None

* with documentation

Terms To Know

aneurysm. Circumscribed dilation or outpouching of an artery wall, often containing blood clots and connecting directly with the lumen of the artery.

embolism. Obstruction of a blood vessel resulting from a clot or foreign substance.

hematoma. Tumor-like collection of blood in some part of the body caused by a break in a blood vessel wall, usually as a result of trauma.

37700

37700 Ligation and division of long saphenous vein at saphenofemoral junction, or distal interruptions

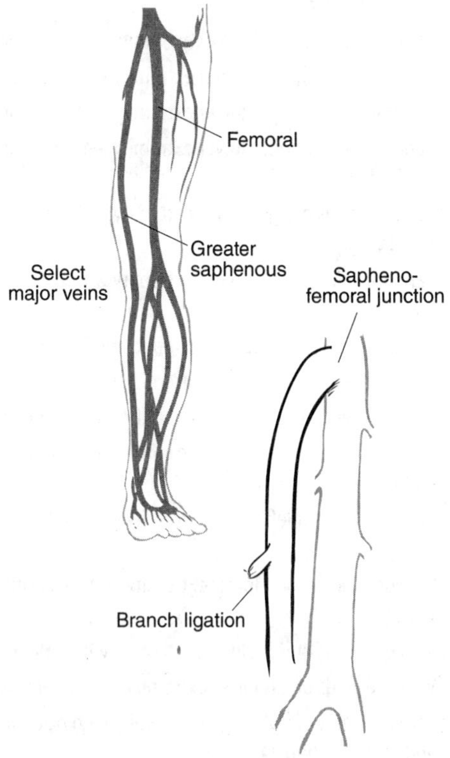

Explanation

Through multiple small incisions in the skin of the upper thigh and along the femoral vein or its branches lower in the thigh, the physician isolates and separates the saphenous vein at the point it joins the femoral vein or at several points farther down the leg. The physician affixes vessel clamps and ligates sections of the saphenous vein along the leg as necessary. Once the ligations are completed, each skin incision is repaired with a layered closure.

Coding Tips

This is a unilateral procedure. If performed bilaterally, some payers require that the service be reported twice with modifier 50 appended to the second code, while others require identification of the service only once with modifier 50 appended. Check with individual payers. Modifier 50 identifies a procedure performed identically on the opposite side of the body (mirror image). Do not report 37700 with 37718 or 37722. For injection of a sclerosing solution, spider veins (telangiectasia), see 36468. For injection of a sclerosing solution for larger veins, see 36470–36471.

ICD-10-CM Diagnostic Codes

I80.01	Phlebitis and thrombophlebitis of superficial vessels of right lower extremity ☑
I80.02	Phlebitis and thrombophlebitis of superficial vessels of left lower extremity ☑
I80.03	Phlebitis and thrombophlebitis of superficial vessels of lower extremities, bilateral ☑
I80.11	Phlebitis and thrombophlebitis of right femoral vein ☑
I80.12	Phlebitis and thrombophlebitis of left femoral vein ☑
I80.13	Phlebitis and thrombophlebitis of femoral vein, bilateral ☑

I80.291 Phlebitis and thrombophlebitis of other deep vessels of right lower extremity ☑
I80.292 Phlebitis and thrombophlebitis of other deep vessels of left lower extremity ☑
I80.293 Phlebitis and thrombophlebitis of other deep vessels of lower extremity, bilateral ☑
I83.011 Varicose veins of right lower extremity with ulcer of thigh ☑
I83.012 Varicose veins of right lower extremity with ulcer of calf ☑
I83.013 Varicose veins of right lower extremity with ulcer of ankle ☑
I83.014 Varicose veins of right lower extremity with ulcer of heel and midfoot ☑
I83.015 Varicose veins of right lower extremity with ulcer other part of foot ☑
I83.018 Varicose veins of right lower extremity with ulcer other part of lower leg ☑
I83.021 Varicose veins of left lower extremity with ulcer of thigh ☑
I83.022 Varicose veins of left lower extremity with ulcer of calf ☑
I83.023 Varicose veins of left lower extremity with ulcer of ankle ☑
I83.024 Varicose veins of left lower extremity with ulcer of heel and midfoot ☑
I83.025 Varicose veins of left lower extremity with ulcer other part of foot ☑
I83.028 Varicose veins of left lower extremity with ulcer other part of lower leg ☑
I83.11 Varicose veins of right lower extremity with inflammation ☑
I83.12 Varicose veins of left lower extremity with inflammation ☑
I83.211 Varicose veins of right lower extremity with both ulcer of thigh and inflammation ☑
I83.212 Varicose veins of right lower extremity with both ulcer of calf and inflammation ☑
I83.213 Varicose veins of right lower extremity with both ulcer of ankle and inflammation ☑
I83.214 Varicose veins of right lower extremity with both ulcer of heel and midfoot and inflammation ☑
I83.215 Varicose veins of right lower extremity with both ulcer other part of foot and inflammation ☑
I83.218 Varicose veins of right lower extremity with both ulcer of other part of lower extremity and inflammation ☑
I83.221 Varicose veins of left lower extremity with both ulcer of thigh and inflammation ☑
I83.222 Varicose veins of left lower extremity with both ulcer of calf and inflammation ☑
I83.223 Varicose veins of left lower extremity with both ulcer of ankle and inflammation ☑
I83.224 Varicose veins of left lower extremity with both ulcer of heel and midfoot and inflammation ☑
I83.225 Varicose veins of left lower extremity with both ulcer other part of foot and inflammation ☑
I83.228 Varicose veins of left lower extremity with both ulcer of other part of lower extremity and inflammation ☑
I83.811 Varicose veins of right lower extremity with pain ☑
I83.812 Varicose veins of left lower extremity with pain ☑
I83.813 Varicose veins of bilateral lower extremities with pain ☑
I83.891 Varicose veins of right lower extremity with other complications ☑
I83.892 Varicose veins of left lower extremity with other complications ☑
I83.893 Varicose veins of bilateral lower extremities with other complications ☑
I83.91 Asymptomatic varicose veins of right lower extremity ☑
I83.92 Asymptomatic varicose veins of left lower extremity ☑
I83.93 Asymptomatic varicose veins of bilateral lower extremities ☑
I87.2 Venous insufficiency (chronic) (peripheral)

AMA: 37700 2018,Mar,3; 2018,Jan,8; 2017,Jan,8; 2016,Jan,13; 2015,Jan,16; 2014,Jan,11

Relative Value Units/Medicare Edits

Non-Facility RVU	Work	PE	MP	Total
37700	3.82	2.38	0.87	7.07
Facility RVU	**Work**	**PE**	**MP**	**Total**
37700	3.82	2.38	0.87	7.07

	FUD	Status	MUE	Modifiers				IOM Reference
37700	90	A	1(2)	51	50	N/A	N/A	None

* with documentation

Terms To Know

clamp. Tool used to grip, compress, join, or fasten body parts.

incision. Act of cutting into tissue or an organ.

ligation. Tying off a blood vessel or duct with a suture or a soft, thin wire.

telangiectasia. Permanent dilation of capillaries, arterioles, or venules that appears as focal red lesions on the skin or mucous membranes.

ulcer. Open sore or excavating lesion of skin or the tissue on the surface of an organ from the sloughing of chronically inflamed and necrosing tissue.

varicose vein. Abnormal, permanently distended or stretched vein.

37718-37722

37718 Ligation, division, and stripping, short saphenous vein
37722 Ligation, division, and stripping, long (greater) saphenous veins from saphenofemoral junction to knee or below

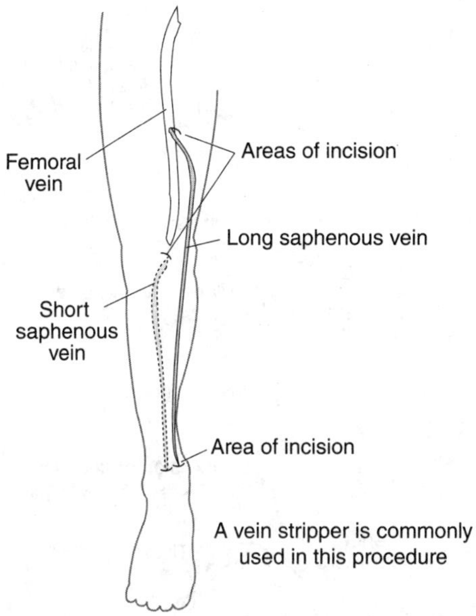

Explanation

The physician makes a skin incision in the upper thigh or upper leg exposing the short saphenous vein (37718) or the long saphenous veins (37722). Additional skin incisions are made at the knee and the ankle and along the leg as necessary. A long wire is threaded through the length of the vein and brought out at the ankle. The vein is tied to the end of the wire and the wire is pulled out along with the vein. Once the vein has been removed, the skin incisions are repaired with layered closures. The leg is wrapped with an elastic pressure dressing postoperatively.

Coding Tips

These are unilateral procedures. If performed bilaterally, some payers require that the service be reported twice with modifier 50 appended to the second code, while others require identification of the service only once with modifier 50 appended. Check with individual payers. Modifier 50 identifies a procedure performed identically on the opposite side of the body (mirror image). Ligation, division, and stripping of the greater saphenous vein are reported with 37722; for the short saphenous vein, report 37718. Do not report 37718 with 37735 or 37780. Do not report 37722 with 37700 or 37735.

ICD-10-CM Diagnostic Codes

I80.01	Phlebitis and thrombophlebitis of superficial vessels of right lower extremity ☑
I80.02	Phlebitis and thrombophlebitis of superficial vessels of left lower extremity ☑
I80.03	Phlebitis and thrombophlebitis of superficial vessels of lower extremities, bilateral ☑
I80.11	Phlebitis and thrombophlebitis of right femoral vein ☑
I80.12	Phlebitis and thrombophlebitis of left femoral vein ☑
I80.13	Phlebitis and thrombophlebitis of femoral vein, bilateral ☑
I80.291	Phlebitis and thrombophlebitis of other deep vessels of right lower extremity ☑
I80.292	Phlebitis and thrombophlebitis of other deep vessels of left lower extremity ☑
I80.293	Phlebitis and thrombophlebitis of other deep vessels of lower extremity, bilateral ☑
I83.011	Varicose veins of right lower extremity with ulcer of thigh ☑
I83.012	Varicose veins of right lower extremity with ulcer of calf ☑
I83.013	Varicose veins of right lower extremity with ulcer of ankle ☑
I83.014	Varicose veins of right lower extremity with ulcer of heel and midfoot ☑
I83.015	Varicose veins of right lower extremity with ulcer other part of foot ☑
I83.018	Varicose veins of right lower extremity with ulcer other part of lower leg ☑
I83.021	Varicose veins of left lower extremity with ulcer of thigh ☑
I83.022	Varicose veins of left lower extremity with ulcer of calf ☑
I83.023	Varicose veins of left lower extremity with ulcer of ankle ☑
I83.024	Varicose veins of left lower extremity with ulcer of heel and midfoot ☑
I83.025	Varicose veins of left lower extremity with ulcer other part of foot ☑
I83.028	Varicose veins of left lower extremity with ulcer other part of lower leg ☑
I83.11	Varicose veins of right lower extremity with inflammation ☑
I83.12	Varicose veins of left lower extremity with inflammation ☑
I83.211	Varicose veins of right lower extremity with both ulcer of thigh and inflammation ☑
I83.212	Varicose veins of right lower extremity with both ulcer of calf and inflammation ☑
I83.213	Varicose veins of right lower extremity with both ulcer of ankle and inflammation ☑
I83.214	Varicose veins of right lower extremity with both ulcer of heel and midfoot and inflammation ☑
I83.215	Varicose veins of right lower extremity with both ulcer other part of foot and inflammation ☑
I83.218	Varicose veins of right lower extremity with both ulcer of other part of lower extremity and inflammation ☑
I83.221	Varicose veins of left lower extremity with both ulcer of thigh and inflammation ☑
I83.222	Varicose veins of left lower extremity with both ulcer of calf and inflammation ☑
I83.223	Varicose veins of left lower extremity with both ulcer of ankle and inflammation ☑
I83.224	Varicose veins of left lower extremity with both ulcer of heel and midfoot and inflammation ☑
I83.225	Varicose veins of left lower extremity with both ulcer other part of foot and inflammation ☑
I83.228	Varicose veins of left lower extremity with both ulcer of other part of lower extremity and inflammation ☑
I83.811	Varicose veins of right lower extremity with pain ☑
I83.812	Varicose veins of left lower extremity with pain ☑
I83.813	Varicose veins of bilateral lower extremities with pain ☑
I83.891	Varicose veins of right lower extremity with other complications ☑
I83.892	Varicose veins of left lower extremity with other complications ☑
I83.893	Varicose veins of bilateral lower extremities with other complications ☑

I83.91 Asymptotic varicose veins of right lower extremity ☑
I83.92 Asymptomatic varicose veins of left lower extremity ☑
I83.93 Asymptomatic varicose veins of bilateral lower extremities ☑
I87.2 Venous insufficiency (chronic) (peripheral)

AMA: **37718** 2018,Mar,3; 2018,Jan,8; 2017,Jan,8; 2014,Jan,11 **37722** 2018,Mar,3; 2018,Jan,8; 2017,Jan,8; 2014,Jan,11

Relative Value Units/Medicare Edits

Non-Facility RVU	Work	PE	MP	Total
37718	7.13	3.68	1.64	12.45
37722	8.16	3.66	1.9	13.72
Facility RVU	**Work**	**PE**	**MP**	**Total**
37718	7.13	3.68	1.64	12.45
37722	8.16	3.66	1.9	13.72

	FUD	Status	MUE	Modifiers				IOM Reference
37718	90	A	1(2)	51	50	62*	N/A	None
37722	90	A	1(2)	51	50	62*	N/A	

* with documentation

Terms To Know

ligation. Tying off a blood vessel or duct with a suture or a soft, thin wire.

ulcer. Open sore or excavating lesion of skin or the tissue on the surface of an organ from the sloughing of chronically inflamed and necrosing tissue.

varicose vein. Abnormal, permanently distended or stretched vein.

37735

37735 Ligation and division and complete stripping of long or short saphenous veins with radical excision of ulcer and skin graft and/or interruption of communicating veins of lower leg, with excision of deep fascia

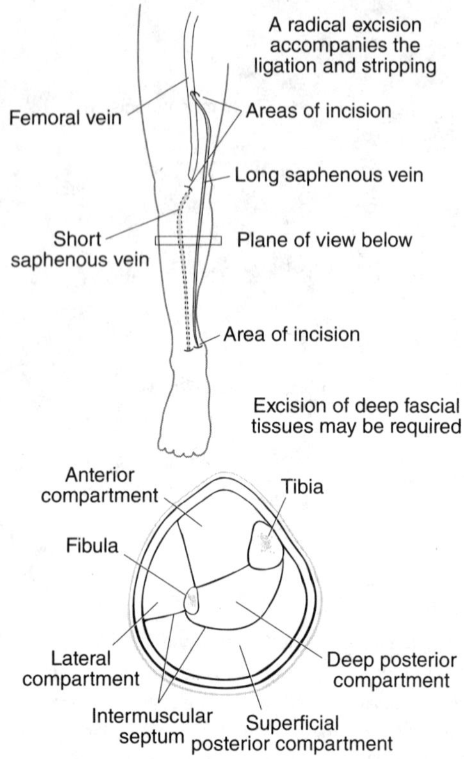

Explanation

The physician makes a skin incision in the upper thigh and the upper leg exposing the long and short saphenous veins. Additional skin incisions are made at the ankle and along the leg as necessary. A long wire is passed through the length of the vein and brought out at the ankle. Each vein is tied to the end of the wire and the vein is pulled out along with the wire. The physician uses a scalpel to remove the skin ulcer from the leg. The ulcer site is covered with a piece of skin that has been shaved from another part of the patient's body. Veins that connect superficial veins with deep veins may be tied off. The tough, fibrous envelope containing the muscle of the leg is split and removed at points where the superficial and deep veins connect. The skin incisions are repaired with layered closures. The leg is wrapped with an elastic pressure dressing postoperatively.

Coding Tips

This is a unilateral procedure. If performed bilaterally, some payers require that the service be reported twice with modifier 50 appended to the second code, while others require identification of the service only once with modifier 50 appended. Check with individual payers. Modifier 50 identifies a procedure performed identically on the opposite side of the body (mirror image). This code includes any debridement performed by the physician. For ligation and division and complete stripping of saphenous veins without excision of ulcer, skin grafting, or interruption of communicating veins, see 37700–37722. Do not report 37735 with 37700, 37718, 37722, or 37780. For injection of a sclerosing solution, spider veins (telangiectasia), see 36468. For injection of a sclerosing solution for larger veins, see 36470–36471.

ICD-10-CM Diagnostic Codes

I83.011 Varicose veins of right lower extremity with ulcer of thigh ☑
I83.012 Varicose veins of right lower extremity with ulcer of calf ☑
I83.013 Varicose veins of right lower extremity with ulcer of ankle ☑
I83.014 Varicose veins of right lower extremity with ulcer of heel and midfoot ☑
I83.015 Varicose veins of right lower extremity with ulcer other part of foot ☑
I83.11 Varicose veins of right lower extremity with inflammation ☑
I83.211 Varicose veins of right lower extremity with both ulcer of thigh and inflammation ☑
I83.212 Varicose veins of right lower extremity with both ulcer of calf and inflammation ☑
I83.213 Varicose veins of right lower extremity with both ulcer of ankle and inflammation ☑
I83.214 Varicose veins of right lower extremity with both ulcer of heel and midfoot and inflammation ☑
I83.811 Varicose veins of right lower extremity with pain ☑
I83.891 Varicose veins of right lower extremity with other complications ☑
I83.91 Asymptomatic varicose veins of right lower extremity ☑
I87.2 Venous insufficiency (chronic) (peripheral)
L97.111 Non-pressure chronic ulcer of right thigh limited to breakdown of skin ☑
L97.112 Non-pressure chronic ulcer of right thigh with fat layer exposed ☑
L97.113 Non-pressure chronic ulcer of right thigh with necrosis of muscle ☑
L97.114 Non-pressure chronic ulcer of right thigh with necrosis of bone ☑
L97.115 Non-pressure chronic ulcer of right thigh with muscle involvement without evidence of necrosis ☑
L97.116 Non-pressure chronic ulcer of right thigh with bone involvement without evidence of necrosis ☑
L97.211 Non-pressure chronic ulcer of right calf limited to breakdown of skin ☑
L97.212 Non-pressure chronic ulcer of right calf with fat layer exposed ☑
L97.213 Non-pressure chronic ulcer of right calf with necrosis of muscle ☑
L97.214 Non-pressure chronic ulcer of right calf with necrosis of bone ☑
L97.215 Non-pressure chronic ulcer of right calf with muscle involvement without evidence of necrosis ☑
L97.216 Non-pressure chronic ulcer of right calf with bone involvement without evidence of necrosis ☑
L97.311 Non-pressure chronic ulcer of right ankle limited to breakdown of skin ☑
L97.312 Non-pressure chronic ulcer of right ankle with fat layer exposed ☑
L97.313 Non-pressure chronic ulcer of right ankle with necrosis of muscle ☑
L97.314 Non-pressure chronic ulcer of right ankle with necrosis of bone ☑
L97.315 Non-pressure chronic ulcer of right ankle with muscle involvement without evidence of necrosis ☑
L97.316 Non-pressure chronic ulcer of right ankle with bone involvement without evidence of necrosis ☑
L97.411 Non-pressure chronic ulcer of right heel and midfoot limited to breakdown of skin ☑
L97.412 Non-pressure chronic ulcer of right heel and midfoot with fat layer exposed ☑
L97.413 Non-pressure chronic ulcer of right heel and midfoot with necrosis of muscle ☑
L97.414 Non-pressure chronic ulcer of right heel and midfoot with necrosis of bone ☑
L97.415 Non-pressure chronic ulcer of right heel and midfoot with muscle involvement without evidence of necrosis ☑
L97.416 Non-pressure chronic ulcer of right heel and midfoot with bone involvement without evidence of necrosis ☑
L97.525 Non-pressure chronic ulcer of other part of left foot with muscle involvement without evidence of necrosis ☑
L97.526 Non-pressure chronic ulcer of other part of left foot with bone involvement without evidence of necrosis ☑
L97.825 Non-pressure chronic ulcer of other part of left lower leg with muscle involvement without evidence of necrosis ☑
L97.826 Non-pressure chronic ulcer of other part of left lower leg with bone involvement without evidence of necrosis ☑

AMA: 37735 2018,Mar,3; 2018,Jan,8; 2017,Jan,8; 2016,Jan,13; 2015,Jan,16; 2014,Jan,11

Relative Value Units/Medicare Edits

Non-Facility RVU	Work	PE	MP	Total
37735	10.9	3.33	2.52	16.75
Facility RVU	**Work**	**PE**	**MP**	**Total**
37735	10.9	3.33	2.52	16.75

	FUD	Status	MUE	Modifiers				IOM Reference
37735	90	A	1(2)	51	50	62*	N/A	None

* with documentation

Terms To Know

debridement. Removal of dead or contaminated tissue and foreign matter from a wound.

fascia. Fibrous sheet or band of tissue that envelops organs, muscles, and groupings of muscles.

graft. Tissue implant from another part of the body or another person.

inflammation. Cytologic and chemical reactions that occur in affected blood vessels and adjacent tissues in response to injury or abnormal stimulation from a physical, chemical, or biologic agent.

ligation. Tying off a blood vessel or duct with a suture or a soft, thin wire.

radical. Extensive surgery.

ulcer. Open sore or excavating lesion of skin or the tissue on the surface of an organ from the sloughing of chronically inflamed and necrosing tissue.

varicose vein. Abnormal, permanently distended or stretched vein.

37760-37761

37760 Ligation of perforator veins, subfascial, radical (Linton type), including skin graft, when performed, open,1 leg

37761 Ligation of perforator vein(s), subfascial, open, including ultrasound guidance, when performed, 1 leg

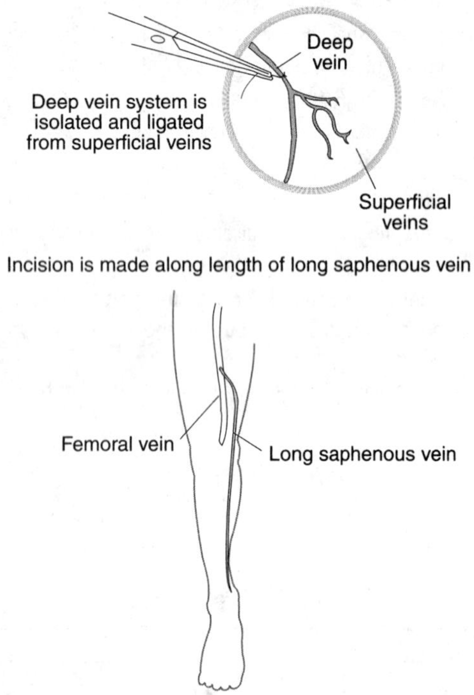

Explanation

The physician performs a radical (Linton type) subfascial ligation (tying) of the perforator veins in 37760 and an open subfascial perforator vein ligation in 37761. Through incisions along the course of the saphenous vein, the veins connecting the deep and superficial veins of the leg are isolated. They are ligated, isolating the two systems along the course of the leg. The incisions may be sutured or covered with skin grafts taken from another part of the patient's body. Code 37760 includes skin grafts, when performed, and code 37761 includes the use of ultrasonic guidance, when performed. Both codes report a procedure involving one leg.

Coding Tips

These are unilateral procedures. If performed bilaterally, some payers require the service be reported twice with modifier 50 appended to the second code, while others require identification of the service only once with modifier 50 appended. Check with individual payers. Modifier 50 identifies a procedure performed identically on the opposite side of the body (mirror image). This code includes any skin graft the physician may perform. For endoscopic ligation of perforator veins, subfascial (SEPS), see 37500. For other treatment of long and/or short saphenous veins, see 37700–37735 and 37780. For injection of a sclerosing solution, spider veins (telangiectasia), see 36468. For injection of a sclerosing solution for larger veins, see 36470–36471. For 37760–37761 codes 76937, 76942, 76998, and 93971 are not separately reportable.

ICD-10-CM Diagnostic Codes

I83.011 Varicose veins of right lower extremity with ulcer of thigh ☑
I83.012 Varicose veins of right lower extremity with ulcer of calf ☑
I83.013 Varicose veins of right lower extremity with ulcer of ankle ☑
I83.014 Varicose veins of right lower extremity with ulcer of heel and midfoot ☑
I83.015 Varicose veins of right lower extremity with ulcer other part of foot ☑
I83.018 Varicose veins of right lower extremity with ulcer other part of lower leg ☑
I83.021 Varicose veins of left lower extremity with ulcer of thigh ☑
I83.022 Varicose veins of left lower extremity with ulcer of calf ☑
I83.023 Varicose veins of left lower extremity with ulcer of ankle ☑
I83.024 Varicose veins of left lower extremity with ulcer of heel and midfoot ☑
I83.025 Varicose veins of left lower extremity with ulcer other part of foot ☑
I83.028 Varicose veins of left lower extremity with ulcer other part of lower leg ☑
I83.10 Varicose veins of unspecified lower extremity with inflammation
I83.11 Varicose veins of right lower extremity with inflammation ☑
I83.12 Varicose veins of left lower extremity with inflammation ☑
I83.211 Varicose veins of right lower extremity with both ulcer of thigh and inflammation ☑
I83.212 Varicose veins of right lower extremity with both ulcer of calf and inflammation ☑
I83.213 Varicose veins of right lower extremity with both ulcer of ankle and inflammation ☑
I83.214 Varicose veins of right lower extremity with both ulcer of heel and midfoot and inflammation ☑
I83.215 Varicose veins of right lower extremity with both ulcer other part of foot and inflammation ☑
I83.218 Varicose veins of right lower extremity with both ulcer of other part of lower extremity and inflammation ☑
I83.221 Varicose veins of left lower extremity with both ulcer of thigh and inflammation ☑
I83.222 Varicose veins of left lower extremity with both ulcer of calf and inflammation ☑
I83.223 Varicose veins of left lower extremity with both ulcer of ankle and inflammation ☑
I83.224 Varicose veins of left lower extremity with both ulcer of heel and midfoot and inflammation ☑
I83.225 Varicose veins of left lower extremity with both ulcer other part of foot and inflammation ☑
I83.228 Varicose veins of left lower extremity with both ulcer of other part of lower extremity and inflammation ☑
I83.811 Varicose veins of right lower extremity with pain ☑
I83.812 Varicose veins of left lower extremity with pain ☑
I83.813 Varicose veins of bilateral lower extremities with pain ☑
I83.891 Varicose veins of right lower extremity with other complications ☑
I83.892 Varicose veins of left lower extremity with other complications ☑
I83.893 Varicose veins of bilateral lower extremities with other complications ☑
I83.90 Asymptomatic varicose veins of unspecified lower extremity
I83.91 Asymptomatic varicose veins of right lower extremity ☑
I83.92 Asymptomatic varicose veins of left lower extremity ☑
I83.93 Asymptomatic varicose veins of bilateral lower extremities ☑

AMA: **37760** 2018,Mar,3; 2018,Jan,8; 2017,Jan,8; 2016,Jan,13; 2015,Jan,16; 2014,Jan,11 **37761** 2018,Mar,3; 2018,Jan,8; 2017,Jan,8; 2016,Jan,13; 2015,Jan,16; 2014,Jan,11

Relative Value Units/Medicare Edits

Non-Facility RVU	Work	PE	MP	Total
37760	10.78	4.84	2.46	18.08
37761	9.13	4.49	2.03	15.65
Facility RVU	**Work**	**PE**	**MP**	**Total**
37760	10.78	4.84	2.46	18.08
37761	9.13	4.49	2.03	15.65

	FUD	Status	MUE	Modifiers				IOM Reference
37760	90	A	1(2)	51	50	62*	N/A	None
37761	90	A	1(2)	51	50	62*	80	

* with documentation

Terms To Know

fascia. Fibrous sheet or band of tissue that envelops organs, muscles, and groupings of muscles.

graft. Tissue implant from another part of the body or another person.

inflammation. Cytologic and chemical reactions that occur in affected blood vessels and adjacent tissues in response to injury or abnormal stimulation from a physical, chemical, or biologic agent.

ligation. Tying off a blood vessel or duct with a suture or a soft, thin wire.

sclerose. To become hard or firm and indurated from increased formation of connective tissue or disease.

ulcer. Open sore or excavating lesion of skin or the tissue on the surface of an organ from the sloughing of chronically inflamed and necrosing tissue.

37765-37766

37765 Stab phlebectomy of varicose veins, 1 extremity; 10-20 stab incisions

37766 more than 20 incisions

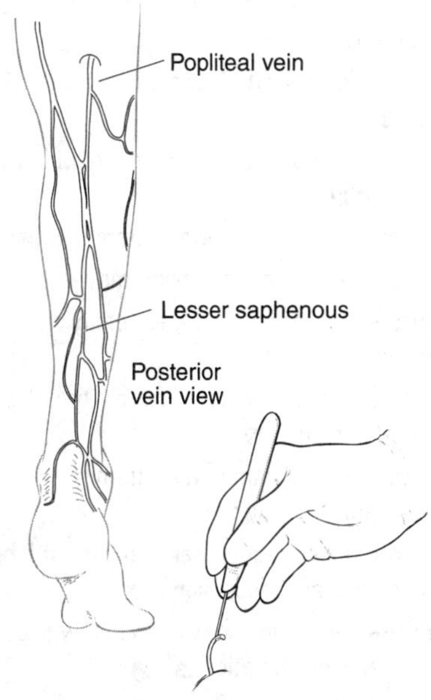

Stab incisions are made over the varicose vein and a hooked device retrieves the section of vein

Explanation

Stab phlebectomy for varicose veins is an ambulatory procedure that permits removal of nearly any incompetent vein below the saphenofemoral and saphenopopliteal junction. The varicose veins are identified with an indelible marking pen while the patient is standing. The patient is placed supine for further marking. Diluted lidocaine is injected into the tissues in large volumes until the perivenous tissues are engorged and distended with the anesthetic. Regional nerve blocks may be used for extensive areas. Tiny stab incisions are made with a scalpel or 18-gauge needle. The varicose vein is dissected with the phlebectomy hook. The vein is undermined along its course, all fibroadipose attachments to the vein are freed, and the vein is grasped with the hook and removed with mosquito forceps. Hemostasis is achieved by applying local compression to the veins already removed. The varicose vein is progressively extracted from one stab incision to the next. No skin closure is needed. Bandages are applied. Large pads are placed along the site of vein removal and covered with an inelastic bandage, followed by a second bandage of highly elastic material. Report 37765 when 10 to 20 stab incisions are made and 37766 when more than 20 are reported.

Coding Tips

For open ligation of subfascial or radical perforator veins, see 37760; for endoscopic ligation of perforator veins, subfascial (SEPS), see 37500. If a stab phlebectomy is performed with less than 10 incisions, see 37799.

ICD-10-CM Diagnostic Codes

I83.011	Varicose veins of right lower extremity with ulcer of thigh ☑
I83.012	Varicose veins of right lower extremity with ulcer of calf ☑
I83.013	Varicose veins of right lower extremity with ulcer of ankle ☑
I83.014	Varicose veins of right lower extremity with ulcer of heel and midfoot ☑
I83.015	Varicose veins of right lower extremity with ulcer other part of foot ☑

I83.018 Varicose veins of right lower extremity with ulcer other part of lower leg ☑
I83.021 Varicose veins of left lower extremity with ulcer of thigh ☑
I83.022 Varicose veins of left lower extremity with ulcer of calf ☑
I83.023 Varicose veins of left lower extremity with ulcer of ankle ☑
I83.024 Varicose veins of left lower extremity with ulcer of heel and midfoot ☑
I83.025 Varicose veins of left lower extremity with ulcer other part of foot ☑
I83.028 Varicose veins of left lower extremity with ulcer other part of lower leg ☑
I83.11 Varicose veins of right lower extremity with inflammation ☑
I83.12 Varicose veins of left lower extremity with inflammation ☑
I83.211 Varicose veins of right lower extremity with both ulcer of thigh and inflammation ☑
I83.212 Varicose veins of right lower extremity with both ulcer of calf and inflammation ☑
I83.213 Varicose veins of right lower extremity with both ulcer of ankle and inflammation ☑
I83.214 Varicose veins of right lower extremity with both ulcer of heel and midfoot and inflammation ☑
I83.215 Varicose veins of right lower extremity with both ulcer other part of foot and inflammation ☑
I83.218 Varicose veins of right lower extremity with both ulcer of other part of lower extremity and inflammation ☑
I83.221 Varicose veins of left lower extremity with both ulcer of thigh and inflammation ☑
I83.222 Varicose veins of left lower extremity with both ulcer of calf and inflammation ☑
I83.223 Varicose veins of left lower extremity with both ulcer of ankle and inflammation ☑
I83.224 Varicose veins of left lower extremity with both ulcer of heel and midfoot and inflammation ☑
I83.225 Varicose veins of left lower extremity with both ulcer other part of foot and inflammation ☑
I83.228 Varicose veins of left lower extremity with both ulcer of other part of lower extremity and inflammation ☑
I83.811 Varicose veins of right lower extremity with pain ☑
I83.812 Varicose veins of left lower extremity with pain ☑
I83.813 Varicose veins of bilateral lower extremities with pain ☑
I83.891 Varicose veins of right lower extremity with other complications ☑
I83.892 Varicose veins of left lower extremity with other complications ☑
I83.893 Varicose veins of bilateral lower extremities with other complications ☑
I83.91 Asymptomatic varicose veins of right lower extremity ☑
I83.92 Asymptomatic varicose veins of left lower extremity ☑
I83.93 Asymptomatic varicose veins of bilateral lower extremities ☑

AMA: **37765** 2018,Mar,3; 2018,Jan,8; 2017,Jan,8; 2016,Nov,3; 2016,Jan,13; 2015,Jan,16; 2014,Oct,6; 2014,Jan,11 **37766** 2018,Mar,3; 2018,Jan,8; 2017,Jan,8; 2016,Nov,3; 2016,Jan,13; 2015,Jan,16; 2014,Oct,6; 2014,Jan,11; 2013,Sep,17

Relative Value Units/Medicare Edits

Non-Facility RVU	Work	PE	MP	Total
37765	7.71	9.24	1.57	18.52
37766	9.66	10.4	1.95	22.01
Facility RVU	**Work**	**PE**	**MP**	**Total**
37765	7.71	3.68	1.57	12.96
37766	9.66	4.21	1.95	15.82

	FUD	Status	MUE	Modifiers				IOM Reference
37765	90	A	1(2)	51	50	62*	N/A	None
37766	90	A	1(2)	51	50	62*	N/A	

* with documentation

Terms To Know

forceps. Tool used for grasping or compressing tissue.

hemostasis. Interruption of blood flow or the cessation or arrest of bleeding.

incision. Act of cutting into tissue or an organ.

supine. Lying on the back.

ulcer. Open sore or excavating lesion of skin or the tissue on the surface of an organ from the sloughing of chronically inflamed and necrosing tissue.

varicose vein. Abnormal, permanently distended or stretched vein.

37780

37780 Ligation and division of short saphenous vein at saphenopopliteal junction (separate procedure)

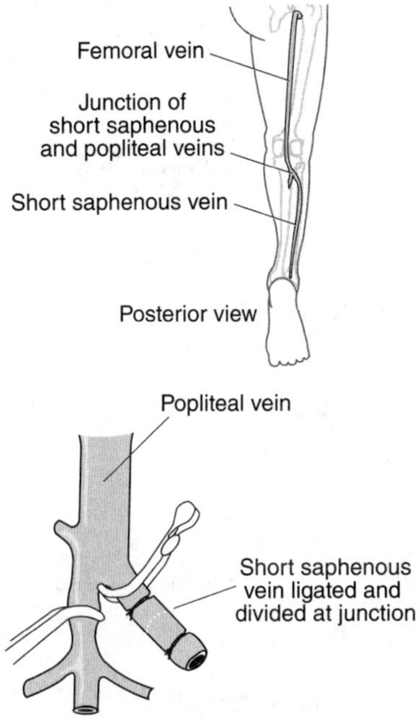

Explanation

The physician makes an incision in the skin overlying the short saphenous vein at its junction with the saphenopopliteal vein at the knee. The vessels are dissected and ties are placed around the short saphenous vein which is divided between the ties. Once the ties are in place and the vein has been divided, the skin incision is repaired with a layered closure.

Coding Tips

This separate procedure by definition is usually a component of a more complex service and is not identified separately. When performed alone or with other unrelated procedures/services, it may be reported. If performed alone, list the code; if performed with other procedures/services, list the code and append modifier 59 or an X{EPSU} modifier. This is a unilateral procedure. If performed bilaterally, some payers require that the service be reported twice with modifier 50 appended to the second code, while others require identification of the service only once with modifier 50 appended. Check with individual payers. Modifier 50 identifies a procedure performed identically on the opposite side of the body (mirror image). For other treatment of long or short saphenous veins, see 37700–37735. For injection of a sclerosing solution, spider veins (telangiectasia), see 36468. For injection of a sclerosing solution for larger veins, see 36470–36471.

ICD-10-CM Diagnostic Codes

I80.221 Phlebitis and thrombophlebitis of right popliteal vein ☑
I80.222 Phlebitis and thrombophlebitis of left popliteal vein ☑
I80.223 Phlebitis and thrombophlebitis of popliteal vein, bilateral ☑
I80.291 Phlebitis and thrombophlebitis of other deep vessels of right lower extremity ☑
I80.292 Phlebitis and thrombophlebitis of other deep vessels of left lower extremity ☑
I80.293 Phlebitis and thrombophlebitis of other deep vessels of lower extremity, bilateral ☑
I83.011 Varicose veins of right lower extremity with ulcer of thigh ☑
I83.012 Varicose veins of right lower extremity with ulcer of calf ☑
I83.013 Varicose veins of right lower extremity with ulcer of ankle ☑
I83.014 Varicose veins of right lower extremity with ulcer of heel and midfoot ☑
I83.015 Varicose veins of right lower extremity with ulcer other part of foot ☑
I83.018 Varicose veins of right lower extremity with ulcer other part of lower leg ☑
I83.021 Varicose veins of left lower extremity with ulcer of thigh ☑
I83.022 Varicose veins of left lower extremity with ulcer of calf ☑
I83.023 Varicose veins of left lower extremity with ulcer of ankle ☑
I83.024 Varicose veins of left lower extremity with ulcer of heel and midfoot ☑
I83.025 Varicose veins of left lower extremity with ulcer other part of foot ☑
I83.028 Varicose veins of left lower extremity with ulcer other part of lower leg ☑
I83.11 Varicose veins of right lower extremity with inflammation ☑
I83.12 Varicose veins of left lower extremity with inflammation ☑
I83.211 Varicose veins of right lower extremity with both ulcer of thigh and inflammation ☑
I83.212 Varicose veins of right lower extremity with both ulcer of calf and inflammation ☑
I83.213 Varicose veins of right lower extremity with both ulcer of ankle and inflammation ☑
I83.214 Varicose veins of right lower extremity with both ulcer of heel and midfoot and inflammation ☑
I83.215 Varicose veins of right lower extremity with both ulcer other part of foot and inflammation ☑
I83.218 Varicose veins of right lower extremity with both ulcer of other part of lower extremity and inflammation ☑
I83.221 Varicose veins of left lower extremity with both ulcer of thigh and inflammation ☑
I83.222 Varicose veins of left lower extremity with both ulcer of calf and inflammation ☑
I83.223 Varicose veins of left lower extremity with both ulcer of ankle and inflammation ☑
I83.224 Varicose veins of left lower extremity with both ulcer of heel and midfoot and inflammation ☑
I83.225 Varicose veins of left lower extremity with both ulcer other part of foot and inflammation ☑
I83.228 Varicose veins of left lower extremity with both ulcer of other part of lower extremity and inflammation ☑
I83.811 Varicose veins of right lower extremity with pain ☑
I83.812 Varicose veins of left lower extremity with pain ☑
I83.813 Varicose veins of bilateral lower extremities with pain ☑
I83.891 Varicose veins of right lower extremity with other complications ☑
I83.892 Varicose veins of left lower extremity with other complications ☑
I83.893 Varicose veins of bilateral lower extremities with other complications ☑
I83.91 Asymptomatic varicose veins of right lower extremity ☑
I83.92 Asymptomatic varicose veins of left lower extremity ☑
I83.93 Asymptomatic varicose veins of bilateral lower extremities ☑
I87.2 Venous insufficiency (chronic) (peripheral)

AMA: **37780** 2018,Jan,8; 2017,Jan,8; 2016,Jan,13; 2015,Jan,16; 2014,Jan,11

Relative Value Units/Medicare Edits

Non-Facility RVU	Work	PE	MP	Total
37780	3.93	1.91	0.91	6.75
Facility RVU	**Work**	**PE**	**MP**	**Total**
37780	3.93	1.91	0.91	6.75

	FUD	Status	MUE	Modifiers				IOM Reference
37780	90	A	1(2)	51	50	62*	N/A	None

* with documentation

Terms To Know

dissect. Cut apart or separate tissue for surgical purposes or for visual or microscopic study.

ligation. Tying off a blood vessel or duct with a suture or a soft, thin wire.

sclerose. To become hard or firm and indurated from increased formation of connective tissue or disease.

telangiectasia. Permanent dilation of capillaries, arterioles, or venules that appears as focal red lesions on the skin or mucous membranes.

ulcer. Open sore or excavating lesion of skin or the tissue on the surface of an organ from the sloughing of chronically inflamed and necrosing tissue.

varicose vein. Abnormal, permanently distended or stretched vein.

37785

37785 Ligation, division, and/or excision of varicose vein cluster(s), 1 leg

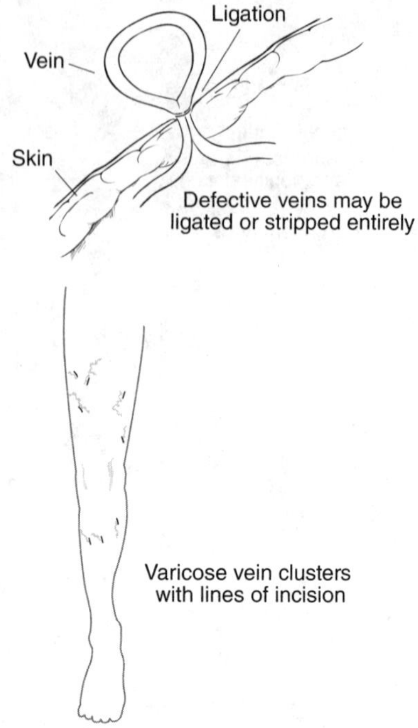

Explanation

The physician ligates, divides, and/or excises varicose vein cluster(s) in one leg. The physician makes small incisions in the skin over localized areas of superficial varicose veins along the leg. These veins are isolated and dissected free of neighboring tissue, tied with sutures and divided, or stripped out bluntly. Pressure is applied over the site to stop bleeding. All incisions are repaired with a layered closure. The legs are wrapped in an elastic pressure dressing postoperatively.

Coding Tips

This is a unilateral procedure. If performed bilaterally, some payers require that the service be reported twice with modifier 50 appended to the second code, while others require identification of the service only once with modifier 50 appended. Check with individual payers. Modifier 50 identifies a procedure performed identically on the opposite side of the body (mirror image). For initial treatment of varicose veins, see 37700–37780. For injection of a sclerosing solution, spider veins (telangiectasia), see 36468. For injection of a sclerosing solution for larger veins, see 36470–36471.

ICD-10-CM Diagnostic Codes

I83.011	Varicose veins of right lower extremity with ulcer of thigh ☑
I83.012	Varicose veins of right lower extremity with ulcer of calf ☑
I83.013	Varicose veins of right lower extremity with ulcer of ankle ☑
I83.014	Varicose veins of right lower extremity with ulcer of heel and midfoot ☑
I83.015	Varicose veins of right lower extremity with ulcer other part of foot ☑
I83.018	Varicose veins of right lower extremity with ulcer other part of lower leg ☑
I83.021	Varicose veins of left lower extremity with ulcer of thigh ☑
I83.022	Varicose veins of left lower extremity with ulcer of calf ☑
I83.023	Varicose veins of left lower extremity with ulcer of ankle ☑

I83.024	Varicose veins of left lower extremity with ulcer of heel and midfoot ☑
I83.025	Varicose veins of left lower extremity with ulcer other part of foot ☑
I83.028	Varicose veins of left lower extremity with ulcer other part of lower leg ☑
I83.11	Varicose veins of right lower extremity with inflammation ☑
I83.12	Varicose veins of left lower extremity with inflammation ☑
I83.211	Varicose veins of right lower extremity with both ulcer of thigh and inflammation ☑
I83.212	Varicose veins of right lower extremity with both ulcer of calf and inflammation ☑
I83.213	Varicose veins of right lower extremity with both ulcer of ankle and inflammation ☑
I83.214	Varicose veins of right lower extremity with both ulcer of heel and midfoot and inflammation ☑
I83.215	Varicose veins of right lower extremity with both ulcer other part of foot and inflammation ☑
I83.218	Varicose veins of right lower extremity with both ulcer of other part of lower extremity and inflammation ☑
I83.221	Varicose veins of left lower extremity with both ulcer of thigh and inflammation ☑
I83.222	Varicose veins of left lower extremity with both ulcer of calf and inflammation ☑
I83.223	Varicose veins of left lower extremity with both ulcer of ankle and inflammation ☑
I83.224	Varicose veins of left lower extremity with both ulcer of heel and midfoot and inflammation ☑
I83.225	Varicose veins of left lower extremity with both ulcer other part of foot and inflammation ☑
I83.228	Varicose veins of left lower extremity with both ulcer of other part of lower extremity and inflammation ☑
I83.811	Varicose veins of right lower extremity with pain ☑
I83.812	Varicose veins of left lower extremity with pain ☑
I83.813	Varicose veins of bilateral lower extremities with pain ☑
I83.891	Varicose veins of right lower extremity with other complications ☑
I83.892	Varicose veins of left lower extremity with other complications ☑
I83.893	Varicose veins of bilateral lower extremities with other complications ☑
I83.91	Asymptomatic varicose veins of right lower extremity ☑
I83.92	Asymptomatic varicose veins of left lower extremity ☑
I83.93	Asymptomatic varicose veins of bilateral lower extremities ☑

AMA: 37785 2018,Jan,8; 2017,Jan,8; 2016,Jan,13; 2015,Jan,16; 2014,Jan,11

Relative Value Units/Medicare Edits

Non-Facility RVU	Work	PE	MP	Total
37785	3.93	5.25	0.89	10.07
Facility RVU	**Work**	**PE**	**MP**	**Total**
37785	3.93	2.63	0.89	7.45

	FUD	Status	MUE	Modifiers				IOM Reference
37785	90	A	1(2)	51	50	N/A	N/A	None

* with documentation

37788-37790

37788 Penile revascularization, artery, with or without vein graft

37790 Penile venous occlusive procedure

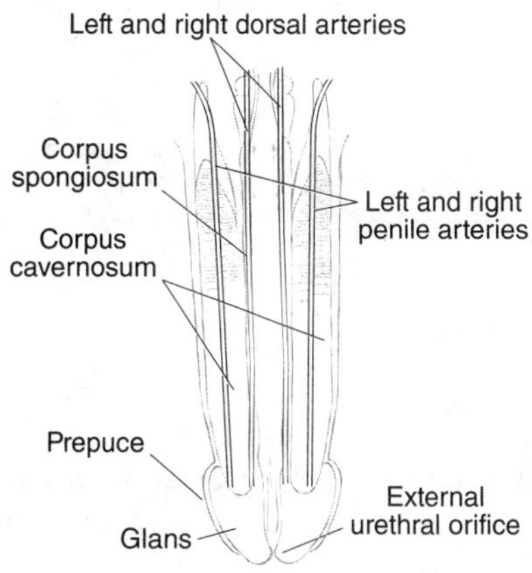

A penile artery is revascularized, with or without vein graft technique

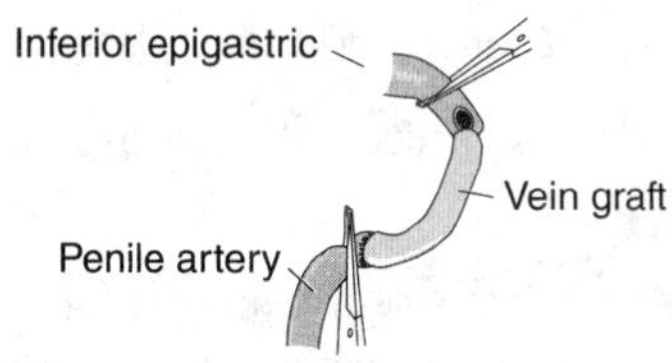

Explanation

Through an incision in the skin near the base of the penis, the physician isolates the penile artery and separates it from critical structures. In 37788, a neighboring artery in the groin or lower abdomen is also isolated and dissected and a vessel clamp applied. The end of the neighboring artery is sewn into the penile artery in an end-to-side fashion, or a piece of harvested vein may be used to connect the two arteries to establish an adequate blood flow to the penis. The clamps are removed and incision is repaired with a layered closure. In 37790, through an inguinoscrotal incision, lateral to the root of the penis, and along the spermatic cord, the physician exposes the suspensory ligaments and detaches them from the pubic bone, The physician incises the superficial layer of Buck's fascia, exposing and suture-ligating each leaking vein. A segment of deep dorsal vein is dissected, ligated at both ends, and resected. The physician reattaches the suspensory ligaments and when the procedure is complete, closes the skin incision with a layered closure.

Coding Tips

Angioscopy during therapeutic intervention is listed separately; see 35400. Any vein graft harvest is not reported separately.

ICD-10-CM Diagnostic Codes

N50.1	Vascular disorders of male genital organs
N50.89	Other specified disorders of the male genital organs
N50.9	Disorder of male genital organs, unspecified
N51	Disorders of male genital organs in diseases classified elsewhere
N52.02	Corporo-venous occlusive erectile dysfunction
N52.03	Combined arterial insufficiency and corporo-venous occlusive erectile dysfunction

AMA: 37788 2014,Jan,11 **37790** 2014,Jan,11

● New ▲ Revised + Add On AMA: CPT Assist [Resequenced] ☑ Laterality

Relative Value Units/Medicare Edits

Non-Facility RVU	Work	PE	MP	Total
37788	23.33	10.66	2.59	36.58
37790	8.43	4.73	0.93	14.09
Facility RVU	**Work**	**PE**	**MP**	**Total**
37788	23.33	10.66	2.59	36.58
37790	8.43	4.73	0.93	14.09

	FUD	Status	MUE	Modifiers				IOM Reference
37788	90	A	1(2)	51	N/A	62*	80	None
37790	90	A	1(2)	51	N/A	N/A	80*	

* with documentation

Terms To Know

angioscopy. Visualization of capillary blood vessels with a microscope, or the inside of a blood vessel with a fiberoptic-equipped catheter.

graft. Tissue implant from another part of the body or another person.

harvest. Removal of cells or tissue from their native site to be used as a graft or transplant to another part of the donor's body or placed into another person.

ligate. To tie off a blood vessel or duct with a suture or a soft, thin wire (ligature wire).

organic impotence. Organic erectile dysfunction in which there is partial or complete failure to attain or maintain erection until completion of intercourse. Organic impotence most often involves a vascular problem of the penis, particularly in older males. Underlying factors may include arteriosclerosis, diabetes, trauma to the arteries, or a venous leak.

revascularization. Restoration of blood flow and oxygen supply to a body part. This may apply to an extremity, the heart, or penis.

vascular. Pertaining to blood vessels.

38300-38305

38300 Drainage of lymph node abscess or lymphadenitis; simple
38305 extensive

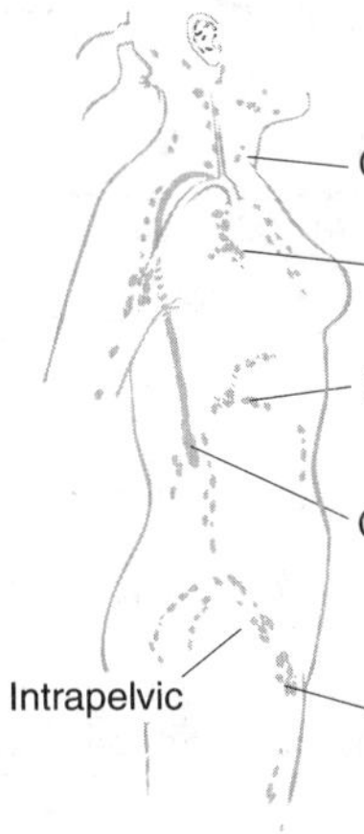

Explanation

The physician performs this procedure to drain inflamed lymph nodes. The physician makes an incision over the affected lymph node and the abscess or infection is drained. The wound is irrigated and closed with sutures or Steri-strips. Report 38305 if the procedure is extensive.

Coding Tips

These are bilateral procedures and as such are reported once even if the procedure is performed on both sides. When 38300 or 38305 is performed with another separately identifiable procedure, the highest dollar value code is listed as the primary procedure and subsequent procedures are appended with modifier 51. For injection for sentinel node identification, see 38792. For imaging guidance, see 76942, 77012, and 77021. For fine needle aspiration, see 10021 For fine needle aspiration, see 10004-10012 and 10021.

ICD-10-CM Diagnostic Codes

A18.2	Tuberculous peripheral lymphadenopathy
A51.49	Other secondary syphilitic conditions
I88.0	Nonspecific mesenteric lymphadenitis
I88.1	Chronic lymphadenitis, except mesenteric
I88.8	Other nonspecific lymphadenitis
I89.8	Other specified noninfective disorders of lymphatic vessels and lymph nodes
L04.0	Acute lymphadenitis of face, head and neck
L04.1	Acute lymphadenitis of trunk
L04.2	Acute lymphadenitis of upper limb
L04.3	Acute lymphadenitis of lower limb
L04.8	Acute lymphadenitis of other sites
R59.0	Localized enlarged lymph nodes
R59.1	Generalized enlarged lymph nodes

AMA: **38300** 2014,Jan,11 **38305** 2014,Jan,11

Relative Value Units/Medicare Edits

Non-Facility RVU	Work	PE	MP	Total
38300	2.36	6.27	0.57	9.2
38305	6.68	5.71	1.61	14.0
Facility RVU	**Work**	**PE**	**MP**	**Total**
38300	2.36	2.93	0.57	5.86
38305	6.68	5.71	1.61	14.0

	FUD	Status	MUE	Modifiers				IOM Reference
38300	10	A	1(3)	51	N/A	N/A	N/A	None
38305	90	A	1(3)	51	N/A	N/A	N/A	

* with documentation

Terms To Know

abscess. Circumscribed collection of pus resulting from bacteria, frequently associated with swelling and other signs of inflammation.

infection. Presence of microorganisms in body tissues that may result in cellular damage.

irrigate. Washing out, lavage.

lymph nodes. Bean-shaped structures along the lymphatic vessels that intercept and destroy foreign materials in the tissue and bloodstream.

lymphadenitis. Inflammation or enlargement of the lymph nodes.

38381

38381 Suture and/or ligation of thoracic duct; thoracic approach

The thoracic duct is a major drainage channel of the lymphatic system. It enters near the junction of the left internal jugular and subclavian veins

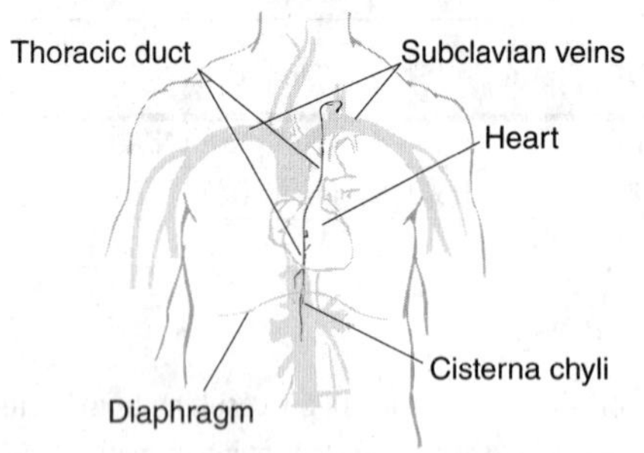

The thoracic duct is accessed by a thoracic incision and is ligated or sutured

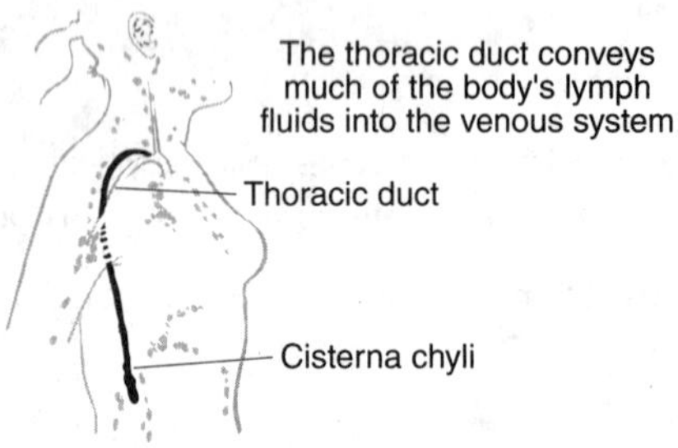

Explanation

The thoracic duct is sutured or ligated. The thoracic duct is a tubular structure, approximately 2 to 3 mm in diameter, that originates in the cisterna chyli, which lies above the second lumbar vertebral body. It ascends on the right, anterior to the vertebral bodies, entering the chest through the aortic hiatus. At the fourth or fifth thoracic vertebra, it crosses to the left and empties into the left jugulosubclavian venous junction. Tears or injury can occur in any segment (cervical, thoracic, abdominal) and the approach is dependent on the site of the leak. An incision is made in the left neck, right or left chest, or abdomen. The involved compartment is drained of all effluent and the leak identified. The duct is ligated a few centimeters below the leak and also a few centimeters above it. Dry gauze is placed at the site of the leak to ensure that the ligation has completely sealed the leak. When it has been determined that the leak is completely sealed, the gauze is removed and glue or other sealant is applied to the area. If the leak is repaired by thoracotomy, chest tubes are placed. Incisions are closed. Report 38381 for a thoracic approach.

Coding Tips

When 38381 is performed with another separately identifiable procedure, the highest dollar value code is listed as the primary procedure, and subsequent procedures are appended with modifier 51.

ICD-10-CM Diagnostic Codes

I89.8	Other specified noninfective disorders of lymphatic vessels and lymph nodes
S27.898A	Other injury of other specified intrathoracic organs, initial encounter

AMA: 38381 2014,Jan,11

Relative Value Units/Medicare Edits

Non-Facility RVU	Work	PE	MP	Total
38381	13.38	6.71	3.12	23.21
Facility RVU	**Work**	**PE**	**MP**	**Total**
38381	13.38	6.71	3.12	23.21

	FUD	Status	MUE	Modifiers				IOM Reference
38381	90	A	1(2)	51	N/A	62*	80	None

* with documentation

Terms To Know

closure. Repairing an incision or wound by suture or other means.

dissect. Cut apart or separate tissue for surgical purposes or for visual or microscopic study.

fistula. Abnormal tube-like passage between two body cavities or organs or from an organ to the outside surface.

incision. Act of cutting into tissue or an organ.

ligation. Tying off a blood vessel or duct with a suture or a soft, thin wire.

lymphadenitis. Inflammation or enlargement of the lymph nodes.

lymphangitis. Inflammation of the lymph channels most often caused by streptococcus.

lymphoma. Tumors occurring in the lymphoid tissues that are most commonly malignant.

malignant. Any condition tending to progress toward death, specifically an invasive tumor with a loss of cellular differentiation that has the ability to spread or metastasize to other body areas.

secondary. Second in order of occurrence or importance, or appearing during the course of another disease or condition.

suture. Numerous stitching techniques employed in wound closure.

38746

\+ **38746** Thoracic lymphadenectomy by thoracotomy, mediastinal and regional lymphadenectomy (List separately in addition to code for primary procedure)

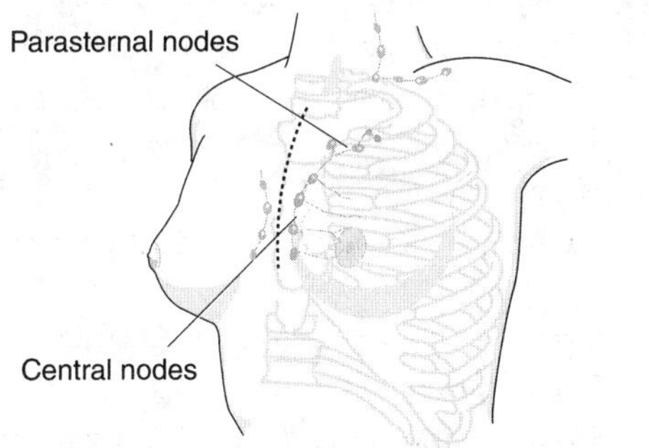

Typical access incision for thoracic lymphadenectomy

Explanation

The physician performs a regional and mediastinal lymphadenectomy via an open approach. Using a scalpel, the surgeon makes a long incision around the side of the chest between two of the ribs. The incision is carried through all of the tissue layers into the chest cavity. Rib spreaders are inserted into the wound and the ribs are spread apart exposing the lung, the heart, and other structures. Alternately, the chest cavity can be opened and the operation performed through a vertical incision in the center of the chest through the sternum. The skin incision is carried down to the sternum bone and a saw is used to split the sternum. With the sternum split in half, the chest is entered by spreading the sternum apart with a set of rib spreaders. Lymph nodes near the lungs, around the heart, and behind the trachea are removed. The area is irrigated and the retractors are removed. If applicable, the sternotomy is repaired using wires to bring the two halves of the sternum together, and the operative wound is closed by sutures or staples.

Coding Tips

Report 38746 in addition to 21601, 31760, 31766, 31786, 32096-32200, 32220-32320, 32440-32491, 32503-32505, 33025, 33030, 33050-33130, 39200-39220, 39560, 39561, 43101, 43112, 43117, 43118, 43122, 43123, 43351, 60270, or 60505. For thoracoscopic mediastinal and regional lymphadenectomy, see 32674.

ICD-10-CM Diagnostic Codes

This/these CPT code(s) are add on code(s). See the primary procedure code that this code is performed with for your ICD-10-CM code selections. Diagnostic code(s) would be the same as the actual procedure performed.

AMA: 38746 2019,Feb,8; 2018,Jan,8; 2017,Jan,8; 2016,Jan,13; 2015,Jan,16; 2014,May,3; 2014,Jan,11

Relative Value Units/Medicare Edits

Non-Facility RVU	Work	PE	MP	Total
38746	4.12	1.16	0.95	6.23
Facility RVU	**Work**	**PE**	**MP**	**Total**
38746	4.12	1.16	0.95	6.23

	FUD	Status	MUE	Modifiers				IOM Reference
38746	N/A	A	1(2)	N/A	N/A	62*	80	None

* with documentation

39000-39010

39000 Mediastinotomy with exploration, drainage, removal of foreign body, or biopsy; cervical approach

39010 transthoracic approach, including either transthoracic or median sternotomy

The mediastinum describes tissues and organs bounded by lungs, spinal column, and sternum. Exploration, drainage, or removal of a foreign body or a biopsy is performed

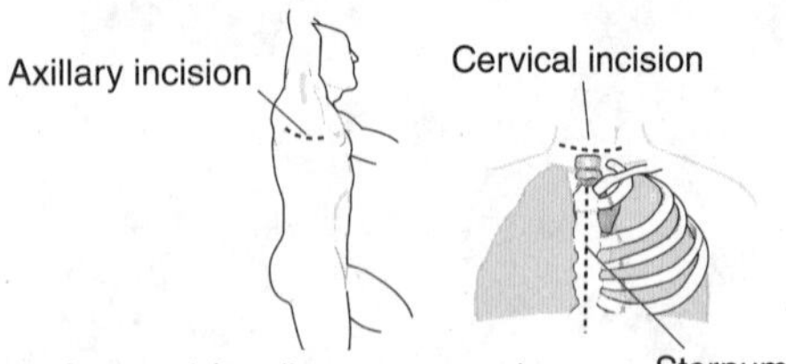

A sternal (median sternotomy) or axillary incision is employed

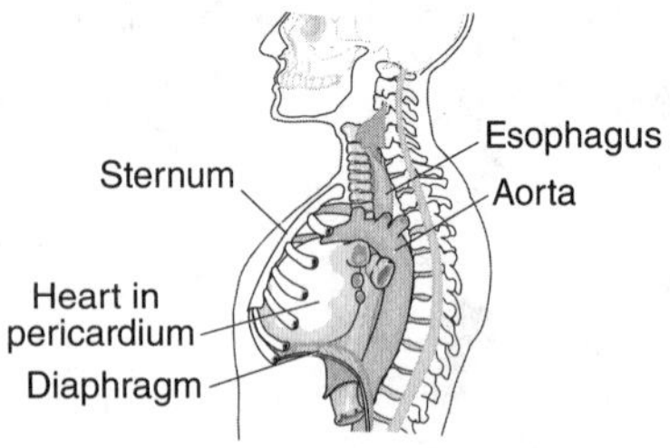

The heart, pericardium, bases of great vessels, trachea, bronchi, esophagus, thymus, thoracic lymph nodes, thoracic duct, and phrenic and vagus nerves are all part of the mediastinum

Explanation

The physician makes an incision, low in the front of the neck, pulling back the sternomastoid muscles and the cranial vessels to the side and drawing the trachea and thyroid to the center. The space behind the esophagus is exposed. The foreign body is removed, biopsy of any abnormal mass performed, and Penrose drains are placed. The incision is closed with sutures or staples. Report 39010 if using a transthoracic approach.

Coding Tips

When 39000 or 39010 is performed with another separately identifiable procedure, the highest dollar value code is listed as the primary procedure and subsequent procedures are appended with modifier 51. Do not report 39010 with 33955, 33956, 33963, or 33964. For mediastinoscopy, with or without biopsy, see 39401. For video-assisted thoracic surgery (VATS) pericardial biopsy, see 32604.

ICD-10-CM Diagnostic Codes

A15.4	Tuberculosis of intrathoracic lymph nodes
C33	Malignant neoplasm of trachea
C34.01	Malignant neoplasm of right main bronchus ☑
C34.02	Malignant neoplasm of left main bronchus ☑
C34.11	Malignant neoplasm of upper lobe, right bronchus or lung ☑
C34.12	Malignant neoplasm of upper lobe, left bronchus or lung ☑
C34.2	Malignant neoplasm of middle lobe, bronchus or lung
C34.31	Malignant neoplasm of lower lobe, right bronchus or lung ☑
C34.32	Malignant neoplasm of lower lobe, left bronchus or lung ☑
C34.81	Malignant neoplasm of overlapping sites of right bronchus and lung ☑
C34.82	Malignant neoplasm of overlapping sites of left bronchus and lung ☑
C37	Malignant neoplasm of thymus
C38.0	Malignant neoplasm of heart
C38.1	Malignant neoplasm of anterior mediastinum
C38.2	Malignant neoplasm of posterior mediastinum
C38.8	Malignant neoplasm of overlapping sites of heart, mediastinum and pleura
C45.0	Mesothelioma of pleura
C77.1	Secondary and unspecified malignant neoplasm of intrathoracic lymph nodes
C78.01	Secondary malignant neoplasm of right lung ☑
C78.02	Secondary malignant neoplasm of left lung ☑
C78.1	Secondary malignant neoplasm of mediastinum
C78.2	Secondary malignant neoplasm of pleura
C7A.090	Malignant carcinoid tumor of the bronchus and lung
C7A.091	Malignant carcinoid tumor of the thymus
C81.02	Nodular lymphocyte predominant Hodgkin lymphoma, intrathoracic lymph nodes
C81.12	Nodular sclerosis Hodgkin lymphoma, intrathoracic lymph nodes
C81.22	Mixed cellularity Hodgkin lymphoma, intrathoracic lymph nodes
C81.32	Lymphocyte depleted Hodgkin lymphoma, intrathoracic lymph nodes
C81.42	Lymphocyte-rich Hodgkin lymphoma, intrathoracic lymph nodes
C81.72	Other Hodgkin lymphoma, intrathoracic lymph nodes
C82.02	Follicular lymphoma grade I, intrathoracic lymph nodes
C82.12	Follicular lymphoma grade II, intrathoracic lymph nodes
C82.32	Follicular lymphoma grade IIIa, intrathoracic lymph nodes
C82.52	Diffuse follicle center lymphoma, intrathoracic lymph nodes
C82.62	Cutaneous follicle center lymphoma, intrathoracic lymph nodes
C82.82	Other types of follicular lymphoma, intrathoracic lymph nodes
C83.02	Small cell B-cell lymphoma, intrathoracic lymph nodes
C83.12	Mantle cell lymphoma, intrathoracic lymph nodes
C83.32	Diffuse large B-cell lymphoma, intrathoracic lymph nodes
C83.52	Lymphoblastic (diffuse) lymphoma, intrathoracic lymph nodes
C83.72	Burkitt lymphoma, intrathoracic lymph nodes
C84.02	Mycosis fungoides, intrathoracic lymph nodes
C84.12	Sezary disease, intrathoracic lymph nodes
C84.Z2	Other mature T/NK-cell lymphomas, intrathoracic lymph nodes
C85.22	Mediastinal (thymic) large B-cell lymphoma, intrathoracic lymph nodes
C85.82	Other specified types of non-Hodgkin lymphoma, intrathoracic lymph nodes
D02.1	Carcinoma in situ of trachea
D02.21	Carcinoma in situ of right bronchus and lung ☑
D02.22	Carcinoma in situ of left bronchus and lung ☑
D02.3	Carcinoma in situ of other parts of respiratory system
D14.2	Benign neoplasm of trachea
D14.31	Benign neoplasm of right bronchus and lung ☑
D14.32	Benign neoplasm of left bronchus and lung ☑
D15.0	Benign neoplasm of thymus
D15.2	Benign neoplasm of mediastinum

D19.0	Benign neoplasm of mesothelial tissue of pleura
D38.1	Neoplasm of uncertain behavior of trachea, bronchus and lung
D38.2	Neoplasm of uncertain behavior of pleura
D38.3	Neoplasm of uncertain behavior of mediastinum
D38.4	Neoplasm of uncertain behavior of thymus
D3A.090	Benign carcinoid tumor of the bronchus and lung
D3A.091	Benign carcinoid tumor of the thymus
J85.3	Abscess of mediastinum
J86.0	Pyothorax with fistula
J91.0	Malignant pleural effusion
J98.51	Mediastinitis
J98.59	Other diseases of mediastinum, not elsewhere classified
S21.321A	Laceration with foreign body of right front wall of thorax with penetration into thoracic cavity, initial encounter ☑
S21.322A	Laceration with foreign body of left front wall of thorax with penetration into thoracic cavity, initial encounter ☑
S21.341A	Puncture wound with foreign body of right front wall of thorax with penetration into thoracic cavity, initial encounter ☑
S21.342A	Puncture wound with foreign body of left front wall of thorax with penetration into thoracic cavity, initial encounter ☑
S21.421A	Laceration with foreign body of right back wall of thorax with penetration into thoracic cavity, initial encounter ☑
S21.422A	Laceration with foreign body of left back wall of thorax with penetration into thoracic cavity, initial encounter ☑
S21.441A	Puncture wound with foreign body of right back wall of thorax with penetration into thoracic cavity, initial encounter ☑
S21.442A	Puncture wound with foreign body of left back wall of thorax with penetration into thoracic cavity, initial encounter ☑

AMA: 39000 2014,Jan,11 **39010** 2018,Jan,8; 2017,Jan,8; 2016,Jan,13; 2015,Jul,3; 2015,Jan,16; 2014,Jan,11; 2014,Jan,5; 2013,Jan,6-8

Relative Value Units/Medicare Edits

Non-Facility RVU	Work	PE	MP	Total
39000	7.57	5.14	1.65	14.36
39010	13.19	6.55	2.99	22.73
Facility RVU	**Work**	**PE**	**MP**	**Total**
39000	7.57	5.14	1.65	14.36
39010	13.19	6.55	2.99	22.73

	FUD	Status	MUE	Modifiers				IOM Reference
39000	90	A	1(2)	51	N/A	62*	80	None
39010	90	A	1(2)	51	N/A	62*	80	

* with documentation

Terms To Know

abscess. Circumscribed collection of pus resulting from bacteria, frequently associated with swelling and other signs of inflammation.

hemorrhage syndrome. Fulminating meningococcal septicemia occurring in children younger than 10 years of age with vomiting, cyanosis, diarrhea, purpura, convulsions, circulatory collapse, meningitis, and hemorrhaging into adrenal glands.

39200

39200 Resection of mediastinal cyst

The mediastinum is the mass of tissues and organs bounded by lungs, spinal column, and sternum

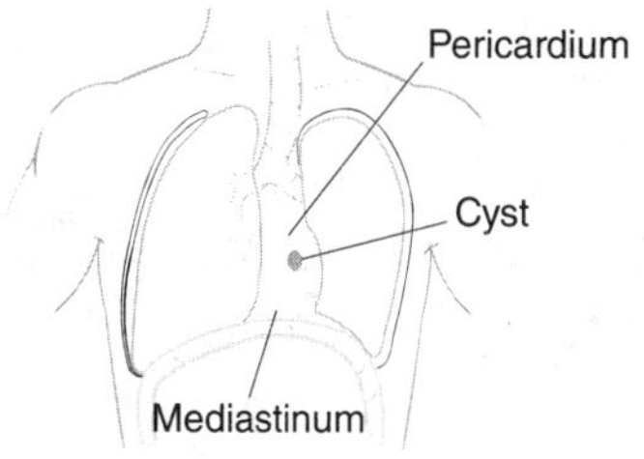

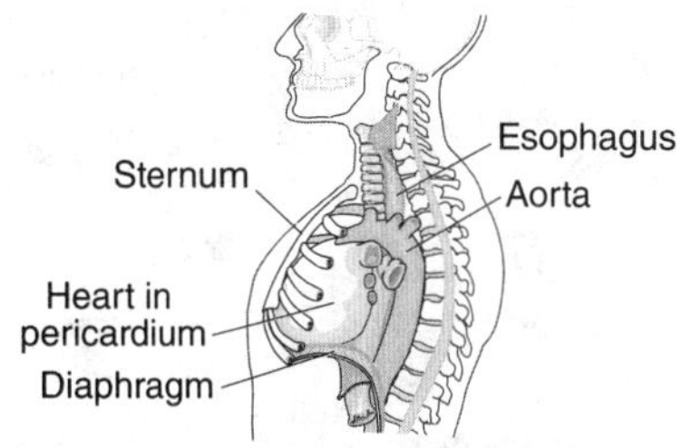

The heart, pericardium, bases of great vessels, trachea, bronchi, esophagus, thymus, thoracic lymph nodes, thoracic duct, and phrenic and vagus nerves are all part of the mediastinum

Explanation

The physician makes an incision from in front of the axilla just below the nipple line. The incision extends below the tip of the shoulder blade and ascends to halfway between the spinal column and the shoulder blade. The physician exposes the rib cage, retracting muscles. A rib spreader is used to ease access to the thoracic cavity. The cyst is located and removed. The rib spreader is removed, and the wound is closed with sutures or staples.

Coding Tips

This procedure may also be performed endoscopically. For thoracoscopic (endoscopic) excision of a mediastinal cyst, tumor, or mass, see 32662. For mediastinotomy with exploration, drainage, removal of foreign body, or biopsy, thoracic approach, see 39010; cervical approach, see 39000.

ICD-10-CM Diagnostic Codes

Q34.1	Congenital cyst of mediastinum

AMA: 39200 2014,Jan,11

Relative Value Units/Medicare Edits

Non-Facility RVU	Work	PE	MP	Total
39200	15.09	6.62	3.58	25.29
Facility RVU	**Work**	**PE**	**MP**	**Total**
39200	15.09	6.62	3.58	25.29

	FUD	Status	MUE	Modifiers				IOM Reference
39200	90	A	1(2)	51	N/A	62*	80	None

* with documentation

39220

39220 Resection of mediastinal tumor

The mediastinum is the mass of tissues and organs bounded by lungs, spinal column, and sternum

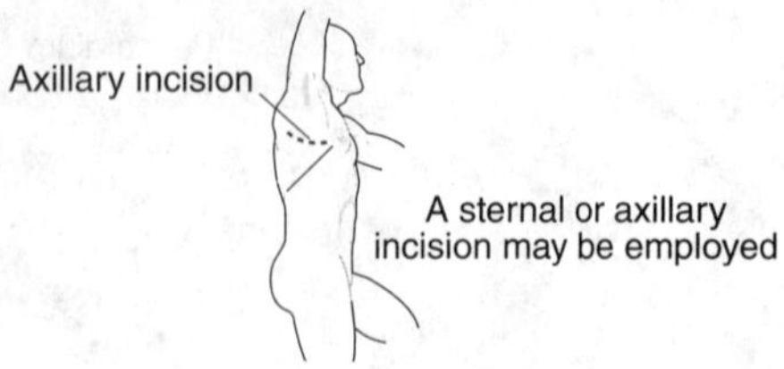

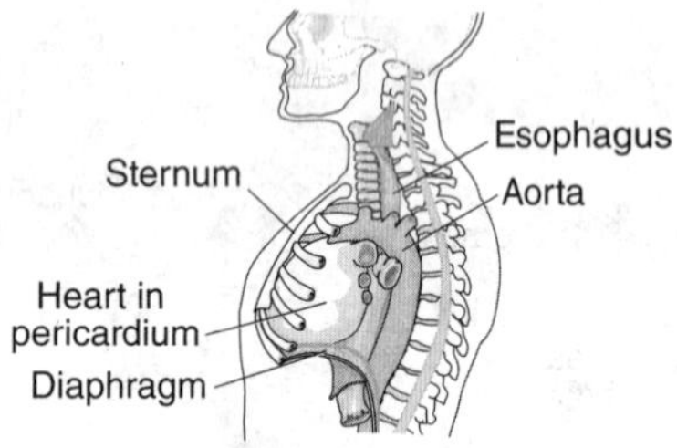

The heart, pericardium, bases of great vessels, trachea, bronchi, esophagus, thymus, thoracic lymph nodes, thoracic duct, and phrenic and vagus nerves are all part of the mediastinum

Explanation

The physician makes an incision from in front of the axilla just below the nipple line. The incision extends below the tip of the shoulder blade and ascends to halfway between the spinal column and the shoulder blade. The physician exposes the rib cage by cutting through the muscles. The chest cavity is entered between the ribs by using a rib spreader. The tumor is located and dissected from the surrounding tissue. The wound is closed using sutures or staples.

Coding Tips

This procedure may be performed endoscopically. For thoracoscopic (endoscopic) resection of a mediastinal cyst, tumor, or mass, see 32662. For mediastinotomy with exploration, drainage, removal of foreign body, or biopsy, thoracic approach, see 39010; cervical approach, see 39000. For resection of a mediastinal cyst, see 39200.

ICD-10-CM Diagnostic Codes

C38.1	Malignant neoplasm of anterior mediastinum
C38.2	Malignant neoplasm of posterior mediastinum
C38.3	Malignant neoplasm of mediastinum, part unspecified
C38.8	Malignant neoplasm of overlapping sites of heart, mediastinum and pleura
D15.2	Benign neoplasm of mediastinum
D38.3	Neoplasm of uncertain behavior of mediastinum

AMA: **39220** 2014,Jan,11

Relative Value Units/Medicare Edits

Non-Facility RVU	Work	PE	MP	Total
39220	19.55	8.88	4.35	32.78
Facility RVU	**Work**	**PE**	**MP**	**Total**
39220	19.55	8.88	4.35	32.78

	FUD	Status	MUE	Modifiers				IOM Reference
39220	90	A	1(2)	51	N/A	62*	80	None

* with documentation

Terms To Know

axillary. Area under the arm.

benign. Mild or nonmalignant in nature.

biopsy. Tissue or fluid removed for diagnostic purposes through analysis of the cells in the biopsy material.

dissect. Cut apart or separate tissue for surgical purposes or for visual or microscopic study.

excision. Surgical removal of an organ or tissue.

incision. Act of cutting into tissue or an organ.

malignant. Any condition tending to progress toward death, specifically an invasive tumor with a loss of cellular differentiation that has the ability to spread or metastasize to other body areas.

manubrium. Sternum.

mediastinotomy. Incision into the mediastinum for purposes of exploration, foreign body removal, drainage, or biopsy.

mediastinum. Collection of organs and tissues that separate the pleural sacs. Located between the sternum and spine above the diaphragm, it contains the heart and great vessels, trachea and bronchi, esophagus, thymus, lymph nodes, and nerves.

neoplasm. New abnormal growth, tumor.

tumor. Pathological swelling or enlargement; a neoplastic growth of uncontrolled, abnormal multiplication of cells.

39401-39402

39401 Mediastinoscopy; includes biopsy(ies) of mediastinal mass (eg, lymphoma), when performed

39402 with lymph node biopsy(ies) (eg, lung cancer staging)

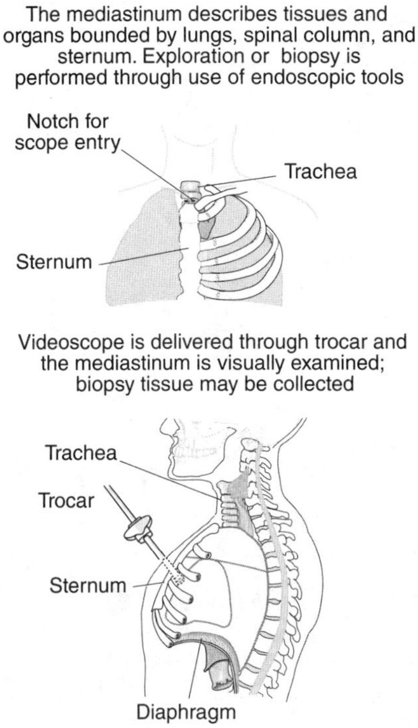

Explanation

The physician performs a mediastinoscopy. The physician makes a small incision in the notch above the sternum. The mediastinoscope is inserted and explorations are carried out between the trachea and the major vessels. The mediastinal lymph nodes, thymus, and thyroid are visualized and a biopsy(ies) may be performed through the mediastinoscope during the procedure. The scope is removed and the incision is closed with sutures or Steri-strips. Report 39401 for biopsy of a mediastinal mass. Report 39402 for a biopsy of the lymph nodes.

Coding Tips

For thoracoscopy, diagnostic, lungs, pericardial sac, mediastinal and pleural space without biopsy, see 32601; pericardial sac with biopsy, see 32604; and mediastinal space with biopsy, see 32606. For thoracoscopy, surgical with excision of mediastinal cyst, tumor, or mass, see 32662. For mediastinotomy with exploration, drainage, removal of foreign body, or biopsy, thoracic approach, see 39010; cervical approach, see 39000. For resection of a mediastinal cyst, see 39200. For resection of a mediastinal tumor, see 39220.

ICD-10-CM Diagnostic Codes

A15.4	Tuberculosis of intrathoracic lymph nodes
A15.8	Other respiratory tuberculosis
C33	Malignant neoplasm of trachea
C34.01	Malignant neoplasm of right main bronchus ☑
C34.02	Malignant neoplasm of left main bronchus ☑
C34.11	Malignant neoplasm of upper lobe, right bronchus or lung ☑
C34.12	Malignant neoplasm of upper lobe, left bronchus or lung ☑
C34.2	Malignant neoplasm of middle lobe, bronchus or lung
C34.31	Malignant neoplasm of lower lobe, right bronchus or lung ☑
C34.32	Malignant neoplasm of lower lobe, left bronchus or lung ☑
C34.81	Malignant neoplasm of overlapping sites of right bronchus and lung ☑
C34.82	Malignant neoplasm of overlapping sites of left bronchus and lung ☑
C37	Malignant neoplasm of thymus
C38.1	Malignant neoplasm of anterior mediastinum
C38.2	Malignant neoplasm of posterior mediastinum
C38.4	Malignant neoplasm of pleura
C38.8	Malignant neoplasm of overlapping sites of heart, mediastinum and pleura
C45.0	Mesothelioma of pleura
C78.01	Secondary malignant neoplasm of right lung ☑
C78.02	Secondary malignant neoplasm of left lung ☑
C78.1	Secondary malignant neoplasm of mediastinum
C78.2	Secondary malignant neoplasm of pleura
C7A.090	Malignant carcinoid tumor of the bronchus and lung
C7A.091	Malignant carcinoid tumor of the thymus
C81.02	Nodular lymphocyte predominant Hodgkin lymphoma, intrathoracic lymph nodes
C81.12	Nodular sclerosis Hodgkin lymphoma, intrathoracic lymph nodes
C81.22	Mixed cellularity Hodgkin lymphoma, intrathoracic lymph nodes
C81.42	Lymphocyte-rich Hodgkin lymphoma, intrathoracic lymph nodes
C82.02	Follicular lymphoma grade I, intrathoracic lymph nodes
C82.12	Follicular lymphoma grade II, intrathoracic lymph nodes
C82.32	Follicular lymphoma grade IIIa, intrathoracic lymph nodes
C82.42	Follicular lymphoma grade IIIb, intrathoracic lymph nodes
C82.52	Diffuse follicle center lymphoma, intrathoracic lymph nodes
C82.62	Cutaneous follicle center lymphoma, intrathoracic lymph nodes
C82.82	Other types of follicular lymphoma, intrathoracic lymph nodes
C83.02	Small cell B-cell lymphoma, intrathoracic lymph nodes
C83.32	Diffuse large B-cell lymphoma, intrathoracic lymph nodes
C83.52	Lymphoblastic (diffuse) lymphoma, intrathoracic lymph nodes
C83.72	Burkitt lymphoma, intrathoracic lymph nodes
C83.82	Other non-follicular lymphoma, intrathoracic lymph nodes
C84.02	Mycosis fungoides, intrathoracic lymph nodes
C84.12	Sezary disease, intrathoracic lymph nodes
C84.Z2	Other mature T/NK-cell lymphomas, intrathoracic lymph nodes
C85.22	Mediastinal (thymic) large B-cell lymphoma, intrathoracic lymph nodes
C85.82	Other specified types of non-Hodgkin lymphoma, intrathoracic lymph nodes
C96.Z	Other specified malignant neoplasms of lymphoid, hematopoietic and related tissue
D02.1	Carcinoma in situ of trachea
D02.21	Carcinoma in situ of right bronchus and lung ☑
D02.22	Carcinoma in situ of left bronchus and lung ☑
D02.3	Carcinoma in situ of other parts of respiratory system
D14.2	Benign neoplasm of trachea
D14.31	Benign neoplasm of right bronchus and lung ☑
D14.32	Benign neoplasm of left bronchus and lung ☑
D15.0	Benign neoplasm of thymus
D15.2	Benign neoplasm of mediastinum

D19.0	Benign neoplasm of mesothelial tissue of pleura
D38.1	Neoplasm of uncertain behavior of trachea, bronchus and lung
D38.2	Neoplasm of uncertain behavior of pleura
D38.3	Neoplasm of uncertain behavior of mediastinum
D38.4	Neoplasm of uncertain behavior of thymus
D3A.090	Benign carcinoid tumor of the bronchus and lung
D3A.091	Benign carcinoid tumor of the thymus
D86.0	Sarcoidosis of lung
D86.1	Sarcoidosis of lymph nodes
D86.2	Sarcoidosis of lung with sarcoidosis of lymph nodes
E32.8	Other diseases of thymus
J91.0	Malignant pleural effusion
J98.51	Mediastinitis
R22.2	Localized swelling, mass and lump, trunk
R59.0	Localized enlarged lymph nodes
R59.1	Generalized enlarged lymph nodes

AMA: 39401 2018,Jan,8; 2017,Jan,8; 2016,Jun,4 **39402** 2018,Jan,8; 2017,Jan,8; 2016,Jun,4

Relative Value Units/Medicare Edits

Non-Facility RVU	Work	PE	MP	Total
39401	5.44	2.24	1.28	8.96
39402	7.25	2.77	1.71	11.73
Facility RVU	**Work**	**PE**	**MP**	**Total**
39401	5.44	2.24	1.28	8.96
39402	7.25	2.77	1.71	11.73

	FUD	Status	MUE	Modifiers				IOM Reference
39401	0	A	1(3)	51	N/A	N/A	N/A	None
39402	0	A	1(3)	51	N/A	N/A	N/A	

* with documentation

Terms To Know

pleura. One of the two membranes that surround the lungs. The visceral pleura encases the lung and the parietal pleura lines the inner chest walls.

thymus. Lymphoid organ located in the front of the upper mediastinum, composed of two symmetrical pyramid-shaped lobes, that is the site where T-lymphocytes are produced.

thyroid. Endocrine gland located in the front of the lower neck composed of two lobes on either side of the trachea, responsible for secreting and storing the thyroid hormones that regulate metabolism.

trachea. Tube descending from the larynx and branching into the right and left main bronchi.

tuberculosis. Bacterial infection that typically spreads by inhalation of an airborne agent that usually attacks the lungs, but may also affect other organs.

39501

39501 Repair, laceration of diaphragm, any approach

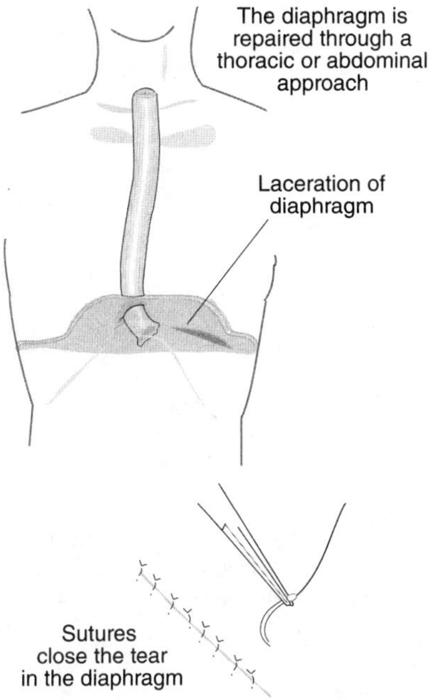

Explanation

The physician makes an abdominal or chest incision and exposes a tear in the diaphragm. The tear is repaired with nonabsorbable sutures. Occasionally, the tear may be so extensive that an artificial patch is used to repair defects or reinforce sutures. The incision is closed with sutures or staples, and a dressing is applied.

Coding Tips

When 39501 is performed with another separately identifiable procedure, the highest dollar value code is listed as the primary procedure, and subsequent procedures are appended with modifier 51.

ICD-10-CM Diagnostic Codes

S27.802A	Contusion of diaphragm, initial encounter
S27.803A	Laceration of diaphragm, initial encounter
S27.808A	Other injury of diaphragm, initial encounter
S27.809A	Unspecified injury of diaphragm, initial encounter

AMA: 39501 2018,Jan,8; 2017,Jan,8; 2016,Jan,13; 2015,Jan,16; 2014,Jan,11; 2014,Dec,16; 2014,Dec,16

Relative Value Units/Medicare Edits

Non-Facility RVU	Work	PE	MP	Total
39501	13.98	7.52	3.15	24.65
Facility RVU	**Work**	**PE**	**MP**	**Total**
39501	13.98	7.52	3.15	24.65

	FUD	Status	MUE	Modifiers				IOM Reference
39501	90	A	1(3)	51	N/A	62*	80	None

* with documentation

39540-39541

39540 Repair, diaphragmatic hernia (other than neonatal), traumatic; acute
39541 chronic

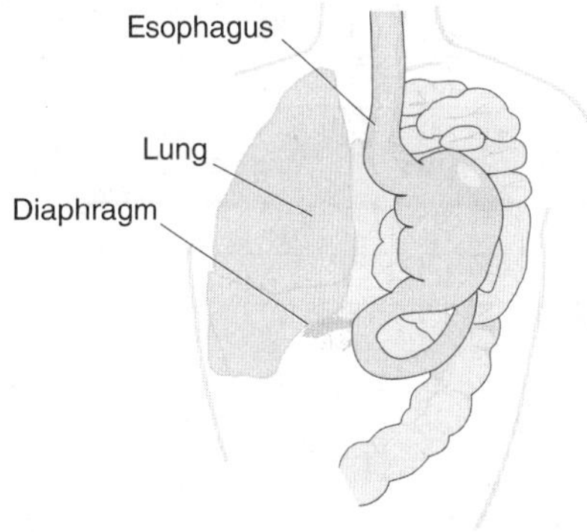

A traumatic or other defect of the diaphragm can allow abdominal contents to herniate into the thoracic cavity

Explanation

A massive injury in the diaphragm is repaired, allowing organs to protrude into the chest cavity. The physician makes an incision into the chest or abdomen. The abdominal contents are drawn back into the abdomen, and the hole in the diaphragm is exposed. The opening is closed with sutures or by insertion of a patch. The tear is repaired with nonabsorbable sutures. The incision is closed with sutures or staples. Report 39541 if the hernia is chronic.

Coding Tips

Diaphragmatic hernias, also referred to as hiatus or sliding hiatal hernias, are caused by a defect in the diaphragm, which allows a portion of the stomach to protrude above the diaphragm. These conditions are differentiated by the type of condition, including acute traumatic condition (39540) or a chronic condition (39541). To report repair of an esophageal hiatus hernia, also referred to as a paraesophageal hernia, see 43334–43337.

ICD-10-CM Diagnostic Codes

K44.0	Diaphragmatic hernia with obstruction, without gangrene
K44.1	Diaphragmatic hernia with gangrene
K44.9	Diaphragmatic hernia without obstruction or gangrene
S27.802A	Contusion of diaphragm, initial encounter
S27.803A	Laceration of diaphragm, initial encounter
S27.808A	Other injury of diaphragm, initial encounter
S27.809A	Unspecified injury of diaphragm, initial encounter

AMA: 39540 2018,Jan,8; 2017,Jan,8; 2016,Jan,13; 2015,Jan,16; 2014,Jan,11
39541 2018,Jan,8; 2017,Jan,8; 2016,Jan,13; 2015,Jan,16; 2014,Jan,11

Relative Value Units/Medicare Edits

Non-Facility RVU	Work	PE	MP	Total
39540	14.57	7.28	3.35	25.2
39541	15.75	7.85	3.65	27.25
Facility RVU	**Work**	**PE**	**MP**	**Total**
39540	14.57	7.28	3.35	25.2
39541	15.75	7.85	3.65	27.25

	FUD	Status	MUE	Modifiers				IOM Reference
39540	90	A	1(2)	51	N/A	62*	80	None
39541	90	A	1(2)	51	N/A	62*	80	

* with documentation

Terms To Know

acute. Sudden, severe.

chronic. Persistent, continuing, or recurring.

diaphragm. Muscular wall separating the thorax and its structures from the abdomen.

gangrene. Death of tissue, usually resulting from a loss of vascular supply, followed by a bacterial attack or onset of disease.

hernia. Protrusion of a body structure through tissue.

incision. Act of cutting into tissue or an organ.

obstruction. Blockage that prevents normal function of the valve or structure.

open wound. Opening or break of the skin.

suture. Numerous stitching techniques employed in wound closure.

39545

39545 Imbrication of diaphragm for eventration, transthoracic or transabdominal, paralytic or nonparalytic

The diaphragm is the muscular wall separating the thorax from the abdominal cavity

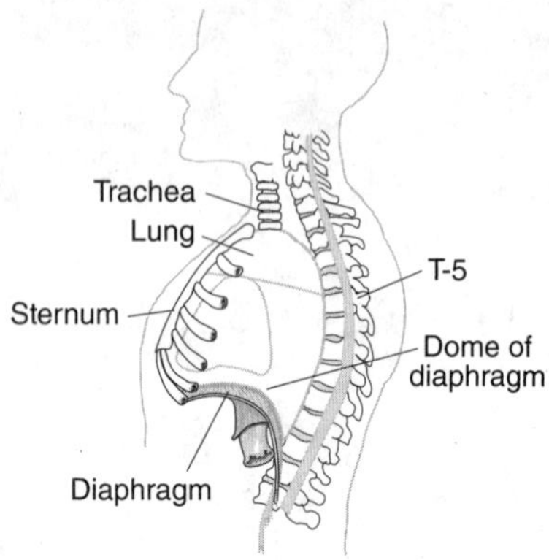

Schematic showing diaphragm

Eventration is an abnormal elevation of the dome of the diaphragm. It may occur as a result of paralysis of the phrenic nerve

Explanation

The physician makes an incision across the chest or abdomen. The abdominal contents are drawn back into the abdomen, and the diaphragm is exposed. The connective tissue is used to stitch folds or tucks into the diaphragm to restore it to its original position. The incision is closed with sutures or staples.

Coding Tips

Eventration of the diaphragm is a condition where the dome of the diaphragm is elevated, usually due to phrenic nerve paralysis. Imbrication restores the diaphragm to its normal position by the creation of a series of folds in the diaphragm. For repair of a diaphragmatic hernia (other than neonatal), traumatic, acute, see 39540; chronic, see 39541.

ICD-10-CM Diagnostic Codes

J98.6	Disorders of diaphragm
K44.0	Diaphragmatic hernia with obstruction, without gangrene
K44.1	Diaphragmatic hernia with gangrene
K44.9	Diaphragmatic hernia without obstruction or gangrene
Q79.0	Congenital diaphragmatic hernia
Q79.1	Other congenital malformations of diaphragm

AMA: 39545 2018,Jan,8; 2017,Jan,8; 2016,Jan,13; 2015,Jan,16; 2014,Jan,11

Relative Value Units/Medicare Edits

Non-Facility RVU	Work	PE	MP	Total
39545	14.67	7.68	3.36	25.71
Facility RVU	**Work**	**PE**	**MP**	**Total**
39545	14.67	7.68	3.36	25.71

	FUD	Status	MUE	Modifiers				IOM Reference
39545	90	A	1(2)	51	N/A	62*	80	None

* with documentation

43101

43101 Excision of lesion, esophagus, with primary repair; thoracic or abdominal approach

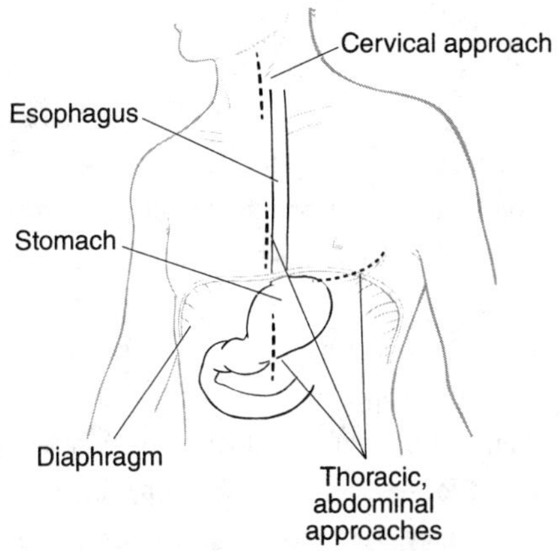

A lesion in the esophagus is removed through a thoracic or abdominal approach

Explanation

The physician removes a lesion in the esophagus. For a thoracic approach, the physician incises and dissects the left posterior chest wall to access the esophagus. For an abdominal approach, the physician makes an upper midline abdominal incision to access the esophagus transhiatally. The physician excises the lesion. The remaining esophageal borders are sutured together. The incision is closed with sutured layers.

Coding Tips

The approach is considered inherent to the procedure and should not be reported separately. For partial esophagectomy, see 43117–43123. For total or partial esophagectomy, without reconstruction (any approach), see 43124.

ICD-10-CM Diagnostic Codes

C15.3	Malignant neoplasm of upper third of esophagus
C15.4	Malignant neoplasm of middle third of esophagus
C15.5	Malignant neoplasm of lower third of esophagus
C15.8	Malignant neoplasm of overlapping sites of esophagus
D00.1	Carcinoma in situ of esophagus
D13.0	Benign neoplasm of esophagus
K22.10	Ulcer of esophagus without bleeding
K22.11	Ulcer of esophagus with bleeding
K22.8	Other specified diseases of esophagus
K23	Disorders of esophagus in diseases classified elsewhere
S27.818A	Other injury of esophagus (thoracic part), initial encounter
T28.1XXA	Burn of esophagus, initial encounter
T28.6XXA	Corrosion of esophagus, initial encounter

AMA: **43101** 2018,Jan,8; 2017,Jan,8; 2016,Jan,13; 2015,Jan,16; 2014,Jan,11

Relative Value Units/Medicare Edits

Non-Facility RVU	Work	PE	MP	Total
43101	17.07	8.01	4.06	29.14
Facility RVU	**Work**	**PE**	**MP**	**Total**
43101	17.07	8.01	4.06	29.14

	FUD	Status	MUE	Modifiers				IOM Reference
43101	90	A	1(3)	51	N/A	62*	80	None

* with documentation

Terms To Know

benign. Mild or nonmalignant in nature.

carcinoma in situ. Malignancy that arises from the cells of the vessel, gland, or organ of origin that remains confined to that site or has not invaded neighboring tissue.

excision. Surgical removal of an organ or tissue.

incision. Act of cutting into tissue or an organ.

lesion. Area of damaged tissue that has lost continuity or function, due to disease or trauma. Lesions may be located on internal structures such as the brain, nerves, or kidneys, or visible on the skin.

malignant. Any condition tending to progress toward death, specifically an invasive tumor with a loss of cellular differentiation that has the ability to spread or metastasize to other body areas.

secondary. Second in order of occurrence or importance, or appearing during the course of another disease or condition.

● New ▲ Revised + Add On AMA: CPT Assist [Resequenced] ☑ Laterality

43112

43112 Total or near total esophagectomy, with thoracotomy; with pharyngogastrostomy or cervical esophagogastrostomy, with or without pyloroplasty (ie, McKeown esophagectomy or tri-incisional esophagectomy)

Esophagus is divided at the cervical level (shown) or at its origin in the pharynx and is discarded

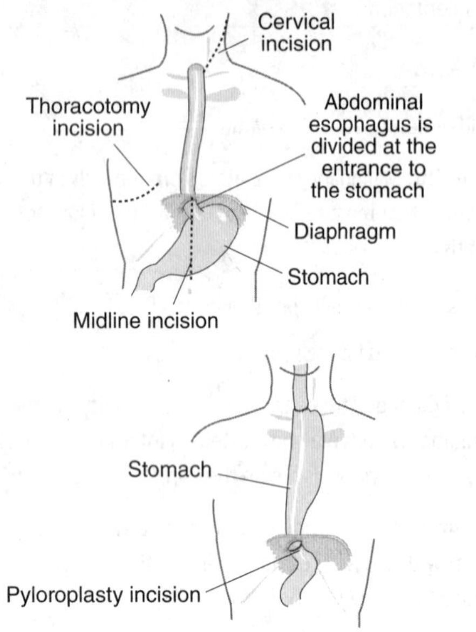

The esophagus is removed and the stomach is pulled up and attached to the remaining esophagus or to the pharynx

Explanation

The esophagus is removed through abdominal, chest, and neck incisions and replaced with stomach. The physician makes a midline abdominal incision. The stomach is dissected free of surrounding structures and the esophagus is mobilized as it passes through the diaphragm to the stomach. The physician makes an incision in the right chest between the ribs and exposes the esophagus. The esophagus is mobilized under direct vision in the chest from the diaphragm to the neck. A longitudinal incision is made in the left or right neck and the esophagus is identified and mobilized in the neck. The esophagus is divided at its junction with the stomach and in the neck and the esophagus is removed. The stomach is pulled through the middle of the chest into the neck and the stomach is connected to the stump of the esophagus in the neck. The incisions are closed. This procedure is also referred to as the McKeown procedure or the tri-incisional esophagectomy.

Coding Tips

The approach is considered inherent to the procedure and should not be reported separately. If a pyloroplasty is performed, it is also not reported separately. If this procedure is performed with colon interposition or small bowel reconstruction, see 43113.

ICD-10-CM Diagnostic Codes

C15.3	Malignant neoplasm of upper third of esophagus
C15.4	Malignant neoplasm of middle third of esophagus
C15.5	Malignant neoplasm of lower third of esophagus
C15.8	Malignant neoplasm of overlapping sites of esophagus
C49.A1	Gastrointestinal stromal tumor of esophagus
K21.0	Gastro-esophageal reflux disease with esophagitis
K21.9	Gastro-esophageal reflux disease without esophagitis
K22.0	Achalasia of cardia
K22.10	Ulcer of esophagus without bleeding
K22.11	Ulcer of esophagus with bleeding
K22.3	Perforation of esophagus
K22.8	Other specified diseases of esophagus
K23	Disorders of esophagus in diseases classified elsewhere
K31.1	Adult hypertrophic pyloric stenosis
Q39.3	Congenital stenosis and stricture of esophagus
Q39.5	Congenital dilatation of esophagus
Q39.6	Congenital diverticulum of esophagus
Q39.8	Other congenital malformations of esophagus
Q40.0	Congenital hypertrophic pyloric stenosis
S27.812A	Contusion of esophagus (thoracic part), initial encounter
S27.813A	Laceration of esophagus (thoracic part), initial encounter
S27.818A	Other injury of esophagus (thoracic part), initial encounter
T28.1XXA	Burn of esophagus, initial encounter
T28.6XXA	Corrosion of esophagus, initial encounter
T54.3X1A	Toxic effect of corrosive alkalis and alkali-like substances, accidental (unintentional), initial encounter
T54.3X3A	Toxic effect of corrosive alkalis and alkali-like substances, assault, initial encounter

AMA: 43112 2018,Jul,7; 2018,Jan,8; 2017,Jan,8; 2016,Jan,13; 2015,Jan,16; 2014,Jan,11; 2013,Aug,13

Relative Value Units/Medicare Edits

Non-Facility RVU	Work	PE	MP	Total
43112	62.0	24.9	14.75	101.65
Facility RVU	**Work**	**PE**	**MP**	**Total**
43112	62.0	24.9	14.75	101.65

	FUD	Status	MUE	Modifiers				IOM Reference
43112	90	A	1(2)	51	N/A	62	80	None

* with documentation

43113

43113 Total or near total esophagectomy, with thoracotomy; with colon interposition or small intestine reconstruction, including intestine mobilization, preparation, and anastomosis(es)

Esophagus is divided at the cervical level (shown) or at its origin in the pharynx and removed

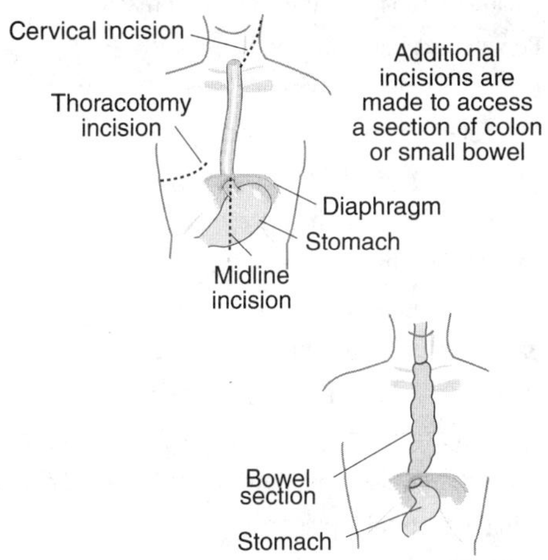

Resected bowel is attached to the stomach and remaining portion of the esophagus or pharynx

Explanation

The physician removes the esophagus through abdominal, chest and neck incisions and replaces the esophagus with colon or small bowel. The physician makes a midline abdominal incision. The stomach is dissected free of surrounding structures and the esophagus is mobilized as it passes through the diagram to the stomach. The physician makes an incision in the right chest between the ribs and exposes the esophagus. The esophagus is mobilized under direct vision in the chest from the diaphragm to the neck. The esophagus is divided at its junction with the stomach and in the neck and the esophagus is removed. The physician selects an appropriate segment of colon or small bowel. The bowel is divided proximal and distal to this segment and the bowel ends are reapproximated. The selected segment of colon or small bowel is pulled through the middle section of the chest and connected to the stump of the esophagus in the neck and to the stomach in the abdomen. The incisions are closed.

Coding Tips

The approach is considered inherent to the procedure and should not be reported separately. If an operating microscope is utilized during anastomosis, report 69990 in addition to the primary procedure. However, head gear (e.g., loupes or binoculars) is considered an integral part of this procedure.

ICD-10-CM Diagnostic Codes

C15.3	Malignant neoplasm of upper third of esophagus
C15.4	Malignant neoplasm of middle third of esophagus
C15.5	Malignant neoplasm of lower third of esophagus
C15.8	Malignant neoplasm of overlapping sites of esophagus
C49.A1	Gastrointestinal stromal tumor of esophagus
K22.4	Dyskinesia of esophagus
K22.8	Other specified diseases of esophagus
K23	Disorders of esophagus in diseases classified elsewhere
Q39.5	Congenital dilatation of esophagus
Q39.6	Congenital diverticulum of esophagus
Q39.8	Other congenital malformations of esophagus
S27.812A	Contusion of esophagus (thoracic part), initial encounter
S27.813A	Laceration of esophagus (thoracic part), initial encounter
S27.818A	Other injury of esophagus (thoracic part), initial encounter
T28.1XXA	Burn of esophagus, initial encounter
T28.6XXA	Corrosion of esophagus, initial encounter
T54.3X1A	Toxic effect of corrosive alkalis and alkali-like substances, accidental (unintentional), initial encounter
T54.3X3A	Toxic effect of corrosive alkalis and alkali-like substances, assault, initial encounter

AMA: **43113** 2014,Jan,11

Relative Value Units/Medicare Edits

Non-Facility RVU	Work	PE	MP	Total
43113	80.06	27.29	19.48	126.83
Facility RVU	**Work**	**PE**	**MP**	**Total**
43113	80.06	27.29	19.48	126.83

	FUD	Status	MUE	Modifiers				IOM Reference
43113	90	A	1(2)	51	N/A	62	80	None

* with documentation

Terms To Know

anastomosis. Surgically created connection between ducts, blood vessels, or bowel segments to allow flow from one to the other.

distal. Located farther away from a specified reference point or the trunk.

interposition. Placement between objects.

proximal. Located closest to a specified reference point, usually the midline or trunk.

resect. Cutting out or removing a portion or all of a bone, organ, or other structure.

43117

43117 Partial esophagectomy, distal two-thirds, with thoracotomy and separate abdominal incision, with or without proximal gastrectomy; with thoracic esophagogastrostomy, with or without pyloroplasty (Ivor Lewis)

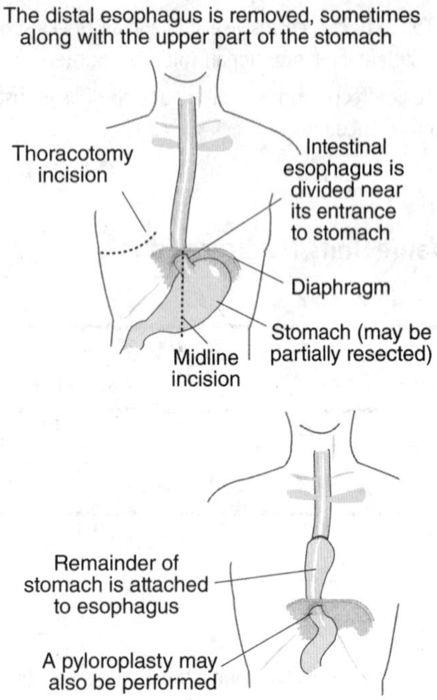

Explanation

The physician removes the distal esophagus and possibly the proximal stomach through abdominal and chest incisions and replaces the esophagus with the remaining stomach. The physician makes a midline abdominal incision. The stomach is dissected free of surrounding structures and the esophagus is mobilized as it passes through the diaphragm to the stomach. The esophagus is divided at its connection to the stomach or the stomach may be divided near its middle portion. Next, a right chest incision is made between the ribs to expose the esophagus. The distal esophagus is mobilized under direct vision and divided above its diseased segment. The distal esophagus and attached proximal stomach are then removed. The remaining stomach is pulled into the chest and connected to the stump of the proximal esophagus. Drains are placed into the chest near the new anastomosis and the incisions are closed.

Coding Tips

Partial esophagectomy procedures are defined by site. This code reports procedures on the distal (lower) two-thirds of the esophagus. The approach is considered inherent to the procedure and should not be reported separately. Distal esophagectomy procedures include proximal gastrectomy when performed. If an operating microscope is utilized during anastomosis, report 69990 in addition to the primary procedure. However, head gear (e.g., loupes or binoculars) is considered an integral part of this procedure. If this procedure is performed with colon interposition or small bowel reconstruction, see 43118. For partial esophagectomy of the cervical (proximal one-third) esophagus, see 43116. For partial esophagectomy, distal two-thirds, by thoracic approach only with esophagogastrostomy, with or without pyloroplasty, see 43121. For partial esophagectomy by thoracoabdominal or abdominal approach with esophagogastrostomy, with or without pyloroplasty, see 43122.

ICD-10-CM Diagnostic Codes

C15.3	Malignant neoplasm of upper third of esophagus
C15.4	Malignant neoplasm of middle third of esophagus
C15.5	Malignant neoplasm of lower third of esophagus
C15.8	Malignant neoplasm of overlapping sites of esophagus
C16.0	Malignant neoplasm of cardia
C49.A1	Gastrointestinal stromal tumor of esophagus
C7A.092	Malignant carcinoid tumor of the stomach
D3A.092	Benign carcinoid tumor of the stomach
K22.10	Ulcer of esophagus without bleeding
K22.11	Ulcer of esophagus with bleeding
K22.4	Dyskinesia of esophagus
K22.5	Diverticulum of esophagus, acquired
K22.70	Barrett's esophagus without dysplasia
K22.710	Barrett's esophagus with low grade dysplasia
K22.711	Barrett's esophagus with high grade dysplasia
K22.8	Other specified diseases of esophagus
K23	Disorders of esophagus in diseases classified elsewhere
K25.2	Acute gastric ulcer with both hemorrhage and perforation
K31.1	Adult hypertrophic pyloric stenosis
Q39.5	Congenital dilatation of esophagus
Q39.6	Congenital diverticulum of esophagus
Q39.8	Other congenital malformations of esophagus
S27.812A	Contusion of esophagus (thoracic part), initial encounter
S27.813A	Laceration of esophagus (thoracic part), initial encounter
S27.818A	Other injury of esophagus (thoracic part), initial encounter
T28.1XXA	Burn of esophagus, initial encounter
T28.6XXA	Corrosion of esophagus, initial encounter

AMA: 43117 2014,Jan,11

Relative Value Units/Medicare Edits

Non-Facility RVU	Work	PE	MP	Total
43117	57.5	23.24	13.65	94.39
Facility RVU	**Work**	**PE**	**MP**	**Total**
43117	57.5	23.24	13.65	94.39

	FUD	Status	MUE	Modifiers				IOM Reference
43117	90	A	1(2)	51	N/A	62	80	None

* with documentation

43118

43118 Partial esophagectomy, distal two-thirds, with thoracotomy and separate abdominal incision, with or without proximal gastrectomy; with colon interposition or small intestine reconstruction, including intestine mobilization, preparation, and anastomosis(es)

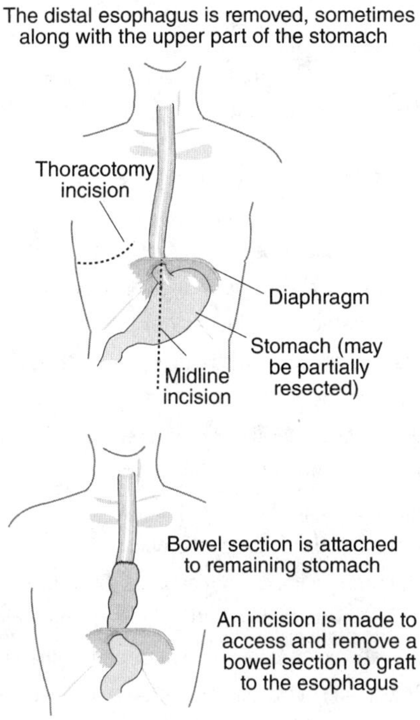

Explanation

The physician removes the distal esophagus and possibly proximal stomach through abdominal and chest incisions and replaces the esophagus with colon or small bowel. The physician makes a midline abdominal incision. The stomach is dissected free of surrounding structures and the esophagus is mobilized as it passes through the diaphragm to the stomach. The esophagus is divided at its connection to the stomach or the stomach may be divided near its middle portion. An appropriate segment of colon or small bowel is selected and the bowel is divided proximal and distal to this segment and the bowel ends re-approximated. One end of the selected bowel segment is connected to the remaining stomach and the other end is placed through the diaphragm into the chest. A right chest incision is made between the ribs to expose the esophagus. The distal esophagus is mobilized under direct vision and divided above its diseased segment. The distal esophagus and attached proximal stomach are removed. The remaining end of the segment of colon or small bowel that has been attached to the stomach is pulled into the chest and connected to the stump of the proximal esophagus. Drains are placed into the chest near the new anastomosis and the incisions are closed.

Coding Tips

Partial esophagectomy procedures are defined by site. This code reports procedures on the distal (lower) two-thirds of the esophagus. The approach is considered inherent to the procedure and should not be reported separately. Distal esophagectomy procedures include proximal gastrectomy when performed. If an operating microscope is utilized during anastomosis, report 69990 in addition to the primary procedure. However, head gear (e.g., loupes or binoculars) is considered an integral part of this procedure. When only a single incision, thoracoabdominal or abdominal, is made to perform this procedure, report 43123. For partial esophagectomy of the cervical (proximal one-third) esophagus, see 43116. For partial esophagectomy, distal two-thirds, by thoracic approach with separate abdominal incision (Ivor Lewis procedure), see 43117; by thoracic approach only, see 43121; by thoracoabdominal or abdominal approach, see 43122.

ICD-10-CM Diagnostic Codes

C15.3	Malignant neoplasm of upper third of esophagus
C15.4	Malignant neoplasm of middle third of esophagus
C15.5	Malignant neoplasm of lower third of esophagus
C15.8	Malignant neoplasm of overlapping sites of esophagus
C16.0	Malignant neoplasm of cardia
C49.A1	Gastrointestinal stromal tumor of esophagus
C7A.092	Malignant carcinoid tumor of the stomach
D3A.092	Benign carcinoid tumor of the stomach
K22.10	Ulcer of esophagus without bleeding
K22.11	Ulcer of esophagus with bleeding
K22.4	Dyskinesia of esophagus
K22.5	Diverticulum of esophagus, acquired
K22.70	Barrett's esophagus without dysplasia
K22.710	Barrett's esophagus with low grade dysplasia
K22.711	Barrett's esophagus with high grade dysplasia
K22.8	Other specified diseases of esophagus
K23	Disorders of esophagus in diseases classified elsewhere
K25.0	Acute gastric ulcer with hemorrhage
K25.2	Acute gastric ulcer with both hemorrhage and perforation
K25.3	Acute gastric ulcer without hemorrhage or perforation
K25.4	Chronic or unspecified gastric ulcer with hemorrhage
Q39.5	Congenital dilatation of esophagus
Q39.6	Congenital diverticulum of esophagus
Q39.8	Other congenital malformations of esophagus
S27.812A	Contusion of esophagus (thoracic part), initial encounter
S27.813A	Laceration of esophagus (thoracic part), initial encounter
S27.818A	Other injury of esophagus (thoracic part), initial encounter
T28.1XXA	Burn of esophagus, initial encounter
T28.6XXA	Corrosion of esophagus, initial encounter

AMA: **43118** 2014,Jan,11

Relative Value Units/Medicare Edits

Non-Facility RVU	Work	PE	MP	Total
43118	67.07	22.47	16.16	105.7
Facility RVU	**Work**	**PE**	**MP**	**Total**
43118	67.07	22.47	16.16	105.7

	FUD	Status	MUE	Modifiers				IOM Reference
43118	90	A	1(2)	51	N/A	62	80	None

* with documentation

43121

43121 Partial esophagectomy, distal two-thirds, with thoracotomy only, with or without proximal gastrectomy, with thoracic esophagogastrostomy, with or without pyloroplasty

The distal esophagus is removed, sometimes along with the upper part of the stomach

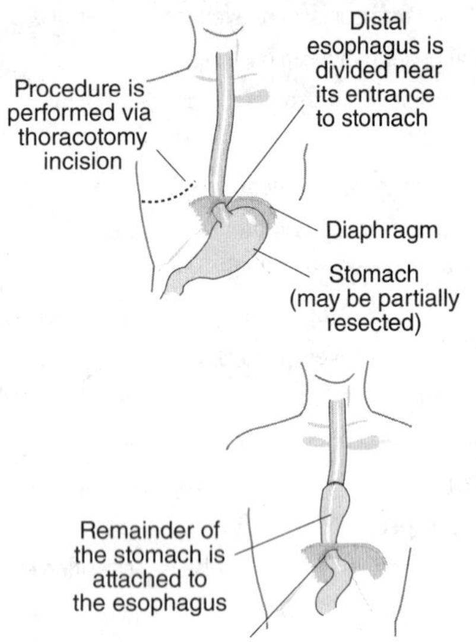

A pyloroplasty may also be performed

Explanation

The physician removes the affected part of the esophagus and proximal stomach and reattaches the remaining stomach to the esophageal stump. The physician accesses the esophagus through a right posterolateral thoracotomy; no abdominal incision is made. The physician resects the affected portion of the distal esophagus and sometimes a portion of the proximal stomach. The resected area is removed. The stomach or gastric remnant is pulled into the thorax and sutured to the esophageal stump. If the stomach is used as the esophageal conduit, a pyloroplasty may be performed to open the pyloric sphincter. The incision is sutured in layers.

Coding Tips

Partial esophagectomy procedures are defined by site. This code reports procedures on the distal (lower) two-thirds of the esophagus. The approach is considered inherent to the procedure and should not be reported separately. Distal esophagectomy procedures include proximal gastrectomy when performed. If an operating microscope is utilized during anastomosis, report 69990 in addition to the primary procedure. However, head gear (e.g., loupes or binoculars) is considered an integral part of this procedure. For partial esophagectomy of the cervical (proximal one-third) esophagus, see 43116. For partial esophagectomy, distal two-thirds, by thoracic approach only with separate abdominal incision, with esophagogastrostomy, with or without pyloroplasty (Ivor Lewis procedure), see 43117. For partial esophagectomy, distal two-thirds, by thoracic approach only with separate abdominal incision, with colon interposition or small intestine reconstruction, see 43118. For partial esophagectomy by thoracoabdominal or abdominal approach with esophagogastrostomy, with or without pyloroplasty, see 43122.

ICD-10-CM Diagnostic Codes

C15.3	Malignant neoplasm of upper third of esophagus
C15.4	Malignant neoplasm of middle third of esophagus
C15.5	Malignant neoplasm of lower third of esophagus
C15.8	Malignant neoplasm of overlapping sites of esophagus
C16.0	Malignant neoplasm of cardia
C49.A1	Gastrointestinal stromal tumor of esophagus
C7A.092	Malignant carcinoid tumor of the stomach
D3A.092	Benign carcinoid tumor of the stomach
K22.10	Ulcer of esophagus without bleeding
K22.11	Ulcer of esophagus with bleeding
K22.2	Esophageal obstruction
K22.3	Perforation of esophagus
K22.4	Dyskinesia of esophagus
K22.70	Barrett's esophagus without dysplasia
K22.710	Barrett's esophagus with low grade dysplasia
K22.711	Barrett's esophagus with high grade dysplasia
K22.8	Other specified diseases of esophagus
K23	Disorders of esophagus in diseases classified elsewhere
K25.0	Acute gastric ulcer with hemorrhage
K25.2	Acute gastric ulcer with both hemorrhage and perforation
K25.3	Acute gastric ulcer without hemorrhage or perforation
K25.4	Chronic or unspecified gastric ulcer with hemorrhage
K31.1	Adult hypertrophic pyloric stenosis
Q39.5	Congenital dilatation of esophagus
Q39.6	Congenital diverticulum of esophagus
Q39.8	Other congenital malformations of esophagus
S27.812A	Contusion of esophagus (thoracic part), initial encounter
S27.813A	Laceration of esophagus (thoracic part), initial encounter
S27.818A	Other injury of esophagus (thoracic part), initial encounter
T28.1XXA	Burn of esophagus, initial encounter
T28.6XXA	Corrosion of esophagus, initial encounter

AMA: **43121** 2014,Jan,11

Relative Value Units/Medicare Edits

Non-Facility RVU	Work	PE	MP	Total
43121	51.43	19.3	12.27	83.0
Facility RVU	**Work**	**PE**	**MP**	**Total**
43121	51.43	19.3	12.27	83.0

	FUD	Status	MUE	Modifiers				IOM Reference
43121	90	A	1(2)	51	N/A	62	80	None

* with documentation

43122

43122 Partial esophagectomy, thoracoabdominal or abdominal approach, with or without proximal gastrectomy; with esophagogastrostomy, with or without pyloroplasty

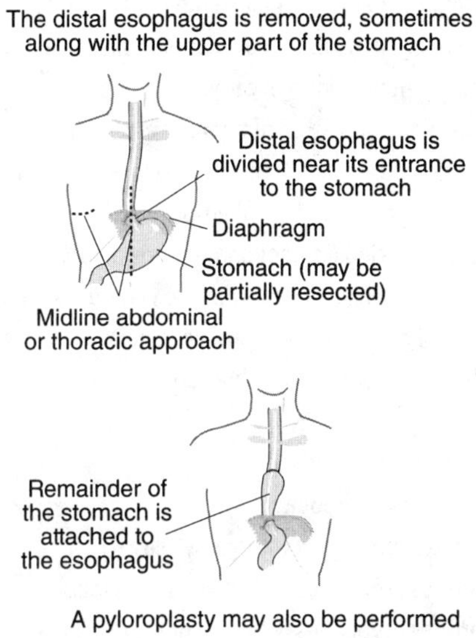

Explanation

The physician removes the distal esophagus and possibly proximal stomach through a combined abdominal and chest incision and replaces the esophagus with the remaining stomach. The physician makes a midline abdominal incision. The stomach is dissected free of surrounding structures and the esophagus is mobilized as it passes through the diaphragm to the stomach. The esophagus is divided proximally above the diseased area and distally at its junction with the stomach or the middle portion of the stomach may be divided. The distal esophagus and attached proximal stomach are removed. The remaining stomach is connected to the stump of the esophagus. The incision is closed.

Coding Tips

Partial esophagectomy procedures are defined by site. Even though it is not specifically stated in the procedure definition, because the approach is thoracoabdominal or abdominal, this code reports procedures on the distal esophagus. The approach is considered inherent to the procedure and should not be reported separately. Distal esophagectomy procedures include proximal gastrectomy when performed. If an operating microscope is utilized during anastomosis, report 69990 in addition to the primary procedure. However, head gear (e.g., loupes or binoculars) is considered an integral part of this procedure. For partial esophagectomy of the cervical (proximal one-third) esophagus, see 43116. For partial esophagectomy, distal two-thirds, by thoracic approach only with separate abdominal incision, with esophagogastrostomy, with or without pyloroplasty (Ivor Lewis procedure), see 43117. For partial esophagectomy, distal two-thirds, by thoracic approach only with separate abdominal incision, with colon interposition or small intestine reconstruction, see 43118. For partial esophagectomy, distal two-thirds, by thoracic approach only with esophagogastrostomy, with or without pyloroplasty, see 43121.

ICD-10-CM Diagnostic Codes

C15.3	Malignant neoplasm of upper third of esophagus
C15.4	Malignant neoplasm of middle third of esophagus
C15.5	Malignant neoplasm of lower third of esophagus
C15.8	Malignant neoplasm of overlapping sites of esophagus
C16.0	Malignant neoplasm of cardia
C49.A1	Gastrointestinal stromal tumor of esophagus
C7A.092	Malignant carcinoid tumor of the stomach
D00.1	Carcinoma in situ of esophagus
D3A.092	Benign carcinoid tumor of the stomach
K21.9	Gastro-esophageal reflux disease without esophagitis
K22.10	Ulcer of esophagus without bleeding
K22.11	Ulcer of esophagus with bleeding
K22.2	Esophageal obstruction
K22.3	Perforation of esophagus
K22.4	Dyskinesia of esophagus
K22.70	Barrett's esophagus without dysplasia
K22.710	Barrett's esophagus with low grade dysplasia
K22.711	Barrett's esophagus with high grade dysplasia
K22.8	Other specified diseases of esophagus
K23	Disorders of esophagus in diseases classified elsewhere
K25.0	Acute gastric ulcer with hemorrhage
K25.2	Acute gastric ulcer with both hemorrhage and perforation
K25.3	Acute gastric ulcer without hemorrhage or perforation
K25.4	Chronic or unspecified gastric ulcer with hemorrhage
K31.1	Adult hypertrophic pyloric stenosis
Q39.5	Congenital dilatation of esophagus
Q39.6	Congenital diverticulum of esophagus
Q39.8	Other congenital malformations of esophagus
S27.812A	Contusion of esophagus (thoracic part), initial encounter
S27.813A	Laceration of esophagus (thoracic part), initial encounter
S27.818A	Other injury of esophagus (thoracic part), initial encounter
T28.1XXA	Burn of esophagus, initial encounter
T28.6XXA	Corrosion of esophagus, initial encounter

AMA: **43122** 2014,Jan,11

Relative Value Units/Medicare Edits

Non-Facility RVU	Work	PE	MP	Total
43122	44.18	19.6	10.33	74.11
Facility RVU	**Work**	**PE**	**MP**	**Total**
43122	44.18	19.6	10.33	74.11

	FUD	Status	MUE	Modifiers				IOM Reference
43122	90	A	1(2)	51	N/A	62*	80	None

* with documentation

43123

43123 Partial esophagectomy, thoracoabdominal or abdominal approach, with or without proximal gastrectomy; with colon interposition or small intestine reconstruction, including intestine mobilization, preparation, and anastomosis(es)

The diseased esophagus is removed, sometimes along with the upper part of the stomach

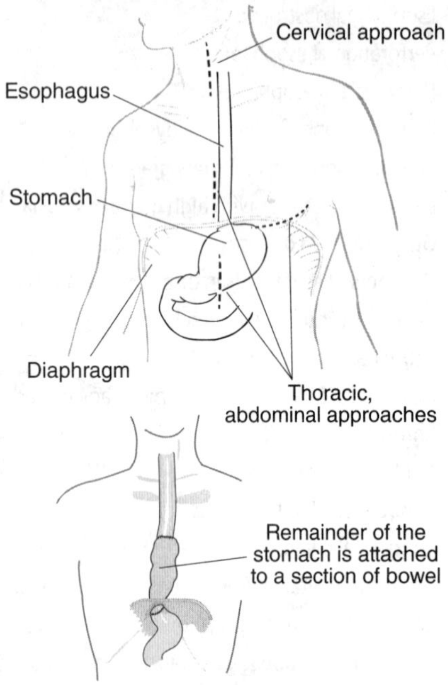

A midline abdominal incision is made to access and remove a bowel section to graft to the esophagus

Explanation

The physician removes the distal esophagus and possibly the proximal stomach through a combined abdominal and chest incision and replaces the esophagus with colon or small bowel. The physician makes a midline abdominal incision that may extend onto the chest between the ribs. The stomach is dissected free of surrounding structures and the esophagus is mobilized as it passes through the diaphragm to the stomach. The esophagus is divided proximally above the diseased area and distally at its junction with the stomach or the middle portion of the stomach may be divided. The distal esophagus and attached stomach are removed. An appropriate segment of colon or small bowel is selected. The bowel is divided proximal and distal to the segment and the bowel ends are re- approximated. The selected segment of bowel is connected proximally to the remaining esophageal stump and distally to the remaining stomach. The incision is closed.

Coding Tips

Partial esophagectomy procedures are defined by site. Even though it is not specifically stated in the procedure definition, because the approach is thoracoabdominal or abdominal, this code reports procedures on the distal esophagus. The approach is considered inherent to the procedure and should not be reported separately. Distal esophagectomy procedures include proximal gastrectomy when performed. If an operating microscope is utilized during anastomosis, report 69990 in addition to the primary procedure. However, head gear (e.g., loupes or binoculars) is considered an integral part of this procedure. For partial esophagectomy of the cervical (proximal one-third) esophagus, see 43116. For partial esophagectomy, distal two-thirds, by thoracic approach only with separate abdominal incision (Ivor Lewis procedure), see 43117; by thoracic approach only with separate abdominal incision, with colon interposition or small intestine reconstruction, see 43118; by thoracic approach only, see 43121; by thoracoabdominal or abdominal approach, see 43122.

ICD-10-CM Diagnostic Codes

C15.3	Malignant neoplasm of upper third of esophagus
C15.4	Malignant neoplasm of middle third of esophagus
C15.5	Malignant neoplasm of lower third of esophagus
C15.8	Malignant neoplasm of overlapping sites of esophagus
C16.0	Malignant neoplasm of cardia
C49.A1	Gastrointestinal stromal tumor of esophagus
C7A.092	Malignant carcinoid tumor of the stomach
D00.1	Carcinoma in situ of esophagus
D3A.092	Benign carcinoid tumor of the stomach
K21.9	Gastro-esophageal reflux disease without esophagitis
K22.10	Ulcer of esophagus without bleeding
K22.11	Ulcer of esophagus with bleeding
K22.2	Esophageal obstruction
K22.3	Perforation of esophagus
K22.4	Dyskinesia of esophagus
K22.70	Barrett's esophagus without dysplasia
K22.710	Barrett's esophagus with low grade dysplasia
K22.711	Barrett's esophagus with high grade dysplasia
K22.8	Other specified diseases of esophagus
K23	Disorders of esophagus in diseases classified elsewhere
K25.0	Acute gastric ulcer with hemorrhage
K25.1	Acute gastric ulcer with perforation
K25.2	Acute gastric ulcer with both hemorrhage and perforation
K25.3	Acute gastric ulcer without hemorrhage or perforation
K25.4	Chronic or unspecified gastric ulcer with hemorrhage
K31.1	Adult hypertrophic pyloric stenosis
Q39.5	Congenital dilatation of esophagus
Q39.6	Congenital diverticulum of esophagus
Q39.8	Other congenital malformations of esophagus
S27.812A	Contusion of esophagus (thoracic part), initial encounter
S27.813A	Laceration of esophagus (thoracic part), initial encounter
S27.818A	Other injury of esophagus (thoracic part), initial encounter
T28.1XXA	Burn of esophagus, initial encounter
T28.6XXA	Corrosion of esophagus, initial encounter

AMA: **43123** 2014,Jan,11

Relative Value Units/Medicare Edits

Non-Facility RVU	Work	PE	MP	Total
43123	83.12	28.15	20.25	131.52
Facility RVU	**Work**	**PE**	**MP**	**Total**
43123	83.12	28.15	20.25	131.52

	FUD	Status	MUE	Modifiers				IOM Reference
43123	90	A	1(2)	51	N/A	62*	80	None

* with documentation

43135

43135 Diverticulectomy of hypopharynx or esophagus, with or without myotomy; thoracic approach

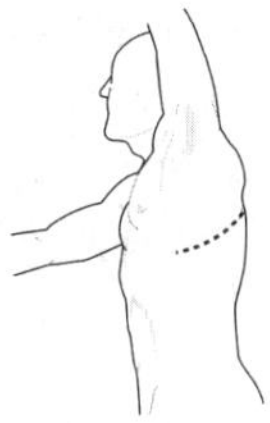

Posterolateral thoracotomy incision

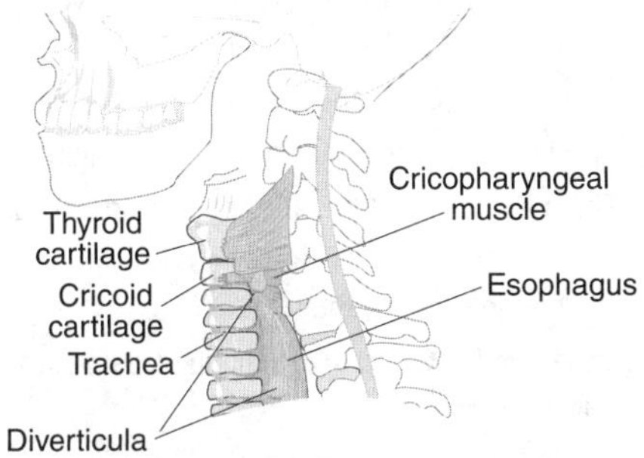

A diverticulum of the hypopharynx or upper esophagus is removed by thoracotomy

Explanation

The physician removes a diverticulum from the hypopharynx or esophagus. A diverticulum is a pouch that occurs normally or because of a defect in the muscular membrane. The physician incises and dissects the left posterior chest wall. The physician may dissect or incise the cricopharyngeous muscle to expose the diverticulum. If a myotomy is necessary, the physician makes a vertical incision through the cricopharyngeous muscle. The physician clamps the diverticulum and closes using sutures or staples. The operative incision is closed with sutured layers.

Coding Tips

The approach is considered inherent to the procedure and should not be reported separately. For excision of a lesion, esophagus, with primary repair, thoracic or abdominal approach, see 43101.

ICD-10-CM Diagnostic Codes

K22.2	Esophageal obstruction
K22.5	Diverticulum of esophagus, acquired
Q38.7	Congenital pharyngeal pouch
Q39.5	Congenital dilatation of esophagus
Q39.6	Congenital diverticulum of esophagus
Q39.8	Other congenital malformations of esophagus
Q39.9	Congenital malformation of esophagus, unspecified
R13.11	Dysphagia, oral phase
R13.13	Dysphagia, pharyngeal phase
R13.14	Dysphagia, pharyngoesophageal phase
R13.19	Other dysphagia

AMA: 43135 2018,Jan,8; 2017,Jan,8; 2016,Jan,13; 2015,Jan,16; 2014,Jan,11

Relative Value Units/Medicare Edits

Non-Facility RVU	Work	PE	MP	Total
43135	26.17	10.37	6.22	42.76
Facility RVU	**Work**	**PE**	**MP**	**Total**
43135	26.17	10.37	6.22	42.76

	FUD	Status	MUE	Modifiers				IOM Reference
43135	90	A	1(3)	51	N/A	62*	80	None

* with documentation

Terms To Know

acquired. Produced by outside influences and not by genetics or birth defect.

anomaly. Irregularity in the structure or position of an organ or tissue.

clamp. Tool used to grip, compress, join, or fasten body parts.

congenital. Present at birth, occurring through heredity or an influence during gestation up to the moment of birth.

excision. Surgical removal of an organ or tissue.

incision. Act of cutting into tissue or an organ.

myotomy. Surgical cutting of a muscle to gain access to underlying tissues or for therapeutic reasons.

suture. Numerous stitching techniques employed in wound closure.

buried suture. Continuous or interrupted suture placed under the skin for a layered closure.

continuous suture. Running stitch with tension evenly distributed across a single strand to provide a leakproof closure line.

interrupted suture. Series of single stitches with tension isolated at each stitch, in which all stitches are not affected if one becomes loose, and the isolated sutures cannot act as a wick to transport an infection.

purse-string suture. Continuous suture placed around a tubular structure and tightened, to reduce or close the lumen.

retention suture. Secondary stitching that bridges the primary suture, providing support for the primary repair; a plastic or rubber bolster may be placed over the primary repair and under the retention sutures.

43310-43312

43310 Esophagoplasty (plastic repair or reconstruction), thoracic approach; without repair of tracheoesophageal fistula
43312 with repair of tracheoesophageal fistula

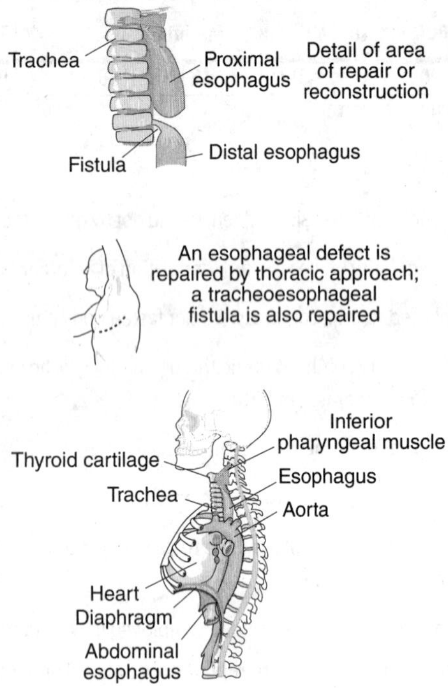

Explanation

The physician repairs a defect in the esophagus using plastic repair or reconstruction. The physician makes a thoracic incision to access the esophagus. In 43310, the defect is identified and repaired. For 43312, the physician also transects the tracheoesophageal fistula. The physician closes the tracheal opening and repairs the esophagus. The incision is sutured in layers.

Coding Tips

The approach is considered inherent to the procedure and should not be reported separately.

ICD-10-CM Diagnostic Codes

C15.3	Malignant neoplasm of upper third of esophagus
C15.4	Malignant neoplasm of middle third of esophagus
C15.5	Malignant neoplasm of lower third of esophagus
C15.8	Malignant neoplasm of overlapping sites of esophagus
D00.1	Carcinoma in situ of esophagus
D13.0	Benign neoplasm of esophagus
J95.04	Tracheo-esophageal fistula following tracheostomy
K22.10	Ulcer of esophagus without bleeding
K22.11	Ulcer of esophagus with bleeding
K22.2	Esophageal obstruction
K22.3	Perforation of esophagus
K22.4	Dyskinesia of esophagus
K22.5	Diverticulum of esophagus, acquired
K22.6	Gastro-esophageal laceration-hemorrhage syndrome
K22.70	Barrett's esophagus without dysplasia
K22.710	Barrett's esophagus with low grade dysplasia
K22.711	Barrett's esophagus with high grade dysplasia
K22.8	Other specified diseases of esophagus
K44.0	Diaphragmatic hernia with obstruction, without gangrene
K44.1	Diaphragmatic hernia with gangrene
K44.9	Diaphragmatic hernia without obstruction or gangrene
Q39.0	Atresia of esophagus without fistula
Q39.1	Atresia of esophagus with tracheo-esophageal fistula
Q39.2	Congenital tracheo-esophageal fistula without atresia
Q39.3	Congenital stenosis and stricture of esophagus
Q39.4	Esophageal web
Q40.1	Congenital hiatus hernia
Q40.8	Other specified congenital malformations of upper alimentary tract
S27.812A	Contusion of esophagus (thoracic part), initial encounter
S27.813A	Laceration of esophagus (thoracic part), initial encounter
S27.818A	Other injury of esophagus (thoracic part), initial encounter
T18.190A	Other foreign object in esophagus causing compression of trachea, initial encounter
T18.198A	Other foreign object in esophagus causing other injury, initial encounter

AMA: 43310 2014,Jan,11; 2013,Jan,11-12 **43312** 2014,Jan,11; 2013,Jan,11-12

Relative Value Units/Medicare Edits

Non-Facility RVU	Work	PE	MP	Total
43310	26.26	10.52	6.24	43.02
43312	29.25	10.11	6.95	46.31
Facility RVU	**Work**	**PE**	**MP**	**Total**
43310	26.26	10.52	6.24	43.02
43312	29.25	10.11	6.95	46.31

	FUD	Status	MUE	Modifiers				IOM Reference
43310	90	A	1(2)	51	N/A	62*	80	None
43312	90	A	1(2)	51	N/A	62*	80	

* with documentation

43320

43320 Esophagogastrostomy (cardioplasty), with or without vagotomy and pyloroplasty, transabdominal or transthoracic approach

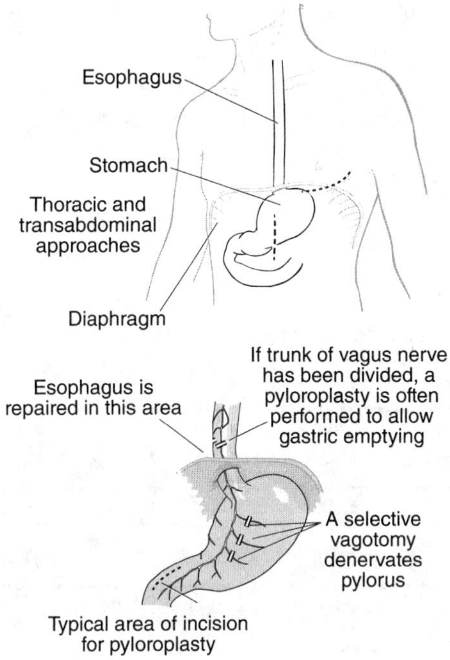

Explanation

The physician performs a plastic repair of the lower esophagus where it joins the upper area (cardia) of the stomach. The physician may also transect the vagus nerve and/or enlarge the pylorus, the distal portion of the stomach. The physician accesses the esophagus through an upper abdominal or lateral thoracic incision. The diseased portion of the esophagus is resected. An anastomosis between the esophageal stump and the cardiac portion of the stomach is created. If the lesion is secondary to acid reflux, a vagotomy may be performed. The anterior and posterior trunks of the vagus nerve are transected to decrease acid production. If the gastric outlet area is decreased, a pyloroplasty may be performed to enlarge the pylorus. The incision is repaired in sutured layers.

Coding Tips

The approach is considered inherent to the procedure and should not be reported separately.

ICD-10-CM Diagnostic Codes

C15.3	Malignant neoplasm of upper third of esophagus
C15.4	Malignant neoplasm of middle third of esophagus
C15.5	Malignant neoplasm of lower third of esophagus
C16.0	Malignant neoplasm of cardia
C7A.092	Malignant carcinoid tumor of the stomach
D00.1	Carcinoma in situ of esophagus
D00.2	Carcinoma in situ of stomach
I85.00	Esophageal varices without bleeding
I85.01	Esophageal varices with bleeding
I85.10	Secondary esophageal varices without bleeding
I85.11	Secondary esophageal varices with bleeding
K22.0	Achalasia of cardia
K22.10	Ulcer of esophagus without bleeding
K22.11	Ulcer of esophagus with bleeding
K22.2	Esophageal obstruction
K22.3	Perforation of esophagus
K22.70	Barrett's esophagus without dysplasia
K22.710	Barrett's esophagus with low grade dysplasia
K22.711	Barrett's esophagus with high grade dysplasia
Q39.0	Atresia of esophagus without fistula
Q39.1	Atresia of esophagus with tracheo-esophageal fistula
Q39.2	Congenital tracheo-esophageal fistula without atresia
Q39.3	Congenital stenosis and stricture of esophagus
Q39.4	Esophageal web
Q39.5	Congenital dilatation of esophagus
Q39.6	Congenital diverticulum of esophagus
Q39.8	Other congenital malformations of esophagus
S27.812A	Contusion of esophagus (thoracic part), initial encounter
S27.813A	Laceration of esophagus (thoracic part), initial encounter
S27.818A	Other injury of esophagus (thoracic part), initial encounter
T18.190A	Other foreign object in esophagus causing compression of trachea, initial encounter
T18.198A	Other foreign object in esophagus causing other injury, initial encounter

AMA: **43320** 2014,Jan,11; 2013,Jan,11-12

Relative Value Units/Medicare Edits

Non-Facility RVU	Work	PE	MP	Total
43320	23.31	11.61	5.65	40.57
Facility RVU	**Work**	**PE**	**MP**	**Total**
43320	23.31	11.61	5.65	40.57

	FUD	Status	MUE	Modifiers				IOM Reference
43320	90	A	1(2)	51	N/A	62*	80	None

* with documentation

Terms To Know

anastomosis. Surgically created connection between ducts, blood vessels, or bowel segments to allow flow from one to the other.

cardia. Portion of the stomach next to and surrounding the cardiac esophageal opening.

fistula. Abnormal tube-like passage between two body cavities or organs or from an organ to the outside surface.

lateral. Located away from the medial plane or farther away from the middle of the body.

pyloroplasty. Enlargement and reconstruction of the lower portion of the stomach opening into the duodenum performed after vagotomy to speed gastric emptying and treat duodenal ulcers.

transection. Transverse dissection; to cut across a long axis; cross section.

vagotomy. Division of the vagus nerves, interrupting impulses resulting in lower gastric acid production and hastening gastric emptying. Used in the treatment of chronic gastric, pyloric, and duodenal ulcers that can cause severe pain and difficulties in eating and sleeping.

43331

43331 Esophagomyotomy (Heller type); thoracic approach

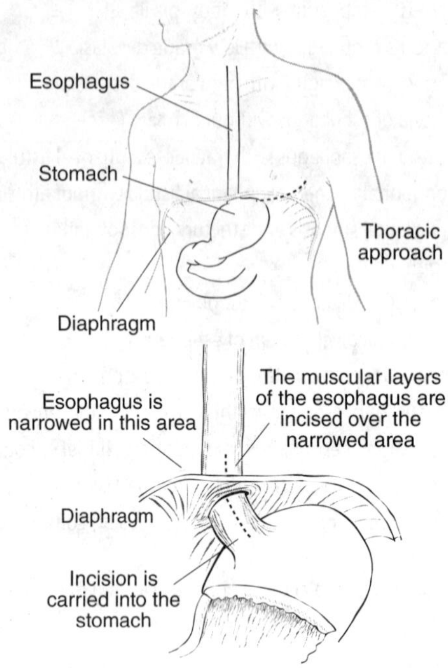

The muscle tissues of the esophagus are incised with the incision carried into the stomach musculature. This relaxes the stricture in the esophagus

Explanation

The esophagus is repaired using a fundic flap. The physician accesses the esophagus through a thoracic incision. The physician makes an incision into the muscular layers of the distal esophagus and cardia of the stomach (myotomy), leaving a gastric fundic flap. The flap is pulled up along the esophagus and sutured onto the margins of the myotomy. Repair of a hiatal hernia is performed by restoring the herniated portion of the stomach back to the abdomen, then narrowing the hiatal opening of the diaphragm by suturing the left and right crura together. All incisions are sutured in layers.

Coding Tips

The approach is considered inherent to the procedure and should not be reported separately.

ICD-10-CM Diagnostic Codes

C15.3	Malignant neoplasm of upper third of esophagus
C15.4	Malignant neoplasm of middle third of esophagus
C15.5	Malignant neoplasm of lower third of esophagus
C15.8	Malignant neoplasm of overlapping sites of esophagus
K21.0	Gastro-esophageal reflux disease with esophagitis
K21.9	Gastro-esophageal reflux disease without esophagitis
K22.0	Achalasia of cardia
K22.10	Ulcer of esophagus without bleeding
K22.11	Ulcer of esophagus with bleeding
K22.2	Esophageal obstruction
K22.3	Perforation of esophagus
K22.5	Diverticulum of esophagus, acquired
K22.6	Gastro-esophageal laceration-hemorrhage syndrome
K22.70	Barrett's esophagus without dysplasia
K22.710	Barrett's esophagus with low grade dysplasia
K22.711	Barrett's esophagus with high grade dysplasia
K22.8	Other specified diseases of esophagus
K23	Disorders of esophagus in diseases classified elsewhere
K44.0	Diaphragmatic hernia with obstruction, without gangrene
K44.9	Diaphragmatic hernia without obstruction or gangrene
Q39.5	Congenital dilatation of esophagus
Q39.6	Congenital diverticulum of esophagus
Q39.8	Other congenital malformations of esophagus
Q79.0	Congenital diaphragmatic hernia
Q79.1	Other congenital malformations of diaphragm

AMA: 43331 2018,Jan,8; 2017,Jan,8; 2016,Jan,13; 2015,Jan,16; 2014,Jan,11; 2013,Jan,11-12

Relative Value Units/Medicare Edits

Non-Facility RVU	Work	PE	MP	Total
43331	23.06	10.31	5.47	38.84
Facility RVU	**Work**	**PE**	**MP**	**Total**
43331	23.06	10.31	5.47	38.84

	FUD	Status	MUE	Modifiers				IOM Reference
43331	90	A	1(2)	51	N/A	62*	80	None

* with documentation

Terms To Know

hiatal hernia. Protrusion of an abdominal organ, usually the stomach, through the esophageal opening within the diaphragm and occurring in two types: the sliding hiatal hernia and the paraesophageal hernia.

incision. Act of cutting into tissue or an organ.

malignant. Any condition tending to progress toward death, specifically an invasive tumor with a loss of cellular differentiation that has the ability to spread or metastasize to other body areas.

myotomy. Surgical cutting of a muscle to gain access to underlying tissues or for therapeutic reasons.

stenosis. Narrowing or constriction of a passage.

stricture. Narrowing of an anatomical structure.

43341

43341 Esophagojejunostomy (without total gastrectomy); thoracic approach

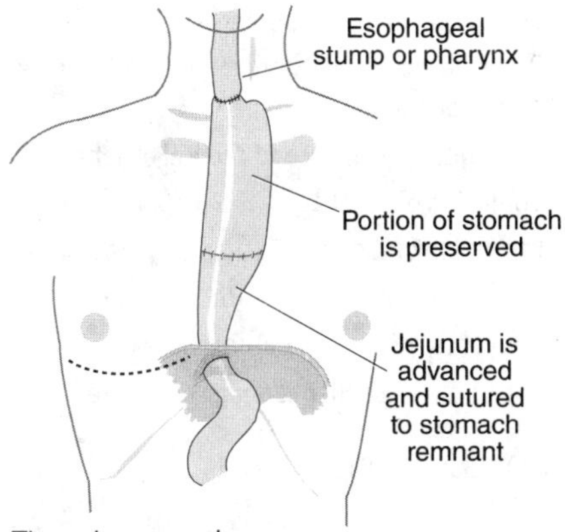

Thoracic approach

Explanation

The physician removes the affected esophagus and stomach, using the remaining stomach and jejunum to restore gastrointestinal continuity. The physician accesses the esophagus and stomach through a thoracic incision. The physician resects the affected part of the esophagus. The stomach is advanced through the hiatus and sutured to the esophageal remnant. The antral portion of the stomach is excised and the proximal jejunum is sutured to the gastric remnant. The distal end of the duodenum is anastomosed to the jejunum; the proximal end of the duodenum is sutured closed to form a blind pouch. The incision is sutured in layers.

Coding Tips

The approach is considered inherent to the procedure and should not be reported separately.

ICD-10-CM Diagnostic Codes

C15.3	Malignant neoplasm of upper third of esophagus
C15.4	Malignant neoplasm of middle third of esophagus
C15.5	Malignant neoplasm of lower third of esophagus
C15.8	Malignant neoplasm of overlapping sites of esophagus
C16.0	Malignant neoplasm of cardia
C16.1	Malignant neoplasm of fundus of stomach
C16.2	Malignant neoplasm of body of stomach
C16.3	Malignant neoplasm of pyloric antrum
C16.4	Malignant neoplasm of pylorus
C16.8	Malignant neoplasm of overlapping sites of stomach
C7A.092	Malignant carcinoid tumor of the stomach
D13.0	Benign neoplasm of esophagus
D13.1	Benign neoplasm of stomach
D3A.092	Benign carcinoid tumor of the stomach
K21.0	Gastro-esophageal reflux disease with esophagitis
K22.2	Esophageal obstruction

AMA: 43341 2014,Jan,11; 2013,Jan,11-12

Relative Value Units/Medicare Edits

Non-Facility RVU	Work	PE	MP	Total
43341	24.23	10.63	5.74	40.6
Facility RVU	**Work**	**PE**	**MP**	**Total**
43341	24.23	10.63	5.74	40.6

	FUD	Status	MUE	Modifiers				IOM Reference
43341	90	A	1(2)	51	N/A	62*	80	None

* with documentation

Terms To Know

anastomosis. Surgically created connection between ducts, blood vessels, or bowel segments to allow flow from one to the other.

duodenum. First portion of the small intestine connected to the stomach at the pylorus and extending to the jejunum.

gastrectomy. Surgical excision of all or part of the stomach.

jejunum. Highly vascular upper two-fifths of the small intestine, extending from the duodenum to the ileum.

ulcer. Open sore or excavating lesion of skin or the tissue on the surface of an organ from the sloughing of chronically inflamed and necrosing tissue.

43351

43351 Esophagostomy, fistulization of esophagus, external; thoracic approach

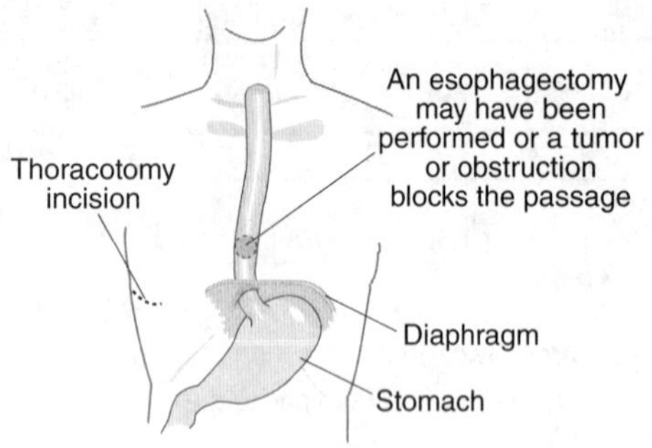

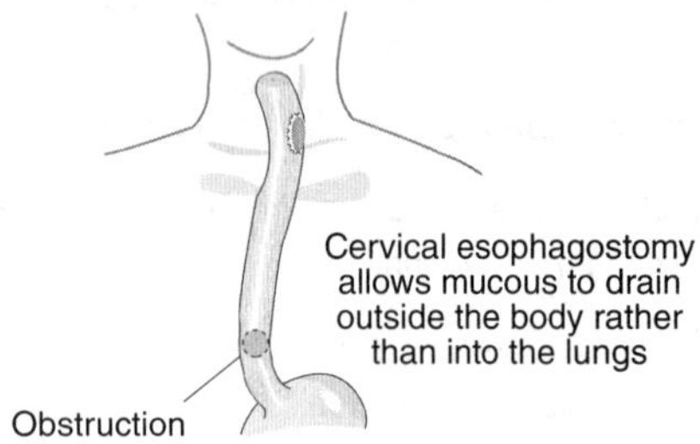

Explanation

The physician connects the esophagus to the exterior of the body, creating a fistula for drainage. The physician uses a lateral thoracotomy to access the esophagus. The physician makes an incision in the esophagus or the esophageal stump. The proximal limb of the esophagus is exteriorized and sutured into place, creating a connection from the exterior of the body to the esophageal lumen for mucus drainage. The incision is sutured in layers.

Coding Tips

Fistulization involves the surgical creation of a communication between two sites, in this case the esophagus and the exterior body. Do not confuse this code with fistula repairs, which should be reported with 43420–43425. The approach is considered inherent to the procedure and should not be reported separately.

ICD-10-CM Diagnostic Codes

C15.3	Malignant neoplasm of upper third of esophagus
C15.4	Malignant neoplasm of middle third of esophagus
C15.5	Malignant neoplasm of lower third of esophagus
C15.8	Malignant neoplasm of overlapping sites of esophagus
J86.0	Pyothorax with fistula
K22.0	Achalasia of cardia
K22.2	Esophageal obstruction
K22.3	Perforation of esophagus
K22.4	Dyskinesia of esophagus
K22.5	Diverticulum of esophagus, acquired
K22.6	Gastro-esophageal laceration-hemorrhage syndrome
K22.8	Other specified diseases of esophagus
Q39.0	Atresia of esophagus without fistula
Q39.1	Atresia of esophagus with tracheo-esophageal fistula
S11.21XA	Laceration without foreign body of pharynx and cervical esophagus, initial encounter
S11.22XA	Laceration with foreign body of pharynx and cervical esophagus, initial encounter
S11.23XA	Puncture wound without foreign body of pharynx and cervical esophagus, initial encounter
S11.24XA	Puncture wound with foreign body of pharynx and cervical esophagus, initial encounter
S11.25XA	Open bite of pharynx and cervical esophagus, initial encounter
S27.812A	Contusion of esophagus (thoracic part), initial encounter
S27.813A	Laceration of esophagus (thoracic part), initial encounter
S27.818A	Other injury of esophagus (thoracic part), initial encounter
T28.1XXA	Burn of esophagus, initial encounter
T28.6XXA	Corrosion of esophagus, initial encounter

AMA: 43351 2014,Jan,11; 2013,Jan,11-12

Relative Value Units/Medicare Edits

Non-Facility RVU	Work	PE	MP	Total
43351	22.05	10.83	5.23	38.11
Facility RVU	**Work**	**PE**	**MP**	**Total**
43351	22.05	10.83	5.23	38.11

	FUD	Status	MUE	Modifiers				IOM Reference
43351	90	A	1(2)	51	N/A	62*	80	None

* with documentation

Terms To Know

duodenum. First portion of the small intestine connected to the stomach at the pylorus and extending to the jejunum.

esophagus. Muscular tube that carries swallowed liquids and foods from the pharynx to the stomach.

gastrectomy. Surgical excision of all or part of the stomach.

jejunum. Highly vascular upper two-fifths of the small intestine, extending from the duodenum to the ileum.

43415

43415 Suture of esophageal wound or injury; transthoracic or transabdominal approach

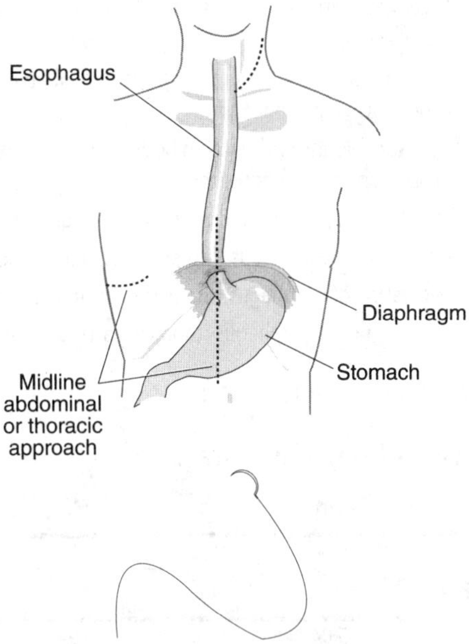

A wound or injury to the esophagus is accessed and sutured

Explanation

The physician sutures a wound or injury to the esophagus. The physician accesses the esophagus through a thoracic or transabdominal approach. The physician exposes the affected segment of the esophagus, which is repaired by suturing. The incision is sutured in layers.

Coding Tips

Additional procedures performed are reported separately. When 43415 is performed with another separately identifiable procedure, the highest dollar value code is listed as the primary procedure, and subsequent procedures are appended with modifier 51. If the procedure is completed through an operating microscope, report 69990 in addition to the primary procedure. However, head gear (e.g., loupes or binoculars) is considered an integral part of this procedure.

ICD-10-CM Diagnostic Codes

K22.6	Gastro-esophageal laceration-hemorrhage syndrome
S11.21XA	Laceration without foreign body of pharynx and cervical esophagus, initial encounter
S11.22XA	Laceration with foreign body of pharynx and cervical esophagus, initial encounter
S11.23XA	Puncture wound without foreign body of pharynx and cervical esophagus, initial encounter
S11.24XA	Puncture wound with foreign body of pharynx and cervical esophagus, initial encounter
S11.25XA	Open bite of pharynx and cervical esophagus, initial encounter
S27.812A	Contusion of esophagus (thoracic part), initial encounter
S27.813A	Laceration of esophagus (thoracic part), initial encounter
S27.818A	Other injury of esophagus (thoracic part), initial encounter
T28.1XXA	Burn of esophagus, initial encounter
T28.6XXA	Corrosion of esophagus, initial encounter

AMA: 43415 2014,Jan,11; 2013,Jan,11-12

Relative Value Units/Medicare Edits

Non-Facility RVU	Work	PE	MP	Total
43415	44.88	19.28	10.5	74.66
Facility RVU	**Work**	**PE**	**MP**	**Total**
43415	44.88	19.28	10.5	74.66

	FUD	Status	MUE	Modifiers				IOM Reference
43415	90	A	1(3)	51	N/A	62*	80	None

* with documentation

Terms To Know

hemorrhage syndrome. Fulminating meningococcal septicemia occurring in children younger than 10 years of age with vomiting, cyanosis, diarrhea, purpura, convulsions, circulatory collapse, meningitis, and hemorrhaging into adrenal glands.

laceration. Tearing injury; a torn, ragged-edged wound.

open wound. Opening or break of the skin.

suture. Numerous stitching techniques employed in wound closure.

buried suture. Continuous or interrupted suture placed under the skin for a layered closure.

continuous suture. Running stitch with tension evenly distributed across a single strand to provide a leakproof closure line.

interrupted suture. Series of single stitches with tension isolated at each stitch, in which all stitches are not affected if one becomes loose, and the isolated sutures cannot act as a wick to transport an infection.

purse-string suture. Continuous suture placed around a tubular structure and tightened, to reduce or close the lumen.

retention suture. Secondary stitching that bridges the primary suture, providing support for the primary repair; a plastic or rubber bolster may be placed over the primary repair and under the retention sutures.

43425

43425 Closure of esophagostomy or fistula; transthoracic or transabdominal approach

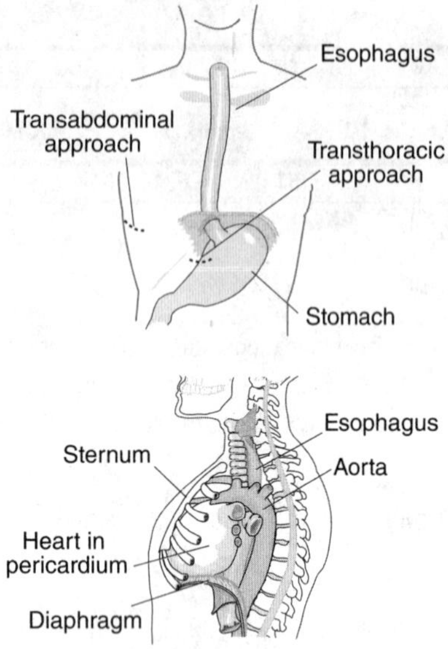

An esophagostomy or esophageal fistula is repaired

Explanation

The physician closes an opening in the esophagus and returns it to its natural position. The physician accesses the defect through a midline abdominal incision or a thoracic incision. The physician closes the opening with sutures and repositions the esophagus to its normal anatomical position. The incision is sutured in layers.

Coding Tips

The approach is considered inherent to the procedure and should not be reported separately. For fistulization of the esophagus, see 43351. For repair of an esophageal hiatal hernia, see 43332 and 43333. For transthoracic repair of a diaphragmatic hernia, see 43334 and 43335.

ICD-10-CM Diagnostic Codes

J86.0	Pyothorax with fistula
K20.0	Eosinophilic esophagitis
K21.0	Gastro-esophageal reflux disease with esophagitis
K22.0	Achalasia of cardia
K22.10	Ulcer of esophagus without bleeding
K22.11	Ulcer of esophagus with bleeding
K22.3	Perforation of esophagus
K22.4	Dyskinesia of esophagus
K22.5	Diverticulum of esophagus, acquired
K22.70	Barrett's esophagus without dysplasia
K22.710	Barrett's esophagus with low grade dysplasia
K22.711	Barrett's esophagus with high grade dysplasia
K22.8	Other specified diseases of esophagus
K23	Disorders of esophagus in diseases classified elsewhere
Q39.1	Atresia of esophagus with tracheo-esophageal fistula
Q39.2	Congenital tracheo-esophageal fistula without atresia
Q39.3	Congenital stenosis and stricture of esophagus
Q39.4	Esophageal web
Q39.8	Other congenital malformations of esophagus
S11.21XA	Laceration without foreign body of pharynx and cervical esophagus, initial encounter
S11.22XA	Laceration with foreign body of pharynx and cervical esophagus, initial encounter
S11.23XA	Puncture wound without foreign body of pharynx and cervical esophagus, initial encounter
S11.24XA	Puncture wound with foreign body of pharynx and cervical esophagus, initial encounter
S11.25XA	Open bite of pharynx and cervical esophagus, initial encounter
S27.812A	Contusion of esophagus (thoracic part), initial encounter
S27.813A	Laceration of esophagus (thoracic part), initial encounter
S27.818A	Other injury of esophagus (thoracic part), initial encounter

AMA: 43425 2014,Jan,11; 2013,Jan,11-12

Relative Value Units/Medicare Edits

Non-Facility RVU	Work	PE	MP	Total
43425	25.04	10.85	5.94	41.83
Facility RVU	**Work**	**PE**	**MP**	**Total**
43425	25.04	10.85	5.94	41.83

	FUD	Status	MUE	Modifiers				IOM Reference
43425	90	A	1(3)	51	N/A	62*	80	None

* with documentation

Terms To Know

achalasia. Failure of the smooth muscles within the gastrointestinal tract to relax at points of junction; most commonly referring to the esophagogastric sphincter's failure to relax when swallowing.

congenital. Present at birth, occurring through heredity or an influence during gestation up to the moment of birth.

dyskinesia of esophagus. Difficult or impaired voluntary muscle movement of the esophagus.

fistula. Abnormal tube-like passage between two body cavities or organs or from an organ to the outside surface.

incision. Act of cutting into tissue or an organ.

malignant. Any condition tending to progress toward death, specifically an invasive tumor with a loss of cellular differentiation that has the ability to spread or metastasize to other body areas.

vesicoureteral reflux. Urine passage from the bladder flows backward up into the ureter and kidneys that can lead to bacterial infection and an increase in hydrostatic pressure, causing kidney damage.

49425-49427

49425 Insertion of peritoneal-venous shunt
49426 Revision of peritoneal-venous shunt
49427 Injection procedure (eg, contrast media) for evaluation of previously placed peritoneal-venous shunt

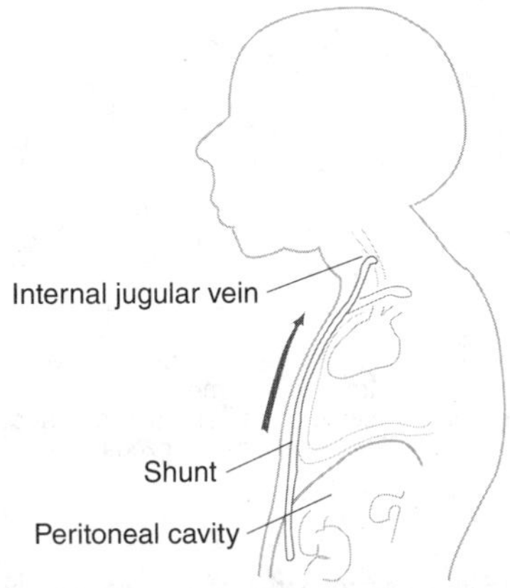

A shunt is prepared and inserted, revised, or injection performed to evaluate shunt function from the peritoneal cavity to a major vein

Explanation

In 49425, the physician places a peritoneal-venous shunt. The physician makes a small lateral upper abdominal incision. Dissection is carried through the abdominal wall layers, the peritoneum is entered and the peritoneal end of the catheter is inserted into the peritoneal cavity and sutured into place. A subcutaneous tunnel is created from the abdominal incision up to the neck and the catheter is pulled through the tunnel into the neck. A counter incision is made in the neck over the internal jugular vein and the venous end of the catheter is inserted into the jugular vein. The incisions are closed. In 49426, the peritoneal-venous shunt is revised. The physician may remove the shunt by incisions over the venous and peritoneal insertion sites with a subcutaneous tunnel created from the abdominal incision up to the neck where the catheter is pulled through the tunnel into the neck. A counter incision is made in the neck over the internal jugular vein and the venous end of the catheter is inserted into the jugular vein. Alternately, the physician may make an incision over the dysfunctional end of the shunt and replace that portion of the shunt and insert it back into the peritoneal cavity or jugular vein. In 49427, the physician injects contrast into a peritoneo-venous shunt. The physician injects contrast material through the skin into the reservoir of the peritoneo-venous shunt. Radiography is used to visualize the flow of contrast through the shunt into the peritoneal and venous ends for evaluation.

Coding Tips

For shunt patency test, see 78291. For radiological supervision and interpretation of an injection procedure performed to evaluate previously placed peritoneal-venous shunt, see 75809 or 78291.

ICD-10-CM Diagnostic Codes

B25.2	Cytomegaloviral pancreatitis
K68.11	Postprocedural retroperitoneal abscess
K70.11	Alcoholic hepatitis with ascites
K70.31	Alcoholic cirrhosis of liver with ascites
K71.51	Toxic liver disease with chronic active hepatitis with ascites
K74.0	Hepatic fibrosis
K74.69	Other cirrhosis of liver
K85.00	Idiopathic acute pancreatitis without necrosis or infection
K85.01	Idiopathic acute pancreatitis with uninfected necrosis
K85.02	Idiopathic acute pancreatitis with infected necrosis
K85.10	Biliary acute pancreatitis without necrosis or infection
K85.11	Biliary acute pancreatitis with uninfected necrosis
K85.12	Biliary acute pancreatitis with infected necrosis
K85.20	Alcohol induced acute pancreatitis without necrosis or infection
K85.21	Alcohol induced acute pancreatitis with uninfected necrosis
K85.22	Alcohol induced acute pancreatitis with infected necrosis
K85.30	Drug induced acute pancreatitis without necrosis or infection
K85.31	Drug induced acute pancreatitis with uninfected necrosis
K85.32	Drug induced acute pancreatitis with infected necrosis
K85.80	Other acute pancreatitis without necrosis or infection
K86.0	Alcohol-induced chronic pancreatitis
K86.1	Other chronic pancreatitis
K86.2	Cyst of pancreas
K86.3	Pseudocyst of pancreas
K86.81	Exocrine pancreatic insufficiency
K86.89	Other specified diseases of pancreas
K87	Disorders of gallbladder, biliary tract and pancreas in diseases classified elsewhere
R18.0	Malignant ascites
R18.8	Other ascites
T81.41XA	Infection following a procedure, superficial incisional surgical site, initial encounter
T81.42XA	Infection following a procedure, deep incisional surgical site, initial encounter
T81.43XA	Infection following a procedure, organ and space surgical site, initial encounter
T81.44XA	Sepsis following a procedure, initial encounter
T81.49XA	Infection following a procedure, other surgical site, initial encounter
T82.818A	Embolism due to vascular prosthetic devices, implants and grafts, initial encounter
T82.828A	Fibrosis due to vascular prosthetic devices, implants and grafts, initial encounter
T82.838A	Hemorrhage due to vascular prosthetic devices, implants and grafts, initial encounter
T82.848A	Pain due to vascular prosthetic devices, implants and grafts, initial encounter
T82.856A	Stenosis of peripheral vascular stent, initial encounter
T82.858A	Stenosis of other vascular prosthetic devices, implants and grafts, initial encounter
T82.868A	Thrombosis due to vascular prosthetic devices, implants and grafts, initial encounter
Z45.2	Encounter for adjustment and management of vascular access device

AMA: 49425 2014,Jan,11; 2013,Jan,11-12 **49426** 2014,Jan,11; 2013,Jan,11-12 **49427** 2014,Jan,11; 2013,Jan,11-12

Abdomen

Relative Value Units/Medicare Edits

Non-Facility RVU	Work	PE	MP	Total
49425	12.22	6.45	2.18	20.85
49426	10.41	5.23	2.22	17.86
49427	0.89	0.31	0.12	1.32
Facility RVU	**Work**	**PE**	**MP**	**Total**
49425	12.22	6.45	2.18	20.85
49426	10.41	5.23	2.22	17.86
49427	0.89	0.31	0.12	1.32

	FUD	Status	MUE	Modifiers				IOM Reference
49425	90	A	1(2)	51	N/A	62*	80	None
49426	90	A	1(3)	51	N/A	N/A	N/A	
49427	0	A	1(3)	51	N/A	N/A	80*	

* with documentation

Terms To Know

patency. State of a tube-like structure or conduit being open and unobstructed.

peritoneum. Strong, continuous membrane that forms the lining of the abdominal and pelvic cavity. The parietal peritoneum, or outer layer, is attached to the abdominopelvic walls and the visceral peritoneum, or inner layer, surrounds the organs inside the abdominal cavity.

shunt. Surgically created passage between blood vessels or other natural passages, such as an arteriovenous anastomosis, to divert or bypass blood flow from the normal channel.

49428-49429

49428 Ligation of peritoneal-venous shunt
49429 Removal of peritoneal-venous shunt

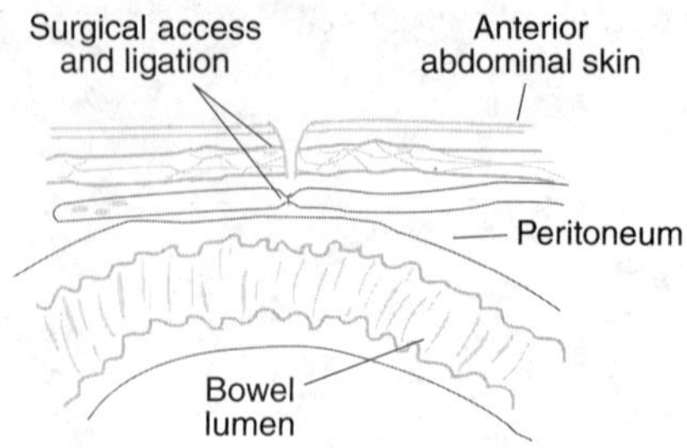

Access is usually by incising the skin over the percutaneous tunnel. This measure is often the simplest way to close off the shunt and assess the body's ability to absorb the excess fluids

Explanation

In 49428, the physician performs ligation of a previously placed peritoneo-venous shunt. The physician makes an incision over the path of the shunt. The shunt tubing under the incision is isolated and ligated with sutures. The incision is closed. In 49429, the physician performs removal of a peritoneal venous shunt. An incision is made over the abdominal insertion site of the shunt. The shunt is dissected from surrounding scar tissue and removed from the abdominal cavity. The fascia and peritoneum of the abdominal insertion site is closed. Usually, the venous end of the catheter can be removed by placing traction on the shunt through the abdominal incision and pulling it through the subcutaneous tunnel. If necessary, a second incision is made over the venous insertion site and the catheter removed from the jugular vein. The incisions are closed.

Coding Tips

For revision of peritoneal-venous shunt, see 49426. For an injection procedure for evaluation of a previously placed peritoneal-venous shunt, see 49427.

ICD-10-CM Diagnostic Codes

K68.11	Postprocedural retroperitoneal abscess
R18.0	Malignant ascites
R18.8	Other ascites
R50.82	Postprocedural fever
T81.41XA	Infection following a procedure, superficial incisional surgical site, initial encounter
T81.42XA	Infection following a procedure, deep incisional surgical site, initial encounter
T81.43XA	Infection following a procedure, organ and space surgical site, initial encounter
T81.44XA	Sepsis following a procedure, initial encounter
T81.49XA	Infection following a procedure, other surgical site, initial encounter
T82.818A	Embolism due to vascular prosthetic devices, implants and grafts, initial encounter
T82.828A	Fibrosis due to vascular prosthetic devices, implants and grafts, initial encounter
T82.838A	Hemorrhage due to vascular prosthetic devices, implants and grafts, initial encounter
T82.848A	Pain due to vascular prosthetic devices, implants and grafts, initial encounter

T82.856A Stenosis of peripheral vascular stent, initial encounter

T82.858A Stenosis of other vascular prosthetic devices, implants and grafts, initial encounter

T82.868A Thrombosis due to vascular prosthetic devices, implants and grafts, initial encounter

T82.898A Other specified complication of vascular prosthetic devices, implants and grafts, initial encounter

Z45.2 Encounter for adjustment and management of vascular access device

AMA: **49428** 2014,Jan,11; 2013,Jan,11-12 **49429** 2014,Jan,11; 2013,Jan,11-12

Relative Value Units/Medicare Edits

Non-Facility RVU	Work	PE	MP	Total
49428	6.87	3.98	1.66	12.51
49429	7.44	4.07	1.8	13.31
Facility RVU	**Work**	**PE**	**MP**	**Total**
49428	6.87	3.98	1.66	12.51
49429	7.44	4.07	1.8	13.31

	FUD	Status	MUE	Modifiers				IOM Reference
49428	10	A	1(2)	51	N/A	N/A	N/A	None
49429	10	A	1(2)	51	N/A	N/A	N/A	

* with documentation

Terms To Know

complication. Condition arising after the beginning of observation and treatment that modifies the course of the patient's illness or the medical care required, or an undesired result or misadventure in medical care.

dissection. Separating by cutting tissue or body structures apart.

fascia. Fibrous sheet or band of tissue that envelops organs, muscles, and groupings of muscles.

ligation. Tying off a blood vessel or duct with a suture or a soft, thin wire.

peritoneal cavity. Space between the lining of the abdominal wall, or parietal peritoneum, and the surface layer of the abdominal organs, or visceral peritoneum. It contains a thin, watery fluid that keeps the peritoneal surfaces moist.

peritoneum. Strong, continuous membrane that forms the lining of the abdominal and pelvic cavity. The parietal peritoneum, or outer layer, is attached to the abdominopelvic walls and the visceral peritoneum, or inner layer, surrounds the organs inside the abdominal cavity.

peritonitis. Inflammation and infection within the peritoneal cavity, the space between the membrane lining the abdominopelvic walls and covering the internal organs.

shunt. Surgically created passage between blood vessels or other natural passages, such as an arteriovenous anastomosis, to divert or bypass blood flow from the normal channel.

49435

\+ **49435** Insertion of subcutaneous extension to intraperitoneal cannula or catheter with remote chest exit site (List separately in addition to code for primary procedure)

The catheter is extended and exits the chest

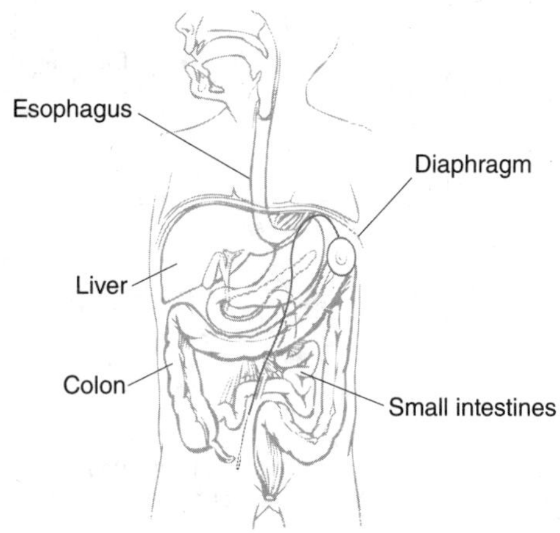

Explanation

A permanent, subcutaneous intraperitoneal catheter is lengthened with an extension and brought to the surface of the skin during the primary procedure in which a catheter/cannula is established. In the primary procedure, the physician makes a small abdominal incision, opens the peritoneum, and establishes the cannula. In 49435, the physician fits an extension to the cannula and tunnels subcutaneously to accommodate the extension. The physician makes a separate incision in the chest as an exit site for the extension. The extension is brought out through the skin and may be attached to the drug delivery system. The operative incision is closed.

Coding Tips

Report 49435 in addition to 49324 or 49421.

ICD-10-CM Diagnostic Codes

This/these CPT code(s) are add on code(s). See the primary procedure code that this code is performed with for your ICD-10-CM code selections. Diagnostic code(s) would be the same as the actual procedure performed.

AMA: **49435** 2014,Jan,11; 2013,Jan,11-12

Relative Value Units/Medicare Edits

Non-Facility RVU	Work	PE	MP	Total
49435	2.25	0.68	0.52	3.45
Facility RVU	**Work**	**PE**	**MP**	**Total**
49435	2.25	0.68	0.52	3.45

	FUD	Status	MUE	Modifiers				IOM Reference
49435	N/A	A	1(2)	N/A	N/A	62*	80	None

* with documentation

49436

49436 Delayed creation of exit site from embedded subcutaneous segment of intraperitoneal cannula or catheter

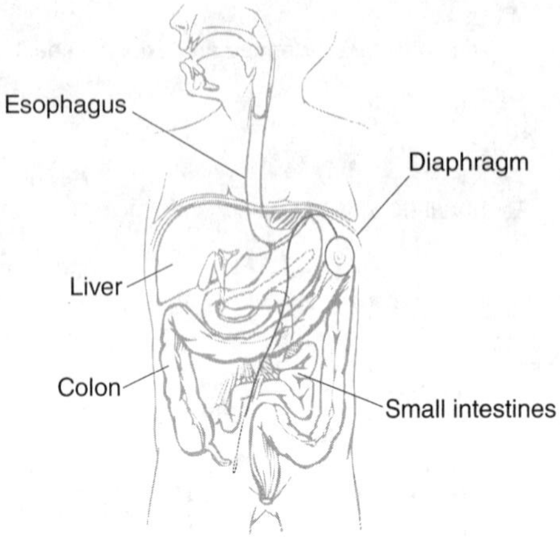

An exit site for the intraperitoneal catheter is created in a subsequent operative session

Explanation

A previously implanted, permanent subcutaneous intraperitoneal catheter is brought to the surface of the skin. The physician makes a small abdominal incision, opens the peritoneum, and locates the end of the existing intraperitoneal cannula. An extension may be fitted to the existing cannula. The physician makes a separate incision as an exit site for the cannula. The cannula is brought out through the skin and may be attached to the drug delivery system. The operative incision is closed.

Coding Tips

For laparoscopic insertion of intraperitoneal cannula or catheter, see 49324. For revision of previously placed intraperiteonal cannula or catheter with removal of intraluminal obstructive material if performed, see 49325; with omentectomy, see 49326. For insertion of subcutaneous extension at time of laparoscopic placement of intraperitoneal catheter, see 49435.

ICD-10-CM Diagnostic Codes

K68.11 Postprocedural retroperitoneal abscess
T81.41XA Infection following a procedure, superficial incisional surgical site, initial encounter
T81.42XA Infection following a procedure, deep incisional surgical site, initial encounter
T81.43XA Infection following a procedure, organ and space surgical site, initial encounter
T81.44XA Sepsis following a procedure, initial encounter
T81.49XA Infection following a procedure, other surgical site, initial encounter
T82.818A Embolism due to vascular prosthetic devices, implants and grafts, initial encounter
T82.828A Fibrosis due to vascular prosthetic devices, implants and grafts, initial encounter
T82.838A Hemorrhage due to vascular prosthetic devices, implants and grafts, initial encounter
T82.848A Pain due to vascular prosthetic devices, implants and grafts, initial encounter
T82.858A Stenosis of other vascular prosthetic devices, implants and grafts, initial encounter
T82.868A Thrombosis due to vascular prosthetic devices, implants and grafts, initial encounter
T82.898A Other specified complication of vascular prosthetic devices, implants and grafts, initial encounter

AMA: **49436** 2014,Jan,11; 2013,Jan,11-12

Relative Value Units/Medicare Edits

Non-Facility RVU	Work	PE	MP	Total
49436	2.72	2.01	0.63	5.36
Facility RVU	**Work**	**PE**	**MP**	**Total**
49436	2.72	2.01	0.63	5.36

	FUD	Status	MUE	Modifiers				IOM Reference
49436	10	A	1(2)	51	N/A	62*	80	None

* with documentation

Terms To Know

cannula. Tube inserted into a blood vessel, duct, or body cavity to facilitate passage.

catheter. Flexible tube inserted into an area of the body for introducing or withdrawing fluid.

peritoneal cavity. Space between the lining of the abdominal wall, or parietal peritoneum, and the surface layer of the abdominal organs, or visceral peritoneum. It contains a thin, watery fluid that keeps the peritoneal surfaces moist.

subcutaneous. Below the skin.

49904-49906

49904 Omental flap, extra-abdominal (eg, for reconstruction of sternal and chest wall defects)

\+ **49905** Omental flap, intra-abdominal (List separately in addition to code for primary procedure)

49906 Free omental flap with microvascular anastomosis

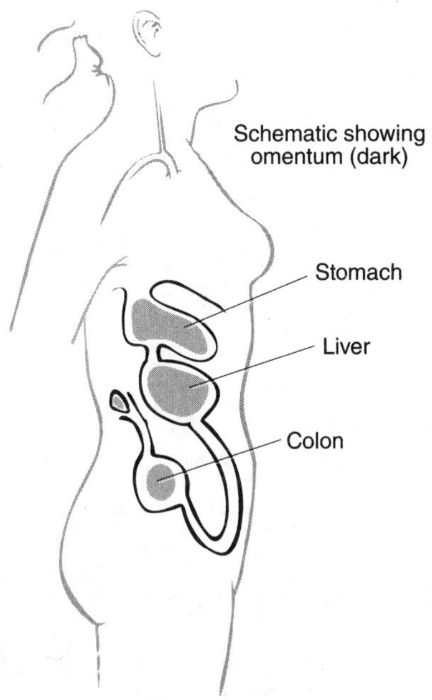

A flap of omentum is used in an extraabdominal repair, such as of the chest wall

Explanation

The physician mobilizes an omental flap for reconstruction of a defect. The surgical recipient site of the flap is prepared. An upper abdominal transverse or midline incision is made. A laparotomy and manual exploration of the abdominal cavity is done first and the omentum and transverse colon are delivered from the cavity. The omentum is dissected from the transverse colon from left to right and small vessels are ligated. When completely separated from the transverse colon, the omentum is dissected from the stomach with careful clamping, division, and ligation of vessels. The omentum is fully mobilized and pedicled on the right or left gastroepiploic vessel, depending on the purpose. More incisions and tunneling may be necessary to bring the flap into its new location to fill a defect. The flap may be used as a pedicled transposition flap or a free microvascular transfer flap. Report 49904 when the flap is transpositioned to repair an extra-abdominal defect, such as chest wounds after radiation and mastectomy or lower extremity trauma wounds. Report 49905 when the omental flap is repositioned to repair a defect intra-abdominally. Report 49906 when the omentum is used as a free vascularized transfer flap to repair defects such as hemifacial atrophy. Microvascular anastomosis is performed to maintain blood flow to the omental flap. The abdominal incision is closed. If a separate split-thickness skin graft is required for omental coverage, it is done immediately and applied directly over the omentum and a dressing is applied.

Coding Tips

Report 49905 separately in addition to the primary procedure. Do not report 69990 in addition to 49906 as the operating microscope is considered an inclusive component of the surgery.

ICD-10-CM Diagnostic Codes

S21.111A	Laceration without foreign body of right front wall of thorax without penetration into thoracic cavity, initial encounter ☑
S21.112A	Laceration without foreign body of left front wall of thorax without penetration into thoracic cavity, initial encounter ☑
S21.121A	Laceration with foreign body of right front wall of thorax without penetration into thoracic cavity, initial encounter ☑
S21.122A	Laceration with foreign body of left front wall of thorax without penetration into thoracic cavity, initial encounter ☑
S21.131A	Puncture wound without foreign body of right front wall of thorax without penetration into thoracic cavity, initial encounter ☑
S21.132A	Puncture wound without foreign body of left front wall of thorax without penetration into thoracic cavity, initial encounter ☑
S21.141A	Puncture wound with foreign body of right front wall of thorax without penetration into thoracic cavity, initial encounter ☑
S21.142A	Puncture wound with foreign body of left front wall of thorax without penetration into thoracic cavity, initial encounter ☑
S21.151A	Open bite of right front wall of thorax without penetration into thoracic cavity, initial encounter ☑
S21.152A	Open bite of left front wall of thorax without penetration into thoracic cavity, initial encounter ☑
S28.1XXA	Traumatic amputation (partial) of part of thorax, except breast, initial encounter
S29.021A	Laceration of muscle and tendon of front wall of thorax, initial encounter
S31.112A	Laceration without foreign body of abdominal wall, epigastric region without penetration into peritoneal cavity, initial encounter
S31.115A	Laceration without foreign body of abdominal wall, periumbilic region without penetration into peritoneal cavity, initial encounter
S31.120A	Laceration of abdominal wall with foreign body, right upper quadrant without penetration into peritoneal cavity, initial encounter ☑
S31.121A	Laceration of abdominal wall with foreign body, left upper quadrant without penetration into peritoneal cavity, initial encounter ☑
S31.122A	Laceration of abdominal wall with foreign body, epigastric region without penetration into peritoneal cavity, initial encounter
S31.123A	Laceration of abdominal wall with foreign body, right lower quadrant without penetration into peritoneal cavity, initial encounter ☑
S31.124A	Laceration of abdominal wall with foreign body, left lower quadrant without penetration into peritoneal cavity, initial encounter ☑
S31.125A	Laceration of abdominal wall with foreign body, periumbilic region without penetration into peritoneal cavity, initial encounter
S31.131A	Puncture wound of abdominal wall without foreign body, left upper quadrant without penetration into peritoneal cavity, initial encounter ☑
S31.132A	Puncture wound of abdominal wall without foreign body, epigastric region without penetration into peritoneal cavity, initial encounter
S31.133A	Puncture wound of abdominal wall without foreign body, right lower quadrant without penetration into peritoneal cavity, initial encounter ☑

Abdomen

S31.134A Puncture wound of abdominal wall without foreign body, left lower quadrant without penetration into peritoneal cavity, initial encounter ☑

S31.135A Puncture wound of abdominal wall without foreign body, periumbilic region without penetration into peritoneal cavity, initial encounter

S31.140A Puncture wound of abdominal wall with foreign body, right upper quadrant without penetration into peritoneal cavity, initial encounter ☑

S31.141A Puncture wound of abdominal wall with foreign body, left upper quadrant without penetration into peritoneal cavity, initial encounter ☑

S31.143A Puncture wound of abdominal wall with foreign body, right lower quadrant without penetration into peritoneal cavity, initial encounter ☑

S31.144A Puncture wound of abdominal wall with foreign body, left lower quadrant without penetration into peritoneal cavity, initial encounter ☑

S31.150A Open bite of abdominal wall, right upper quadrant without penetration into peritoneal cavity, initial encounter ☑

S31.151A Open bite of abdominal wall, left upper quadrant without penetration into peritoneal cavity, initial encounter ☑

S31.152A Open bite of abdominal wall, epigastric region without penetration into peritoneal cavity, initial encounter

S31.153A Open bite of abdominal wall, right lower quadrant without penetration into peritoneal cavity, initial encounter ☑

S31.154A Open bite of abdominal wall, left lower quadrant without penetration into peritoneal cavity, initial encounter ☑

S31.155A Open bite of abdominal wall, periumbilic region without penetration into peritoneal cavity, initial encounter

T21.31XA Burn of third degree of chest wall, initial encounter

T21.71XA Corrosion of third degree of chest wall, initial encounter

AMA: **49904** 2014,Jan,11; 2013,Jan,11-12 **49905** 2018,Jan,8; 2017,Jan,8; 2016,Jan,13; 2015,Jan,16; 2014,Jan,11; 2013,Jan,11-12 **49906** 2018,Jan,8; 2017,Jan,8; 2016,Jan,13; 2016,Feb,12; 2015,Jan,16; 2014,Jan,11; 2013,Jan,11-12

Relative Value Units/Medicare Edits

Non-Facility RVU	Work	PE	MP	Total
49904	22.35	13.92	4.69	40.96
49905	6.54	2.32	1.39	10.25
49906	0.0	0.0	0.0	0.0
Facility RVU	**Work**	**PE**	**MP**	**Total**
49904	22.35	13.92	4.69	40.96
49905	6.54	2.32	1.39	10.25
49906	0.0	0.0	0.0	0.0

	FUD	Status	MUE	Modifiers				IOM Reference
49904	90	A	1(3)	51	N/A	62*	N/A	None
49905	N/A	A	1(3)	N/A	N/A	62	80	
49906	90	C	1(3)	51	N/A	62*	N/A	

* with documentation

Abdomen

60270

60270 Thyroidectomy, including substernal thyroid; sternal split or transthoracic approach

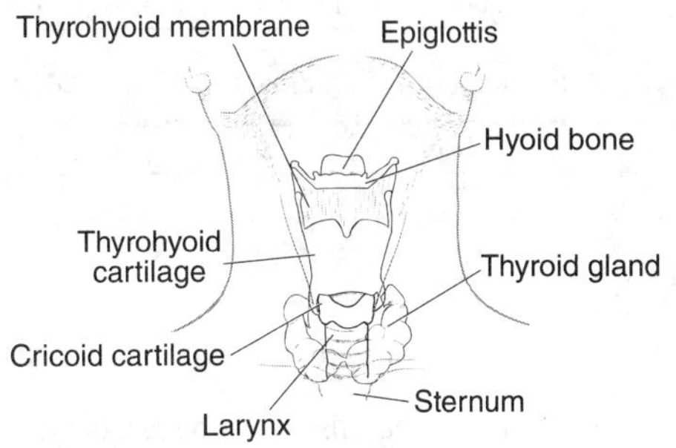

The thyroid gland is removed, including portions that occur below the sternum

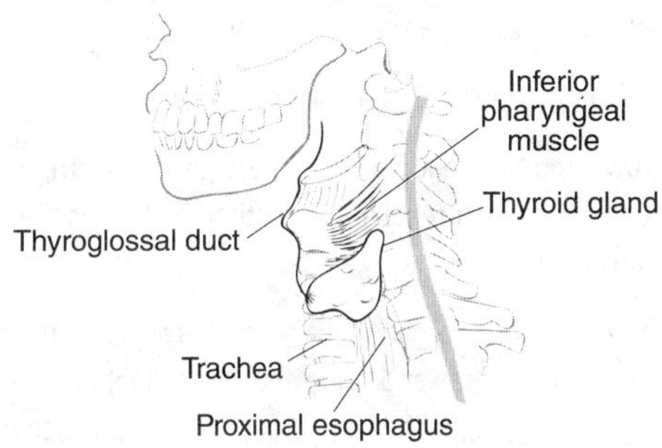

Explanation

The physician removes the thyroid, including the substernal thyroid gland. The physician exposes the thyroid via sternal split or transthoracic approach. The platysmas is divided and the strap muscles separated in the midline. The thyroid gland is mobilized and the superior and inferior thyroid vessels are ligated. The parathyroid glands are preserved and the thyroid is resected free of the trachea and removed. Any substernal thyroid is bluntly dissected. Upper sternal incision may be necessary for complete excision of substernal thyroid. The platysmas and skin are closed.

Coding Tips

The approach is considered inherent to the procedure and should not be reported separately.

ICD-10-CM Diagnostic Codes

C73	Malignant neoplasm of thyroid gland
C79.89	Secondary malignant neoplasm of other specified sites
D09.3	Carcinoma in situ of thyroid and other endocrine glands
D09.8	Carcinoma in situ of other specified sites
D34	Benign neoplasm of thyroid gland
D44.0	Neoplasm of uncertain behavior of thyroid gland
E01.0	Iodine-deficiency related diffuse (endemic) goiter
E04.0	Nontoxic diffuse goiter
E04.1	Nontoxic single thyroid nodule
E04.2	Nontoxic multinodular goiter
E04.8	Other specified nontoxic goiter
E05.00	Thyrotoxicosis with diffuse goiter without thyrotoxic crisis or storm
E05.01	Thyrotoxicosis with diffuse goiter with thyrotoxic crisis or storm
E05.10	Thyrotoxicosis with toxic single thyroid nodule without thyrotoxic crisis or storm
E05.11	Thyrotoxicosis with toxic single thyroid nodule with thyrotoxic crisis or storm
E05.20	Thyrotoxicosis with toxic multinodular goiter without thyrotoxic crisis or storm
E05.21	Thyrotoxicosis with toxic multinodular goiter with thyrotoxic crisis or storm
E05.30	Thyrotoxicosis from ectopic thyroid tissue without thyrotoxic crisis or storm

AMA: 60270 2018,Jan,8; 2017,Jan,8; 2016,Jan,13; 2015,Jan,16; 2014,Jan,11

Relative Value Units/Medicare Edits

Non-Facility RVU	Work	PE	MP	Total
60270	23.2	11.69	4.55	39.44
Facility RVU	**Work**	**PE**	**MP**	**Total**
60270	23.2	11.69	4.55	39.44

	FUD	Status	MUE	Modifiers				IOM Reference
60270	90	A	1(2)	51	N/A	62*	80	None

* with documentation

Terms To Know

dissection. Separating by cutting tissue or body structures apart.

excision. Surgical removal of an organ or tissue.

goiter. Abnormal enlargement of the thyroid gland commonly caused by a deficiency of dietary iodine.

incision. Act of cutting into tissue or an organ.

ligate. To tie off a blood vessel or duct with a suture or a soft, thin wire (ligature wire).

lymphoma. Tumors occurring in the lymphoid tissues that are most commonly malignant.

malignant. Any condition tending to progress toward death, specifically an invasive tumor with a loss of cellular differentiation that has the ability to spread or metastasize to other body areas.

60505

60505 Parathyroidectomy or exploration of parathyroid(s); with mediastinal exploration, sternal split or transthoracic approach

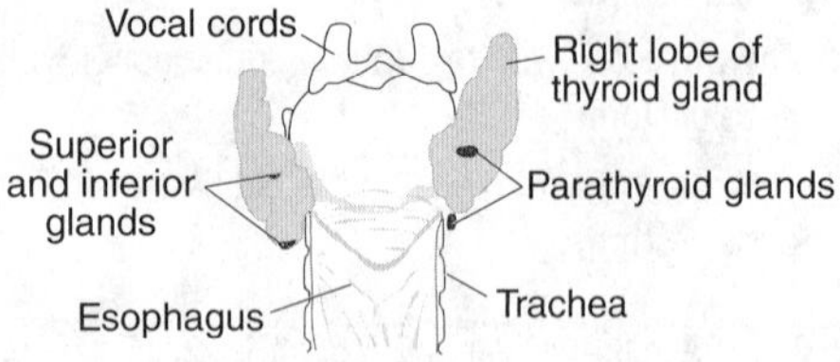

Posterior view of parathyroid glands

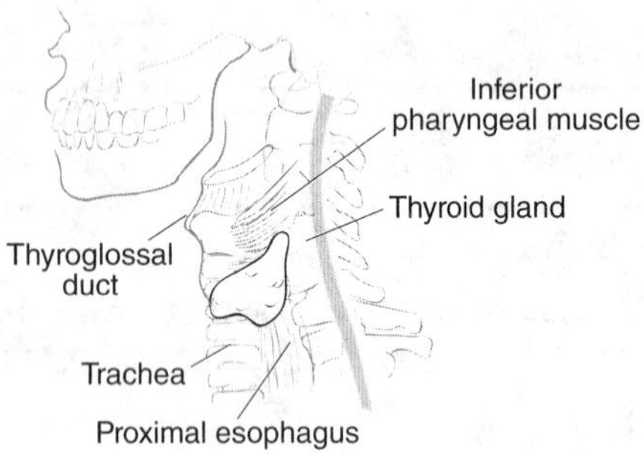

Parathyroid glands are removed or merely explored and biopsied. Usually four glands occur (two per thyroid lobe)

Explanation

The physician removes or explores the parathyroids, glands adjacent to the thyroids with mediastinal exploration, sternal split or transthoracic approach. The physician exposes the thyroid via a sternal split or transthoracic approach. The parathyroid glands are identified and tissue is excised for separately reportable pathological examination. The mediastinum is explored. The parathyroid may be removed; usually a port remains following excision. The platysmas and skin are closed.

Coding Tips

The approach is considered inherent to the procedure and should not be reported separately.

ICD-10-CM Diagnostic Codes

C75.0	Malignant neoplasm of parathyroid gland
D35.1	Benign neoplasm of parathyroid gland
D44.2	Neoplasm of uncertain behavior of parathyroid gland
E20.0	Idiopathic hypoparathyroidism
E20.1	Pseudohypoparathyroidism
E20.9	Hypoparathyroidism, unspecified
E21.0	Primary hyperparathyroidism
E21.1	Secondary hyperparathyroidism, not elsewhere classified
E21.2	Other hyperparathyroidism
E83.51	Hypocalcemia
E83.52	Hypercalcemia

AMA: 60505 2018,Jan,8; 2017,Jan,8; 2016,Jan,13; 2015,Jan,16; 2014,Jan,11

Relative Value Units/Medicare Edits

Non-Facility RVU	Work	PE	MP	Total
60505	23.06	12.72	4.38	40.16
Facility RVU	**Work**	**PE**	**MP**	**Total**
60505	23.06	12.72	4.38	40.16

	FUD	Status	MUE	Modifiers				IOM Reference
60505	90	A	1(3)	51	N/A	62*	80	None

* with documentation

Terms To Know

benign. Mild or nonmalignant in nature.

carcinoma in situ. Malignancy that arises from the cells of the vessel, gland, or organ of origin that remains confined to that site or has not invaded neighboring tissue.

excision. Surgical removal of an organ or tissue.

exploration. Examination for diagnostic purposes.

malignant. Any condition tending to progress toward death, specifically an invasive tumor with a loss of cellular differentiation that has the ability to spread or metastasize to other body areas.

mediastinum. Collection of organs and tissues that separate the pleural sacs. Located between the sternum and spine above the diaphragm, it contains the heart and great vessels, trachea and bronchi, esophagus, thymus, lymph nodes, and nerves.

platysma. Muscle originating from the neck region attached to the mandible that opens the jaw.

secondary. Second in order of occurrence or importance, or appearing during the course of another disease or condition.

60521-60522

60521 Thymectomy, partial or total; sternal split or transthoracic approach, without radical mediastinal dissection (separate procedure)

60522 sternal split or transthoracic approach, with radical mediastinal dissection (separate procedure)

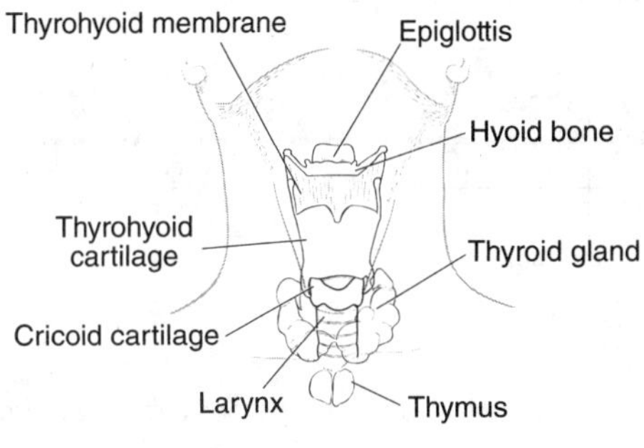

The thymus is removed, either partially or in total

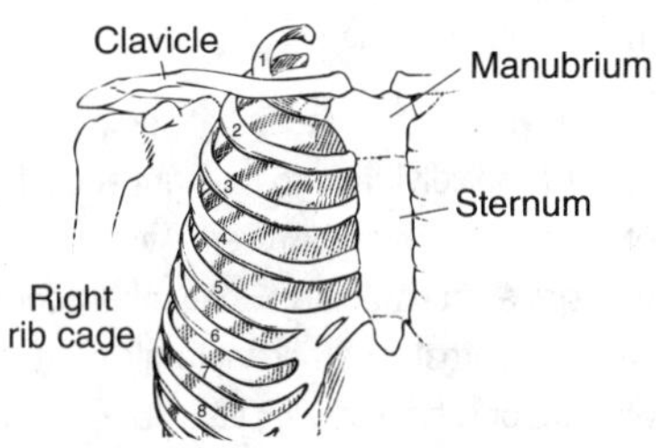

Explanation

The physician removes part or all of the thymus gland. The physician exposes the thymus via a sternal split or transthoracic approach. The sternum is retracted and strap muscles separated. The superior lobe of the thymus is separated from the inferior aspect of the thyroid. The blood supply to the thymus is divided and the thymus is dissected free from the pericardium and removed. In 60522, the mediastinum is dissected. In both procedures, the incision is closed.

Coding Tips

Note that 60521 and 60522, separate procedures by definition, are usually components of a more complex service and are not identified separately. When performed alone or with other unrelated procedures/services, they may be reported. If performed alone, list the code; if performed with other procedures/services, list the code and append modifier 59 or an X{EPSU} modifier. The approach is considered inherent to the procedure and should not be reported separately. For thoracoscopic video-assisted thoracic surgery (VATS), thymectomy, see 32673.

ICD-10-CM Diagnostic Codes

C37	Malignant neoplasm of thymus
C7A.091	Malignant carcinoid tumor of the thymus
D15.0	Benign neoplasm of thymus
D38.4	Neoplasm of uncertain behavior of thymus
D3A.091	Benign carcinoid tumor of the thymus
D49.89	Neoplasm of unspecified behavior of other specified sites
G70.01	Myasthenia gravis with (acute) exacerbation

AMA: 60521 2018,Jan,8; 2017,Jan,8; 2016,Jan,13; 2015,Jan,16; 2014,Jan,11
60522 2014,Jan,11

Relative Value Units/Medicare Edits

Non-Facility RVU	Work	PE	MP	Total
60521	19.18	8.83	4.4	32.41
60522	23.48	10.66	5.37	39.51
Facility RVU	**Work**	**PE**	**MP**	**Total**
60521	19.18	8.83	4.4	32.41
60522	23.48	10.66	5.37	39.51

	FUD	Status	MUE	Modifiers				IOM Reference
60521	90	A	1(2)	51	N/A	62*	80	None
60522	90	A	1(2)	51	N/A	62*	80	

* with documentation

Terms To Know

anomaly. Irregularity in the structure or position of an organ or tissue.

benign. Mild or nonmalignant in nature.

congenital. Present at birth, occurring through heredity or an influence during gestation up to the moment of birth.

dissection. Separating by cutting tissue or body structures apart.

excision. Surgical removal of an organ or tissue.

incision. Act of cutting into tissue or an organ.

malignant. Any condition tending to progress toward death, specifically an invasive tumor with a loss of cellular differentiation that has the ability to spread or metastasize to other body areas.

pericardium. Thin and slippery case in which the heart lies that is lined with fluid so that the heart is free to pulse and move as it beats.

secondary. Second in order of occurrence or importance, or appearing during the course of another disease or condition.

60600-60605

60600 Excision of carotid body tumor; without excision of carotid artery
60605 with excision of carotid artery

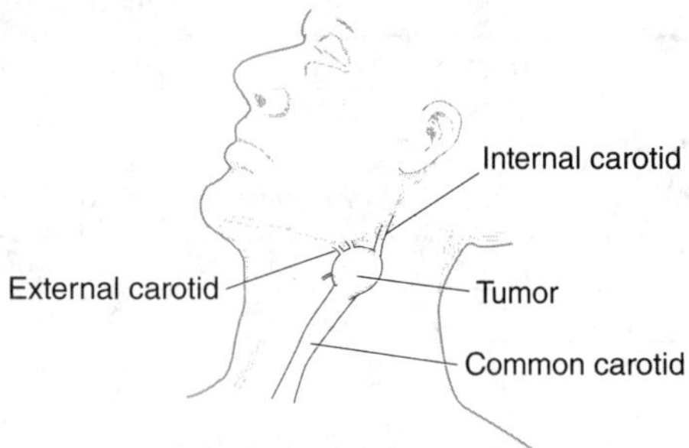

Schematic showing tumor at bifurcation of carotid artery

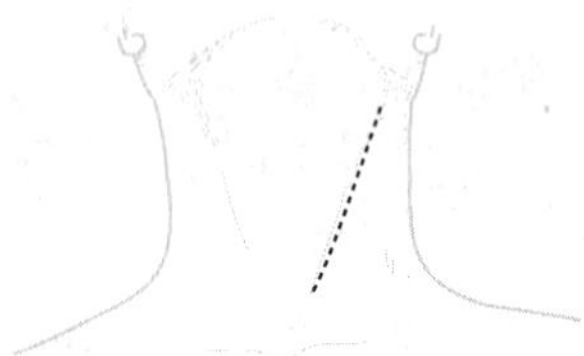

Typical incision to access the carotid body

Explanation

This physician removes a tumor from a small epithelioid structure (carotid body) just above the bifurcation of the carotid. The physician exposes the carotid body via an incision anterior to the sternocleidomastoid. After dissection down to the carotid sheath, the vein is retracted and the carotid bifurcation exposed. The blood supply to the tumor is ligated and the tumor resected. The incision is closed. Report 60605 if the carotid body tumor excision is performed with excision of the carotid artery.

Coding Tips

When 60600 or 60605 is performed with another separately identifiable procedure, the highest dollar value code is listed as the primary procedure, and subsequent procedures are appended with modifier 51.

ICD-10-CM Diagnostic Codes

C75.4	Malignant neoplasm of carotid body
D35.5	Benign neoplasm of carotid body

AMA: 60600 2014,Jan,11 **60605** 2018,Sep,9; 2017,Sep,13; 2016,Sep,8; 2016,Oct,10; 2016,Nov,8; 2016,Jul,10; 2014,Jan,11

Relative Value Units/Medicare Edits

Non-Facility RVU	Work	PE	MP	Total
60600	25.09	9.26	5.28	39.63
60605	31.96	8.61	7.39	47.96
Facility RVU	**Work**	**PE**	**MP**	**Total**
60600	25.09	9.26	5.28	39.63
60605	31.96	8.61	7.39	47.96

	FUD	Status	MUE	Modifiers				IOM Reference
60600	90	A	1(3)	51	N/A	62*	80	100-03,20.18
60605	90	A	1(3)	51	N/A	62*	80	

* with documentation

Terms To Know

artery. Vessel through which oxygenated blood passes away from the heart to any part of the body.

benign. Mild or nonmalignant in nature.

bifurcation. Point of division into two separate branches or structures, such as the site where the trachea divides into the right and left main bronchi or the common carotid artery becomes the external and internal carotid arteries. For diagnostic purposes, a bifurcation is a congenital anomaly that results in an imperfect closure of an organ or other anatomical structure, such as the ureter, renal pelvis, hard or soft palate, lip, etc.

carotid body tumor. Benign growth that forms at the fork of the common carotid artery causing symptoms such as dizziness due to its effect on carotid body functions.

dissection. Separating by cutting tissue or body structures apart.

excision. Surgical removal of an organ or tissue.

incision. Act of cutting into tissue or an organ.

ligation. Tying off a blood vessel or duct with a suture or a soft, thin wire.

malignant. Any condition tending to progress toward death, specifically an invasive tumor with a loss of cellular differentiation that has the ability to spread or metastasize to other body areas.

neoplasm. New abnormal growth, tumor.

resection. Surgical removal of a part or all of an organ or body part.

secondary. Second in order of occurrence or importance, or appearing during the course of another disease or condition.

tumor. Pathological swelling or enlargement; a neoplastic growth of uncontrolled, abnormal multiplication of cells.

64415-64416

▲ **64415** Injection(s), anesthetic agent(s) and/or steroid; brachial plexus
▲ **64416** brachial plexus, continuous infusion by catheter (including catheter placement)

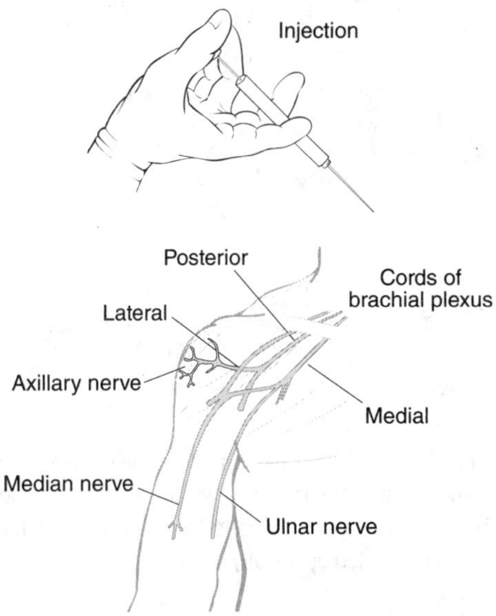

An anesthetic agent is injected to block the brachial plexus, a group of nerves serving the arm and upper thorax

Explanation

The physician injects one or more anesthetic agents and/or steroids near the brachial plexus to relieve pain and inflammation in 64415. The physician draws a local anesthetic and/or steroid into a syringe and injects it into a targeted area near the brachial plexus, approached in one of three locations: intrascalene, supraclavicular, or axillary. In 64416, continuous infusion of local anesthetic and/or steroid through a catheter is done to provide a nerve block lasting longer than the block effect achieved through a single injection. An indwelling catheter is placed and positioned so as to provide anesthesia to the brachial plexus. An infusion pump is connected to the catheter to supply a continuous flow of infused agent at a set rate. The infusion system may be used for regional surgical anesthesia when general anesthesia is not required and for postoperative pain management. Catheter placement is included in 64416 and is not reported separately.

Coding Tips

These are unilateral procedures. If performed bilaterally, some payers require that the service be reported twice with modifier 50 appended to the second code while others require identification of the service only once with modifier 50 appended. Check with individual payers. Supplies used when providing this procedure may be reported with the appropriate HCPCS Level II J2400 code. Check with the specific payer to determine coverage. Imaging guidance and localization may be reported separately. For anesthesia by injection performed by a different provider, see 01991 and 01992.

ICD-10-CM Diagnostic Codes

G54.0	Brachial plexus disorders
G56.41	Causalgia of right upper limb ☑
G56.42	Causalgia of left upper limb ☑
G56.43	Causalgia of bilateral upper limbs ☑
G90.511	Complex regional pain syndrome I of right upper limb ☑
G90.512	Complex regional pain syndrome I of left upper limb ☑
G90.513	Complex regional pain syndrome I of upper limb, bilateral ☑
M12.511	Traumatic arthropathy, right shoulder ☑
M12.512	Traumatic arthropathy, left shoulder ☑
M25.511	Pain in right shoulder ☑
M25.512	Pain in left shoulder ☑
M25.521	Pain in right elbow ☑
M25.522	Pain in left elbow ☑
M25.541	Pain in joints of right hand ☑
M25.542	Pain in joints of left hand ☑
M50.13	Cervical disc disorder with radiculopathy, cervicothoracic region
M54.12	Radiculopathy, cervical region
M54.13	Radiculopathy, cervicothoracic region
M54.2	Cervicalgia
M79.11	Myalgia of mastication muscle
M79.12	Myalgia of auxiliary muscles, head and neck
M79.18	Myalgia, other site
M79.601	Pain in right arm ☑
M79.602	Pain in left arm ☑
M79.621	Pain in right upper arm ☑
M79.622	Pain in left upper arm ☑
M79.631	Pain in right forearm ☑
M79.632	Pain in left forearm ☑
M79.641	Pain in right hand ☑
M79.642	Pain in left hand ☑
M79.644	Pain in right finger(s) ☑
M79.645	Pain in left finger(s) ☑
M79.7	Fibromyalgia
S13.4XXA	Sprain of ligaments of cervical spine, initial encounter
S13.8XXA	Sprain of joints and ligaments of other parts of neck, initial encounter
S16.1XXA	Strain of muscle, fascia and tendon at neck level, initial encounter
S43.421A	Sprain of right rotator cuff capsule, initial encounter ☑
S43.422A	Sprain of left rotator cuff capsule, initial encounter ☑

AMA: 64415 2018,Jan,8; 2017,Jan,8; 2016,Jan,13; 2015,Jan,16; 2014,Jan,11; 2013,Jan,13-14 **64416** 2018,Jan,8; 2017,Jan,8; 2016,Jan,13; 2015,Jan,16; 2014,Jan,11; 2013,Jan,13-14

Relative Value Units/Medicare Edits

Non-Facility RVU	Work	PE	MP	Total
64415	1.48	1.78	0.12	3.38
64416	1.81	0.33	0.14	2.28
Facility RVU	**Work**	**PE**	**MP**	**Total**
64415	1.48	0.27	0.12	1.87
64416	1.81	0.33	0.14	2.28

	FUD	Status	MUE	Modifiers				IOM Reference
64415	0	A	1(3)	51	50	N/A	N/A	None
64416	0	A	1(2)	51	50	N/A	N/A	

* with documentation

92950

92950 Cardiopulmonary resuscitation (eg, in cardiac arrest)

Explanation

Cardiopulmonary arrest occurs when the patient's heart and lungs suddenly stop. In a clinical setting, cardiopulmonary resuscitation, the attempt at restarting the heart and lungs, is usually directed by a physician or another health care provider who is certified in Advanced Cardiac Life Support (ACLS). The patient's lungs are ventilated by mouth-to-mouth breathing or by a bag and mask. The patient's circulation is assisted using external chest compression. An electronic defibrillator may be used to shock the heart into restarting. Medications used to restart the heart include epinephrine and lidocaine.

Coding Tips

See also critical care services, 99291–99292, and neonatal and pediatric critical care services, 99468–99476. For critical care services provided during transport of a pediatric patient, see 99466–99467. For resuscitation services provided in the delivery or birthing room, see 99465.

ICD-10-CM Diagnostic Codes

I46.2	Cardiac arrest due to underlying cardiac condition
I46.8	Cardiac arrest due to other underlying condition
J80	Acute respiratory distress syndrome
J95.1	Acute pulmonary insufficiency following thoracic surgery
J95.2	Acute pulmonary insufficiency following nonthoracic surgery
J95.3	Chronic pulmonary insufficiency following surgery
J95.821	Acute postprocedural respiratory failure
J95.822	Acute and chronic postprocedural respiratory failure
J96.01	Acute respiratory failure with hypoxia
J96.02	Acute respiratory failure with hypercapnia
J96.21	Acute and chronic respiratory failure with hypoxia
J96.22	Acute and chronic respiratory failure with hypercapnia
P29.81	Cardiac arrest of newborn
R06.03	Acute respiratory distress

AMA: 92950 2018,Jan,8; 2018,Feb,11; 2017,Jan,8; 2016,Jan,13; 2015,Jan,16; 2014,Jan,11

Relative Value Units/Medicare Edits

Non-Facility RVU	Work	PE	MP	Total
92950	4.0	4.56	0.36	8.92
Facility RVU	**Work**	**PE**	**MP**	**Total**
92950	4.0	0.99	0.36	5.35

	FUD	Status	MUE	Modifiers				IOM Reference
92950	0	A	2(3)	N/A	N/A	N/A	80*	None

* with documentation

Terms To Know

cardiac arrest. Sudden, unexpected cessation of cardiac action, including absence of heart sounds and/or blood pressure.

respiratory distress syndrome. Premature neonates with respiratory distress and associated with reduced amounts of lung surfactant. Frequently fatal.

92953

92953 Temporary transcutaneous pacing

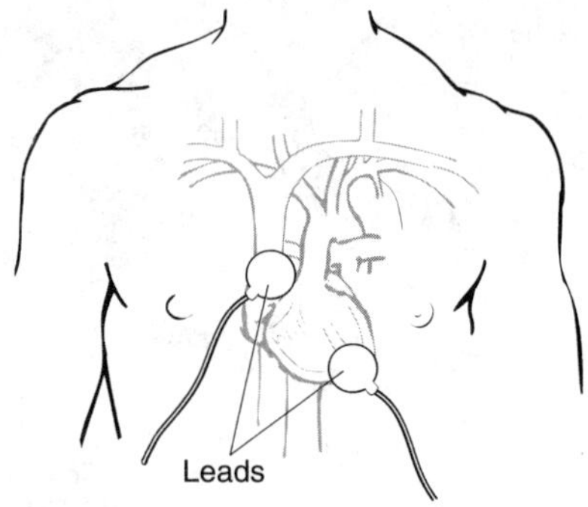

The heart is paced using transcutaneous leads (skin mounted)

Explanation

A temporary pacemaker is placed on the patient's heart to regulate heartbeats considered dangerously irregular. The physician applies electrodes to the chest wall. The electrodes give small electronic shocks through the chest to pace the heart as controlled by the physician.

Coding Tips

When medically necessary, report moderate (conscious) sedation provided by the performing physician with 99151-99153. When provided by another physician, report 99155-99157. When temporary pacing is done under physician direction from a remote location (e.g., hospital to ambulance or rescue personnel outside the hospital), report 99288 and not 92953. Temporary transcutaneous pacing is considered a component of critical care services. Do not report 92953 with 99291 or 99292. For temporary transvenous pacing, see 33210 and 33211.

ICD-10-CM Diagnostic Codes

I44.1	Atrioventricular block, second degree
I44.2	Atrioventricular block, complete
I45.2	Bifascicular block
I45.3	Trifascicular block
I49.5	Sick sinus syndrome
R00.1	Bradycardia, unspecified

AMA: 92953 2019,Aug,8; 2018,Jan,8; 2018,Feb,11; 2017,Jan,8; 2016,Jan,13; 2015,Jan,16; 2014,May,4; 2014,Jan,11

Relative Value Units/Medicare Edits

Non-Facility RVU	Work	PE	MP	Total
92953	0.01	0.01	0.01	0.03
Facility RVU	**Work**	**PE**	**MP**	**Total**
92953	0.01	0.01	0.01	0.03

	FUD	Status	MUE	Modifiers				IOM Reference
92953	0	A	2(3)	N/A	N/A	N/A	80*	None

* with documentation

92960-92961

92960 Cardioversion, elective, electrical conversion of arrhythmia; external
92961 internal (separate procedure)

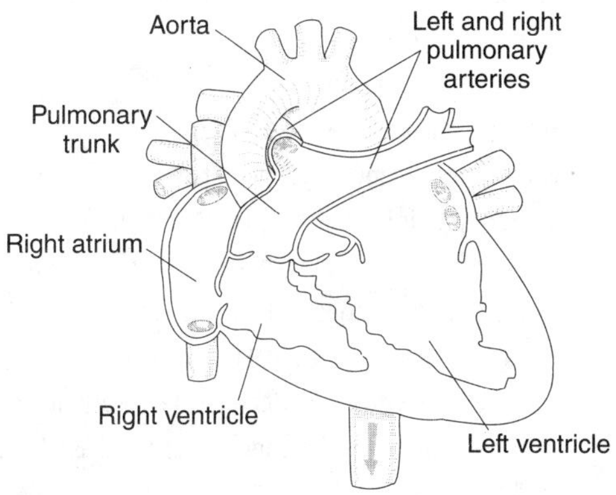

Explanation

The physician may administer an electronic shock to the patient's chest to regulate heartbeats considered dangerously irregular. The physician uses a defibrillator machine and places two paddles on the patient's chest and/or back. A measured electric shock is delivered through the chest to the heart to convert the heartbeat to a regular rhythm. Report 92960 for external cardioversion and 92961 when the procedure is performed internally.

Coding Tips

When medically necessary, report moderate (conscious) sedation provided by the performing physician with 99151-99153. When provided by another physician report 99155-99157. Note that 92961, a separate procedure by definition, is usually a component of a more complex service and is not identified separately. When performed alone or with other unrelated procedures/services, it may be reported. If performed alone, list the code; if performed with other procedures/services, list the code and append modifier 59 or an X{EPSU} modifier. Do not report 92961 with 93282-93284, 93287, 93289, 93295, 93296, 93618-93624, 93631, 93640-96342, 93650, 93653-93657, or 93662.

ICD-10-CM Diagnostic Codes

I44.0	Atrioventricular block, first degree
I44.1	Atrioventricular block, second degree
I44.2	Atrioventricular block, complete
I44.39	Other atrioventricular block
I44.4	Left anterior fascicular block
I44.5	Left posterior fascicular block
I44.69	Other fascicular block
I45.0	Right fascicular block
I45.19	Other right bundle-branch block
I45.2	Bifascicular block
I45.3	Trifascicular block
I45.4	Nonspecific intraventricular block
I45.5	Other specified heart block
I45.6	Pre-excitation syndrome
I45.81	Long QT syndrome
I45.89	Other specified conduction disorders
I47.0	Re-entry ventricular arrhythmia
I47.1	Supraventricular tachycardia
I47.2	Ventricular tachycardia
I48.0	Paroxysmal atrial fibrillation
I48.11	Longstanding persistent atrial fibrillation
I48.19	Other persistent atrial fibrillation
I48.21	Permanent atrial fibrillation
I48.3	Typical atrial flutter
I48.4	Atypical atrial flutter
I49.01	Ventricular fibrillation
I49.02	Ventricular flutter
I49.1	Atrial premature depolarization
I49.2	Junctional premature depolarization
I49.3	Ventricular premature depolarization
I49.49	Other premature depolarization
I49.5	Sick sinus syndrome
I49.8	Other specified cardiac arrhythmias

AMA: 92960 2018,Jan,8; 2018,Feb,11; 2017,Jan,8; 2016,Jan,13; 2015,Jan,16; 2014,Jan,11 **92961** 2018,Jan,8; 2018,Feb,11; 2017,Jan,8; 2016,Jan,13; 2015,Jan,16; 2015,Feb,3; 2014,Jan,11

Relative Value Units/Medicare Edits

Non-Facility RVU	Work	PE	MP	Total
92960	2.0	2.37	0.14	4.51
92961	4.34	1.91	0.98	7.23
Facility RVU	**Work**	**PE**	**MP**	**Total**
92960	2.0	0.99	0.14	3.13
92961	4.34	1.91	0.98	7.23

	FUD	Status	MUE	Modifiers				IOM Reference
92960	0	A	2(3)	N/A	N/A	N/A	80*	None
92961	0	A	1(3)	N/A	N/A	N/A	N/A	

* with documentation

Terms To Know

anomalous atrioventricular excitation. Pre-excitation associated with paroxysmal tachycardia or atrial fibrillation with a short P-R interval on EKG and an early delta wave. The normal conduction pathway is bypassed.

arrhythmias. Heart disorder of rhythm or rate, due to an electrical conduction system malfunction.

atrioventricular block. Condition in which there is a disturbance of electrical conduction, such as a delay, intermittence, or absence in the transmission of an impulse from the atria to the ventricles and categorized according to degree of severity.

supraventricular tachycardia. Rapid beating of the heart, usually pertains to more than 100 beats per minute and can be as high as 250 beats per minute. SVT is caused by abnormal electrical impulses originating at the AV node or above it in the atria (upper chambers) of the heart.

92970-92971

92970 Cardioassist-method of circulatory assist; internal
92971 external

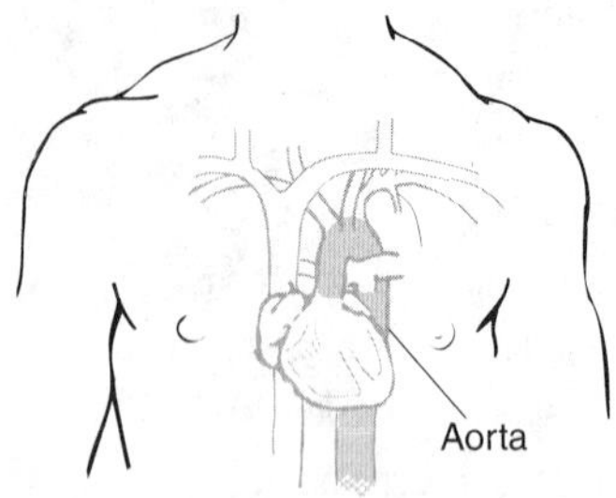

Internal circulatory assist involves accessing the aorta by catheter or cannula and inserting a blood flow assist device

External circulatory assist trousers

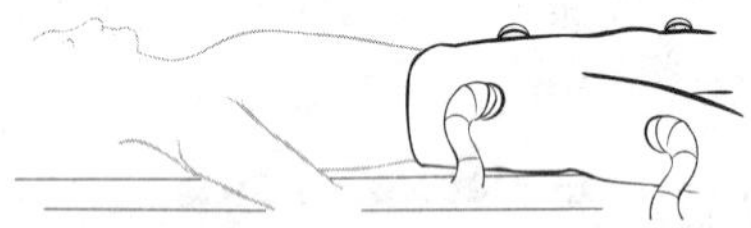

The trousers are rhythmically inflated and deflated, from the toes proximally toward the heart. The action improves venous return while reducing cardiac workload

Explanation

In 92970, in internal circulatory assist, the femoral artery is cannulated and a catheter with balloon or other device is inserted into the aorta. Various devices may be used to assist circulation. This code should be reported for the internal insertion of such a device, but should not be used to report intra-aortic balloon pump (IABP) or implantation of ventricular assist devices that are reported elsewhere. In 92971, devices are placed at the outside of the body to assist circulation. One example of external circulatory assist is Military Anti-Shock Trousers (MAST), which apply counterpressure around the legs and abdomen. The artificial peripheral resistance helps coronary perfusion. In a related procedure, pressure cuffs are used to assist circulation. The patient is placed on a treatment table where their lower extremities are wrapped in a series of three compressive air cuffs, which inflate and deflate in synchronization with the patient's cardiac cycle. During diastole the three sets of air cuffs are inflated sequentially (distal to proximal) compressing the vascular beds within the muscles of the calves, lower thighs, and upper thighs. This action results in an increase in diastolic pressure, generation of retrograde arterial blood flow, and an increase in venous return. The cuffs are deflated simultaneously just prior to systole, which produces a rapid drop in vascular impedance, a decrease in ventricular workload, and an increase in cardiac output. The augmented diastolic pressure and retrograde aortic flow appear to improve myocardial perfusion, while systolic unloading appears to reduce cardiac workload and oxygen requirements. The increased venous return coupled with enhanced systolic flow appears to increase cardiac output.

Coding Tips

For balloon atrial-septostomy, see 92992. For placement of catheters for use in circulatory assist devices such as intra-aortic balloon pump, see 33970.

ICD-10-CM Diagnostic Codes

I11.0	Hypertensive heart disease with heart failure
I13.0	Hypertensive heart and chronic kidney disease with heart failure and stage 1 through stage 4 chronic kidney disease, or unspecified chronic kidney disease
I13.2	Hypertensive heart and chronic kidney disease with heart failure and with stage 5 chronic kidney disease, or end stage renal disease
I16.0	Hypertensive urgency
I16.1	Hypertensive emergency
I50.1	Left ventricular failure, unspecified
I50.21	Acute systolic (congestive) heart failure
I50.22	Chronic systolic (congestive) heart failure
I50.23	Acute on chronic systolic (congestive) heart failure
I50.31	Acute diastolic (congestive) heart failure
I50.32	Chronic diastolic (congestive) heart failure
I50.33	Acute on chronic diastolic (congestive) heart failure
I50.41	Acute combined systolic (congestive) and diastolic (congestive) heart failure
I50.42	Chronic combined systolic (congestive) and diastolic (congestive) heart failure
I50.43	Acute on chronic combined systolic (congestive) and diastolic (congestive) heart failure
I50.811	Acute right heart failure
I50.812	Chronic right heart failure
I50.813	Acute on chronic right heart failure
I50.814	Right heart failure due to left heart failure
I50.82	Biventricular heart failure
I50.83	High output heart failure
I50.84	End stage heart failure
I97.110	Postprocedural cardiac insufficiency following cardiac surgery
I97.111	Postprocedural cardiac insufficiency following other surgery
I97.120	Postprocedural cardiac arrest following cardiac surgery
I97.121	Postprocedural cardiac arrest following other surgery
I97.130	Postprocedural heart failure following cardiac surgery
I97.131	Postprocedural heart failure following other surgery
I97.190	Other postprocedural cardiac functional disturbances following cardiac surgery
I97.191	Other postprocedural cardiac functional disturbances following other surgery
I97.710	Intraoperative cardiac arrest during cardiac surgery
I97.711	Intraoperative cardiac arrest during other surgery
I97.790	Other intraoperative cardiac functional disturbances during cardiac surgery
I97.791	Other intraoperative cardiac functional disturbances during other surgery
I97.88	Other intraoperative complications of the circulatory system, not elsewhere classified
I97.89	Other postprocedural complications and disorders of the circulatory system, not elsewhere classified
R57.0	Cardiogenic shock

AMA: 92970 2018,Feb,11 **92971** 2018,Feb,11

Relative Value Units/Medicare Edits

Non-Facility RVU	Work	PE	MP	Total
92970	3.51	1.19	0.82	5.52
92971	1.77	0.75	0.39	2.91
Facility RVU	**Work**	**PE**	**MP**	**Total**
92970	3.51	1.19	0.82	5.52
92971	1.77	0.75	0.39	2.91

	FUD	Status	MUE	Modifiers				IOM Reference
92970	0	A	1(3)	N/A	N/A	N/A	80*	None
92971	0	A	1(3)	N/A	N/A	N/A	80*	

* with documentation

Terms To Know

cannula. Tube inserted into a blood vessel, duct, or body cavity to facilitate passage.

cardiac output. Measurement of the volume of blood ejected by the heart ventricle that is usually measured by a catheter with an opening in the right atrium and pulmonary artery.

catheter. Flexible tube inserted into an area of the body for introducing or withdrawing fluid.

diastole. Relaxation period of the heart muscle between the first and second heart sounds, during which the chambers, particularly the ventricles, are filling in between contractions.

perfusion. Act of pouring over or through, especially the passage of a fluid through the vessels of a specific organ.

peripheral. Outside of a structure or organ.

retrograde. Moving against the usual direction of flow.

septostomy. Surgical creation of a septal defect or opening.

systole. Contraction phase of the heart, especially of the ventricles, in which blood is driven through the aorta and pulmonary artery to circulate through the lungs and out to the rest of the body. Indicated physically by the first sound of the heart and by the arterial pulse.

92986-92990

92986 Percutaneous balloon valvuloplasty; aortic valve
92987 mitral valve
92990 pulmonary valve

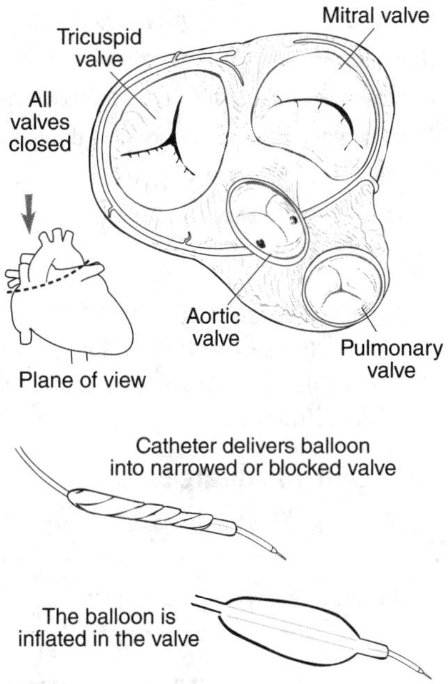

Explanation

The physician performs a percutaneous valvuloplasty. The physician makes a small incision in the arm or leg. Two catheters are placed: a central venous catheter and a second catheter threaded up to the heart. The physician inflates a balloon at the tip of the second catheter to open the blocked valve. The catheters are removed. Pressure is placed over the incision for 20 to 30 minutes to stem bleeding. The patient is observed for a period afterward. Report 92986 if the procedure is performed on the aortic valve; 92987 if the procedure is performed on the mitral valve; and 92990 if the procedure is performed on the pulmonary valve.

Coding Tips

When medically necessary, report moderate (conscious) sedation provided by the performing physician with 99151-99153. When provided by another physician report 99155-99157. For open mitral valvuloplasty, see 33425-33427. For closed heart valvuloplasty, see 33470-33471.

ICD-10-CM Diagnostic Codes

I05.0	Rheumatic mitral stenosis
I05.1	Rheumatic mitral insufficiency
I05.2	Rheumatic mitral stenosis with insufficiency
I05.8	Other rheumatic mitral valve diseases
I06.0	Rheumatic aortic stenosis
I06.1	Rheumatic aortic insufficiency
I06.2	Rheumatic aortic stenosis with insufficiency
I06.8	Other rheumatic aortic valve diseases
I08.0	Rheumatic disorders of both mitral and aortic valves
I08.8	Other rheumatic multiple valve diseases
I09.89	Other specified rheumatic heart diseases
I34.0	Nonrheumatic mitral (valve) insufficiency
I34.1	Nonrheumatic mitral (valve) prolapse

I34.2	Nonrheumatic mitral (valve) stenosis
I34.8	Other nonrheumatic mitral valve disorders
I35.0	Nonrheumatic aortic (valve) stenosis
I35.1	Nonrheumatic aortic (valve) insufficiency
I35.2	Nonrheumatic aortic (valve) stenosis with insufficiency
I35.8	Other nonrheumatic aortic valve disorders
I37.0	Nonrheumatic pulmonary valve stenosis
I37.1	Nonrheumatic pulmonary valve insufficiency
I37.2	Nonrheumatic pulmonary valve stenosis with insufficiency
I37.8	Other nonrheumatic pulmonary valve disorders
Q22.1	Congenital pulmonary valve stenosis
Q23.1	Congenital insufficiency of aortic valve
Q23.3	Congenital mitral insufficiency

AMA: **92986** 2018,Jan,8; 2018,Feb,11; 2017,Jan,8; 2016,Jan,13; 2015,Jan,16; 2015,Feb,3; 2014,Jan,11; 2013,Jan,6-8 **92987** 2018,Jan,8; 2018,Feb,11; 2017,Jan,8; 2016,Jan,13; 2015,Feb,3 **92990** 2018,Jan,8; 2018,Feb,11; 2017,Jan,8; 2016,Jan,13; 2015,Jul,10; 2015,Feb,3

Relative Value Units/Medicare Edits

Non-Facility RVU	Work	PE	MP	Total
92986	22.6	10.57	5.21	38.38
92987	23.38	10.92	5.29	39.59
92990	18.27	9.04	4.31	31.62
Facility RVU	**Work**	**PE**	**MP**	**Total**
92986	22.6	10.57	5.21	38.38
92987	23.38	10.92	5.29	39.59
92990	18.27	9.04	4.31	31.62

	FUD	Status	MUE	Modifiers				IOM Reference
92986	90	A	1(2)	51	N/A	N/A	80*	None
92987	90	A	1(2)	51	N/A	N/A	80*	
92990	90	A	1(2)	51	N/A	N/A	80*	

* with documentation

Terms To Know

aortic insufficiency. Malfunction of the aortic valve resulting in backflow of blood into the ventricle.

aortic valve. Heart valve, comprising three cusps, that divides the left ventricle and the aorta.

balloon catheter. Any catheter equipped with an inflatable balloon at the end to hold it in place in a body cavity or to be used for dilation of a vessel lúmen.

mitral valve. Valve with two cusps that is between the left atrium and left ventricle of the heart.

pulmonary valve. Valve with three cusps between the right ventricle and the pulmonary artery.

valvuloplasty. Surgical repair of a valve.

92992

92992 Atrial septectomy or septostomy; transvenous method, balloon (eg, Rashkind type) (includes cardiac catheterization)

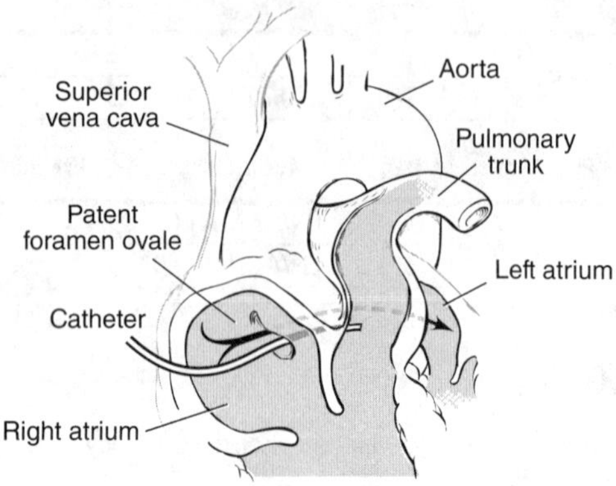

Depiction of patent foramen ovale. The procedure involves placing a catheter through the foramen ovale and enlarging the opening to allow mixing of blood between the atria. A balloon catheter may be used, or a cutting device may be required to create an opening (septostomy)

Explanation

Certain congenital heart defects, particularly those involving transposition of the great vessels, require surgical creation or enlargement of an opening in the interatrial septum (wall) that separates the upper right and left chambers of the heart. The physician makes a small incision in the arm or leg. Two catheters are placed—a central venous catheter and a second catheter threaded up to the heart. When the foramen ovale has not closed, a deflated balloon (Rashkind-type) is passed through the foramen ovale, inflated, and pulled through the atrial septum, enlarging the opening and improving oxygenation of the blood. When the septum is intact, the deflated balloon (Rashkind-type) is passed from the right atrium through the septum to the left atrium, inflated, and withdrawn, creating an interatrial septal defect and improving oxygenation of the blood. The catheters are removed. Pressure is placed over the incision for 20 to 30 minutes to stem bleeding. A cardiac catheterization may be included. The patient is observed for a period afterward.

Coding Tips

Do not report cardiac catheterization services separately as they are included in this procedure. For atrial septectomy or septostomy by blade method (Park septostomy), see 92993.

ICD-10-CM Diagnostic Codes

Q20.0	Common arterial trunk
Q20.1	Double outlet right ventricle
Q20.3	Discordant ventriculoarterial connection
Q21.3	Tetralogy of Fallot
Q21.8	Other congenital malformations of cardiac septa
Q22.0	Pulmonary valve atresia
Q22.4	Congenital tricuspid stenosis
Q22.6	Hypoplastic right heart syndrome
Q22.8	Other congenital malformations of tricuspid valve
Q23.8	Other congenital malformations of aortic and mitral valves
Q24.8	Other specified congenital malformations of heart
Q25.0	Patent ductus arteriosus

Q25.21	Interruption of aortic arch
Q25.29	Other atresia of aorta
Q25.5	Atresia of pulmonary artery
Q26.2	Total anomalous pulmonary venous connection

AMA: 92992 2018,Jan,8; 2018,Feb,11; 2017,Jan,8; 2016,Jul,3; 2016,Jan,13; 2015,Jan,16; 2014,Jan,11

Relative Value Units/Medicare Edits

Non-Facility RVU	Work	PE	MP	Total
92992	0.0	0.0	0.0	0.0
Facility RVU	**Work**	**PE**	**MP**	**Total**
92992	0.0	0.0	0.0	0.0

	FUD	Status	MUE	Modifiers				IOM Reference
92992	90	C	1(2)	51	N/A	N/A	80	None

* with documentation

Terms To Know

atresia. Congenital closure or absence of a tubular organ or an opening to the body surface.

atrial septal defect. Cardiac anomaly consisting of a patent opening in the atrial septum due to a fusion failure, classified as ostium secundum type, ostium primum defect, or endocardial cushion defect.

congenital. Present at birth, occurring through heredity or an influence during gestation up to the moment of birth.

Rashkind procedure. Transvenous balloon atrial septectomy or septostomy performed by cardiac catheterization. A balloon catheter is inserted into the heart either to create or enlarge an opening in the interatrial septal wall.

septostomy. Surgical creation of a septal defect or opening.

septum. Anatomical partition or dividing wall.

stenosis. Narrowing or constriction of a passage.

transposition. Removal or exchange from one side to another; change of position from one place to another.

92993

92993 Atrial septectomy or septostomy; blade method (Park septostomy) (includes cardiac catheterization)

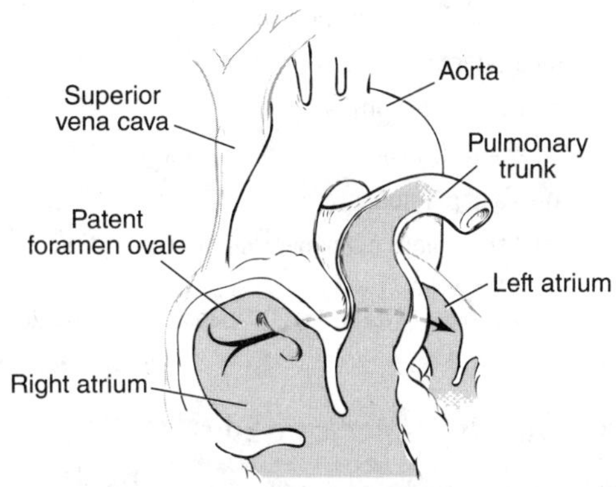

Depiction of patent foramen ovale. The procedure involves placing a catheter through the foramen ovale and enlarging the opening to allow mixing of blood between the atria

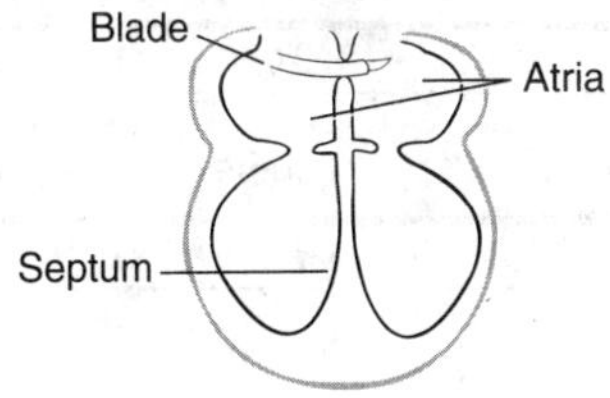

Explanation

The purpose of this procedure is to increase blood flow across the atrial septum in children with certain forms of cyanotic congenital heart disease. This procedure is used as an alternative to the Rashkind procedure (balloon method of atrial septostomy), typically in infants older than 1 month of age. The physician makes a small incision in the femoral vein. The physician places a transseptal sheath in the right femoral vein using standard methods, advancing the sheath to the superior vena cava under fluoroscopic or echocardiographic guidance. The physician uses a transseptal needle to cross the atrial septum, entering the left atrium. The physician introduces a guidewire into the left atrium and removes the transseptal catheter while leaving the wire in place. The physician advances a septostomy catheter over the wire into the left atrium. This catheter has a retracted blade, which the physician extends. The physician pulls the blade slowly across the atrial septum from the left into the right atrium, under fluoroscopic or echocardiographic guidance. The physician may make several passes with the blade catheter in this fashion. The physician removes the septostomy catheter and venous sheath. Pressure is placed over the incision for 20 to 30 minutes to stem bleeding. The patient is observed for a period afterward.

Coding Tips

Do not report cardiac catheterization services separately as they are included in this procedure. For atrial septectomy or septostomy, balloon method (Rashkind type), see 92992.

ICD-10-CM Diagnostic Codes

Q20.0	Common arterial trunk
Q20.1	Double outlet right ventricle
Q20.3	Discordant ventriculoarterial connection
Q21.3	Tetralogy of Fallot
Q21.8	Other congenital malformations of cardiac septa

Q22.0	Pulmonary valve atresia
Q22.4	Congenital tricuspid stenosis
Q22.6	Hypoplastic right heart syndrome
Q22.8	Other congenital malformations of tricuspid valve
Q23.8	Other congenital malformations of aortic and mitral valves
Q24.8	Other specified congenital malformations of heart
Q25.0	Patent ductus arteriosus
Q25.21	Interruption of aortic arch
Q25.29	Other atresia of aorta
Q25.5	Atresia of pulmonary artery
Q26.2	Total anomalous pulmonary venous connection

AMA: **92993** 2018,Jan,8; 2018,Feb,11; 2017,Jan,8; 2016,Jul,3; 2016,Jan,13; 2015,Jan,16; 2014,Jan,11

Relative Value Units/Medicare Edits

Non-Facility RVU	Work	PE	MP	Total
92993	0.0	0.0	0.0	0.0
Facility RVU	**Work**	**PE**	**MP**	**Total**
92993	0.0	0.0	0.0	0.0

	FUD	Status	MUE	Modifiers				IOM Reference
92993	90	C	1(2)	51	N/A	N/A	80	None

* with documentation

Terms To Know

atresia. Congenital closure or absence of a tubular organ or an opening to the body surface.

atrial septal defect. Cardiac anomaly consisting of a patent opening in the atrial septum due to a fusion failure, classified as ostium secundum type, ostium primum defect, or endocardial cushion defect.

congenital. Present at birth, occurring through heredity or an influence during gestation up to the moment of birth.

fluoroscopy. Radiology technique that allows visual examination of part of the body or a function of an organ using a device that projects an x-ray image on a fluorescent screen.

guidewire. Flexible metal instrument designed to lead another instrument in its proper course.

septostomy. Surgical creation of a septal defect or opening.

92997-92998

92997 Percutaneous transluminal pulmonary artery balloon angioplasty; single vessel

\+ **92998** each additional vessel (List separately in addition to code for primary procedure)

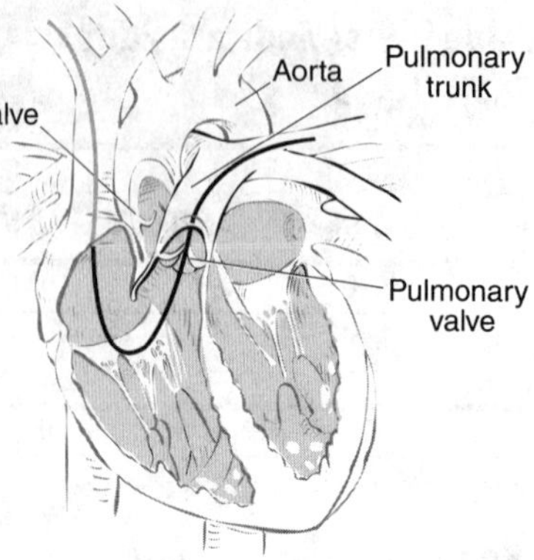

A pulmonary artery is approached transluminally by percutaneous entry. Balloon angioplasty is performed

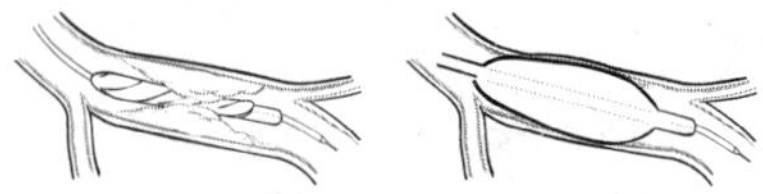

Explanation

The purpose of this procedure is to use a balloon to expand a narrowed pulmonary artery. The physician places an introducer sheath in the femoral vein, using percutaneous puncture. The physician places an angioplasty catheter through the introducer sheath into the femoral vein and advances it under fluoroscopic guidance to the right ventricle and out into the main pulmonary artery. The physician advances the angioplasty balloon into the narrowed pulmonary artery, using injections of x-ray contrast material to guide the way. In 92998, following single vessel percutaneous transluminal pulmonary artery balloon angioplasty, the physician redirects the balloon angioplasty catheter to an additional pulmonary artery. The physician may change to a different sized balloon catheter if the additional pulmonary artery is of a different size. For both procedures, the physician inflates the balloon to expand the pulmonary artery, sometimes using several balloon inflations. The physician removes the catheter and sheath from the femoral vein. Pressure is placed on the wound for 20 to 30 minutes to stem bleeding.

Coding Tips

Report 75741 or 75743 for the radiological supervision and interpretation, when appropriate. If intravascular ultrasound is used, report 37252-37253.

ICD-10-CM Diagnostic Codes

I26.01	Septic pulmonary embolism with acute cor pulmonale
I26.02	Saddle embolus of pulmonary artery with acute cor pulmonale
I26.09	Other pulmonary embolism with acute cor pulmonale
I26.90	Septic pulmonary embolism without acute cor pulmonale
I26.92	Saddle embolus of pulmonary artery without acute cor pulmonale
I26.93	Single subsegmental pulmonary embolism without acute cor pulmonale
I26.94	Multiple subsegmental pulmonary emboli without acute cor pulmonale

I26.99	Other pulmonary embolism without acute cor pulmonale
I28.8	Other diseases of pulmonary vessels
Q21.3	Tetralogy of Fallot
Q24.3	Pulmonary infundibular stenosis
Q25.5	Atresia of pulmonary artery
Q25.6	Stenosis of pulmonary artery
Q25.71	Coarctation of pulmonary artery
Q25.72	Congenital pulmonary arteriovenous malformation
Q25.79	Other congenital malformations of pulmonary artery

AMA: **92997** 2018,Jan,8; 2018,Feb,11; 2017,Jul,3; 2017,Jan,8; 2016,Mar,5; 2016,Jan,13; 2015,Feb,3 **92998** 2018,Jan,8; 2018,Feb,11; 2017,Jul,3; 2017,Jan,8; 2016,Mar,5; 2016,Jan,13; 2015,Feb,3

Relative Value Units/Medicare Edits

Non-Facility RVU	Work	PE	MP	Total
92997	11.98	4.27	2.84	19.09
92998	5.99	2.05	1.4	9.44
Facility RVU	**Work**	**PE**	**MP**	**Total**
92997	11.98	4.27	2.84	19.09
92998	5.99	2.05	1.4	9.44

	FUD	Status	MUE	Modifiers				IOM Reference
92997	0	A	1(2)	51	N/A	N/A	80*	None
92998	N/A	A	2(3)	N/A	N/A	N/A	80*	

* with documentation

Terms To Know

embolism. Obstruction of a blood vessel resulting from a clot or foreign substance.

fluoroscopy. Radiology technique that allows visual examination of part of the body or a function of an organ using a device that projects an x-ray image on a fluorescent screen.

infarction. Area of necrosis in tissue, due to ischemia from lack of circulation, usually from a thrombus or an embolus.

percutaneous. Through the skin.

transluminal balloon angioplasty. Balloon-tipped catheter is placed within a narrowed artery or vein and the balloon is inflated to stretch the vessel to a larger diameter for increased blood flow.

[92920, 92921]

92920 Percutaneous transluminal coronary angioplasty; single major coronary artery or branch

\+ **92921** Percutaneous transluminal coronary angioplasty; each additional branch of a major coronary artery (List separately in addition to code for primary procedure)

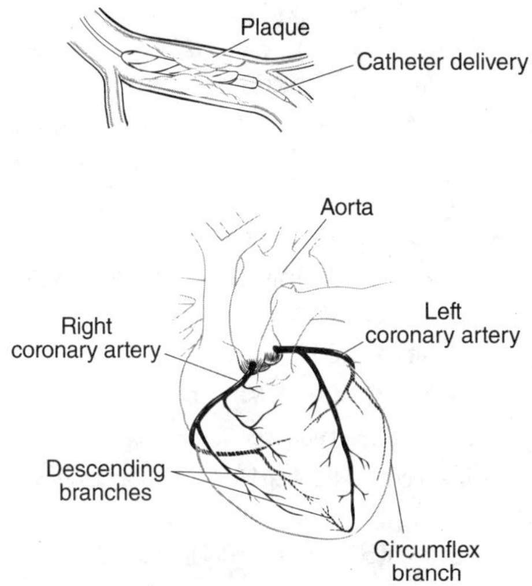

Percutaneous angioplasty of one or more major coronary arteries

Explanation

The physician makes a small incision in the arm or leg to access the artery for placement of two catheters. A central venous catheter is inserted through the femoral or brachial artery and a second catheter with a balloon tip is threaded up to the heart and into an obstructed native coronary artery. The physician inflates the balloon at the tip of the second catheter to flatten plaque obstructing the artery against the walls of the coronary artery. If sufficient results are not obtained after the first inflation, the physician may reinflate the balloon for a longer period of time or at greater pressure. The catheters are removed. Pressure is placed over the incision for 20 to 30 minutes to stop bleeding. Report 92920 for each angioplasty performed on a single major coronary artery or branch. Report 92921 for each additional branch of the major coronary artery treated during percutaneous coronary intervention.

Coding Tips

When medically necessary, report moderate (conscious) sedation provided by the performing physician with 99151-99153. When provided by another physician, report 99155-99157. Report 92921 in addition to 92920, 92924, 92928, 92933, 92937, 92941, or 92943. Diagnostic coronary angiography performed at the time of the procedure may be reported in certain instances, such as when no prior catheter-based angiography study has been performed or a significant change in the patient's condition has occurred since the time of a prior study. Diagnostic coronary angiography services reported at the same surgical session as a percutaneous revascularization service may be reported separately. Only one base code from the percutaneous coronary intervention (PCI) codes should be reported for revascularization of a major coronary artery and its branches or revascularization of a bypass graft. The PCI base codes are 92920, 92924, 92928, 92933, 92937, 92941, and 92943, and the most intensive service for the target vessel should be selected. Services performed on additional branches should be reported using the add-on codes throughout the section. See CPT section guidelines for details on hierarchy and examples. Medicare and some other payers may require HCPCS Level II codes C9600–C9601 be reported for these services if drug eluting stents are used.

ICD-10-CM Diagnostic Codes

I20.0	Unstable angina
I21.01	ST elevation (STEMI) myocardial infarction involving left main coronary artery
I21.02	ST elevation (STEMI) myocardial infarction involving left anterior descending coronary artery
I21.09	ST elevation (STEMI) myocardial infarction involving other coronary artery of anterior wall
I21.11	ST elevation (STEMI) myocardial infarction involving right coronary artery
I21.19	ST elevation (STEMI) myocardial infarction involving other coronary artery of inferior wall
I21.21	ST elevation (STEMI) myocardial infarction involving left circumflex coronary artery
I21.29	ST elevation (STEMI) myocardial infarction involving other sites
I21.4	Non-ST elevation (NSTEMI) myocardial infarction
I21.A1	Myocardial infarction type 2
I22.0	Subsequent ST elevation (STEMI) myocardial infarction of anterior wall
I22.1	Subsequent ST elevation (STEMI) myocardial infarction of inferior wall
I22.2	Subsequent non-ST elevation (NSTEMI) myocardial infarction
I22.8	Subsequent ST elevation (STEMI) myocardial infarction of other sites
I24.0	Acute coronary thrombosis not resulting in myocardial infarction
I24.1	Dressler's syndrome
I24.8	Other forms of acute ischemic heart disease
I25.110	Atherosclerotic heart disease of native coronary artery with unstable angina pectoris
I25.111	Atherosclerotic heart disease of native coronary artery with angina pectoris with documented spasm
I25.118	Atherosclerotic heart disease of native coronary artery with other forms of angina pectoris
I25.2	Old myocardial infarction
I25.3	Aneurysm of heart
I25.41	Coronary artery aneurysm
I25.42	Coronary artery dissection
I25.5	Ischemic cardiomyopathy
I25.6	Silent myocardial ischemia
I25.710	Atherosclerosis of autologous vein coronary artery bypass graft(s) with unstable angina pectoris
I25.711	Atherosclerosis of autologous vein coronary artery bypass graft(s) with angina pectoris with documented spasm
I25.718	Atherosclerosis of autologous vein coronary artery bypass graft(s) with other forms of angina pectoris
I25.720	Atherosclerosis of autologous artery coronary artery bypass graft(s) with unstable angina pectoris
I25.721	Atherosclerosis of autologous artery coronary artery bypass graft(s) with angina pectoris with documented spasm
I25.728	Atherosclerosis of autologous artery coronary artery bypass graft(s) with other forms of angina pectoris
I25.730	Atherosclerosis of nonautologous biological coronary artery bypass graft(s) with unstable angina pectoris
I25.731	Atherosclerosis of nonautologous biological coronary artery bypass graft(s) with angina pectoris with documented spasm
I25.738	Atherosclerosis of nonautologous biological coronary artery bypass graft(s) with other forms of angina pectoris
I25.750	Atherosclerosis of native coronary artery of transplanted heart with unstable angina
I25.760	Atherosclerosis of bypass graft of coronary artery of transplanted heart with unstable angina
I25.761	Atherosclerosis of bypass graft of coronary artery of transplanted heart with angina pectoris with documented spasm
I25.768	Atherosclerosis of bypass graft of coronary artery of transplanted heart with other forms of angina pectoris
I25.790	Atherosclerosis of other coronary artery bypass graft(s) with unstable angina pectoris
I25.791	Atherosclerosis of other coronary artery bypass graft(s) with angina pectoris with documented spasm
I25.798	Atherosclerosis of other coronary artery bypass graft(s) with other forms of angina pectoris
I25.810	Atherosclerosis of coronary artery bypass graft(s) without angina pectoris
I25.812	Atherosclerosis of bypass graft of coronary artery of transplanted heart without angina pectoris
I25.82	Chronic total occlusion of coronary artery
I25.84	Coronary atherosclerosis due to calcified coronary lesion
I25.89	Other forms of chronic ischemic heart disease
R57.0	Cardiogenic shock
R94.31	Abnormal electrocardiogram [ECG] [EKG]
T82.211A	Breakdown (mechanical) of coronary artery bypass graft, initial encounter
T82.212A	Displacement of coronary artery bypass graft, initial encounter
T82.213A	Leakage of coronary artery bypass graft, initial encounter
T82.218A	Other mechanical complication of coronary artery bypass graft, initial encounter
T82.818A	Embolism due to vascular prosthetic devices, implants and grafts, initial encounter
T82.828A	Fibrosis due to vascular prosthetic devices, implants and grafts, initial encounter
T82.838A	Hemorrhage due to vascular prosthetic devices, implants and grafts, initial encounter
T82.848A	Pain due to vascular prosthetic devices, implants and grafts, initial encounter
T82.858A	Stenosis of other vascular prosthetic devices, implants and grafts, initial encounter
T82.868A	Thrombosis due to vascular prosthetic devices, implants and grafts, initial encounter
T82.898A	Other specified complication of vascular prosthetic devices, implants and grafts, initial encounter

AMA: **92920** 2018,Jan,8; 2018,Feb,11; 2017,Jul,3; 2017,Jan,8; 2016,Jan,13; 2015,Jan,16; 2014,Dec,6; 2013,Jan,3-5 **92921** 2018,Jan,8; 2018,Feb,11; 2017,Jul,3; 2017,Jan,8; 2016,Jan,13; 2015,Jan,16; 2014,Sep,13; 2014,Dec,6; 2013,Jan,3-5

Relative Value Units/Medicare Edits

Non-Facility RVU	Work	PE	MP	Total
92920	9.85	3.39	2.25	15.49
92921	0.0	0.0	0.0	0.0
Facility RVU	**Work**	**PE**	**MP**	**Total**
92920	9.85	3.39	2.25	15.49
92921	0.0	0.0	0.0	0.0

	FUD	Status	MUE	Modifiers				IOM Reference
92920	0	A	3(3)	51	N/A	N/A	80*	None
92921	N/A	B	6(2)	N/A	N/A	N/A	N/A	

* with documentation

Terms To Know

angiography. Radiographic imaging of the arteries.

angioplasty. Reconstruction or repair of a diseased or damaged blood vessel.

angioplasty balloon. Balloon-tipped medical device used to clear the blockage of an artery. After insertion into the clogged artery, the balloon is inflated to expand a narrowing arterial section.

revascularization. Restoration of blood flow and oxygen supply to a body part. This may apply to an extremity, the heart, or penis.

[92924, 92925]

92924 Percutaneous transluminal coronary atherectomy, with coronary angioplasty when performed; single major coronary artery or branch

\+ **92925** Percutaneous transluminal coronary atherectomy, with coronary angioplasty when performed; each additional branch of a major coronary artery (List separately in addition to code for primary procedure)

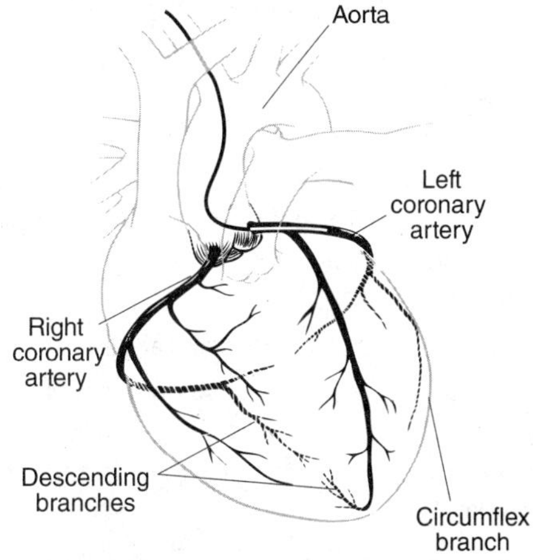

A coronary artery is approached transluminally by a percutaneous entry. Atherosclerotic deposits in the vessel are removed, mechanically or by other methods

Explanation

The physician removes the atherosclerotic plaque blocking a native coronary artery. The physician makes a small incision in the arm or leg to access the artery for placement of two catheters. A central venous catheter is inserted through the femoral or brachial artery and a second catheter threaded up to the coronary artery blockage. The plaque is removed using a rotary cutter introduced through a catheter under radiographic guidance. The blockage may also require subsequent inflation of the balloon on the tip of the second catheter to flatten any remaining plaque. The catheters are removed. Pressure is placed over the incision for 20 to 30 minutes to stop bleeding. Report 92924 for each atherectomy performed on a single major coronary artery or branch. Report 92925 for each additional branch of the major coronary artery treated during percutaneous coronary intervention.

Coding Tips

When medically necessary, report moderate (conscious) sedation provided by the performing physician with 99151-99153. When provided by another physician, report 99155-99157. Report 92925 in addition to 92924, 92928, 92933, 92937, 92941, or 92943. Diagnostic coronary angiography performed at the time of the procedure may be reported in certain instances, such as when no prior catheter-based angiography study has been performed or a significant change in the patient's condition has occurred since the time of a prior study. Diagnostic coronary angiography services reported at the same surgical session as a percutaneous revascularization service may be reported separately. Only one base code from the percutaneous coronary intervention (PCI) codes should be reported for revascularization of a major coronary artery and its branches or revascularization of a bypass graft. The PCI base codes are 92920, 92924, 92928, 92933, 92937, 92941, and 92943, and the most intensive service for the target vessel should be selected. Services performed on additional branches should be reported using the add-on codes throughout the section. See CPT section guidelines for details on hierarchy and examples.

Medicare and some other payers may require HCPCS Level II codes C9602–C9603 be reported for these services if drug eluting stents are used.

ICD-10-CM Diagnostic Codes

I20.0	Unstable angina
I21.01	ST elevation (STEMI) myocardial infarction involving left main coronary artery
I21.02	ST elevation (STEMI) myocardial infarction involving left anterior descending coronary artery
I21.09	ST elevation (STEMI) myocardial infarction involving other coronary artery of anterior wall
I21.11	ST elevation (STEMI) myocardial infarction involving right coronary artery
I21.19	ST elevation (STEMI) myocardial infarction involving other coronary artery of inferior wall
I21.21	ST elevation (STEMI) myocardial infarction involving left circumflex coronary artery
I21.29	ST elevation (STEMI) myocardial infarction involving other sites
I21.4	Non-ST elevation (NSTEMI) myocardial infarction
I22.0	Subsequent ST elevation (STEMI) myocardial infarction of anterior wall
I22.1	Subsequent ST elevation (STEMI) myocardial infarction of inferior wall
I22.2	Subsequent non-ST elevation (NSTEMI) myocardial infarction
I22.8	Subsequent ST elevation (STEMI) myocardial infarction of other sites
I24.0	Acute coronary thrombosis not resulting in myocardial infarction
I24.1	Dressler's syndrome
I24.8	Other forms of acute ischemic heart disease
I25.10	Atherosclerotic heart disease of native coronary artery without angina pectoris
I25.110	Atherosclerotic heart disease of native coronary artery with unstable angina pectoris
I25.111	Atherosclerotic heart disease of native coronary artery with angina pectoris with documented spasm
I25.118	Atherosclerotic heart disease of native coronary artery with other forms of angina pectoris
I25.2	Old myocardial infarction
I25.3	Aneurysm of heart
I25.41	Coronary artery aneurysm
I25.42	Coronary artery dissection
I25.5	Ischemic cardiomyopathy
I25.6	Silent myocardial ischemia
I25.750	Atherosclerosis of native coronary artery of transplanted heart with unstable angina
I25.82	Chronic total occlusion of coronary artery
I25.84	Coronary atherosclerosis due to calcified coronary lesion
I25.89	Other forms of chronic ischemic heart disease
I25.9	Chronic ischemic heart disease, unspecified
R57.0	Cardiogenic shock
R94.31	Abnormal electrocardiogram [ECG] [EKG]
T82.211A	Breakdown (mechanical) of coronary artery bypass graft, initial encounter
T82.212A	Displacement of coronary artery bypass graft, initial encounter
T82.213A	Leakage of coronary artery bypass graft, initial encounter
T82.218A	Other mechanical complication of coronary artery bypass graft, initial encounter
T82.818A	Embolism due to vascular prosthetic devices, implants and grafts, initial encounter
T82.828A	Fibrosis due to vascular prosthetic devices, implants and grafts, initial encounter
T82.838A	Hemorrhage due to vascular prosthetic devices, implants and grafts, initial encounter
T82.848A	Pain due to vascular prosthetic devices, implants and grafts, initial encounter
T82.858A	Stenosis of other vascular prosthetic devices, implants and grafts, initial encounter
T82.868A	Thrombosis due to vascular prosthetic devices, implants and grafts, initial encounter
T82.898A	Other specified complication of vascular prosthetic devices, implants and grafts, initial encounter

AMA: 92924 2018,Jan,8; 2018,Feb,11; 2017,Jul,3; 2017,Jan,8; 2016,Jan,13; 2015,Jan,16; 2014,Dec,6; 2013,Jan,3-5 **92925** 2018,Jan,8; 2018,Feb,11; 2017,Jul,3; 2017,Jan,8; 2016,Jan,13; 2015,Jan,16; 2014,Sep,13; 2014,Dec,6; 2013,Jan,3-5

Relative Value Units/Medicare Edits

Non-Facility RVU	Work	PE	MP	Total
92924	11.74	4.02	2.72	18.48
92925	0.0	0.0	0.0	0.0
Facility RVU	**Work**	**PE**	**MP**	**Total**
92924	11.74	4.02	2.72	18.48
92925	0.0	0.0	0.0	0.0

	FUD	Status	MUE	Modifiers				IOM Reference
92924	0	A	2(3)	51	N/A	N/A	80*	None
92925	N/A	B	6(2)	N/A	N/A	N/A	N/A	

* with documentation

Terms To Know

angiography. Radiographic imaging of the arteries.

angioplasty balloon. Balloon-tipped medical device used to clear the blockage of an artery. After insertion into the clogged artery, the balloon is inflated to expand a narrowing arterial section.

percutaneous transluminal coronary angioplasty. Procedure used to treat coronary artery obstruction. A balloon catheter is placed in the affected artery and the balloon is inflated to flatten the plaque against the wall of the artery and open the obstruction.

plaque. Accumulation of a soft sticky substance on the teeth largely composed of bacteria and its byproducts.

stent. Tube to provide support in a body cavity or lumen.

[92928, 92929]

92928 Percutaneous transcatheter placement of intracoronary stent(s), with coronary angioplasty when performed; single major coronary artery or branch

\+ **92929** Percutaneous transcatheter placement of intracoronary stent(s), with coronary angioplasty when performed; each additional branch of a major coronary artery (List separately in addition to code for primary procedure)

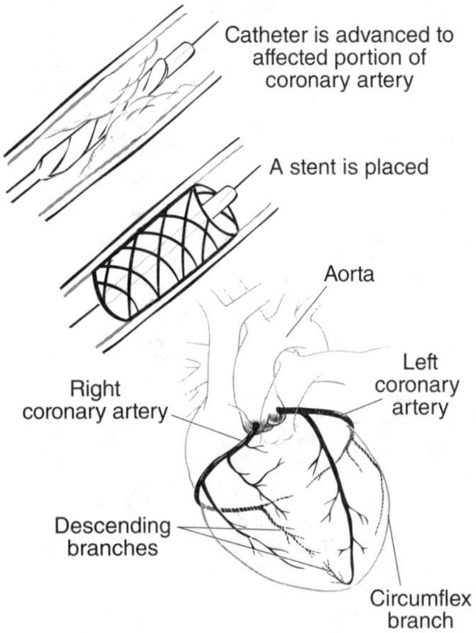

Explanation

A stent is used to hold open a blocked or collapsed native artery in the heart. The physician makes a small incision in the arm or leg to access the artery for placement of two catheters. A central venous catheter is inserted through the femoral or brachial artery and a second catheter is threaded up to the affected coronary artery. An obstruction may be treated first by inflating a balloon at the tip of the second catheter (PTCA) to flatten the obstruction. A stent is introduced through a catheter, placed under radiographic guidance, and expanded to fit the lumen of the artery by inflating the balloon on the second catheter. The catheters are removed. Pressure is placed over the incision for 20 to 30 minutes to stop the bleeding. Report 92928 for each stent placement performed on a single major coronary artery or branch. Report 92929 for each additional branch of the major coronary artery stented during percutaneous coronary intervention.

Coding Tips

When medically necessary, report moderate (conscious) sedation provided by the performing physician with 99151-99153. When provided by another physician, report 99155-99157. Report 92929 in addition to 92928, 92933, 92937, 92941, or 92943. Diagnostic coronary angiography performed at the time of the procedure may be reported in certain instances, such as when no prior catheter-based angiography study has been performed or a significant change in the patient's condition has occurred since the time of a prior study. Diagnostic coronary angiography services reported at a different surgical session as a percutaneous revascularization service may be reported separately. Only one base code from the percutaneous coronary intervention (PCI) codes should be reported for revascularization of a major coronary artery and its branches or revascularization of a bypass graft. The PCI base codes are 92920, 92924, 92928, 92933, 92937, 92941, and 92943, and the most intensive service for the target vessel should be selected. Services performed on additional branches should be reported using the add-on codes throughout the section. See CPT section guidelines for details on hierarchy and examples.

ICD-10-CM Diagnostic Codes

I20.0	Unstable angina
I21.01	ST elevation (STEMI) myocardial infarction involving left main coronary artery
I21.02	ST elevation (STEMI) myocardial infarction involving left anterior descending coronary artery
I21.09	ST elevation (STEMI) myocardial infarction involving other coronary artery of anterior wall
I21.11	ST elevation (STEMI) myocardial infarction involving right coronary artery
I21.19	ST elevation (STEMI) myocardial infarction involving other coronary artery of inferior wall
I21.21	ST elevation (STEMI) myocardial infarction involving left circumflex coronary artery
I21.29	ST elevation (STEMI) myocardial infarction involving other sites
I21.4	Non-ST elevation (NSTEMI) myocardial infarction
I21.A1	Myocardial infarction type 2
I22.0	Subsequent ST elevation (STEMI) myocardial infarction of anterior wall
I22.1	Subsequent ST elevation (STEMI) myocardial infarction of inferior wall
I22.2	Subsequent non-ST elevation (NSTEMI) myocardial infarction
I22.8	Subsequent ST elevation (STEMI) myocardial infarction of other sites
I24.0	Acute coronary thrombosis not resulting in myocardial infarction
I24.1	Dressler's syndrome
I24.8	Other forms of acute ischemic heart disease
I25.10	Atherosclerotic heart disease of native coronary artery without angina pectoris
I25.110	Atherosclerotic heart disease of native coronary artery with unstable angina pectoris
I25.111	Atherosclerotic heart disease of native coronary artery with angina pectoris with documented spasm
I25.118	Atherosclerotic heart disease of native coronary artery with other forms of angina pectoris
I25.119	Atherosclerotic heart disease of native coronary artery with unspecified angina pectoris
I25.2	Old myocardial infarction
I25.3	Aneurysm of heart
I25.41	Coronary artery aneurysm
I25.42	Coronary artery dissection
I25.5	Ischemic cardiomyopathy
I25.6	Silent myocardial ischemia
I25.750	Atherosclerosis of native coronary artery of transplanted heart with unstable angina
I25.82	Chronic total occlusion of coronary artery
I25.84	Coronary atherosclerosis due to calcified coronary lesion
I25.89	Other forms of chronic ischemic heart disease
I25.9	Chronic ischemic heart disease, unspecified
R57.0	Cardiogenic shock
R94.31	Abnormal electrocardiogram [ECG] [EKG]
T82.211A	Breakdown (mechanical) of coronary artery bypass graft, initial encounter

Medicine

T82.212A	Displacement of coronary artery bypass graft, initial encounter
T82.213A	Leakage of coronary artery bypass graft, initial encounter
T82.218A	Other mechanical complication of coronary artery bypass graft, initial encounter
T82.818A	Embolism due to vascular prosthetic devices, implants and grafts, initial encounter
T82.828A	Fibrosis due to vascular prosthetic devices, implants and grafts, initial encounter
T82.838A	Hemorrhage due to vascular prosthetic devices, implants and grafts, initial encounter
T82.848A	Pain due to vascular prosthetic devices, implants and grafts, initial encounter
T82.858A	Stenosis of other vascular prosthetic devices, implants and grafts, initial encounter
T82.868A	Thrombosis due to vascular prosthetic devices, implants and grafts, initial encounter
T82.898A	Other specified complication of vascular prosthetic devices, implants and grafts, initial encounter

AMA: 92928 2018,Jan,8; 2018,Feb,11; 2017,Jul,3; 2017,Jan,6; 2017,Jan,8; 2017,Feb,14; 2016,Jan,13; 2015,Jan,16; 2014,Sep,13; 2014,Mar,13; 2014,Jan,3; 2014,Dec,6; 2013,Jan,3-5 **92929** 2018,Jan,8; 2018,Feb,11; 2017,Jul,3; 2017,Jan,8; 2017,Jan,6; 2016,Jan,13; 2015,Jan,16; 2014,Sep,13; 2014,Dec,6; 2013,Jan,3-5

Relative Value Units/Medicare Edits

Non-Facility RVU	Work	PE	MP	Total
92928	10.96	3.76	2.52	17.24
92929	0.0	0.0	0.0	0.0
Facility RVU	**Work**	**PE**	**MP**	**Total**
92928	10.96	3.76	2.52	17.24
92929	0.0	0.0	0.0	0.0

	FUD	Status	MUE	Modifiers				IOM Reference
92928	0	A	3(3)	51	N/A	N/A	80*	None
92929	N/A	B	6(2)	N/A	N/A	N/A	N/A	

* with documentation

Terms To Know

percutaneous transluminal coronary angioplasty. Procedure used to treat coronary artery obstruction. A balloon catheter is placed in the affected artery and the balloon is inflated to flatten the plaque against the wall of the artery and open the obstruction.

revascularization. Restoration of blood flow and oxygen supply to a body part. This may apply to an extremity, the heart, or penis.

[92933, 92934]

92933 Percutaneous transluminal coronary atherectomy, with intracoronary stent, with coronary angioplasty when performed; single major coronary artery or branch

+ **92934** Percutaneous transluminal coronary atherectomy, with intracoronary stent, with coronary angioplasty when performed; each additional branch of a major coronary artery (List separately in addition to code for primary procedure)

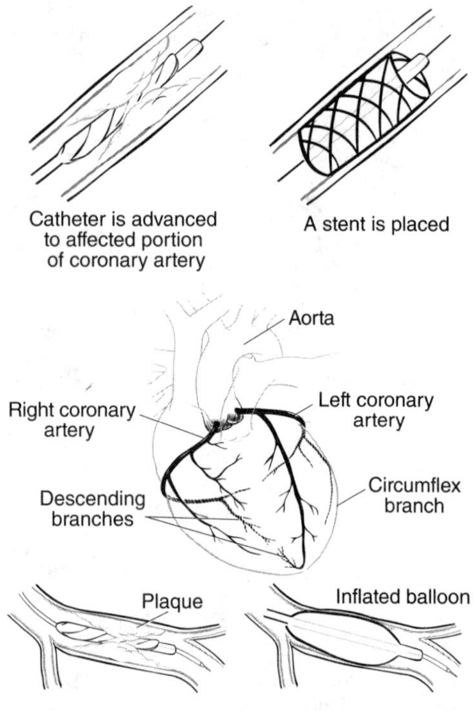

A balloon may be inflated or other intravascular therapy may accompany the procedure

Explanation

A stent is used to hold open a blocked native coronary artery. The physician makes a small incision in the arm or leg to access the artery for placement of two catheters. A central venous catheter is inserted through the femoral or brachial artery and a second catheter is threaded up to the affected coronary artery. Any obstruction is treated first by using a rotary cutter (atherectomy) to flatten or remove the obstruction. The obstruction may also be treated by inflating a balloon at the tip of the second catheter (PTCA). A stent is introduced through a catheter, placed under radiographic guidance, and expanded to fit the lumen of the artery by inflating the balloon on the second catheter. The catheters are removed. Pressure is placed over the incision for 20 to 30 minutes to stop the bleeding. Report 92933 for each atherectomy with stent placement performed on a single major coronary artery or branch. Report 92934 for each additional branch of the major coronary artery treated with atherectomy and stent during percutaneous coronary intervention.

Coding Tips

When medically necessary, report moderate (conscious) sedation provided by the performing physician with 99151-99153. When provided by another physician, report 99155-99157. Report 92934 in addition to 92933, 92937, 92941, or 92943. Diagnostic coronary angiography performed at the time of the procedure may be reported in certain instances, such as when no prior catheter-based angiography study has been performed or a significant change in the patient's condition has occurred since the time of a prior study.

Diagnostic coronary angiography services reported at the same surgical session as a percutaneous revascularization service may be reported separately. Only one base code from the percutaneous coronary intervention (PCI) codes should be reported for revascularization of a major coronary artery and its branches or revascularization of a bypass graft. The PCI base codes are 92920, 92924, 92928, 92933, 92937, 92941, and 92943, and the most intensive service for the target vessel should be selected. Services performed on additional branches should be reported using the add-on codes throughout the section. See CPT section guidelines for details on hierarchy and examples.

ICD-10-CM Diagnostic Codes

I20.0	Unstable angina
I21.01	ST elevation (STEMI) myocardial infarction involving left main coronary artery
I21.02	ST elevation (STEMI) myocardial infarction involving left anterior descending coronary artery
I21.09	ST elevation (STEMI) myocardial infarction involving other coronary artery of anterior wall
I21.11	ST elevation (STEMI) myocardial infarction involving right coronary artery
I21.19	ST elevation (STEMI) myocardial infarction involving other coronary artery of inferior wall
I21.21	ST elevation (STEMI) myocardial infarction involving left circumflex coronary artery
I21.29	ST elevation (STEMI) myocardial infarction involving other sites
I21.4	Non-ST elevation (NSTEMI) myocardial infarction
I21.A1	Myocardial infarction type 2
I22.0	Subsequent ST elevation (STEMI) myocardial infarction of anterior wall
I22.1	Subsequent ST elevation (STEMI) myocardial infarction of inferior wall
I22.2	Subsequent non-ST elevation (NSTEMI) myocardial infarction
I22.8	Subsequent ST elevation (STEMI) myocardial infarction of other sites
I24.0	Acute coronary thrombosis not resulting in myocardial infarction
I24.1	Dressler's syndrome
I24.8	Other forms of acute ischemic heart disease
I25.10	Atherosclerotic heart disease of native coronary artery without angina pectoris
I25.110	Atherosclerotic heart disease of native coronary artery with unstable angina pectoris
I25.111	Atherosclerotic heart disease of native coronary artery with angina pectoris with documented spasm
I25.118	Atherosclerotic heart disease of native coronary artery with other forms of angina pectoris
I25.119	Atherosclerotic heart disease of native coronary artery with unspecified angina pectoris
I25.2	Old myocardial infarction
I25.3	Aneurysm of heart
I25.41	Coronary artery aneurysm
I25.42	Coronary artery dissection
I25.5	Ischemic cardiomyopathy
I25.6	Silent myocardial ischemia
I25.750	Atherosclerosis of native coronary artery of transplanted heart with unstable angina
I25.82	Chronic total occlusion of coronary artery
I25.84	Coronary atherosclerosis due to calcified coronary lesion
I25.89	Other forms of chronic ischemic heart disease
I25.9	Chronic ischemic heart disease, unspecified
R57.0	Cardiogenic shock
R94.31	Abnormal electrocardiogram [ECG] [EKG]
T82.211A	Breakdown (mechanical) of coronary artery bypass graft, initial encounter
T82.212A	Displacement of coronary artery bypass graft, initial encounter
T82.213A	Leakage of coronary artery bypass graft, initial encounter
T82.218A	Other mechanical complication of coronary artery bypass graft, initial encounter
T82.818A	Embolism due to vascular prosthetic devices, implants and grafts, initial encounter
T82.828A	Fibrosis due to vascular prosthetic devices, implants and grafts, initial encounter
T82.838A	Hemorrhage due to vascular prosthetic devices, implants and grafts, initial encounter
T82.848A	Pain due to vascular prosthetic devices, implants and grafts, initial encounter
T82.858A	Stenosis of other vascular prosthetic devices, implants and grafts, initial encounter
T82.868A	Thrombosis due to vascular prosthetic devices, implants and grafts, initial encounter
T82.898A	Other specified complication of vascular prosthetic devices, implants and grafts, initial encounter

AMA: 92933 2018,Jan,8; 2018,Feb,11; 2017,Jul,3; 2017,Jan,8; 2016,Jan,13; 2015,Jan,16; 2014,Dec,6; 2013,Jan,3-5 **92934** 2018,Jan,8; 2018,Feb,11; 2017,Jul,3; 2017,Jan,8; 2016,Jan,13; 2015,Jan,16; 2014,Sep,13; 2014,Dec,6; 2013,Jan,3-5

Relative Value Units/Medicare Edits

Non-Facility RVU	Work	PE	MP	Total
92933	12.29	4.21	2.84	19.34
92934	0.0	0.0	0.0	0.0
Facility RVU	**Work**	**PE**	**MP**	**Total**
92933	12.29	4.21	2.84	19.34
92934	0.0	0.0	0.0	0.0

	FUD	Status	MUE	Modifiers				IOM Reference
92933	0	A	2(3)	51	N/A	N/A	80*	None
92934	N/A	B	6(2)	N/A	N/A	N/A	N/A	

* with documentation

Terms To Know

atherectomy. Surgical removal of arterial plaque from inside an artery. The procedure may be performed percutaneously, using a special catheter with a high-speed burr at the tip to bore through the sclerotic deposits, or transluminally by open incision.

revascularization. Restoration of blood flow and oxygen supply to a body part. This may apply to an extremity, the heart, or penis.

[92937, 92938]

92937 Percutaneous transluminal revascularization of or through coronary artery bypass graft (internal mammary, free arterial, venous), any combination of intracoronary stent, atherectomy and angioplasty, including distal protection when performed; single vessel

\+ **92938** Percutaneous transluminal revascularization of or through coronary artery bypass graft (internal mammary, free arterial, venous), any combination of intracoronary stent, atherectomy and angioplasty, including distal protection when performed; each additional branch subtended by the bypass graft (List separately in addition to code for primary procedure)

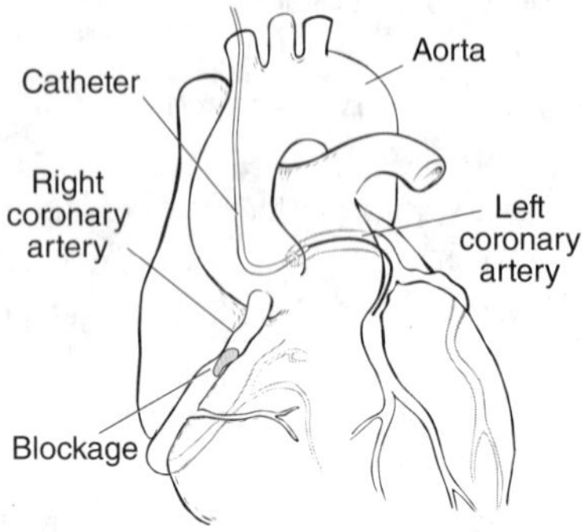

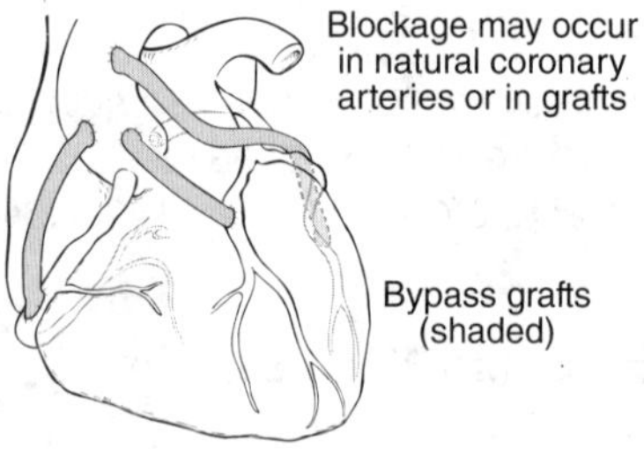

Explanation

The use of one or any combination of angioplasty, atherectomy, or stent placement is performed to restore a blocked coronary artery bypass graft (CABG). The physician makes a small incision in the arm or leg to access the artery for placement of two catheters. A central venous catheter is inserted through the femoral or brachial artery and a second catheter is threaded up to the affected graft. The obstruction may be treated by using a rotary cutter (atherectomy) to flatten or remove the obstruction, inflating a balloon at the tip of the second catheter (PTCA), or introducing a stent that is expanded to fit the lumen of the artery. The catheters are removed. Pressure is placed over the incision for 20 to 30 minutes to stop the bleeding. Report 92937 for treatment of the first CABG. Report 92938 for each additional graft treated.

Coding Tips

When medically necessary, report moderate (conscious) sedation provided by the performing physician with 99151-99153. When provided by another physician, report 99155-99157. Report 92938 in addition to 92937. Diagnostic coronary angiography performed at the time of the procedure may be reported in certain instances, such as when no prior catheter-based angiography study has been performed or a significant change in the patient's condition has occurred since the time of a prior study. Diagnostic coronary angiography services reported at the same surgical session as a percutaneous revascularization service may be reported separately. Only one base code from the percutaneous coronary intervention (PCI) codes should be reported for revascularization of a major coronary artery and its branches or revascularization of a bypass graft. The PCI base codes are 92920, 92924, 92928, 92933, 92937, 92941, and 92943, and the most intensive service for the target vessel should be selected. Services performed on additional branches should be reported using the add-on codes throughout the section. See CPT section guidelines for details on hierarchy and examples. Medicare and some other payers may require HCPCS Level II codes C9604–C9605 be reported for these services if drug eluting stents are used.

ICD-10-CM Diagnostic Codes

I20.0	Unstable angina
I21.01	ST elevation (STEMI) myocardial infarction involving left main coronary artery
I21.02	ST elevation (STEMI) myocardial infarction involving left anterior descending coronary artery
I21.09	ST elevation (STEMI) myocardial infarction involving other coronary artery of anterior wall
I21.11	ST elevation (STEMI) myocardial infarction involving right coronary artery
I21.19	ST elevation (STEMI) myocardial infarction involving other coronary artery of inferior wall
I21.21	ST elevation (STEMI) myocardial infarction involving left circumflex coronary artery
I21.29	ST elevation (STEMI) myocardial infarction involving other sites
I21.4	Non-ST elevation (NSTEMI) myocardial infarction
I21.A1	Myocardial infarction type 2
I22.0	Subsequent ST elevation (STEMI) myocardial infarction of anterior wall
I22.1	Subsequent ST elevation (STEMI) myocardial infarction of inferior wall
I22.2	Subsequent non-ST elevation (NSTEMI) myocardial infarction
I22.8	Subsequent ST elevation (STEMI) myocardial infarction of other sites
I24.0	Acute coronary thrombosis not resulting in myocardial infarction
I24.1	Dressler's syndrome
I24.8	Other forms of acute ischemic heart disease
I25.10	Atherosclerotic heart disease of native coronary artery without angina pectoris
I25.110	Atherosclerotic heart disease of native coronary artery with unstable angina pectoris
I25.111	Atherosclerotic heart disease of native coronary artery with angina pectoris with documented spasm
I25.2	Old myocardial infarction
I25.3	Aneurysm of heart
I25.41	Coronary artery aneurysm
I25.42	Coronary artery dissection
I25.5	Ischemic cardiomyopathy
I25.6	Silent myocardial ischemia
I25.710	Atherosclerosis of autologous vein coronary artery bypass graft(s) with unstable angina pectoris
I25.711	Atherosclerosis of autologous vein coronary artery bypass graft(s) with angina pectoris with documented spasm
I25.718	Atherosclerosis of autologous vein coronary artery bypass graft(s) with other forms of angina pectoris
I25.720	Atherosclerosis of autologous artery coronary artery bypass graft(s) with unstable angina pectoris

I25.721 Atherosclerosis of autologous artery coronary artery bypass graft(s) with angina pectoris with documented spasm

I25.728 Atherosclerosis of autologous artery coronary artery bypass graft(s) with other forms of angina pectoris

I25.730 Atherosclerosis of nonautologous biological coronary artery bypass graft(s) with unstable angina pectoris

I25.731 Atherosclerosis of nonautologous biological coronary artery bypass graft(s) with angina pectoris with documented spasm

I25.738 Atherosclerosis of nonautologous biological coronary artery bypass graft(s) with other forms of angina pectoris

I25.750 Atherosclerosis of native coronary artery of transplanted heart with unstable angina

I25.760 Atherosclerosis of bypass graft of coronary artery of transplanted heart with unstable angina

I25.761 Atherosclerosis of bypass graft of coronary artery of transplanted heart with angina pectoris with documented spasm

I25.768 Atherosclerosis of bypass graft of coronary artery of transplanted heart with other forms of angina pectoris

I25.790 Atherosclerosis of other coronary artery bypass graft(s) with unstable angina pectoris

I25.791 Atherosclerosis of other coronary artery bypass graft(s) with angina pectoris with documented spasm

I25.798 Atherosclerosis of other coronary artery bypass graft(s) with other forms of angina pectoris

I25.810 Atherosclerosis of coronary artery bypass graft(s) without angina pectoris

I25.812 Atherosclerosis of bypass graft of coronary artery of transplanted heart without angina pectoris

I25.82 Chronic total occlusion of coronary artery

I25.84 Coronary atherosclerosis due to calcified coronary lesion

I25.89 Other forms of chronic ischemic heart disease

I25.9 Chronic ischemic heart disease, unspecified

R57.0 Cardiogenic shock

R94.31 Abnormal electrocardiogram [ECG] [EKG]

T82.211A Breakdown (mechanical) of coronary artery bypass graft, initial encounter

T82.212A Displacement of coronary artery bypass graft, initial encounter

T82.213A Leakage of coronary artery bypass graft, initial encounter

T82.218A Other mechanical complication of coronary artery bypass graft, initial encounter

T82.529A Displacement of unspecified cardiac and vascular devices and implants, initial encounter

T82.539A Leakage of unspecified cardiac and vascular devices and implants, initial encounter

T82.818A Embolism due to vascular prosthetic devices, implants and grafts, initial encounter

T82.828A Fibrosis due to vascular prosthetic devices, implants and grafts, initial encounter

T82.838A Hemorrhage due to vascular prosthetic devices, implants and grafts, initial encounter

T82.848A Pain due to vascular prosthetic devices, implants and grafts, initial encounter

T82.858A Stenosis of other vascular prosthetic devices, implants and grafts, initial encounter

T82.868A Thrombosis due to vascular prosthetic devices, implants and grafts, initial encounter

T82.898A Other specified complication of vascular prosthetic devices, implants and grafts, initial encounter

AMA: **92937** 2018,Jan,8; 2018,Feb,11; 2017,Jul,3; 2017,Jan,8; 2017,Feb,14; 2016,Jan,13; 2015,Jan,16; 2014,Mar,13; 2014,Dec,6; 2013,Jan,3-5 **92938** 2018,Jan,8; 2018,Feb,11; 2017,Jul,3; 2017,Jan,8; 2016,Jan,13; 2015,Jan,16; 2014,Sep,13; 2014,Mar,13; 2014,Dec,6; 2013,Jan,3-5

Relative Value Units/Medicare Edits

Non-Facility RVU	Work	PE	MP	Total
92937	10.95	3.75	2.53	17.23
92938	0.0	0.0	0.0	0.0
Facility RVU	**Work**	**PE**	**MP**	**Total**
92937	10.95	3.75	2.53	17.23
92938	0.0	0.0	0.0	0.0

	FUD	Status	MUE	Modifiers				IOM Reference
92937	0	A	2(3)	51	N/A	N/A	80*	None
92938	N/A	B	6(3)	N/A	N/A	N/A	N/A	

* with documentation

Terms To Know

angioplasty. Reconstruction or repair of a diseased or damaged blood vessel.

atherectomy. Surgical removal of arterial plaque from inside an artery. The procedure may be performed percutaneously, using a special catheter with a high-speed burr at the tip to bore through the sclerotic deposits, or transluminally by open incision.

bypass graft. Surgically created alternative blood vessel used to reroute blood flow around an area of obstruction or disease.

revascularization. Restoration of blood flow and oxygen supply to a body part. This may apply to an extremity, the heart, or penis.

stent. Tube to provide support in a body cavity or lumen.

[92941]

92941 Percutaneous transluminal revascularization of acute total/subtotal occlusion during acute myocardial infarction, coronary artery or coronary artery bypass graft, any combination of intracoronary stent, atherectomy and angioplasty, including aspiration thrombectomy when performed, single vessel

Revascularization of occlusion in native or bypass coronary artery

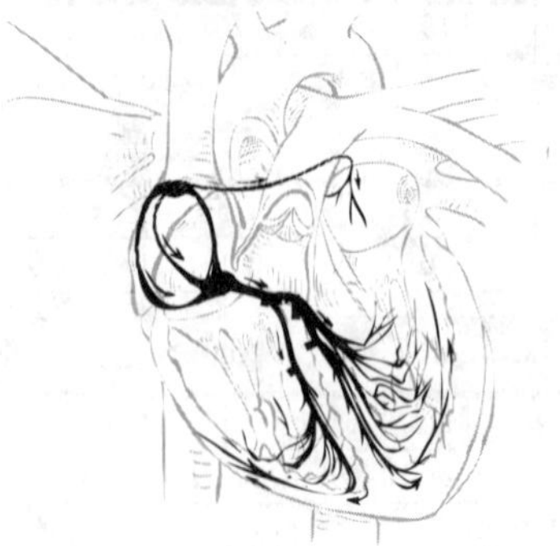

Explanation

The use of one or any combination of angioplasty, atherectomy, or stent placement is performed to restore an acutely blocked coronary artery bypass graft (CABG) or native coronary artery during an acute myocardial infarction. The physician makes a small incision in the arm or leg to access the artery for placement of two catheters. A central venous catheter is inserted through the femoral or brachial artery and a second catheter is threaded up to the affected vessel or graft. The obstruction may be treated by using a rotary cutter (atherectomy) to flatten or remove the obstruction, inflating a balloon at the tip of the second catheter (PTCA), or introducing a stent that is expanded to fit the lumen of the artery. The catheters are removed. Pressure is placed over the incision for 20 to 30 minutes to stop the bleeding.

Coding Tips

When medically necessary, report moderate (conscious) sedation provided by the performing physician with 99151-99153. When provided by another physician, report 99155-99157. Diagnostic coronary angiography performed at the time of the procedure may be reported in certain instances, such as when no prior catheter-based angiography study has been performed or a significant change in the patient's condition has occurred since the time of a prior study. Diagnostic coronary angiography services reported at the same surgical session as a percutaneous revascularization service may be reported separately. Only one base code from the percutaneous coronary intervention (PCI) codes should be reported for revascularization of a major coronary artery and its branches or revascularization of a bypass graft. The PCI base codes are 92920, 92924, 92928, 92933, 92937, 92941, and 92943, and the most intensive service for the target vessel should be selected. Services performed on additional branches should be reported using the add-on codes throughout the section. See CPT section guidelines for details on hierarchy and examples. Code 92941 reports a single vessel. For additional vessels treated, see 92920–92938, 92943, or 92944. Medicare and some other payers may require HCPCS Level II code C9606 be reported for this service if drug eluting stents are used.

ICD-10-CM Diagnostic Codes

I20.0	Unstable angina
I21.01	ST elevation (STEMI) myocardial infarction involving left main coronary artery
I21.02	ST elevation (STEMI) myocardial infarction involving left anterior descending coronary artery
I21.09	ST elevation (STEMI) myocardial infarction involving other coronary artery of anterior wall
I21.11	ST elevation (STEMI) myocardial infarction involving right coronary artery
I21.19	ST elevation (STEMI) myocardial infarction involving other coronary artery of inferior wall
I21.21	ST elevation (STEMI) myocardial infarction involving left circumflex coronary artery
I21.29	ST elevation (STEMI) myocardial infarction involving other sites
I21.4	Non-ST elevation (NSTEMI) myocardial infarction
I21.A1	Myocardial infarction type 2
I22.0	Subsequent ST elevation (STEMI) myocardial infarction of anterior wall
I22.1	Subsequent ST elevation (STEMI) myocardial infarction of inferior wall
I22.2	Subsequent non-ST elevation (NSTEMI) myocardial infarction
I22.8	Subsequent ST elevation (STEMI) myocardial infarction of other sites
I24.0	Acute coronary thrombosis not resulting in myocardial infarction
I24.8	Other forms of acute ischemic heart disease
I25.10	Atherosclerotic heart disease of native coronary artery without angina pectoris
I25.110	Atherosclerotic heart disease of native coronary artery with unstable angina pectoris
I25.111	Atherosclerotic heart disease of native coronary artery with angina pectoris with documented spasm
I25.5	Ischemic cardiomyopathy
I25.6	Silent myocardial ischemia
I25.710	Atherosclerosis of autologous vein coronary artery bypass graft(s) with unstable angina pectoris
I25.711	Atherosclerosis of autologous vein coronary artery bypass graft(s) with angina pectoris with documented spasm
I25.718	Atherosclerosis of autologous vein coronary artery bypass graft(s) with other forms of angina pectoris
I25.720	Atherosclerosis of autologous artery coronary artery bypass graft(s) with unstable angina pectoris
I25.721	Atherosclerosis of autologous artery coronary artery bypass graft(s) with angina pectoris with documented spasm
I25.728	Atherosclerosis of autologous artery coronary artery bypass graft(s) with other forms of angina pectoris
I25.730	Atherosclerosis of nonautologous biological coronary artery bypass graft(s) with unstable angina pectoris
I25.731	Atherosclerosis of nonautologous biological coronary artery bypass graft(s) with angina pectoris with documented spasm
I25.738	Atherosclerosis of nonautologous biological coronary artery bypass graft(s) with other forms of angina pectoris
I25.750	Atherosclerosis of native coronary artery of transplanted heart with unstable angina
I25.760	Atherosclerosis of bypass graft of coronary artery of transplanted heart with unstable angina
I25.761	Atherosclerosis of bypass graft of coronary artery of transplanted heart with angina pectoris with documented spasm
I25.768	Atherosclerosis of bypass graft of coronary artery of transplanted heart with other forms of angina pectoris

Medicine

I25.790	Atherosclerosis of other coronary artery bypass graft(s) with unstable angina pectoris
I25.791	Atherosclerosis of other coronary artery bypass graft(s) with angina pectoris with documented spasm
I25.798	Atherosclerosis of other coronary artery bypass graft(s) with other forms of angina pectoris
I25.810	Atherosclerosis of coronary artery bypass graft(s) without angina pectoris
I25.812	Atherosclerosis of bypass graft of coronary artery of transplanted heart without angina pectoris
I25.82	Chronic total occlusion of coronary artery
I25.84	Coronary atherosclerosis due to calcified coronary lesion
I25.89	Other forms of chronic ischemic heart disease
T82.818A	Embolism due to vascular prosthetic devices, implants and grafts, initial encounter
T82.828A	Fibrosis due to vascular prosthetic devices, implants and grafts, initial encounter
T82.838A	Hemorrhage due to vascular prosthetic devices, implants and grafts, initial encounter
T82.848A	Pain due to vascular prosthetic devices, implants and grafts, initial encounter
T82.858A	Stenosis of other vascular prosthetic devices, implants and grafts, initial encounter
T82.868A	Thrombosis due to vascular prosthetic devices, implants and grafts, initial encounter
T82.898A	Other specified complication of vascular prosthetic devices, implants and grafts, initial encounter

AMA: 92941 2018,Jan,8; 2018,Feb,11; 2017,Jul,3; 2017,Jan,8; 2017,Feb,14; 2016,Jan,13; 2015,Jan,16; 2014,Mar,13; 2014,Jan,3; 2014,Dec,6; 2013,Jan,3-5

Relative Value Units/Medicare Edits

Non-Facility RVU	Work	PE	MP	Total
92941	12.31	4.23	2.85	19.39
Facility RVU	**Work**	**PE**	**MP**	**Total**
92941	12.31	4.23	2.85	19.39

	FUD	Status	MUE	Modifiers				IOM Reference
92941	0	A	1(3)	51	N/A	N/A	80*	None

* with documentation

Terms To Know

atherectomy. Surgical removal of arterial plaque from inside an artery. The procedure may be performed percutaneously, using a special catheter with a high-speed burr at the tip to bore through the sclerotic deposits, or transluminally by open incision.

revascularization. Restoration of blood flow and oxygen supply to a body part. This may apply to an extremity, the heart, or penis.

[92943, 92944]

92943 Percutaneous transluminal revascularization of chronic total occlusion, coronary artery, coronary artery branch, or coronary artery bypass graft, any combination of intracoronary stent, atherectomy and angioplasty; single vessel

\+ **92944** Percutaneous transluminal revascularization of chronic total occlusion, coronary artery, coronary artery branch, or coronary artery bypass graft, any combination of intracoronary stent, atherectomy and angioplasty; each additional coronary artery, coronary artery branch, or bypass graft (List separately in addition to code for primary procedure)

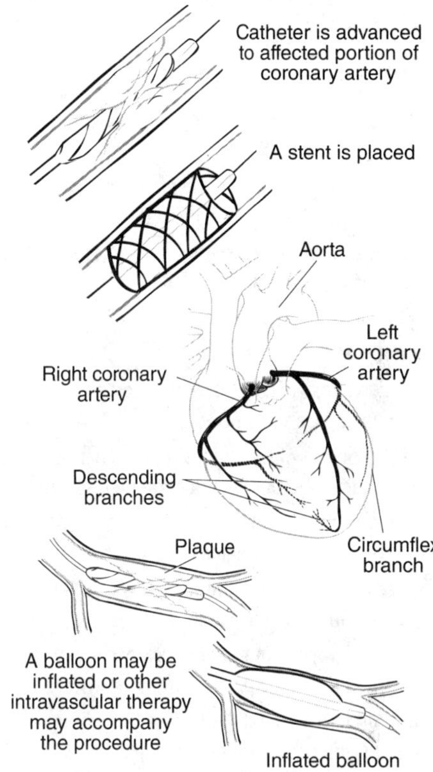

Explanation

The use of one or any combination of angioplasty, atherectomy, or stent placement is performed to restore a chronic totally blocked coronary artery bypass graft (CABG) or native coronary artery. The physician makes a small incision in the arm or leg to access the artery for placement of two catheters. A central venous catheter is inserted through the femoral or brachial artery and a second catheter is threaded up to the affected vessel or graft. The obstruction may be treated by using a rotary cutter (atherectomy) to flatten or remove the obstruction, inflating a balloon at the tip of the second catheter (PTCA), or introducing a stent that is expanded to fit the lumen of the artery. The catheters are removed. Pressure is placed over the incision for 20 to 30 minutes to stop the bleeding. Report 92943 for the treatment of the first native artery or CABG. Report 92944 for each additional graft or vessel treated.

Coding Tips

When medically necessary, report moderate (conscious) sedation provided by the performing physician with 99151-99153. When provided by another physician, report 99155-99157. Report 92944 in addition to 92924, 92928, 92933, 92937, 92941, and 92943. Diagnostic coronary angiography performed at the time of the procedure may be reported in certain instances, such as when no prior catheter-based angiography study has been performed or a

Medicine

significant change in the patient's condition has occurred since the time of a prior study. Diagnostic coronary angiography services reported at the same surgical session as a percutaneous revascularization service may be reported separately. Only one base code from the percutaneous coronary intervention (PCI) codes should be reported for revascularization of a major coronary artery and its branches or revascularization of a bypass graft. The PCI base codes are 92920, 92924, 92928, 92933, 92937, 92941, and 92943, and the most intensive service for the target vessel should be selected. Services performed on additional branches should be reported using the add-on codes throughout the section. See CPT section guidelines for details on hierarchy and examples. For transcatheter placement of a radiation delivery device for coronary intravascular brachytherapy, see 92974. For intravascular application of a radioelement, see 77770–77772. Medicare and some other payers may require HCPCS Level II codes C9607–C9608 be reported for these services if drug eluting stents are used.

ICD-10-CM Diagnostic Codes

I25.110	Atherosclerotic heart disease of native coronary artery with unstable angina pectoris
I25.111	Atherosclerotic heart disease of native coronary artery with angina pectoris with documented spasm
I25.118	Atherosclerotic heart disease of native coronary artery with other forms of angina pectoris
I25.5	Ischemic cardiomyopathy
I25.6	Silent myocardial ischemia
I25.710	Atherosclerosis of autologous vein coronary artery bypass graft(s) with unstable angina pectoris
I25.711	Atherosclerosis of autologous vein coronary artery bypass graft(s) with angina pectoris with documented spasm
I25.718	Atherosclerosis of autologous vein coronary artery bypass graft(s) with other forms of angina pectoris
I25.720	Atherosclerosis of autologous artery coronary artery bypass graft(s) with unstable angina pectoris
I25.721	Atherosclerosis of autologous artery coronary artery bypass graft(s) with angina pectoris with documented spasm
I25.728	Atherosclerosis of autologous artery coronary artery bypass graft(s) with other forms of angina pectoris
I25.730	Atherosclerosis of nonautologous biological coronary artery bypass graft(s) with unstable angina pectoris
I25.731	Atherosclerosis of nonautologous biological coronary artery bypass graft(s) with angina pectoris with documented spasm
I25.738	Atherosclerosis of nonautologous biological coronary artery bypass graft(s) with other forms of angina pectoris
I25.760	Atherosclerosis of bypass graft of coronary artery of transplanted heart with unstable angina
I25.761	Atherosclerosis of bypass graft of coronary artery of transplanted heart with angina pectoris with documented spasm
I25.768	Atherosclerosis of bypass graft of coronary artery of transplanted heart with other forms of angina pectoris
I25.790	Atherosclerosis of other coronary artery bypass graft(s) with unstable angina pectoris
I25.791	Atherosclerosis of other coronary artery bypass graft(s) with angina pectoris with documented spasm
I25.798	Atherosclerosis of other coronary artery bypass graft(s) with other forms of angina pectoris
I25.810	Atherosclerosis of coronary artery bypass graft(s) without angina pectoris
I25.812	Atherosclerosis of bypass graft of coronary artery of transplanted heart without angina pectoris
I25.82	Chronic total occlusion of coronary artery
I25.84	Coronary atherosclerosis due to calcified coronary lesion
I25.89	Other forms of chronic ischemic heart disease

AMA: 92943 2018,Jan,8; 2018,Feb,11; 2017,Jul,3; 2017,Jan,8; 2016,Jan,13; 2015,Jan,16; 2014,Dec,6; 2013,Jan,3-5 **92944** 2018,Jan,8; 2018,Feb,11; 2017,Jul,3; 2017,Jan,8; 2016,Jan,13; 2015,Jan,16; 2014,Sep,13; 2014,Dec,6; 2013,Jan,3-5

Relative Value Units/Medicare Edits

Non-Facility RVU	Work	PE	MP	Total
92943	12.31	4.23	2.84	19.38
92944	0.0	0.0	0.0	0.0
Facility RVU	**Work**	**PE**	**MP**	**Total**
92943	12.31	4.23	2.84	19.38
92944	0.0	0.0	0.0	0.0

	FUD	Status	MUE	Modifiers				IOM Reference
92943	0	A	2(3)	51	N/A	N/A	80*	None
92944	N/A	B	3(3)	N/A	N/A	N/A	N/A	

* with documentation

Terms To Know

atherectomy. Surgical removal of arterial plaque from inside an artery. The procedure may be performed percutaneously, using a special catheter with a high-speed burr at the tip to bore through the sclerotic deposits, or transluminally by open incision.

bypass graft. Surgically created alternative blood vessel used to reroute blood flow around an area of obstruction or disease.

revascularization. Restoration of blood flow and oxygen supply to a body part. This may apply to an extremity, the heart, or penis.

[92973]

\+ **92973** Percutaneous transluminal coronary thrombectomy mechanical (List separately in addition to code for primary procedure)

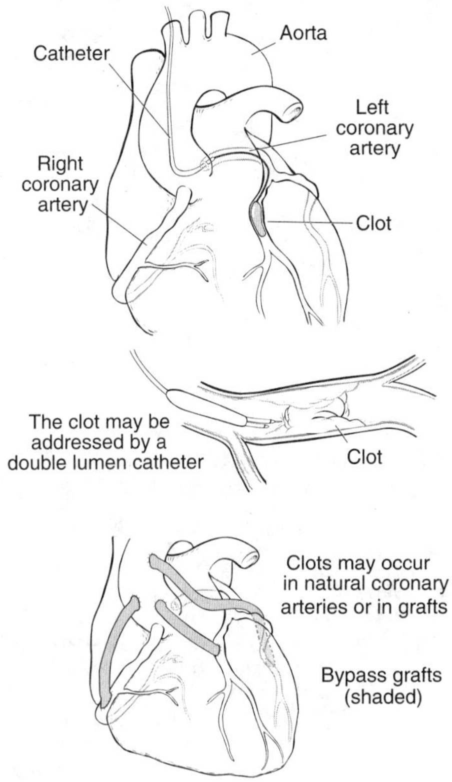

Explanation

The physician percutaneously removes a blood clot from a native or grafted coronary artery. A double lumen catheter is passed to the area of the clot. A high-pressure saline stream (via a pump) is introduced through a lumen that has multiple jet orifices located at the distal tip. The low-pressure zone created by the jets causes the clot to break up into small pieces and be pushed through the catheter with a force that drives debris from the thrombus through the other lumen (exhaust) and out of the body. The procedure is useful to clear fatty and degenerated arteries and to modify plaques in preparation for more definitive treatment with adjunctive balloon angioplasty or stenting.

Coding Tips

When medically necessary, report moderate (conscious) sedation provided by the performing physician with 99151-99153. When provided by another physician, report 99155-99157. Report 92973 in addition to 92920, 92924, 92928, 92933, 92937, 92941, 92943, 92975, 93454–93461, 93563, or 93564. For intravascular radioelement application, see 77770–77772.

ICD-10-CM Diagnostic Codes

This/these CPT code(s) are add on code(s). See the primary procedure code that this code is performed with for your ICD-10-CM code selections. Diagnostic code(s) would be the same as the actual procedure performed.

AMA: 92973 2018,Jan,8; 2018,Feb,11; 2017,Jan,8; 2017,Feb,14; 2016,Jan,13; 2015,Jan,16; 2014,Jan,11; 2014,Dec,6

Relative Value Units/Medicare Edits

Non-Facility RVU	Work	PE	MP	Total
92973	3.28	1.12	0.75	5.15
Facility RVU	**Work**	**PE**	**MP**	**Total**
92973	3.28	1.12	0.75	5.15

	FUD	Status	MUE	Modifiers				IOM Reference
92973	N/A	A	2(3)	N/A	N/A	N/A	80*	None

* with documentation

Terms To Know

catheterization. Use or insertion of a tubular device into a duct, blood vessel, hollow organ, or body cavity for injecting or withdrawing fluids for diagnostic or therapeutic purposes.

lumen. Space inside an intestine, artery, vein, duct, or tube.

moderate sedation. Medically controlled state of depressed consciousness, with or without analgesia, while maintaining the patient's airway, protective reflexes, and ability to respond to stimulation or verbal commands.

thrombectomy. Removal of a clot (thrombus) from a blood vessel utilizing various methods.

[92974]

+ **92974** Transcatheter placement of radiation delivery device for subsequent coronary intravascular brachytherapy (List separately in addition to code for primary procedure)

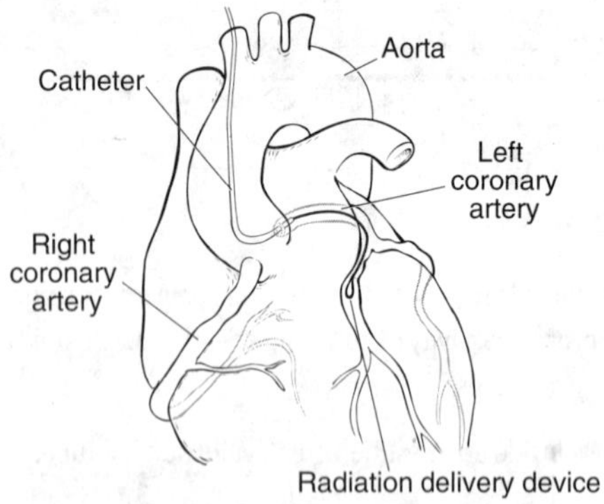

A radiation delivery device is introduced transcatheterally into a coronary artery

Explanation

Using an X-ray machine in a cardiac catheterization laboratory, the physician places the delivery catheter in the coronary artery at the site of the in-stent restenosis (reblockage in the artery). The transfer delivery device is connected to the delivery catheter; the transfer delivery device is used to deliver the radioactive seeds to the location. There are various methods for transcatheter placement, but commonly the methods involve the use of a guiding catheter. The radioactive seeds are positioned at the location for an appropriate length of time to administer radiation to the artery. At the completion of the radiation treatment, the radioactive seeds are returned to the transfer device.

Coding Tips

When medically necessary, report moderate (conscious) sedation provided by the performing physician with 99151-99153. When provided by another physician, report 99155-99157. Report 92974 in addition to 92920, 92924, 92928, 92933, 92937, 92941, 92943, and 93454–93461. For intravascular radioelement application, see 77770–77772.

ICD-10-CM Diagnostic Codes

This/these CPT code(s) are add on code(s). See the primary procedure code that this code is performed with for your ICD-10-CM code selections. Diagnostic code(s) would be the same as the actual procedure performed.

AMA: **92974** 2018,Jan,8; 2018,Feb,11; 2017,Jan,8; 2017,Feb,14; 2016,Jan,13; 2015,Jan,16; 2014,Jan,11; 2014,Dec,6

Relative Value Units/Medicare Edits

Non-Facility RVU	Work	PE	MP	Total
92974	3.0	1.02	0.7	4.72
Facility RVU	**Work**	**PE**	**MP**	**Total**
92974	3.0	1.02	0.7	4.72

	FUD	Status	MUE	Modifiers				IOM Reference
92974	N/A	A	1(3)	N/A	N/A	N/A	80*	None

* with documentation

[92975, 92977]

92975 Thrombolysis, coronary; by intracoronary infusion, including selective coronary angiography

92977 Thrombolysis, coronary; by intravenous infusion

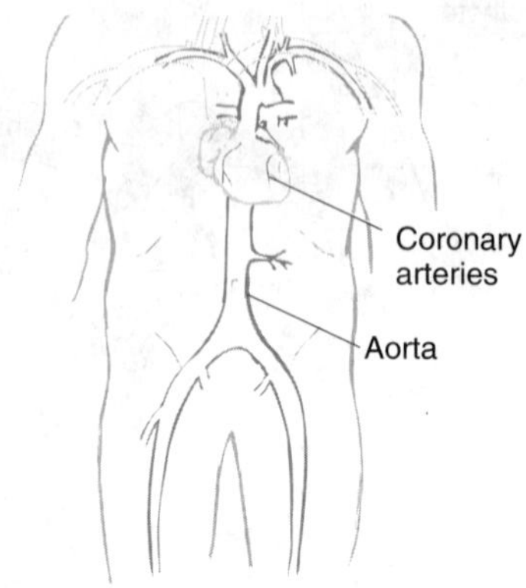

Coronary arteries are accessed transcatheterally and an infusion of thrombolytic agent is released near a thrombus of a coronary artery

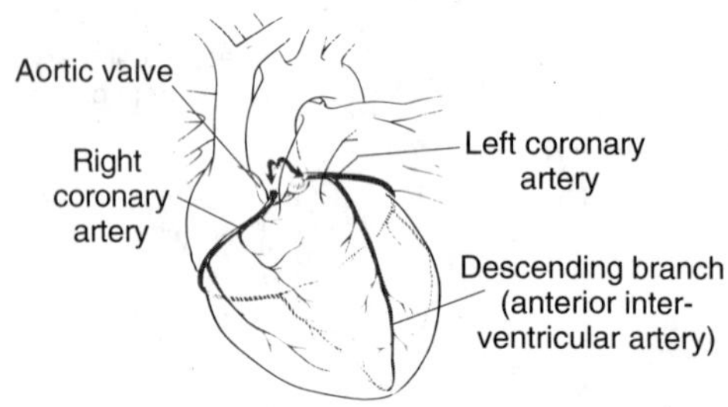

Explanation

In 92975, the physician places a hollow catheter in the aorta from the arm or leg via a small incision. Using fluoroscopic guidance, the physician advances the catheter tip to the coronary artery to be treated and confirms the presence of thrombus (blood clot) in the artery by injecting contrast material through the catheter into the artery. In 92977, a catheter equipped with an infusion tip is threaded into the vessel. The physician infuses a thrombolytic agent (e.g., urokinase) into the affected artery in order to dissolve the thrombus. The physician may perform contrast injections to assess the size and extent of the thrombus after infusion of the thrombolytic agent. The catheter is removed from the patient's body. Pressure is placed over the incision to stem bleeding. The patient is observed for a period afterward.

Coding Tips

When medically necessary, report moderate (conscious) sedation provided by the performing physician with 99151-99153. When provided by another physician, report 99155-99157. For thrombolysis of vessels other than coronary, see 37211–37214. For cerebral thrombolysis, see 37195.

ICD-10-CM Diagnostic Codes

I21.01 ST elevation (STEMI) myocardial infarction involving left main coronary artery

I21.02 ST elevation (STEMI) myocardial infarction involving left anterior descending coronary artery

I21.09 ST elevation (STEMI) myocardial infarction involving other coronary artery of anterior wall

I21.11 ST elevation (STEMI) myocardial infarction involving right coronary artery
I21.19 ST elevation (STEMI) myocardial infarction involving other coronary artery of inferior wall
I21.21 ST elevation (STEMI) myocardial infarction involving left circumflex coronary artery
I21.29 ST elevation (STEMI) myocardial infarction involving other sites
I21.4 Non-ST elevation (NSTEMI) myocardial infarction
I21.A1 Myocardial infarction type 2
I22.0 Subsequent ST elevation (STEMI) myocardial infarction of anterior wall
I22.1 Subsequent ST elevation (STEMI) myocardial infarction of inferior wall
I22.2 Subsequent non-ST elevation (NSTEMI) myocardial infarction
I22.8 Subsequent ST elevation (STEMI) myocardial infarction of other sites
I24.0 Acute coronary thrombosis not resulting in myocardial infarction
I25.110 Atherosclerotic heart disease of native coronary artery with unstable angina pectoris
I25.111 Atherosclerotic heart disease of native coronary artery with angina pectoris with documented spasm
I25.118 Atherosclerotic heart disease of native coronary artery with other forms of angina pectoris
I25.710 Atherosclerosis of autologous vein coronary artery bypass graft(s) with unstable angina pectoris
I25.711 Atherosclerosis of autologous vein coronary artery bypass graft(s) with angina pectoris with documented spasm
I25.718 Atherosclerosis of autologous vein coronary artery bypass graft(s) with other forms of angina pectoris
I25.720 Atherosclerosis of autologous artery coronary artery bypass graft(s) with unstable angina pectoris
I25.721 Atherosclerosis of autologous artery coronary artery bypass graft(s) with angina pectoris with documented spasm
I25.728 Atherosclerosis of autologous artery coronary artery bypass graft(s) with other forms of angina pectoris
I25.730 Atherosclerosis of nonautologous biological coronary artery bypass graft(s) with unstable angina pectoris
I25.731 Atherosclerosis of nonautologous biological coronary artery bypass graft(s) with angina pectoris with documented spasm
I25.738 Atherosclerosis of nonautologous biological coronary artery bypass graft(s) with other forms of angina pectoris
I25.760 Atherosclerosis of bypass graft of coronary artery of transplanted heart with unstable angina
I25.761 Atherosclerosis of bypass graft of coronary artery of transplanted heart with angina pectoris with documented spasm
I25.768 Atherosclerosis of bypass graft of coronary artery of transplanted heart with other forms of angina pectoris
I25.790 Atherosclerosis of other coronary artery bypass graft(s) with unstable angina pectoris
I25.791 Atherosclerosis of other coronary artery bypass graft(s) with angina pectoris with documented spasm
I25.798 Atherosclerosis of other coronary artery bypass graft(s) with other forms of angina pectoris
I25.82 Chronic total occlusion of coronary artery

AMA: 92975 2018,Feb,11 **92977** 2018,Feb,11

Relative Value Units/Medicare Edits

Non-Facility RVU	Work	PE	MP	Total
92975	6.99	2.41	1.58	10.98
92977	0.0	1.46	0.12	1.58
Facility RVU	**Work**	**PE**	**MP**	**Total**
92975	6.99	2.41	1.58	10.98
92977	0.0	1.46	0.12	1.58

	FUD	Status	MUE	Modifiers				IOM Reference
92975	0	A	1(3)	51	N/A	N/A	80*	None
92977	N/A	A	1(3)	N/A	N/A	N/A	80*	

* with documentation

Terms To Know

aneurysm. Circumscribed dilation or outpouching of an artery wall, often containing blood clots and connecting directly with the lumen of the artery.

infusion. Introduction of a therapeutic fluid, other than blood, into the bloodstream.

myocardial infarction. Obstruction of circulation to the heart, resulting in necrosis.

selective placement. Introduction and manipulation of a catheter or guidewire within a vascular tree or family into a specified target area that is identified and monitored by radiographic imaging in order to carry out a diagnostic or therapeutic procedure.

thrombolytic agent. Drugs or other substances used to dissolve blood clots in blood vessels or in tubes that have been placed into the body.

[92978, 92979]

\+ **92978** Endoluminal imaging of coronary vessel or graft using intravascular ultrasound (IVUS) or optical coherence tomography (OCT) during diagnostic evaluation and/or therapeutic intervention including imaging supervision, interpretation and report; initial vessel (List separately in addition to code for primary procedure)

\+ **92979** Endoluminal imaging of coronary vessel or graft using intravascular ultrasound (IVUS) or optical coherence tomography (OCT) during diagnostic evaluation and/or therapeutic intervention including imaging supervision, interpretation and report; each additional vessel (List separately in addition to code for primary procedure)

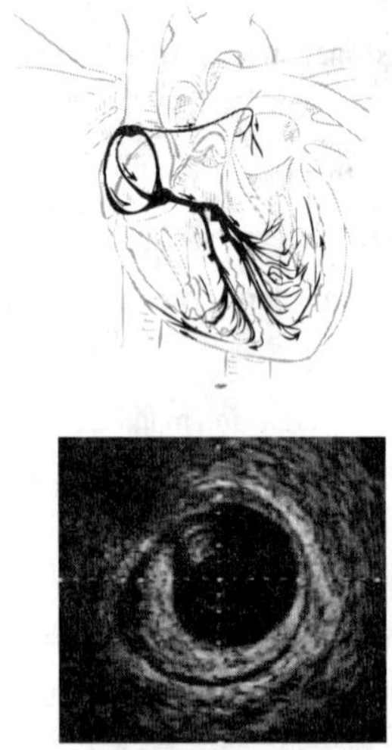

An intravascular ultrasound is used during a diagnostic study of a coronary vessel or coronary artery graft

Explanation

Intravascular ultrasound (IVUS) or optical coherence tomography (OCT) may be used for endoluminal imaging during diagnostic evaluation of a coronary vessel or graft. It may also be used before and after a therapeutic intervention on a coronary vessel or graft to assess patency and integrity of the vessel or graft. A needle is inserted through the skin and into a blood vessel. A guidewire is threaded through the needle into a coronary blood vessel or graft. The needle is removed. An intravascular ultrasound catheter is placed over the guidewire. The ultrasound probe is used to obtain images from inside the vessel to assess area and extent of disease prior to interventional therapy, as well as adequacy of therapy after interventional therapy. The ultrasound probe provides a two-dimensional, cross-sectional view of the vessel or graft as the probe is advanced and withdrawn along the area of interest. When the ultrasound examination is complete, the catheter is removed. OCT utilizes light instead of sound to provide cross-sectional images in high resolution within the lumen. Report 92978 for the initial vessel or graft. In 92979, the physician advances the ultrasound catheter into additional vessels or grafts to assess patency and structure. The catheter and guidewire are removed and pressure is applied over the puncture site to stop bleeding.

Coding Tips

When medically necessary, report moderate (conscious) sedation provided by the performing physician with 99151-99153. When provided by another physician, report 99155-99157. Report 92978 in addition to 92920, 92924, 92928, 92933, 92937, 92941, 92943, 92975, 93454–93461, 93563, and 93564. Use 92979 in addition to 92978. Transducer manipulation and repositioning within the specific vessel being examined both before and after therapeutic intervention is considered integral to the intravascular ultrasound service and should not be reported separately. Report 92978 once per encounter and 92979 once per additional vessel.

ICD-10-CM Diagnostic Codes

This/these CPT code(s) are add on code(s). See the primary procedure code that this code is performed with for your ICD-10-CM code selections. Diagnostic code(s) would be the same as the actual procedure performed.

AMA: 92978 2018,Jan,8; 2018,Feb,11; 2017,Jan,8; 2016,Jan,13; 2015,Jan,16; 2014,Jan,11; 2014,Dec,6; 2013,Dec,16 **92979** 2018,Jan,8; 2018,Feb,11; 2017,Jan,8; 2016,Jan,13; 2015,Jan,16; 2014,Jan,11; 2014,Dec,6; 2013,Dec,16

Relative Value Units/Medicare Edits

Non-Facility RVU	Work	PE	MP	Total
92978	0.0	0.0	0.0	0.0
92979	0.0	0.0	0.0	0.0
Facility RVU	**Work**	**PE**	**MP**	**Total**
92978	0.0	0.0	0.0	0.0
92979	0.0	0.0	0.0	0.0

	FUD	Status	MUE	Modifiers				IOM Reference
92978	N/A	C	1(3)	N/A	N/A	N/A	80*	None
92979	N/A	C	2(3)	N/A	N/A	N/A	80*	

* with documentation

Terms To Know

diagnostic procedures. Procedure performed on a patient to obtain information to assess the medical condition of the patient or to identify a disease and to determine the nature and severity of an illness or injury.

intravascular. Within a blood vessel.

therapeutic procedure. Manner of effecting change through the application of clinical skills and/or services that attempt to improve function.

ultrasound. Imaging using ultra-high sound frequency bounced off body structures.

93355

93355 Echocardiography, transesophageal (TEE) for guidance of a transcatheter intracardiac or great vessel(s) structural intervention(s) (eg,TAVR, transcatheter pulmonary valve replacement, mitral valve repair, paravalvular regurgitation repair, left atrial appendage occlusion/closure, ventricular septal defect closure) (peri-and intra-procedural), real-time image acquisition and documentation, guidance with quantitative measurements, probe manipulation, interpretation, and report, including diagnostic transesophageal echocardiography and, when performed, administration of ultrasound contrast, Doppler, color flow, and 3D

Anatomy

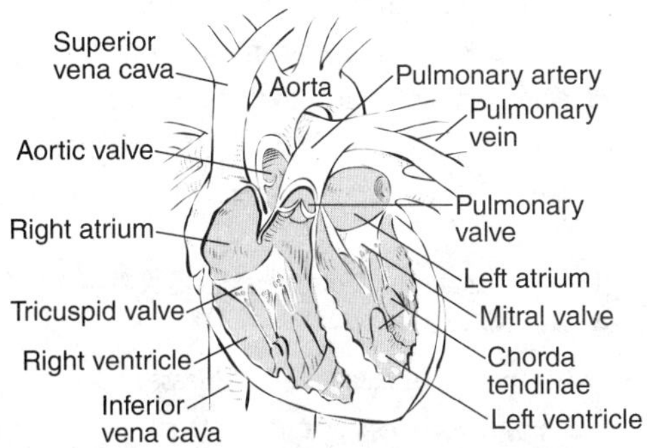

Explanation

Transesophageal echocardiography (TEE) is an invasive technique whereby the transducer is placed at the tip of an endoscope and introduced into the patient's esophagus as guidance for procedures performed on intracardiac or other great vessels and structures. The transducer sends sound waves to the heart and collects the echoes that bounce back. These echoes become high-quality moving pictures that show up on a computer screen. TEE provides high-quality, real-time images of the beating heart and mediastinal structures. This code reports the guidance during the procedure(s), as well as measurements of the surrounding structures. It includes probe navigation, image acquisition, and physician's interpretation and report. Diagnostic TEE is included and contrast administration, Doppler, color flow, and 3D images, when performed, are also included.

Coding Tips

Report this code when performed during transcatheter intracardiac therapy. It is reported only one time per interventional procedure and only by a provider not performing the intervention. For placement of a transesophageal probe by a different provider, see 93313. Do not report 93355 with 76376, 76377, 93312–93318, 93320, 93321, or 93325.

ICD-10-CM Diagnostic Codes

I05.0	Rheumatic mitral stenosis
I05.1	Rheumatic mitral insufficiency
I05.2	Rheumatic mitral stenosis with insufficiency
I05.8	Other rheumatic mitral valve diseases
I06.0	Rheumatic aortic stenosis
I06.1	Rheumatic aortic insufficiency
I06.2	Rheumatic aortic stenosis with insufficiency
I08.0	Rheumatic disorders of both mitral and aortic valves
I08.8	Other rheumatic multiple valve diseases
I34.0	Nonrheumatic mitral (valve) insufficiency
I34.1	Nonrheumatic mitral (valve) prolapse
I34.2	Nonrheumatic mitral (valve) stenosis
I34.8	Other nonrheumatic mitral valve disorders
I35.0	Nonrheumatic aortic (valve) stenosis
I35.1	Nonrheumatic aortic (valve) insufficiency
I35.2	Nonrheumatic aortic (valve) stenosis with insufficiency
I35.8	Other nonrheumatic aortic valve disorders
I36.0	Nonrheumatic tricuspid (valve) stenosis
I36.1	Nonrheumatic tricuspid (valve) insufficiency
I36.2	Nonrheumatic tricuspid (valve) stenosis with insufficiency
I36.8	Other nonrheumatic tricuspid valve disorders
I37.0	Nonrheumatic pulmonary valve stenosis
I37.1	Nonrheumatic pulmonary valve insufficiency
I37.2	Nonrheumatic pulmonary valve stenosis with insufficiency
I37.8	Other nonrheumatic pulmonary valve disorders
Q21.0	Ventricular septal defect
Q21.3	Tetralogy of Fallot
Q21.4	Aortopulmonary septal defect
Q21.8	Other congenital malformations of cardiac septa
Q22.0	Pulmonary valve atresia
Q22.1	Congenital pulmonary valve stenosis
Q22.3	Other congenital malformations of pulmonary valve
Q22.4	Congenital tricuspid stenosis
Q22.6	Hypoplastic right heart syndrome
Q22.8	Other congenital malformations of tricuspid valve
Q23.0	Congenital stenosis of aortic valve
Q23.1	Congenital insufficiency of aortic valve
Q23.2	Congenital mitral stenosis
Q23.3	Congenital mitral insufficiency
Q23.8	Other congenital malformations of aortic and mitral valves
Q24.8	Other specified congenital malformations of heart
T82.01XA	Breakdown (mechanical) of heart valve prosthesis, initial encounter
T82.02XA	Displacement of heart valve prosthesis, initial encounter
T82.03XA	Leakage of heart valve prosthesis, initial encounter
T82.09XA	Other mechanical complication of heart valve prosthesis, initial encounter
T82.6XXA	Infection and inflammatory reaction due to cardiac valve prosthesis, initial encounter

AMA: **93355** 2018,Feb,11

Relative Value Units/Medicare Edits

Non-Facility RVU	Work	PE	MP	Total
93355	4.66	1.6	0.31	6.57
Facility RVU	**Work**	**PE**	**MP**	**Total**
93355	4.66	1.6	0.31	6.57

	FUD	Status	MUE	Modifiers				IOM Reference
93355	N/A	A	1(3)	N/A	N/A	N/A	80*	None

* with documentation

Medicine

93451

93451 Right heart catheterization including measurement(s) of oxygen saturation and cardiac output, when performed

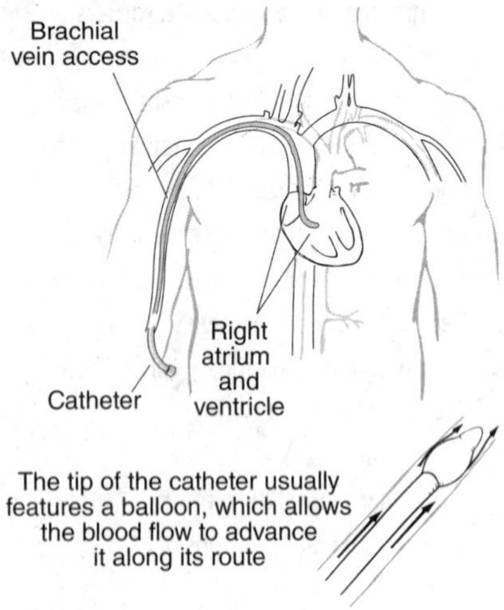

Right side catheterization usually takes pressure measurements at several sites

Explanation

The physician threads a catheter to the heart, most frequently through an introducing sheath placed percutaneously into the femoral vein. However, the physician may elect to use the subclavian, internal jugular, or antecubital vein instead. The catheter is threaded into the right atrium, through the tricuspid valve into the right ventricle, and across the pulmonary valve into the pulmonary arteries. ECG monitoring for the entirety of the procedure is included, as are intracardiac or intravascular pressure recordings, cardiac output and oxygen saturation measurements, and final evaluation and procedure report. This code applies to catheterizing the heart's right side only.

Coding Tips

When medically necessary, report moderate (conscious) sedation provided by the performing physician with 99151-99153. When provided by another physician, report 99155-99157. Right heart catheterization includes placement of the catheter into the right-side heart chambers or structures (right atrium, right ventricle, pulmonary artery, and wedge), specimen collection for blood gas measurements, and cardiac output measurements. For right heart catheterization performed in addition to other cardiac catheterizations, see 93453, 93456, 93457, 93460, or 93461. For placement of a flow directed catheter (Swan-Ganz) for hemodynamic monitoring not performed in addition to other cardiac catheterization procedures, see 93503. Report right ventricular or right atrial angiogram (93566) in addition to right heart catheterization when performed. This procedure includes introduction, positioning, and repositioning (when utilized) of the catheter within the vessel; recording of intracardiac and/or intravascular pressure; and final report evaluation. Additionally, all roadmapping angiography for catheter placement, as well as injections and imaging, are included. Report separately contrast injections and imaging that is separately indicated within a specific CPT code. Do not separately report contrast injections to view the access site when placing a closure device or the placement of the closure device at the vessel access site. Do not report 93451 with 33289, 93453, 93456, 93457, 93460, or 93461. Code 93451 may be reported in addition to 33274 and 33275 only if the catheterization is performed for reasons distinct from the leadless pacemaker procedure. Do not report 93451 with 33418, 0345T, 0483T, 0484T, 0544T, or 0545T for diagnostic right catheterization intrinsic to the valve repair or annulus reconstruction.

ICD-10-CM Diagnostic Codes

I05.0	Rheumatic mitral stenosis
I05.1	Rheumatic mitral insufficiency
I05.2	Rheumatic mitral stenosis with insufficiency
I05.8	Other rheumatic mitral valve diseases
I06.0	Rheumatic aortic stenosis
I06.1	Rheumatic aortic insufficiency
I06.2	Rheumatic aortic stenosis with insufficiency
I06.8	Other rheumatic aortic valve diseases
I07.0	Rheumatic tricuspid stenosis
I07.1	Rheumatic tricuspid insufficiency
I07.2	Rheumatic tricuspid stenosis and insufficiency
I07.8	Other rheumatic tricuspid valve diseases
I08.0	Rheumatic disorders of both mitral and aortic valves
I08.1	Rheumatic disorders of both mitral and tricuspid valves
I08.2	Rheumatic disorders of both aortic and tricuspid valves
I08.3	Combined rheumatic disorders of mitral, aortic and tricuspid valves
I08.8	Other rheumatic multiple valve diseases
I09.81	Rheumatic heart failure
I09.89	Other specified rheumatic heart diseases
I21.01	ST elevation (STEMI) myocardial infarction involving left main coronary artery
I21.02	ST elevation (STEMI) myocardial infarction involving left anterior descending coronary artery
I21.09	ST elevation (STEMI) myocardial infarction involving other coronary artery of anterior wall
I21.11	ST elevation (STEMI) myocardial infarction involving right coronary artery
I21.19	ST elevation (STEMI) myocardial infarction involving other coronary artery of inferior wall
I21.21	ST elevation (STEMI) myocardial infarction involving left circumflex coronary artery
I21.29	ST elevation (STEMI) myocardial infarction involving other sites
I21.4	Non-ST elevation (NSTEMI) myocardial infarction
I21.A1	Myocardial infarction type 2
I22.0	Subsequent ST elevation (STEMI) myocardial infarction of anterior wall
I22.1	Subsequent ST elevation (STEMI) myocardial infarction of inferior wall
I22.2	Subsequent non-ST elevation (NSTEMI) myocardial infarction
I22.8	Subsequent ST elevation (STEMI) myocardial infarction of other sites
I23.0	Hemopericardium as current complication following acute myocardial infarction
I23.1	Atrial septal defect as current complication following acute myocardial infarction
I23.2	Ventricular septal defect as current complication following acute myocardial infarction
I25.3	Aneurysm of heart
I25.5	Ischemic cardiomyopathy
I25.89	Other forms of chronic ischemic heart disease
I26.01	Septic pulmonary embolism with acute cor pulmonale
I26.02	Saddle embolus of pulmonary artery with acute cor pulmonale

I26.09	Other pulmonary embolism with acute cor pulmonale
I26.90	Septic pulmonary embolism without acute cor pulmonale
I26.92	Saddle embolus of pulmonary artery without acute cor pulmonale
I26.93	Single subsegmental pulmonary embolism without acute cor pulmonale
I26.94	Multiple subsegmental pulmonary emboli without acute cor pulmonale
I26.99	Other pulmonary embolism without acute cor pulmonale
I27.0	Primary pulmonary hypertension
I27.21	Secondary pulmonary arterial hypertension
I27.22	Pulmonary hypertension due to left heart disease
I27.23	Pulmonary hypertension due to lung diseases and hypoxia
I27.24	Chronic thromboembolic pulmonary hypertension
I27.29	Other secondary pulmonary hypertension
I27.81	Cor pulmonale (chronic)
I27.83	Eisenmenger's syndrome
I34.0	Nonrheumatic mitral (valve) insufficiency
I34.1	Nonrheumatic mitral (valve) prolapse
I34.2	Nonrheumatic mitral (valve) stenosis
I34.8	Other nonrheumatic mitral valve disorders
I35.0	Nonrheumatic aortic (valve) stenosis
I35.1	Nonrheumatic aortic (valve) insufficiency
I35.2	Nonrheumatic aortic (valve) stenosis with insufficiency
I35.8	Other nonrheumatic aortic valve disorders
I36.0	Nonrheumatic tricuspid (valve) stenosis
I36.1	Nonrheumatic tricuspid (valve) insufficiency
I36.2	Nonrheumatic tricuspid (valve) stenosis with insufficiency
I36.8	Other nonrheumatic tricuspid valve disorders
I37.0	Nonrheumatic pulmonary valve stenosis
I37.1	Nonrheumatic pulmonary valve insufficiency
I37.2	Nonrheumatic pulmonary valve stenosis with insufficiency
I37.8	Other nonrheumatic pulmonary valve disorders
I38	Endocarditis, valve unspecified
I39	Endocarditis and heart valve disorders in diseases classified elsewhere
I40.0	Infective myocarditis
I40.1	Isolated myocarditis
I40.8	Other acute myocarditis
I42.0	Dilated cardiomyopathy
I42.1	Obstructive hypertrophic cardiomyopathy
I42.2	Other hypertrophic cardiomyopathy
I42.3	Endomyocardial (eosinophilic) disease
I42.4	Endocardial fibroelastosis
I42.5	Other restrictive cardiomyopathy
I42.6	Alcoholic cardiomyopathy
I42.7	Cardiomyopathy due to drug and external agent
I42.8	Other cardiomyopathies
I43	Cardiomyopathy in diseases classified elsewhere
I46.2	Cardiac arrest due to underlying cardiac condition
I46.8	Cardiac arrest due to other underlying condition
I50.1	Left ventricular failure, unspecified
I50.21	Acute systolic (congestive) heart failure
I50.22	Chronic systolic (congestive) heart failure
I50.23	Acute on chronic systolic (congestive) heart failure
I50.31	Acute diastolic (congestive) heart failure
I50.32	Chronic diastolic (congestive) heart failure
I50.33	Acute on chronic diastolic (congestive) heart failure
I50.41	Acute combined systolic (congestive) and diastolic (congestive) heart failure
I50.42	Chronic combined systolic (congestive) and diastolic (congestive) heart failure
I50.43	Acute on chronic combined systolic (congestive) and diastolic (congestive) heart failure
I50.811	Acute right heart failure
I50.812	Chronic right heart failure
I50.813	Acute on chronic right heart failure
I50.814	Right heart failure due to left heart failure
I50.82	Biventricular heart failure
I50.83	High output heart failure
I50.84	End stage heart failure
I50.9	Heart failure, unspecified
I51.0	Cardiac septal defect, acquired
R57.0	Cardiogenic shock
R57.1	Hypovolemic shock
R57.8	Other shock

AMA: 93451 2019,Mar,6; 2019,Jun,3; 2018,Jan,8; 2018,Feb,11; 2018,Dec,10; 2018,Dec,10; 2017,Jul,3; 2017,Jan,8; 2017,Dec,13; 2016,Mar,5; 2016,Jan,13; 2015,Sep,3; 2015,Jan,16; 2014,Jul,3; 2014,Jan,11; 2013,May,12

Relative Value Units/Medicare Edits

Non-Facility RVU	Work	PE	MP	Total
93451	2.47	19.18	0.49	22.14
Facility RVU	**Work**	**PE**	**MP**	**Total**
93451	2.47	19.18	0.49	22.14

	FUD	Status	MUE	Modifiers				IOM Reference
93451	0	A	1(3)	51	N/A	N/A	80*	None

* with documentation

Terms To Know

cardiac output. Measurement of the volume of blood ejected by the heart ventricle that is usually measured by a catheter with an opening in the right atrium and pulmonary artery.

catheterization. Use or insertion of a tubular device into a duct, blood vessel, hollow organ, or body cavity for injecting or withdrawing fluids for diagnostic or therapeutic purposes.

93452

93452 Left heart catheterization including intraprocedural injection(s) for left ventriculography, imaging supervision and interpretation, when performed

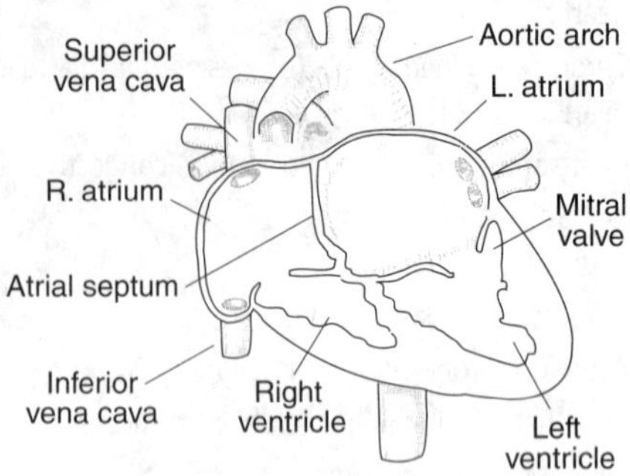

Left heart is catheterized

Explanation

The physician threads a catheter to the heart, most frequently through an introducing sheath placed percutaneously into the femoral, brachial, or axillary artery using retrograde technique. Using this technique, the catheter passes through the aortic valve into the left ventricle. Intracardiac and intravascular pressures are recorded. Left ventricular injections may be performed for left ventriculography; the physician injects dye through a previously placed catheter threaded through a central line into the left ventricle or atrium to evaluate function with fluoroscopy. Imaging supervision and interpretation, when performed, are included in this code, as is any required repositioning of catheters.

Coding Tips

When medically necessary, report moderate (conscious) sedation provided by the performing physician with 99151-99153. When provided by another physician, report 99155-99157. This procedure includes placement of the catheter into the left-side heart chambers or structures (left ventricle, left atrium) and left ventricular injection when utilized. Intraprocedural injections for left ventricular/atrial angiogram and imaging supervision and interpretation are also included. Do not report 93503 in addition to other diagnostic cardiac cath codes. When left heart catheterization is performed via transapical puncture into the left ventricle or transseptal puncture into the septum, report 93462 in addition to 93452, 93453, 93458–93461, 93653, and 93654. This procedure includes introduction, positioning, and repositioning (when utilized) of the catheter within the vessel; recording of intracardiac and/or intravascular pressure; and final report evaluation. All roadmapping angiography for catheter placement, as well as injections and imaging, are also included. Report separately contrast injections and imaging that is separately indicated within a specific CPT code. Do not separately report contrast injections to view the access site when placing a closure device or the placement of the closure device at the vessel access site. Do not report 93452 with 93453, 93458–93461, 0408T-0411T, or 0414T-0415T. Do not report 93452 with 33418, 0345T, 0483T, 0484T, 0544T, or 0545T for diagnostic left catheterization intrinsic to the valve repair or annulus reconstruction.

ICD-10-CM Diagnostic Codes

C38.0	Malignant neoplasm of heart
D15.1	Benign neoplasm of heart
I05.0	Rheumatic mitral stenosis
I05.1	Rheumatic mitral insufficiency
I06.0	Rheumatic aortic stenosis
I06.1	Rheumatic aortic insufficiency
I07.0	Rheumatic tricuspid stenosis
I07.1	Rheumatic tricuspid insufficiency
I09.81	Rheumatic heart failure
I20.0	Unstable angina
I20.1	Angina pectoris with documented spasm
I21.01	ST elevation (STEMI) myocardial infarction involving left main coronary artery
I21.02	ST elevation (STEMI) myocardial infarction involving left anterior descending coronary artery
I21.11	ST elevation (STEMI) myocardial infarction involving right coronary artery
I21.21	ST elevation (STEMI) myocardial infarction involving left circumflex coronary artery
I21.4	Non-ST elevation (NSTEMI) myocardial infarction
I21.A1	Myocardial infarction type 2
I22.0	Subsequent ST elevation (STEMI) myocardial infarction of anterior wall
I22.1	Subsequent ST elevation (STEMI) myocardial infarction of inferior wall
I22.2	Subsequent non-ST elevation (NSTEMI) myocardial infarction
I23.1	Atrial septal defect as current complication following acute myocardial infarction
I23.2	Ventricular septal defect as current complication following acute myocardial infarction
I23.3	Rupture of cardiac wall without hemopericardium as current complication following acute myocardial infarction
I23.7	Postinfarction angina
I24.0	Acute coronary thrombosis not resulting in myocardial infarction
I24.1	Dressler's syndrome
I25.10	Atherosclerotic heart disease of native coronary artery without angina pectoris
I25.110	Atherosclerotic heart disease of native coronary artery with unstable angina pectoris
I25.111	Atherosclerotic heart disease of native coronary artery with angina pectoris with documented spasm
I25.2	Old myocardial infarction
I25.3	Aneurysm of heart
I25.41	Coronary artery aneurysm
I25.5	Ischemic cardiomyopathy
I25.6	Silent myocardial ischemia
I25.710	Atherosclerosis of autologous vein coronary artery bypass graft(s) with unstable angina pectoris
I25.711	Atherosclerosis of autologous vein coronary artery bypass graft(s) with angina pectoris with documented spasm
I25.720	Atherosclerosis of autologous artery coronary artery bypass graft(s) with unstable angina pectoris
I25.721	Atherosclerosis of autologous artery coronary artery bypass graft(s) with angina pectoris with documented spasm
I25.730	Atherosclerosis of nonautologous biological coronary artery bypass graft(s) with unstable angina pectoris
I25.731	Atherosclerosis of nonautologous biological coronary artery bypass graft(s) with angina pectoris with documented spasm
I25.750	Atherosclerosis of native coronary artery of transplanted heart with unstable angina

Medicine

I25.751	Atherosclerosis of native coronary artery of transplanted heart with angina pectoris with documented spasm
I25.760	Atherosclerosis of bypass graft of coronary artery of transplanted heart with unstable angina
I25.761	Atherosclerosis of bypass graft of coronary artery of transplanted heart with angina pectoris with documented spasm
I25.810	Atherosclerosis of coronary artery bypass graft(s) without angina pectoris
I25.812	Atherosclerosis of bypass graft of coronary artery of transplanted heart without angina pectoris
I25.82	Chronic total occlusion of coronary artery
I25.84	Coronary atherosclerosis due to calcified coronary lesion
I27.0	Primary pulmonary hypertension
I27.23	Pulmonary hypertension due to lung diseases and hypoxia
I27.24	Chronic thromboembolic pulmonary hypertension
I27.81	Cor pulmonale (chronic)
I27.83	Eisenmenger's syndrome
I34.1	Nonrheumatic mitral (valve) prolapse
I34.2	Nonrheumatic mitral (valve) stenosis
I35.0	Nonrheumatic aortic (valve) stenosis
I35.1	Nonrheumatic aortic (valve) insufficiency
I36.0	Nonrheumatic tricuspid (valve) stenosis
I36.1	Nonrheumatic tricuspid (valve) insufficiency
I37.0	Nonrheumatic pulmonary valve stenosis
I37.1	Nonrheumatic pulmonary valve insufficiency
I46.2	Cardiac arrest due to underlying cardiac condition
I50.21	Acute systolic (congestive) heart failure
I50.22	Chronic systolic (congestive) heart failure
I50.23	Acute on chronic systolic (congestive) heart failure
I50.31	Acute diastolic (congestive) heart failure
I50.32	Chronic diastolic (congestive) heart failure
I50.33	Acute on chronic diastolic (congestive) heart failure
I50.811	Acute right heart failure
I50.812	Chronic right heart failure
I50.813	Acute on chronic right heart failure
I50.814	Right heart failure due to left heart failure
I50.82	Biventricular heart failure
I50.83	High output heart failure
I50.84	End stage heart failure
R57.0	Cardiogenic shock
R57.1	Hypovolemic shock
T80.0XXA	Air embolism following infusion, transfusion and therapeutic injection, initial encounter
T82.817A	Embolism due to cardiac prosthetic devices, implants and grafts, initial encounter
T82.818A	Embolism due to vascular prosthetic devices, implants and grafts, initial encounter

AMA: **93452** 2018,Jan,8; 2018,Feb,11; 2017,Jul,3; 2017,Jan,8; 2016,Jan,13; 2015,Jan,16; 2014,Jul,3; 2014,Jan,11; 2013,May,12; 2013,Jan,6-8

Relative Value Units/Medicare Edits

Non-Facility RVU	Work	PE	MP	Total
93452	4.5	19.22	0.88	24.6
Facility RVU	**Work**	**PE**	**MP**	**Total**
93452	4.5	19.22	0.88	24.6

	FUD	Status	MUE	Modifiers				IOM Reference
93452	0	A	1(3)	51	N/A	N/A	80*	None

* with documentation

Terms To Know

angiogram. Radiographic image of the arteries. Imaging may be performed to study the vasculature of any given organ, body system, or area of circulation such as the brain, heart, chest, kidneys, limbs, gastrointestinal tract, aorta, and pulmonary circulation to visualize the formation and the function of the blood vessels to detect problems such as a blockage or stricture.

aortic valve. Heart valve, comprising three cusps, that divides the left ventricle and the aorta.

fluoroscopy. Radiology technique that allows visual examination of part of the body or a function of an organ using a device that projects an x-ray image on a fluorescent screen.

supervision and interpretation. Radiology services that usually contain an invasive component and are reported by the radiologist for supervision of the procedure and the personnel involved with performing the examination, reading the film, and preparing the written report.

ventriculogram. Interventional procedure that demonstrates the contractility of the cardiac ventricles by serial recording of the distribution of intravenously injected radionuclide or that of radiographic contrast medium injected through an intracardiac catheter.

93453

93453 Combined right and left heart catheterization including intraprocedural injection(s) for left ventriculography, imaging supervision and interpretation, when performed

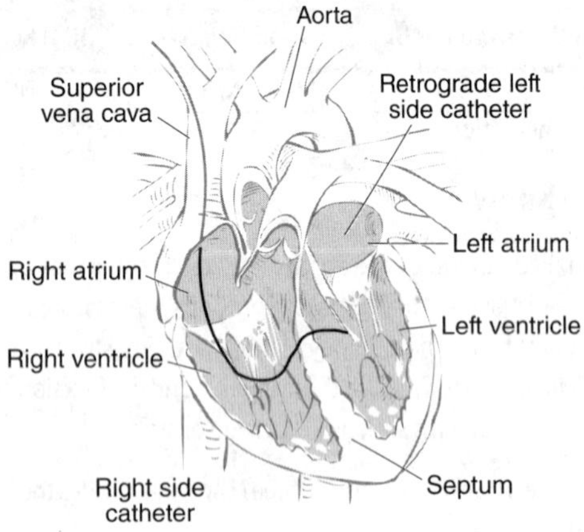

Both sides of the heart are catheterized

Explanation

This procedure is performed to evaluate both right and left heart function. To accomplish right heart catheterization, the physician threads a catheter through an introducing sheath placed percutaneously into the femoral, subclavian, internal jugular, or antecubital vein. The catheter is threaded into the right atrium, through the tricuspid valve into the right ventricle, and across the pulmonary valve into the pulmonary arteries. Left heart catheterization is also performed, in this case using retrograde technique. The catheter is inserted through an introducing sheath placed percutaneously into the femoral, brachial, or axillary artery. The catheter is passed through the aortic valve into the left ventricle. Intracardiac and intravascular pressures are recorded. Left ventricular injections may be performed for left ventriculography; the physician injects dye through a previously placed catheter threaded through a central line into the left ventricle or atrium to evaluate function with fluoroscopy. Imaging supervision and interpretation, when performed, are included in this code, as is any required repositioning of catheters.

Coding Tips

When medically necessary, report moderate (conscious) sedation provided by the performing physician with 99151-99153. When provided by another physician, report 99155-99157. Right heart catheterization includes placement of the catheter into the right-side heart chambers or structures (right atrium, right ventricle, pulmonary artery, and wedge), specimen collection for blood gas measurements, and cardiac output measurements. For right heart catheterization performed in addition to other cardiac catheterizations, see 93453, 93456, 93457, 93460, or 93461. When placement of a flow directed catheter (Swan-Ganz) for hemodynamic monitoring is not performed in addition to other cardiac catheterization procedures, see 93503. Report right ventricular or right atrial angiogram (93566) in addition to right heart catheterization when performed. Left heart catheterization includes placement of the catheter into the left-side heart chambers or structures (left ventricle, left atrium) and left ventricular injection when utilized. Intraprocedural injections for left ventricular/atrial angiogram and imaging supervision and interpretation are also included. Do not report 93503 in addition to other diagnostic cardiac cath codes. This procedure includes introduction, positioning, and repositioning (when utilized) of the catheter within the vessel; recording of intracardiac and/or intravascular pressure; and final report evaluation. All roadmapping angiography for catheter placement, as well as injections and imaging, are also included. Report separately contrast injections and imaging that are separately indicated within a specific CPT code. Do not separately report contrast injections to view the access site when placing a closure device or the placement of the closure device at the vessel access site. Do not report 93453 with 93451, 93452, 93456–93461, 0408T-0411T, or 0414T-0415T. Do not report 93453 with 33418, 0345T, 0483T, 0484T, 0544T, or 0545T for diagnostic left and right catheterization intrinsic to the valve repair or annulus reconstruction. Code 93453 may be reported in addition to 33274 and 33275 only if the catheterization is performed for reasons distinct from the leadless pacemaker procedure.

ICD-10-CM Diagnostic Codes

C38.0	Malignant neoplasm of heart
I05.0	Rheumatic mitral stenosis
I05.1	Rheumatic mitral insufficiency
I06.0	Rheumatic aortic stenosis
I06.1	Rheumatic aortic insufficiency
I07.0	Rheumatic tricuspid stenosis
I07.1	Rheumatic tricuspid insufficiency
I09.81	Rheumatic heart failure
I20.0	Unstable angina
I20.1	Angina pectoris with documented spasm
I21.01	ST elevation (STEMI) myocardial infarction involving left main coronary artery
I21.02	ST elevation (STEMI) myocardial infarction involving left anterior descending coronary artery
I21.21	ST elevation (STEMI) myocardial infarction involving left circumflex coronary artery
I21.4	Non-ST elevation (NSTEMI) myocardial infarction
I21.A1	Myocardial infarction type 2
I22.0	Subsequent ST elevation (STEMI) myocardial infarction of anterior wall
I22.1	Subsequent ST elevation (STEMI) myocardial infarction of inferior wall
I22.2	Subsequent non-ST elevation (NSTEMI) myocardial infarction
I23.0	Hemopericardium as current complication following acute myocardial infarction
I23.1	Atrial septal defect as current complication following acute myocardial infarction
I23.2	Ventricular septal defect as current complication following acute myocardial infarction
I23.3	Rupture of cardiac wall without hemopericardium as current complication following acute myocardial infarction
I23.7	Postinfarction angina
I24.0	Acute coronary thrombosis not resulting in myocardial infarction
I24.1	Dressler's syndrome
I25.110	Atherosclerotic heart disease of native coronary artery with unstable angina pectoris
I25.111	Atherosclerotic heart disease of native coronary artery with angina pectoris with documented spasm
I25.2	Old myocardial infarction
I25.3	Aneurysm of heart
I25.41	Coronary artery aneurysm
I25.5	Ischemic cardiomyopathy
I25.6	Silent myocardial ischemia

I25.710	Atherosclerosis of autologous vein coronary artery bypass graft(s) with unstable angina pectoris
I25.711	Atherosclerosis of autologous vein coronary artery bypass graft(s) with angina pectoris with documented spasm
I25.82	Chronic total occlusion of coronary artery
I25.84	Coronary atherosclerosis due to calcified coronary lesion
I26.01	Septic pulmonary embolism with acute cor pulmonale
I26.02	Saddle embolus of pulmonary artery with acute cor pulmonale
I26.90	Septic pulmonary embolism without acute cor pulmonale
I26.92	Saddle embolus of pulmonary artery without acute cor pulmonale
I27.0	Primary pulmonary hypertension
I27.21	Secondary pulmonary arterial hypertension
I27.24	Chronic thromboembolic pulmonary hypertension
I27.81	Cor pulmonale (chronic)
I27.83	Eisenmenger's syndrome
I34.0	Nonrheumatic mitral (valve) insufficiency
I34.1	Nonrheumatic mitral (valve) prolapse
I34.2	Nonrheumatic mitral (valve) stenosis
I35.0	Nonrheumatic aortic (valve) stenosis
I35.1	Nonrheumatic aortic (valve) insufficiency
I36.0	Nonrheumatic tricuspid (valve) stenosis
I36.1	Nonrheumatic tricuspid (valve) insufficiency
I37.0	Nonrheumatic pulmonary valve stenosis
I37.1	Nonrheumatic pulmonary valve insufficiency
I40.0	Infective myocarditis
I40.1	Isolated myocarditis
I42.0	Dilated cardiomyopathy
I42.1	Obstructive hypertrophic cardiomyopathy
I42.3	Endomyocardial (eosinophilic) disease
I42.4	Endocardial fibroelastosis
I42.6	Alcoholic cardiomyopathy
I50.23	Acute on chronic systolic (congestive) heart failure
I50.33	Acute on chronic diastolic (congestive) heart failure
I50.813	Acute on chronic right heart failure
I50.814	Right heart failure due to left heart failure
I50.82	Biventricular heart failure
I50.83	High output heart failure
I50.84	End stage heart failure
I51.0	Cardiac septal defect, acquired
R57.0	Cardiogenic shock
R57.1	Hypovolemic shock
T80.0XXA	Air embolism following infusion, transfusion and therapeutic injection, initial encounter
T82.817A	Embolism due to cardiac prosthetic devices, implants and grafts, initial encounter
T82.818A	Embolism due to vascular prosthetic devices, implants and grafts, initial encounter

AMA: 93453 2019,Mar,6; 2019,Jun,3; 2018,Jan,8; 2018,Feb,11; 2017,Jul,3; 2017,Jan,8; 2016,Mar,5; 2016,Jan,13; 2015,Sep,3; 2015,Jan,16; 2014,Jul,3; 2014,Jan,11; 2013,May,12; 2013,Jan,6-8

Relative Value Units/Medicare Edits

Non-Facility RVU	Work	PE	MP	Total
93453	5.99	24.69	1.24	31.92
Facility RVU	**Work**	**PE**	**MP**	**Total**
93453	5.99	24.69	1.24	31.92

	FUD	Status	MUE	Modifiers				IOM Reference
93453	0	A	1(3)	51	N/A	N/A	80*	None

* with documentation

Terms To Know

catheterization. Use or insertion of a tubular device into a duct, blood vessel, hollow organ, or body cavity for injecting or withdrawing fluids for diagnostic or therapeutic purposes.

left heart. Area of the heart consisting of the left atrium and left ventricle.

retrograde. Moving against the usual direction of flow.

right heart. Areas of the right heart, including the right atrium and right ventricle.

93454

93454 Catheter placement in coronary artery(s) for coronary angiography, including intraprocedural injection(s) for coronary angiography, imaging supervision and interpretation;

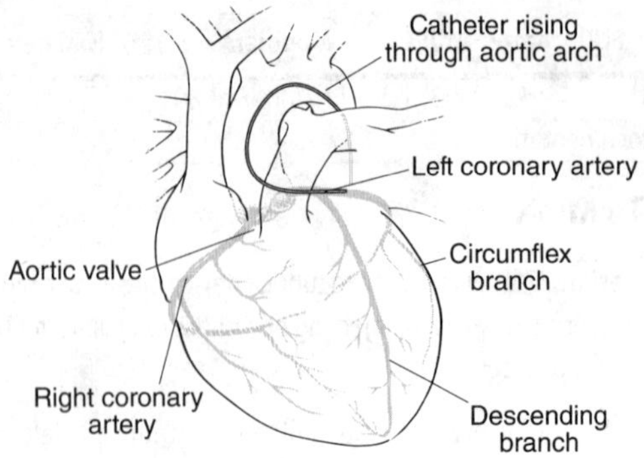

The catheter may enter the coronary grafts, but does not cross the aortic valve into the left ventricle

Explanation

The physician performs a catheter placement in one or more coronary arteries for coronary angiography, without concomitant left heart catheterization. The physician places an introducer sheath in an artery, typically the femoral artery, using percutaneous puncture. The physician advances an angiography catheter through the introducer sheath into the ascending aorta and advances it, under fluoroscopic guidance, to the opening of the coronary artery. The physician injects radiopaque contrast material through the catheter into the vessel while recording a cineangiogram. The physician removes the catheter and sheath from the femoral artery. Pressure is placed on the wound for 20 to 30 minutes to stem bleeding. This code includes imaging supervision and interpretation, as well as any required repositioning of catheters.

Coding Tips

When medically necessary, report moderate (conscious) sedation provided by the performing physician with 99151-99153. When provided by another physician, report 99155-99157. This procedure includes placement of the catheter into the coronary arteries involving selective placement of the native coronary artery origin in order to perform coronary angiogram. Codes 93454–93461, for other than congenital conditions, include intraprocedural injection and imaging when performing coronary angiogram. For right ventricle/atrium angiograms performed in addition to cardiac catheterization (93451–93461, 93530–93533), report 93566. For aortography, see 93567. For pulmonary angiogram, see 93568. Do not report 93454 with 33418, 0345T, 0483T, 0484T, 0544T, or 0545T for coronary angiography intrinsic to the valve repair or annulus reconstruction.

ICD-10-CM Diagnostic Codes

I20.0	Unstable angina
I20.1	Angina pectoris with documented spasm
I20.8	Other forms of angina pectoris
I21.01	ST elevation (STEMI) myocardial infarction involving left main coronary artery
I21.02	ST elevation (STEMI) myocardial infarction involving left anterior descending coronary artery
I21.09	ST elevation (STEMI) myocardial infarction involving other coronary artery of anterior wall
I21.11	ST elevation (STEMI) myocardial infarction involving right coronary artery
I21.19	ST elevation (STEMI) myocardial infarction involving other coronary artery of inferior wall
I21.21	ST elevation (STEMI) myocardial infarction involving left circumflex coronary artery
I21.29	ST elevation (STEMI) myocardial infarction involving other sites
I21.4	Non-ST elevation (NSTEMI) myocardial infarction
I21.A1	Myocardial infarction type 2
I22.0	Subsequent ST elevation (STEMI) myocardial infarction of anterior wall
I22.1	Subsequent ST elevation (STEMI) myocardial infarction of inferior wall
I22.2	Subsequent non-ST elevation (NSTEMI) myocardial infarction
I22.8	Subsequent ST elevation (STEMI) myocardial infarction of other sites
I24.0	Acute coronary thrombosis not resulting in myocardial infarction
I24.8	Other forms of acute ischemic heart disease
I25.10	Atherosclerotic heart disease of native coronary artery without angina pectoris
I25.110	Atherosclerotic heart disease of native coronary artery with unstable angina pectoris
I25.111	Atherosclerotic heart disease of native coronary artery with angina pectoris with documented spasm
I25.118	Atherosclerotic heart disease of native coronary artery with other forms of angina pectoris
I25.3	Aneurysm of heart
I25.41	Coronary artery aneurysm
I25.5	Ischemic cardiomyopathy
I25.6	Silent myocardial ischemia
I25.82	Chronic total occlusion of coronary artery
I25.84	Coronary atherosclerosis due to calcified coronary lesion
I25.89	Other forms of chronic ischemic heart disease
I42.0	Dilated cardiomyopathy
I42.1	Obstructive hypertrophic cardiomyopathy
I42.2	Other hypertrophic cardiomyopathy
I42.8	Other cardiomyopathies
I43	Cardiomyopathy in diseases classified elsewhere
I50.1	Left ventricular failure, unspecified
I50.21	Acute systolic (congestive) heart failure
I50.22	Chronic systolic (congestive) heart failure
I50.23	Acute on chronic systolic (congestive) heart failure
I50.31	Acute diastolic (congestive) heart failure
I50.32	Chronic diastolic (congestive) heart failure
I50.33	Acute on chronic diastolic (congestive) heart failure
I50.41	Acute combined systolic (congestive) and diastolic (congestive) heart failure
I50.42	Chronic combined systolic (congestive) and diastolic (congestive) heart failure
I50.43	Acute on chronic combined systolic (congestive) and diastolic (congestive) heart failure
I50.811	Acute right heart failure
I50.812	Chronic right heart failure
I50.813	Acute on chronic right heart failure
I50.814	Right heart failure due to left heart failure
I50.82	Biventricular heart failure

I50.83	High output heart failure
I50.84	End stage heart failure
I51.7	Cardiomegaly

AMA: 93454 2018,Jan,8; 2018,Feb,11; 2017,Jan,8; 2017,Feb,14; 2016,Mar,5; 2016,Jan,13; 2015,Jan,16; 2014,Jul,3; 2014,Jan,11; 2014,Dec,6; 2013,May,12

Relative Value Units/Medicare Edits

Non-Facility RVU	Work	PE	MP	Total
93454	4.54	19.38	0.93	24.85
Facility RVU	**Work**	**PE**	**MP**	**Total**
93454	4.54	19.38	0.93	24.85

	FUD	Status	MUE	Modifiers				IOM Reference
93454	0	A	1(3)	51	N/A	N/A	80*	None

* with documentation

Terms To Know

angiogram. Radiographic image of the arteries. Imaging may be performed to study the vasculature of any given organ, body system, or area of circulation such as the brain, heart, chest, kidneys, limbs, gastrointestinal tract, aorta, and pulmonary circulation to visualize the formation and the function of the blood vessels to detect problems such as a blockage or stricture.

catheterization. Use or insertion of a tubular device into a duct, blood vessel, hollow organ, or body cavity for injecting or withdrawing fluids for diagnostic or therapeutic purposes.

concomitant. Occurring at the same time, accompanying.

congenital. Present at birth, occurring through heredity or an influence during gestation up to the moment of birth.

radiopaque dye. Medium injected into the body that is impenetrable by x-rays.

supervision and interpretation. Radiology services that usually contain an invasive component and are reported by the radiologist for supervision of the procedure and the personnel involved with performing the examination, reading the film, and preparing the written report.

93455

93455 Catheter placement in coronary artery(s) for coronary angiography, including intraprocedural injection(s) for coronary angiography, imaging supervision and interpretation; with catheter placement(s) in bypass graft(s) (internal mammary, free arterial, venous grafts) including intraprocedural injection(s) for bypass graft angiography

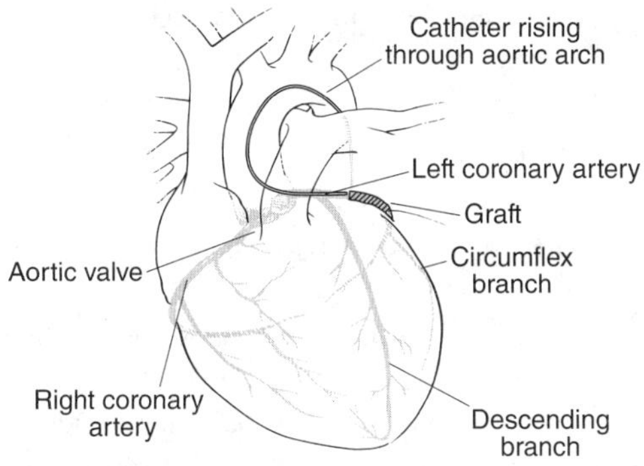

The catheter may enter the coronary grafts, but does not cross the aortic valve into the left ventricle

Explanation

The physician performs a catheter placement in one or more coronary arteries and bypass grafts (i.e., internal mammary, free arterial venous grafts) for coronary and bypass graft angiography, without concomitant left heart catheterization. The physician places an introducer sheath in an artery, typically the femoral artery, using percutaneous puncture. The physician advances an angiography catheter through the introducer sheath into the ascending aorta and advances it, under fluoroscopic guidance, to the opening of the coronary artery or the bypass graft. The physician injects radiopaque contrast material through the catheter into the vessel while recording a cineangiogram. The physician removes the catheter and sheath from the femoral artery. Pressure is placed on the wound for 20 to 30 minutes to stem bleeding. This code includes imaging supervision and interpretation, as well as any required repositioning of catheters.

Coding Tips

When medically necessary, report moderate (conscious) sedation provided by the performing physician with 99151-99153. When provided by another physician, report 99155-99157. This procedure includes placement of the catheter into the coronary arteries involving selective placement of the native coronary artery origin in order to perform coronary angiogram. Codes 93454–93461, for other than congenital conditions, include intraprocedural injection and imaging when performing coronary angiogram. These procedures (93455, 93457, 93459, 93461) include intraprocedural injections and imaging supervision and interpretation for bypass graft angiogram. Do not report 93563–93565 in addition to 93452–93461. Do not report 93455 with 33418, 0345T, 0483T, 0484T, 0544T, or 0545T for coronary angiography intrinsic to the valve repair or annulus reconstruction. Placement of the catheter in bypass grafts (venous, internal mammary, free arterial graft) involves selective placement of the graft origin for bypass angiogram and is most often performed in addition to coronary angiogram of native vessels.

ICD-10-CM Diagnostic Codes

I20.0	Unstable angina
I20.1	Angina pectoris with documented spasm
I20.8	Other forms of angina pectoris
I21.01	ST elevation (STEMI) myocardial infarction involving left main coronary artery

Medicine

I21.02	ST elevation (STEMI) myocardial infarction involving left anterior descending coronary artery
I21.09	ST elevation (STEMI) myocardial infarction involving other coronary artery of anterior wall
I21.11	ST elevation (STEMI) myocardial infarction involving right coronary artery
I21.19	ST elevation (STEMI) myocardial infarction involving other coronary artery of inferior wall
I21.21	ST elevation (STEMI) myocardial infarction involving left circumflex coronary artery
I21.29	ST elevation (STEMI) myocardial infarction involving other sites
I21.4	Non-ST elevation (NSTEMI) myocardial infarction
I21.A1	Myocardial infarction type 2
I22.0	Subsequent ST elevation (STEMI) myocardial infarction of anterior wall
I22.1	Subsequent ST elevation (STEMI) myocardial infarction of inferior wall
I22.2	Subsequent non-ST elevation (NSTEMI) myocardial infarction
I22.8	Subsequent ST elevation (STEMI) myocardial infarction of other sites
I24.0	Acute coronary thrombosis not resulting in myocardial infarction
I24.8	Other forms of acute ischemic heart disease
I25.10	Atherosclerotic heart disease of native coronary artery without angina pectoris
I25.110	Atherosclerotic heart disease of native coronary artery with unstable angina pectoris
I25.111	Atherosclerotic heart disease of native coronary artery with angina pectoris with documented spasm
I25.118	Atherosclerotic heart disease of native coronary artery with other forms of angina pectoris
I25.3	Aneurysm of heart
I25.41	Coronary artery aneurysm
I25.5	Ischemic cardiomyopathy
I25.6	Silent myocardial ischemia
I25.710	Atherosclerosis of autologous vein coronary artery bypass graft(s) with unstable angina pectoris
I25.711	Atherosclerosis of autologous vein coronary artery bypass graft(s) with angina pectoris with documented spasm
I25.718	Atherosclerosis of autologous vein coronary artery bypass graft(s) with other forms of angina pectoris
I25.720	Atherosclerosis of autologous artery coronary artery bypass graft(s) with unstable angina pectoris
I25.721	Atherosclerosis of autologous artery coronary artery bypass graft(s) with angina pectoris with documented spasm
I25.728	Atherosclerosis of autologous artery coronary artery bypass graft(s) with other forms of angina pectoris
I25.730	Atherosclerosis of nonautologous biological coronary artery bypass graft(s) with unstable angina pectoris
I25.731	Atherosclerosis of nonautologous biological coronary artery bypass graft(s) with angina pectoris with documented spasm
I25.738	Atherosclerosis of nonautologous biological coronary artery bypass graft(s) with other forms of angina pectoris
I25.750	Atherosclerosis of native coronary artery of transplanted heart with unstable angina
I25.751	Atherosclerosis of native coronary artery of transplanted heart with angina pectoris with documented spasm
I25.758	Atherosclerosis of native coronary artery of transplanted heart with other forms of angina pectoris
I25.760	Atherosclerosis of bypass graft of coronary artery of transplanted heart with unstable angina
I25.761	Atherosclerosis of bypass graft of coronary artery of transplanted heart with angina pectoris with documented spasm
I25.768	Atherosclerosis of bypass graft of coronary artery of transplanted heart with other forms of angina pectoris
I25.790	Atherosclerosis of other coronary artery bypass graft(s) with unstable angina pectoris
I25.791	Atherosclerosis of other coronary artery bypass graft(s) with angina pectoris with documented spasm
I25.798	Atherosclerosis of other coronary artery bypass graft(s) with other forms of angina pectoris
I25.810	Atherosclerosis of coronary artery bypass graft(s) without angina pectoris
I25.812	Atherosclerosis of bypass graft of coronary artery of transplanted heart without angina pectoris
I25.82	Chronic total occlusion of coronary artery
I25.84	Coronary atherosclerosis due to calcified coronary lesion
I25.89	Other forms of chronic ischemic heart disease
I42.0	Dilated cardiomyopathy
I42.1	Obstructive hypertrophic cardiomyopathy
I42.2	Other hypertrophic cardiomyopathy
I42.8	Other cardiomyopathies
I43	Cardiomyopathy in diseases classified elsewhere
I50.1	Left ventricular failure, unspecified
I50.21	Acute systolic (congestive) heart failure
I50.22	Chronic systolic (congestive) heart failure
I50.23	Acute on chronic systolic (congestive) heart failure
I50.31	Acute diastolic (congestive) heart failure
I50.32	Chronic diastolic (congestive) heart failure
I50.33	Acute on chronic diastolic (congestive) heart failure
I50.41	Acute combined systolic (congestive) and diastolic (congestive) heart failure
I50.42	Chronic combined systolic (congestive) and diastolic (congestive) heart failure
I50.43	Acute on chronic combined systolic (congestive) and diastolic (congestive) heart failure
I50.811	Acute right heart failure
I50.812	Chronic right heart failure
I50.813	Acute on chronic right heart failure
I50.814	Right heart failure due to left heart failure
I50.82	Biventricular heart failure
I50.83	High output heart failure
I50.84	End stage heart failure
I51.7	Cardiomegaly

AMA: 93455 2018,Jan,8; 2018,Feb,11; 2017,Jan,8; 2016,Mar,5; 2016,Jan,13; 2015,Jan,16; 2014,Jul,3; 2014,Jan,11; 2014,Dec,6; 2013,May,12

Relative Value Units/Medicare Edits

Non-Facility RVU	Work	PE	MP	Total
93455	5.29	22.26	1.09	28.64
Facility RVU	**Work**	**PE**	**MP**	**Total**
93455	5.29	22.26	1.09	28.64

	FUD	Status	MUE	Modifiers				IOM Reference
93455	0	A	1(3)	51	N/A	N/A	80*	None

* with documentation

Terms To Know

angina pectoris. Sudden chest pain due to a lack of oxygen within the heart muscles.

angioplasty. Reconstruction or repair of a diseased or damaged blood vessel.

atherosclerosis. Buildup of yellowish plaques composed of cholesterol and lipoid material within the arteries.

autologous. Tissue, cells, or structure obtained from the same individual.

bypass graft. Surgically created alternative blood vessel used to reroute blood flow around an area of obstruction or disease.

catheter. Flexible tube inserted into an area of the body for introducing or withdrawing fluid.

fluoroscopy. Radiology technique that allows visual examination of part of the body or a function of an organ using a device that projects an x-ray image on a fluorescent screen.

nonautogenous. Derived from a source other than the same individual or recipient (e.g., cells, tissue, blood vessels, and other organs donated from another human).

93456-93457

93456 Catheter placement in coronary artery(s) for coronary angiography, including intraprocedural injection(s) for coronary angiography, imaging supervision and interpretation; with right heart catheterization

93457 with catheter placement(s) in bypass graft(s) (internal mammary, free arterial, venous grafts) including intraprocedural injection(s) for bypass graft angiography and right heart catheterization

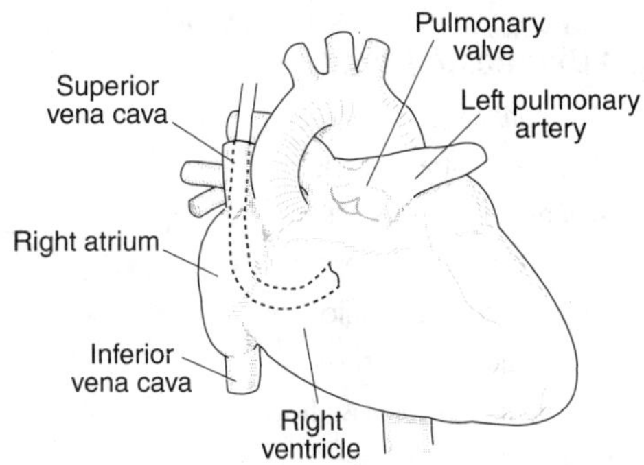

Introduction of a catheter into the right side of the heart

Explanation

The physician performs a catheter placement in one or more coronary arteries for coronary angiography, without concomitant left heart catheterization. The physician places an introducer sheath in an artery, typically the femoral artery, using percutaneous puncture. The physician advances an angiography catheter through the introducer sheath into the ascending aorta and advances it, under fluoroscopic guidance, to the opening of the coronary artery. The physician injects radiopaque contrast material through the catheter into the vessel while recording a cineangiogram. The physician removes the catheter and sheath from the femoral artery. Pressure is placed on the wound for 20 to 30 minutes to stem bleeding. These codes include imaging supervision and interpretation, as well as any required repositioning of catheters. Code 93456 includes right heart catheterization, in which the catheter is threaded into the right atrium, through the tricuspid valve into the right ventricle, and across the pulmonary valve into the pulmonary arteries. Code 93457 includes catheter placement in one or more bypass grafts for angiography, in addition to the right heart catheterization. Intracardiac or intravascular pressure recordings are included in these codes, as are cardiac output and oxygen saturation measurements, and final evaluation and procedure report.

Coding Tips

When medically necessary, report moderate (conscious) sedation provided by the performing physician with 99151-99153. When provided by another physician, report 99155-99157. These procedures include placement of the catheter into the coronary arteries involving selective placement of the native coronary artery origin in order to perform coronary angiogram. Codes 93454–93461, other than congenital conditions, include intraprocedural injection and imaging when performing coronary angiogram. Right heart catheterization includes placement of the catheter into the right-side heart chambers or structures (right atrium, right ventricle, pulmonary artery, and wedge), specimen collection for blood gas measurements, and cardiac output measurements. Report right ventricular or right atrial angiogram (93566) in addition to right heart catheterization when performed. Procedures 93455, 93457, 93459, and 93461 include intraprocedural injections and imaging supervision and interpretation for bypass graft angiogram. Placement of the catheter in bypass grafts (venous, internal mammary, free arterial graft) involves selective placement of the graft origin for bypass angiogram and is most often performed in addition to coronary angiogram of native vessels. For pharmacologic administration in addition to a cardiac catheterization procedure for re-evaluating hemodynamic measurements and responses, report 93463 with 93451–93453 and 93456–93461. These codes may be reported in addition to 33274 and 33275 only if the catheterization is performed for reasons distinct from the leadless pacemaker procedure. Do not report 93563–93565 with 93452–93461. Do not report 93456 or 93457 with 33418, 0345T, 0483T, 0484T, 0544T, or 0545T for diagnostic coronary angiography or right heart catheterization intrinsic to the valve repair or annulus reconstruction.

ICD-10-CM Diagnostic Codes

C38.0	Malignant neoplasm of heart
I05.0	Rheumatic mitral stenosis
I05.1	Rheumatic mitral insufficiency
I06.0	Rheumatic aortic stenosis
I06.1	Rheumatic aortic insufficiency
I07.0	Rheumatic tricuspid stenosis
I07.1	Rheumatic tricuspid insufficiency
I09.81	Rheumatic heart failure
I20.0	Unstable angina
I21.01	ST elevation (STEMI) myocardial infarction involving left main coronary artery
I21.02	ST elevation (STEMI) myocardial infarction involving left anterior descending coronary artery
I21.21	ST elevation (STEMI) myocardial infarction involving left circumflex coronary artery
I21.4	Non-ST elevation (NSTEMI) myocardial infarction
I21.A1	Myocardial infarction type 2
I22.0	Subsequent ST elevation (STEMI) myocardial infarction of anterior wall
I22.1	Subsequent ST elevation (STEMI) myocardial infarction of inferior wall
I22.2	Subsequent non-ST elevation (NSTEMI) myocardial infarction
I23.7	Postinfarction angina
I24.0	Acute coronary thrombosis not resulting in myocardial infarction
I24.1	Dressler's syndrome
I25.10	Atherosclerotic heart disease of native coronary artery without angina pectoris
I25.110	Atherosclerotic heart disease of native coronary artery with unstable angina pectoris
I25.111	Atherosclerotic heart disease of native coronary artery with angina pectoris with documented spasm
I25.3	Aneurysm of heart
I25.41	Coronary artery aneurysm
I25.5	Ischemic cardiomyopathy
I25.6	Silent myocardial ischemia
I25.82	Chronic total occlusion of coronary artery
I25.84	Coronary atherosclerosis due to calcified coronary lesion
I26.01	Septic pulmonary embolism with acute cor pulmonale
I26.02	Saddle embolus of pulmonary artery with acute cor pulmonale
I26.90	Septic pulmonary embolism without acute cor pulmonale
I26.92	Saddle embolus of pulmonary artery without acute cor pulmonale
I27.0	Primary pulmonary hypertension
I27.21	Secondary pulmonary arterial hypertension
I27.22	Pulmonary hypertension due to left heart disease
I27.23	Pulmonary hypertension due to lung diseases and hypoxia
I27.24	Chronic thromboembolic pulmonary hypertension
I27.81	Cor pulmonale (chronic)
I27.83	Eisenmenger's syndrome
I34.0	Nonrheumatic mitral (valve) insufficiency
I34.1	Nonrheumatic mitral (valve) prolapse
I34.2	Nonrheumatic mitral (valve) stenosis
I35.0	Nonrheumatic aortic (valve) stenosis
I35.1	Nonrheumatic aortic (valve) insufficiency
I36.0	Nonrheumatic tricuspid (valve) stenosis
I36.1	Nonrheumatic tricuspid (valve) insufficiency
I37.0	Nonrheumatic pulmonary valve stenosis
I37.1	Nonrheumatic pulmonary valve insufficiency
I40.0	Infective myocarditis
I40.1	Isolated myocarditis
I42.0	Dilated cardiomyopathy
I42.1	Obstructive hypertrophic cardiomyopathy
I42.3	Endomyocardial (eosinophilic) disease
I42.4	Endocardial fibroelastosis
I42.6	Alcoholic cardiomyopathy
I50.23	Acute on chronic systolic (congestive) heart failure
I50.33	Acute on chronic diastolic (congestive) heart failure
I50.813	Acute on chronic right heart failure
I50.814	Right heart failure due to left heart failure
I50.82	Biventricular heart failure
I50.83	High output heart failure
I50.84	End stage heart failure
I51.7	Cardiomegaly
R57.0	Cardiogenic shock
R57.1	Hypovolemic shock

AMA: **93456** 2019,Mar,6; 2019,Jun,3; 2018,Jan,8; 2018,Feb,11; 2017,Jul,3; 2017,Jan,8; 2016,Mar,5; 2016,Jan,13; 2015,Sep,3; 2015,Jan,16; 2014,Jul,3; 2014,Jan,11; 2014,Dec,6; 2013,May,12 **93457** 2019,Mar,6; 2019,Jun,3; 2018,Jan,8; 2018,Feb,11; 2017,Jan,8; 2016,Mar,5; 2016,Jan,13; 2015,Sep,3; 2015,Jan,16; 2014,Jul,3; 2014,Jan,11; 2014,Dec,6; 2013,May,12

Relative Value Units/Medicare Edits

Non-Facility RVU	Work	PE	MP	Total
93456	5.9	24.37	1.2	31.47
93457	6.64	27.18	1.36	35.18
Facility RVU	**Work**	**PE**	**MP**	**Total**
93456	5.9	24.37	1.2	31.47
93457	6.64	27.18	1.36	35.18

	FUD	Status	MUE	Modifiers				IOM Reference
93456	0	A	1(3)	51	N/A	N/A	80*	None
93457	0	A	1(3)	51	N/A	N/A	80*	

* with documentation

93458-93459

93458 Catheter placement in coronary artery(s) for coronary angiography, including intraprocedural injection(s) for coronary angiography, imaging supervision and interpretation; with left heart catheterization including intraprocedural injection(s) for left ventriculography, when performed

93459 with left heart catheterization including intraprocedural injection(s) for left ventriculography, when performed, catheter placement(s) in bypass graft(s) (internal mammary, free arterial, venous grafts) with bypass graft angiography

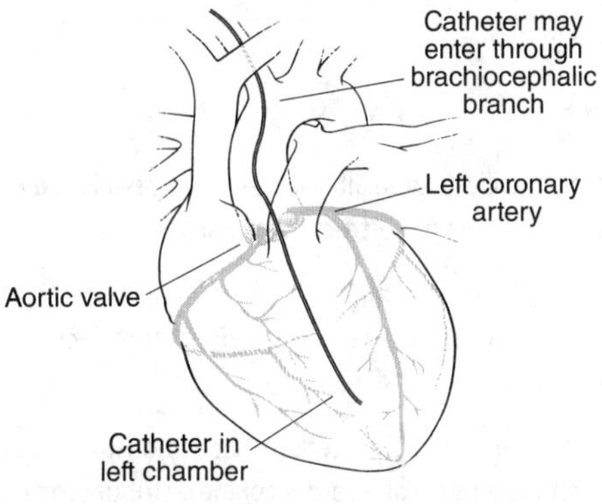

The catheter crosses the aortic valve and enters the left ventricle of the heart

Explanation

The physician places a catheter into one or more coronary arteries for coronary angiography. The physician threads a catheter to the heart, most frequently through an introducing sheath placed percutaneously into the femoral, brachial, or axillary artery using retrograde technique. The catheter passes through the aortic valve into the left ventricle. Intracardiac and intravascular pressures are recorded. Left ventricular injections may be performed for left ventriculography; the physician injects dye through a previously placed catheter threaded through a central line into the left ventricle or atrium to evaluate function with fluoroscopy. Code 93459 includes catheter placement in one or more bypass grafts with bypass graft angiography. The physician removes the catheter and sheath from the femoral artery. Pressure is placed on the wound for 20 to 30 minutes to stem bleeding. These codes include imaging supervision and interpretation, as well as any required repositioning of catheters.

Coding Tips

When medically necessary, report moderate (conscious) sedation provided by the performing physician with 99151-99153. When provided by another physician, report 99155-99157. These procedures include placement of the catheter into the coronary arteries involving selective placement of the native coronary artery origin in order to perform coronary angiogram. Codes 93454–93461, for other than congenital conditions, include intraprocedural injection and imaging when performing coronary angiogram. These procedures include placement of the catheter into the left-side heart chambers or structures (left ventricle, left atrium) and left ventricular injection when utilized. Intraprocedural injections for left ventricular/atrial angiogram and imaging supervision and interpretation are also included. Do not report 93503 in addition to other diagnostic cardiac cath codes. For left heart catheterization that is performed via transapical puncture into the left ventricle or transseptal puncture into the septum, report 93462 in addition to 93452, 93453, 93458–93461, 93653, and 93654. Right heart catheterization includes placement of the catheter into the right-side heart chambers or structures (right atrium, right ventricle, pulmonary artery, and wedge), specimen collection for blood gas measurements, and cardiac output measurements. Report right ventricular or right atrial angiogram (93566) in addition to right heart catheterization when performed. Procedures 93455, 93457, 93459, and 93461 include intraprocedural injections and imaging supervision and interpretation for bypass graft angiogram. Do not report 93563–93565 with 93452–93461. Placement of the catheter in bypass grafts (venous, internal mammary, free arterial graft) involves selective placement of the graft origin for bypass angiogram and is most often performed in addition to coronary angiogram of native vessels. For pharmacologic administration in addition to a cardiac catheterization procedure for re-evaluating hemodynamic measurements and responses, report 93463 in addition to 93451–93453 and 93456–93461. Do not report these codes with 0408T-0411T or 0414T-0415T. Do not report 93458 or 93459 with 33418, 0345T, 0483T, 0484T, 0544T, or 0545T for diagnostic coronary angiography or left heart catheterization intrinsic to the valve repair or annulus reconstruction.

ICD-10-CM Diagnostic Codes

C38.0	Malignant neoplasm of heart
I05.0	Rheumatic mitral stenosis
I05.1	Rheumatic mitral insufficiency
I06.0	Rheumatic aortic stenosis
I06.1	Rheumatic aortic insufficiency
I07.0	Rheumatic tricuspid stenosis
I07.1	Rheumatic tricuspid insufficiency
I09.81	Rheumatic heart failure
I20.0	Unstable angina
I20.8	Other forms of angina pectoris
I21.01	ST elevation (STEMI) myocardial infarction involving left main coronary artery
I21.02	ST elevation (STEMI) myocardial infarction involving left anterior descending coronary artery
I21.09	ST elevation (STEMI) myocardial infarction involving other coronary artery of anterior wall
I21.11	ST elevation (STEMI) myocardial infarction involving right coronary artery
I21.19	ST elevation (STEMI) myocardial infarction involving other coronary artery of inferior wall
I21.21	ST elevation (STEMI) myocardial infarction involving left circumflex coronary artery
I21.4	Non-ST elevation (NSTEMI) myocardial infarction
I21.A1	Myocardial infarction type 2
I22.0	Subsequent ST elevation (STEMI) myocardial infarction of anterior wall
I22.1	Subsequent ST elevation (STEMI) myocardial infarction of inferior wall
I22.2	Subsequent non-ST elevation (NSTEMI) myocardial infarction
I23.7	Postinfarction angina
I24.0	Acute coronary thrombosis not resulting in myocardial infarction
I24.1	Dressler's syndrome
I25.10	Atherosclerotic heart disease of native coronary artery without angina pectoris
I25.110	Atherosclerotic heart disease of native coronary artery with unstable angina pectoris
I25.111	Atherosclerotic heart disease of native coronary artery with angina pectoris with documented spasm
I25.118	Atherosclerotic heart disease of native coronary artery with other forms of angina pectoris

Medicine

I25.2 Old myocardial infarction
I25.3 Aneurysm of heart
I25.41 Coronary artery aneurysm
I25.5 Ischemic cardiomyopathy
I25.6 Silent myocardial ischemia
I25.82 Chronic total occlusion of coronary artery
I25.84 Coronary atherosclerosis due to calcified coronary lesion
I26.01 Septic pulmonary embolism with acute cor pulmonale
I26.02 Saddle embolus of pulmonary artery with acute cor pulmonale
I26.90 Septic pulmonary embolism without acute cor pulmonale
I26.92 Saddle embolus of pulmonary artery without acute cor pulmonale
I27.0 Primary pulmonary hypertension
I27.81 Cor pulmonale (chronic)
I27.83 Eisenmenger's syndrome
I34.0 Nonrheumatic mitral (valve) insufficiency
I34.1 Nonrheumatic mitral (valve) prolapse
I34.2 Nonrheumatic mitral (valve) stenosis
I35.0 Nonrheumatic aortic (valve) stenosis
I35.1 Nonrheumatic aortic (valve) insufficiency
I35.2 Nonrheumatic aortic (valve) stenosis with insufficiency
I36.0 Nonrheumatic tricuspid (valve) stenosis
I36.1 Nonrheumatic tricuspid (valve) insufficiency
I37.0 Nonrheumatic pulmonary valve stenosis
I37.1 Nonrheumatic pulmonary valve insufficiency
I42.0 Dilated cardiomyopathy
I42.1 Obstructive hypertrophic cardiomyopathy
I50.23 Acute on chronic systolic (congestive) heart failure
I50.33 Acute on chronic diastolic (congestive) heart failure
I50.43 Acute on chronic combined systolic (congestive) and diastolic (congestive) heart failure
I50.813 Acute on chronic right heart failure
I50.814 Right heart failure due to left heart failure
I50.82 Biventricular heart failure
I50.83 High output heart failure
I50.84 End stage heart failure
I51.7 Cardiomegaly
R57.0 Cardiogenic shock
R57.1 Hypovolemic shock
T80.0XXA Air embolism following infusion, transfusion and therapeutic injection, initial encounter
T82.817A Embolism due to cardiac prosthetic devices, implants and grafts, initial encounter
T82.818A Embolism due to vascular prosthetic devices, implants and grafts, initial encounter

AMA: 93458 2018,Jan,8; 2018,Feb,11; 2017,Jul,3; 2017,Jan,8; 2016,Mar,5; 2016,Jan,13; 2015,Sep,3; 2015,Jan,16; 2014,Jul,3; 2014,Jan,11; 2014,Dec,6; 2013,May,12; 2013,Jan,6-8 **93459** 2018,Jan,8; 2018,Feb,11; 2017,Jul,3; 2017,Jan,8; 2016,Mar,5; 2016,Jan,13; 2015,Sep,3; 2015,Jan,16; 2014,Jul,3; 2014,Jan,11; 2014,Dec,6; 2013,May,12; 2013,Jan,6-8

Relative Value Units/Medicare Edits

Non-Facility RVU	Work	PE	MP	Total
93458	5.6	22.74	1.16	29.5
93459	6.35	24.74	1.31	32.4
Facility RVU	**Work**	**PE**	**MP**	**Total**
93458	5.6	22.74	1.16	29.5
93459	6.35	24.74	1.31	32.4

	FUD	Status	MUE	Modifiers				IOM Reference
93458	0	A	1(3)	51	N/A	N/A	80*	None
93459	0	A	1(3)	51	N/A	N/A	80*	

* with documentation

Terms To Know

bypass graft. Surgically created alternative blood vessel used to reroute blood flow around an area of obstruction or disease.

fluoroscopy. Radiology technique that allows visual examination of part of the body or a function of an organ using a device that projects an x-ray image on a fluorescent screen.

ventriculogram. Interventional procedure that demonstrates the contractility of the cardiac ventricles by serial recording of the distribution of intravenously injected radionuclide or that of radiographic contrast medium injected through an intracardiac catheter.

93460-93461

93460 Catheter placement in coronary artery(s) for coronary angiography, including intraprocedural injection(s) for coronary angiography, imaging supervision and interpretation; with right and left heart catheterization including intraprocedural injection(s) for left ventriculography, when performed

93461 with right and left heart catheterization including intraprocedural injection(s) for left ventriculography, when performed, catheter placement(s) in bypass graft(s) (internal mammary, free arterial, venous grafts) with bypass graft angiography

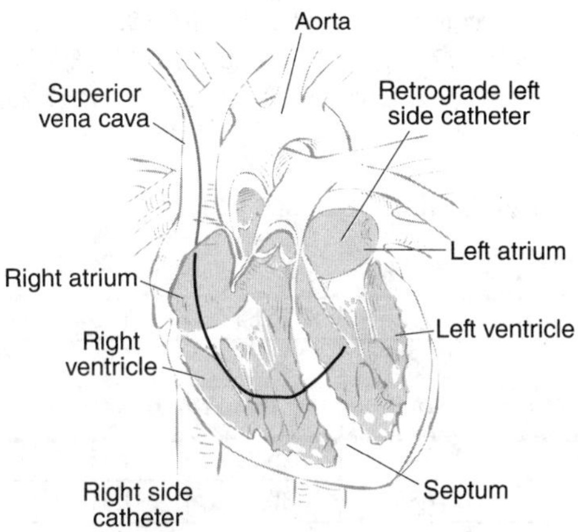

Both sides of the heart are catheterized with left ventriculogram

Explanation

The physician places a catheter in one or more coronary arteries for coronary angiography. In 93460, right and left heart function is evaluated. To accomplish right heart catheterization, the physician threads a catheter through an introducing sheath placed percutaneously into the femoral, subclavian, internal jugular, or antecubital vein. The catheter is threaded into the right atrium, through the tricuspid valve into the right ventricle, and across the pulmonary valve into the pulmonary arteries. Left heart catheterization is also performed, in this case using retrograde technique. The catheter is inserted through an introducing sheath placed percutaneously into the femoral, brachial, or axillary artery. The catheter is passed through the aortic valve into the left ventricle. Intracardiac and intravascular pressures are recorded. Left ventricular injections may be performed for left ventriculography; the physician injects dye through a previously placed catheter threaded through a central line into the left ventricle or atrium to evaluate function with fluoroscopy. Code 93461 includes catheter placement in one or more bypass grafts for angiography. The physician removes the catheter and sheath from the femoral artery. Pressure is placed on the wound for 20 to 30 minutes to stem bleeding. These codes include imaging supervision and interpretation, as well as any required repositioning of catheters.

Coding Tips

When medically necessary, report moderate (conscious) sedation provided by the performing physician with 99151-99153. When provided by another physician, report 99155-99157. These procedures include placement of the catheter into the coronary arteries involving selective placement of the native coronary artery origin in order to perform coronary angiogram. Codes 93454–93461, for other than congenital conditions, include intraprocedural injection and imaging when performing coronary angiogram. Right heart catheterization includes placement of the catheter into the right-side heart chambers or structures (right atrium, right ventricle, pulmonary artery, and wedge), specimen collection for blood gas measurements, and cardiac output measurements. Report right ventricular or right atrial angiogram (93566) in addition to right heart catheterization when performed. These procedures include placement of the catheter into the left-side heart chambers or structures (left ventricle, left atrium) and left ventricular injection when utilized. Intraprocedural injections for left ventricular/atrial angiogram and imaging supervision and interpretation are also included. For left heart catheterization performed via transapical puncture into the left ventricle or transseptal puncture into the septum, report 93462 with 93452, 93453, 93458–93461, 93653, and 93654. Procedures 93455, 93457, 93459, and 93461 include intraprocedural injections and imaging supervision and interpretation for bypass graft angiogram. Placement of the catheter in bypass grafts (venous, internal mammary, free arterial graft) involves selective placement of the graft origin for bypass angiogram and is most often performed in addition to coronary angiogram of native vessels. For pharmacologic administration in addition to a cardiac catheterization procedure for re-evaluating hemodynamic measurements and responses, report 93463 with 93451–93453 and 93456–93461. These codes may be reported in addition to 33274 and 33275 only if the catheterization is performed for reasons distinct from the leadless pacemaker procedure. Do not report 93563–93565 with 93452–93461, 0408T-0411T, or 0414T-0415T. Do not report 93460 or 93461 with 33418, 0345T, 0483T, 0484T, 0544T, or 0545T for diagnostic coronary angiography or left and right heart catheterization intrinsic to the valve repair or annulus reconstruction.

ICD-10-CM Diagnostic Codes

C38.0	Malignant neoplasm of heart
I05.0	Rheumatic mitral stenosis
I05.1	Rheumatic mitral insufficiency
I06.0	Rheumatic aortic stenosis
I06.1	Rheumatic aortic insufficiency
I07.0	Rheumatic tricuspid stenosis
I07.1	Rheumatic tricuspid insufficiency
I08.3	Combined rheumatic disorders of mitral, aortic and tricuspid valves
I09.81	Rheumatic heart failure
I20.0	Unstable angina
I20.1	Angina pectoris with documented spasm
I21.01	ST elevation (STEMI) myocardial infarction involving left main coronary artery
I21.02	ST elevation (STEMI) myocardial infarction involving left anterior descending coronary artery
I21.09	ST elevation (STEMI) myocardial infarction involving other coronary artery of anterior wall
I21.11	ST elevation (STEMI) myocardial infarction involving right coronary artery
I21.19	ST elevation (STEMI) myocardial infarction involving other coronary artery of inferior wall
I21.21	ST elevation (STEMI) myocardial infarction involving left circumflex coronary artery
I21.4	Non-ST elevation (NSTEMI) myocardial infarction
I21.A1	Myocardial infarction type 2
I22.0	Subsequent ST elevation (STEMI) myocardial infarction of anterior wall
I22.1	Subsequent ST elevation (STEMI) myocardial infarction of inferior wall
I22.2	Subsequent non-ST elevation (NSTEMI) myocardial infarction
I23.0	Hemopericardium as current complication following acute myocardial infarction

I23.1	Atrial septal defect as current complication following acute myocardial infarction
I23.2	Ventricular septal defect as current complication following acute myocardial infarction
I23.3	Rupture of cardiac wall without hemopericardium as current complication following acute myocardial infarction
I23.7	Postinfarction angina
I24.0	Acute coronary thrombosis not resulting in myocardial infarction
I24.1	Dressler's syndrome
I25.10	Atherosclerotic heart disease of native coronary artery without angina pectoris
I25.110	Atherosclerotic heart disease of native coronary artery with unstable angina pectoris
I25.111	Atherosclerotic heart disease of native coronary artery with angina pectoris with documented spasm
I25.2	Old myocardial infarction
I25.3	Aneurysm of heart
I25.41	Coronary artery aneurysm
I25.5	Ischemic cardiomyopathy
I25.6	Silent myocardial ischemia
I25.82	Chronic total occlusion of coronary artery
I25.84	Coronary atherosclerosis due to calcified coronary lesion
I26.01	Septic pulmonary embolism with acute cor pulmonale
I26.02	Saddle embolus of pulmonary artery with acute cor pulmonale
I26.90	Septic pulmonary embolism without acute cor pulmonale
I26.92	Saddle embolus of pulmonary artery without acute cor pulmonale
I27.0	Primary pulmonary hypertension
I27.81	Cor pulmonale (chronic)
I27.83	Eisenmenger's syndrome
I34.0	Nonrheumatic mitral (valve) insufficiency
I34.1	Nonrheumatic mitral (valve) prolapse
I34.2	Nonrheumatic mitral (valve) stenosis
I35.0	Nonrheumatic aortic (valve) stenosis
I35.1	Nonrheumatic aortic (valve) insufficiency
I35.2	Nonrheumatic aortic (valve) stenosis with insufficiency
I36.0	Nonrheumatic tricuspid (valve) stenosis
I36.1	Nonrheumatic tricuspid (valve) insufficiency
I37.0	Nonrheumatic pulmonary valve stenosis
I37.1	Nonrheumatic pulmonary valve insufficiency
I40.0	Infective myocarditis
I40.1	Isolated myocarditis
I42.0	Dilated cardiomyopathy
I42.1	Obstructive hypertrophic cardiomyopathy
I42.3	Endomyocardial (eosinophilic) disease
I42.4	Endocardial fibroelastosis
I42.6	Alcoholic cardiomyopathy
I50.23	Acute on chronic systolic (congestive) heart failure
I50.33	Acute on chronic diastolic (congestive) heart failure
I50.813	Acute on chronic right heart failure
I50.814	Right heart failure due to left heart failure
I50.82	Biventricular heart failure
I50.83	High output heart failure
I50.84	End stage heart failure
I51.7	Cardiomegaly
R57.0	Cardiogenic shock
R57.1	Hypovolemic shock
T80.0XXA	Air embolism following infusion, transfusion and therapeutic injection, initial encounter
T82.817A	Embolism due to cardiac prosthetic devices, implants and grafts, initial encounter
T82.818A	Embolism due to vascular prosthetic devices, implants and grafts, initial encounter

AMA: **93460** 2019,Mar,6; 2019,Jun,3; 2018,Jan,8; 2018,Feb,11; 2017,Jul,3; 2017,Jan,8; 2016,Mar,5; 2016,Jan,13; 2015,Sep,3; 2015,Jan,16; 2014,Jul,3; 2014,Jan,11; 2014,Dec,6; 2013,May,12; 2013,Jan,6-8 **93461** 2019,Mar,6; 2019,Jun,3; 2018,Jan,8; 2018,Feb,11; 2017,Jul,3; 2017,Jan,8; 2016,Mar,5; 2016,Jan,13; 2015,Sep,3; 2015,Jan,16; 2014,Jul,3; 2014,Jan,11; 2014,Dec,6; 2013,May,12; 2013,Jan,6-8

Relative Value Units/Medicare Edits

Non-Facility RVU	Work	PE	MP	Total
93460	7.1	26.85	1.45	35.4
93461	7.85	30.61	1.61	40.07
Facility RVU	**Work**	**PE**	**MP**	**Total**
93460	7.1	26.85	1.45	35.4
93461	7.85	30.61	1.61	40.07

	FUD	Status	MUE	Modifiers				IOM Reference
93460	0	A	1(3)	51	N/A	N/A	80*	None
93461	0	A	1(3)	51	N/A	N/A	80*	

* with documentation

Terms To Know

angiogram. Radiographic image of the arteries. Imaging may be performed to study the vasculature of any given organ, body system, or area of circulation such as the brain, heart, chest, kidneys, limbs, gastrointestinal tract, aorta, and pulmonary circulation to visualize the formation and the function of the blood vessels to detect problems such as a blockage or stricture.

supervision and interpretation. Radiology services that usually contain an invasive component and are reported by the radiologist for supervision of the procedure and the personnel involved with performing the examination, reading the film, and preparing the written report.

93462

\+ **93462** Left heart catheterization by transseptal puncture through intact septum or by transapical puncture (List separately in addition to code for primary procedure)

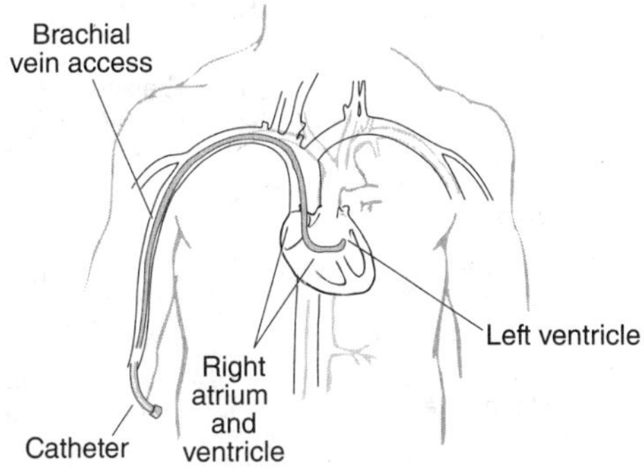

Explanation

Transseptal catheterization involves passing a catheter from the right femoral vein into the right atrium. The interatrial wall or septum is punctured and the catheter is passed into either the left atrium or left ventricle. When the left atrium is accessed, the catheter may be further advanced through the mitral valve and into the left ventricle. The transapical or direct left ventricular puncture involves using a large bore needle to puncture the chest wall directly into the left ventricular cavity. These methods are used when the patient has had valve replacement and the left heart cannot be accessed any other way.

Coding Tips

When medically necessary, report moderate (conscious) sedation provided by the performing physician with 99151-99153. When provided by another physician, report 99155-99157. This procedure includes placement of the catheter into the left-side heart chambers or structures (left ventricle, left atrium) and left ventricular injection when utilized. Intraprocedural injections for left ventricular/atrial angiogram and imaging supervision and interpretation are also included. Report 93462 in addition to 33477, 93452, 93453, 93458–93461, 93582, 93653, and 93654. Do not report 93462 with 93656. Do not report 93462 with 0345T or 0544T unless transapical puncture is performed.

ICD-10-CM Diagnostic Codes

This/these CPT code(s) are add on code(s). See the primary procedure code that this code is performed with for your ICD-10-CM code selections. Diagnostic code(s) would be the same as the actual procedure performed.

AMA: 93462 2018,Jan,8; 2018,Feb,11; 2017,Sep,3; 2017,Jul,3; 2017,Jan,8; 2016,Jan,13; 2015,Sep,3; 2015,Jan,16; 2014,Jul,3; 2014,Jan,11; 2013,May,12; 2013,Jun,6-8

Relative Value Units/Medicare Edits

Non-Facility RVU	Work	PE	MP	Total
93462	3.73	1.53	0.85	6.11
Facility RVU	**Work**	**PE**	**MP**	**Total**
93462	3.73	1.53	0.85	6.11

	FUD	Status	MUE	Modifiers				IOM Reference
93462	N/A	A	1(3)	N/A	N/A	N/A	80*	None

* with documentation

93463

\+ **93463** Pharmacologic agent administration (eg, inhaled nitric oxide, intravenous infusion of nitroprusside, dobutamine, milrinone, or other agent) including assessing hemodynamic measurements before, during, after and repeat pharmacologic agent administration, when performed (List separately in addition to code for primary procedure)

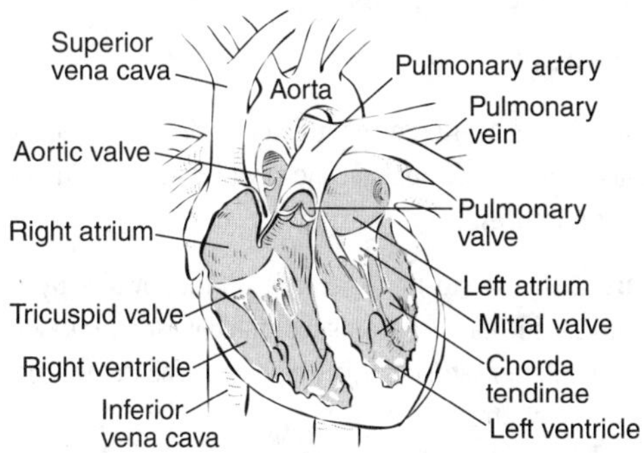

Explanation

The physician administers a pharmacologic agent to invoke stress on coronary vessels in order to measure blood flow through and around the heart. This produces the same result as physical exercise. Arteries become enlarged as the body increases physical activity that requires more oxygen. When plaque is present within a vessel, it does not allow for this enlargement. This slows the ability of the oxygenated blood to reach the necessary organs, which can lead to ischemia.

Coding Tips

When medically necessary, report moderate (conscious) sedation provided by the performing physician with 99151-99153. When provided by another physician, report 99155-99157. Report 93463 in addition to 33477, 93451–93453, 93456–93461, 93530–93533, 93580, and 93581. For pharmacologic administration in addition to a cardiac catheterization procedure for re-evaluating hemodynamic measurements and responses, report 93463 with 93451–93453 and 93456–93461. Do not report 93463 for intracoronary administration of pharmacologic administration with percutaneous coronary procedures, intracoronary assessment of pressures, flow and resistance, or intracoronary imaging procedures. Do not report 93463 with 92920–92944, 92975, or 92977.

ICD-10-CM Diagnostic Codes

This/these CPT code(s) are add on code(s). See the primary procedure code that this code is performed with for your ICD-10-CM code selections. Diagnostic code(s) would be the same as the actual procedure performed.

AMA: 93463 2018,Jan,8; 2018,Feb,11; 2017,Jan,8; 2016,Jan,13; 2015,Jan,16; 2014,Jul,3; 2014,Jan,11; 2014,Dec,6

Relative Value Units/Medicare Edits

Non-Facility RVU	Work	PE	MP	Total
93463	2.0	0.69	0.13	2.82
Facility RVU	**Work**	**PE**	**MP**	**Total**
93463	2.0	0.69	0.13	2.82

	FUD	Status	MUE	Modifiers				IOM Reference
93463	N/A	A	1(3)	N/A	N/A	N/A	80*	None

* with documentation

Terms To Know

catheterization. Use or insertion of a tubular device into a duct, blood vessel, hollow organ, or body cavity for injecting or withdrawing fluids for diagnostic or therapeutic purposes.

dobutamine. Drug used to increase cardiac output by directly stimulating beta 1 receptors to increase myocardial contractility and stroke volume. Often used supportively after cardiac surgery or in heart failure. May be sold under the brand name Dobutrex.

ischemia. Deficiency in blood supply causing tissues to be deprived of oxygen, resulting from trauma, mechanical or functional constriction of blood vessels, or a physical obstruction.

percutaneous. Through the skin.

pharmacological agent. Drug used to produce a chemical effect.

prophylactic. Agent or treatment measure intended to prevent or ward off a disease condition.

therapeutic. Act meant to alleviate a medical or mental condition.

93464

\+ **93464** Physiologic exercise study (eg, bicycle or arm ergometry) including assessing hemodynamic measurements before and after (List separately in addition to code for primary procedure)

Arteries of the Heart

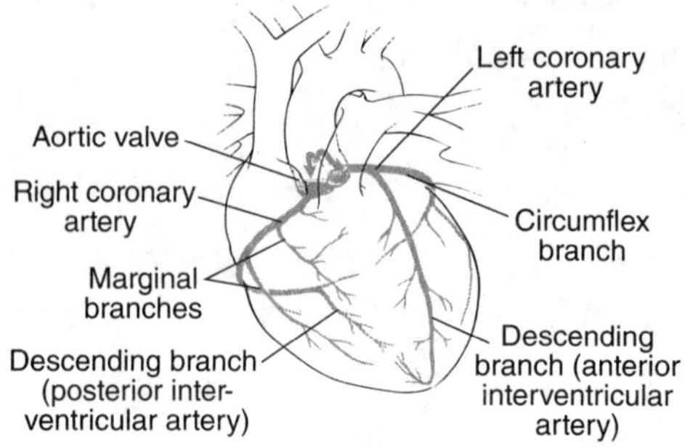

Explanation

The physician monitors a patient during physiologic exercise (e.g., stationary bicycle) to measure blood flow through and around the heart. During periods of exercise, the arteries become enlarged to allow increased blood flow to supply greater levels of oxygen to the necessary vessels and organs. When plaque is present within a vessel, it does not allow for this enlargement. The oxygenated blood's ability to reach the necessary organs is decreased, which can lead to ischemia. This study is often conducted when narrowing of a coronary artery is discovered during a cardiac catheter procedure.

Coding Tips

When medically necessary, report moderate (conscious) sedation provided by the performing physician with 99151-99153. When provided by another physician, report 99155-99157. This code is reported only one time per catheterization procedure. Report 93464 in addition to 33477, 93451–93453, 93456–93461, and 93530–93533. For pharmacologic agent administration, see 93463. For bundle of His recording, see 93600.

ICD-10-CM Diagnostic Codes

This/these CPT code(s) are add on code(s). See the primary procedure code that this code is performed with for your ICD-10-CM code selections. Diagnostic code(s) would be the same as the actual procedure performed.

AMA: 93464 2018,Jan,8; 2018,Feb,11; 2017,Jan,8; 2016,Jan,13; 2015,Jan,16; 2014,Jul,3; 2014,Jan,11

Relative Value Units/Medicare Edits

Non-Facility RVU	Work	PE	MP	Total
93464	1.8	5.16	0.08	7.04
Facility RVU	**Work**	**PE**	**MP**	**Total**
93464	1.8	5.16	0.08	7.04

	FUD	Status	MUE	Modifiers				IOM Reference
93464	N/A	A	1(3)	N/A	N/A	N/A	80*	None

* with documentation

Medicine

93503

93503 Insertion and placement of flow directed catheter (eg, Swan-Ganz) for monitoring purposes

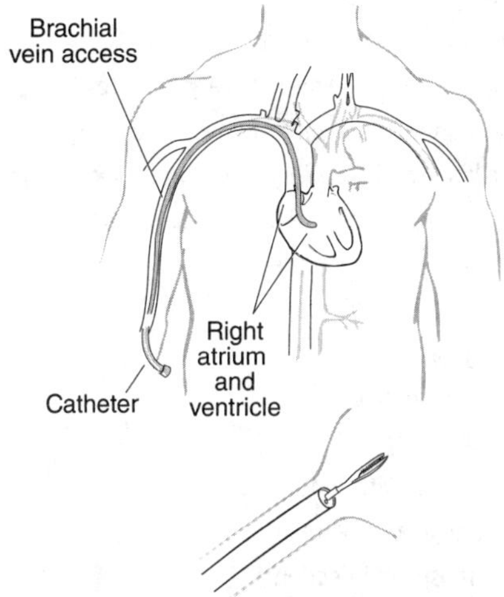

A biopsy tome is inserted through the catheter and several tiny tissue samples are collected from the walls of the heart

Explanation

The physician threads a catheter to the right heart through a central intravenous line often inserted up the femoral vein to take blood samples, pressure and electrical recordings, and/or other tests. This code applies to the insertion of a flow directed catheter, such as the Swan-Ganz device, used for measuring pressure and related parameters.

Coding Tips

As exempt from modifier 51, 93503 has not been designated in CPT as an add-on service/procedure. However, codes identified as exempt from modifier 51 are not subject to multiple procedure rules. No reimbursement reduction or modifier 51 is applied. For subsequent monitoring, see 99356–99357.

ICD-10-CM Diagnostic Codes

I05.0	Rheumatic mitral stenosis
I05.1	Rheumatic mitral insufficiency
I05.2	Rheumatic mitral stenosis with insufficiency
I05.8	Other rheumatic mitral valve diseases
I06.0	Rheumatic aortic stenosis
I06.1	Rheumatic aortic insufficiency
I06.2	Rheumatic aortic stenosis with insufficiency
I06.8	Other rheumatic aortic valve diseases
I07.0	Rheumatic tricuspid stenosis
I07.1	Rheumatic tricuspid insufficiency
I07.2	Rheumatic tricuspid stenosis and insufficiency
I07.8	Other rheumatic tricuspid valve diseases
I08.0	Rheumatic disorders of both mitral and aortic valves
I08.1	Rheumatic disorders of both mitral and tricuspid valves
I08.2	Rheumatic disorders of both aortic and tricuspid valves
I08.3	Combined rheumatic disorders of mitral, aortic and tricuspid valves
I08.8	Other rheumatic multiple valve diseases
I09.0	Rheumatic myocarditis
I09.81	Rheumatic heart failure
I09.89	Other specified rheumatic heart diseases
I20.0	Unstable angina
I21.01	ST elevation (STEMI) myocardial infarction involving left main coronary artery
I21.02	ST elevation (STEMI) myocardial infarction involving left anterior descending coronary artery
I21.09	ST elevation (STEMI) myocardial infarction involving other coronary artery of anterior wall
I21.11	ST elevation (STEMI) myocardial infarction involving right coronary artery
I21.19	ST elevation (STEMI) myocardial infarction involving other coronary artery of inferior wall
I21.21	ST elevation (STEMI) myocardial infarction involving left circumflex coronary artery
I21.29	ST elevation (STEMI) myocardial infarction involving other sites
I21.4	Non-ST elevation (NSTEMI) myocardial infarction
I21.A1	Myocardial infarction type 2
I22.0	Subsequent ST elevation (STEMI) myocardial infarction of anterior wall
I22.1	Subsequent ST elevation (STEMI) myocardial infarction of inferior wall
I22.2	Subsequent non-ST elevation (NSTEMI) myocardial infarction
I22.8	Subsequent ST elevation (STEMI) myocardial infarction of other sites
I25.10	Atherosclerotic heart disease of native coronary artery without angina pectoris
I25.110	Atherosclerotic heart disease of native coronary artery with unstable angina pectoris
I25.710	Atherosclerosis of autologous vein coronary artery bypass graft(s) with unstable angina pectoris
I25.720	Atherosclerosis of autologous artery coronary artery bypass graft(s) with unstable angina pectoris
I25.730	Atherosclerosis of nonautologous biological coronary artery bypass graft(s) with unstable angina pectoris
I25.750	Atherosclerosis of native coronary artery of transplanted heart with unstable angina
I25.760	Atherosclerosis of bypass graft of coronary artery of transplanted heart with unstable angina
I25.790	Atherosclerosis of other coronary artery bypass graft(s) with unstable angina pectoris
I26.01	Septic pulmonary embolism with acute cor pulmonale
I26.02	Saddle embolus of pulmonary artery with acute cor pulmonale
I26.09	Other pulmonary embolism with acute cor pulmonale
I26.90	Septic pulmonary embolism without acute cor pulmonale
I26.92	Saddle embolus of pulmonary artery without acute cor pulmonale
I26.99	Other pulmonary embolism without acute cor pulmonale
I27.0	Primary pulmonary hypertension
I27.21	Secondary pulmonary arterial hypertension
I27.22	Pulmonary hypertension due to left heart disease
I27.23	Pulmonary hypertension due to lung diseases and hypoxia
I27.24	Chronic thromboembolic pulmonary hypertension
I27.29	Other secondary pulmonary hypertension
I27.81	Cor pulmonale (chronic)

I27.82 Chronic pulmonary embolism
I27.83 Eisenmenger's syndrome
I27.89 Other specified pulmonary heart diseases
I31.4 Cardiac tamponade
I34.0 Nonrheumatic mitral (valve) insufficiency
I34.1 Nonrheumatic mitral (valve) prolapse
I34.2 Nonrheumatic mitral (valve) stenosis
I34.8 Other nonrheumatic mitral valve disorders
I35.0 Nonrheumatic aortic (valve) stenosis
I35.1 Nonrheumatic aortic (valve) insufficiency
I35.2 Nonrheumatic aortic (valve) stenosis with insufficiency
I35.8 Other nonrheumatic aortic valve disorders
I36.0 Nonrheumatic tricuspid (valve) stenosis
I36.1 Nonrheumatic tricuspid (valve) insufficiency
I36.2 Nonrheumatic tricuspid (valve) stenosis with insufficiency
I36.8 Other nonrheumatic tricuspid valve disorders
I37.0 Nonrheumatic pulmonary valve stenosis
I37.1 Nonrheumatic pulmonary valve insufficiency
I37.2 Nonrheumatic pulmonary valve stenosis with insufficiency
I37.8 Other nonrheumatic pulmonary valve disorders
I39 Endocarditis and heart valve disorders in diseases classified elsewhere
I40.0 Infective myocarditis
I40.1 Isolated myocarditis
I40.8 Other acute myocarditis
I41 Myocarditis in diseases classified elsewhere
I46.2 Cardiac arrest due to underlying cardiac condition
I46.8 Cardiac arrest due to other underlying condition
I50.1 Left ventricular failure, unspecified
I50.21 Acute systolic (congestive) heart failure
I50.22 Chronic systolic (congestive) heart failure
I50.23 Acute on chronic systolic (congestive) heart failure
I50.31 Acute diastolic (congestive) heart failure
I50.32 Chronic diastolic (congestive) heart failure
I50.33 Acute on chronic diastolic (congestive) heart failure
I50.41 Acute combined systolic (congestive) and diastolic (congestive) heart failure
I50.42 Chronic combined systolic (congestive) and diastolic (congestive) heart failure
I50.43 Acute on chronic combined systolic (congestive) and diastolic (congestive) heart failure
I50.811 Acute right heart failure
I50.812 Chronic right heart failure
I50.813 Acute on chronic right heart failure
I50.814 Right heart failure due to left heart failure
I50.82 Biventricular heart failure
I50.83 High output heart failure
I50.84 End stage heart failure
I97.110 Postprocedural cardiac insufficiency following cardiac surgery
I97.111 Postprocedural cardiac insufficiency following other surgery
I97.120 Postprocedural cardiac arrest following cardiac surgery
I97.121 Postprocedural cardiac arrest following other surgery
I97.130 Postprocedural heart failure following cardiac surgery
I97.131 Postprocedural heart failure following other surgery
I97.190 Other postprocedural cardiac functional disturbances following cardiac surgery
I97.191 Other postprocedural cardiac functional disturbances following other surgery
J81.0 Acute pulmonary edema
J81.1 Chronic pulmonary edema
M32.11 Endocarditis in systemic lupus erythematosus
N17.0 Acute kidney failure with tubular necrosis
N17.1 Acute kidney failure with acute cortical necrosis
N17.2 Acute kidney failure with medullary necrosis
N17.8 Other acute kidney failure
P29.81 Cardiac arrest of newborn
R57.0 Cardiogenic shock
R57.1 Hypovolemic shock
R57.8 Other shock
R65.21 Severe sepsis with septic shock
T86.22 Heart transplant failure
T86.23 Heart transplant infection
T86.31 Heart-lung transplant rejection
T86.32 Heart-lung transplant failure
T86.33 Heart-lung transplant infection
T86.39 Other complications of heart-lung transplant

AMA: 93503 2018,Jan,8; 2018,Feb,11; 2017,Jan,8; 2016,Jan,13; 2015,Jan,16; 2014,Jan,11

Relative Value Units/Medicare Edits

Non-Facility RVU	Work	PE	MP	Total
93503	2.0	0.38	0.17	2.55
Facility RVU	**Work**	**PE**	**MP**	**Total**
93503	2.0	0.38	0.17	2.55

	FUD	Status	MUE	Modifiers				IOM Reference
93503	0	A	2(3)	N/A	N/A	N/A	80*	None

* with documentation

Medicine

93505

93505 Endomyocardial biopsy

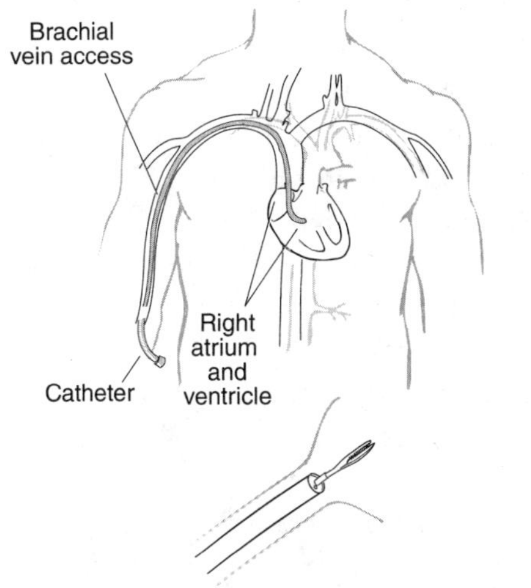

A biopsy tome is inserted through the catheter and several tiny tissue samples are collected from the walls of the heart

Explanation

The physician threads a catheter to the heart through a central intravenous line often inserted up the femoral vein to take tissue samples of the heart's septum.

Coding Tips

When medically necessary, report moderate (conscious) sedation provided by the performing physician with 99151-99153. When provided by another physician report 99155-99157. This code includes all biopsy specimens obtained from one or more endomyocardial sites. Report 76932 in addition to 93505 when ultrasonic guidance is used to obtain the biopsy. For transcatheter placement of a radiation delivery device in coronary intravascular brachytherapy, see 92974. For application of intravascular radioelements, see 77770–77772.

ICD-10-CM Diagnostic Codes

A18.84	Tuberculosis of heart
A52.03	Syphilitic endocarditis
B37.6	Candidal endocarditis
C38.0	Malignant neoplasm of heart
C79.89	Secondary malignant neoplasm of other specified sites
D15.1	Benign neoplasm of heart
D48.7	Neoplasm of uncertain behavior of other specified sites
D49.89	Neoplasm of unspecified behavior of other specified sites
I01.1	Acute rheumatic endocarditis
I25.2	Old myocardial infarction
I25.3	Aneurysm of heart
I33.0	Acute and subacute infective endocarditis
I40.0	Infective myocarditis
I40.1	Isolated myocarditis
I40.8	Other acute myocarditis
I41	Myocarditis in diseases classified elsewhere
I42.0	Dilated cardiomyopathy
I42.1	Obstructive hypertrophic cardiomyopathy
I42.2	Other hypertrophic cardiomyopathy
I42.3	Endomyocardial (eosinophilic) disease
I42.7	Cardiomyopathy due to drug and external agent
I42.8	Other cardiomyopathies
M32.11	Endocarditis in systemic lupus erythematosus
T86.21	Heart transplant rejection
T86.22	Heart transplant failure
T86.31	Heart-lung transplant rejection
T86.32	Heart-lung transplant failure

AMA: 93505 2018,Jan,8; 2018,Feb,11; 2017,Jan,8; 2017,Dec,13; 2016,Jan,13; 2015,Jan,16; 2014,Jan,11

Relative Value Units/Medicare Edits

Non-Facility RVU	Work	PE	MP	Total
93505	4.12	15.01	0.82	19.95
Facility RVU	**Work**	**PE**	**MP**	**Total**
93505	4.12	15.01	0.82	19.95

	FUD	Status	MUE	Modifiers				IOM Reference
93505	0	A	1(2)	51	N/A	N/A	80*	None

* with documentation

Terms To Know

biopsy. Tissue or fluid removed for diagnostic purposes through analysis of the cells in the biopsy material.

catheterization. Use or insertion of a tubular device into a duct, blood vessel, hollow organ, or body cavity for injecting or withdrawing fluids for diagnostic or therapeutic purposes.

diagnostic procedures. Procedure performed on a patient to obtain information to assess the medical condition of the patient or to identify a disease and to determine the nature and severity of an illness or injury.

fluoroscopy. Radiology technique that allows visual examination of part of the body or a function of an organ using a device that projects an x-ray image on a fluorescent screen.

intravascular. Within a blood vessel.

moderate sedation. Medically controlled state of depressed consciousness, with or without analgesia, while maintaining the patient's airway, protective reflexes, and ability to respond to stimulation or verbal commands.

septum. Anatomical partition or dividing wall.

ultrasound. Imaging using ultra-high sound frequency bounced off body structures.

 ● New ▲ Revised + Add On AMA: CPT Assist [Resequenced] ☑ Laterality

93530

93530 Right heart catheterization, for congenital cardiac anomalies

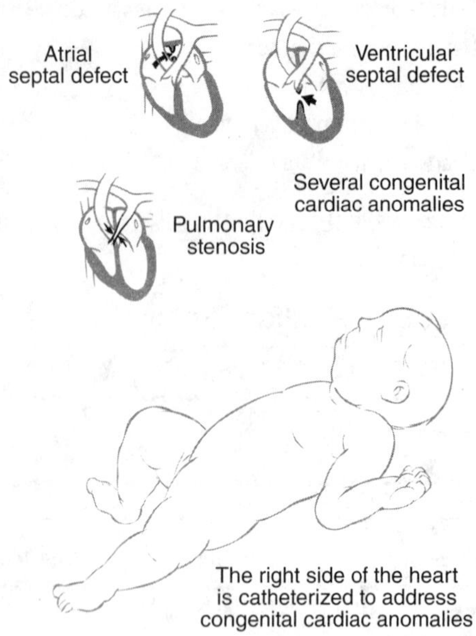

Explanation

The physician performs a right heart catheterization for congenital cardiac anomalies. The physician investigates congenital cardiac anomalies by measuring pressures, taking blood samples for oximetry, and/or injecting contrast to assess chamber size and function. The physician places an introducer sheath in a vein (typically, the femoral vein) using percutaneous puncture. The physician places a lumen catheter through the introducer sheath into the femoral vein and advances it, under fluoroscopic guidance, to the heart chamber receiving venous circulation. The physician may use the fluid filled catheter to record intracardiac pressures, withdraw blood samples, or inject radiopaque contrast material. The physician removes the catheter and sheath from the femoral vein. Pressure is placed on the wound for 20 to 30 minutes to stem bleeding.

Coding Tips

When medically necessary, report moderate (conscious) sedation provided by the performing physician with 99151-99153. When provided by another physician, report 99155-99157. Contrast injections are reported separately, see 93563–93568. Do not report 93530 with 33289. Code 93530 may be reported in addition to 33274 and 33275 only if the catheterization is performed for reasons distinct from the leadless pacemaker procedure.

ICD-10-CM Diagnostic Codes

Q20.0	Common arterial trunk
Q20.1	Double outlet right ventricle
Q20.2	Double outlet left ventricle
Q20.3	Discordant ventriculoarterial connection
Q20.4	Double inlet ventricle
Q20.5	Discordant atrioventricular connection
Q20.8	Other congenital malformations of cardiac chambers and connections
Q21.0	Ventricular septal defect
Q21.1	Atrial septal defect
Q21.3	Tetralogy of Fallot
Q23.3	Congenital mitral insufficiency
Q23.4	Hypoplastic left heart syndrome
Q23.8	Other congenital malformations of aortic and mitral valves
Q24.0	Dextrocardia
Q24.1	Levocardia
Q24.2	Cor triatriatum
Q24.3	Pulmonary infundibular stenosis
Q24.4	Congenital subaortic stenosis
Q24.5	Malformation of coronary vessels
Q24.6	Congenital heart block
Q24.8	Other specified congenital malformations of heart
Q25.0	Patent ductus arteriosus
Q25.1	Coarctation of aorta
Q25.21	Interruption of aortic arch
Q25.29	Other atresia of aorta
Q25.3	Supravalvular aortic stenosis
Q25.41	Absence and aplasia of aorta
Q25.42	Hypoplasia of aorta
Q25.43	Congenital aneurysm of aorta
Q25.44	Congenital dilation of aorta
Q25.45	Double aortic arch
Q25.46	Tortuous aortic arch
Q25.47	Right aortic arch
Q25.48	Anomalous origin of subclavian artery
Q25.49	Other congenital malformations of aorta
Q25.5	Atresia of pulmonary artery
Q25.6	Stenosis of pulmonary artery
Q25.71	Coarctation of pulmonary artery
Q25.72	Congenital pulmonary arteriovenous malformation
Q25.79	Other congenital malformations of pulmonary artery

AMA: 93530 2019,Mar,6; 2019,Jun,3; 2018,Jan,8; 2018,Feb,11; 2017,Jul,3; 2017,Jan,8; 2016,Mar,5; 2016,Jan,13; 2015,Sep,3; 2015,Jan,16; 2014,Jul,3; 2014,Jan,11; 2013,May,12

Relative Value Units/Medicare Edits

Non-Facility RVU	Work	PE	MP	Total
93530	0.0	0.0	0.0	0.0
Facility RVU	**Work**	**PE**	**MP**	**Total**
93530	0.0	0.0	0.0	0.0

	FUD	Status	MUE	Modifiers				IOM Reference
93530	0	C	1(3)	51	N/A	N/A	80*	None

* with documentation

Terms To Know

anomaly. Irregularity in the structure or position of an organ or tissue.

atresia. Congenital closure or absence of a tubular organ or an opening to the body surface.

sheath. Covering enclosing an organ or part.

93531

93531 Combined right heart catheterization and retrograde left heart catheterization, for congenital cardiac anomalies

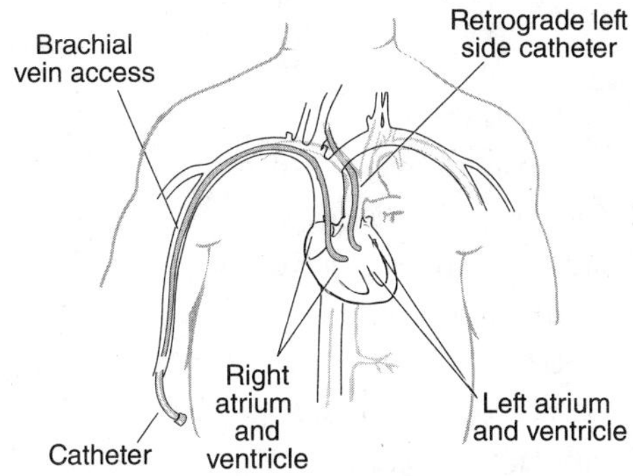

A combined right side catheterization and retrograde left side catheterization is performed to address congenital cardiac anomalies

Explanation

The physician performs combined right heart catheterization and retrograde left heart catheterization to investigate congenital cardiac anomalies. The physician places an introducer sheath in a vein (typically, the femoral vein) using percutaneous puncture. The physician places a lumen catheter through the introducer sheath into the femoral vein and advances it, under fluoroscopic guidance, to the heart chamber receiving venous circulation. The physician places an introducer sheath in an artery (typically, the femoral artery) using percutaneous puncture. The physician places a lumen catheter through the introducer sheath into the femoral artery and advances it, under fluoroscopic guidance, through the aorta to the heart chamber providing arterial circulation. The physician may use the fluid filled catheters to record intracardiac pressures, withdraw blood samples, or inject radiopaque contrast material. The physician removes the catheters and sheaths from the femoral vessels. Pressure is placed on the wound for 20 to 30 minutes to stem bleeding.

Coding Tips

Contrast injections are reported separately, see 93563–93568. Do not report 93531 with 33289. Code 93531 may be reported in addition to 33274 and 33275 only if the catheterization is performed for reasons distinct from the leadless pacemaker procedure.

ICD-10-CM Diagnostic Codes

Q20.0	Common arterial trunk
Q20.1	Double outlet right ventricle
Q20.2	Double outlet left ventricle
Q20.3	Discordant ventriculoarterial connection
Q20.4	Double inlet ventricle
Q20.5	Discordant atrioventricular connection
Q20.8	Other congenital malformations of cardiac chambers and connections
Q21.0	Ventricular septal defect
Q21.1	Atrial septal defect
Q21.3	Tetralogy of Fallot
Q23.3	Congenital mitral insufficiency
Q23.4	Hypoplastic left heart syndrome
Q23.8	Other congenital malformations of aortic and mitral valves
Q24.0	Dextrocardia
Q24.1	Levocardia
Q24.2	Cor triatriatum
Q24.3	Pulmonary infundibular stenosis
Q24.4	Congenital subaortic stenosis
Q24.5	Malformation of coronary vessels
Q24.6	Congenital heart block
Q24.8	Other specified congenital malformations of heart
Q25.0	Patent ductus arteriosus
Q25.1	Coarctation of aorta
Q25.21	Interruption of aortic arch
Q25.29	Other atresia of aorta
Q25.3	Supravalvular aortic stenosis
Q25.41	Absence and aplasia of aorta
Q25.42	Hypoplasia of aorta
Q25.43	Congenital aneurysm of aorta
Q25.44	Congenital dilation of aorta
Q25.45	Double aortic arch
Q25.46	Tortuous aortic arch
Q25.47	Right aortic arch
Q25.48	Anomalous origin of subclavian artery
Q25.49	Other congenital malformations of aorta
Q25.5	Atresia of pulmonary artery
Q25.6	Stenosis of pulmonary artery
Q25.71	Coarctation of pulmonary artery
Q25.72	Congenital pulmonary arteriovenous malformation
Q25.79	Other congenital malformations of pulmonary artery

AMA: 93531 2019,Mar,6; 2019,Jun,3; 2018,Jan,8; 2018,Feb,11; 2017,Jul,3; 2017,Jan,8; 2016,Mar,5; 2016,Jan,13; 2015,Sep,3; 2015,Jan,16; 2014,Jul,3; 2014,Jan,11

Relative Value Units/Medicare Edits

Non-Facility RVU	Work	PE	MP	Total
93531	0.0	0.0	0.0	0.0
Facility RVU	**Work**	**PE**	**MP**	**Total**
93531	0.0	0.0	0.0	0.0

	FUD	Status	MUE	Modifiers				IOM Reference
93531	0	C	1(3)	51	N/A	N/A	80*	None

* with documentation

Terms To Know

atresia. Congenital closure or absence of a tubular organ or an opening to the body surface.

fluoroscopy. Radiology technique that allows visual examination of part of the body or a function of an organ using a device that projects an x-ray image on a fluorescent screen.

radiopaque dye. Medium injected into the body that is impenetrable by x-rays.

93532

93532 Combined right heart catheterization and transseptal left heart catheterization through intact septum with or without retrograde left heart catheterization, for congenital cardiac anomalies

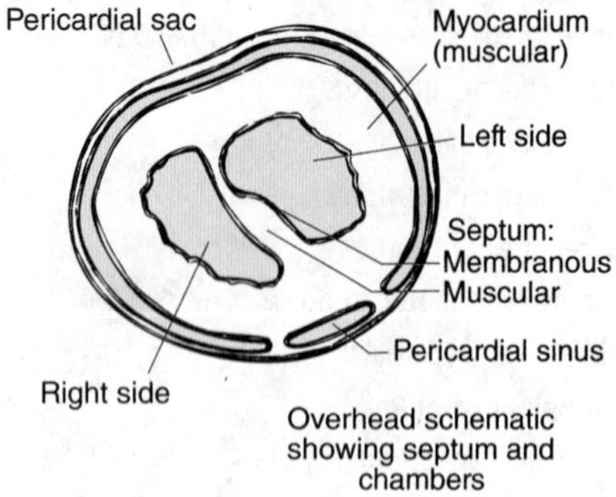

The septum of the heart is muscular and contains natural passages between the chambers, such as the foramen ovale, or anomalous passages that occur as defects

Explanation

The purpose of this procedure is to investigate congenital cardiac anomalies by measuring pressures, taking blood samples for oximetry, and/or injecting contrast to assess chamber size and function. The physician places an introducer sheath in a vein (typically, the femoral vein) using percutaneous puncture. The physician places a lumen catheter through the introducer sheath into the femoral vein and advances it, under fluoroscopic guidance, to the heart chamber receiving venous circulation. The physician exchanges this catheter over a wire for a transseptal puncture needle, dilator, and sheath. The physician advances the transseptal puncture apparatus to the right atrium and punctures the intraatrial septum with the needle. The physician advances the needle, dilator, and transseptal sheath into the left atrium. The physician may also perform retrograde left heart catheterization as follows. The physician places an introducer sheath and lumen catheter in an artery (typically, the femoral artery) using percutaneous puncture. The physician advances the lumen catheter, under fluoroscopic guidance, through the aorta to the heart chamber providing arterial circulation. The physician may use the fluid filled catheters to record intracardiac pressures, withdraw blood samples, or inject radiopaque contrast material. The physician removes the catheters and sheaths from the femoral vessels. Pressure is placed on the wound for 20 to 30 minutes to stem bleeding.

Coding Tips

Contrast injections are reported separately, see 93563–93568. Do not report 93532 with 33289. Code 93532 may be reported in addition to 33274 and 33275 only if the catheterization is performed for reasons distinct from the leadless pacemaker procedure.

ICD-10-CM Diagnostic Codes

Q20.0 Common arterial trunk
Q20.1 Double outlet right ventricle
Q20.2 Double outlet left ventricle
Q20.3 Discordant ventriculoarterial connection
Q20.4 Double inlet ventricle
Q20.5 Discordant atrioventricular connection
Q20.8 Other congenital malformations of cardiac chambers and connections
Q21.0 Ventricular septal defect
Q21.1 Atrial septal defect
Q21.3 Tetralogy of Fallot
Q23.3 Congenital mitral insufficiency
Q23.4 Hypoplastic left heart syndrome
Q23.8 Other congenital malformations of aortic and mitral valves
Q24.0 Dextrocardia
Q24.1 Levocardia
Q24.2 Cor triatriatum
Q24.3 Pulmonary infundibular stenosis
Q24.4 Congenital subaortic stenosis
Q24.5 Malformation of coronary vessels
Q24.6 Congenital heart block
Q24.8 Other specified congenital malformations of heart
Q25.0 Patent ductus arteriosus
Q25.1 Coarctation of aorta
Q25.21 Interruption of aortic arch
Q25.29 Other atresia of aorta
Q25.3 Supravalvular aortic stenosis
Q25.41 Absence and aplasia of aorta
Q25.42 Hypoplasia of aorta
Q25.43 Congenital aneurysm of aorta
Q25.44 Congenital dilation of aorta
Q25.45 Double aortic arch
Q25.46 Tortuous aortic arch
Q25.47 Right aortic arch
Q25.48 Anomalous origin of subclavian artery
Q25.49 Other congenital malformations of aorta
Q25.5 Atresia of pulmonary artery
Q25.6 Stenosis of pulmonary artery
Q25.71 Coarctation of pulmonary artery
Q25.72 Congenital pulmonary arteriovenous malformation
Q25.79 Other congenital malformations of pulmonary artery

AMA: 93532 2019,Mar,6; 2019,Jun,3; 2018,Jan,8; 2018,Feb,11; 2017,Jul,3; 2017,Jan,8; 2016,Mar,5; 2016,Jan,13; 2015,Sep,3; 2015,Jan,16; 2014,Jul,3; 2014,Jan,11

Relative Value Units/Medicare Edits

Non-Facility RVU	Work	PE	MP	Total
93532	0.0	0.0	0.0	0.0
Facility RVU	**Work**	**PE**	**MP**	**Total**
93532	0.0	0.0	0.0	0.0

	FUD	Status	MUE	Modifiers				IOM Reference
93532	0	C	1(3)	51	N/A	N/A	80*	None

* with documentation

93533

93533 Combined right heart catheterization and transseptal left heart catheterization through existing septal opening, with or without retrograde left heart catheterization, for congenital cardiac anomalies

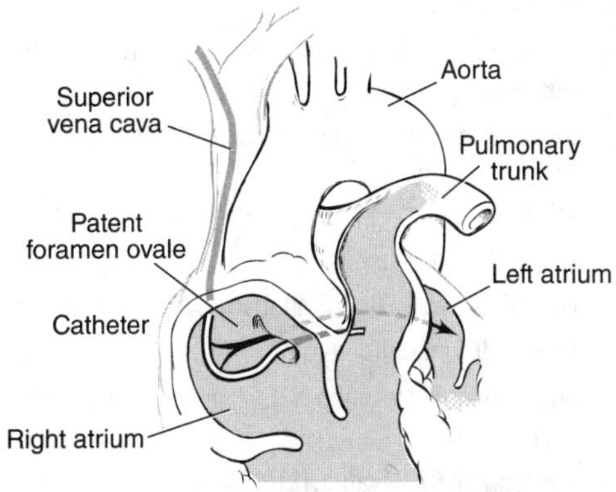

The septum of the heart is muscular and contains natural passages between the chambers, such as the foramen ovale, or anomalous passages that occur as defects

Explanation

The purpose of this procedure is to investigate congenital cardiac anomalies by measuring pressures, taking blood samples for oximetry, and/or injecting contrast to assess chamber size and function. The physician places an introducer sheath in a vein (typically, the femoral vein) using percutaneous puncture. The physician places a lumen catheter through the introducer sheath into the femoral vein and advances it, under fluoroscopic guidance, to the heart chamber receiving venous circulation. The physician directs this catheter through an existing septal opening into the left atrium. The physician may also perform retrograde left heart catheterization as follows. The physician places an introducer sheath and lumen catheter in an artery (typically, the femoral artery) using percutaneous puncture. The physician advances the lumen catheter, under fluoroscopic guidance, through the aorta to the heart chamber providing arterial circulation. The physician may use the fluid filled catheters to record intracardiac pressures, withdraw blood samples, or inject radiopaque contrast material. The physician removes the catheters and sheaths from the femoral vessels. Pressure is placed on the wound for 20 to 30 minutes to stem bleeding.

Coding Tips

Contrast injections are reported separately, see 93563–93568. Do not report 93533 with 33289. Code 93533 may be reported in addition to 33274 and 33275 only if the catheterization is performed for reasons distinct from the leadless pacemaker procedure.

ICD-10-CM Diagnostic Codes

Q20.0	Common arterial trunk
Q20.1	Double outlet right ventricle
Q20.2	Double outlet left ventricle
Q20.3	Discordant ventriculoarterial connection
Q20.4	Double inlet ventricle
Q20.5	Discordant atrioventricular connection
Q20.8	Other congenital malformations of cardiac chambers and connections
Q21.0	Ventricular septal defect
Q21.1	Atrial septal defect
Q21.3	Tetralogy of Fallot
Q23.3	Congenital mitral insufficiency
Q23.4	Hypoplastic left heart syndrome
Q23.8	Other congenital malformations of aortic and mitral valves
Q24.0	Dextrocardia
Q24.1	Levocardia
Q24.2	Cor triatriatum
Q24.3	Pulmonary infundibular stenosis
Q24.4	Congenital subaortic stenosis
Q24.5	Malformation of coronary vessels
Q24.6	Congenital heart block
Q24.8	Other specified congenital malformations of heart
Q25.0	Patent ductus arteriosus
Q25.1	Coarctation of aorta
Q25.21	Interruption of aortic arch
Q25.29	Other atresia of aorta
Q25.3	Supravalvular aortic stenosis
Q25.41	Absence and aplasia of aorta
Q25.42	Hypoplasia of aorta
Q25.43	Congenital aneurysm of aorta
Q25.44	Congenital dilation of aorta
Q25.45	Double aortic arch
Q25.46	Tortuous aortic arch
Q25.47	Right aortic arch
Q25.48	Anomalous origin of subclavian artery
Q25.49	Other congenital malformations of aorta
Q25.5	Atresia of pulmonary artery
Q25.6	Stenosis of pulmonary artery
Q25.71	Coarctation of pulmonary artery
Q25.72	Congenital pulmonary arteriovenous malformation
Q25.79	Other congenital malformations of pulmonary artery

AMA: 93533 2019,Mar,6; 2019,Jun,3; 2018,Jan,8; 2018,Feb,11; 2017,Jul,3; 2017,Jan,8; 2016,Mar,5; 2016,Jan,13; 2015,Sep,3; 2015,Jan,16; 2014,Jul,3; 2014,Jan,11

Relative Value Units/Medicare Edits

Non-Facility RVU	Work	PE	MP	Total
93533	0.0	0.0	0.0	0.0
Facility RVU	**Work**	**PE**	**MP**	**Total**
93533	0.0	0.0	0.0	0.0

	FUD	Status	MUE	Modifiers				IOM Reference
93533	0	C	1(3)	51	N/A	N/A	80*	None

* with documentation

Terms To Know

tetralogy of Fallot. Specific combination of congenital cardiac defects: obstruction of the right ventricular outflow tract with pulmonary stenosis, interventricular septal defect, malposition of the aorta, overriding the interventricular septum and receiving blood from both the venous and arterial systems, and enlargement of the right ventricle.

93561-93562

93561 Indicator dilution studies such as dye or thermodilution, including arterial and/or venous catheterization; with cardiac output measurement (separate procedure)

93562 subsequent measurement of cardiac output

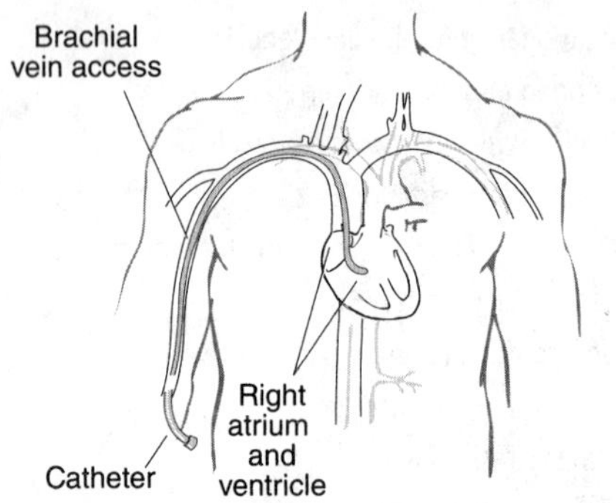

The physician threads a catheter through a central line leading to the heart and performs indicator dilution studies

Explanation

Indicator dilution studies use a technique based on the principle that the volume of a fluid within a container can be determined by adding a known quantity of an indicator to the fluid and measuring the concentration of the indicator after it has completely mixed with the fluid. A time-concentration curve arises and the area of the inscribed curve is calculated. The physician threads a catheter through a central line leading to the heart and dye, such as nontoxic, water-soluble indocyanine green, or a thermal indicator, usually iced saline, is injected. In the thermodilution method, cardiac output is measured by a computer using an equation that incorporates body temperature, injection volume and temperature, time, and other calculated ratios over a denominator of the integral of the change in blood temperature during the cold injection, reflected by the area of the inscribed curve. Report 93562 if a subsequent cardiac output measurement is taken.

Coding Tips

When medically necessary, report moderate (conscious) sedation provided by the performing physician with 99151-99153. When provided by another physician, report 99155-99157. Do not report 93561 and 93562 with cardiac catheterization codes 93451–93462 or 93582 for closure of patent ductus arteriosus. For radioisotope method of cardiac output, see 78472, 78473, or 78481.

ICD-10-CM Diagnostic Codes

I05.0	Rheumatic mitral stenosis
I05.1	Rheumatic mitral insufficiency
I06.0	Rheumatic aortic stenosis
I06.1	Rheumatic aortic insufficiency
I07.0	Rheumatic tricuspid stenosis
I07.1	Rheumatic tricuspid insufficiency
I09.81	Rheumatic heart failure
I11.0	Hypertensive heart disease with heart failure
I13.0	Hypertensive heart and chronic kidney disease with heart failure and stage 1 through stage 4 chronic kidney disease, or unspecified chronic kidney disease
I13.2	Hypertensive heart and chronic kidney disease with heart failure and with stage 5 chronic kidney disease, or end stage renal disease
I16.0	Hypertensive urgency
I16.1	Hypertensive emergency
I21.01	ST elevation (STEMI) myocardial infarction involving left main coronary artery
I21.02	ST elevation (STEMI) myocardial infarction involving left anterior descending coronary artery
I21.11	ST elevation (STEMI) myocardial infarction involving right coronary artery
I21.21	ST elevation (STEMI) myocardial infarction involving left circumflex coronary artery
I21.4	Non-ST elevation (NSTEMI) myocardial infarction
I21.A1	Myocardial infarction type 2
I22.0	Subsequent ST elevation (STEMI) myocardial infarction of anterior wall
I22.1	Subsequent ST elevation (STEMI) myocardial infarction of inferior wall
I22.2	Subsequent non-ST elevation (NSTEMI) myocardial infarction
I23.1	Atrial septal defect as current complication following acute myocardial infarction
I23.2	Ventricular septal defect as current complication following acute myocardial infarction
I25.5	Ischemic cardiomyopathy
I26.01	Septic pulmonary embolism with acute cor pulmonale
I26.02	Saddle embolus of pulmonary artery with acute cor pulmonale
I26.90	Septic pulmonary embolism without acute cor pulmonale
I30.0	Acute nonspecific idiopathic pericarditis
I30.1	Infective pericarditis
I31.0	Chronic adhesive pericarditis
I31.1	Chronic constrictive pericarditis
I31.3	Pericardial effusion (noninflammatory)
I31.4	Cardiac tamponade
I33.0	Acute and subacute infective endocarditis
I34.0	Nonrheumatic mitral (valve) insufficiency
I34.1	Nonrheumatic mitral (valve) prolapse
I34.2	Nonrheumatic mitral (valve) stenosis
I35.0	Nonrheumatic aortic (valve) stenosis
I35.1	Nonrheumatic aortic (valve) insufficiency
I36.0	Nonrheumatic tricuspid (valve) stenosis
I36.1	Nonrheumatic tricuspid (valve) insufficiency
I37.0	Nonrheumatic pulmonary valve stenosis
I37.1	Nonrheumatic pulmonary valve insufficiency
I40.0	Infective myocarditis
I40.1	Isolated myocarditis
I42.0	Dilated cardiomyopathy
I42.1	Obstructive hypertrophic cardiomyopathy
I42.3	Endomyocardial (eosinophilic) disease
I42.4	Endocardial fibroelastosis
I42.6	Alcoholic cardiomyopathy
I50.23	Acute on chronic systolic (congestive) heart failure
I50.33	Acute on chronic diastolic (congestive) heart failure

I50.43	Acute on chronic combined systolic (congestive) and diastolic (congestive) heart failure
I51.0	Cardiac septal defect, acquired
I51.7	Cardiomegaly
I97.110	Postprocedural cardiac insufficiency following cardiac surgery
I97.111	Postprocedural cardiac insufficiency following other surgery
I97.130	Postprocedural heart failure following cardiac surgery
I97.131	Postprocedural heart failure following other surgery
M32.11	Endocarditis in systemic lupus erythematosus
M32.12	Pericarditis in systemic lupus erythematosus
Q20.0	Common arterial trunk
Q20.1	Double outlet right ventricle
Q20.2	Double outlet left ventricle
Q20.3	Discordant ventriculoarterial connection
Q20.4	Double inlet ventricle
Q20.5	Discordant atrioventricular connection
Q20.6	Isomerism of atrial appendages
Q21.0	Ventricular septal defect
Q21.1	Atrial septal defect
Q21.3	Tetralogy of Fallot
Q21.4	Aortopulmonary septal defect
Q23.2	Congenital mitral stenosis
Q23.3	Congenital mitral insufficiency
Q23.4	Hypoplastic left heart syndrome
Q24.2	Cor triatriatum
Q24.4	Congenital subaortic stenosis
Q25.0	Patent ductus arteriosus
Q25.1	Coarctation of aorta
Q25.21	Interruption of aortic arch
Q25.41	Absence and aplasia of aorta
Q25.42	Hypoplasia of aorta
Q25.43	Congenital aneurysm of aorta
Q25.44	Congenital dilation of aorta
Q25.45	Double aortic arch
Q25.46	Tortuous aortic arch
Q25.47	Right aortic arch
Q25.48	Anomalous origin of subclavian artery
Q25.5	Atresia of pulmonary artery
Q25.6	Stenosis of pulmonary artery
Q25.71	Coarctation of pulmonary artery
Q25.72	Congenital pulmonary arteriovenous malformation
Q26.1	Persistent left superior vena cava
Q26.2	Total anomalous pulmonary venous connection
Q26.3	Partial anomalous pulmonary venous connection
Q26.5	Anomalous portal venous connection
Q26.6	Portal vein-hepatic artery fistula
R57.0	Cardiogenic shock
R57.1	Hypovolemic shock

AMA: 93561 2019,Aug,8; 2018,Jan,8; 2018,Feb,11; 2017,Jan,8; 2016,Jan,13; 2015,Jan,16; 2014,Jul,3; 2014,Jan,11 **93562** 2019,Aug,8; 2018,Jan,8; 2018,Feb,11; 2017,Jan,8; 2016,Jan,13; 2015,Jan,16; 2014,May,4; 2014,Jul,3; 2014,Jan,11

Relative Value Units/Medicare Edits

Non-Facility RVU	Work	PE	MP	Total
93561	0.0	0.0	0.0	0.0
93562	0.0	0.0	0.0	0.0
Facility RVU	**Work**	**PE**	**MP**	**Total**
93561	0.0	0.0	0.0	0.0
93562	0.0	0.0	0.0	0.0

	FUD	Status	MUE	Modifiers				IOM Reference
93561	N/A	C	1(3)	N/A	N/A	N/A	80*	None
93562	N/A	C	1(3)	N/A	N/A	N/A	80*	

* with documentation

Terms To Know

anesthesia. Loss of feeling or sensation, usually induced to permit the performance of surgery or other painful procedures.

cardiac output. Measurement of the volume of blood ejected by the heart ventricle that is usually measured by a catheter with an opening in the right atrium and pulmonary artery.

catheterization. Use or insertion of a tubular device into a duct, blood vessel, hollow organ, or body cavity for injecting or withdrawing fluids for diagnostic or therapeutic purposes.

central venous catheter. Catheter positioned in the superior vena cava or right atrium and introduced through a large vein, such as the jugular or subclavian, and used to measure venous pressure or administer fluids or medication.

dilution. Concentration reduction of a mixture or solution by adding more fluid.

moderate sedation. Medically controlled state of depressed consciousness, with or without analgesia, while maintaining the patient's airway, protective reflexes, and ability to respond to stimulation or verbal commands.

venous. Relating to the veins.

93563

+ 93563 Injection procedure during cardiac catheterization including imaging supervision, interpretation, and report; for selective coronary angiography during congenital heart catheterization (List separately in addition to code for primary procedure)

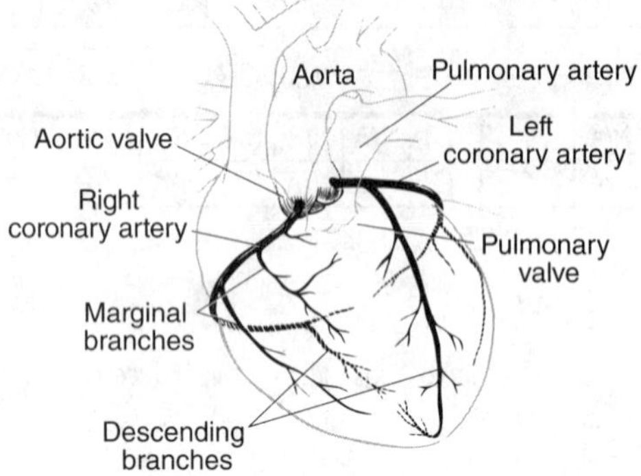

The coronary vessels visualized

Explanation

The physician injects dye into the coronary arteries to evaluate function during congenital heart catheterization procedures. Any required repositioning of catheters or use of automatic power injectors is included in this procedure, as is imaging supervision, interpretation, and report.

Coding Tips

When medically necessary, report moderate (conscious) sedation provided by the performing physician with 99151-99153. When provided by another physician, report 99155-99157. Report 93563 in addition to 93530–93533. This procedure includes any radiological supervision, interpretation, and report. Contrast administration performed during cardiac catheterization for congenital conditions is reported separately with 93563–93568. Injection procedures for right ventricular, right atrial, aortic, or pulmonary angiogram performed with cardiac catheterizations are reported separately with 93566–93568. Report 93567 for supravalvular ascending aortogram done at the same session as cardiac catheterization. Report 93568 with right heart catheterization codes when done at the same session as a pulmonary angiogram. Injection procedures do not include catheter placement when applicable; however, repositioning of the catheter and automatic power injections should not be reported separately. Do not report 93563–93565 with 93452–93461. Do not report 93563 with 33418, 0345T, 0483T, 0484T, 0544T, or 0545T for coronary angiography intrinsic to the valve repair or annulus reconstruction.

ICD-10-CM Diagnostic Codes

This/these CPT code(s) are add on code(s). See the primary procedure code that this code is performed with for your ICD-10-CM code selections.

AMA: **93563** 2018,Jan,8; 2018,Feb,11; 2017,Jan,8; 2016,Mar,5; 2016,Jan,13; 2015,Jan,16; 2014,Jan,11; 2014,Dec,6; 2013,Jan,6-8

Relative Value Units/Medicare Edits

Non-Facility RVU	Work	PE	MP	Total
93563	1.11	0.38	0.2	1.69
Facility RVU	**Work**	**PE**	**MP**	**Total**
93563	1.11	0.38	0.2	1.69

	FUD	Status	MUE	Modifiers				IOM Reference
93563	N/A	A	1(3)	N/A	N/A	N/A	80*	None

* with documentation

Terms To Know

aortography. Radiographic visualization of the aorta and its branches by injecting contrast medium through percutaneous puncture or catheterization technique.

catheterization. Use or insertion of a tubular device into a duct, blood vessel, hollow organ, or body cavity for injecting or withdrawing fluids for diagnostic or therapeutic purposes.

congenital anomaly. Abnormality that is present at birth that may be the result of genetic factors, teratogens, or other conditions that affect the fetus in utero. The abnormalities may be readily apparent at birth or may remain undiscovered until some point after birth.

contrast material. Any internally administered substance that has a different opacity from soft tissue on radiography or computed tomograph; includes barium, used to opacify parts of the gastrointestinal tract; water-soluble iodinated compounds, used to opacify blood vessels or the genitourinary tract; may refer to air occurring naturally or introduced into the body; also, paramagnetic substances used in magnetic resonance imaging. Substances may also be documented as contrast agent or contrast medium.

supervision and interpretation. Radiology services that usually contain an invasive component and are reported by the radiologist for supervision of the procedure and the personnel involved with performing the examination, reading the film, and preparing the written report.

93564

\+ **93564** Injection procedure during cardiac catheterization including imaging supervision, interpretation, and report; for selective opacification of aortocoronary venous or arterial bypass graft(s) (eg, aortocoronary saphenous vein, free radial artery, or free mammary artery graft) to one or more coronary arteries and in situ arterial conduits (eg, internal mammary), whether native or used for bypass to one or more coronary arteries during congenital heart catheterization, when performed (List separately in addition to code for primary procedure)

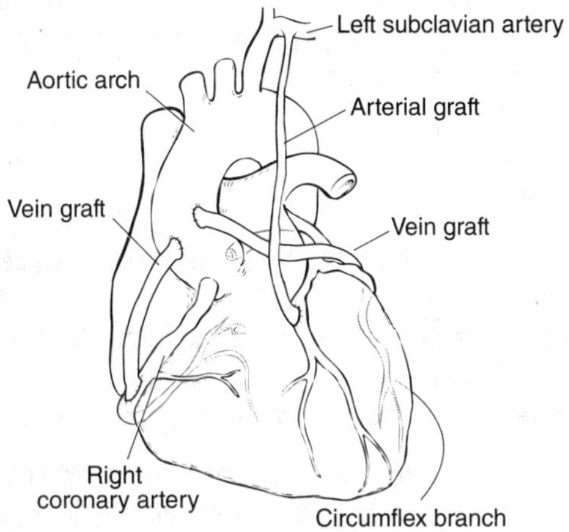

Explanation

The physician injects dye into the coronary arteries to evaluate function during congenital heart catheterization procedures. This code is used when the physician chooses to visualize a specific aortocoronary vessel bypass graft that communicates with other coronary arteries or conduits. Any required repositioning of catheters or use of automatic power injectors is included in this procedure, as is imaging supervision, interpretation, and report.

Coding Tips

When medically necessary, report moderate (conscious) sedation provided by the performing physician with 99151-99153. When provided by another physician, report 99155-99157. Report 93564 in addition to 93530–93533. This procedure includes any radiological supervision, interpretation, and report. Contrast administration performed during cardiac catheterization for congenital conditions is reported separately with 93563–93568. Report 93567 for supravalvular ascending aortogram done at the same session as cardiac catheterization. Injection procedures do not include catheter placement when applicable; however, repositioning of the catheter and automatic power injections should not be reported separately. Do not report 93564 with 93452–93461. Do not report 93564 with 33418, 0345T, 0483T, 0484T, 0544T, or 0545T for coronary angiography intrinsic to the valve repair or annulus reconstruction.

ICD-10-CM Diagnostic Codes

This/these CPT code(s) are add on code(s). See the primary procedure code that this code is performed with for your ICD-10-CM code selections.

AMA: 93564 2018,Jan,8; 2018,Feb,11; 2017,Jan,8; 2016,Mar,5; 2016,Jan,13; 2015,Jan,16; 2014,Jan,11; 2014,Dec,6; 2013,Jan,6-8

Relative Value Units/Medicare Edits

Non-Facility RVU	Work	PE	MP	Total
93564	1.13	0.39	0.27	1.79
Facility RVU	**Work**	**PE**	**MP**	**Total**
93564	1.13	0.39	0.27	1.79

	FUD	Status	MUE	Modifiers				IOM Reference
93564	N/A	A	1(3)	N/A	N/A	N/A	80*	None

* with documentation

Terms To Know

aortography. Radiographic visualization of the aorta and its branches by injecting contrast medium through percutaneous puncture or catheterization technique.

bypass graft. Surgically created alternative blood vessel used to reroute blood flow around an area of obstruction or disease.

catheter. Flexible tube inserted into an area of the body for introducing or withdrawing fluid.

conduit. Surgically created channel for the passage of fluids.

in situ. Located in the natural position or contained within the origin site, not spread into neighboring tissue.

injection. Forcing a liquid substance into a body part such as a joint or muscle.

instillation. Administering a liquid slowly over time, drop by drop.

supervision and interpretation. Radiology services that usually contain an invasive component and are reported by the radiologist for supervision of the procedure and the personnel involved with performing the examination, reading the film, and preparing the written report.

Medicine

93565-93566

+ **93565** Injection procedure during cardiac catheterization including imaging supervision, interpretation, and report; for selective left ventricular or left atrial angiography (List separately in addition to code for primary procedure)
+ **93566** for selective right ventricular or right atrial angiography (List separately in addition to code for primary procedure)

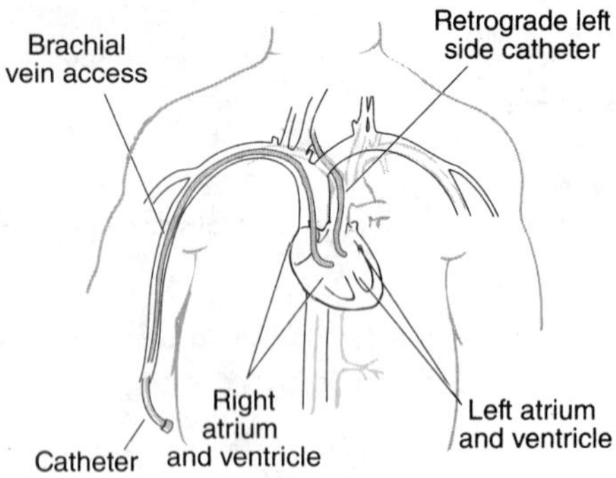

Catheters are placed into the right or left side of the heart

Explanation

The physician injects dye into the coronary arteries to evaluate function during heart catheterization procedures. Code 93565 is specific to the visualization of the left atrium or ventricle during catheterization procedures for congenital anomalies, while 93566 reports that associated with the right atrium or ventricle and may be associated with catheterization procedures for congenital or noncongenital indications. These codes do not report the introduction of catheters, but do include any required repositioning of catheters or use of automatic power injectors, as well as radiological supervision, interpretation, and report.

Coding Tips

When medically necessary, report moderate (conscious) sedation provided by the performing physician with 99151-99153. When provided by another physician, report 99155-99157. Report 93565 in addition to 93530–93533. Report 93566 in addition to 93530–93533 and 93451–93461. These procedures include any radiological supervision, interpretation, and report. Contrast administration performed during cardiac catheterization for congenital conditions is reported separately with 93563–93568. Injection procedures for right ventricular, right atrial, aortic, or pulmonary angiogram performed with cardiac catheterizations are reported separately with 93566–93568. For right ventricular or right atrial angiogram performed during the same session as a cardiac catheterization, report 93566 in addition to the applicable catheterization codes: 93451, 93453, 93456, 93457, 93460, or 93461. Injection procedures do not include catheter placement when applicable; however, repositioning of the catheter and automatic power injections should not be reported separately. Do not report 93565 with 93452–93461. Do not report 93566 with 33274 or 33275 for right ventriculography performed with leadless pacemaker insertion or removal. Do not report 93566 with 0545T for right ventricular or right atrial angiography intrinsic to annulus reconstruction.

ICD-10-CM Diagnostic Codes

This/these CPT code(s) are add on code(s). See the primary procedure code that this code is performed with for your ICD-10-CM code selections. Diagnostic code(s) would be the same as the actual procedure performed.

AMA: **93565** 2018,Jan,8; 2018,Feb,11; 2017,Jan,8; 2016,Jan,13; 2015,Jan,16; 2014,Jan,11; 2013,Jan,6-8 **93566** 2019,Mar,6; 2018,Jan,8; 2018,Feb,11; 2017,Jan,8; 2016,May,5; 2016,Mar,5; 2016,Jan,13; 2016,Aug,5; 2015,May,3; 2015,Jan,16; 2014,Jan,11; 2013,Jan,6-8

Relative Value Units/Medicare Edits

Non-Facility RVU	Work	PE	MP	Total
93565	0.86	0.3	0.15	1.31
93566	0.86	3.33	0.19	4.38
Facility RVU	**Work**	**PE**	**MP**	**Total**
93565	0.86	0.3	0.15	1.31
93566	0.86	0.3	0.19	1.35

	FUD	Status	MUE	Modifiers				IOM Reference
93565	N/A	A	1(3)	N/A	N/A	N/A	80*	None
93566	N/A	A	1(3)	N/A	N/A	N/A	80*	

* with documentation

Terms To Know

angiogram. Radiographic image of the arteries. Imaging may be performed to study the vasculature of any given organ, body system, or area of circulation such as the brain, heart, chest, kidneys, limbs, gastrointestinal tract, aorta, and pulmonary circulation to visualize the formation and the function of the blood vessels to detect problems such as a blockage or stricture.

catheterization. Use or insertion of a tubular device into a duct, blood vessel, hollow organ, or body cavity for injecting or withdrawing fluids for diagnostic or therapeutic purposes.

contrast material. Any internally administered substance that has a different opacity from soft tissue on radiography or computed tomograph; includes barium, used to opacify parts of the gastrointestinal tract; water-soluble iodinated compounds, used to opacify blood vessels or the genitourinary tract; may refer to air occurring naturally or introduced into the body; also, paramagnetic substances used in magnetic resonance imaging. Substances may also be documented as contrast agent or contrast medium.

supervision and interpretation. Radiology services that usually contain an invasive component and are reported by the radiologist for supervision of the procedure and the personnel involved with performing the examination, reading the film, and preparing the written report.

93567-93568

\+ **93567** Injection procedure during cardiac catheterization including imaging supervision, interpretation, and report; for supravalvular aortography (List separately in addition to code for primary procedure)

\+ **93568** for pulmonary angiography (List separately in addition to code for primary procedure)

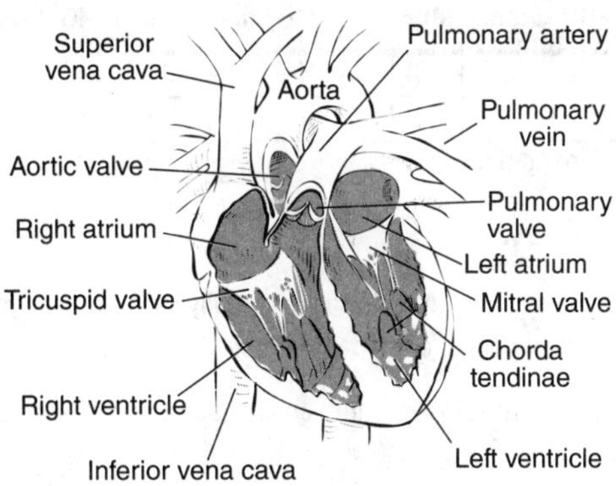

Injection for supravalvular aortography or pulmonary angiography

Explanation

The physician injects dye into the coronary arteries to evaluate function during congenital or noncongenital heart catheterization procedures. Code 93567 is specific to the visualization of the valves just above the aorta and its branches, while 93568 is specific to that of the pulmonary vessels. These codes do not report the introduction of catheters, but do include any required repositioning of catheters or use of automatic power injectors, as well as radiological supervision, interpretation, and report.

Coding Tips

When medically necessary, report moderate (conscious) sedation provided by the performing physician with 99151-99153. When provided by another physician, report 99155-99157. Report 93567 in addition to 93451–93461 or 93530–93533. Report 93568 in addition to 93451, 93453, 93456, 93457, 93460, 93461, 93530–93533, 93582, or 93583. Do not report 93568 with 33289. These procedures include any radiological supervision, interpretation, and report. Contrast administration performed during cardiac catheterization for congenital conditions is reported separately with 93563–93568. Injection procedures for right ventricular, right atrial, aortic, or pulmonary angiogram performed with cardiac catheterizations are reported separately with 93567–93568. Report 93567 for supravalvular ascending aortogram done at the same session as cardiac catheterization. Report 93568 with right heart catheterization codes when done at the same session as a pulmonary angiogram. Injection procedures do not include catheter placement when applicable; however, repositioning of the catheter and automatic power injections should not be reported separately.

ICD-10-CM Diagnostic Codes

This/these CPT code(s) are add on code(s). See the primary procedure code that this code is performed with for your ICD-10-CM code selections. Diagnostic code(s) would be the same as the actual procedure performed.

AMA: **93567** 2018,Jan,8; 2018,Feb,11; 2017,Jan,8; 2016,Mar,5; 2016,Jan,13; 2015,Jan,16; 2014,Jan,11; 2013,Jan,6-8 **93568** 2019,Jun,3; 2019,Apr,10; 2018,Jan,8; 2018,Feb,11; 2017,Jan,8; 2016,Mar,5; 2016,Jan,13; 2015,Jan,16; 2014,Jan,11; 2013,Jan,6-8

Relative Value Units/Medicare Edits

Non-Facility RVU	Work	PE	MP	Total
93567	0.97	2.52	0.22	3.71
93568	0.88	2.9	0.19	3.97
Facility RVU	**Work**	**PE**	**MP**	**Total**
93567	0.97	0.34	0.22	1.53
93568	0.88	0.31	0.19	1.38

	FUD	Status	MUE	Modifiers				IOM Reference
93567	N/A	A	1(3)	N/A	N/A	N/A	80*	None
93568	N/A	A	1(3)	N/A	N/A	N/A	80*	

* with documentation

Terms To Know

aortography. Radiographic visualization of the aorta and its branches by injecting contrast medium through percutaneous puncture or catheterization technique.

congenital. Present at birth, occurring through heredity or an influence during gestation up to the moment of birth.

contrast material. Any internally administered substance that has a different opacity from soft tissue on radiography or computed tomograph; includes barium, used to opacify parts of the gastrointestinal tract; water-soluble iodinated compounds, used to opacify blood vessels or the genitourinary tract; may refer to air occurring naturally or introduced into the body; also, paramagnetic substances used in magnetic resonance imaging. Substances may also be documented as contrast agent or contrast medium.

supra. Above.

valve. Fold or membrane within a body canal or passageway that prevents backflow of fluids running through it.

93571-93572

+ **93571** Intravascular Doppler velocity and/or pressure derived coronary flow reserve measurement (coronary vessel or graft) during coronary angiography including pharmacologically induced stress; initial vessel (List separately in addition to code for primary procedure)
+ **93572** each additional vessel (List separately in addition to code for primary procedure)

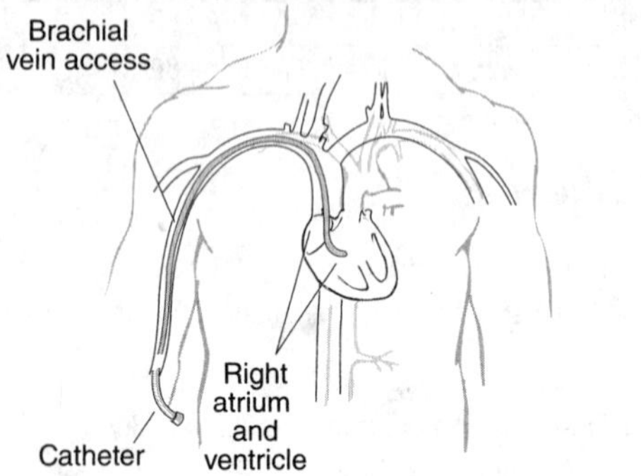

The physician threads a catheter through a central line leading to the heart and performs intravascular Doppler velocity and/or pressure derived coronary flow reserve measurement of a coronary vessel or graft

Explanation

A diagnostic angiography is the x-ray visualization of the heart and blood vessels after the introduction of a radiopaque contrast medium. Testing for patient hypersensitivity to the iodine content of the medium is advised before the radiopaque substance is used. The physician injects the contrast medium into a catheter inserted into a peripheral artery and threaded through the vessel to the visceral site. A Doppler ultrasound records blood velocity and pressure by measuring the frequency of ultrasonic waves reflected from moving surface. This code reports the Doppler measurements of the initial vessel; a second code reports the primary coronary angiography procedure. Report 93572 for each additional vessel beyond the initial vessel.

Coding Tips

When medically necessary, report moderate (conscious) sedation provided by the performing physician with 99151-99153. When provided by another physician, report 99155-99157. Report 93571 in addition to 92920, 92924, 92928, 92933, 92937, 92941, 92943, 92975, 93454–93461, 93563, or 93564. Use 93572 in addition to 93571. Do not report 93571 or 93572 in addition to 0523T. Any required manipulation or repositioning of the Doppler transducer within the specific vessel being examined is included and should not be reported separately.

ICD-10-CM Diagnostic Codes

This/these CPT code(s) are add on code(s). See the primary procedure code that this code is performed with for your ICD-10-CM code selections. Diagnostic code(s) would be the same as the actual procedure performed.

AMA: 93571 2018,Jan,8; 2018,Feb,11; 2017,Jan,8; 2016,Jan,13; 2015,May,10; 2015,Jan,16; 2015,Dec,18; 2014,Jan,11; 2014,Dec,6 **93572** 2018,Jan,8; 2018,Feb,11; 2017,Jan,8; 2016,Jan,13; 2015,May,10; 2015,Jan,16; 2015,Dec,18; 2014,Jan,11; 2014,Dec,6

Relative Value Units/Medicare Edits

Non-Facility RVU	Work	PE	MP	Total
93571	0.0	0.0	0.0	0.0
93572	0.0	0.0	0.0	0.0
Facility RVU	**Work**	**PE**	**MP**	**Total**
93571	0.0	0.0	0.0	0.0
93572	0.0	0.0	0.0	0.0

	FUD	Status	MUE	Modifiers				IOM Reference
93571	N/A	C	1(3)	N/A	N/A	N/A	80*	None
93572	N/A	C	2(3)	N/A	N/A	N/A	80*	

* with documentation

Terms To Know

anesthesia. Loss of feeling or sensation, usually induced to permit the performance of surgery or other painful procedures.

catheter. Flexible tube inserted into an area of the body for introducing or withdrawing fluid.

doppler. Ultrasonography used to augment two-dimensional images by registering velocity. When emitted sound waves reflect back off a moving object, the frequency of the reflected sound waves varies in relation to the speed of the moving object and may be used in many different procedures.

echography. Radiographic imaging that uses sound waves reflected off the different densities of anatomic structures to create images.

intravascular. Within a blood vessel.

moderate sedation. Medically controlled state of depressed consciousness, with or without analgesia, while maintaining the patient's airway, protective reflexes, and ability to respond to stimulation or verbal commands.

93580

93580 Percutaneous transcatheter closure of congenital interatrial communication (ie, Fontan fenestration, atrial septal defect) with implant

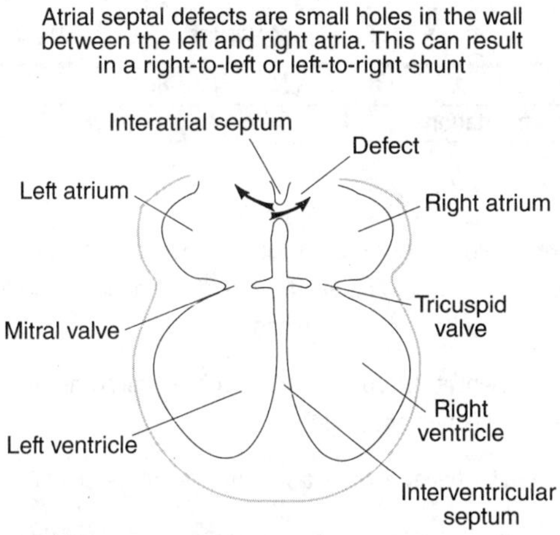

Posterior schematic showing atrial septal defect

Explanation

A congenital atrial septal defect is closed percutaneously by catheter. This procedure may be performed on infants or adults, usually under moderate sedation. After heparinization is induced, a combined right and left heart catheterization is undertaken through the existing septal opening. Contrast material is injected for atrial and ventricular angiograms to map the anatomy. Using a specialized catheter, the atrial defect is crossed from the right atrium into the left. The catheter is threaded into the upper left pulmonary vein. A guidewire is inserted, the catheter is removed, and a balloon is threaded over the guidewire into position across the defect and inflated with low pressure. The "stretched" diameter of the defect is measured. Testing is carried out to ensure that the repair will remain hemodynamically stable by occluding the defect temporarily with the balloon while taking right-side pressures and saturation measurements. A dilator and sheath holding the device are advanced over the guidewire and positioned in the left atrium. Positioning is checked using echocardiography or fluoroscopy before releasing the device. The implant is deployed across the atrial opening and positioning is checked again. Any leaks, abnormal placement, or an improperly sized device may require removal of the implant and placement of a second device. The catheters and guidewires are removed.

Coding Tips

This procedure includes a right heart catheterization and injection of contrast for atrial and ventricular angiograms. Do not report 93580 with 93451–93453, 93455–93461, 93530–93533, or 93564–93566 with 93580. For echocardiographic services performed with 93580, see 93303–93317 and 93662 as appropriate.

ICD-10-CM Diagnostic Codes

Q21.1	Atrial septal defect
Q21.2	Atrioventricular septal defect

AMA: 93580 2018,Jan,8; 2018,Feb,11; 2017,Jan,8; 2016,Jan,13; 2015,Jan,16; 2014,Jan,11

Relative Value Units/Medicare Edits

Non-Facility RVU	Work	PE	MP	Total
93580	17.97	6.51	3.97	28.45
Facility RVU	**Work**	**PE**	**MP**	**Total**
93580	17.97	6.51	3.97	28.45

	FUD	Status	MUE	Modifiers				IOM Reference
93580	0	A	1(3)	51	N/A	N/A	80*	None

* with documentation

Terms To Know

angiography. Radiographic imaging of the arteries. Imaging may be performed to study the vasculature of any given organ, body system, or area of circulation such as the brain, heart, chest, kidneys, limbs, gastrointestinal tract, aorta, and pulmonary circulation to visualize the formation and the function of the blood vessels to detect problems such as a blockage or stricture. A catheter is inserted through an accessible blood vessel and the artery is injected with a radiopaque contrast material after which x-rays are taken.

anomaly. Irregularity in the structure or position of an organ or tissue.

atria. Two upper chambers of the heart. The left and right atria are divided by the septum, a muscular wall.

catheterization. Use or insertion of a tubular device into a duct, blood vessel, hollow organ, or body cavity for injecting or withdrawing fluids for diagnostic or therapeutic purposes.

congenital. Present at birth, occurring through heredity or an influence during gestation up to the moment of birth.

fluoroscopy. Radiology technique that allows visual examination of part of the body or a function of an organ using a device that projects an x-ray image on a fluorescent screen.

implant. Material or device inserted or placed within the body for therapeutic, reconstructive, or diagnostic purposes.

septum. Anatomical partition or dividing wall.

Medicine

● New ▲ Revised + Add On AMA: CPT Assist [Resequenced] ☑ Laterality

93581

93581 Percutaneous transcatheter closure of a congenital ventricular septal defect with implant

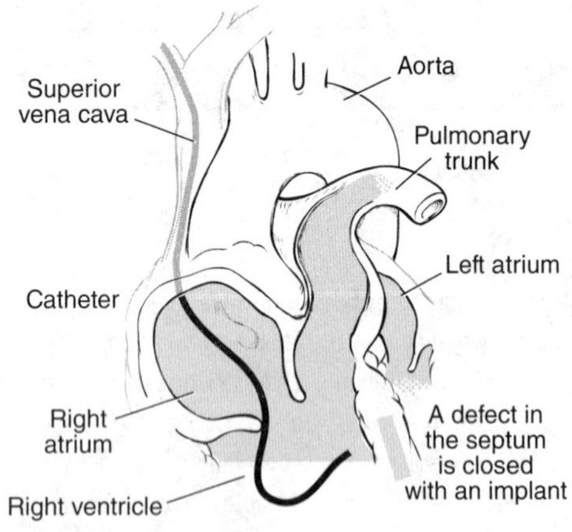

A ventricular septal defect (VSD) is addressed transcatheterally inserted percutaneously. Closure is accomplished using an implant

Explanation

A congenital ventricular septal defect is closed percutaneously by catheter. The patient is given local anesthesia and the femoral artery and vein are cannulated. A guidewire and catheter are inserted and advanced through the ventricular septum, into the right ventricle, and across the tricuspid valve into the right atrium. A separate venous sheath is placed in the jugular vein to allow passage of a snare catheter. The snare is advanced into the atrium and grasps the free wire or catheter that was threaded through the ventricular septal defect. This provides a through-and-through from the femoral vein to the ventricular septal defect and out the jugular. The jugular end is used to pass a dilator and sheath over the defect for the positioning of the occlusive device into the left ventricle. The sheath must be in the exact position with its tip in the left ventricle for delivery of the occlusive device. If necessary, traction is used at the opposite end to secure the sheath as the dilator is removed. If the sheath is displaced during removal of the dilator, the dilator is reinserted for correct positioning. Once the sheath is in place and the dilator removed, the delivery catheter loaded with an occlusive device is advanced to the center of the right atrium. The device is advanced out of the delivery catheter and into the tip of the sheath. It is gently advanced so that the distal legs are in the left ventricle and the center of the device is in the defect. A slight withdrawing of the sheath causes the distal legs to open within the left ventricle. Further withdrawal of the sheath allows the proximal legs to open in the right ventricle. The occlusion is confirmed with angiography and the delivery system and catheters are removed.

Coding Tips

This procedure includes a right heart catheterization and injection of contrast for atrial and ventricular angiograms. Do not report 93581 with 93451–93453, 93455–93461, 93530–93533, or 93564–93566. For echocardiographic services performed in addition to 93581, see 93303–93317 and 93662 as appropriate.

ICD-10-CM Diagnostic Codes

Q21.0 Ventricular septal defect

AMA: **93581** 2018,Jan,8; 2018,Feb,11; 2017,Jan,8; 2016,Jan,13; 2015,Jan,16; 2014,Jan,11

Relative Value Units/Medicare Edits

Non-Facility RVU	Work	PE	MP	Total
93581	24.39	8.64	5.74	38.77
Facility RVU	**Work**	**PE**	**MP**	**Total**
93581	24.39	8.64	5.74	38.77

	FUD	Status	MUE	Modifiers				IOM Reference
93581	0	A	1(3)	51	N/A	N/A	80*	None

* with documentation

Terms To Know

cannulation. Insertion of a flexible length of hollow tubing into a blood vessel, duct, or body cavity, usually for extracorporeal circulation or chemotherapy infusion to a particular region of the body.

congenital. Present at birth, occurring through heredity or an influence during gestation up to the moment of birth.

distal. Located farther away from a specified reference point or the trunk.

guidewire. Flexible metal instrument designed to lead another instrument in its proper course.

percutaneous. Through the skin.

proximal. Located closest to a specified reference point, usually the midline or trunk.

septum. Anatomical partition or dividing wall.

snare. Wire used as a loop to excise a polyp or lesion.

ventricular septal defect. Congenital cardiac anomaly resulting in a continual opening in the septum between the ventricles that, in severe cases, causes oxygenated blood to flow back into the lungs, resulting in pulmonary hypertension.

Medicine

93582

93582 Percutaneous transcatheter closure of patent ductus arteriosus

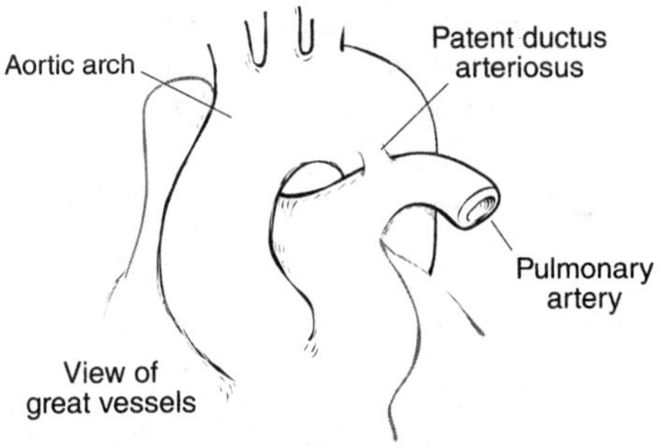

The ductus arteriosus is the natural shunt that bypasses lung circulation in the prenatal phase

Explanation

A patent ductus arteriosus (PDA) is closed using a transcatheter technique. A small incision is made in an extremity artery (usually the femoral artery). The physician threads a catheter through the arteries and heart to the PDA. A coil or other occlusion device is deployed into the PDA via the catheter. An angiography may be performed to check for patency of the closure device. The catheter is removed and the incision is closed.

Coding Tips

When medically necessary, report moderate (conscious) sedation provided by the performing physician with 99151-99153. When provided by another physician, report 99155-99157. This procedure includes catheter placement in the aorta, congenital right and left heart catheterization, as well as aortic arch angiography, if performed, and they may not be reported separately. Do not report 93582 with 36013, 36014, 36200, 75600, 75605, 93451–93461, 93530, 93531, 93532, 93533, or 93567. For other cardiac angiography performed, see 93563–93566 or 93568. For left heart catheterization by transseptal puncture through intact septum or by transapical puncture, see 93462. For repair of patent ductus arteriosus by ligation, see 33820, 33822, or 33824. For intracardiac echocardiography services performed during the procedure, see 93662. Other echocardiographic procedures provided by another individual are reported with 93315–99317.

ICD-10-CM Diagnostic Codes

Q25.0	Patent ductus arteriosus

AMA: 93582 2019,Apr,10; 2018,Jan,8; 2018,Feb,11; 2017,Jan,8; 2016,Jan,13; 2015,Jan,16; 2014,Jul,3

Relative Value Units/Medicare Edits

Non-Facility RVU	Work	PE	MP	Total
93582	12.31	4.19	2.92	19.42
Facility RVU	Work	PE	MP	Total
93582	12.31	4.19	2.92	19.42

	FUD	Status	MUE	Modifiers				IOM Reference
93582	0	A	1(2)	51	N/A	N/A	80*	None

* with documentation

93583

93583 Percutaneous transcatheter septal reduction therapy (eg, alcohol septal ablation) including temporary pacemaker insertion when performed

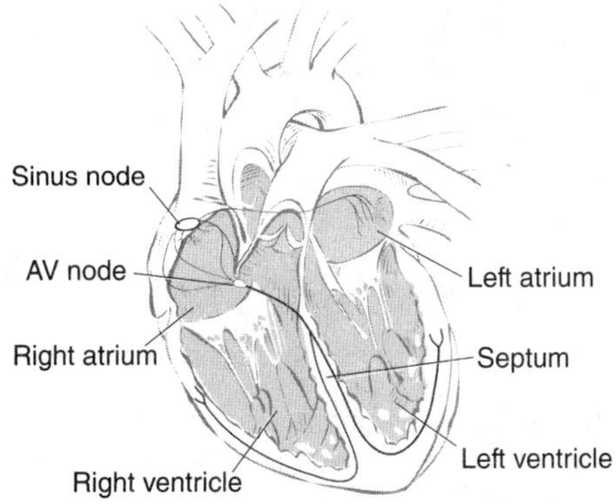

A temporary pacemaker may be placed as part of the procedure

Explanation

Septal reduction therapy, also known as alcohol septal ablation (ASA), is performed to decrease the size of the cardiac septal muscle in patients with hypertrophic cardiomyopathy. A small incision is made in an extremity artery (usually the femoral artery). A catheter is threaded through the arteries to the heart and a coronary angiography is performed to locate the first septal perforator branch of the left anterior descending (LAD) artery. A balloon is inflated within the perforator and contrast is injected to ensure no flow back into the LAD. A slow injection of absolute alcohol is performed until a partial initial response is rendered. The balloon is deflated and an additional coronary angiogram is performed to ensure patency of the LAD. The catheters are removed and the incision is closed.

Coding Tips

When medically necessary, report moderate (conscious) sedation provided by the performing physician with 99151-99153. When provided by another physician, report 99155-99157. This procedure includes insertion of a temporary pacemaker and left heart catheterization. It also includes left anterior descending coronary angiography for the purpose of guiding the intervention. Diagnostic cardiac catheterization may only be separately reported when no prior catheter-based study of the treatment area is available, the prior studies are inadequate, or the patient's condition has changed significantly enough to warrant the additional study. Do not report 93583 with 33210, 33211, 93452, 93453, 93458, 93459, 93460, 93461, 93531, 93532, 93533, or 93565. Do not report 93463 for the injection of alcohol for the procedure. For intracardiac echocardiography services performed during the procedure, see 93662.

ICD-10-CM Diagnostic Codes

I42.1	Obstructive hypertrophic cardiomyopathy
I42.2	Other hypertrophic cardiomyopathy
Q24.8	Other specified congenital malformations of heart

AMA: 93583 2018,Feb,11

Relative Value Units/Medicare Edits

Non-Facility RVU	Work	PE	MP	Total
93583	13.75	4.75	3.14	21.64
Facility RVU	Work	PE	MP	Total
93583	13.75	4.75	3.14	21.64

	FUD	Status	MUE	Modifiers				IOM Reference
93583	0	A	1(2)	51	N/A	N/A	80*	None

* with documentation

Terms To Know

angiography. Radiographic imaging of the arteries.

anomaly. Irregularity in the structure or position of an organ or tissue.

cardiomegaly. Enlargement of the heart due to a thickened heart muscle or an enlarged heart chamber. Cardiomegaly is a result of the heart having to work harder than normal.

cardiomyopathy. General term used to describe a number of conditions of the heart muscle.

congenital. Present at birth, occurring through heredity or an influence during gestation up to the moment of birth.

pacemaker. Implantable cardiac device that controls the heart's rhythm and maintains regular beats by artificial electric discharges. This device consists of the pulse generator with a battery and the electrodes, or leads, which are placed in single or dual chambers of the heart, usually transvenously.

percutaneous. Through the skin.

septum. Anatomical partition or dividing wall.

93590-93592

93590 Percutaneous transcatheter closure of paravalvular leak; initial occlusion device, mitral valve

93591 initial occlusion device, aortic valve

+ **93592** each additional occlusion device (List separately in addition to code for primary procedure)

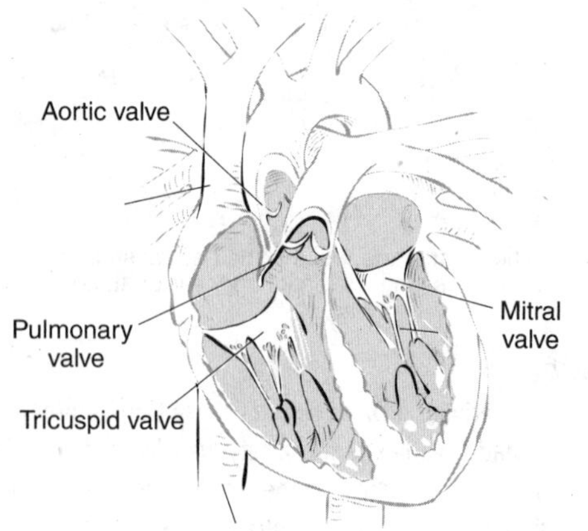

Paravalvular leak is repaired with an occlusion device

Explanation

Percutaneous transcatheter closure of a paravalvular leak (PVL) in the mitral or aortic valve can be achieved by antegrade or retrograde approach. A transesophageal echocardiogram (TEE) for a mitral valve leak or a transthoracic echocardiogram (TTE) for an aortic leak was performed within the previous six months, earlier if the patient was symptomatic. A retrograde transfemoral approach is performed utilizing a catheter and guidewire. Upon crossing the leak, the wire is removed and a stiff wire is inserted along with the device delivery system consisting of a guide catheter or sheath. The wire is removed allowing for advancement and deployment of an occlusion device. In cases where support becomes an issue, a transseptal access and snare may be employed to establish a rail. This entails the snaring of the initial wire within the left atrium or the formation of an apical ventricular rail by left ventricular puncture with the wire crossing the apex. In mitral PVL, if this approach does not achieve the desired results, an antegrade transseptal approach may be used. Upon completion of the procedure for 93590, TEE should indicate fluent leaflets, clear pulmonary veins, and if anterior leak, clear mitral valve. In 93591, the physician must evaluate that the coronary ostia is not covered and leaflets are fluent. For both procedures, the device deployed is dependent upon the defect size. Many closure devices are currently used in these procedures, such as embolization coils, double-umbrella devices, occluders, and plugs approved for other specific defects and may be suitable in most cases. However for PVLs they are limited by size, shape, specific characteristics, and features of delivery system. Report 93592 for each additional occlusion device.

Coding Tips

Report 93592 in addition to 93590 and 93591. Percutaneous access, fluoroscopy, angiography, placement of the access sheath, maneuvering the delivery system to the leak, device deployment, and positioning and repositioning the closure device are included in 93590 and 93591. Additional diagnostic cardiac catheterization procedures unrelated to the PVL closure may be reported separately. Do not report 93590 with 93462 for transseptal puncture but do report transapical puncture (93462) with 93590. Report 93591 with 93462 for transseptal or transapical puncture.

ICD-10-CM Diagnostic Codes

T82.03XA	Leakage of heart valve prosthesis, initial encounter
T82.09XA	Other mechanical complication of heart valve prosthesis, initial encounter
T82.223A	Leakage of biological heart valve graft, initial encounter
T82.228A	Other mechanical complication of biological heart valve graft, initial encounter

AMA: **93590** 2018,Jan,8; 2018,Feb,11; 2017,Sep,3 **93591** 2018,Jan,8; 2018,Feb,11; 2017,Sep,3 **93592** 2018,Jan,8; 2018,Feb,11; 2017,Sep,3

Relative Value Units/Medicare Edits

Non-Facility RVU	Work	PE	MP	Total
93590	21.7	7.98	1.52	31.2
93591	17.97	6.48	1.25	25.7
93592	8.0	2.83	0.56	11.39
Facility RVU	**Work**	**PE**	**MP**	**Total**
93590	21.7	7.98	1.52	31.2
93591	17.97	6.48	1.25	25.7
93592	8.0	2.83	0.56	11.39

	FUD	Status	MUE	Modifiers				IOM Reference
93590	0	A	1(2)	51	N/A	62*	80	None
93591	0	A	1(2)	51	N/A	62	80*	
93592	N/A	A	2(3)	N/A	N/A	62*	80	

* with documentation

Terms To Know

embolization. Placement of a clotting agent, such as a coil, plastic particles, gel, foam, etc., into an area of hemorrhage to stop the bleeding or to block blood flow to a problem area, such as an aneurysm or a tumor.

occlusion. Constriction, closure, or blockage of a passage.

retrograde. Moving against the usual direction of flow.

transcatheter. Procedure or treatment performed via a catheter.

transesophageal echocardiography. Guidance of a small probe into the esophagus under sedation to closely evaluate the heart and blood vessels within the chest.

93600

93600 Bundle of His recording

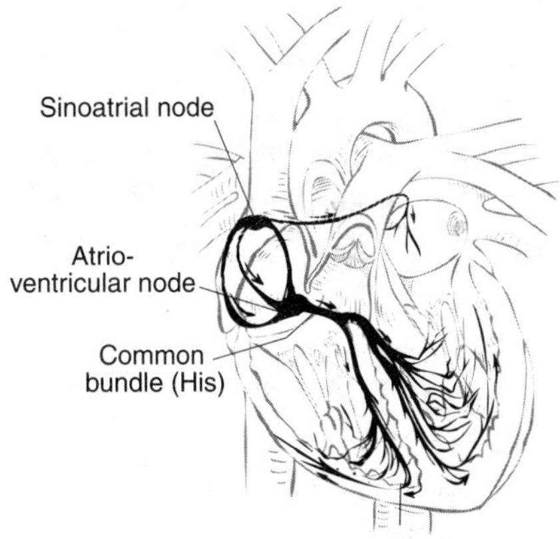

Conduction system of the heart

The His bundle is recorded, typically from the right atria

Explanation

The physician places a venous sheath, usually in a femoral vein, using standard techniques. The physician advances an electrical catheter through the venous sheath and into the right heart under fluoroscopic guidance. The physician attaches the catheter to an electrical recording device to allow depiction of the intracardiac electrograms obtained from electrodes on the catheter tip. The physician moves the catheter tip to the bundle of His, on the anteroseptal tricuspid annulus, and obtains recordings. Alternatively, the physician may obtain similar recordings by placing a catheter into the left ventricular outflow tract via the aorta.

Coding Tips

As exempt from modifier 51, 93600 has not been designated in CPT as an add-on service/procedure. However, codes identified as exempt from modifier 51 are not subject to multiple procedure rules. No reimbursement reduction or modifier 51 is applied. Do not report 93600 with 93619, 93620, 93653, 93654, or 93656. Procedure 93600 has both a technical and professional component. To report only the professional component, append modifier 26. To report only the technical component, append modifier TC. To report the complete procedure (i.e., both the professional and technical components), submit without a modifier. Fluoroscopic guidance is included in electrophysiological procedures and should not be reported separately. Procedure 93600 reports bundle of His recording only. For comprehensive electrophysiologic evaluation with bundle of His recording, see 93619–92622.

ICD-10-CM Diagnostic Codes

I44.0	Atrioventricular block, first degree
I44.1	Atrioventricular block, second degree
I44.2	Atrioventricular block, complete
I44.39	Other atrioventricular block
I44.4	Left anterior fascicular block
I44.5	Left posterior fascicular block
I44.69	Other fascicular block
I45.0	Right fascicular block
I45.19	Other right bundle-branch block
I45.2	Bifascicular block

I45.3 Trifascicular block
I45.4 Nonspecific intraventricular block
I45.5 Other specified heart block
I45.6 Pre-excitation syndrome
I45.89 Other specified conduction disorders
I46.2 Cardiac arrest due to underlying cardiac condition
I46.8 Cardiac arrest due to other underlying condition
I47.0 Re-entry ventricular arrhythmia
I47.1 Supraventricular tachycardia
I47.2 Ventricular tachycardia
I48.0 Paroxysmal atrial fibrillation
I48.11 Longstanding persistent atrial fibrillation
I48.19 Other persistent atrial fibrillation
I48.21 Permanent atrial fibrillation
I48.3 Typical atrial flutter
I48.4 Atypical atrial flutter
I49.01 Ventricular fibrillation
I49.02 Ventricular flutter
I49.1 Atrial premature depolarization
I49.2 Junctional premature depolarization
I49.3 Ventricular premature depolarization
I49.49 Other premature depolarization
I49.5 Sick sinus syndrome
I49.8 Other specified cardiac arrhythmias

AMA: 93600 2018,Jan,8; 2018,Feb,11; 2017,Jan,8; 2016,Jan,13; 2015,Jan,16; 2014,Jan,11; 2014,Apr,3; 2013,Jun,6-8; 2013,Jul,7-9

Relative Value Units/Medicare Edits

Non-Facility RVU	Work	PE	MP	Total
93600	0.0	0.0	0.0	0.0
Facility RVU	Work	PE	MP	Total
93600	0.0	0.0	0.0	0.0

	FUD	Status	MUE	Modifiers				IOM Reference
93600	0	C	1(3)	N/A	N/A	N/A	80*	100-03,20.13

* with documentation

93602

93602 Intra-atrial recording

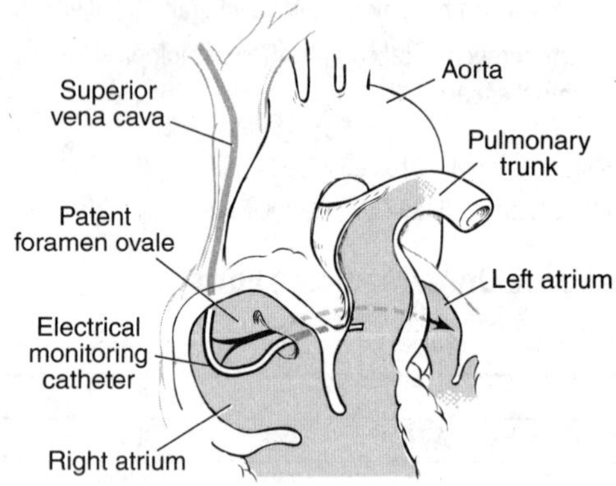

Intraatrial recordings are made. The monitor may be placed in the right atria or the left atria by retrograde approach.The septum may be probed from either side, as well

Explanation

The physician places a venous sheath, usually in a femoral vein, using standard techniques. The physician advances an electrical catheter through the venous sheath and into the right heart under fluoroscopic guidance. The physician attaches the catheter to an electrical recording device to allow depiction of the intracardiac electrograms obtained from electrodes on the catheter tip. The physician moves the catheter tip to the right atrium and obtains recordings. The physician may obtain left atrial recordings by crossing the interatrial septum. Alternatively, the physician may obtain left atrial recordings by placing an arterial catheter into the aorta and crossing both the aortic and mitral valves in a retrograde fashion.

Coding Tips

As exempt from modifier 51, 93602 has not been designated in CPT as an add-on service/procedure. However, codes identified as exempt from modifier 51 are not subject to multiple procedure rules. No reimbursement reduction or modifier 51 is applied. Do not report 93602 with 93619, 93620, 93653, 93654, or 93656. Procedure 93602 has both a technical and professional component. To report only the professional component, append modifier 26. To report only the technical component, append modifier TC. To report the complete procedure (i.e., both the professional and technical components), submit without a modifier. Fluoroscopic guidance is included in electrophysiological procedures and should not be reported separately. Procedure 93602 reports intra-atrial recording only. For comprehensive electrophysiologic evaluation including intra-atrial recording, see 93619–92622.

ICD-10-CM Diagnostic Codes

I44.0 Atrioventricular block, first degree
I44.1 Atrioventricular block, second degree
I44.2 Atrioventricular block, complete
I44.39 Other atrioventricular block
I45.5 Other specified heart block
I45.6 Pre-excitation syndrome
I45.89 Other specified conduction disorders
I48.0 Paroxysmal atrial fibrillation
I48.11 Longstanding persistent atrial fibrillation

I48.19	Other persistent atrial fibrillation
I48.21	Permanent atrial fibrillation
I48.3	Typical atrial flutter
I48.4	Atypical atrial flutter
I49.1	Atrial premature depolarization
I49.5	Sick sinus syndrome
I49.8	Other specified cardiac arrhythmias

AMA: 93602 2018,Jan,8; 2018,Feb,11; 2017,Jan,8; 2016,Jan,13; 2015,Jan,16; 2014,Jan,11; 2014,Apr,3; 2013,Jun,6-8; 2013,Jul,7-9

Relative Value Units/Medicare Edits

Non-Facility RVU	Work	PE	MP	Total
93602	0.0	0.0	0.0	0.0
Facility RVU	**Work**	**PE**	**MP**	**Total**
93602	0.0	0.0	0.0	0.0

	FUD	Status	MUE	Modifiers				IOM Reference
93602	0	C	1(3)	N/A	N/A	N/A	80*	None

* with documentation

Terms To Know

fluoroscopy. Radiology technique that allows visual examination of part of the body or a function of an organ using a device that projects an x-ray image on a fluorescent screen.

retrograde. Moving against the usual direction of flow.

93603

93603 Right ventricular recording

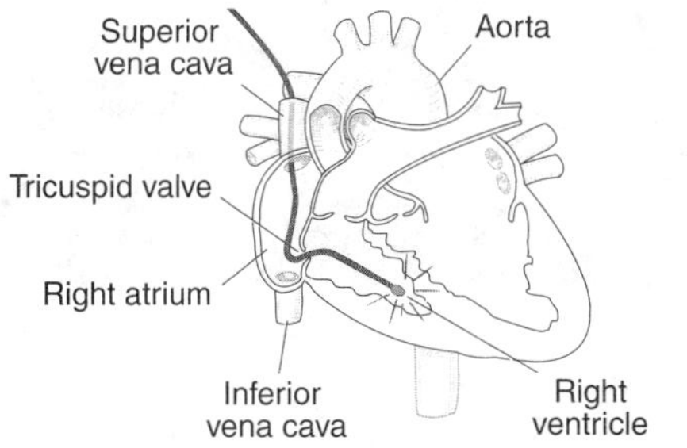

Recordings are collected from the right ventricle

Explanation

The physician places a venous sheath, usually in a femoral vein, using standard techniques. The physician advances an electrical catheter through the venous sheath and into the right heart under fluoroscopic guidance. The physician attaches the catheter to an electrical recording device to allow depiction of the intracardiac electrograms obtained from electrodes on the catheter tip. The physician moves the catheter tip to the right ventricle and obtains recordings.

Coding Tips

As exempt from modifier 51, 93603 has not been designated in CPT as an add-on service/procedure. However, codes identified as exempt from modifier 51 are not subject to multiple procedure rules. No reimbursement reduction or modifier 51 is applied. Do not report 93603 with 93619, 93620, 93653, 93654, or 93656. Procedure 93603 has both a technical and professional component. To report only the professional component, append modifier 26. To report only the technical component, append modifier TC. To report the complete procedure (i.e., both the professional and technical components), submit without a modifier. Fluoroscopic guidance is included in electrophysiological procedures and should not be reported separately. Procedure 93603 reports right ventricular recording only. For comprehensive electrophysiologic evaluation including right ventricular recording, see 93619–92622.

ICD-10-CM Diagnostic Codes

I42.8	Other cardiomyopathies
I44.0	Atrioventricular block, first degree
I44.1	Atrioventricular block, second degree
I44.2	Atrioventricular block, complete
I44.30	Unspecified atrioventricular block
I44.39	Other atrioventricular block
I45.4	Nonspecific intraventricular block
I45.5	Other specified heart block
I45.6	Pre-excitation syndrome
I45.89	Other specified conduction disorders
I45.9	Conduction disorder, unspecified
I47.0	Re-entry ventricular arrhythmia
I47.1	Supraventricular tachycardia
I47.2	Ventricular tachycardia
I49.01	Ventricular fibrillation

I49.02 Ventricular flutter
I49.3 Ventricular premature depolarization

AMA: **93603** 2018,Jan,8; 2018,Feb,11; 2017,Jan,8; 2016,Jan,13; 2015,Jan,16; 2014,Jan,11; 2014,Apr,3; 2013,Jun,6-8; 2013,Jul,7-9

Relative Value Units/Medicare Edits

Non-Facility RVU	Work	PE	MP	Total
93603	0.0	0.0	0.0	0.0
Facility RVU	**Work**	**PE**	**MP**	**Total**
93603	0.0	0.0	0.0	0.0

	FUD	Status	MUE	Modifiers				IOM Reference
93603	0	C	1(3)	N/A	N/A	N/A	80*	None

* with documentation

Terms To Know

atrioventricular block. Condition in which there is a disturbance of electrical conduction, such as a delay, intermittence, or absence in the transmission of an impulse from the atria to the ventricles and categorized according to degree of severity.

electrode. Electric terminal specialized for a particular electrochemical reaction that acts as a medium between a body surface and another instrument, commonly termed a lead.

fluoroscopy. Radiology technique that allows visual examination of part of the body or a function of an organ using a device that projects an x-ray image on a fluorescent screen.

sheath. Covering enclosing an organ or part.

93609

+ 93609 Intraventricular and/or intra-atrial mapping of tachycardia site(s) with catheter manipulation to record from multiple sites to identify origin of tachycardia (List separately in addition to code for primary procedure)

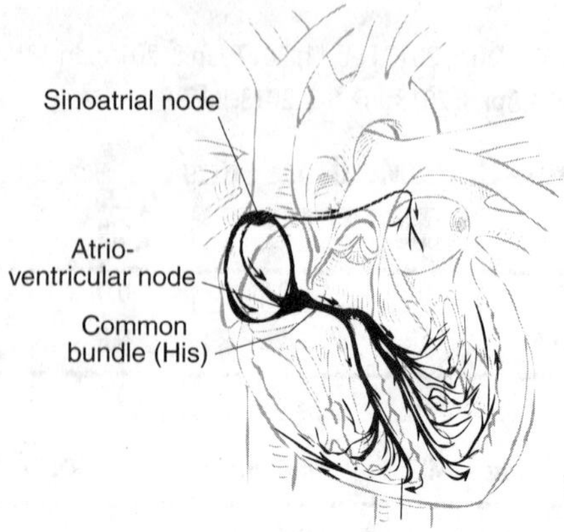

Nerve conduction of the heart

Explanation

The physician places an appropriate arterial or venous sheath, usually femoral, to allow access to the chamber to be mapped. The physician advances an electrical catheter through the sheath and into the appropriate chamber under fluoroscopic guidance. The physician attaches the catheter to an electrical recording device to allow depiction of the intracardiac electrograms obtained from electrodes on the catheter tip. The physician moves the catheter tip throughout the chamber to be mapped and obtains recordings. The physician compares activation times from different sites in order to identify the origin of the tachycardia.

Coding Tips

When medically necessary, report moderate (conscious) sedation provided by the performing physician with 99151-99153. When provided by another physician, report 99155-99157. Report 93609 in addition to 93620, 93653, or 93656. Only one mapping procedure may be reported with a comprehensive electrophysiologic evaluation (93620) or intracardiac catheter ablation (93653). Three-dimensional mapping (93613) is the higher valued service and should be reported instead of 93609 when both are performed. Do not report 93609 with 93613 or 93654. Procedure 93609 has both a technical and professional component. To report only the professional component, append modifier 26. To report only the technical component, append modifier TC. To report the complete procedure (i.e., both the professional and technical components), submit without a modifier. Fluoroscopic guidance is included in electrophysiological procedures and should not be reported separately. Intraventricular and/or intra-atrial mapping is not included in comprehensive electrophysiologic evaluation, see 93620–92622.

ICD-10-CM Diagnostic Codes

This/these CPT code(s) are add on code(s). See the primary procedure code that this code is performed with for your ICD-10-CM code selections. Diagnostic code(s) would be the same as the actual procedure performed.

AMA: **93609** 2018,Jan,8; 2018,Feb,11; 2017,Jan,8; 2016,Jan,13; 2015,Jan,16; 2014,Jan,11; 2014,Apr,3; 2013,Jun,6-8; 2013,Jul,7-9

Relative Value Units/Medicare Edits

Non-Facility RVU	Work	PE	MP	Total
93609	0.0	0.0	0.0	0.0
Facility RVU	**Work**	**PE**	**MP**	**Total**
93609	0.0	0.0	0.0	0.0

	FUD	Status	MUE	Modifiers				IOM Reference
93609	N/A	C	1(3)	N/A	N/A	N/A	80*	None

* with documentation

Terms To Know

ablation. Removal or destruction of tissue by cutting, electrical energy, chemical substances, or excessive heat application.

fluoroscopy. Radiology technique that allows visual examination of part of the body or a function of an organ using a device that projects an x-ray image on a fluorescent screen.

moderate sedation. Medically controlled state of depressed consciousness, with or without analgesia, while maintaining the patient's airway, protective reflexes, and ability to respond to stimulation or verbal commands.

sinoatrial node. Group of cells located on the wall of the right atrium, close to the superior vena cava, that naturally discharge electrical impulses initiating heart contracture. For this reason, it is often referred to as the "physiologic pacemaker."

tachycardia. Excessively rapid beating action of the heart, defined as more than 100 beats per minute for an adult, that is usually defined by its origin (atrial or ventricular) and whether the onset and cessation occurs in sudden attacks (paroxysmal) or in a slow pattern (nonparoxysmal).

93610

93610 Intra-atrial pacing

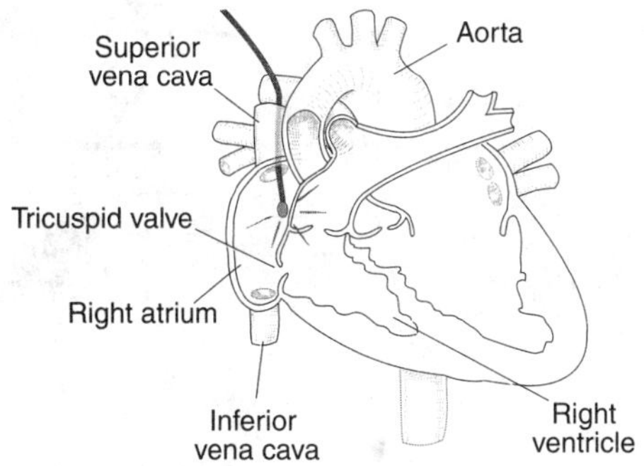

Schematic of right atrial pacing

Explanation

The physician places a venous sheath, usually in a femoral vein, using standard techniques. The physician advances an electrical catheter through the venous sheath and into the right heart under fluoroscopic guidance. The physician attaches the catheter to an electrical pacing device to allow transmission of pacing impulses through the catheter to the right atrium. The physician may pace the left atrium by placing the catheter in the coronary sinus or by crossing the interatrial septum. Alternatively, the physician may pace the left atrium by placing an arterial catheter into the aorta and crossing both the aortic and mitral valves in a retrograde fashion.

Coding Tips

As exempt from modifier 51, 93610 has not been designated in CPT as an add-on service/procedure. However, codes identified as exempt from modifier 51 are not subject to multiple procedure rules. No reimbursement reduction or modifier 51 is applied. Procedure 93610 has both a technical and professional component. To report only the professional component, append modifier 26. To report only the technical component, append modifier TC. To report the complete procedure (i.e., both the professional and technical components), submit without a modifier. Fluoroscopic guidance is included in electrophysiological procedures and should not be reported separately. Do not report 93610 with 93619, 93620, 93653, 93654, or 93656. Procedure 93610 reports intra-atrial pacing only. For comprehensive electrophysiologic evaluation including intra-atrial pacing, see 93619–92622.

ICD-10-CM Diagnostic Codes

I44.0	Atrioventricular block, first degree
I44.1	Atrioventricular block, second degree
I44.2	Atrioventricular block, complete
I44.39	Other atrioventricular block
I48.0	Paroxysmal atrial fibrillation
I48.11	Longstanding persistent atrial fibrillation
I48.19	Other persistent atrial fibrillation
I48.21	Permanent atrial fibrillation
I48.3	Typical atrial flutter
I48.4	Atypical atrial flutter
I49.1	Atrial premature depolarization
I49.5	Sick sinus syndrome

AMA: 93610 2018,Jan,8; 2018,Feb,11; 2017,Jan,8; 2016,Jan,13; 2015,Jan,16; 2014,Jan,11; 2014,Apr,3; 2013,Jun,6-8; 2013,Jul,7-9

Relative Value Units/Medicare Edits

Non-Facility RVU	Work	PE	MP	Total
93610	0.0	0.0	0.0	0.0
Facility RVU	**Work**	**PE**	**MP**	**Total**
93610	0.0	0.0	0.0	0.0

	FUD	Status	MUE	Modifiers				IOM Reference
93610	0	C	1(3)	N/A	N/A	N/A	80*	100-03,20.12

* with documentation

Terms To Know

arrhythmia. Irregular heartbeat.

fibrillation. Spontaneous contraction of individual muscle fibers.

sick sinus syndrome. Range of electrophysiological abnormalities of the heart including sinus bradycardia, sinus arrest, sinus node exit block, chronic atrial fibrillation, and bradycardia-tachycardia syndrome. Most often found in older patients with a history of heart disease, it is distinguished by delayed or failed conduction between the sinus node and atria, due to inadequate sinus node pacemaking or conduction disturbances.

tachycardia. Excessively rapid beating action of the heart, defined as more than 100 beats per minute for an adult, that is usually defined by its origin (atrial or ventricular) and whether the onset and cessation occurs in sudden attacks (paroxysmal) or in a slow pattern (nonparoxysmal).

93612

93612 Intraventricular pacing

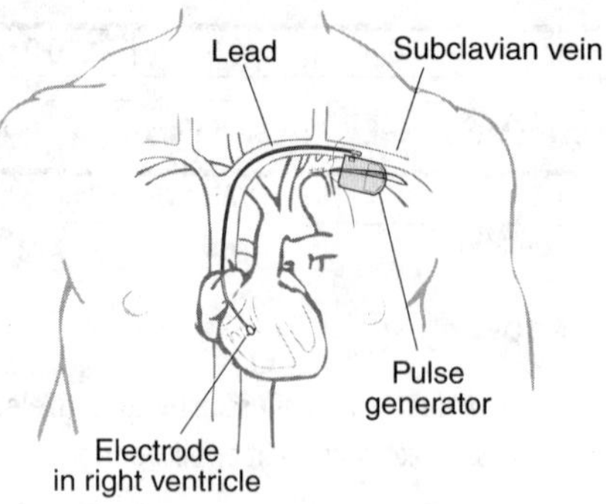

A ventricle of the heart is paced by an electrode positioned within the ventricle. Either left or right ventricle may be addressed according to the description

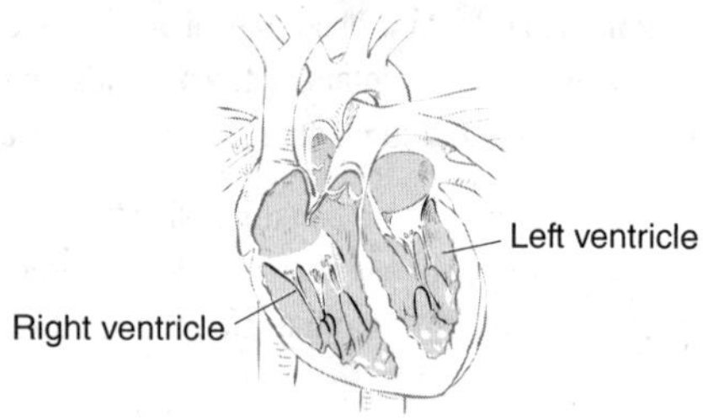

Explanation

The physician places a venous sheath using standard techniques. The physician advances an electrical catheter through the venous sheath and into the right ventricle under fluoroscopic guidance. The physician attaches the catheter to an electrical pacing device to allow transmission of pacing impulses through the catheter to the right ventricle. Alternatively, the physician may pace the left ventricle by placing the catheter in the right atrium, crossing the intraatrial septum and mitral valve. Finally, the physician may pace the left ventricle by advancing a catheter through an arterial sheath, via the aorta, across the aortic valve into the left ventricle.

Coding Tips

As exempt from modifier 51, 93612 has not been designated in CPT as an add-on service/procedure. However, codes identified as exempt from modifier 51 are not subject to multiple procedure rules. No reimbursement reduction or modifier 51 is applied. Procedure 93612 has both a technical and professional component. To report only the professional component, append modifier 26. To report only the technical component, append modifier TC. To report the complete procedure (i.e., both the professional and technical components), submit without a modifier. Fluoroscopic guidance is included in electrophysiological procedures and should not be reported separately. Do not report 93612 with 93619, 93620–93622, 93653, 93654, or 93656. Procedure 93612 reports intraventricular pacing only. For comprehensive electrophysiologic evaluation including intraventricular pacing, see 93619–92622.

ICD-10-CM Diagnostic Codes

I44.0	Atrioventricular block, first degree
I44.1	Atrioventricular block, second degree
I44.2	Atrioventricular block, complete
I44.39	Other atrioventricular block

Medicine

I44.4	Left anterior fascicular block
I44.5	Left posterior fascicular block
I44.69	Other fascicular block
I45.0	Right fascicular block
I45.19	Other right bundle-branch block
I45.2	Bifascicular block
I45.3	Trifascicular block
I45.4	Nonspecific intraventricular block
I47.0	Re-entry ventricular arrhythmia
I47.1	Supraventricular tachycardia
I47.2	Ventricular tachycardia
I49.01	Ventricular fibrillation
I49.02	Ventricular flutter
I49.3	Ventricular premature depolarization

AMA: 93612 2018,Jan,8; 2018,Feb,11; 2017,Jan,8; 2016,Jan,13; 2015,Jan,16; 2014,Jan,11; 2014,Apr,3; 2013,Jun,6-8; 2013,Jul,7-9

Relative Value Units/Medicare Edits

Non-Facility RVU	Work	PE	MP	Total
93612	0.0	0.0	0.0	0.0
Facility RVU	**Work**	**PE**	**MP**	**Total**
93612	0.0	0.0	0.0	0.0

	FUD	Status	MUE	Modifiers				IOM Reference
93612	0	C	1(3)	N/A	N/A	N/A	80*	None

* with documentation

93613

+ 93613 Intracardiac electrophysiologic 3-dimensional mapping (List separately in addition to code for primary procedure)

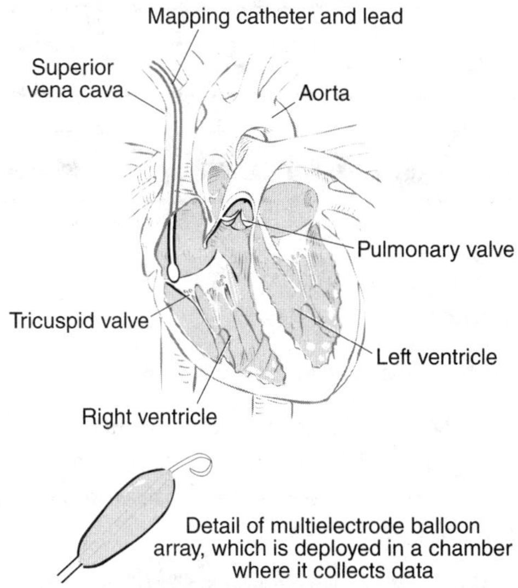

The heart is mapped by an intracardiac electrophysiologic sensor. The study yields three-dimensional views of the area under investigation

Explanation

Electrophysiologic studies use electric stimulation and monitoring in the diagnosis of conduction abnormalities that predispose patients to bradyarrhythmias and to determine a patient's chance of developing ventricular and supraventricular tachyarrhythmias. The physician inserts an electrode catheter percutaneously into the right subclavian vein and, under fluoroscopic guidance, positions the electrode catheter at the right ventricular apex, both for recording and stimulating the right atrium and the right ventricle. For mapping, additional electrode catheters are inserted percutaneously from the right femoral artery and advanced to the specific site to be mapped in conjunction with the primary procedure (93620, 93653, 93656). Ventricular tachycardia is induced by programmed ventricular stimulation from the right and left ventricular apexes. The earliest activation site is determined and the diastolic pressure is recorded on the endocardial activation map during the ventricular tachycardia. Intracardiac electrograms with surface electrocardiograms are simultaneously displayed and recorded on a multichannel oscilloscopic photographic recorder.

Coding Tips

When medically necessary, report moderate (conscious) sedation provided by the performing physician with 99151-99153. When provided by another physician, report 99155-99157. Report 93613 in addition to 93620, 93653, or 93656. Only one mapping procedure may be reported with a comprehensive electrophysiologic evaluation (93620) or intracardiac catheter ablation (93563). Three-dimensional mapping (93613) is the higher valued service and should be reported instead of 93609 when both are performed. Do not report 93613 with 93609 or 93654. Fluoroscopic guidance is included in electrophysiological procedures and should not be reported separately.

ICD-10-CM Diagnostic Codes

This/these CPT code(s) are add on code(s). See the primary procedure code that this code is performed with for your ICD-10-CM code selections. Diagnostic code(s) would be the same as the actual procedure performed.

AMA: **93613** 2018,Jan,8; 2018,Feb,11; 2017,Jan,8; 2016,Jan,13; 2015,Jan,16; 2014,Jan,11; 2014,Apr,3; 2013,Jun,6-8; 2013,Jul,7-9

Relative Value Units/Medicare Edits

Non-Facility RVU	Work	PE	MP	Total
93613	5.23	2.19	1.21	8.63
Facility RVU	**Work**	**PE**	**MP**	**Total**
93613	5.23	2.19	1.21	8.63

	FUD	Status	MUE	Modifiers				IOM Reference
93613	N/A	A	1(3)	N/A	N/A	N/A	80*	None

* with documentation

Terms To Know

dysrhythmia. Abnormality or disturbance in rhythm.

electrophysiologic studies. Electrical stimulation and monitoring to diagnose heart conduction abnormalities that predispose patients to bradyarrhythmias and to determine a patient's chance for developing ventricular and supraventricular tachyarrhythmias.

moderate sedation. Medically controlled state of depressed consciousness, with or without analgesia, while maintaining the patient's airway, protective reflexes, and ability to respond to stimulation or verbal commands.

ventricular tachycardia. Excessively rapid ventricular rhythm of the heart, usually more than 150 beats per minute, with an origin beat generated in the ventricle, commonly from atrioventricular dissociation.

93615-93616

93615 Esophageal recording of atrial electrogram with or without ventricular electrogram(s);

93616 with pacing

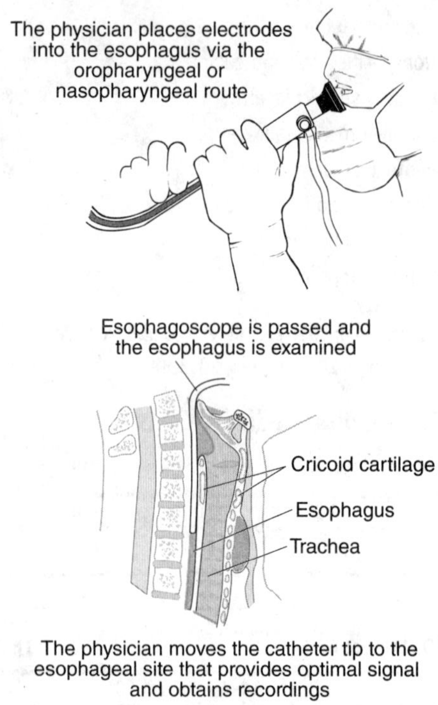

Explanation

The physician places electrodes into the esophagus via an oropharyngeal or nasopharyngeal route. The physician attaches the catheter to an electrical recording device to allow depiction of the esophageal electrograms obtained from electrodes on the catheter tip. The physician moves the catheter tip to the esophageal site that provides the optimal signal and obtains recordings. The physician compares the esophageal and surface electrograms to identify the mechanism of the arrhythmia. Report 93616 when the physician measures the heart's electrical function using a catheter placed into the patient's esophagus. The recording electrode at the end of the probe measures electrical activity of the atrium by pacing with or without recording activity of the ventricle.

Coding Tips

When medically necessary, report moderate (conscious) sedation provided by the performing physician with 99151-99153. When provided by another physician, report 99155-99157. As exempt from modifier 51, 93615 and 93616 have not been designated in CPT as add-on services/procedures. However, codes identified as exempt from modifier 51 are not subject to multiple procedure rules. No reimbursement reduction or modifier 51 is applied. Procedures 93615 and 93616 have both a technical and professional component. To report only the professional component, append modifier 26. To report only the technical component, append modifier TC. To report the complete procedure (i.e., both the professional and technical components), submit without a modifier. Fluoroscopic guidance is included in electrophysiological procedures and should not be reported separately.

ICD-10-CM Diagnostic Codes

I44.0	Atrioventricular block, first degree
I44.1	Atrioventricular block, second degree

I44.2	Atrioventricular block, complete
I44.39	Other atrioventricular block
I45.4	Nonspecific intraventricular block
I45.5	Other specified heart block
I45.6	Pre-excitation syndrome
I45.89	Other specified conduction disorders
I47.0	Re-entry ventricular arrhythmia
I47.1	Supraventricular tachycardia
I47.2	Ventricular tachycardia
I48.0	Paroxysmal atrial fibrillation
I48.11	Longstanding persistent atrial fibrillation
I48.19	Other persistent atrial fibrillation
I48.21	Permanent atrial fibrillation
I48.3	Typical atrial flutter
I48.4	Atypical atrial flutter
I49.01	Ventricular fibrillation
I49.02	Ventricular flutter

AMA: 93615 2018,Jan,8; 2018,Feb,11; 2017,Jan,8; 2016,Jan,13; 2015,Jan,16; 2014,Jan,11 **93616** 2018,Jan,8; 2018,Feb,11; 2017,Jan,8; 2016,Jan,13; 2015,Jan,16; 2014,Jan,11

Relative Value Units/Medicare Edits

Non-Facility RVU	Work	PE	MP	Total
93615	0.0	0.0	0.0	0.0
93616	0.0	0.0	0.0	0.0
Facility RVU	**Work**	**PE**	**MP**	**Total**
93615	0.0	0.0	0.0	0.0
93616	0.0	0.0	0.0	0.0

	FUD	Status	MUE	Modifiers				IOM Reference
93615	0	C	1(3)	N/A	N/A	N/A	80*	None
93616	0	C	1(3)	N/A	N/A	N/A	80*	

* with documentation

Terms To Know

arrhythmias. Heart disorder of rhythm or rate, due to an electrical conduction system malfunction.

dysrhythmia. Abnormality or disturbance in rhythm.

93618

93618 Induction of arrhythmia by electrical pacing

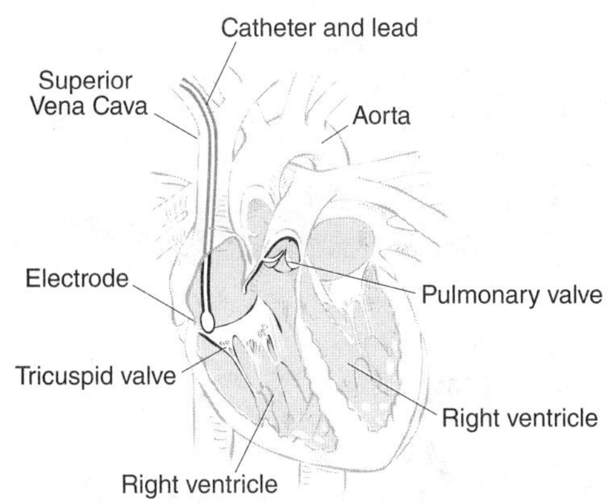

Arrhythmia is induced through electrical pacing. Usually the procedure is performed in conjunction with mapping of an area of the heart

Explanation

The physician places an appropriate arterial or venous sheath, usually femoral, to allow access to the chamber to be studied. The physician advances an electrical catheter through the sheath and into the appropriate chamber under fluoroscopic guidance. The physician attaches the catheter to an electrical pacing device to allow transmission of pacing impulses through the catheter to the heart chamber of interest. The physician stimulates the heart with rapid pacing or programmed electrical stimulation until the arrhythmia is induced.

Coding Tips

When medically necessary, report moderate (conscious) sedation provided by the performing physician with 99151-99153. When provided by another physician, report 99155-99157. As exempt from modifier 51, 93618 has not been designated in CPT as an add-on service/procedure. However, codes identified as exempt from modifier 51 are not subject to multiple procedure rules. No reimbursement reduction or modifier 51 is applied. Procedure 93618 has both a technical and professional component. To report only the professional component, append modifier 26. To report only the technical component, append modifier TC. To report the complete procedure (i.e., both the professional and technical components), submit without a modifier. Fluoroscopic guidance is included in electrophysiological procedures and should not be reported separately. Procedure 93618 reports induction of arrhythmia only. For comprehensive electrophysiologic evaluation, including induction of arrhythmia, see 93620–93622. Do not report 93618 with 93619, 93620–93622, 93653, 93654, or 93656. For intracardiac phonocardiogram, see 93799. Moderate sedation performed with 93618 is considered to be an integral part of the procedure and is not reported separately. However, anesthesia services (00100–01999) may be billed separately when performed by a physician (or other qualified provider) other than the physician performing the procedure.

ICD-10-CM Diagnostic Codes

I45.89	Other specified conduction disorders
I47.0	Re-entry ventricular arrhythmia
I47.1	Supraventricular tachycardia
I47.2	Ventricular tachycardia
I48.0	Paroxysmal atrial fibrillation
I48.11	Longstanding persistent atrial fibrillation

I48.19	Other persistent atrial fibrillation
I48.21	Permanent atrial fibrillation
I48.3	Typical atrial flutter
I48.4	Atypical atrial flutter
I49.01	Ventricular fibrillation
I49.02	Ventricular flutter
I49.1	Atrial premature depolarization
I49.2	Junctional premature depolarization
I49.3	Ventricular premature depolarization
I49.49	Other premature depolarization
I49.5	Sick sinus syndrome
I49.8	Other specified cardiac arrhythmias
R55	Syncope and collapse

AMA: **93618** 2018,Jan,8; 2018,Feb,11; 2017,Jan,8; 2016,Jan,13; 2015,Jan,16; 2014,Jan,11; 2014,Apr,3; 2013,Jun,6-8; 2013,Jul,7-9

Relative Value Units/Medicare Edits

Non-Facility RVU	Work	PE	MP	Total
93618	0.0	0.0	0.0	0.0
Facility RVU	**Work**	**PE**	**MP**	**Total**
93618	0.0	0.0	0.0	0.0

	FUD	Status	MUE	Modifiers				IOM Reference
93618	0	C	1(3)	N/A	N/A	N/A	80*	None

* with documentation

Terms To Know

arrhythmias. Heart disorder of rhythm or rate, due to an electrical conduction system malfunction.

fluoroscopy. Radiology technique that allows visual examination of part of the body or a function of an organ using a device that projects an x-ray image on a fluorescent screen.

93619

93619 Comprehensive electrophysiologic evaluation with right atrial pacing and recording, right ventricular pacing and recording, His bundle recording, including insertion and repositioning of multiple electrode catheters, without induction or attempted induction of arrhythmia

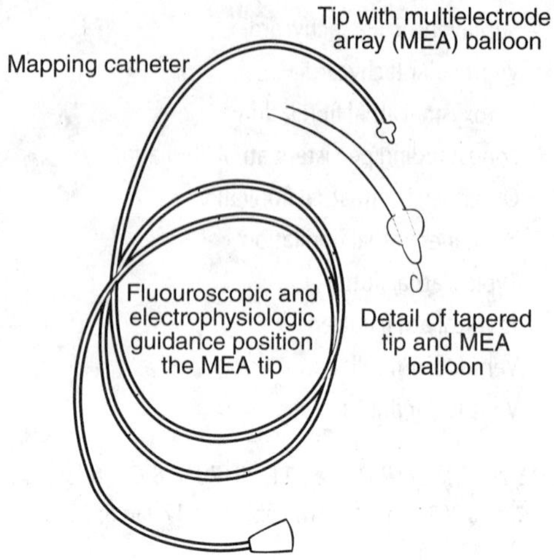

The right atrium and right ventricle are paced and recorded; the His bundle along the septum is recorded without any attempt to induce arrhythmia

Explanation

The physician places three venous sheaths, usually in one or both femoral veins, using standard techniques. The physician advances three electrical catheters through the venous sheaths and into the right heart under fluoroscopic guidance. The physician attaches the three catheters to an electrical recording device to allow depiction of the intracardiac electrograms obtained from electrodes on the catheter tips. The physician moves the tips of the three catheters to the right atrium, the bundle of His, and the right ventricle and obtains recordings.

Coding Tips

When medically necessary, report moderate (conscious) sedation provided by the performing physician with 99151-99153. When provided by another physician, report 99155-99157. Procedure 93619 has both a technical and professional component. To report only the professional component, append modifier 26. To report only the technical component, append modifier TC. To report the complete procedure (i.e., both the professional and technical components), submit without a modifier. Fluoroscopic guidance is included in electrophysiological procedures and should not be reported separately. Do not report 93619 with 93600, 93602, 93603, 93610, 93612, 93618, 93620–93622, or 93653–93657.

ICD-10-CM Diagnostic Codes

I44.0	Atrioventricular block, first degree
I44.1	Atrioventricular block, second degree
I44.2	Atrioventricular block, complete
I44.30	Unspecified atrioventricular block
I44.39	Other atrioventricular block
I44.4	Left anterior fascicular block
I44.5	Left posterior fascicular block
I44.69	Other fascicular block
I45.0	Right fascicular block

I45.19	Other right bundle-branch block
I45.2	Bifascicular block
I45.3	Trifascicular block
I45.4	Nonspecific intraventricular block
I45.5	Other specified heart block
I45.6	Pre-excitation syndrome
I45.89	Other specified conduction disorders
I47.0	Re-entry ventricular arrhythmia
I47.1	Supraventricular tachycardia
I47.2	Ventricular tachycardia
I48.0	Paroxysmal atrial fibrillation
I48.11	Longstanding persistent atrial fibrillation
I48.19	Other persistent atrial fibrillation
I48.21	Permanent atrial fibrillation
I48.3	Typical atrial flutter
I48.4	Atypical atrial flutter
I49.01	Ventricular fibrillation
I49.02	Ventricular flutter
I49.1	Atrial premature depolarization
I49.2	Junctional premature depolarization
I49.3	Ventricular premature depolarization
I49.49	Other premature depolarization
I49.5	Sick sinus syndrome
I49.8	Other specified cardiac arrhythmias
P29.81	Cardiac arrest of newborn
R55	Syncope and collapse

AMA: 93619 2018,Jan,8; 2018,Feb,11; 2017,Jan,8; 2016,Jan,13; 2015,Jan,16; 2014,Jan,11; 2014,Apr,3; 2013,Jun,6-8; 2013,Jul,7-9

Relative Value Units/Medicare Edits

Non-Facility RVU	Work	PE	MP	Total
93619	0.0	0.0	0.0	0.0
Facility RVU	**Work**	**PE**	**MP**	**Total**
93619	0.0	0.0	0.0	0.0

	FUD	Status	MUE	Modifiers				IOM Reference
93619	0	C	1(3)	51	N/A	N/A	80*	100-03,20.12

* with documentation

93620

93620 Comprehensive electrophysiologic evaluation including insertion and repositioning of multiple electrode catheters with induction or attempted induction of arrhythmia; with right atrial pacing and recording, right ventricular pacing and recording, His bundle recording

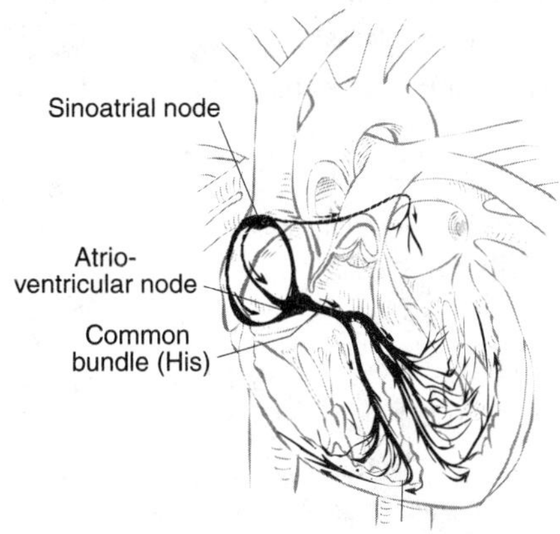

Conduction system of the heart

Explanation

The electrophysiologist places three venous sheaths, usually in one or both femoral veins, using standard techniques. Three electrical catheters are threaded through the venous sheaths and into the right heart under fluoroscopic guidance. The catheters are attached to an electrical recording device to allow depiction of the intracardiac electrograms obtained from electrodes on the catheter tips. The physician moves the tips of the catheters to the high right atrium, the bundle of His, and the right ventricle and obtains recordings. The physician then attaches the catheters to an electrical pacing device to allow transmission of pacing impulses through the catheters to the different heart chambers. The physician stimulates the heart with rapid pacing or programmed electrical stimulation in an attempt to induce an arrhythmia.

Coding Tips

When medically necessary, report moderate (conscious) sedation provided by the performing physician with 99151-99153. When provided by another physician, report 99155-99157. Procedure 93620 has both a technical and professional component. To report only the professional component, append modifier 26. To report only the technical component, append modifier TC. To report the complete procedure (i.e., both the professional and technical components), submit without a modifier. Fluoroscopic guidance is included in electrophysiological procedures and should not be reported separately. Do not report 93620 with 93600, 93602, 93603, 93610, 93612, 93618, 93619, or 93653–93657.

ICD-10-CM Diagnostic Codes

I44.0	Atrioventricular block, first degree
I44.1	Atrioventricular block, second degree
I44.2	Atrioventricular block, complete
I44.39	Other atrioventricular block
I44.4	Left anterior fascicular block
I44.5	Left posterior fascicular block
I44.69	Other fascicular block
I45.0	Right fascicular block
I45.19	Other right bundle-branch block

I45.2	Bifascicular block
I45.3	Trifascicular block
I45.4	Nonspecific intraventricular block
I45.5	Other specified heart block
I45.6	Pre-excitation syndrome
I45.89	Other specified conduction disorders
I46.2	Cardiac arrest due to underlying cardiac condition
I46.8	Cardiac arrest due to other underlying condition
I47.0	Re-entry ventricular arrhythmia
I47.1	Supraventricular tachycardia
I47.2	Ventricular tachycardia
I48.0	Paroxysmal atrial fibrillation
I48.11	Longstanding persistent atrial fibrillation
I48.21	Permanent atrial fibrillation
I48.3	Typical atrial flutter
I48.4	Atypical atrial flutter
I49.01	Ventricular fibrillation
I49.02	Ventricular flutter
I49.1	Atrial premature depolarization
I49.2	Junctional premature depolarization
I49.3	Ventricular premature depolarization
I49.49	Other premature depolarization
I49.5	Sick sinus syndrome
I49.8	Other specified cardiac arrhythmias
P29.81	Cardiac arrest of newborn
R55	Syncope and collapse

AMA: 93620 2018,Jan,8; 2018,Feb,11; 2017,Jan,8; 2016,Jan,13; 2015,Jan,16; 2014,Jan,11; 2014,Apr,3; 2013,Jun,6-8; 2013,Jul,7-9

Relative Value Units/Medicare Edits

Non-Facility RVU	Work	PE	MP	Total
93620	0.0	0.0	0.0	0.0
Facility RVU	**Work**	**PE**	**MP**	**Total**
93620	0.0	0.0	0.0	0.0

	FUD	Status	MUE	Modifiers				IOM Reference
93620	0	C	1(3)	51	N/A	N/A	80*	None

* with documentation

Terms To Know

arrhythmias. Heart disorder of rhythm or rate, due to an electrical conduction system malfunction.

dysrhythmia. Abnormality or disturbance in rhythm.

fluoroscopy. Radiology technique that allows visual examination of part of the body or a function of an organ using a device that projects an x-ray image on a fluorescent screen.

Lown (-Ganong)-Levine syndrome. Electrocardiographic disorder indicated by a short P-R interval with normal duration of the QRS complex.

Medicine

93621

+ 93621 Comprehensive electrophysiologic evaluation including insertion and repositioning of multiple electrode catheters with induction or attempted induction of arrhythmia; with left atrial pacing and recording from coronary sinus or left atrium (List separately in addition to code for primary procedure)

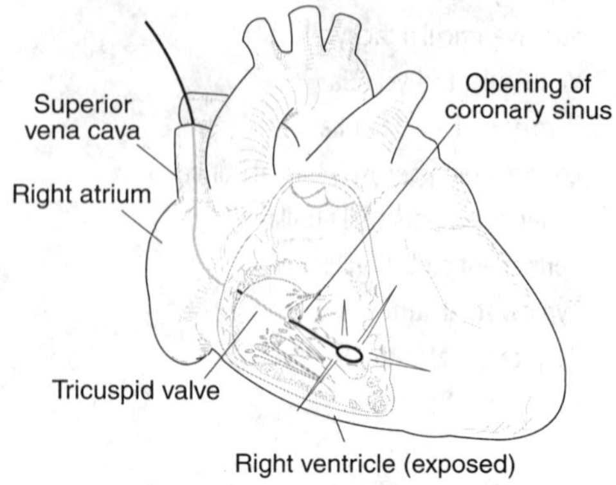

The catheters may be advanced through the venous system and the right side of the heart, or through to the left ventricle via the foramen ovale

Explanation

The physician places four central venous sheaths using standard techniques. Four electrical catheters are threaded through the venous sheaths and into the right heart under fluoroscopic guidance. The catheters are attached to an electrical recording device to allow depiction of the intracardiac electrograms obtained from electrodes on the catheter tips. The physician moves the tips of the catheters to the high right atrium, the bundle of His, the right ventricle, and through the coronary sinus to the left atrium and obtains recordings. The physician attaches the catheters to an electrical pacing device to allow transmission of pacing impulses through the catheters to the different heart chambers. The physician stimulates the heart with rapid pacing or programmed electrical stimulation in an attempt to induce an arrhythmia.

Coding Tips

When medically necessary, report moderate (conscious) sedation provided by the performing physician with 99151-99153. When provided by another physician, report 99155-99157. Report 93621 in addition to 93620, 93653, or 93654. Do not report 93621 with 93656. Procedure 93621 has both a technical and professional component. To report only the professional component, append modifier 26. To report only the technical component, append modifier TC. To report the complete procedure (i.e., both the professional and technical components), submit without a modifier. Fluoroscopic guidance is included in electrophysiological procedures and should not be reported separately.

ICD-10-CM Diagnostic Codes

This/these CPT code(s) are add on code(s). See the primary procedure code that this code is performed with for your ICD-10-CM code selections. Diagnostic code(s) would be the same as the actual procedure performed.

AMA: 93621 2018,Jan,8; 2018,Feb,11; 2017,Jan,8; 2016,Jan,13; 2015,Jan,16; 2014,Jan,11; 2014,Apr,3; 2013,Jun,6-8; 2013,Jul,7-9

Relative Value Units/Medicare Edits

Non-Facility RVU	Work	PE	MP	Total
93621	0.0	0.0	0.0	0.0
Facility RVU	**Work**	**PE**	**MP**	**Total**
93621	0.0	0.0	0.0	0.0

	FUD	Status	MUE	Modifiers				IOM Reference
93621	N/A	C	1(3)	N/A	N/A	N/A	80*	None

* with documentation

Terms To Know

arrhythmia. Irregular heartbeat.

electrophysiologic studies. Electrical stimulation and monitoring to diagnose heart conduction abnormalities that predispose patients to bradyarrhythmias and to determine a patient's chance for developing ventricular and supraventricular tachyarrhythmias.

fluoroscopy. Radiology technique that allows visual examination of part of the body or a function of an organ using a device that projects an x-ray image on a fluorescent screen.

paroxysmal supraventricular tachycardia. Rapid heartbeat that starts above the ventricles and occurs sporadically.

supraventricular tachycardia. Rapid beating of the heart, usually pertains to more than 100 beats per minute and can be as high as 250 beats per minute. SVT is caused by abnormal electrical impulses originating at the AV node or above it in the atria (upper chambers) of the heart.

93622

\+ **93622** Comprehensive electrophysiologic evaluation including insertion and repositioning of multiple electrode catheters with induction or attempted induction of arrhythmia; with left ventricular pacing and recording (List separately in addition to code for primary procedure)

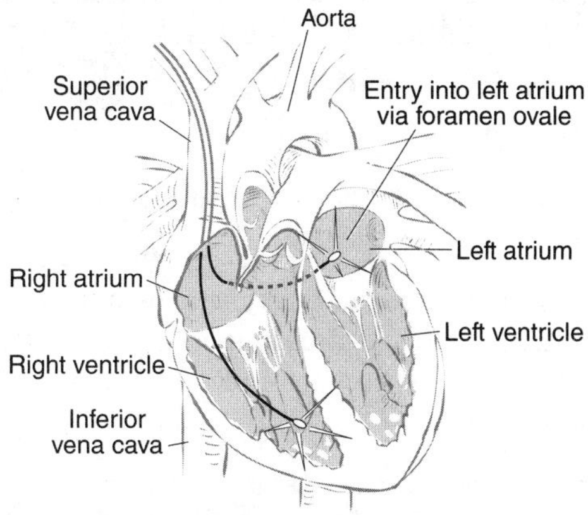

The left ventricle is paced and recorded, either remotely from the right side of the heart or intraventricularly

Explanation

The physician places three central venous sheaths and an arterial sheath using standard techniques. The physician advances four electrical catheters through these sheaths and into the heart under fluoroscopic guidance. The physician attaches the four catheters to an electrical recording device to allow depiction of the intracardiac electrograms obtained from electrodes on the catheter tips. The physician moves the tips of the four catheters to the right atrium, the bundle of His, the right ventricle, and the left ventricle and obtains recordings. The physician may attach the catheters to an electrical pacing device to allow transmission of pacing impulses through the catheters to the different heart chambers. The physician may stimulate the heart with rapid pacing or programmed electrical stimulation in an attempt to induce an arrhythmia.

Coding Tips

When medically necessary, report moderate (conscious) sedation provided by the performing physician with 99151-99153. When provided by another physician, report 99155-99157. Report 93622 in addition to 93620, 93653, or 93656. Do not report 93622 with 93654. Procedure 93622 has both a technical and professional component. To report only the professional component, append modifier 26. To report only the technical component, append modifier TC. To report the complete procedure (i.e., both the professional and technical components), submit without a modifier. Fluoroscopic guidance is included in electrophysiological procedures and should not be reported separately.

ICD-10-CM Diagnostic Codes

This/these CPT code(s) are add on code(s). See the primary procedure code that this code is performed with for your ICD-10-CM code selections. Diagnostic code(s) would be the same as the actual procedure performed.

AMA: 93622 2018,Jan,8; 2018,Feb,11; 2017,Jan,8; 2016,Jan,13; 2015,Jan,16; 2014,Jan,11; 2014,Apr,3; 2013,Jun,6-8; 2013,Jul,7-9

Relative Value Units/Medicare Edits

Non-Facility RVU	Work	PE	MP	Total
93622	0.0	0.0	0.0	0.0
Facility RVU	Work	PE	MP	Total
93622	0.0	0.0	0.0	0.0

	FUD	Status	MUE	Modifiers				IOM Reference
93622	N/A	C	1(3)	N/A	N/A	N/A	80*	None

* with documentation

Terms To Know

arrhythmias. Heart disorder of rhythm or rate, due to an electrical conduction system malfunction.

bundle of His. Bundle of modified cardiac fibers that begins at the atrioventricular node and passes through the right atrioventricular fibrous ring to the interventricular septum, where it divides into two branches. Bundle of His recordings are taken for intracardiac electrograms.

fluoroscopy. Radiology technique that allows visual examination of part of the body or a function of an organ using a device that projects an x-ray image on a fluorescent screen.

Lown (-Ganong)-Levine syndrome. Electrocardiographic disorder indicated by a short P-R interval with normal duration of the QRS complex.

moderate sedation. Medically controlled state of depressed consciousness, with or without analgesia, while maintaining the patient's airway, protective reflexes, and ability to respond to stimulation or verbal commands.

93623

+ 93623 Programmed stimulation and pacing after intravenous drug infusion (List separately in addition to code for primary procedure)

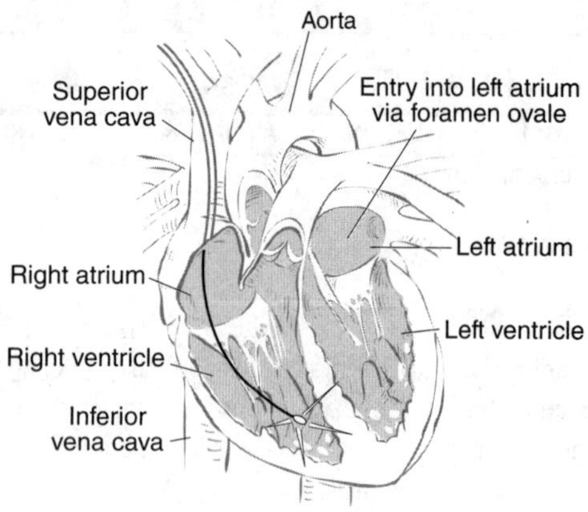

Stimulation and pacing is carried out as specified in previous codes, but an IV drug infusion occurs as a component of this procedure

Explanation

Following a comprehensive electrophysiological study with or without attempted or actual induction of an arrhythmia, before the electrode catheters are removed, an intravenous drug, such as isoproterenol, is infused. The physician attaches the catheter to an electrical pacing device to allow transmission of pacing impulses through the catheter to the heart chamber of interest. The heart is stimulated using rapid pacing or programmed electrical stimulation in an attempt to induce an arrhythmia. This code is reported in addition to the code for the primary electrophysiological procedure.

Coding Tips

Report 93623 in addition to 93610, 93612, 93619, 93620, 93653, 93654, or 93656. Procedure 93623 has both a technical and professional component. To report only the professional component, append modifier 26. To report only the technical component, append modifier TC. To report the complete procedure (i.e., both the professional and technical components), submit without a modifier. Only report 93623 once per day. Fluoroscopic guidance is included in electrophysiological procedures and should not be reported separately.

ICD-10-CM Diagnostic Codes

This/these CPT code(s) are add on code(s). See the primary procedure code that this code is performed with for your ICD-10-CM code selections. Diagnostic code(s) would be the same as the actual procedure performed.

AMA: **93623** 2018,Jan,8; 2018,Feb,11; 2017,Jan,8; 2016,Jan,13; 2015,Jan,16; 2014,Jan,11; 2014,Apr,3; 2013,Jul,7-9

Relative Value Units/Medicare Edits

Non-Facility RVU	Work	PE	MP	Total
93623	0.0	0.0	0.0	0.0
Facility RVU	Work	PE	MP	Total
93623	0.0	0.0	0.0	0.0

	FUD	Status	MUE	Modifiers				IOM Reference
93623	N/A	C	1(3)	N/A	N/A	N/A	80*	None

* with documentation

Terms To Know

arrhythmia induction. Heart disorder of rhythm or rate, due to an electrical conduction system malfunction. A. induction: Intentional performance of cardiac pacing into arrhythmic states at different rates by the introduction of critically timed electrical impulses. This is usually included as part of an intracardiac electrophysiological study to determine where the disruption of the heart's normal pattern of conduction occurs, and help identify the proper treatment or its effectiveness for the patient's rhythm abnormalities.

electrophysiologic studies. Electrical stimulation and monitoring to diagnose heart conduction abnormalities that predispose patients to bradyarrhythmias and to determine a patient's chance for developing ventricular and supraventricular tachyarrhythmias.

intravenous. Within a vein or veins.

93624

93624 Electrophysiologic follow-up study with pacing and recording to test effectiveness of therapy, including induction or attempted induction of arrhythmia

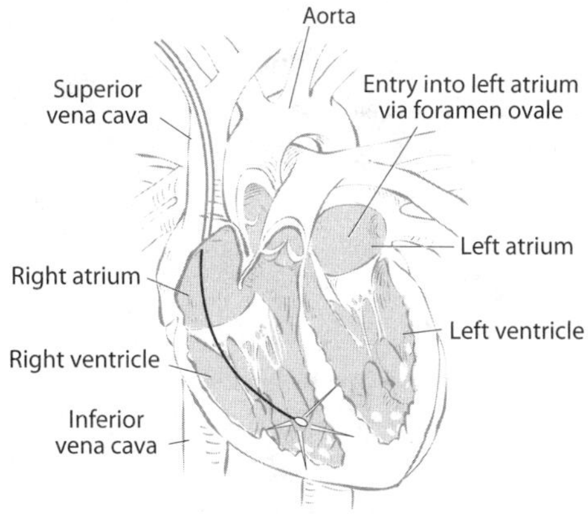

A follow-up EPS is performed with pacing and recording to test the effectiveness of therapy

Explanation

Following administration of therapy (antiarrhythmic drugs, surgery, ablation, etc.), the physician places an appropriate arterial or venous sheath, usually femoral, to allow access to the chamber to be studied. Under fluoroscopic guidance, the physician advances an electrical catheter through the sheath and into the appropriate chamber. An intravenous drug, such as isoproterenol, is infused. The physician attaches the catheter to an electrical pacing device to allow transmission of pacing impulses through the catheter to the heart chamber of interest. The physician stimulates the heart with rapid pacing or programmed electrical stimulation in an attempt to induce an arrhythmia.

Coding Tips

When medically necessary, report moderate (conscious) sedation provided by the performing physician with 99151-99153. When provided by another physician, report 99155-99157. Procedure 93624 has both a technical and professional component. To report only the professional component, append modifier 26. To report only the technical component, append modifier TC. To report the complete procedure (i.e., both the professional and technical components), submit without a modifier. Fluoroscopic guidance is included in electrophysiological procedures and should not be reported separately.

ICD-10-CM Diagnostic Codes

I44.0	Atrioventricular block, first degree
I44.1	Atrioventricular block, second degree
I44.2	Atrioventricular block, complete
I44.39	Other atrioventricular block
I44.4	Left anterior fascicular block
I44.5	Left posterior fascicular block
I44.69	Other fascicular block
I45.0	Right fascicular block
I45.19	Other right bundle-branch block
I45.2	Bifascicular block
I45.3	Trifascicular block
I45.4	Nonspecific intraventricular block
I45.5	Other specified heart block
I45.6	Pre-excitation syndrome

I45.89	Other specified conduction disorders
I46.2	Cardiac arrest due to underlying cardiac condition
I46.8	Cardiac arrest due to other underlying condition
I47.0	Re-entry ventricular arrhythmia
I47.1	Supraventricular tachycardia
I47.2	Ventricular tachycardia
I48.0	Paroxysmal atrial fibrillation
I48.11	Longstanding persistent atrial fibrillation
I48.19	Other persistent atrial fibrillation
I48.21	Permanent atrial fibrillation
I48.3	Typical atrial flutter
I48.4	Atypical atrial flutter
I49.01	Ventricular fibrillation
I49.02	Ventricular flutter
I49.1	Atrial premature depolarization
I49.2	Junctional premature depolarization
I49.3	Ventricular premature depolarization
I49.49	Other premature depolarization
I49.5	Sick sinus syndrome
I49.8	Other specified cardiac arrhythmias

AMA: 93624 2018,Jan,8; 2018,Feb,11; 2017,Jan,8; 2016,Jan,13; 2015,Jan,16; 2014,Jan,11

Relative Value Units/Medicare Edits

Non-Facility RVU	Work	PE	MP	Total
93624	0.0	0.0	0.0	0.0
Facility RVU	**Work**	**PE**	**MP**	**Total**
93624	0.0	0.0	0.0	0.0

	FUD	Status	MUE	Modifiers				IOM Reference
93624	0	C	1(3)	51	N/A	N/A	80*	100-03,20.12

* with documentation

93631

93631 Intra-operative epicardial and endocardial pacing and mapping to localize the site of tachycardia or zone of slow conduction for surgical correction

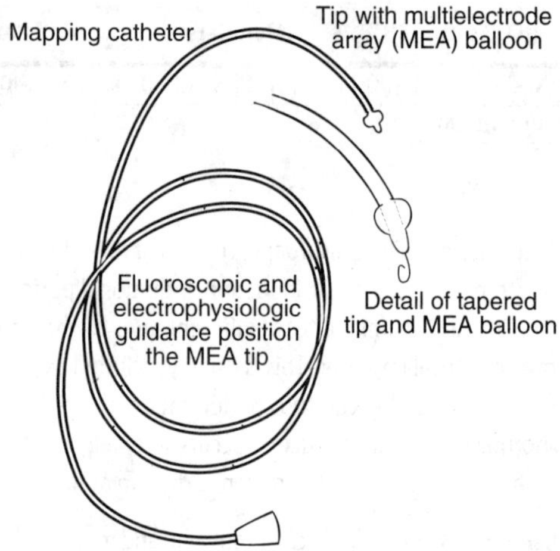

The physician places mapping and pacing catheters inside the heart prior to or during surgery using a standard transvenous approach. The tachycardia site or zone of slow conduction is localized so that it can be surgically corrected

Explanation

The purpose of this procedure is to localize the site of tachycardia during open-heart surgery to allow surgical correction of the tachycardia. The physician may place pacing or mapping catheters inside the heart prior to or during surgery using a standard transvenous approach. Additionally, the surgeon will place electrical probes on the outside (epicardium) of the heart in order to allow additional mapping. The physician attaches the catheters and probes to an electrical recording device to allow depiction of the electrograms obtained from electrodes on the catheter and probe tips. The surgeon's electrical probe can be moved around the outside of the heart to allow comparison of electrical activation times from different regions. The physician may attach the catheters to an electrical pacing device to allow transmission of pacing impulses through the catheters to the different heart chambers. The physician may stimulate the heart with rapid pacing or programmed electrical stimulation in an attempt to induce an arrhythmia.

Coding Tips

As exempt from modifier 51, 93631 has not been designated in CPT as an add-on service/procedure. However, codes identified as exempt from modifier 51 are not subject to multiple procedure rules. No reimbursement reduction or modifier 51 is applied. When an open heart ablation procedure is performed, the cardiothoracic surgeon typically performs the ablation component (33250–33261) and the electrophysiologist performs the pacing and mapping component (93631). Modifiers for multiple procedures, co-surgeons, and assistant surgeons are not reported with the two components because the individual codes describe the separate components that each physician performs. Procedure 93631 has both a technical and professional component. To report only the professional component, append modifier 26. To report only the technical component, append modifier TC. To report the complete procedure (i.e., both the professional and technical components), submit without a modifier.

ICD-10-CM Diagnostic Codes

I45.89	Other specified conduction disorders

I47.0 Re-entry ventricular arrhythmia
I47.1 Supraventricular tachycardia
I47.2 Ventricular tachycardia
I48.0 Paroxysmal atrial fibrillation
I48.11 Longstanding persistent atrial fibrillation
I48.19 Other persistent atrial fibrillation
I48.21 Permanent atrial fibrillation
I48.3 Typical atrial flutter
I48.4 Atypical atrial flutter
I49.01 Ventricular fibrillation
I49.02 Ventricular flutter
I49.1 Atrial premature depolarization
I49.2 Junctional premature depolarization
I49.3 Ventricular premature depolarization
I49.49 Other premature depolarization
I49.5 Sick sinus syndrome
I49.8 Other specified cardiac arrhythmias

AMA: **93631** 2018,Jan,8; 2018,Feb,11; 2017,Jan,8; 2016,Jan,13; 2015,Jan,16; 2014,Jan,11

Relative Value Units/Medicare Edits

Non-Facility RVU	Work	PE	MP	Total
93631	0.0	0.0	0.0	0.0
Facility RVU	**Work**	**PE**	**MP**	**Total**
93631	0.0	0.0	0.0	0.0

	FUD	Status	MUE	Modifiers				IOM Reference
93631	0	C	1(3)	N/A	N/A	N/A	80*	100-03,20.11

* with documentation

93640-93641

93640 Electrophysiologic evaluation of single or dual chamber pacing cardioverter-defibrillator leads including defibrillation threshold evaluation (induction of arrhythmia, evaluation of sensing and pacing for arrhythmia termination) at time of initial implantation or replacement;

93641 with testing of single or dual chamber pacing cardioverter-defibrillator pulse generator

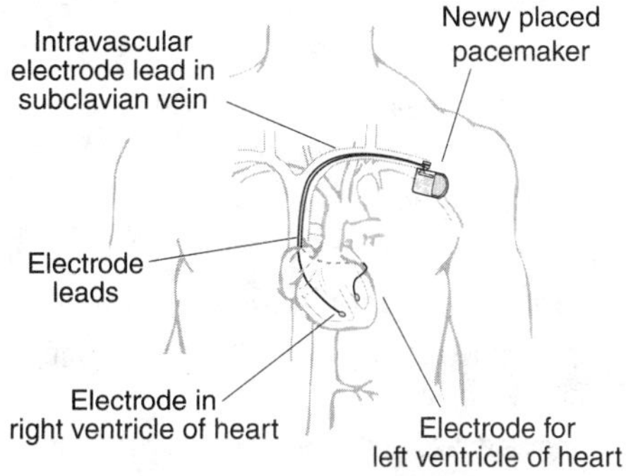

Testing is performed on cardioverter-defibrillator leads and pulse generator to ensure that they are functioning properly

Explanation

The purpose of this study is to ensure that the cardioverter-defibrillator (ICD) leads are positioned well and working properly, to guarantee proper function of this device in the future. Leads are typically placed in the heart via the subclavian vein, but occasionally defibrillation patches are placed on the epicardium or under the skin. To test the leads, the physician records cardiac electrical signals and paces the heart through the leads. The physician may test the leads using the actual ICD or by hooking the leads to an external device. The physician uses the leads to pace the heart into an arrhythmia, such as ventricular tachycardia or fibrillation. The ICD or external device detects the arrhythmia and shocks the heart through the ICD leads. The physician may perform this test with several different levels of shock to ensure that the ICD can reliably terminate the arrhythmia. In 93640, only the leads are tested. In 93641, both the leads and the cardioverter-defibrillator pulse generator are tested.

Coding Tips

When medically necessary, report moderate (conscious) sedation provided by the performing physician with 99151-99153. When provided by another physician, report 99155-99157. Codes 93640 and 93641 are reported in addition to the insertion codes at the time of implantation or replacement of the single or dual chamber pacing cardioverter-defibrillator electrode leads (93640) or pulse generator (93641). Induction of arrhythmia is included in 93640 and 93641. Do not report 93618 separately. Procedures 93640 and 93641 have both a technical and professional component. To report only the professional component, append modifier 26. To report only the technical component, append modifier TC. To report the complete procedure (i.e., both the professional and technical components), submit without a modifier. For subsequent or periodic electronic analysis and/or reprogramming of single or dual chamber pacing cardioverter-defibrillators, see 93282, 93283, 93289, 93292, 93295, and 93642.

ICD-10-CM Diagnostic Codes

I45.89 Other specified conduction disorders
I47.0 Re-entry ventricular arrhythmia

I47.1	Supraventricular tachycardia
I47.2	Ventricular tachycardia
I48.0	Paroxysmal atrial fibrillation
I48.11	Longstanding persistent atrial fibrillation
I48.19	Other persistent atrial fibrillation
I48.21	Permanent atrial fibrillation
I48.3	Typical atrial flutter
I48.4	Atypical atrial flutter
I49.01	Ventricular fibrillation
I49.02	Ventricular flutter
I49.1	Atrial premature depolarization
I49.2	Junctional premature depolarization
I49.3	Ventricular premature depolarization
I49.49	Other premature depolarization
I49.5	Sick sinus syndrome
I49.8	Other specified cardiac arrhythmias
T82.817A	Embolism due to cardiac prosthetic devices, implants and grafts, initial encounter
T82.827A	Fibrosis due to cardiac prosthetic devices, implants and grafts, initial encounter
T82.837A	Hemorrhage due to cardiac prosthetic devices, implants and grafts, initial encounter
T82.847A	Pain due to cardiac prosthetic devices, implants and grafts, initial encounter
T82.857A	Stenosis of other cardiac prosthetic devices, implants and grafts, initial encounter
T82.867A	Thrombosis due to cardiac prosthetic devices, implants and grafts, initial encounter
T82.897A	Other specified complication of cardiac prosthetic devices, implants and grafts, initial encounter
Z45.02	Encounter for adjustment and management of automatic implantable cardiac defibrillator
Z95.810	Presence of automatic (implantable) cardiac defibrillator

AMA: 93640 2018,Jan,8; 2018,Feb,11; 2017,Jan,8; 2016,Jan,13; 2015,Jan,16; 2014,Jan,11 **93641** 2018,Jan,8; 2018,Feb,11; 2017,Jan,8; 2016,Jan,13; 2015,Jan,16; 2014,Jan,11; 2014,Apr,3

Relative Value Units/Medicare Edits

Non-Facility RVU	Work	PE	MP	Total
93640	0.0	0.0	0.0	0.0
93641	0.0	0.0	0.0	0.0
Facility RVU	**Work**	**PE**	**MP**	**Total**
93640	0.0	0.0	0.0	0.0
93641	0.0	0.0	0.0	0.0

	FUD	Status	MUE	Modifiers				IOM Reference
93640	0	C	1(3)	51	N/A	N/A	80*	100-03,20.12
93641	0	C	1(2)	51	N/A	N/A	80*	

* with documentation

93642

93642 Electrophysiologic evaluation of single or dual chamber transvenous pacing cardioverter-defibrillator (includes defibrillation threshold evaluation, induction of arrhythmia, evaluation of sensing and pacing for arrhythmia termination, and programming or reprogramming of sensing or therapeutic parameters)

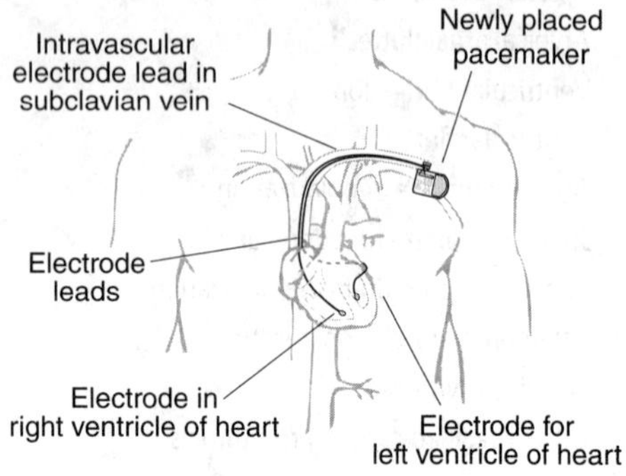

Testing is performed on cardioverter-defibrillator leads and pulse generator to ensure that they are functioning properly

Explanation

The purpose of this study is to ensure that the transvenous pacing cardioverter-defibrillator (ICD) and ICD leads are positioned well and working properly, to guarantee proper function of this device in the future. The physician records cardiac electrical signals from the leads and paces the heart through the leads to determine pacing threshold. The physician uses the ICD pulse generator to pace the heart into an arrhythmia, such as ventricular tachycardia or fibrillation. The ICD detects and terminates the arrhythmia using pacing or shocking the heart through the ICD lead. The physician may reprogram the ICD's treatment parameters to optimize the device function to best treat the patient's arrhythmia.

Coding Tips

When medically necessary, report moderate (conscious) sedation provided by the performing physician with 99151-99153. When provided by another physician, report 99155-99157. Code 93642 reports subsequent or periodic electronic analysis and/or reprogramming of a transvenous pacing cardioverter-defibrillator. When electrophysiologic evaluation of a pacing cardioverter-defibrillator is performed at the time of initial implantation or replacement, report 93640 or 93641 instead of 93642. Procedure 93642 has both a technical and professional component. To report only the professional component, append modifier 26. To report only the technical component, append modifier TC. To report the complete procedure (i.e., both the professional and technical components), submit without a modifier.

ICD-10-CM Diagnostic Codes

I45.89	Other specified conduction disorders
I47.0	Re-entry ventricular arrhythmia
I47.1	Supraventricular tachycardia
I47.2	Ventricular tachycardia
I48.0	Paroxysmal atrial fibrillation
I48.11	Longstanding persistent atrial fibrillation
I48.19	Other persistent atrial fibrillation
I48.21	Permanent atrial fibrillation
I48.3	Typical atrial flutter
I48.4	Atypical atrial flutter

I49.01 Ventricular fibrillation
I49.02 Ventricular flutter
I49.1 Atrial premature depolarization
I49.2 Junctional premature depolarization
I49.3 Ventricular premature depolarization
I49.49 Other premature depolarization
I49.5 Sick sinus syndrome
I49.8 Other specified cardiac arrhythmias
T82.817A Embolism due to cardiac prosthetic devices, implants and grafts, initial encounter
T82.827A Fibrosis due to cardiac prosthetic devices, implants and grafts, initial encounter
T82.837A Hemorrhage due to cardiac prosthetic devices, implants and grafts, initial encounter
T82.847A Pain due to cardiac prosthetic devices, implants and grafts, initial encounter
T82.857A Stenosis of other cardiac prosthetic devices, implants and grafts, initial encounter
T82.867A Thrombosis due to cardiac prosthetic devices, implants and grafts, initial encounter
T82.897A Other specified complication of cardiac prosthetic devices, implants and grafts, initial encounter
Z45.02 Encounter for adjustment and management of automatic implantable cardiac defibrillator
Z95.810 Presence of automatic (implantable) cardiac defibrillator

AMA: **93642** 2018,Jan,8; 2018,Feb,11; 2017,Jan,8; 2016,Jan,13; 2015,Jan,16; 2014,Jan,11; 2014,Apr,3; 2013,Jun,6-8; 2013,Jul,7-9

Relative Value Units/Medicare Edits

Non-Facility RVU	Work	PE	MP	Total
93642	4.63	4.19	0.96	9.78
Facility RVU	**Work**	**PE**	**MP**	**Total**
93642	4.63	4.19	0.96	9.78

	FUD	Status	MUE	Modifiers				IOM Reference
93642	0	A	1(3)	51	N/A	N/A	80*	None

* with documentation

Terms To Know

arrhythmias. Heart disorder of rhythm or rate, due to an electrical conduction system malfunction.

cardioverter-defibrillator. Device that uses both low energy cardioversion or defibrillating shocks and antitachycardia pacing to treat ventricular tachycardia or ventricular fibrillation.

93644

93644 Electrophysiologic evaluation of subcutaneous implantable defibrillator (includes defibrillation threshold evaluation, induction of arrhythmia, evaluation of sensing for arrhythmia termination, and programming or reprogramming of sensing or therapeutic parameters)

Explanation

A study is performed to ensure that the subcutaneous implantable defibrillator system and leads are positioned well and working properly in order to guarantee proper function. The physician records cardiac electrical signals from the leads and paces the heart through the leads to determine pacing threshold. The physician uses the pulse generator to pace the heart into an arrhythmia, such as ventricular tachycardia or fibrillation. The system detects and terminates the arrhythmia using pacing or shocking the heart through the lead. The physician may reprogram the treatment parameters to optimize the device function to best treat the patient's arrhythmia.

Coding Tips

When medically necessary, report moderate (conscious) sedation provided by the performing physician with 99151-99153. When provided by another physician, report 99155-99157. For recurrent electrophysiologic evaluation of device, see 93260 and 93261. Do not report 93644 with 33270 during the same encounter for subcutaneous defibrillator insertion. For electrophysiologic evaluation of single or dual chamber implantable defibrillator leads including threshold evaluation at the time of implant or replacement, see 93640. For electrophysiologic evaluation of a single or dual chamber implantable defibrillator generator at the time of implant or replacement, see 93641. For recurrent analysis and/or reprogramming of single or dual chamber implantable defibrillators, see 93282, 93283, 93289, 93292, 93295, and 93642. For electrophysiologic evaluation of a single or dual chamber transvenous pacing cardioverter-defibrillator, see 93642.

ICD-10-CM Diagnostic Codes

I45.89 Other specified conduction disorders
I47.0 Re-entry ventricular arrhythmia
I47.1 Supraventricular tachycardia
I47.2 Ventricular tachycardia
I48.0 Paroxysmal atrial fibrillation
I48.11 Longstanding persistent atrial fibrillation
I48.19 Other persistent atrial fibrillation
I48.21 Permanent atrial fibrillation
I48.3 Typical atrial flutter
I48.4 Atypical atrial flutter
I49.01 Ventricular fibrillation
I49.02 Ventricular flutter
I49.1 Atrial premature depolarization
I49.2 Junctional premature depolarization
I49.3 Ventricular premature depolarization
I49.49 Other premature depolarization
I49.5 Sick sinus syndrome
I49.8 Other specified cardiac arrhythmias
T82.817A Embolism due to cardiac prosthetic devices, implants and grafts, initial encounter
T82.827A Fibrosis due to cardiac prosthetic devices, implants and grafts, initial encounter

T82.837A	Hemorrhage due to cardiac prosthetic devices, implants and grafts, initial encounter
T82.847A	Pain due to cardiac prosthetic devices, implants and grafts, initial encounter
T82.855A	Stenosis of coronary artery stent, initial encounter
T82.857A	Stenosis of other cardiac prosthetic devices, implants and grafts, initial encounter
T82.867A	Thrombosis due to cardiac prosthetic devices, implants and grafts, initial encounter
T82.897A	Other specified complication of cardiac prosthetic devices, implants and grafts, initial encounter
Z45.02	Encounter for adjustment and management of automatic implantable cardiac defibrillator
Z95.810	Presence of automatic (implantable) cardiac defibrillator

AMA: **93644** 2018,Feb,11

Relative Value Units/Medicare Edits

Non-Facility RVU	Work	PE	MP	Total
93644	3.04	2.49	0.12	5.65
Facility RVU	**Work**	**PE**	**MP**	**Total**
93644	3.04	2.49	0.12	5.65

	FUD	Status	MUE	Modifiers				IOM Reference
93644	0	A	1(3)	51	N/A	N/A	80*	None

* with documentation

Terms To Know

arrhythmia. Irregular heartbeat.

defibrillator system. System that includes a pulse generator and electrodes, implanted in the same manner as the pacemaker systems.

electrophysiologic studies. Electrical stimulation and monitoring to diagnose heart conduction abnormalities that predispose patients to bradyarrhythmias and to determine a patient's chance for developing ventricular and supraventricular tachyarrhythmias.

paroxysmal supraventricular tachycardia. Rapid heartbeat that starts above the ventricles and occurs sporadically.

supraventricular tachycardia. Rapid beating of the heart, usually pertains to more than 100 beats per minute and can be as high as 250 beats per minute. SVT is caused by abnormal electrical impulses originating at the AV node or above it in the atria (upper chambers) of the heart.

93650

93650 Intracardiac catheter ablation of atrioventricular node function, atrioventricular conduction for creation of complete heart block, with or without temporary pacemaker placement

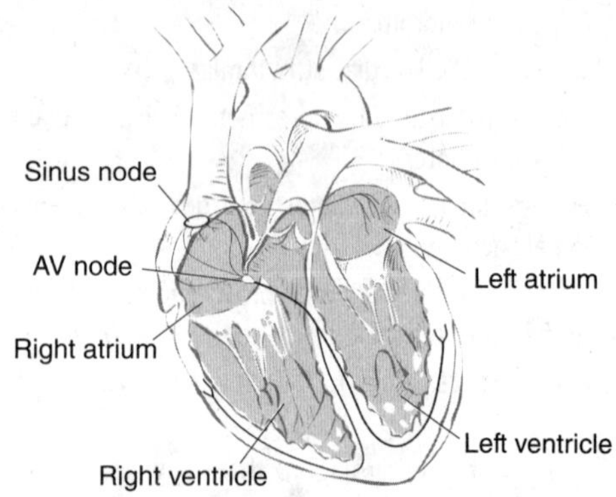

The atrioventricular (AV) node is ablated by intracardiaccatheter. The elimination of AV function is usually to address atrial fibrillation. A temporary pacemaker may be placed as part of the procedure since the result is total stoppage of the heart's electromuscular function

Explanation

The purpose of this procedure is to create complete heart block, usually for control of the ventricular rate during atrial arrhythmias. The physician places a venous sheath, usually in a femoral vein, using standard techniques. The physician advances an electrical catheter through the venous sheath and into the right heart using fluoroscopic guidance. The physician attaches the catheter to an electrical recording device to allow depiction of the intracardiac electrograms obtained from electrodes on the catheter tip. The physician moves the catheter tip to the bundle of His, on the anteroseptal tricuspid annulus, and obtains recordings. Alternatively, the physician may obtain similar recordings by placing a catheter into the left ventricular outflow tract via the aorta. The physician maps the His bundle area and ablates the His bundle by sending cautery (radiofrequency) current through the catheter. The physician may also place a temporary pacing catheter in the right ventricle for this procedure.

Coding Tips

When medically necessary, report moderate (conscious) sedation provided by the performing physician with 99151-99153. When provided by another physician, report 99155-99157. Note that intracardiac catheter ablations are specific to the type of arrhythmia being treated. Code 93650 reports ablation of atrioventricular node function usually performed to control ventricular rate during atrial arrhythmias. For treatment of supraventricular tachycardia by intracardiac ablation, see 93653. For treatment of ventricular tachycardia by intracardiac ablation, see 93654. Fluoroscopic guidance is included in electrophysiological procedures and should not be reported separately.

ICD-10-CM Diagnostic Codes

I48.0	Paroxysmal atrial fibrillation
I48.11	Longstanding persistent atrial fibrillation
I48.19	Other persistent atrial fibrillation
I48.21	Permanent atrial fibrillation
I48.3	Typical atrial flutter
I48.4	Atypical atrial flutter
I48.91	Unspecified atrial fibrillation

I48.92	Unspecified atrial flutter
I49.1	Atrial premature depolarization

AMA: 93650 2018,Jan,8; 2018,Feb,11; 2017,Jan,8; 2016,Jan,13; 2015,Jan,16; 2014,Jan,11

Relative Value Units/Medicare Edits

Non-Facility RVU	Work	PE	MP	Total
93650	10.24	4.59	2.37	17.2
Facility RVU	**Work**	**PE**	**MP**	**Total**
93650	10.24	4.59	2.37	17.2

	FUD	Status	MUE	Modifiers				IOM Reference
93650	0	A	1(2)	51	N/A	N/A	80*	None

* with documentation

Terms To Know

arrhythmias. Heart disorder of rhythm or rate, due to an electrical conduction system malfunction.

atrioventricular block. Condition in which there is a disturbance of electrical conduction, such as a delay, intermittence, or absence in the transmission of an impulse from the atria to the ventricles and categorized according to degree of severity.

cardiac arrest. Sudden, unexpected cessation of cardiac action, including absence of heart sounds and/or blood pressure.

cautery. Destruction or burning of tissue by means of a hot instrument, an electric current, or a caustic chemical, such as silver nitrate.

ventricular tachycardia. Excessively rapid ventricular rhythm of the heart, usually more than 150 beats per minute, with an origin beat generated in the ventricle, commonly from atrioventricular dissociation.

93653-93654

93653 Comprehensive electrophysiologic evaluation including insertion and repositioning of multiple electrode catheters with induction or attempted induction of an arrhythmia with right atrial pacing and recording, right ventricular pacing and recording (when necessary), and His bundle recording (when necessary) with intracardiac catheter ablation of arrhythmogenic focus; with treatment of supraventricular tachycardia by ablation of fast or slow atrioventricular pathway, accessory atrioventricular connection, cavo-tricuspid isthmus or other single atrial focus or source of atrial re-entry

93654 with treatment of ventricular tachycardia or focus of ventricular ectopy including intracardiac electrophysiologic 3D mapping, when performed, and left ventricular pacing and recording, when performed

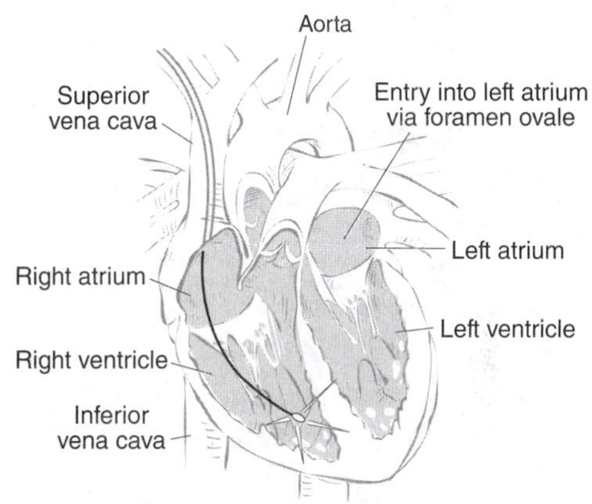

Eletrophysiologic evaluation of right heart

Explanation

Catheter ablation is performed on cardiac tissue. In 93653, ablation is performed on dual atrioventricular nodal pathways, accessory atrioventricular connections, or other atrial foci causing supraventricular tachycardia (SVT). In 93654, ablation is performed on the cardiac tissue causing ventricular tachycardia or ectopy. For either procedure, the physician places three venous sheaths, usually in one or both femoral veins, using standard techniques. The physician advances three electrical catheters through the venous sheaths and into the right heart under fluoroscopic guidance. The three catheters are attached to an electrical recording device to allow depiction of the intracardiac electrograms obtained from electrodes on the catheter tips. The tips of the three catheters are moved to the right atrium, the bundle of His, and the right ventricle and recordings are obtained. Selective destruction (ablation) of cardiac tissue to correct the SVT (93653) or the tachycardia or ectopy (93654) is based on the recordings. Code 93654 also includes the use of three-dimensional mapping software and left ventricle pacing and recording when used.

Coding Tips

When medically necessary, report moderate (conscious) sedation provided by the performing physician with 99151-99153. When provided by another physician, report 99155-99157. Do not report 93653 with 93600–93603, 93610, 93612, 93618–93620, 93642, 93654, or 93656. Do not report 93654 with 93279–93284, 93286–93289, 93600–93603, 93609, 93610, 93612, 93613, 93618–93620, 93622, 93642, 93653, or 93656.

ICD-10-CM Diagnostic Codes

I44.39	Other atrioventricular block

Medicine

I44.4 Left anterior fascicular block
I44.5 Left posterior fascicular block
I44.69 Other fascicular block
I45.0 Right fascicular block
I45.19 Other right bundle-branch block
I45.2 Bifascicular block
I45.3 Trifascicular block
I45.4 Nonspecific intraventricular block
I45.6 Pre-excitation syndrome
I45.89 Other specified conduction disorders
I46.2 Cardiac arrest due to underlying cardiac condition
I46.8 Cardiac arrest due to other underlying condition
I47.0 Re-entry ventricular arrhythmia
I47.1 Supraventricular tachycardia
I47.2 Ventricular tachycardia
I48.0 Paroxysmal atrial fibrillation
I48.11 Longstanding persistent atrial fibrillation
I48.19 Other persistent atrial fibrillation
I48.21 Permanent atrial fibrillation
I48.3 Typical atrial flutter
I48.4 Atypical atrial flutter
I49.01 Ventricular fibrillation
I49.02 Ventricular flutter
I49.2 Junctional premature depolarization
I49.8 Other specified cardiac arrhythmias

AMA: **93653** 2018,Jan,8; 2018,Feb,11; 2017,Jan,8; 2016,Jan,13; 2015,Jan,16; 2014,Apr,3; 2013,Jun,6-8; 2013,Jul,7-9 **93654** 2018,Jan,8; 2018,Feb,11; 2017,Jan,8; 2016,Jan,13; 2015,Jan,16; 2014,Apr,3; 2013,Jun,6-8; 2013,Jul,7-9

Relative Value Units/Medicare Edits

Non-Facility RVU	Work	PE	MP	Total
93653	14.75	6.18	3.43	24.36
93654	19.75	8.27	4.58	32.6
Facility RVU	**Work**	**PE**	**MP**	**Total**
93653	14.75	6.18	3.43	24.36
93654	19.75	8.27	4.58	32.6

	FUD	Status	MUE	Modifiers				IOM Reference
93653	0	A	1(3)	51	N/A	N/A	80*	100-03,20.12
93654	0	A	1(3)	51	N/A	N/A	80*	

* with documentation

93655

+ 93655 Intracardiac catheter ablation of a discrete mechanism of arrhythmia which is distinct from the primary ablated mechanism, including repeat diagnostic maneuvers, to treat a spontaneous or induced arrhythmia (List separately in addition to code for primary procedure)

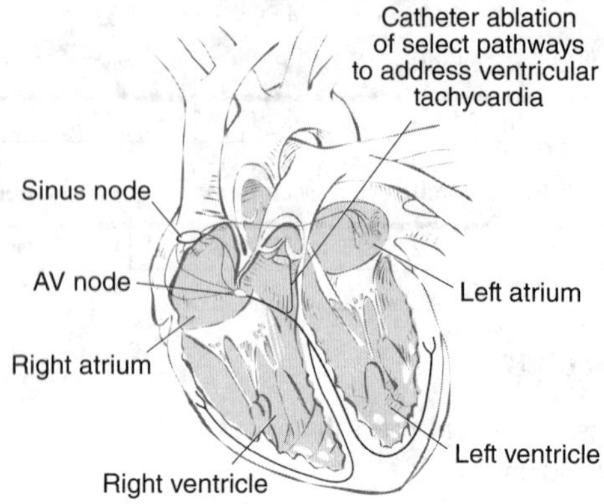

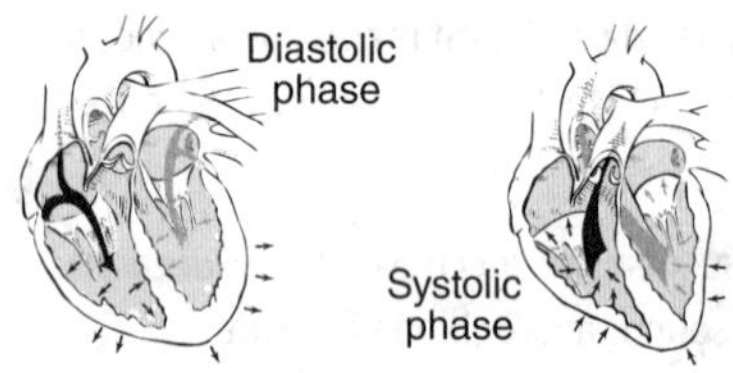

Explanation

After the initial treatment (ablation) for supraventricular or ventricular tachycardia, a postablation evaluation is performed. If there is a new (not previously diagnosed) or different mechanism causing the arrhythmia found on this evaluation, this is recorded and additional cardiac tissue is destroyed via the catheter to correct the newly discovered spontaneous or induced arrhythmia.

Coding Tips

When medically necessary, report moderate (conscious) sedation provided by the performing physician with 99151-99153. When provided by another physician, report 99155-99157. Report 93655 in addition to 93653, 93654, or 93656. This code is used when a separate, non-atrial fibrillation tachycardia has been separately diagnosed following pulmonary vein isolation.

ICD-10-CM Diagnostic Codes

This/these CPT code(s) are add on code(s). See the primary procedure code that this code is performed with for your ICD-10-CM code selections. Diagnostic code(s) would be the same as the actual procedure performed.

AMA: **93655** 2018,Jan,8; 2018,Feb,11; 2017,Jan,8; 2016,Jan,13; 2015,Jan,16; 2014,Apr,3; 2013,Jun,6-8; 2013,Jul,7-9

Relative Value Units/Medicare Edits

Non-Facility RVU	Work	PE	MP	Total
93655	7.5	3.16	1.74	12.4
Facility RVU	**Work**	**PE**	**MP**	**Total**
93655	7.5	3.16	1.74	12.4

	FUD	Status	MUE	Modifiers				IOM Reference
93655	N/A	A	2(3)	N/A	N/A	N/A	80*	None

* with documentation

Terms To Know

ablation. Removal or destruction of a body part or tissue or its function. Ablation may be performed by surgical means, hormones, drugs, radiofrequency, heat, chemical application, or other methods.

arrhythmia. Irregular heartbeat.

bundle branch block. Delay or obstruction of the electrical impulse that makes the heartbeat. Bundle branch block may occur in the right or left bundle branches, and is known as right bundle branch block (RBBB) or left bundle branch block (LBBB).

supraventricular tachycardia. Rapid beating of the heart, usually pertains to more than 100 beats per minute and can be as high as 250 beats per minute. SVT is caused by abnormal electrical impulses originating at the AV node or above it in the atria (upper chambers) of the heart.

ventricular fibrillation. Cardiac arrhythmia in which ventricular myocardial fibers are rapidly and repetitively excited from a random or ectopic focus of electrical impulse, causing the muscle fibers to contract in an erratic manner without corresponding contraction of the ventricles. The condition requires immediate restoration of normal cardiac rhythm, often by electroshock through paddles placed on the chest.

ventricular tachycardia. Excessively rapid ventricular rhythm of the heart, usually more than 150 beats per minute, with an origin beat generated in the ventricle, commonly from atrioventricular dissociation.

93656-93657

93656 Comprehensive electrophysiologic evaluation including transseptal catheterizations, insertion and repositioning of multiple electrode catheters with induction or attempted induction of an arrhythmia including left or right atrial pacing/recording when necessary, right ventricular pacing/recording when necessary, and His bundle recording when necessary with intracardiac catheter ablation of atrial fibrillation by pulmonary vein isolation

Afib

\+ **93657** Additional linear or focal intracardiac catheter ablation of the left or right atrium for treatment of atrial fibrillation remaining after completion of pulmonary vein isolation (List separately in addition to code for primary procedure)

S/P failed catheter ablation

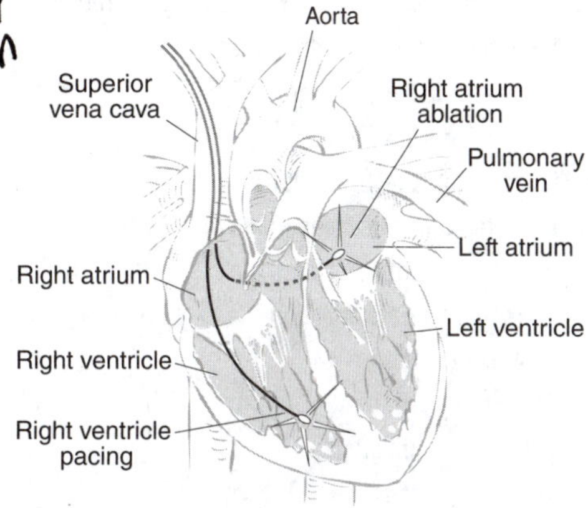

The left ventricle is paced and recorded and the pulmonary vein isolated

Explanation

During ablation by pulmonary vein isolation, also called pulmonary vein antrum isolation (PVAI), cardiac tissue responsible for the electrical irritability that causes atrial fibrillation is found at the opening of each of the four pulmonary veins that terminate in the left atrium. The physician places three venous sheaths, usually in one or both femoral veins, using standard techniques. Three electrical catheters are advanced through the venous sheaths into the right heart under fluoroscopic guidance and the septum is punctured for access to the left atrium. The physician attaches the three catheters to an electrical recording device to allow depiction of the intracardiac electrograms obtained from electrodes on the catheter tips. The tips of the three catheters are moved to the left atrium and selective destruction (ablation) of the cardiac tissue at the opening of the pulmonary veins is performed to correct the atrial fibrillation. The three catheters may also be maneuvered to the bundle of His and the right ventricle for pacing and to obtain recording. Report 93656 for the PVAI procedure. Report 93657 when a postablation evaluation is performed after the initial PVAI and a new (not previously diagnosed) or different mechanism causing the atrial fibrillation is found and ablated.

Coding Tips

When medically necessary, report moderate (conscious) sedation provided by the performing physician with 99151-99153. When provided by another physician, report 99155-99157. Report 93657 in addition to 93656. Do not report 93656 with 93279–93284, 93286–93289, 93462, 93600, 93602, 93603, 93610, 93612, 93618, 93619, 93620, 93621, 93653, or 93654. For treatment of SVT or ventricular tachycardia via intracardiac catheter ablation of arrhythmogenic focus, see 93653 and 93654.

ICD-10-CM Diagnostic Codes

I44.39	Other atrioventricular block
I44.4	Left anterior fascicular block
I44.5	Left posterior fascicular block
I44.69	Other fascicular block
I45.0	Right fascicular block
I45.19	Other right bundle-branch block
I45.2	Bifascicular block
I45.3	Trifascicular block
I45.4	Nonspecific intraventricular block
I45.6	Pre-excitation syndrome
I45.89	Other specified conduction disorders
I46.2	Cardiac arrest due to underlying cardiac condition
I46.8	Cardiac arrest due to other underlying condition
I47.0	Re-entry ventricular arrhythmia
I47.1	Supraventricular tachycardia
I47.2	Ventricular tachycardia
I48.0	Paroxysmal atrial fibrillation
I48.11	Longstanding persistent atrial fibrillation
I48.19	Other persistent atrial fibrillation
I48.21	Permanent atrial fibrillation
I48.3	Typical atrial flutter
I48.4	Atypical atrial flutter
I49.01	Ventricular fibrillation
I49.02	Ventricular flutter
I49.2	Junctional premature depolarization
I49.8	Other specified cardiac arrhythmias

AMA: 93656 2019,Sep,10; 2018,Jan,8; 2018,Feb,11; 2017,Jan,8; 2016,Jan,13; 2015,Jan,16; 2014,Apr,3; 2013,Jun,6-8; 2013,Jul,7-9 **93657** 2019,Sep,10; 2018,Jan,8; 2018,Feb,11; 2017,Jan,8; 2016,Jan,13; 2015,Jan,16; 2014,Apr,3; 2013,Jun,6-8; 2013,Jul,7-9

Relative Value Units/Medicare Edits

Non-Facility RVU	Work	PE	MP	Total
93656	19.77	8.33	4.6	32.7
93657	7.5	3.14	1.74	12.38
Facility RVU	**Work**	**PE**	**MP**	**Total**
93656	19.77	8.33	4.6	32.7
93657	7.5	3.14	1.74	12.38

	FUD	Status	MUE	Modifiers				IOM Reference
93656	0	A	1(3)	51	N/A	N/A	80*	100-03,20.12
93657	N/A	A	1(3)	N/A	N/A	N/A	80*	

* with documentation

93662

+ 93662 Intracardiac echocardiography during therapeutic/diagnostic intervention, including imaging supervision and interpretation (List separately in addition to code for primary procedure)

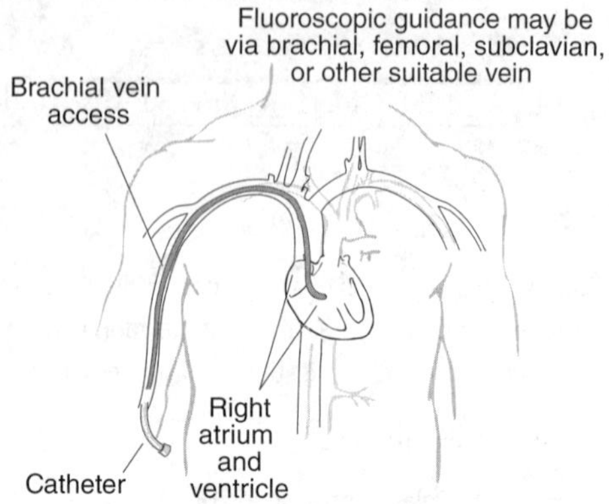

An intracardiac echocardiogram (ICE) is performed during a therapeutic or diagnostic intervention (reported separately)

Explanation

During separately reportable electrophysiologic evaluation or intracardiac catheter ablation of arrhythmogenic focus, intracardiac echocardiography (ICE) is performed. ICE uses intravascular ultrasound imaging systems in the cardiac chambers providing direct endocardial visualization. A single rotating transducer that provides a 360-degree field of view in a plane transverse to the long axis of the catheter is introduced through a long vascular sheath. Access is typically via the femoral vein. The transducer is directed to various sites within the heart. During electrophysiologic evaluation, ICE is used to guide placement of mapping and stimulating catheters. During intracardiac ablation procedures, ICE allows for precise anatomic localization of the ablation catheter tip in relation to endocardial structures. Since the focus of some arrhythmias can be anatomically determined, it also allows the ablative procedure to be performed using anatomic landmarks.

Coding Tips

Report 93662 in addition to 92987, 93453, 93460–93462, 93532, 93580, 93581, 93620, 93621, 93622, 93653, 93654, or 93656. Do not report 93662 with 92961, 0569T, or 0570T. Electrophysiologic evaluation or intracardiac catheter ablation procedures are reported separately.

ICD-10-CM Diagnostic Codes

This/these CPT code(s) are add on code(s). See the primary procedure code that this code is performed with for your ICD-10-CM code selections. Diagnostic code(s) would be the same as the actual procedure performed.

AMA: 93662 2018,Jan,8; 2018,Feb,11; 2017,Jan,8; 2016,Jan,13; 2015,Jan,16; 2014,Jan,11

Relative Value Units/Medicare Edits

Non-Facility RVU	Work	PE	MP	Total
93662	0.0	0.0	0.0	0.0
Facility RVU	**Work**	**PE**	**MP**	**Total**
93662	0.0	0.0	0.0	0.0

	FUD	Status	MUE	Modifiers				IOM Reference
93662	N/A	C	1(3)	N/A	N/A	N/A	80*	None

* with documentation

Terms To Know

ablation. Removal or destruction of a body part or tissue or its function. Ablation may be performed by surgical means, hormones, drugs, radiofrequency, heat, chemical application, or other methods.

catheterization. Use or insertion of a tubular device into a duct, blood vessel, hollow organ, or body cavity for injecting or withdrawing fluids for diagnostic or therapeutic purposes.

diagnostic procedures. Procedure performed on a patient to obtain information to assess the medical condition of the patient or to identify a disease and to determine the nature and severity of an illness or injury.

echography. Radiographic imaging that uses sound waves reflected off the different densities of anatomic structures to create images.

electrophysiologic studies. Electrical stimulation and monitoring to diagnose heart conduction abnormalities that predispose patients to bradyarrhythmias and to determine a patient's chance for developing ventricular and supraventricular tachyarrhythmias.

mitral valve. Valve with two cusps that is between the left atrium and left ventricle of the heart.

therapeutic procedure. Manner of effecting change through the application of clinical skills and/or services that attempt to improve function.

G0248-G0250

G0248 Demonstration, prior to initiation of home INR monitoring, for patient with either mechanical heart valve(s), chronic atrial fibrillation, or venous thromboembolism who meets Medicare coverage criteria, under the direction of a physician; includes: face-to-face demonstration of use and care of the INR monitor, obtaining at least one blood sample, provision of instructions for reporting home INR test results, and documentation of patient's ability to perform testing and report results

G0249 Provision of test materials and equipment for home INR monitoring of patient with either mechanical heart valve(s), chronic atrial fibrillation, or venous thromboembolism who meets Medicare coverage criteria; includes: provision of materials for use in the home and reporting of test results to physician; testing not occurring more frequently than once a week; testing materials, billing units of service include four tests

G0250 Physician review, interpretation, and patient management of home INR testing for patient with either mechanical heart valve(s), chronic atrial fibrillation, or venous thromboembolism who meets Medicare coverage criteria; testing not occurring more frequently than once a week; billing units of service include four tests

Explanation

Patients with a mechanical heart valve, chronic atrial fibrillation, or venous thromboembolism are at risk of developing intracardiac or intravascular thrombi and are frequently managed with long-term use of warfarin anticoagulation. Periodic monitoring is necessary to maintain a therapeutic effect of the anticoagulation treatment and reduce thromboembolic and hemorrhagic events. The use of the internationalized normalized ratio (INR) (rather than the prothrombin time) provides a result that is independent of the laboratory reagents used. The INR is the ratio of the patient's prothrombin time compared to the mean prothrombin time for a group of normal individuals. Patient self-testing and self-management through the use of a home INR monitor improve the time in therapeutic rate and hence clinical outcomes. Portable coagulometers that measure the prothrombin time and calculate the INR with the use of a drop of whole blood allow the patient to do self-testing.

Coding Tips

Medicare covers the use of home PT/INR monitoring when prescribed by a physician and when the patient has been anticoagulated for at least three months before using the home INR device, has undergone a face-to-face educational program on anticoagulation management, has demonstrated the correct use of the device prior to use in the home, continues to correctly use the device, and self-testing with the device does not occur more than once a week. Since G0250 is a professional service furnished by a physician, it is not payable under the outpatient prospective payment services (OPPS).

ICD-10-CM Diagnostic Codes

D68.51	Activated protein C resistance
D68.52	Prothrombin gene mutation
D68.59	Other primary thrombophilia
D68.61	Antiphospholipid syndrome
D68.62	Lupus anticoagulant syndrome
I26.01	Septic pulmonary embolism with acute cor pulmonale
I26.02	Saddle embolus of pulmonary artery with acute cor pulmonale
I26.09	Other pulmonary embolism with acute cor pulmonale
I26.90	Septic pulmonary embolism without acute cor pulmonale
I26.92	Saddle embolus of pulmonary artery without acute cor pulmonale
I26.93	Single subsegmental pulmonary embolism without acute cor pulmonale
I26.94	Multiple subsegmental pulmonary emboli without acute cor pulmonale
I48.0	Paroxysmal atrial fibrillation
I48.11	Longstanding persistent atrial fibrillation
I48.19	Other persistent atrial fibrillation
I48.21	Permanent atrial fibrillation
I80.01	Phlebitis and thrombophlebitis of superficial vessels of right lower extremity ☑
I80.02	Phlebitis and thrombophlebitis of superficial vessels of left lower extremity ☑
I80.03	Phlebitis and thrombophlebitis of superficial vessels of lower extremities, bilateral ☑
I80.11	Phlebitis and thrombophlebitis of right femoral vein ☑
I80.12	Phlebitis and thrombophlebitis of left femoral vein ☑
I80.13	Phlebitis and thrombophlebitis of femoral vein, bilateral ☑
I80.211	Phlebitis and thrombophlebitis of right iliac vein ☑
I80.212	Phlebitis and thrombophlebitis of left iliac vein ☑
I80.213	Phlebitis and thrombophlebitis of iliac vein, bilateral ☑
I80.221	Phlebitis and thrombophlebitis of right popliteal vein ☑
I80.222	Phlebitis and thrombophlebitis of left popliteal vein ☑
I80.223	Phlebitis and thrombophlebitis of popliteal vein, bilateral ☑
I80.231	Phlebitis and thrombophlebitis of right tibial vein ☑
I80.232	Phlebitis and thrombophlebitis of left tibial vein ☑
I80.233	Phlebitis and thrombophlebitis of tibial vein, bilateral ☑
I80.291	Phlebitis and thrombophlebitis of other deep vessels of right lower extremity ☑
I80.292	Phlebitis and thrombophlebitis of other deep vessels of left lower extremity ☑
I80.293	Phlebitis and thrombophlebitis of other deep vessels of lower extremity, bilateral ☑
I80.8	Phlebitis and thrombophlebitis of other sites
I82.0	Budd-Chiari syndrome
I82.1	Thrombophlebitis migrans
I82.220	Acute embolism and thrombosis of inferior vena cava
I82.221	Chronic embolism and thrombosis of inferior vena cava
T80.0XXA	Air embolism following infusion, transfusion and therapeutic injection, initial encounter
T82.817A	Embolism due to cardiac prosthetic devices, implants and grafts, initial encounter
T82.818A	Embolism due to vascular prosthetic devices, implants and grafts, initial encounter
Z95.2	Presence of prosthetic heart valve

Relative Value Units/Medicare Edits

Non-Facility RVU	Work	PE	MP	Total
G0248	0.0	2.0	0.02	2.02
G0249	0.0	2.02	0.01	2.03
G0250	0.18	0.07	0.01	0.26
Facility RVU	**Work**	**PE**	**MP**	**Total**
G0248	0.0	2.0	0.02	2.02
G0249	0.0	2.02	0.01	2.03
G0250	0.18	0.07	0.01	0.26

	FUD	Status	MUE	Modifiers				IOM Reference
G0248	N/A	R	1(2)	N/A	N/A	N/A	80*	None
G0249	N/A	R	3(3)	N/A	N/A	N/A	80*	
G0250	N/A	R	1(2)	N/A	N/A	N/A	80*	

* with documentation

Terms To Know

anticoagulant. Substance that reduces or eradicates the blood's ability to clot.

atrial fibrillation. Cardiac arrhythmia caused by small areas of muscle fibers becoming erratically and spontaneously activated through multiple circuits in uncoordinated phases of depolarization and repolarization.

embolism. Obstruction of a blood vessel resulting from a clot or foreign substance.

thrombosis. Condition arising from the presence or formation of blood clots within a blood vessel that may cause vascular obstruction and insufficient oxygenation.

G0278

G0278 Iliac and/or femoral artery angiography, nonselective, bilateral or ipsilateral to catheter insertion, performed at the same time as cardiac catheterization and/or coronary angiography, includes positioning or placement of the catheter in the distal aorta or ipsilateral femoral or iliac artery, injection of dye, production of permanent images, and radiologic supervision and interpretation (List separately in addition to primary procedure)

Explanation

An iliac artery is radiologically examined using contrast material at the same time as cardiac catheterization. The catheter that has been threaded over the guidewire from the access site is positioned nonselectively in the distal aorta or iliac artery. Contrast medium is injected and a series of permanent images are taken to visualize the vessels and evaluate any abnormalities. The catheter is removed and pressure applied to the site. Radiological supervision and interpretation is included. List this code separately in addition to the code for the main cardiac catheterization procedure.

Coding Tips

Report this procedure with cardiac catheterization codes 93451–93462. An examination of the iliac or femoral vessels is not ordinarily indicated during a cardiac catheterization. However, angiography and interventions on these vessels at the same time as the catheterization may be reported for conditions that would have required investigation and treatments whether or not a cardiac catheterization was performed. To be eligible for Medicare payment, the medical record must substantiate that these services were medically reasonable and necessary in accordance with accepted practice standards. Do not report G0278 if the iliac angiogram is performed only to determine the type of closure.

ICD-10-CM Diagnostic Codes

This/these CPT code(s) are add on code(s). See the primary procedure code that this code is performed with for your ICD-10-CM code selections.

Relative Value Units/Medicare Edits

Non-Facility RVU	Work	PE	MP	Total
G0278	0.25	0.09	0.06	0.4
Facility RVU	**Work**	**PE**	**MP**	**Total**
G0278	0.25	0.09	0.06	0.4

	FUD	Status	MUE	Modifiers				IOM Reference
G0278	N/A	A	1(2)	N/A	N/A	N/A	80*	None

* with documentation

Terms To Know

angiography. Radiographic imaging of the arteries. Imaging may be performed to study the vasculature of any given organ, body system, or area of circulation such as the brain, heart, chest, kidneys, limbs, gastrointestinal tract, aorta, and pulmonary circulation to visualize the formation and the function of the blood vessels to detect problems such as a blockage or stricture. A catheter is inserted through an accessible blood vessel and the artery is injected with a radiopaque contrast material after which x-rays are taken.

HCPCS

G0403-G0405

G0403 Electrocardiogram, routine ECG with 12 leads; performed as a screening for the initial preventive physical examination with interpretation and report

G0404 Electrocardiogram, routine ECG with 12 leads; tracing only, without interpretation and report, performed as a screening for the initial preventive physical examination

G0405 Electrocardiogram, routine ECG with 12 leads; interpretation and report only, performed as a screening for the initial preventive physical examination

Explanation

Electrocardiogram (ECG) services are performed as a component of the initial preventive physical examination provided to a new beneficiary during the first 12 months of Medicare enrollment. Twelve electrodes are placed on a patient's chest to record electrical activity of the heart. A physician interprets the findings. Code G0403 includes interpretation and report of findings; G0404 includes a tracing only, without interpretation and report findings; and G0405 includes interpretation and report only.

Coding Tips

These codes are billable when it is a result of a referral from an initial preventive physical examination (IPPE).

ICD-10-CM Diagnostic Codes

Z13.6 Encounter for screening for cardiovascular disorders

Relative Value Units/Medicare Edits

Non-Facility RVU	Work	PE	MP	Total
G0403	0.17	0.29	0.02	0.48
G0404	0.0	0.23	0.01	0.24
G0405	0.17	0.06	0.01	0.24
Facility RVU	**Work**	**PE**	**MP**	**Total**
G0403	0.17	0.29	0.02	0.48
G0404	0.0	0.23	0.01	0.24
G0405	0.17	0.06	0.01	0.24

	FUD	Status	MUE	Modifiers				IOM Reference
G0403	N/A	A	1(2)	N/A	N/A	N/A	80*	None
G0404	N/A	A	1(2)	N/A	N/A	N/A	80*	
G0405	N/A	A	1(2)	N/A	N/A	N/A	80*	

* with documentation

HCPCS

G0288

G0288 Reconstruction, computed tomographic angiography of aorta for surgical planning for vascular surgery

Explanation

Report this code for the computer reconstruction of computerized tomography (CT) generated angiographic images of the aorta for the purpose of planning vascular surgery.

Relative Value Units/Medicare Edits

Non-Facility RVU	Work	PE	MP	Total
G0288	0.0	0.91	0.1	1.01
Facility RVU	**Work**	**PE**	**MP**	**Total**
G0288	0.0	0.91	0.1	1.01

G0422-G0423

G0422 Intensive cardiac rehabilitation; with or without continuous ECG monitoring with exercise, per session

G0423 Intensive cardiac rehabilitation; with or without continuous ECG monitoring; without exercise, per session

Explanation

Cardiac rehabilitation is a medically supervised program intended to help people with heart problems. The program includes training and education on the risk factors of heart disease, such as smoking, high blood pressure, and lack of exercise. Encouragement is given to adopt a healthy lifestyle by increasing physical activity, developing stress coping techniques, and adopting a healthy diet. The program may or may not include exercise and continuous ECG monitoring. Intensive cardiac rehabilitation (ICR) sessions are limited to 72 one-hour sessions, up to six sessions per day, over a period of up to 18 weeks.

Relative Value Units/Medicare Edits

Non-Facility RVU	Work	PE	MP	Total
G0422	1.77	1.41	0.1	3.28
G0423	1.77	1.41	0.1	3.28
Facility RVU	**Work**	**PE**	**MP**	**Total**
G0422	1.77	1.41	0.1	3.28
G0423	1.77	1.41	0.1	3.28

G0446

G0446 Annual, face-to-face intensive behavioral therapy for cardiovascular disease, individual, 15 minutes

Explanation

Annual intensive behavioral therapy for cardiovascular disease for risk reduction is reported with this code. Risk reduction includes encouraging aspirin therapy for the primary prevention of cardiovascular disease when the benefits outweigh the risks for men ages 45 to 70 years and women 55 to 79 years; screening for high blood pressure for patients 18 years and older; and intensive behavioral counseling to promote a healthy diet for adults with hyperlipidemia, hypertension, advancing age, and any other risk factors for cardiovascular and diet-related chronic disease. Behavioral counseling interventions should include the following Five A's approach that has been adopted by the United States Preventive Services Task Force (USPSTF): Assess: Ask about/assess behavioral health risk(s) and factors affecting choice of behavior and change goals/methods; Advise: Give clear, specific, and personalized behavior change advice, including information about personal health harms and benefits; Agree: collaboratively select appropriate treatment goals and methods based on the patient's interest in and willingness to change the behavior; Assist: Using behavior change techniques (self-help and/or counseling), aid the patient in achieving agreed-upon goals by acquiring the skills, confidence, and social/environmental supports for behavior change, supplemented with adjunctive medical treatments when appropriate; Arrange: Schedule follow-up contacts (in person or by telephone) to provide ongoing assistance/support and to adjust the treatment plan as needed, including referral to more intensive or specialized treatment.

Relative Value Units/Medicare Edits

Non-Facility RVU	Work	PE	MP	Total
G0446	0.45	0.26	0.03	0.74
Facility RVU	**Work**	**PE**	**MP**	**Total**
G0446	0.45	0.19	0.03	0.67

G0447

G0447 Face-to-face behavioral counseling for obesity, 15 minutes

Explanation

Behavioral counseling for obesity is reported with this code. The United States Preventive Services Task Force (USPSTF) considers body mass index (BMI) a good indication of morbidity and mortality as a result of being overweight or obesity. BMI is calculated using the following formula: BMI = (weight in pounds / (height in inches x height in inches)) x 703. Obese adults are considered those that have a BMI >=30 kg/m2. Behavioral counseling and behavior modification can be an effective combination to produce moderate, sustainable weight loss. The patients should have the following services: screening for obesity using BMI, assessment of food and nutritional intake, and counseling to include diet and exercise. Behavioral counseling interventions should include the following Five A's approach that has been developed by the United States Preventive Services Task Force (USPSTF): Assess: Ask about/assess behavioral health risk(s) and factors affecting choice of behavior and change goals/methods; Advise: Give clear, specific, and personalized behavior change advice, including information about personal health harms and benefits; Agree: collaboratively select appropriate treatment goals and methods based on the patient's interest in and willingness to change the behavior; Assist: Using behavior change techniques (self-help and/or counseling), aid the patient in achieving agreed-upon goals by acquiring the skills, confidence, and social/environmental supports for behavior change, supplemented with adjunctive medical treatments when appropriate; Arrange: Schedule follow-up contacts (in person or by telephone) to provide ongoing assistance/support and to adjust the treatment plan as needed, including referral to more intensive or specialized treatment.

Relative Value Units/Medicare Edits

Non-Facility RVU	Work	PE	MP	Total
G0447	0.45	0.25	0.03	0.73
Facility RVU	**Work**	**PE**	**MP**	**Total**
G0447	0.45	0.19	0.03	0.67

G9157

G9157 Transesophageal Doppler used for cardiac monitoring

Explanation

Transesophageal Doppler is an ultrasound diagnostic procedure that uses low energy sound waves to provide noninvasive visualization. This code is specific to Medicare coverage of transesophageal Doppler monitoring of cardiac output for ventilated patients in the ICU and operative patients with a need for intraoperative fluid optimization. This service is only covered in a hospital setting or ambulatory surgical center and is included in the Inpatient Prospective Payment System payment.

Relative Value Units/Medicare Edits

Non-Facility RVU	Work	PE	MP	Total
G9157	2.2	0.39	0.17	2.76
Facility RVU	**Work**	**PE**	**MP**	**Total**
G9157	2.2	0.39	0.17	2.76

Q0035

Q0035 Cardiokymography

Explanation

Cardiokymography involves the use of a noninvasive device to record the anterior left ventricle segmental wall motion. The device typically consists of a 5 cm diameter capacitive plate transducer as part of a high-frequency, low-power oscillator with recording probe. Changes in wall motion affect the magnetic field and thus the oscillatory frequency, which is then recorded on a multichannel analog waveform polygraph. Medicare and most payers cover this type of test only as an adjunct to electrocardiographic stress testing to evaluate coronary artery disease and only when specific clinical indications are present. For male patients there must be atypical angina pectoris or nonischemic chest pain. For female patients, there must be angina, either typical or atypical.

Relative Value Units/Medicare Edits

Non-Facility RVU	Work	PE	MP	Total
Q0035	0.17	0.38	0.02	0.57
Facility RVU	**Work**	**PE**	**MP**	**Total**
Q0035	0.17	0.38	0.02	0.57

36400

36400 Venipuncture, younger than age 3 years, necessitating the skill of a physician or other qualified health care professional, not to be used for routine venipuncture; femoral or jugular vein

Explanation

A needle is inserted through the skin to puncture the femoral or jugular vein of a child younger than age 3. The needle is inserted into the vein and used for the withdrawal of blood for diagnostic study or for the therapeutic infusion of intravenous medication. A soft flexible catheter may be placed for prolonged therapy. Once the procedure is complete, the needle or catheter is withdrawn and pressure is applied over the puncture site to control bleeding. Use this code for venipuncture when it necessitates the skill of a physician or other qualified health care professional. Do not use this code when routine venipuncture is performed.

Relative Value Units/Medicare Edits

Non-Facility RVU	Work	PE	MP	Total
36400	0.38	0.35	0.02	0.75
Facility RVU	**Work**	**PE**	**MP**	**Total**
36400	0.38	0.13	0.02	0.53

36405-36406

36405 Venipuncture, younger than age 3 years, necessitating the skill of a physician or other qualified health care professional, not to be used for routine venipuncture; scalp vein

36406 other vein

Explanation

A needle is inserted through the skin to puncture a vein of a child younger than age 3. In 36405, the scalp vein is punctured and in 36406, a vein other than the femoral, jugular, or scalp vein is used. The needle is inserted into the vein and used for the withdrawal of blood or for the therapeutic infusion of intravenous medication. A soft flexible catheter may be placed for prolonged therapy. Once the procedure is complete, the needle or catheter is withdrawn and pressure is applied over the puncture site to control bleeding. Use these codes when venipuncture necessitates the skill of a physician or other qualified health care professional. Do not use these codes when routine venipuncture is performed.

Relative Value Units/Medicare Edits

Non-Facility RVU	Work	PE	MP	Total
36405	0.31	0.33	0.02	0.66
36406	0.18	0.28	0.01	0.47
Facility RVU	**Work**	**PE**	**MP**	**Total**
36405	0.31	0.11	0.02	0.44
36406	0.18	0.06	0.01	0.25

36410

36410 Venipuncture, age 3 years or older, necessitating the skill of a physician or other qualified health care professional (separate procedure), for diagnostic or therapeutic purposes (not to be used for routine venipuncture)

Explanation

A needle is inserted through the skin to puncture a vein of a person 3 years of age or older. The needle is inserted into the vein and used for the withdrawal of blood for diagnostic study or for the therapeutic infusion of intravenous medication. A soft flexible catheter may be placed for prolonged therapy. Once the procedure is complete, the needle or catheter is withdrawn and pressure is applied over the puncture site to control bleeding. Use this code when the venipuncture necessitates the skills of a physician or other qualified health care professional. Do not use this code when routine venipuncture is performed.

Relative Value Units/Medicare Edits

Non-Facility RVU	Work	PE	MP	Total
36410	0.18	0.29	0.02	0.49
Facility RVU	**Work**	**PE**	**MP**	**Total**
36410	0.18	0.07	0.02	0.27

36415-36416

36415 Collection of venous blood by venipuncture

36416 Collection of capillary blood specimen (eg, finger, heel, ear stick)

Explanation

A needle is inserted into the skin over a vein to puncture the blood vessel and withdraw blood for venous collection in 36415. In 36416, a prick is made into the finger, heel, or ear and capillary blood that pools at the puncture site is collected in a pipette. In either case, the blood is used for diagnostic study and no catheter is placed.

Relative Value Units/Medicare Edits

Non-Facility RVU	Work	PE	MP	Total
36415	0.0	0.0	0.0	0.0
36416	0.0	0.0	0.0	0.0
Facility RVU	**Work**	**PE**	**MP**	**Total**
36415	0.0	0.0	0.0	0.0
36416	0.0	0.0	0.0	0.0

36420-36425

36420 Venipuncture, cutdown; younger than age 1 year
36425 age 1 or over

Explanation

The physician makes an incision in the skin directly over the vessel and dissects the area surrounding the vein. A needle is passed into the vein for the withdrawal of blood or for the infusion of intravenous medication of a patient under 12 months of age (in 36420) or over 12 months of age (in 36425). A catheter may be left behind. Once the procedure is complete, the incision is repaired with a layered closure.

Relative Value Units/Medicare Edits

Non-Facility RVU	Work	PE	MP	Total
36420	1.01	0.18	0.16	1.35
36425	0.76	0.3	0.1	1.16
Facility RVU	**Work**	**PE**	**MP**	**Total**
36420	1.01	0.18	0.16	1.35
36425	0.76	0.3	0.1	1.16

36430

36430 Transfusion, blood or blood components

Explanation

The physician transfuses blood or blood components to a patient. The physician establishes venous access with a needle and catheter and transfuses the blood products.

Relative Value Units/Medicare Edits

Non-Facility RVU	Work	PE	MP	Total
36430	0.0	0.97	0.02	0.99
Facility RVU	**Work**	**PE**	**MP**	**Total**
36430	0.0	0.97	0.02	0.99

36440

36440 Push transfusion, blood, 2 years or younger

Explanation

The physician performs a push transfusion on a child 2 years old and under. The physician calculates the amount of blood to be transfused and slowly injects it into the patient using a needle or existing catheter.

Relative Value Units/Medicare Edits

Non-Facility RVU	Work	PE	MP	Total
36440	1.03	0.36	0.07	1.46
Facility RVU	**Work**	**PE**	**MP**	**Total**
36440	1.03	0.36	0.07	1.46

36510

36510 Catheterization of umbilical vein for diagnosis or therapy, newborn

Explanation

The physician catheterizes the umbilical vein for diagnostic or therapeutic purposes. The physician cleanses the umbilical cord stump and locates the umbilical vein. A catheter is inserted in the vein for reasons including blood sampling or administering medication.

Relative Value Units/Medicare Edits

Non-Facility RVU	Work	PE	MP	Total
36510	1.09	1.18	0.07	2.34
Facility RVU	**Work**	**PE**	**MP**	**Total**
36510	1.09	0.38	0.07	1.54

36660

36660 Catheterization, umbilical artery, newborn, for diagnosis or therapy

Explanation

The physician catheterizes an umbilical artery in a newborn for diagnostic or therapeutic purposes. The physician prepares the umbilical artery and passes a catheter sheath inside the lumen for arterial access. The catheter is attached to a pressure line that maintains patency of the arterial lumen. The access is used for diagnostic or therapeutic purposes, allowing the drawing of blood for tests or instillation of medication.

Relative Value Units/Medicare Edits

Non-Facility RVU	Work	PE	MP	Total
36660	1.4	0.49	0.09	1.98
Facility RVU	**Work**	**PE**	**MP**	**Total**
36660	1.4	0.49	0.09	1.98

71045-71048

71045 Radiologic examination, chest; single view
71046 2 views
71047 3 views
71048 4 or more views

Explanation

In 71045, a single x-ray is taken of the patient's chest. Report 71046 for two views; 71047 for three views; and 71048 for four or more views.

Relative Value Units/Medicare Edits

Non-Facility RVU	Work	PE	MP	Total
71045	0.18	0.5	0.02	0.7
71046	0.22	0.65	0.02	0.89
71047	0.27	0.83	0.02	1.12
71048	0.31	0.88	0.02	1.21
Facility RVU	**Work**	**PE**	**MP**	**Total**
71045	0.18	0.5	0.02	0.7
71046	0.22	0.65	0.02	0.89
71047	0.27	0.83	0.02	1.12
71048	0.31	0.88	0.02	1.21

74018-74021

74018 Radiologic examination, abdomen; 1 view
74019 2 views
74021 3 or more views

Explanation

In 74018, a single x-ray is taken of the patient's abdomen. Because an abdominal x-ray usually precedes another diagnostic imaging procedure, it is not coded separately unless performed as a separately identifiable examination. Report 74019 for two views and 74021 for three or more views.

Relative Value Units/Medicare Edits

Non-Facility RVU	Work	PE	MP	Total
74018	0.18	0.6	0.02	0.8
74019	0.23	0.73	0.02	0.98
74021	0.27	0.83	0.03	1.13
Facility RVU	**Work**	**PE**	**MP**	**Total**
74018	0.18	0.6	0.02	0.8
74019	0.23	0.73	0.02	0.98
74021	0.27	0.83	0.03	1.13

75557-75559

75557 Cardiac magnetic resonance imaging for morphology and function without contrast material;

75559 with stress imaging

Explanation

Cardiac magnetic resonance imaging (MRI) is a radiation-free, noninvasive technique that produces high quality, detailed, three-dimensional imaging of complex congenital heart defects, as well as functional cardiac analysis. MRI uses the natural magnetic properties of the hydrogen atoms in our bodies that emit radiofrequency signals when exposed to radio waves within a strong electromagnetic field. These signals are processed and converted by the computer into high-resolution images. Patients with metallic or electronic implants or foreign bodies cannot be exposed to MRI. The patient must remain still while lying on a motorized table within the large, circular MRI tunnel. A sedative may be administered. Imaging is performed by obtaining tomographic cuts from the base to the apex and/or the interior to the posterior in order to interrogate the entire heart. Function studies may include observation of the atria and/or ventricles, qualitative and quantitative assessment of ventricular function, and obtaining numerical values for ejection fraction (EF) ventricular volumes, ventricular mass, and cardiac output. Code 75557 describes the observation of the cardiac function and morphology without administration of a contrast agent. Report 75559 if stress imaging is included. Following dobutamine injection, which mimics the effects of exercise on the heart and induces ischemia, the physician evaluates the left ventricular wall's ability to move during physical stress.

Relative Value Units/Medicare Edits

Non-Facility RVU	Work	PE	MP	Total
75557	2.35	6.69	0.12	9.16
75559	2.95	9.68	0.14	12.77
Facility RVU	**Work**	**PE**	**MP**	**Total**
75557	2.35	6.69	0.12	9.16
75559	2.95	9.68	0.14	12.77

75561-75565

75561 Cardiac magnetic resonance imaging for morphology and function without contrast material(s), followed by contrast material(s) and further sequences;

75563 with stress imaging

\+ **75565** Cardiac magnetic resonance imaging for velocity flow mapping (List separately in addition to code for primary procedure)

Explanation

Cardiac magnetic resonance imaging (MRI) is a radiation-free, noninvasive technique that produces high quality, detailed, three-dimensional imaging of complex congenital heart defects, as well as functional cardiac analysis. MRI uses the natural magnetic properties of the hydrogen atoms in our bodies that emit radiofrequency signals when exposed to radio waves within a strong electromagnetic field. These signals are processed and converted by the computer into high-resolution images. Patients with metallic or electronic implants or foreign bodies cannot be exposed to MRI. The patient must remain still while lying on a motorized table within the large, circular MRI tunnel. A sedative may be administered. Images are first obtained without contrast materials, followed by administration of contrast materials and further sequences. Imaging is performed by obtaining tomographic cuts from the base to the apex and/or the interior to the posterior in order to interrogate the entire heart. Function studies may include observation of the atria and/or ventricles, qualitative and quantitative assessment of ventricular function, and obtaining numerical values for ejection fraction (EF) ventricular volumes, ventricular mass, and cardiac output. Report 75561 for observation of cardiac function and morphology. Report 75563 if stress imaging is included. Following dobutamine injection, which mimics the effects of exercise on the heart and induces ischemia, the physician evaluates the left ventricular wall's ability to move during physical stress. If velocity flow mapping is performed, report 75565 in addition to the code for the primary procedure.

Relative Value Units/Medicare Edits

Non-Facility RVU	Work	PE	MP	Total
75561	2.6	9.29	0.14	12.03
75563	3.0	11.12	0.14	14.26
75565	0.25	1.25	0.01	1.51
Facility RVU	**Work**	**PE**	**MP**	**Total**
75561	2.6	9.29	0.14	12.03
75563	3.0	11.12	0.14	14.26
75565	0.25	1.25	0.01	1.51

75898

75898 Angiography through existing catheter for follow-up study for transcatheter therapy, embolization or infusion, other than for thrombolysis

Explanation

Angiography is performed during or following transcatheter infusion or embolization through the existing catheter to reassess the therapy's effectiveness. A radiopaque contrast medium is injected through the catheter and by fluoroscopic images recorded of the vessel, the radiologist interprets the status of the blood vessel and the effectiveness of treatment rendered.

Relative Value Units/Medicare Edits

Non-Facility RVU	Work	PE	MP	Total
75898	0.0	0.0	0.0	0.0
Facility RVU	**Work**	**PE**	**MP**	**Total**
75898	0.0	0.0	0.0	0.0

75989

75989 Radiological guidance (ie, fluoroscopy, ultrasound, or computed tomography), for percutaneous drainage (eg, abscess, specimen collection), with placement of catheter, radiological supervision and interpretation

Explanation

Fluoroscopic, ultrasonic, or CT guidance may be used for percutaneous drainage of an abscess or to obtain a specimen and place a tube or catheter. Once the abscess is located, the skin is punctured with a needle to begin draining. A catheter may be advanced over a guidewire inserted through the needle and into the abscess cavity. The tract to the outside is dilated to facilitate placing a percutaneous drainage tube. The cavity is aspirated and the drainage tube placed at the lowest point to ensure complete drainage. The drainage tube is secured to suction drainage. This code reports the radiological supervision and interpretation only for this procedure.

Relative Value Units/Medicare Edits

Non-Facility RVU	Work	PE	MP	Total
75989	1.19	2.14	0.09	3.42
Facility RVU	**Work**	**PE**	**MP**	**Total**
75989	1.19	2.14	0.09	3.42

76120-76125

76120 Cineradiography/videoradiography, except where specifically included

\+ **76125** Cineradiography/videoradiography to complement routine examination (List separately in addition to code for primary procedure)

Explanation

Cineradiography uses high speed x-ray films to take a series of images of an organ or system in motion such as the vocal cords or heart. These images taken in exposure ranges of nanoseconds to milliseconds are like the individual frames of a motion picture. This allows the movement to be frozen and tracked very minutely to gather information about time-varying characteristics. Use 76120 when performed alone and not specifically included as part of the procedure. Use 76125 when cineradiography is performed in conjunction with a routine exam.

Relative Value Units/Medicare Edits

Non-Facility RVU	Work	PE	MP	Total
76120	0.38	2.46	0.03	2.87
76125	0.0	0.0	0.0	0.0
Facility RVU	**Work**	**PE**	**MP**	**Total**
76120	0.38	2.46	0.03	2.87
76125	0.0	0.0	0.0	0.0

76604

76604 Ultrasound, chest (includes mediastinum), real time with image documentation

Explanation

Diagnostic ultrasound is an imaging technique bouncing sound waves far above the level of human perception through interior body structures. The sound waves pass through different densities of tissue and reflect back to a receiving unit at varying speeds. The unit converts the waves to electrical pulses that are immediately displayed in picture form on screen. Real time scanning displays structure images and movement with time. This code reports ultrasound and real time for the chest, including the mediastinum.

Relative Value Units/Medicare Edits

Non-Facility RVU	Work	PE	MP	Total
76604	0.55	1.92	0.04	2.51
Facility RVU	**Work**	**PE**	**MP**	**Total**
76604	0.55	1.92	0.04	2.51

76700-76705

76700 Ultrasound, abdominal, real time with image documentation; complete

76705 limited (eg, single organ, quadrant, follow-up)

Explanation

Diagnostic ultrasound is an imaging technique bouncing sound waves far above the level of human perception through interior body structures. The sound waves pass through different densities of tissue and reflect back to a receiving unit at varying speeds. The unit converts the waves to electrical pulses that are immediately displayed in picture form on screen. Real time scanning displays structure images and movement with time. Report 76700 for ultrasound and real time of the entire abdomen and 76705 for a single quadrant or organ of the abdomen.

Relative Value Units/Medicare Edits

Non-Facility RVU	Work	PE	MP	Total
76700	0.81	2.57	0.05	3.43
76705	0.59	1.93	0.04	2.56
Facility RVU	**Work**	**PE**	**MP**	**Total**
76700	0.81	2.57	0.05	3.43
76705	0.59	1.93	0.04	2.56

76706

76706 Ultrasound, abdominal aorta, real time with image documentation, screening study for abdominal aortic aneurysm (AAA)

Explanation

Screening ultrasound of the abdominal aorta with real time image documentation is the imaging technique of bouncing sound waves far above the level of human perception through interior body structures. The sound waves pass through different densities of tissue and reflect back to a receiving unit at varying speeds. The unit converts the waves to electrical pulses that are immediately displayed in picture form on screen. Real time scanning gathers and displays structural images and movement with time. This procedure is used as a tool to evaluate for abdominal aortic aneurysms (AAA) by viewing how the flow of blood moves through the abdominal aorta, which shows defects within the artery typical for an AAA. The U.S. Preventive Services Task Force has suggested screening be performed on men ages 65 to 75 who are or have been smokers, as well as men age 60 and older with family history of AAA.

Relative Value Units/Medicare Edits

Non-Facility RVU	Work	PE	MP	Total
76706	0.55	2.61	0.04	3.2
Facility RVU	**Work**	**PE**	**MP**	**Total**
76706	0.55	2.61	0.04	3.2

76932

76932 Ultrasonic guidance for endomyocardial biopsy, imaging supervision and interpretation

Explanation

The physician takes a biopsy of muscle tissue from within the heart guided by ultrasound. Ultrasound is an imaging technique bouncing sound waves far above the level of human perception through interior body structures. The sound waves pass through different densities of tissue and reflect back to a receiving unit, which converts the waves to electrical pulses that are immediately displayed in picture form on screen. The physician threads a biopsy catheter to the heart through a central intravenous line often inserted into the femoral vein and takes tissue samples of the heart's septum. This code reports the imaging supervision and interpretation only for this procedure.

Relative Value Units/Medicare Edits

Non-Facility RVU	Work	PE	MP	Total
76932	0.0	0.0	0.0	0.0
Facility RVU	**Work**	**PE**	**MP**	**Total**
76932	0.0	0.0	0.0	0.0

76937

\+ **76937** Ultrasound guidance for vascular access requiring ultrasound evaluation of potential access sites, documentation of selected vessel patency, concurrent realtime ultrasound visualization of vascular needle entry, with permanent recording and reporting (List separately in addition to code for primary procedure)

Explanation

This is an add-on code to report ultrasound guidance used in conjunction with procedures requiring vascular access. For example: a tunneled, centrally inserted CVAD is inserted without subcutaneous port or pump. The site over the access vein (e.g., subclavian, jugular) is injected with local anesthesia and punctured with a needle or accessed by cutdown approach. A guidewire is inserted. A subcutaneous tunnel is created using a blunt pair of forceps or sharp tunneling tools, over the clavicle from the anterior chest wall to the venotomy site, which is dilated to the right size. The catheter is passed through this tunnel over the guidewire and into the target vein. Report 76937 for the ultrasound guidance used for this procedure, including the evaluation of potential vascular access sites or the patency of selected vessels; guidance during needle entry and catheter manipulation; and verification of final catheter positioning. This code includes permanent recording and reporting.

Relative Value Units/Medicare Edits

Non-Facility RVU	Work	PE	MP	Total
76937	0.3	0.64	0.02	0.96
Facility RVU	**Work**	**PE**	**MP**	**Total**
76937	0.3	0.64	0.02	0.96

76978-76979

76978 Ultrasound, targeted dynamic microbubble sonographic contrast characterization (non-cardiac); initial lesion

\+ **76979** each additional lesion with separate injection (List separately in addition to code for primary procedure)

Explanation

Contrast-enhanced ultrasound (CEUS) imaging using microbubbles as an intravascular contrast agent has shown to be extremely effective in measuring blood flow in the heart and other organs; imaging blood perfusion in organs; describing and defining lesions, particularly focal liver lesions; and evaluating therapy responses. Microbubbles are approximately the same size as a red blood cell and are made up of a gas (e.g., perfluoro gas) enclosed with a phospholipid shell and have the ability to reflect ultrasound waves, enhance the reflections of the ultrasound waves, and create a unique image. There is a variety of microbubble contrast agents that vary based on the shell and gas core composition, as well as whether they are targeted or untargeted. Currently, all FDA-approved microbubbles are considered "untargeted," meaning they are used in clinics today; "targeted" microbubbles are in preclinical development. The microbubbles are administered using a small bolus or via continuous intravenous infusion into the circulation system and remain in the bloodstream for about five minutes. The technician directs the ultrasound waves to the area being evaluated; once the microbubbles pass into the ultrasound waves, the microbubbles produce a "fingerprint-like" harmonic reverberating sound within the ultrasound field vastly different from surrounding tissue that can be detected using microbubble-specific software. The system subsequently produces a contrast-enhanced real-time image. Microbubbles as a contrast agent are better tolerated over MR and CT agents, do not have as many side-effects and, when present, the side effects are typically less severe, and are not as toxic to the kidneys. Report 76978 for the initial lesion targeted and 76979 for each additional lesion with separate injection.

Relative Value Units/Medicare Edits

Non-Facility RVU	Work	PE	MP	Total
76978	1.62	7.45	0.11	9.18
76979	0.85	5.33	0.05	6.23
Facility RVU	**Work**	**PE**	**MP**	**Total**
76978	1.62	7.45	0.11	9.18
76979	0.85	5.33	0.05	6.23

77001

\+ **77001** Fluoroscopic guidance for central venous access device placement, replacement (catheter only or complete), or removal (includes fluoroscopic guidance for vascular access and catheter manipulation, any necessary contrast injections through access site or catheter with related venography radiologic supervision and interpretation, and radiographic documentation of final catheter position) (List separately in addition to code for primary procedure)

Explanation

This code reports the fluoroscopic guidance for placement, replacement, or removal of a central venous access device (CVAD) to be used in conjunction with the code for the procedure. For example, a tunneled, centrally inserted CVAD is inserted without subcutaneous port or pump. The site over the access vein (e.g., subclavian, jugular) is injected with local anesthesia and punctured with a needle or accessed by cutdown approach. A guidewire is inserted. A subcutaneous tunnel is created using a blunt pair of forceps or sharp tunneling tools over the clavicle from the anterior chest wall to the venotomy site, which is dilated to the right size. The catheter is passed through this tunnel over the guidewire and into the target vein. Fluoroscopy is used throughout the procedure to guide catheter placement and to check the positioning of the catheter tip. This code includes any contrast injections done through the access site or through the catheter with the necessary corresponding radiological supervision and interpretation of the venography, and the radiographic check of final catheter position.

Relative Value Units/Medicare Edits

Non-Facility RVU	Work	PE	MP	Total
77001	0.38	2.13	0.04	2.55
Facility RVU	**Work**	**PE**	**MP**	**Total**
77001	0.38	2.13	0.04	2.55

77002

\+ **77002** Fluoroscopic guidance for needle placement (eg, biopsy, aspiration, injection, localization device) (List separately in addition to code for primary procedure)

Explanation

Fluoroscopic guidance produces x-ray images shown on a screen to assist in visualization of the anatomy, instrument insertion, and/or contrast. This code is specifically reported when utilized for needle biopsy or fine needle aspiration. A cutting biopsy or fine needle is inserted into the target area and the position reaffirmed by fluoroscopy. This is done for an internal mass or lesion that has been positively identified by other diagnostic imaging performed earlier.

Relative Value Units/Medicare Edits

Non-Facility RVU	Work	PE	MP	Total
77002	0.54	2.28	0.04	2.86
Facility RVU	**Work**	**PE**	**MP**	**Total**
77002	0.54	2.28	0.04	2.86

78414

78414 Determination of central c-v hemodynamics (non-imaging) (eg, ejection fraction with probe technique) with or without pharmacologic intervention or exercise, single or multiple determinations

Explanation

Measurement of central cardiovascular hemodynamics, such as left ventricular ejection fraction, is performed noninvasively using a scintillation probe. Using chest x-rays or echocardiography, the proper location for the probe is marked on the chest wall. An intravenous bolus of radiotracer and/or exercise may be introduced. The probe is applied and the variations in left ventricular volume changes are recorded and measured.

Relative Value Units/Medicare Edits

Non-Facility RVU	Work	PE	MP	Total
78414	0.0	0.0	0.0	0.0
Facility RVU	**Work**	**PE**	**MP**	**Total**
78414	0.0	0.0	0.0	0.0

78428

78428 Cardiac shunt detection

Explanation

For detecting right to left cardiac shunts, radiolabeled macroaggregated albumin is used, which is trapped by the lungs and will be identified in the systemic circulation if a right to left shunt is present. For left to right shunts, the first pass technique is used. A bolus of radionuclide is injected and rapid image frames are acquired as it moves in the venous system through the chambers of the heart. Early recirculation detected would identify a left to right shunt.

Relative Value Units/Medicare Edits

Non-Facility RVU	Work	PE	MP	Total
78428	0.78	4.45	0.06	5.29
Facility RVU	**Work**	**PE**	**MP**	**Total**
78428	0.78	4.45	0.06	5.29

78445

78445 Non-cardiac vascular flow imaging (ie, angiography, venography)

Explanation

Nuclear imaging for non-cardiac vascular flow studies may be performed to test for arterial or venous peripheral vascular diseases or injuries, graft patency, and even catheter malfunctions. In radionuclide angiography, for example, red blood cells from the patient are tagged with radioactivity and injected intravenously. A scintillation camera positioned over the arterial area of interest detects the radioactivity in the blood and takes a series of dynamic images every 2 to 3 seconds immediately after injection, followed by static images. These are recorded on computer and/or film to be studied at different frame rates, times, and intensities. Normal flow is demonstrated as swift and unimpeded. Luminal narrowing or widening, blood flow obstructions and occlusions, and extraluminal accumulation of the radioactive cells can be visualized for diagnostic purposes.

Relative Value Units/Medicare Edits

Non-Facility RVU	Work	PE	MP	Total
78445	0.49	4.82	0.07	5.38
Facility RVU	**Work**	**PE**	**MP**	**Total**
78445	0.49	4.82	0.07	5.38

78451-78452

78451 Myocardial perfusion imaging, tomographic (SPECT) (including attenuation correction, qualitative or quantitative wall motion, ejection fraction by first pass or gated technique, additional quantification, when performed); single study, at rest or stress (exercise or pharmacologic)

78452 multiple studies, at rest and/or stress (exercise or pharmacologic) and/or redistribution and/or rest reinjection

Explanation

For tomographic myocardial perfusion imaging, the patient receives an intravenous injection of a radionuclide, usually thallium or technetium-99m, which localizes only in nonischemic tissue. SPECT (single photon emission computed tomographic) images of the heart are taken immediately to identify areas of perfusion vs. infarction. SPECT imaging differs from planar imaging by using a single or multiple-head camera that rotates around the patient to give three-dimensional tomographic imaging of the heart displayed in thin slices. In the nonstress version of the procedure, radionuclide is injected and images are taken without stress induction. In 78451, a single study is performed at rest or stress. If the test is to be done at a stress condition, it is induced with the standard treadmill exercise test or pharmacologically with the infusion of a vasodilator. In 78452, multiple studies are done at rest and/or stress with a second injection of radionuclide given again in the redistribution and/or resting phase just prior to resting images being taken. These codes also include attenuation correction (AC), which provides a more accurate diagnostic image for diagnosing defects or infarcted areas by raising the importance of radioactivity distribution counts arising from certain areas. For instance, counts from the anterior wall may be reduced or impeded by the presence of the breast. These codes also include qualitative or quantitative wall motion, ejection fraction (EF) by first pass or gated technique, and additional quantification, when performed.

Relative Value Units/Medicare Edits

Non-Facility RVU	Work	PE	MP	Total
78451	1.38	8.29	0.1	9.77
78452	1.62	11.86	0.12	13.6
Facility RVU	**Work**	**PE**	**MP**	**Total**
78451	1.38	8.29	0.1	9.77
78452	1.62	11.86	0.12	13.6

78453-78454

78453 Myocardial perfusion imaging, planar (including qualitative or quantitative wall motion, ejection fraction by first pass or gated technique, additional quantification, when performed); single study, at rest or stress (exercise or pharmacologic)

78454 multiple studies, at rest and/or stress (exercise or pharmacologic) and/or redistribution and/or rest reinjection

Explanation

For planar myocardial perfusion imaging, stress is induced with the standard treadmill exercise test or pharmacologically with the infusion of a vasodilator, if the test is to be done at stress conditions. The patient receives an intravenous injection of a radionuclide, usually thallium or technetium-99m, which localizes only in nonischemic tissue. Planar images of the heart are scanned immediately with a gamma camera that detects the radiation in the heart tissue to identify areas of infarction. In the nonstress version of the procedure, radionuclide is injected and images taken without stress induction. In 78453, a single study is performed at rest or stress. In 78454, multiple procedures are done at rest and/or at stress with a second injection of radionuclide given again in the redistribution or resting phase just prior to resting images being taken. For tests performed during pharmacological or exercise-induced stress, report the appropriate stress testing code. These codes also include qualitative or quantitative wall motion, ejection fraction (EF) by first pass or gated technique, and additional quantification, when performed.

Relative Value Units/Medicare Edits

Non-Facility RVU	Work	PE	MP	Total
78453	1.0	7.69	0.09	8.78
78454	1.34	11.1	0.12	12.56
Facility RVU	**Work**	**PE**	**MP**	**Total**
78453	1.0	7.69	0.09	8.78
78454	1.34	11.1	0.12	12.56

78456

78456 Acute venous thrombosis imaging, peptide

Explanation

Diagnostic nuclear imaging for acute venous thrombosis imaging uses radiolabeled peptides. Peptides are short-string proteins that attach to platelets, which are essential in blood clotting, and localize at sites where clots are present or beginning to form. Images from a scintillation, or gamma camera, are taken by detecting the gamma radiation from the radiotracer in the peptides attached to the blood component and these images can identify clots as soon as 10 minutes after the injection. Usually another set of images is done after 60 to 90 minutes following the injection as the image quality tends to improve with time after the injection. If a scan showed significantly increased uptake in any region of one leg compared to the other, or more intense uptake on delayed imaging, deep venous thrombosis is suspected.

Relative Value Units/Medicare Edits

Non-Facility RVU	Work	PE	MP	Total
78456	1.0	7.85	0.08	8.93
Facility RVU	**Work**	**PE**	**MP**	**Total**
78456	1.0	7.85	0.08	8.93

78457-78458

78457 Venous thrombosis imaging, venogram; unilateral
78458 bilateral

Explanation

A diagnostic nuclear venogram is done to identify the presence and location of thrombi (blood clots) within the venous system. An intravenous injection of a radiopharmaceutical into one or both extremities, most often the legs, is first performed. This is followed by rapid sequence imaging as the radiopharmaceutical passes through the venous system. Unilateral imaging for venous thrombosis is reported with 78457; bilateral imaging is reported with 78458. Bilateral studies may be performed even when only one leg is symptomatic for deep-vein thrombus as the normal extremity if used for comparison purposes.

Relative Value Units/Medicare Edits

Non-Facility RVU	Work	PE	MP	Total
78457	0.77	4.65	0.1	5.52
78458	0.9	4.94	0.08	5.92
Facility RVU	**Work**	**PE**	**MP**	**Total**
78457	0.77	4.65	0.1	5.52
78458	0.9	4.94	0.08	5.92

78459 [78429]

▲ **78459** Myocardial imaging, positron emission tomography (PET), metabolic evaluation study (including ventricular wall motion[s] and/or ejection fraction[s], when performed), single study;

● **78429** Myocardial imaging, positron emission tomography (PET), metabolic evaluation study (including ventricular wall motion[s] and/or ejection fraction[s], when performed), single study; with concurrently acquired computed tomography transmission scan

Explanation

In 78459, the cardiac muscle is imaged using data received from positron-emitting radionuclides administered to the patient by intravenous injection. The collision of the positrons emitted by the radionuclide with the negatively-charged electrons normally present in tissue is computer-synthesized to produce an image, usually in color. This image shows the presence or absence of ischemic or fibrotic cardiac tissue and allows evaluation of metabolic functioning of cardiac tissue. A test to determine the percentage of blood that is pumped out of a filled ventricle with each heartbeat, known as the ejection fraction, may also be undertaken at this time, as well as evaluation of ventricular wall motion. In 78429, a computed tomography (CT) scan is performed concurrently with the above-described PET study utilizing a combination PET/CT camera. Data sets obtained from the CT and PET are joined electronically by the scanner's computer system and can be viewed interactively by the clinician on a workstation, combining both excellent anatomic detail and physiologic information regarding metabolic activity.

Relative Value Units/Medicare Edits

Non-Facility RVU	Work	PE	MP	Total
78429				
78459	0.0	0.0	0.0	0.0
Facility RVU	**Work**	**PE**	**MP**	**Total**
78429				
78459	0.0	0.0	0.0	0.0

78466-78469

78466 Myocardial imaging, infarct avid, planar; qualitative or quantitative
78468 with ejection fraction by first pass technique
78469 tomographic SPECT with or without quantification

Explanation

A radionuclide is injected intravenously that localizes in recently (under 72-hours) infarcted myocardial tissue. Multiple cardiac images are obtained between one and four hours after injection of the isotope. The location and extent of infarct can be determined by the presence of the radionuclide in the heart tissue. In 78468, first-pass technique is utilized. In first-pass technique, a bolus of Technetium-99m or other radionuclide is injected and visualized as it moves through the venous system into the right atrium, right ventricle, pulmonary artery, lungs, left atrium, left ventricle, and aorta. Several cardia cycles are generally observed. Ejection fraction measurements from both the right and left ventricle are calculated by determining the change in radioactivity over time. In 78469, SPECT images are obtained. SPECT images are tomographic reconstructions derived from a single- or multiple-head gamma camera that rotates around the patient. Tomographic imaging displays the heart in thin slices allowing better separation of myocardial and nonmyocardial structures. SPECT imaging is helpful in identifying small infarcts that are sometimes missed using planar imaging alone.

Relative Value Units/Medicare Edits

Non-Facility RVU	Work	PE	MP	Total
78466	0.69	4.92	0.06	5.67
78468	0.8	5.01	0.07	5.88
78469	0.92	5.52	0.06	6.5
Facility RVU	**Work**	**PE**	**MP**	**Total**
78466	0.69	4.92	0.06	5.67
78468	0.8	5.01	0.07	5.88
78469	0.92	5.52	0.06	6.5

78472-78473

78472 Cardiac blood pool imaging, gated equilibrium; planar, single study at rest or stress (exercise and/or pharmacologic), wall motion study plus ejection fraction, with or without additional quantitative processing

78473 multiple studies, wall motion study plus ejection fraction, at rest and stress (exercise and/or pharmacologic), with or without additional quantification

Explanation

Radionuclide, which will adhere to the patient's red blood cells, is injected intravenously for cardiac blood pool imaging. Multiple images of the heart, synchronized with the electrocardiographic RR interval (ECG gated), are taken several minutes later, after the radionuclide has spread through the blood pool. These images are computer synthesized and data is generated to produce a video display of cardiac wall motion, calculation of left ventricular ejection fractions, and images based on computer manipulation of the data received. In 78472, the procedure is performed as a single study at rest or stress, not both; in 78473, the procedure is performed at both rest and stress. For tests performed during pharmacological or exercise-induced stress, report the appropriate stress testing code also.

Relative Value Units/Medicare Edits

Non-Facility RVU	Work	PE	MP	Total
78472	0.98	5.53	0.08	6.59
78473	1.47	6.76	0.09	8.32
Facility RVU	**Work**	**PE**	**MP**	**Total**
78472	0.98	5.53	0.08	6.59
78473	1.47	6.76	0.09	8.32

78481-78483

78481 Cardiac blood pool imaging (planar), first pass technique; single study, at rest or with stress (exercise and/or pharmacologic), wall motion study plus ejection fraction, with or without quantification

78483 multiple studies, at rest and with stress (exercise and/or pharmacologic), wall motion study plus ejection fraction, with or without quantification

Explanation

A bolus of radionuclide is injected intravenously for cardiac blood pool imaging, first pass technique. As the radioisotope passes through the cardiac chambers, rapid sequence imaging and computer generation of data and images is done to produce a video display of cardiac wall motion, calculation of ventricular ejection fractions, and images based on computer manipulation of the data received. This technique provides information about the functional status of the heart at rest or in response to stress. In 78481, the procedure is performed as a single study at rest or stress, not both; in 78483, the procedure is performed at rest and stress. For tests performed during pharmacological or exercise-induced stress, report the appropriate stress testing code also.

Relative Value Units/Medicare Edits

Non-Facility RVU	Work	PE	MP	Total
78481	0.98	4.01	0.07	5.06
78483	1.47	5.28	0.08	6.83
Facility RVU	**Work**	**PE**	**MP**	**Total**
78481	0.98	4.01	0.07	5.06
78483	1.47	5.28	0.08	6.83

78491, 78492

▲ **78491** Myocardial imaging, positron emission tomography (PET), perfusion study (including ventricular wall motion[s] and/or ejection fraction[s], when performed); single study, at rest or stress (exercise or pharmacologic)

▲ **78492** multiple studies at rest and stress (exercise or pharmacologic)

Explanation

The cardiac muscle is imaged using data received from positron-emitting radionuclides administered to the patient by intravenous injection. The collision of the positrons emitted by the radionuclide with the negatively-charged electrons normally present in tissue is computer-synthesized to produce an image, usually in color, which shows the presence or absence of perfusion into normal or ischemic cardiac tissue. A determination of the percentage of blood that is pumped out of a filled ventricle with each heartbeat, known as the ejection fraction, may also be made at this time, as well as evaluation of ventricular wall motion. Report 78491 if the procedure is performed as a single study at rest or during exercise or pharmacologic-induced stress. Report 78492 for multiple studies at rest and during exercise or pharmacologic-induced stress.

Relative Value Units/Medicare Edits

Non-Facility RVU	Work	PE	MP	Total
78491	0.0	0.0	0.0	0.0
78492	0.0	0.0	0.0	0.0
Facility RVU	**Work**	**PE**	**MP**	**Total**
78491	0.0	0.0	0.0	0.0
78492	0.0	0.0	0.0	0.0

[78430, 78431]

● **78430** Myocardial imaging, positron emission tomography (PET), perfusion study (including ventricular wall motion[s] and/or ejection fraction[s], when performed); single study, at rest or stress (exercise or pharmacologic), with concurrently acquired computed tomography transmission scan

● **78431** Myocardial imaging, positron emission tomography (PET), perfusion study (including ventricular wall motion[s] and/or ejection fraction[s], when performed); multiple studies at rest and stress (exercise or pharmacologic), with concurrently acquired computed tomography transmission scan

Explanation

The cardiac muscle is imaged using data received from positron-emitting radionuclides administered to the patient by intravenous injection. The collision of the positrons emitted by the radionuclide with the negatively-charged electrons normally present in tissue is computer-synthesized to produce an image, usually in color, which shows the presence or absence of perfusion into normal or ischemic cardiac tissue. A determination of the percentage of blood that is pumped out of a filled ventricle with each heartbeat, known as the ejection fraction, may also be made at this time, as well as evaluation of ventricular wall motion. A computed tomography (CT) scan is performed concurrently with the aforementioned PET study utilizing a combination PET/CT camera. Data sets obtained from the CT and PET are joined electronically by the scanner's computer system and can be viewed interactively by the clinician on a work station, combining both excellent anatomic detail and pertinent physiologic information. Report 78430 if the procedure is performed as a single study at rest or during exercise or pharmacologic-induced stress. Report 78431 for multiple studies at rest and during exercise or pharmacologic-induced stress.

Relative Value Units/Medicare Edits

Non-Facility RVU	Work	PE	MP	Total
78430				
78431				
Facility RVU	**Work**	**PE**	**MP**	**Total**
78430				
78431				

[78432, 78433]

● **78432** Myocardial imaging, positron emission tomography (PET), combined perfusion with metabolic evaluation study (including ventricular wall motion[s] and/or ejection fraction[s], when performed), dual radiotracer (eg, myocardial viability);

● **78433** Myocardial imaging, positron emission tomography (PET), combined perfusion with metabolic evaluation study (including ventricular wall motion[s] and/or ejection fraction[s], when performed), dual radiotracer (eg, myocardial viability); with concurrently acquired computed tomography transmission scan

Explanation

In 78432, a myocardial viability study is undertaken using dual radiotracers such as rubidium-82 (to measure blood flow) and 18F-fluorodeoxyglucose or FDG (to measure whether heart muscle cells are alive) that are administered to the patient by intravenous injection. The collision of the positrons emitted by the radionuclide with the negatively-charged electrons normally present in tissue is computer-synthesized to produce an image, usually in color, which shows the presence or absence of ischemic or fibrotic cardiac tissue and allows evaluation of its metabolic functioning. It also reveals the presence or absence of perfusion into these tissues. A determination of the percentage of blood that is pumped out of a filled ventricle with each heartbeat, known as the ejection fraction, may also be made at this time, as well as evaluation of ventricular wall motion. The procedure is performed to assess myocardial viability. In 78433, a computed tomography (CT) scan is performed concurrently with the above-described PET study utilizing a combination PET/CT camera. Data sets obtained from the CT and PET are joined electronically by the scanner's computer system and can be viewed interactively by the clinician on a workstation, combining both excellent anatomic detail and pertinent physiologic information.

Relative Value Units/Medicare Edits

Non-Facility RVU	Work	PE	MP	Total
78432				
78433				
Facility RVU	**Work**	**PE**	**MP**	**Total**
78432				
78433				

[78434]

+● **78434** Absolute quantitation of myocardial blood flow (AQMBF), positron emission tomography (PET), rest and pharmacologic stress (List separately in addition to code for primary procedure)

Explanation

The physician performs absolute quantitation of myocardial blood flow during rest and pharmacologic stress using positron emission tomography (PET). Absolute quantitation of myocardial blood flow (MBF) by PET is an established method and superior tool in the detection, analysis, and management of epicardial and microvascular coronary artery disease (CAD) and provides clinicians the ability to measure, in a noninvasive manner, MBF in milliliters per minute, per gram of tissue. Positron emission tomography is a radionuclide imaging technique for noninvasive quantification of MBF. The process of evaluating myocardial perfusion is a key aspect in diagnosing and determining outcomes for cases of suspected or known CAD. Resting MBF is the total amount of blood flow received by the myocardium per minute, per gram of tissue and may be impacted by a myriad of factors including, but not limited to, the patient's age, gender, blood pressure, and heart rate. Normal values for MBF at rest range from 0.6 to 1.3 mL/min/g. Stress MBF, also referred to as hyperemic blood flow, describes the highest amount of blood flow that can be provided to the heart during the topmost period of vasodilation of the heart's vascular bed. Typically, to reach this maximum vasodilation, the patient receives vasodilators or inotropic agents via IV to simulate stress as well as a cold pressor test (CPT) and mental stress tests. Stress MBF may be impacted by a number of factors including, but not limited to, caffeine, increased microvascular tone and resistance, and coronary risk factors. Report 78434 in addition to the code for the primary procedure.

Relative Value Units/Medicare Edits

Non-Facility RVU	Work	PE	MP	Total
78434				
Facility RVU	**Work**	**PE**	**MP**	**Total**
78434				

78494

78494 Cardiac blood pool imaging, gated equilibrium, SPECT, at rest, wall motion study plus ejection fraction, with or without quantitative processing

Explanation

Radionuclide, which will adhere to the patient's red blood cells, is injected intravenously for cardiac blood pool imaging, gated equilibrium. Multiple SPECT (single photon emission computed tomography) images of the heart, synchronized with the electrocardiographic RR interval (ECG gated), are taken several minutes later, after the radionuclide has spread through the blood pool. These SPECT images are taken by a rotating single or multiple-head camera for three-dimensional views of cross-sectional slices and provide better contrast in imaging and greater accuracy than planar scans. The SPECT images are computer synthesized and data is generated to produce a video display of cardiac wall motion, calculation of ventricular ejection fractions, and images based on computer manipulation of the data received.

Relative Value Units/Medicare Edits

Non-Facility RVU	Work	PE	MP	Total
78494	1.19	5.24	0.08	6.51
Facility RVU	**Work**	**PE**	**MP**	**Total**
78494	1.19	5.24	0.08	6.51

78496

+ **78496** Cardiac blood pool imaging, gated equilibrium, single study, at rest, with right ventricular ejection fraction by first pass technique (List separately in addition to code for primary procedure)

Explanation

A bolus of radionuclide is injected intravenously for cardiac blood pool imaging with right ventricular ejection fraction by first pass technique. As the radioisotope in the venous system passes through the cardiac chambers, rapid sequence imaging, synchronized with the electrocardiographic RR interval (ECG gated), is done. This first pass technique provides information for right ventricular ejection fraction calculation not possible with static gated images which do not show right ventricular count in isolation. This test for functional status of the heart is done as a single study at rest in addition to the primary procedure.

Relative Value Units/Medicare Edits

Non-Facility RVU	Work	PE	MP	Total
78496	0.5	0.72	0.03	1.25
Facility RVU	**Work**	**PE**	**MP**	**Total**
78496	0.5	0.72	0.03	1.25

80051

80051 Electrolyte panel This panel must include the following: Carbon dioxide (bicarbonate) (82374) Chloride (82435) Potassium (84132) Sodium (84295)

Explanation

An electrolyte panel includes the following tests: carbon dioxide (82374), chloride (82435), potassium (84132), and sodium (84295). Blood specimen is obtained by venipuncture. See specific codes for additional information about the listed tests.

Relative Value Units/Medicare Edits

Non-Facility RVU	Work	PE	MP	Total
80051	0.0	0.0	0.0	0.0
Facility RVU	**Work**	**PE**	**MP**	**Total**
80051	0.0	0.0	0.0	0.0

80061

80061 Lipid panel This panel must include the following: Cholesterol, serum, total (82465) Lipoprotein, direct measurement, high density cholesterol (HDL cholesterol) (83718) Triglycerides (84478)

Explanation

A lipid panel includes the following tests: total serum cholesterol (82465), high-density cholesterol (HDL cholesterol) by direct measurement (83718), and triglycerides (84478). Blood specimen is obtained by venipuncture. See specific codes for additional information about the listed tests.

Relative Value Units/Medicare Edits

Non-Facility RVU	Work	PE	MP	Total
80061	0.0	0.0	0.0	0.0
Facility RVU	**Work**	**PE**	**MP**	**Total**
80061	0.0	0.0	0.0	0.0

80162-80163

80162 Digoxin; total
80163 free

Explanation

This digitalis glycoside or digoxin has numerous trade names: Crystodigin, Purodigin, Lanoxin, etc. The drugs are used principally to treat conditions surrounding congestive heart failure, such as arrhythmias, atrial fibrillation, and tachycardia. Test specimens may be drawn during peak and trough periods, which is shortly after administration of digitalis and again just before the next administration when serum concentration is at its lowest. Method for total digoxin (80162) is high performance liquid chromatography (HPLC) or gas liquid chromatography (GLC) and is used to determine dosage. Free digoxin levels are useful in determining digoxin toxicity. A protein-free ultrafiltrate is prepared from the patient's serum, and the digoxin in the ultrafiltrate (free digoxin) is measured by fluorescence polarization immunoassay. Report 80162 for total serum levels and 80163 when free digoxin is assayed.

Relative Value Units/Medicare Edits

Non-Facility RVU	Work	PE	MP	Total
80162	0.0	0.0	0.0	0.0
80163	0.0	0.0	0.0	0.0
Facility RVU	**Work**	**PE**	**MP**	**Total**
80162	0.0	0.0	0.0	0.0
80163	0.0	0.0	0.0	0.0

81000

81000 Urinalysis, by dip stick or tablet reagent for bilirubin, glucose, hemoglobin, ketones, leukocytes, nitrite, pH, protein, specific gravity, urobilinogen, any number of these constituents; non-automated, with microscopy

Explanation

This type of test may be ordered by the brand name product and the analytes tested. Although, screens are considered to show the presence of an analyte (qualitative), some newer products are semi-quantitative. Many are plastic strips that contain sites impregnated with chemicals that react with urine when the strip is dipped into a specimen. The result is a color change that is compared against a standardized chart. Most strips will test for numerous analytes, as well as for pH and specific gravity. Tablets work in a similar fashion. A drop of urine is placed on the tablet and a chemical reaction causes a color change that is compared to a standard chart. Usually, only a single analyte is under consideration, per tablet. Code 81000 involves a manual (nonautomated) test and includes a microscopic examination. Microscopy involves examination of the urine sediments or solids. The urine is first centrifuged in a graduated tube to concentrate the sediments. Samples (either wet or dry) are examined, usually under both high and low power, and abnormal constituents are noted. These may include a wide range of biological abnormalities, such as blood cells, casts, and bacteria, as well as chemical anomalies, such as crystals.

Relative Value Units/Medicare Edits

Non-Facility RVU	Work	PE	MP	Total
81000	0.0	0.0	0.0	0.0
Facility RVU	**Work**	**PE**	**MP**	**Total**
81000	0.0	0.0	0.0	0.0

 ● New ▲ Revised + Add On [Resequenced] © 2019 Optum360, LLC

81001

81001 Urinalysis, by dip stick or tablet reagent for bilirubin, glucose, hemoglobin, ketones, leukocytes, nitrite, pH, protein, specific gravity, urobilinogen, any number of these constituents; automated, with microscopy

Explanation

This type of test may be ordered by the type of processor used and the analytes tested. The testing methodology is similar to the manual strips, except that the color change caused by the chemical reaction with urine is processed and read mechanically. The strip is exposed to the urine sample and is mechanically fed through a processor that reads the colors emitted by the reaction. The unit will be calibrated according to international standards and readings have a high degree of accuracy. The result may be displayed on a monitor, but is always printed or recorded in some form. Code 81001 also includes microscopy. Microscopy involves examination of the urine sediments or solids. The urine is first centrifuged in a graduated tube to concentrate the sediments. Samples (wet or dry) are examined, usually under both high and low power, and abnormal constituents are noted. These may include a wide range of biological abnormalities, such as blood cells, casts, and bacteria, as well as chemical anomalies, such as crystals.

Relative Value Units/Medicare Edits

Non-Facility RVU	Work	PE	MP	Total
81001	0.0	0.0	0.0	0.0
Facility RVU	Work	PE	MP	Total
81001	0.0	0.0	0.0	0.0

81002

81002 Urinalysis, by dip stick or tablet reagent for bilirubin, glucose, hemoglobin, ketones, leukocytes, nitrite, pH, protein, specific gravity, urobilinogen, any number of these constituents; non-automated, without microscopy

Explanation

This type of test may be ordered by the brand name product and the analytes tested. Although usually considered screens to show the presence of an analyte (qualitative), some newer products are semi-quantitative. Many are plastic strips that contain sites impregnated with chemicals that react with urine when the strip is dipped into a specimen. The result is a color change that is compared against a standardized chart. Most strips will test for numerous analytes, as well as for pH and specific gravity. Tablets work in a similar fashion. A drop of urine is placed on the tablet and a chemical reaction causes a color change that is compared to a standard chart. Usually only a single analyte is under consideration per tablet, however. Code 81002 does not include a microscopic examination of the urine sample or its components.

Relative Value Units/Medicare Edits

Non-Facility RVU	Work	PE	MP	Total
81002	0.0	0.0	0.0	0.0
Facility RVU	Work	PE	MP	Total
81002	0.0	0.0	0.0	0.0

81003

81003 Urinalysis, by dip stick or tablet reagent for bilirubin, glucose, hemoglobin, ketones, leukocytes, nitrite, pH, protein, specific gravity, urobilinogen, any number of these constituents; automated, without microscopy

Explanation

This type of test may be ordered by the type of processor used and the analytes tested. The testing methodology is similar to the manual strips, except that the color change caused by the chemical reaction with urine is processed and read mechanically. The strip is exposed to the urine sample and is fed through a processor that reads the colors emitted by the reaction. The unit will be calibrated according to international standards and readings have a high degree of accuracy. The result may be displayed on a monitor, but is always printed or recorded in some form. Code 81003 does not include a microscopic examination of the urine sample or its components.

Relative Value Units/Medicare Edits

Non-Facility RVU	Work	PE	MP	Total
81003	0.0	0.0	0.0	0.0
Facility RVU	Work	PE	MP	Total
81003	0.0	0.0	0.0	0.0

82465

82465 Cholesterol, serum or whole blood, total

Explanation

Cholesterol level is a risk indicator for atherosclerosis and myocardial infarction. Blood specimen is obtained by venipuncture. Method is enzymatic. This test reports total cholesterol in serum or whole blood.

Relative Value Units/Medicare Edits

Non-Facility RVU	Work	PE	MP	Total
82465	0.0	0.0	0.0	0.0
Facility RVU	Work	PE	MP	Total
82465	0.0	0.0	0.0	0.0

82550

82550 Creatine kinase (CK), (CPK); total

Explanation

This test may be requested as creatine kinase (CK) or creatine phosphokinase (CPK). Blood specimen is obtained by venipuncture. Method is enzymatic, kinetic, or spectrophotometry. This code reports total CK. Creatine kinase is an enzyme found in striated muscle and it is released following injury. Elevated CK levels are primarily associated with myocardial infarction, trauma and surgery, but CK levels may be elevated with a number of other conditions as well.

Relative Value Units/Medicare Edits

Non-Facility RVU	Work	PE	MP	Total
82550	0.0	0.0	0.0	0.0
Facility RVU	Work	PE	MP	Total
82550	0.0	0.0	0.0	0.0

82552

82552 Creatine kinase (CK), (CPK); isoenzymes

Explanation

This test may be requested as creatine kinase (CK) isoenzymes or creatine phosphokinase (CPK) isoenzymes. Method is electrophoresis (EP), column ion-exchange chromatography. Creatine kinase consists of three isoenzymes, each of which is composed of two units, muscle (MM), brain (BB), or muscle and brain (MB). CK1 (BB) is found primarily in the brain and smooth muscle, CK2 (MB) in cardiac muscle, and CK3 (MM) in skeletal muscle. Because elevated

CK levels are indicative of injury to the cells, quantifying the levels of each isoenzyme may assist in pinpointing the injured site.

Relative Value Units/Medicare Edits

Non-Facility RVU	Work	PE	MP	Total
82552	0.0	0.0	0.0	0.0
Facility RVU	Work	PE	MP	Total
82552	0.0	0.0	0.0	0.0

82553

82553 Creatine kinase (CK), (CPK); MB fraction only

Explanation

This test may be requested as creatine kinase (CK) MB fraction, creatine phosphokinase (CPK) MB fraction, or CK2. Methods include immunochemical, fluorometric radial partition, microparticle enzyme immunoassay, immunoenzymetric, or chemiluminometric. Creatine kinase consists of three isoenzymes, which are each composed of two units, muscle (MM), brain (BB), or muscle and brain (MB). CK1 (BB) is found primarily in the brain and smooth muscle, CK2 (MB) in cardiac muscle, and CK3 (MM) in skeletal muscle. This code tests for the MB or CK2 fraction only.

Relative Value Units/Medicare Edits

Non-Facility RVU	Work	PE	MP	Total
82553	0.0	0.0	0.0	0.0
Facility RVU	Work	PE	MP	Total
82553	0.0	0.0	0.0	0.0

82554

82554 Creatine kinase (CK), (CPK); isoforms

Explanation

This test may be requested as CK isoforms or CPK isoforms. Blood specimen is obtained by venipuncture. Methods include electrophoresis (EP), high performance liquid chromatography (HPLC), and isoelectric focusing (IEF). Creatine kinase consists of three isoenzymes, which are each composed of two units, muscle (MM), brain (BB), or muscle and brain (MB). CK1 (BB) is found primarily in the brain and smooth muscle, CK2 (MB) in cardiac muscle, and CK3 (MM) in skeletal muscle. These isoenzymes can be further subdivided into isoforms which are designated by the isoenzyme (MM, MB, BB) followed by a number (e.g., 1, 2, 3) Examples include CK-MB1, CK-MB2.

Relative Value Units/Medicare Edits

Non-Facility RVU	Work	PE	MP	Total
82554	0.0	0.0	0.0	0.0
Facility RVU	Work	PE	MP	Total
82554	0.0	0.0	0.0	0.0

82800

82800 Gases, blood, pH only

Explanation

This test may be requested as blood pH. Blood pH is tested to identify acidemia or alkalemia. Arterial puncture is preferred, but venipuncture may also be performed. Method is glass pH electrode or potentiometry.

Relative Value Units/Medicare Edits

Non-Facility RVU	Work	PE	MP	Total
82800	0.0	0.0	0.0	0.0
Facility RVU	Work	PE	MP	Total
82800	0.0	0.0	0.0	0.0

82803-82805

82803 Gases, blood, any combination of pH, pCO2, pO2, CO2, HCO3 (including calculated O2 saturation);

82805 with O2 saturation, by direct measurement, except pulse oximetry

Explanation

These tests may be requested as arterial blood gases (ABGs). Blood gases are usually requested to evaluate disturbances of acid-base balance, which may be caused by respiratory or metabolic disorders. Blood specimen is obtained by arterial puncture. Code 82803 reports any combination of pH, pCO2, pO2, CO2, and HCO3, including calculated O2 saturation. Code 82805 reports any combination of the same gases, but O2 saturation is performed by direct measurement. Method is selective electrode, potentiometry, or spectrophotometry (O2 saturation).

Relative Value Units/Medicare Edits

Non-Facility RVU	Work	PE	MP	Total
82803	0.0	0.0	0.0	0.0
82805	0.0	0.0	0.0	0.0
Facility RVU	Work	PE	MP	Total
82803	0.0	0.0	0.0	0.0
82805	0.0	0.0	0.0	0.0

82810

82810 Gases, blood, O2 saturation only, by direct measurement, except pulse oximetry

Explanation

This test may be requested as O2. Oxygen saturation is the percent of the oxygen in the blood that combines with hemoglobin. Blood specimen is obtained by arterial puncture. Method is spectrophotometry.

Relative Value Units/Medicare Edits

Non-Facility RVU	Work	PE	MP	Total
82810	0.0	0.0	0.0	0.0
Facility RVU	Work	PE	MP	Total
82810	0.0	0.0	0.0	0.0

82820

82820 Hemoglobin-oxygen affinity (pO2 for 50% hemoglobin saturation with oxygen)

Explanation

This test may be requested as oxygen, P50 or as pO2, P50. This test is performed to measure the affinity of hemoglobin for oxygen, which allows evaluation of oxygen delivery to body tissues. Blood specimen is obtained by arterial puncture. Method is spectrophotometry or potentiometry.

Relative Value Units/Medicare Edits

Non-Facility RVU	Work	PE	MP	Total
82820	0.0	0.0	0.0	0.0
Facility RVU	**Work**	**PE**	**MP**	**Total**
82820	0.0	0.0	0.0	0.0

82948

82948 Glucose; blood, reagent strip

Explanation

This test is used to monitor disorders of carbohydrate metabolism. Blood specimen is obtained by finger stick. A drop of blood is placed on the reagent strip for a specified amount of time. When the prescribed amount of time has elapsed, the strip is blotted and the reagent strip is compared to a color chart. Method is reagent strip with visual comparison.

Relative Value Units/Medicare Edits

Non-Facility RVU	Work	PE	MP	Total
82948	0.0	0.0	0.0	0.0
Facility RVU	**Work**	**PE**	**MP**	**Total**
82948	0.0	0.0	0.0	0.0

83036-83037

83036 Hemoglobin; glycosylated (A1C)
83037 glycosylated (A1C) by device cleared by FDA for home use

Explanation

These tests may also be known as HbA1C. A blood specimen is collected. Glycosylated hemoglobin levels reflect the average level of glucose in the blood over a three-month period. Methods may include high-performance liquid chromatography and ion exchange chromatography (83036) or FDA approved home monitoring device (83037).

Relative Value Units/Medicare Edits

Non-Facility RVU	Work	PE	MP	Total
83036	0.0	0.0	0.0	0.0
83037	0.0	0.0	0.0	0.0
Facility RVU	**Work**	**PE**	**MP**	**Total**
83036	0.0	0.0	0.0	0.0
83037	0.0	0.0	0.0	0.0

83615

83615 Lactate dehydrogenase (LD), (LDH);

Explanation

This test may also be ordered as LD or LDH. The test is a measure of LD or LDH, which is found in many body tissues, particularly the heart, liver, red blood cells, and kidneys. Methods used are lactate to pyruvate or pyruvate to lactate. This test may be ordered for a wide variety of disorders, including renal diseases and congestive heart failure.

Relative Value Units/Medicare Edits

Non-Facility RVU	Work	PE	MP	Total
83615	0.0	0.0	0.0	0.0
Facility RVU	**Work**	**PE**	**MP**	**Total**
83615	0.0	0.0	0.0	0.0

83625

83625 Lactate dehydrogenase (LD), (LDH); isoenzymes, separation and quantitation

Explanation

This test may be ordered as LDH isoenzymes or LD isoenzymes. Three serial blood specimens are collected at 6-8 hour intervals to detect changes in the LD isoenzymes. Shifts in the values of five clinically significant LD fractions monitored over time create diagnostic patterns that correlate with diseases such as myocardial infarction, renal infarction and hepatic congestion. This allows for the differential diagnosis of numerous conditions. Method is by electrophoresis or immunochemical methods, including immunoprecipitation. This test may be ordered for a wide variety of reasons, and results may point to numerous diagnoses.

Relative Value Units/Medicare Edits

Non-Facility RVU	Work	PE	MP	Total
83625	0.0	0.0	0.0	0.0
Facility RVU	**Work**	**PE**	**MP**	**Total**
83625	0.0	0.0	0.0	0.0

83701

83701 Lipoprotein, blood; high resolution fractionation and quantitation of lipoproteins including lipoprotein subclasses when performed (eg, electrophoresis, ultracentrifugation)

Explanation

This test may be referred to as Type III fractionation. Type III hyperlipoproteinemia is an inherited disorder whereby both the cholesterol and triglycerides show high plasma concentrations. This particular test is usually performed following previous tests to further isolate abnormal beta-lipoproteins. The patient is told to fast. Blood is drawn by venipuncture. The test may be performed by various methods including ultracentrifugation or electrophoresis. Ultracentrifugation is more common and is considered the traditional standard for accuracy in high-density lipoproteins (HDL) subclass quantitation.

Relative Value Units/Medicare Edits

Non-Facility RVU	Work	PE	MP	Total
83701	0.0	0.0	0.0	0.0
Facility RVU	**Work**	**PE**	**MP**	**Total**
83701	0.0	0.0	0.0	0.0

83718

83718 Lipoprotein, direct measurement; high density cholesterol (HDL cholesterol)

Explanation

This test may be requested as HDL, HDLC, or HDL cholesterol. Lipoproteins are compounds composed of lipids bound to proteins, which are transported through the blood. High-density lipoprotein (HDL) is frequently referred to as "good cholesterol," or "friendly lipid," as it is responsible for decreasing plaque deposits in blood vessels. High levels of HDL decrease the risk of premature coronary artery disease. This code reports direct measurement only, normally performed using an enzymatic or precipitation method.

Relative Value Units/Medicare Edits

Non-Facility RVU	Work	PE	MP	Total
83718	0.0	0.0	0.0	0.0
Facility RVU	Work	PE	MP	Total
83718	0.0	0.0	0.0	0.0

83719

83719 Lipoprotein, direct measurement; VLDL cholesterol

Explanation

This test measures VLDL, the lipoprotein that carries triglycerides in the blood. The test is useful to determine a patient's risk of arteriosclerotic occlusive disease, as well as other cholesterol-related disorders. The method used is electrophoresis and may first involve ultracentrifugation.

Relative Value Units/Medicare Edits

Non-Facility RVU	Work	PE	MP	Total
83719	0.0	0.0	0.0	0.0
Facility RVU	Work	PE	MP	Total
83719	0.0	0.0	0.0	0.0

83721

83721 Lipoprotein, direct measurement; LDL cholesterol

Explanation

This test may also be referred to as LDL-C. It measures the amount of low-density lipoprotein (LDL), also known as "bad cholesterol." The test is useful to determine the patient's risk of coronary heart disease (CHD), among other disorders. Method may be by precipitation procedure with results derived by the Friedewald formula.

Relative Value Units/Medicare Edits

Non-Facility RVU	Work	PE	MP	Total
83721	0.0	0.0	0.0	0.0
Facility RVU	Work	PE	MP	Total
83721	0.0	0.0	0.0	0.0

83789

83789 Mass spectrometry and tandem mass spectrometry (eg, MS, MS/MS, MALDI, MS-TOF, QTOF), non-drug analyte(s) not elsewhere specified, qualitative or quantitative, each specimen

Explanation

This test identifies the presence of (qualitative), and measures the amount of (quantifies), specific analytes in protein. Specimen varies. Method is mass spectrometry (MS). The test is used for identifying the chemical makeup and structure of a substance. Tandem MS (MS/MS) is one type of MS using sequential analysis to provide structural information by establishing relationships between substances. Others include quadrupole/time-of-flight (Q/TOF) and matrix-assisted laser desorption/ionization (MALDI). This test assists in identifying the chemical makeup and structure of a substance, analyzing viruses, sequencing and analyzing peptides and proteins, and providing information on such life-threatening diseases as AIDS and various types of skin cancers as well as quantifies (measures) the amount of analyte in the specimen.

Relative Value Units/Medicare Edits

Non-Facility RVU	Work	PE	MP	Total
83789	0.0	0.0	0.0	0.0
Facility RVU	Work	PE	MP	Total
83789	0.0	0.0	0.0	0.0

84132

84132 Potassium; serum, plasma or whole blood

Explanation

This test may be requested as K or K+. Potassium is the major electrolyte found in intracellular fluids. Potassium influences skeletal and cardiac muscle activity. Very small fluctuations outside the normal range may cause significant health risk, including muscle weakness and cardiac arrhythmias. Blood specimen is serum, plasma, or whole blood. Methods include atomic absorption spectrometry (AAS), ion-selective electrode (ISE), and flame emission spectroscopy (FES).

Relative Value Units/Medicare Edits

Non-Facility RVU	Work	PE	MP	Total
84132	0.0	0.0	0.0	0.0
Facility RVU	Work	PE	MP	Total
84132	0.0	0.0	0.0	0.0

84450

84450 Transferase; aspartate amino (AST) (SGOT)

Explanation

This test is usually referred to as aspartate aminotransferase (AST) or as serum glutamic oxaloacetic transaminase (SGOT). AST is an enzyme found primarily in heart muscle and the liver. Serum levels are low unless there is cellular damage, at which time large amounts are released into circulation. AST levels are increased following acute myocardial infarction (MI). Liver disease may also cause elevated levels of AST. Blood specimen is serum or plasma. Method is spectrophotometry, kinetic assay, and enzymatic.

Relative Value Units/Medicare Edits

Non-Facility RVU	Work	PE	MP	Total
84450	0.0	0.0	0.0	0.0
Facility RVU	Work	PE	MP	Total
84450	0.0	0.0	0.0	0.0

84478

84478 Triglycerides

Explanation

This test may be requested as trig. Triglycerides are blood lipids that are transported through the circulatory system by lipoproteins. Triglycerides contribute to atherosclerosis and other arterial diseases. Blood specimen is serum or plasma. Method is enzymatic or colorimetry.

Relative Value Units/Medicare Edits

Non-Facility RVU	Work	PE	MP	Total
84478	0.0	0.0	0.0	0.0
Facility RVU	Work	PE	MP	Total
84478	0.0	0.0	0.0	0.0

84512

84512 Troponin, qualitative

Explanation

This may also be known as troponin regulatory complex. The specimen is plasma. Cardiac troponins are markers for myocardial muscle damage. Qualitative tests (positive/negative results) are primarily used to rule-in or rule-out myocardial infarction. Several bedside, point-of-care type assays are available. Methods are radioimmunoassay, enzyme-linked immunosorbent assay, and immunoenzymatic assay may also be seen.

Relative Value Units/Medicare Edits

Non-Facility RVU	Work	PE	MP	Total
84512	0.0	0.0	0.0	0.0
Facility RVU	Work	PE	MP	Total
84512	0.0	0.0	0.0	0.0

85002

85002 Bleeding time

Explanation

This test may be ordered as a bleeding time or as an Ivy bleeding time. A small, superficial wound is nicked in the patient's forearm. Essentially, the amount of time it takes for the wound to stop bleeding is recorded at bedside. The Ivy bleeding time test is one standardized method. All methods are manual or point of care. A bleeding time is a rough measure of platelet (thrombocyte) function. The test is often performed on a preoperative patient.

Relative Value Units/Medicare Edits

Non-Facility RVU	Work	PE	MP	Total
85002	0.0	0.0	0.0	0.0
Facility RVU	Work	PE	MP	Total
85002	0.0	0.0	0.0	0.0

85004

85004 Blood count; automated differential WBC count

Explanation

This test may be ordered as a blood count with automated differential. The specimen is whole blood. Method is automated cell counter. The blood count typically includes a measurement of normal cell constituents including white blood cells or leukocytes, red blood cells, and platelets. In addition, this test includes a differential count of the white blood cells or "diff" in which the following leukocytes are differentiated and counted automatically: neutrophils or granulocytes, lymphocytes, monocytes, eosinophils, and basophils.

Relative Value Units/Medicare Edits

Non-Facility RVU	Work	PE	MP	Total
85004	0.0	0.0	0.0	0.0
Facility RVU	Work	PE	MP	Total
85004	0.0	0.0	0.0	0.0

85007

85007 Blood count; blood smear, microscopic examination with manual differential WBC count

Explanation

This test may be ordered as a manual blood smear examination, RBC smear, peripheral blood smear, or RBC morphology with manual WBC differential. The specimen is whole blood. The method is manual testing. A blood smear is prepared and microscopically examined for the presence of normal cell constituents, including white blood cells, red blood cells, and platelets. A manual differential of white blood cells is included in which the following leukocytes are differentiated: neutrophils or granulocytes, lymphocytes, monocytes, eosinophils, and basophils.

Relative Value Units/Medicare Edits

Non-Facility RVU	Work	PE	MP	Total
85007	0.0	0.0	0.0	0.0
Facility RVU	Work	PE	MP	Total
85007	0.0	0.0	0.0	0.0

85008

85008 Blood count; blood smear, microscopic examination without manual differential WBC count

Explanation

This test may be ordered as a manual blood smear examination, RBC smear, peripheral blood smear, or RBC morphology without differential WBC count. The specimen is whole blood. This method is manual testing. A blood smear is prepared and microscopically examined for the presence of normal cell constituents, including white blood cells, red blood cells, and platelets. The white blood cell and platelet or thrombocyte counts are estimated and red cell morphology is commented on if abnormal.

Relative Value Units/Medicare Edits

Non-Facility RVU	Work	PE	MP	Total
85008	0.0	0.0	0.0	0.0
Facility RVU	Work	PE	MP	Total
85008	0.0	0.0	0.0	0.0

85009

85009 Blood count; manual differential WBC count, buffy coat

Explanation

This test may be ordered as a buffy coat differential or as a differential WBC count, buffy coat. Specimen is whole blood. Other collection types (e.g., finger stick or heel stick) do not yield the volume of blood required for this test. Method is manual testing. The whole blood is centrifuged to concentrate the white blood cells, and a manual WBC differential is performed in which the following leukocytes are differentiated: neutrophils or granulocytes, lymphocytes, monocytes, eosinophils, and basophils. This test is usually performed when the number of WBCs or leukocytes is abnormally low and the presence of abnormal white cells (e.g., blasts or cancer cells) is suspected clinically.

Relative Value Units/Medicare Edits

Non-Facility RVU	Work	PE	MP	Total
85009	0.0	0.0	0.0	0.0
Facility RVU	Work	PE	MP	Total
85009	0.0	0.0	0.0	0.0

85013

85013 Blood count; spun microhematocrit

Explanation

This test may be ordered as a microhematocrit, a spun microhematocrit, or a "spun crit." The specimen (whole blood) is by finger stick or heel stick in infants. The sample is placed in a tube and into a microcentrifuge device. The vials can be read manually against a chart for the volume of packed red cells or a digital reader in the centrifuge device. A spun microhematocrit only reports the volume of packed red cells. It is typically performed at sites where limited testing is available, the patient is a very difficult blood draw, or on infants.

Relative Value Units/Medicare Edits

Non-Facility RVU	Work	PE	MP	Total
85013	0.0	0.0	0.0	0.0
Facility RVU	Work	PE	MP	Total
85013	0.0	0.0	0.0	0.0

85014

85014 Blood count; hematocrit (Hct)

Explanation

This test may be ordered as a hematocrit, Hmt, or Hct. The specimen is whole blood. Method is automated cell counter. The hematocrit or volume of packed red cells (VPRC) in the blood sample is calculated by multiplying the red blood cell count or RBC times the mean corpuscular volume or MCV.

Relative Value Units/Medicare Edits

Non-Facility RVU	Work	PE	MP	Total
85014	0.0	0.0	0.0	0.0
Facility RVU	Work	PE	MP	Total
85014	0.0	0.0	0.0	0.0

85018

85018 Blood count; hemoglobin (Hgb)

Explanation

This test may be ordered as hemoglobin, Hgb, or hemoglobin concentration. The specimen is whole blood. Method is usually automated cell counter but a manual method is seen in labs with a limited test menu and blood bank drawing stations. Hemoglobin is an index of the oxygen-carrying capacity of the blood.

Relative Value Units/Medicare Edits

Non-Facility RVU	Work	PE	MP	Total
85018	0.0	0.0	0.0	0.0
Facility RVU	Work	PE	MP	Total
85018	0.0	0.0	0.0	0.0

85025

85025 Blood count; complete (CBC), automated (Hgb, Hct, RBC, WBC and platelet count) and automated differential WBC count

Explanation

This test may be ordered as a complete automated blood count (CBC). The specimen is whole blood. Method is automated cell counter. This code includes the measurement of erythrocytes (red blood cells or RBC), leukocytes (white blood cells or WBC), hemoglobin, hematocrit (volume of packed red blood cells or VPRC), platelet or thrombocyte count, and indices (mean corpuscular hemoglobin or MCH, mean corpuscular hemoglobin concentration or MCHC, mean corpuscular volume or MCV, and red cell distribution width or RDW). In addition, this test includes an automated differential of white blood cells or "diff" in which the following leukocytes will be differentiated: neutrophils or granulocytes, lymphocytes, monocytes, eosinophils and basophils.

Relative Value Units/Medicare Edits

Non-Facility RVU	Work	PE	MP	Total
85025	0.0	0.0	0.0	0.0
Facility RVU	Work	PE	MP	Total
85025	0.0	0.0	0.0	0.0

85027

85027 Blood count; complete (CBC), automated (Hgb, Hct, RBC, WBC and platelet count)

Explanation

This test may be ordered as a complete automated blood count (CBC). The specimen is whole blood. Method is automated cell counter. This code includes the measurement of erythrocytes (red blood cells or RBC), leukocytes (white blood cells or WBC), hemoglobin, hematocrit (volume of packed red blood cells or VPRC), platelet or thrombocyte count, and indices (mean corpuscular hemoglobin or MCH, mean corpuscular hemoglobin concentration or MCHC, mean corpuscular volume or MCV, and red cell distribution width or RDW). Report 85027 if the complete CBC, or automated blood count, is done without the differential WBC count.

Relative Value Units/Medicare Edits

Non-Facility RVU	Work	PE	MP	Total
85027	0.0	0.0	0.0	0.0
Facility RVU	Work	PE	MP	Total
85027	0.0	0.0	0.0	0.0

85032

85032 Blood count; manual cell count (erythrocyte, leukocyte, or platelet) each

Explanation

This code reports a manual cell count done for red blood cells (erythrocytes), white blood cells (leukocytes), or platelets (thrombocytes), each. The specimen is whole blood. The method is manual examination and counting.

Relative Value Units/Medicare Edits

Non-Facility RVU	Work	PE	MP	Total
85032	0.0	0.0	0.0	0.0
Facility RVU	Work	PE	MP	Total
85032	0.0	0.0	0.0	0.0

85041

85041 Blood count; red blood cell (RBC), automated

Explanation

This test may be ordered as red blood cell count or RBC. The specimen is by whole blood. Method is automated cell counter.

Relative Value Units/Medicare Edits

Non-Facility RVU	Work	PE	MP	Total
85041	0.0	0.0	0.0	0.0
Facility RVU	**Work**	**PE**	**MP**	**Total**
85041	0.0	0.0	0.0	0.0

85044

85044 Blood count; reticulocyte, manual

Explanation

This test may be ordered as a manual reticulocyte count or as a manual "retic." The specimen is whole blood. Method is manual. A blood smear is prepared and stained with a dye that highlights the reticulum in the immature red blood cells, or the reticulocytes. The reticulocytes reported as a percentage of total red blood cells.

Relative Value Units/Medicare Edits

Non-Facility RVU	Work	PE	MP	Total
85044	0.0	0.0	0.0	0.0
Facility RVU	**Work**	**PE**	**MP**	**Total**
85044	0.0	0.0	0.0	0.0

85045

85045 Blood count; reticulocyte, automated

Explanation

This test may be ordered as an automated reticulocyte count, an "auto retic," or a reticulocyte by flow cytometry. The specimen is whole blood. Method is automated cell counter or flow cytometer. Reticulocytes are immature red blood cells that still contain mitochondria and ribosomes. The reticulocytes are reported as a percentage of total red blood cells.

Relative Value Units/Medicare Edits

Non-Facility RVU	Work	PE	MP	Total
85045	0.0	0.0	0.0	0.0
Facility RVU	**Work**	**PE**	**MP**	**Total**
85045	0.0	0.0	0.0	0.0

85337

85337 Thrombomodulin

Explanation

This test may be ordered as a thrombomodulin assay. The specimen is plasma. The method is usually automated coagulation instrument but may be manual. Thrombomodulin is a protein involved in activation of the clot dissolution or lysis process.

Relative Value Units/Medicare Edits

Non-Facility RVU	Work	PE	MP	Total
85337	0.0	0.0	0.0	0.0
Facility RVU	**Work**	**PE**	**MP**	**Total**
85337	0.0	0.0	0.0	0.0

85348

85348 Coagulation time; other methods

Explanation

This test may be ordered as a clotting time. The specimen is whole blood finger stick or, in infants, heel stick. Methods vary, as the formal description implies. Point-of-care testing often involves a hand held instrument that gives some measurement of whole blood clotting time.

Relative Value Units/Medicare Edits

Non-Facility RVU	Work	PE	MP	Total
85348	0.0	0.0	0.0	0.0
Facility RVU	**Work**	**PE**	**MP**	**Total**
85348	0.0	0.0	0.0	0.0

85396

85396 Coagulation/fibrinolysis assay, whole blood (eg, viscoelastic clot assessment), including use of any pharmacologic additive(s), as indicated, including interpretation and written report, per day

Explanation

A coagulation/fibrinolysis assay is done on whole blood to assess the viscoelastic properties of blood as it clots. Information about the kinetics of clot formation and growth and the strength and stability of the formed clot provides a more global assessment about hemostatic function as a whole dynamic process. The interaction between fibrinogen, platelets, and the protein coagulation process are measured in viscoelastic assays as clotting happens, and followed through to clot lysis. This is invaluable in surgical circumstances for patients who have been treated with anticoagulants, or are suspected of thromboembolic disease.

Relative Value Units/Medicare Edits

Non-Facility RVU	Work	PE	MP	Total
85396	0.37	0.19	0.02	0.58
Facility RVU	**Work**	**PE**	**MP**	**Total**
85396	0.37	0.19	0.02	0.58

85576

85576 Platelet, aggregation (in vitro), each agent

Explanation

This test may be ordered as a platelet aggregation study, or as an in vitro platelet aggregation study. Specimen is collected plasma. The method may be platelet aggregometer. Platelet function is measured by observing the amount of platelet clumping that occurs when certain chemicals are added to a solution of platelets. The test is an in vitro enactment of the platelet aggregation that occurs naturally at the site of vascular injury. The test may be used to detect von Willebrand's disease or other inherited platelet disjunction diseases.

Relative Value Units/Medicare Edits

Non-Facility RVU	Work	PE	MP	Total
85576	0.0	0.0	0.0	0.0
Facility RVU	**Work**	**PE**	**MP**	**Total**
85576	0.0	0.0	0.0	0.0

85610

85610 Prothrombin time;

Explanation

This test may be ordered as a prothrombin time (PT), a prothrombin, or as simply PT. The specimen is plasma. Method is one-stage using an automated device. The prothrombin time is prolonged when deficiencies of coagulation factors II, V, VII, or X are present. More commonly, this test monitors the effectiveness of the anticoagulant drug Coumadin or warfarin, prescribed to patients who have had blood clots or myocardial infarction.

Relative Value Units/Medicare Edits

Non-Facility RVU	Work	PE	MP	Total
85610	0.0	0.0	0.0	0.0
Facility RVU	**Work**	**PE**	**MP**	**Total**
85610	0.0	0.0	0.0	0.0

85611

85611 Prothrombin time; substitution, plasma fractions, each

Explanation

This test may be ordered as a diluted prothrombin time (PT), a prothrombin 1:1, or as plasma diluted PT. The specimen is plasma. Addition or dilution with normal plasma differentiates between a clotting factor deficiency and a circulating anticoagulant. Prolonged prothrombin times due to a clotting factor deficiency will shorten to normal with the addition of normal plasma while a prolonged prothrombin time due to a circulating anticoagulant may increase with the addition of normal plasma.

Relative Value Units/Medicare Edits

Non-Facility RVU	Work	PE	MP	Total
85611	0.0	0.0	0.0	0.0
Facility RVU	**Work**	**PE**	**MP**	**Total**
85611	0.0	0.0	0.0	0.0

85651

85651 Sedimentation rate, erythrocyte; non-automated

Explanation

This test may be ordered as an erythrocyte sedimentation rate (ESR), a Westergren sedimentation rate, Wintrobe sedimentation rate, or simply as a "sed rate." The specimen is whole blood. This test is a non-specific screening test for a number of diseases including anemia, disorders of protein production such as multiple myeloma, other conditions that alter the size and/or shape of red cells or erythrocytes, and to screen diseases that cause an increase or decrease in the amount of protein in the plasma. Further studies are often launched by ESR results. The method is manual. A variety of procedures have been used over time to study sedimentation rate. A common one performed manually is the Westergren tube.

Relative Value Units/Medicare Edits

Non-Facility RVU	Work	PE	MP	Total
85651	0.0	0.0	0.0	0.0
Facility RVU	**Work**	**PE**	**MP**	**Total**
85651	0.0	0.0	0.0	0.0

85652

85652 Sedimentation rate, erythrocyte; automated

Explanation

This test may be ordered as a Zeta sedimentation rate or as a Zeta sed rate. Specimen is whole blood. Method is centrifugation; this is an automated test. This test is a non-specific screening test for a number of diseases including anemia, disorders of protein production such as multiple myeloma, and other conditions that alter the size and/or shape of red cells or erythrocytes. This test may also be used to screen diseases that cause an increase or decrease in the amount of protein in the plasma or liquid portion of the blood.

Relative Value Units/Medicare Edits

Non-Facility RVU	Work	PE	MP	Total
85652	0.0	0.0	0.0	0.0
Facility RVU	**Work**	**PE**	**MP**	**Total**
85652	0.0	0.0	0.0	0.0

85730

85730 Thromboplastin time, partial (PTT); plasma or whole blood

Explanation

This test may be ordered as a partial thromboplastin time or PTT, or as an activated partial thromboplastin time or APTT. The specimen is plasma. The method is automated coagulation instrument. The partial thromboplastin time is prolonged when deficiencies of coagulation factors VIII, IX, XI, and XII are present. This test is used to monitor the effectiveness of the anticoagulant drug heparin, which is prescribed for patients who have had blood clots or heart attacks.

Relative Value Units/Medicare Edits

Non-Facility RVU	Work	PE	MP	Total
85730	0.0	0.0	0.0	0.0
Facility RVU	**Work**	**PE**	**MP**	**Total**
85730	0.0	0.0	0.0	0.0

85732

85732 Thromboplastin time, partial (PTT); substitution, plasma fractions, each

Explanation

This test may be ordered as a diluted partial thromboplastin time, a PTT or APTT 1:1, or as a plasma diluted PTT or APTT. The specimen is plasma. The method is automated coagulation instrument. Addition of or dilution with normal plasma differentiates between a clotting factor deficiency and a circulating anticoagulant. Prolonged partial thromboplastin times due to a clotting factor deficiency will shorten to normal with the addition of normal plasma while a prolonged PTT due to a circulating anticoagulant may increase with the addition of normal plasma.

Relative Value Units/Medicare Edits

Non-Facility RVU	Work	PE	MP	Total
85732	0.0	0.0	0.0	0.0
Facility RVU	**Work**	**PE**	**MP**	**Total**
85732	0.0	0.0	0.0	0.0

86147

86147 Cardiolipin (phospholipid) antibody, each Ig class

Explanation

This test may also be ordered as antiphospholipid antibody or anticardiolipin antibodies (ACA). The specimen is serum. Method is enzyme-linked immunoassay (ELISA). The test may be used to classify patients with recurrent venous or arterial thrombosis, thrombocytopenia (low platelet count), recurrent fetal loss, and acquired valvular heart disease, and systemic lupus erythematosus (SLE).

Relative Value Units/Medicare Edits

Non-Facility RVU	Work	PE	MP	Total
86147	0.0	0.0	0.0	0.0
Facility RVU	**Work**	**PE**	**MP**	**Total**
86147	0.0	0.0	0.0	0.0

86590

86590 Streptokinase, antibody

Explanation

This test is commonly ordered as ASO. The specimen is serum. The test is useful for detection of antibody to an extracellular antigenic product of group A streptococci and commonly used to detect previous exposure to group A strep. The test may be performed by latex agglutination or enzyme-linked immunosorbent assay (ELISA).

Relative Value Units/Medicare Edits

Non-Facility RVU	Work	PE	MP	Total
86590	0.0	0.0	0.0	0.0
Facility RVU	**Work**	**PE**	**MP**	**Total**
86590	0.0	0.0	0.0	0.0

86828-86829

86828 Antibody to human leukocyte antigens (HLA), solid phase assays (eg, microspheres or beads, ELISA, flow cytometry); qualitative assessment of the presence or absence of antibody(ies) to HLA Class I and Class II HLA antigens

86829 qualitative assessment of the presence or absence of antibody(ies) to HLA Class I or Class II HLA antigens

Explanation

These tests are commonly used to predict the histocompatibility between a patient and a donor to predict and prevent graft versus host disease (GVHD) or transplanted organ rejection. Human leukocyte antigens (HLA) are a group of genes found on chromosome 6. There are two types of HLA: class I and class II. The higher number of anti-HLA antibodies the higher the chance of a reaction to donor tissue. The specimen is blood. The method is enzyme-linked immunosorbent assay (ELISA) technique and the use of fluorescent beads with HLA molecules bound to their surface, which can be used in conventional flow cytometry or in conjunction with Luminex instrumentation. Report 86828 if the presence or absence of both HLA class I and II antibodies are assessed. Report 86829 when only one HLA class antibody is qualified.

Relative Value Units/Medicare Edits

Non-Facility RVU	Work	PE	MP	Total
86828	0.0	0.0	0.0	0.0
86829	0.0	0.0	0.0	0.0
Facility RVU	**Work**	**PE**	**MP**	**Total**
86828	0.0	0.0	0.0	0.0
86829	0.0	0.0	0.0	0.0

87086-87088

87086 Culture, bacterial; quantitative colony count, urine

87088 with isolation and presumptive identification of each isolate, urine

Explanation

These codes report the performance of a urine bacterial culture with a calibrated inoculating device so that a colony count accurately correlates with the number of organisms in the urine. In 87088, isolation and presumptive identification of bacteria recovered from the sample is done by means of identifying colony morphology, subculturing organisms to selective media and the performance of a gram stain or other simple test to identify bacteria to the genus level. There are several automated systems that detect the presence of bacteria using colorimetric, radiometric, or spectrophotometric means. In 87086, quantified colony count numbers within the urine sample are measured.

Relative Value Units/Medicare Edits

Non-Facility RVU	Work	PE	MP	Total
87086	0.0	0.0	0.0	0.0
87088	0.0	0.0	0.0	0.0
Facility RVU	**Work**	**PE**	**MP**	**Total**
87086	0.0	0.0	0.0	0.0
87088	0.0	0.0	0.0	0.0

87181

87181 Susceptibility studies, antimicrobial agent; agar dilution method, per agent (eg, antibiotic gradient strip)

Explanation

A susceptibility study is performed to determine the susceptibility of a bacterium to an antibiotic. The methodology is agar diffusion (the E test is a method of agar diffusion). The specific antibiotics could be chosen and limited. The test is reported per antibiotic tested. The agar dilution is reported as minimum inhibitory concentration (MIC), which is a method of measuring the exact amount of antibiotic needed to inhibit an organism.

Relative Value Units/Medicare Edits

Non-Facility RVU	Work	PE	MP	Total
87181	0.0	0.0	0.0	0.0
Facility RVU	**Work**	**PE**	**MP**	**Total**
87181	0.0	0.0	0.0	0.0

87271

87271 Infectious agent antigen detection by immunofluorescent technique; Cytomegalovirus, direct fluorescent antibody (DFA)

Explanation

A cytomegalovirus is detected by direct fluorescent antibody (DFA) staining technique. The presence of the infectious agent microorganism is detected indirectly when the fluorescent reaction of the dye is seen under a special microscope. The cytomegalovirus is isolated in cell culture for the test. Specimens include throat swabs, CSF, and blood samples. A cytomegalovirus is any virus in the Betaherpesvirinae subfamily.

Relative Value Units/Medicare Edits

Non-Facility RVU	Work	PE	MP	Total
87271	0.0	0.0	0.0	0.0
Facility RVU	**Work**	**PE**	**MP**	**Total**
87271	0.0	0.0	0.0	0.0

90471-90472

90471 Immunization administration (includes percutaneous, intradermal, subcutaneous, or intramuscular injections); 1 vaccine (single or combination vaccine/toxoid)

+ **90472** each additional vaccine (single or combination vaccine/toxoid) (List separately in addition to code for primary procedure)

Explanation

A physician, nurse, or medical assistant administers an injectable (percutaneous, intradermal, subcutaneous, or intramuscular) immunization to the patient. It may be a single vaccine or a combination vaccine/toxoid in one immunization administration (e.g., diphtheria, pertussis, and tetanus toxoids are in a single DPT immunization). Report 90471 for one vaccine and 90472 for each additional vaccine (single or combination vaccine/toxoid).

Relative Value Units/Medicare Edits

Non-Facility RVU	Work	PE	MP	Total
90471	0.17	0.29	0.01	0.47
90472	0.15	0.2	0.01	0.36
Facility RVU	**Work**	**PE**	**MP**	**Total**
90471	0.17	0.29	0.01	0.47
90472	0.15	0.2	0.01	0.36

90657-90658

90657 Influenza virus vaccine, trivalent (IIV3), split virus, 0.25 mL dosage, for intramuscular use

90658 Influenza virus vaccine, trivalent (IIV3), split virus, 0.5 mL dosage, for intramuscular use

Explanation

These codes report the supply of the vaccine only. A vaccine produces active immunization by inducing the immune system to build its own antibodies against specific microorganisms/viruses. The body retains memory of the antibody production pattern for long-term protection. A split virus suspension of three (two influenza A and one influenza B) (IIV3) of the most prevalent strains of influenza is prepared for intramuscular use. Report 90657 for a 0.25 mL dose and 90658 for a 0.5 mL dose. The vaccine induces active immunity to the highly contagious infection of the respiratory tract caused by a myxovirus and transmitted by airborne droplet infection. Report these codes with the appropriate administration code.

Relative Value Units/Medicare Edits

Non-Facility RVU	Work	PE	MP	Total
90657	0.0	0.0	0.0	0.0
90658	0.0	0.0	0.0	0.0
Facility RVU	**Work**	**PE**	**MP**	**Total**
90657	0.0	0.0	0.0	0.0
90658	0.0	0.0	0.0	0.0

[90674]

90674 Influenza virus vaccine, quadrivalent (ccIIV4), derived from cell cultures, subunit, preservative and antibiotic free, 0.5 mL dosage, for intramuscular use

Explanation

A vaccine produces active immunization by inducing the immune system to build its own antibodies against specific microorganisms/viruses. The body retains memory of the antibody production pattern for long-term protection. A suspension of the prevalent strain of influenza virus that has been derived from cell cultures is prepared for intramuscular use. Cell culture-derived vaccines are those in which the virus is grown in mammalian cells rather than egg-derived. The vaccine provides active immunity to the highly contagious infection of the respiratory tract caused by a myxovirus and transmitted by airborne droplet infection. This vaccine (ccIIV4) is preservative and antibiotic-free. This code reports a subunit in a .50 mL dose and should be reported with the appropriate administration code.

Relative Value Units/Medicare Edits

Non-Facility RVU	Work	PE	MP	Total
90674	0.0	0.0	0.0	0.0
Facility RVU	**Work**	**PE**	**MP**	**Total**
90674	0.0	0.0	0.0	0.0

90732

90732 Pneumococcal polysaccharide vaccine, 23-valent (PPSV23), adult or immunosuppressed patient dosage, when administered to individuals 2 years or older, for subcutaneous or intramuscular use

Explanation

This code reports supply of a vaccine only. A vaccine produces active immunization by inducing the immune system to build its own antibodies against specific microorganisms/viruses. The body retains memory of these antibody production patterns for long-term protection. This code reports a pneumococcal polysaccharide vaccine, 23-valent (PPSV23), adult or immunosuppressed patient dosage, for subcutaneous or intramuscular administration to patients 2 years of age or older. Report this code with the appropriate administration code.

Relative Value Units/Medicare Edits

Non-Facility RVU	Work	PE	MP	Total
90732	0.0	0.0	0.0	0.0
Facility RVU	**Work**	**PE**	**MP**	**Total**
90732	0.0	0.0	0.0	0.0

93000-93010

93000 Electrocardiogram, routine ECG with at least 12 leads; with interpretation and report

93005 tracing only, without interpretation and report

93010 interpretation and report only

Explanation

Multiple electrodes are placed on a patient's chest to record the electrical activity of the heart. A physician interprets the findings. Report 93000 for the combined technical and professional components of an ECG; 93005 for the technical component only; and 93010 for the professional component only.

Relative Value Units/Medicare Edits

Non-Facility RVU	Work	PE	MP	Total
93000	0.17	0.29	0.02	0.48
93005	0.0	0.23	0.01	0.24
93010	0.17	0.06	0.01	0.24
Facility RVU	**Work**	**PE**	**MP**	**Total**
93000	0.17	0.29	0.02	0.48
93005	0.0	0.23	0.01	0.24
93010	0.17	0.06	0.01	0.24

93015-93018

93015 Cardiovascular stress test using maximal or submaximal treadmill or bicycle exercise, continuous electrocardiographic monitoring, and/or pharmacological stress; with supervision, interpretation and report
93016 supervision only, without interpretation and report
93017 tracing only, without interpretation and report
93018 interpretation and report only

Explanation

A continuous recording of electrical activity of the heart is acquired by an assistant supervised by a qualified health care professional while the patient is exercising on a treadmill or bicycle and/or given medicines. The stress on the heart during the test is monitored. Code 93015 includes the test, supervision, and interpretation of the report; 93016 includes only the supervision of the test; 93017 includes performing the test only; and 93018 is reported for the interpretation of a previously performed test.

Relative Value Units/Medicare Edits

Non-Facility RVU	Work	PE	MP	Total
93015	0.75	1.22	0.04	2.01
93016	0.45	0.16	0.02	0.63
93017	0.0	0.95	0.01	0.96
93018	0.3	0.11	0.01	0.42
Facility RVU	**Work**	**PE**	**MP**	**Total**
93015	0.75	1.22	0.04	2.01
93016	0.45	0.16	0.02	0.63
93017	0.0	0.95	0.01	0.96
93018	0.3	0.11	0.01	0.42

93024

93024 Ergonovine provocation test

Explanation

The purpose of the study is to evaluate for coronary artery spasm. If ergonovine is not available, certain other ergot medications may be infused for the same purpose. Following baseline coronary angiography (coded elsewhere), the physician infuses gradually escalating doses of ergonovine into a peripheral vein, while monitoring for chest discomfort and electrocardiographic changes. Repeat angiography is performed during ergonovine infusion to assess the size of the coronary lumen. If the patient develops symptomatic coronary spasm, the physician may directly infuse vasodilating medications through the intracoronary catheter to relieve the problem.

Relative Value Units/Medicare Edits

Non-Facility RVU	Work	PE	MP	Total
93024	1.17	1.89	0.06	3.12
Facility RVU	**Work**	**PE**	**MP**	**Total**
93024	1.17	1.89	0.06	3.12

93025

93025 Microvolt T-wave alternans for assessment of ventricular arrhythmias

Explanation

T-Wave Alternans testing is an electrocardiographic method of measuring the alternating electrical amplitude from beat to beat on an electrocardiogram and is used as a method of evaluating ventricular arrhythmia risk. Microvolt T-wave alternans can be measured during exercise or pharmacologic stress, or during cardiac pacing, using a spectral analytic method with equipment that is able to detect as little as one microvolt of T-wave alternans. In electrode placement for a 12-lead ECG, the health care provider positions the leads on the wrists and ankles or shoulders and groins. Left leg electrodes are placed below the heart (but not on the chest), preferably below the umbilicus. The sensing electrodes look at the inferior surface of the heart, the left or lateral side of the heart, and at the right side of the heart.

Relative Value Units/Medicare Edits

Non-Facility RVU	Work	PE	MP	Total
93025	0.75	3.44	0.04	4.23
Facility RVU	**Work**	**PE**	**MP**	**Total**
93025	0.75	3.44	0.04	4.23

93040-93042

93040 Rhythm ECG, 1-3 leads; with interpretation and report
93041 tracing only without interpretation and report
93042 interpretation and report only

Explanation

An assistant records the electrical activity of the heart by placing one to three electrodes on a patient's chest in a predetermined pattern. Report 93040 when the physician interprets the report. Report 93041 when only the tracing is performed. Report 93042 when a physician interprets a previously acquired report.

Relative Value Units/Medicare Edits

Non-Facility RVU	Work	PE	MP	Total
93040	0.15	0.19	0.02	0.36
93041	0.0	0.15	0.01	0.16
93042	0.15	0.04	0.01	0.2
Facility RVU	**Work**	**PE**	**MP**	**Total**
93040	0.15	0.19	0.02	0.36
93041	0.0	0.15	0.01	0.16
93042	0.15	0.04	0.01	0.2

93050

93050 Arterial pressure waveform analysis for assessment of central arterial pressures, includes obtaining waveform(s), digitization and application of nonlinear mathematical transformations to determine central arterial pressures and augmentation index, with interpretation and report, upper extremity artery, non-invasive

Explanation

Blood pressure pulse wave analysis measures the blood pressure at the heart rather than in the arm as with traditional blood pressure cuffs, as well as providing information regarding the interaction of the heart and blood vessels. The brachial blood pressure is obtained to calibrate the radial pressure waveform. The pressure sensor wand (tonometer) is placed on the wrist where the strongest pulse is present. The pressure waveforms are transmitted and displayed on a data collection screen on a computer. After there is at least 10 seconds of data displayed, the data is captured. The data reflects average central aortic waveform, pressure measurements, and central parameters, as well as reference ranges. The augmentation index can be acquired by direct measurement or acquired pressure waveforms. This index is a percentage of pressure from systolic rise over pressure waves. The nonlinear mathematical transformation can be utilized to differentiate between active and rest blood pressure coinciding with the systolic and diastolic process. This code includes the digitization of the data, as well as the use of nonlinear mathematical transformation to determine pressure, augmentation index, and the provider interpretation and report.

Relative Value Units/Medicare Edits

Non-Facility RVU	Work	PE	MP	Total
93050	0.17	0.27	0.02	0.46
Facility RVU	**Work**	**PE**	**MP**	**Total**
93050	0.17	0.27	0.02	0.46

93224-93227

93224 External electrocardiographic recording up to 48 hours by continuous rhythm recording and storage; includes recording, scanning analysis with report, review and interpretation by a physician or other qualified health care professional

93225 recording (includes connection, recording, and disconnection)

93226 scanning analysis with report

93227 review and interpretation by a physician or other qualified health care professional

Explanation

The purpose of this study is to evaluate the patient's ambient heart rhythm during a full daily cycle. The physician or other qualified health care professional instructs the patient in the use of an external electrocardiographic (ECG) recorder, also known as a Holter monitor. A technician places ECG leads on the patient's chest, and the patient wears the recorder for up to 48 hours. During this time, there is continuous rhythm recording and storage. The patient returns the device, and the recorded heart rhythm is played back into digital format by a technician. The technician uses a scanning methodology to classify different ECG waveforms and to generate a report. The generated report describes the overall rhythm and significant arrhythmias. Code 93224 reports the recording, scanning analysis with report, provider review of the data, and the provision of a final interpretation in a report. Code 93225 reports the recording only, which includes connection, recording of data, and disconnection. Code 93226 reports only the scanning analysis with report. Code 93227 reports only the provider review and interpretation.

Relative Value Units/Medicare Edits

Non-Facility RVU	Work	PE	MP	Total
93224	0.52	1.95	0.04	2.51
93225	0.0	0.72	0.01	0.73
93226	0.0	1.02	0.01	1.03
93227	0.52	0.21	0.02	0.75
Facility RVU	**Work**	**PE**	**MP**	**Total**
93224	0.52	1.95	0.04	2.51
93225	0.0	0.72	0.01	0.73
93226	0.0	1.02	0.01	1.03
93227	0.52	0.21	0.02	0.75

93228-93229

93228 External mobile cardiovascular telemetry with electrocardiographic recording, concurrent computerized real time data analysis and greater than 24 hours of accessible ECG data storage (retrievable with query) with ECG triggered and patient selected events transmitted to a remote attended surveillance center for up to 30 days; review and interpretation with report by a physician or other qualified health care professional

93229 technical support for connection and patient instructions for use, attended surveillance, analysis and transmission of daily and emergent data reports as prescribed by a physician or other qualified health care professional

Explanation

Mobile cardiovascular telemetry (MCT) uses external electrodes placed on the patient's body to continuously record electrocardiographic rhythm. Data segments are transmitted to a remote surveillance location by phone signal (cellular or landline); this is accomplished automatically and does not require patient intervention. Selected rhythm segments may be triggered for transmission automatically by rapid and slow heart rates or by the patient during a symptomatic episode. Data are analyzed continuously in real time. A remote technician responds to the alerts from the external device, reviewing the data and notifying the physician or other qualified health care professional depending on the stipulated criteria. Report 93228 for provider review and interpretation with report and 93229 for technical support, which includes connection, instructions to the patient for use, attended surveillance, analysis, and transmission of daily and emergent data reports per provider protocol. These codes may be reported only once per 30-day period.

Relative Value Units/Medicare Edits

Non-Facility RVU	Work	PE	MP	Total
93228	0.52	0.19	0.03	0.74
93229	0.0	19.89	0.06	19.95
Facility RVU	**Work**	**PE**	**MP**	**Total**
93228	0.52	0.19	0.03	0.74
93229	0.0	19.89	0.06	19.95

93268-93272

93268 External patient and, when performed, auto activated electrocardiographic rhythm derived event recording with symptom-related memory loop with remote download capability up to 30 days, 24-hour attended monitoring; includes transmission, review and interpretation by a physician or other qualified health care professional

93270 recording (includes connection, recording, and disconnection)

93271 transmission and analysis

93272 review and interpretation by a physician or other qualified health care professional

Explanation

The purpose of this study is to evaluate the patient's ambient heart rhythm during symptoms. The physician or other qualified health care professional instructs the patient in the use of an external rhythm monitor. A technician places ECG leads on the patient's chest, and the monitor uses a symptom-related memory loop mechanism with remote download capability up to 30 days to record the patient's rhythm. During symptoms, the patient activates the monitor by pressing a button. The resulting recording includes ECG activity prior to and during symptoms. The patient uses the device to transmit the recording over the telephone line, allowing a rhythm printout to be generated. The provider reviews and interprets this rhythm strip. Code 93268 reports transmission and provider review and interpretation. Code 93270 reports the recording only (including connection, recording, and disconnection). Code 93271 reports transmission download and analysis. Code 93272 reports only the provider review and interpretation.

Relative Value Units/Medicare Edits

Non-Facility RVU	Work	PE	MP	Total
93268	0.52	5.14	0.04	5.7
93270	0.0	0.25	0.01	0.26
93271	0.0	4.71	0.01	4.72
93272	0.52	0.18	0.02	0.72
Facility RVU	**Work**	**PE**	**MP**	**Total**
93268	0.52	5.14	0.04	5.7
93270	0.0	0.25	0.01	0.26
93271	0.0	4.71	0.01	4.72
93272	0.52	0.18	0.02	0.72

93278

93278 Signal-averaged electrocardiography (SAECG), with or without ECG

Explanation

Electrodes placed on a patient's chest record the heart's electrical activity. This technique uses signal-averaged electrocardiography (SAECG) and may include a standard electrocardiogram.

Relative Value Units/Medicare Edits

Non-Facility RVU	Work	PE	MP	Total
93278	0.25	0.6	0.02	0.87
Facility RVU	**Work**	**PE**	**MP**	**Total**
93278	0.25	0.6	0.02	0.87

[93264]

93264 Remote monitoring of a wireless pulmonary artery pressure sensor for up to 30 days, including at least weekly downloads of pulmonary artery pressure recordings, interpretation(s), trend analysis, and report(s) by a physician or other qualified health care professional

Explanation

A pulmonary pressure monitoring system, a device comprised of a battery-free sensor such as the CardioMEMS™, permits ongoing monitoring and measurement of a patient's heartrate as well as systolic, diastolic, and mean pressures in a patient diagnosed with non-rhythm related cardiac conditions (i.e., heart failure). Pulmonary arterial pressure (PAP) readings transmitted from an internally implanted sensor to a wireless electronic unit are subsequently transmitted to an internet-based file server or monitored by a surveillance technician with results sent to an online portal that can be accessed by the patient's treating health care provider. Through accurate monitoring of patients diagnosed with heart failure (HF) for exacerbations, it is possible to minimize the need for additional hospitalizations and the associated complications and allow for early pharmacological intervention.

Relative Value Units/Medicare Edits

Non-Facility RVU	Work	PE	MP	Total
93264	0.7	0.69	0.05	1.44
Facility RVU	**Work**	**PE**	**MP**	**Total**
93264	0.7	0.27	0.05	1.02

93279-93281

93279 Programming device evaluation (in person) with iterative adjustment of the implantable device to test the function of the device and select optimal permanent programmed values with analysis, review and report by a physician or other qualified health care professional; single lead pacemaker system or leadless pacemaker system in one cardiac chamber

93280 dual lead pacemaker system

93281 multiple lead pacemaker system

Explanation

A programming device evaluation is performed in person in order to test the device's function and select the most favorable permanent programmed values. Patients with previously implanted pacemakers require periodic programming device evaluations. This diagnostic procedure includes a face-to-face assessment of all device functions. Components that must be evaluated in order to assign a code from this range include the battery, leads, capture and sensing function, heart rhythm, and programmed parameters. Stored and measured data regarding these components are retrieved using an office, hospital, or emergency room instrument. This information is assessed to discern battery voltage, lead impedance, and settings for rhythm treatment and tachycardia detection, as well as to determine the pacemaker's current programming. If necessary, the sensing value and rate response, upper and lower heart rates, AV intervals, pacing voltage and pulse duration, and diagnostics are adjusted. These codes include physician or other qualified health care professional review, interpretation, and report, and are assigned per procedure. Report 93279 for evaluation of a single-lead pacemaker or leadless system (one in which there is pacing and sensing function in only one chamber of the heart). Report 93280 for evaluation of a dual-lead device (one with pacing and sensing function in only two chambers). Report 93281 for evaluation of a multiple-lead device (one with pacing and sensing function in three or more chambers).

Relative Value Units/Medicare Edits

Non-Facility RVU	Work	PE	MP	Total
93279	0.65	0.88	0.03	1.56
93280	0.77	1.02	0.04	1.83
93281	0.85	1.08	0.04	1.97
Facility RVU	**Work**	**PE**	**MP**	**Total**
93279	0.65	0.88	0.03	1.56
93280	0.77	1.02	0.04	1.83
93281	0.85	1.08	0.04	1.97

93282-93284

93282 Programming device evaluation (in person) with iterative adjustment of the implantable device to test the function of the device and select optimal permanent programmed values with analysis, review and report by a physician or other qualified health care professional; single lead transvenous implantable defibrillator system

93283 dual lead transvenous implantable defibrillator system

93284 multiple lead transvenous implantable defibrillator system

Explanation

A programming device evaluation is performed in person in order to test the device's function and select the most favorable permanent programmed values. Patients with transvenous implantable defibrillator systems require periodic programming device evaluations. This diagnostic procedure includes a face-to-face assessment of all device functions. Components that must be evaluated in order to assign a code from this range include the battery, leads, programmed parameters, presence or absence of therapy for ventricular tachyarrhythmias, and heart rhythm. Stored and measured data regarding these components are retrieved using an office, hospital, or emergency room instrument. This information is assessed to discern battery voltage, lead impedance, and settings for rhythm treatment and tachycardia detection, as well as to determine the defibrillator's current programming. If necessary, the sensing value and sensor rate response, upper and lower heart rates, AV intervals, pacing voltage and pulse duration, and diagnostics are adjusted. Ventricular tachycardia detection and therapies may also be altered. These codes include physician or other qualified health care professional review, interpretation, and report, and are assigned per procedure. Report 93282 for evaluation of a single-lead system (one in which there is pacing and sensing function in only one chamber of the heart). Report 93283 for evaluation of a dual-lead device (one with pacing and sensing function in only two chambers). Report 93284 for evaluation of a multiple-lead device (one with pacing and sensing function in three or more chambers).

Relative Value Units/Medicare Edits

Non-Facility RVU	Work	PE	MP	Total
93282	0.85	1.01	0.04	1.9
93283	1.15	1.19	0.05	2.39
93284	1.25	1.28	0.06	2.59
Facility RVU	**Work**	**PE**	**MP**	**Total**
93282	0.85	1.01	0.04	1.9
93283	1.15	1.19	0.05	2.39
93284	1.25	1.28	0.06	2.59

[93260]

93260 Programming device evaluation (in person) with iterative adjustment of the implantable device to test the function of the device and select optimal permanent programmed values with analysis, review and report by a physician or other qualified health care professional; implantable subcutaneous lead defibrillator system

Explanation

A programming device evaluation is performed in person in order to test the device's function and select the most favorable permanent programmed values. Patients with previously placed subcutaneous implantable defibrillator systems require periodic programming device evaluations. This diagnostic procedure includes a face-to-face assessment of all device functions, including analysis, review, and report by a physician or other qualified health care professional. Components that must be evaluated in order to assign a code from this range include the battery, leads, capture and sensing function, heart rhythm, and programmed parameters. Stored and measured data regarding these components are retrieved using an office, hospital, or emergency room instrument. This information is assessed to discern battery voltage, lead impedance, and settings, as well as to determine the system's current programming. If necessary, the parameters are reprogrammed.

Relative Value Units/Medicare Edits

Non-Facility RVU	Work	PE	MP	Total
93260	0.85	1.04	0.04	1.93
Facility RVU	**Work**	**PE**	**MP**	**Total**
93260	0.85	1.04	0.04	1.93

93285

93285 Programming device evaluation (in person) with iterative adjustment of the implantable device to test the function of the device and select optimal permanent programmed values with analysis, review and report by a physician or other qualified health care professional; subcutaneous cardiac rhythm monitor system

Explanation

A programming device evaluation is performed in person in order to test the device's function and select the most favorable permanent programmed values. Patients with previously placed subcutaneous cardiac rhythm monitor systems require periodic programming device evaluations. This diagnostic procedure includes a face-to-face assessment of all device functions. Components that must be evaluated include heartrate and rhythm during recorded episodes (patient-initiated and device algorithm detected events), as well as programmed parameters. Stored and measured data are retrieved using an office, hospital, or emergency room instrument. This information is assessed to discern current programming and to evaluate specific aspects of the device's function. If necessary, the bradycardia and tachycardia detection criteria are adjusted. This code includes physician or other qualified health care professional review, interpretation, and report, and is assigned per procedure.

Relative Value Units/Medicare Edits

Non-Facility RVU	Work	PE	MP	Total
93285	0.52	0.82	0.03	1.37
Facility RVU	**Work**	**PE**	**MP**	**Total**
93285	0.52	0.82	0.03	1.37

93286-93287

93286 Peri-procedural device evaluation (in person) and programming of device system parameters before or after a surgery, procedure, or test with analysis, review and report by a physician or other qualified health care professional; single, dual, or multiple lead pacemaker system, or leadless pacemaker system

93287 single, dual, or multiple lead implantable defibrillator system

Explanation

A programming device evaluation is performed in person in order to test the device's function and select the most favorable permanent programmed values. Patients with a previously implanted pacemaker or defibrillator systems may require adjustment of the device to patient-specific settings prior to a surgery, test, or procedure. The device system data is interrogated to evaluate the battery, leads, and sensors, as well as the stored patient and system measurements. If necessary, the device is programmed to settings appropriate for the surgery, test, or procedure. A postprocedure evaluation and programming may also be performed, with adjustments as required. Report 93286 for evaluation of a single-, dual-, or multiple-lead implantable pacemaker system or leadless pacemaker system. Report 93287 for evaluation of a single-, dual-, or multiple-lead implantable defibrillator system. Both codes include physician or other qualified health care professional analysis, review, and report.

Relative Value Units/Medicare Edits

Non-Facility RVU	Work	PE	MP	Total
93286	0.3	0.67	0.02	0.99
93287	0.45	0.74	0.03	1.22
Facility RVU	**Work**	**PE**	**MP**	**Total**
93286	0.3	0.67	0.02	0.99
93287	0.45	0.74	0.03	1.22

93288-93292 [93261]

93288 Interrogation device evaluation (in person) with analysis, review and report by a physician or other qualified health care professional, includes connection, recording and disconnection per patient encounter; single, dual, or multiple lead pacemaker system, or leadless pacemaker system

93289 single, dual, or multiple lead transvenous implantable defibrillator system, including analysis of heart rhythm derived data elements

93261 Interrogation device evaluation (in person) with analysis, review and report by a physician or other qualified health care professional, includes connection, recording and disconnection per patient encounter; implantable subcutaneous lead defibrillator system

93290 implantable cardiovascular physiologic monitor system, including analysis of 1 or more recorded physiologic cardiovascular data elements from all internal and external sensors

93291 subcutaneous cardiac rhythm monitor system, including heart rhythm derived data analysis

93292 wearable defibrillator system

Explanation

Patients with a previously implanted device, such as a cardiac pacemaker, transvenous implantable defibrillator, implantable cardiovascular monitor (ICM), or subcutaneous cardiac rhythm monitor system require periodic interrogation device evaluations. This diagnostic procedure includes a face-to-face assessment of all device functions. Components that must be evaluated in order to assign 93288 include the battery, capture and sensing function, heart rhythm, and programmed parameters of a single-, dual-, multiple-lead, or leadless pacemaker system. Code 93289 requires evaluation of the battery, lead(s), capture and sensing function, heart rhythm derived elements, presence or absence of therapy for ventricular tachyarrhythmias, and programmed parameters of a single-, dual-, or multiple-lead transvenous implantable defibrillator system. Code 93290 requires analysis of at least one recorded physiologic cardiovascular data element obtained from internal or external sensors and evaluation of programmed parameters of an ICM. Code 93291 requires evaluation of heartrate and rhythm during recorded episodes (patient-initiated and device algorithm detected events), as well as evaluation of programmed parameters of a subcutaneous cardiac rhythm monitor system. Code 93292 reports an interrogation device evaluation of a wearable defibrillation system. Code 93261 reports interrogation device evaluation of an implantable subcutaneous lead defibrillator system. These codes include physician or other qualified health care professional analysis, review, and report. They also include connection, recording, and disconnection, and are assigned per procedure.

Relative Value Units/Medicare Edits

Non-Facility RVU	Work	PE	MP	Total
93261	0.74	0.99	0.04	1.77
93288	0.43	0.79	0.03	1.25
93289	0.75	0.91	0.04	1.7
93290	0.43	0.73	0.03	1.19
93291	0.37	0.68	0.02	1.07
93292	0.43	0.68	0.03	1.14
Facility RVU	**Work**	**PE**	**MP**	**Total**
93261	0.74	0.99	0.04	1.77
93288	0.43	0.79	0.03	1.25
93289	0.75	0.91	0.04	1.7
93290	0.43	0.73	0.03	1.19
93291	0.37	0.68	0.02	1.07
93292	0.43	0.68	0.03	1.14

93293

93293 Transtelephonic rhythm strip pacemaker evaluation(s) single, dual, or multiple lead pacemaker system, includes recording with and without magnet application with analysis, review and report(s) by a physician or other qualified health care professional, up to 90 days

Explanation

Patients with previously implanted pacemakers require periodic analysis of pacemaker function. A pacemaker may be implanted to control a patient's irregular heartbeat. This code applies to transtelephonic pacemaker monitoring, a form of evaluation in which the patient sends a rhythm strip over the telephone using a transmitter. This transmission is recorded by a receiving location using a receiver/recorder. The rhythm strip is recorded with and without a magnet being applied over the pacemaker and is assessed for heart rate and rhythm, as well as atrial and ventricular capture and sensing (if observed). The pacemaker's battery status is also determined. Code 93293 may be reported for a single, dual, or multiple lead pacemaker system, and includes physician or other qualified health care professional analysis, review, and report. This code should be reported only once per 90-day period.

Relative Value Units/Medicare Edits

Non-Facility RVU	Work	PE	MP	Total
93293	0.31	1.15	0.02	1.48
Facility RVU	**Work**	**PE**	**MP**	**Total**
93293	0.31	1.15	0.02	1.48

93294-93296

93294 Interrogation device evaluation(s) (remote), up to 90 days; single, dual, or multiple lead pacemaker system, or leadless pacemaker system with interim analysis, review(s) and report(s) by a physician or other qualified health care professional

93295 single, dual, or multiple lead implantable defibrillator system with interim analysis, review(s) and report(s) by a physician or other qualified health care professional

93296 single, dual, or multiple lead pacemaker system, leadless pacemaker system, or implantable defibrillator system, remote data acquisition(s), receipt of transmissions and technician review, technical support and distribution of results

Explanation

Patients with a previously implanted device, such as a cardiac pacemaker or implantable defibrillator, require periodic interrogation device evaluations. These codes report remote evaluations only and apply to single-, dual-, multiple-lead or leadless devices. Code 93294 reports the remote evaluation of a pacemaker system with interim physician or other qualified health care professional analysis, review, and report. Components that must be evaluated in order to assign this code include the battery, lead(s), capture and sensing function, heart rhythm, and programmed parameters. Code 93295 reports the remote evaluation of an implantable defibrillator system with interim physician or other qualified health care professional analysis, review, and report. Required evaluation components include the battery, lead(s), capture and sensing function, heart rhythm derived elements, presence or absence of therapy for ventricular tachyarrhythmias, and programmed parameters. Code 93296 reports the acquisition of remote data, transmission receipt and technician review, technical support, and result distribution and applies to pacemaker and defibrillator systems. Codes from this range may be reported only once per 90-day period.

Relative Value Units/Medicare Edits

Non-Facility RVU	Work	PE	MP	Total
93294	0.6	0.23	0.04	0.87
93295	0.74	0.47	0.05	1.26
93296	0.0	0.71	0.01	0.72
Facility RVU	**Work**	**PE**	**MP**	**Total**
93294	0.6	0.23	0.04	0.87
93295	0.74	0.47	0.05	1.26
93296	0.0	0.71	0.01	0.72

93297-93298

93297 Interrogation device evaluation(s), (remote) up to 30 days; implantable cardiovascular physiologic monitor system, including analysis of 1 or more recorded physiologic cardiovascular data elements from all internal and external sensors, analysis, review(s) and report(s) by a physician or other qualified health care professional

93298 subcutaneous cardiac rhythm monitor system, including analysis of recorded heart rhythm data, analysis, review(s) and report(s) by a physician or other qualified health care professional

Explanation

Patients with a previously implanted device, such as an implantable cardiovascular physiologic monitor (ICM) or subcutaneous cardiac rhythm monitor system, require periodic interrogation device evaluations. These codes report remote evaluations only and may be reported once per 30-day period. Report 93297 for the remote evaluation of an ICM, which includes the analysis of at least one recorded physiologic cardiovascular data element obtained from internal or external sensors. Physician or other qualified health care professional analysis, review, and report are also included. Report 93298 for the analysis of recorded heart rhythm data; this code also includes the provider's review and report.

Relative Value Units/Medicare Edits

Non-Facility RVU	Work	PE	MP	Total
93297	0.52	0.2	0.03	0.75
93298	0.52	0.2	0.03	0.75
Facility RVU	**Work**	**PE**	**MP**	**Total**
93297	0.52	0.2	0.03	0.75
93298	0.52	0.2	0.03	0.75

93303-93304

93303 Transthoracic echocardiography for congenital cardiac anomalies; complete

93304 follow-up or limited study

Explanation

Transducers are placed on the patient's chest to record an echocardiograph, which uses ultrasound to visualize the heart's function, blood flow, valves, and chambers. Report 93303 for a complete evaluation for congenital defects. Report 93304 for a follow-up or a limited evaluation for congenital defects.

Relative Value Units/Medicare Edits

Non-Facility RVU	Work	PE	MP	Total
93303	1.3	5.28	0.07	6.65
93304	0.75	3.74	0.04	4.53
Facility RVU	**Work**	**PE**	**MP**	**Total**
93303	1.3	5.28	0.07	6.65
93304	0.75	3.74	0.04	4.53

93306-93308

93306 Echocardiography, transthoracic, real-time with image documentation (2D), includes M-mode recording, when performed, complete, with spectral Doppler echocardiography, and with color flow Doppler echocardiography

93307 Echocardiography, transthoracic, real-time with image documentation (2D), includes M-mode recording, when performed, complete, without spectral or color Doppler echocardiography

93308 Echocardiography, transthoracic, real-time with image documentation (2D), includes M-mode recording, when performed, follow-up or limited study

Explanation

This is a noninvasive study that uses ultrasound to visualize the heart's function, blood flow, valves, and chambers. Two-dimensional echocardiography, also referred to as real-time imaging, is performed using multiple transducers or a rotating transducer, and these images are recorded on videotape. Computer reconstruction provides the two-dimensional image of specific planes of the heart. M-mode, when performed, provides additional detail of specific portions of the heart. A stationary ultrasound beam is directed at the area of the heart requiring additional study. Report 93306 for a complete evaluation that includes spectral and color flow Doppler, which provide information regarding intracardiac blood flow and hemodynamics. Report 93307 for a complete evaluation but without spectral or color flow Doppler. Report 93308 for a follow-up or limited study.

Relative Value Units/Medicare Edits

Non-Facility RVU	Work	PE	MP	Total
93306	1.5	4.27	0.07	5.84
93307	0.92	3.01	0.04	3.97
93308	0.53	2.22	0.03	2.78
Facility RVU	**Work**	**PE**	**MP**	**Total**
93306	1.5	4.27	0.07	5.84
93307	0.92	3.01	0.04	3.97
93308	0.53	2.22	0.03	2.78

93312-93314

93312 Echocardiography, transesophageal, real-time with image documentation (2D) (with or without M-mode recording); including probe placement, image acquisition, interpretation and report

93313 placement of transesophageal probe only

93314 image acquisition, interpretation and report only

Explanation

Transesophageal echocardiograph (TEE) is an invasive technique whereby the transducer is placed at the tip of an endoscope and introduced into the patient's esophagus to record a two-dimensional echocardiograph. This set of codes should be used for TEE used to diagnose cardiac sources of emboli, prosthetic heart valve malfunction, endocarditis, aortic dissection, cardiac tumors, and valvular heart disease excluding congenital heart disease. Code 93312 applies to a complete evaluation including probe placement, image acquisition, and the physician's interpretation. Report 93313 for probe placement only. Report 93314 for image acquisition, physician interpretation, and report only.

Relative Value Units/Medicare Edits

Non-Facility RVU	Work	PE	MP	Total
93312	2.3	4.56	0.11	6.97
93313	0.26	0.05	0.02	0.33
93314	1.85	4.69	0.19	6.73
Facility RVU	**Work**	**PE**	**MP**	**Total**
93312	2.3	4.56	0.11	6.97
93313	0.26	0.05	0.02	0.33
93314	1.85	4.69	0.19	6.73

93315-93317

93315 Transesophageal echocardiography for congenital cardiac anomalies; including probe placement, image acquisition, interpretation and report

93316 placement of transesophageal probe only

93317 image acquisition, interpretation and report only

Explanation

Transesophageal echocardiograph (TEE) is an invasive technique whereby the transducer is placed at the tip of an endoscope and introduced into the patient's esophagus to record a two-dimensional echocardiograph. This set of codes should be used for TEE used to diagnose cardiac sources of emboli, prosthetic heart valve malfunction, endocarditis, aortic dissection, cardiac tumors, and valvular heart disease excluding congenital heart disease. The set of codes is specific to evaluations for congenital defects. Code 93315 applies to a complete evaluation for congenital defects including probe placement, image acquisition, and the physician's interpretation. Report 93316 for probe placement only. Report 93317 for image acquisition, physician interpretation, and report only.

Relative Value Units/Medicare Edits

Non-Facility RVU	Work	PE	MP	Total
93315	0.0	0.0	0.0	0.0
93316	0.6	0.14	0.05	0.79
93317	0.0	0.0	0.0	0.0
Facility RVU	**Work**	**PE**	**MP**	**Total**
93315	0.0	0.0	0.0	0.0
93316	0.6	0.14	0.05	0.79
93317	0.0	0.0	0.0	0.0

93318

93318 Echocardiography, transesophageal (TEE) for monitoring purposes, including probe placement, real time 2-dimensional image acquisition and interpretation leading to ongoing (continuous) assessment of (dynamically changing) cardiac pumping function and to therapeutic measures on an immediate time basis

Explanation

Transesophageal echocardiograph (TEE) is an invasive technique whereby the transducer is placed at the tip of an endoscope and introduced into the patient's esophagus to record a two-dimensional echocardiograph. TEE provides high-quality, real-time images of the beating heart and mediastinal structures. This code reports ongoing hemodynamic monitoring using TEE. TEE may be used to monitor critically ill patients in the intensive care unit as well as patients in certain operative settings. In both the intensive care unit and the operating room, it is used to monitor cardiac function including cardiac preload, contractility, and valve function in patients with acute hemodynamic decompensation. In addition, TEE may also be used to assess and monitor mediastinal, heart, lung, and aortic injury resulting from blunt chest trauma even in patients undergoing other life-saving procedures.

Relative Value Units/Medicare Edits

Non-Facility RVU	Work	PE	MP	Total
93318	0.0	0.0	0.0	0.0
Facility RVU	**Work**	**PE**	**MP**	**Total**
93318	0.0	0.0	0.0	0.0

93320-93321

+ **93320** Doppler echocardiography, pulsed wave and/or continuous wave with spectral display (List separately in addition to codes for echocardiographic imaging); complete

+ **93321** follow-up or limited study (List separately in addition to codes for echocardiographic imaging)

Explanation

Transducers are placed on a patient's chest to record a Doppler echocardiograph, which uses ultrasound to visualize blood flow velocity, direction, and type of flow in different locations in the heart. Doppler studies can be displayed on a strip chart or video recorder. Report 93320 for a complete evaluation and 93321 for limited or follow-up studies.

Relative Value Units/Medicare Edits

Non-Facility RVU	Work	PE	MP	Total
93320	0.38	1.12	0.01	1.51
93321	0.15	0.6	0.01	0.76
Facility RVU	**Work**	**PE**	**MP**	**Total**
93320	0.38	1.12	0.01	1.51
93321	0.15	0.6	0.01	0.76

93325

+ **93325** Doppler echocardiography color flow velocity mapping (List separately in addition to codes for echocardiography)

Explanation

The technique for Doppler color flow velocity mapping is similar to that of other echocardiographs with transducers being placed on the patient's chest to record cardiac activity. Color Doppler is two-dimensional Doppler in which the signal is encoded with color to more clearly identify flow direction. List 93325 separately in addition to the code for echocardiography (76825, 76826, 76827, 76828, 93303, 93304, 93308, 93312, 93314, 93315, 93317, 93350, and 93351).

Relative Value Units/Medicare Edits

Non-Facility RVU	Work	PE	MP	Total
93325	0.07	0.64	0.0	0.71
Facility RVU	**Work**	**PE**	**MP**	**Total**
93325	0.07	0.64	0.0	0.71

93350-93352

93350 Echocardiography, transthoracic, real-time with image documentation (2D), includes M-mode recording, when performed, during rest and cardiovascular stress test using treadmill, bicycle exercise and/or pharmacologically induced stress, with interpretation and report;

93351 including performance of continuous electrocardiographic monitoring, with supervision by a physician or other qualified health care professional

+ **93352** Use of echocardiographic contrast agent during stress echocardiography (List separately in addition to code for primary procedure)

Explanation

Transducers are placed on a patient's chest to record a two-dimensional echocardiograph, which uses ultrasound to visualize the heart's function, blood flow, valves, and chambers. In 93350, the echocardiography is completed while the patient is at rest and exercising on a treadmill or stationary bicycle with or without medication and includes M-mode recording, when performed. Code 93351 also includes the performance of continuous electrocardiographic monitoring with supervision by the physician or other qualified health care professional. Code 93352 is assigned as an additional code to report the use of an echocardiographic contrast agent during the stress test and should not be reported more than once per stress echocardiogram. Supply of the contrast agent and/or the drugs used in pharmacologic stress are reported separately in addition to these procedure codes.

Relative Value Units/Medicare Edits

Non-Facility RVU	Work	PE	MP	Total
93350	1.46	3.79	0.06	5.31
93351	1.75	4.74	0.08	6.57
93352	0.19	0.74	0.02	0.95
Facility RVU	**Work**	**PE**	**MP**	**Total**
93350	1.46	3.79	0.06	5.31
93351	1.75	4.74	0.08	6.57
93352	0.19	0.74	0.02	0.95

[93356]

+● **93356** Myocardial strain imaging using speckle tracking-derived assessment of myocardial mechanics (List separately in addition to codes for echocardiography imaging)

Explanation

Myocardial strain imaging, also referred to as echocardiographic strain imaging or deformation (lengthening, shortening, or thickening) imaging, was initially utilized as a feature of Doppler imaging where velocity information is regenerated into strain rate. New technology, known as speckle tracking echocardiography (STE), utilizes image-processing algorithms to track areas of interest. Used in conjunction with two-dimensional or three-dimensional echocardiography for determining the multidirectional components of left ventricular (LV) deformation, these areas contain blocks of 20 to 40 pixels that contain constant patterns referred to as speckles. These markers or fingerprints are helpful in outlining irregularities by comprehensive assessment of regional myocardial function, specifically by discriminating between active and passive myocardial wall movement. Strain rate data assists in early detection of myocardial dysfunction and is beneficial in therapeutic decisions and follow-up of previous cardiac surgery. Report 93356 in addition to applicable codes for echocardiography imaging.

Relative Value Units/Medicare Edits

Non-Facility RVU	Work	PE	MP	Total
93356				
Facility RVU	**Work**	**PE**	**MP**	**Total**
93356				

93660

93660 Evaluation of cardiovascular function with tilt table evaluation, with continuous ECG monitoring and intermittent blood pressure monitoring, with or without pharmacological intervention

Explanation

The purpose of this procedure is to evaluate the patient's susceptibility to neurocardiogenic syncope. The physician secures the patient to the tilt table and attaches ECG leads to the chest. The physician also attaches an intermittent blood pressure monitor. The physician tilts the table, with the patient on it, and monitors the patient's symptoms, heart rhythm, and blood pressure. The physician may infuse medication, such as isoproterenol, through a standard intravenous catheter and repeat the tilt test.

Relative Value Units/Medicare Edits

Non-Facility RVU	Work	PE	MP	Total
93660	1.89	2.53	0.09	4.51
Facility RVU	**Work**	**PE**	**MP**	**Total**
93660	1.89	2.53	0.09	4.51

93668

93668 Peripheral arterial disease (PAD) rehabilitation, per session

Explanation

An exercise physiologist or nurse supervises rehabilitation exercises in a patient diagnosed with peripheral arterial disease (PAD). Rehabilitation for PAD is provided using either a motorized treadmill or a track. The patient is supervised during physical exercise sessions lasting between 45-60 minutes in order to achieve symptom-limited claudication. The supervising provider monitors the patient's claudication threshold and other cardiovascular limitations and adjusts the level of activity in order to reduce claudication symptoms and increase exercise tolerance.

Relative Value Units/Medicare Edits

Non-Facility RVU	Work	PE	MP	Total
93668	0.0	0.47	0.03	0.5
Facility RVU	**Work**	**PE**	**MP**	**Total**
93668	0.0	0.47	0.03	0.5

93701

93701 Bioimpedance-derived physiologic cardiovascular analysis

Explanation

Bioimpedance is a noninvasive, continuous measurement of blood flow, respiration, and other cardiopulmonary dynamics, using a patient's thorax as an impedance transducer. The health care provider attaches the patient to the bioimpedance system with solid-gel electrodes placed along the widest dimension of the thorax. The electrical bioimpedance measurement current is passed through the thorax in a direction parallel with the spine between a pair of electrodes placed on the upper neck and a pair of electrodes placed on the upper abdomen. On its way through the thorax, the measurement current seeks the shortest and the most conductive pathway. As a result, the majority of the thoracic electrical bioimpedance (TEB) measurement current flows through the thoracic aorta and superior and inferior vena. The measurement current produces a high-frequency voltage across the impedance of the thorax, sensed by two other pairs of electrodes placed at the beginning of the thorax and the end of the thorax. The sensing electrodes also detect the ECG signal. The heart rate is derived from the R-R intervals of the ECG signal.

Relative Value Units/Medicare Edits

Non-Facility RVU	Work	PE	MP	Total
93701	0.0	0.7	0.01	0.71
Facility RVU	**Work**	**PE**	**MP**	**Total**
93701	0.0	0.7	0.01	0.71

93702

93702 Bioimpedance spectroscopy (BIS), extracellular fluid analysis for lymphedema assessment(s)

Explanation

Bioimpedance spectroscopy (BIS) is an accurate, reproducible, and noninvasive method that detects alterations in extracellular fluid volume differences between the limbs using a device called an impedance plethysmograph. Skin electrodes are applied to the limb. A small alternating current is passed through the limb via these electrodes, and the impedance (opposition) to the current's flow is measured. This measurement is subsequently converted to fluid levels. Differences in extracellular fluid levels between the limbs can be an early indication of lymphedema (swelling from fluid buildup caused by inadequate functioning of the lymphatic system).

Relative Value Units/Medicare Edits

Non-Facility RVU	Work	PE	MP	Total
93702	0.0	3.55	0.02	3.57
Facility RVU	**Work**	**PE**	**MP**	**Total**
93702	0.0	3.55	0.02	3.57

93724

93724 Electronic analysis of antitachycardia pacemaker system (includes electrocardiographic recording, programming of device, induction and termination of tachycardia via implanted pacemaker, and interpretation of recordings)

Explanation

Patients with previously implanted pacemakers require periodic analysis of pacemaker function. This code applies to routine electronic analysis of pacemakers used to control irregularly fast heartbeats (antitachycardial) and includes electrocardiogram, programming, tests, and physician interpretation of the tests.

Relative Value Units/Medicare Edits

Non-Facility RVU	Work	PE	MP	Total
93724	4.88	2.82	0.19	7.89
Facility RVU	**Work**	**PE**	**MP**	**Total**
93724	4.88	2.82	0.19	7.89

93740

93740 Temperature gradient studies

Explanation

Temperature gradient studies assess heart or circulatory functions by contrasting temperatures of certain vessels via an intravenous catheter.

Relative Value Units/Medicare Edits

Non-Facility RVU	Work	PE	MP	Total
93740	0.16	0.06	0.01	0.23
Facility RVU	**Work**	**PE**	**MP**	**Total**
93740	0.16	0.06	0.01	0.23

93745

93745 Initial set-up and programming by a physician or other qualified health care professional of wearable cardioverter-defibrillator includes initial programming of system, establishing baseline electronic ECG, transmission of data to data repository, patient instruction in wearing system and patient reporting of problems or events

Explanation

The physician or other qualified health care professional performs initial set-up and programming of a wearable cardioverter-defibrillator. A wearable cardioverter-defibrillator is an external device that includes a monitor, electrodes, and an alarm contained in a vest-like garment that is worn 24 hours a day by the patient. The wearable cardioverter-defibrillator is used to detect, monitor, and treat life-threatening tachycardia and fibrillation that can lead to sudden cardiac arrest and death. The wearable cardioverter-defibrillator works by restoring a normal rhythm using low frequency shocks (cardioversion) or by returning a fast, disordered rhythm to normal rhythm by means of high-energy shock(s) (defibrillation). This code reports the initial programming of the system by the provider that includes establishing a baseline ECG. The initial set-up also includes verifying data transmission to a data repository, patient instruction on wearing the device, and patient reporting of events or problems with the device.

Relative Value Units/Medicare Edits

Non-Facility RVU	Work	PE	MP	Total
93745	0.0	0.0	0.0	0.0
Facility RVU	**Work**	**PE**	**MP**	**Total**
93745	0.0	0.0	0.0	0.0

93750

93750 Interrogation of ventricular assist device (VAD), in person, with physician or other qualified health care professional analysis of device parameters (eg, drivelines, alarms, power surges), review of device function (eg, flow and volume status, septum status, recovery), with programming, if performed, and report

Explanation

Patients with a previously implanted ventricular assist device (VAD) require periodic interrogation of the device. Code 93750 reports a diagnostic procedure that is performed in person and includes a face-to-face assessment of all device functions. Components that must be evaluated include device parameters (alarms, drivelines, and power surges) and a review of the device function (flow/volume status, septum status, and recovery). This code includes physician or other qualified health care professional analysis, review, and report. It also includes device programming, if performed.

Relative Value Units/Medicare Edits

Non-Facility RVU	Work	PE	MP	Total
93750	0.92	0.58	0.08	1.58
Facility RVU	**Work**	**PE**	**MP**	**Total**
93750	0.92	0.32	0.08	1.32

93770

93770 Determination of venous pressure

Explanation

Venous blood pressure is measured to assess heart and circulatory system functions. This code applies to the peripheral measurement.

Relative Value Units/Medicare Edits

Non-Facility RVU	Work	PE	MP	Total
93770	0.16	0.06	0.01	0.23
Facility RVU	**Work**	**PE**	**MP**	**Total**
93770	0.16	0.06	0.01	0.23

93784-93790

▲ **93784** Ambulatory blood pressure monitoring, utilizing report-generating software, automated, worn continuously for 24 hours or longer; including recording, scanning analysis, interpretation and report

▲ **93786** recording only

▲ **93788** scanning analysis with report

▲ **93790** review with interpretation and report

Explanation

A patient's ambient blood pressure is evaluated during a 24-hour period. A technician attaches the blood pressure monitor to the patient, who wears the monitor continuously for 24 hours. During this period, the device obtains blood pressure measurements and records them on automated report-generating software. Ambulatory blood pressure monitoring (ABPM) may be useful for patients with suspected masked or white coat hypertension. Report 93784 for the complete procedure, including interpretation and report. Report 93786 for the recording only. Report 93788 when a technician scans the data and generates a data summary. Report 93790 for review and interpretation of the data and a subsequent report of the findings.

Relative Value Units/Medicare Edits

Non-Facility RVU	Work	PE	MP	Total
93784	0.38	1.1	0.03	1.51
93786	0.0	0.82	0.01	0.83
93788	0.0	0.14	0.01	0.15
93790	0.38	0.14	0.01	0.53
Facility RVU	**Work**	**PE**	**MP**	**Total**
93784	0.38	1.1	0.03	1.51
93786	0.0	0.82	0.01	0.83
93788	0.0	0.14	0.01	0.15
93790	0.38	0.14	0.01	0.53

93792-93793

93792 Patient/caregiver training for initiation of home international normalized ratio (INR) monitoring under the direction of a physician or other qualified health care professional, face-to-face, including use and care of the INR monitor, obtaining blood sample, instructions for reporting home INR test results, and documentation of patient's/caregiver's ability to perform testing and report results

93793 Anticoagulant management for a patient taking warfarin, must include review and interpretation of a new home, office, or lab international normalized ratio (INR) test result, patient instructions, dosage adjustment (as needed), and scheduling of additional test(s), when performed

Explanation

Home and outpatient international normalized ratio (INR) monitoring is anticoagulant management of warfarin therapy, including ordering, review, and interpretation of new INR test results; patient instructions; and dosage adjustments, as appropriate. In 93792, face-to-face, clinician-directed training is started for the patient and/or caregiver for in-home INR monitoring to include proper use and care of the INR monitoring device, instructions for obtaining blood samples, and reporting INR test results. A documented determination as to the patient's and/or caregiver's ability to adequately perform testing and reporting is also required. Report 93793 for review and interpretation of a new home, office, or lab INR test result with instructions and dosage modifications, as necessary, as well as the scheduling of any additional tests, when performed.

Relative Value Units/Medicare Edits

Non-Facility RVU	Work	PE	MP	Total
93792	0.0	1.46	0.02	1.48
93793	0.18	0.15	0.01	0.34
Facility RVU	**Work**	**PE**	**MP**	**Total**
93792	0.0	1.46	0.02	1.48
93793	0.18	0.15	0.01	0.34

93797-93798

93797 Physician or other qualified health care professional services for outpatient cardiac rehabilitation; without continuous ECG monitoring (per session)

93798 with continuous ECG monitoring (per session)

Explanation

Patients with severe cardiac disease, particularly those who have had myocardial infarctions, surgery on the coronary vessels, and other occlusive coronary artery diseases, often require outpatient rehabilitation. A physician or other qualified health care professional supervises outpatient cardiac rehabilitation in areas of exercise, diet, and related modalities. Report 93798 when continuous electrocardiogram monitoring is provided.

Relative Value Units/Medicare Edits

Non-Facility RVU	Work	PE	MP	Total
93797	0.18	0.27	0.01	0.46
93798	0.28	0.42	0.02	0.72
Facility RVU	**Work**	**PE**	**MP**	**Total**
93797	0.18	0.06	0.01	0.25
93798	0.28	0.1	0.02	0.4

 ● New ▲ Revised + Add On [Resequenced]

93880-93882

93880 Duplex scan of extracranial arteries; complete bilateral study
93882 unilateral or limited study

Explanation

The physician or an assistant performs a Duplex ultrasound scan, which is a combination of real-time and Doppler studies of the extracranial arteries in the head and neck to evaluate vascular blood flow in relation to blockage. Ultrasound uses high frequency sound waves to provide an image. Report 93880 when the procedure is performed on both sides of the head and neck. Report 93882 when a unilateral (one side of the head or neck) or limited study is performed.

Relative Value Units/Medicare Edits

Non-Facility RVU	Work	PE	MP	Total
93880	0.8	4.81	0.09	5.7
93882	0.5	3.06	0.08	3.64
Facility RVU	**Work**	**PE**	**MP**	**Total**
93880	0.8	4.81	0.09	5.7
93882	0.5	3.06	0.08	3.64

93886-93888

93886 Transcranial Doppler study of the intracranial arteries; complete study
93888 limited study

Explanation

The physician or an assistant performs a Doppler ultrasound scan of the intracranial arteries in the head and neck to evaluate vascular blood flow in relation to blockage. Code 93886 applies to a complete study of the intracranial arteries. Code 93888 applies to a limited study of the intracranial arteries.

Relative Value Units/Medicare Edits

Non-Facility RVU	Work	PE	MP	Total
93886	0.91	6.68	0.08	7.67
93888	0.5	3.91	0.06	4.47
Facility RVU	**Work**	**PE**	**MP**	**Total**
93886	0.91	6.68	0.08	7.67
93888	0.5	3.91	0.06	4.47

93890

93890 Transcranial Doppler study of the intracranial arteries; vasoreactivity study

Explanation

The physician performs a vasoreactivity transcranial Doppler study of the intracranial arteries to identify cerebrovascular disease. Transcranial Doppler is a noninvasive ultrasound technology used to evaluate blood flow in the major intracranial arteries. Vasoreactivity, also referred to as vasomotor reactivity, measures changes in blood flow velocity in response to pharmacologic or other agent. A Doppler ultrasound scan of the intracranial arteries is performed and flow velocity measured. A pharmacologic or other agent is administered and Doppler ultrasound scan is again performed and flow velocity measured. Changes in blood flow velocity in the intracranial arteries are compared and analyzed.

Relative Value Units/Medicare Edits

Non-Facility RVU	Work	PE	MP	Total
93890	1.0	6.74	0.08	7.82
Facility RVU	**Work**	**PE**	**MP**	**Total**
93890	1.0	6.74	0.08	7.82

93892-93893

93892 Transcranial Doppler study of the intracranial arteries; emboli detection without intravenous microbubble injection
93893 emboli detection with intravenous microbubble injection

Explanation

The physician performs a transcranial Doppler study of the intracranial arteries for detection of emboli. Transcranial Doppler is a noninvasive ultrasound technology used to evaluate blood flow in the major intracranial arteries. A new application of transcranial Doppler includes the classification and quantification of intracranial emboli. Intracranial circulating microemboli appear as high intensity transient signals in the transcranial Doppler waveform. Report 93892 if the study is performed without intravenous microbubble injection. Report 93893 if the study is performed with intravenous microbubble injection. Transcranial Doppler studies described as "with contrast" are performed with intravenous microbubble injection. The bubbles serve to enhance ultrasound signals thus enabling better visualization of the intracranial arteries.

Relative Value Units/Medicare Edits

Non-Facility RVU	Work	PE	MP	Total
93892	1.15	7.55	0.11	8.81
93893	1.15	8.57	0.09	9.81
Facility RVU	**Work**	**PE**	**MP**	**Total**
93892	1.15	7.55	0.11	8.81
93893	1.15	8.57	0.09	9.81

93895

93895 Quantitative carotid intima media thickness and carotid atheroma evaluation, bilateral

Explanation

Carotid intima media thickness (IMT) study is a noninvasive assessment performed on the common carotid artery bilaterally. The measurements of the inner two artery layers, the intima and the media, are used as risk factor indicators for atherosclerosis and coronary heart disease. This test is performed by scanning with high-resolution B mode ultrasonography and using computer enhancement and analysis to determine the thickness of the intima and media of the carotid artery. The results evaluate for any thickening or signs of anatomical changes from early atherosclerotic disease.

Relative Value Units/Medicare Edits

Non-Facility RVU	Work	PE	MP	Total
93895	0.0	0.0	0.0	0.0
Facility RVU	**Work**	**PE**	**MP**	**Total**
93895	0.0	0.0	0.0	0.0

93922-93923

93922 Limited bilateral noninvasive physiologic studies of upper or lower extremity arteries, (eg, for lower extremity: ankle/brachial indices at distal posterior tibial and anterior tibial/dorsalis pedis arteries plus bidirectional, Doppler waveform recording and analysis at 1-2 levels, or ankle/brachial indices at distal posterior tibial and anterior tibial/dorsalis pedis arteries plus volume plethysmography at 1-2 levels, or ankle/brachial indices at distal posterior tibial and anterior tibial/dorsalis pedis arteries with, transcutaneous oxygen tension measurement at 1-2 levels)

93923 Complete bilateral noninvasive physiologic studies of upper or lower extremity arteries, 3 or more levels (eg, for lower extremity: ankle/brachial indices at distal posterior tibial and anterior tibial/dorsalis pedis arteries plus segmental blood pressure measurements with bidirectional Doppler waveform recording and analysis, at 3 or more levels, or ankle/brachial indices at distal posterior tibial and anterior tibial/dorsalis pedis arteries plus segmental volume plethysmography at 3 or more levels, or ankle/brachial indices at distal posterior tibial and anterior tibial/dorsalis pedis arteries plus segmental transcutaneous oxygen tension measurements at 3 or more levels), or single level study with provocative functional maneuvers (eg, measurements with postural provocative tests, or measurements with reactive hyperemia)

Explanation

The physician or assistant physician evaluates the arteries of the arms or legs to check blood flow in relation to blockage. In one method, the physician places a transducer on each leg at a prescribed level and measures the change in blood-handling characteristics during constriction by pneumatic cuffs. The technique is similar to constriction and measuring of tension in the vascular system, but the medium may change. Report 93922 applies for ultrasound, plethysmography, and oxygen tension measurements in a bilateral evaluation limited to one or two levels. When a unilateral study of one to two levels is performed, report 93922 with modifier 52. This code is also applicable to a unilateral study when three or more levels are recorded or if provocative functional maneuvers are performed. Report 93923 for a complete bilateral study of three or more levels or a single-level study with provocative functional maneuvers.

Relative Value Units/Medicare Edits

Non-Facility RVU	Work	PE	MP	Total
93922	0.25	2.15	0.04	2.44
93923	0.45	3.26	0.07	3.78
Facility RVU	**Work**	**PE**	**MP**	**Total**
93922	0.25	2.15	0.04	2.44
93923	0.45	3.26	0.07	3.78

93924

93924 Noninvasive physiologic studies of lower extremity arteries, at rest and following treadmill stress testing, (ie, bidirectional Doppler waveform or volume plethysmography recording and analysis at rest with ankle/brachial indices immediately after and at timed intervals following performance of a standardized protocol on a motorized treadmill plus recording of time of onset of claudication or other symptoms, maximal walking time, and time to recovery) complete bilateral study

Explanation

The physician or assistant evaluates the arteries of the legs to check blood flow in relation to blockage. This code applies to ultrasound and oxygen tension measurements in a bilateral evaluation that occurs before and after a treadmill stress test.

Relative Value Units/Medicare Edits

Non-Facility RVU	Work	PE	MP	Total
93924	0.5	4.1	0.07	4.67
Facility RVU	**Work**	**PE**	**MP**	**Total**
93924	0.5	4.1	0.07	4.67

93925-93926

93925 Duplex scan of lower extremity arteries or arterial bypass grafts; complete bilateral study

93926 unilateral or limited study

Explanation

The physician or assistant evaluates the arteries of the legs bilaterally to check blood flow in relation to blockage by use of Duplex ultrasonography, which is a combination of real-time and Doppler studies. Code 93925 refers to a complete bilateral study. Code 93926 applies to studies of one leg or limited areas of both legs.

Relative Value Units/Medicare Edits

Non-Facility RVU	Work	PE	MP	Total
93925	0.8	6.35	0.1	7.25
93926	0.5	3.69	0.07	4.26
Facility RVU	**Work**	**PE**	**MP**	**Total**
93925	0.8	6.35	0.1	7.25
93926	0.5	3.69	0.07	4.26

93930-93931

93930 Duplex scan of upper extremity arteries or arterial bypass grafts; complete bilateral study

93931 unilateral or limited study

Explanation

A diagnostic study is performed on the upper extremity arteries or arterial bypass grafts. A duplex scan involves a two-dimensional ultrasonic scan, which provides a two-dimensional display of the structure. Code 93930 reports a procedure performed on both arms (complete bilateral study). Code 93931 applies to studies of one arm or limited areas of both arms.

Relative Value Units/Medicare Edits

Non-Facility RVU	Work	PE	MP	Total
93930	0.8	4.92	0.1	5.82
93931	0.5	3.07	0.06	3.63
Facility RVU	**Work**	**PE**	**MP**	**Total**
93930	0.8	4.92	0.1	5.82
93931	0.5	3.07	0.06	3.63

93970-93971

93970 Duplex scan of extremity veins including responses to compression and other maneuvers; complete bilateral study

93971 unilateral or limited study

Explanation

The physician or assistant performs a Duplex ultrasound scan, which is a combination of real-time and Doppler studies, of the veins in the arms or legs to evaluate vascular blood flow in relation to blockage. Code 93970 applies to complete responses to compression and other tests on both sides (complete bilateral study). Code 93971 applies to complete responses to compression and other tests and includes one side or limited areas of both sides.

Relative Value Units/Medicare Edits

Non-Facility RVU	Work	PE	MP	Total
93970	0.7	4.74	0.08	5.52
93971	0.45	2.92	0.05	3.42
Facility RVU	**Work**	**PE**	**MP**	**Total**
93970	0.7	4.74	0.08	5.52
93971	0.45	2.92	0.05	3.42

93975-93976

93975 Duplex scan of arterial inflow and venous outflow of abdominal, pelvic, scrotal contents and/or retroperitoneal organs; complete study

93976 limited study

Explanation

The physician or assistant performs a Duplex ultrasound scan, which is a combination of real-time and Doppler studies, of the arteries and veins in the abdominal, pelvic, or genitorectal areas to evaluate vascular blood flow in relation to blockage. Code 93975 applies to a complete bilateral evaluation. Code 93976 applies to a limited evaluation.

Relative Value Units/Medicare Edits

Non-Facility RVU	Work	PE	MP	Total
93975	1.16	6.6	0.12	7.88
93976	0.8	3.78	0.06	4.64
Facility RVU	**Work**	**PE**	**MP**	**Total**
93975	1.16	6.6	0.12	7.88
93976	0.8	3.78	0.06	4.64

93978-93979

93978 Duplex scan of aorta, inferior vena cava, iliac vasculature, or bypass grafts; complete study

93979 unilateral or limited study

Explanation

The physician or assistant performs a Duplex ultrasound scan, which is a combination of real-time and Doppler studies, of the arteries and veins in the aorta, inferior vena cava, or iliac areas to evaluate vascular blood flow in relation to blockage. Code 93978 applies to a complete bilateral evaluation. Code 93979 applies to one side or limited areas of both sides.

Relative Value Units/Medicare Edits

Non-Facility RVU	Work	PE	MP	Total
93978	0.8	4.43	0.11	5.34
93979	0.5	2.83	0.07	3.4
Facility RVU	**Work**	**PE**	**MP**	**Total**
93978	0.8	4.43	0.11	5.34
93979	0.5	2.83	0.07	3.4

93980-93981

93980 Duplex scan of arterial inflow and venous outflow of penile vessels; complete study

93981 follow-up or limited study

Explanation

The physician performs a Duplex ultrasound scan, producing real-time images integrating B-mode two-dimensional structure with Doppler mapping or imaging of motion with time, of the arteries and veins in the penis to evaluate vascular blood flow in and out of the penis in relation to blockages. Report 93980 for a complete evaluation and 93981 for a follow-up or a limited study.

Relative Value Units/Medicare Edits

Non-Facility RVU	Work	PE	MP	Total
93980	1.25	2.22	0.06	3.53
93981	0.44	1.67	0.04	2.15
Facility RVU	**Work**	**PE**	**MP**	**Total**
93980	1.25	2.22	0.06	3.53
93981	0.44	1.67	0.04	2.15

93985-93986

● **93985** Duplex scan of arterial inflow and venous outflow for preoperative vessel assessment prior to creation of hemodialysis access; complete bilateral study

● **93986** complete unilateral study

Explanation

The physician performs a Duplex ultrasound scan, producing real-time images integrating B-mode two-dimensional structure with Doppler mapping or imaging of motion with time for preoperative assessment of vascular blood flow prior to the creation of a hemodialysis access. This assessment includes the arterial inflow and venous outflow. Native arteriovenous fistula (AVF) is the preferred vascular access for hemodialysis patients, lasting longer and having fewer complications than grafts and central venous catheters. The use of the Doppler ultrasound (DUS) in preoperative vascular mapping enables identification of vessels that are most appropriate for fistula construction. Report 93985 for a complete bilateral study and 93986 for a complete unilateral study.

Relative Value Units/Medicare Edits

Non-Facility RVU	Work	PE	MP	Total
93985				
93986				
Facility RVU	**Work**	**PE**	**MP**	**Total**
93985				
93986				

93990

93990 Duplex scan of hemodialysis access (including arterial inflow, body of access and venous outflow)

Explanation

The physician performs a Duplex ultrasound scan, producing real-time images integrating B-mode two-dimensional structure with Doppler mapping or imaging of motion with time, of a hemodialysis access site, including the arterial inflow, body of the access site or device, and venous outflow, to evaluate vascular blood flow in relation to blockage.

Relative Value Units/Medicare Edits

Non-Facility RVU	Work	PE	MP	Total
93990	0.5	3.82	0.1	4.42
Facility RVU	**Work**	**PE**	**MP**	**Total**
93990	0.5	3.82	0.1	4.42

94002-94004

94002 Ventilation assist and management, initiation of pressure or volume preset ventilators for assisted or controlled breathing; hospital inpatient/observation, initial day

94003 hospital inpatient/observation, each subsequent day

94004 nursing facility, per day

Explanation

A mechanical ventilator is applied with a mask over the nose and mouth or through a tube placed into the trachea for patients requiring help breathing due to a lung disorder. Intermittent positive pressure breathing uses positive pressure during the inspiration phase of breathing. Code 94002 applies to ventilation assistance using adjustments in volume and pressure on the initial day of treatment in a hospital to an inpatient or observation patient and 94003 is reported for ventilation assistance to a hospital inpatient or observation patient provided on subsequent days. Ventilation assistance and management provided to a nursing facility patient is reported with 94004 on a per day basis.

Relative Value Units/Medicare Edits

Non-Facility RVU	Work	PE	MP	Total
94002	1.99	0.49	0.16	2.64
94003	1.37	0.41	0.11	1.89
94004	1.0	0.32	0.08	1.4
Facility RVU	**Work**	**PE**	**MP**	**Total**
94002	1.99	0.49	0.16	2.64
94003	1.37	0.41	0.11	1.89
94004	1.0	0.32	0.08	1.4

94150

94150 Vital capacity, total (separate procedure)

Explanation

This procedure measures the largest volume of air a patient can expire from his lungs. The patient amount of air inhaled and exhaled is measured and calculated with body size to determine the capacity of the lungs. This test is important for determining the threshold of capacity needed for vitality in patients with compromised respiration. For men, this is typically four to five liters; for women, this is normally three to four liters. It is normally performed as a part of a larger procedure and should only be billed separately when performed alone.

Relative Value Units/Medicare Edits

Non-Facility RVU	Work	PE	MP	Total
94150	0.07	0.63	0.02	0.72
Facility RVU	**Work**	**PE**	**MP**	**Total**
94150	0.07	0.63	0.02	0.72

94617

94617 Exercise test for bronchospasm, including pre- and post-spirometry, electrocardiographic recording(s), and pulse oximetry

Explanation

An exercise-induced bronchospasm (EIB) test is performed to diagnose EIB based on the difference in lung function postexercise rather than on symptoms. Bronchospasm, an occurrence that happens when the lungs shrink during exercise, makes it difficult to breathe. The clinician conducts a pre- and post-spirometry test that measures the amount of air a patient inhales and how much air is being exhaled. An EIB test typically involves rapidly increasing the intensity of the exercise, such as cycling or running, over a period of about two to four minutes duration in order to have the patient reach a high rate of breathing dry air via the use of a nasal clip. Exercise is continued until the patient's heartrate is 80 to 90 percent of the predicted maximum or once the patient's breathing reaches 68, 72, or 73 (17.5 to 21 times FEV1). The patient has to maintain this level for an additional four to six minutes. Studies have shown that running helps reach these targets faster than any other type of exercise. Measurement of the patient's oxygen level by pulse oximetry and an electrocardiography (ECG, EKG) are performed to monitor the heart.

Relative Value Units/Medicare Edits

Non-Facility RVU	Work	PE	MP	Total
94617	0.7	1.91	0.05	2.66
Facility RVU	**Work**	**PE**	**MP**	**Total**
94617	0.7	1.91	0.05	2.66

94618-94621

94618 Pulmonary stress testing (eg, 6-minute walk test), including measurement of heart rate, oximetry, and oxygen titration, when performed

94621 Cardiopulmonary exercise testing, including measurements of minute ventilation, CO2 production, O2 uptake, and electrocardiographic recordings

Explanation

In 94618, a pulmonary exercise stress test is performed to determine how much air is moving in and out of the lungs during exercise and to establish where breathing problems are occurring, since they may be in the lungs, heart, or circulation. An exercise stress test is done with the patient riding a stationary bike (ergometer) or walking on a treadmill. Heartrate, breathing, and blood pressure are monitored before beginning the exercise. Basic ventilation studies are performed with a spirometer and recording device as the patient breathes through a mouthpiece and connecting tube while a nose clip prevents nasal breathing. Measurement of the patient's oxygen level by pulse oximetry is included, as well as oxygen titration and heartrate, when performed. In 94621, cardiopulmonary exercise testing is performed. Electrodes are placed on the upper body to monitor the heart. Throughout the process, blood samples may be taken to measure oxygen uptake and carbon dioxide waste products in the blood, as well as other tests including minute ventilation and an electrocardiogram (ECG, EKG).

Relative Value Units/Medicare Edits

Non-Facility RVU	Work	PE	MP	Total
94618	0.48	0.45	0.03	0.96
94621	1.42	3.04	0.08	4.54
Facility RVU	**Work**	**PE**	**MP**	**Total**
94618	0.48	0.45	0.03	0.96
94621	1.42	3.04	0.08	4.54

[95943]

95943 Simultaneous, independent, quantitative measures of both parasympathetic function and sympathetic function, based on time-frequency analysis of heart rate variability concurrent with time-frequency analysis of continuous respiratory activity, with mean heart rate and blood pressure measures, during rest, paced (deep) breathing, Valsalva maneuvers, and head-up postural change

Explanation

An electronic blood pressure monitor is placed on a patient to test the parasympathetic and sympathetic nervous system's ability to regulate blood pressure. The patient is placed supine and the heart rate variability, blood pressure measurements, and respiratory activity are monitored and the mean heart rate is calculated. These measurements are taken during rest, deep breathing, the Valsalva maneuver (expelling air against a closed glottis), and head up postural change. Autonomic testing utilizing beat-to-beat recording or tilt table testing is reported elsewhere.

Relative Value Units/Medicare Edits

Non-Facility RVU	Work	PE	MP	Total
95943	0.0	0.0	0.0	0.0
Facility RVU	**Work**	**PE**	**MP**	**Total**
95943	0.0	0.0	0.0	0.0

96160-96161

96160 Administration of patient-focused health risk assessment instrument (eg, health hazard appraisal) with scoring and documentation, per standardized instrument

96161 Administration of caregiver-focused health risk assessment instrument (eg, depression inventory) for the benefit of the patient, with scoring and documentation, per standardized instrument

Explanation

A provision in the Patient Protection and Affordable Care Act of 2010 (ACA) established a Medicare Wellness Visit, which included a Health Risk Assessment (HRA) and customized wellness or prevention plan. HRAs are typically completed by a patient or caregiver prior to the encounter with a physician or other qualified health care professional, but can involve the assistance of the clinician and/or staff members. The HRA tool is purposefully designed to be brief, straightforward, and easy to comprehend with questions such as patient demographic information, personal and/or family history, a self-assessment of how the patient interprets his/her health to be, risk factors, biometric measurements, and compliance. Completion of the HRA tool takes approximately 20 minutes and may be done via the internet or on a paper-based document. Assessments that emphasize a patient or caregiver focus may be referred to as HRA plus assessments and as such should be person centered and culturally appropriate in all areas, including, but not limited to, the assessment instrument, the administration process of the assessment, clinician communication with the patient regarding findings, as well as followup and monitoring. Additionally, the patient-focused HRA takes into consideration the importance of care support services over and above the health care system; for example, by family members, community support services, or even in the workplace setting where the individual receiving care is not deemed to be a "patient." An emphasis is also placed on cultural competency as means of limited health disparities through respect of the patient's beliefs and understanding the mental and physical ways a patient can experience illness and health and working together to establish a health plan. Another area of patient-focused care involves areas of importance to patients as consumers, such as convenience as well as increasing outcomes that matter to patients; for example, improved quality of life and function. Similarly, caregiver-focused assessment tools serve to identify areas of concern such as stress levels, depression, and the burdens placed on the caregiver. HRAs contribute to the goals of the government to drive health improvements, quality of life, and value for the health care delivery system in the United States. Report 96160 for administration of a patient-focused health risk assessment tool and 96161 for administration of a caregiver-focused assessment tool. Both codes include scoring and documentation of the assessment tool.

Relative Value Units/Medicare Edits

Non-Facility RVU	Work	PE	MP	Total
96160	0.0	0.09	0.0	0.09
96161	0.0	0.09	0.0	0.09
Facility RVU	**Work**	**PE**	**MP**	**Total**
96160	0.0	0.09	0.0	0.09
96161	0.0	0.09	0.0	0.09

96360-96361

96360 Intravenous infusion, hydration; initial, 31 minutes to 1 hour

\+ **96361** each additional hour (List separately in addition to code for primary procedure)

Explanation

A physician or an assistant under direct physician supervision infuses a hydration solution (prepackaged fluid and electrolytes) for 31 minutes to one hour through an intravenous catheter inserted by needle into a patient's vein or by infusion through an existing indwelling intravascular access catheter or port. Report 96361 for each additional hour beyond the first hour. Intravenous infusion for hydration lasting 30 minutes or less is not reported.

Relative Value Units/Medicare Edits

Non-Facility RVU	Work	PE	MP	Total
96360	0.17	0.88	0.02	1.07
96361	0.09	0.28	0.01	0.38
Facility RVU	**Work**	**PE**	**MP**	**Total**
96360	0.17	0.88	0.02	1.07
96361	0.09	0.28	0.01	0.38

96365-96368

96365 Intravenous infusion, for therapy, prophylaxis, or diagnosis (specify substance or drug); initial, up to 1 hour

\+ **96366** each additional hour (List separately in addition to code for primary procedure)

\+ **96367** additional sequential infusion of a new drug/substance, up to 1 hour (List separately in addition to code for primary procedure)

\+ **96368** concurrent infusion (List separately in addition to code for primary procedure)

Explanation

A physician or an assistant under direct physician supervision injects or infuses a therapeutic, prophylactic (preventive), or diagnostic medication other than chemotherapy or other highly complex drugs or biologic agents via intravenous route. Infusions are administered through an intravenous catheter inserted by needle into a patient's vein or by injection or infusion through an existing indwelling intravascular access catheter or port. Report 96365 for the initial hour and 96366 for each additional hour. Report 96367 for each additional sequential infusion of a different substance or drug, up to one hour, and 96368 for each concurrent infusion of substances other than chemotherapy or other highly complex drugs or biologic agents.

Relative Value Units/Medicare Edits

Non-Facility RVU	Work	PE	MP	Total
96365	0.21	1.77	0.04	2.02
96366	0.18	0.42	0.01	0.61
96367	0.19	0.67	0.02	0.88
96368	0.17	0.41	0.01	0.59
Facility RVU	**Work**	**PE**	**MP**	**Total**
96365	0.21	1.77	0.04	2.02
96366	0.18	0.42	0.01	0.61
96367	0.19	0.67	0.02	0.88
96368	0.17	0.41	0.01	0.59

96369-96371

96369 Subcutaneous infusion for therapy or prophylaxis (specify substance or drug); initial, up to 1 hour, including pump set-up and establishment of subcutaneous infusion site(s)

\+ **96370** each additional hour (List separately in addition to code for primary procedure)

\+ **96371** additional pump set-up with establishment of new subcutaneous infusion site(s) (List separately in addition to code for primary procedure)

Explanation

A physician or an assistant under direct physician supervision infuses a therapeutic or prophylactic (preventive) medication other than chemotherapy or other highly complex drug or biologic agent via a subcutaneous route. Indications for subcutaneous infusion may include coma, dysphagia, nausea/vomiting, intestinal obstruction, malabsorption, or extreme weakness. Infusions are administered through a needle inserted beneath the skin; common infusion sites include the upper arm, shoulder, abdomen, and thigh. Report 96369 for infusions lasting longer than 15 minutes and up to one hour. This code includes pump set-up and the establishment of subcutaneous infusion sites. Report 96370 for each additional hour and 96371 for an additional pump set-up with the establishment of new subcutaneous infusion sites. Codes 96369 and 96371 should be reported only once per encounter.

Relative Value Units/Medicare Edits

Non-Facility RVU	Work	PE	MP	Total
96369	0.21	4.46	0.02	4.69
96370	0.18	0.25	0.01	0.44
96371	0.0	1.84	0.0	1.84
Facility RVU	**Work**	**PE**	**MP**	**Total**
96369	0.21	4.46	0.02	4.69
96370	0.18	0.25	0.01	0.44
96371	0.0	1.84	0.0	1.84

96372-96376

96372 Therapeutic, prophylactic, or diagnostic injection (specify substance or drug); subcutaneous or intramuscular

96373 intra-arterial

96374 intravenous push, single or initial substance/drug

\+ **96375** each additional sequential intravenous push of a new substance/drug (List separately in addition to code for primary procedure)

\+ **96376** each additional sequential intravenous push of the same substance/drug provided in a facility (List separately in addition to code for primary procedure)

Explanation

The physician or an assistant under direct physician supervision administers a therapeutic, prophylactic, or diagnostic substance by subcutaneous or intramuscular injection (96372), intra-arterial injection (96373), or by push into an intravenous catheter or intravascular access device (96374 for a single or initial substance, 96375 for each additional sequential IV push of a new substance, and 96376 for each additional sequential IV push of the same substance after 30 minutes have elapsed). The push technique involves an infusion of less than 15 minutes. Code 96376 may be reported only by facilities.

Relative Value Units/Medicare Edits

Non-Facility RVU	Work	PE	MP	Total
96372	0.17	0.29	0.01	0.47
96373	0.17	0.35	0.01	0.53
96374	0.18	0.9	0.02	1.1
96375	0.1	0.36	0.01	0.47
96376	0.0	0.0	0.0	0.0
Facility RVU	**Work**	**PE**	**MP**	**Total**
96372	0.17	0.29	0.01	0.47
96373	0.17	0.35	0.01	0.53
96374	0.18	0.9	0.02	1.1
96375	0.1	0.36	0.01	0.47
96376	0.0	0.0	0.0	0.0

99026-99027

99026 Hospital mandated on call service; in-hospital, each hour

99027 out-of-hospital, each hour

Explanation

The code reports the time for hospital mandated on call service provided by the physician. This code does not include prolonged physician attendance time for standby services or the time spent performing other reportable procedures or services. Report 99026 for each hour of hospital mandated on call service spent in the hospital and 99027 for each hour of hospital mandated on call service spent outside the hospital.

Relative Value Units/Medicare Edits

Non-Facility RVU	Work	PE	MP	Total
99026	0.0	0.0	0.0	0.0
99027	0.0	0.0	0.0	0.0
Facility RVU	**Work**	**PE**	**MP**	**Total**
99026	0.0	0.0	0.0	0.0
99027	0.0	0.0	0.0	0.0

99190-99192

99190 Assembly and operation of pump with oxygenator or heat exchanger (with or without ECG and/or pressure monitoring); each hour

99191 45 minutes

99192 30 minutes

Explanation

The health care provider assembles and operates a pump with an oxygenator or heat exchanger. Report 99190 to identify each hour; 99191 to report 45 minutes; and 99192 to report 30 minutes.

Relative Value Units/Medicare Edits

Non-Facility RVU	Work	PE	MP	Total
99190	0.0	0.0	0.0	0.0
99191	0.0	0.0	0.0	0.0
99192	0.0	0.0	0.0	0.0
Facility RVU	**Work**	**PE**	**MP**	**Total**
99190	0.0	0.0	0.0	0.0
99191	0.0	0.0	0.0	0.0
99192	0.0	0.0	0.0	0.0

99195

99195 Phlebotomy, therapeutic (separate procedure)

Explanation

The health care provider draws blood from the patient to right dramatically imbalanced blood levels (i.e., hemoglobin, potassium salts). The procedure is similar to drawing blood from a donor, but a number of pints may be taken to reduce the imbalance. Blood removal is performed under a physician's direction.

Relative Value Units/Medicare Edits

Non-Facility RVU	Work	PE	MP	Total
99195	0.0	2.8	0.06	2.86
Facility RVU	**Work**	**PE**	**MP**	**Total**
99195	0.0	2.8	0.06	2.86

0085T

0085T Breath test for heart transplant rejection

Explanation

A marker for heart transplant rejection, the breath methylated alkane contour (BMAC) is administered as a lab test. Heart transplant rejection is accompanied by oxidative stress that degrades membrane polyunsaturated fatty acids, evolving alkanes, and methylalkanes. These are excreted in the form of volatile organic compounds (VOC). To evaluate VOC, a breath sample is taken. Breath VOCs are analyzed using gas chromatography and mass spectrometry. The BMAC is derived based on the abundance of C4-C20 alkanes and monomethylalkanes.

0126T

0126T Common carotid intima-media thickness (IMT) study for evaluation of atherosclerotic burden or coronary heart disease risk factor assessment

Explanation

An intima-media thickness (IMT) study is performed on the common carotid artery. The measurements of the inner two artery layers, the intima and the media, are used as risk factor indicators for atherosclerosis and coronary heart disease. This noninvasive test is performed by scanning with high-resolution B mode ultrasonography and using computer enhancement and analysis to determine the thickness of the intima and media of the carotid artery. The results evaluate for any thickening or signs of anatomical changes from early atherosclerotic disease.

0234T-0238T

0234T Transluminal peripheral atherectomy, open or percutaneous, including radiological supervision and interpretation; renal artery
0235T visceral artery (except renal), each vessel
0236T abdominal aorta
0237T brachiocephalic trunk and branches, each vessel
0238T iliac artery, each vessel

Explanation

The physician treats a stenosed artery percutaneously or via open surgical incision to relieve a blockage. In the percutaneous approach, a needle punctures the skin at the access site and is followed by a guidewire and an introducer sheath to protect and enclose the opening. A series of catheters and guidewires are inserted until the stenosed area has been traversed. An atherectomy catheter is manipulated to the study area and activated to cut or drill a channel through the plaque lesion and reopen the artery. Contrast medium is injected to fluoroscopically visualize the degree of luminal opening. The process may be repeated with a larger diameter catheter if necessary. In the open surgical approach, the physician creates a femoral cutdown incision to expose one of the femoral arteries. The physician punctures the femoral artery with a large needle and passes a guidewire via the needle into the artery. The physician removes the needle while leaving the guidewire in place, enlarges the arterial opening slightly with a blade, and slides an introducer sheath over the guidewire into the arterial lumen. The physician slides a guidewire through the atherectomy catheter or device and inserts the guidewire/atherectomy catheter combination through the introducer sheath into the stenosed vessel. The atherectomy device is fluoroscopically positioned at the area of stenosis and then activated to remove the stenotic tissue. The physician rechecks the diameter of the lesion by angiography. Several passes with the atherectomy device may be required. The physician removes the atherectomy catheter, guidewire, and introducer sheath, closing the femoral arteriotomy with suture. Report 0234T when the blockage occurs in the renal artery; 0235T in a visceral artery; 0236T in the abdominal aorta; 0237T in the brachiocephalic trunk and branches; and 0238T in the iliac artery.

0266T-0268T

0266T Implantation or replacement of carotid sinus baroreflex activation device; total system (includes generator placement, unilateral or bilateral lead placement, intra-operative interrogation, programming, and repositioning, when performed)
0267T lead only, unilateral (includes intra-operative interrogation, programming, and repositioning, when performed)
0268T pulse generator only (includes intra-operative interrogation, programming, and repositioning, when performed)

Explanation

A carotid sinus baroreflex activation system is implanted for refractory hypertension. The baroreflex sends signals to the brain to naturally regulate blood pressure. The insertion of this system allows the signals to be triggered artificially, causing the body to lower blood pressure. An incision is made below the clavicle to form a pocket for the baroreflex activation generator. Incisions on each side of the neck are made to place the electrodes directly on the carotid sinuses, which control the baroreflex. The leads (wires) attached to the electrodes are tunneled beneath the skin to the generator pocket and connected to the generator. The generator is secured within the surgically created pocket and the system is tested. All incisions are closed routinely. Report 0266T for insertion or replacement of the entire carotid sinus baroreflex activation system (generator and leads); report 0267T for unilateral lead insertion(s) or replacement; and report 0268T for insertion or replacement of the pulse generator only. These codes include intraoperative interrogation, programming, and repositioning.

0269T-0271T

0269T Revision or removal of carotid sinus baroreflex activation device; total system (includes generator placement, unilateral or bilateral lead placement, intra-operative interrogation, programming, and repositioning, when performed)

0270T lead only, unilateral (includes intra-operative interrogation, programming, and repositioning, when performed)

0271T pulse generator only (includes intra-operative interrogation, programming, and repositioning, when performed)

Explanation

A carotid sinus baroreflex activation system is implanted for refractory hypertension. The baroreflex sends signals to the brain to naturally regulate blood pressure. The insertion of this system allows the signals to be triggered artificially, causing the body to lower blood pressure. There are two components to a baroreflex activation system: a generator, which is positioned in a pocket below the clavicle, and electrodes (leads), one placed on each carotid sinus in the neck. Report 0269T for revision or removal of the entire carotid sinus baroreflex activation system (generator and leads); report 0270T for unilateral lead revision or removal; and report 0271T for revision or removal of the pulse generator only. These codes include intraoperative interrogation, programming, and repositioning.

0272T-0273T

0272T Interrogation device evaluation (in person), carotid sinus baroreflex activation system, including telemetric iterative communication with the implantable device to monitor device diagnostics and programmed therapy values, with interpretation and report (eg, battery status, lead impedance, pulse amplitude, pulse width, therapy frequency, pathway mode, burst mode, therapy start/stop times each day);

0273T with programming

Explanation

The purpose of these studies is to ensure that the carotid sinus baroreflex activation system is positioned well and working properly in order to guarantee proper function of the system in the future. A carotid sinus baroreflex activation system is implanted for refractory hypertension. The baroreflex sends signals to the brain to naturally regulate blood pressure. The insertion of this system allows the signals to be triggered artificially, causing the body to lower blood pressure. There are two components to a baroreflex activation system: a generator, which is positioned in a pocket below the clavicle, and electrodes (leads), one placed on each carotid sinus in the neck. The physician interrogates the device using the wireless programmer and collects and reports information including battery status, lead impedance, pulse amplitude and width, therapy frequency, pathway and burst modes, and therapy start and stop times. This interrogation must be performed in person. Report 0272T for the evaluation and 0273T if programming is performed in addition to the evaluation.

0295T-0298T

0295T External electrocardiographic recording for more than 48 hours up to 21 days by continuous rhythm recording and storage; includes recording, scanning analysis with report, review and interpretation

0296T recording (includes connection and initial recording)

0297T scanning analysis with report

0298T review and interpretation

Explanation

The purpose of this study is to evaluate the patient's ambient heart rhythm during a full daily cycle. The physician or other qualified health care provider instructs the patient in the use of an external electrocardiographic (ECG) recorder, also known as a Holter monitor. A technician places ECG leads on the patient's chest, and the patient wears the recorder for 48 hours to 21 days. During this time there is continuous rhythm recording and storage. The patient returns the device and the recorded heart rhythm is played back into digital format by a technician. The technician uses a scanning methodology to classify different ECG waveforms and to generate a report. The generated report describes the overall rhythm and significant arrhythmias. Code 0295T reports the recording, scanning analysis with report, provider review of the data, and the provision of a final interpretation in a report. Code 0296T reports the recording only, which includes connection, recording of data, and disconnection. Code 0297T reports only the scanning analysis with report. Code 0298T reports only the provider review and interpretation.

0331T-0332T

0331T Myocardial sympathetic innervation imaging, planar qualitative and quantitative assessment;

0332T with tomographic SPECT

Explanation

Myocardial sympathetic innervation imaging is performed to help assess cardiac nerve activity in patients with heart failure. Iodine meta-iodobenzylguanidine (MIBG) is injected intravenously. Planar images are taken at 15 minutes (early) and four hours (late) after injection to test the MIBG concentration levels in the myocardial sympathetic nerve endings. Qualitative and quantitative studies are performed using the average count per pixel and decrease in counts between early and late images. Report 0332T if single-photon emission computed tomography imaging is performed after the early and late planar images.

0338T-0339T

0338T Transcatheter renal sympathetic denervation, percutaneous approach including arterial puncture, selective catheter placement(s) renal artery(ies), fluoroscopy, contrast injection(s), intraprocedural roadmapping and radiological supervision and interpretation, including pressure gradient measurements, flush aortogram and diagnostic renal angiography when performed; unilateral

0339T bilateral

Explanation

A small incision is made over the femoral artery and a catheter with an electrode on the tip is inserted. Using fluoroscopic guidance, the catheter is maneuvered to the renal artery. The catheter is connected to a radiofrequency generator that delivers lower powered, precisely focused bursts of energy to disrupt the surrounding renal nerves and reduce the renal contribution to central blood pressure elevation. Report 0338T for a unilateral procedure and 0339T when performed bilaterally.

0342T

0342T Therapeutic apheresis with selective HDL delipidation and plasma reinfusion

Explanation

Therapeutic apheresis with selective high-density lipoprotein (HDL) delipidation and plasma reinfusion is a procedure in which plasma is removed from the body by apheresis, processed through a delipidation device, and returned to the patient. This technique may be employed to reduce atherosclerosis development in cardiovascular disease. Vascular access is established. A bag of the patient's blood is collected and the plasma is separated from the rest of the blood constituents. The red blood cells may be returned to the bloodstream. The plasma is treated, removing the cholesterol from HDL (good cholesterol), which results in what is known as pre-beta-HDL. This pre-beta-HDL infused plasma is considered delipidated plasma. The delipidated plasma is infused back into the patient once a week for seven weeks.

0345T

0345T Transcatheter mitral valve repair percutaneous approach via the coronary sinus

Explanation

A percutaneous mitral valve repair is performed. The right atrium of the heart is accessed using a catheter inserted in the internal jugular or subclavian vein. The coronary sinus is located and intubated with the compressed device within a sheath. An anchor, which resembles and functions much like a stent, on one end of the device is placed in the great cardiac vein and another is placed at the coronary sinus ostium and expanded holding them in place. The anchors are connected by a bridge or wire. The bridge is made of dissolvable material that dissipates over time and pulls the anchors together closing the mitral annulus. If the wire technique is used, the wire is pulled to bring the anchors closer together to shorten the mitral annulus before the anchors are expanded. Coronary compression may be assessed by angiogram and tension of the anchors adjusted. The sheath and catheter are removed and any wounds closed.

0381T-0382T

0381T External heart rate and 3-axis accelerometer data recording up to 14 days to assess changes in heart rate and to monitor motion analysis for the purposes of diagnosing nocturnal epilepsy seizure events; includes report, scanning analysis with report, review and interpretation by a physician or other qualified health care professional

0382T review and interpretation only

Explanation

This epilepsy seizure event monitor is utilized as a more cost-effective monitoring device to record seizure activity, particularly documenting the occurrences. It provides an automated account of activity that is more stable than handwritten entries by the patient. The monitor sensor attaches to the patient by a patch that feeds into the monitor, recording and documenting ECG motion that is transmitted to a main terminal and from there sent to the nurse or guardian if abnormal activity is discovered. This type of monitor is considered investigational. Report 0381T for the recording, including report, analysis, review, and interpretation. Report 0382T for the review and interpretation only. These codes report up to 14 days of recording.

0383T-0384T

0383T External heart rate and 3-axis accelerometer data recording from 15 to 30 days to assess changes in heart rate and to monitor motion analysis for the purposes of diagnosing nocturnal epilepsy seizure events; includes report, scanning analysis with report, review and interpretation by a physician or other qualified health care professional

0384T review and interpretation only

Explanation

This epilepsy seizure event monitor is utilized as a more cost-effective monitoring device to record seizure activity, particularly documenting the occurrences. It provides an automated account of activity that is more stable than handwritten entries by the patient. The monitor attaches to the patient by a patch that feeds into the monitor, recording and documenting ECG motion that is transmitted to a main terminal and from there sent to the nurse or guardian if abnormal activity is discovered. This type of monitor is considered investigational. Report 0383T for the recording, including report, analysis, review, and interpretation. Report 0384T for the review and interpretation only. These codes report 15 to 30 days of data recording.

0385T-0386T

0385T External heart rate and 3-axis accelerometer data recording more than 30 days to assess changes in heart rate and to monitor motion analysis for the purposes of diagnosing nocturnal epilepsy seizure events; includes report, scanning analysis with report, review and interpretation by a physician or other qualified health care professional

0386T review and interpretation only

Explanation

This epilepsy seizure event monitor is utilized as a more cost-effective monitoring device to record seizure activity, particularly documenting the occurrences. It provides an automated account of activity that is more stable than handwritten entries by the patient. The monitor attaches to the patient by a patch that feeds into the monitor, recording and documenting ECG motion that is transmitted to a main terminal and from there sent to the nurse or guardian if abnormal activity is discovered. This type of monitor is considered investigational. Report 0385T for the recording, including report, analysis, review, and interpretation. Report 0386T for the review and interpretation only. These codes report more than 30 days of data recording.

0408T-0411T

0408T Insertion or replacement of permanent cardiac contractility modulation system, including contractility evaluation when performed, and programming of sensing and therapeutic parameters; pulse generator with transvenous electrodes

0409T pulse generator only

0410T atrial electrode only

0411T ventricular electrode only

Explanation

Cardiac contractility modulation (CCM) is utilized to improve ventricular pump function and for patients who have normal QRS duration. The device consists of a programmable and rechargeable generator, powered by a lithium battery. The patient is given local anesthesia and the device is implanted within a pocket on the right side of the chest below the collarbone with an electrode fixed on the carotid sinus. One incision allows access to the cervical vagal nerve with another incision made for insertion of the right ventricular electrode. The vagal electrode is connected to the generator via subcutaneous tunnel. This unit includes three standard leads placed transvenously into the right side of the heart: one in the right atrium for sensing and two in the right ventricle for sensing and delivery of impulses. These impulses do not change the cardiac sequence (rhythm), but instead modify contractility by sending high-energy impulses to the myocardium during the refractory period. The unit allows the patient the ability to recharge the battery with an external charger that operates transcutaneously. This is required once a week and typically takes about 90 minutes. Programming and interrogation follows the same process as a pacemaker. Report 0408T for insertion or replacement of the entire system, including evaluation and programming when performed; 0409T for insertion or replacement of the pulse generator only; 0410T for insertion or replacement of the atrial electrode only; and 0411T for insertion or replacement of the ventricular electrode only.

0412T-0413T

0412T Removal of permanent cardiac contractility modulation system; pulse generator only

0413T transvenous electrode (atrial or ventricular)

Explanation

In 0412T, the physician removes a cardiac contractility modulation (CCM) system. The pocket is opened. The existing system is disconnected from the wire and removed. In 0413T, the electrodes are removed (atrial or ventricular). Previous insertion incisions may be reopened for removal of electrodes, which are disconnected from the generator as well as the vagal nerve, right atrium, and right ventricle.

0414T

0414T Removal and replacement of permanent cardiac contractility modulation system pulse generator only

Explanation

The physician removes and replaces a cardiac contractility modulation (CCM) system generator. The pocket is opened. The existing system is disconnected form the wire and removed. The electrodes remain in position and a new CCM system is inserted into the pocket. The electrodes are connected to the new system and tested. The pocket is closed.

0415T

0415T Repositioning of previously implanted cardiac contractility modulation transvenous electrode, (atrial or ventricular lead)

Explanation

The physician repositions a previously implanted cardiac contractility modulation transvenous electrode (atrial or ventricular lead). The physician gains access transvenously with imaging guidance and the electrode is repositioned. Depending on the extent of the work, the electrode may require reconnection to the generator, which would be tested for appropriate function. The incisions are closed.

0416T

0416T Relocation of skin pocket for implanted cardiac contractility modulation pulse generator

Explanation

The physician relocates a cardiac contractility modulation (CCM) system generator due to complications from the original generator placement. The pocket is opened and the generator is removed. A new pocket is formed within the subcutaneous tissue in close proximity of the existing electrodes. The electrodes are brought through a new subcutaneous tunnel into the new pocket. The old pocket is closed. The new or existing generator is inserted into the pocket and the electrodes are attached and tested. The pocket is closed.

0417T-0418T

0417T Programming device evaluation (in person) with iterative adjustment of the implantable device to test the function of the device and select optimal permanent programmed values with analysis, including review and report, implantable cardiac contractility modulation system

0418T Interrogation device evaluation (in person) with analysis, review and report, includes connection, recording and disconnection per patient encounter, implantable cardiac contractility modulation system

Explanation

A programming device evaluation (0417T) or interrogation (0418T) is performed in person in order to test the device's function and select the most favorable permanent programmed values. Patients with previously implanted cardiac contractility modulation (CCM) systems require periodic programming device evaluations. These diagnostic procedures include a face-to-face assessment of all device functions. Components that must be evaluated in order to assign a code from this range include the battery, leads, capture and sensing function, and programmed parameters. Stored and measured data regarding these components are retrieved using an office, hospital, or emergency room instrument. This information is assessed to discern battery voltage, lead impedance, and settings, as well as to determine the device's current programming. In 0417T, if necessary, the sensing value and rate response, upper and lower heart rates, impulses, and diagnostics are adjusted. These codes include physician or other qualified health care professional analysis, review, interpretation, and report, and are assigned per procedure. They also include connection, recording, and disconnection.

0439T

\+ **0439T** Myocardial contrast perfusion echocardiography, at rest or with stress, for assessment of myocardial ischemia or viability (List separately in addition to code for primary procedure)

Explanation

Myocardial contrast perfusion echocardiography is used to examine myocardial microcirculation. Intravenous infusion of contrast containing microbubbles that exist primarily within the vascular space and maintain intravascular characteristics similar to red blood cells is utilized. Injection of contrast into the venous system may also be used since the microbubbles will continue circulating for approximately three to five minutes after injection. Low intensity ultrasound is necessary in order to avoid destroying the microbubbles. The perfusion is analyzed as the microbubbles are destroyed with a burst of high intensity ultrasound and the rate of restoration is evaluated as the microbubbles flow back into myocardial circulation. This evaluation can determine the velocity and peak myocardial signal intensity allowing for quantification of any changes. This imaging provides improved resolution that enables the physician to detect perfusion defects that may not be seen in lower resolution imaging.

0451T-0454T

0451T Insertion or replacement of a permanently implantable aortic counterpulsation ventricular assist system, endovascular approach, and programming of sensing and therapeutic parameters; complete system (counterpulsation device, vascular graft, implantable vascular hemostatic seal, mechano-electrical skin interface and subcutaneous electrodes)

0452T aortic counterpulsation device and vascular hemostatic seal

0453T mechano-electrical skin interface

0454T subcutaneous electrode

Explanation

Implantable counterpulsation devices are exceeding limitations of traditional left ventricular assist devices (LVAD) by reducing the amount of energy utilized within the left ventricle, pulling on LV reserves for systolic function, improving LV performance, retaining velocity of blood flow, and maintaining heart stability. These devices are built to assist the heart in pumping blood through the body by assisting in the outflow from the left side of the heart into the aorta. The device is inserted in the aorta by creating a subclavian arterial graft and subcutaneous pocket where the mechano-electrical interface is placed. This interface gathers ECG signals and transmits them to the external control unit. The control unit can determine the area of the "dicrotic notch," the moment in the cardiac cycle when pressure dips in conjunction with the closure of the aortic valve, initiating the process of compressed air through the system to inflate the counterpulsation device. Upon diastole conclusion, the device suctions out the air via the same circuit. These devices are for long term use and utilize a vascular graft and hemostatic seal, mechano-electrical skin interface, and subcutaneous electrodes. The Symphony brand device is an example of an implantable device that is deployed endovascularly and sits within a pacemaker like pocket on the right side of the chest. This device incorporates a pump sac connected to the patient's circulation by a vascular graft that is adhered to the subclavian artery. A line is tunneled out through the skin and connected to the control unit or console. Report 0451T for insertion or replacement of the entire system; 0452T for insertion or replacement of the aortic counterpulsation device and vascular hemostatic seal (blocks blood flow and establishes an area allowing the blood to clot); 0453T for insertion or replacement of the mechano-electrical skin interface; and 0454T for insertion or replacement of the subcutaneous electrode.

0455T-0458T

0455T Removal of permanently implantable aortic counterpulsation ventricular assist system; complete system (aortic counterpulsation device, vascular hemostatic seal, mechano-electrical skin interface and electrodes)
0456T aortic counterpulsation device and vascular hemostatic seal
0457T mechano-electrical skin interface
0458T subcutaneous electrode

Explanation

In 0455T, the physician removes an implantable aortic counterpulsation ventricular assist system. The pocket is opened. The existing system is disconnected from the electrodes and removed. The device is removed from the aorta, along with all components of the system. The pocket is closed. Report 0456T for removal of the counterpulsation device and vascular hemostatic seal; 0457T for removal of the mechano-electrical skin interface; and 0458T for removal of the subcutaneous electrode.

0459T

0459T Relocation of skin pocket with replacement of implanted aortic counterpulsation ventricular assist device, mechano-electrical skin interface and electrodes

Explanation

The physician relocates the skin pocket and replaces the counterpulsation device, mechano-electrical skin interface, and electrodes due to complications or infection from the original device and/or components. The pocket is opened and the device is removed. The old pocket is closed and a new pocket is formed within the subcutaneous tissue. Electrodes are replaced through the subcutaneous tunnel. The new device is inserted into the pocket and the electrodes are attached and tested. The pocket is closed.

0460T-0461T

0460T Repositioning of previously implanted aortic counterpulsation ventricular assist device; subcutaneous electrode
0461T aortic counterpulsation device

Explanation

The physician repositions the subcutaneous electrode (0460T) or counterpulsation device (0461T). This is done when the system does not function due to improper placement of the electrode or counterpulsation device. The electrode and/or counterpulsation device is tested to ensure they are not defective, but simply in the wrong place. The electrode and/or counterpulsation device is reattached to the interface in its new position and tested again.

0462T

0462T Programming device evaluation (in person) with iterative adjustment of the implantable mechano-electrical skin interface and/or external driver to test the function of the device and select optimal permanent programmed values with analysis, including review and report, implantable aortic counterpulsation ventricular assist system, per day

Explanation

A programming device evaluation is performed in person in order to test the device's function and select the most favorable permanent programmed values. Patients with previously implanted aortic counterpulsation ventricular assist systems require periodic programming device evaluations. This diagnostic procedure includes a face-to-face assessment of all device functions. Components that must be evaluated in order to assign this code include iterative adjustment of the implantable mechano-skin interface and/or external unit and programmed parameters. This code includes physician or other qualified health care professional review and report and is assigned on a per day basis.

0463T

0463T Interrogation device evaluation (in person) with analysis, review and report, includes connection, recording and disconnection per patient encounter, implantable aortic counterpulsation ventricular assist system, per day

Explanation

Patients with previously implanted aortic counterpulsation ventricular assist systems require periodic interrogation device evaluations. This diagnostic procedure includes a face-to-face assessment of all device functions. This code includes physician or other qualified health care professional analysis, review, interpretation, and report. This evaluation includes connection, recording, and disconnection and is assigned on a per day basis.

0466T-0468T

\+ **0466T** Insertion of chest wall respiratory sensor electrode or electrode array, including connection to pulse generator (List separately in addition to code for primary procedure)
0467T Revision or replacement of chest wall respiratory sensor electrode or electrode array, including connection to existing pulse generator
0468T Removal of chest wall respiratory sensor electrode or electrode array

Explanation

Chest wall respiratory sensor electrodes or electrode arrays may be used in conjunction with an implantable cardiac device, such as a pacemaker or defibrillator, allowing for monitoring of respiration waveforms and a generator programmed to evaluate patterns including motion detection to assist in evaluation of various respiratory conditions. The physician inserts a chest wall respiratory sensor electrode/electrode array in 0466T. In 0467T, the physician revises or replaces the respiratory sensor electrode/electrode array. The physician incises the skin above the array and locates it. Following location, the physician replaces or revises the array, connects it to the existing pulse generator, and closes any incisions with sutures. In 0468T, the physician removes the respiratory sensor electrode/electrode array. The physician incises the skin above the unit. After locating the array, the physician removes it and closes the incision with sutures.

0475T-0478T

0475T Recording of fetal magnetic cardiac signal using at least 3 channels; patient recording and storage, data scanning with signal extraction, technical analysis and result, as well as supervision, review, and interpretation of report by a physician or other qualified health care professional
0476T patient recording, data scanning, with raw electronic signal transfer of data and storage
0477T signal extraction, technical analysis, and result
0478T review, interpretation, report by physician or other qualified health care professional

Explanation

The magnetic field created from electrical activity in the fetal heart is measured in a noninvasive technique that uses microfabricated optically pumped magnetometer (OPM) technology that works to fit the patient's abdomen at any stage of pregnancy. Individual sensors are inserted into a flexible belt-shaped holder, which is connected to light sources and electronics that are placed outside of a magnetically shielded room via optical and electrical cabling as fetal cardiac signals have only a very small magnitude. Two sensor belts are placed over a pregnant patient's abdomen and one over her chest. Recordings from the fetal magnetocardiogram placed over the patient's abdomen contains the mother's cardiac signal, which often dominates the fetal heart signals; to address this, orthogonal projection and independent component analysis signal processing methods are applied in order to obtain only fetal signals. In addition, the fetal heartrate is also removed from the fetal magnetocardiogram. These tests offer a lower cost means of evaluating certain kinds of fetal silent heart arrhythmias that may not be detected using standard echocardiography. Report 0475T for a complete test recording the fetal magnetic cardiac signal using a minimum of three channels with patient recording and storage, data scanning with signal extraction, analysis, and results including review, supervision, and interpretation from a physician or other qualified health care professional. Report 0476T for recording, data scanning, and raw electronic signal transfer of data and storage. Report 0477T for signal extraction, technical analysis, and result only. Report 0478T for review and interpretation by the clinician.

0483T-0484T

0483T Transcatheter mitral valve implantation/replacement (TMVI) with prosthetic valve; percutaneous approach, including transseptal puncture, when performed

0484T transthoracic exposure (eg, thoracotomy, transapical)

Explanation

The physician performs transcatheter mitral valve implantation or replacement (TMVI). Mitral regurgitation (MR) is a condition that may be treated with transcatheter mitral valve implantation or replacement (TMVI/TMVR) in patients who are at high risk for open heart surgery. In 0483T, the procedure is performed via a percutaneous approach and includes a transseptal puncture, when performed. Under general anesthesia, the physician makes an incision over a lower extremity vessel, usually the femoral vein. A catheter with a specially designed prosthesis is maneuvered through the vessels to the heart under fluoroscopic imaging guidance. The catheter is threaded through the inferior vena cava to the right atrium where the interatrial wall or septum is punctured to access the left atrium. When the left atrium is accessed, the catheter is further advanced through the mitral valve and to the left ventricle. A stent-based prosthesis is implanted within the mitral annulus. In 0484T, under general anesthesia, the physician makes a left lateral mini-thoracotomy. The transapical puncture involves using a large bore needle to puncture the chest wall directly into the left ventricular cavity. A small incision is made between ribs (usually the fifth or sixth intercostal space) on the lower left side of the patient's chest to achieve direct access to the heart. A catheter is inserted following the guidewire to the mitral valve. A balloon is inflated to compress the native valve. The self-expanding prosthesis is introduced through the catheter, partially uncovered. Once in the left atrium, the catheter is deployed and secured using polyethylene tether fastened to an epicardial pad. Pledgeted sutures are placed. The tether tension is modified after the prosthesis has been deployed to ensure optimal placement of the device but also to limit movement of it within the annulus. No cardiopulmonary bypass or rapid ventricular pacing is required during the procedure. These procedures include vascular access, catheterization, balloon valvuloplasty, deploying the valve, repositioning the valve as needed, temporary pacemaker insertion for rapid pacing, and access site closure, when performed. Angiography, radiological supervision and interpretation, intraprocedural roadmapping to guide TMVI (e.g., contrast injections, fluoroscopy), left ventriculography (e.g., to assess mitral regurgitation for guidance of TMVI), and completion angiography are also included.

0497T-0498T

0497T External patient-activated, physician- or other qualified health care professional-prescribed, electrocardiographic rhythm derived event recorder without 24 hour attended monitoring; in-office connection

0498T review and interpretation by a physician or other qualified health care professional per 30 days with at least one patient-generated triggered event

Explanation

In 0497T, the patient is connected to an external patient-activated cardiac event recorder device, also known as an ambulatory electrocardiographic (ECG) device, as prescribed by the physician or other qualified health care professional to monitor the symptoms of arrhythmia (irregular heartbeats) or other cardiac irregularities. A cardiac event recorder is a portable, battery operated, patient-controlled device that records the electrical activity of the patient's heart at the time the patient is experiencing symptoms. A technician places ECG leads on the patient's chest, and the monitor uses a symptom-related memory loop mechanism with remote download capability up to 30 days to record the patient's rhythm. During symptoms, the patient activates the monitor by pressing a button. Once the device has made a recording of the event, it stores the data for transmission to a data receiving center or to the physician via a telephone. The recording includes ECG activity prior to and during symptoms. Some of the information that the physician can gain from the patient wearing this device includes, but is not limited to, whether or not medications prescribed for irregular heart rhythms are working, if a pacemaker or implantable cardioverter defibrillator (ICD) is functioning correctly, and to help diagnose patients who are presenting with symptoms such as chest pain, lightheadedness, or fainting episodes. Devices may be worn on the wrist and the patient puts the device against the chest when an event occurs prior to pressing the record button or may be worn on the chest using electrodes to attach the device. Instructions for appropriate placement of the device are provided. After an event occurs, the patient typically places the mouthpiece portion of the telephone to the front of the device to transmit the data. Based on review of the data, the patient may be instructed to return to the clinic or facility to be seen by a physician. Report 0498T when the physician or other qualified health care professional reviews and interprets data every 30 days with a minimum of one patient-generated triggered event during that time period.

0501T-0504T

0501T Noninvasive estimated coronary fractional flow reserve (FFR) derived from coronary computed tomography angiography data using computation fluid dynamics physiologic simulation software analysis of functional data to assess the severity of coronary artery disease; data preparation and transmission, analysis of fluid dynamics and simulated maximal coronary hyperemia, generation of estimated FFR model, with anatomical data review in comparison with estimated FFR model to reconcile discordant data, interpretation and report

0502T data preparation and transmission

0503T analysis of fluid dynamics and simulated maximal coronary hyperemia, and generation of estimated FFR model

0504T anatomical data review in comparison with estimated FFR model to reconcile discordant data, interpretation and report

Explanation

A proprietary noninvasive fractional flow reserve technology called HeartFlow® FFRct is used to assist a physician in evaluating the degree of coronary artery disease (CAD) that a patient has, including how a CAD blockage can affect blood flow to the heart, with much greater accuracy based on combining anatomy (coronary CT angiogram) and physiology (HeartFlow FFRct). This technology allows clinicians to personalize a patient's care plan and reduce the likelihood of needing more invasive procedures. The patient undergoes a coronary computed tomography (CT) angiogram. Data from this test is securely uploaded from the hospital's system to a cloud server. The HeartFlow process creates a personalized, digital, three-dimensional representation of the patient's coronary arteries and employs robust algorithms to help determine and replicate coronary blood flow. The model can also determine any potential effect of blockages on coronary blood flow. Once the process is complete, the physician receives the patient's results through a secure web interface and selects the best treatment course for the patient. Report 0501T for the noninvasive FFR process with interpretation and report. Report 0502T for data preparation and transmission only. Report 0503T for analysis of fluid dynamics, simulated maximal coronary hyperemia, and generation of estimated FFR model. Report 0504T for an anatomical data review comparison to estimated FFR model for reconciliation of discordant data, including interpretation and review.

[0523T]

+ **0523T** Intraprocedural coronary fractional flow reserve (FFR) with 3D functional mapping of color-coded FFR values for the coronary tree, derived from coronary angiogram data, for real-time review and interpretation of possible atherosclerotic stenosis(es) intervention (List separately in addition to code for primary procedure)

Explanation

Noninvasive 3-dimensional (3-D) fractional flow reserve (FFR) enabled interpretation is performed during a coronary angiography procedure for possible atherosclerotic stenosis as an aid to the physician in making a determination for whether a percutaneous coronary intervention (PCI) is indicated and whether revascularization occurs in each angiography procedure performed. Medically recognized standards generally recommend that revascularization by percutaneous coronary intervention (PCI) is to be performed when the patient's stenosis of >50 percent is observed of the left main (LM) stem or proximal left anterior descending (LAD) coronary artery during angiography, the patient has one remaining patent vessel, or the patient suffers from two- or three-vessel disease with a left ventricular ejection fraction <40 percent. The Cathworks FFRangio™ System is a proprietary FFR platform that accurately conveys evidence-based multi-vessel physiologic measurements to enable the physician to confirm whether or not to proceed with intraprocedural PCI therapy.

0505T

0505T Endovenous femoral-popliteal arterial revascularization, with transcatheter placement of intravascular stent graft(s) and closure by any method, including percutaneous or open vascular access, ultrasound guidance for vascular access when performed, all catheterization(s) and intraprocedural roadmapping and imaging guidance necessary to complete the intervention, all associated radiological supervision and interpretation, when performed, with crossing of the occlusive lesion in an extraluminal fashion

Explanation

Endovenous femoral-popliteal arterial revascularization (i.e., femoral popliteal bypass surgery) is a procedure used to treat femoral artery disease. The procedure involves going around the blocked area of the femoral artery, which is the main artery in the leg, using an intravascular stent graft via an open or percutaneous approach. The patient is placed supine on the operating table and an IV is started; additional catheters may also be placed in the neck or collarbone areas and/or wrist areas to allow for heart and blood pressure monitoring and blood draws. A heart monitor is also used to evaluate heart activity. Local anesthesia, general anesthesia, and/or sedation may be used. Antibiotics may be administered via the IV for infection prevention. Ultrasound guidance may be used to guide access to the vascular site. The site is cleansed using an antiseptic solution. The physician makes an incision in the leg with the site determined based on which arteries are being bypassed. A prosthetic graft or leg vein is used to circumvent the area damaged by the disease or injury. After the graft has been attached, blood flow to the leg may be confirmed via arteriogram. Blood pressure medications are continued post-surgery to ensure pressures remain within normal range. The incision is closed and a dressing applied. Ultrasound and other imaging guidance, all radiological supervision and interpretation, and all catheterizations are included in this service and are not reported separately when performed.

0515T-0522T

0515T Insertion of wireless cardiac stimulator for left ventricular pacing, including device interrogation and programming, and imaging supervision and interpretation, when performed; complete system (includes electrode and generator [transmitter and battery])

0516T electrode only

0517T pulse generator component(s) (battery and/or transmitter) only

0518T Removal of only pulse generator component(s) (battery and/or transmitter) of wireless cardiac stimulator for left ventricular pacing

0519T Removal and replacement of wireless cardiac stimulator for left ventricular pacing; pulse generator component(s) (battery and/or transmitter)

0520T pulse generator component(s) (battery and/or transmitter), including placement of a new electrode

0521T Interrogation device evaluation (in person) with analysis, review and report, includes connection, recording, and disconnection per patient encounter, wireless cardiac stimulator for left ventricular pacing

0522T Programming device evaluation (in person) with iterative adjustment of the implantable device to test the function of the device and select optimal permanent programmed values with analysis, including review and report, wireless cardiac stimulator for left ventricular pacing

Explanation

Wireless cardiac stimulator systems are made up of two components. The first component is a wireless endocardial left ventricular electrode that is implanted in the artery of the left ventricular wall. The electrode is wirelessly powered via ultrasound pulses originating from a transmitter implanted into one of two subcutaneous pockets created on the chest wall. The second component is a pulse generator, which is also comprised of two separate elements: a transmitter and a battery. The battery is housed in the other chest wall pocket. The battery and the electrode are connected via a subcutaneously tunneled cable. This system provides biventricular pacing by sensing right ventricular pacing output from a previously placed conventional device (i.e., pacemaker or defibrillator using uni- or biventricular leads) that subsequently transmits an ultrasound pulse to the wireless electrode inserted onto the left ventricle endocardium resulting in a left ventricular pacing pulse emission. Patients with these systems require programming and interrogation of both the conventional and wireless devices. Report 0515T for insertion of the complete wireless cardiac stimulation system, including the programming and interrogation and all echocardiography and imaging, when performed. Report 0516T for insertion of the electrode only; 0517T for insertion of the pulse generator only (battery and/or transmitter). Removal of the battery or transmitter only is reported using 0518T; removal with replacement of the battery or transmitter is reported using 0519T. When the generator and/or battery are removed and replaced with a new electrode, report 0520T. Report 0521T for interrogation evaluation, including analysis, review. Report 0522T for programming, including analysis, review, and report.

0524T

0524T Endovenous catheter directed chemical ablation with balloon isolation of incompetent extremity vein, open or percutaneous, including all vascular access, catheter manipulation, diagnostic imaging, imaging guidance and monitoring

Explanation

Endovascular catheter-directed chemical ablation with balloon isolation (i.e., balloon sclerotherapy) describes treatment of varicose veins in an extremity by incorporating two familiar procedures: sclerotherapy and balloon catheterization as a minimally invasive and cost-effective treatment option. Traditional catheter-based endovenous sclerotherapy can often have negative effects to the overall body system resulting from the combination of air and the sclerosing agent. The physician uses a double lumen balloon catheter as a means of separating or isolating venous blood, allowing the physician to use the minimal amount of sclerosing agent needed while removing the excess amounts and subsequently limiting the potential for systemic risk. Vein occlusion occurs when the physician carefully retracts the expanded balloon containing the captured sclerotherapeutic agent in between.

0525T-0527T

0525T Insertion or replacement of intracardiac ischemia monitoring system, including testing of the lead and monitor, initial system programming, and imaging supervision and interpretation; complete system (electrode and implantable monitor)

0526T electrode only

0527T implantable monitor only

Explanation

An intracardiac ischemia monitoring system analyzes and records cardiac data to detect ischemic events. If an ischemic event is occurring, the device sends out auditory, visual, and vibrational alerts to the patient to seek medical care immediately. Access to the central caval veins is obtained through the subclavian vein or jugular vein. The vein is penetrated with a large needle and a guidewire is passed through. A fluoroscope is used to guide a standard pacemaker intracardiac lead to the right ventricular apex. A pocket for an implantable device (IMD) that analyzes and records the cardiac data is created and the lead is tested. The lead is connected to the IMD and the subcutaneous pocket is closed. Report 0525T for insertion or replacement of the complete system (electrode and implantable monitor). Report 0526T for insertion or replacement of the electrode only; report 0527T for implantable monitor only. All imaging, including supervision and interpretation, is included in these services.

0528T-0529T

0528T Programming device evaluation (in person) of intracardiac ischemia monitoring system with iterative adjustment of programmed values, with analysis, review, and report

0529T Interrogation device evaluation (in person) of intracardiac ischemia monitoring system with analysis, review, and report

Explanation

An intracardiac ischemia monitoring system analyzes and records cardiac data to detect ischemic events. If an ischemic event is occurring, the device sends out auditory, visual, and vibrational alerts to the patient to seek medical care immediately. In 0528T, a programming device evaluation is performed in person in order to test the functioning of the device and to select the most favorable permanent programming values. Patients with previously implanted monitoring systems require periodic programming device evaluations. This diagnostic procedure includes a face-to-face assessment of all device functions. Stored and measured data regarding these components are retrieved using an office, hospital, or emergency department instrument. This information is assessed in order to discern lead impedance and settings for detection, as well as to determine the system's current programming. If necessary, sensing values and diagnostics are adjusted. In 0529T, only an in-person device interrogation (extraction of data accumulated in a medical device) is performed, accessing the stored and measured data. Both of these codes include clinician analysis, review, and report.

0530T-0532T

0530T Removal of intracardiac ischemia monitoring system, including all imaging supervision and interpretation; complete system (electrode and implantable monitor)

0531T electrode only

0532T implantable monitor only

Explanation

An intracardiac ischemia monitoring system analyzes and records cardiac data to detect ischemic events. If an ischemic event is occurring, the device sends out auditory, visual, and vibrational alerts to the patient to seek medical care immediately. In 0530T, the subcutaneous pocket incision is reopened and the complete system (electrode and implantable monitor) is disconnected from the cardiac lead and removed. The lead is dissected from the scar tissue that has formed around it. Once the lead is completely freed, it is removed. Report 0531T for electrode removal only and 0532T when only the implantable monitor is removed.

0543T

● **0543T** Transapical mitral valve repair, including transthoracic echocardiography, when performed, with placement of artificial chordae tendineae

Explanation

This procedure describes treatment for patients with mitral regurgitation, a progressive condition where the mitral valve does not close appropriately resulting in blood leaking back through the mitral valve. The surgeon performs a thoracotomy and places a proprietary system designed for use when the patient's native chordae tendineae (tough, tendinous type strands of the heart) become elongated or rupture from the disease process. The system contains expandable "jaws" that are used to hold the mitral valve leaflet or cusp and an average of three to four artificial chordae are inserted around the edge of the leaflet in order to rehang the prolapsed leaflet. Transesophageal echocardiography (TEE) is used as guidance to reduce the amount of blood leaking back into the mitral valve by varying the lengths of the artificial chordae. Once the appropriate level has been determined, the chordae are fastened to a small piece of absorbent material and attached to the outer layer of the heart wall.

0544T-0545T

● **0544T** Transcatheter mitral valve annulus reconstruction, with implantation of adjustable annulus reconstruction device, percutaneous approach including transseptal puncture

● **0545T** Transcatheter tricuspid valve annulus reconstruction with implantation of adjustable annulus reconstruction device, percutaneous approach

Explanation

The physician performs a transcatheter mitral valve annulus reconstruction with the implantation of an adjustable annulus reconstructive device. A proprietary system is used in these procedures, comprised of three components: the implant catheter (IC) itself, a guide catheter (GC), and a transseptal steerable sheath (TSS). The implant is made of a contraction wire with a covering made of a polyester fabric that is secured along the back annulus of the mitral valve by stainless steel anchors. Once fastened down, the implant is contracted under fluoroscopy and echocardiography imaging in order to reach the optimum constraint and amount of valvular regurgitation. The surgeon accesses the mitral valve using a percutaneous, catheter-delivered approach going through the femoral vein and the inferior vena cava. A transseptal puncture under transesophageal echocardiography (TEE) imaging is performed to identify the interatrial septum over the back middle mitral commissure, the area where the posterior leaflets or cusps are located. A transseptal steerable sheath (TSS) is introduced into the left atrium using a guidewire and the implant delivery system is advanced through the TSS and into the left atrium. It is positioned to line up with the top of the IC near the front lateral trigone using TEE guidance. Anchors are moved through the fabric of the implant and into the annular tissue to ensure the implant is securely fastened. Once secure, the tip of the IC continues to be moved along to each continuous point of anchoring on the commissure. When the last anchor is positioned in the trigone near the posterior medial commissure, the implant is disconnected from the IC with an average of 12 to 17 anchors required based on the length of the implant. Typically, this system and treatment is most often used for patients with functional mitral regurgitation (FMR) and more recently functional tricuspid regurgitation (FTR). Angiography, all radiological supervision and interpretation, intraprocedural road mapping, ventriculography required for device implantation, and adjustment are included. Report 0545T for reconstruction of the tricuspid valve annulus with an implanted adjustable annulus reconstruction device in a similar manner.

0553T

- ● **0553T** Percutaneous transcatheter placement of iliac arteriovenous anastomosis implant, inclusive of all radiological supervision and interpretation, intraprocedural roadmapping, and imaging guidance necessary to complete the intervention

Explanation

This procedure is performed for treatment of uncontrolled hypertension, which is defined as a systolic blood pressure reading of 150 or greater. Systolic pressure is the upper number represented in the blood pressure fraction (i.e., 120/80) and describes the degree of force imposed on blood vessels when the heart contracts. This condition is often seen in older patients with hardening of blood vessels and is largely associated with heart attacks, strokes, and congestive heart failure. In addition, it is not typically responsive to usual pharmacological approaches. Using a small proprietary implant similar in size to a paper clip called a ROX® coupler, the stent-like device is placed in the upper thigh between the iliac artery and vein transferring a small amount of blood from the artery to the vein and subsequently relieving the pressure in the artery. The implant is placed via a standard transcatheter procedure under fluoroscopic guidance in an angiography or endovascular catheterization lab and requires only local anesthesia. Radiological supervision and interpretation, intraprocedural road mapping, and imaging guidance are included in the procedure and are not reported separately.

0559T-0560T

- ● **0559T** Anatomic model 3D-printed from image data set(s); first individually prepared and processed component of an anatomic structure
- + ● **0560T** each additional individually prepared and processed component of an anatomic structure (List separately in addition to code for primary procedure)

Explanation

These codes describe the creation of three-dimensional (3D) printed models of individually prepared and processed elements of anatomic structures, such as bones, arteries, veins, nerves, ureters, muscles, tendons, ligaments, joints, visceral organs, and the brain. Models may be comprised of one or more distinct parts and incorporate various colors and materials. Uses of 3D-printed anatomic models are continuing to increase for a number of applications including, but not limited to, surgery planning, preparing and practicing for the procedure, training and education of health care professionals, and for patient education.

0561T-0562T

- ● **0561T** Anatomic guide 3D-printed and designed from image data set(s); first anatomic guide
- + ● **0562T** each additional anatomic guide (List separately in addition to code for primary procedure)

Explanation

Three-dimensional (3D) printed cutting or drilling guides are patient-specific surgery guides combining individualized imaging information that is used by the surgeon to navigate a procedure. Each guide is a sole, distinctive tool created to be an exact fit to the patient's natural anatomy customized to precisely match every intervention aspect, such as position and angles that mirror the actual surgery. The use of guides saves considerable time and resources; the predictability permitted by the guides allows for greater confidence in the operation room, which subsequently improves patient outcomes. In some cases, the surgery may require the use of a 3D-printed model and cutting or drilling guide for the same patient.

0569T-0570T

- ● **0569T** Transcatheter tricuspid valve repair, percutaneous approach; initial prosthesis
- + ● **0570T** each additional prosthesis during same session (List separately in addition to code for primary procedure)

Explanation

The physician performs a transcatheter tricuspid valve repair utilizing a percutaneous approach. Transcatheter devices currently in clinical testing include annuloplasty devices (suture, direct, or ring), coaptation devices, and heterotopic caval valve implantation. In one repair method, the surgeon accesses the tricuspid valve using a percutaneous, catheter-delivered approach through the left subclavian or axillary vein. An expandable, foam-filled balloon spacer is advanced through a sheath introducer and is stabilized by a rail that is anchored at the right ventricular apex. This device is intended to reduce the regurgitant orifice area by reducing malcoaptation of the tricuspid leaflets. Report 0569T for the initial prosthesis and 0570T for each additional prosthesis used during the same session.

0571T-0574T, 0580T

- ● **0571T** Insertion or replacement of implantable cardioverter-defibrillator system with substernal electrode(s), including all imaging guidance and electrophysiological evaluation (includes defibrillation threshold evaluation, induction of arrhythmia, evaluation of sensing for arrhythmia termination, and programming or reprogramming of sensing or therapeutic parameters), when performed
- ● **0572T** Insertion of substernal implantable defibrillator electrode
- ● **0573T** Removal of substernal implantable defibrillator electrode
- ● **0574T** Repositioning of previously implanted substernal implantable defibrillator-pacing electrode
- ● **0580T** Removal of substernal implantable defibrillator pulse generator only

Explanation

The physician inserts or replaces an implantable substernal cardioverter-defibrillator system, which consists of a pulse generator and at least one substernal electrode. Under appropriate anesthesia, the physician creates a subcutaneous pocket over the lateral rib cage and places the generator. Without entering the pericardial cavity, the electrode is tunneled subcutaneously and placed into the substernal anterior mediastinum, where it performs defibrillation and pacing as needed. All imaging guidance is included, as is the electrophysiological evaluation, which includes evaluation of the defibrillation threshold, arrhythmia induction, evaluation of sensing for termination of arrhythmia, and programming/reprogramming of sensing or therapeutic parameters. Report 0571T for insertion or replacement of the entire system. Report 0572T for insertion of the electrode only and 0573T for removal of the electrode only. Report 0574T for repositioning of a previously implanted defibrillator-pacing electrode. Report 0580T for removal of the pulse generator only. Refer to CPT guidelines in this section for specific instructions regarding concurrent removal and replacement.

0575T-0576T

- **0575T** Programming device evaluation (in person) of implantable cardioverter-defibrillator system with substernal electrode, with iterative adjustment of the implantable device to test the function of the device and select optimal permanent programmed values with analysis, review and report by a physician or other qualified health care professional
- **0576T** Interrogation device evaluation (in person) of implantable cardioverter-defibrillator system with substernal electrode, with analysis, review and report by a physician or other qualified health care professional, includes connection, recording and disconnection per patient encounter

Explanation

A physician or other qualified health care provider performs device evaluations of an implantable cardioverter-defibrillator system with substernal electrode. In 0575T, a programming device evaluation is performed, consisting of repetitive adjustments of the device to test function and select optimal permanent programmed values. In 0576T, an interrogation device evaluation is performed, which includes connection, recording, and disconnection per patient encounter. These codes include analysis, review, and report.

0577T

- **0577T** Electrophysiological evaluation of implantable cardioverter-defibrillator system with substernal electrode (includes defibrillation threshold evaluation, induction of arrhythmia, evaluation of sensing for arrhythmia termination, and programming or reprogramming of sensing or therapeutic parameters)

Explanation

A physician or other qualified health care provider performs an electrophysiological evaluation of an implantable cardioverter-defibrillator system with substernal electrode. This includes evaluation of defibrillation threshold, arrhythmia induction, evaluation of sensing for arrhythmia termination, and programming or reprogramming of sensing or therapeutic parameters.

0578T-0579T

- **0578T** Interrogation device evaluation(s) (remote), up to 90 days, substernal lead implantable cardioverter-defibrillator system with interim analysis, review(s) and report(s) by a physician or other qualified health care professional
- **0579T** Interrogation device evaluation(s) (remote), up to 90 days, substernal lead implantable cardioverter-defibrillator system, remote data acquisition(s), receipt of transmissions and technician review, technical support and distribution of results

Explanation

These codes report remote (up to 90 days) evaluations of a substernal lead implantable cardioverter-defibrillator system. In 0578T, a physician or other qualified health care professional provides interim analysis with review and report. In 0579T, included components are remote data acquisition, receipt of transmissions and technician review, technical support, and distribution of results. These codes may be reported once per 90 days.

Correct Coding Initiative Update 25.3

❖Indicates Mutually Exclusive Edit

0085T 36591-36592, 96523

0126T 36591-36592, 96523

0234T 01924-01926, 0213T, 0216T, 11000-11006, 11042-11047, 34713-34716, 34812, 34820, 34833-34834, 35201-35206, 35226-35236, 35256-35266, 35286, 36000, 36002-36005, 36400-36410, 36420-36430, 36440, 36500, 36591-36592, 36600-36640, 37184, 43752, 49000-49002, 51701-51703, 61645-61650, 62320-62327, 64400-64410, 64413-64435, 64445-64450, 64461, 64463, 64479, 64483, 64486-64490, 64493, 64505, 64510-64530, 69990, 75893, 76000, 76942, 76970, 76998, 77002, 93000-93010, 93040-93042, 93050, 93318, 93355, 94002, 94200, 94250, 94680-94690, 94770, 95812-95816, 95819, 95822, 95829, 95955, 96360, 96365, 96372, 96374-96377, 96523, 97597-97598, 97602, 99155, 99156, 99157, 99446-99449, 99451-99452, G0471

0235T 01924-01926, 0213T, 0216T, 11000-11006, 11042-11047, 34713-34716, 34812, 34820, 34833-34834, 35201-35206, 35226-35236, 35256-35266, 35286, 36000, 36002-36005, 36400-36410, 36420-36430, 36440, 36500, 36591-36592, 36600-36640, 37184, 43752, 49000-49002, 51701-51703, 61645-61650, 62320-62327, 64400-64410, 64413-64435, 64445-64450, 64461, 64463, 64479, 64483, 64486-64490, 64493, 64505, 64510-64530, 69990, 75726, 75736, 75774, 75893, 76000, 76942, 76970, 76998, 77002, 93000-93010, 93040-93042, 93050, 93318, 93355, 94002, 94200, 94250, 94680-94690, 94770, 95812-95816, 95819, 95822, 95829, 95955, 96360, 96365, 96372, 96374-96377, 96523, 97597-97598, 97602, 99155, 99156, 99157, 99446-99449, 99451-99452, G0471

0236T 01924-01926, 0213T, 0216T, 11000-11006, 11042-11047, 32551, 32556-32557, 34713-34716, 34812, 34820, 34833-34834, 35201-35206, 35226-35236, 35256-35266, 35286, 36000, 36002-36005, 36400-36410, 36420-36430, 36440, 36500, 36591-36592, 36600-36640, 37184, 43752, 49000-49002, 51701-51703, 61645-61650, 62320-62327, 64400-64410, 64413-64435, 64445-64450, 64461, 64463, 64479, 64483, 64486-64490, 64493, 64505, 64510-64530, 69990, 75600, 75605, 75625, 75630, 75635, 75893, 76000, 76942, 76970, 76998, 77002, 93000-93010, 93040-93042, 93050, 93318, 93355, 94002, 94200, 94250, 94680-94690, 94770, 95812-95816, 95819, 95822, 95829, 95955, 96360, 96365, 96372, 96374-96377, 96523, 97597-97598, 97602, 99155, 99156, 99157, 99446-99449, 99451-99452, G0471

0237T 01924-01926, 0213T, 0216T, 11000-11006, 11042-11047, 34715-34716, 34834, 35201-35206, 35226-35236, 35256-35266, 35286, 36000, 36002-36005, 36400-36410, 36420-36430, 36440, 36500, 36591-36592, 36600-36640, 37184, 43752, 51701-51703, 61645-61650, 62320-62327, 64400-64410, 64413-64435, 64445-64450, 64461, 64463, 64479, 64483, 64486-64490, 64493, 64505, 64510-64530, 69990, 75605, 75710, 75716, 75893, 76000, 76942, 76970, 76998, 77002, 93000-93010, 93040-93042, 93050, 93318, 93355, 94002, 94200, 94250, 94680-94690, 94770, 95812-95816, 95819, 95822, 95829, 95955, 96360, 96365, 96372, 96374-96377, 96523, 97597-97598, 97602, 99155, 99156, 99157, 99446-99449, 99451-99452, G0471

0238T 01924, 11000-11006, 11042-11047, 35201-35206, 35226-35236, 35256-35266, 35286, 36000, 36002-36005, 36400-36410, 36420-36430, 36440, 36500, 36591-36592, 36600-36640, 43752, 51701-51703, 61650, 62320-62327, 64400-64410, 64413-64435, 64445-64450, 64461, 64463, 64479, 64483, 64486-64490, 64493, 64505, 64510-64530, 69990, 75630, 75635, 75710, 75716, 75736, 75774, 75893, 76000, 76942, 76970, 76998, 77002, 93000-93010, 93040-93042, 93050, 93318, 93355, 94002, 94200, 94250, 94680-94690, 94770, 95812-95816, 95819, 95822, 95829, 95955, 96360, 96365, 96372, 96374-96377, 96523, 97597-97598, 97602, 99155, 99156, 99157, 99446-99449, 99451-99452, G0471

0266T 0213T, 0216T, 0228T, 0230T, 0267T-0273T, 11000-11006, 11042-11047, 36000, 36400-36410, 36420-36430, 36440, 36591-36592, 36600, 36640, 43752, 51701-51703, 61650, 62320-62327, 64400-64410, 64413-64435, 64445-64450, 64461, 64463, 64479, 64483, 64486-64490, 64493, 64505, 64510-64530, 69990, 93000-93010, 93040-93042, 93318, 93355, 94002, 94200, 94250, 94680-94690, 94770, 95812-95816, 95819, 95822, 95829, 95955, 96360, 96365, 96372, 96374-96377, 96523, 97597-97598, 97602, 99155, 99156, 99157, 99446-99449, 99451-99452, G0471

0267T 0213T, 0216T, 0228T, 0230T, 0270T, 0272T-0273T, 11000-11006, 11042-11047, 36000, 36400-36410, 36420-36430, 36440, 36591-36592, 36600, 36640, 43752, 51701-51703, 61650, 62320-62327, 64400-64410, 64413-64435, 64445-64450, 64461, 64463, 64479, 64483, 64486-64490, 64493, 64505, 64510-64530, 69990, 93000-93010, 93040-93042, 93318, 93355, 94002, 94200, 94250, 94680-94690, 94770, 95812-95816, 95819, 95822, 95829, 95955, 96360, 96365, 96372, 96374-96377, 96523, 97597-97598, 97602, 99155, 99156, 99157, 99446-99449, 99451-99452, G0471

0268T 0213T, 0216T, 0228T, 0230T, 0270T-0273T, 11000-11006, 11042-11047, 36000, 36400-36410, 36420-36430, 36440, 36591-36592, 36600, 36640, 43752, 51701-51703, 61650, 62320-62327, 64400-64410, 64413-64435, 64445-64450, 64461, 64463, 64479, 64483, 64486-64490, 64493, 64505, 64510-64530, 69990, 93000-93010, 93040-93042, 93318, 93355, 94002, 94200, 94250, 94680-94690, 94770, 95812-95816, 95819, 95822, 95829, 95955, 96360, 96365, 96372, 96374-96377, 96523, 97597-97598, 97602, 99155, 99156, 99157, 99446-99449, 99451-99452, G0471

0269T 0213T, 0216T, 0228T, 0230T, 0267T-0268T, 0270T-0273T, 11000-11006, 11042-11047, 36000, 36400-36410, 36420-36430, 36440, 36591-36592, 36600, 36640, 43752, 51701-51703, 61650, 62320-62327, 64400-64410, 64413-64435, 64445-64450, 64461, 64463, 64479, 64483, 64486-64490, 64493, 64505, 64510-64530, 69990, 93000-93010, 93040-93042, 93318, 93355, 94002, 94200, 94250, 94680-94690, 94770, 95812-95816, 95819, 95822, 95829, 95955, 96360, 96365, 96372, 96374-96377, 96523, 97597-97598, 97602, 99155, 99156, 99157, 99446-99449, 99451-99452, G0471

0270T 0213T, 0216T, 0228T, 0230T, 0272T-0273T, 11000-11006, 11042-11047, 36000, 36400-36410, 36420-36430, 36440, 36591-36592, 36600, 36640, 43752, 51701-51703, 61650, 62320-62327, 64400-64410, 64413-64435, 64445-64450, 64461, 64463, 64479, 64483, 64486-64490, 64493, 64505, 64510-64530, 69990, 93000-93010, 93040-93042, 93318, 93355, 94002, 94200, 94250, 94680-94690, 94770, 95812-95816, 95819, 95822, 95829, 95955, 96360, 96365, 96372, 96374-96377, 96523, 97597-97598, 97602, 99155, 99156, 99157, 99446-99449, 99451-99452, G0471

0271T 0213T, 0216T, 0228T, 0230T, 0267T, 0270T, 0272T-0273T, 11000-11006, 11042-11047, 36000, 36400-36410, 36420-36430, 36440, 36591-36592, 36600, 36640, 43752, 51701-51703, 61650, 62320-62327, 64400-64410, 64413-64435, 64445-64450, 64461, 64463, 64479, 64483, 64486-64490, 64493, 64505, 64510-64530, 69990, 93000-93010, 93040-93042, 93318, 93355, 94002, 94200, 94250, 94680-94690, 94770, 95812-95816, 95819, 95822, 95829, 95955, 96360, 96365, 96372, 96374-96377, 96523, 97597-97598, 97602, 99155, 99156, 99157, 99446-99449, 99451-99452, G0471

0272T 0213T, 0216T, 0228T, 0230T, 36000, 36400-36410, 36420-36430, 36440, 36591-36592, 36600, 36640, 43752, 51701-51703, 61650, 62320-62327, 64400-64410, 64413-64435, 64445-64450, 64461, 64463, 64479, 64483, 64486-64490, 64493, 64505, 64510-64530, 69990, 93000-93010, 93040-93042, 93318, 93355, 94002, 94200, 94250, 94680-94690, 94770, 95812-95816, 95819, 95822, 95829, 95955, 96360, 96365, 96372, 96374-96377, 96523, 99155, 99156, 99157, 99446-99449, 99451-99452, G0471

0273T 0213T, 0216T, 0228T, 0230T, 0272T, 36000, 36400-36410, 36420-36430, 36440, 36591-36592, 36600, 36640, 43752, 51701-51703, 61650, 62320-62327, 64400-64410, 64413-64435, 64445-64450, 64461, 64463, 64479, 64483, 64486-64490, 64493, 64505, 64510-64530, 69990, 93000-93010, 93040-93042, 93318, 93355, 94002, 94200, 94250, 94680-94690, 94770, 95812-95816, 95819, 95822, 95829, 95955, 96360, 96365, 96372, 96374-96377, 96523, 99155, 99156, 99157, 99446-99449, 99451-99452, G0471

0295T 0296T-0298T, 0497T-0498T, 36591-36592, 92920✦, 92924✦, 92928✦, 92933✦, 92937✦, 92941-92943✦, 93000-93010, 93040-93042, 94774-94777, 96523, 99453-99454, C9600-C9607✦

0296T 0497T-0498T, 36591-36592, 92920✦, 92924✦, 92928✦, 92933✦, 92937✦, 92941-92943✦, 93000-93010, 93040-93042, 94774-94777, 96523, 99453-99454, C9600-C9607✦

0297T 0497T-0498T, 36591-36592, 92920✦, 92924✦, 92928✦, 92933✦, 92937✦, 92941-92943✦, 93000-93010, 93040-93042, 94774-94777, 96523, 99453-99454, C9600-C9607✦

0298T 0497T-0498T, 36591-36592, 92920✦, 92924✦, 92928✦, 92933✦, 92937✦, 92941-92943✦, 93000-93010, 93040-93042, 94774-94777, 96523, 99453-99454, C9600-C9607✦

0331T 36000, 36005, 36410, 36591-36592, 76000, 76376-76377, 96360, 96365, 96372, 96374-96377, 96523

0332T 0331T, 36000, 36005, 36410, 36591-36592, 76000, 76376-76377, 96360, 96365, 96372, 96374-96377, 96523

0338T 0213T, 0216T, 0228T, 0230T, 12001-12007, 12011-12057, 13100-13133, 13151-13153, 35201-35206, 35226-35236, 35256-35266, 35286, 36000, 36140, 36160-36200, 36245-36248, 36251-36254, 36400-36410, 36420-36430, 36440, 36591-36592, 36600, 36640, 43752, 51701-51703, 61650, 62320-62327, 64400-64410, 64413-64435, 64445-64450, 64461, 64463, 64479, 64483, 64486-64490, 64493, 64505, 64510-64530, 69990, 75625, 75630, 76000, 77002, 92012-92014, 93000-93010, 93040-93042, 93050, 93318, 93355, 94002, 94200, 94250, 94680-94690, 94770, 95812-95816, 95819, 95822, 95829, 95955, 96360, 96365, 96372, 96374-96377, 96523, 99155, 99156, 99157, 99211-99223, 99231-99255, 99291-99292, 99304-99310, 99315-99316, 99334-99337, 99347-99350, 99374-99375, 99377-99378, 99446-99449, 99451-99452, G0269-G0471

0339T 0213T, 0216T, 0228T, 0230T, 0338T, 12001-12007, 12011-12057, 13100-13133, 13151-13153, 35201-35206, 35226-35236, 35256-35266, 35286, 36000, 36140, 36160-36200, 36245-36248, 36251-36254, 36400-36410, 36420-36430, 36440, 36591-36592, 36600, 36640, 43752, 51701-51703, 61650, 62320-62327, 64400-64410, 64413-64435, 64445-64450, 64461, 64463, 64479, 64483, 64486-64490, 64493, 64505, 64510-64530, 69990, 75625, 75630, 76000, 77002, 92012-92014, 93000-93010, 93040-93042, 93050, 93318, 93355, 94002, 94200, 94250, 94680-94690, 94770, 95812-95816, 95819, 95822, 95829, 95955, 96360, 96365, 96372, 96374-96377, 96523, 99155, 99156, 99157, 99211-99223, 99231-99255, 99291-99292, 99304-99310, 99315-99316, 99334-99337, 99347-99350, 99374-99375, 99377-99378, 99446-99449, 99451-99452, G0269-G0471

0342T 0213T, 0216T, 0228T, 0230T, 12001-12007, 12011-12057, 13100-13133, 13151-13153, 36000, 36400-36410, 36420-36430, 36440, 36591-36592, 36600, 36640, 43752, 51701-51703, 61650, 62320-62327, 64400-64410, 64413-64435, 64445-64450, 64461, 64463, 64479, 64483, 64486-64490, 64493, 64505, 64510-64530, 69990, 92012-92014, 93000-93010, 93040-93042, 93318, 93355, 94002, 94200, 94250, 94680-94690, 94770, 95812-95816, 95819, 95822, 95829, 95955, 96360, 96365, 96372, 96374-96377, 96523, 99155, 99156, 99157, 99211-99223, 99231-99255, 99291-99292, 99304-99310, 99315-99316, 99334-99337, 99347-99350, 99374-99375, 99377-99378, G0463-G0471

0345T 01920, 01924, 01926, 0213T, 0216T, 0228T, 0230T, 0484T✦, 12001-12007, 12011-12057, 13100-13133, 13151-13153, 32554-32557, 33210-33211, 33310-33315, 35201-35207, 35211-35286, 36000, 36010, 36013-36100, 36140, 36160-36200, 36400-36410, 36420-36430, 36440, 36500, 36555-36556, 36568-36569, 36572-36573, 36591-36592, 36600-36640, 43752, 51701-51703, 61650, 62320-62327, 64400-64410, 64413-64435, 64445-64450, 64461, 64463, 64479, 64483, 64486-64490, 64493, 64505, 64510-64530, 69990, 75600, 75605, 75625, 75630, 75710, 75716, 75741, 75743, 75746, 75756, 75893, 76000, 76496, 76942, 76970, 76998, 77002, 78635, 92012-92014, 92961, 93000-93010, 93040-93042, 93050, 93306-93308, 93312-93325, 93355, 93451-93462, 93503, 93530-93533, 93561-93565, 93567, 94002, 94200, 94250, 94680-94690, 94770, 95812-95816, 95819, 95822, 95829, 95955, 96360, 96365, 96372-96377, 96523, 99155, 99156, 99157, 99211-99223, 99231-99255, 99291-99292, 99304-99310, 99315-99316, 99334-99337, 99347-99350, 99374-99375, 99377-99378, 99446-99449, 99451-99452, G0269-J2001

0381T 0382T, 36591-36592, 96523, 99453-99454

0382T 36591-36592, 96523, 99453-99454

0383T 0381T-0382T, 0384T, 36591-36592, 96523, 99453-99454

0384T 0381T-0382T, 36591-36592, 96523, 99453-99454

0385T 0381T-0384T, 0386T, 36591-36592, 96523, 99453-99454

0386T 0381T-0384T, 36591-36592, 96523, 99453-99454

0408T 00530, 00534, 0213T, 0216T, 0228T, 0230T, 0409T-0411T, 0414T-0418T, 0525T, 0526T-0527T, 0528T, 0529T, 11000-11006, 11042-11047, 12001-12007, 12011-12057, 13100-13133, 13151-13153, 35201-35206, 35226-35236, 35256-35266, 35286, 36000, 36005-36013, 36140, 36400-36410, 36420-36430, 36440, 36555-36556, 36568-36569, 36572-36573, 36591-36592, 36600, 36640, 43752, 51701-51703, 61650, 62320-62327, 64400-64410, 64413-64435, 64445-64450, 64461, 64463, 64479, 64483, 64486-64490, 64493, 64505, 64510-64530, 69990, 76000, 76942, 76970, 76998, 77001-77002, 92012-92014, 92960-92961, 93000-93010, 93040-93042, 93260-93261, 93286-93287, 93318, 93355, 93452-93453, 93458-93461, 93600-93603, 93610-93612, 94002, 94200, 94250, 94680-94690, 94770, 95812-95816, 95819, 95822, 95829, 95955, 96360, 96365, 96372, 96374-96377, 96523, 97597-97598, 97602, 99155, 99156, 99157, 99211-99223, 99231-99255, 99291-99292, 99304-99310, 99315-99316, 99334-99337, 99347-99350, 99374-99375, 99377-99378, 99446-99449, 99451-99452, 99495-99496, G0463-G0471

0409T 00530, 00534, 0213T, 0216T, 0228T, 0230T, 0412T, 0416T-0418T, 0525T, 0526T-0527T, 0528T, 0529T-0532T, 11000-11006, 11042-11047, 12001-12007, 12011-12057, 13100-13133, 13151-13153, 33275, 36000, 36005, 36400-36410, 36420-36430, 36440, 36591-36592, 36600, 36640, 43752, 51701-51703, 61650, 62320-62327, 64400-64410, 64413-64435, 64445-64450, 64461, 64463, 64479, 64483, 64486-64490, 64493, 64505, 64510-64530, 69990, 76000, 76942, 76970, 76998, 77002, 92012-92014, 92960-92961, 93000-93010, 93040-93042, 93260-93261, 93286-93287, 93318, 93355, 93452-93453, 93458-93461, 93600-93603,

93610-93612, 94002, 94200, 94250, 94680-94690, 94770, 95812-95816, 95819, 95822, 95829, 95955, 96360, 96365, 96372, 96374-96377, 96523, 97597-97598, 97602, 99155, 99156, 99157, 99211-99223, 99231-99255, 99291-99292, 99304-99310, 99315-99316, 99334-99337, 99347-99350, 99374-99375, 99377-99378, 99446-99449, 99451-99452, 99495-99496, G0463-G0471

0410T 00530, 00534, 0213T, 0216T, 0228T, 0230T, 0409T, 0414T-0418T, 0525T, 0526T-0527T, 0528T, 0529T, 11000-11006, 11042-11047, 12001-12007, 12011-12057, 13100-13133, 13151-13153, 35201-35206, 35226-35236, 35256-35266, 35286, 36000, 36005-36013, 36140, 36400-36410, 36420-36430, 36440, 36555-36556, 36568-36569, 36572-36573, 36591-36592, 36600, 36640, 43752, 51701-51703, 61650, 62320-62327, 64400-64410, 64413-64435, 64445-64450, 64461, 64463, 64479, 64483, 64486-64490, 64493, 64505, 64510-64530, 69990, 76000, 76942, 76970, 76998, 77001-77002, 92012-92014, 92960-92961, 93000-93010, 93040-93042, 93260-93261, 93286-93287, 93318, 93355, 93452-93453, 93458-93461, 93600-93603, 93610-93612, 94002, 94200, 94250, 94680-94690, 94770, 95812-95816, 95819, 95822, 95829, 95955, 96360, 96365, 96372, 96374-96377, 96523, 97597-97598, 97602, 99155, 99156, 99157, 99211-99223, 99231-99255, 99291-99292, 99304-99310, 99315-99316, 99334-99337, 99347-99350, 99374-99375, 99377-99378, 99446-99449, 99451-99452, 99495-99496, G0463-G0471

0411T 00530, 00534, 0213T, 0216T, 0228T, 0230T, 0409T, 0414T-0418T, 0525T, 0526T-0527T, 0528T, 0529T, 11000-11006, 11042-11047, 12001-12007, 12011-12057, 13100-13133, 13151-13153, 35201-35206, 35226-35236, 35256-35266, 35286, 36000, 36005-36013, 36140, 36400-36410, 36420-36430, 36440, 36555-36556, 36568-36569, 36572-36573, 36591-36592, 36600, 36640, 43752, 51701-51703, 61650, 62320-62327, 64400-64410, 64413-64435, 64445-64450, 64461, 64463, 64479, 64483, 64486-64490, 64493, 64505, 64510-64530, 69990, 76000, 76942, 76970, 76998, 77001-77002, 92012-92014, 92960-92961, 93000-93010, 93040-93042, 93260-93261, 93286-93287, 93318, 93355, 93452-93453, 93458-93461, 93600-93603, 93610-93612, 94002, 94200, 94250, 94680-94690, 94770, 95812-95816, 95819, 95822, 95829, 95955, 96360, 96365, 96372, 96374-96377, 96523, 97597-97598, 97602, 99155, 99156, 99157, 99211-99223, 99231-99255, 99291-99292, 99304-99310, 99315-99316, 99334-99337, 99347-99350, 99374-99375, 99377-99378, 99446-99449, 99451-99452, 99495-99496, G0463-G0471

0412T 00530, 00534, 0213T, 0216T, 0228T, 0230T, 0415T, 0417T-0418T, 0525T, 0526T-0527T, 0528T, 0529T, 11000-11006, 11042-11047, 12001-12007, 12011-12057, 13100-13133, 13151-13153, 36000, 36005, 36400-36410, 36420-36430, 36440, 36591-36592, 36600, 36640, 43752, 51701-51703, 61650, 62320-62327, 64400-64410, 64413-64435, 64445-64450, 64461, 64463, 64479, 64483, 64486-64490, 64493, 64505, 64510-64530, 69990, 76000, 76942, 76970, 76998, 77002, 92012-92014, 92960-92961, 93000-93010, 93040-93042, 93260-93261, 93318, 93355, 94002, 94200, 94250, 94680-94690, 94770, 95812-95816, 95819, 95822, 95829, 95955, 96360, 96365, 96372, 96374-96377, 96523, 97597-97598, 97602, 99155, 99156, 99157, 99211-99223, 99231-99255, 99291-99292, 99304-99310, 99315-99316, 99334-99337, 99347-99350, 99374-99375, 99377-99378, 99446-99449, 99451-99452, 99495-99496, G0463-G0471

0413T 00530, 00534, 0213T, 0216T, 0228T, 0230T, 0415T-0418T, 0525T, 0526T-0527T, 0528T, 0529T, 11000-11006, 11042-11047, 12001-12007, 12011-12057, 13100-13133, 13151-13153, 35201-35206, 35226-35236, 35256-35266, 35286, 36000, 36005-36013, 36140, 36400-36410, 36420-36430, 36440, 36555-36556, 36568-36569, 36572-36573, 36591-36592, 36600, 36640, 43752, 51701-51703, 61650, 62320-62327, 64400-64410, 64413-64435, 64445-64450, 64461, 64463, 64479, 64483, 64486-64490, 64493, 64505, 64510-64530, 69990, 76000, 76942, 76970, 76998, 77001-77002, 92012-92014, 92960-92961, 93000-93010, 93040-93042, 93260-93261, 93318, 93355, 94002, 94200, 94250, 94680-94690, 94770, 95812-95816, 95819, 95822, 95829, 95955, 96360, 96365, 96372, 96374-96377, 96523, 97597-97598, 97602, 99155, 99156, 99157, 99211-99223, 99231-99255, 99291-99292, 99304-99310, 99315-99316, 99334-99337, 99347-99350, 99374-99375, 99377-99378, 99446-99449, 99451-99452, 99495-99496, G0463-G0471

0414T 00530, 00534, 0213T, 0216T, 0228T, 0230T, 0409T, 0412T, 0415T-0418T, 0525T, 0526T-0527T, 0528T, 0529T-0532T, 11000-11006, 11042-11047, 12001-12007, 12011-12057, 13100-13133, 13151-13153, 36000, 36005, 36400-36410, 36420-36430, 36440, 36591-36592, 36600, 36640, 43752, 51701-51703, 61650, 62320-62327, 64400-64410, 64413-64435, 64445-64450, 64461, 64463, 64479, 64483, 64486-64490, 64493, 64505, 64510-64530, 69990, 76000, 76942, 76970, 76998, 77002, 92012-92014, 93000-93010, 93040-93042, 93260-93261, 93286-93287, 93318, 93355, 93452-93453, 93458-93461, 93600-93603, 93610-93612, 94002, 94200, 94250, 94680-94690, 94770, 95812-95816, 95819, 95822, 95829, 95955, 96360, 96365, 96372, 96374-96377, 96523, 97597-97598, 97602, 99155, 99156, 99157, 99211-99223, 99231-99255, 99291-99292, 99304-99310, 99315-99316, 99334-99337, 99347-99350, 99374-99375, 99377-99378, 99446-99449, 99451-99452, 99495-99496, G0463-G0471

0415T 00530, 00540, 0213T, 0216T, 0228T, 0230T, 0416T-0418T, 0525T, 0526T-0527T, 0528T, 0529T, 12001-12007, 12011-12057, 13100-13133, 13151-13153, 35201-35206, 35226-35236, 35256-35266, 35286, 36000, 36005-36013, 36140, 36400-36410, 36420-36430, 36440, 36555-36556, 36568-36569, 36572-36573, 36591-36592, 36600, 36640, 43752, 51701-51703, 61650, 62320-62327, 64400-64410, 64413-64435, 64445-64450, 64461, 64463, 64479, 64483, 64486-64490, 64493, 64505, 64510-64530, 69990, 76000, 76942, 76970, 76998, 77001-77002, 92012-92014, 92960-92961, 93000-93010, 93040-93042, 93260-93261, 93286-93287, 93318, 93355, 93452-93453, 93458-93461, 93600-93603, 93610-93612, 94002, 94200, 94250, 94680-94690, 94770, 95812-95816, 95819, 95822, 95829, 95955, 96360, 96365, 96372, 96374-96377, 96523, 99155, 99156, 99157, 99211-99223, 99231-99255, 99291-99292, 99304-99310, 99315-99316, 99334-99337, 99347-99350, 99374-99375, 99377-99378, 99446-99449, 99451-99452, 99495-99496, G0463-G0471

0416T 00530, 00534, 0213T, 0216T, 0228T, 0230T, 0412T❖, 0417T-0418T, 0525T, 0526T-0527T, 0528T, 0529T, 10060-10061, 10140, 10180, 11000-11006, 11042-11047, 12001-12007, 12011-12057, 13100-13133, 13151-13153, 36000, 36005, 36400-36410, 36420-36430, 36440, 36591-36592, 36600, 36640, 43752, 51701-51703, 61650, 62320-62327, 64400-64410, 64413-64435, 64445-64450, 64461, 64463, 64479, 64483, 64486-64490, 64493, 64505, 64510-64530, 69990, 76000, 76942, 76970, 76998, 77002, 92012-92014, 92960-92961, 93000-93010, 93040-93042, 93260-93261, 93318, 93355, 94002, 94200, 94250, 94680-94690, 94770, 95812-95816, 95819, 95822, 95829, 95955, 96360, 96365, 96372, 96374-96377, 96523, 97597-97598, 97602, 99155, 99156, 99157, 99211-99223, 99231-99255, 99291-99292, 99304-99310, 99315-99316, 99334-99337, 99347-99350, 99374-99375, 99377-99378, 99446-99449, 99451-99452, 99495-99496, G0463-G0471

0417T 0295T-0298T, 0418T, 0497T-0498T, 36591-36592, 93000-93010, 93040-93042, 93224-93229, 93268, 93270-93272, 96523, 99446-99449, 99451-99452

0418T 0295T-0298T, 0497T-0498T, 36591-36592, 93000-93010, 93040-93042, 93224-93229, 93268, 93270-93272, 96523, 99446-99449, 99451-99452

0439T 36591-36592, 96523

0451T 0213T, 0216T, 0228T, 0230T, 0452T-0458T, 0460T-0463T, 0523T, 11000-11006, 11042-11047, 12001-12007, 12011-12057, 13100-13133, 13151-13153, 32100, 32551, 32556-32557, 33210-33211, 33254-33256, 33310-33315, 33967❖, 33970❖, 33973-33974❖, 34715-34716, 35201-35207, 35211-35286, 35511, 35612, 36000, 36002-36010, 36140, 36200, 36215-36218, 36221-36228, 36245-36248, 36400-36410, 36420-36430, 36440, 36591-36592, 36600, 36640, 39000-39010, 43752, 51701-51703, 62320-62327, 64400-64410, 64413-64435, 64445-64450, 64461-64463, 64479-64505, 64510-64530, 69990, 75600, 75605, 75625, 75630, 75635, 75705, 75710, 75716, 75726, 75731, 75733, 75736, 75741, 75743, 75746, 75756, 75774, 76000, 76936-76937, 76942, 76970, 76998, 77001-77002, 77011-77012, 77021, 92012-92014, 93000-93010, 93040-93042, 93318, 93355, 93451-93464, 93503-93505, 93530-93533, 93561-93572, 94002, 94200, 94250, 94680-94690, 94770, 95812-95816, 95819, 95822, 95829, 95955, 96360-96368, 96372, 96374-96377, 96523, 97597-97598, 97602, 99155, 99156, 99157, 99211-99223, 99231-99255, 99291-99292, 99304-99310, 99315-99316, 99334-99337, 99347-99350, 99374-99375, 99377-99378, 99446-99449, 99451-99452, 99495-99496, G0463-G0471

0452T 0213T, 0216T, 0228T, 0230T, 0453T-0458T❖, 0461T-0463T, 0523T, 11000-11006, 11042-11047, 12001-12007, 12011-12057, 13100-13133, 13151-13153, 32100, 32551, 32556-32557, 33210-33211, 33254-33256, 33310-33315, 33967❖, 33970❖, 33973-33974❖, 34715-34716, 35201-35207, 35211-35286, 35511, 35612, 36000, 36002-36010, 36140, 36200, 36215-36218, 36221-36228, 36245-36248, 36400-36410, 36420-36430, 36440, 36591-36592, 36600, 36640, 39000-39010, 43752, 51701-51703, 62320-62327, 64400-64410, 64413-64435, 64445-64450, 64461-64463, 64479-64505, 64510-64530, 69990, 75600, 75605, 75625, 75630, 75635, 75705, 75710, 75716, 75726, 75731, 75733, 75736, 75741, 75743, 75746, 75756, 75774, 76000, 76936-76937, 76942, 76970, 76998, 77001-77002, 77011-77012, 77021, 92012-92014, 93000-93010, 93040-93042, 93318, 93355, 93451-93464, 93503-93505, 93530-93533, 93561-93572, 94002, 94200, 94250, 94680-94690, 94770, 95812-95816, 95819, 95822, 95829, 95955, 96360-96368, 96372, 96374-96377, 96523, 97597-97598, 97602, 99155, 99156, 99157, 99211-99223, 99231-99255, 99291-99292, 99304-99310, 99315-99316, 99334-99337, 99347-99350, 99374-99375, 99377-99378, 99446-99449, 99451-99452, 99495-99496, G0463-G0471

0453T 0213T, 0216T, 0228T, 0230T, 0454T-0458T❖, 0462T-0463T, 0523T, 11000-11006, 11042-11047, 12001-12007, 12011-12057, 13100-13133, 13151-13153, 32100, 32551, 32556-32557, 33210-33211, 33254-33256, 33310-33315, 33967❖, 33970❖, 33973-33974❖, 36000, 36002-36010, 36140, 36200, 36215-36218, 36221-36228, 36245-36248, 36400-36410, 36420-36430, 36440, 36591-36592, 36600, 36640, 39000-39010, 43752, 51701-51703, 62320-62327, 64400-64410, 64413-64435, 64445-64450, 64461-64463, 64479-64505, 64510-64530, 69990, 75600, 75605, 75625, 75630, 75635, 75705, 75710, 75716, 75726, 75731, 75733, 75736, 75741, 75743, 75746, 75756, 75774, 76000, 76936-76937, 76942, 76970, 76998, 77001-77002, 77011-77012, 77021, 92012-92014, 93000-93010, 93040-93042, 93318, 93355, 93451-93464, 93503-93505, 93530-93533, 93561-93572, 94002, 94200, 94250, 94680-94690, 94770, 95812-95816, 95819, 95822, 95829, 95955, 96360-96368, 96372, 96374-96377, 96523, 97597-97598, 97602, 99155, 99156, 99157, 99211-99223, 99231-99255, 99291-99292, 99304-99310, 99315-99316, 99334-99337, 99347-99350, 99374-99375, 99377-99378, 99446-99449, 99451-99452, 99495-99496, G0463-G0471

0454T 0213T, 0216T, 0228T, 0230T, 0455T-0458T, 0460T-0463T, 0523T, 11000-11006, 11042-11047, 12001-12007, 12011-12057, 13100-13133, 13151-13153, 32100, 32551, 32556-32557, 33210-33211, 33254-33256, 33310-33315, 33973, 36000, 36002-36010, 36140, 36200, 36215-36218, 36221-36228, 36245-36248, 36400-36410, 36420-36430, 36440, 36591-36592, 36600, 36640, 39000-39010, 43752, 51701-51703, 62320-62327, 64400-64410, 64413-64435, 64445-64450, 64461-64463, 64479-64505, 64510-64530, 69990, 75600, 75605, 75625, 75630, 75635, 75705, 75710, 75716, 75726, 75731, 75733, 75736, 75741, 75743, 75746, 75756, 75774, 76000, 76936-76937, 76942, 76970, 76998, 77001-77002, 77011-77012, 77021, 92012-92014, 93000-93010, 93040-93042, 93318, 93355, 93451-93464, 93503-93505, 93530-93533, 93561-93572, 94002, 94200, 94250, 94680-94690, 94770, 95812-95816, 95819, 95822, 95829, 95955, 96360-96368, 96372, 96374-96377, 96523, 97597-97598, 97602, 99155, 99156, 99157, 99211-99223, 99231-99255, 99291-99292, 99304-99310, 99315-99316, 99334-99337, 99347-99350, 99374-99375, 99377-99378, 99446-99449, 99451-99452, 99495-99496, G0463-G0471

0455T 0213T, 0216T, 0228T, 0230T, 0456T-0458T, 0462T-0463T, 0523T, 11000-11006, 11042-11047, 12001-12007, 12011-12057, 13100-13133, 13151-13153, 32100, 32551, 32556-32557, 33210-33211, 33254-33256, 33310-33315, 33320-33330, 33335, 33974, 34715-34716, 35201-35207, 35211-35286, 35511, 35612, 36000, 36002-36010, 36140, 36200, 36215-36218, 36221-36228, 36245-36248, 36400-36410, 36420-36430, 36440, 36591-36592, 36600, 36640, 39000-39010, 43752, 51701-51703, 62320-62327, 64400-64410, 64413-64435, 64445-64450, 64461-64463, 64479-64505, 64510-64530, 69990, 75600, 75605, 75625, 75630, 75635, 75705, 75710, 75716, 75726, 75731, 75733, 75736, 75741, 75743, 75746, 75756, 75774, 76000, 76936-76937, 76942, 76970, 76998, 77001-77002, 77011-77012, 77021, 92012-92014, 93000-93010, 93040-93042, 93318, 93355, 93451-93464, 93503-93505, 93530-93533, 93561-93572, 94002, 94200, 94250, 94680-94690, 94770, 95812-95816, 95819, 95822, 95829, 95955, 96360-96368, 96372, 96374-96377, 96523, 97597-97598, 97602, 99155, 99156, 99157, 99211-99223, 99231-99255, 99291-99292, 99304-99310, 99315-99316, 99334-99337, 99347-99350, 99374-99375, 99377-99378, 99446-99449, 99451-99452, 99495-99496, G0463-G0471

0456T 0213T, 0216T, 0228T, 0230T, 0457T-0458T❖, 0462T-0463T, 0523T, 11000-11006, 11042-11047, 12001-12007, 12011-12057, 13100-13133, 13151-13153, 32100, 32551, 32556-32557, 33210-33211, 33254-33256, 33310-33315, 33320-33330, 33335, 33974, 34715-34716, 35201-35207, 35211-35286, 35511, 35612, 36000, 36002-36010, 36140, 36200, 36215-36218, 36221-36228, 36245-36248, 36400-36410, 36420-36430, 36440, 36591-36592, 36600, 36640, 39000-39010, 43752, 51701-51703, 62320-62327, 64400-64410, 64413-64435, 64445-64450, 64461-64463, 64479-64505, 64510-64530, 69990, 75600, 75605, 75625, 75630, 75635, 75705, 75710, 75716, 75726, 75731, 75733, 75736, 75741, 75743, 75746, 75756, 75774, 76000, 76936-76937, 76942, 76970, 76998, 77001-77002, 77011-77012, 77021, 92012-92014, 93000-93010, 93040-93042, 93318, 93355, 93451-93464, 93503-93505, 93530-93533, 93561-93572, 94002, 94200, 94250, 94680-94690, 94770, 95812-95816, 95819, 95822, 95829, 95955, 96360-96368, 96372, 96374-96377, 96523, 97597-97598, 97602, 99155, 99156, 99157, 99211-99223, 99231-99255, 99291-99292, 99304-99310, 99315-99316, 99334-99337, 99347-99350, 99374-99375, 99377-99378, 99446-99449, 99451-99452, 99495-99496, G0463-G0471

0457T 0213T, 0216T, 0228T, 0230T, 0458T❖, 0462T-0463T, 0523T, 11000-11006, 11042-11047, 12001-12007, 12011-12057, 13100-13133, 13151-13153, 32100, 32551, 32556-32557, 33210-33211, 33254-33256, 33310-33315, 33320-33330, 33335, 33974, 36000, 36002-36010, 36140, 36200, 36215-36218, 36221-36228, 36245-36248, 36400-36410, 36420-36430, 36440, 36591-36592, 36600, 36640, 39000-39010, 43752, 51701-51703, 62320-62327, 64400-64410, 64413-64435, 64445-64450, 64461-64463, 64479-64505, 64510-64530, 69990, 75600, 75605, 75625,

75630, 75635, 75705, 75710, 75716, 75726, 75731, 75733, 75736, 75741, 75743, 75746, 75756, 75774, 76000, 76936-76937, 76942, 76970, 76998, 77001-77002, 77011-77012, 77021, 92012-92014, 93000-93010, 93040-93042, 93318, 93355, 93451-93464, 93503-93505, 93530-93533, 93561-93572, 94002, 94200, 94250, 94680-94690, 94770, 95812-95816, 95819, 95822, 95829, 95955, 96360-96368, 96372, 96374-96377, 96523, 97597-97598, 97602, 99155, 99156, 99157, 99211-99223, 99231-99255, 99291-99292, 99304-99310, 99315-99316, 99334-99337, 99347-99350, 99374-99375, 99377-99378, 99446-99449, 99451-99452, 99495-99496, G0463-G0471

0458T 0213T, 0216T, 0228T, 0230T, 0462T-0463T, 0523T, 11000-11006, 11042-11047, 12001-12007, 12011-12057, 13100-13133, 13151-13153, 32100, 32551, 32556-32557, 33210-33211, 33254-33256, 33310-33315, 33320-33330, 33335, 33974, 36000, 36002-36010, 36140, 36200, 36215-36218, 36221-36228, 36245-36248, 36400-36410, 36420-36430, 36440, 36591-36592, 36600, 36640, 39000-39010, 43752, 51701-51703, 62320-62327, 64400-64410, 64413-64435, 64445-64450, 64461-64463, 64479-64505, 64510-64530, 69990, 75600, 75605, 75625, 75630, 75635, 75705, 75710, 75716, 75726, 75731, 75733, 75736, 75741, 75743, 75746, 75756, 75774, 76000, 76936-76937, 76942, 76970, 76998, 77001-77002, 77011-77012, 77021, 92012-92014, 93000-93010, 93040-93042, 93318, 93355, 93451-93464, 93503-93505, 93530-93533, 93561-93572, 94002, 94200, 94250, 94680-94690, 94770, 95812-95816, 95819, 95822, 95829, 95955, 96360-96368, 96372, 96374-96377, 96523, 97597-97598, 97602, 99155, 99156, 99157, 99211-99223, 99231-99255, 99291-99292, 99304-99310, 99315-99316, 99334-99337, 99347-99350, 99374-99375, 99377-99378, 99446-99449, 99451-99452, 99495-99496, G0463-G0471

0459T 00530, 00534, 0213T, 0216T, 0228T, 0230T, 0412T❖, 0417T-0418T, 0451T-0458T, 0460T-0463T, 0523T, 0525T, 0526T-0527T, 0528T, 0529T, 10060-10061, 10140, 10180, 11000-11006, 11042-11047, 12001-12007, 12011-12057, 13100-13133, 13151-13153, 35201-35206, 35211-35216, 35226-35246, 35256-35276, 35286, 35511, 35612, 36000, 36002-36010, 36013-36014, 36140, 36160-36200, 36215-36218, 36221-36228, 36245-36248, 36400-36410, 36420-36430, 36440, 36591-36592, 36600, 36640, 43752, 51701-51703, 61650, 62320-62327, 64400-64410, 64413-64435, 64445-64450, 64461-64463, 64479-64505, 64510-64530, 69990, 75600, 75605, 75625, 75630, 75635, 75705, 75710, 75716, 75726, 75731, 75733, 75736, 75741, 75743, 75746, 75756, 75774, 76000, 76936-76937, 76942, 76970, 76998, 77001-77002, 77011-77012, 77021, 92012-92014, 92960-92961, 93000-93010, 93040-93042, 93260-93261, 93318, 93355, 93451-93464, 93503-93505, 93530-93533, 93561-93572, 94002, 94200, 94250, 94680-94690, 94770, 95812-95816, 95819, 95822, 95829, 95955, 96360-96368, 96372, 96374-96377, 96523, 97597-97598, 97602, 99155, 99156, 99157, 99211-99223, 99231-99255, 99291-99292, 99304-99310, 99315-99316, 99334-99337, 99347-99350, 99374-99375, 99377-99378, 99446-99449, 99451-99452, 99495-99496, G0463-G0471

0460T 00530, 00534, 0213T, 0216T, 0228T, 0230T, 0412T❖, 0417T-0418T, 0462T-0463T, 0523T, 0525T, 0526T-0527T, 0528T, 0529T, 10060-10061, 10140, 10180, 11000-11006, 11042-11047, 12001-12007, 12011-12057, 13100-13133, 13151-13153, 35201-35206, 35211-35216, 35226-35246, 35256-35276, 35286, 35511, 35612, 36000, 36002-36010, 36013-36014, 36140, 36160-36200, 36215-36218, 36221-36228, 36245-36248, 36400-36410, 36420-36430, 36440, 36591-36592, 36600, 36640, 43752, 51701-51703, 61650, 62320-62327, 64400-64410, 64413-64435, 64445-64450, 64461-64463, 64479-64505, 64510-64530, 69990, 75600, 75605, 75625, 75630, 75635, 75705, 75710, 75716, 75726, 75731, 75733, 75736, 75741, 75743, 75746, 75756, 75774, 76000, 76936-76937, 76942, 76970, 76998, 77001-77002, 77011-77012, 77021, 92012-92014, 92960-92961, 93000-93010, 93040-93042, 93260-93261, 93318, 93355, 93451-93464, 93503-93505, 93530-93533, 93561-93572, 94002, 94200, 94250, 94680-94690, 94770, 95812-95816, 95819, 95822, 95829, 95955, 96360-96368, 96372, 96374-96377, 96523, 97597-97598, 97602, 99155, 99156, 99157, 99211-99223, 99231-99255, 99291-99292, 99304-99310, 99315-99316, 99334-99337, 99347-99350, 99374-99375, 99377-99378, 99446-99449, 99451-99452, 99495-99496, G0463-G0471

0461T 00530, 00534, 0213T, 0216T, 0228T, 0230T, 0412T❖, 0417T-0418T, 0460T❖, 0462T-0463T, 0523T, 0525T, 0526T-0527T, 0528T, 0529T, 10060-10061, 10140, 10180, 11000-11006, 11042-11047, 12001-12007, 12011-12057, 13100-13133, 13151-13153, 35201-35206, 35211-35216, 35226-35246, 35256-35276, 35286, 35511, 35612, 36000, 36002-36010, 36013-36014, 36140, 36160-36200, 36215-36218, 36221-36228, 36245-36248, 36400-36410, 36420-36430, 36440, 36591-36592, 36600, 36640, 43752, 51701-51703, 61650, 62320-62327, 64400-64410, 64413-64435, 64445-64450, 64461-64463, 64479-64505, 64510-64530, 69990, 75600, 75605, 75625, 75630, 75635, 75705, 75710, 75716, 75726, 75731, 75733, 75736, 75741, 75743, 75746, 75756, 75774, 76000, 76936-76937, 76942, 76970, 76998, 77001-77002, 77011-77012, 77021, 92012-92014, 92960-92961, 93000-93010, 93040-93042, 93260-93261, 93318, 93355, 93451-93464, 93503-93505, 93530-93533, 93561-93572, 94002, 94200, 94250, 94680-94690, 94770, 95812-95816, 95819, 95822, 95829, 95955, 96360-96368, 96372, 96374-96377, 96523, 97597-97598, 97602, 99155, 99156, 99157, 99211-99223, 99231-99255, 99291-99292, 99304-99310, 99315-99316, 99334-99337, 99347-99350, 99374-99375, 99377-99378, 99446-99449, 99451-99452, 99495-99496, G0463-G0471

0462T 0295T-0298T, 0463T, 0497T-0498T, 0522T-0523T, 36000, 36002-36010, 36200, 36215-36218, 36221-36228, 36591-36592, 75600, 75605, 75625, 75630, 75635, 75705, 75710, 75716, 75726, 75731, 75733, 75736, 75741, 75743, 75746, 75756, 75774, 76000, 76936-76937, 77001-77002, 77011-77012, 77021, 93000-93010, 93040-93042, 93224-93229, 93268, 93270-93272, 93285-93288, 93291, 93451-93464, 93503-93505, 93530-93533, 93561-93572, 96523, 99446-99449, 99451-99452

0463T 0295T-0298T, 0497T-0498T, 0521T❖, 0523T, 36000, 36002-36010, 36200, 36215-36218, 36221-36228, 36591-36592, 75600, 75605, 75625, 75630, 75635, 75705, 75710, 75716, 75726, 75731, 75733, 75736, 75741, 75743, 75746, 75756, 75774, 76000, 76936-76937, 77001-77002, 77011-77012, 77021, 93000-93010, 93040-93042, 93224-93229, 93264, 93268, 93270-93272, 93286, 93291, 93296, 93299, 93451-93464, 93503-93505, 93530-93533, 93561-93572, 96523, 99446-99449, 99451-99452

0466T 0213T, 0216T, 0228T, 0230T, 0333T, 0464T, 12001-12007, 12011-12057, 13100-13133, 13151-13153, 36000, 36400-36410, 36420-36430, 36440, 36591-36592, 36600, 36640, 43752, 51701-51703, 61885, 61888, 62320-62327, 64400-64410, 64413-64435, 64445-64450, 64461-64463, 64479-64505, 64510-64530, 69990, 92012-92014, 92585, 93000-93010, 93040-93042, 93318, 93355, 94002, 94200, 94250, 94680-94690, 94770, 95812-95816, 95819, 95822, 95829, 95860-95870, 95907-95913, 95925-95933, 95937-95940, 95955, 96360-96368, 96372, 96374-96377, 96523, 99155, 99156, 99157, 99211-99223, 99231-99255, 99291-99292, 99304-99310, 99315-99316, 99334-99337, 99347-99350, 99374-99375, 99377-99378, 99446-99449, 99451-99452, 99495-99496, G0453-G0471

0467T 0213T, 0216T, 0228T, 0230T, 0333T, 0464T, 0466T, 0468T, 11000-11006, 11042-11047, 12001-12007, 12011-12057, 13100-13133, 13151-13153, 36000, 36400-36410, 36420-36430, 36440, 36591-36592, 36600, 36640, 43752, 51701-51703, 61888, 62320-62327, 64400-64410, 64413-64435,

64445-64450, 64461-64463, 64479-64505, 64510-64530, 64568, 64570, 69990, 92012-92014, 92585, 93000-93010, 93040-93042, 93318, 93355, 94002, 94200, 94250, 94680-94690, 94770, 95812-95816, 95819, 95822, 95829, 95860-95870, 95907-95913, 95925-95933, 95937-95940, 95955, 96360-96368, 96372, 96374-96377, 96523, 97597-97598, 97602, 99155, 99156, 99157, 99211-99223, 99231-99255, 99291-99292, 99304-99310, 99315-99316, 99334-99337, 99347-99350, 99374-99375, 99377-99378, 99446-99449, 99451-99452, 99495-99496, G0453-G0471

0468T 0213T, 0216T, 0228T, 0230T, 0333T, 0464T, 0466T, 11000-11006, 11042-11047, 12001-12007, 12011-12057, 13100-13133, 13151-13153, 36000, 36400-36410, 36420-36430, 36440, 36591-36592, 36600, 36640, 43752, 51701-51703, 61888, 62320-62327, 64400-64410, 64413-64435, 64445-64450, 64461-64463, 64479-64505, 64510-64530, 64568, 69990, 92012-92014, 92585, 93000-93010, 93040-93042, 93318, 93355, 94002, 94200, 94250, 94680-94690, 94770, 95812-95816, 95819, 95822, 95829, 95860-95870, 95907-95913, 95925-95933, 95937-95940, 95955, 96360-96368, 96372, 96374-96377, 96523, 97597-97598, 97602, 99155, 99156, 99157, 99211-99223, 99231-99255, 99291-99292, 99304-99310, 99315-99316, 99334-99337, 99347-99350, 99374-99375, 99377-99378, 99446-99449, 99451-99452, 99495-99496, G0453-G0471

0475T 0476T-0478T, 36591-36592, 76970, 96523, 99453-99454

0476T 36591-36592, 76970, 96523, 99453-99454

0477T 36591-36592, 96523, 99453-99454

0478T 36591-36592, 96523, 99453-99454

0483T 01920, 01924, 01926, 0213T, 0216T, 0228T, 0230T, 0345T❖, 12001-12007, 12011-12057, 13100-13133, 13151-13153, 32554-32557, 33210-33211, 33254-33256, 33310-33315, 35201-35207, 35211-35286, 36000, 36010-36100, 36140, 36160-36200, 36215-36217, 36245-36247, 36400-36410, 36420-36430, 36440, 36500, 36555-36556, 36568-36569, 36572-36573, 36591-36592, 36600-36640, 43752, 51701-51703, 62320-62327, 64400-64410, 64413-64435, 64445-64450, 64461-64463, 64479-64505, 64510-64530, 69990, 75600, 75605, 75625, 75630, 75710, 75716, 75741, 75743, 75746, 75756, 75893, 76000, 76496, 76942, 76970, 76998, 77002, 78635, 92012-92014, 92961, 93000-93010, 93040-93042, 93306-93308, 93312-93325, 93355, 93451-93462, 93503, 93530-93533, 93561-93565, 93567, 93590, 93592, 94002, 94200, 94250, 94680-94690, 94770, 95812-95816, 95819, 95822, 95829, 95955, 96360-96368, 96372-96377, 96523, 99155, 99156, 99157, 99211-99223, 99231-99255, 99291-99292, 99304-99310, 99315-99316, 99334-99337, 99347-99350, 99374-99375, 99377-99378, 99446-99449, 99451-99452, G0269-J2001

0484T 01920, 01924, 01926, 0213T, 0216T, 0228T, 0230T, 11000-11006, 11042-11047, 12001-12007, 12011-12057, 13100-13133, 13151-13153, 20680, 21750, 32100, 32551, 32554-32557, 33140, 33210-33211, 33254-33256, 33310-33315, 35201-35207, 35211-35286, 36000, 36010-36100, 36140, 36160-36200, 36215-36217, 36245-36247, 36400-36410, 36420-36430, 36440, 36500, 36555-36556, 36568-36569, 36572-36573, 36591-36592, 36600-36640, 39000-39010, 43752, 51701-51703, 62320-62327, 64400-64410, 64413-64435, 64445-64450, 64461-64463, 64479-64505, 64510-64530, 69990, 75600, 75605, 75625, 75630, 75710, 75716, 75741, 75743, 75746, 75756, 75893, 76000, 76496, 76942, 76970, 76998, 77002, 78635, 92012-92014, 92961, 93000-93010, 93040-93042, 93306-93308, 93312-93325, 93355, 93451-93462, 93503, 93530-93533, 93561-93565, 93567, 93590, 93592, 94002, 94200, 94250, 94680-94690, 94770, 95812-95816, 95819, 95822, 95829, 95955, 96360-96368, 96372-96377, 96523, 97597-97598, 97602, 99155, 99156, 99157, 99211-99223, 99231-99255, 99291-99292, 99304-99310, 99315-99316, 99334-99337, 99347-99350, 99374-99375, 99377-99378, 99446-99449, 99451-99452, G0269-J2001

0497T 36591-36592, 93000-93010, 93040-93042, 94774-94777, 96523, 99453-99454

0498T 36591-36592, 93000-93010, 93040-93042, 94774-94777, 96523, 99453-99454

0501T 0502T, 0503T-0504T, 0523T, 36591-36592, 76376-76377, 96523

0502T 0523T, 36591-36592, 76376-76377, 96523

0503T 0523T, 36591-36592, 76376-76377, 96523

0504T 0523T, 36591-36592, 76376-76377, 96523

0505T 01924, 11000-11006, 11042-11047, 12001-12007, 12011-12057, 13100-13133, 13151-13153, 34713-34716, 34812-34820, 34833-34834, 35201-35206, 35226-35236, 35256-35266, 35286, 35302-35303, 36000, 36002-36012, 36140, 36160-36200, 36245-36247, 36400-36410, 36420-36430, 36440, 36500, 36591-36592, 36600-36640, 37186, 37224-37227, 37236-37239, 37246-37249, 43752, 51701-51703, 62320-62327, 64400-64410, 64413-64435, 64445-64450, 64461-64463, 64479-64505, 64510-64530, 69990, 75630, 75710, 75716, 75736, 75774, 75893, 76000, 76937, 76942, 76970, 76998, 77002, 92012-92014, 93000-93010, 93040-93042, 93050, 93318, 93355, 94002, 94200, 94250, 94680-94690, 94770, 95812-95816, 95819, 95822, 95829, 95955, 96360-96368, 96372, 96374-96377, 96523, 97597-97598, 97602, 99155, 99156, 99157, 99211-99223, 99231-99255, 99291-99292, 99304-99310, 99315-99316, 99334-99337, 99347-99350, 99374-99375, 99377-99378, 99446-99449, 99451-99452, 99495-99496, G0269-J2001

0515T 00530, 00534, 0213T, 0216T, 0228T, 0230T, 0462T-0463T, 0516T, 0517T, 0518T, 0519T, 0520T, 0521T-0522T, 11000-11006, 11042-11047, 12001-12007, 12011-12057, 13100-13133, 13151-13153, 32100, 33206-33208, 33210-33218, 33220-33229, 33230-33231, 33233-33238, 33240-33241, 33243-33244, 33249, 33262-33264, 33270-33275, 35201-35207, 35211-35286, 36000, 36100, 36140, 36160-36200, 36215-36217, 36221, 36400-36410, 36420-36430, 36440, 36555-36556, 36568-36569, 36591-36592, 36600, 36640, 39010, 43752, 51701-51703, 62320-62327, 64400-64410, 64413-64435, 64445-64450, 64461-64463, 64479-64505, 64510-64530, 69990, 76000, 76380, 76937, 76942, 76970, 76998, 77001-77002, 77012, 77021, 92012-92014, 92960-92961, 93000-93010, 93040-93042, 93260-93261, 93279, 93280, 93281-93299, 93303-93304, 93306-93308, 93312-93355, 93452-93453, 93458-93461, 93531-93533, 93565, 93600-93603, 93610-93612, 94002, 94200, 94250, 94680-94690, 94770, 95812-95816, 95819, 95822, 95829, 95955, 96360-96368, 96372, 96374-96377, 96523, 97597-97598, 97602, 99155, 99156, 99157, 99211-99223, 99231-99255, 99291-99292, 99304-99310, 99315-99316, 99334-99337, 99347-99350, 99374-99375, 99377-99378, 99446-99449, 99495-99496, G0448-G0471

0516T 00530, 00534, 0213T, 0216T, 0228T, 0230T, 0462T-0463T, 0517T, 0518T, 0519T, 0520T, 0521T-0522T, 11000-11006, 11042-11047, 12001-12007, 12011-12057, 13100-13133, 13151-13153, 33206-33207, 33210-33216, 33218, 33221-33229, 33230-33231, 33233-33238, 33240-33241, 33243-33244, 33249, 33270-33273, 33275, 35201-35207, 35211-35286, 36000, 36100, 36140, 36160-36200, 36215-36217, 36221, 36400-36410, 36420-36430, 36440, 36555-36556, 36568-36569, 36591-36592, 36600, 36640, 43752, 51701-51703, 62320-62327, 64400-64410, 64413-64435, 64445-64450, 64461-64463, 64479-64505, 64510-64530, 69990, 76000, 76380, 76937, 76942, 76970, 76998, 77001-77002, 77012, 77021, 92012-92014, 92960-92961, 93000-93010, 93040-93042, 93260-93261, 93279, 93280, 93281-93299, 93303-93304, 93306-93308, 93312-93355, 93452-93453, 93458-93461, 93531-93533, 93565, 93600-93603, 93610-93612, 94002, 94200, 94250, 94680-94690, 94770, 95812-95816, 95819, 95822, 95829, 95955, 96360-96368, 96372, 96374-96377, 96523, 97597-97598, 97602, 99155, 99156,

99157, 99211-99223, 99231-99255, 99291-99292, 99304-99310, 99315-99316, 99334-99337, 99347-99350, 99374-99375, 99377-99378, 99446-99449, 99495-99496, G0448-G0471

0517T 00530, 00534, 0213T, 0216T, 0228T, 0230T, 0462T-0463T, 0518T, 0519T, 0520T, 0521T-0522T, 11000-11006, 11042-11047, 12001-12007, 12011-12057, 13100-13133, 13151-13153, 33206-33208, 33210-33218, 33220-33229, 33230-33231, 33233-33238, 33240-33241, 33243-33244, 33249, 33270-33275, 36000, 36005, 36400-36410, 36420-36430, 36440, 36591-36592, 36600, 36640, 43752, 51701-51703, 62320-62327, 64400-64410, 64413-64435, 64445-64450, 64461-64463, 64479-64505, 64510-64530, 69990, 76000, 76380, 76937, 76942, 76970, 76998, 77002, 77012, 77021, 92012-92014, 92960-92961, 93000-93010, 93040-93042, 93260-93261, 93279, 93280, 93281-93299, 93303-93304, 93306-93308, 93312-93355, 93600-93603, 93610-93612, 94002, 94200, 94250, 94680-94690, 94770, 95812-95816, 95819, 95822, 95829, 95955, 96360-96368, 96372, 96374-96377, 96523, 97597-97598, 97602, 99155, 99156, 99157, 99211-99223, 99231-99255, 99291-99292, 99304-99310, 99315-99316, 99334-99337, 99347-99350, 99374-99375, 99377-99378, 99446-99449, 99495-99496, G0463-G0471

0518T 00530, 00534, 0213T, 0216T, 0228T, 0230T, 0462T-0463T, 0521T-0522T, 11000-11006, 11042-11047, 12001-12007, 12011-12057, 13100-13133, 13151-13153, 33210-33211, 33215, 36000, 36005, 36400-36410, 36420-36430, 36440, 36591-36592, 36600, 36640, 43752, 51701-51703, 62320-62327, 64400-64410, 64413-64435, 64445-64450, 64461-64463, 64479-64505, 64510-64530, 69990, 76000, 76380, 76937, 76942, 76970, 76998, 77002, 77012, 77021, 92012-92014, 92960-92961, 93000-93010, 93040-93042, 93260-93261, 93279, 93280, 93281-93299, 93303-93304, 93306-93308, 93312-93355, 94002, 94200, 94250, 94680-94690, 94770, 95812-95816, 95819, 95822, 95829, 95955, 96360-96368, 96372, 96374-96377, 96523, 97597-97598, 97602, 99155, 99156, 99157, 99211-99223, 99231-99255, 99291-99292, 99304-99310, 99315-99316, 99334-99337, 99347-99350, 99374-99375, 99377-99378, 99446-99449, 99495-99496, G0463-G0471

0519T 00530, 00534, 0213T, 0216T, 0228T, 0230T, 0462T-0463T, 0518T, 0521T-0522T, 11000-11006, 11042-11047, 12001-12007, 12011-12057, 13100-13133, 13151-13153, 33210-33211, 33215-33217, 33230-33231, 33240-33241, 36000, 36005, 36400-36410, 36420-36430, 36440, 36591-36592, 36600, 36640, 43752, 51701-51703, 62320-62327, 64400-64410, 64413-64435, 64445-64450, 64461-64463, 64479-64505, 64510-64530, 69990, 76000, 76380, 76937, 76942, 76970, 76998, 77002, 77012, 77021, 92012-92014, 93000-93010, 93040-93042, 93260-93261, 93279, 93280, 93281-93299, 93303-93304, 93306-93308, 93312-93355, 93600-93603, 93610-93612, 94002, 94200, 94250, 94680-94690, 94770, 95812-95816, 95819, 95822, 95829, 95955, 96360-96368, 96372, 96374-96377, 96523, 97597-97598, 97602, 99155, 99156, 99157, 99211-99223, 99231-99255, 99291-99292, 99304-99310, 99315-99316, 99334-99337, 99347-99350, 99374-99375, 99377-99378, 99446-99449, 99495-99496, G0463-G0471

0520T 00530, 00534, 0213T, 0216T, 0228T, 0230T, 0462T-0463T, 0518T, 0519T, 0521T-0522T, 11000-11006, 11042-11047, 12001-12007, 12011-12057, 13100-13133, 13151-13153, 32100, 33210-33211, 33215-33217, 33223-33226, 33230-33231, 33240, 33262-33264, 35201-35207, 35211-35286, 36000, 36100, 36140, 36160-36200, 36215-36217, 36221, 36400-36410, 36420-36430, 36440, 36555-36556, 36568-36569, 36591-36592, 36600, 36640, 39010, 43752, 51701-51703, 62320-62327, 64400-64410, 64413-64435, 64445-64450, 64461-64463, 64479-64505, 64510-64530, 69990, 76000, 76380, 76937, 76942, 76970, 76998, 77001-77002, 77012, 77021, 92012-92014, 92960-92961, 93000-93010, 93040-93042, 93260-93261, 93279, 93280, 93281-93299, 93303-93304, 93306-93308, 93312-93355, 93452-93453, 93458-93461, 93531-93533, 93565, 93600-93603, 93610-93612, 94002, 94200, 94250, 94680-94690, 94770, 95812-95816, 95819, 95822, 95829, 95955, 96360-96368, 96372, 96374-96377, 96523, 97597-97598, 97602, 99155, 99156, 99157, 99211-99223, 99231-99255, 99291-99292, 99304-99310, 99315-99316, 99334-99337, 99347-99350, 99374-99375, 99377-99378, 99446-99449, 99495-99496, G0448-G0471

0521T 0295T-0298T, 0462T, 0497T-0498T, 36591-36592, 93000-93010, 93040-93042, 93224-93229, 93261, 93268, 93270-93272, 93279, 93280, 93286-93287, 93291, 93294, 93296-93299, 96523, 99446-99449

0522T 0295T-0298T, 0463T, 0497T-0498T, 0521T, 36591-36592, 93000-93010, 93040-93042, 93224-93229, 93261, 93268, 93270-93272, 93285-93289, 93291, 93745, 96523, 99446-99449

0523T 0213T, 0216T, 0228T, 0230T, 12001-12007, 12011-12057, 13100-13133, 13151-13153, 33210-33211, 36000, 36400-36410, 36420-36430, 36440, 36591-36592, 36600, 36640, 43752, 51701-51703, 62320-62327, 64400-64410, 64413-64435, 64445-64450, 64461-64463, 64479-64505, 64510-64530, 69990, 76376-76377, 92012-92014, 93000-93010, 93040-93042, 93318, 93355, 94002, 94200, 94250, 94680-94690, 94770, 95812-95816, 95819, 95822, 95829, 95955, 96360-96368, 96372, 96374-96377, 96523, 99155, 99156, 99157, 99211-99223, 99231-99255, 99291-99292, 99304-99310, 99315-99316, 99334-99337, 99347-99350, 99374-99375, 99377-99378, 99446-99449

0524T 0213T, 0216T, 0228T, 0230T, 12001-12007, 12011-12057, 13100-13133, 13151-13153, 29581, 35201-35207, 35211-35286, 36000, 36002-36012, 36400-36410, 36420-36430, 36440, 36474, 36476, 36479, 36591-36592, 36600, 36640, 37241, 43752, 51701-51703, 62320-62327, 64400-64410, 64413-64435, 64445-64450, 64461-64463, 64479-64505, 64510-64530, 69990, 75894, 76000, 76380, 76937, 76940, 76942, 76970, 76998, 77002, 77012-77013, 77021-77022, 92012-92014, 93000-93010, 93040-93042, 93318, 93355, 93970-93971, 94002, 94200, 94250, 94680-94690, 94770, 95812-95816, 95819, 95822, 95829, 95955, 96360-96368, 96372, 96374-96377, 96523, 99155, 99156, 99157, 99211-99223, 99231-99255, 99291-99292, 99304-99310, 99315-99316, 99334-99337, 99347-99350, 99374-99375, 99377-99378, 99446-99449, 99495-99496, G0463-J2001

0525T 00530, 00534, 0213T, 0216T, 0228T, 0230T, 0295T-0298T, 0417T-0418T, 0462T-0463T, 0526T-0527T, 0528T, 0529T, 11000-11006, 11042-11047, 12001-12007, 12011-12057, 13100-13133, 13151-13153, 36000, 36005-36013, 36140, 36400-36410, 36420-36430, 36440, 36555-36556, 36568-36569, 36591-36592, 36600, 36640, 43752, 51701-51703, 61650, 62320-62327, 64400-64410, 64413-64435, 64445-64450, 64461, 64463, 64479, 64483, 64486-64490, 64493, 64505, 64510-64530, 69990, 76000, 76942, 76970, 76998, 77001-77002, 92960-92961, 93000-93010, 93040-93042, 93050, 93224-93229, 93268, 93270-93272, 93279, 93285-93286, 93288, 93290-93293, 93296-93297, 93299, 93318, 93355, 93602, 94002, 94200, 94250, 94680-94690, 94770, 95812-95816, 95819, 95822, 95829, 95955, 96360, 96365, 96372, 96374-96377, 96523, 97597-97598, 97602, 99155, 99156, 99157, 99446-99449, G0471

0526T 00530, 00534, 0213T, 0216T, 0228T, 0230T, 0295T-0298T, 0417T-0418T, 0462T-0463T, 0528T, 0529T, 11000-11006, 11042-11047, 12001-12007, 12011-12057, 13100-13133, 13151-13153, 36000, 36005-36013, 36140, 36400-36410, 36420-36430, 36440, 36555-36556, 36568-36569, 36591-36592, 36600, 36640, 43752, 51701-51703, 61650, 62320-62327, 64400-64410, 64413-64435, 64445-64450, 64461, 64463, 64479, 64483, 64486-64490, 64493, 64505, 64510-64530, 69990, 76000, 76942, 76970, 76998, 77001-77002, 92960-92961, 93000-93010, 93040-93042, 93224-93229, 93268, 93270-93272, 93279, 93285-93286, 93288, 93290-93293, 93296-93297, 93299, 93318, 93355, 94002, 94200,

94250, 94680-94690, 94770, 95812-95816, 95819, 95822, 95829, 95955, 96360, 96365, 96372, 96374-96377, 96523, 97597-97598, 97602, 99155, 99156, 99157, 99446-99449, G0471

0527T 00530, 00534, 0213T, 0216T, 0228T, 0230T, 0295T-0298T, 0417T-0418T, 0462T-0463T, 0526T, 0528T, 0529T, 11000-11006, 11042-11047, 12001-12007, 12011-12057, 13100-13133, 13151-13153, 36000, 36005, 36400-36410, 36420-36430, 36440, 36591-36592, 36600, 36640, 43752, 51701-51703, 61650, 62320-62327, 64400-64410, 64413-64435, 64445-64450, 64461, 64463, 64479, 64483, 64486-64490, 64493, 64505, 64510-64530, 69990, 76000, 76942, 76970, 76998, 92960-92961, 93000-93010, 93040-93042, 93224-93229, 93268, 93270-93272, 93279, 93285-93286, 93288, 93290-93293, 93296-93297, 93299, 93318, 93355, 94002, 94200, 94250, 94680-94690, 94770, 95812-95816, 95819, 95822, 95829, 95955, 96360, 96365, 96372, 96374-96377, 96523, 97597-97598, 97602, 99155, 99156, 99157, 99446-99449, G0471

0528T 0295T-0298T, 0418T, 0463T, 0529T, 36591-36592, 93000-93010, 93040-93042, 93224-93229, 93268, 93270-93272, 93285-93288, 93291, 96523, 99446-99449

0529T 36591-36592, 93000-93010, 93286, 93296, 93299, 96523, 99446-99449

0530T 00530, 00534, 0213T, 0216T, 0228T, 0230T, 0415T-0418T, 0462T-0463T, 0528T, 0529T, 11000-11006, 11042-11047, 12001-12007, 12011-12057, 13100-13133, 13151-13153, 33210-33211, 33215, 36000, 36005-36013, 36140, 36400-36410, 36420-36430, 36440, 36555-36556, 36568-36569, 36591-36592, 36600, 36640, 43752, 51701-51703, 61650, 62320-62327, 64400-64410, 64413-64435, 64445-64450, 64461, 64463, 64479, 64483, 64486-64490, 64493, 64505, 64510-64530, 69990, 76000, 76942, 76970, 76998, 77001-77002, 92960-92961, 93000-93010, 93040-93042, 93260-93261, 93279, 93280, 93281-93299, 93318, 93355, 94002, 94200, 94250, 94680-94690, 94770, 95812-95816, 95819, 95822, 95829, 95955, 96360, 96365, 96372, 96374-96377, 96523, 97597-97598, 97602, 99155, 99156, 99157, 99446-99449, G0471

0531T 00530, 00534, 0213T, 0216T, 0228T, 0230T, 0415T-0418T, 0462T-0463T, 0528T, 0529T, 11000-11006, 11042-11047, 12001-12007, 12011-12057, 13100-13133, 13151-13153, 33210-33211, 33215, 36000, 36005-36013, 36140, 36400-36410, 36420-36430, 36440, 36555-36556, 36568-36569, 36591-36592, 36600, 36640, 43752, 51701-51703, 61650, 62320-62327, 64400-64410, 64413-64435, 64445-64450, 64461, 64463, 64479, 64483, 64486-64490, 64493, 64505, 64510-64530, 69990, 76000, 76942, 76970, 76998, 77001-77002, 92960-92961, 93000-93010, 93040-93042, 93260-93261, 93279, 93280, 93281-93299, 93318, 93355, 94002, 94200, 94250, 94680-94690, 94770, 95812-95816, 95819, 95822, 95829, 95955, 96360, 96365, 96372, 96374-96377, 96523, 97597-97598, 97602, 99155, 99156, 99157, 99446-99449, G0471

0532T 00530, 00534, 0213T, 0216T, 0228T, 0230T, 0415T-0418T, 0462T-0463T, 0528T, 0529T, 11000-11006, 11042-11047, 12001-12007, 12011-12057, 13100-13133, 13151-13153, 33210-33211, 33215, 36000, 36005-36013, 36140, 36400-36410, 36420-36430, 36440, 36555-36556, 36568-36569, 36591-36592, 36600, 36640, 43752, 51701-51703, 61650, 62320-62327, 64400-64410, 64413-64435, 64445-64450, 64461, 64463, 64479, 64483, 64486-64490, 64493, 64505, 64510-64530, 69990, 76000, 76942, 76970, 76998, 77001-77002, 92960-92961, 93000-93010, 93040-93042, 93260-93261, 93279, 93280, 93281-93299, 93318, 93355, 94002, 94200, 94250, 94680-94690, 94770, 95812-95816, 95819, 95822, 95829, 95955, 96360, 96365, 96372, 96374-96377, 96523, 97597-97598, 97602, 99155, 99156, 99157, 99446-99449, G0471

0543T No CCI edits apply to this code.

0544T No CCI edits apply to this code.

0545T No CCI edits apply to this code.

0553T No CCI edits apply to this code.

0559T No CCI edits apply to this code.

0560T No CCI edits apply to this code.

0561T No CCI edits apply to this code.

0562T No CCI edits apply to this code.

0569T No CCI edits apply to this code.

0570T No CCI edits apply to this code.

0571T No CCI edits apply to this code.

0572T No CCI edits apply to this code.

0573T No CCI edits apply to this code.

0574T No CCI edits apply to this code.

0575T No CCI edits apply to this code.

0576T No CCI edits apply to this code.

0577T No CCI edits apply to this code.

0578T No CCI edits apply to this code.

0579T No CCI edits apply to this code.

0580T No CCI edits apply to this code.

20101 0213T, 0216T, 0228T, 0230T, 11000, 11042-11044, 12001-12007, 12011-12057, 13100-13133, 13151-13152, 13160, 36000, 36400-36410, 36420-36430, 36440, 36591-36592, 36600, 36640, 43752, 51701-51703, 62320-62327, 64400-64410, 64413-64435, 64445-64450, 64461-64463, 64479-64505, 64510-64530, 69990, 92012-92014, 93000-93010, 93040-93042, 93318, 93355, 94002, 94200, 94250, 94680-94690, 94770, 95812-95816, 95819, 95822, 95829, 95955, 96360-96368, 96372, 96374-96377, 96523, 97597-97598, 97602-97608, 99155, 99156, 99157, 99211-99223, 99231-99255, 99291-99292, 99304-99310, 99315-99316, 99334-99337, 99347-99350, 99374-99375, 99377-99378, 99446-99449, 99451-99452, 99495-99496, G0168-J2001

20985 0213T, 0216T, 36000, 36410, 36591-36592, 61650, 62324-62327, 64415-64417, 64450, 64486-64490, 64493, 69990, 76000, 76380, 76942, 76970, 76998, 77001-77002, 77011-77012, 77021, 96360, 96365, 96372, 96374-96377, 96523

21501 0213T, 0216T, 0228T, 0230T, 10030, 10060, 10140, 10160, 12001-12007, 12011-12057, 13100-13133, 13151-13153, 20100-20101, 21555, 35800, 36000, 36400-36410, 36420-36430, 36440, 36591-36592, 36600, 36640, 43752, 49185, 49424, 51701-51703, 62320-62327, 64400-64410, 64413-64435, 64445-64450, 64461-64463, 64479-64505, 64510-64530, 69990, 92012-92014, 93000-93010, 93040-93042, 93318, 93355, 94002, 94200, 94250, 94680-94690, 94770, 95812-95816, 95819, 95822, 95829, 95955, 96360-96368, 96372, 96374-96377, 96523, 97597-97598, 97602-97608, 99155, 99156, 99157, 99211-99223, 99231-99255, 99291-99292, 99304-99310, 99315-99316, 99334-99337, 99347-99350, 99374-99375, 99377-99378, 99446-99449, 99451-99452, 99495-99496, G0463-J2001

21502 0213T, 0216T, 0228T, 0230T, 10030, 10060, 10140, 10160, 11000-11006, 11010-11011, 11042-11047, 12001-12007, 12011-12057, 13100-13133, 13151-13153, 20101, 20220, 21501, 36000, 36400-36410, 36420-36430, 36440, 36591-36592, 36600, 36640, 43752, 51701-51703, 62320-62327, 64400-64410, 64413-64435, 64445-64450, 64461-64463, 64479-64505, 64510-64530, 69990, 92012-92014, 93000-93010, 93040-93042, 93318, 93355, 94002, 94200, 94250, 94680-94690, 94770, 95812-95816, 95819, 95822, 95829, 95955, 96360-96368, 96372, 96374-96377, 96523, 97597-97598, 97602-97608, 99155, 99156, 99157, 99211-99223, 99231-99255, 99291-99292, 99304-99310,

99315-99316, 99334-99337, 99347-99350, 99374-99375, 99377-99378, 99446-99449, 99451-99452, 99495-99496, G0463-G0471

21510 00550, 0213T, 0216T, 0228T, 0230T, 10030, 10060, 10140, 10160, 11010-11011, 12001-12007, 12011-12057, 13100-13133, 13151-13153, 20101, 20615, 36000, 36400-36410, 36420-36430, 36440, 36591-36592, 36600, 36640, 43752, 51701-51703, 62320-62327, 64400-64410, 64413-64435, 64445-64450, 64461-64463, 64479-64505, 64510-64530, 69990, 92012-92014, 93000-93010, 93040-93042, 93318, 93355, 94002, 94200, 94250, 94680-94690, 94770, 95812-95816, 95819, 95822, 95829, 95955, 96360-96368, 96372, 96374-96377, 96523, 97597-97598, 97602-97608, 99155, 99156, 99157, 99211-99223, 99231-99255, 99291-99292, 99304-99310, 99315-99316, 99334-99337, 99347-99350, 99374-99375, 99377-99378, 99446-99449, 99451-99452, 99495-99496, G0463-G0471

21550 0213T, 0216T, 0228T, 0230T, 10005, 10007, 10009, 10011, 10021, 10030, 10060, 10140, 10160, 12001-12007, 12011-12057, 13100-13133, 13151-13153, 20100, 36000, 36400-36410, 36420-36430, 36440, 36591-36592, 36600, 36640, 38500, 38531, 43752, 51701-51703, 62320-62327, 64400-64410, 64413-64435, 64445-64450, 64461-64463, 64479-64505, 64510-64530, 69990, 92012-92014, 93000-93010, 93040-93042, 93318, 93355, 94002, 94200, 94250, 94680-94690, 94770, 95812-95816, 95819, 95822, 95829, 95955, 96360-96368, 96372, 96374-96377, 96523, 99155, 99156, 99157, 99211-99223, 99231-99255, 99291-99292, 99304-99310, 99315-99316, 99334-99337, 99347-99350, 99374-99375, 99377-99378, 99446-99449, 99451-99452, 99495-99496, G0463-J2001

21552 0213T, 0216T, 0228T, 0230T, 10005, 10007, 10009, 10011, 10021, 10030, 10060, 10140, 10160, 11000-11006, 11010-11012❖, 11042-11047, 12001-12007, 12011-12057, 13100-13133, 13151-13153, 21501, 21550, 21555, 36000, 36400-36410, 36420-36430, 36440, 36591-36592, 36600, 36640, 38500-38520❖, 38531-38555❖, 38700❖, 38720❖, 38724❖, 43752, 51701-51703, 62320-62327, 64400-64410, 64413-64435, 64445-64450, 64461-64463, 64479-64505, 64510-64530, 69990, 92012-92014, 93000-93010, 93040-93042, 93318, 93355, 94002, 94200, 94250, 94680-94690, 94770, 95812-95816, 95819, 95822, 95829, 95955, 96360-96368, 96372, 96374-96377, 96523, 97597-97598, 97602, 99155, 99156, 99157, 99211-99223, 99231-99255, 99291-99292, 99304-99310, 99315-99316, 99334-99337, 99347-99350, 99374-99375, 99377-99378, 99446-99449, 99451-99452, 99495-99496, G0463-J2001

21554 0213T, 0216T, 0228T, 0230T, 10005, 10007, 10009, 10011, 10021, 10030, 10060, 10140, 10160, 11000-11006, 11010-11012❖, 11042-11047, 12001-12007, 12011-12057, 13100-13133, 13151-13153, 21501, 21550-21552, 21555-21556, 36000, 36400-36410, 36420-36430, 36440, 36591-36592, 36600, 36640, 38500-38520❖, 38531-38555❖, 38700❖, 38720❖, 38724❖, 43752, 51701-51703, 62320-62327, 64400-64410, 64413-64435, 64445-64450, 64461-64463, 64479-64505, 64510-64530, 69990, 92012-92014, 93000-93010, 93040-93042, 93318, 93355, 94002, 94200, 94250, 94680-94690, 94770, 95812-95816, 95819, 95822, 95829, 95955, 96360-96368, 96372, 96374-96377, 96523, 97597-97598, 97602, 99155, 99156, 99157, 99211-99223, 99231-99255, 99291-99292, 99304-99310, 99315-99316, 99334-99337, 99347-99350, 99374-99375, 99377-99378, 99446-99449, 99451-99452, 99495-99496, G0463-G0471

21555 0228T, 0230T, 10005, 10007, 10009, 10011, 10021, 10030, 10060, 10140, 10160, 11000-11006, 11010-11012❖, 11042-11047, 12001-12007, 12011-12057, 13100-13133, 13151-13153, 21550, 36000, 36400-36410, 36420-36430, 36440, 36591-36592, 36600, 36640, 38500-38520❖, 38531-38555❖, 38700❖, 38720❖, 38724❖, 43752, 51701-51703, 62320-62327, 64400-64410, 64413-64435, 64445-64450, 64461-64463, 64479-64505, 64510-64530, 69990, 92012-92014, 93000-93010, 93040-93042, 93318, 93355, 94002, 94200, 94250, 94680-94690, 94770, 95812-95816, 95819, 95822, 95829, 95955, 96360-96368, 96372, 96374-96377, 96523, 97597-97598, 97602, 99155, 99156, 99157, 99211-99223, 99231-99255, 99291-99292, 99304-99310, 99315-99316, 99334-99337, 99347-99350, 99374-99375, 99377-99378, 99446-99449, 99451-99452, 99495-99496, G0463-J2001

21556 0228T, 0230T, 10005, 10007, 10009, 10011, 10021, 10030, 10060, 10140, 10160, 11000-11006, 11010-11012❖, 11042-11047, 12001-12007, 12011-12057, 13100-13133, 13151-13153, 21501, 21550-21552, 21555, 36000, 36400-36410, 36420-36430, 36440, 36591-36592, 36600, 36640, 38500-38520❖, 38531-38555❖, 38700❖, 38720❖, 38724❖, 43752, 51701-51703, 62320-62327, 64400-64410, 64413-64435, 64445-64450, 64461-64463, 64479-64505, 64510-64530, 69990, 92012-92014, 93000-93010, 93040-93042, 93318, 93355, 94002, 94200, 94250, 94680-94690, 94770, 95812-95816, 95819, 95822, 95829, 95955, 96360-96368, 96372, 96374-96377, 96523, 97597-97598, 97602, 99155, 99156, 99157, 99211-99223, 99231-99255, 99291-99292, 99304-99310, 99315-99316, 99334-99337, 99347-99350, 99374-99375, 99377-99378, 99446-99449, 99451-99452, 99495-99496, G0463-G0471

21557 0213T, 0216T, 0228T, 0230T, 10005, 10007, 10009, 10011, 10021, 10030, 10060, 10140, 10160, 11000-11006, 11010-11012❖, 11042-11047, 12001-12007, 12011-12057, 13100-13133, 13151-13153, 21501, 21550-21556, 36000, 36400-36410, 36420-36430, 36440, 36591-36592, 36600, 36640, 38500-38520❖, 38531-38555❖, 38700❖, 38720❖, 38724❖, 43752, 51701-51703, 62320-62327, 64400-64410, 64413-64435, 64445-64450, 64461-64463, 64479-64505, 64510-64530, 69990, 92012-92014, 93000-93010, 93040-93042, 93318, 93355, 94002, 94200, 94250, 94680-94690, 94770, 95812-95816, 95819, 95822, 95829, 95955, 96360-96368, 96372, 96374-96377, 96523, 97597-97598, 97602, 99155, 99156, 99157, 99211-99223, 99231-99255, 99291-99292, 99304-99310, 99315-99316, 99334-99337, 99347-99350, 99374-99375, 99377-99378, 99446-99449, 99451-99452, 99495-99496, G0463-G0471

21558 0213T, 0216T, 0228T, 0230T, 10005, 10007, 10009, 10011, 10021, 10030, 10060, 10140, 10160, 11000-11006, 11010-11012❖, 11042-11047, 12001-12007, 12011-12057, 13100-13133, 13151-13153, 21501, 21550-21557, 36000, 36400-36410, 36420-36430, 36440, 36591-36592, 36600, 36640, 38500-38520❖, 38531-38555❖, 38700❖, 38720❖, 38724❖, 43752, 51701-51703, 62320-62327, 64400-64410, 64413-64435, 64445-64450, 64461-64463, 64479-64505, 64510-64530, 69990, 92012-92014, 93000-93010, 93040-93042, 93318, 93355, 94002, 94200, 94250, 94680-94690, 94770, 95812-95816, 95819, 95822, 95829, 95955, 96360-96368, 96372, 96374-96377, 96523, 97597-97598, 97602, 99155, 99156, 99157, 99211-99223, 99231-99255, 99291-99292, 99304-99310, 99315-99316, 99334-99337, 99347-99350, 99374-99375, 99377-99378, 99446-99449, 99451-99452, 99495-99496, G0463-G0471

21600 0213T, 0216T, 0228T, 0230T, 11000-11006, 11012❖, 11042-11047, 12001-12007, 12011-12057, 13100-13133, 13151-13153, 21610, 35820, 36000, 36400-36410, 36420-36430, 36440, 36591-36592, 36600, 36640, 43752, 49010, 51701-51703, 62320-62327, 64400-64410, 64413-64435, 64445-64450, 64461-64463, 64479-64505, 64510-64530, 69990, 92012-92014, 93000-93010, 93040-93042, 93318, 93355, 94002, 94200, 94250, 94680-94690, 94770, 95812-95816, 95819, 95822, 95829, 95955, 96360-96368, 96372, 96374-96377, 96523, 97597-97598, 97602, 99155, 99156, 99157, 99211-99223, 99231-99255, 99291-99292, 99304-99310, 99315-99316, 99334-99337, 99347-99350, 99374-99375, 99377-99378, 99446-99449, 99451-99452, 99495-99496, G0463-G0471

21601 No CCI edits apply to this code.

21602 No CCI edits apply to this code.

21603 No CCI edits apply to this code.

21610 0213T, 0216T, 0228T, 0230T, 11000-11006, 11042-11047, 12001-12007, 12011-12057, 13100-13133, 13151-13153, 20101, 36000, 36400-36410, 36420-36430, 36440, 36591-36592, 36600, 36640, 37616, 43752, 51701-51703, 62320-62327, 64400-64410, 64413-64435, 64445-64450, 64461-64463, 64479-64505, 64510-64530, 69990, 92012-92014, 93000-93010, 93040-93042, 93318, 93355, 94002, 94200, 94250, 94680-94690, 94770, 95812-95816, 95819, 95822, 95829, 95955, 96360-96368, 96372, 96374-96377, 96523, 97597-97598, 97602, 99155, 99156, 99157, 99211-99223, 99231-99255, 99291-99292, 99304-99310, 99315-99316, 99334-99337, 99347-99350, 99374-99375, 99377-99378, 99446-99449, 99451-99452, 99495-99496, G0463-G0471

21615 0213T, 0216T, 0228T, 0230T, 11000-11006, 11042-11047, 12001-12007, 12011-12057, 13100-13133, 13151-13153, 20101, 21600, 21610, 36000, 36400-36410, 36420-36430, 36440, 36591-36592, 36600, 36640, 43752, 51701-51703, 62320-62327, 64400-64410, 64413-64435, 64445-64450, 64461-64463, 64479-64505, 64510-64530, 69990, 92012-92014, 93000-93010, 93040-93042, 93318, 93355, 94002, 94200, 94250, 94680-94690, 94770, 95812-95816, 95819, 95822, 95829, 95955, 96360-96368, 96372, 96374-96377, 96523, 97597-97598, 97602, 99155, 99156, 99157, 99211-99223, 99231-99255, 99291-99292, 99304-99310, 99315-99316, 99334-99337, 99347-99350, 99374-99375, 99377-99378, 99446-99449, 99451-99452, 99495-99496, G0463-G0471

21616 0213T, 0216T, 0228T, 0230T, 11000-11006, 11042-11047, 12001-12007, 12011-12057, 13100-13133, 13151-13153, 20101, 21600, 21610-21615, 36000, 36400-36410, 36420-36430, 36440, 36591-36592, 36600, 36640, 43752, 51701-51703, 62320-62327, 64400-64410, 64413-64435, 64445-64450, 64461-64463, 64479-64505, 64510-64530, 69990, 92012-92014, 93000-93010, 93040-93042, 93318, 93355, 94002, 94200, 94250, 94680-94690, 94770, 95812-95816, 95819, 95822, 95829, 95955, 96360-96368, 96372, 96374-96377, 96523, 97597-97598, 97602, 99155, 99156, 99157, 99211-99223, 99231-99255, 99291-99292, 99304-99310, 99315-99316, 99334-99337, 99347-99350, 99374-99375, 99377-99378, 99446-99449, 99451-99452, 99495-99496, G0463-G0471

21620 00550, 0213T, 0216T, 0228T, 0230T, 11000-11006, 11012✦, 11042-11047, 12001-12007, 12011-12057, 13100-13133, 13151-13153, 20101, 20220-20225, 20240-20245, 21750, 35820, 36000, 36400-36410, 36420-36430, 36440, 36591-36592, 36600, 36640, 43752, 51701-51703, 62320-62327, 64400-64410, 64413-64435, 64445-64450, 64461-64463, 64479-64505, 64510-64530, 69990, 92012-92014, 93000-93010, 93040-93042, 93318, 93355, 94002, 94200, 94250, 94680-94690, 94770, 95812-95816, 95819, 95822, 95829, 95955, 96360-96368, 96372, 96374-96377, 96523, 97597-97598, 97602, 99155, 99156, 99157, 99211-99223, 99231-99255, 99291-99292, 99304-99310, 99315-99316, 99334-99337, 99347-99350, 99374-99375, 99377-99378, 99446-99449, 99451-99452, 99495-99496, G0463-G0471

21627 00550, 0213T, 0216T, 0228T, 0230T, 11012✦, 12001-12007, 12011-12057, 13100-13133, 13151-13153, 20101, 20500, 20670-20680, 35820, 36000, 36400-36410, 36420-36430, 36440, 36591-36592, 36600, 36640, 43752, 51701-51703, 62320-62327, 64400-64410, 64413-64435, 64445-64450, 64461-64463, 64479-64505, 64510-64530, 69990, 92012-92014, 93000-93010, 93040-93042, 93318, 93355, 94002, 94200, 94250, 94680-94690, 94770, 95812-95816, 95819, 95822, 95829, 95955, 96360-96368, 96372, 96374-96377, 96523, 99155, 99156, 99157, 99211-99223, 99231-99255, 99291-99292, 99304-99310, 99315-99316, 99334-99337, 99347-99350, 99374-99375, 99377-99378, 99446-99449, 99451-99452, 99495-99496, G0463-G0471

21630 00550, 0213T, 0216T, 0228T, 0230T, 10030, 10060, 10140, 10160, 11000-11006, 11042-11047, 12001-12007, 12011-12057, 13100-13133, 13151-13153, 20101, 20650, 20670-20680, 21600, 21620-21627, 21750, 35820, 36000, 36400-36410, 36420-36430, 36440, 36591-36592, 36600, 36640, 43752, 51701-51703, 62320-62327, 64400-64410, 64413-64435, 64445-64450, 64461-64463, 64479-64505, 64510-64530, 69990, 92012-92014, 93000-93010, 93040-93042, 93318, 93355, 94002, 94200, 94250, 94680-94690, 94770, 95812-95816, 95819, 95822, 95829, 95955, 96360-96368, 96372, 96374-96377, 96523, 97597-97598, 97602, 99155, 99156, 99157, 99211-99223, 99231-99255, 99291-99292, 99304-99310, 99315-99316, 99334-99337, 99347-99350, 99374-99375, 99377-99378, 99446-99449, 99451-99452, 99495-99496, G0463-G0471

21632 00550, 0213T, 0216T, 0228T, 0230T, 10030, 10060, 10140, 10160, 11000-11006, 11042-11047, 12001-12007, 12011-12057, 13100-13133, 13151-13153, 20101, 20650, 20670-20680, 21600, 21620-21630, 21750, 36000, 36400-36410, 36420-36430, 36440, 36591-36592, 36600, 36640, 43752, 51701-51703, 62320-62327, 64400-64410, 64413-64435, 64445-64450, 64461-64463, 64479-64505, 64510-64530, 69990, 92012-92014, 93000-93010, 93040-93042, 93318, 93355, 94002, 94200, 94250, 94680-94690, 94770, 95812-95816, 95819, 95822, 95829, 95955, 96360-96368, 96372, 96374-96377, 96523, 97597-97598, 97602, 99155, 99156, 99157, 99211-99223, 99231-99255, 99291-99292, 99304-99310, 99315-99316, 99334-99337, 99347-99350, 99374-99375, 99377-99378, 99446-99449, 99451-99452, 99495-99496, G0463-G0471

21700 0213T, 0216T, 0228T, 0230T, 11000-11006, 11012✦, 11042-11047, 12001-12007, 12011-12057, 13100-13133, 13151-13153, 36000, 36400-36410, 36420-36430, 36440, 36591-36592, 36600, 36640, 43752, 51701-51703, 62320-62327, 64400-64410, 64413-64435, 64445-64450, 64461-64463, 64479-64505, 64510-64530, 69990, 92012-92014, 93000-93010, 93040-93042, 93318, 93355, 94002, 94200, 94250, 94680-94690, 94770, 95812-95816, 95819, 95822, 95829, 95955, 96360-96368, 96372, 96374-96377, 96523, 97597-97598, 97602, 99155, 99156, 99157, 99211-99223, 99231-99255, 99291-99292, 99304-99310, 99315-99316, 99334-99337, 99347-99350, 99374-99375, 99377-99378, 99446-99449, 99451-99452, 99495-99496, G0463-J2001

21705 0213T, 0216T, 0228T, 0230T, 11000-11006, 11042-11047, 12001-12007, 12011-12057, 13100-13133, 13151-13153, 21700, 36000, 36400-36410, 36420-36430, 36440, 36591-36592, 36600, 36640, 43752, 51701-51703, 62320-62327, 64400-64410, 64413-64435, 64445-64450, 64461-64463, 64479-64505, 64510-64530, 69990, 92012-92014, 93000-93010, 93040-93042, 93318, 93355, 94002, 94200, 94250, 94680-94690, 94770, 95812-95816, 95819, 95822, 95829, 95955, 96360-96368, 96372, 96374-96377, 96523, 97597-97598, 97602, 99155, 99156, 99157, 99211-99223, 99231-99255, 99291-99292, 99304-99310, 99315-99316, 99334-99337, 99347-99350, 99374-99375, 99377-99378, 99446-99449, 99451-99452, 99495-99496, G0463-G0471

21740 0213T, 0216T, 0228T, 0230T, 12001-12007, 12011-12057, 13100-13133, 13151-13153, 21600, 21610, 21620, 21742-21743, 29000-29015, 29035-29058, 29200, 36000, 36400-36410, 36420-36430, 36440, 36591-36592, 36600, 36640, 43752, 51701-51703, 62320-62327, 64400-64410, 64413-64435, 64445-64450, 64461-64463, 64479-64505, 64510-64530, 69990, 92012-92014, 93000-93010, 93040-93042, 93318, 93355, 94002, 94200, 94250, 94680-94690, 94770, 95812-95816, 95819, 95822, 95829, 95955, 96360-96368, 96372, 96374-96377, 96523, 99155, 99156, 99157, 99211-99223, 99231-99255, 99291-99292, 99304-99310, 99315-99316, 99334-99337, 99347-99350, 99374-99375, 99377-99378, 99446-99449, 99451-99452, 99495-99496, G0463-G0471

21742 0213T, 0216T, 0228T, 0230T, 12001-12007, 12011-12057, 13100-13133, 13151-13153, 21610, 29000-29015, 29035-29058, 29200, 32601, 32604, 32606-32609, 36000, 36400-36410, 36420-36430, 36440, 36591-36592, 36600, 36640, 43752, 51701-51703, 62320-62327, 64400-64410,

64413-64435, 64445-64450, 64461-64463, 64479-64505, 64510-64530, 69990, 92012-92014, 93000-93010, 93040-93042, 93318, 93355, 94002, 94200, 94250, 94680-94690, 94770, 95812-95816, 95819, 95822, 95829, 95955, 96360-96368, 96372, 96374-96377, 96523, 99155, 99156, 99157, 99211-99223, 99231-99255, 99291-99292, 99304-99310, 99315-99316, 99334-99337, 99347-99350, 99374-99375, 99377-99378, 99446-99449, 99451-99452, 99495-99496, G0463-G0471

21743 0213T, 0216T, 0228T, 0230T, 12001-12007, 12011-12057, 13100-13133, 13151-13153, 21610, 21742❖, 29000-29015, 29035-29058, 29200, 32601, 32604, 32606-32609, 36000, 36400-36410, 36420-36430, 36440, 36591-36592, 36600, 36640, 43752, 51701-51703, 62320-62327, 64400-64410, 64413-64435, 64445-64450, 64461-64463, 64479-64505, 64510-64530, 69990, 92012-92014, 93000-93010, 93040-93042, 93318, 93355, 94002, 94200, 94250, 94680-94690, 94770, 95812-95816, 95819, 95822, 95829, 95955, 96360-96368, 96372, 96374-96377, 96523, 99155, 99156, 99157, 99211-99223, 99231-99255, 99291-99292, 99304-99310, 99315-99316, 99334-99337, 99347-99350, 99374-99375, 99377-99378, 99446-99449, 99451-99452, 99495-99496, G0463-G0471

21750 00550, 0213T, 0216T, 0228T, 0230T, 11000-11006, 11042-11047, 12001-12007, 12011-12057, 13100-13133, 13151-13153, 20650, 20670-20680, 21627, 35820, 36000, 36400-36410, 36420-36430, 36440, 36591-36592, 36600, 36640, 43752, 51701-51703, 62320-62327, 64400-64410, 64413-64435, 64445-64450, 64461-64463, 64479-64505, 64510-64530, 69990, 92012-92014, 93000-93010, 93040-93042, 93318, 93355, 94002, 94200, 94250, 94680-94690, 94770, 95812-95816, 95819, 95822, 95829, 95955, 96360-96368, 96372, 96374-96377, 96523, 97597-97598, 97602, 99155, 99156, 99157, 99211-99223, 99231-99255, 99291-99292, 99304-99310, 99315-99316, 99334-99337, 99347-99350, 99374-99375, 99377-99378, 99446-99449, 99451-99452, 99495-99496, G0463-G0471

21811 0213T, 0216T, 0228T, 0230T, 12001-12007, 12011-12057, 13100-13133, 13151-13153, 20650, 20690, 20692, 20696, 29200, 29700-29710, 32601, 36000, 36400-36410, 36420-36430, 36440, 36591-36592, 36600, 36640, 43752, 51701-51703, 62320-62327, 64400-64410, 64413-64435, 64445-64450, 64461-64463, 64479-64505, 64510-64530, 69990, 92012-92014, 93000-93010, 93040-93042, 93318, 93355, 94002, 94200, 94250, 94680-94690, 94770, 95812-95816, 95819, 95822, 95829, 95955, 96360-96368, 96372, 96374-96377, 96523, 97597-97598, 97602-97608, 99155, 99156, 99157, 99211-99223, 99231-99255, 99291-99292, 99304-99310, 99315-99316, 99334-99337, 99347-99350, 99374-99375, 99377-99378, 99446-99449, 99451-99452, 99495-99496, G0463-G0471

21812 0213T, 0216T, 0228T, 0230T, 12001-12007, 12011-12057, 13100-13133, 13151-13153, 20650, 20690, 20692, 20696, 21811, 29200, 29700-29710, 32601, 36000, 36400-36410, 36420-36430, 36440, 36591-36592, 36600, 36640, 43752, 51701-51703, 62320-62327, 64400-64410, 64413-64435, 64445-64450, 64461-64463, 64479-64505, 64510-64530, 69990, 92012-92014, 93000-93010, 93040-93042, 93318, 93355, 94002, 94200, 94250, 94680-94690, 94770, 95812-95816, 95819, 95822, 95829, 95955, 96360-96368, 96372, 96374-96377, 96523, 97597-97598, 97602-97608, 99155, 99156, 99157, 99211-99223, 99231-99255, 99291-99292, 99304-99310, 99315-99316, 99334-99337, 99347-99350, 99374-99375, 99377-99378, 99446-99449, 99451-99452, 99495-99496, G0463-G0471

21813 0213T, 0216T, 0228T, 0230T, 12001-12007, 12011-12057, 13100-13133, 13151-13153, 20650, 20690, 20692, 20696, 21811-21812, 29200, 29700-29710, 32601, 36000, 36400-36410, 36420-36430, 36440, 36591-36592, 36600, 36640, 43752, 51701-51703, 62320-62327, 64400-64410, 64413-64435, 64445-64450, 64461-64463, 64479-64505, 64510-64530, 69990, 92012-92014, 93000-93010, 93040-93042, 93318, 93355, 94002, 94200, 94250, 94680-94690, 94770, 95812-95816, 95819, 95822, 95829, 95955, 96360-96368, 96372, 96374-96377, 96523, 97597-97598, 97602-97608, 99155, 99156, 99157, 99211-99223, 99231-99255, 99291-99292, 99304-99310, 99315-99316, 99334-99337, 99347-99350, 99374-99375, 99377-99378, 99446-99449, 99451-99452, 99495-99496, G0463-G0471

21820 00550, 0213T, 0216T, 0228T, 0230T, 12001-12007, 12011-12057, 13100-13133, 13151-13153, 21750, 29200, 29700-29710, 36000, 36400-36410, 36420-36430, 36440, 36591-36592, 36600, 36640, 43752, 51701-51703, 62320-62327, 64400-64410, 64413-64435, 64445-64450, 64461-64463, 64479-64505, 64510-64530, 69990, 92012-92014, 93000-93010, 93040-93042, 93318, 93355, 94002, 94200, 94250, 94680-94690, 94770, 95812-95816, 95819, 95822, 95829, 95955, 96360-96368, 96372, 96374-96377, 96523, 97597-97598, 97602-97608, 99155, 99156, 99157, 99211-99223, 99231-99255, 99291-99292, 99304-99310, 99315-99316, 99334-99337, 99347-99350, 99374-99375, 99377-99378, 99446-99449, 99451-99452, 99495-99496, G0463-G0471

21825 00550, 0213T, 0216T, 0228T, 0230T, 12001-12007, 12011-12057, 13100-13133, 13151-13153, 20650, 20690, 20692, 20696-20697, 21750, 21820, 29200, 29700-29710, 36000, 36400-36410, 36420-36430, 36440, 36591-36592, 36600, 36640, 43752, 51701-51703, 62320-62327, 64400-64410, 64413-64435, 64445-64450, 64461-64463, 64479-64505, 64510-64530, 69990, 92012-92014, 93000-93010, 93040-93042, 93318, 93355, 94002, 94200, 94250, 94680-94690, 94770, 95812-95816, 95819, 95822, 95829, 95955, 96360-96368, 96372, 96374-96377, 96523, 97597-97598, 97602-97608, 99155, 99156, 99157, 99211-99223, 99231-99255, 99291-99292, 99304-99310, 99315-99316, 99334-99337, 99347-99350, 99374-99375, 99377-99378, 99446-99449, 99451-99452, 99495-99496, G0463-G0471

31500 00320, 00326, 12001-12007, 12011-12057, 13100-13133, 13151-13153, 31505, 31510-31531, 31536-31541, 31560-31578, 36000, 36400-36410, 36420-36430, 36440, 36591-36592, 36600, 36640, 43752, 51701-51703, 64461-64463, 64486-64495, 69990, 71045-71047, 92012-92014, 92502, 93000-93010, 93040-93042, 93318, 93355, 94002, 94200, 94250, 94680-94690, 94770, 95812-95816, 95819, 95822, 95829, 95955, 96360-96368, 96372, 96374-96377, 96523, 99155, 99156, 99157, 99211-99223, 99231-99255, 99291-99292, 99304-99310, 99315-99316, 99334-99337, 99347-99350, 99374-99375, 99377-99378, 99446-99449, 99451-99452, 99495-99496, G0463-J2001

31515 00326, 0213T, 0216T, 0228T, 0230T, 12001-12007, 12011-12057, 13100-13133, 13151-13153, 31505, 31575❖, 36000, 36400-36410, 36420-36430, 36440, 36591-36592, 36600, 36640, 43752, 51701-51703, 62320-62327, 64400-64410, 64413-64435, 64445-64450, 64461-64463, 64479-64505, 64510-64530, 69990, 76000, 77001-77002, 92012-92014, 92502, 92511, 93000-93010, 93040-93042, 93318, 93355, 94002, 94200, 94250, 94680-94690, 94770, 95812-95816, 95819, 95822, 95829, 95955, 96360-96368, 96372, 96374-96377, 96523, 99155, 99156, 99157, 99211-99223, 99231-99255, 99291-99292, 99304-99310, 99315-99316, 99334-99337, 99347-99350, 99374-99375, 99377-99378, 99446-99449, 99451-99452, 99495-99496, G0463-J2001

31520 00320, 00326, 0213T, 0216T, 0228T, 0230T, 12001-12007, 12011-12057, 13100-13133, 13151-13153, 31505, 31575❖, 36000, 36400-36410, 36420-36430, 36440, 36591-36592, 36600, 36640, 43752, 51701-51703, 62320-62327, 64400-64410, 64413-64435, 64445-64450, 64461-64463, 64479-64505, 64510-64530, 69990, 76000, 77001-77002, 92012-92014, 92502, 92511, 93000-93010, 93040-93042, 93318, 93355, 94002, 94200, 94250, 94680-94690, 94770, 95812-95816, 95819, 95822, 95829, 95955, 96360-96368, 96372, 96374-96377, 96523, 99155,

99156, 99157, 99211-99223, 99231-99255, 99291-99292, 99304-99310, 99315-99316, 99334-99337, 99347-99350, 99374-99375, 99377-99378, 99446-99449, 99451-99452, 99495-99496, G0463-G0471

31525 00320, 00326, 0213T, 0216T, 0228T, 0230T, 12001-12007, 12011-12057, 13100-13133, 13151-13153, 31505, 31575❖, 36000, 36400-36410, 36420-36430, 36440, 36591-36592, 36600, 36640, 42800, 42806, 43752, 51701-51703, 62320-62327, 64400-64410, 64413-64435, 64445-64450, 64461-64463, 64479-64505, 64510-64530, 69990, 76000, 77001-77002, 92012-92014, 92502, 92511, 93000-93010, 93040-93042, 93318, 93355, 94002, 94200, 94250, 94680-94690, 94770, 95812-95816, 95819, 95822, 95829, 95955, 96360-96368, 96372, 96374-96377, 96523, 99155, 99156, 99157, 99211-99223, 99231-99255, 99291-99292, 99304-99310, 99315-99316, 99334-99337, 99347-99350, 99374-99375, 99377-99378, 99446-99449, 99451-99452, 99495-99496, G0463-J2001

31526 00320, 00326, 0213T, 0216T, 0228T, 0230T, 12001-12007, 12011-12057, 13100-13133, 13151-13153, 31505, 31575❖, 36000, 36400-36410, 36420-36430, 36440, 36591-36592, 36600, 36640, 43752, 51701-51703, 62320-62327, 64400-64410, 64413-64435, 64445-64450, 64461-64463, 64479-64505, 64510-64530, 69990, 76000, 77001-77002, 92012-92014, 92502, 92511, 93000-93010, 93040-93042, 93318, 93355, 94002, 94200, 94250, 94680-94690, 94770, 95812-95816, 95819, 95822, 95829, 95955, 96360-96368, 96372, 96374-96377, 96523, 99155, 99156, 99157, 99211-99223, 99231-99255, 99291-99292, 99304-99310, 99315-99316, 99334-99337, 99347-99350, 99374-99375, 99377-99378, 99446-99449, 99451-99452, 99495-99496, G0463-G0471

31527 00326, 0213T, 0216T, 0228T, 0230T, 11000-11006, 11042-11047, 12001-12007, 12011-12057, 13100-13133, 13151-13153, 31505, 31525, 31575❖, 36000, 36400-36410, 36420-36430, 36440, 36591-36592, 36600, 36640, 43752, 51701-51703, 62320-62327, 64400-64410, 64413-64435, 64445-64450, 64461-64463, 64479-64505, 64510-64530, 69990, 76000, 77001-77002, 92012-92014, 92502, 92511, 93000-93010, 93040-93042, 93318, 93355, 94002, 94200, 94250, 94680-94690, 94770, 95812-95816, 95819, 95822, 95829, 95955, 96360-96368, 96372, 96374-96377, 96523, 97597-97598, 97602, 99155, 99156, 99157, 99211-99223, 99231-99255, 99291-99292, 99304-99310, 99315-99316, 99334-99337, 99347-99350, 99374-99375, 99377-99378, 99446-99449, 99451-99452, 99495-99496, G0463-G0471

31528 00320, 00326, 0213T, 0216T, 0228T, 0230T, 12001-12007, 12011-12057, 13100-13133, 13151-13153, 31505, 31525, 31529❖, 31575❖, 36000, 36400-36410, 36420-36430, 36440, 36591-36592, 36600, 36640, 43752, 51701-51703, 62320-62327, 64400-64410, 64413-64435, 64445-64450, 64461-64463, 64479-64505, 64510-64530, 69990, 76000, 77001-77002, 92012-92014, 92502, 92511, 93000-93010, 93040-93042, 93318, 93355, 94002, 94200, 94250, 94680-94690, 94770, 95812-95816, 95819, 95822, 95829, 95955, 96360-96368, 96372, 96374-96377, 96523, 99155, 99156, 99157, 99211-99223, 99231-99255, 99291-99292, 99304-99310, 99315-99316, 99334-99337, 99347-99350, 99374-99375, 99377-99378, 99446-99449, 99451-99452, 99495-99496, G0463-G0471

31529 00320, 00326, 0213T, 0216T, 0228T, 0230T, 12001-12007, 12011-12057, 13100-13133, 13151-13153, 31505, 31525, 31575❖, 36000, 36400-36410, 36420-36430, 36440, 36591-36592, 36600, 36640, 43752, 51701-51703, 62320-62327, 64400-64410, 64413-64435, 64445-64450, 64461-64463, 64479-64505, 64510-64530, 69990, 76000, 77001-77002, 92012-92014, 92502, 92511, 93000-93010, 93040-93042, 93318, 93355, 94002, 94200, 94250, 94680-94690, 94770, 95812-95816, 95819, 95822, 95829, 95955, 96360-96368, 96372, 96374-96377, 96523, 99155, 99156, 99157, 99211-99223, 99231-99255, 99291-99292, 99304-99310, 99315-99316, 99334-99337, 99347-99350, 99374-99375, 99377-99378, 99446-99449, 99451-99452, 99495-99496, G0463-G0471

31592 00520, 0213T, 0216T, 0228T, 0230T, 11000-11006, 11042-11047, 12001-12007, 12011-12057, 13100-13133, 13151-13153, 14040-14041, 14301, 15574, 15620, 15650, 15733, 15756, 15760, 20926, 31600-31601, 31780-31781❖, 31800, 31820-31830, 36000, 36400-36410, 36420-36430, 36440, 36591-36592, 36600, 36640, 43752, 51701-51703, 62320-62327, 64400-64410, 64413-64435, 64445-64450, 64461-64463, 64479-64505, 64510-64530, 69990, 92012-92014, 92502, 93000-93010, 93040-93042, 93318, 93355, 94002, 94200, 94250, 94680-94690, 94770, 95812-95816, 95819, 95822, 95829, 95955, 96360-96368, 96372, 96374-96377, 96523, 97597-97598, 97602, 99155, 99156, 99157, 99211-99223, 99231-99255, 99291-99292, 99304-99310, 99315-99316, 99334-99337, 99347-99350, 99374-99375, 99377-99378, 99446-99449, 99451-99452, 99495-99496, G0463-J2001

31600 00320, 00326, 00520, 0213T, 0216T, 0228T, 0230T, 12001-12007, 12011-12057, 13100-13133, 13151-13153, 31603-31605, 31622, 31634, 31647, 36000, 36400-36410, 36420-36430, 36440, 36591-36592, 36600, 36640, 43752, 51701-51703, 62320-62327, 64400-64410, 64413-64435, 64445-64450, 64461-64463, 64479-64505, 64510-64530, 69990, 92012-92014, 92502, 93000-93010, 93040-93042, 93318, 93355, 94002, 94200, 94250, 94680-94690, 94770, 95812-95816, 95819, 95822, 95829, 95955, 96360-96368, 96372, 96374-96377, 96523, 99155, 99156, 99157, 99211-99223, 99231-99255, 99291-99292, 99304-99310, 99315-99316, 99334-99337, 99347-99350, 99374-99375, 99377-99378, 99446-99449, 99451-99452, 99495-99496, G0463-G0471

31601 00320, 00326, 00520, 0213T, 0216T, 0228T, 0230T, 12001-12007, 12011-12057, 13100-13133, 13151-13153, 31605, 36000, 36400-36410, 36420-36430, 36440, 36591-36592, 36600, 36640, 43752, 51701-51703, 62320-62327, 64400-64410, 64413-64435, 64445-64450, 64461-64463, 64479-64505, 64510-64530, 69990, 92012-92014, 92502, 93000-93010, 93040-93042, 93318, 93355, 94002, 94200, 94250, 94680-94690, 94770, 95812-95816, 95819, 95822, 95829, 95955, 96360-96368, 96372, 96374-96377, 96523, 99155, 99156, 99157, 99211-99223, 99231-99255, 99291-99292, 99304-99310, 99315-99316, 99334-99337, 99347-99350, 99374-99375, 99377-99378, 99446-99449, 99451-99452, 99495-99496, G0463-G0471

31603 00320, 00326, 00520, 0213T, 0216T, 0228T, 0230T, 12001-12007, 12011-12057, 13100-13133, 13151-13153, 31525-31526, 31575, 31610❖, 31613-31614❖, 36000, 36400-36410, 36420-36430, 36440, 36591-36592, 36600, 36640, 43752, 51701-51703, 62320-62327, 64400-64410, 64413-64435, 64445-64450, 64461-64463, 64479-64505, 64510-64530, 69990, 92012-92014, 92502, 93000-93010, 93040-93042, 93318, 93355, 94002, 94200, 94250, 94680-94690, 94770, 95812-95816, 95819, 95822, 95829, 95955, 96360-96368, 96372, 96374-96377, 96523, 99155, 99156, 99157, 99211-99223, 99231-99255, 99291-99292, 99304-99310, 99315-99316, 99334-99337, 99347-99350, 99374-99375, 99377-99378, 99446-99449, 99451-99452, 99495-99496, G0463-G0471

31605 00320, 00326, 00520, 0213T, 0216T, 0228T, 0230T, 12001-12007, 12011-12057, 13100-13133, 13151-13153, 31603❖, 31610❖, 31613-31614❖, 36000, 36400-36410, 36420-36430, 36440, 36591-36592, 36600, 36640, 43752, 51701-51703, 62320-62327, 64400-64410, 64413-64435, 64445-64450, 64461-64463, 64479-64505, 64510-64530, 69990, 92012-92014, 92502, 93000-93010, 93040-93042, 93318, 93355, 94002, 94200, 94250, 94680-94690, 94770, 95812-95816, 95819, 95822, 95829, 95955, 96360-96368, 96372, 96374-96377, 96523, 99155, 99156, 99157, 99211-99223, 99231-99255, 99291-99292, 99304-99310, 99315-99316, 99334-99337, 99347-99350,

99374-99375, 99377-99378, 99446-99449, 99451-99452, 99495-99496, G0463-G0471

31610 00320, 00326, 00520, 0213T, 0216T, 0228T, 0230T, 12001-12007, 12011-12057, 13100-13133, 13151-13153, 31600-31601, 36000, 36400-36410, 36420-36430, 36440, 36591-36592, 36600, 36640, 43752, 51701-51703, 62320-62327, 64400-64410, 64413-64435, 64445-64450, 64461-64463, 64479-64505, 64510-64530, 69990, 92012-92014, 92502, 93000-93010, 93040-93042, 93318, 93355, 94002, 94200, 94250, 94680-94690, 94770, 95812-95816, 95819, 95822, 95829, 95955, 96360-96368, 96372, 96374-96377, 96523, 99155, 99156, 99157, 99211-99223, 99231-99255, 99291-99292, 99304-99310, 99315-99316, 99334-99337, 99347-99350, 99374-99375, 99377-99378, 99446-99449, 99451-99452, 99495-99496, G0463-G0471

31611 00320, 00326, 00520, 0213T, 0216T, 0228T, 0230T, 11000-11006, 11042-11047, 12001-12007, 12011-12057, 13100-13133, 13151-13153, 31525-31526, 31575, 31600-31601, 31614❖, 36000, 36400-36410, 36420-36430, 36440, 36591-36592, 36600, 36640, 43752, 51701-51703, 62320-62327, 64400-64410, 64413-64435, 64445-64450, 64461-64463, 64479-64505, 64510-64530, 69990, 92012-92014, 92502, 93000-93010, 93040-93042, 93318, 93355, 94002, 94200, 94250, 94680-94690, 94770, 95812-95816, 95819, 95822, 95829, 95955, 96360-96368, 96372, 96374-96377, 96523, 97597-97598, 97602, 99155, 99156, 99157, 99211-99223, 99231-99255, 99291-99292, 99304-99310, 99315-99316, 99334-99337, 99347-99350, 99374-99375, 99377-99378, 99446-99449, 99451-99452, 99495-99496, G0463-G0471

31612 00320, 00326, 00520, 0213T, 0216T, 0228T, 0230T, 12001-12007, 12011-12057, 13100-13133, 13151-13153, 31525-31526, 31575, 31600-31605❖, 31610-31611❖, 31613-31614❖, 36000, 36400-36410, 36420-36430, 36440, 36591-36592, 36600, 36640, 43752, 51701-51703, 62320-62327, 64400-64410, 64413-64435, 64445-64450, 64461-64463, 64479-64505, 64510-64530, 69990, 89220, 92012-92014, 92502, 93000-93010, 93040-93042, 93318, 93355, 94002, 94200, 94250, 94680-94690, 94770, 95812-95816, 95819, 95822, 95829, 95955, 96360-96368, 96372, 96374-96377, 96523, 99155, 99156, 99157, 99211-99223, 99231-99255, 99291-99292, 99304-99310, 99315-99316, 99334-99337, 99347-99350, 99374-99375, 99377-99378, 99446-99449, 99451-99452, 99495-99496, G0463-J2001

31613 00320, 00326, 00520, 0213T, 0216T, 0228T, 0230T, 11000-11006, 11042-11047, 12001-12007, 12011-12057, 13100-13133, 13151-13153, 31525-31526, 31575, 31600-31601, 31610-31611❖, 36000, 36400-36410, 36420-36430, 36440, 36591-36592, 36600, 36640, 43752, 51701-51703, 62320-62327, 64400-64410, 64413-64435, 64445-64450, 64461-64463, 64479-64505, 64510-64530, 69990, 92012-92014, 92502, 93000-93010, 93040-93042, 93318, 93355, 94002, 94200, 94250, 94680-94690, 94770, 95812-95816, 95819, 95822, 95829, 95955, 96360-96368, 96372, 96374-96377, 96523, 97597-97598, 97602, 99155, 99156, 99157, 99211-99223, 99231-99255, 99291-99292, 99304-99310, 99315-99316, 99334-99337, 99347-99350, 99374-99375, 99377-99378, 99446-99449, 99451-99452, 99495-99496, G0463-G0471

31614 00320, 00326, 00520, 0213T, 0216T, 0228T, 0230T, 11000-11006, 11042-11047, 12001-12007, 12011-12057, 13100-13133, 13151-13153, 31515, 31525-31526, 31575, 31600-31601, 31610❖, 31613, 36000, 36400-36410, 36420-36430, 36440, 36591-36592, 36600, 36640, 43752, 51701-51703, 62320-62327, 64400-64410, 64413-64435, 64445-64450, 64461-64463, 64479-64505, 64510-64530, 69990, 92012-92014, 92502, 93000-93010, 93040-93042, 93318, 93355, 94002, 94200, 94250, 94680-94690, 94770, 95812-95816, 95819, 95822, 95829, 95955, 96360-96368, 96372, 96374-96377, 96523, 97597-97598, 97602, 99155, 99156, 99157, 99211-99223, 99231-99255, 99291-99292, 99304-99310, 99315-99316, 99334-99337, 99347-99350, 99374-99375, 99377-99378, 99446-99449, 99451-99452, 99495-99496, G0463-G0471

31615 00320, 00326, 00520, 0213T, 0216T, 0228T, 0230T, 12001-12007, 12011-12057, 13100-13133, 13151-13153, 31525-31526, 31575, 31610❖, 31622-31625❖, 31628-31631❖, 31635❖, 31640-31648❖, 31651❖, 31660-31661❖, 31717❖, 31720-31725, 36000, 36400-36410, 36420-36430, 36440, 36591-36592, 36600, 36640, 43752, 51701-51703, 62320-62327, 64400-64410, 64413-64435, 64445-64450, 64461-64463, 64479-64505, 64510-64530, 69990, 76000, 77001-77002, 89220, 92012-92014, 93000-93010, 93040-93042, 93318, 93355, 94002, 94200, 94250, 94680-94690, 94770, 95812-95816, 95819, 95822, 95829, 95955, 96360-96368, 96372, 96374-96377, 96523, 99155, 99156, 99157, 99211-99223, 99231-99255, 99291-99292, 99304-99310, 99315-99316, 99334-99337, 99347-99350, 99374-99375, 99377-99378, 99446-99449, 99451-99452, 99495-99496, G0463-J2001

31622 00520, 0213T, 0216T, 0228T, 0230T, 12001-12007, 12011-12057, 13100-13133, 13151-13153, 31231, 31525, 31535, 31575, 31717, 31720-31725, 36000, 36400-36410, 36420-36430, 36440, 36591-36592, 36600, 36640, 43752, 51701-51703, 62320-62327, 64400-64410, 64413-64435, 64445-64450, 64461-64463, 64479-64505, 64510-64530, 69990, 76000, 77001-77002, 89220, 92012-92014, 92511, 93000-93010, 93040-93042, 93318, 93355, 94002, 94200, 94250, 94680-94690, 94770, 95812-95816, 95819, 95822, 95829, 95955, 96360-96368, 96372, 96374-96377, 96523, 99155, 99156, 99157, 99211-99223, 99231-99255, 99291-99292, 99304-99310, 99315-99316, 99334-99337, 99347-99350, 99374-99375, 99377-99378, 99446-99449, 99451-99452, 99495-99496, G0463-J2001

31623 00520, 00528-00529, 0213T, 0216T, 0228T, 0230T, 12001-12007, 12011-12057, 13100-13133, 13151-13153, 31231, 31525-31526, 31535, 31575, 31622, 31634, 31647, 31717, 31720-31725, 36000, 36400-36410, 36420-36430, 36440, 36591-36592, 36600, 36640, 43752, 51701-51703, 62320-62327, 64400-64410, 64413-64435, 64445-64450, 64461-64463, 64479-64505, 64510-64530, 69990, 76000, 77001-77002, 89220, 92012-92014, 92511, 93000-93010, 93040-93042, 93318, 93355, 94002, 94200, 94250, 94680-94690, 94770, 95812-95816, 95819, 95822, 95829, 95955, 96360-96368, 96372, 96374-96377, 96523, 99155, 99156, 99157, 99211-99223, 99231-99255, 99291-99292, 99304-99310, 99315-99316, 99334-99337, 99347-99350, 99374-99375, 99377-99378, 99446-99449, 99451-99452, 99495-99496, G0463-J2001

31624 00520, 00528-00529, 0213T, 0216T, 0228T, 0230T, 12001-12007, 12011-12057, 13100-13133, 13151-13153, 31231, 31525-31526, 31535, 31575, 31622, 31634, 31647, 31717, 31720-31725, 36000, 36400-36410, 36420-36430, 36440, 36591-36592, 36600, 36640, 43752, 51701-51703, 62320-62327, 64400-64410, 64413-64435, 64445-64450, 64461-64463, 64479-64505, 64510-64530, 69990, 76000, 77001-77002, 89220, 92012-92014, 92511, 93000-93010, 93040-93042, 93318, 93355, 94002, 94200, 94250, 94680-94690, 94770, 95812-95816, 95819, 95822, 95829, 95955, 96360-96368, 96372, 96374-96377, 96523, 99155, 99156, 99157, 99211-99223, 99231-99255, 99291-99292, 99304-99310, 99315-99316, 99334-99337, 99347-99350, 99374-99375, 99377-99378, 99446-99449, 99451-99452, 99495-99496, G0463-J2001

31625 00520, 0213T, 0216T, 0228T, 0230T, 10005, 10007, 10009, 10011, 10021, 12001-12007, 12011-12057, 13100-13133, 13151-13153, 31231, 31525-31526, 31535, 31575, 31622, 31634, 31647, 31717, 31720-31725, 36000, 36400-36410, 36420-36430, 36440, 36591-36592, 36600, 36640, 43752, 51701-51703, 62320-62327, 64400-64410, 64413-64435, 64445-64450, 64461-64463, 64479-64505, 64510-64530, 69990, 76000, 77001-77002, 89220, 92012-92014, 92511, 93000-93010, 93040-93042, 93318, 93355, 94002, 94200, 94250, 94680-94690,

94770, 95812-95816, 95819, 95822, 95829, 95955, 96360-96368, 96372, 96374-96377, 96523, 99155, 99156, 99157, 99211-99223, 99231-99255, 99291-99292, 99304-99310, 99315-99316, 99334-99337, 99347-99350, 99374-99375, 99377-99378, 99446-99449, 99451-99452, 99495-99496, G0463-J2001

31626 00520, 00528-00529, 0213T, 0216T, 0228T, 0230T, 10035-10036❖, 12001-12007, 12011-12057, 13100-13133, 13151-13153, 31231, 31525-31526, 31535, 31575, 31615❖, 31622, 31634, 31643❖, 31647, 31717, 31720-31725, 36000, 36400-36410, 36420-36430, 36440, 36591-36592, 36600, 36640, 43752, 51701-51703, 62320-62327, 64400-64410, 64413-64435, 64445-64450, 64461-64463, 64479-64505, 64510-64530, 69990, 76000, 77001-77002, 89220, 92012-92014, 92511, 93000-93010, 93040-93042, 93318, 93355, 94002, 94200, 94250, 94680-94690, 94770, 95812-95816, 95819, 95822, 95829, 95955, 96360-96368, 96372, 96374-96377, 96523, 99155, 99156, 99157, 99211-99223, 99231-99255, 99291-99292, 99304-99310, 99315-99316, 99334-99337, 99347-99350, 99374-99375, 99377-99378, 99446-99449, 99451-99452, 99495-99496, G0463-J2001

31627 0213T, 0216T, 0228T, 0230T, 36000, 36400-36410, 36420-36430, 36440, 36591-36592, 36600, 36640, 43752, 51701-51703, 61650, 62320-62327, 64400-64410, 64413-64435, 64445-64450, 64461, 64463, 64479, 64483, 64486-64490, 64493, 64505, 64510-64530, 69990, 76000, 76376-76377, 77001-77002, 93000-93010, 93040-93042, 93318, 93355, 94002, 94200, 94250, 94680-94690, 94770, 95812-95816, 95819, 95822, 95829, 95955, 96360, 96365, 96372, 96374-96377, 96523, 99155, 99156, 99157, G0471

31628 00520, 0213T, 0216T, 0228T, 0230T, 10005, 10007, 10009, 10011, 10021, 12001-12007, 12011-12057, 13100-13133, 13151-13153, 31231, 31525-31526, 31535-31541, 31575, 31622, 31625, 31634, 31647, 31717, 31720-31725, 36000, 36400-36410, 36420-36430, 36440, 36591-36592, 36600, 36640, 43752, 51701-51703, 62320-62327, 64400-64410, 64413-64435, 64445-64450, 64461-64463, 64479-64505, 64510-64530, 69990, 76000, 77001-77002, 89220, 92012-92014, 92511, 93000-93010, 93040-93042, 93318, 93355, 94002, 94200, 94250, 94680-94690, 94770, 95812-95816, 95819, 95822, 95829, 95955, 96360-96368, 96372, 96374-96377, 96523, 99155, 99156, 99157, 99211-99223, 99231-99255, 99291-99292, 99304-99310, 99315-99316, 99334-99337, 99347-99350, 99374-99375, 99377-99378, 99446-99449, 99451-99452, 99495-99496, G0463-J2001

31629 00520, 0213T, 0216T, 0228T, 0230T, 10005, 10007, 10009, 10011, 10021, 12001-12007, 12011-12057, 13100-13133, 13151-13153, 31231, 31525-31526, 31535-31541, 31575, 31622, 31625, 31634, 31647, 31717, 31725, 36000, 36400-36410, 36420-36430, 36440, 36591-36592, 36600, 36640, 43752, 51701-51703, 62320-62327, 64400-64410, 64413-64435, 64445-64450, 64461-64463, 64479-64505, 64510-64530, 69990, 76000, 77001-77002, 89220, 92012-92014, 92511, 93000-93010, 93040-93042, 93318, 93355, 94002, 94200, 94250, 94680-94690, 94770, 95812-95816, 95819, 95822, 95829, 95955, 96360-96368, 96372, 96374-96377, 96523, 99155, 99156, 99157, 99211-99223, 99231-99255, 99291-99292, 99304-99310, 99315-99316, 99334-99337, 99347-99350, 99374-99375, 99377-99378, 99446-99449, 99451-99452, 99495-99496, G0463-J2001

31630 00520, 0213T, 0216T, 0228T, 0230T, 12001-12007, 12011-12057, 13100-13133, 13151-13153, 31231, 31525-31526, 31535-31541, 31575, 31622, 31634, 31647, 31717, 31720-31725, 36000, 36400-36410, 36420-36430, 36440, 36591-36592, 36600, 36640, 43752, 51701-51703, 62320-62327, 64400-64410, 64413-64435, 64445-64450, 64461-64463, 64479-64505, 64510-64530, 69990, 76000, 77001-77002, 89220, 92012-92014, 92511, 93000-93010, 93040-93042, 93318, 93355, 94002, 94200, 94250, 94680-94690, 94770, 95812-95816, 95819, 95822, 95829, 95955, 96360-96368, 96372, 96374-96377, 96523, 99155, 99156, 99157, 99211-99223, 99231-99255, 99291-99292, 99304-99310, 99315-99316, 99334-99337, 99347-99350, 99374-99375, 99377-99378, 99446-99449, 99451-99452, 99495-99496, G0463-G0471

31631 00520, 0213T, 0216T, 0228T, 0230T, 12001-12007, 12011-12057, 13100-13133, 13151-13153, 31231, 31525-31526, 31535-31541, 31575, 31622, 31630, 31634, 31647, 31717, 31720-31725, 36000, 36400-36410, 36420-36430, 36440, 36591-36592, 36600, 36640, 43752, 51701-51703, 62320-62327, 64400-64410, 64413-64435, 64445-64450, 64461-64463, 64479-64505, 64510-64530, 69990, 76000, 77001-77002, 89220, 92012-92014, 92511, 93000-93010, 93040-93042, 93318, 93355, 94002, 94200, 94250, 94680-94690, 94770, 95812-95816, 95819, 95822, 95829, 95955, 96360-96368, 96372, 96374-96377, 96523, 99155, 99156, 99157, 99211-99223, 99231-99255, 99291-99292, 99304-99310, 99315-99316, 99334-99337, 99347-99350, 99374-99375, 99377-99378, 99446-99449, 99451-99452, 99495-99496, G0463-G0471

31632 10005, 10007, 10009, 10011, 10021, 36591-36592, 77001, 89220, 96523

31633 10005, 10007, 10009, 10011, 10021, 36591-36592, 77001, 89220, 96523

31634 00520, 0213T, 0216T, 12001-12007, 12011-12057, 13100-13133, 13151-13153, 31231, 31525-31526, 31535, 31575, 31615❖, 31622, 31717, 31720-31725, 36000, 36400-36410, 36420-36430, 36440, 36591-36592, 36600, 36640, 43752, 51701-51703, 62320-62327, 64400-64410, 64413-64435, 64445-64450, 64461-64463, 64479-64505, 64510-64530, 69990, 76000, 77002, 89220, 92012-92014, 92511, 93000-93010, 93040-93042, 93318, 93355, 94002, 94200, 94250, 94680-94690, 94770, 95812-95816, 95819, 95822, 95829, 95955, 96360-96368, 96372, 96374-96377, 96523, 99155, 99156, 99157, 99211-99223, 99231-99255, 99291-99292, 99304-99310, 99315-99316, 99334-99337, 99347-99350, 99374-99375, 99377-99378, 99446-99449, 99451-99452, 99495-99496, G0463-J2001

31635 00520, 0213T, 0216T, 0228T, 0230T, 11000-11006, 11042-11047, 12001-12007, 12011-12057, 13100-13133, 13151-13153, 31231, 31525-31526, 31535-31541, 31575, 31622, 31634, 31647-31648❖, 31717, 31720-31725, 36000, 36400-36410, 36420-36430, 36440, 36591-36592, 36600, 36640, 43752, 51701-51703, 62320-62327, 64400-64410, 64413-64435, 64445-64450, 64461-64463, 64479-64505, 64510-64530, 69990, 76000, 77001-77002, 89220, 92012-92014, 92511, 93000-93010, 93040-93042, 93318, 93355, 94002, 94200, 94250, 94680-94690, 94770, 95812-95816, 95819, 95822, 95829, 95955, 96360-96368, 96372, 96374-96377, 96523, 97597-97598, 97602, 99155, 99156, 99157, 99211-99223, 99231-99255, 99291-99292, 99304-99310, 99315-99316, 99334-99337, 99347-99350, 99374-99375, 99377-99378, 99446-99449, 99451-99452, 99495-99496, G0463-G0471

31636 00520, 0213T, 0216T, 0228T, 0230T, 12001-12007, 12011-12057, 13100-13133, 13151-13153, 31231, 31525-31526, 31535-31541, 31575, 31615❖, 31622, 31630, 31634, 31647, 31717, 31720-31725, 36000, 36400-36410, 36420-36430, 36440, 36591-36592, 36600, 36640, 43752, 51701-51703, 62320-62327, 64400-64410, 64413-64435, 64445-64450, 64461-64463, 64479-64505, 64510-64530, 69990, 76000, 77001-77002, 92012-92014, 92511, 93000-93010, 93040-93042, 93318, 93355, 94002, 94200, 94250, 94680-94690, 94770, 95812-95816, 95819, 95822, 95829, 95955, 96360-96368, 96372, 96374-96377, 96523, 99155, 99156, 99157, 99211-99223, 99231-99255, 99291-99292, 99304-99310, 99315-99316, 99334-99337, 99347-99350, 99374-99375, 99377-99378, 99446-99449, 99451-99452, 99495-99496, G0463-G0471

31637 36591-36592, 77001, 96523

31638 00520, 0213T, 0216T, 0228T, 0230T, 11000-11006, 11042-11047, 12001-12007, 12011-12057, 13100-13133, 13151-13153, 31231, 31525-31526, 31535-31541, 31575, 31615❖, 31622, 31630-31631❖, 31634, 31636❖, 31647, 31717, 31720-31725, 36000, 36400-36410, 36420-36430, 36440, 36591-36592, 36600, 36640, 43752, 51701-51703, 62320-62327, 64400-64410, 64413-64435, 64445-64450, 64461-64463, 64479-64505, 64510-64530, 69990, 76000, 77001-77002, 92012-92014, 92511, 93000-93010, 93040-93042, 93318, 93355, 94002, 94200, 94250, 94680-94690, 94770, 95812-95816, 95819, 95822, 95829, 95955, 96360-96368, 96372, 96374-96377, 96523, 97597-97598, 97602, 99155, 99156, 99157, 99211-99223, 99231-99255, 99291-99292, 99304-99310, 99315-99316, 99334-99337, 99347-99350, 99374-99375, 99377-99378, 99446-99449, 99451-99452, 99495-99496, G0463-G0471

31640 00520, 0213T, 0216T, 0228T, 0230T, 11000-11006, 11042-11047, 12001-12007, 12011-12057, 13100-13133, 13151-13153, 31231, 31525-31526, 31535-31541, 31575, 31622, 31625, 31634, 31647, 31660-31661❖, 31717, 31720-31725, 36000, 36400-36410, 36420-36430, 36440, 36591-36592, 36600, 36640, 43752, 51701-51703, 62320-62327, 64400-64410, 64413-64435, 64445-64450, 64461-64463, 64479-64505, 64510-64530, 69990, 76000, 77001-77002, 89220, 92012-92014, 92511, 93000-93010, 93040-93042, 93318, 93355, 94002, 94200, 94250, 94680-94690, 94770, 95812-95816, 95819, 95822, 95829, 95955, 96360-96368, 96372, 96374-96377, 96523, 97597-97598, 97602, 99155, 99156, 99157, 99211-99223, 99231-99255, 99291-99292, 99304-99310, 99315-99316, 99334-99337, 99347-99350, 99374-99375, 99377-99378, 99446-99449, 99451-99452, 99495-99496, G0463-G0471

31641 00520, 0213T, 0216T, 0228T, 0230T, 11000-11006, 11042-11047, 12001-12007, 12011-12057, 13100-13133, 13151-13153, 31231, 31525-31526, 31535-31541, 31575, 31622, 31625, 31634, 31640❖, 31647, 31651, 31717, 31720, 36000, 36400-36410, 36420-36430, 36440, 36591-36592, 36600, 36640, 43752, 51701-51703, 62320-62327, 64400-64410, 64413-64435, 64445-64450, 64461-64463, 64479-64505, 64510-64530, 69990, 76000, 77001-77002, 89220, 92012-92014, 92511, 93000-93010, 93040-93042, 93318, 93355, 94002, 94200, 94250, 94680-94690, 94770, 95812-95816, 95819, 95822, 95829, 95955, 96360-96368, 96372, 96374-96377, 96523, 97597-97598, 97602, 99155, 99156, 99157, 99211-99223, 99231-99255, 99291-99292, 99304-99310, 99315-99316, 99334-99337, 99347-99350, 99374-99375, 99377-99378, 99446-99449, 99451-99452, 99495-99496, G0463-G0471

31643 00520, 00528-00529, 0213T, 0216T, 0228T, 0230T, 12001-12007, 12011-12057, 13100-13133, 13151-13153, 31231, 31525-31526, 31535, 31575, 31622, 31634, 31647, 31717, 31720-31725, 36000, 36400-36410, 36420-36430, 36440, 36591-36592, 36600, 36640, 43752, 51701-51703, 62320-62327, 64400-64410, 64413-64435, 64445-64450, 64461-64463, 64479-64505, 64510-64530, 69990, 76000, 77001-77002, 89220, 92012-92014, 92511, 93000-93010, 93040-93042, 93318, 93355, 94002, 94200, 94250, 94680-94690, 94770, 95812-95816, 95819, 95822, 95829, 95955, 96360-96368, 96372, 96374-96377, 96523, 99155, 99156, 99157, 99211-99223, 99231-99255, 99291-99292, 99304-99310, 99315-99316, 99334-99337, 99347-99350, 99374-99375, 99377-99378, 99446-99449, 99451-99452, 99495-99496, G0463-G0471

31645 00520, 0213T, 0216T, 0228T, 0230T, 12001-12007, 12011-12057, 13100-13133, 13151-13153, 31231, 31525-31526, 31535, 31540, 31575, 31622, 31634, 31647, 31717, 31720-31725, 36000, 36400-36410, 36420-36430, 36440, 36591-36592, 36600, 36640, 43752, 51701-51703, 62320-62327, 64400-64410, 64413-64435, 64445-64450, 64461-64463, 64479-64505, 64510-64530, 69990, 76000, 77001-77002, 89220, 92012-92014, 92511, 93000-93010, 93040-93042, 93318, 93355, 94002, 94200, 94250, 94680-94690, 94770, 95812-95816, 95819, 95822, 95829, 95955, 96360-96368, 96372, 96374-96377, 96523, 99155, 99156, 99157, 99211-99223, 99231-99255, 99291-99292, 99304-99310, 99315-99316, 99334-99337, 99347-99350, 99374-99375, 99377-99378, 99446-99449, 99451-99452, 99495-99496, G0463-J2001

31646 00520, 0213T, 0216T, 0228T, 0230T, 12001-12007, 12011-12057, 13100-13133, 13151-13153, 31231, 31525-31526, 31535-31541, 31575, 31622, 31634, 31645❖, 31647, 31717, 31720-31725, 36000, 36400-36410, 36420-36430, 36440, 36591-36592, 36600, 36640, 43752, 51701-51703, 62320-62327, 64400-64410, 64413-64435, 64445-64450, 64461-64463, 64479-64505, 64510-64530, 69990, 76000, 77001-77002, 89220, 92012-92014, 92511, 93000-93010, 93040-93042, 93318, 93355, 94002, 94200, 94250, 94680-94690, 94770, 95812-95816, 95819, 95822, 95829, 95955, 96360-96368, 96372, 96374-96377, 96523, 99155, 99156, 99157, 99211-99223, 99231-99255, 99291-99292, 99304-99310, 99315-99316, 99334-99337, 99347-99350, 99374-99375, 99377-99378, 99446-99449, 99451-99452, 99495-99496, G0463-J2001

31717 00520, 0213T, 0216T, 0228T, 0230T, 10005, 10007, 10009, 10011, 10021, 12001-12007, 12011-12057, 13100-13133, 13151-13153, 36000, 36400-36410, 36420-36430, 36440, 36591-36592, 36600, 36640, 43752, 51701-51703, 62320-62327, 64400-64410, 64413-64435, 64445-64450, 64461-64463, 64479-64505, 64510-64530, 69990, 89220, 92012-92014, 93000-93010, 93040-93042, 93318, 93355, 94002, 94200, 94250, 94680-94690, 94770, 95812-95816, 95819, 95822, 95829, 95955, 96360-96368, 96372, 96374-96377, 96523, 99155, 99156, 99157, 99211-99223, 99231-99255, 99291-99292, 99304-99310, 99315-99316, 99334-99337, 99347-99350, 99374-99375, 99377-99378, 99446-99449, 99451-99452, 99495-99496, G0463-J2001

31720 00520, 0213T, 0216T, 0228T, 0230T, 12001-12007, 12011-12057, 13100-13133, 13151-13153, 36000, 36400-36410, 36420-36430, 36440, 36591-36592, 36600, 36640, 43752, 51701-51703, 62320-62327, 64400-64410, 64413-64435, 64445-64450, 64461-64463, 64479-64505, 64510-64530, 69990, 89220, 92012-92014, 93000-93010, 93040-93042, 93318, 93355, 94002, 94200, 94250, 94680-94690, 94770, 95812-95816, 95819, 95822, 95829, 95955, 96360-96368, 96372, 96374-96377, 96523, 99155, 99156, 99157, 99211-99223, 99231-99255, 99291-99292, 99304-99310, 99315-99316, 99334-99337, 99347-99350, 99374-99375, 99377-99378, 99446-99449, 99451-99452, 99495-99496, G0463-G0471

31725 00520, 0213T, 0216T, 0228T, 0230T, 12001-12007, 12011-12057, 13100-13133, 13151-13153, 36000, 36400-36410, 36420-36430, 36440, 36591-36592, 36600, 36640, 43752, 51701-51703, 62320-62327, 64400-64410, 64413-64435, 64445-64450, 64461-64463, 64479-64505, 64510-64530, 69990, 89220, 92012-92014, 93000-93010, 93040-93042, 93318, 93355, 94002, 94200, 94250, 94680-94690, 94770, 95812-95816, 95819, 95822, 95829, 95955, 96360-96368, 96372, 96374-96377, 96523, 99155, 99156, 99157, 99211-99223, 99231-99255, 99291-99292, 99304-99310, 99315-99316, 99334-99337, 99347-99350, 99374-99375, 99377-99378, 99446-99449, 99451-99452, 99495-99496, G0463-G0471

31730 00520, 0213T, 0216T, 0228T, 0230T, 12001-12007, 12011-12057, 13100-13133, 13151-13153, 36000, 36400-36410, 36420-36430, 36440, 36591-36592, 36600, 36640, 43752, 51701-51703, 62320-62327, 64400-64410, 64413-64435, 64445-64450, 64461-64463, 64479-64505, 64510-64530, 69990, 92012-92014, 92502, 93000-93010, 93040-93042, 93318, 93355, 94002, 94200, 94250, 94680-94690, 94770, 95812-95816, 95819, 95822, 95829, 95955, 96360-96368, 96372, 96374-96377, 96523, 99155, 99156, 99157, 99211-99223, 99231-99255, 99291-99292, 99304-99310, 99315-99316, 99334-99337, 99347-99350, 99374-99375, 99377-99378, 99446-99449, 99451-99452, 99495-99496, G0463-J2001

31760 00520, 0213T, 0216T, 0228T, 0230T, 11000-11006, 11042-11047, 12001-12007, 12011-12057, 13100-13133, 13151-13153, 31805, 36000, 36400-36410, 36420-36430, 36440, 36591-36592, 36600, 36640, 39000-39010, 43752, 51701-51703, 62320-62327, 64400-64410, 64413-64435, 64445-64450, 64461-64463, 64479-64505, 64510-64530, 69990, 92012-92014, 93000-93010, 93040-93042, 93318, 93355, 94002, 94200, 94250, 94680-94690, 94770, 95812-95816, 95819, 95822, 95829, 95955, 96360-96368, 96372, 96374-96377, 96523, 97597-97598, 97602, 99155, 99156, 99157, 99211-99223, 99231-99255, 99291-99292, 99304-99310, 99315-99316, 99334-99337, 99347-99350, 99374-99375, 99377-99378, 99446-99449, 99451-99452, 99495-99496, G0463-G0471

31770 00520, 0213T, 0216T, 0228T, 0230T, 11000-11006, 11042-11047, 12001-12007, 12011-12057, 13100-13133, 13151-13153, 31775❖, 32100, 36000, 36400-36410, 36420-36430, 36440, 36591-36592, 36600, 36640, 39000-39010, 43752, 51701-51703, 62320-62327, 64400-64410, 64413-64435, 64445-64450, 64461-64463, 64479-64505, 64510-64530, 69990, 92012-92014, 93000-93010, 93040-93042, 93318, 93355, 94002, 94200, 94250, 94680-94690, 94770, 95812-95816, 95819, 95822, 95829, 95955, 96360-96368, 96372, 96374-96377, 96523, 97597-97598, 97602, 99155, 99156, 99157, 99211-99223, 99231-99255, 99291-99292, 99304-99310, 99315-99316, 99334-99337, 99347-99350, 99374-99375, 99377-99378, 99446-99449, 99451-99452, 99495-99496, G0463-G0471

31775 00520, 0213T, 0216T, 0228T, 0230T, 11000-11006, 11042-11047, 12001-12007, 12011-12057, 13100-13133, 13151-13153, 32100, 36000, 36400-36410, 36420-36430, 36440, 36591-36592, 36600, 36640, 39000-39010, 43752, 51701-51703, 62320-62327, 64400-64410, 64413-64435, 64445-64450, 64461-64463, 64479-64505, 64510-64530, 69990, 92012-92014, 93000-93010, 93040-93042, 93318, 93355, 94002, 94200, 94250, 94680-94690, 94770, 95812-95816, 95819, 95822, 95829, 95955, 96360-96368, 96372, 96374-96377, 96523, 97597-97598, 97602, 99155, 99156, 99157, 99211-99223, 99231-99255, 99291-99292, 99304-99310, 99315-99316, 99334-99337, 99347-99350, 99374-99375, 99377-99378, 99446-99449, 99451-99452, 99495-99496, G0463-G0471

31781 00520, 0213T, 0216T, 0228T, 0230T, 11000-11006, 11042-11047, 12001-12007, 12011-12057, 13100-13133, 13151-13153, 32100, 36000, 36400-36410, 36420-36430, 36440, 36591-36592, 36600, 36640, 39000-39010, 43752, 51701-51703, 62320-62327, 64400-64410, 64413-64435, 64445-64450, 64461-64463, 64479-64505, 64510-64530, 69990, 92012-92014, 93000-93010, 93040-93042, 93318, 93355, 94002, 94200, 94250, 94680-94690, 94770, 95812-95816, 95819, 95822, 95829, 95955, 96360-96368, 96372, 96374-96377, 96523, 97597-97598, 97602, 99155, 99156, 99157, 99211-99223, 99231-99255, 99291-99292, 99304-99310, 99315-99316, 99334-99337, 99347-99350, 99374-99375, 99377-99378, 99446-99449, 99451-99452, 99495-99496, G0463-G0471

31786 00520, 0213T, 0216T, 0228T, 0230T, 11000-11006, 11042-11047, 12001-12007, 12011-12057, 13100-13133, 13151-13153, 31805, 32100, 36000, 36400-36410, 36420-36430, 36440, 36591-36592, 36600, 36640, 39000-39010, 43752, 51701-51703, 62320-62327, 64400-64410, 64413-64435, 64445-64450, 64461-64463, 64479-64505, 64510-64530, 69990, 92012-92014, 93000-93010, 93040-93042, 93318, 93355, 94002, 94200, 94250, 94680-94690, 94770, 95812-95816, 95819, 95822, 95829, 95955, 96360-96368, 96372, 96374-96377, 96523, 97597-97598, 97602, 99155, 99156, 99157, 99211-99223, 99231-99255, 99291-99292, 99304-99310, 99315-99316, 99334-99337, 99347-99350, 99374-99375, 99377-99378, 99446-99449, 99451-99452, 99495-99496, G0463-G0471

31805 00520, 0213T, 0216T, 0228T, 0230T, 12001-12007, 12011-12057, 13100-13133, 13151-13153, 32100, 36000, 36400-36410, 36420-36430, 36440, 36591-36592, 36600, 36640, 39000-39010, 43752, 51701-51703, 62320-62327, 64400-64410, 64413-64435, 64445-64450, 64461-64463, 64479-64505, 64510-64530, 69990, 92012-92014, 93000-93010, 93040-93042, 93318, 93355, 94002, 94200, 94250, 94680-94690, 94770, 95812-95816, 95819, 95822, 95829, 95955, 96360-96368, 96372, 96374-96377, 96523, 99155, 99156, 99157, 99211-99223, 99231-99255, 99291-99292, 99304-99310, 99315-99316, 99334-99337, 99347-99350, 99374-99375, 99377-99378, 99446-99449, 99451-99452, 99495-99496, G0463-G0471

31820 00520, 0213T, 0216T, 0228T, 0230T, 11000-11006, 11042-11047, 12001-12007, 12011-12057, 13100-13133, 13151-13153, 31830❖, 36000, 36400-36410, 36420-36430, 36440, 36591-36592, 36600, 36640, 43752, 51701-51703, 62320-62327, 64400-64410, 64413-64435, 64445-64450, 64461-64463, 64479-64505, 64510-64530, 69990, 92012-92014, 92502, 93000-93010, 93040-93042, 93318, 93355, 94002, 94200, 94250, 94680-94690, 94770, 95812-95816, 95819, 95822, 95829, 95955, 96360-96368, 96372, 96374-96377, 96523, 97597-97598, 97602, 99155, 99156, 99157, 99211-99223, 99231-99255, 99291-99292, 99304-99310, 99315-99316, 99334-99337, 99347-99350, 99374-99375, 99377-99378, 99446-99449, 99451-99452, 99495-99496, G0463-J2001

31825 00520, 0213T, 0216T, 0228T, 0230T, 11000-11006, 11042-11047, 12001-12007, 12011-12057, 13100-13133, 13151-13153, 31820, 36000, 36400-36410, 36420-36430, 36440, 36591-36592, 36600, 36640, 43752, 51701-51703, 62320-62327, 64400-64410, 64413-64435, 64445-64450, 64461-64463, 64479-64505, 64510-64530, 69990, 92012-92014, 92502, 93000-93010, 93040-93042, 93318, 93355, 94002, 94200, 94250, 94680-94690, 94770, 95812-95816, 95819, 95822, 95829, 95955, 96360-96368, 96372, 96374-96377, 96523, 97597-97598, 97602, 99155, 99156, 99157, 99211-99223, 99231-99255, 99291-99292, 99304-99310, 99315-99316, 99334-99337, 99347-99350, 99374-99375, 99377-99378, 99446-99449, 99451-99452, 99495-99496, G0463-J2001

32035 0213T, 0216T, 0228T, 0230T, 11000-11006, 11042-11047, 12001-12007, 12011-12057, 13100-13133, 13151-13153, 32036❖, 32096-32098, 32220-32225, 32551, 32556-32557, 32601, 32607-32609, 32900, 36000, 36400-36410, 36420-36430, 36440, 36591-36592, 36600, 36640, 43752, 51701-51703, 62320-62327, 64400-64410, 64413-64435, 64445-64450, 64461-64463, 64479-64505, 64510-64530, 69990, 92012-92014, 93000-93010, 93040-93042, 93318, 93355, 94002, 94200, 94250, 94680-94690, 94770, 95812-95816, 95819, 95822, 95829, 95955, 96360-96368, 96372, 96374-96377, 96523, 97597-97598, 97602, 99155, 99156, 99157, 99211-99223, 99231-99255, 99291-99292, 99304-99310, 99315-99316, 99334-99337, 99347-99350, 99374-99375, 99377-99378, 99446-99449, 99451-99452, 99495-99496, G0463-G0471

32036 0213T, 0216T, 0228T, 0230T, 12001-12007, 12011-12057, 13100-13133, 13151-13153, 32096-32098, 32220-32225, 32551, 32556-32557, 32601, 32607-32609, 36000, 36400-36410, 36420-36430, 36440, 36591-36592, 36600, 36640, 43752, 51701-51703, 62320-62327, 64400-64410, 64413-64435, 64445-64450, 64461-64463, 64479-64505, 64510-64530, 69990, 92012-92014, 93000-93010, 93040-93042, 93318, 93355, 94002, 94200, 94250, 94680-94690, 94770, 95812-95816, 95819, 95822, 95829, 95955, 96360-96368, 96372, 96374-96377, 96523, 99155, 99156, 99157, 99211-99223, 99231-99255, 99291-99292, 99304-99310, 99315-99316, 99334-99337, 99347-99350, 99374-99375, 99377-99378, 99446-99449, 99451-99452, 99495-99496, G0463-G0471

32096 0213T, 0216T, 0228T, 0230T, 10005, 10007, 10009, 10011, 10021, 11000-11006, 11042-11047, 12001-12007, 12011-12057, 13100-13133, 13151-13153, 20101, 21600, 31622, 31634, 31647, 32098-32100, 32220-32225, 32310, 32405❖, 32551, 32556-32601, 32607-32609, 36000, 36400-36410, 36420-36430, 36440, 36591-36592, 36600, 36640, 43752, 51701-51703, 62320-62327, 64400-64410, 64413-64435, 64445-64450, 64461-64463, 64479-64505, 64510-64530, 69990,

92012-92014, 93000-93010, 93040-93042, 93318, 93355, 94002, 94200, 94250, 94680-94690, 94770, 95812-95816, 95819, 95822, 95829, 95955, 96360-96368, 96372, 96374-96377, 96523, 97597-97598, 97602, 99155, 99156, 99157, 99211-99223, 99231-99255, 99291-99292, 99304-99310, 99315-99316, 99334-99337, 99347-99350, 99374-99375, 99377-99378, 99446-99449, 99451-99452, 99495-99496, G0463-G0471

32097 0213T, 0216T, 0228T, 0230T, 10005, 10007, 10009, 10011, 10021, 11000-11006, 11042-11047, 12001-12007, 12011-12057, 13100-13133, 13151-13153, 20101, 21600, 31622, 31634, 31647, 32096*, 32098-32100, 32220-32225, 32310, 32405*, 32551, 32556-32601, 32607-32609, 36000, 36400-36410, 36420-36430, 36440, 36591-36592, 36600, 36640, 43752, 51701-51703, 62320-62327, 64400-64410, 64413-64435, 64445-64450, 64461-64463, 64479-64505, 64510-64530, 69990, 92012-92014, 93000-93010, 93040-93042, 93318, 93355, 94002, 94200, 94250, 94680-94690, 94770, 95812-95816, 95819, 95822, 95829, 95955, 96360-96368, 96372, 96374-96377, 96523, 97597-97598, 97602, 99155, 99156, 99157, 99211-99223, 99231-99255, 99291-99292, 99304-99310, 99315-99316, 99334-99337, 99347-99350, 99374-99375, 99377-99378, 99446-99449, 99451-99452, 99495-99496, G0463-G0471

32098 0213T, 0216T, 0228T, 0230T, 10005, 10007, 10009, 10011, 10021, 11000-11006, 11042-11047, 12001-12007, 12011-12057, 13100-13133, 13151-13153, 20101, 21600, 31622, 31634, 31647, 32100, 32220-32225, 32310, 32400*, 32405*, 32551, 32556-32601, 32607-32609, 36000, 36400-36410, 36420-36430, 36440, 36591-36592, 36600, 36640, 43752, 51701-51703, 62320-62327, 64400-64410, 64413-64435, 64445-64450, 64461-64463, 64479-64505, 64510-64530, 69990, 92012-92014, 93000-93010, 93040-93042, 93318, 93355, 94002, 94200, 94250, 94680-94690, 94770, 95812-95816, 95819, 95822, 95829, 95955, 96360-96368, 96372, 96374-96377, 96523, 97597-97598, 97602, 99155, 99156, 99157, 99211-99223, 99231-99255, 99291-99292, 99304-99310, 99315-99316, 99334-99337, 99347-99350, 99374-99375, 99377-99378, 99446-99449, 99451-99452, 99495-99496, G0463-G0471

32100 0213T, 0216T, 0228T, 0230T, 11000-11006, 11042-11047, 12001-12007, 12011-12057, 13100-13133, 13151-13153, 20101, 21600, 31622, 31634, 31647, 32200, 32215, 32225, 32310, 32551, 32556-32601, 32607-32609, 36000, 36400-36410, 36420-36430, 36440, 36591-36592, 36600, 36640, 43752, 51701-51703, 62320-62327, 64400-64410, 64413-64435, 64445-64450, 64461-64463, 64479-64505, 64510-64530, 69990, 92012-92014, 93000-93010, 93040-93042, 93318, 93355, 94002, 94200, 94250, 94680-94690, 94770, 95812-95816, 95819, 95822, 95829, 95955, 96360-96368, 96372, 96374-96377, 96523, 97597-97598, 97602, 99155, 99156, 99157, 99211-99223, 99231-99255, 99291-99292, 99304-99310, 99315-99316, 99334-99337, 99347-99350, 99374-99375, 99377-99378, 99446-99449, 99451-99452, 99495-99496, G0463-G0471

32110 0213T, 0216T, 0228T, 0230T, 11000-11006, 11042-11047, 12001-12007, 12011-12057, 13100-13133, 13151-13153, 20101, 31622, 31634, 31647, 32096-32100, 32200, 32220-32225, 32551, 32556-32601, 32607-32609, 36000, 36400-36410, 36420-36430, 36440, 36591-36592, 36600, 36640, 43752, 51701-51703, 62320-62327, 64400-64410, 64413-64435, 64445-64450, 64461-64463, 64479-64505, 64510-64530, 69990, 92012-92014, 93000-93010, 93040-93042, 93318, 93355, 94002, 94200, 94250, 94680-94690, 94770, 95812-95816, 95819, 95822, 95829, 95955, 96360-96368, 96372, 96374-96377, 96523, 97597-97598, 97602, 99155, 99156, 99157, 99211-99223, 99231-99255, 99291-99292, 99304-99310, 99315-99316, 99334-99337, 99347-99350, 99374-99375, 99377-99378, 99446-99449, 99451-99452, 99495-99496, G0463-G0471

32120 0213T, 0216T, 0228T, 0230T, 11000-11006, 11042-11047, 12001-12007, 12011-12057, 13100-13133, 13151-13153, 20101, 31622, 31634, 31647, 32096-32100, 32110*, 32215-32225, 32551, 32556-32557, 32601, 32607-32609, 36000, 36400-36410, 36420-36430, 36440, 36591-36592, 36600, 36640, 43752, 51701-51703, 62320-62327, 64400-64410, 64413-64435, 64445-64450, 64461-64463, 64479-64505, 64510-64530, 69990, 92012-92014, 93000-93010, 93040-93042, 93318, 93355, 94002, 94200, 94250, 94680-94690, 94770, 95812-95816, 95819, 95822, 95829, 95955, 96360-96368, 96372, 96374-96377, 96523, 97597-97598, 97602, 99155, 99156, 99157, 99211-99223, 99231-99255, 99291-99292, 99304-99310, 99315-99316, 99334-99337, 99347-99350, 99374-99375, 99377-99378, 99446-99449, 99451-99452, 99495-99496, G0463-G0471

32124 0213T, 0216T, 0228T, 0230T, 11000-11006, 11042-11047, 12001-12007, 12011-12057, 13100-13133, 13151-13153, 20101, 31622, 31634, 31647, 32096-32100, 32200, 32215-32225, 32551, 32556-32601, 32607-32609, 32654, 32940*, 36000, 36400-36410, 36420-36430, 36440, 36591-36592, 36600, 36640, 43752, 51701-51703, 62320-62327, 64400-64410, 64413-64435, 64445-64450, 64461-64463, 64479-64505, 64510-64530, 69990, 92012-92014, 93000-93010, 93040-93042, 93318, 93355, 94002, 94200, 94250, 94680-94690, 94770, 95812-95816, 95819, 95822, 95829, 95955, 96360-96368, 96372, 96374-96377, 96523, 97597-97598, 97602, 99155, 99156, 99157, 99211-99223, 99231-99255, 99291-99292, 99304-99310, 99315-99316, 99334-99337, 99347-99350, 99374-99375, 99377-99378, 99446-99449, 99451-99452, 99495-99496, G0463-G0471

32140 0213T, 0216T, 0228T, 0230T, 11000-11006, 11042-11047, 12001-12007, 12011-12057, 13100-13133, 13151-13153, 20101, 31622, 31634, 31647, 32096-32100, 32200, 32215-32225, 32551, 32556-32601, 32607-32609, 32654, 36000, 36400-36410, 36420-36430, 36440, 36591-36592, 36600, 36640, 43752, 51701-51703, 62320-62327, 64400-64410, 64413-64435, 64445-64450, 64461-64463, 64479-64505, 64510-64530, 69990, 92012-92014, 93000-93010, 93040-93042, 93318, 93355, 94002, 94200, 94250, 94680-94690, 94770, 95812-95816, 95819, 95822, 95829, 95955, 96360-96368, 96372, 96374-96377, 96523, 97597-97598, 97602, 99155, 99156, 99157, 99211-99223, 99231-99255, 99291-99292, 99304-99310, 99315-99316, 99334-99337, 99347-99350, 99374-99375, 99377-99378, 99446-99449, 99451-99452, 99495-99496, G0463-G0471

32141 0213T, 0216T, 0228T, 0230T, 11000-11006, 11042-11047, 12001-12007, 12011-12057, 13100-13133, 13151-13153, 20101, 31622, 31634, 31647, 32096-32100, 32200, 32215-32225, 32551, 32556-32601, 32607-32609, 32654, 36000, 36400-36410, 36420-36430, 36440, 36591-36592, 36600, 36640, 43752, 51701-51703, 62320-62327, 64400-64410, 64413-64435, 64445-64450, 64461-64463, 64479-64505, 64510-64530, 69990, 92012-92014, 93000-93010, 93040-93042, 93318, 93355, 94002, 94200, 94250, 94680-94690, 94770, 95812-95816, 95819, 95822, 95829, 95955, 96360-96368, 96372, 96374-96377, 96523, 97597-97598, 97602, 99155, 99156, 99157, 99211-99223, 99231-99255, 99291-99292, 99304-99310, 99315-99316, 99334-99337, 99347-99350, 99374-99375, 99377-99378, 99446-99449, 99451-99452, 99495-99496, G0463-G0471

32150 0213T, 0216T, 0228T, 0230T, 11000-11006, 11042-11047, 12001-12007, 12011-12057, 13100-13133, 13151-13153, 20101, 31622, 31634, 31647, 32096-32100, 32200, 32215-32225, 32551, 32556-32601, 32607-32609, 32654, 36000, 36400-36410, 36420-36430, 36440, 36591-36592, 36600, 36640, 43752, 51701-51703, 62320-62327, 64400-64410, 64413-64435, 64445-64450, 64461-64463, 64479-64505, 64510-64530, 69990, 92012-92014, 93000-93010, 93040-93042, 93318, 93355, 94002, 94200, 94250, 94680-94690, 94770, 95812-95816, 95819, 95822, 95829, 95955, 96360-96368, 96372, 96374-96377, 96523, 97597-97598, 97602, 99155, 99156, 99157, 99211-99223, 99231-99255, 99291-99292, 99304-99310, 99315-99316, 99334-99337, 99347-99350, 99374-99375, 99377-99378, 99446-99449, 99451-99452, 99495-99496, G0463-G0471

32151 0213T, 0216T, 0228T, 0230T, 11000-11006, 11042-11047, 12001-12007, 12011-12057, 13100-13133, 13151-13153, 20101, 31622, 31634, 31647, 32096-32100, 32200, 32215-32225, 32551, 32556-32562, 32654, 36000, 36400-36410, 36420-36430, 36440, 36591-36592, 36600, 36640, 43752, 51701-51703, 62320-62327, 64400-64410, 64413-64435, 64445-64450, 64461-64463, 64479-64505, 64510-64530, 69990, 92012-92014, 93000-93010, 93040-93042, 93318, 93355, 94002, 94200, 94250, 94680-94690, 94770, 95812-95816, 95819, 95822, 95829, 95955, 96360-96368, 96372, 96374-96377, 96523, 97597-97598, 97602, 99155, 99156, 99157, 99211-99223, 99231-99255, 99291-99292, 99304-99310, 99315-99316, 99334-99337, 99347-99350, 99374-99375, 99377-99378, 99446-99449, 99451-99452, 99495-99496, G0463-G0471

32160 0213T, 0216T, 0228T, 0230T, 11000-11006, 11042-11047, 12001-12007, 12011-12057, 13100-13133, 13151-13153, 20101, 31622, 31634, 31647, 32096-32100, 32215-32225, 32551, 32556-32557, 32601, 32607-32609, 32654, 36000, 36400-36410, 36420-36430, 36440, 36591-36592, 36600, 36640, 43752, 51701-51703, 62320-62327, 64400-64410, 64413-64435, 64445-64450, 64461-64463, 64479-64505, 64510-64530, 69990, 92012-92014, 93000-93010, 93040-93042, 93318, 93355, 94002, 94200, 94250, 94680-94690, 94770, 95812-95816, 95819, 95822, 95829, 95955, 96360-96368, 96372, 96374-96377, 96523, 97597-97598, 97602, 99155, 99156, 99157, 99211-99223, 99231-99255, 99291-99292, 99304-99310, 99315-99316, 99334-99337, 99347-99350, 99374-99375, 99377-99378, 99446-99449, 99451-99452, 99495-99496, G0463-G0471

32200 0213T, 0216T, 0228T, 0230T, 12001-12007, 12011-12057, 13100-13133, 13151-13153, 20101, 32035-32036, 32551, 32556-32557, 32601, 32607-32609, 36000, 36400-36410, 36420-36430, 36440, 36591-36592, 36600, 36640, 43752, 49405, 51701-51703, 62320-62327, 64400-64410, 64413-64435, 64445-64450, 64461-64463, 64479-64505, 64510-64530, 69990, 92012-92014, 93000-93010, 93040-93042, 93318, 93355, 94002, 94200, 94250, 94680-94690, 94770, 95812-95816, 95819, 95822, 95829, 95955, 96360-96368, 96372, 96374-96377, 96523, 99155, 99156, 99157, 99211-99223, 99231-99255, 99291-99292, 99304-99310, 99315-99316, 99334-99337, 99347-99350, 99374-99375, 99377-99378, 99446-99449, 99451-99452, 99495-99496, G0463-G0471

32215 0213T, 0216T, 0228T, 0230T, 12001-12007, 12011-12057, 13100-13133, 13151-13153, 20101, 32551, 32556-32601, 32607-32609, 36000, 36400-36410, 36420-36430, 36440, 36591-36592, 36600, 36640, 43752, 49185✧, 51701-51703, 62320-62327, 64400-64410, 64413-64435, 64445-64450, 64461-64463, 64479-64505, 64510-64530, 69990, 92012-92014, 93000-93010, 93040-93042, 93318, 93355, 94002, 94200, 94250, 94680-94690, 94770, 95812-95816, 95819, 95822, 95829, 95955, 96360-96368, 96372, 96374-96377, 96523, 99155, 99156, 99157, 99211-99223, 99231-99255, 99291-99292, 99304-99310, 99315-99316, 99334-99337, 99347-99350, 99374-99375, 99377-99378, 99446-99449, 99451-99452, 99495-99496, G0463-G0471

32220 0213T, 0216T, 0228T, 0230T, 12001-12007, 12011-12057, 13100-13133, 13151-13153, 20101, 32100, 32310, 32551, 32556-32601, 32607-32609, 36000, 36400-36410, 36420-36430, 36440, 36591-36592, 36600, 36640, 43752, 51701-51703, 62320-62327, 64400-64410, 64413-64435, 64445-64450, 64461-64463, 64479-64505, 64510-64530, 69990, 92012-92014, 93000-93010, 93040-93042, 93318, 93355, 94002, 94200, 94250, 94680-94690, 94770, 95812-95816, 95819, 95822, 95829, 95955, 96360-96368, 96372, 96374-96377, 96523, 99155, 99156, 99157, 99211-99223, 99231-99255, 99291-99292, 99304-99310, 99315-99316, 99334-99337, 99347-99350, 99374-99375, 99377-99378, 99446-99449, 99451-99452, 99495-99496, G0463-G0471

32225 0213T, 0216T, 0228T, 0230T, 12001-12007, 12011-12057, 13100-13133, 13151-13153, 20101, 32556-32601, 32607-32609, 36000, 36400-36410, 36420-36430, 36440, 36591-36592, 36600, 36640, 43752, 51701-51703, 62320-62327, 64400-64410, 64413-64435, 64445-64450, 64461-64463, 64479-64505, 64510-64530, 69990, 92012-92014, 93000-93010, 93040-93042, 93318, 93355, 94002, 94200, 94250, 94680-94690, 94770, 95812-95816, 95819, 95822, 95829, 95955, 96360-96368, 96372, 96374-96377, 96523, 99155, 99156, 99157, 99211-99223, 99231-99255, 99291-99292, 99304-99310, 99315-99316, 99334-99337, 99347-99350, 99374-99375, 99377-99378, 99446-99449, 99451-99452, 99495-99496, G0463-G0471

32310 0213T, 0216T, 0228T, 0230T, 11000-11006, 11042-11047, 12001-12007, 12011-12057, 13100-13133, 13151-13153, 20101, 32225, 32551, 32556-32601, 32607-32609, 36000, 36400-36410, 36420-36430, 36440, 36591-36592, 36600, 36640, 43752, 51701-51703, 62320-62327, 64400-64410, 64413-64435, 64445-64450, 64461-64463, 64479-64505, 64510-64530, 69990, 92012-92014, 93000-93010, 93040-93042, 93318, 93355, 94002, 94200, 94250, 94680-94690, 94770, 95812-95816, 95819, 95822, 95829, 95955, 96360-96368, 96372, 96374-96377, 96523, 97597-97598, 97602, 99155, 99156, 99157, 99211-99223, 99231-99255, 99291-99292, 99304-99310, 99315-99316, 99334-99337, 99347-99350, 99374-99375, 99377-99378, 99446-99449, 99451-99452, 99495-99496, G0463-G0471

32320 0213T, 0216T, 0228T, 0230T, 11000-11006, 11042-11047, 12001-12007, 12011-12057, 13100-13133, 13151-13153, 20101, 32100, 32225, 32310, 32551, 32556-32601, 32607-32609, 36000, 36400-36410, 36420-36430, 36440, 36591-36592, 36600, 36640, 43752, 51701-51703, 62320-62327, 64400-64410, 64413-64435, 64445-64450, 64461-64463, 64479-64505, 64510-64530, 69990, 92012-92014, 93000-93010, 93040-93042, 93318, 93355, 94002, 94200, 94250, 94680-94690, 94770, 95812-95816, 95819, 95822, 95829, 95955, 96360-96368, 96372, 96374-96377, 96523, 97597-97598, 97602, 99155, 99156, 99157, 99211-99223, 99231-99255, 99291-99292, 99304-99310, 99315-99316, 99334-99337, 99347-99350, 99374-99375, 99377-99378, 99446-99449, 99451-99452, 99495-99496, G0463-G0471

32400 0213T, 0216T, 0228T, 0230T, 10005, 10007, 10009, 10011, 10021, 12001-12007, 12011-12057, 13100-13133, 13151-13153, 20101, 32551, 32556-32557, 32601, 32607-32609, 36000, 36400-36410, 36420-36430, 36440, 36591-36592, 36600, 36640, 43752, 51701-51703, 62320-62327, 64400-64410, 64413-64435, 64445-64450, 64461-64463, 64479-64505, 64510-64530, 69990, 88172, 92012-92014, 93000-93010, 93040-93042, 93318, 93355, 94002, 94200, 94250, 94680-94690, 94770, 95812-95816, 95819, 95822, 95829, 95955, 96360-96368, 96372, 96374-96377, 96523, 99155, 99156, 99157, 99211-99223, 99231-99255, 99291-99292, 99304-99310, 99315-99316, 99334-99337, 99347-99350, 99374-99375, 99377-99378, 99446-99449, 99451-99452, 99495-99496, G0463-J2001

32405 0213T, 0216T, 0228T, 0230T, 10005, 10007, 10009, 10011, 10021, 12001-12007, 12011-12057, 13100-13133, 13151-13153, 20101, 32551, 32601, 32607-32609, 36000, 36400-36410, 36420-36430, 36440, 36591-36592, 36600, 36640, 43752, 51701-51703, 62320-62321, 62324-62327, 64400-64410, 64413-64435, 64445-64450, 64461-64463, 64479-64505, 64510-64530, 69990, 88172, 92012-92014, 93000-93010, 93040-93042, 93318, 93355, 94002, 94200, 94250, 94680-94690, 94770, 95812-95816, 95819, 95822, 95829, 95955, 96360-96368, 96372, 96374-96377, 96523, 99155, 99156, 99157, 99211-99223, 99231-99255, 99291-99292, 99304-99310, 99315-99316, 99334-99337, 99347-99350, 99374-99375, 99377-99378, 99446-99449, 99451-99452, 99495-99496, G0463-J2001

32440 0213T, 0216T, 0228T, 0230T, 11000-11006, 11042-11047, 12001-12007, 12011-12057, 13100-13133, 13151-13153, 20101, 31622-31625, 31626,

31634, 31643-31645, 31647, 32096-32100, 32110, 32124-32151, 32215, 32480-32484, 32486-32488*, 32491*, 32505-32506, 32551, 32601, 32607-32609, 32666-32667, 32810-32815, 32994-32998, 36000, 36400-36410, 36420-36430, 36440, 36591-36592, 36600, 36640, 39010, 39220, 43752, 51701-51703, 62320-62327, 64400-64410, 64413-64435, 64445-64450, 64461-64463, 64479-64505, 64510-64530, 64620, 69990, 92012-92014, 93000-93010, 93040-93042, 93318, 93355, 94002, 94200, 94250, 94680-94690, 94770, 95812-95816, 95819, 95822, 95829, 95955, 96360-96368, 96372, 96374-96377, 96523, 97597-97598, 97602, 99155, 99156, 99157, 99211-99223, 99231-99255, 99291-99292, 99304-99310, 99315-99316, 99334-99337, 99347-99350, 99374-99375, 99377-99378, 99446-99449, 99451-99452, 99495-99496, G0463-G0471

32442 0213T, 0216T, 0228T, 0230T, 11000-11006, 11042-11047, 12001-12007, 12011-12057, 13100-13133, 13151-13153, 20101, 31622-31625, 31626, 31634, 31643-31645, 31647, 32096-32100, 32110, 32124-32151, 32215, 32440, 32480-32484, 32503-32506, 32551, 32556-32557, 32601, 32607-32609, 32666-32667, 32810, 32994-32998, 36000, 36400-36410, 36420-36430, 36440, 36591-36592, 36600, 36640, 39010, 39220, 43752, 51701-51703, 62320-62327, 64400-64410, 64413-64435, 64445-64450, 64461-64463, 64479-64505, 64510-64530, 64620, 69990, 92012-92014, 93000-93010, 93040-93042, 93318, 93355, 94002, 94200, 94250, 94680-94690, 94770, 95812-95816, 95819, 95822, 95829, 95955, 96360-96368, 96372, 96374-96377, 96523, 97597-97598, 97602, 99155, 99156, 99157, 99211-99223, 99231-99255, 99291-99292, 99304-99310, 99315-99316, 99334-99337, 99347-99350, 99374-99375, 99377-99378, 99446-99449, 99451-99452, 99495-99496, G0463-G0471

32445 0213T, 0216T, 0228T, 0230T, 11000-11006, 11042-11047, 12001-12007, 12011-12057, 13100-13133, 13151-13153, 20101, 31622-31625, 31626, 31634, 31643-31645, 31647, 32096-32100, 32110, 32124-32151, 32215, 32440-32442*, 32480-32484, 32488*, 32503-32506, 32551, 32556-32557, 32601, 32607-32609, 32666-32667, 32810-32815, 32994-32998, 36000, 36400-36410, 36420-36430, 36440, 36591-36592, 36600, 36640, 39010, 39220, 43752, 51701-51703, 62320-62327, 64400-64410, 64413-64435, 64445-64450, 64461-64463, 64479-64505, 64510-64530, 64620, 69990, 92012-92014, 93000-93010, 93040-93042, 93318, 93355, 94002, 94200, 94250, 94680-94690, 94770, 95812-95816, 95819, 95822, 95829, 95955, 96360-96368, 96372, 96374-96377, 96523, 97597-97598, 97602, 99155, 99156, 99157, 99211-99223, 99231-99255, 99291-99292, 99304-99310, 99315-99316, 99334-99337, 99347-99350, 99374-99375, 99377-99378, 99446-99449, 99451-99452, 99495-99496, G0463-G0471

32480 0213T, 0216T, 0228T, 0230T, 11000-11006, 11042-11047, 12001-12007, 12011-12057, 13100-13133, 13151-13153, 20101, 31622-31625, 31626, 31634, 31643-31645, 31647, 32096-32100, 32110, 32124-32151, 32215, 32484*, 32486-32488*, 32505-32506, 32551, 32556-32557, 32601, 32607-32609, 32666-32667, 32810-32815, 32994-32998, 35820, 36000, 36400-36410, 36420-36430, 36440, 36591-36592, 36600, 36640, 39010, 43752, 51701-51703, 62320-62327, 64400-64410, 64413-64435, 64445-64450, 64461-64463, 64479-64505, 64510-64530, 64620, 69990, 92012-92014, 93000-93010, 93040-93042, 93318, 93355, 94002, 94200, 94250, 94680-94690, 94770, 95812-95816, 95819, 95822, 95829, 95955, 96360-96368, 96372, 96374-96377, 96523, 97597-97598, 97602, 99155, 99156, 99157, 99211-99223, 99231-99255, 99291-99292, 99304-99310, 99315-99316, 99334-99337, 99347-99350, 99374-99375, 99377-99378, 99446-99449, 99451-99452, 99495-99496, G0463-G0471

32482 0213T, 0216T, 0228T, 0230T, 11000-11006, 11042-11047, 12001-12007, 12011-12057, 13100-13133, 13151-13153, 20101, 31622-31625, 31626, 31634, 31643-31645, 31647, 32096-32100, 32110, 32124-32151, 32215, 32480, 32484*, 32486*, 32505-32507*, 32551, 32556-32557, 32601, 32607-32609, 32666-32667, 32810-32815, 32994-32998, 36000, 36400-36410, 36420-36430, 36440, 36591-36592, 36600, 36640, 39010, 39220, 43752, 51701-51703, 62320-62327, 64400-64410, 64413-64435, 64445-64450, 64461-64463, 64479-64505, 64510-64530, 64620, 69990, 92012-92014, 93000-93010, 93040-93042, 93318, 93355, 94002, 94200, 94250, 94680-94690, 94770, 95812-95816, 95819, 95822, 95829, 95955, 96360-96368, 96372, 96374-96377, 96523, 97597-97598, 97602, 99155, 99156, 99157, 99211-99223, 99231-99255, 99291-99292, 99304-99310, 99315-99316, 99334-99337, 99347-99350, 99374-99375, 99377-99378, 99446-99449, 99451-99452, 99495-99496, G0463-G0471

32484 0213T, 0216T, 0228T, 0230T, 11000-11006, 11042-11047, 12001-12007, 12011-12057, 13100-13133, 13151-13153, 20101, 31622-31625, 31626, 31634, 31643-31645, 31647, 32096-32100, 32110, 32124-32151, 32215, 32486-32488*, 32505-32507*, 32551, 32556-32557, 32601, 32607-32609, 32666-32667, 32810-32815, 32994-32998, 36000, 36400-36410, 36420-36430, 36440, 36591-36592, 36600, 36640, 39010, 39220, 43752, 51701-51703, 62320-62327, 64400-64410, 64413-64435, 64445-64450, 64461-64463, 64479-64505, 64510-64530, 64620, 69990, 92012-92014, 93000-93010, 93040-93042, 93318, 93355, 94002, 94200, 94250, 94680-94690, 94770, 95812-95816, 95819, 95822, 95829, 95955, 96360-96368, 96372, 96374-96377, 96523, 97597-97598, 97602, 99155, 99156, 99157, 99211-99223, 99231-99255, 99291-99292, 99304-99310, 99315-99316, 99334-99337, 99347-99350, 99374-99375, 99377-99378, 99446-99449, 99451-99452, 99495-99496, G0463-G0471

32486 0213T, 0216T, 0228T, 0230T, 11000-11006, 11042-11047, 12001-12007, 12011-12057, 13100-13133, 13151-13153, 20101, 31622-31625, 31626, 31634, 31643-31645, 31647, 32096-32100, 32110, 32124-32151, 32215, 32442-32445*, 32488*, 32503-32507*, 32551, 32556-32557, 32601, 32607-32609, 32666-32667, 32810-32815, 32994-32998, 36000, 36400-36410, 36420-36430, 36440, 36591-36592, 36600, 36640, 39010, 39220, 43752, 51701-51703, 62320-62327, 64400-64410, 64413-64435, 64445-64450, 64461-64463, 64479-64505, 64510-64530, 64620, 69990, 92012-92014, 93000-93010, 93040-93042, 93318, 93355, 94002, 94200, 94250, 94680-94690, 94770, 95812-95816, 95819, 95822, 95829, 95955, 96360-96368, 96372, 96374-96377, 96523, 97597-97598, 97602, 99155, 99156, 99157, 99211-99223, 99231-99255, 99291-99292, 99304-99310, 99315-99316, 99334-99337, 99347-99350, 99374-99375, 99377-99378, 99446-99449, 99451-99452, 99495-99496, G0463-G0471

32488 0213T, 0216T, 0228T, 0230T, 11000-11006, 11042-11047, 12001-12007, 12011-12057, 13100-13133, 13151-13153, 20101, 31622-31625, 31626, 31634, 31643-31645, 31647, 32096-32100, 32110, 32124-32151, 32215, 32442*, 32503-32507*, 32551, 32556-32557, 32601, 32607-32609, 32666-32667, 32810-32815, 32994-32998, 36000, 36400-36410, 36420-36430, 36440, 36591-36592, 36600, 36640, 39010, 39220, 43752, 51701-51703, 62320-62327, 64400-64410, 64413-64435, 64445-64450, 64461-64463, 64479-64505, 64510-64530, 64620, 69990, 92012-92014, 93000-93010, 93040-93042, 93318, 93355, 94002, 94200, 94250, 94680-94690, 94770, 95812-95816, 95819, 95822, 95829, 95955, 96360-96368, 96372, 96374-96377, 96523, 97597-97598, 97602, 99155, 99156, 99157, 99211-99223, 99231-99255, 99291-99292, 99304-99310, 99315-99316, 99334-99337, 99347-99350, 99374-99375, 99377-99378, 99446-99449, 99451-99452, 99495-99496, G0463-G0471

32491 0213T, 0216T, 0228T, 0230T, 11000-11006, 11042-11047, 12001-12007, 12011-12057, 13100-13133, 13151-13153, 31622, 31634, 31645, 31647, 32096-32100, 32110-32151, 32200, 32215-32225, 32310, 32320-32400, 32442-32445*, 32488*, 32505-32506, 32551, 32556-32601, 32607-32609, 32650-32656, 32666-32667, 32672, 32820, 32905, 32940, 32960-32998, 36000, 36400-36410, 36420-36430, 36440, 36591-36592, 36600, 36640, 39010, 43752, 51701-51703, 62320-62327, 64400-64410, 64413-64435, 64445-64450, 64461-64463, 64479-64505, 64510-64530, 69990, 92012-92014, 93000-93010, 93040-93042, 93318, 93355, 94002,

94200, 94250, 94680-94690, 94770, 95812-95816, 95819, 95822, 95829, 95955, 96360-96368, 96372, 96374-96377, 96523, 97597-97598, 97602, 99155, 99156, 99157, 99211-99223, 99231-99255, 99291-99292, 99304-99310, 99315-99316, 99334-99337, 99347-99350, 99374-99375, 99377-99378, 99446-99449, 99451-99452, 99495-99496, G0463-G0471

32501 11000-11006, 11042-11047, 32994, 32998, 36591-36592, 96523, 97597-97598, 97602

32503 0213T, 0216T, 0228T, 0230T, 11000-11006, 11042-11047, 12001-12007, 12011-12057, 13100-13133, 13151-13153, 19260-19272, 20101, 31622, 31634, 31647, 32096-32100, 32110, 32124-32151, 32440❖, 32480-32484❖, 32491❖, 32505-32506, 32551, 32554-32557, 32601, 32607-32609, 32666-32667, 32820, 32900, 32994, 32998, 36000, 36400-36410, 36420-36430, 36440, 36591-36592, 36600, 36640, 43752, 51701-51703, 62320-62327, 64400-64410, 64413-64435, 64445-64450, 64461-64463, 64479-64505, 64510-64530, 69990, 92012-92014, 93000-93010, 93040-93042, 93318, 93355, 94002, 94200, 94250, 94680-94690, 94770, 95812-95816, 95819, 95822, 95829, 95955, 96360-96368, 96372, 96374-96377, 96523, 97597-97598, 97602, 99155, 99156, 99157, 99211-99223, 99231-99255, 99291-99292, 99304-99310, 99315-99316, 99334-99337, 99347-99350, 99374-99375, 99377-99378, 99446-99449, 99451-99452, 99495-99496, G0463-G0471

32504 0213T, 0216T, 0228T, 0230T, 11000-11006, 11042-11047, 12001-12007, 12011-12057, 13100-13133, 13151-13153, 19260-19272, 20101, 31622, 31634, 31647, 32096-32100, 32110, 32124-32151, 32440❖, 32480-32484❖, 32491❖, 32505-32506, 32551, 32554-32557, 32601, 32607-32609, 32666-32667, 32820, 32900, 32994, 32998, 36000, 36400-36410, 36420-36430, 36440, 36591-36592, 36600, 36640, 43752, 51701-51703, 62320-62327, 64400-64410, 64413-64435, 64445-64450, 64461-64463, 64479-64505, 64510-64530, 69990, 92012-92014, 93000-93010, 93040-93042, 93318, 93355, 94002, 94200, 94250, 94680-94690, 94770, 95812-95816, 95819, 95822, 95829, 95955, 96360-96368, 96372, 96374-96377, 96523, 97597-97598, 97602, 99155, 99156, 99157, 99211-99223, 99231-99255, 99291-99292, 99304-99310, 99315-99316, 99334-99337, 99347-99350, 99374-99375, 99377-99378, 99446-99449, 99451-99452, 99495-99496, G0463-G0471

32505 0213T, 0216T, 0228T, 0230T, 11000-11006, 11042-11047, 12001-12007, 12011-12057, 13100-13133, 13151-13153, 20101, 21600, 31622, 31645, 32096-32100, 32110, 32124-32151, 32220-32225, 32310, 32551, 32556-32601, 32607-32609, 32810-32815, 32994, 32998, 35820, 36000, 36400-36410, 36420-36430, 36440, 36591-36592, 36600, 36640, 39010,

32507 0213T, 0216T, 0228T, 0230T, 11000-11006, 11042-11047, 20101, 31645, 32096-32100, 32110, 32124-32151, 32505-32506, 32551, 32556-32557, 32601, 32607-32609, 32666-32667, 32810-32815, 32994, 32998, 35820, 36000, 36400-36410, 36420-36430, 36440, 36591-36592, 36600, 36640, 39010, 43752, 51701-51703, 61650, 62320-62327, 64400-64410, 64413-64435, 64445-64450, 64461, 64463, 64479, 64483, 64486-64490, 64493, 64505, 64510-64530, 64620, 69990, 93000-93010, 93040-93042, 93318, 93355, 94002, 94200, 94250, 94680-94690, 94770, 95812-95816, 95819, 95822, 95829, 95955, 96360, 96365, 96372, 96374-96377, 96523, 97597-97598, 97602, 99155, 99156, 99157, G0471

32540 0213T, 0216T, 0228T, 0230T, 11000-11006, 11042-11047, 12001-12007, 12011-12057, 13100-13133, 13151-13153, 32096-32100, 32110, 32124-32151, 32220-32225, 32551, 32556-32557, 32601, 32607-32609, 32810, 36000, 36400-36410, 36420-36430, 36440, 36591-36592, 36600, 36640, 43752, 51701-51703, 62320-62327, 64400-64410, 64413-64435, 64445-64450, 64461-64463, 64479-64505, 64510-64530, 69990, 92012-92014, 93000-93010, 93040-93042, 93318, 93355, 94002, 94200, 94250, 94680-94690, 94770, 95812-95816, 95819, 95822, 95829, 95955, 96360-96368, 96372, 96374-96377, 96523, 97597-97598, 97602, 99155, 99156, 99157, 99211-99223, 99231-99255, 99291-99292, 99304-99310, 99315-99316, 99334-99337, 99347-99350, 99374-99375, 99377-99378, 99446-99449, 99451-99452, 99495-99496, G0463-G0471

32550 0213T, 0216T, 0228T, 0230T, 11000-11006, 11042-11047, 12001-12007, 12011-12057, 13100-13133, 13151-13153, 32551, 32555-32556, 32560-32562❖, 36000, 36400-36410, 36420-36430, 36440, 36591-36592, 36600, 36640, 43752, 62320-62327, 64400-64410, 64413-64435, 64445-64450, 64461-64463, 64479-64505, 64510-64530, 69990, 71045-71047, 76000, 76380, 76942, 76970, 76998, 77001-77002, 77012, 92012-92014, 93000-93010, 93040-93042, 93318, 93355, 94002, 94200, 94250, 94680-94690, 94770, 95812-95816, 95819, 95822, 95829, 95955, 96360-96368, 96372, 96374-96377, 96523, 97597-97598, 97602, 99155, 99156, 99157, 99211-99223, 99231-99255, 99291-99292, 99304-99310, 99315-99316, 99334-99337, 99347-99350, 99374-99375, 99377-99378, 99446-99449, 99451-99452, 99495-99496, G0463

32551 0213T, 0216T, 0228T, 0230T, 12001-12007, 12011-12057, 13100-13133, 13151-13153, 36000, 36400-36410, 36420-36430, 36440, 36591-36592, 36600, 36640, 43752, 49185, 49423-49424, 62320-62327, 64400-64410, 64413-64435, 64445-64450, 64461-64463, 64479-64505, 64510-64530,

IMPORTANT

Note: The following URL and password will provide you with access to download and view the complete list of CCI edits:

https://www.optum360coding.com/productupdates

2020 password: CODING20

Please note that you should log in each quarter to ensure you receive the most current updates. An email reminder will also be sent to you when the updates are available.

CPT Index

● New ▲ Revised + Add On AMA: CPT Assist [Resequenced]

 ● New ▲ Revised + Add On AMA: CPT Assist[Resequenced]

E

● New ▲ Revised + Add On AMA: CPT Assist [Resequenced]

H

J

K

L

M

CPT Index

 ● New ▲ Revised + Add On AMA: CPT Assist [Resequenced]

● New ▲ Revised + Add On AMA: CPT Assist [Resequenced]

S

T

● New ▲ Revised + Add On AMA: CPT Assist [Resequenced]

W

X

Y